Principles and Practice of Transplant Infectious Diseases

Amar Safdar
Editor

Principles and Practice of Transplant Infectious Diseases

Springer

Editor
Amar Safdar
Clinical Associate Professor of Medicine
Texas Tech University Health Sciences Center El Paso
Paul L. Foster School of Medicine
El Paso, TX
USA

ISBN 978-1-4939-9032-0 ISBN 978-1-4939-9034-4 (eBook)
https://doi.org/10.1007/978-1-4939-9034-4

This Springer imprint is published by the registered company Springer Science+Business Media, LLC part of Springer Nature.
The registered company address is: 233 Spring Street, New York, NY 10013, U.S.A.

This book is dedicated to my parents, Taj & Safdar, for enduring inspiration and tenacity of purpose.

Preface

In pursuit of recognizing the risk of infection in patients undergoing transplantation, prescient cognizance requires sagacious understanding of hosts' home and healthcare environment, factors pertaining to the level of immune suppression that may have accumulated overtime, and, importantly, recent alterations in immune function resulting from additional immunosuppressive treatments such as donor lymphocyte transfusion, antineoplastic therapy, and immune modulatory biologic drugs and medical disorders like graft-versus-host disease, donor allograft rejection, posttransplant opportunistic malignancies, recrudescent or newly acquired cytomegalovirus infection, and relapsed hematologic neoplasms.

It is prudent to establish a targeted approach toward diagnosis, an approach which portends recognition of the true etiology with the help of assiduous investigation based on patient-specific vulnerability for infection. Special consideration needs to be placed upon the possibility of noninfectious processes that clinically are often difficult to distinguish from infection or sepsis-like syndrome. Toxicity due to commonly used drugs in the posttransplant period, thromboembolic events, acute engraftment syndrome, postsurgical deep tissue and body cavity hematoma, tissue ischemia and necrosis, opportunistic malignancies, and the potential for less common paraneoplastic disorders including tumor fever may initially present as a nonspecific acute febrile illness, with or without features suggestive of systemic inflammatory response syndrome. Similarly, a host of noninfectious maladies involving the skin and skin structures, brain, orointestinal tract, liver, kidneys, and lungs may clinically resemble infection. It is important to take into account that such processes may occur concurrently or sequentially in patients with a known infection diagnosis. Furthermore, in immunosuppressed patients after hematopoietic or solid organ allograft transplantation, plurality of simultaneously occurring infections makes selection of targeted, pathogen-specific empiric therapy a daunting task.

Individuals' genetic haecceity and its influence on susceptibility or inherent resistance to certain infections is evolving. Once validated and available for clinical use, this has the potential to reliably identify select subgroups of transplant recipients that are additionally vulnerable to specific infection(s). Infection prevention and empiric or preemptive treatment strategies in such patients may advance from the putative and arbitrary risk profiles presently in use.

This volume aims to provide a comprehensive and in-depth review of the issues pertaining to infectious diseases in patients undergoing transplantation.

El Paso, TX, USA — Amar Safdar, MD

Contents

Contributors

Cybele Lara R. Abad Section of Infectious Diseases, Department of Medicine, University of the Philippines, Philippine General Hospital, Manila, Philippines

Peter Abrams MedStar Georgetown University Hospital, MedStar Georgetown Transplant Institute, Washington, DC, USA

Samuel L. Aitken Infectious Diseases, The University of Texas MD Anderson Cancer Center, Division of Pharmacy, Houston, TX, USA

Barbara D. Alexander Duke University Medical Center, Departments of Medicine and Pathology, Division of Infectious Diseases and International Health, Durham, NC, USA

Jerry Altshuler The Mount Sinai Hospital, Department of Pharmacy, New York, NY, USA

Donald Armstrong Infectious Disease Service, Memorial Sloan-Kettering Cancer Center, New York, NY, USA

Cornell University Medical College (ret), New York, NY, USA

Infectious Disease Society of America, Albuquerque, NM, USA

Robin K. Avery Division of Infectious Disease, Johns Hopkins, Baltimore, MD, USA

Jenny S. Ayala Hospice and Palliative Medicine, Hospital Medicine, White Plains Hospital, White Plains, NY, USA

N. Esther Babady Department of Laboratory Medicine, Clinical Microbiology Service, Memorial Sloan-Kettering Cancer Center, New York, NY, USA

Lindsey R. Baden Division of Infectious Diseases, Brigham and Women's Hospital, Dana-Farber Cancer Institute, Harvard Medical School, Boston, MA, USA

Merav Bar Fred Hutchinson Cancer Research Center, Clinical Research Division, Seattle, WA, USA

Gerard R. Barber Department of Pharmacy Services, University of Colorado Hospital, University of Colorado, Skaggs School of Pharmacy and Pharmaceutical Sciences, Aurora, CO, USA

Maura Barry University of Vermont College of Medicine, University of Vermont Medical Center, Division of Hematology & Oncology, Burlington, VT, USA

Brian G. Blackburn Stanford University Medical Center, Palo Alto, CA, USA

Division of Infectious Diseases and Geographic Medicine, Stanford University School of Medicine, Stanford, CA, USA

Emily A. Blumberg Division of Infectious Diseases, Perelman School of Medicine at the University of Pennsylvania, Philadelphia, PA, USA

Hospital of the University of Pennsylvania, Perelman School of Medicine at the University of Pennsylvania, Department of Medicine, Philadelphia, PA, USA

Michael Boeckh Fred Hutchinson Cancer Research Center, University of Washington Medical Center, Washington, DC, USA

Justin M. Broyles Department of Plastic and Reconstructive Surgery, The Johns Hopkins Hospital, Baltimore, MD, USA

Richard E. Champlin MD Anderson Cancer Center, Department of Stem Cell Transplantation and Cellular Therapy, Houston, TX, USA

Sunandana Chandra Northwestern University Feinberg School of Medicine, Division of Hematology & Oncology, Chicago, IL, USA

Pearlie P. Chong Division of Infectious Diseases, Department of Medicine, and the William J. von Liebig Transplant Center, Mayo Clinic College of Medicine, Mayo Clinic, Rochester, MN, USA

University of North Carolina at Chapel Hill, Division of Infectious Diseases, Chapel Hill, NC, USA

Sunwen Chou Oregon Health and Science University, Division of Infectious Diseases, Portland, OR, USA

Ana Ciurea Department of Dermatology, The University of Texas, MD Anderson Cancer Center, Houston, TX, USA

Heather E. Clauss Section of Infectious Diseases, Department of Medicine, Temple University School of Medicine, Philadelphia, PA, USA

Temple University, Philadelphia, PA, USA

Temple University Hospital, Department of Infectious Diseases, Philadelphia, PA, USA

Valerie Cluzet Division of Infectious Diseases, Perelman School of Medicine at the University of Pennsylvania, Philadelphia, PA, USA

Health Quest Medical Practice, Department of Infectious Diseases, Poughkeepsie, NY, USA

Matthew Cooper MedStar Georgetown Transplant Institute, Washington, DC, USA

Scott Cutro Department of Infectious Disease, The Southeast Permanente Medical Group, Kaiser Permanente, Atlanta, GA, USA

Charles L. Daley Division of Mycobacterial and Respiratory Infections, National Jewish Health and University of Colorado, Denver, CO, USA

Lara Danziger-Isakov Pediatric Infectious Diseases, Immunocompromised Host Infectious Disease, Cincinnati Children's Hospital Medical Center, Cincinnati, OH, USA

William K. Decker Department of Pathology and Immunology, Baylor College of Medicine, Houston, TX, USA

Stan Deresinski Stanford University School of Medicine, Department of Medicine, Division of Infectious Diseases and Geographic Medicine, Stanford, CA, USA

Burton F. Dickey Department of Pulmonary Medicine, University of Texas MD Anderson Cancer Center, Houston, TX, USA

Yanina Dubrovskaya NYU Langone Medical Center, NYU Langone Health, Department of Pharmacy, New York, NY, USA

Simon Frédéric Dufresne Hôpital Maisonneuve-Rosemont, Université de Montréal, Department of Infectious Diseases and Medical Microbiology, Montréal, QC, Canada

Herbert L. DuPont, MD Baylor St. Luke's Medical Center, Department of Research, Houston, TX, USA

Program in Infectious Diseases, University of Texas School of Public Health, Houston, TX, USA

Kelsey Research Foundation, Houston, TX, USA

Baylor College of Medicine, Houston, TX, USA

University of Texas School of Medicine Houston, Houston, TX, USA

Marlene L. Durand Department of Ophthalmology, Harvard Medical School, Massachusetts Eye and Ear Infirmary, Boston, MA, USA

Department of Medicine, Infectious Disease Unit, Massachusetts General Hospital, Boston, MA, USA

Infectious Disease Service, Massachusetts Eye and Ear Infirmary, Boston, MA, USA

Thomas M. Fishbein Georgetown University Hospital, Transplant Institute, Washington, DC, USA

Graeme N. Forrest Division of Infectious Diseases, Portland VA Medical Center and Oregon Health and Science University, Portland, OR, USA

Alison G. Freifeld Infectious Diseases Division, University of Nebraska Medical Center, Omaha, NE, USA

Benjamin E. Gewurz Brigham and Women's Hospital, Division of Infectious Diseases, Department of Medicine, Boston, MA, USA

Raffaele Girlanda Georgetown University Hospital, Department Transplant Surgery, Washington, DC, USA

Chad R. Gordon Department of Plastic and Reconstructive Surgery, The Johns Hopkins Hospital, Baltimore, MD, USA

David E. Griffith University of Texas Health Science Center, Tyler, TX, USA

Heartland National TB Center, Tyler, TX, USA

Chadi A. Hage Indiana University School of Medicine, Pulmonary-Critical Care, Thoracic Transplantation Program, Methodist Professional Center-2, Indianapolis, IN, USA

Morgan Hakki Oregon Health and Science University, Division of Infectious Diseases, Portland, OR, USA

Matthew M. Halpert Department of Pathology and Immunology, Baylor College of Medicine, Houston, TX, USA

Christopher N. Hampton Department of Pathology and Immunology, Baylor College of Medicine, Huffington Center on Aging, Houston, TX, USA

Stephen Harold, MD, MPH Baylor St. Luke's Medical Center, Department of Research, Houston, TX, USA

Andrés F. Henao-Martínez Division of Infectious Diseases, Department of Medicine, University of Colorado Denver, Aurora, CO, USA

Dora Y. Ho Division of Infectious Diseases and Geographic Medicine, Stanford University School of Medicine, Stanford, CA, USA

Harold W. Horowitz New University School of Medicine, Division of Infectious Diseases and Immunology, New York, NY, USA

Weill Cornell Medicine, New York—Presbyterian—Brooklyn Methodist Hospital, Department of Medicine, Division of Infectious Diseases, Brooklyn, NY, USA

Shirish Huprikar The Mount Sinai Hospital, Icahn School of Medicine at Mount Sinai, New York, NY, USA

Kenneth B. Hymes Hematology, Coagulation, and Medical Oncology, Laura and Isaac Perlmutter Cancer Center, NYU Langone Health, New York, NY, USA

Sharon Hymes Department of Dermatology, The University of Texas, MD Anderson Cancer Center, Houston, TX, USA

Samantha E. Jacobs Transplantation-Oncology Infectious Diseases Program, Division of Infectious Diseases, Weill Cornell Medicine, New York, NY, USA

Transplant Infectious Diseases Program, Division of Infectious Diseases, Icahn School of Medicine at Mount Sinai, Department of Medicine, New York, NY, USA

Alexander Z. Jow Division of Gastroenterology, Mid-Atlantic Kaiser Permanente Medical Group, Springfield, VA, USA

Aspasia Katragkou Transplantation-Oncology Infectious Diseases Program, New York-Presbyterian/Weill Cornell Medical Center, New York, NY, USA

3rd Department of Pediatrics, Aristotle University, Hippokration Hospital, Thessaloniki, Greece

Nationwide Children's Hospital, Department of Pediatric Infectious Diseases, Columbus, OH, USA

Carol A. Kauffman University of Michigan Medical School, Infectious Diseases Section, Veterans Affairs Ann Arbor Healthcare System, Ann Arbor, MI, USA

Partow Kebriaei MD Anderson Cancer Center, Department of Stem Cell Transplantation and Cellular Therapy, Houston, TX, USA

Vanaja Konduri Department of Pathology and Immunology, Baylor College of Medicine, Houston, TX, USA

Robert M. Kotloff Department of Pulmonary Medicine, Respiratory Institute, Cleveland Clinic, Cleveland, OH, USA

Camille Nelson Kotton Transplant and Immunocompromised Host Infectious Diseases, Division of Infectious Diseases, Massachusetts General Hospital, Travelers' Advice and Immunization Center, Division of Infectious Diseases, Massachusetts General Hospital, Harvard Medical School, Boston, MA, USA

Carrie L. Kovarik Departments of Medicine and Dermatology, Perelman School of Medicine at the University of Pennsylvania, Philadelphia, PA, USA

Yeon Joo Lee Department of Internal Medicine, Infectious Diseases Service, Memorial Sloan Kettering Cancer Center, New York, NY, USA

Weill Cornell Medical College, Cornell University, New York, NY, USA

Dan Liang Department of Pathology and Immunology, Baylor College of Medicine, Houston, TX, USA

Catherine Liu Fred Hutchinson Cancer Research Center, University of Washington Medical Center, Washington, DC, USA

Ann-Marie Lobo Department of Ophthalmology and Visual Sciences, Illinois Eye and Ear Infirmary, University of Illinois at Chicago, Chicago, IL, USA

Bennett Lorber Section of Infectious Diseases, Department of Medicine, Temple University School of Medicine, Philadelphia, PA, USA

Temple University, Philadelphia, PA, USA

Temple University Hospital, Department of Infectious Diseases, Philadelphia, PA, USA

Joseph Lowy NYU Langone Health, NYU Medical School, Department of Medicine, New York, NY, USA

Nell S. Lurain Rush University Medical Center, Department of Immunology/Microbiology, Chicago, IL, USA

Johan Maertens Department of Hematology, Acute Leukemia and Stem Cell Transplantation Unit, University Hospital Gasthuisberg, K. U. Leuven, Leuven, Belgium

Dennis G. Maki Section of Infectious Diseases, Department of Medicine, University of Wisconsin-Madison, School of Medicine and Public Health, and the William S. Middleton Memorial Veterans Hospital, Madison, WI, USA

Kieren A. Marr Johns Hopkins University, Department of Medicine, Baltimore, MD, USA

Melanie Maslow New York University School of Medicine, New York, NY, USA

Matthew W. McCarthy Weill Cornell Medicine, Department of General Internal Medicine, New York, NY, USA

Man Yee Merl Smilow Cancer Hospital at Yale-New Haven Health, Department of Pharmacy, New Haven, CT, USA

Jonathan Merola Department of Surgery, Yale School of Medicine, Yale-New Haven Hospital, New Haven, CT, USA

Robert G. Micheletti Departments of Medicine and Dermatology, Perelman School of Medicine at the University of Pennsylvania, Philadelphia, PA, USA

Benjamin A. Miko Columbia University Medical Center, Division of Infectious Diseases, Department of Medicine, New York, NY, USA

Elizabeth Ann Misch University of Wisconsin Hospital, Department of Medicine, Division of Allergy and Infectious Disease, Madison, WI, USA

University of Wisconsin-Madison, School of Medicine and Public Health, Department of Medicine, Madison, WI, USA

Sheila Mitsuma Massachusetts General Hospital, Division of Infectious Diseases, Boston, MA, USA

Robert M. Mocharla Division of Gastroenterology, NYU School of Medicine, Department of Internal Medicine, New York, NY, USA

B. Sharmila Mohanraj MedStar Georgetown University Hospital, Department of Infectious Diseases and Travel Medicine, Washington, DC, USA

José G. Montoya Division of Infectious Diseases and Geographic Medicine, Stanford University School of Medicine, Stanford, CA, USA

Palo Alto Medical Foundation Toxoplasma Serology Laboratory, National Reference Center for the Study and Diagnosis of Toxoplasmosis, Palo Alto, CA, USA

Stanford University Medical Center, Palo Alto, CA, USA

Megan K. Morales University of Maryland School of Medicine, Institute of Human Virology/ Department of Infectious Diseases, Baltimore, MD, USA

Scott W. Mueller Department of Clinical Pharmacy, University of Colorado Hospital, University of Colorado, Skaggs School of Pharmacy and Pharmaceutical Sciences, Aurora, CO, USA

Lior Nesher Infectious Disease Institute, Faculty of Health Sciences, Ben-Gurion University of the Negev, Beer Sheba, Israel

Soroka University Medical Center affiliated with Faculty of Health Sciences Ben-Gurion University of the Negev, Infectious Disease Institute, Beer Sheba, Israel

Marcio Nucci University Hospital, Universidade Federal do Rio de Janeiro, Rio de Janeiro, RJ, Brazil

Hospital Universitário Clementino Fraga Filho, Department of Internal Medicine – Hematology, Rio de Janeiro, RJ, Brazil

Lucy O'Connor Transplantation-Oncology Infectious Diseases Program, New York-Presbyterian/Weill Cornell Medical Center, New York, NY, USA

University of Manchester School of Medicine, Manchester, UK

John Papadopoulos Department of Pharmacy, Division of Pharmacotherapy, NYU Langone Medical Center, New York, NY, USA

Genovefa Papanicolaou Department of Internal Medicine, Infectious Diseases Service, Memorial Sloan Kettering Cancer Center, New York, NY, USA

Weill Cornell Medical College, Cornell University, New York, NY, USA

Memorial Sloan Kettering Cancer Center, Memorial Hospital, Department of Medicine, New York, NY, USA

Marcus R. Pereira Department of Medicine – Infectious Diseases, Columbia University Medical Center, New York, NY, USA

John R. Perfect Duke University Medical Center, Departments of Medicine and Pathology, Division of Infectious Diseases and International Health, Durham, NC, USA

David S. Perlin Public Health Research Institute, Rutgers Biomedical and Health Sciences, Rutgers New Jersey Medical School, Newark, NJ, USA

Jennifer A. Philips Division of Infectious Diseases, Department of Medicine, Washington University School of Medicine, St. Louis, MO, USA

Julie V. Philley University of Texas Health Science Center at Tyler, Department of Pulmonary and Critical Care Medicine, Tyler, TX, USA

Michael Phillips New University School of Medicine, Division of Infectious Diseases and Immunology, New York, NY, USA

Didier Pittet Infection Control Programme and WHO Collaborating Centre on Patient Safety, University of Geneva Hospitals and Faculty of Medicine, Geneva, Switzerland

Michelle Limei Poon National University Hospital, Department of Hematology Oncology, Singapore, Singapore

Cynthia Portal-Celhay Division of Infectious Diseases, Department of Medicine, NYU Langone Medical Center, NYU School of Medicine, New York, NY, USA

Stephanie M. Pouch Division of Infectious Diseases, Emory University, Atlanta, GA, USA

Amol S. Rangnekar MedStar Georgetown University Hospital, MedStar Georgetown Transplant Institute, Washington, DC, USA

Raymund R. Razonable Division of Infectious Diseases, Department of Medicine, and the William J. von Liebig Center for Transplantation and Clinical Regeneration, College of Medicine, Mayo Clinic, Rochester, MN, USA

Emmanuel Roilides 3rd Department of Pediatrics, Hippokration Hospital, School of Health Sciences, Aristotle University of Thessaloniki, Thessaloniki, Greece

Kenneth V. I. Rolston Department of Infectious Diseases, Infection Control & Employee Health, The University of Texas MD Anderson Cancer Center, Houston, TX, USA

Axel Rosengart Cedars-Sinai Medical Center, Departments of Neurology, Neurosurgery and Biomedical Sciences, Los Angeles, CA, USA

Amar Safdar Clinical Associate Professor of Medicine, Texas Tech University Health Sciences Center El Paso, Paul L. Foster School of Medicine, El Paso, TX, USA

Nasia Safdar Section of Infectious Diseases, Department of Medicine, University of Wisconsin-Madison, School of Medicine and Public Health, and the William S. Middleton Memorial Veterans Hospital, Madison, WI, USA

Michael J. Satlin Transplantation-Oncology Infectious Diseases Program, Division of Infectious Diseases, Weill Cornell Medicine, New York, NY, USA

Jennifer L. Saullo Duke University Medical Center, Department of Medicine, Division of Infectious Diseases and International Health, Durham, NC, USA

Joanna M. D. Schaenman Division of Infectious Diseases, David Geffen School of Medicine at UCLA, Los Angeles, CA, USA

Kelly E. Schoeppler Department of Pharmacy Services, University of Colorado Health, University of Colorado, Skaggs School of Pharmacy and Pharmaceutical Sciences, Aurora, CO, USA

Marco R. Scipione Department of Pharmacy, Memorial Sloan Kettering Cancer Center, New York, NY, USA

Brian Scully Columbia University Medical Center, Division of Infectious Diseases, Department of Medicine, New York, NY, USA

Susan K. Seo Department of Medicine, Infectious Disease Service, Memorial Sloan-Kettering Cancer Center, New York, NY, USA

Shmuel Shoham Johns Hopkins University School of Medicine, Department of Infectious Diseases, Baltimore, MD, USA

Amy Sievers Dana-Farber Cancer Institute, Division of Medical Oncology, Boston, MA, USA

Samuel H. Sigal Division of Gastroenterology and Hepatology, Department of Medicine, Albert Einstein College of Medicine, Montefiore Medical Center, Bronx, NY, USA

Maria Simitsopoulou Research Infectious Disease Laboratory, 3rd Department Pediatrics, Aristotle University School of Medicine, Hippokration Hospital, Thessaloniki, Greece

Lucia Sobrin Department of Ophthalmology, Harvard Medical School, Massachusetts Eye and Ear Infirmary, Boston, MA, USA

Kevin M. Soriano Georgetown University Hospital, Department of Infectious Diseases, Washington, DC, USA

Brad Spellberg Los Angeles County+University of Southern California (LAC+USC) Medical Center, Los Angeles, CA, USA

Division of Infectious Diseases, Keck School of Medicine at USC, Los Angeles, CA, USA

Lynne Strasfeld Oregon Health and Science University, Division of Infectious Diseases, Portland, OR, USA

Susanna K. Tan Stanford University School of Medicine, Department of Medicine, Division of Infectious Diseases and Geographic Medicine, Stanford, CA, USA

Yi-Wei Tang Department of Laboratory Medicine, Clinical Microbiology Service, Memorial Sloan-Kettering Cancer Center, New York, NY, USA

Weill Cornell Medical College, Cornell University, New York, NY, USA

Joseph G. Timpone Jr. MedStar Georgetown University Hospital, Division of Infectious Diseases and Travel Medicine, Washington, DC, USA

Gaurav Trikha Division of Infectious Diseases, University of Florida College of Medicine, Gainesville, FL, USA

University of Florida Health Shands Hospital, Division of Hematology/Oncology, Department of Medicine, Gainesville, FL, USA

Nicholas Vander Els Pulmonary Service, Memorial Sloan- Kettering Cancer Center, New York, NY, USA

Pascalis Vergidis University Hospital of South Manchester, University of Manchester, Department of Medicine, Manchester, UK

Jesse J. Waggoner Emory University School of Medicine, Department of Medicine, Division of Infectious Diseases, Atlanta, GA, USA

Thomas J. Walsh Transplantation-Oncology Infectious Diseases Program, New York-Presbyterian/Weill Cornell Medical Center, New York, NY, USA

Department of Pediatrics, New York-Presbyterian/Weill Cornell Medical Center, New York, NY, USA

Department of Microbiology and Immunology, New York-Presbyterian/Weill Cornell Medical Center, New York, NY, USA

Transplant Infectious Diseases Program, Division of Infectious Diseases, Icahn School of Medicine at Mount Sinai, New York, NY, USA

David M. Weinstock Dana-Farber Cancer Institute, Harvard Medical School, Division of Medical Oncology, Boston, MA, USA

L. Joseph Wheat MiraVista Diagnostics, Indianapolis, IN, USA

Kathryn Whitaker Division of Infectious Diseases, Perelman School of Medicine at the University of Pennsylvania, Philadelphia, PA, USA

Hospital at the University of Pennsylvania, Philadelphia, PA, USA

John R. Wingard University of Florida, Division of Hematology/Oncology, Department of Medicine, Gainesville, FL, USA

Belinda Yen-Lieberman Pathology and Laboratory Medicine Institute, Cleveland Clinic, Department of Laboratory Medicine, Cleveland, OH, USA

Jasmine Zain City of Hope National Medical Center, Department of Hematology/Hematopoietic Cell Transplantation, Duarte, CA, USA

Sara A. M. Zerbel UnityPoint Health-Meriter, Department of Performance Improvement, Madison, WI, USA

Walter Zingg Infection Control Programme and WHO Collaborating Centre on Patient Safety, University of Geneva Hospitals and Faculty of Medicine, Geneva, Switzerland

Part I

Principles of Transplantation and Overview of Infectious Diseases

Infections in Transplantation: Introduction and Overview

1

Amar Safdar

Transplantation remains a pioneering scientific innovation that has a significant impact on restoring well-being for patients and benefit society as a whole. Blood and marrow hematopoietic stem cells have become accepted and, in some instances, established approach to treat incurable neoplastic diseases and congenital disorders of immune system [1]. Similarly, use of allografts in patients with end-stage organ disease involving the liver, kidneys, intestines, heart, and lungs has provided a possibility for continuation of life and a potential for patients to integrate and resume participation in their communities [2]. Recent advances in limb, integument, and face transplantation underscore the substantial leap forward in restoring normalcy for individuals with devastating and often catastrophic physical encumbrance [3, 4].

In patients undergoing solid organ transplantation, advancement in understanding the complex interplay within various facets of immune response against the transplanted allogeneic tissue that recipients' immune system fails to recognize as "self" has resulted in encouraging long-term outcomes [5]. These achievements in decoding higher mammalian immunity underscore the recent progress made in development and implementation of refined strategies to harness potentially devastating immune rejection of the implanted solid organ allograft [6]. The antirejection strategies, as expected, involve a delicate balance that favors preservation of a functioning allograft and aims at limit severity of drug-induced suppression of recipients' immune function, which is crucial for the surveillance against various neoplastic processes; conventional and opportunistic infections.

A similar, albeit an opposing role of undesired immune response comes into play in patients undergoing hematopoietic blood and marrow stem cell transplantation from a foreign donor. The conflict arises from aforementioned disconnect between immune recognition of self versus nonself [7, 8]. These transplanted stem cells install foreign effector immune cells in the recipient, and if remain unabated, the resulting graft-versus-host disease is capable of unleashing potentially ruinous systemic inflammation resulting in irreversible tissue damage and death [7]. The stem cell graft restores immunity and functional marrow in patients in need for myeloablative antineoplastic therapy. Furthermore, it is the foreign, graft-mediated, adaptive cancer immune surveillance that has now been widely recognized as the pivotal feature that sustains cancer in remission following successful allogeneic hematopoietic stem cell transplantation. This feature of stem cell graft-assisted antitumor response is recognized as "graft-versus-leukemia or graft-versus-tumor effect." Donor-derived adaptive antitumor immunity is an important objective of allogeneic stem cell transplantation, especially in patients with hematologic malignancies, and forms the bases for donor lymphocyte infusions to treat cancer recurrences during posttransplant period [9]. As in patients following solid organ transplants, in recipients of allogeneic HSCT, anti-GVHD therapy is assessed and continuously refined to achieve the lowest possible cumulative iatrogenic immune suppression required to prevent or treat GVHD, whereas an earnest attempt is made for preservation of recipients' immune function such that the risk of conventional and opportunistic infections and malignancies do not overwhelm the projected efficacy and feasibility of these lifesaving procedures.

A number of agents have been successfully used for prevention and treatment of graft-versus-host disease and solid organ allograft rejection [8, 10]. Severity of immune dysfunction is in most instance a direct consequence of treatment with these agents that are commonly prescribed

A. Safdar (✉)
Clinical Associate Professor of Medicine, Texas Tech University Health Sciences Center El Paso, Paul L. Foster School of Medicine, El Paso, TX, USA
e-mail: amar.safdar@cidimmunology.com

A. Safdar (ed.), *Principles and Practice of Transplant Infectious Diseases*, https://doi.org/10.1007/978-1-4939-9034-4_1

as combination drug regimens. Cyclosporine was the first major breakthrough in this regard; subsequent generation calcineurin inhibitors (CNI) have improved therapeutic index although resultant severe immune suppression and the risk for opportunistic infection like CMV, BK virus, and certain posttransplant cancers question the therapeutic feasibility for agents such as tacrolimus, especially in patients with low risk for allograft-related complications. Serious infections due to cytomegalovirus including viremia and end-organ disease, BK virus viremia, viruria, and BK virus allograft nephropathy with risk for potential graft compromise, rare progressive multifocal leukoencephalopathy due to polyomavirus, higher potential for opportunist cancers such as Kaposi's sarcoma, EBV lymphoproliferative disorders among others, are well-recognized limitations in individuals given tacrolimus for extended duration with doses leading to prolong high serum drug concentration [11]. Experience with sirolimus, a macrolide xenobiotic that induces potent immune suppression via inhibition of mechanistic target of rapamycin (mTOR; a conserved threonine and serine protein kinase) was associated with lower incidence of CMV infection in solid organ transplant recipients. This protective antiviral effect of mTOR inhibitors against BK virus nephropathy after renal transplantation has not been noted consistently. Additionally, antitumor properties of mTOR inhibitors may favorably influence the lower incidence and risk for posttransplant malignancies in recipients of solid organ allografts, especially those with a profile that indicates low risk for graft rejection [12].

Monoclonal antibodies against T- and B-cell pathways have also gained prominence, as potential treatment options. Alemtuzumab (Campath) is a monoclonal antibody that targets C52 antigen expressed on all lymphocytes. Treatment with Campath results in profound lymphocyte depletion. The drug-induced immune suppression may last for up to 9 months, although maximum degree of lymphopenia is noted between 8 and 9 weeks after therapy. As part of HSCT preparatory condition regimen, treatment with alemtuzumab was associated with reduced risk for GVHD following allogeneic hematopoietic stem cell transplantation [13].

In kidney transplant recipients, the risk for organ rejection was low in patients given alemtuzumab; however, this benefit was mainly observed in patients that were at a low risk for allograft rejection [14]. Other trials are underway with the aim to explore regimen(s) that may spare CNI (tacrolimus) for the prevention of allograft rejection.

Humanized monoclonal antibody rituximab that targets CD20 antigen expressed prominently and selectively on B lymphocytes forms the cornerstone for treatment of solid organ antibody-mediated renal allograft rejection. It is also considered the standard of care for the treatment of posttransplant B-cell lymphoproliferative disorders [15].

Systemic glucocorticoids have maintained relevance in drug cocktails given to prevent and treat solid organ graft rejection and GVHD. Since the early observation enabled addition of corticosteroids to successfully reduce cyclosporine dose that was traditionally needed to prevent rejection of transplanted allograft, this observation was regarded as a major breakthrough and forged the path for preservation of transplanted organs without serious, life-threatening CNI toxicity. Detailed discussion regarding immunosuppressive agents for prevention and treatment of allograft rejection is provided in chapters throughout this book.

A keen understanding of patients' underlying immune defect(s) is the knowledge cornerstone, essential for optimizing infection risk stratification, assessing need for preventive, preemptive or empiric antimicrobial therapy. This information serves as an imperative in establishing meaningful patient-centered management and infection prevention paradigm [16, 17]. Table 1.1 provides an outline for such a relationship between underlying immune defects and susceptibility for particular group of pathogens. It is also important to note that a combination of unrelated immune defects may overlap. Furthermore, such patients may present with multiple infections concurrently, sequentially, or in close proximity to a primary infection episode, with a variety of conventional and opportunistic microorganisms.

An extensive exposure to hospital environment poses risk for transplant recipients to acquire infections that may not respond to conventional antimicrobial drugs. The recent interest in exploring the potential influence of perturbation and reorganization of hosts' microbial flora or microbiota resulting from extensive exposure to healthcare environment, broad-spectrum antimicrobial drugs among other factors, has yielded greater insight into a field that was largely underappreciated for decades. Altered orointestinal microbiota has been proposed in limited observational studies to influence the risk for acquiring infection, recurrence of previously resolved infection, suboptimum response to antimicrobial therapy, and importantly, long-term viability of the transplanted allograft [18–20]. The possibility of noninfectious complications and their potential relationship with altered hosts' microbiota are currently under investigation.

An important approach in the assessment of transplant patients lends from the understanding and knowledge of temporal relationship for the risk of infection that may occur during various clinical phases after transplantation procedure (Table 1.2, with Figs. 1.1, 1.2, 1.3, 1.4, 1.5, and 1.6). For example, patients with long-standing chronic GVHD are

Table 1.1 Infections in transplant patients in relationship with the underlying immune defects

Immune defect	Bacteria	Yeasts and dimorphic fungi	Filamentous molds	Viruses	Parasites
Granulocytopenia	*Staphylococcus aureus*	*Candida* spp.	Hyalohyphomycetes (hyaline or clear wall)	Herpes simplex virus type I and II	
[ANC < 500 cell/ml]	*Streptococcus pneumoniae*	*Candida albicans*[a]	*Aspergillus fumigatus*	Varicella zoster virus	
	Streptococcus gp A, and gp B	Non-*albicans* *Candida* spp.	*Aspergillus flavus*		
	Enterococci including VRE[b]	*Candida glabrata*[c]	*Aspergillus niger*		
	Coagulase-negative *Staphylococcus*[d]	*Candida krusei*[e]	*Aspergillus terreus*[f]		
	Enterobacteriaceae	*Candida parapsilosis*[g]	*Aspergillus nidulans*		
	Escherichia coli	*Candida guilliermondii*[g]	Non-*Aspergillus* hyalohyphomycetes		
	Klebsiella species	Non-*Candida* yeasts[h]	*Fusarium* spp.[i]		
	Enterobacter spp.	*Trichosporon asahii*	*Paecilomyces*		
	Proteus spp.	*Saprochaete capitata*[j]	Mucormycoses		
	Citrobacter spp.	*Saccharomyces*	*Mucorales species*[k]		
	Serratia spp.	*Magnusiomyces capitatus*	Dematiaceous (black or melanin pigmented) molds		
	Nonfermentative gram-negative bacteria	*Rhodotorula mucilaginosa*	*Alternaria*, *Bipolaris*, *Curvularia*, *Exserohilum* spp.		
	Pseudomonas aeruginosa	*Wickerhamomyces anomalus*	*Pseudallescheria boydii*		
	Stenotrophomonas maltophilia	*Pichia kudriavzevii*	*Scedosporium apiospermum*		
	Acinetobacter species	*Cyberlindnera fabianii*	*Scedosporium prolificans*		
	Achromobacter spp.	*Kodamaea ohmeri*			
		Lodderomyces elongisporus			
		Pseudozyma			
Cellular immune defects	*Nocardia asteroides complex*	*Cryptococcus neoformans*	*Aspergillus spp*	Human cytomegalovirus	*Toxoplasma gondii*
	Salmonella typhimurium	Endemic mycoses	Non-*Aspergillus* hyalohyphomycetes	Respiratory viruses	*Strongyloides stercoralis*[l]
	Salmonella enteritidis	*Histoplasma capsulatum*	*Pneumocystis jirovecii*	Influenza A and influenza B	*Microsporidium* spp.
	Rhodococcus equi	*Coccidioides immitis*	Dematiaceous (black pigmented wall) molds	Respiratory syncytial virus	*Cryptosporidium*
	Rhodococcus bronchialis	*Blastomyces dermatitidis*	Mucormycoses	Parainfluenza type-3	*Microspora* spp.
	Listeria monocytogenes	*Paracoccidioides brasiliensis*	*Cryptococcus neoformans*	Adenovirus	*Cyclospora* spp.
	Mycobacterium tuberculosis		Endemic mycoses	Human coronavirus HKU1, NL63, OC43 and C229E[m]	*Leishmania donovani*[n]
	Nontuberculous mycobacteria		*Histoplasma capsulatum*	Corona virus, SARS, MERS[o]	*Leishmania infantum*[p]
	Legionella spp.		*Coccidioides immitis*	Human metapneumovirus[q]	
	Yersinia spp.		*Blastomyces dermatitidis*	Varicella	
	Campylobacter jejuni[r]		*Paracoccidioides brasiliensis*	Varicella zoster virus	
				Human herpes virus 6	
				Parvovirus B19	
				Hantavirus	

(continued)

Table 1.1 (continued)

Immune defect	Bacteria	Yeasts and dimorphic fungi	Filamentous molds	Viruses	Parasites
Humoral immune defects	Encapsulated bacteria			Varicella zoster virus[s]	*Giardia lamblia*
	Streptococcus pneumoniae			Echovirus and other enteroviruses	*Babesia microti*
	Haemophilus influenzae				
	Neisseria meningitidis				
	Campylobacter jejuni				
Splenectomy and functional hyposplenism	Encapsulated bacteria				*Giardia lamblia*
	Streptococcus pneumoniae				*Babesia microti*
	Haemophilus influenzae				
	Neisseria meningitidis				
	Capnocytophaga canimorsus				
Mixed immune defects	*Streptococcus pneumoniae*		*Pneumocystis jirovecii*	Respiratory viruses	*Toxoplasma gondii*
	Staphylococcus aureus		*Aspergillus* spp.	Adenovirus	*Strongyloides stercoralis*
	Haemophilus influenzae		*Candida* spp.	Varicella zoster virus	
	Klebsiella pneumonia		*Cryptococcus neoformans*		
	Pseudomonas aeruginosa		Mucormycoses		
	Acinetobacter spp.		Endemic mycoses		
	Enterobacter spp.		Dematiaceous (black) molds		
	Stenotrophomonas maltophilia				
	Nocardia asteroides complex				
	Listeria monocytogenes				
	Legionella spp.				
	Campylobacter jejuni				

Patients with mixed immune defects include recipients of allogeneic hematopoietic stem cell transplant; patients receiving treatment for acute or chronic graft-versus-host disease; acute or chronic solid organ allograft rejection

Abbreviations: VRE vancomycin-resistant enterococci, *SARS* severe acute respiratory syndrome, *MERS* Middle East respiratory syndrome

[a]In the past two decades, the prevalence of non-albicans invasive candidiasis is seen in excess of *Candida albicans* infections; the emergence of invasive disease due to *Candida auris* with limited susceptibility to currently used antifungal drugs is a challenge

[b]Certain transplant units across the USA have seen a high level of VRE colonization and subsequent risk for invasive disease; these infections are often a surrogate and reflect hosts' high-risk status

[c]Increasing reports of echinocandin resistance among clinical isolates of *C. glabrata* is an alarming trend, where this to become more prominent in the future

[d]Among CoNS group of bacteria, an emerging and recently described highly virulent *Staphylococcus lugdunensis* causes tissue-destructive infections similar to *S. aureus* with an emphasis on necrotizing and difficult-to-treat endocarditis

[e]*Candida krusei* is intrinsically nonsusceptible to fluconazole and to some extent itraconazole; these yeasts are uniformly susceptible to the broad-spectrum triazoles such as voriconazole, posaconazole, and isavuconazonium sulfate

[f]*Aspergillus terreus* is the only clinically relevant *Aspergillus* species that exhibit variable degree of resistance to amphotericin B, thereby increasing the probability of failure to amphotericin-based therapy

[g]*Candida parapsilosis* and *C. guilliermondii* have demonstrated less inherent in vitro susceptibility to the echinocandins; alternative antifungal agents are suggested to treat such infections

[h]Non-*Candida* and non-Cryptococcal yeasts are rare cause of fungemia seen mainly in patients with severe immune dysfunction and those with chronic lung disease

[i]*Fusarium* spp. infections are now increasingly attributed to food-related intestinal tract colonization and invasive disease during periods of severe immune suppression, such as profound and prolonged neutropenia, especially in patients with extensive orointestinal mucosal disruption; other filamentous fungal pathogens from food are *Aspergillus* and *Mucor* spp. Rare organisms linked to food and food products include *Lichtheimia*, *Curvularia*, *Phoma*, *Trichoderma*, *Alternaria*, *Acremonium*, *Paecilomyces*, *Penicillium*, *Achaetomium*, *Amesia*, *Botryotrichum*, *Chaetomium*, *Dichotomopilus*; *Microascus*, *Scopulariopsis*, and *Wallemia*. *Mucor circinelloides* was isolated from yogurt samples and presumed to cause illness in >200 consumers

Table 1.1 (continued)

[j]*Geotrichum capitatum* is now named *Saprochaete capitata*
[k]Mucormycoses in transplant recipients remain an uncommon cause of invasive fungal disease, although patients with voriconazole breakthrough mold disease have significantly higher probability of mucormycosis
[l]*Strongyloides stercoralis* may lead to serious, life-threatening hyperinfection syndrome in patients with marked cellular immune defects following allogeneic allograft transplantation, albeit, this remains a rare complication in patients undergoing transplantation even in the endemic regions
[m]These strains of human coronavirus may cause potentially serious lower respiratory tract disease in the immunocompromised host
[n]*L. donovani* and *L. infantum* may lead to serious visceral leishmaniasis in patients with profound cellular immune defects; *L. donovani* is seen in Africa and Asia
[o]These novel outbreak stains of coronavirus have been observed to cause serious illness in immunosuppressed patients and those with diabetes mellitus, ischemic heart disease, or end-stage kidney disease
[p]*L. infantum* is seen in Africa, Europe, Mediterranean, Central and South America
[q]Systemic extrapulmonary infection including viral encephalitis along with viral pneumonitis in allogeneic stem cell transplant recipients has been noted to cause devastating and life-threatening illness
[r]The incidence of campylobacter disease in AIDS patients is 40-fold higher than in the general population; patients with humoral and cellular immune defects are considered susceptible; it is important to recognize the serious sequelae such as Guillain-Barre syndrome, and reactive arthritis may follow acute infection episode in a small group of patients
[s]VZV is rarely associated with systemic dissemination in patients with humoral immune defects or even those with mixed immune dysfunctions

Table 1.2 Infections in recipients of allogeneic hematopoietic stem cell transplantation

Pathogens	Pretransplant disease or high-risk exposure-related infections	Pre-engraftment during neutropenia (0–30 days)	Post-engraftment including acute GVHD (30–100 days)	Posttransplant including chronic GVHD (>100 days)	Posttransplant seasonal community-onset infections
Bacteria	*Streptococcus pneumoniae*[a]	*Staphylococcus aureus*[b]	GPB and GNB bacteremia[c]	Encapsulated bacteria[d]	Community acquired pneumonia
	Staphylococcus aureus[b]	Coagulase-negative staphylococcus[e]	*Listeria monocytogenes*[f]	GPB and GNB bacteremia[c]	Community onset sinusitis
	Coagulase-negative staphylococcus[e]	*Enterobacteriaceae*[g]	Nocardiosis[h]	*Listeria monocytogenes*	Community onset or travel-related enterocolits
	Enterobacteriaceae[g]	*Escherichia coli*		Nocardiosis	Community onset urinary tract infection including pyelonephritis
	Escherichia coli	*Klebsiella pneumoniae and Klebsiella oxytoca*			Community onset *Clostridium difficile*-associated diarrhea
	Klebsiella pneumoniae and Klebsiella oxytoca	Nonfermentative gram-negatives[i]			
	Nonfermentative gram-negatives[i]	*Pseudomonas aeruginosa*			
	Pseudomonas aeruginosa	*Stenotrophomonas maltophilia*			
	Stenotrophomonas maltophilia	*Clostridium difficile*-associated diarrhea[j]			
	Clostridium difficile-associated diarrhea[j]				
Mycobacteria	*M. tuberculosis*[k]			Reactivation of latent tuberculosis	
	M. kansasii[l]			Relapse of previously treated *M. kansasii* infection	
	Nontuberculous mycobacteria			New or relapse MAC infection[m]	
	Rapid-growing mycobacteria				
	Slow-growing mycobacteria				

(continued)

Table 1.2 (continued)

Pathogens	Pretransplant disease or high-risk exposure-related infections	Pre-engraftment during neutropenia (0–30 days)	Post-engraftment including acute GVHD (30–100 days)	Posttransplant including chronic GVHD (>100 days)	Posttransplant seasonal community-onset infections
Viruses	Herpes simplex type 1 and II	Herpes simplex type I and II	Cytomegalovirus[n]	Cytomegalovirus[o]	Influenza A and B[p]
	Human cytomegalovirus[q]	Varicella zoster virus[r]	Human herpesvirus[s]	Human herpesvirus 6[s]	Parainfluenza
	Varicella zoster virus	Cytomegalovirus[t]	Adenovirus[u]	Adenovirus[u]	RSV[v]
		Human herpesvirus 6[s]	BK virus cystitis[w]	Epstein-Barr virus PTLD[x]	hMPV[y]
		Adenovirus[u]	Epstein-Barr virus PTLD[x]	Parvovirus B 19[z]	hCoV[aa]
				BK virus cystitis[w]	
				JC virus PML[ab]	
Molds and yeasts	Invasive aspergillosis	*Candida fungemia*[ac]	Invasive aspergillosis[ad]	Invasive aspergillosis[ae]	
	Endemic mycosis	Invasive aspergillosis and rare molds[af]	Invasive candidiasis[ag]	Invasive candidiasis[ah]	
	Cryptococcal disease		*Pneumocystis jirovecii*[ai]	*Pneumocystis jirovecii*	
	Invasive candidiasis		Zygomycosis[aj]	Zygomycosis[aj]	
			Fusariosis[ak]	Fusariosis[ak]	
			Dematiaceous (melanin pigmented) molds[al]	Dematiaceous (melanin pigmented) molds[al]	
			Cryptococcal disease[am]	Cryptococcal disease[am]	
Parasites	*Toxoplasma gondii*		*Toxoplasma gondii*[an]	*Toxoplasma gondii*[an]	
	Strongyloidiasis[ao]		Strongyloidiasis[ap]	Strongyloidiasis[ap]	
	Chagas disease[aq]		Chagas disease	Chagas disease	
	Leishmaniasis[ar]		Leishmaniasis	Leishmaniasis	

[a]Pneumococcus is the leading cause of community-onset bacterial pneumonia, and patients with hematologic malignancies, especially those with cancer or antineoplastic therapy-related humoral immune dysfunction and various other medical comorbid conditions such as diabetes mellitus, chronic structural lung diseases like emphysema, end-stage kidney disease, and cirrhosis of liver to name a few, are at risk for potentially severe systemic disease

[b]The emergence and global spread of community-acquired methicillin-resistant *S. aureus* has made empiric use of anti-staphylococcal penicillin's obsolete

[c]Catheter-related bloodstream infection, extensive healthcare environment exposure and hospital-acquired pathogens, persistent mucositis, orointestinal or cutaneous hyper-acute and acute GVHD, and accelerated iatrogenic immune suppression including need for high-dose corticosteroids are salient factors that promote invasive bacterial infections during this period. Pretransplant colonization due to VRE, MRSA, or MDR GNB including MRD Pseudomonas, ESBL-producing *Enterobacteriaceae*, and some food-borne fungi such as Fusarium spp., especially in transplant unit located in certain geographic areas, are thought to promote infections due to these pathogens

[d]Hyposplenism after HSCT is a late complication and commonly attributed to late-onset acute GVHD, most frequently noted in patients with chronic GVHD. It is however important to recognize that a number of allogeneic HSCT recipients without clinical diagnosis of GVHD may have functional hyposplenism and are at risk for severe, systemic infection due to encapsulated bacteria

[e]Indwelling prosthetic devices including intravascular access catheters; surgical drains; implanted prosthesis such as heart valves, joints, biliary, bronchial, urinary tract stents; and other various implantable surgical devices promote infections due to CoNS and *Candida* spp. that commonly colonizes the skin and genitourinary and orointestinal tracts

[f]Listeria bacteremia and meningitis are rare complications in patients receiving TMP-SMX prophylaxis for PCP. The incidence of bacterial meningitis is 30-fold higher in HSCT recipients compared with persons without HSCT. As expected, patients undergoing allograft stem cell transplant are at a significant higher risk compared with those undergoing autologous HSCT (70 vs. 16 per 100 000 patients per year). In HSCT recipients *Streptococcus pneumoniae* is the most common pathogen associated with bacterial meningitis, *Neisseria meningitidis*, *Streptococcus mitis*, listeriosis may be rarely seen

[g]Increasing frequency of multidrug-resistant strains to fluorinated quinolones and regional high prevalence of extended-spectrum beta-lactamases producing GNB including carbapenem-resistant *Enterobacteriaceae* has seriously curtailed treatment options for such infections. *Enterobacteriaceae* include *Salmonella* spp., *Escherichia coli*, *Yersinia pestis*, *Klebsiella* spp., *Shigella*, *Proteus*, *Enterobacter*, *Serratia*, and *Citrobacter*

[h]CNS nocardiosis is difficult to distinguish from brain toxoplasmosis, tuberculosis, aspergillosis and other neurotropic clear (hyaline) and black mold infections, and CNS lymphoma

[i]Nonfermentative gram-negatives include *Pseudomonas aeruginosa*, *Burkholderia cepacia*, *Stenotrophomonas maltophilia*, *Acinetobacter baumannii*, other *Acinetobacter* spp., *Alcaligenes* and *Achromobacter* spp., and emerging cases of *Sphingomonas paucimobilis*. Inherent or acquired drug resistance is a major concern in selection of effective empiric therapy for pathogens in this group, which may either lack the drug target site or produce extended-spectrum hydrolyzing enzymes aginst a variety of commonly used antimicrobials; these bacteria may also exhibit phenotypes with reduced expression of outer membrane porins and/or heightened expression of efflux pumps among other mechanisms for antimicrobial drug resistance

[j]Orointestinal mucositis increases the risk of CDAD and so does exposure to broad-spectrum antimicrobials and possibly antineoplastic chemotherapy-induced alteration in hosts' intestinal protective anaerobic microbiota

Table 1.2 (continued)

[k]It now considered standard of care to perform interferon-gamma release assays for diagnosis of latent tuberculosis infection; treatment with isoniazid is considered gold standard and should be administered for a minimum of 6 months prior to the transplantation procedure, with the aim to prevent active tuberculosis infection during the post-transplant period. Such infections tend to be more serious and, due to potential drug toxicity and drug-drug interaction, often difficult to treat after allograft transplantation

[l]*M. kansasii* leads to clinical disease indistinguishable from *M. tuberculosis* infection; risk for infection relapse, drug resistance, and infection recalcitrance are reason for longer duration of therapy

[m]In a recent study from South Korea, in 7342 SOT and 1266 HSCT recipients, 22 patients developed NTM after a median 2 years following transplantation. *Mycobacterium avium-intracellulare* complex was the most common pathogen isolated; nodular bronchiectasis (~80%) was common presentation. A near 70% response to antimicrobial therapy in this group was encouraging. However, disseminated NTM including MAC disease in severely immunosuppressed patients following high-risk allogeneic HSCT may occasionally present as salvage therapy-refractroy recalcitrant bacteremia with high fatality

[n]Risk of CMV infection is highest in CMV-seronegative recipients in whom allograft is given from a CMV-seropositive donor. Ganciclovir prophylaxis effectively prevents CMV disease in high-risk patients during the first 100 days after allogeneic HSCT

[o]Late CMV disease is associated with high mortality rate nearing 45% and seen 170 median days after HSCT. It is important to recognize that close to 40% of patients that respond to the initial episode of late posttransplant CMV infection will develop a second CMV episode within a median of 11–12 weeks. Three months after HSCT, patients with positive CMV-pp65 antigenemia; post-engraftment severe lymphopenia of less than 100 lymphocytes/mm^3, especially those with helper T-cell lymphocytopenia of less than 50 cells/mm^3; presence of GVHD; and those with undetectable CMV-specific T-cell responses are at higher risk for late CMV end-organ disease. Furthermore, after 100 days following transplantation, presence of CMV viremia or pp65 antigenemia and severe lymphopenia endorsed by less than 300 lymphocytes/mm^3 is considered strong predictors for late CMV disease and death

[p]Most frequently detected viruses in symptomatic HSCT or SOT recipients with URTI are picornaviruses (~40%), such as rhinovirus and enterovirus, whereas coronavirus and influenza are isolated in nearly 20% of such patients, each. Influenza URTIs similar to RSV and unlike parainfluenza virus infections have the potential for progression to the lower respiratory tract. Viral pneumonitis is a serious complication in patients following allogeneic stem cell transplantation. It is important to recognize that hosts' immune response to influenza infection garners a high IFN-gamma state resulting in a transient increased susceptibility for secondary bacterial infections like pneumococcus, *S. aureus*, and *Pseudomonas* spp. The resulting superimposed bacterial pneumonia may precipitate life-threatening sepsis and respiratory failure. Furthermore, RTVIs are recognized as fostering enhanced susceptibility for invasive fungal lung disease during early and late transplant periods

[q]Serologic evaluation of the donor and recipient for latent CMV infection is the cornerstone during pretransplant assessment. Dissonance between D+ and R- CMV serology is the most important complicating factors during early and late posttransplant period. Antiviral prophylaxis, preemptive and empiric therapy approaches are based on CMV serologic disparities

[r]It is standard to provide prophylaxis for HSV and VZV during preparatory conditioning regimen and continue during the early post-HSCT period. Prophylaxis may have to be extended in patients with acute GVHD, cancer recurrence, patients undergoing high-risk transplantation procedure, and those with primary or secondary allograft compromise

[s]HHV-6 high-grade viremia by DNA analysis has been associated with central nervous system (CNS) dysfunction, although viral interstitial/alveolar pneumonitis is not an uncommon disease attributed to HHV6 infection following allogeneic HSCT. HHV6 may also present as limbic encephalitis with subcortical temporal lobe seizure activity presenting as memory loss and insomnia. Febrile partial or complete myelosuppression and/or skin rash should alert the physicians regarding HHV6 as a potential treatable cause of secondary stem cell allograft loss. Viral gastroduodenitis, colitis, and pericarditis are other clinical manifestations attributed to HHV6 infection in this vulnerable population. An association with post-HSCT HHV6 viremia with delayed monocyte and platelet engraftment, increased platelet transfusion requirements, risk for high-grade GVHD, and all-cause mortality needs further evaluation

[t]Early CMV low-grade viremia was observed by the use of ultrasensitive nucleic assays, within 3–4 weeks after high-risk allogeneic stem cell graft transplantation

[u]The incidence of adenovirus disease ranges from 3% to as high as 47% in high-risk pediatric allogeneic HSCT recipients. Patients undergoing T-cell-depleted stem cell grafts and those with acute graft-versus-host disease are also at increased risk for severe life-threatening adenovirus disseminated disease, which is a well-recognized complication in patients with persistent peripheral blood lymphocyte counts of <300 cells/mm^3. Infection involves respiratory (viral pneumonitis), gastrointestinal (colitis, including hemorrhagic colitis) tracts, and hepatitis;patients may present with posttransplant hemorrhagic cystitis. Adenovirus dissemination represents severity of underlying immune defect and is seen in 10–20% of patients with end-organ viral disease, except in patients with adenovirus cystitis, where disseminated adenoviral disease is seldom observed

[v]Long-term (>30 days) viral shedding is not uncommon in patients following allogeneic HSCT; RSV is notable RTVI in this regard. The 80 days of median duration of viral shedding may extend to just under a year in some allogeneic transplant recipients. This potential for pronged viral shedding warrants heightened awareness and strict adherence to appropriate precautions to prevent nosocomial RSV transmission to other vulnerable hospitalized patients. In the pediatric HSCT recipients, RSV infection within 60 days after transplant, patients given systemic corticosteroids within a week prior to the onset of RSV infection and the need for assisted mechanical ventilation were significant predictors for subsequent complications and death

[w]The BK virus was first isolated in 1971; after primary childhood infection, persistent BKV infection occurs within renal tubular cells and the urothelium. Viral reactivation in the recipients of kidney and allogeneic HSCT usually presents as allograft nephropathy and hemorrhagic cystitis, respectively. Presently, reduction in drug-induced immune suppression, when possible, and supportive care are the only viable treatment option; direct antiviral drug against BKV remains elusive

[x]EBV influence over B-cell malignant clones may act through different mechanisms of transcriptional regulation and possibly variance in genetic mechanisms that eventually determined viral latency during early EBV infection and EBV-host interaction

[y]The incidence of hMPV infection was similar to the incidence of RSV or parainfluenza virus UTRIs in patients undergoing HSCT. hMPV infections are notable for low risk of progression to the LRT. Serious systemic hMPV disease including viral encephalitis has been reported. Overall, these infections are well-tolerated, albeit hMPV pneumonitis in severely immunosuppressed stem cell allograft recipients may result in serious life-threatening lung disease

(continued)

Table 1.2 (continued)

[z]Parvo B19 infection may present as pure red cell aplasia after allogeneic HSCT

[aa]hCoV similar to hMPV is a common RTV. Serotypes associated with disease in transplant population include hCoV-OC43 followed by NL63, HKU1; 229E is less common. Unlike hMPV, these infections have a higher likelihood for progressing to the LRT, which often presents as subclinical, mild to moderate viral illness. In an observation among HSCT recipients, hCoV infection resulted in a notable number (~20%) of hospitalizations. In concert with hMPV infection, despite presence of severe immune suppression, hCoV-related confirmed deaths in allogeneic HSCT recipients remain less than 5%. Approximately one-third of transplant patients with hCoV infection may have infection due to other RTVs such as human bocavirus (HBoV). HBoV is an uncommon RTV in transplant patients and often (> 80%) seen with other RTVs. HBoV rarely causes LRTI; most infections are well-tolerated despite, transplant-related severe immune suppression

[ab]John Cunningham virus (JCV)-associated progressive multifocal leukoencephalopathy (PML) is an uncommon disease in patients undergoing allogeneic HSCT. In a report from Israel, 20 of 40 patients (24%) with JCV reactivation had persistent viremia after receiving myeloablative and nonmyeloablative pretransplant conditioning. PML was diagnosed in two patients with persistent JCV viremia, 96 and 127 days after HSCT. Advanced age was a significant predictor of JCV reactivation; 70% of these allogeneic HSCT recipients with persistent viral reactivation had died. Identifying high-risk patients with persistent JCV reactivation, especially those with incremental levels of viremia, may benefit from reduced drug-induced immune suppression for prevention of JCV leukoencephalopathy. PML continues to remain a devastating, albeit rare post-transplant infectious complication. *Artesunate*, an antimalarial drug that showed potent ex vivo activity against HHV-6, however, clinical response to artesunate in HSCT recipients with JCV-PML, has not been encouraging

[ac]Candidemia is seen in patients with severe pre-engraftment neutropenia (absolute neutrophil count <500 cell/microliter) that extends longer than 5 days. The increase in non-*albicans Candida* spp. is mainly due to *C. glabrata*, although patients following HSCT are also at risk for *C. krusei* infection. Emergence of echinocandin resistance among clinical *C. glabrata* isolates is concerning. For patients with *C. parapsilosis* infection, it is recommended to use antifungal drugs other than echinocandin class. The emergence of MDR *Candida auris* infections in transplant population makes selection of empiric anti-yeast therapy more challenging

[ad]Genetic susceptibility for IA include mutations in Dectin-1 and DC-SIGN among other well recognized risk factors such as high-risk allogeneic HSCT, CMV and respiratory virus infection, and positive *Aspergillus* PCR. It was recently noted that presence of three of the aforementioned factors generated a 57% probability for developing IA. In patients with no risk factors, the probability of IA was 2%, compared to ~80% in patients with four or more such risk factors

[ae]CMV reactivation after stem cell allograft transplantation increases the risk for IFD during the late transplant period. Unlike the risk factors for early IFD such as AML (HR 3), HLA antigen-mismatched donor graft (HR 3.4); HSCT recipients with lymphoma (HR 8.5), CMV reactivation (HR 5.5), and severe neutropenia (HR 3.5) are considered prominent risk factors for late-onset IFD. Patients with pretransplant IgG responses against *Aspergillus* proteins indicating significant fungal colonization or ongoing subclinical *Aspergillus* infections before preparatory conditioning regimen has commenced needs further clinical validation. Evaluation of 5589 HSCT recipients at a comprehensive cancer center between 1985 and 1999 showed increased incidence of IA after 1992 and remained high during that decade. The authors also reported increasing frequency of non-*Aspergillus* molds such as *Fusarium* spp. and mucormycosis in the late 1990s. These non-*Aspergillus* molds were prominent in patients undergoing multiple transplants. Most cases of mucormycosis were seen during the late transplant period, especially in patients with chronic GVHD. In patients undergoing nonmyeloablative HSCT, presence of severe acute GVHD, chronic extensive GVHD, and CMV infection are prominent risk factors for IFD

[af]Invasive aspergillosis is a complication seen in patients with delayed (>2 weeks) recovery of peripheral blood granulocyte count. Patients receiving high-dose systemic corticosteroids are also at an increased risk. *Aspergillus fumigatus* remains the most prevalent mold to cause invasive human disease, including in patients undergoing HSCT. Infections caused by *Scedosporium* and *Fusarium* spp. are occasionally seen in hematopoietic stem cell allograft recipients and commonly present during the period(s) of severe and prolonged neutropenia

[ag]Routine blood cultures have low sensitivity for diagnosis of fungemia. Carbohydrate biomarker (1, 3)-β-d-glucan has emerged as a useful laboratory test for the diagnosis of invasive yeast and mold disease. Furthermore, it may be used to monitor response to systemic antifungal therapy and infection relapse

[ah]Post-HSCT recovery of antigen-specific T lymphocyte-mediated immune response against CMV and *Candida albicans* is regarded as critical during the early and the late transplant period. Most patients develop antigen-specific T-cell response early in the transplant period which is derived from clones of both donor and recipient stem cell origin. Reconstitution of immune response via antigen-specific T lymphocytes of recipient origin is weakened in patients with GVHD. Incidence of IC during the 1st year after nonmyeloablative (5%) and myeloablative transplant conditioning is lower than that for IA (14%). Echinocandin nonsusceptible *Candida* spp. infection has been recently recognized as an emerging challenge in providing care for these highly vulnerable patients

[ai]PCP is a serious OI in transplant patients with severe cellular immune defect(s). Routine anti-PCP prophylaxis breakthrough infections are rare; although in patients receiving aerosolized pentamidine, atypical upper lung PCP may occasionally occur

[aj]Invasive zygomycosis or mucormycosis may occur disproportionally more frequently in patients on voriconazole prophylaxis and those with sinuorbital invasive mold disease. In transplant patients, the overall prevalence is less than 8% among all invasive fungal infections

[ak]Nearly half of the patients with disseminated fusariosis have evidence of fungemia, and close to 80% may exhibit multiple (>10–15) papular skin lesions with a necrotic center that is indistinguishable from ecthyma gangrenosum due to *Staphylococcus aureus* or disseminated *Pseudomonas* spp. infection

[al]Dematiaceous or melanin pigmented molds are associated with chronic localized infections and prevalent in certain geographic regions. In transplant patients, disseminated infections may occur; neurotropism is an important feature of these infections, and treatment with older antifungal drugs such as amphotericin B and early generation triazole-based compounds was associated with high rates of treatment failure

[am]The cumulative incidence of CNS infection following HSCT is <1% within first 30 days, 2% within 3 months, and 5% after 5 years following transplantation. Significantly high risk of CNS infection 5 years after CBT (8%) vs. matched related HSCT (2%) is important to note for the purpose of risk stratification. CNS fungal (35%) and viral (32%) infections are prominent, whereas toxoplasmosis and bacterial infection are seen in just over 10% of the patients. Aspergillosis is common (67%) followed by *Cryptococcus neoformans* (17%). CNS infection in transplant population is associated with high mortality (59%), and low (20%) 5-year overall survival

Table 1.2 (continued)

[an]Donor-derived toxoplasmosis has been reported along with cases of brucellosis in the endemic regions, along with West Nile virus infection, rabies, Chagas disease, and rare cases of lymphocytic choriomeningitis virus infection

[ao]*Strongyloides stercoralis* (pinworm or threadworms and *Enterobius vermiculari*) in the underdeveloped countries where fecal contamination of soil and water is common; evaluation of allogeneic transplant candidates requires serologic evaluation for exposure and if present, appropriate treatment should be completed for intestinal subclinical parasitic infestation prior to the trasnplantation procedure

[ap]In patients with extensive T-cell immune defects, *Strongyloides stercoralis* may cause accelerated autoinfection. Hyperinfection pulmonary syndrome in such patients is almost always fatal. Screening serology tests for the presence of strongyloidiasis by enzyme-linked immunosorbent assay after allogeneic HSCT may be falsely negative; and stool ova and parasite examination, in the absence of accelerated autoinfection during the pretransplant, is also riddled with low sensitivity

[aq]American trypanosomiasis caused by *Trypanosoma cruzi* needs to be assessed in patients planned to undergo allograft transplant procedure from endemic regions

[ar]Leishmania is transmitted by the bite of certain species of sand flies and presents as cutaneous (common) and visceral (uncommon and severe) disease; pretransplant evaluation should include serologic testing for prior exposure to these parasites in appropriate patients with high risk for prior exposure

Abbreviations: GVHD graft-versus-host disease, *HSV* herpes simplex virus 1 and 2, *CMV* cytomegalovirus, *VZV* varicella zoster virus, *HHV6* human herpesvirus 6, *EBV* Epstein-Barr virus, *CoNS* coagulase-negative *Staphylococcus*, *CDAD Clostridium difficile*-associated diarrhea, *GPB* gram-positive bacteria, *GNB* gram-negative bacteria, *HSCT* hematopoietic stem cell transplantation, *RSV* respiratory syncytial virus, *hMPV human metapneumovirus*, *hCoV* human coronavirus hypervirulent subtypes NL63 and HKU1, *PML* progressive multifocal leukoencephalopathy, *EBV-PTLD* Epstein-Barr virus-associated B-cell lymphoproliferative disorder, *HR* hazard ratio, *IFD* invasive fungal disease, *IA* invasive aspergillosis, *IC* invasive candidiasis, *SOT* solid organ transplant, *URTI* upper respiratory tract infection, *LRTI* lower respiratory tract infections, *RTV* respiratory tract virus, *RTVIs* respiratory tract viral infections, *hCoV* human coronavirus

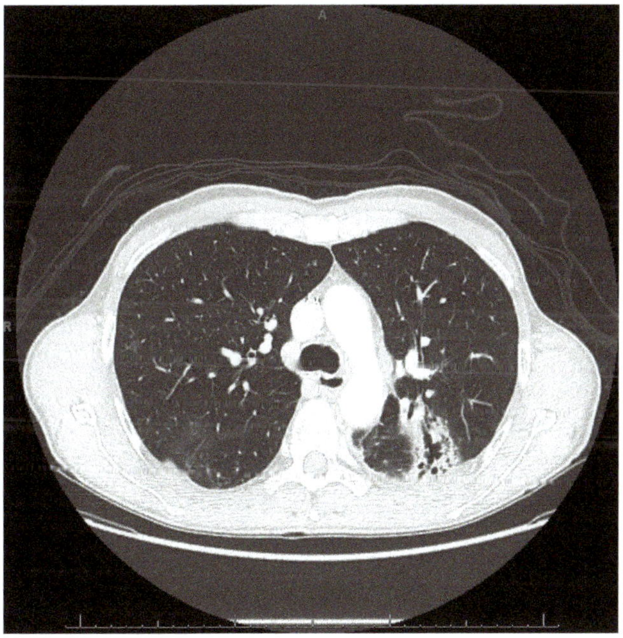

Fig. 1.1 CT scan of lungs without intravenous contrast showing necrotizing left lung *Pseudomonas* infection in a patient following HSCT. The differential for this thick-walled irregular cavitary lesion is broad and includes other bacterial infection such as *Klebsiella* spp., *Stenotrophomonas maltophilia*, *Staphylococcus aureus*, *Streptococcus pneumoniae*, *Escherichia coli*, *Nocardia* spp.; *Mycobacterium tuberculosis* and nontuberculous mycobacterial infections. Cavitary rapidly growing cancers may have similar presentation, whereas viral infections including cytomegalovirus and adenovirus seldom present with such features. Other than suppurative necrosis of the lung, ischemic necrosis, i.e. pulmonary infarction, should also be considered. Tissue invasive mold lung disease may also have comparable radiographic presentation

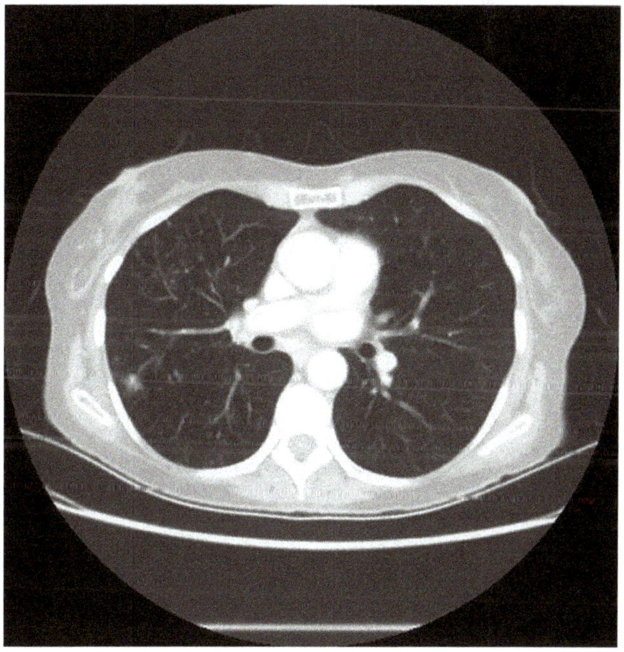

Fig. 1.2 CT scan of lungs without intravenous contrast showing tree-in-bud appearance due to pulmonary *Mycobacterium avium* complex disease mostly involving the right lung demonstrating multiple areas of centrilobular nodules with a linear branching pattern. Endobronchial tuberculosis may present with such a radiographic finding, wherein patients with acutely developed tree-in-bud infiltrates bacterial or viral (CMV) etiology may also be entertained. It is important to note that bronchiectasis is the prominent radiographic presentation of *Mycobacterium avium* complex infection in patients undergoing transplantation. Rarely carcinomatous endarteritis due to breast or gastric cancer; bronchovascular interstitial infiltration due to lymphoma, leukemia, and sarcoidosis may have similar presentation. Scedosporium lung disease and pulmonary fusariosis may occassionally have nodular peribrochovascular distribution

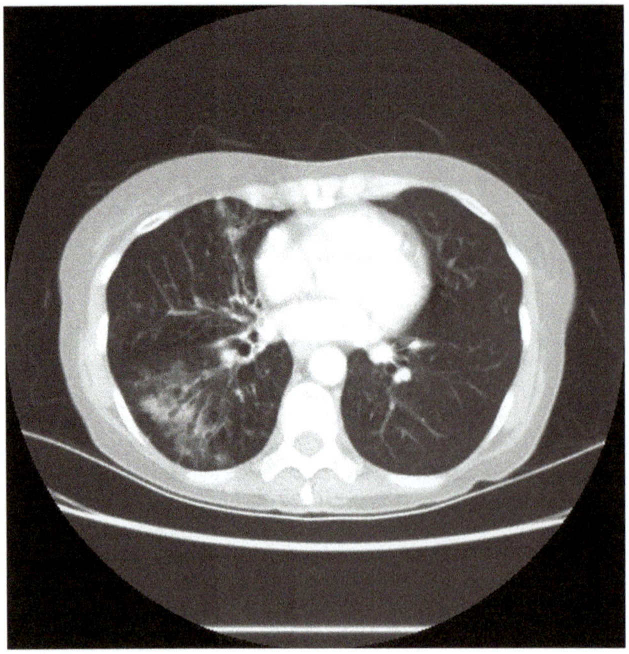

Fig. 1.3 CT scan of lungs without intravenous contrast showing right lung *Mycobacterium kansasii* pneumonia with peribronchial thickening that could be mistaken for CMV pneumonitis and *Mycobacterium tuberculosis*, among other lung infections in a patients following allogeneic HSCT

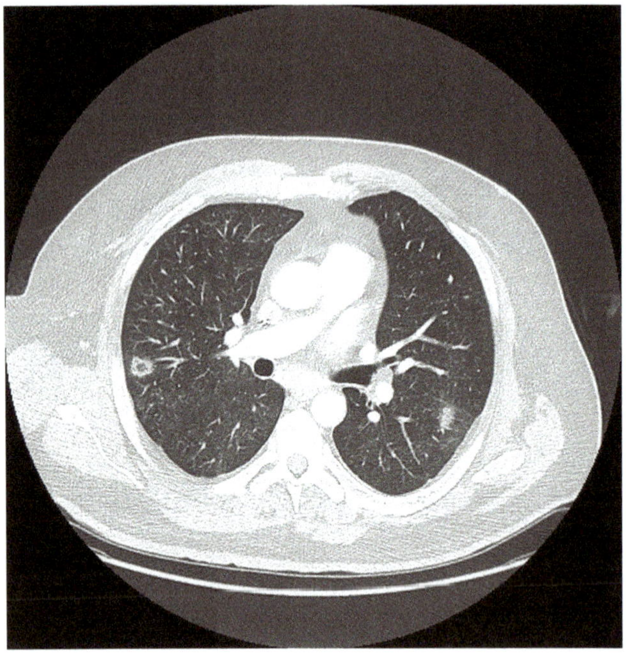

Fig. 1.4 CT scan of lungs without intravenous contrast showing bilateral nodular zygomycosis in a patient following allogeneic HSCT while receiving voriconazole prophylaxis. The right lung nodule with a central cavity cannot be radiographically excluded from other causes of nodular pneumonia such as invasive pulmonary aspergillosis, *Fusarium* spp., and other mold lung disease. Among bacteria, *Nocardia* spp. is a concern in allograft transplant recipients with such radiographic presentation. Primary lung lymphoma may have similar presentation. Rarely, patients with relapse acute leukemia in the post HSCT period may present with atypical pulmonary infiltrates

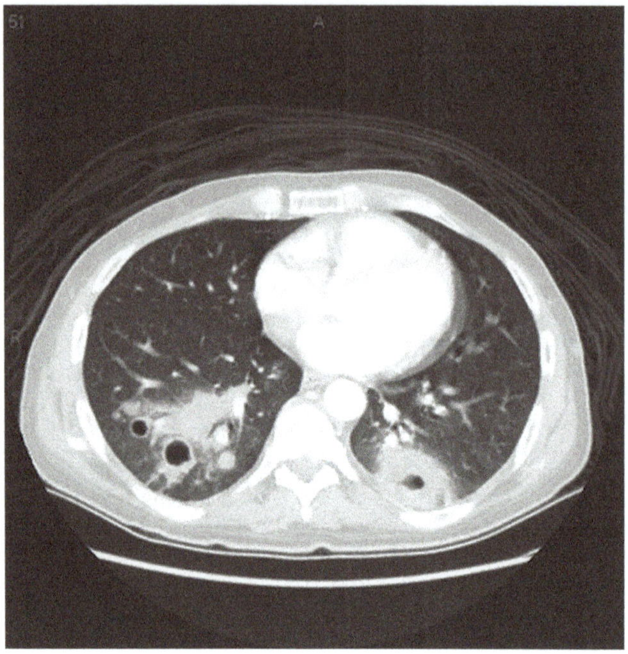

Fig. 1.5 CT scan of lungs without intravenous contrast showing cavitary pneumonia with dense consolidation involving both lower lobes in a patient with GVHD, who developed infection due to dematiaceous mold following allogeneic HSCT. In the differential diagnosis, necrotizing bacterial, clear (hyaline) and black (melanin pigmented) mold infections should also be considered along with multifocal pulmonary nocardiosis

at an additional risk for infections that are often seen in asplenic patients or those with functional hyposplenism. Patients with chronic GVHD are not only at an increased risk for systemic fungal disease like invasive aspergillosis or herpes virus reactivation herald by CMV viremia; additionally, encapsulated bacteria such as outlined in Table 1.1 may also be included in the risk profile during evaluation of such patients.

Patients receiving treatment for acute GVHD after allogeneic HSCT have heightened risk for invasive aspergillosis and infections due to other filamentous molds. Unlike the first risk period for invasive mold disease in allogeneic stem cell recipients, which coincides with the period of pre-engraftment severe neutropenia, patients with acute and chronic GVHD are seldom neutropenic.

Table 1.3 illustrates the salient features of infection risk and their association with the type of stem cell graft, pretransplant conditioning preparatory regimens, and drugs commonly used in the prevention of GVHD. Cord blood stem cells are regarded as a major breakthrough for source that yields a steady supply of hematopoietic stem cells, especially among patients with difficult to find, immunologically (HLA-matched) compatible hematopoietic stem cell graft [18]. Cord blood stem cells have a limited number of nucleated cells that are adequate for children. In adults

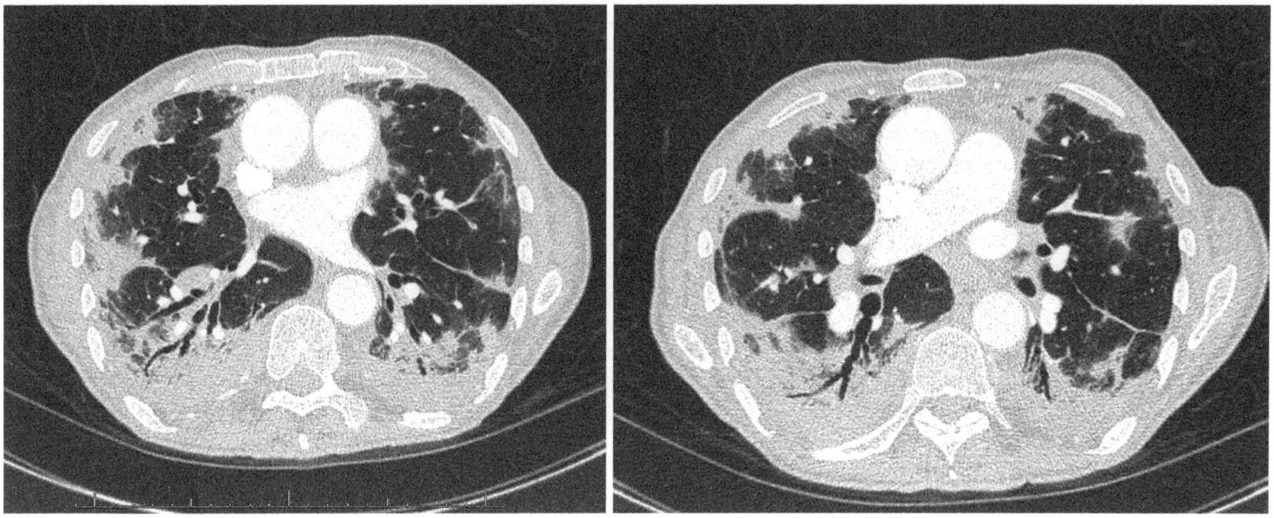

Fig. 1.6 CT scan of lungs without intravenous contrast showing cryptogenic organising pneumonia in a patient following allogeneic HSCT that may be mistaken for fibrosing subacute infection due to endemic mycosis among other causes of subacute lung infection

due to larger body surface area, transplantation with less than optimum number of stem cells complicate posttransplant period with issues such as inadequate and delayed neutrophil engraftment and peripheral blood cell count recovery, precarious graft stability, and, similar to recipients of T-cell-depleted grafts, a higher risk for infections associated with severe and prolonged neutropenia or those observed during GVHD (Tables 1.1 and 1.2). Various strategies are being explored to assuage this limitation including transplantation with cord blood grafts from more than one donor and ex vivo expansion of a single donor cord blood graft to increase the yield of nucleated cells [21]. In a review of 100 cord blood transplants at a comprehensive cancer center in Houston, Texas, the infection incidence rate ratio, which was total infection episodes per days at risk (survival after CBT) × 100, was 2.4 times higher in adult patients compared with children [22]. It was important to note that risk of infection was even greater (three times higher) in adults with neutropenia and was 1.9 times higher in patients with GVHD when compared with children undergoing CBT procedure [22].

It is considered essential to create a comprehensive infection assessment strategy that takes into account and recognizes the local issues at a particular transplant unit and its unique patient population. Such an approach requires cognizance of existing influences that may promote risk for infection including local and regional infection trends, patterns in pathogen prevalence and drug susceptibility profiles. Continued vigilance regarding emergent pathogens and ever-changing infection risk profile with advances in transplant procedures and drug-induced immune suppression are of paramount importance in providing care for the highly vulnerable transplant population.

A variety of noninfectious conditions may clinically and radiographically emulate an infectious process. Among these noninfectious maladies, those involving the skin and the lungs are the great imitators; when present, they are difficult to clinically distinguish from infections such as cellulitis or pneumonia. Two chapters in this volume are dedicated to provide an in-depth discussion on these topics.

An approach for establishing correct diagnosis for opportunistic infections is based on the maxim "when uncertain, obtain a tissue sample." A diligent adjudication is the central tenet in establishing accurate diagnosis for the immunologically vulnerable patients, in whom proclivity for atypical disease presentation further complicates ascertaining correct and timely diagnosis. Inaccurate diagnosis under the old dispensation of serologic and culture-based system may lead to inappropriate and ineffective treatment, worsening patients' morbidity, risk for further complications, and death. Therefore, focused yet comprehensive differential diagnoses, which encompasses etiology of infections and noninfectious causes that may mimic an infectious process including but not limited to drug toxicity; de novo malignancies or post transplant cancer recurrence; typical or atypical presentation of lymphoproliferative disorders; immune-inflammatory diseases like GVHD; and tissue infiltrative processes such as solid allograft rejection among others may greatly improve the guidance for an optimized management approach in patients undergoing lifesaving, stem cell and solid organ allograft transplantation.

Table 1.3 Relationship between infection risk and HSCT variables

Stem cell source, preparatory conditioning regimens, and GVHD prophylaxis	Immune defects	Infections
Allogeneic vs. autologous graft	Allograft recipient exhibits gradual recovery of cellular and adaptive immune function	Pre-engraftment neutropenia, if longer than 7–14 days, increases the risk for invasive candidiasis and IMD
	Innate immune function aided by cellular and acellular antimicrobial defense is to recover early after transplantation, especially in patients undergoing conventional autologous and nonmyeloablative HSCT. It is heralded by granulocyte engraftment and posttransplant resolution of neutropenia	IFD heightened risk coincides with the peak incidence of acute and chronic GVHD
	Complements and antimicrobial peptides reconstitute early after transplantation	Severe respiratory viral infections are also problematic in patients given systemic corticosteroids and immunosuppressive therapy for GVHD
	Patients with persistent severe thrombocytopenia that may follow in high-risk allogeneic stem cell recipients may continue to exhibit reduced host defense due to suboptimum thrombin-releasable antimicrobial peptides from platelets including platelet factor 4, RANTES, connective tissue-activating peptide 3, platelet basic protein, thymosin β-4, fibrinopeptide B, and fibrinopeptide A. The impact of depleted platelet-assisted immune defense and potentially higher susceptibility for infection in HSCT recipients with severe thrombocytopenia is not certain	CMV, less commonly HHV6, and disseminated adenovirus are encountered in patients with profound defects in anti-CMV and other antiviral pathogen-specific, effector cellular immune response
	Myeloid and plasmacytoid dendritic cells are recovered within 60 days after allogeneic HSCT to pretransplant levels, unless patients develop acute GVHD, in which case this recovery is significantly delayed. However, it may take a year or longer to achieve normal functional DC cell population after undergoing allogeneic stem cell transplantation. Plasmacytoid DCs are important for regulation and maintenance of immune tolerance and defense against viruses. The myeloid DCs serve as APCs that are pivotal in eliciting pathogen-directed cellular adaptive immune response	
	Recovery of NK cells in most patients undergoing allogeneic HSCT occurs usually 45 days after transplantation. These innate immune effector cells can directly lyse virus-infected cells and provide antineoplastic immune surveillance. NK cells are an important, readily available, albeit transient source of IFNγ and GM-CSF. The chemokines such as MIP-1α, MIP-1β, IL-8, and RANTES play a critical role in adaptive immune modulation. It was notable that lack of qualitative NK cell recovery in patients with T-cell-depleted transplant may render them less effective for prolonged periods	

Table 1.3 (continued)

Stem cell source, preparatory conditioning regimens, and GVHD prophylaxis	Immune defects	Infections
Unrelated donor or mismatched stem cell graft	Unrelated donor grafts are more frequently associated with severe GVHD and/or graft rejection compared with sibling donor stem cell allograft transplants	Mismatched and unrelated donor stem cell allograft transplants carry a significant risk for serious life-threatening infections seen in the late (6–18 months) post-transplant period. CMV infection and acute GVHD contribute significantly toward this risk. The late fatal infections include pneumonia, sepsis, central nervous system infection, and disseminated varicella
	Slow reconstitution of adaptive cellular helper and cytotoxic immunity, which is further delayed in patients requiring treatment for acute GVHD	IA 6 months after transplantation was associated with chronic GVHD and CMV disease
	Humoral immune response may not fully recover in patients with chronic GVHD	*Fusarium* spp. IFD is threefold higher in patients undergoing HLA-mismatched vs. HLA-matched HSCT; most cases occur 48 median days after transplantation. The trimodal distribution similar to IA coincides with pre-engraftment neutropenia; 60 days and over 1 year after transplant, corresponding with the incidence of acute and chronic GVHD, respectively
	Bone marrow as the source of stem cells and treatment with high-dose corticosteroids delay recovery of functional T-cell-based immunity for 3 months or longer after transplantation	Persistent neutropenia similar to that seen in cases with disseminated *Scedosporium* spp. infection and other invasive mold disease after allogeneic HSCT was the prominent prognosticator for death in patients with fusariosis
		It has also been recognized that subclinical CMV reactivation in patients while on ganciclovir prophylaxis or preemptive therapy appears to be a potent stimulator of T-cell function after transplantation
		Other serious infections include EBV-PTLD, disseminated HHV-6, and disseminated adenovirus infections
Peripheral blood stem cell graft vs. bone marrow stem cells	Faster neutrophil engraftment	The rate of severe and proven infections following stem cell engraftment was ≥twofold higher in patients in whom bone marrow SCT was given compared with those undergoing transplantation with PBSC allografts
	Blood stem cell grafts have higher lymphocyte subset counts, which, in most part, account for fewer infectious complications during the posttransplant period	HLA-matched, related-donor peripheral blood stem cells appear to lend protection against IA during early transplant period compared with those undergoing similar bone marrow stem cell allograft transplants
	Late transplant immune suppression due to chronic GVHD may occur	The greatest benefit of PBSC vs. BMSC has been noted in the risk profile for IFD, whereas for bacterial infections such benefit is intermediate, and it is least for viral infections

(continued)

Table 1.3 (continued)

Stem cell source, preparatory conditioning regimens, and GVHD prophylaxis	Immune defects	Infections
Cord blood stem cell graft	Slower neutrophil engraftment resulting in prolonged neutropenia in adult CBT recipients continues to be a serious limitation for this stem cell donor source	Cord blood stem cell transplantation increases the risk of early (<40 days) IAs
	Adult patients require a higher number of total nucleated cells and CD34+ progenitors than are often present in a cord blood unit, yielding to instability of the allograft even after successful engraftment. To mitigate these limitations, especially in adults, strategies to expand selected subpopulations of stem cell within the cord blood unit and transplantation of multiunit CB are currently being explored	CBT recipients had a higher incidence of severe bacterial infections within 100 days after transplantation; however, 3 years after CBT, risks of severe bacterial and other infections are comparable to patients undergoing BMT or peripheral blood allogeneic HSCT
	Slower restitution of T-cell pathogen-specific, cellular immune response as cord blood T-cells are predominantly naïve and exhibit suboptimum T-cell proliferation and IFN-gamma production in response to an insult or exposure to a foreign antigen. This inherent cellular dysfunction in CBS grafts appears to reflect defect(s) in signal transduction pathway(s)	CMV infection and/or presence of acute GVHD significantly increases the risk for IA
	Furthermore, T-cell dysfunction may also arise from prominence of Treg population in CBS with potent suppressor function compared with moderate Treg population in adult donor-derived stem cell grafts	Most (>90%) IFD similar to bacterial infections are seen within 100 days after transplantation
	Hypogammaglobulinemia and other B-cell dysfunction may occur in patients with chronic GVHD	Nearly half of the early fungal infections may be noted within the first 30 days after CBT
	Risk of graft rejection and severe acute GVHD have been comparable to that observed following PBSC or BMSC transplants; this is despite high degree of HLA antigen donor-recipient disparity in most adult patients undergoing CBT	CMV and varicella zoster virus infections after 100 days following CBT are mostly seen in patients with chronic GVHD
	Graft-versus-leukemia/lymphoma effect in CBT recipients has also been comparable to conventional stem cell graft transplants	Patients who recover peripheral blood lymphocyte count following successful CBT engraftment are at a significantly low risk for serious systemic infections
T-cell-depleted stem cell graft	Higher risk for graft rejection may be an issue	These patients have a higher risk of infections during the prolonged pre-engraftment neutropenia
	Slower reconstitution of cellular and humoral immunity	The risk factors for IA noted in allogeneic HSCT recipients include T-cell-depleted or DC34-selected stem cell grafts, treatment with systemic corticosteroids, GVHD, presence of severe lymphocytopenia, and neutropenia
	CD8 cells recover rapidly, whereas helper T-cells and B lymphocyte recovery remain significantly stunted for 1 year or longer after T lymphocyte-depleted stem cell graft transplantation	CMV infection and end-organ disease; LRTI due to RTVs are now recognized as important predictors for IA and other IFD during post-engraftment period
	Natural killer cells also make early and sustained recovery after transplantation	
	Despite T-cell-depleted PBSC grafts having higher numbers of mononuclear cells and granulocyte-macrophage units compared with BM grafts, recovery in B lymphocyte and T-cell subpopulations has not been dissimilar, in either group	
	These patients also exhibit a subnormal level of primed T-cell repertoire. Prominent lymphocyte population in such stem cell grafts is composed of naïve/unprimed T-cells. Primed T lymphocytes including activated helper T-cells that are an important and sustained source of IFN-gamma, a critical cytokine in targeted intracellular neutralization of various pathogens	
	Hypogammaglobulinemia has not been an issue in patients undergoing T-cell-depleted vs. conventional stem cell transplantation	

Table 1.3 (continued)

Stem cell source, preparatory conditioning regimens, and GVHD prophylaxis	Immune defects	Infections
Nonmyeloablative stem cell transplantation	Faster neutrophil engraftment following reduced intensive preparatory regimen	Patients with chronic lymphocytic leukemia (138 episodes/100 person-years) and recipients of matched unrelated donor graft (128 episodes/100 person-years) had higher risk of infection after NMT
	Blood stem cell recipients have higher lymphocyte subset counts and account for fewer infectious complications during posttransplant period	Nearly half of the CMV viremia is noted between 31 and 100 days after transplantation. CMV infection as expected is mostly encountered after the resolution of neutropenia
	Substantially reduced incidence of GVHD, especially severe grade III–IV acute GVHD	Close to 80% of IFI are late transplant infections that are diagnosed 100 days after NMT and associated with unacceptably high mortality (~80%). Presence of GVHD and treatment with systemic corticosteroids significantly increases the risk for IFD in such patients
	Late transplant immune suppression due to chronic GVHD may occur	
	B-cell dysfunction, when present, is often represented as deficiencies of immunoglobulin subclasses rather than severe hypogammaglobulinemia	The risk of IA after NMT appears to increase with time, while well-under 10% within 1 year after HSCT, the overall risk increases to around 10% at 2 years and close to 15% 3 years after transplantation. Patients with GVHD involving the intestinal tract show a significant risk for IA after NMT
	As in all transplant recipients including those undergoing autologous SCT, B-cell hyporesponsiveness is clinically demonstrated as reduced immunogenicity for convention vaccines. Response to protein conjugate vaccines tends to be superior compared with response elicited by pure polysaccharide and other complex sugar immunogens. Superior conjugate vaccine construct requires restitution of cellular immune response and a functional antigen presentation process	GVHD treatment with daclizumab further enhances the risk for IA. Daclizumab is a humanized monoclonal antibody that binds to CD25, the alpha subunit of the IL-2 T-cell receptor resulting in severe iatrogenic drug-induced cellular immune suppression
	Adults with rapid engraftment of NMT become full donor T-cell chimeras within 6 months after transplantation. In contrast to children, quantitative B-cell recovery in adults is usually delayed until 1 year after HSCT. It was interesting that immune reconstitution occurs faster in children undergoing NMT who exhibit extended duration of mixed hematopoietic chimerism, whereas in adults, reconstitution is more gradual despite rapid donor stem cell engraftment and T-cell chimerism	

(continued)

Table 1.3 (continued)

Stem cell source, preparatory conditioning regimens, and GVHD prophylaxis	Immune defects	Infections
Total body irradiation and chemotherapy-induced mucositis	Radiation exposure and highly active antineoplastic drugs kill rapidly proliferating cancer cells. The rapidly dividing normal orointestinal epithelial cells also sustain unintended damage that may clinically present in patients with severe and potentially life-threatening mucositis	Patients with severe mucositis, especially those with mucosal ulcerations, have threefold higher risk for α-hemolytic streptococcal bacteremia compared with those without ulcerative mucositis following HSCT. In such patients, presence of oral ulcerations significantly increases the length of hospitalization by nearly 1 week
	Various strategies including recombinant human keratinocyte growth factor among others are being explored to mitigate this serious debilitating complication commonly seen in the early posttransplant period	Similarly, presence of orointestinal mucositis has been associated with the risk for neutropenic enterocolitis or typhlitis and CDAD
	Initial phase of chemotherapy-induced stomatotoxicity is infiltration of tissue with inflammatory cells and vascular congestion, followed by epithelial cell damage resulting in ulceration; risk for bacterial and less often yeast invasion resulting in systemic infection. Patients who survive this phase are expected to make full recovery	The risk of fungemia due to *Candida* spp. may also be increased in such patients
	Divergent cytokine response plays an important role in the risk, severity, and duration of mucositis as does hosts' genetic predisposition	Patients with intestinal VRE colonization and mucosal disruption heighten the risk for systemic invasion and risk of VRE bloodstream infection
		Later TBI complication between 12 and 136 months after treatment is mostly noninfectious and includes restrictive lung disease (~8%) and altered pulmonary diffusing capacity (~12%); pulmonary complications had been statistically higher in patients with GVHD and those who underwent high-dose (15 MV vs. 9 MV) energy beam radiation therapy. Ocular complications are noted in nearly 30% of patients on long-term follow-up and include cataract and dry eye syndrome (~15% each), whereas keratitis is seldom seen
Antithymocyte globulin	ATG is polyclonal human antilymphocyte globulins that result in multifaceted immunomodulation and are shown to reduce the incidence of solid organ graft rejection and GVHD following allogeneic HSCT	The incidence of EBV-related complications was twice as high (~7%) in patients undergoing non-HLA-matched vs. HLA-matched allograft stem cell transplants. This risk was significantly higher (>20%) in patients given antithymocyte globulin versus those in whom this treatment was not given (<2%). In HSCT recipient with persistent EBV reactivation, just above 80% developed EBV-related PTLD suggested targeted surveillance
	ATG in vivo depletes proinflammatory cytotoxic T-cells in the peripheral blood via complement-dependent cell lysis, and peripheral lymphoid tissue T-cell depletion occurs via cell activation and apoptosis	Febrile illness, CMV infection, and hematologic abnormalities are known complications in patients treated with ATG
	ATG downregulates expression of the α-chain of the IL-2 receptor (CD25), which is expressed on activated T lymphocytes thereby interrupting an important signal for cell proliferation	
	Modulation of key cell surface molecules such as integrins and intercellular adhesion molecules that facilitate and regulate lymphocyte interactions with the endothelium. Chemotaxis is effected by interference with CXCR4 and stromal cell-derived factor-1α-driven lymphocyte migration	
	ATG induces apoptosis in B-cell lineages	
	It promotes and expands functionally immunosuppressive regulatory T-cells	

Abbreviations: *GVHD* graft-versus-host disease, *CMV* cytomegalovirus, *DC* dendritic cells, *NK* natural killer, *PML* JC virus-associated progressive multifocal leukoencephalopathy, *PTLD* Epstein-Barr virus-associated B-cell lymphoproliferative disorders, *IFD* invasive fungal disease, *CDAD Clostridium difficile*-associated diarrhea, *CBT* cord blood stem cell transplantation, *IA* invasive aspergillosis, *IC* invasive candidiasis, *Treg* regulatory T-cells, *HSCT* hematopoietic stem cell transplantation, *IMD* invasive mold disease, *HHV6* human herpes virus 6, *RANTES* regulated on activation, normal T-cell expressed and secreted, *APC* antigen-presenting cells, *IFNγ* interferon gamma, *NTM* nonmyeloablative transplant, NST, *GM-CSF* granulocyte-macrophage colony-stimulating factor, *CBS* cord blood stem cells, *BMSC* bone marrow stem cells, *PBSC* peripheral blood stem cells, *LRTI* lower respiratory tract infection, *SCT* stem cell transplant, *HLA* human leukocyte antigen

References

1. Singh AK, McGuirk JP. Allogeneic stem cell transplantation: a historical and scientific overview. Cancer Res. 2016;76:6445–51.
2. Sass DA, Doyle AM. Liver and kidney transplantation: a half-century historical perspective. Med Clin North Am. 2016;100:435–48.
3. Roche NA, Blondeel PN, Van Lierde KM, Vermeersch HF. Facial transplantation: history and update. Acta Chir Belg. 2015;115:99–103.
4. Garrett GL, Beegun I, D'souza A. Facial transplantation: historical developments and future directions. J Laryngol Otol. 2015;129:206–11.
5. Sá H, Leal R, Rosa MS. Renal transplant immunology in the last 20 years: a revolution towards graft and patient survival improvement. Int Rev Immunol. 2017;36:182–203.
6. Chinen J, Notarangelo LD, Shearer WT. Advances in basic and clinical immunology in 2014. J Allergy Clin Immunol. 2015;135:1132–41.
7. Brent L. Transplantation tolerance – a historical introduction. Immunology. 2016;147:267–8.
8. Boieri M, Shah P, Dressel R, Inngjerdingen M. The role of animal models in the study of hematopoietic stem cell transplantation and GvHD: a historical overview. Front Immunol. 2016;30(7):333.
9. Cichocki F, Verneris MR, Cooley S, Bachanova V, Brunstein CG, Blazar BR, et al. The past, present, and future of NK cells in hematopoietic cell transplantation and adoptive transfer. Curr Top Microbiol Immunol. 2016;395:225–43.
10. Meirelles Júnior RF, Salvalaggio P, Rezende MB, Evangelista AS, Guardia BD, Matielo CE, et al. Liver transplantation: history, outcomes and perspectives. Einstein (Sao Paulo). 2015;13:149–52.
11. Grinyó JM, Cruzado JM. Mycophenolate mofetil and sirolimus combination in renal transplantation. Am J Transplant. 2006;6:1991–9.
12. Stallone G, Schena A, Infante B, Di Paolo S, Loverre A, Maggio G, et al. Sirolimus for Kaposi's sarcoma in renal-transplant recipients. N Engl J Med. 2005;352:1317–23.
13. Faulkner RD, Craddock C, Byrne JL, Mahendra P, Haynes AP, Prentice HG, et al. BEAM-alemtuzumab reduced-intensity allogeneic stem cell transplantation for lymphoproliferative diseases: GVHD, toxicity, and survival in 65 patients. Blood. 2004;103:428–34.
14. Hanaway MJ, Woodle ES, Mulgaonkar S, Peddi VR, Kaufman DB, First MR, et al. Alemtuzumab induction in renal transplantation. N Engl J Med. 2011;364:1909–19.
15. Choquet S, Leblond V, Herbrecht R, Socié G, Stoppa AM, Vandenberghe P, et al. Efficacy and safety of rituximab in B-cell post-transplantation lymphoproliferative disorders: results of a prospective multicenter phase 2 study. Blood. 2006;107:3053–7.
16. Safdar A, Armstrong D. Infectious morbidity in critically ill patients with cancer. Crit Care Clin. 2001;17:531–70.
17. Safdar A, Armstrong D. Infections in patients with hematologic neoplasms and hematopoietic stem cell transplantation: neutropenia, humoral, and splenic defects. Clin Infect Dis. 2011;53:798–806.
18. Weber D, Jenq RR, Peled JU, Taur Y, Hiergeist A, Koestler J, et al. Microbiota disruption induced by early use of broad-spectrum antibiotics is an independent risk factor of outcome after allogeneic stem cell transplantation. Biol Blood Marrow Transplant. 2017;23:845–52.
19. Galloway-Pena JR, Jenq RR, Shelburne SA. Can consideration of the microbiome improve antimicrobial utilization and treatment outcomes in the oncology patient? Clin Cancer Res. 2017;23(13):3263–8.
20. Lee YJ, Arguello EP, Jenq RR, Littmann E, Kim GJ, Miller LC, et al. Protective factors in the intestinal microbiome against clostridium difficile infection in recipients of allogeneic hematopoietic stem cell transplantation. J Infect Dis. 2017;215:1117–23. [Epub ahead of print] PubMed PMID: 28329030.
21. Kiernan J, Damien P, Monaghan M, Shorr R, McIntyre L, Fergusson D, et al. Clinical studies of ex vivo expansion to accelerate engraftment after umbilical cord blood transplantation: a systematic review. Transfus Med Rev. 2017;31:173–82.
22. Safdar A, Rodriguez GH, De Lima MJ, Petropoulos D, Chemaly RF, Worth LL, et al. Infections in 100 cord blood transplantations: spectrum of early and late posttransplant infections in adult and pediatric patients 1996-2005. Medicine (Baltimore). 2007;86:324–33.

Infections in Heart, Lung, and Heart-Lung Transplantation

2

Andrés F. Henao-Martínez and José G. Montoya

Historical Perspective

We have conceived the human heart as the main source of our deep emotions and feelings. A place where our very conscious resides as portrayed by Edgar Allan Poe in his famous *The Tell-Tale Heart* short story: "I felt that I must scream or die! And now—again!—hark! Louder! Louder! Louder! Louder!" Dr. John Gibbon Jr. used for the first time in 1953 a heart-lung respirator to keep a patient alive while performing heart surgery. Dr. Norman Shumway at Stanford developed and perfected the first surgical technique leading to heart transplantation surgery. After Dr. Christian Barnard's first orthotopic heart transplant in December 1967, and Dr. Shumway first heart transplant in the United States in January 1968, heart transplantation became a standard therapeutic option for life-threatening congestive failure and started to be performed in the hundreds over the next following years at different centers. Heart transplant surgery faced complications due in part to rejection and infection. However, the development of more selective immunosuppressive therapy and improvements in prevention, detection, and treatment of infections allowed for heart transplant surgery to increase rapidly worldwide.

Four thousand and ninety six heart (3529 adults) transplants were reported to the International Society of Heart and Lung Transplant Registry (ISHL) in 2011 [1]. The landscape of infection affecting heart transplant patients has been shaped by different factors: (A) implementation of more selective calcineurin-based immunosuppressive protocols, (B) lessened immunosuppressive induction regimens, (C) the institution of antimicrobial prophylaxis resulting in a significant decrease or delay in the emergence of major infections episodes including *P. jirovecii* (PCP), *Nocardia* spp., *Listeria spp.*, *Toxoplasma gondii*, cytomegalovirus, toxoplasmosis, cytomegalovirus (CMV), herpes simplex virus (CMV), varicella zoster virus (VZV), and invasive fungal infections, (D) introduction of novel diagnostic technology facilitating earlier recognition and treatment of infections, (E) expansion in the criteria to select donors and recipients to include various scenarios dealing with HBV, HCV, and HIV infections [2], and (F) shift toward predominantly Gram-positive bacterial infections and multiresistant bacteria in recent years [3–5].

A Stanford team lead by Dr. Bruce Reitz performed a Lung transplantation as a combined heart-lung transplant procedure in 1981 [6]. Shortly after, thoracic surgeons optimized the single- and double-lung transplant procedures. Improvement of surgical techniques, especially bronchial anastomosis and evolution of flush perfusion lung preservation, decreased the perioperative bronchial complications substantially. Similarly to heart transplantation, improvements in immunosuppressive regimens, antimicrobial prophylaxis, and graft preservation led to enhancement in survival among lung transplant recipients. In contrast to cardiac, lung transplantation has faced the challenge of infections unique to the transplant of this organ. Mold infections of the anastomotic site, host versus graft disease, and serious infections with *Mycobacterium abscessus*, *Chlamydia* spp., bronchiolitis, and *Burkholderia cepacia* complex are among infectious complications rarely observed in other transplant patients [7].

Transplantation of thoracic organs has improved the quality of life and prevented the death of thousands of

A. F. Henao-Martínez
Department of Medicine, Division of Infectious Diseases, University of Colorado Denver, Aurora, CO, USA
e-mail: andres.henaomartinez@ucdenver.edu

J. G. Montoya (✉)
Division of Infectious Diseases and Geographic Medicine, Stanford University School of Medicine, Stanford, CA, USA

Palo Alto Medical Foundation Toxoplasma Serology Laboratory, National Reference Center for the Study and Diagnosis of Toxoplasmosis, Palo Alto, CA, USA
e-mail: gilberto@stanford.edu

A. Safdar (ed.), *Principles and Practice of Transplant Infectious Diseases*, https://doi.org/10.1007/978-1-4939-9034-4_2

individuals worldwide. Graft survival and life expectancy have been markedly improved in these patients due to the introduction of more optimal immunosuppression, antimicrobial prophylaxis, and diagnostic technology allowing the earlier diagnosis and treatment of infection and rejection. Finally, further control of infection is likely to result from implementation of new approaches to assess the net state of immunosuppression in these patients.

Epidemiology

Infection was recognized as a major threat to thoracic transplantation from the early inception days [8]. There are several factors predisposing thoracic transplant recipients to infections: (A) factors present before transplantation: age, presence of comorbidities (e.g., chronic kidney disease, diabetes mellitus, cancer, etc.), nutrition status, latent infections, colonization with healthcare-associated organisms, and occult community-acquired infections; (B) factors during the surgery: duration of the transplant procedure, graft injury including ischemic time, colonization or latent infection of the graft, surgical instrumentation (e.g., mechanical ventilation, invasive devices such as catheters, drains, Foley catheters, etc.), ICU stay, and need for re-interventions; and (C) factors present after transplant: degree of immunosuppression, CMV infection, and rejections (Table 2.1).

Table 2.1 Clinical features modifying infection risk in transplantation

Before transplantation
Age
Comorbidities: diabetes mellitus, chronic kidney disease, cancer, etc.
Nutrition status
Latent infections or occult community-acquired infections
Colonization with healthcare-associated organisms
During transplantation
Duration of the transplant procedure
Graft injury
Ischemic time
Anastomosis site in lung transplant
Denervation of allograft (e.g., diminished cough reflex)
Lymphatic drainage disruption
Colonization or latent infection of the graft
Surgical instrumentation (e.g., mechanical ventilation)
ICU stay
Need for re-interventions
After transplantation
Immunosuppression
CMV infection
Rejections

Heart Transplant Infections

A total of 4096 heart transplants were performed in 2011. Heart transplant recipients have an average age of 54 years and are predominantly man (76%). They have a significant history of smoking (46%) and hypertension (45%) and have cardiomyopathy (54%) followed by coronary artery disease (37%) as the leading causes of transplant [1]. The historical (pediatric and adult transplants between 1982 and 2011) 1-year, 5-year, and 10-year survival rates are 81%, 69%, and 50%, respectively. Overall median survival is 11 years, but it increases up to 13 years for those surviving the first year after transplantation. Although not associated with increased posttransplant mortality, infections before transplant can affect up to 25% of heart transplant candidates. Being bronchitis and soft tissue infections, the more commonly present [9]. Despite no major changes in the distribution of causes of death since 1994, infections remained a predominant factor of mortality during the first 3 years after transplant. It contributes with up to almost 20% of causes of death [3]. The global incidence of infections in heart transplant ranges between 30% and 60% and the associated mortality between 4% and 15% [10]. The incidence of infection measured as major infectious episodes per patient has steadily declined from 2.83 in the early 1970s to 0.81 in the early 2000s [3, 8, 11]. The most frequent type of infection is bacterial (44%), followed by viral (42%), fungal including *Pneumocystis jirovecii* (14%), and protozoa (0.6%). Unfavorable functional outcomes are observed in patients who developed infections in the first year of transplant, mainly associated with bloodstream, CMV, and lung infections [12]. Pulmonary and central nervous system (CNS) infections are independent predictors of mortality among heart transplant recipients. Reactivation of latent parasitic infections residing in extra-cardiac tissues in the host or transmitted in the transplanted heart is an important consideration. The classic example is the reactivation of *Trypanosoma cruzi*. Chagas disease is a vector-borne illness transmitted by triatomine bugs, and it is endemic in Latin America. The ethnicity or origin of either the donor or the recipient from these regions should raise the concern for possible reactivation. Chagas reactivation was documented in 38.8% of cases in a cohort of Brazilian heart transplant recipients, where Chagas cardiomyopathy was the second most common indication for transplant (34.9%) [13]. Chagas can also reactivate from the transplanted heart procured from a seropositive donor and transplanted into a seronegative recipient. Although with a substantial decreased on its prevalence in the most recent eras, toxoplasmosis is another important consideration in this setting. Similarly to Chagas, *Toxoplasma gondii*—also with a predilection to invade the myocardium—can be transmitted by reactivation of quiescent cysts in the recipient or the transplanted heart [14].

Lung and Heart-Lung Transplant Infections

By 2011, 3640 adults received lung transplantation, the highest reported number of procedures up to that date, driven mainly by the increase of double-lung transplants. Double-lung transplant is indicated for septic lung diseases (e.g., cystic fibrosis). Around 66% of recipients were aged 45–65 years old. The most frequent indications for transplant were COPD (34%), followed by interstitial lung disease (ILD) (24%), bronchiectasis associated with cystic fibrosis (CF) (17%), and α1AT deficiency-related COPD (6%) [15]. The overall (from 1994 to 2011) 1-year, 5-year, and 10-year survival rates among lung recipients are 79%, 53%, and 31%, respectively. Overall median survival is 5.6 years. Lung transplants from CMV seronegative donors have better survival rates than from CMV seropositive donor. Thirty-day mortality was led by graft failure (24.7%) and non-CMV infections (19.6%). During the remainder of the year, non-CMV infections were the leading cause of death (35.6%). Infection is still prominent as the cause of death following the first year of transplant after bronchiolitis obliterans syndrome (BOS)/chronic lung rejection or graft failure [15]. Other infections complications historically present among the ten primary causes of death within the first year include sepsis, pneumonia, and fungal infections [16]. High lung allocation score (LAS) at the time of transplantation is associated with a lower 1-year survival and higher rates of infections among lung transplant recipients [17].

Sixty-three adult Heart-Lung transplantations were reported to the ISHL registry in 2011. Sixty-six percent of recipients were in the group range from 18 to 49 years old. Sixty-three percent of the indications were for congenital heart disease and idiopathic pulmonary arterial hypertension. Heart-lung transplant for CF was higher in Europe and other centers compared to North American. When compared to lung only transplants, short-term survival was worse, but long-term survival was better for the heart-lung transplant recipients. Their 1-year, 5-year, and 10-year survival rates were 63%, 44%, and 31%, respectively. The median survival was 3.3 years and 10 years for those surviving the first year. Similarly, they have graft failure (27%), technical complications (21.9%), and non-CMV infections (17.8%) as leading causes of death during the first 30 days posttransplant. Non-CMV infections (35.1%) were the top cause of death after 1 month and within 1 year of transplant. After the first year, BOS/late graft failure and non-CMV infections were the predominant causes of death [15]. Among other risk factors for mortality in lung transplantation are cystic fibrosis, nosocomial infections, and mechanical ventilation before transplant [18].

Infections in lung transplant recipients are predominantly bacterial (48%), viral (35%), fungal (13%), and mycobacterial (4%) [19]. In 60%, the infection site is pulmonary. Risk factors for infection vary by the type of organism. Mechanical ventilation (MV) for >5 days immediately following transplant surgery and isolation of *Staphylococcus aureus* (SA) from airway cultures in the recipient were considered risk factors for invasive SA infections in a retrospective study of patients with lung and heart-lung transplants [20]. Likewise, risk factors for the development of healthcare-associated infections with Gram-negative organisms, *Aspergillus*, *Legionella*, and MRSA (methicillin-resistant *Staphylococcus aureus*), include prolonging MV, renal failure, use of ATG (antithymocyte globulin), and recurrent rejections episodes [21]. Additionally, α-1-antitrypsin deficiency and repeat transplantation are also risk factors for nosocomial infections. *Mycobacterium tuberculosis* transmission from lung donors with latent infection has been documented in highly endemic areas [22]. Colonization with MDR organisms (*Pseudomonas aeruginosa*, *Burkholderia*, *Acinetobacter*, nontuberculous mycobacteria (NTM), and *Scedosporium*) before transplant—especially important in CF patients—can predict the development of challenging infections to treat after transplant [23].

Pretransplant Evaluation of Recipients and Donors

Pretransplant Screening of Recipients

Patients should undergo a comprehensive evaluation of potential infectious complications associated with transplantation. A detailed medical history including previous vaccinations, history of past infections, exposures (geographical, occupational, animal, etc.), travel, and foreign-born status among others should be obtained.

Clinicians shuold perform routine serologies for the detection of pathogen-specific IgG for CMV, HSV, EBV (VCA), VZV, hepatitis B (HBsAg, HBsAb, HBcAb), HIV, hepatitis C, and syphilis. Toxoplasma IgG should also be performed in heart and heart-lung transplant candidates. Additionally, we recommend to obtain UA, urine culture, CXR, and tuberculin skin test (TST), or a Quantiferon assay. In lung and heart-lung transplant candidates, sputum should be cultured for bacterial, fungal, and AFB studies.

Some centers advocate the screening of patients for colonization with MDR (multidrug resistant) bacteria such as MRSA and VRE (vancomycin resistant *Enterococci*), which it may have an impact on the type of antibacterial prophylaxis used preoperatively or the empirical antibiotics should sepsis develop in the immediate postoperative period. In potential lung recipients, previous respiratory colonization with MDR *Pseudomonas*, especially in CF patients, should not exclude them from transplant [24]. On the other hand, if colonization with *B. cenocepacia* (genomovar III) in CF is present transplant is relatively contraindicated [25, 26].

Checking for endemic fungi such as *Coccidioides immitis* or for the parasites *Trypanosoma cruzi*, *Strongyloides stercoralis*, and *Leishmania* spp. is indicated in the presence of the appropriate risk factors [27–31].

Histoplasma capsulatum has reactivated during immunosuppressive therapy [32]. Infections after solid organ transplantation (SOT) are rare and attributable to transmission from the donor [33]. Furthermore, latent histoplasmosis can be present with negative serologies and treatment after transplant carries a good outcome. Therefore the role of screening for histoplasmosis is of questionable significance [34].

Pretransplant Screening of Donors

The type of evaluation may change if the donor is alive or deceased depending on the available time to collect the samples. Similarly to recipients, donors should undertake a comprehensive assessment including a complete history, assessment of risk factors, exposures, immunizations, and previous or current infections. Donors should be screened for HIV, hepatitis B/C, syphilis, and tuberculosis. Furthermore, we recommend to obtain serologies for CMV, EBV, HSV, VZV, and *Toxoplasma gondii*, and for HTLV-1/HTLV-2 in endemic areas. In high-risk donors, the use of nucleic acid amplification tests (NAAT) for HBV, HCV, and HIV should be considered. Additionally, blood cultures to document an occult bacteremia are recommended. In lung transplant donors, we recommend obtaining respiratory cultures through bronchoscopy to detect colonizing organisms and target them to prevent invasive infections in the donor. Culturing the media of the allograft during acquisition or processing have been advocated to reduce the risk of mycotic aneurysms among kidney transplant recipients, which may apply to other SOT [35]. Screening of donors for endemic mycosis is not well established. On the other hand, heart transplant donors should be screened for Chagas if the donor was born in Latin America [29]. Finally, it is important to highlight the increase recognition of emerging, unusual viral infections such as West Nile virus, lymphocytic choriomeningitis virus, rabies, and different human coronaviruses [34, 36]. Testing for those organisms should be done based on individual assessments. Table 2.2 describes and summarizes the diagnostic workup recommend among donors and recipients.

Table 2.2 Infectious screening during transplantation

Diagnostic workup among donors and recipients
Routine tests obtained among donors and recipients:
Viral test: HIV Elisa, hepatitis C antibody, HBV (HBsAg, HBcAb total, HBsAb), IgG antibody for CMV, HSV, EBV VCA, VZV
Bacterial: Treponemal antibody (e.g., EIAs, FTA-ABS), QFN assay or PPD
Parasite: Toxoplasmosis IgG (routinely indicated for heart transplant patients)
Other screening to consider among donors or recipients in the presence of specific risk factors:
Viral: NAAT for HIV, HCV, HBV in high-risk donors. HTLV-1/HTLV-2 in donors from endemic areas
Bacterial:
Recipients: UA, urine culture, CXR, and sputum culture.
Optional: To consider screen for colonization with MDR organisms (MRSA or VRE)
Donors: Blood cultures, allograft media culture, and bronchoscopy with culture from respiratory specimens in lung donors
Parasite: Ortho EIA and Abbott Prism Chagas test to screen for *Trypanosoma cruzi* in donors or recipients from Latin America. *Strongyloides stercoralis* and *Leishmania* spp. serologies should be obtained in recipients in the presence of appropriate geographic risk factors
Fungal: EIA for coccidioidal antibodies or complement fixing antibodies for cocci

Abbreviations: NAAT Nucleic acid amplification test, *CXR* chest X-ray, *MDR* multidrug resistant, *EIA* enzyme-linked immunosorbent assay

Prevention of Infections

Immunizations

Immunization should be optimized before transplantation since the recipient will have better chances to mount an adequate immune response [37]. The advisory committee on immunization practices (ACIP) [38] and the guidelines for immunizations in solid organ transplantation [39] recommend inactivated influenza vaccine annually. Tetanus, diphtheria, and acellular pertussis (Tdap) should be administered to all adults who have not previously received Tdap or have an unknown status. Varicella vaccination with two doses in patients without evidence of immunity or a single dose of zoster vaccination, inactivated polio vaccine, hepatitis A/B, HPV (three series through 26 years of age), and meningococcal and pneumococcal vaccines should be administered [38]. It is remarkably important to vaccinate all household members as well. BCG and rabies vaccines can be considered under some extenuating or exposure-related indications. See Table 2.3.

Avoidance of Exposures

Education of the patient and the family members is a cornerstone to establishing effective preventive measures. Emphasis should be enforced about hand hygiene and food handling.

Table 2.3 Immunizations recommendations during transplantation

Recommended vaccines among heart, lung, and heart-lung recipients
Annual inactivated influenza vaccine
Tdap (should be administered to all adults who have not previously received Tdap or have an unknown status)
VZV (two series) in patients without evidence of immunity
Zoster vaccine should be given in varicella-positive candidates age ≥60 years and considered in candidates aged 50–59 (>4 weeks before transplant)
Inactivated polio
Hepatitis A series
Hepatitis B series
HPV (three series through 26 years of age)
Pneumococcal: Pneumococcal conjugate 13-valent (PCV13) followed by pneumococcal polysaccharide 23 (PPSV23) vaccine 8 weeks later (If PPSV23 was received first; PCV13 should be given at least 1 year after)
Meningococcal conjugate vaccine
Under special circumstances: Rabies and BCG

Additionally, potential sources of bacteria, fungi (e.g., *Aspergillus*), and toxoplasmosis such as plants and flowers, cleaning pet's litter or cages, eating uncooked meat, acquiring new pets, construction areas, farming, barnyard activities, and smoking marihuana should be avoided. If those recreational or occupational exposures are unavoidable; appropriate gear, such gloves, must be worn. Education about possible community exposures is also important. Close contacts with persons with fevers or rash potentially infected with VZV, herpes zoster, or influenza should be circumvented as well. Patients should cook all meals thoroughly, wash all fruits and vegetables, and shun all unpasteurized products. Safe sex practices are recommended. If any foreign travel is planned, seeking evaluation in a specialized travel clinic is advisable.

Prophylaxis

Guidelines for the management of surgical antimicrobial prophylaxis list cefazolin (2 g, 3 g for patients with weight >120 Kg every 4 h) as the recommended regimen for heart, lung, and heart-lung transplantation surgery. Clindamycin (900 mg every 6 h) or vancomycin (15 mg/kg) can be substituted as alternative agents in beta-lactam allergic patients [40, 41]. This recommendation can be adjusted individually, based on local hospital surveillance data or previous knowledge of colonizing organisms (e.g., addition of aztreonam, gentamicin, or a single-quinolone dose). However, the widespread use of quinolones may increase the resurgence of antimicrobial resistance. The antibiotic should be administered within 60 min before surgical incision (within 120 min for vancomycin or quinolones) and to be continued for 24–48 h in heart transplants and 48–72 h and no longer than 7 days in lung and heart-lung transplant recipients. Recommendation to continue antibacterial prophylaxis until chest and mediastinal tubes are removed lacks sufficient evidence. Redosing will depend on the procedure duration and associated blood loss.

The recipient does not need treatment if a localized infection was present in the donor, except during meningitis where concomitant bacteremia often coexist. In meningitis and bacteremia, it is prudent to treat the recipient for 2–4 weeks [34].

Indications for antifungal prophylaxis in heart transplant recipients are not clear. A systemic review showed no benefit of antifungal therapy to prevent invasive fungal infections in transplants recipients other than liver [42]. Although a prospective cohort of heart transplant recipients showed targeted prophylaxis—an echinocandin for a median of 30 days with the presence of at least one risk factor for invasive aspergillosis (IA) (reoperation, cytomegalovirus disease, posttransplantation hemodialysis, and another patient with IA in the program 2 months before or after the procedure)—was highly effective and safe in preventing IA episodes [43], no consensus exists for universal antifungal prophylaxis in heart transplant recipients. Most centers have adopted antifungal prophylaxis including inhaled amphotericin B, oral itraconazole, or IV targeted echinocandin prophylaxis.

In lung and lung-heart transplant recipients, fungal prophylaxis should be considered, especially if pretransplantation respiratory cultures either from the donor lung or recipient airways shows *Aspergillus* or *Candida*. One approach is to use inhaled amphotericin B (50 or 100 mg in extubated or intubated patients, respectively) daily until 4 days after transplant and then weekly until hospital discharge in patients with no known colonization [44, 45]. If a mold has been isolated, voriconazole is recommended up to 4 months after transplant. Although evidence and efficacy need to be confirmed, combination antifungal prophylaxis therapies is used at some centers [46].

Pneumocystis jiroveci prophylaxis is done with trimethoprim-sulfamethoxazole (TMP-SMX) for 6 months, up to 1 year. Some centers extend the PJP prophylaxis to lifelong. TMP-SMX also confers protection against *Toxoplasma*, *Nocardia*, and *Listeria* species infections. Alternatively, dapsone, inhaled pentamidine, or atovaquone can be used in patients with a history of sulfa allergy. TMP-SMX is recommended at many centers for lifelong in toxoplasmosis seronegative recipients of seropositive cardiac donors (*Toxoplasma* D+/R−) [11].

CMV prevention is recommended to all D+/R− and R+ patients. There are two common strategies for CMV prevention: antiviral prophylaxis and preemptive therapy. Both approaches possess similar success rate and their advantages and disadvantages [47]. Guidelines recommend valganciclovir or intravenous ganciclovir as the preferred antivirals. Oral ganciclovir is an option in heart transplant patients, although it possesses a low oral bioavailability and therefore the theoretical risk of increased resistance. Often, CMV immune globulin is used as an adjunctive agent. In heart recipients, prophylaxis is recommended for 3–6 months in D+/R− and 3 months in R+. In lung and heart-lung recipients, the duration of prophylaxis is 12 months and 6–12 months in D+/R− and R+ recipients, respectively [48]. In D−/R− patients, otherwise not receiving CMV active agents, antiviral prophylaxis against other herpes viruses, such as HSV and VZV, should be considered. Use of oral CMX001 (oral liposomal formulation of cidofovir) in hematopoietic-cell transplants reduced CMV-related events and may have a potential role in preventing CMV in other transplant settings [49]. Refer to Table 2.4 for a list of prophylaxis recommendations.

Table 2.4 Antimicrobial prophylaxis

Prophylaxis in heart, lung, and heart-lung transplant
Bacterial[a]:
Preferred: Cefazolin 2 g (3 g for patients with weight >120 Kg). Redose every 4 h for extended procedure time and significant blood loss
Alternative: Vancomycin 15 mg/kg or clindamycin, 900 mg IV
CMV prophylaxis[b]:
Valganciclovir, 900 mg PO once daily
IV ganciclovir, 5 mg/kg IV once daily
Oral ganciclovir (heart transplant), 1 gr PO three times a day
Consider adjuvant therapy with CMV immune globulin
Pneumocystis jiroveci:
TMP-SMX, one single tablet a day or one double-strength tablet three to seven times a week for 6–12 months
Alternatively, dapsone (100 mg PO daily); inhaled pentamidine (300 mg/dose monthly) or atovaquone (1500 mg PO once daily) can be used
Other: In D–/R– patients, otherwise not receiving CMV prophylaxis, consider acyclovir to prevent HSV/VZV reactivation
Prophylaxis in heart transplants
Parasitic:
Consider lifelong TMP-SMX in toxoplasmosis mismatch recipients (D+/R–)
CMV prophylaxis:
Doses as above. Duration: 3–6 months in D+/R– and 3 months in R+ recipients
Fungal (optional):
IV echinocandin daily for 30 days in the presence of IA risk factors
Prophylaxis in lung and heart-lung transplants
Bacterial:
Consider the addition of aztreonam, gentamycin, or a single-quinolone dose in the presence of previous respiratory cultures positive for Gram negatives
CMV prophylaxis[b]:
Doses as above. Duration: 12 months in D+/R– and 6–12 months in R+ recipients
Fungal:
Negative pretransplant respiratory cultures: Inhaled *amphotericin B*, 50 or 100 mg in extubated or intubated patients, respectively, daily until 4 days after transplant and then weekly until hospital discharge
Positive pretransplant respiratory cultures for *Aspergillus*: *voriconazole*, 6 mg/kg every 12 h for 2 doses; followed by maintenance dose of 4 mg/kg every 12 h, is recommended up to 4 months after transplant. Maintenance dose can be achieved with oral voriconazole 200 mg PO every 12 h

Abbreviation: IA Invasive aspergillosis

[a]The antibiotic should be administered within 60 min before surgical incision (within 120 min for vancomycin or quinolones) and to be continued for 24–48 h in heart transplants and 48–72 h and no longer than 7 days in lung and heart-lung transplant recipients

[b]Doses of valganciclovir, ganciclovir, and other antibiotics may require adjustment for renal function

Risk of Infection Posttransplantation

<1 Month

This period is characterized more commonly for nosocomial, bacterial infections. Thus, the bacterial organisms present are often MDR (e.g., VRE, MRSA). In heart transplant recipients, skin and soft tissue infections (SSTI), surgical site infection, and mediastinitis are of concern during this period. Likewise, lung and lung-heart transplant recipients may develop infections related to previous respiratory colonization (*Pseudomonas, Aspergillus*). Other significant infections include aspiration pneumonitis, healthcare- and ventilator-associated pneumonia, catheter-related bloodstream infections (CRBSI), nosocomial UTIs, and *Clostridium difficile* colitis. Donor-derived infections during this period can be present and will include HSV, lymphocytic choriomeningitis virus (LCMV), rhabdovirus (rabies), West Nile virus (WNV), and HIV. *Toxoplasma gondii* and *Trypanosoma cruzi* are also serious donor-derived infections in heart transplant recipients that can develop within the first 6 months posttransplantation [50].

1–6 Months

During this period, reactivation of latent infections usually occurs. Hence, bacterial infections such as those caused by *Nocardia asteroides*, *Listeria monocytogenes*, and *Mycobacteria tuberculosis* typically occur. Additionally, fungal infections by *Aspergillus* spp., *Cryptococcus neoformans*, and *P. jiroveci* and parasitic by *Toxoplasma gondii*, *Leishmania* spp., *Strongyloides*, and *Trypanosoma cruzi* can also be seen. Viral infections present during this period include herpesviruses (HSV, VZV, CMV, and EBV) and adenovirus.

>6 Months

Development of infections after 6 months are predominantly community-acquired pneumonia and urinary tract infections. Other diseases include *Aspergillus* and *Mucor* species, *Nocardia*, *Rhodococcus*, and late viral infections including CMV, hepatitis B and C, JC polyomavirus infection, post-transplant lymphoproliferative disorder (PTLD), HSV encephalitis, and viral community-acquired infections (e.g., coronavirus, West Nile virus, influenza).

Monitoring

Infections

It is important to recognize transplant recipients as a patient population with increased susceptibility to infections and have a low threshold to perform diagnostic workup in the presence of any concerning signs or symptoms. Infections monitoring is also done in a structured way when preemptive therapy for CMV is in place (as opposed to universal prophylaxis). Protocols vary by the transplant center but, usually, implies a weekly CMV PCR or pp65 Ag monitoring [51]. Likewise, monitoring of cell-mediated immunity (CMI) using a Quantiferon-CMV assay may be useful predicting late-onset CMV disease once CMV prophylaxis has been stopped [52]. CMI also have been monitored for EBV using an enzyme-linked immunoSpot assay [53].

Immunoglobulin G (IgG), C3, IgG2 levels, and NK cell counts have been proposed as an attempt to identify the risk of infection in heart transplant recipients within the first year [54].

Drug-Drug Interactions

Significant drug-drug interactions exist among antimicrobial and immunosuppressive agents. Patient medication list should be reviewed carefully. CTP3A4 strong inducers such as nafcillin reduce tacrolimus serum concentrations. In contrast, azoles such as fluconazole can result in increased levels of tacrolimus or cyclosporine. For voriconazole, the dose of tacrolimus needs to be reduced by two-thirds [55] and the cyclosporine dose by 50% [56]. Rifamycins can have an opposite drug-drug interaction by decreasing the concentrations of prednisone, cyclosporine, tacrolimus, sirolimus, and mycophenolate mofetil (MMF) [57, 58]. Likewise, tacrolimus administration along with quinolones may cause QT prolongation [59].

Infections in Heart Transplantation

Infecting Microbial Agents

Bacterial

In heart transplant patients, bacterial infections have similar clinical manifestations commonly observed in other patient populations. However, clinical signs may be subtle or absent (e.g., afebrile). They are the most frequent type of infections in this setting, reaching up to 50% of all infections [3]. The most common are pulmonary infections followed by bacteremias, mediastinal, and skin infections. *Staphylococcus aureus*—predominantly methicillin-resistant—can cause SSTI, ventilator-associated pneumonia, mediastinitis, CRBSI, other forms of bacteremia, and osteomyelitis. In contrast, coagulase-negative *Staphylococcus* is more commonly associated with CRBSI. Among Gram-negative bacteria, *Pseudomonas aeruginosa* is common, usually of pulmonary origin. *Escherichia coli* is the primary causal organism of UTIs. Extended-spectrum β-lactamase (ESBL)-producing *Klebsiella pneumoniae*, *Escherichia coli*, *Klebsiella oxytoca*, and *Citrobacter freundii* are also found in 2.2% of heart transplant recipients [60].

Nocardia species are well recognized as an opportunistic pathogen in this setting. Although relatively rare in heart transplant recipients (frequency <1%), *Nocardia* is only second in frequency in heart transplant after lung transplant recipients [61–63]. Pertinent-independent risk factors associated with the development of this infection in SOT include high-dose steroids, history of CMV disease, and high levels of calcineurin inhibitors [62]. With the almost universal prophylaxis with TMP-SMX, *Nocardia* infection is less common and often present late, usually after 1 year posttransplant [63]. When they occurred, they affect the lung predominantly, which is the port of entry for disseminated infections and CNS invasion. Also, it can cause skin nodules and abscesses. *Listeria monocytogenes* can also be seen in heart transplant recipients and can count for a significant proportion of the bacterial meningitis cases in this setting [64]. Additionally, myocarditis and myocardial abscesses with this organism have also been documented [65]. *Mycobacterium tuberculosis* and nontuberculous mycobacteria (NTM), although, documented to occur in heart transplantation, are rare in the United States [66, 67]. However, it is important to recognize that the development of tuberculosis (TB) can be more prevalent in some endemic regions and often present with extrapulmonary involvement [68, 69]. *Legionellosis* and *Rhodococcus equi* with mainly pulmonary manifestations (pneumonia, pulmonary infiltrates, or cavitation) are another significant infections among heart transplant recipients [70].

Fungal

Fungal infections excluding PCP represent around 4.0% of all the infections. From them, invasive mold infections (IMI) are a significant contribution to morbidity and mortality among heart transplant recipients. The incidence in this population can reach 10 per 1000 person-years, and its associated mortality is approximately 17% [71]. *Aspergillus* represents up to 65% of all IMI. Its median time of onset is about 46 days, although late presentation (>90 days) has been more recently recognized associated with receipt of sirolimus in conjunction with tacrolimus for refractory rejection or cardiac allograft vasculopathy [72]. The most common clinical presentation for aspergillosis includes fever, cough, and single or multiple pulmonary nodules [73]. Extrapulmonary manifestations include spondylodiscitis, infective endocarditis, mediastinitis, endophthalmitis, and brain and cutaneous abscesses [74–78]. Dissemination tends to affect the CNS in a good proportion of the cases. Mucormycosis is the second most frequent mold affecting heart transplant recipients. *Mucor*, along with other non-*Aspergillus* molds (e.g., *Scedosporium*, *Ochroconis gallopava*), are associated with disseminated infections, CNS involvement, and poorer outcomes [79, 80]. *Pneumocystis jiroveci* (PCP)—although with a marked reduction in incidence with the introduction of universal prophylaxis—is still a significant pathogen and cases may occur late after heart transplant. Cryptococcosis, although infrequent among SOT patients, has its higher incidence in heart transplant recipients [81]. Usually, its manifestations present late and affect the lungs and the CNS predominantly. Histoplasmosis and coccidioidomycosis occurred typically in the first year after transplant. Antigenuria was the most sensitive diagnostic test in SOT for histoplasmosis [82]. Finally, *Candida* infections are an important cause of morbidity and mortality as well. Rate of colonization is higher than in the general population [83]. *Candida* most commonly causes an oral mucosa infection. Although there has been a decline of invasive infections over time, these do occur and typically in the form of bloodstream infections secondary to catheter-related infections, tracheobronchitis, or disseminated disease [84]. Additionally, other confined end-organ injuries such as endophthalmitis and esophagitis can also be seen.

Viral

CMV infection is of critical importance among SOT. In heart transplant recipients, CMV has been inconsistently associated with cardiac allograft vasculopathy [85]. Furthermore, CMV leads to upregulation of pro-inflammatory cytokines, increase procoagulant response, left ventricular dysfunction, allograft rejection, and an increase of opportunistic infections [86]. The greatest risk for developing CMV disease is CMV-negative recipients of CMV-positive organs (D+/R−), followed by D+/R+ and D−/R+. A clinical report estimated that the rate of *infections* in heart transplant ranges between 9% and 35%, and *disease* is present in around 25% of patients [87]. The clinical manifestations are not unique to heart transplant recipients and include a CMV syndrome (fevers, myalgias, arthralgias, malaise, leukopenia, and thrombocytopenia). CMV-associated end-organ injury in this setting includes most frequently pneumonitis and gastrointestinal disease [10]. Other manifestations comprise myelosuppression, hepatitis, and pancreatitis. In contrast to the high frequency observed in AIDS patients, chorioretinitis in heart transplant patients is relatively rare [87]. Guidelines on CMV diagnosis and managements are discussed in more detail in Chap. 55 and also have been published elsewhere [88]. Other herpes viruses are of important consideration as well. EBV-associated T-cell PTLDs are more frequent in heart transplant recipients (0.4%) than in other SOT patients [89]. PTLD is a significant contributor to morbidity and mortality in the pediatric heart transplant population [90]. Human T-lymphotropic virus type I (HTLV1), human herpes virus (HHV)-6, HHV-7, and HHV-8 might play a role in EBV(−) T-cell PTLDs as well. Herpes viruses can manifest, as in other hosts, as mucocutaneous lesions for HSV, herpes zoster for VZV, infectious mononucleosis in the case of EBV, Kaposi sarcoma for HHV-8, and encephalitis for HHV-6/7. Hepatitis, colitis, pneumonitis, and gastrointestinal disease have also been attributed to dissemination with certain herpes viruses. Herpes viruses can present with disseminated skin lesions (with or without vesicle formation) and fever of unknown origin.

Adenovirus has been associated with rejection, ventricular dysfunction, coronary vasculopathy, and the need for retransplantation. The current standard treatment for adenovirus is cidofovir, but outcomes are not optimal [91].

Chronic hepatitis without an identifiable cause should prompt testing for hepatitis E virus (HEV). Chronic HEV infection leads to the rapid development of fibrosis. HEV testing should be done with RNA PCR due to a delay in the antibody response. We recommend decreased immunosuppression and ribavirin therapy for 3 months [92, 93]. Other less common manifestation that should be considered under the correct epidemiologic risk factors include HTLV-1/HTLV-2-associated myelopathy, rabies, lymphocytic choriomeningitis virus, subacute measles encephalitis, mumps (associated parotitis, orchitis, vestibular neuritis, and allograft involvement), dengue virus, orf virus, human coronavirus, and influenza [36].

Parasitic

Cardiac transplant itself is one the predictors for development of toxoplasmosis [94]. Other associated risk factors include negative serum status before transplant, diagnosis of cytomegalovirus (CMV) infection, and high-dose prednisone. Toxoplasmosis can be transmitted by the donor heart (D+/R−, especially during the first 3 months) or can reactivate from the recipient (>3 months). Most of the infections developed during the first 6 months posttransplant and are predominantly primary infections. About 22% of infected patients had a disseminated infection carrying an estimated 17% mortality. Toxoplasmosis can manifest otherwise with myocarditis, encephalitis, pneumonitis, or chorioretinitis. Diagnosis requires identification of tissue cysts surrounded by an abnormal inflammatory response, detection of *Toxoplasma* DNA in body fluids by PCR, or positive *Toxoplasma*-specific immunohistochemistry in affected organs. Posttransplant serological tests are not helpful for diagnosis and may be misleading since results may change or not regardless of the presence of toxoplasmosis [95]. The preferred treatment regimen is a combination of pyrimethamine with sulfadiazine [96].

Advanced Chagasic cardiomyopathy is a primary indication for heart transplantation in some centers [13]. *Trypanosoma cruzi*, the causal organism of Chagas disease, can be transmitted up to 75% of the time from infected heart donors (D+/R−) [97]. Additionally, Chagas disease can reactivate from the donor once immunosuppression is in place (R+). The reactivation rate can range between 22% and 90% in recipients with chronic chagasic cardiomyopathy undergoing heart transplant [98–100]. Additional risk factors for reactivation include rejection episodes, neoplasms, and use of MMF [98]. The mean onset of symptoms is approximately 112 days [101]. Once manifested, Chagas can present with nonspecific symptoms such as fever, malaise, anorexia, hepatosplenomegaly, and lymphadenopathy. Myocarditis, pericarditis, and encephalitis are also seen. Reactivation can mimic rejection and exhibits congestive heart failure, AV block and skin manifestations such as nodules and panniculitis. Increased eosinophil count and anemia can be indirect indicators of reactivation [102]. Diagnosis is made with the visualization of circulating trypomastigotes in peripheral blood. Additionally, blood and tissue PCR can be used. Tissue amastigotes can be seen in biopsy H&E preparations (Fig. 2.1). Finally, serologies are a crucial aspect in the diagnosis especially if seroconversion have been documented. In asymptomatic individuals, when the diagnosis of Chagas has been established in the donor, monitoring should be instituted with weekly blood *T. cruzi* PCR and microscopy [29]. Preferred antitrypanosomal therapy consists on benznidazole. Nifurtimox is an alternative treatment option. Posaconazole has anti-parasitic activity but carries high failure rates [103, 104]. GI disease with *Isospora* (*Cystoisospora*) *belli*, *Cryptosporidium*, *Cyclospora*, and *Microsporidia* has been reported to affect SOT recipients. Microsporidiosis can manifest with disseminated disease: fever, keratoconjunctivitis, CNS involvement, cholangitis, cough, and thoracic/abdominal pain [94]. Other rare parasitic infections affecting heart transplants include leishmaniasis, strongyloidiasis, and free-living amoebas [94, 105].

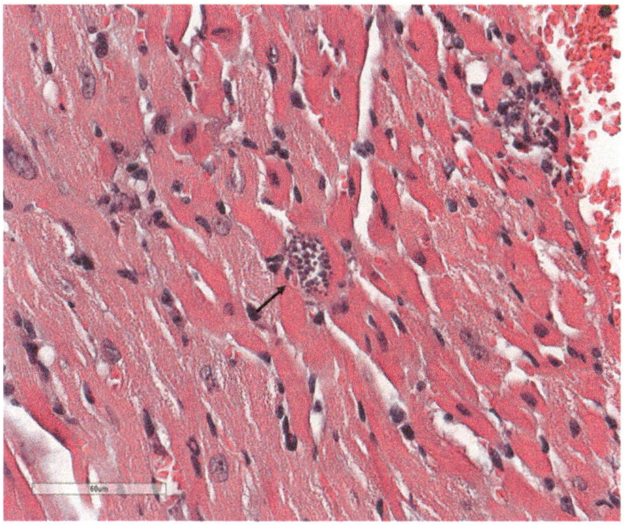

Fig. 2.1 *Trypanosoma cruzi* amastigote in heart tissue (H&E stain, 400×)

Sites and Types of Infection

Skin, Soft Tissue, and Bone

The rate of surgical site infections (SSI)—sternal wound infections—in patients receiving antimicrobial prophylaxis ranged from 5.8% to 8.8% following heart transplant procedures [41]. Heart transplantation itself is an independent risk factor for SSIs. Other risk factors include age, prophylaxis with ciprofloxacin alone, positive wire cultures, female gender, previous left ventricular assist device (VAD) placement, BMI >30 kg/m^2, previous cardiac procedures, and inotropic support for hemodynamic instability [41, 106]. Similarly to other hosts, *Staphylococcus* species are the predominant organism causing SSTIs. MRSA can reach up to 21% of the cases. Gram-positive organisms: VRE (*E. faecalis*), coagulase-negative staphylococci, and other *Enterococcus* species are other etiologic agents. Candida and selected gram negatives such as *Enterobacteriaceae*, *P. aeruginosa*, and *Stenotrophomonas maltophilia* can cause SSIs as well [107]. Sternal osteomyelitis often complicates deep SSI. Additionally, sternal wound infections by NTM and fungi such as *Aspergillus* and *Scedosporium* have been documented [108, 109]. Herpes zoster is also an important consideration and source of morbidity. Herpes zoster (HZ) is found as a complication in 19–22% of the patients with a median time of presentation ranging from 0.73 to 2.10 years [64, 110]. Close to half may develop postherpetic neuralgia. Multi-dermatome involvement, zoster ophthalmicus, and meningoencephalitis are also described. Exposure to MMF is an independent risk factor. Conversely, CMV prophylaxis reduces the risk for HZ.

Bloodstream

Bloodstream infections (BSIs) are a risk factor for mortality among heart transplant recipients. Likewise, SOT recipient status is an independent risk factor for developing bacteremia [111]. In heart transplant recipients; the rate of BSI ranged between 16% and 24%. The median onset is about 51–191 days, and the sources are in order of frequency: lower respiratory tract, urinary tract, and CRBSI. Gram-negative bacteria were more commonly isolated. They are in order of appearance *E. coli*, *P. aeruginosa*, and *K. pneumoniae*. More common Gram-positive bacteria were *S. aureus*, *S. epidermidis*, *E. faecalis*, and *L. monocytogenes*. Directly attributable mortality is 12.2%. Among the identifiable independent risk factors to develop BSI are hemodialysis, prolonged intensive care unit stay, and viral infections [112, 113]. Infective endocarditis (IE) is seen more frequently among heart transplant recipients than in the general population. With IE occurred, it most commonly involves the mitral and tricuspid valves and *Staphylococcus aureus* and *Aspergillus* are the main etiologic organisms. The main predisposing factors in this setting are believed to be the frequent use of vascular indwelling catheters and the frequency of endomyocardial biopsies [114]. *Staphylococcus aureus* bacteremia in heart transplant recipients ranges from 10% to 38% [11, 115]. The sources of SA bacteremia in SOT are CRBSI (30%), pneumonia (24%), wound (14%), endocarditis (10%), intra-abdominal infections (9%), bone and joint (7%), cardiac devices (3%), UTI (1%), and SSTI (1%) [115].

Chest

Immediately following heart transplant and during the 1st month, patients are more susceptible to develop pneumonia, most of which are healthcare or ventilator associated and therefore caused by nosocomial organisms such as MRSA, *Pseudomonas aeruginosa*, and other Gram negatives including *Acinetobacter* and ESBL-*Enterobacteriaceas*. Pneumonia is one the major contributors to mortality in the early postoperative period. Pneumonia-related mortality approaches 15% [116]. After the 1st month, interstitial pneumonia and pneumonitis can develop, and the differential includes herpesviruses (HSV, CMV, VZV) and respiratory syncytial virus (RSV), *Toxoplasma gondii* and *Pneumocystis jiroveci.* Pulmonary nodules with or without cavitation can be caused by fungi such as coccidioidomycosis, aspergillosis, mucormycosis, cryptococcosis; bacterial including actinomycosis, tuberculosis, atypical mycobacterial infections, *Nocardia*, *Rhodococcus equi*, and Gram-negative bacilli; and noninfectious causes like pulmonary infarction or lymphoproliferative disorders [117, 118]. Pulmonary nodules are seen in about 10% of the patients, and the median detection time is about 66 days. The associated symptoms are fever and cough. The most frequent etiology is *Aspergillus* followed by *Nocardia*, and *Rhodococcus*. CMV is an exceedingly rare cause of pulmonary nodules. The diagnostic approach with the higher yield is transthoracic fine needle aspiration followed by bronchoalveolar lavage and transtracheal aspiration [118]. Community-acquired pneumonia caused by *Streptococcus pneumonia*, *Legionella* spp., mycoplasma, and influenza is another source of morbidity [10].

Mediastinitis is a common complication in this setting. In patients receiving antimicrobial prophylaxis, mediastinitis develops in 3–7% of the patients [107, 119]. A CT scan is usually necessary to determine the extension of the infection. MRSA *Staphylococcus epidermidis*, Gram-negative bacteria, and *Aspergillus fumigatus* are frequently found as the causal organisms [120]. Antimicrobial therapy should be accompanied by aggressive surgical debridement [121].

Abdominal/Genitourinary

There are not distinctive abdominal-pelvic complications among heart transplant recipients. *Clostridium difficile* is a common hospital-related cause of diarrhea associated with the use of antimicrobials. Other etiology for diarrhea secondary to acute gastroenteritis can present in a protracted way in this setting. Listeria infection can present as a febrile gastroenteritis illness as well. Nontyphoid *Salmonella* infection has been described to complicate the early postoperative period in a center in Taiwan [122]. Acute cholecystitis can affect heart transplant recipients advocating to have a low threshold to use ultrasound as a screening method [123]. Acute pancreatitis with abscess formation has also been described [124]. As pointed above, hepatitis E can present with persistently abnormal liver tests.

Although less frequent than in kidney transplant recipients, urinary tract infections are an important cause of morbidity. UTIs are predisposed by Foley catheters. The organisms most commonly involved are Gram-negative bacteria, *Enterococcus*, and *Candida*. Polyomavirus nephropathy by BK virus has been described in heart transplant recipients and might be a contributor to chronic kidney disease [125].

Central Nervous System

The need for urgent transplantation and multiple transfusions are independently associated with infectious, neurologic complications. Its overall mortality can reach 12% [64]. Donor-derived meningoencephalitides affecting heart transplant recipients usually manifest within the first 30 days. These infections include West Nile virus, arenaviruses (e.g., LCMV), and rabies. WNV can manifest with a Guillain-Barré-like axonopathy with cerebrospinal fluid (CSF) pleocytosis. In addition to meningitis or encephalitis, ataxia, myelitis, optic neuritis, polyradiculitis, and seizures can also be observed [126]. WNV can be also acquired by the recipient in the community or through blood transfusions and present at a later time [127]. Other infectious forms of meningitis and encephalitis that can present after the 1st month include listeriosis, *Streptococcus pneumoniae*, *Trypanosoma cruzi*, *Toxoplasma*, HHV-6, and disseminated herpes virus infections (CMV, VZV, HSV, and EBV) [128–130]. The absence of appropriate primary prophylaxis or monitoring increases their risk. *Aspergillus* causes the majority of brain abscess. Additionally *Toxoplasma*, tuberculosis, *Listeria* spp., *Cryptococcus neoformans*, *Scedosporium* spp., and *Nocardia* can also be causative agents [129]. Concomitant pulmonary involvement is common, particularly for those whose portal of entry is the respiratory tract.

Progressive multifocal leukoencephalopathy (PML), a demyelinating disease caused by the reactivation of JC virus, has a usual median onset of 27 months. It carries a marked high case fatality rate and a median survival of 6.4 months in SOT [131]. The use of rituximab as an antirejection treatment seems to confer an increased risk for PML [132]. HTLV-1-associated myelopathy (HAM) has been described as well in SOT.

Infections in Lung and Heart-Lung Transplantation

Infecting Microbial Agents

Bacterial

Bacterial infections are the most common type of infections among lung and lung-heart transplant recipients. The anatomic site most frequently affected is the respiratory tract, usually manifested with pneumonia, sinusitis, or tracheobronchitis. Previous colonization, healthcare associated, and procedures related are the primary sources. For patients with cystic fibrosis (CF), knowledge of previous colonization results may provide some diagnostic and therapeutic advantages. *Pseudomonas aeruginosa* is a predominant colonizing pathogen in CF. However, *Acinetobacter baumannii*, *Burkholderia* species, *Stenotrophomonas maltophilia*, *Achromobacter xylosoxidans*, NTM, *Pandorea*, and *Ralstonia* are also observed [23]. Furthermore, pathogens that are known to cause nosocomial pneumonia during the 1st month include *Staphylococcus aureus*, *Pseudomonas aeruginosa*, other Gram negatives (*Klebsiella pneumoniae*, *Enterobacter cloacae*, *Serratia marcescens*, *Escherichia coli*, *Acinetobacter* species), and anaerobes.

Gram-positive bacteria are a common source of infections making up to 40% of them [133]. The most common sites affected were the respiratory tract, followed by bacteremia, skin, wound, and catheter related. The pathogens more frequently identified are *Staphylococcus* species (77%), *Enterococcus* species (12%), *Streptococcus* species (6%), *Pneumococcus* (4%), and *Eubacterium lentum* (1%). *Staphylococcus aureus* infection can develop up to 20% of lung recipients. SA commonly causes pneumonia, followed by tracheobronchitis, bacteremia, intrathoracic infections, and SSTIs [20]. *Streptococcus pneumoniae* is community acquired and present with pneumonia, usually after 6 months posttransplant. *Pseudomonas aeruginosa* has high rates of colonization (up to 40%) and disease (30%) [134]. Other significant bacterial infections that may present after the 1st month are *Mycobacterium tuberculosis*, NTM, *Nocardia*, *Rhodococcus*, and *Legionella*. Isolation of NTM in lung transplant recipients without evidence of disease is not associated with increased mortality [135]. Nocardiosis can occur in about 2% of the lung transplant recipients. The median time of onset ranges from 14.3 to 34.1 months [136, 137]. *Nocardia asteroides*, *N. farcinica*, *N. nova*, and *N. brasiliensis* have been reported. *N. farcinica* appears to carry worse outcomes. This infection can present as a breakthrough in the presence of trimethoprim-sulfamethoxazole for *P. jiroveci* prophylaxis, although the isolates may remain susceptible. Mortality has been reported to range between 18% and 40%. The native lung is more frequently affected in single-lung transplant recipients. Nodules are the more prevalent radiographic finding. Extrapulmonary involvement affecting the skin and brain can be seen. Hypogammaglobulinemia and neutropenia seem to confer additional risk factors for nocardiosis in this setting [137].

Fungal

Fungal infections are frequent complications in lung and lung-heart transplant. They present in about 15–35% and carry an overall mortality close to 60% [138]. *Aspergillus* and *Candida* are the most frequent causative agents. Other important fungi include *Cryptococcus* spp., mucormycosis, endemic fungi (*Histoplasma*, *Coccidioides*, and *Blastomyces* spp.), *Scedosporium* spp., *Fusarium* spp., and dematiaceous molds. Candida infections are prominent during the 1st month after transplantation. It can be one of the most common causes of BSI in this setting [139]. Although colonization of the upper airways and gastrointestinal tract is common, *Candida* additionally can cause mucocutaneous disease, tracheobronchitis, anastomosis site infections, CRBSI, and disseminated disease. *Aspergillus* spp. lead as the cause of invasive fungal infections. Its attack rate of infection is almost ten times compared to that in other SOT patients (estimated incidence of 6% among lung transplant recipients) [140, 141]. *A. fumigatus* is the most common species, but *A. terreus*, *A. flavus*, and *A. niger* have been described as well. The main predisposing risk factors in this setting are intense immunosuppression, previous colonization with *Aspergillus* spp., airway ischemia, and BOS. Single-lung transplant possesses the greatest risk to developing an invasive *Aspergillus* infection carrying a higher mortality than double-lung and heart-lung transplant recipients. Single-lung recipients are usually older and more likely to have COPD as the indication for transplantation [140]. *Aspergillus* infections can present as tracheobronchitis, pneumonia, or disseminated disease. Extrapulmonary involvement includes sinusitis, CNS or orbits infections, and vertebral osteomyelitis. Aids in the diagnosis can include surveillance bronchoscopies (bronchoalveolar lavage stain and culture; biopsy), chest CT and serum/BAL galactomannan, beta-D-glucan, and PCR. The presence of pulmonary nodular lesions in invasive infections can carry better outcomes [142]. Voriconazole is the treatment of choice. It is important to note that immune reconstitution inflammatory syndrome (IRIS) can develop at a median of 56 days in 7% of treated lung transplant recipients [143]. In *Aspergillus* tracheobronchitis, nebulized amphotericin B and debridement of the bronchial anastomosis are important adjuvant measures to systemic antifungal therapy [144, 145]. *Pneumocystis jirovecii* pneumonia manifests from 1 to 6 months. Its incidence has been reduced dramatically with universal TMP/SMX prophylaxis. Cryptococcosis with a rate of 2% in lung transplant recipients presents with pulmonary involvement, but dissemination with meningitis can occur. Furthermore, *Cryptococcus* skin manifestations like cellulitis and *Cryptococcus*-associated IRIS have been documented [146, 147].

Viral

Viral infections are a common cause of morbidity among lung transplant recipients. The most common viruses are (1) CMV among the herpes viruses and (2) community-acquired respiratory viruses. As in other SOT recipients, the higher risk to develop CMV infection is among D+/R−, followed by D+/R+, D−/R+, and D−/R−. This last scenario carries less than 5% of risk [48, 148]. Lung transplant recipients possess higher risk for CMV than other SOT with an estimated incidence of 30–86% [87]. The lung is considered a primary reservoir for CMV latency, and abundant lymphocytic tissue surrounds the transplanted organ. Additionally, the use of antilymphocyte antibodies to treat rejection or for immunosuppression and other herpesviruses infections are additional risk factors for CMV disease [149]. Interferon (IFN)-γ (+874T/T) polymorphism increases IFN levels and may be a predisposition for CMV disease [150]. CMV is significantly associated with BOS, which reduces survival after the first year posttransplant [151]. CMV disease is most commonly manifested by pneumonitis or viral syndrome and less frequently with gastrointestinal disease. Among lung transplant recipients, ganciclovir-resistant CMV carries an increased morbidity and mortality [152].

Infections with community-acquired respiratory viruses ranged from 7.7% to 64%. These infections are associated with increased risk to develop pneumonia, graft dysfunction manifested by lung function loss, BOS, high calcineurin inhibitor blood levels, and increase mortality [153–155]. These viruses include influenza, parainfluenza, respiratory syncytial virus (RSV), coronaviruses, human rhinovirus, adenovirus, human metapneumoviruses, and bocaviruses. The hospitalization rates are higher for influenza and parainfluenza (50% and 17%, respectively) [154]. Symptoms are usually nonspecific. Diagnosis often requires detection of viral nucleoprotein antigens in nasopharyngeal swabs or bronchoalveolar lavage (BAL) by enzyme immunoassay or fluorescent antibody or the amplification of nucleic acid by PCR. Ribavirin may possess activity against *Paramyxoviruses* (RSV, *Metapneumovirus*, and parainfluenza). Ribavirin is administered inhaled, orally, or intravenously. Oseltamivir or zanamivir is the treatment choice of influenza A or B [156]. Adamantanes (amantadine and rimantadine) are not active against influenza B, and there is a marked increase resistance among influenza A strains [156]. Similarly to other SOT recipients, DNA viruses like non-CMV herpesviruses (HSV-1,-2), VZV, HHV 6,-7,-8, and EBV are a source of significant morbidity including but not limited to CMV-negative viral syndrome, rash, pneumonitis, hepatitis, and encephalitis [157]. Lastly, polyomavirus such as BK virus (BKV), JC virus (JCV), and simian virus 40 (SV40)—although frequently encountered in lung transplant recipients with an unclear causality—may cause worsening renal function or survival [158]. PTLD is also a well-recognized complication. A trend toward late PTLD presentation (>1 year) has been documented where B symptoms are more predominant as well as extra-graft involvement [159].

Parasitic

As other immunosuppressive states, certain parasitic infections can complicate lung and heart-lung transplants recipients. It is critical to elicit a detailed history and geographic risk factors to determine the risk of acquisition and the potential etiologic agent. Toxoplasmosis can result from primary infection or reactivation of previous latent infections. Toxoplasmosis can develop in patients with negative epidemiological history for cat ownership or consumption of undercooked meat. In patients with primary toxoplasmosis, nonspecific symptoms such as fever, lymphadenopathy, or organ injury may be present. Reactivation can cause encephalitis with or without space-occupying brain lesions, seizures, chorioretinitis, fever of unknown origin, pneumonitis, myocarditis, and rash. Although cases of the lung fluke, *Paragonimus westermani* have not been reported in lung transplantation, it can be a potential threat in endemic areas where this organism is endemic. Other parasites that can target the lung in immunosuppressive states include *Echinococcus*, *Schistosoma*, and *Strongyloides stercoralis* [160]. Strongyloidiasis can present as hyperinfection syndrome [161]. *Leishmania*, although infrequently seen, has been reported among lung and lung-heart recipients [30]. Free-living amoebas can affect this population as well. Amoebic granulomatous dermatitis and disseminated infection presenting with ulcerative skin lesions, respiratory failure, and seizures have been described in lung transplant recipients [162, 163]. Finally, alimentary protozoa, including *Cryptosporidium*, which present with diarrhea and may elevate tacrolimus levels [164], and microsporidia, which present with unusual manifestations like myositis or granulomatous interstitial nephritis, affects lung transplant recipients [165, 166].

Sites and Types of Infection

Skin, Soft Tissue, and Bone

The overall rate of SSIs is about 13% with a significant proportion of infections being organ or space occupying (72%), deep incisional (17%), and superficial (10%) [18, 41]. Independent risk factors to develop SSI are diabetes, female donor, prolonged ischemic time, and the number of red blood cells transfusion during the perioperative period [167]. SSIs are associated with a 35% mortality within the first year of transplantation. The most common organisms found to cause

SSI or mediastinitis are *P. aeruginosa*, *Candida* species, *S. aureus* (including MRSA), *Enterococcus*, coagulase-negative *Staphylococci*, *Burkholderia cepacia*, *E. coli*, *Proteus mirabilis*, *Serratia marcescens*, *Acinetobacter baumannii*, *Enterobacter cloacae*, and *Klebsiella* species. There is a correlation in up to 33% of the patients' SSI causative organisms with previous pathogens colonizing recipients' native lungs at the time of the transplant [167]. The median onset is 25 days after lung transplant [167]. Although rare, NTM can cause SSI infections among lung transplant recipients. The most frequently encountered are *Mycobacterium avium* complex followed by *Mycobacterium abscessus* and *Mycobacterium gordonae*. NTM SSI infections can be complicated by progressive disseminated disease or requirement of lifelong suppressive therapy [135]. Other organisms such as *Mycoplasma hominis* and *Lactobacillus* spp. have also been described. Deep infections can affect up to 5% of the patients. Sternal osteomyelitis can reach up to 6% of these deep infections. Causative organisms for sternal osteomyelitis include *Pseudomonas aeruginosa*, *Serratia marcescens*, and *Scedosporium*. Non-sternal osteomyelitis affecting the calcaneus bone has complicated a disseminated infection with *Aspergillus fumigatus* [168].

Bloodstream

Bloodstream infections (BSIs) occur with an estimated rate of 25% among lung transplant recipients. A major proportion of BSIs occur in the early posttransplant period. BSIs infections are significantly associated with worse survival [139, 169]. The most common organisms encountered are *Staphylococcus aureus*, *Pseudomonas aeruginosa*, and *Candida* [139]. *Pseudomonas aeruginosa* BSI—predominantly present during the transplant hospitalization period and more commonly affecting CF patients—is followed in frequency by *Burkholderia cepacia* and *Candida albicans*. Conversely, *Staphylococcus aureus* was the predominant organism after transplantation discharge. In an estimated 70% of BSI, the source was pulmonary, followed in frequency by CRBSI, gastrointestinal infection, peritonitis, and UTI. A pulmonary source of bacteremia in SOT often develops into septic shock [170]. Although unusual, cases of *Aspergillus fumigatus* endocarditis have been described following lung transplantation [171]. Often patients had CF as the underlying lung disease and a median of 8 ± 6 months presentation. This complication carries a high mortality and often requires a combination of antifungal therapy with valvular replacement surgery.

Chest

Infectious complications related to the chest cavity include mediastinitis, cardiac (pericarditis and myocarditis), lung parenchyma infections (nodular infiltrates, cavitation, or pneumonia), bronchial anastomosis infections, and pleural space infections (bronchopleural fistula and empyema). Empyema followed by mediastinitis and pericarditis, in addition to surgical wound infections and sternal osteomyelitis, is the most frequent deep SSI complications affecting the chest cavity. Empyema presents in around of 3.6% of cases. It occurs during the first 6 months after transplantation (median 46 ± 39 days) carrying an estimated mortality of 28.6% [172]. Most common organisms found are *Staphylococcus* spp., *E. coli*, *Enterobacter* spp., *Klebsiella* spp., *Mycoplasma hominis*, VRE, and *Candida*. Furthermore, *Mycobacterium abscessus* was isolated as a rare causative agent of empyema as well [173]. The degree of immunosuppression, reduced renal function, previous sternotomy, and re-exploration due to bleeding are listed as potential risk factors for mediastinitis [119]. There is an increased prevalence of mediastinitis caused by Gram negatives and fungi among lung transplant recipients. Causative organisms for mediastinitis are similar to SSI and are listed above. Infectious pericarditis can be present up to 6% of the patients (isolated organisms include MSSA, *Mycoplasma hominis*, and *Scedosporium prolificans*) [167, 174, 175]. Due to their high fatal rate, fungal bronchial anastomotic infections are critical to recognize.

Pneumonia is believed to affect around 21% of lung recipients and 40% of heart-lung recipients. Nosocomial organisms cause early pneumonia as in other posttransplant settings. The donor's lung seems to be the primary source for pneumonic infections, although the recipients' upper airways or sinuses are also potential sources. Preoperative colonization with Gram-negative rods and colonized infected donor bronchus or perfusate are recognized risk factors for pneumonia. Likewise, pretransplantation colonizing microorganisms from suppurative lung disease are associated with pneumonia development posttransplant [176]. The most common causal organisms are *Pseudomonas aeruginosa*, *Staphylococcus aureus*, and *Aspergillus* spp. Other pathogens include bacteria such as *B. cepacia*, *Enterobacter* species, *S. maltophilia*, *Klebsiella* species, *S. epidermidis*, and *E. coli*, and fungi such as *Fusarium* spp., *Cryptococcus neoformans*, and *Paracoccidioides brasiliensis* [176]. After the 1st month, pneumonia can present as local infiltrates, diffuse interstitial infiltrates, and nodules with or without cavitation. This type of presentation may aid in the possible causative microorganism. The list of potential pathogens is extensive and includes in addition to the already mentioned *Nocardia*, *Chlamydia pneumonia*, *Legionella*, TB, NTM, *Pneumocystis jirovecii*, *Rhodococcus*, herpesviruses (CMV, HSV, and VZV), respiratory viruses, endemic fungi (e.g., histoplasmosis), mucormycosis, and *Scedosporium* spp. [177–179].

Abdominal/Genitourinary

Similarly to other SOT, common infectious complications affecting the gastrointestinal or genitourinary tract include *Clostridium difficile* colitis and UTIs. Intra-abdominal complication carries an overall increase mortality [180]. Frequent GI symptoms presenting posttransplant are diarrhea which can affect almost 30% of lung transplant recipients and abdominal pain. Abdominal pain should prompt further investigation for potential intra-abdominal causes. In the pediatric population, the possibility of PTLD should be investigated since it carries a high mortality [181]. Other described infectious intra-abdominal complications include digestive perforation (seen in 6%) [182], retroperitoneal abscesses, cholecystitis, perianal abscesses, esophagitis, pancreatitis, pancreatic abscesses, hepatitis, diverticulitis, appendicitis, CMV colitis, megacolon, and colon rupture [180, 183, 184]. In developing countries, persistently abnormal liver enzymes should prompt testing for HEV. HEV RNA should be used for screening. Oral ribavirin seems to be safe and effective in this setting [185].

Central Nervous System (CNS)

CNS symptoms developing during the 1st month following lung or heart-lung transplantation should trigger the concern for donor-derived viral infections. LCMV often is accompanied by CSF normal to low glucose, marked elevated protein, and mild pleocytosis [36]. Although with unclear benefit, ribavirin has been used. Donor-transmitted rabies is an uncommon but neurologic devastating complication that occurs within the first 30 days of transplant. Lung transplantation has been described as a potential causal mechanism [186]. Other organisms known to cause meningitis in lung transplant recipients are *Cryptococcus*, tuberculosis, WNV, and herpesviruses [187, 188]. Diagnosis of WNV in this setting requires nuclear acid amplification due to the unreliability of serologic testing. *Scedosporium apiospermum* infections often cause dissemination including CNS abscesses in addition to pulmonary involvement among lung transplant recipients [189]. It is important to differentiate from other molds, since amphotericin B is ineffective against *Scedosporium* spp. In severe cases or refractory disease without an appropriate surgical debridement, the addition of terbinafine to voriconazole may prove to be useful [190]. Other recognized organisms causing occupying brain lesions are *Fusarium*, *Nocardia*, *Aspergillus*, toxoplasmosis, *Cryptococcus neoformans*, *Listeria*, and *Cladophialophora bantiana* [191–193]. PML, a late manifestation, can be associated with intensified immunosuppression or rituximab. Cidofovir followed by mirtazapine can be considered as a form of therapy for PML.

Conclusions

Infections in heart, lung, and heart-lung transplant recipients are a complex, dynamic, and evolving process. Many factors such as demographics, timing, type of transplant, anatomy, and microbiology, among others, interplay in the development of these fatal complications. Pertinent recognition and treatment of these infections improve transplantation outcomes.

Acknowledgments No funding agencies had any role in the preparation, review, or approval of this paper. The views expressed in this paper are those of the authors and do not necessarily represent the views of the University of Colorado Denver or Stanford University. No conflict of interests was reported by Andrés F. Henao-Martínez and José G. Montoya.

References

1. Lund LH, Edwards LB, Kucheryavaya AY, Dipchand AI, Benden C, Christie JD, et al. The registry of the international society for heart and lung transplantation: thirtieth official adult heart transplant report—2013; focus theme: age. J Heart Lung Transplant. 2013;32(10):951–64.
2. Durante-Mangoni E, Casillo R, Pinto D, Caianiello C, Albisinni R, Caprioli V, et al. Heart transplantation during active infective endocarditis: case report and review of the literature. Transplant Proc. 2011;43(1):304–6.
3. Haddad F, Deuse T, Pham M, Khazanie P, Rosso F, Luikart H, et al. Changing trends in infectious disease in heart transplantation. J Heart Lung Transplant. 2010;29(3):306–15.
4. Munoz-Price LS, Poirel L, Bonomo RA, Schwaber MJ, Daikos GL, Cormican M, et al. Clinical epidemiology of the global expansion of *Klebsiella pneumoniae* carbapenemases. Lancet Infect Dis. 2013;13(9):785–96.
5. Woodford N, Livermore DM. Infections caused by Gram-positive bacteria: a review of the global challenge. J Infect. 2009;59(Suppl 1):S4–16.
6. Reitz BA, Wallwork JL, Hunt SA, Pennock JL, Billingham ME, Oyer PE, et al. Heart-lung transplantation. N Engl J Med. 1982;306(10):557–64.
7. De Soyza A, Meachery G, Hester KL, Nicholson A, Parry G, Tocewicz K, et al. Lung transplantation for patients with cystic fibrosis and Burkholderia cepacia complex infection: a single-center experience. J Heart Lung Transplant. 2010;29(12):1395–404.
8. Stinson EB, Bieber CP, Griepp RB, Clark DA, Shumway NE, Remington JS. Infectious complications after cardiac transplantation in man. Ann Intern Med. 1971;74(1):22–36.
9. Gonzalez-Padilla M, Caston JJ, Vidal E, Arizon JM, Segura C, Montejo M, et al. Epidemiology and clinical impact of infection in patients awaiting heart transplantation. Int J Infect Dis. 2013;17(9):e681–5.
10. Gurgui M, Munoz P. Infection in heart transplantation. Enferm Infecc Microbiol Clin. 2007;25(9):587–97. quiz 98
11. Montoya JG, Giraldo LF, Efron B, Stinson EB, Gamberg P, Hunt S, et al. Infectious complications among 620 consecutive heart transplant patients at Stanford University Medical Center. Clin Infect Dis. 2001;33(5):629–40.
12. van de Beek D, Kremers WK, Del Pozo JL, Daly RC, Edwards BS, McGregor CG, et al. Effect of infectious diseases on outcome after heart transplant. Mayo Clin Proc. 2008;83(3):304–8.
13. Godoy HL, Guerra CM, Viegas RF, Dinis RZ, Branco JN, Neto VA, et al. Infections in heart transplant recipients in Brazil: the challenge of Chagas' disease. J Heart Lung Transplant. 2010;29(3): 286–90.
14. Carlos, Gomez SHT, Gould K, Valantine H, Montoya JG. Diagnosis and management of infectious diseases in cardiothoracic transplantation and mechanical circulatory support. ISHLT Monograph Series. 5. Elsevier; 2011. p. 1–10.

15. Yusen RD, Christie JD, Edwards LB, Kucheryavaya AY, Benden C, Dipchand AI, et al. The registry of the international society for heart and lung transplantation: thirtieth adult lung and heart-lung transplant report—2013; focus theme: age. J Heart Lung Transplant. 2013;32(10):965–78.
16. Cai J. Thoracic transplantation in the United States: an analysis of UNOS registry data. Clin Transpl. 2006;1:41–56.
17. Russo MJ, Iribarne A, Hong KN, Davies RR, Xydas S, Takayama H, et al. High lung allocation score is associated with increased morbidity and mortality following transplantation. Chest. 2010;137(3):651–7.
18. Mattner F, Fischer S, Weissbrodt H, Chaberny IF, Sohr D, Gottlieb J, et al. Post-operative nosocomial infections after lung and heart transplantation. J Heart Lung Transplant. 2007;26(3):241–9.
19. Parada MT, Alba A, Sepulveda C. Early and late infections in lung transplantation patients. Transplant Proc. 2010;42(1):333–5.
20. Shields RK, Clancy CJ, Minces LR, Kwak EJ, Silveira FP, Abdel Massih RC, et al. *Staphylococcus aureus* infections in the early period after lung transplantation: epidemiology, risk factors, and outcomes. J Heart Lung Transplant. 2012;31(11):1199–206.
21. Speich R, van der Bij W. Epidemiology and management of infections after lung transplantation. Clin Infect Dis. 2001;33(Suppl 1):S58–65.
22. Singh N, Paterson DL. Mycobacterium tuberculosis infection in solid-organ transplant recipients: impact and implications for management. Clin Infect Dis. 1998;27(5):1266–77.
23. Shoham S, Shah PD. Impact of multidrug-resistant organisms on patients considered for lung transplantation. Infect Dis Clin N Am. 2013;27(2):343–58.
24. Aris RM, Gilligan PH, Neuringer IP, Gott KK, Rea J, Yankaskas JR. The effects of panresistant bacteria in cystic fibrosis patients on lung transplant outcome. Am J Respir Crit Care Med. 1997;155(5):1699–704.
25. Alexander BD, Petzold EW, Reller LB, Palmer SM, Davis RD, Woods CW, et al. Survival after lung transplantation of cystic fibrosis patients infected with Burkholderia cepacia complex. Am J Transplant. 2008;8(5):1025–30.
26. Boussaud V, Guillemain R, Grenet D, Coley N, Souilamas R, Bonnette P, et al. Clinical outcome following lung transplantation in patients with cystic fibrosis colonised with Burkholderia cepacia complex: results from two French centres. Thorax. 2008;63(8):732–7.
27. Fitzpatrick MA, Caicedo JC, Stosor V, Ison MG. Expanded infectious diseases screening program for Hispanic transplant candidates. Transpl Infect Dis. 2010;12(4):336–41.
28. Vikram HR, Dosanjh A, Blair JE. Coccidioidomycosis and lung transplantation. Transplantation. 2011;92(7):717–21.
29. Chin-Hong PV, Schwartz BS, Bern C, Montgomery SP, Kontak S, Kubak B, et al. Screening and treatment of chagas disease in organ transplant recipients in the United States: recommendations from the chagas in transplant working group. Am J Transplant. 2011;11(4):672–80.
30. Morales P, Torres JJ, Salavert M, Peman J, Lacruz J, Sole A. Visceral leishmaniasis in lung transplantation. Transplant Proc. 2003;35(5):2001–3.
31. Roxby AC, Gottlieb GS, Limaye AP. Strongyloidiasis in transplant patients. Clin Infect Dis. 2009;49(9):1411–23.
32. Jain VV, Evans T, Peterson MW. Reactivation histoplasmosis after treatment with anti-tumor necrosis factor alpha in a patient from a nonendemic area. Respir Med. 2006;100(7):1291–3.
33. Luong ML, Morrissey O, Husain S. Assessment of infection risks prior to lung transplantation. Curr Opin Infect Dis. 2010;23(6):578–83.
34. Fischer SA, Avery RK. Screening of donor and recipient prior to solid organ transplantation. Am J Transplant. 2009;9(Suppl 4):S7–18.
35. Matignon M, Botterel F, Audard V, Dunogue B, Dahan K, Lang P, et al. Outcome of renal transplantation in eight patients with Candida sp. contamination of preservation fluid. Am J Transplant. 2008;8(3):697–700.
36. Waggoner JJ, Soda EA, Deresinski S. Rare and emerging viral infections in transplant recipients. Clin Infect Dis. 2013;57(8):1182–8.
37. Gangappa S, Kokko KE, Carlson LM, Gourley T, Newell KA, Pearson TC, et al. Immune responsiveness and protective immunity after transplantation. Transpl Int. 2008;21(4):293–303.
38. Bridges CB, Woods L, Coyne-Beasley T. Advisory Committee on Immunization Practices (ACIP) recommended immunization schedule for adults aged 19 years and older – United States, 2013. MMWR Surveill Summ. 2013;62(Suppl 1):9–19.
39. Rubin LG, Levin MJ, Ljungman P, Davies EG, Avery R, Tomblyn M, et al. 2013 IDSA clinical practice guideline for vaccination of the immunocompromised host. Clin Infect Dis. 2014;58(3):309–18.
40. Soave R. Prophylaxis strategies for solid-organ transplantation. Clin Infect Dis. 2001;33(Suppl 1):S26–31.
41. Bratzler DW, Dellinger EP, Olsen KM, Perl TM, Auwaerter PG, Bolon MK, et al. Clinical practice guidelines for antimicrobial prophylaxis in surgery. Am J Health Syst Pharm. 2013;70(3):195–283.
42. Playford EG, Webster AC, Sorell TC, Craig JC. Antifungal agents for preventing fungal infections in solid organ transplant recipients. Cochrane Database Syst Rev. 2004;(3):CD004291.
43. Munoz P, Valerio M, Palomo J, Giannella M, Yanez JF, Desco M, et al. Targeted antifungal prophylaxis in heart transplant recipients. Transplantation. 2013;96(7):664–9.
44. Drew RH, Dodds Ashley E, Benjamin DK Jr, Duane Davis R, Palmer SM, Perfect JR. Comparative safety of amphotericin B lipid complex and amphotericin B deoxycholate as aerosolized antifungal prophylaxis in lung-transplant recipients. Transplantation. 2004;77(2):232–7.
45. Palmer SM, Drew RH, Whitehouse JD, Tapson VF, Davis RD, McConnell RR, et al. Safety of aerosolized amphotericin B lipid complex in lung transplant recipients. Transplantation. 2001;72(3):545–8.
46. Avery RK. Antifungal prophylaxis in lung transplantation. Semin Respir Crit Care Med. 2011;32(6):717–26.
47. Beam E, Razonable RR. Cytomegalovirus in solid organ transplantation: epidemiology, prevention, and treatment. Curr Infect Dis Rep. 2012;14(6):633–41.
48. Razonable RR, Humar A. Cytomegalovirus in solid organ transplantation. Am J Transplant. 2013;13(Suppl 4):93–106.
49. Marty FM, Winston DJ, Rowley SD, Vance E, Papanicolaou GA, Mullane KM, et al. CMX001 to prevent cytomegalovirus disease in hematopoietic-cell transplantation. N Engl J Med. 2013;369(13):1227–36.
50. Fishman JA. Infection in solid-organ transplant recipients. N Engl J Med. 2007;357(25):2601–14.
51. Humar A, Snydman D. Cytomegalovirus in solid organ transplant recipients. Am J Transplant. 2009;9(Suppl 4):S78–86.
52. Kumar D, Chernenko S, Moussa G, Cobos I, Manuel O, Preiksaitis J, et al. Cell-mediated immunity to predict cytomegalovirus disease in high-risk solid organ transplant recipients. Am J Transplant. 2009;9(5):1214–22.
53. Ritta M, Costa C, Sinesi F, Sidoti F, Di Nauta A, Mantovani S, et al. Evaluation of Epstein-Barr virus-specific immunologic response in solid organ transplant recipients with an enzyme-linked ImmunoSpot assay. Transplant Proc. 2013;45(7):2754–7.
54. Sarmiento E, del Pozo N, Gallego A, Fernandez-Yanez J, Palomo J, Villa A, et al. Decreased levels of serum complement C3 and natural killer cells add to the predictive value of total immunoglobulin G for severe infection in heart transplant recipients. Transpl Infect Dis. 2012;14(5):526–39.
55. Mori T, Aisa Y, Kato J, Nakamura Y, Ikeda Y, Okamoto S. Drug interaction between voriconazole and calcineurin inhibitors in allo-

geneic hematopoietic stem cell transplant recipients. Bone Marrow Transplant. 2009;44(6):371–4.
56. Romero AJ, Le Pogamp P, Nilsson LG, Wood N. Effect of voriconazole on the pharmacokinetics of cyclosporine in renal transplant patients. Clin Pharmacol Ther. 2002;71(4):226–34.
57. Kuypers DR, Verleden G, Naesens M, Vanrenterghem Y. Drug interaction between mycophenolate mofetil and rifampin: possible induction of uridine diphosphate-glucuronosyltransferase. Clin Pharmacol Ther. 2005;78(1):81–8.
58. Buffington GA, Dominguez JH, Piering WF, Hebert LA, Kauffman HM Jr, Lemann J Jr. Interaction of rifampin and glucocorticoids. Adverse effect on renal allograft function. JAMA. 1976;236(17):1958–60.
59. Kannankeril P, Roden DM, Darbar D. Drug-induced long QT syndrome. Pharmacol Rev. 2010;62(4):760–81.
60. Bui KT, Mehta S, Khuu TH, Ross D, Carlson M, Leibowitz MR, et al. Extended spectrum beta-lactamase-producing Enterobacteriaceae infection in heart and lung transplant recipients and in mechanical circulatory support recipients. Transplantation. 2014;97(5):590–4.
61. Raso-Raso R, Martinez-Dolz LV, Almenar-Bonet L, Navarro-Manchon J, Blanes-Julia M, Salvador-Sanz A. Nocardia infection in heart transplant recipients. Rev Clin Esp. 2010;210(8):389–93.
62. Peleg AY, Husain S, Qureshi ZA, Silveira FP, Sarumi M, Shutt KA, et al. Risk factors, clinical characteristics, and outcome of Nocardia infection in organ transplant recipients: a matched case-control study. Clin Infect Dis. 2007;44(10):1307–14.
63. Peraira JR, Segovia J, Fuentes R, Jimenez-Mazuecos J, Arroyo R, Fuertes B, et al. Pulmonary nocardiosis in heart transplant recipients: treatment and outcome. Transplant Proc. 2003;35(5):2006–8.
64. Munoz P, Valerio M, Palomo J, Fernandez-Yanez J, Fernandez-Cruz A, Guinea J, et al. Infectious and non-infectious neurologic complications in heart transplant recipients. Medicine (Baltimore). 2010;89(3):166–75.
65. Stamm AM, Smith SH, Kirklin JK, McGiffin DC. Listerial myocarditis in cardiac transplantation. Rev Infect Dis. 1990;12(5):820–3.
66. Munoz P, Palomo J, Munoz R, Rodriguez-Creixems M, Pelaez T, Bouza E. Tuberculosis in heart transplant recipients. Clin Infect Dis. 1995;21(2):398–402.
67. Patel R, Roberts GD, Keating MR, Paya CV. Infections due to nontuberculous mycobacteria in kidney, heart, and liver transplant recipients. Clin Infect Dis. 1994;19(2):263–73.
68. Bodro M, Sabe N, Santin M, Cruzado JM, Llado L, Gonzalez-Costello J, et al. Clinical features and outcomes of tuberculosis in solid organ transplant recipients. Transplant Proc. 2012;44(9):2686–9.
69. Chou NK, Wang JL, Chi NH, Wu IH, Huang SC, Chen YS, et al. Tuberculosis after heart transplantation: twenty years of experience in a single center in Taiwan. Transplant Proc. 2008;40(8):2631–3.
70. Horbach I, Fehrenbach FJ. Legionellosis in heart transplant recipients. Infection. 1990;18(6):361–3.
71. Neofytos D, Treadway S, Ostrander D, Alonso CD, Dierberg KL, Nussenblatt V, et al. Epidemiology, outcomes, and mortality predictors of invasive mold infections among transplant recipients: a 10-year, single-center experience. Transpl Infect Dis. 2013;15(3):233–42.
72. Singh N, Limaye AP, Forrest G, Safdar N, Muñoz P, Pursell K, et al. Late-onset invasive aspergillosis in organ transplant recipients in the current era. Med Mycol. 2006;44(5):445–9.
73. Montoya JG, Chaparro SV, Celis D, Cortes JA, Leung AN, Robbins RC, et al. Invasive aspergillosis in the setting of cardiac transplantation. Clin Infect Dis. 2003;37(Suppl 3):S281–92.
74. Galimberti R, Kowalczuk A, Hidalgo Parra I, Gonzalez Ramos M, Flores V. Cutaneous aspergillosis: a report of six cases. Br J Dermatol. 1998;139(3):522–6.
75. Gregory ME, Weir CR, Roberts F, Browne BH. Aspergillus endophthalmitis following orthotopic heart transplant. Can J Ophthalmol. 2009;44(5):607–8.
76. Morio F, Treilhaud M, Lepelletier D, Le Pape P, Rigal JC, Delile L, et al. Aspergillus fumigatus endocarditis of the mitral valve in a heart transplant recipient: a case report. Diagn Microbiol Infect Dis. 2008;62(4):453–6.
77. Byl B, Jacobs F, Antoine M, Depierreux M, Serruys E, Primo G, et al. Mediastinitis caused by Aspergillus fumigatus with ruptured aortic pseudoaneurysm in a heart transplant recipient: case study. Heart Lung. 1993;22(2):145–7.
78. Cortet B, Richard R, Deprez X, Lucet L, Flipo RM, Le Loet X, et al. Aspergillus spondylodiscitis: successful conservative treatment in 9 cases. J Rheumatol. 1994;21(7):1287–91.
79. Husain S, Alexander BD, Munoz P, Avery RK, Houston S, Pruett T, et al. Opportunistic mycelial fungal infections in organ transplant recipients: emerging importance of non-Aspergillus mycelial fungi. Clin Infect Dis. 2003;37(2):221–9.
80. Cardeau-Desangles I, Fabre A, Cointault O, Guitard J, Esposito L, Iriart X, et al. Disseminated Ochroconis gallopava infection in a heart transplant patient. Transpl Infect Dis. 2013;15(3):E115–8.
81. Vilchez RA, Fung J, Kusne S. Cryptococcosis in organ transplant recipients: an overview. Am J Transplant. 2002;2(7):575–80.
82. Assi M, Martin S, Wheat LJ, Hage C, Freifeld A, Avery R, et al. Histoplasmosis after solid organ transplant. Clin Infect Dis. 2013;57(11):1542–9.
83. Ribeiro PM, Bacal F, Koga-Ito CY, Junqueira JC, Jorge AO. Presence of Candida spp. in the oral cavity of heart transplantation patients. J Appl Oral Sci. 2011;19(1):6–10.
84. Schaenman JM, Rosso F, Austin JM, Baron EJ, Gamberg P, Miller J, et al. Trends in invasive disease due to Candida species following heart and lung transplantation. Transpl Infect Dis. 2009;11(2):112–21.
85. Colvin-Adams M, Agnihotri A. Cardiac allograft vasculopathy: current knowledge and future direction. Clin Transplant. 2011;25(2):175–84.
86. Potena L, Valantine HA. Cytomegalovirus-associated allograft rejection in heart transplant patients. Curr Opin Infect Dis. 2007;20(4):425–31.
87. Snydman DR, Limaye AP, Potena L, Zamora MR. Update and review: state-of-the-art management of cytomegalovirus infection and disease following thoracic organ transplantation. Transplant Proc. 2011;43(3 Suppl):S1–S17.
88. Kotton CN, Kumar D, Caliendo AM, Asberg A, Chou S, Danziger-Isakov L, et al. Updated international consensus guidelines on the management of cytomegalovirus in solid-organ transplantation. Transplantation. 2013;96(4):333–60.
89. Herreman A, Dierickx D, Morscio J, Camps J, Bittoun E, Verhoef G, et al. Clinicopathological characteristics of posttransplant lymphoproliferative disorders of T-cell origin: single-center series of nine cases and meta-analysis of 147 reported cases. Leuk Lymphoma. 2013;54(10):2190–9.
90. Manlhiot C, Pollock-Barziv SM, Holmes C, Weitzman S, Allen U, Clarizia NA, et al. Post-transplant lymphoproliferative disorder in pediatric heart transplant recipients. J Heart Lung Transplant. 2010;29(6):648–57.
91. Florescu DF, Kwon JY, Dumitru I. Adenovirus infections in heart transplantation. Cardiol Rev. 2013;21(4):203–6.
92. Koning L, Pas SD, de Man RA, Balk AH, de Knegt RJ, ten Kate FJ, et al. Clinical implications of chronic hepatitis E virus infection in heart transplant recipients. J Heart Lung Transplant. 2013;32(1):78–85.
93. Kamar N, Izopet J, Tripon S, Bismuth M, Hillaire S, Dumortier J, et al. Ribavirin for chronic hepatitis E virus infection in transplant recipients. N Engl J Med. 2014;370(12):1111–20.

94. Coster LO. Parasitic infections in solid organ transplant recipients. Infect Dis Clin N Am. 2013;27(2):395–427.
95. Luft BJ, Naot Y, Araujo FG, Stinson EB, Remington JS. Primary and reactivated toxoplasma infection in patients with cardiac transplants. Clinical spectrum and problems in diagnosis in a defined population. Ann Intern Med. 1983;99(1):27–31.
96. Gallino A, Maggiorini M, Kiowski W, Martin X, Wunderli W, Schneider J, et al. Toxoplasmosis in heart transplant recipients. Eur J Clin Microbiol Infect Dis. 1996;15(5):389–93.
97. Huprikar S, Bosserman E, Patel G, Moore A, Pinney S, Anyanwu A, et al. Donor-derived Trypanosoma cruzi infection in solid organ recipients in the United States, 2001–2011. Am J Transplant. 2013;13(9):2418–25.
98. Campos SV, Strabelli TM, Amato Neto V, Silva CP, Bacal F, Bocchi EA, et al. Risk factors for Chagas' disease reactivation after heart transplantation. J Heart Lung Transplant. 2008;27(6):597–602.
99. Bestetti RB, Theodoropoulos TA. A systematic review of studies on heart transplantation for patients with end-stage Chagas' heart disease. J Card Fail. 2009;15(3):249–55.
100. Fiorelli AI, Santos RH, Oliveira JL Jr, Lourenco-Filho DD, Dias RR, Oliveira AS, et al. Heart transplantation in 107 cases of Chagas' disease. Transplant Proc. 2011;43(1):220–4.
101. Bern C. Chagas disease in the immunosuppressed host. Curr Opin Infect Dis. 2012;25(4):450–7.
102. Theodoropoulos TA, Silva AG, Bestetti RB. Eosinophil blood count and anemia are associated with Trypanosoma cruzi infection reactivation in Chagas' heart transplant recipients. Int J Cardiol. 2010;145(1):55–6.
103. Pinazo MJ, Espinosa G, Cortes-Lletget C, Posada Ede J, Aldasoro E, Oliveira I, et al. Immunosuppression and Chagas disease: a management challenge. PLoS Negl Trop Dis. 2013;7(1):e1965.
104. Molina I, Gómez i Prat J, Salvador F, Treviño B, Sulleiro E, Serre N, et al. Randomized trial of posaconazole and benznidazole for chronic Chagas' disease. N Engl J Med. 2014;370(20):1899–908.
105. Golino A, Duncan JM, Zeluff B, DePriest J, McAllister HA, Radovancevic B, et al. Leishmaniasis in a heart transplant patient. J Heart Lung Transplant. 1992;11(4 Pt 1):820–3.
106. Ramos A, Asensio A, Munez E, Torre-Cisneros J, Blanes M, Carratala J, et al. Incisional surgical infection in heart transplantation. Transpl Infect Dis. 2008;10(4):298–302.
107. Filsoufi F, Rahmanian PB, Castillo JG, Pinney S, Broumand SR, Adams DH. Incidence, treatment strategies and outcome of deep sternal wound infection after orthotopic heart transplantation. J Heart Lung Transplant. 2007;26(11):1084–90.
108. Talbot TR, Hatcher J, Davis SF, Pierson RN 3rd, Barton R, Dummer S. Scedosporium apiospermum pneumonia and sternal wound infection in a heart transplant recipient. Transplantation. 2002;74(11):1645–7.
109. Hummel M, Schuler S, Weber U, Schwertlick G, Hempel S, Theiss D, et al. Aspergillosis with Aspergillus osteomyelitis and diskitis after heart transplantation: surgical and medical management. J Heart Lung Transplant. 1993;12(4):599–603.
110. Koo S, Gagne LS, Lee P, Pratibhu PP, James LM, Givertz MM, et al. Incidence and risk factors for herpes zoster following heart transplantation. Transpl Infect Dis. 2014;16(1):17–25.
111. Parkins MD, Gregson DB, Pitout JD, Ross T, Laupland KB. Population-based study of the epidemiology and the risk factors for Pseudomonas aeruginosa bloodstream infection. Infection. 2010;38(1):25–32.
112. Rodriguez C, Munoz P, Rodriguez-Creixems M, Yanez JF, Palomo J, Bouza E. Bloodstream infections among heart transplant recipients. Transplantation. 2006;81(3):384–91.
113. Hsu RB, Chang CI, Fang CT, Chang SC, Wang SS, Chu SH. Bloodstream infection in heart transplant recipients: 12-year experience at a university hospital in Taiwan. Eur J Cardiothorac Surg. 2011;40(6):1362–7.
114. Sherman-Weber S, Axelrod P, Suh B, Rubin S, Beltramo D, Manacchio J, et al. Infective endocarditis following orthotopic heart transplantation: 10 cases and a review of the literature. Transpl Infect Dis. 2004;6(4):165–70.
115. Malinis MF, Mawhorter SD, Jain A, Shrestha NK, Avery RK, van Duin D. *Staphylococcus aureus* bacteremia in solid organ transplant recipients: evidence for improved survival when compared with nontransplant patients. Transplantation. 2012;93(10):1045–50.
116. Atasever A, Bacakoglu F, Uysal FE, Nalbantgil S, Karyagdi T, Guzelant A, et al. Pulmonary complications in heart transplant recipients. Transplant Proc. 2006;38(5):1530–4.
117. Haddad F, Hunt SA, Perlroth M, Valantine H, Doyle R, Montoya J. Pulmonary nocardiosis in a heart transplant patient: case report and review of the literature. J Heart Lung Transplant. 2007;26(1):93–7.
118. Munoz P, Palomo J, Guembe P, Rodriguez-Creixems M, Gijon P, Bouza E. Lung nodular lesions in heart transplant recipients. J Heart Lung Transplant. 2000;19(7):660–7.
119. Abid Q, Nkere UU, Hasan A, Gould K, Forty J, Corris P, et al. Mediastinitis in heart and lung transplantation: 15 years experience. Ann Thorac Surg. 2003;75(5):1565–71.
120. Senechal M, LePrince P, Tezenas du Montcel S, Bonnet N, Dubois M, El-Serafi M, et al. Bacterial mediastinitis after heart transplantation: clinical presentation, risk factors and treatment. J Heart Lung Transplant. 2004;23(2):165–70.
121. Chou NK, Wang JL, Chi NH, Wu IH, Huang SC, Chen YS, et al. Surgical treatment of mediastinitis after cardiac transplantation. Transplant Proc. 2008;40(8):2629–30.
122. Hsu RB, Lin FY. Nontyphoid Salmonella infection in heart transplant recipients. Am J Med Sci. 2008;336(5):393–6.
123. Menegaux F, Huraux C, Jordi-Galais P, Dorent R, Ghossoub JJ, Pavie A, et al. Cholelithiasis in heart transplant patients. Ann Chir. 2000;125(9):832–7.
124. Oaks TE, Pennock JL, Myers JL, Wisman CB. Survival following rupture of a pancreatic abscess in a heart transplant recipient. J Heart Transplant. 1986;5(2):148–53.
125. Limaye AP, Smith KD, Cook L, Groom DA, Hunt NC, Jerome KR, et al. Polyomavirus nephropathy in native kidneys of non-renal transplant recipients. Am J Transplant. 2005;5(3):614–20.
126. Murtagh B, Wadia Y, Messner G, Allison P, Harati Y, Delgado R. West Nile virus infection after cardiac transplantation. J Heart Lung Transplant. 2005;24(6):774–6.
127. Kumar D, Prasad GV, Zaltzman J, Levy GA, Humar A. Community-acquired West Nile virus infection in solid-organ transplant recipients. Transplantation. 2004;77(3):399–402.
128. Bestetti RB, Rubio FG, Ferraz Filho JR, Goes MJ, de Santi Neto D, Akio F, et al. Trypanosoma cruzi infection reactivation manifested by encephalitis in a Chagas heart transplant recipient. Int J Cardiol. 2013;163(1):e7–8.
129. van de Beek D, Patel R, Daly RC, McGregor CG, Wijdicks EF. Central nervous system infections in heart transplant recipients. Arch Neurol. 2007;64(12):1715–20.
130. Wiesmayr S, Tabarelli W, Stelzmueller I, Nachbaur D, Boesmueller C, Wykypiel H, et al. Listeria meningitis in transplant recipients. Wien Klin Wochenschr. 2005;117(5–6):229–33.
131. Mateen FJ, Muralidharan R, Carone M, van de Beek D, Harrison DM, Aksamit AJ, et al. Progressive multifocal leukoencephalopathy in transplant recipients. Ann Neurol. 2011;70(2):305–22.
132. Loyaga-Rendon RY, Taylor DO, Koval CE. Progressive multifocal leukoencephalopathy in a heart transplant recipient following rituximab therapy for antibody-mediated rejection. Am J Transplant. 2013;13(4):1075–9.
133. Gupta MR, Valentine VG, Walker JE Jr, Lombard GA, LaPlace SG, Seoane L, et al. Clinical spectrum of gram-positive infections in lung transplantation. Transpl Infect Dis. 2009;11(5):424–31.

134. Zeglen S, Wojarski J, Wozniak-Grygiel E, Siola M, Jastrzebski D, Kucewicz-Czech E, et al. Frequency of Pseudomonas aeruginosa colonizations/infections in lung transplant recipients. Transplant Proc. 2009;41(8):3222–4.
135. Knoll BM, Kappagoda S, Gill RR, Goldberg HJ, Boyle K, Baden LR, et al. Non-tuberculous mycobacterial infection among lung transplant recipients: a 15-year cohort study. Transpl Infect Dis. 2012;14(5):452–60.
136. Husain S, McCurry K, Dauber J, Singh N, Kusne S. Nocardia infection in lung transplant recipients. J Heart Lung Transplant. 2002;21(3):354–9.
137. Poonyagariyagorn HK, Gershman A, Avery R, Minai O, Blazey H, Asamoto K, et al. Challenges in the diagnosis and management of Nocardia infections in lung transplant recipients. Transpl Infect Dis. 2008;10(6):403–8.
138. Sole A, Salavert M. Fungal infections after lung transplantation. Curr Opin Pulm Med. 2009;15(3):243–53.
139. Palmer SM, Alexander BD, Sanders LL, Edwards LJ, Reller LB, Davis RD, et al. Significance of blood stream infection after lung transplantation: analysis in 176 consecutive patients. Transplantation. 2000;69(11):2360–6.
140. Singh N, Husain S. Aspergillus infections after lung transplantation: clinical differences in type of transplant and implications for management. J Heart Lung Transplant. 2003;22(3):258–66.
141. Minari A, Husni R, Avery RK, Longworth DL, DeCamp M, Bertin M, et al. The incidence of invasive aspergillosis among solid organ transplant recipients and implications for prophylaxis in lung transplants. Transpl Infect Dis. 2002;4(4):195–200.
142. Singh N, Suarez JF, Avery R, Lass-Florl C, Geltner C, Pasqualotto AC, et al. Risk factors and outcomes in lung transplant recipients with nodular invasive pulmonary aspergillosis. J Inf Secur. 2013;67(1):72–8.
143. Singh N, Suarez JF, Avery R, Lass-Florl C, Geltner C, Pasqualotto AC, et al. Immune reconstitution syndrome-like entity in lung transplant recipients with invasive aspergillosis. Transpl Immunol. 2013;29(1–4):109–13.
144. Hadjiliadis D, Howell DN, Davis RD, Lawrence CM, Rea JB, Tapson VF, et al. Anastomotic infections in lung transplant recipients. Ann Transplant. 2000;5(3):13–9.
145. Walsh TJ, Anaissie EJ, Denning DW, Herbrecht R, Kontoyiannis DP, Marr KA, et al. Treatment of aspergillosis: clinical practice guidelines of the Infectious Diseases Society of America. Clin Infect Dis. 2008;46(3):327–60.
146. Rakvit A, Meyerrose G, Vidal AM, Kimbrough RC, Sarria JC. Cellulitis caused by *Cryptococcus neoformans* in a lung transplant recipient. J Heart Lung Transplant. 2005;24(5):642.
147. Singh N, Lortholary O, Alexander BD, Gupta KL, John GT, Pursell K, et al. An immune reconstitution syndrome-like illness associated with *Cryptococcus neoformans* infection in organ transplant recipients. Clin Infect Dis. 2005;40(12):1756–61.
148. Fishman JA, Emery V, Freeman R, Pascual M, Rostaing L, Schlitt HJ, et al. Cytomegalovirus in transplantation – challenging the status quo. Clin Transplant. 2007;21(2):149–58.
149. Zamora MR. Cytomegalovirus and lung transplantation. Am J Transplant. 2004;4(8):1219–26.
150. Mitsani D, Nguyen MH, Girnita DM, Spichty K, Kwak EJ, Silveira FP, et al. A polymorphism linked to elevated levels of interferon-gamma is associated with an increased risk of cytomegalovirus disease among Caucasian lung transplant recipients at a single center. J Heart Lung Transplant. 2011;30(5):523–9.
151. Paraskeva M, Bailey M, Levvey BJ, Griffiths AP, Kotsimbos TC, Williams TP, et al. Cytomegalovirus replication within the lung allograft is associated with bronchiolitis obliterans syndrome. Am J Transplant. 2011;11(10):2190–6.
152. Minces LR, Nguyen MH, Mitsani D, Shields RK, Kwak EJ, Silveira FP, et al. Ganciclovir-resistant cytomegalovirus (CMV) infections among lung transplant recipients are associated with poor outcomes despite treatment with foscarnet-containing regimens. Antimicrob Agents Chemother. 2014;58(1):128–35.
153. Shalhoub S, Husain S. Community-acquired respiratory viral infections in lung transplant recipients. Curr Opin Infect Dis. 2013;26(4):302–8.
154. Bridevaux PO, Aubert JD, Soccal PM, Mazza-Stalder J, Berutto C, Rochat T, et al. Incidence and outcomes of respiratory viral infections in lung transplant recipients: a prospective study. Thorax. 2014;69(1):32–8.
155. Shah PD, McDyer JF. Viral infections in lung transplant recipients. Semin Respir Crit Care Med. 2010;31(2):243–54.
156. Fiore AE, Fry A, Shay D, Gubareva L, Bresee JS, Uyeki TM. Antiviral agents for the treatment and chemoprophylaxis of influenza – recommendations of the Advisory Committee on Immunization Practices (ACIP). MMWR Recomm Rep. 2011;60(1):1–24.
157. Clark NM, Lynch JP 3rd, Sayah D, Belperio JA, Fishbein MC, Weigt SS. DNA viral infections complicating lung transplantation. Semin Respir Crit Care Med. 2013;34(3):380–404.
158. Thomas LD, Milstone AP, Vilchez RA, Zanwar P, Butel JS, Dummer JS. Polyomavirus infection and its impact on renal function and long-term outcomes after lung transplantation. Transplantation. 2009;88(3):360–6.
159. Muchtar E, Kramer MR, Vidal L, Ram R, Gurion R, Rosenblat Y, et al. Posttransplantation lymphoproliferative disorder in lung transplant recipients: a 15-year single institution experience. Transplantation. 2013;96(7):657–63.
160. Vijayan VK. Parasitic lung infections. Curr Opin Pulm Med. 2009;15(3):274–82.
161. Balagopal A, Mills L, Shah A, Subramanian A. Detection and treatment of Strongyloides hyperinfection syndrome following lung transplantation. Transpl Infect Dis. 2009;11(2):149–54.
162. Walia R, Montoya JG, Visvesvera GS, Booton GC, Doyle RL. A case of successful treatment of cutaneous Acanthamoeba infection in a lung transplant recipient. Transpl Infect Dis. 2007;9(1):51–4.
163. Duarte AG, Sattar F, Granwehr B, Aronson JF, Wang Z, Lick S. Disseminated acanthamoebiasis after lung transplantation. J Heart Lung Transplant. 2006;25(2):237–40.
164. Bonatti H, Barroso LF 2nd, Sawyer RG, Kotton CN, Sifri CD. Cryptosporidium enteritis in solid organ transplant recipients: multicenter retrospective evaluation of 10 cases reveals an association with elevated tacrolimus concentrations. Transpl Infect Dis. 2012;14(6):635–48.
165. Field AS, Paik JY, Stark D, Qiu MR, Morey A, Plit ML, et al. Myositis due to the microsporidian Anncaliia (Brachiola) algerae in a lung transplant recipient. Transpl Infect Dis. 2012;14(2):169–76.
166. Levine DJ, Riley DJ, Jorgensen JH, McClain WD, Tio F, Visvesvara GS, et al. Key diagnostic features of granulomatous interstitial nephritis due to Encephalitozoon cuniculi in a lung transplant recipient. Am J Surg Pathol. 2013;37(3):447–52.
167. Shields RK, Clancy CJ, Minces LR, Shigemura N, Kwak EJ, Silveira FP, et al. Epidemiology and outcomes of deep surgical site infections following lung transplantation. Am J Transplant. 2013;13(8):2137–45.
168. Lodge BA, Ashley ED, Steele MP, Perfect JR. Aspergillus fumigatus empyema, arthritis, and calcaneal osteomyelitis in a lung transplant patient successfully treated with posaconazole. J Clin Microbiol. 2004;42(3):1376–8.
169. Danziger-Isakov LA, Sweet S, Delamorena M, Huddleston CB, Mendeloff E, Debaun MR. Epidemiology of bloodstream infections in the first year after pediatric lung transplantation. Pediatr Infect Dis J. 2005;24(4):324–30.

170. Candel FJ, Grima E, Matesanz M, Cervera C, Soto G, Almela M, et al. Bacteremia and septic shock after solid-organ transplantation. Transplant Proc. 2005;37(9):4097–9.
171. Lazaro M, Ramos A, Ussetti P, Asensio A, Laporta R, Munez E, et al. Aspergillus endocarditis in lung transplant recipients: case report and literature review. Transpl Infect Dis. 2011;13(2):186–91.
172. Nunley DR, Grgurich WF, Keenan RJ, Dauber JH. Empyema complicating successful lung transplantation. Chest. 1999;115(5):1312–5.
173. Fairhurst RM, Kubak BM, Shpiner RB, Levine MS, Pegues DA, Ardehali A. Mycobacterium abscessus empyema in a lung transplant recipient. J Heart Lung Transplant. 2002;21(3):391–4.
174. Sayah DM, Schwartz BS, Kukreja J, Singer JP, Golden JA, Leard LE. Scedosporium prolificans pericarditis and mycotic aortic aneurysm in a lung transplant recipient receiving voriconazole prophylaxis. Transpl Infect Dis. 2013;15(2):E70–4.
175. Mitsani D, Nguyen MH, Silveira FP, Bermudez C, Toyoda Y, Pasculle AW, et al. Mycoplasma hominis pericarditis in a lung transplant recipient: review of the literature about an uncommon but important cardiothoracic pathogen. Transpl Infect Dis. 2010;12(2):146–50.
176. Campos S, Caramori M, Teixeira R, Afonso J Jr, Carraro R, Strabelli T, et al. Bacterial and fungal pneumonias after lung transplantation. Transplant Proc. 2008;40(3):822–4.
177. Bhaskaran A, Hosseini-Moghaddam SM, Rotstein C, Husain S. Mold infections in lung transplant recipients. Semin Respir Crit Care Med. 2013;34(3):371–9.
178. Bangsborg JM, Uldum S, Jensen JS, Bruun BG. Nosocomial legionellosis in three heart-lung transplant patients: case reports and environmental observations. Eur J Clin Microbiol Infect Dis. 1995;14(2):99–104.
179. Glanville AR, Gencay M, Tamm M, Chhajed P, Plit M, Hopkins P, et al. Chlamydia pneumoniae infection after lung transplantation. J Heart Lung Transplant. 2005;24(2):131–6.
180. Miller CB, Malaisrie SC, Patel J, Garrity E, Vigneswaran WT, Gamelli RL. Intraabdominal complications after lung transplantation. J Am Coll Surg. 2006;203(5):653–60.
181. Tai CC, Curtis JL, Szmuszkovicz JR, Horn MV, Ford HR, Woo MS, et al. Abdominal involvement in pediatric heart and lung transplant recipients with posttransplant lymphoproliferative disease increases the risk of mortality. J Pediatr Surg. 2008;43(12):2174–7.
182. Bravo C, Gispert P, Borro JM, de la Torre M, Cifrian Martinez JM, Fernandez Rozas S, et al. Prevalence and management of gastrointestinal complications in lung transplant patients: MITOS study group. Transplant Proc. 2007;39(7):2409–12.
183. Maurer JR. The spectrum of colonic complications in a lung transplant population. Ann Transplant. 2000;5(3):54–7.
184. Augustine SM, Yeo CJ, Buchman TG, Achuff SC, Baumgartner WA. Gastrointestinal complications in heart and in heart-lung transplant patients. J Heart Lung Transplant. 1991;10(4):547–55. discussion 55–6
185. Riezebos-Brilman A, Puchhammer-Stockl E, van der Weide HY, Haagsma EB, Jaksch P, Bejvl I, et al. Chronic hepatitis E infection in lung transplant recipients. J Heart Lung Transplant. 2013;32(3):341–6.
186. Maier T, Schwarting A, Mauer D, Ross RS, Martens A, Kliem V, et al. Management and outcomes after multiple corneal and solid organ transplantations from a donor infected with rabies virus. Clin Infect Dis. 2010;50(8):1112–9.
187. Hiemann NE, Grimmer S, Kemper D, Knosalla C, Hetzer R. Tuberculous meningitis in a lung transplanted patient. Transpl Infect Dis. 2012;14(4):E19–22.
188. Levi ME, Quan D, Ho JT, Kleinschmidt-Demasters BK, Tyler KL, Grazia TJ. Impact of rituximab-associated B-cell defects on West Nile virus meningoencephalitis in solid organ transplant recipients. Clin Transplant. 2010;24(2):223–8.
189. Sahi H, Avery RK, Minai OA, Hall G, Mehta AC, Raina P, et al. Scedosporium apiospermum (Pseudoallescheria boydii) infection in lung transplant recipients. J Heart Lung Transplant. 2007;26(4):350–6.
190. Henao-Martinez AF, Castillo-Mancilla JR, Barron MA, Nichol AC. Combination antifungal therapy in the treatment of Scedosporium apiospermum central nervous system infections. Case Rep Infect Dis. 2013;2013:589490.
191. Levin TP, Baty DE, Fekete T, Truant AL, Suh B. Cladophialophora bantiana brain abscess in a solid-organ transplant recipient: case report and review of the literature. J Clin Microbiol. 2004;42(9):4374–8.
192. Kleinschmidt-Demasters BK. Disseminated Fusarium infection with brain abscesses in a lung transplant recipient. Clin Neuropathol. 2009;28(6):417–21.
193. Hall WA, Martinez AJ, Dummer JS, Griffith BP, Hardesty RL, Bahnson HT, et al. Central nervous system infections in heart and heart-lung transplant recipients. Arch Neurol. 1989;46(2):173–7.

Infections in Liver Transplantation

3

B. Sharmila Mohanraj, Amol S. Rangnekar, and Joseph G. Timpone Jr.

Indications for Liver Transplantation

Orthotopic liver transplantation (LT) is most commonly offered to patients with end-stage liver disease. However, this lifesaving therapy can also be used to successfully treat patients with acute liver failure, primary and some metastatic liver tumors, and selected metabolic conditions (Table 3.1).

Decompensated cirrhosis is defined by the presence of specific complications including jaundice, hepatic encephalopathy, ascites, spontaneous bacterial peritonitis, hepatorenal syndrome, or variceal hemorrhage. Once a patient develops complications of portal hypertension, 5-year survival is <50%. Additionally, patients with cirrhosis may develop life-threatening pulmonary complications such as hepatopulmonary syndrome (HPS) or portopulmonary hypertension (PPH).

The Child-Turcotte-Pugh (CTP) score helps to stratify severity of illness according to a combination of five physiologic and laboratory variables: ascites, hepatic encephalopathy, bilirubin, albumin, and prothrombin time. Patients in CTP class B or C have less than a 60% 2-year survival and should be considered for OLT. The Model for End-Stage Liver Disease (MELD) score is a more simplified and objective method designed to characterize the degree of illness of patients with end-stage liver disease. The MELD score incorporates serum bilirubin, prothrombin time, and creatinine values [1]. Based on its ability to predict survival, the MELD score has been used to prioritize patients on the OLT wait list. It is generally accepted that patients with a MELD score greater than 10 should be referred for liver transplant evaluation, and those with a MELD score of 15 or higher are most likely to derive benefit from OLT [2]. Despite its simplicity, the MELD score does disadvantage a subset of patients who have severely decompensated liver disease but minimally abnormal laboratory results. Recently, serum sodium has been incorporated into the MELD score, i.e., MELD-Na. Hyponatremia is an independent predictor of mortality in patients with decompensated cirrhosis, and diminished serum sodium levels may be a surrogate marker of advanced portal hypertension [3, 4].

Table 3.1 Indications for liver transplantation

Indications
Decompensated hepatic cirrhosis
Biliary cirrhosis (primary biliary cholangitis, primary sclerosing cholangitis, biliary atresia, Alagille syndrome, cystic fibrosis, progressive familial intrahepatic cholestasis)
Hepatocellular carcinoma
Hepatoblastoma
Hemangioendothelioma
Metastatic neuroendocrine tumors
Glycogen storage disease
Neonatal hemochromatosis
Amyloidosis
Hyperoxaluria
Urea cycle defects
Disorders of branch chain amino acids
Acute liver failure
Budd-Chiari syndrome
Polycystic liver disease

Acute liver failure (ALF) is a rare but life-threatening condition, which is manifested by evidence of hepatic injury, coagulopathy, encephalopathy, and absence of underlying cirrhosis in most patients. In Western countries, nearly half of all cases are attributed to acetaminophen overdose. Other less common etiologies include drug injury, viral hepatitis, autoimmune hepatitis, and fulminant Wilson disease. Mortality exceeds 30% with death often occurring within 1 week of presentation. Although a majority of patients with ALF due to acetaminophen toxicity may recover spontaneously, those with ALF due to other etiologies often require OLT to survive [5, 6].

B. S. Mohanraj · J. G. Timpone Jr. (✉)
MedStar Georgetown University Hospital, Division of Infectious Diseases and Travel Medicine, Washington, DC, USA
e-mail: bernardine.r.s.mohanraj@gunet.georgetown.edu; timponej@gunet.georgetown.edu

A. S. Rangnekar
MedStar Georgetown University Hospital, MedStar Georgetown Transplant Institute, Washington, DC, USA
e-mail: amol.s.rangnekar@gunet.georgetown.edu

A. Safdar (ed.), *Principles and Practice of Transplant Infectious Diseases*, https://doi.org/10.1007/978-1-4939-9034-4_3

Certain patients with liver-based metabolic conditions and systemic complications may also benefit from OLT. Examples of these conditions include familial amyloidosis, glycogen storage disease, and primary hyperoxaluria. Although underlying liver synthetic function is preserved, hepatic allograft transplant allows for correction of a specific metabolic deficit in these patients.

As the incidence of hepatocellular carcinoma (HCC) continues to rise, patients with this disease now represent a substantial proportion of liver transplant recipients. Patients with cirrhosis and portal hypertension are unlikely to tolerate hepatic resection of their HCC and are offered OLT in order to improve their recurrence-free survival. Typically, patients with tumor burden within the Milan criteria are considered good candidates for OLT and are typically awarded MELD exception points [7]. More liberal tumor burden criteria have been proposed for transplant, although larger tumor size and number seem to correlate with a higher risk of recurrence [8].

Most patients with cholangiocarcinoma have traditionally not been candidates for liver transplants due to high post-transplant recurrence rates and poor survival. However, recent data suggest that carefully selected patients with isolated unresectable hilar tumors who are treated with neoadjuvant chemotherapy and radiation therapy may have acceptable survival rates after transplant [9]. In general, patients with known intrahepatic cholangiocarcinoma may be candidates for resection but are not typically considered for OLT.

In the USA, patients are prioritized for liver transplantation on the basis of the MELD score. In selected cases, patients with specific complications of liver disease may be eligible for MELD exception scores. MELD exception scores may be standardized, as is the case presently in patients with HCC within Milan criteria, certain pulmonary complications of cirrhosis, and selected metabolic disorders. In specific cases, some patients may be granted MELD exception on an individual basis by the regional review board after taking into account extenuating circumstances.

Contraindications to Liver Transplant

Life-threatening conditions such as severe cardiopulmonary disease or sepsis are generally major contraindications to OLT. Although patients with human immunodeficiency virus (HIV) infection can successfully undergo transplant, those with AIDS are thought to be poor candidates based on their poor health and the risk of additional post-transplant immune suppression. Patients actively using drugs or alcohol are often excluded as well. Many transplant centers have traditionally required abstinence from alcohol for a minimum of 6 months prior to listing, although this requirement has been evolving recently after a significant post-transplant survival benefit was demonstrated in selected patients with severe alcoholic hepatitis [10]. Patients with extrahepatic malignancy, metastatic HCC, or intrahepatic cholangiocarcinoma should not undergo transplant. Patients may also be denied liver transplant on the basis of certain psychosocial factors such as persistent noncompliance with medical care or lack of adequate social support. Relative contraindications to liver transplantation include advanced age, severe obesity, prior abdominal surgeries, and significant mesenteric vascular thromboses.

Pre-transplant infectious disease work-up includes serologic testing to diagnose infectious causes of acute or chronic liver disease such as hepatitis A virus (HAV), hepatitis B virus (HBV), and hepatitis C virus (HCV) and to identify latent infections, which may reactivate in the setting of post-transplant immunosuppression. These include cytomegalovirus (CMV), Epstein-Barr virus (EBV), varicella zoster virus (VZV), rapid plasma regain test for syphilis, and interferon gamma release assay or tuberculin skin test for latent tuberculosis. All patients are screened for HIV. Selected high-risk individuals may undergo testing for coccidioidomycosis, *Trypanosoma cruzi*, or *Strongyloides stercoralis*, depending upon geographic location, travel history, and/or history of exposure to various endemic infections. Pre-transplant dental evaluation is typically mandatory in order to identify and manage potential oral sources of infection after undergoing transplantation. Dental extractions, if warranted, should occur prior to liver transplantation. Immunizations for HAV, HBV, pneumococcus, influenza, diphtheria, tetanus, and pertussis should be administered to appropriate transplant candidates at the time of the pre-transplant evaluation. As there is a contraindication to live vaccines after transplantation, immunization status for measles, mumps, and rubella (MMR) and varicella should also be obtained. The American Association for the Study of Liver Diseases (AASLD) has published online guidelines in 2013 for the evaluation of potential liver transplant recipients which can be found at https://www.aasld.org/publications/practice-guidelines-0.

Based on reasonable short- and long-term outcomes, patients with HIV infection can successfully undergo OLT. Typically, these patients should have well-controlled disease on antiretroviral therapy, with undetectable HIV RNA and absence of active AIDS-associated opportunistic infections or malignancies. CD4+ counts >100 may be a reasonable cutoff in patients with leukopenia due to portal hypertension and splenic sequestration. Other contraindications to liver transplantation may include a history of AIDS-defining opportunistic infection that requires chronic secondary prophylaxis or has limited treatment options such as progressive multifocal leukoencephalopathy (PML), disseminated *Mycobacterium avium* complex, chronic cryptosporidiosis,

EBV and human herpesvirus-8-related lymphoproliferative disorders such as non-Hodgkin's lymphoma and visceral Kaposi's sarcoma (KS), or significant cervical or anal neoplastic disease due to human papillomavirus. Some centers have performed transplants in patients with cutaneous KS. Although recurrence of the malignancy can occur after undergoing transplant surgery, these patients may be managed with mechanistic target of rapamycin (mTOR) inhibitor-based immunosuppressive regimens after OLT based on the antineoplastic effects of these agents.

Several factors may increase the risk for graft loss in HIV+ patients undergoing liver transplants including older donor age, HCV-positive donors, low recipient BMI, and simultaneous liver and kidney transplantation [11]. Of note, these outcomes and predictors of graft loss were identified in older studies of HIV- and HCV-coinfected patients undergoing transplant. Additional studies are needed to determine outcomes in an era of improved HCV therapy and specifically in non-coinfected patients requiring transplant.

Types of Liver Transplantation

The majority of liver transplants in the Western world utilize whole organ allografts from deceased donors. However, alternative options such as split deceased donor grafts or partial living donor grafts are used occasionally. In the USA, living donor liver transplantation (LDLT) currently accounts for less than 5% of all liver transplants, although in other parts of the world, LDLT is utilized more frequently.

Most deceased donors are considered on the basis of donation after brain death (DBD). Occasionally donation after circulatory death (DCD) can be considered. DCD donors are characterized by the absence of systemic circulation along with irreversible apnea and unresponsiveness. The main risk associated with DCD is organ ischemia and the potential for biliary epithelial injury. Initial results of the experience with DCD OLT were marked by increased rates of ischemic cholangiopathy, a condition which can lead to recurrent cholangitis, graft loss requiring retransplantation, or death [12, 13]. However, some centers have reported similar patient and graft survival with DCD and DBD donors, particularly with the use of donors less than 40 years old, and minimization of cold and warm ischemia times [14, 15].

LDLT offers the advantage of allowing for expedited access to transplantation at a time before the recipient develops advanced liver failure while simultaneously increasing the donor pool. However, these benefits must be balanced against the potential risks of morbidity and death for the donor.

In order to be considered for LDLT in the USA, patients must already be listed for deceased donor liver transplantation (DDLT). Selected recipients with low MELD score and significant hepatic decompensation, HCC, or other complications of advanced liver disease such as primary sclerosing cholangitis with recurrent episodes of ascending cholangitis or polycystic liver disease are typically good candidates for LDLT. Conversely, patients with higher MELD scores and severe hepatic decompensation usually have limited survival and a shorter anticipated waiting time for transplant. As compared to patient undergoing DDLT, LDLT recipients may have a significantly higher rate of complications and need for retransplantation, although adjusted long-term survival appears to be similar [16, 17]. As such, careful recipient selection is critical. Contraindications to LDLT may include significant mesenteric vascular thrombosis, severe portal hypertension, need for simultaneous renal transplantation, or retransplantation. An additional consideration is matching donor and recipient body size. Specifically, a graft weight-to-body weight ratio of 0.8% is recommended to avoid the development of small-for-size syndrome, a condition marked by the development of hyperbilirubinemia, intractable ascites, coagulopathy, renal failure, and extended duration of hepatic encephalopathy. Biliary complications tend to occur with higher frequency in LDLT recipients, although rates are lower in centers with higher volume living donor, partial hepatic graft transplantation [18].

Deceased donor livers may also be split to maximize yield for recipients. As with LDLT, adequate graft weight for the recipient must be determined prior to transplant. Most commonly deceased donor livers are split so as to offer the left lateral segment to a pediatric recipient and the remaining allograft to an adult recipient.

Donor Selection

In the USA, the majority of liver donation occurs after brain death. The criteria to determine initial DBD donor eligibility include complete apnea, brainstem areflexia, cerebral unresponsiveness, and evidence of irreversible and permanent loss of central nervous system function [19, 20]. The diagnosis can often be determined based on clinical examination and noninvasive testing such as electroencephalography, evoked cerebral potentials, and transcranial Doppler ultrasonography [21, 22].

Absolute contraindications to organ donation include most extrahepatic malignancies and transmissible infections associated with high risk of mortality. Specifically, donors with active extracranial or hematologic malignancies are not considered suitable for organ donation. However, patients with primary brain tumors without extracranial metastases may be considered as donors for transplant. Donors with fungemia, mycobacterial disease, disseminated resistant bacterial infections, and prion disease are typically excluded from donation.

Once a donor is considered suitable based on these preliminary criteria, additional information is required. Initial donor-recipient matching is determined based primarily on blood type and graft size, although multiple other factors are evaluated prior to transplantation. An ideal donor would meet the following criteria: age less than 50 years, hemodynamic stability, absence of significant chronic disease, systemic infection, malignancy, or abdominal trauma.

However, since only a limited number of donors meet these parameters, transplant providers have liberalized exclusion criteria in an effort to increase the donor pool. Extended criteria donor grafts refer to those from donors with older age, higher degree of hepatic steatosis, history of malignancy, active viral or bacterial infection, or history of trauma. Traditionally, older donor age was considered a risk factor for graft failure, primarily based on increased risk for chronic vascular disease, significant comorbidities, and potentially more hepatic steatosis in elderly donors. However, more recent experiences suggest that donor age alone may not be a predictor of graft outcome. In fact, older donors even greater than 80 years old may be used with reasonable success if other donor risk factors such as hepatic steatosis and cold ischemia time can be minimized [23–25]. The use of older donors in recipients with HCV infection has traditionally correlated with increased graft loss. This finding may become less relevant in the modern era of improved HCV direct antiviral therapy, as HCV infection can be successfully eradicated in the majority of HCV-seropositive recipients either before or soon after liver transplantation.

Hepatic steatosis can be quantified by biopsy of the donor liver. Grafts with mild macrovesicular steatosis (<30%) are routinely used with good graft outcomes. In contrast, severe macrovesicular steatosis (>60%) within the donor graft increases the risk of primary nonfunction and is usually a contraindication for use of the organ [26, 27]. The donor risk index (DRI) predicts liver graft failure based on specific donor characteristics and transplant factors including age, race, height, cause of death, partial or split organ, DCD status, cold ischemia time, and sharing outside of a local donor service area [28].

All organ donors undergo nucleic acid testing (NAT) to rule out specific transmissible viral infections such as HIV, HBV, or HCV. In general there is a finite, albeit low, risk of viral transmission from the average donor. A study of organ procurement organizations in the USA has reported HIV and HCV prevalence rates of 0.1% and 3.5%, respectively, in donors with normal risk. Among high-risk donors, the prevalence of HIV and HCV was higher (0.5% and 18%, respectively). A model based on these known prevalence numbers estimates the incidence of undetected viremia as being 1 in 60,000 for HIV and 1 in 5000 for HCV in normal-risk donors. Among high-risk donors, the incidence may rise to 1 in 12,000 for HIV and 1 in 1000 for HCV [29].

The US Public Health Service (PHS) has developed specific criteria to classify donors as being at increased risk for recent HIV, HBV, or HCV infection [30]. These criteria include factors such as high-risk sexual behaviors and prior injection drug use. The specific PHS criteria for high-risk donors established in 2013 include:

1. High-risk sexual behavior within the preceding 12 months (people who have had sex with a person known or suspected to have HIV, HBV, or HCV infections, men who had sex with men [MSM], women who have had sex with an MSM, people who have had sex in exchange for money or drugs, people who have had sex with a person who had sex in exchange for money or drugs, people who have had sex with a person that has injected drugs by intravenous, intramuscular, or subcutaneous route for nonmedical reasons)
2. High-risk children (a child who is ≤18 months of age and born to a mother known to be infected with or at increased risk for HIV, HBV, or HCV infections, a child who has been breastfed within the preceding 12 months and a mother known to be infected with, or at increased risk for, HIV infection)
3. People who have injected drugs by intravenous, intramuscular, or subcutaneous route for nonmedical reasons in the preceding 12 months
4. People who have been in lockup, jail, prison, or a juvenile correctional facility for more than 72 h in the preceding 12 months
5. People who have been newly diagnosed with or have been treated for syphilis, gonorrhea, chlamydia, or genital ulcers in the preceding 12 months
6. People who have been on hemodialysis in the preceding 12 months (increased risk for recent HCV infection only) [30]

Recipients of organs from PHS high-risk donors typically receive separate counseling about the potentially increased risk of viral transmission. All transplant recipients undergo pre-transplant testing for HIV, HBV, and HCV. Post-transplant serologic surveillance within the first year after transplant is recommended to exclude new infections in recipients of organs from PHS high-risk donors.

While patients with positive hepatitis B surface antigen are excluded from donation, selected patients with isolated positive hepatitis B core antibody (HBcAb+) may be considered as suitable donors. Initial evaluation requires excluding underlying hepatic fibrosis in case the donor had prior hepatitis B infection. If the graft is found to be suitable for donation, there is still a risk of viral transmission to the recipient. Risk of HBV infection in the recipient depends largely on whether the recipient has immunity against HBV. Specifically, although infection rates are low in hepatitis B surface antibody (HBsAb) positive/HBcAb+ recipients, they may be as high as 76% in recipients with both negative HBsAb and HBcAb [31]. As such, the recipient of a liver allograft from a HBcAb+ donor will usually receive oral antiviral medication with or without hepatitis B immune globulin (HBIG) for prophylaxis. The use of lamivudine for prophylaxis has reduced the risk of infection to less than 4%, and the use of newer agents such as tenofovir and entecavir with lower rates of resistance may result in even lower infection rates among OLT recipients from isolated HBcAb+ donors. The addition of HBIG to oral antiviral agents may not provide additional benefit in this setting [32].

HCV-seropositive (+) donor livers are used in HCV-seropositive recipients. Assuming the absence of significant hepatic fibrosis in the donor liver, the use of HCV+ donors for HCV+ recipients can be considered and does not appear to affect patient survival, graft survival, or severity of HCV recurrence following transplantation [33].

Experience with HIV-seropositive (+) donors in organ transplantation is limited at this time. In 2013, the USA enacted the HIV Organ Policy Equity Act which allowed for the transplantation of HIV+ organs into HIV+ recipients. Initial reports of liver transplantation with HIV+ donors suggest good short-term outcomes.

Surgical Approaches to Liver Transplantation

The abdomen is typically opened with a bilateral subcostal incision with midline extension. To begin the recipient hepatectomy, the falciform and gastrohepatic ligaments are divided. The liver can then be lifted to expose the porta hepatis. Subsequently the hepatic artery, bile duct, and portal vein are sequentially divided. The patient is often placed on veno-venous bypass during this time. The suprahepatic and infrahepatic vena cava are clamped, and the recipient's liver is removed en bloc with the excluded portion of the vena cava. The gallbladder is removed along with the liver. Back-table preparation of the allograft typically occurs during the recipient hepatectomy. The allograft is then placed into the recipient, and the vena cava and portal venous anastomoses are created. The allograft is reperfused, and systemic bypass is discontinued. After reperfusion of the allograft, the arterial and biliary anastomoses are completed.

In certain cases, variant anatomy may require alteration in the creation of vascular or biliary anastomoses. An arterial conduit can be used if the recipient hepatic artery is insufficient. Roux-en-Y hepaticojejunostomy is considered in select cases such as when the recipient common duct is diminutive or large biliary collateral veins are present. Patients with primary sclerosing cholangitis typically require Roux-en-Y hepaticojejunostomy. In the past, T tubes were used in the case of donor-recipient duct size mismatch. However, their use has declined significantly in recent years due to the risk of complications including bile leak. Many centers will now consider closing a portion of the larger duct with suture prior to creating the biliary anastomosis.

An alternative to vena cava exclusion is the piggyback technique. In this situation, the hepatic artery, common duct, and portal vein are divided in the typical fashion. However, instead of clamping the vena cava and removing the liver en bloc with the vena cava, the surgeon instead dissects the liver surface off of the vena cava. The hepatic veins are clamped and divided, and the recipient liver is removed without disrupting the recipient vena cava. Longitudinal incisions are made in the recipient and donor vena cavas to allow for creation of a cavo-caval anastomosis. Potential benefits of the piggyback technique include decreased warm ischemia time, reduced blood transfusions requirements, and less need for veno-venous bypass. Piggyback reconstruction may increase the risk of developing hepatic venous outflow obstruction and subsequent Budd-Chiari syndrome.

Surgical Complications Resulting in Infection

Multiple surgical complications after LT may predispose to the development of infection. Hepatic artery thrombosis (HAT) is the most common vascular complication after OLT, with a 4% incidence reported in adult recipients [34]. HAT can be classified as early or late occurring before or after 4 weeks following transplantation. Early HAT may present in three distinct ways. The most severe presentation is fulminant hepatic failure, which is marked by acute rise in liver enzymes, encephalopathy, coagulopathy, and often sepsis. Other patients with HAT can present subacutely with ischemic injury to the bile ducts which predominantly rely on perfusion by the hepatic artery. These patients will subsequently develop biliary complications including strictures, acute cholangitis, hepatic abscesses, or recurrent episodes of bacteremia. A final group of patients with HAT may be asymptomatic and diagnosed incidentally.

HAT can be identified on Doppler ultrasound, although either radiographic or conventional angiography is often required to confirm the diagnosis. Patients with HAT and fulminant hepatic failure require management of sepsis including broad-spectrum antibiotics and prompt retransplantation. Less symptomatic patients can be taken to the operating room for hepatic artery revision and possible thrombectomy or managed non-operatively with catheter-directed thrombolysis. Patients who present with biliary complications of late HAT typically will develop a progressive course marked by recurrent cholangitis and other complications of biliary obstruction. In the short term, they can be managed with endoscopic or percutaneous biliary drainage and antibiotics during episodes of acute cholangitis. However, many of these patients will ultimately require retransplantation.

Biliary complications occur frequently with an average incidence of up to 25% reported in some series. Many types of complications may occur including anastomotic and non-anastomotic biliary strictures, bile leak, biliary abscess, obstruction due to stones or casts, or acute cholangitis. The majority of biliary complications occur in the first 3 months after transplant, although biliary strictures may present several years post-LT. Approximately 80% of biliary strictures are at the site of anastomosis, but later presentations of non-anastomotic strictures may occur as a consequence of DCD organ use, older donor age, technical factors at the time of arterial anastomosis, HAT, hepatic artery stenosis, prolonged cold ischemia time, CMV infection, ABO blood group mismatch, or recurrent primary sclerosing cholangitis [35–37]. LDLT and split liver recipients are at increased risk for biliary complications as compared to DDLT recipients due to the cut surface of the liver and potentially more delicate biliary anastomoses. Most biliary structures are managed with endoscopic retrograde cholangiopancreatography (ERCP) or percutaneous biliary drainage. In patients with persistent anastomotic strictures despite repeated endoscopic therapy, surgical revision may be considered.

Intra-abdominal hemorrhage can occur in the early post-transplant period with a reported prevalence as high as 20%. Preexisting coagulopathy and diminished hepatic synthetic function are associated with a higher risk of bleeding. Initial management is typically supportive, but reoperation may be required in up to 15% of cases if bleeding persists. However, a source of hemorrhage may be identified in only half of such cases [38].

Immunosuppressive Regimens in Liver Transplantation

The alloimmune response after LT is primarily T-cell mediated. The role of donor-specific antibodies and the concept of antibody-mediated rejection require further study but generally appear to be rare. Currently, induction immunosuppression with T-cell-depleting agents, such as thymoglobulin, is not used routinely after OLT. On Day 1, liver transplant recipients receive 500–1000 mg of methylprednisolone followed by a taper and conversion to prednisone. Initially, recipients are maintained on a multidrug regimen including a calcineurin inhibitor (CNI) such as tacrolimus, an antimetabolite agent such as mycophenolate, and corticosteroids.

CNIs serve as the backbone of immunosuppression regimens for most patients after liver transplantation. Most centers use tacrolimus as the preferred CNI. Direct comparisons between tacrolimus and cyclosporine after OLT have revealed lower rates of acute rejection and improved patient and graft survival with the use of tacrolimus [39–41]. CNIs are associated with nephrotoxicity, neurotoxicity, hypertension, and hyperlipidemia. Alopecia and hyperglycemia are more often seen with tacrolimus use, while hirsutism and gingival hyperplasia are more commonly associated with cyclosporine. Patients with acute liver failure and decompensated cirrhosis with severe hepatic encephalopathy may be more prone to neurotoxicity from these agents. As such, introduction of the CNI may be delayed until the patient is awake. CNIs are metabolized by the cytochrome p450 system; therefore, their serum concentration may be affected by several other commonly used medications. CNI levels and drug exposure will decrease with concurrent use of certain antiepileptic medications, rifampin, alcohol, and St. John wort. In contrast, CNI levels and drug exposure will increase with the use of macrolide antibiotics, azole and triazole-based antifungals, verapamil, and grapefruit juice.

In selected patients, mTOR inhibitors such as sirolimus or everolimus may also be used, often to minimize potential toxicities from a CNI-based regimen. Everolimus is FDA approved for use with a low-dose CNI in patients after liver transplantation, while sirolimus is not approved by FDA for use in patients undergoing liver transplants, and occasionally used off-label in select patients. The use of mTOR inhibitors within the first 30 days after liver transplant is discouraged due to the risk of hepatic artery thrombosis and impaired wound healing. Some studies suggest that early initiation of mTOR inhibitors within 90 days of OLT may lead to increased preservation of renal function [42–44]. The recommendation for concurrent use of a low-dose CNI is based on a higher risk of acute rejection for patients on mTOR monotherapy. Additionally, mTOR inhibitors do exhibit some anti-neoplastic activity and have been shown to reduce the risk of recurrent cutaneous squamous cell carcinoma after renal transplantation [45]. It is not clear that mTOR inhibitors improve long-term post-transplant recurrence risk in regard to HCC [46, 47]. Besides the risk of hepatic artery thrombosis and impaired wound healing, other common adverse effects associated with mTOR inhibitors include oral ulcers, edema, proteinuria, hyperlipidemia, and bone marrow suppression.

Mycophenolate, an antimetabolite agent, is commonly used in conjunction with a CNI in patients after liver transplantation and allows for more rapid discontinuation of corticosteroids. In many patients, mycophenolate is withdrawn within the first year after transplant; however, prolonged use may be indicated in order to minimize adverse effects of CNIs, such as nephrotoxicity [48]. Additionally, some centers maintain patients transplanted for autoimmune liver diseases on mycophenolate for a longer duration given the increased risk of acute rejection or recurrent autoimmune disease after OLT. The use of mycophenolate in pregnancy is contraindicated based on an increased risk of pregnancy loss and congenital malformations. Azathioprine may be a substitute for mycophenolate at some centers.

Glucocorticoids, usually prednisone, have multiple inhibitory effects on hosts' immune responses mediated by both innate and adaptive T and B cells. Due to their numerous side effects, most centers attempt to rapidly taper and wean patients off prednisone as soon as possible, often within the first 6 months after transplantation. Long-term low-dose prednisone has been utilized in patients with pre-transplant autoimmune liver disease. Since steroids increase HCV replication, abrupt changes in steroids, such as rapid withdrawal or bolus dosing for rejection, may be associated with worse outcomes [49].

Humanized monoclonal antibodies against the IL-2 receptor can be used in order to delay initiation of a CNI, particularly to avoid the immediate risk of nephrotoxicity or neurotoxicity. The use of daclizumab has demonstrated low rejection rates and improved renal function without an increase in CMV or other infections [50]. In 2009, daclizumab was removed from the market for commercial reasons. Basiliximab is commercially available and occasionally used clinically, although published data regarding the use of this immune modulator in liver transplant recipients are limited.

Management of Rejection in Liver Transplantation

Acute cellular rejection (ACR) occurs in up to 25% of OLT recipients, with the majority of cases occurring within the first month after transplant [51]. Antibody-mediated rejection is thought to be an uncommon phenomenon in this solid organ allograft transplant population. The risk of ACR after 1-year post-transplant declines to 10% and is potentially associated with poor compliance with antirejection medication. Early ACR does not seem to affect graft survival, but late ACR has been associated with an increased risk of developing chronic rejection and graft loss [52]. In many cases, the initial suspicion for ACR arises when elevated liver enzymes are discovered. Symptoms including fever or jaundice are less common, particularly if ACR is identified early. Liver biopsy is required to make the diagnosis of ACR, which is defined by a triad of mixed cell portal inflammation, endotheliitis, and ductulitis [53]. The majority of cases of ACR can be managed with corticosteroid therapy. Typically a high dose of methylprednisolone 500–1000 mg daily is given intravenously for 1–3 days with a subsequent taper. Patients with refractory ACR can be managed with either a second course of steroids or less often thymoglobulin. Thymoglobulin, a polyclonal antibody preparation directed against lymphocytes, is administered intravenously for up to 5 days with careful monitoring of white blood cell and platelet counts. All patients generally receive oral antimicrobial prophylaxis for CMV and *Pneumocystis jirovecii* when treated for ACR.

Chronic rejection (CR) occurs in less than 5% of OLT recipients in the modern era. Prior ACR, autoimmune liver disease, and CMV infection all may predispose to development of CR. Patients with CR typically present with laboratory evidence of cholestasis and may be jaundiced. As opposed to in ACR, steroid therapy is not beneficial in the management of CR. Options for management include increasing the dose of tacrolimus or the use of additional immunosuppressants such as mycophenolate mofetil or an mTOR inhibitor. Despite maximal medical therapy, many patients with CR will ultimately require retransplantation [54].

Infectious Complications in Patients with Chronic Liver Disease and Cirrhosis

Cirrhosis represents a state of progressive hepatic fibrosis with marked distortion of the hepatic architecture and development of regenerative nodules. The liver plays an important role in the hosts' immunity against bacterial pathogens; therefore, the development of chronic liver disease and cirrhosis renders such patients to an increased risk for infections. Thus, liver transplant candidates represent a unique patient population that is highly vulnerable to multiple infectious complications affecting the pre-transplant course. In addition, chronic liver disease and cirrhosis are associated with increased morbidity and mortality, due to gastrointestinal and variceal bleeding, severe and recurring ascites, hepatic encephalopathy, hepatorenal and hepatopulmonary syndromes, bile secretion impairment, and severe coagulopathy. Infections play an important role in the overall morbidity and prognosis for persons with chronic liver disease including cirrhosis and may contribute to 30–50% mortality [55]. Bacterial infections are noted at the time of hospitalization or during the course of hospital stay in 25–35% of patients with cirrhosis [56]. It is estimated that there is a 15% hospital mortality for cirrhotic patients who develop an infection episode [55]. In patients with cirrhosis, it is estimated that 30% are community-acquired infection, and the remainder are healthcare-onset infections. Approximately 35–40% of these healthcare-acquired infections will occur >48 h after hospital admission, which places these patients at an increased risk for infections due to multidrug-resistant organisms (MDROs) [56, 57].

Overview of Liver Function and Its Contribution to Host Defense

The liver is an organ that plays an important role in the metabolism, synthesis, and the storage of nutrients and proteins. The liver produces the majority of the body's proteins and therefore has pivotal synthetic functions such as metabolism and synthesis of amino acids, carbohydrates, fatty acids, lipoproteins, plasma proteins like albumin, transport proteins, protease inhibitors, fibrinogen, clotting factors, and complements. The liver also serves as a center of detoxification, removing or degrading toxic components from the circulation. In order for the liver to accomplish these functions, the hepatocyte must extract nutrients, waste, and toxic products from the blood that circulate through the liver within its sinusoids. The liver is continuously exposed to dietary ingredients consisting of exogenous molecules and micronutrients, environmental products, and byproducts of the gastrointestinal microbiota. The blood from the gastrointestinal and mesenteric circulation enters the liver via the portal vein and mixes with oxygen-rich blood from the systemic circulation via the hepatic artery and ultimately drains into the liver sinusoids. It is estimated that 80% of the hepatic blood flow within the liver arises from the gastrointestinal tract through the portal circulation [58]. Therefore, hepatocytes are exposed to a mixture of portal venous and arterial blood. The sinusoids are lined with liver sinusoidal endothelial cells that contain fenestrations to facilitate passage of the blood to reach the hepatocytes [58]. The hepatocytes are constantly exposed to foreign and immunogenic antigens and environmental toxins and those produced by the endogenous orointestinal microbiota. This constant exposure could result in untamed systemic immune activation; however, the liver plays a critical role in regulation and maintenance of immunologic and inflammatory homeostasis [58].

In addition to metabolism and synthesis, the hepatocytes play an important role in host defense. Their contribution to host immunity includes the production of complement and antimicrobial proteins, acute phase proteins in response to infection, and antigen presentation to T cells [58]. The liver is also a lymphoid organ with unique immunological properties. The liver-specific macrophages, known as Kupffer cells, line the luminal surface of the hepatic sinusoids and are an important part of the reticuloendothelial system (RES). The Kupffer cells in the liver comprise 90% of the body's tissue macrophages and make up one-third of the parenchymal cells in the liver [59]. Both the Kupffer cells and the hepatocytes contain pattern recognition receptors (PRR) which can bind to microbe-associated molecular patterns and damage-associated molecular patterns that originate from the gastrointestinal tract through the portal circulation [60–62]. These molecular patterns are then phagocytized by the Kupffer cells or hepatocytes and are removed and cleared from the circulation. These local processes of removal and degradation by the Kupffer cells and the hepatocytes serve a protective role to prevent systemic immune activation as a result of antigens and byproducts from the gastrointestinal tract [58]. These properties ensure an efficient innate defense against intestinal organisms and toxins and confer a particular capacity for preservation of immune tolerance. The normal liver is therefore considered to be immune tolerant or "tolerogenic." This is best supported by the observations that liver transplant recipients can reduce and also wean their immunosuppressive therapy in up to 20% of the patients, compared to recipients of other solid organ transplant [63].

On the other hand, with regard to host defense, the Kupffer cells of the liver play a key role in the removal of bacteria and their endotoxins from the bloodstream, as well as producing local inflammatory cytokines. Their presence within the vascular sinusoids provides an effective first line of defense against infections via the hematogenous route and bacterial translocation from the gastrointestinal tract.

Immunologic Dysfunction in Cirrhosis

In patients with cirrhosis, this crucial hepatic immunologic homeostasis is severely disrupted. Additionally, a milieu of dysregulated systemic pro-inflammatory cytokine response can result in further organ damage, especially in cirrhotic patients with systemic infection or sepsis [57]. The immunopathogenesis seen in cirrhosis is quite complex and is outlined in Fig. 3.1. In general, the clearance of bacteria and bacterial endotoxins by the Kupffer cells is impaired in patients with cirrhosis due to portosystemic shunting. The immunologic dysfunction associated with cirrhosis is further augmented by compromised liver synthetic function, malnutrition, stress catabolism, and also lifestyle factors, such as alcohol consumption. Chronic liver disease and cirrhosis are associated with alterations and/or deficiencies in all of the host defense mechanisms. In addition to depressed host immunity, these patients are at increased risk for exposure to healthcare-acquired infections due to their frequent need for hospitalization to manage the many complications associated with chronic and end-stage liver disease.

The key host factors that contribute to an increased risk of infection in patients with cirrhosis include (1) alterations in the intestinal microbiota and the intestinal mucosal barrier; (2) depression of activity by Kupffer cells and RES; (3) suboptimum opsonic activity in serum and the ascitic fluid; (4) neutrophil dysfunction with decreased phagocytosis and chemotaxis; and (5) decreased production and abnormalities in complement pathways, pattern recognition receptors, and C-reactive protein [57].

In recent years there has been an increased appreciation of the importance of the normal gut microbiota which contributes to both the host's metabolic and immunologic functions. The majority of the gut microbiota is comprised of obligate anaerobes within the phylum *Firmicutes* (specifically *Clostridia* spp. and Gram-negative anaerobes such as the *Bacteroides* spp.). In the bowel of healthy subjects, Gram-negative bacteria are present in relatively low numbers as compared with the obligate anaerobes, whereas

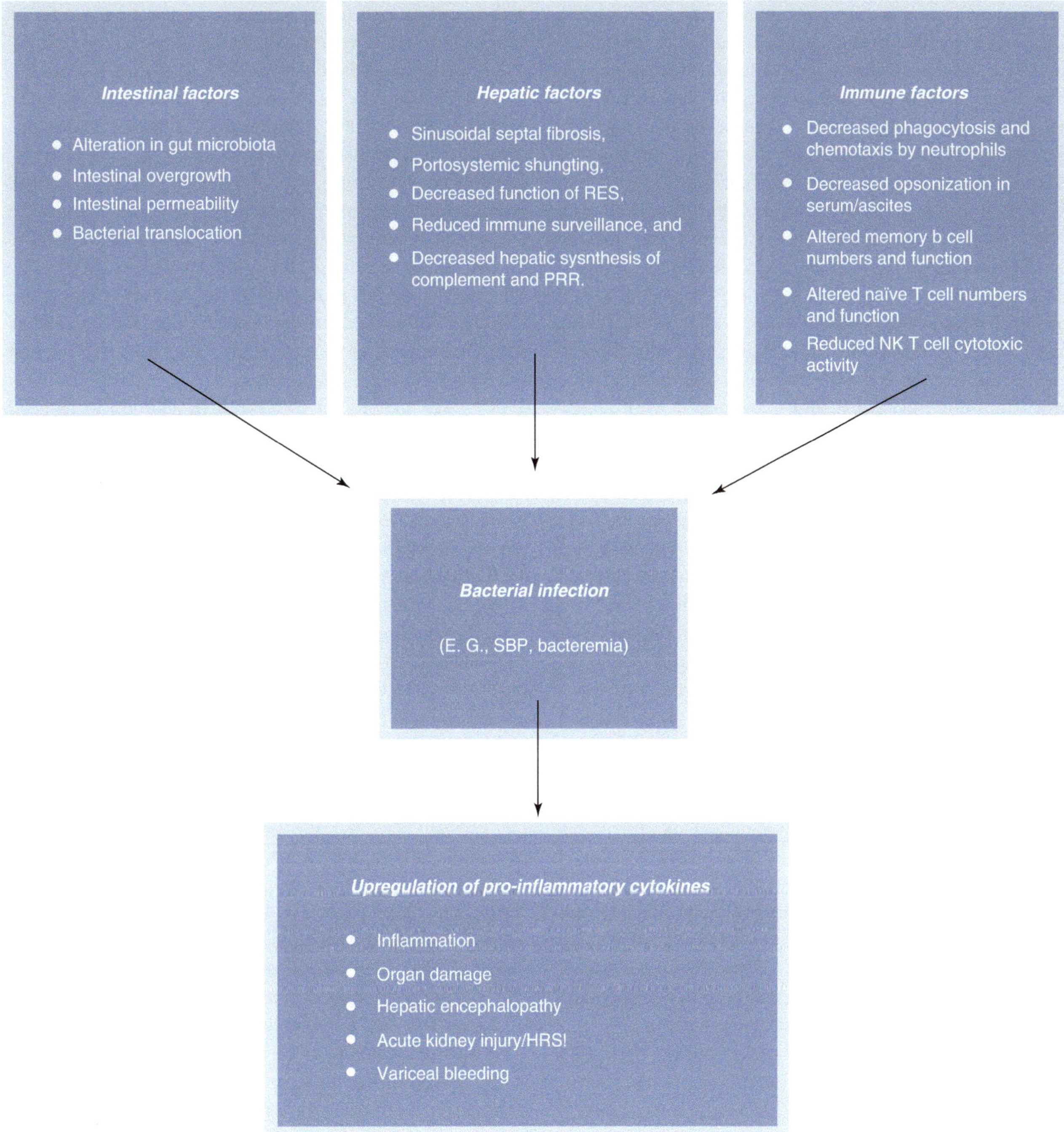

Fig. 3.1 Immunologic dysfunction associated with cirrhosis. PRR, pattern recognision receptors. SBP, spontaneous bacterial peritonitis. HRS, hepato-renal syndrome

with cirrhosis, the proportion of Gram-negative bacteria is more prominent. Alterations in the composition of the gut microbiota are well recognized in patients with cirrhosis, with an increase in colonization by the Proteobacteria that are predominantly Gram-negative enteric bacteria [64]. Spontaneous infections with Gram-negative bacilli are common in patients with cirrhosis, and it is proposed that this is mainly due to bacterial translocation from the gastrointestinal tract that has undergone alteration in the gut microbiota. Bacterial translocation occurs when bacteria or yeast migrate to the mesenteric lymph nodes and into the portosystemic circulation [57]. In animal experiments, oral administration of radiolabeled *E. coli* was detected within the intestinal lumen, mesenteric lymph nodes, and the ascitic fluid in mice with cirrhosis [65], supporting the possible mechanism of enhanced bacterial translocation that may also occur in patients with cirrhosis. Additionally, Gram-negative bacilli are demonstrated to be more efficient in translocating across bowel lumen when compared to obligate anaerobes in a murine experimental model [66], providing further evidence for clinical observations that Gram-negative enteric bacilli are the most common cause of infection in patients with chronic end-stage liver disease and systemic infections due to anaerobes are seldom seen. Other factors that contribute to the bacterial translocation of pathogenic bacteria in cirrhosis include intestinal bacterial overgrowth and increased intestinal permeability [64]. Intestinal overgrowth and alterations in the gut microbiota appear to correlate with the Child-Pugh score; higher prevalence of bacterial overgrowth has been observed in patients with Child-Pugh classes B and C compared with patients having class A liver disease [67, 68]. Moreover, intestinal bacterial overgrowth has been associated with a diagnosis of minimal hepatic encephalopathy and supports the use of nonabsorbable rifaximin in the treatment and prevention of hepatic encephalopathy in such patients [68]. It has also been shown that there is a higher bacterial burden of pathogenic *E. coli* in stool cultures in patients with cirrhosis and those with early-stage hepatic encephalopathy [69]. Normal hosts have tight junctions between mucosal and epithelial cells, which limit translocation of bacteria and bacterial products. Patients with cirrhosis have alterations in tight junction or desmosome proteins that compromise the physiologic barrier and may result in increased bacterial translocation [70, 71]. Additionally, intestinal bacterial access to the gut epithelial cells may be facilitated by deficiencies in IgA, bile lipids, and antimicrobial peptides that are notably observed in patients with advanced cirrhosis [64, 72, 73]. Therefore, changes in the gut microbiota, coupled with the increased intestinal permeability, particularly in cirrhotic patients with ascites greatly enhance the risk for bacterial translocation due to aerobic Gram-negative bacteria resulting in spontaneous bacterial peritonitis and bloodstream infections.

Cirrhosis is associated with both sinusoidal and septal fibrosis which results in portosystemic shunting. Patients with cirrhosis have depressed RES-Kupffer cell function, which can further promote translocation of bacterial pathogens and their endotoxins, thus reducing immune surveillance by the Kupffer cells/RES and allowing these pathogens access to the bloodstream [74]. Toll-like receptors (TLRs) are expressed on the surface of macrophages including Kupffer cells and can recognize and bind to bacterial products including endotoxins. Alterations in the TLRs and nucleotide-binding oligomerization domain (NOD) 2 gene via minor genetic polymorphisms may result in decreased affinity of TLR for Gram-negative bacilli lipopolysaccharide further enhancing the risk for bacterial infections in patients with cirrhosis [75, 76]. Furthermore, it has been demonstrated that simultaneous variations in the NOD 2 and TLR genes are associated with increased risk for spontaneous bacterial peritonitis, as well as an increase in surrogate markers for intestinal permeability in patients with cirrhosis [77]. It appears that genetic polymorphisms may contribute to the risk of spontaneous bacterial peritonitis and other bacterial infections in patients with chronic liver disease and cirrhosis.

Patients with cirrhosis experience both generalized immunodeficiency and systemic immune activation with the production of pro-inflammatory cytokines, also referred to as cirrhosis-associated immune dysfunction (CAID) [77]. There are numerous immunologic deficits that contribute to CAID and ultimately risk of systemic infection. In patients with cirrhosis, there is an overall reduction of circulating immune cells, and this is most notable for neutrophils, naïve T cells, and memory B cells [78]. In addition to reduced numbers of immune cells, there is a cellular dysfunction, including reduced phagocytic and chemotactic properties of neutrophils, reduced phagocytic activity of monocytes, hypoproliferative response to mitogens by T and B cells, and reduced natural killer cell cytotoxic activity [79–82]. Stunted TNFα production and HLA-DR expression have also been noted in cirrhotic patients with acute decompensation, such as sepsis, and referred to as "immune paralysis" [83].

Finally, as cirrhosis affects the synthetic function of the liver, the production of both complement and pattern recognition receptors (PRRs) are diminished [84]. Several important soluble PRRs produced by the liver include C-reactive protein, lipopolysaccharide-binding protein, peptidoglycan recognition protein, and soluble CD14, which activate complement associated opsonization cascade [85, 86]. Reduction in complement and PRR synthesis decreases bactericidal function of phagocytic cells in patients with cirrhosis [87]. Specifically, decreased concentrations of C3, C4, and CH50 result in suboptimal opsonic activity in both serum and ascitic fluid and have been recognized as an important risk factor that is associated with increased susceptibility to bacterial infections [88, 89]. Bactericidal functions of neutrophils are compromised resulting from decreased circulating cells in the peripheral blood due to splenic sequestration, decreased chemotaxis, and phagocytosis [88]. In patients with cirrhosis, neutrophils have reduced microbicidal activity owing to diminished intracellular superoxide production and myeloperoxidase activity [90]. Additionally, neutrophil dysfunction can be further exacerbated by alcohol consumption further suppressing phagocytosis and increasing the risk of bacterial infection [91].

In summary, the immunologic and synthetic function of the liver plays an important role in immune surveillance and immunologic homeostasis. Patients with advanced liver disease awaiting liver transplantation are a vulnerable population due to hepatic structural abnormalities, reduced production of critical immuno-protective proteins, reduced circulating immune cells, and impaired function of these cells. This overwhelming acquired immunodeficiency in patients with end-stage liver disease is further augmented by the frequent exposure to the healthcare setting, placing these patients at risk for numerous infectious complications prior to undergoing hepatic allograft transplantation.

Clinical Aspects of Infections in Patients with Chronic Liver Disease and Cirrhosis

As a result of CAID, infectious complications are extremely common in patients with chronic liver disease and may be the cause of mortality in up to 50% of these patients [92–94]. The most common types of infections are spontaneous bacterial peritonitis (SBP), UTI, pneumonia, bloodstream infections, and skin and soft tissue infections [95, 96]. The bacteriologic causes of these infections are predominantly (~75%) due to Gram-negative bacilli (GNB); Gram-positive organisms and anaerobes account for 20% and 3%, respectively [97]. It is estimated that 64% of these infections may be due to drug-resistant bacteria [98]. Infection in patients with cirrhosis can exacerbate liver failure and precipitate end-organ damage at other sites [99]. Due to the dysregulation of the pro-inflammatory cytokine response in patients with cirrhosis, sepsis carries a mortality rate of 26–44%. Infection can cause acute decompensation in individuals with chronic liver failure, which can result in worsening hepatic encephalopathy. Acute kidney injury with hepatorenal syndrome, acute lung injury with ARDS, and severe coagulopathy with gastrointestinal bleeding can all be precipitated by bacterial infections in patients with cirrhosis [62].

Spontaneous bacterial peritonitis is a common infection in cirrhotic patients with ascites. Severe, potentially life-threatening SBP that requires hospitalization often noted in patients with advanced liver disease may be associated with 31% mortality [59]. SBP is characterized by the spontaneous infection of ascitic fluid in the absence of an intra-abdominal source of infection. The pathogenesis of SBP is caused by bacterial translocation from the intestinal tract in the setting of portosystemic shunting. The most common organism isolated from peritoneal fluid is *Escherichia coli*. In a large series of 519 patients with SBP, the prevalence of culture-positive organisms included *E. coli* (43%), *Klebsiella pneumoniae* (11%), *Streptococcus pneumoniae* (9%), other streptococcal species (19%), other *Enterobacteriaceae* (4%), *Staphylococcus* species (3%), and *Pseudomonas aeruginosa* (1%), and 10% were miscellaneous organisms [100]. Another study noted that in the setting of norfloxacin prophylaxis for SBP, viridans group streptococci were prominent streptococcal isolates followed by group B *Streptococcus*, *Streptococcus pneumoniae*, and *Streptococcus bovis*, emphasizing the increasing importance of streptococcal species breakthrough infection as a cause of SBP in patients receiving fluoroquinolone prophylaxis [101]. Guidelines and recommendations for the diagnosis, management, and prevention of SBP have been published and are updated by the American Association for the Study of Liver Diseases (AASLD) [102]. After SBP, UTIs are the next common site of infection in patients with cirrhosis. As in other patient populations, urinary catheters are an important risk factor for such infections, and as expected, GNB are common causative pathogens.

Patients with cirrhosis are at increased risk for community-acquired pneumonia (CAP), healthcare-acquired pneumonia (HCAP), and aspiration pneumonia. As patients with cirrhosis have both complement and B-cell defects, they are at increased risk for infections due to encapsulated organisms such as *Streptococcus pneumoniae*, *Haemophilus influenzae*, and *Klebsiella pneumoniae*. Additionally, these patients are more likely to have concurrent bacteremia and have multilobar involvement compared with CAP in the general population [103]. The depressed cellular immune response associated with cirrhosis also places these patients at increased risk for legionellosis. These patients require frequent hospitalization, and therefore they are at increased risk for HCAP. Hepatic encephalopathy is a risk factor for HCAP, because these patients have decreased mental status and are at risk for aspiration of oropharyngeal contents that often are colonized by Gram-negative enteric bacilli. Empiric treatment for HCAP should include coverage for *Pseudomonas aeruginosa* and other drug-resistant GNB, as well as MRSA. Patients with cirrhosis are at increased risk for aspiration events in the setting of altered mental status due to hepatic encephalopathy or excessive alcohol consumption, which places them at risk for lower respiratory tract infections [104]. Additionally, the periodontal disease that is seen in alcoholic patients provides a favorable environment for both anaerobes and *Klebsiella pneumoniae* colonization, which can lead to lower respiratory tract infection during aspiration events [67, 105]. It is well recognized that patients with chronic alcoholism are at an increased risk for community-acquired pneumonia due to *S. pneumoniae*; a study reported that alcohol abuse was also a risk factor for CAP and septic shock due to *Pseudomonas aeruginosa* and *Acinetobacter* species [106]. It is important to note that the latter two infections are uncommon in patients with alcoholic cirrhosis unless these patients have extensive prior healthcare exposure including stays in the intensive care unit or need for mechanical ventilatory support; other risk factors include leukopenia or neutropenia.

Bloodstream infections can occur as a result of bacterial translocation from the gastrointestinal tract; Gram-negative enteric bacilli, enterococci, and *Streptococcus* spp. are common pathogens [58, 107]. It has been reported that bacteremia or SBP can complicate gastrointestinal bleeding in 17–45% of the episodes [108]. The management of esophageal varices involves esophageal variceal ligation (EVL) and esophageal variceal sclerotherapy (EVS); both of these procedures may increase the risk for transient bacteremia. In a meta-analysis, the overall rate of bacteremia following these procedures was 13%; bacteremia was significantly more common after EVS (17%) compared with EVL (6%) [109]. The most common cause of transient bacteremia associated with EVS and EVL includes alpha-hemolytic *Streptococcus* and coagulase-negative staphylococci [110, 111]. As with other hospitalized patients, invasive procedures such as indwelling central venous catheters place these patients at increased risk for bloodstream infections due to *Staphylococcus aureus* including MRSA and coagulase-negative staphylococci. Presence of cirrhosis was noted as an independent risk factor for the development of spontaneous bacteremia due to group B *Streptococcus* [112].

Hepatic hydrothorax is another complication of cirrhosis, and this can evolve into spontaneous bacterial empyema. Spontaneous bacterial empyema may be seen in 10–20% of patients with hepatic hydrothorax, and like SBP, these infections are primarily due to Gram-negative enteric bacilli [113–115].

Skin and soft tissue infections including necrotizing fasciitis have been reported in patients with cirrhosis. In patients with end-stage liver disease, generalized edema, especially involving the lower extremities, is not uncommon; furthermore, suboptimal personal hygiene and malnutrition place these patients at increased risk for relapsing skin and soft tissue infections. The common causative agents are *Staphylococcus aureus*, including CA- and HA-MRSA, and β-hemolytic *Streptococcus* including group B *Streptococcus*; GNB infections have also been reported [62]. Other rare causes of skin and soft tissue infections due to *Vibrio vulnificus* and *Aeromonas hydrophila* may be seen more often in patients with cirrhosis compared with the general population.

Specific Pathogens

Patients with chronic liver disease exhibit CAID due to decreased complement levels, less effective phagocytic activity and chemotaxis, "bypass" of the reticuloendothelial system due to portosystemic shunting, and availability of free iron that promotes growth of particular organisms.

Iron is bound to proteins such as hemoglobin, ferritin, transferrin, and lactoferrin, which maintain a low level of free iron that inhibits sustained bacterial growth. The liver plays a key role in iron metabolism, and this can be significantly disrupted in patients with chronic liver disease and cirrhosis. While this disruption in iron homeostasis is most notable in hemochromatosis, it has also been reported in patients with alcoholic liver disease, nonalcoholic fatty liver disease, and chronic hepatitis C infection. Cirrhosis is associated with decreased synthetic function, including the production of hepcidin, an important regulatory peptide for iron metabolism. In response to infection and inflammation, there is increased production of hepcidin, which decreases the availability of free iron, resulting in induced hypoferremia. The decreased levels of free iron by hepcidin have important antimicrobial properties, by creating an environment that does not support bacterial growth. Animal models of hepcidin-deficient mice showed increased susceptibility to infection with *Vibrio vulnificus*. Therefore, suggesting that reduced production of hepcidin in patients with chronic liver disease and cirrhosis contributes greatly to their susceptibility to specific pathogens [116–118].

Noteworthy pathogens that are more common in patients with chronic liver disease and cirrhosis, as compared to the general population, include *E. coli*, *Vibrio* spp., *Aeromonas hydrophila*, *Plesiomonas shigelloides*, *Yersinia* spp., *Salmonella* spp., *Listeria monocytogenes*, *Mycobacterium tuberculosis*, and the invasive molds like *Aspergillus fumigatus* and *Rhizopus* spp. These organisms are able to take advantage of the immunodeficiency associated with chronic liver disease and cirrhosis; additionally high free iron levels provide favorable growth environment for such organisms [62, 79, 119].

The *Vibrio* spp., including *V. vulnificus*, *V. cholera*, and *V. parahaemolyticus*, can cause severe infection in patients with chronic liver disease and those with cirrhosis. *Vibrio vulnificus* is a Gram-negative, halophilic noncholera *Vibrio* species that is a common organism isolated from estuarine and marine environments and has been associated with gastroenteritis, skin and soft tissue infections with hemorrhagic bullae, and bacteremia resulting in severe sepsis and death. Impaired iron metabolism and increased iron availability appear to underlie the pathogenicity of *V. vulnificus* invasive disease [120–122]. Common coastal sites where *V. vulnificus* is endemic include the Chesapeake Bay and the Gulf Coast. Most patients (90%) with *V. vulnificus* bacteremia have a history of consuming raw or undercooked shellfish specifically oysters, whereas skin and soft tissue infections are associated with the handling of raw seafood or direct inoculation due to recreational exposure to marine environment [84, 123, 124]. Gastroenteritis is the most common clinical manifestation, cellulitis with hemorrhagic bullae, and less commonly seen necrotizing fasciitis has also been reported. Patients with chronic liver disease or cirrhosis can present with primary *V. vulnificus* bacteremia associated with multiple hemorrhagic bullae and septic shock. In case series, *V. vulnificus* bacteremia carries a mortality of 40%, with an extremely poor prognosis in patients with septic shock at the time of presentation [83–86, 125]. Therefore, it is recommended that persons with chronic liver disease should avoid consuming raw undercooked shellfish and exposure to marine water.

Aeromonas species are GNB that are isolated predominantly from fresh water. *Aeromonas hydrophila* is the most common species and mainly presents as gastroenteritis. A rapidly progressive cellulitis or necrotizing fasciitis may rarely occur in such patients following exposure to fresh water. Bacteremia due to *Aeromonas* spp. is more common in patients with underlying cirrhosis and was associated with a 36% crude mortality [126]. In the same series, *Aeromonas* bacteremia, cirrhosis was the common underlying disease. *Aeromonas* SBP is an uncommon illness that may be observed during the summer months and associated with a diarrheal illness [127]. *Plesiomonas shigelloides* is also a GNB which can be acquired by the ingestion of raw or undercooked shellfish. It has been associated with gastroenteritis and in rare instances SBP [128, 129]. It may have a propensity to cause severe disease in iron overload conditions such as hemochromatosis.

The *Yersinia* spp., *Y. enterocolitica*, and *Y. pseudotuberculosis* are Gram-negative enteric bacilli that are also ferrophilic. Therefore, patients with cirrhosis and hemochromatosis are at risk for these gastrointestinal pathogens, which can be transmitted by undercooked pork products. In rare instances, *Yersinia enterocolitica* bacteremia has been associated with blood transfusions [130].

Listeria monocytogenes are Gram-positive bacilli that may be acquired via the ingestion of infected processed and canned food products or unpasteurized milk and products made from raw milk such as certain variety of cheese. The most important risk factor for invasive *L. monocytogenes* infection is depressed cellular immunity; availability of free iron in the hosts has been recognized as an important determinant of *Listeria* pathogenicity and virulence. Hence *L. monocytogenes* infections have been described in patients with hemochromatosis and cirrhosis [131–133]. Bacteremia and meningitis are the common clinical presentations of *L. monocytogenes* invasive disease.

Infections due to *Mycobacterium tuberculosis*, *Aspergillus fumigatus*, and *Rhizopus* spp. can rarely complicate the course of patients with chronic liver disease and cirrhosis due to the underlying immunodeficiency coupled with the alteration in iron homeostasis [62, 79, 80, 82].

Infectious Complications in Liver Transplant Recipients

Epidemiology

The incidence of infection after liver transplantation (LT) is particularly high compared to other solid organ transplants, likely due to the complexity of the procedure, risk of abdominal contamination, and especially due to poor medical status of many allograft recipients with end-stage liver disease. Although mortality has markedly improved post-LT (), it is estimated that up to two-thirds of all LT patients suffer at least one episode of infection [134].

The risk of infection post-transplant is primarily determined by epidemiologic exposures including donor-derived, recipient-derived, healthcare-acquired, and community-acquired pathogens – and the patient's net state of immunosuppression. The net state of immunosuppression is based on multiple factors and includes the level of pharmacologic immunosuppression, underlying host factors, surgical procedures and other medical interventions, and viral infections (such as CMV). This is a complex interaction, and it generally varies predictably over time, based on typical protocols for antirejection immunosuppressive therapy and prophylactic strategies. Consequently, the risk of infection post solid organ transplant is traditionally subdivided into three distinct intervals: from surgery to 1 month post-transplant, 1 month to 6–12 months post-transplant, and beyond 6–12 months post-transplant [135, 136].

Pre-transplant Screening for Infections

Pre-transplant screening of both potential donors and recipients can help prevent infectious complications in multiple ways: by identifying contraindications to transplant, by detecting latent or occult active infections, and by stratifying risk for future infections and allowing appropriate preventive steps such as prophylactic antimicrobials or vaccination. Historically, screening approaches have differed widely between organ procurement organizations within the USA and internationally [137, 138]. With greater experience and ability to diagnose transplant-related infections, there is now an established subset of infections that are routinely screened for in most cases. Most transplant centers' screening protocols require and perform the following tests in donors and recipients prior to transplantation and include human immunodeficiency virus (HIV) antibody, HSV (herpes simplex) IgG antibody (at some centers), cytomegalovirus (CMV) IgG antibody, hepatitis C virus (HCV) antibody, hepatitis B virus (HBV) surface antigen (HBsAg), hepatitis B core antibody (HBcAb IgM and IgG, or total core antibody), hepatitis B surface antibody (HBsAb), rapid plasma reagin (RPR), toxoplasma antibody (especially in heart recipients), Epstein-Barr virus (EBV) antibody (EBV VCA IgG, IgM), varicella zoster virus (VZV) antibody, purified protein derivative (PPD) or interferon gamma release assay (IGRA) for latent TB infection in recipients, *Strongyloides* serology (for recipients from endemic areas), *Coccidioides* serology (for recipients from endemic areas), *Trypanosoma cruzi* serology (for donors and recipients from endemic areas), serologies for tetanus, diphtheria, measles, mumps, and pneumococcal titers as an aid to pre-transplant immunization (at some centers).

Some optional screening measures include West Nile virus serology or NAT HHV-8 serology and BK serology in kidney donor and recipients. NAT for HIV, HCV, and HBV is also performed and is of increasing importance especially in donors with high-risk social behaviors.

However, screening practices can still vary by transplant center [139]. Caregivers may choose to expand screening tests based on epidemiological or clinical factors on a case-by-case basis. Presurgical testing for LT is generally similar to protocols for other solid organ transplants; however, addressing potential latent *Mycobacterium tuberculosis* infection (LTBI) in candidate recipients raises some specific challenges.

Immunocompromised states may confer a weakened ability to react to tuberculin skin tests (TSTs) and interferon gamma release assays (IGRAs), decreasing the sensitivity of these tests when screening for *Mycobacterium tuberculosis* (MTb) [140, 141]. Individuals with cirrhosis are known to have impaired immune responses, including altered T-cell-dependent functions, which may affect the sensitivity of MTb testing [142]. There is no gold standard for latent MTb diagnosis, and all current tests have questionable accuracy for immunocompromised hosts. However, they do have high specificity and, thus, are still a valuable tool for minimizing the risk of active tuberculosis infection for many patients after undergoing transplantation [143–145]. Although there is limited research on the use of these tests specifically in individuals prior to transplantation, 2013 guidelines from the American Society of Transplantation recommend standard TST for all transplant candidates, with consideration of a second boosting TST 2 weeks later for those who initially test negative; this can potentially reveal a positive test for patients with remote exposure [146]. IGRAs are also recommended as an alternative to TST and may be preferable for convenience at most transplant centers. The use of an IGRA for screening for LTBI is favored in the setting where a patient has received a prior BCG vaccine, as an IGRA is more specific than a TST in this instance. The QuantiFERON-TB Gold In-Tube test (QFT) (Cellestis, Australia) has been compared to the TST for diagnosis of latent tuberculosis infection in candidates being considered for LT, and of note, indeterminate QFT results were more likely in patients with higher MELD scores [145]. There is some evidence that the T-SPOT TB test (Oxford Immunotec Ltd) may have slightly higher sensitivity than the QuantiFERON-Gold In-Tube test [147].

Treatment for LTBI also poses a unique challenge for pre-LT candidates, given the hepatotoxic potential of the treatment options. Completion of treatment before transplantation is ideal to best minimize the risk of developing active tuberculosis infection. With careful monitoring, even compensated cirrhotic individuals can complete the treatment safely [148, 149]. If exposure to MTb is suspected to be recent (i.e., if the candidate had recent conversion of their TST or IGRA from negative to positive), early treatment is especially favored, as risk for MTb activation is highest during the initial 1–2 years post exposure [150]. However, for candidates with advanced decompensated liver disease, it is usually advisable to defer treatment till after transplant when the patient is deemed stable from a liver function standpoint, to minimize the risk of fulminant hepatotoxicity.

There are two standard treatment options for LTBI in pre-liver transplant candidates: isoniazid for 9 months or rifampin for 4 months. The risk for hepatotoxicity has not been shown to be significantly different between the two drugs for this population [145]. Due to the contraindicated drug interactions between rifampin and many immunosuppressants, rifampin is not recommended following transplantation. The coadministration of rifampin with tacrolimus results in decreased drug exposure of tacrolimus. Twelve weeks of directly observed therapy with isoniazid and rifapentine is a third approved regimen for LTBI in the general population; however, as it has not been studied in the LT population, it is not recommended in these cases. Additionally, rifapentine is similar to rifampin in its effect on tacrolimus drug exposure. A randomized prospective study sought to investigate the efficacy and safety of 9 months of levofloxacin prophylaxis in LT candidates; however, the study was terminated early due to an 18% rate of severe tenosynovitis in the levofloxacin arm [151].

Timeline for Infectious Complications from Transplant Procedure to 1 Month After Transplantation

Bacterial and Healthcare-Acquired Infections

In the first month post-LT, infections are most often healthcare associated and bacterial in origin, similar to the infection risks for immunocompetent hosts undergoing other hepatobiliary procedures. A variety of factors are associated with an increased risk for bacterial infection. These factors include older age, length of preoperative stay, CMV infection, duration of surgery, retransplantation, volume of transfused blood products, preoperative MELD and CTP scores, bilioenteric anastomosis, technical complications (e.g., biliary leak, HAT), renal replacement therapy, and hyperglycemia [152]. Intra-abdominal infections are most common due to the technical nature of the surgery. The bile duct has no natural collaterals, being supplied only arterially, as opposed to the liver, which has dual circulation through the portal system. The biliary epithelium is thus more vulnerable to hypoperfusion during transplantation or resulting from hepatic artery thrombosis (HAT). A 30-year review at one center found a 14% rate of biliary complications post-LT, including anastomotic and non-anastomotic strictures, bile leaks, and cholangitis. Elevated MELD, HAT, and elevated donor creatinine suspected to reflect altered metabolic factors at the site of anastomosis, which may impair healing, were all significant risk factors for anastomotic biliary complications [153]. Biliary complication may in turn lead to further infectious complications, such as hepatic and intra-abdominal abscesses. A 10-year retrospective study at a large transplant center diagnosed hepatic abscess post-LT at a rate of 4.8 per 1000 transplant patient-years [154]. In the same study, HAT was confirmed to be a significant predisposing factor for hepatic abscess. Management of infectious biliary complications warrants antibiotic coverage for enteric Gram-negative organisms and anaerobes, as well as healthcare-associated bacteria based on the patient's history. Source control may necessitate drainage, endoscopic intervention, surgical repair or in severe cases, retransplantation.

After intra-abdominal infections, the lungs are the second most frequent site of infectious complication post-LT. A retrospective study of deceased donor hepatic allograft recipients found an incidence of 10 episodes of ventilator-associated pneumonia per 1000 days of mechanical ventilation. *Enterobacteriaceae* accounted for 79% of bacterial etiologic agents. Both intra-abdominal infection and pneumonia can be complicated by concurrent bacteremia. A multicenter retrospective study found bloodstream infections complicated 29% of LT recipients in the first year after transplantation, with 52% of infections occurring within the first 100 days [155].

Surgical wound infections are third common infectious complications during this period, followed by urinary tract infections and other healthcare-associated infections (HAIs) [150]. Risk factors identified for surgical site infection include prolonged operative time, large-volume blood transfusion, biliary leak, retransplantation, dialysis, and CMV infection [156, 157].

Antibiotic resistance has become an increasing problem for treating HAIs. In 2014, the CDC found that 14% of HAIs in short-term acute care hospitals were caused by 1 of 6 major antibiotic-resistant threat bacteria [158]. The most recent survey of HAIs from the National Healthcare Safety Network from 2011 to 2014 further showed that resistance patterns continue to change over time [159]. Antibiotic resistance is particularly a concern for liver transplant recipients who are likely to have had prior antibiotic exposures as a result of numerous hospitalizations associated with the complications of chronic liver disease in the pre-transplant period. A study of 300 liver transplant recipients found 88 suffered at least 1 infection in the early 30-day post-transplant period; and of these, 78 (89%) were due to drug-resistant bacteria [159]. The multidrug-resistant organisms (MDROs) most commonly encountered in LT recipients include extended β-lactamase-producing *Enterobacteriaceae* (ESBL), MDR *Pseudomonas aeruginosa*, carbapenem-resistant *Acinetobacter baumannii* (CR-AB), carbapenem-resistant *Enterobacteriaceae* (CRE), vancomycin-resistant *Enterococcus* (VRE), and methicillin-resistant *Staphylococcus aureus* (MRSA) [160].

The most common MDROs associated with ESBL production are *Klebsiella pneumoniae* and *E. coli*. Although it appears that ESBL-producing organisms may be more common in kidney transplant recipients, often as an etiology for UTIs, LT recipients are also at risk for these organisms and have been reported in 5.5–7% [161–163]. In a large solid organ transplant cohort, 53% of the *Klebsiella pneumoniae* isolates were ESBL producing, and the highest risks were seen in kidney transplant recipients, especially those requiring post-transplant renal replacement therapy [162]. Infections due to ESBL-producing organisms in solid organ transplant recipients have been noted to be associated with mortality that ranged from 5% to 20% [162, 164, 165]. Carbapenems are the preferred treatment of choice for serious infections due to ESBL-producing *Klebsiella pneumoniae* and *E. coli*.

Pseudomonas aeruginosa has many resistance mechanisms and therefore demonstrates lack of susceptibility to a variety of antibiotics in liver transplant recipients. MDR *Pseudomonas* was the causative pathogen for healthcare-associated pneumonia (HCAP) in 18% of LT recipients [166]. Bloodstream infections due to *P. aeruginosa* have occurred in up to 10% of LT recipients, and 50% of these isolates are multidrug resistant. Treatment of MDR *Pseudomonas aeruginosa* can be quite challenging in LT; clinicians may often need to resort to nephrotoxic agents such as the aminoglycosides and the polymyxins. The role of cephalosporin ß-lactamase combinations such as ceftolozane/tazobactam and ceftazidime/avibactam may offer additional options for MDR *Pseudomonas*; however, data in the solid organ transplant patient population for these newer antimicrobial drugs is lacking.

Infections due to carbapenem-resistant Acinetobacter baumannii have been reported with increasing frequency in LT recipients, and appear to predominantly occur in the setting of HCAP and bloodstream infections. Bloodstream infections due to *Acinetobacter baumannii* have been reported to be as high as 24% in LT recipients, with over 50% of these isolates being caused by carbapenem-resistant *A. baumannii* [167–169]. *Acinetobacter* infections in LT recipients can carry a poor prognosis with inhospital mortality rates that may exceed 50% [168, 170, 171]. As with MDR *Pseudomonas*, treatment options are limited and include the polymyxins, such as colistin, and addition of aminoglycosides. Other options include minocycline, tigecycline, and ampicillin/sulbactam, as the β-lactamase inhibitor, sulbactam, has intrinsic activity against *A. baumannii*.

Recently, infections due to carbapenem-resistant *Enterobacteriaceae* (CRE) have been identified in solid organ transplant centers. Although there are multiple patterns of carbapenem resistance, the majority of cases in the USA are due to type A carbapenemases – specifically carbapenem-resistant *Klebsiella pneumoniae* (CRKP). Rates of CRKP have been reported between 6.6% and 12.9% in patients undergoing liver transplantation, although 1 transplant center has noted a rate as high as 23% [172–174]. In general, the most common sites of infections due to CRKP in LT recipients include surgical site, organ space, HAP, and UTI [172]. Mortality associated with CRKP infections in LT recipients ranges from 18% to as high as 80% [172, 174–176]. Another cohort of solid organ transplant patients found that infection with CRKP was independently associated with higher mortality (HR 5.562 [CI 95% 1.186–26.088]) [177]. In addition to traditional risk factors associated with CRKP infections in other patient populations, pre-transplant colonization with CRKP can place such patients at an increased risk for CRKP infections following transplantation [175, 176]. Despite this risk, there are currently no absolute contraindications to exclude donors that are colonized with CRKP. Treatment of LT recipients who developed CRE or CRKP infections is quite complicated, often requires combination antimicrobial therapy, and can also be associated with drug toxicity. Agents that have been used include the polymyxins such as colistin, aminoglycosides, and tigecycline along with or without a carbapenem agent. Although fosfomycin can be considered for treatment of uncomplicated UTIs due to CRE, the intravenous formulation is not available in the USA. One case report of complicated extensively drug-resistant (XDR) *Klebsiella pneumoniae* bacteremia during early post-transplant period necessitated addition of IV fosfomycin as an investigational drug to a multidrug regimen [178]. The role of the newer β-lactamase agents such as ceftazidime/avibactam and meropenem/vaborbactam is yet to be defined for the management of serious infections due to CRE and CRKP.

Infection and colonization by vancomycin-resistant *Enterococcus* (VRE) have been well characterized in pre-liver transplant candidates and in patients following liver transplantation. In the USA, the estimated rates of VRE colonization, prior to and after transplantation, were 16% and 22%, respectively [179]. There is wide variation in the prevalence of VRE colonization in LT candidates and liver transplant recipients, depending upon the transplant center and the patient population studied, and ranges from 0% to 44% [180–182]. In a prospective surveillance study, pre-transplant VRE colonization was found to be associated with an increased risk for VRE infections after transplantation and associated with higher morbidity as measured by ICU stay and length of hospitalization; however, VRE colonization did not result in increased mortality. On the other hand, the acquisition of VRE colonization post-LT was associated with increased morbidity and mortality compared with LT recipients with no evidence of VRE colonization [183]. The risk factors that are associated with VRE infection include prior antibiotic exposure, prolonged hospitalization, interventional procedures or complications of the biliary tract, and surgical re-exploration [161]. Common sites of VRE infection in the LT recipient include intra-abdominal, organ space, hepatobiliary, surgical site, bloodstream, and the urinary tract. Mortality due to VRE infections in LT recipients has previously been reported to be as high as 82%; this was, however, at a time when limited treatment options for VRE were available [184]. The use of linezolid and daptomycin, agents that have activity against such drug-resistant bacterial strains, has improved patient outcomes, although a 37.6% mortality has been reported in solid organ transplant recipients treated with linezolid for VRE infections [185].

Infections due to MRSA have been declining in the LT population, likely because of improved infection prevention practices such as strict implementation of hand hygiene, development of bundles for central venous catheter insertion and management, perioperative surgical site antiseptic policies, the use of daily chlorhexidine washes for select group of patients, and adherence to contact isolation policies [186]. A meta-analysis noted that there was 8.5% and 9.4% prevalence of MRSA colonization in pre- and post-liver transplant recipients, respectively. Additionally, pre- and post-transplant colonization was associated with six- to eleven-fold higher probability for subsequent development of MRSA invasive disease [179]. A single-center study reported 23% MRSA infection in LT recipients over an 8-year period; central vascular catheters, surgical wound, intra-abdominal space, and the lung were the most common sites of infection. Furthermore, the authors noted a 21% 30-day mortality in patients with MRSA infections [187]. Vancomycin continues to be the mainstay of treatment against MRSA; daptomycin and linezolid are being used with increasing frequency in select high-risk patients. Ceftaroline, the first cephalosporin with activity against MRSA, is approved for skin and soft tissue infections, and bacterial pneumonia, and may offer an alternative treatment option for MRSA infections in the LT patient population pending further clinical data.

The growing threat of MDRO infections in LT recipients can certainly affect patient outcomes. Therefore, emphasis on infection prevention and antibiotic stewardship is vital to limit further increases in antibiotic-resistant HAIs in patients undergoing a transplantation procedure [188]. This multidisciplinary approach has been shown to decrease surgical site infection rates by 52% in solid organ transplant recipients [189].

Infection due to *Clostridium difficile* has become an important healthcare-acquired pathogen with high morbidity and risk of death. The combined effect of potent immunosuppression and broad-spectrum antibiotic exposure increases the risk of *Clostridium difficile*-associated colitis during the early post-LT period. In a retrospective study of 1340 solid organ transplant recipients, the cumulative incidence of *C. difficile* colitis was highest (3%) in liver allograft recipients [190]. In a series of 467 LT recipients, incidence was 8%, with the majority of cases occurring within the first month following transplantation [191]. Another single-center retrospective study observed an incidence of 14% for *C. difficile* infection over a mean follow-up time of 1.8 years after LT; 41% of these cases occurred within 1 week after transplantation. The authors reported that most patients with *C. difficile* colitis had fever, whereas white blood cell count was less than 12,000 cells per μL [192].

Fungal Infections

In addition to bacterial infections, *Candida* spp. are a significant pathogen in the early post-transplant period. In a prospective multicenter investigation of invasive fungal infections following solid organ transplantation, 639 such cases among nearly 17,000 patients under surveillance were observed during the 6-year study period. Liver allograft recipients were at a high risk (41%) among this large cohort of SOT recipients. Fungemia was prominent (44%) disease presentation followed by intra-abdominal infection (14%). *Candida albicans* and *Candida glabrata* species constituted the majority of infections (46% and 24%, respectively) [193].

In the general population, the known risk factors for developing invasive *Candida* infection include extended treatment with broad-spectrum antibiotics, presence of central venous catheter, use of total parenteral nutrition, presence of severe neutropenia (ANC <500 cells per μL), diabetes mellitus, renal replacement therapy, mechanical ventilation, and intensive care stay. In transplant patients, recent CMV infection, primary graft failure, early surgical re-exploration, and colonization with *Candida* spp. during pre- and early post-transplant period are additional risk factors of invasive candidiasis. In LT recipients specifically, choledochojejunostomy is associated with a higher risk of invasive candidiasis compared to a choledochocholedochostomy anastomosis, as the former requires opening of the bowel [194]. Also, prophylaxis for spontaneous bacterial peritonitis with fluoroquinolones has been found to be an independent risk factor for invasive candidiasis in patients undergoing LT [195].

Diagnosis of invasive *Candida* infection is definitive when cultured from a sterile site; however, routine blood cultures lack optimal sensitivity, and often diagnosis can be missed or delayed. Detection of β-D-glucan, a polysaccharide component of fungal cell walls, can be a useful adjunctive test. However, in a multicenter analysis among LT recipients, β-D-glucan was not a reliable test for the diagnosis of invasive fungal disease [196]. Treatment for *Candida* spp. infection in liver transplant recipients is similar to the general population [197]. Source control, including removing central venous catheters when determined as the source of fungemia, remains important for successful clearance of fungemia.

Given the high frequency of invasive *Candida* infection in LT population, antifungal prophylaxis after transplant surgery may be considered among patients at increased risk for fungal disease. A randomized, double-blind, placebo-controlled trial of fluconazole prophylaxis vs. no antifungal prophylaxis after LT demonstrated a decreased rate of fungal colonization and both superficial and invasive fungal infection, although no difference in mortality was found [198]. Current guidelines recommend stratification based on specific risk factors. Patients are deemed high risk for invasive candidiasis, if they have ≥2 of the following conditions: prolonged or repeat operation, retransplantation, renal failure, ≥40 units of cellular blood products, choledochojejunostomy, or *Candida* spp. colonization in the perioperative period [188]. In one series including 30 pre-LT candidates, 81% were found to have *Candida* carriage in gastrointestinal tract [199]. High-risk patients are recommended to be treated with an antifungal medication. Fluconazole 400 mg daily is sufficient for most *Candida* spp. coverage, though, notably, prevalence of non-*albicans Candida* spp. have increased and such infections are associated with higher mortality in the immunosuppressed host [194]. Duration of antifungal prophylaxis may vary by transplant center; however, 4-week duration is common. Prophylaxis may be extended based on ongoing risk factors. Recipients at low risk for invasive fungal infection may be observed without antifungal prophylaxis [200].

While *Candida* spp. constitute the majority of fungal infections during early post-LT period, *Aspergillus* spp. infections are rare, albeit a significant, pathogen. In case series and retrospective reviews, the incidence of invasive aspergillosis (IA) after LT may vary from 1% to 10% [201–203]. A multicenter surveillance network of transplant patients found an 11% incidence of IA over 5 years post-LT [204]. Multiple factors have been correlated with an increased risk of IA after transplantation. Retransplantation and the need for renal replacement therapy have the highest association [205]. It is theorized that injury to the hepatic reticuloendothelial phagocytes and alteration of platelet-mediated inflammation seen in patients with hepatic dysfunction increase susceptibility to tissue-invasive *Aspergillus* spp. infection [206, 207]. Renal failure may directly impact granulocyte and macrophage function or may be a marker for other predisposing factors in critically ill patients. Other factors that increase risk for IA in the initial 90 days post-LT include urgent transplantation, CMV infection, prolonged intensive care unit stay, additional surgery, and multiple invasive bacterial infections [208].

Historically, IA was most common in the first 90 days post-LT and may occur within 30 days after transplant surgery in patients at particularly high risk. However, recent analysis has found a slight shift in the diagnosis of IA to later post-transplantation period (>90 days) [209]. This is speculated to be due to improved overall management of transplant patients, ranging from surgical techniques to improved infection prevention and surveillance protocols. In addition, CMV infection is a known risk factor for IA, and prophylaxis against CMV may have also contributed to shift the timing of IA. Recent cases also demonstrated significantly lower mortality than in the past from >90% down to 60%; however, IA associated with early retransplantation still carries a high mortality [205, 210].

Clinically, pulmonary IA is the most common manifestation followed by disseminated disease. Diagnosis can be challenging, as cultures have low sensitivity, since isolation of *Aspergillus* spp. in respiratory tract culture samples in most patients represent fungal colonization. Serum fungal assays such as galactomannan and β-D-glucan are increasingly utilized to help confirm or rule out IA; however, accuracy and reliability of these assays remain uncertain [195]. Positive *Aspergillus* antigen from bronchoalveolar fluid has been shown to have high specificity in lung transplant recipients [211]. A combination of clinical, microbiological, and radiographic findings along with hosts' susceptibility for these infections should be considered in making diagnosis of IA in patients following LT.

Treatment of IA in liver transplant recipients is similar to the general population, as outlined in the Infectious Diseases Society of America guidelines [212]. Given the high mortality and difficulty in ascertaining correct IA diagnosis in highly susceptible transplant patients, it is recommended to initiate anti-mold therapy when IA is strongly suspected, while work-up including tissue biopsy is in progress. Voriconazole is the drug of choice for primary IA; drug interactions may warrant modified dosing for certain antirejection drugs. Concomitant reduction of immunosuppression is ideal if feasible. Adjunctive surgery may be warranted in select cases. Duration is variable, but a minimum of 12 weeks is typically recommended; however, this should be extended based on clinical and radiographic treatment response, extent of the disease, and level of net immune suppression.

While universal prophylaxis for IA is not routinely recommended following solid organ transplantation, high-risk LT recipients have been shown to benefit from it [179, 200]. This targeted prophylaxis is correlated with decreased rates of IA and appears to be cost-effective. One retrospective single-center review found administering 90 days of voriconazole prophylaxis to high-risk patients post-LT had an institutional cost of 5.6% of the predicted cost for treating IA [213]. The best choice of prophylactic antifungal is not clear. Prior studies have investigated echinocandins, liposomal amphotericin B, and voriconazole [214–216]. Echinocandins are a common choice, given their ease of single daily dosing, minimal toxicity, and drug-drug interaction. The most suitable choice for anti-mold prophylaxis may vary depending on the clinical context.

Donor-Derived Infections

Unexpected donor-derived infections are a rare occurrence with an estimated incidence of 0.2% in solid organ transplant recipients [217]. As a result of current screening and prophylaxis practices, many viruses such as HIV, CMV, EBV, HBV, and HCV are identified early during the procurement period of the donor, and therefore, appropriate graft acceptance, infection surveillance, and when applicable treatment can ensue in the recipient. Unexpected donor-derived infections, although uncommon, can be an important complication particularly in the early post-transplant period. In addition to routine pre-transplant screening of the donor whether living or cadaveric allografts by history and laboratory screening, the procuring surgeon should carefully inspect the organ and donor for signs of infection by thorough physical examination. Surveillance cultures are typically sent that include blood, urine, and sputum samples. Peritoneal cultures may be warranted in cases of enterotomy and ascitic contamination to guide postsurgical antibiotic coverage [218]. Active infection in the cadaveric donor is not necessarily an absolute contraindication for transplantation; targeted antibiotics often can mitigate the risk. However, decisions are made on a case-by-case basis. Liver transplant recipients are particularly vulnerable to acquire bacterial infections via the allograft harvested from a donor with bacteremia; this possibly is related to the large tissue and vascular volume of the liver compared to other solid organ transplants [219]. Antibiotic prophylaxis may need to be extended in high-risk scenarios, such as donors with infective endocarditis and meningitis [220]. If an active bacteremia is diagnosed in the donor, the liver may still be used safely, provided that the donor has received appropriate treatment for the infection for 48 h and that the recipient receives at least 14 days of targeted treatment against that infection following transplantation [217, 221]. Guidelines suggest that for virulent pathogens that can cause endovascular infections such as *Staphylococcus aureus* and *Pseudomonas aeruginosa*, 2–4 weeks of antibiotic therapy should be considered although prolonged course of antibiotic therapy in recipients of such allografts has not been clinically validated [222]. Isolation of bacteria at a distant tissue site, such as in sputum or urine, usually does not necessitate antibiotic therapy in recipients of such donor allografts, with the exception of liver grafts from donors with confirmed or suspected bacterial pneumonia or pyelonephritis [222]. In some infections, such as severe encephalitis of unclear etiology, allografts are typically excluded outright [223].

In addition to bacterial etiologies, reported donor-transmitted infections in LT have run the gamut and have included viruses, fungi, and parasites [224]. Uncommon diseases may be challenging to diagnose, and donor origin among other possible exposure and potential infection transmission history should be considered for atypical post-transplant infection. Some less common viral infections that have resulted in allograft infection transmission include West Nile virus, lymphocytic choriomeningitis virus (LCMV), and rabies; these viruses have been associated with devastating neurologic morbidity and mortality in recipients of solid organ transplantation [139, 225, 226].

The most common fungal pathogens that can be transmitted from donor to recipient are *Candida* species, *Coccidioides immitis*, and *Cryptococcus neoformans* [222]. *Candida* can be derived from the organ donor, although transmission of *Candida* spp. to recipients occurs more typically from contamination during the organ procurement and preservation process [227–229]. Although donor transmission of any endemic mycoses is possible, donor screening for *Coccidioides immitis* is the only fungal serology that is routinely obtained in donors from endemic regions. Prophylaxis with an azole antifungal agent is recommended for LT recipients whose donor has a documented positive *Coccidioides* serology [226]. Recently, reports of infections due to *Cryptococcus neoformans* occurring in the early post-transplant period have raised possibility of potential donor transmission of the dimorphic fungal infection [226, 230–232]. Donor transmission of *Mycobacterium tuberculosis* has been well documented in the solid organ transplant population [217, 233]. Patients with active tuberculosis infection should not be considered for organ donation; however, latent tuberculous infection in a donor is not considered contraindication for organ procurement and transplantation. In this setting, treatment of latent tuberculous infection in the recipient will mitigate the risk of developing active tuberculosis after LT.

Strongyloides stercoralis and *Trypanosoma cruzi*, the causative agents of Chagas disease, are the most common parasites that have been associated with donor-transmitted parasitic infections. In the solid organ transplant recipient, *Strongyloides* can lead to accelerated intestinal infection increasing the risk for polymicrobial bacteremia and bacterial meningitis due to enteric Gram-negative bacilli (GNB) or the rare devastating *Strongyloides* hyperinfection syndrome, which is associated with rapidly progressive respiratory failure and death. As a result, donor screening with *Strongyloides* serology should be performed in donors from endemic regions such as tropics, subtropics, and Appalachia, USA; if serology is positive, recipients should be treated with ivermectin [234, 235]. *Trypanosoma cruzi* donor-derived infection is more problematic in patients undergoing heart transplantation; donor serologic screening for *T. cruzi* should be considered for liver allograft donors from endemic regions including Mexico and Central and South America. If a donor is positive for *T. cruzi* serology, there is no clear contraindication for liver transplantation, as long as the LT recipient undergoes regular surveillance for parasitemia. Preemptive treatment with benznidazole is initiated for patients with a positive *T. cruzi* PCR assay [236, 237].

Stored pre-transplant serum from both donor and recipient can be used to test and help confirm allograft-transmitted infection. Close collaboration with the national transplant authorities, the local organ procurement organizations, and appropriate public health agencies is vital for tracking these infections and to notify all other organ recipients from such donors.

Opportunistic Infections 1 to 6–12 Months After Liver Transplantation

After the first month, surgical recovery is well underway, and nosocomial infections become less prevalent. However, iatrogenic antirejection drug-induced immunosuppression is still high, and thus opportunistic infections are considered especially common from 1 month to 6–12 months after LT. Without prophylaxis, herpesviruses such as herpes simplex virus 1 and 2, varicella zoster virus, and cytomegalovirus, and environmental fungi like *Pneumocystis jirovecii* are important pathogens.

Cytomegalovirus (CMV) is the most important viral infection in LT recipients and contributes to significant morbidity and mortality in this patient population. CMV can manifest from asymptomatic viremia, to a syndrome associated with fevers and pancytopenia, to invasive target organ disease. In LT recipients, the gastrointestinal tract is the most common site of CMV involvement and can present as esophagitis, gastritis, and enterocolitis but can also involve other sites such as the lungs [238]. CMV has a predilection to involve the allograft, and therefore CMV hepatitis is an extremely common manifestation in LT recipients and can sometimes be confused with allograft rejection [239]. The incidence of CMV infection in LT recipients varies depending upon the risk group studied, with rates of 18–29% overall; however, it has been reported to be as high as 65% in the high-risk donor-recipient mismatch (D+/R−) [240–243]. The use of CMV prophylaxis with ganciclovir or valganciclovir in LT recipients for at least 3 months post-transplantation has reduced the incidence in the D+/R− subgroup to 12–30% [241, 243–246]. Historically, in LT recipients who do not receive CMV prophylaxis, CMV infection occurs within 3–6 months from the time of liver transplantation, which correlates with the period of maximal immunosuppression. However, in the setting of CMV prophylaxis, LT recipients can experience delayed-onset (also referred to as late-onset) CMV disease – after CMV prophylaxis has been discontinued – often occurring >6 months from the time of transplant [247, 248]. Delayed-onset CMV infection in LT recipients is more likely to cause tissue-invasive disease as compared to early-onset disease [248].

As CMV is an immunomodulatory virus, it has numerous indirect effects on the liver allograft. CMV can upregulate alloreactive T cells, and it can precipitate allograft rejection. In LT recipients, it has been thought to be associated with the vanishing bile duct syndrome, chronic ductopenic allograft rejection, cholestasis, and ultimately allograft failure [249–252]. Chronic CMV infection, in the setting of immunosuppression, may be related to atrophy of the biliary ducts and the development of allograft arteriopathy that is seen with chronic allograft failure [253]. It is also postulated that as CMV can invade the vascular endothelium, it may be responsible for hepatic artery thrombosis [254, 255]. Finally, CMV infection can further augment the immunosuppression of transplant patients and places LT recipients at increased risk for bacterial, viral, and fungal infections, as well as increased risk for EBV-associated post-transplant lymphoproliferative disorder (PTLD) [256–258].

Risk factors for CMV infection include CMV D+/R− mismatch, lymphocyte-depleting agents such as thymoglobulin and alemtuzumab, high-dose mycophenolate mofetil, genetic polymorphisms in the toll-like receptor 2 gene, allograft rejection, and retransplantation [259, 260]. Initial infection is significantly more likely to cause symptomatic illness than reactivation [261]. There are two accepted strategies for prevention. Universal prophylaxis with valganciclovir is one approach and has the added benefit of prophylaxis against other herpesviruses. A duration of 3–6 months of prophylaxis is typical but may be extended based on clinical factors [262]. Alternatively, a preemptive approach utilizes weekly monitoring for CMV antigenemia or PCR, with prompt initiation of treatment for early replication; this strategy may be preferable for avoiding drug toxicity. There is no definitive recommendation of one approach over the other, although universal prophylaxis is preferred in high-risk transplantations – specifically CMV D+/R− allograft mismatches. A meta-analysis comparing the two in the LT population found no difference in the incidence of CMV disease. Using indirect comparison, there was also no difference in acute cellular rejection or mortality between the two groups, but a decreased incidence of graft loss with universal prophylaxis was found [263]. Treatment of CMV infection with either oral valganciclovir or intravenous ganciclovir in LT recipients is similar to other SOT recipients. Resistance to ganciclovir is rare, but more likely in patients with past prolonged use of ganciclovir [264].

Pneumocystis jirovecii is ubiquitous in the environment but transforms to a common respiratory pathogen for the immunosuppressed. Without prophylaxis, the incidence of infection in LT recipients has been found to vary from 1% to 11% [265]. Clinical presentation in SOT recipients is similar to individuals with human immunodeficiency virus (HIV), though the acuity of symptoms is typically thought to be more severe in non-HIV patients. Treatment approach is also similar to HIV patients, with trimethoprim-sulfamethoxazole (TMP/SMX) being the drug of choice and adjunctive steroids a consideration based on hypoxemia [266]. Prophylaxis against *Pneumocystis* is routinely recommended for the first 6–12 months in all SOT patients and may be extended as needed based on ongoing risk [267]. TMP/SMX is the first choice for prophylaxis and has the added benefit of helping to prevent other opportunistic pathogens, such as *Toxoplasma gondii*, *Listeria monocytogenes*, *Nocardia* spp., *Isospora*, *Cyclospora*, and some bacterial agents.

With prophylaxis for the most prevalent infections being standard, their incidences have overall been reduced, but can still occur, typically after the prophylactic course has ended. Endemic fungi and *Mycobacterial* spp. including *M. tuberculosis* are also not uncommon pathogens during this post-transplant period. During the time of maximal immunosuppression (1–6 months after transplantation), reactivation of endemic mycoses can occur but oftentimes present later after transplantation and may be due to exogenous infection. *Cryptococcus neoformans* is the third most common fungal infection in solid organ transplant recipients, with an incidence that ranges from 0.2% to 5% [268, 269]. In general, cryptococcosis is a late infectious complication, occurring a median of 16–21 months after transplantation, although in liver and lung transplant recipients, it can present earlier – within 12 months post-transplantation [269–271]. The most common sites of infection are the lungs and the central nervous system, although cutaneous, liver, kidney, and osteoarticular involvement can also occur. Disseminated and extrapulmonary cryptococcosis has been reported in 50–75% of solid organ transplant recipients [271–273]. Liver transplant recipients have a sixfold increase risk for disseminated disease as compared to other types of transplant recipients [269]. The diagnosis and management of cryptococcosis in solid organ transplant recipients have been extrapolated from other patient populations (such as HIV) and retrospective/observational experience and are available as practice guidelines from the Infectious Diseases Society of America and the AST Infectious Diseases Community of Practice. Initial treatment with a lipid preparation of amphotericin B and flucytosine, followed by fluconazole maintenance treatment, is recommended [269, 274].

The true incidence of endemic mycoses in the solid organ transplant population is not well defined, but infections due to *Histoplasma capsulatum*, *Coccidioides immitis/posadasii*, and *Blastomyces dermatitidis* have been well recognized. All of these infections can occur as a result of reactivation or as an exogenous new infection. *Histoplasma capsulatum* is a soil-based pathogen which has been well recognized to be endemic in the Ohio-Mississippi River Valley region of the USA. Histoplasmosis is a relatively uncommon infection in solid organ transplant recipients, with an incidence of <1%, even in endemic regions. Histoplasmosis usually presents within the first 2 years after transplant, but there can be wide variability regarding the time of presentation [275–278]. In solid organ transplant recipients, it presents as progressive disseminated histoplasmosis that includes pulmonary and extrapulmonary manifestations such as hepatosplenomegaly, pancytopenia, and gastrointestinal and mucosal involvement. Coccidioidomycosis is endemic in the southwestern states including Southern California, as well as Mexico, and Central America. Most cases occur within the first year of transplant, with a reported incidence of 1.4–6.9% in endemic regions [279]. Due to depressed cellular immunity in solid organ transplant recipients, severe pneumonia, as well as dissemination to skin, bones, joints, meninges, and organ allograft can occur [280–283]. Patients with a prior history of coccidioidomycosis or a positive *Coccidioides* serology prior to transplantation should receive fluconazole prophylaxis after transplantation [280]. The endemic regions for blastomycosis include the Midwest, south central and southeastern regions of the USA, and provinces of Canada along the waterways. Blastomycosis is rare in solid organ transplant recipients, and an incidence of only 0.14% was noted over a 16-year observational period [284]. The treatment for the endemic mycoses includes a lipid preparation of amphotericin B and the azoles, and recommendations and guidelines for the diagnosis and management have been established [280].

Overall, a range of opportunistic infections may occur during this time of high immunosuppression post-LT, warranting a broad differential for patients presenting with infectious symptoms [285].

Community-Acquired/Late Infections

Beyond 6–12 months, graft function has ideally stabilized, and immunosuppressive medications can slowly be minimized. This decreases the net state of immunosuppression and consequently the risk of opportunistic infections; however, there is always some ongoing risk. Infections during this phase are typically community-acquired. A 5-year study at a large transplant center found a prevalence of 183 hospitalizations for infectious complications post-LT, with 145 (79%) occurring in the post-6-month period. The same study found respiratory infections to be the most frequent etiology overall for solid organ recipients, accounting for 26.9% of late infections. The next most common etiologies were sepsis/bacteremia (13.1%), liver/biliary tract (12.4%), genitourinary (12.2%), CMV (7.5%), and fever of unknown origin (8%) [286]. Community-acquired infections in post-transplant patients may also present with more severe clinical manifestations [287]. Less common pathogens, such as fungi, parasites, and mycobacteria, are also seen in the post-6-month period, sometimes related to diminished vigilance for environmental exposure prevention over time. Infections due to *Nocardia* spp. are relatively uncommon, with an overall incidence of 0.7–3.5% in solid organ transplant recipients and only a reported incidence of 0.1% in LT recipients [288–290]. The median time to the onset of *Nocardia* infection in a European cohort was 17.5 months after transplantation, and infection was associated with corticosteroid use, tacrolimus use, and elevated calcineurin trough levels within the preceding month; interestingly, the use of TMP/SMX was not protective [291]. Recently there has been an emergence of non-*Aspergillus* mold infections in the solid organ transplant patient population. The occurrence of these mold infections can have a bimodal distribution, and in one study, 37.8% occurred within 6 months of diagnosis, and 33% occurred >2 years from the time of transplantation. In that same study, the median time to development of an invasive mold infection in the LT recipients was 81 days [292]. The most common non-*Aspergillus* molds were the *Mucorales*, *Fusarium* spp., and *Scedosporium* spp. The most common sites of infection for these molds were the lungs, sinuses, skin, and dissemination to the central nervous system. The dematiaceous molds that include *Exophiala*, *Alternaria*, *Dactylaria*, *Curvularia*, *Cladophialophora*, *Verruconis gallopava*, and others have been reported in the solid organ transplant populations as case reports and small case series [293]. This group of molds most often manifests as skin and soft tissue infections but can disseminate to the central nervous system. In one case series, the median time to onset was 22 months after transplantation, and the cutaneous presentation was associated with a good outcome [294].

Viral infections associated with the presence of chronic immunosuppression can also occur and include late-onset CMV infection, EBV-associated PTLD, JC virus infection associated with progressive multifocal leukoencephalopathy (PML), and HHV-8 infection associated with Kaposi's sarcoma. Liver transplant recipients have an intermediate risk for the development of EBV-associated PTLD as compared to other solid organ transplant recipients. One center reported an incidence of PTLD in 6.3% of their pediatric LT recipients and an incidence of 1.2% in the adult LT recipients [295]. The cumulative incidence of PTLD in LT recipients has been estimated to be 1–2% over 5 years [296]. The highest risk factors for EBV-associated PTLD is due to primary infection as a result of an EBV D+/R− mismatch, in addition to a higher level of immunosuppression [297]. While the majority of cases occur within 1 year of transplantation, a 0.25% incidence has been noted in LT recipients at 1 year. Guidelines and recommendations have been established for the monitoring, diagnosis, and management of EBV-associated PTLD [298].

Infection with *Mycobacterium tuberculosis* (MTb) can occur during the period of maximal immunosuppression and well beyond that time period. Treatment of active MTb in all solid organ recipients poses a challenge for drug dosing, due to the strong interaction between rifampin (and other rifamycins) and calcineurin inhibitors or rapamycin. For LT recipients in particular, the likelihood of drug-induced hepatotoxicity is increased, warranting careful medication management [298]. Substitution of one or more first-line drugs may be needed, based on the liver function at baseline and during the course of treatment; frequent lab monitoring and consultation with a MTb expert is advised [143]. Directly observed therapy is generally preferred for transplant recipients and is vital when alternative regimens are employed. Some experts recommend a minimum 9-month treatment course for all solid organ transplant patients, due to a concern for increased mortality with shorter courses [299].

Individuals with chronic allograft dysfunction requiring higher maintenance immunosuppression should be considered at ongoing high risk for opportunistic disease and thus continued on appropriate prophylaxis as necessary.

Prophylaxis/Prevention of Infections

As detailed above, there are standard screening recommendations and protocols for prophylaxis against the most common opportunistic pathogens, particularly *P. jirovecii*, *CMV*, and *Candida* spp. Vaccination is another crucial prevention strategy. Despite the clear preventive benefits, vaccination rates have been suboptimal in LT recipients [300]. Due to chronic immune dysfunction, patients with advanced liver disease may have diminished antibody response to vaccination [301]. Consequently, it is advisable to administer vaccines as early as indicated [302]. Live vaccines are generally contraindicated post-transplant.

National guidelines for perioperative antibiotics recommend piperacillin-tazobactam or cefotaxime plus ampicillin as standard prophylaxis in liver transplantation; however, individual centers may vary their protocol [303]. A 4-year single-center review found that 53% of surgical site infections were caused by multidrug-resistant bacteria, emphasizing the need for a tailored prophylactic approach, based on patients' histories and local antibiotic resistance patterns [157].

Relapse of HBV and HCV Post-liver Transplantation

HBV reinfection rates of the allograft were previously reported to range between 80% and 100% in the 1980s. Based on 2-year graft survival of only 50%, many centers discontinued offering OLT in this population for a time [304]. Additionally, in the absence of antiviral therapy, some patients have developed fibrosing cholestatic hepatitis, a rapidly progressive and often fatal condition [305]. However, the introduction of HBIG and antiviral medications in the late 1980s has significantly improved post-transplant survival in such patients.

There are several risk factors for HBV reinfection after liver transplant. Patients at higher risk include those with positive hepatitis B e antigen (HBeAg), negative HBeAg but high HBV DNA level, or history of pre-transplant antiviral drug resistance. Patients at lower risk include those with cirrhosis and low HBV DNA level with or without antiviral medication, coinfection with hepatitis delta virus (HDV), or fulminant HBV infection [306].

Subclinical HBV reactivation has been reported in HBsAg-negative and HBcAb-positive recipients who have received livers from HBsAg-negative and HBcAb-negative recipients. However, this low-grade viral replication has not been associated with the development of positive HBsAg or active viral hepatitis. Therefore, antiviral therapy is not indicated in this scenario [307].

HCV infection recurs in the allograft in greater than 95% of HCV+ liver allograft recipients [308]. Advanced donor age and high-intensity immunosuppression such as the use of bolus steroids or thymoglobulin can influence the severity of HCV recurrence after OLT [309, 310]. Although the course of HCV recurrence may be variable after liver transplant; up to 20% of patients develop allograft cirrhosis within 5 years of transplantation [311]. HCV+ recipients have demonstrated lower patient and graft survival when compared to patients transplanted for other indications. HIV coinfection has also correlated with diminished post-transplant survival. Fibrosing cholestatic hepatitis is a rapidly progressive condition that develops in 5–10% of HCV+ liver transplant recipients, at times within the first year after transplant, and often leads to diminished survival [312]. Differentiating recurrent HCV from ACR can be difficult due to overlapping histologic features, but certain findings such as lobular or interface hepatitis and lymphoid follicles may be more suggestive of HCV infection.

HBV Prophylaxis

All patients with HBV infection prior to transplantation should be continued on antiviral therapy after undergoing OLT. Additionally, patients without HBV infection who receive livers from isolated HBcAb+ donors should also be started on antiviral therapy. Most often either entecavir or tenofovir are utilized, and the choice of a specific agent is made based on prior treatment history and side effect profiles of individual antiviral drug.

The role of HBIG in the current era remains unclear. Prior to the discovery of potent antiviral agents, HBIG was often used long-term as standard prophylaxis with reduction in the risk for HBV recurrence [313]. However, high-dose intravenous HBIG is expensive and may not provide additional benefit compared to the use of oral antiviral agents alone, especially in low-risk patients. In high-risk patients, HBIG may be discontinued after 1 year following transplantation.

HCV Treatment Post-liver Transplantation

Ideally, most patients with HCV should be treated with antiviral therapy prior to transplant. However, pre-transplant antiviral therapy may be difficult to tolerate and less effective in patients with decompensated cirrhosis. Specifically, the use of protease inhibitors for HCV is generally not recommended in patients with decompensated cirrhosis.

Currently, there are several options for treatment of genotype 1 HCV in post-OLT patients. Ledipasvir/sofosbuvir combination therapy after OLT with weight-based ribavirin for 24 weeks has been associated with a 96% SVR12 rate in patients with Metavir fibrosis stage F0 to F3 or those with compensated cirrhosis. In patients with decompensated cirrhosis, SVR rates range between 60% and 88% depending on degree of hepatic impairment [314]. Simeprevir and sofosbuvir with or without ribavirin for 12–24 weeks has been associated with SVR12 rates greater than 80% in both cirrhotic and non-cirrhotic patients [315, 316]. Daclatasvir in combination with sofosbuvir with or without ribavirin for 24 weeks after OLT demonstrated a 91% SVR12 rate in patients with severe recurrent HCV infection. The SVR12 rate was notably lower when daclatasvir was administered with simeprevir with or without ribavirin for 24 weeks [317]. The fixed-dose PrOD combination (paritaprevir, ritonavir, ombitasvir, dasabuvir) with ribavirin for 24 weeks resulted in a 96% SVR24 rate in patients with mild fibrosis, in whom the treatment commenced after transplantation [318]. CNI troughs must be monitored carefully with the use of simeprevir or paritaprevir. Newer regimens including elbasvir/grazoprevir and sofosbuvir/velpatasvir have yet to be studied in liver transplant population with HCV infection.

There are limited data for non-genotype 1 HCV infection in patients undergoing OLT. Daclatasvir in conjunction with sofosbuvir with or without ribavirin can be used in patients with genotype 2 or 3 HCV infection. Patients with genotype 4 HCV can be managed with either ledipasvir/sofosbuvir given with or without ribavirin or daclatasvir and sofosbuvir along with or without ribavirin. Sofosbuvir/velpatasvir has pangenotypic coverage and may be another option, although data in OLT recipients have yet to be reported.

Other Hepatitis Virus Infections After Transplantation

Hepatitis A Infection After Liver Transplant

Hepatitis A virus (HAV) is contracted through a fecal-oral route. Although most patients with HAV experience a self-limited course, acute liver failure may develop in less than 1% of infected individuals. Patients over 50 years of age and those with other chronic liver diseases are at higher risk to develop fulminant liver failure [319]. Accordingly, it is generally recommended that patients with chronic liver disease, including cirrhosis, should be vaccinated in the pre-transplant setting. Despite vaccination, a subset of anti-HAV IgG+ patients may lose anti-HAV IgG antibodies within the first 2 years after liver transplantation [320]. Whether loss of the anti-HAV IgG antibodies correlates with true loss of immunity and need for booster immunization(s) remains unclear. HAV vaccine is safe to administer in the post-transplant setting, although serologic response is often lower than seen in patients vaccinated prior to undergoing allograft transplantation [321]. Assuring receipt of two vaccine doses and deferring vaccination to a later time when the patient is on a lower level of immunosuppression may improve serologic response in patients requiring further vaccine doses after transplantation [322, 323]. The specific implications of HAV infection in patients undergoing liver transplantation are not well described. However, as this patient population tends to be older, and may develop chronic liver disease following OLT, the risk for severe HAV infection may be greater. Additionally, chronic drug-induced immunosuppression may promote HAV replication by subverting hosts' immune surveillance.

Hepatitis E Infection After Liver Transplant

Infection from the hepatitis E virus (HEV) was previously thought to be an uncommon disease in Western countries. Past reports had described a self-limited illness, which is noted more often in developing regions in Asia and Sub-Saharan Africa. However, HEV is being increasingly diagnosed in Europe and the USA, particularly over the past decade. Complications such as fulminant liver failure or severe hepatic decompensation have been described in a small minority of patients, particularly those who are pregnant or have chronic liver disease [324–326].

Traditionally, HEV transmission has been attributed to consumption of contaminated water and/or food, including pork products or venison. Due to its perceived rarity, most Western countries have not routinely tested blood or organ donors for HEV. However, a case of HEV transmission during blood transfusion was described in a patient following liver transplantation [327]. Additionally, there have been reports of potential cases of liver allograft-transmitted HEV infection with subsequent development of chronic hepatitis and cirrhosis of the transplanted allograft [328, 329].

In most immunocompetent individuals, HEV tends to cause an acute infection that resolves spontaneously. In contrast, chronic HEV infection defined as persistence of viral infection for greater than 3 months has been described in greater than 60% of solid organ transplant recipients following a primary HEV infection during the post-transplant period [330]. Among solid organ transplant (SOT), recipients of liver allografts are considered at highest risk for chronic HEV infection. Most infections are due to HEV genotype 3. In such patients, persistent HEV infection after transplantation may increase the risk for rapidly progressive hepatic fibrosis which may ultimately result in graft failure [331]. Extrahepatic manifestations of HEV infection such as cryoglobulinemia have also been reported in patients, including those who have undergone solid organ transplantation [332].

Studies from France have shown that incidence of HEV in patients undergoing OLT ranges between 2.8 and 4.8 per 100 person years [333, 334]. Due to the variable sensitivity of HEV-IgM assays and delayed IgG response after transplantation, HEV RNA may be a more useful test for the diagnosis of chronic HEV infection in such patients [335]. Furthermore, it is important to note that SOT recipients may still contract new HEV infection despite the presence of pre-transplant anti-HEV seropositivity [126].

Diagnosis of new HEV infection after transplantation should prompt a reduction in antirejection drug-related immune suppression; nearly a third of transplant recipients may resolve HEV chronic infection with this measure alone [123]. Specific immunosuppressive medications may correlate with risk of HEV persistence in transplant patients. In vitro studies have demonstrated increased HEV replication in the setting of tacrolimus, cyclosporine, and mTOR inhibitors [336, 337]. However, in one clinical study, liver or kidney transplant recipients who developed chronic HEV infection were more likely to have been on tacrolimus rather than cyclosporine [123]. In contrast, in vitro studies have demonstrated that mycophenolate mofetil reduces HEV replication, and this finding has been correlated in a clinical study where heart transplant patients taking mycophenolate mofetil were more likely to clear post-transplant HEV infection [338]. Corticosteroid use does not appear to affect HEV replication [129].

Patients with persistent HEV infection even after reduction of immunosuppression are candidates for antiviral therapy. In solid organ transplant recipients, ribavirin at a dose of 8 mg/kg given for at least 3 months can lead to sustained virologic response in the majority of patients [339]. Dose adjustments may be necessary based on renal function and during the course of therapy if patients develop medication-induced anemia. Smaller studies have demonstrated that PEG-interferon alpha over a 3–12 month period may lead to viral clearance, although treatment is associated with significant adverse effects and may precipitate graft rejection [340, 341].

Acknowledgments The authors express their deepest appreciation to Jonathan Kumar for his assistance with manuscript preparation.

References

1. Kamath PS, Wiesner RH, Malinchoc M, et al. A model to predict survival in patients with end-stage liver disease. Hepatology. 2001;33(2):464–70.
2. Merion RM, Schaubel DE, Dykstra DM, et al. The survival benefit of liver transplantation. Am J Transplant. 2005;5(2):307–13.
3. Angeli P, Wong F, Watson H, et al. Hyponatremia in cirrhosis: results of a patient population survey. Hepatology. 2006;44(6): 1535–42.
4. Kim WR, Biggins SW, Kremers WK, et al. Hyponatremia and mortality among patients on the liver-transplant waiting list. N Engl J Med. 2008;359(10):1018–26.
5. Ostapowicz G, Fontana RJ, Schiodt FV, et al. Results of a prospective study of acute liver failure at 17 tertiary care centers in the United States. Ann Intern Med. 2002;137(12):947–54.
6. Larson AM, Polson J, Fontana RJ, et al. Acetaminophen-induced acute liver failure: results of a United States multicenter, prospective study. Hepatology. 2005;42(6):1364–72.
7. Mazzaferro V, Regalia E, Doci R, et al. Liver transplantation for the treatment of small hepatocellular carcinomas in patients with cirrhosis. N Engl J Med. 1996;334(11):693–9.
8. Yao FY. Liver transplantation for hepatocellular carcinoma: beyond the Milan criteria. Am J Transplant. 2008;8(10):1982–9.
9. Darwish Murad S, Kim WR, Harnois DM, et al. Efficacy of neoadjuvant chemoradiation, followed by liver transplantation for perihilar cholangiocarcinoma at 12 US centers. Gastroenterology. 2012;143(1):88–98.
10. Mathurin P, Moreno C, Samuel D, et al. Early liver transplantation for severe alcoholic hepatitis. N Engl J Med. 2011;365(19):1790–800.
11. Terrault NA, Roland ME, Schiano T, et al. Outcomes of liver transplant recipients with hepatitis C and human immunodeficiency virus coinfection. Liver Transpl. 2012;18(6):716–26.
12. Abt PL, Desai NM, Crawford MD, et al. Survival following liver transplantation from controlled non-heart-beating donors: an increased incidence of biliary complications. Transplantation. 2004;239:87–92.
13. Manzarbeitia CY, Ortiz JA, Jeon H, et al. Long-term outcome of controlled non-heart-beating donor liver transplantation. Transplantation. 2004;78:211–5.
14. Mateo R, Cho Y, Singh G, et al. Risk factors for graft survival after liver transplantation from donation after cardiac death donors: an analysis of OPTN/UNOS data. Am J Transplant. 2006;6:791–6.
15. Lee KW, Simpkins CE, Montgomery RA, et al. Factors affecting graft survival after liver transplantation from donation after cardiac death donors. Transplantation. 2006;82:1683–8.
16. Freise CE, Gillespie BW, Koffron AJ, et al. Recipient morbidity after living and deceased donor liver transplantation: findings from the A2ALL retrospective cohort study. Am J Transplant. 2008;8(12):2569–79.
17. Olthoff KM, Smith AR, Abecassis M, et al. Defining long-term outcomes with living donor liver transplantation in North America. Ann Surg. 2015;262(3):465–75.

18. Wan P, Yu X, Xia Q. Operative outcomes of adult living donor liver transplantation and deceased donor liver transplantation: a systematic review and meta-analysis. Liver Transpl. 2014;20(4):425–36.
19. A definition of irreversible coma Report of the Ad Hoc Committee of the Harvard Medical School to Examine the Definition of Brain Death. JAMA. 1968;2015:337–40.
20. Guidelines for the determination of death Report of the medical consultants on the diagnosis of death to the President's Commission for the Study of Ethical Problems in Medicine and Biomedical and Behavioral Research. JAMA. 1981;246:2184–6.
21. Guideline three: minimum technical standards for EEG recording in suspected cerebral death. J Clinical Neurophysiol. 1994;11:10–3.
22. Roper AH, Kehne SM, Weschler L. Transcranial Doppler in brain death. Neurology. 1987;37:1733–5.
23. Wall WJ, Mimeault R, Grant DR, et al. The use of older donor livers for hepatic transplantation. Transplantation. 1990;49:377–81.
24. Cescon M, Grazi GL, Cucchetti A. Improving the outcome of liver transplantation with very old donors with updated selection and management criteria. Liver Transpl. 2000;14:672–9.
25. Nardo B, Masetti M, Urbani L, et al. Liver transplantation from donors aged 80 years and over: pushing the limit. Am J Transplant. 2004;4:1139–47.
26. Veretemati M, Sabatella G, Minola E. Morphometric analysis of primary graft non-function in liver transplantation. Histopathology. 2005;46:451–9.
27. Imber CJ, St Peter SD, Handa A, et al. Hepatic steatosis and its relationship to transplantation. Liver Transpl. 2002;8:415–23.
28. Feng S, Goodrich NP, Bragg-Gresham JL, et al. Characteristics associated with liver graft failure: the concept of a donor risk index. Am J Transplant. 2006;6:783–90.
29. Ellingson K, Seem D, Nowicki M, et al. Estimated risk of human immunodeficiency virus and hepatitis C virus infection among potential organ donors from 17 organ procurement organizations in the United States. Am J Transplant. 2011;11:1201–8.
30. Seem DL, Lee I, Umscheid CA, et al. PHS guideline for reducing human immunodeficiency virus, hepatitis B virus, and hepatitis C virus transmission through organ transplantation. Public Health Rep. 2013;128:247–343.
31. Munoz SJ. Use of hepatitis B core antibody-positive donors for liver transplantation. Liver Transpl. 2002;8(10 Suppl 1):S82–7.
32. Saab S, Waterman B, Chi AC, et al. Comparison of different immunoprophylaxis regimens after liver transplantation with hepatitis B core antibody-positive donors: a systematic review. Liver Transpl. 2010;16(3):300–7.
33. Vargas HE, Laskus T, Wang LF, et al. Outcome of liver transplantation in hepatitis C virus-infected patients who received hepatitis C virus-infected grafts. Gastroenterology. 1999;117(1):149–53.
34. Duffy JP, Hong JC, Farmer DG, et al. Vascular complications of orthotopic liver transplantation: experience in more than 4,200 patients. J Am Coll Surg. 2009;208(5):896–903.
35. Welling TH, Heidt DG, Englesbe MJ, et al. Biliary complications following liver transplantation in the model for end-stage liver disease era: effect of donor, recipient, and technical factors. Liver Transpl. 2008;14(1):73–80.
36. Jay CL, Lyuksemburg V, Ladner DP, et al. Ischemic cholangiopathy after controlled donation after cardiac death liver transplantation: a meta-analysis. Ann Surg. 2011;253(2):259–64.
37. Dacha S, Barad A, Martin J, et al. Association of hepatic artery stenosis and biliary strictures in liver transplant recipients. Liver Transpl. 2011;17(7):849–54.
38. Motschman TL, Taswell HF, Brecher ME, et al. Intraoperative blood loss and patient and graft survival in orthotopic liver transplantation: their relationship to clinical and laboratory data. Mayo Clin Proc. 1989;64(3):346–55.
39. U.S. Multicenter FK506 Liver Study Group. A comparison of tacrolimus (FK506) and cyclosporine for immunosuppression in liver transplantation. The U.S. Multicenter FK506 Liver Study Group. N Engl J Med. 1994;331(17):1110–5.
40. O'Grady JG, Burroughs A, Hardy P, et al. Tacrolimus versus microemulsified ciclosporin in liver transplantation: the TMC randomised controlled trial. Lancet. 2002;360(9340):1119–25.
41. McAlister VC, Haddad E, Renouf E, et al. Cyclosporin versus tacrolimus as primary immunosuppressant after liver transplantation: a meta-analysis. Am J Transplant. 2006;6(7):1578–85.
42. Asrani SK, Leise MD, West CP, et al. Use of sirolimus in liver transplant recipients with renal insufficiency: a systematic review and meta-analysis. Hepatology. 2010;52(4):1360–70.
43. Rogers CC, Johnson SR, Mandelbrot DA, et al. Timing of sirolimus conversion influences recovery of renal function in liver transplant recipients. Clin Transpl. 2009;23(6):887–96.
44. Sterneck M, Kaiser GM, Richter N, et al. Everolimus and early calcineurin inhibitor withdrawal: 3-year results from a randomized trial in liver transplantation. Am J Transplant. 2014;14(3):701–10.
45. Euvrard S, Morelon E, Rostaing L, et al. Sirolimus and secondary skin-cancer prevention in kidney transplantation. N Engl J Med. 2012;367(4):329–39.
46. Zimmerman MA, Trotter JF, Wachs M, et al. Sirolimus-based immunosuppression following liver transplantation for hepatocellular carcinoma. Liver Transpl. 2008;14(5):633–8.
47. Geissler EK, Schnitzbauer AA, Zulke C, et al. Sirolimus use in liver transplant recipients with hepatocellular carcinoma: a randomized, multicenter, open-label phase 3 trial. Transplantation. 2016;100(1):116–25.
48. Lake J, Patel D, David K, et al. The association between MMF and risk of progressive renal dysfunction and death in adult liver transplant recipients with HCV. Clin Transpl. 2009;23(1):108–15.
49. Vivarelli M, Burra P, La Barba G, et al. Influence of steroids on HCV recurrence after liver transplantation: a prospective study. J Hepatol. 2007;47(6):793–8.
50. Eckhoff DE, McGuire B, Sellers M, et al. The safety and efficacy of a two-dose daclizumab (zenapax) induction therapy in liver transplant recipients. Transplantation. 2000;69(9):1867–72.
51. Wiesner RH, Menon KV. Late hepatic allograft dysfunction. Liver Transpl. 2001;7(11 Supple 1):S60–73.
52. Thurairajah PH, Carbone M, Bridgestock H, et al. Late acute liver allograft rejection; a study of its natural history and graft survival in the current era. Transplantation. 2013;95(7):955–9.
53. Banff schema for grading liver allograft rejection: an international consensus document. Hepatology. 1997;25(3):658–63.
54. Wiesner RH, Batts KP, Krom RA. Severe ductopenic rejection following liver transplantation: incidence, time of onset, risk factors, treatment, and outcome. Liver Transpl Surg. 1999;5(5):388–400.
55. Wong F, Bernardi M, Balk R, et al. Sepsis in cirrhosis: report on the 7th meeting of the International Ascites Club. Gut. 2005;54:718–25.
56. Fernandez J, Arroyo V. Bacterial infections in cirrhosis: a growing problem with significant implications. Clin Liver Dis. 2013;2:102–5.
57. Bunchorntavakul C, Chamroonkul N, Chavalitdhamrong D. Bacterial infections in cirrhosis: a critical review and practical guidance. World J Hepatol. 2016;8(6):307–21.
58. Robinson MW, Harmon C, O'Farrelly C. Liver immunology and its role in inflammation and homeostasis. Cell Mol Immunol. 2016;13(3):267–76.
59. Bilzer M, Roggel F, Gerbes AL. Role of Kupffer cells in host defense and liver disease. Liver Int. 2006;26:1175–86.
60. Janeway CA. The immune system evolved to discriminate infectious nonself from noninfectious self. Immunol Today. 1992;13:11–6.
61. Takeuchi O, Akira S. Pattern recognition receptors and inflammation. Cell. 2010;140:805–20.
62. Kubes P, Mehal WZ. Sterile inflammation in the liver. Gastroenterology. 2012;143:1158–72.
63. Crispe IN. Immune tolerance in liver disease. Hepatology. 2014;60:2109–17.

64. Goel A, Gupta M, Aggarwal R. Gut microbiota and liver disease. J Gastroenterol Hepatol. 2014;29(6):1139–48.
65. Teltschik Z, Wiest R, Beisner J, et al. Intestinal bacterial translocation in rats with cirrhosis is related to compromised Paneth cell antimicrobial host defense. Hepatology. 2012;55:1154–63.
66. Steffen EK, Berg RD, Deitch EA. Comparison of translocation rates of various indigenous bacteria from the gastrointestinal tract to the mesenteric lymph node. J Infect Dis. 1988;157:1032–8.
67. Lakshmi CP, Ghoshal UC, Kumar S, et al. Frequency and factors associated with small intestinal bacterial overgrowth in patients with cirrhosis of the liver and extra hepatic portal venous obstruction. Dig Dis Sci. 2010;55:1142–8.
68. Gupta A, Dhiman RK, Kumari S, et al. Role of small intestinal bacterial overgrowth and delayed gastrointestinal transit time in cirrhotic patients with minimal hepatic encephalopathy. J Hepatol. 2010;53:849–55.
69. Liu Q, Duan ZP, Ha DK, et al. Symbiotic modulation of gut flora: effect on minimal hepatic encephalopathy in patients with cirrhosis. Hepatology. 2004;39:1441–9.
70. Assimakopoulos SF, Tsamandas AC, Tsiaoussis GI, et al. Altered intestinal tight junctions' expression in patients with liver cirrhosis: a pathogenetic mechanism of intestinal hyperpermeability. Eur J Clin Investig. 2012;42:439–46.
71. Assimakopoulos SF. Uncovering the molecular events associated with increased intestinal permeability in liver cirrhosis: the pivotal role of enterocyte tight junctions and future perspectives. J Hepatol. 2013;59:1144–6.
72. Saitoh O, Sugi K, Lojima K, et al. Increased prevalence of intestinal inflammation in patients with liver cirrhosis. World J Gastroenterol. 1999;5:391–6.
73. Lorenzo-Zuniga V, Bartoli R, Planas R, et al. Oral bile acids reduce bacterial overgrowth, bacterial translocation, and endotoxemia in cirrhotic rats. Hepatology. 2003;37:551–7.
74. Jenne CN, Kubes P. Immune surveillance by the liver. Nat Immunol. 2013;14(10):996–1006.
75. Guarner-Argente C, Sánchez E, Vidal S, et al. Toll-like receptor 4 D299G polymorphism and the incidence of infections in cirrhotic patients. Aliment Pharmacol Ther. 2010;31:1192–9.
76. Nischalke HD, Berger C, Aldenhoff K, et al. Toll-like receptor (TLR) 2 promoter and intron 2 polymorphisms are associated with increased risk for spontaneous bacterial peritonitis in liver cirrhosis. J Hepatol. 2011;55:1010–6.
77. Jalan R, Fernandez J, Wiest R, et al. Bacterial infections in cirrhosis: a position statement based on the EASL special conference 2013. J Hepatol. 2014;60:1310–24.
78. Tritto G, Bechlis Z, Stadlbauer V, et al. Evidence of neutrophil functional defect despite inflammation in stable cirrhosis. J Hepatol. 2011;55:574–81.
79. Doi H, Iyer TK, Carpenter E, et al. Dysfunctional B-cell activation in cirrhosis resulting from hepatitis C infection associated with disappearance of CD27-positive B-cell population. Hepatology. 2012;55:709–19.
80. Tian Z, Chen Y, Gao B. Natural killer cells in liver disease. Hepatology. 2013;57:1654–62.
81. Lario M, Munoz L, Ubeda M, et al. Defective thymopoiesis and poor peripheral homeostatic replenishment of T-helper cells cause T-cell lymphopenia in cirrhosis. J Hepatol. 2013;59:723–30.
82. Laso FJ, Madruga JI, Giron JA, et al. Decreased natural killer cytotoxic activity in chronic alcoholism is associated with alcohol liver disease but not active ethanol consumption. Hepatology. 1997;25:1096–100.
83. Wasmuth HE, Kunz D, Yagmur E, et al. Patients with acute on chronic liver failure display "sepsis like" immune paralysis. J Hepatol. 2005;42:195–201.
84. Gao B, Jeong WI, Tian Z. Liver: an organ with predominant innate immunity. Hepatology. 2008;47(2):729–36.
85. Ramadori G, Christ B. Cytokines and the hepatic acute-phase response. Semin Liver Dis. 1999;19(2):141–55.
86. Liu C, Xu Z, Gupta D, et al. Peptidoglycan recognition proteins: a novel family of four human innate immunity pattern recognition molecules. J Biol Chem. 2001;276(37):34686–94.
87. Albillos A, Lario M, Álvarez-Mon M. Cirrhosis-associated immune dysfunction: distinctive features and clinical relevance. J Hepatol. 2014;61:1385–96.
88. Runyon BA, Morrissey RL, Hoefs JC, et al. Opsonic activity of human ascitic fluid: a potentially important protective mechanism against spontaneous bacterial peritonitis. Hepatology. 1985;5(4):634–7.
89. Runyon BA. Patients with deficient ascitic fluid opsonic activity are predisposed to spontaneous bacterial peritonitis. Hepatology. 1988;8(3):632–5.
90. Rajkovic IA, Williams R. Abnormalities of neutrophil phagocytosis, intracellular killing and metabolic activity in alcoholic cirrhosis and hepatitis. Hepatology. 1986;6(2):252–62.
91. Szabo G, Saha B. Alcohol's effect on host defense. Alcohol Res. 2015;37(2):159–70.
92. Tandon P, Garcia-Tsao G. Bacterial infections, sepsis, and multiorgan failure in cirrhosis. Semin Liver Dis. 2008;28(1):26–42.
93. Bonnel AR, Bunchorntavakul C, Reddy KR. Immune dysfunction and infections in patients with cirrhosis. Clin Gastroenterol Hepatol. 2011;9:727–38.
94. Barnes PF, Arevalo C, Chan LS, Wong SF, Reynolds TB. A prospective evaluation of bacteremic patients with chronic liver disease. Hepatology. 1988;8:1099–103.
95. Fernández J, Navasa M, Gómez J, Colmenero J, Vila J, Arroyo V, Rodés J. Bacterial infections in cirrhosis: epidemiological changes with invasive procedures and norfloxacin prophylaxis. Hepatology. 2002;35:140–8.
96. Caly WR, Strauss E. A prospective study of bacterial infections in patients with cirrhosis. J Hepatol. 1993;18(3):353–8.
97. Brann OS. Infectious complications of cirrhosis. Curr Gastroenterol Rep. 2001;3:285–92.
98. Merli M, Lucidi C, Giannelli V, Giusto M, Riggio O, Falcone M, et al. Cirrhotic patients are at risk for health care-associated bacterial infections. Clin Gastroenterol Hepatol. 2010;8:979–85.
99. Bunchorntavakul C, Chavalitdhamrong D. Bacterial infections other than spontaneous bacterial peritonitis in cirrhosis. World J Hepatol. 2012;4:158–68.
100. McHutchison JG, Runyon BA. Spontaneous bacterial Peritonitis. In: Surawicz CM, Owen RL, editors. Gastrointestinal and hepatic infections. Philadelphia: WB Saunders; 1995. p. 455.
101. Bert F, Noussair L, Lambert-Zechovsky N, Valla D. Viridans group streptococci: an underestimated cause of spontaneous bacterial peritonitis in cirrhotic patients with ascites. Eur J Gastroenterol Hepatol. 2005;17:929–3.
102. Runyon BA. Introduction to the revised American Association for the Study of Liver Diseases Practice Guideline management of adult patients with ascites due to cirrhosis 2012. Hepatology. 2013;57:1651.
103. Mandell LA, Wunderink RG, Anzueto A, Bartlett JG, Campbell GD, Dean NC, et al. Infectious Diseases Society of America/American Thoracic Society consensus guidelines on the management of community-acquired pneumonia in adults. Clin Infect Dis. 2007;44(Suppl 2):S27–72.
104. Happel KI, Nelson S. Alcohol, immunosuppression, and the lung. Proc Am Thorac Soc. 2005;2:428–32.
105. Fuxench-Lopez Z, Ramirez-Ronda CH. Pharyngeal flora in ambulatory alcoholic patients: prevalence of gram-negative bacilli. Arch Intern Med. 1978;138:1815–6.
106. Marik PE. The clinical features of severe community-acquired pneumonia presenting as septic shock. Norasept II Study Investigators. J Crit Care. 2000;15:85–90.

107. Campillo B, Richardet JP, Kheo T, et al. Nosocomial spontaneous bacterial peritonitis and bacteremia in cirrhotic patients: impact of isolate type on prognosis and characteristics of infection. Clin Infect Dis. 2002;35:1–10.
108. Bernard B, Grangé JD, Khac EN, et al. Antibiotic prophylaxis for the prevention of bacterial infections in cirrhotic patients with gastrointestinal bleeding: a meta-analysis. Hepatology. 1999;29:1655–61.
109. Jia Y, Dwivedi A, Elhanafi S, et al. Low risk of bacteremia after endoscopic variceal therapy for esophageal varices: a systematic review and meta-analysis. Endosc Int Open. 2015;3(5): E409–17.
110. Sauerbruch T, Holl J, Ruckdeschel G, et al. Bacteremia associated with endoscopic sclerotherapy of oesophageal varices. Endoscopy. 1985;17(5):170–2.
111. Maulaz EB, de Mattos AA, Pereira-Lima J, et al. Bacteremia in cirrhotic patients submitted to endoscopic band ligation of esophageal varices. Arq Gastroenterol. 2003;40(3):166–72.
112. Cho SY, Kang CI, Kim J, et al. Association of liver cirrhosis with group B streptococcal bacteremia in non-pregnant adults. J Infect. 2013;67(6):617–9.
113. Xiol X, Castellví JM, Guardiola J, et al. Spontaneous bacterial empyema in cirrhotic patients: a prospective study. Hepatology. 1996;23:719–23.
114. Chen TA, Lo GH, Lai KH. Risk factors for spontaneous bacterial empyema in cirrhotic patients with hydrothorax. J Chin Med Assoc. 2003;66:579–86.
115. Chen CH, Shih CM, Chou JW, et al. Outcome predictors of cirrhotic patients with spontaneous bacterial empyema. Liver Int. 2011;31:417–24.
116. Michels K, Nemeth E, Ganz T, et al. Hepcidin and host defense against infectious diseases. PLoS Pathog. 2015;11:e1004998.
117. Milic S, Mikolasevic I, Orlic L, et al. The role of iron and iron overload in chronic liver disease. Med Sci Monit. 2016;22:2144–51.
118. Arezes J, Jung G, Gabayan V, et al. Hepcidin-induced hypoferremia is a critical host defense mechanism against the siderophilic bacterium Vibrio vulnificus. Cell Host Microbe. 2015;17(1):47–57.
119. Khan FA, Fisher MA, Khakis RA. Association of hemochromatosis with infectious diseases: expanding spectrum. Int J Infect Dis. 2007;11(6):482–7.
120. Blake PA, Merson MH, Weaver RE, et al. Disease caused by a marine Vibrio. Clinical characteristics and epidemiology. N Engl J Med. 1979;300:1.
121. Dechet AM, Yu PA, Koram N. Non-foodborne Vibrio infections: an important cause of morbidity and mortality in the United States, 1997–2006. Clin Infect Dis. 2008;46:970.
122. Tacket CO, Brenner F, Blake PA. Clinical features and an epidemiological study of Vibrio vulnificus infections. J Infect Dis. 1984;149:558.
123. Jones MK, Oliver JD. Vibrio vulnificus: disease and pathogenesis. Infect Immun. 2009;77:1723.
124. Yoder JS, Hlavsa MC, Craun GF, et al. Surveillance for waterborne disease and outbreaks associated with recreational water use and other aquatic facility-associated health events – United States, 2005–2006. MMWR Surveill Summ. 2008;57:1.
125. Liu JW, Lee IK, Tang HJ, et al. Prognostic factors and antibiotics in Vibrio vulnificus septicemia. Arch Intern Med. 2006;166(19):2117.
126. Ko WC, Chuang YC. Aeromonas bacteremia: review of 59 episodes. Clin Infect Dis. 1995;20:1298–304.
127. Choi JP, Lee SO, Kwon HH, et al. Clinical significance of spontaneous Aeromonas bacterial peritonitis in cirrhotic patients: a matched case-control study. Clin Infect Dis. 2008;47(1):66–72.
128. Alcañiz JP, de Cuenca Morón B, Gómez Rubio M, et al. Spontaneous bacterial peritonitis due to Plesiomonas shigelloides. Am J Gastroenterol. 1995;90:1529–30.
129. Patel S, Gandhi D, Mehta V, et al. Plesiomonas shigelloides: an extremely rare cause of spontaneous bacterial peritonitis. Acta Gastroenterol Belg. 2016;79(1):52–3.
130. Centers for Disease Control and Prevention (CDC). Red blood cell transfusions contaminated with Yersinia enterocolitica – United States, 1991–1996, and initiation of a national study to detect bacteria-associated transfusion reactions. MMWR Morb Mortal Wkly Rep. 1997;46:553.
131. van Asbeck BS, Verbrugh HA, van Oost BA, et al. *Listeria monocytogenes* meningitis and decreased phagocytosis associated with iron overload. Br Med J (Clin Res Ed). 1982;284(6315):524.
132. Mossey RT, Sondheimer J. Listeriosis in patients with long-term hemodialysis and transfusional iron overload. Am J Med. 1985;79:397.
133. Mook P, O'Brien SJ, Gillespie IA. Concurrent conditions and human listeriosis, England, 1999–2009. Emerg Infect Dis. 2011;17:38.
134. Winston DJ, Emmanouilides C, Busuttil RW. Infections in liver transplant recipients. Clin Infect Dis. 1995;21:1077–91.
135. Fishman JA. Infection in solid-organ transplant recipients. N Engl J Med. 2007;357(25):2601–14.
136. Fishman JA. Infection in organ transplantation. Am J Transplant. 2017;17(4):856–79.
137. Domen RE, Nelson KA. Results of a survey of infectious disease testing practices by organ procurement organization in the United States. Transplantation. 1997;63(12):1790–4.
138. Delmonico FL, Snydman DR. Organ donor screening for infectious diseases: review of practice and implications for transplantation. Transplantation. 1998;65(5):603–10.
139. Fischer SA, Lu K, the AST Infectious Diseases Community of Practice. Screening of donor and recipient in solid organ transplantation. Am J Transplant. 2013;13:9–21.
140. Cohn DL, O'Brien RJ, Geiter LJ, et al. Targeted tuberculin testing and treatment of latent tuberculosis infection. American Thoracic Society. MMWR Recomm Rep. 2000;49(RR-6):1–51.
141. Mazurek GH, Jerob J, Vernon A, et al. Updated guidelines for using interferon gamma release assays to detect mycobacterium tuberculosis infection – United States, 2010. MMWR Recomm Rep. 2010;59(RR05):1–25.
142. Schirren CA, Jung MC, Zachoval R, et al. Analysis of T-cell activation pathways in patients with liver cirrhosis, impaired delayed hypersensitivity and other T-cell dependent functions. Clin Exp Immunol. 1997;108:144–50.
143. Lindemann M, Dioury Y, Beckebaum S, et al. Diagnosis of tuberculosis infection in patients awaiting liver transplantation. Hum Immunol. 2009;70:24–8.
144. Casas S, Munoz L, Moure R, et al. Comparison of the 2-step tuberculin skin test and the quantiFERON-TB gold in-tube test for the screening of tuberculosis infection before liver transplantation. Liver Transpl. 2011;17(10):1205–11.
145. Theodoropoulos N, Lanternier F, Rassiwala J, et al. Use of the QuantiFERON-TB gold interferon-gamma release assay for screening transplant candidates: a single-center retrospective study. Transpl Infect Dis. 2012;14(1):1–8.
146. Subramanian AK, Morris MI, the AST Infectious Diseases Community of Practice. Mycobacterium tuberculosis infections in solid organ transplantation. Am J Transplant. 2013;13: 68–76.
147. Pai M, Zwerling A, Menzies D. Systematic review: T-cell-based assays for the diagnosis of latent tuberculosis infection: an update. Ann Intern Med. 2008;149:177–84.
148. Jhang AW, Tran T, Bui L, et al. Safety of treatment of latent tuberculosis infection in compensated cirrhotic patients during transplant candidacy period. Transplantation. 2007;83:1557–62.
149. Singh N, Wagener MM, Gayowski T. Safety and efficacy of isoniazid chemoprophylaxis administered during liver transplant

candidacy for the prevention of post-transplant tuberculosis. Transplantation. 2002;74:892–5.
150. Centers for Disease Control and Prevention. Targeted tuberculin testing and treatment of latent tuberculosis infection. MMWR. 2000;49(No.RR-6):7.
151. Torre-Cisneros J, San-Juan R, Rosso-Fernández CM, et al. Tuberculosis prophylaxis with levofloxacin in liver transplant patients is associated with a high incidence of tenosynovitis: safety analysis of a multicenter randomized trial. Clin Infect Dis. 2015;60(11):1642–9.
152. Del Pilar Hernandez M, Martin P, Simkins J. Infectious complications after liver transplantation. Gastroenterol Hepatol. 2015;11(11):741–53.
153. Kaltenborn A, Gutcke A, Gwiasda J, et al. Biliary complications following liver transplantation: single center experience over three decades and recent risk factors. World J Hepatol. 2017;9(3):147–54.
154. Tachopoulou OA, Vogt DP, Henderson JM, et al. Hepatic abscess after liver transplantation: 1990–2000. Transplantation. 2003;72(1):79–83.
155. Santos CA, Hotchkiss RS, Chapman WC, et al. Epidemiology of bloodstream infections in a multicenter retrospective cohort of liver transplant recipients. Transplant Dir. 2016;2(3):e67.
156. Freire MP, Soares Oshiro IC, Bonazzi PR, et al. Surgical site infections in liver transplant recipients in the model for end-stage liver disease era: an analysis of the epidemiology, risk factors, and outcomes. Liver Transpl. 2013;19(9):1011–9.
157. Viehman JA, Clancy CJ, Clarke L, et al. Surgical site infections after liver transplantation: emergence of multidrug-resistant bacteria and implications for prophylaxis and treatment strategies. Transplantation. 2016;100:2107–14.
158. Weiner LM, Fridkin SK, Aponte-Torres Z, et al. Vital signs: preventing antibiotic-resistant infections in hospitals – United States, 2014. Am J Transplant. 2016;16(7):2224–30.
159. Weiner LM, Webb AK, Limbago B, et al. Antimicrobial-resistant pathogens associated with healthcare-associated infections: summary of data reported to the National Healthcare Safety Network at the Centers for Disease Control and Prevention, 2011–2014. Infect Control Hosp Epidemiol. 2016;37(11):1288–301.
160. van Duin D, van Delden C, the AST Infectious Diseases Community of Practice. Multidrug-resistant gram-negative bacteria infections in solid organ transplantation. Am J Transplant. 2013;13(suppl 4):31–41.
161. Santoro-Lopes G, de Gouvêa EF. Multidrug-resistant bacterial infections after liver transplantation: an ever-growing challenge. World J Gastroenterol. 2014;20(20):6201–10.
162. Linares L, Cervera C, Hoyo I, et al. *Klebsiella pneumoniae* infection in solid organ transplant recipients: epidemiology and antibiotic resistance. Transplant Proc. 2010;42(8):2941–3.
163. Bert F, Larroque B, Paugam-Burtz C, et al. Pretransplant fecal carriage of extended-spectrum β-lactamase-producing Enterobacteriaceae and infection after liver transplant, France. Emerg Infect Dis. 2012;18:908–16.
164. Rebuck JA, Olsen KM, Fey PD, et al. Characterization of an outbreak due to extended-spectrum beta-lactamase-producing *Klebsiella pneumoniae* in a pediatric intensive care unit transplant population. Clin Infect Dis. 2000;31:1368–72.
165. Winters HA, Parbhoo RK, Schafer JJ, et al. Extended-spectrum beta-lactamase-producing bacterial infections in adult solid organ transplant recipients. Ann Pharmacother. 2011;45:309–16.
166. Cervera C, Agustí C, Angeles Marcos M, et al. Microbiologic features and outcome of pneumonia in transplanted patients. Diagn Microbiol Infect Dis. 2006;55:47–54.
167. Shi SH, Kong HS, Xu J, et al. Multidrug resistant gram-negative bacilli as predominant bacteremic pathogens in liver transplant recipients. Transpl Infect Dis. 2009;11:405–12.
168. Liu H, Ye Q, Wan Q, et al. Predictors of mortality in solid-organ transplant recipients with infections caused by Acinetobacter baumannii. Ther Clin Risk Manag. 2015;11:1251–7.
169. Ye QF, Zhao J, Wan QQ, et al. Frequency and clinical outcomes of ESKAPE bacteremia in solid organ transplantation and the risk factors for mortality. Transpl Infect Dis. 2014;16:767–74.
170. Shields RK, Clancy CJ, Gillis LM, et al. Epidemiology, clinical characteristics and outcomes of extensively drug-resistant Acinetobacter baumannii infections among solid organ transplant recipients. PLoS One. 2012;7:e52349.
171. Kim YJ, Yoon JH, Kim SI, Hong KW, Kim JI, Choi JY, et al. High mortality associated with Acinetobacter species infection in liver transplant patients. Transplant Proc. 2011;43:2397–9.
172. Pereira MR, Scully BF, Pouch SM, et al. Risk factors and outcomes of carbapenem-resistant *Klebsiella pneumoniae* infections in liver transplant recipients. Liver Transpl. 2015;21:1511–9.
173. Bergamasco MD, Barros O, Barbosa M, et al. Infection with *Klebsiella pneumoniae* carbapenemase (KPC)-producing *K. pneumoniae* in solid organ transplantation. Transpl Infect Dis. 2012;14:198–205.
174. Kalpoe JS, Sonnenberg E, Factor SH, et al. Mortality associated with carbapenem-resistant *Klebsiella pneumoniae* infections in liver transplant recipients. Liver Transpl. 2012;18:468–74.
175. Giannella M, Bartoletti M, Morelli MC, et al. Risk factors for infection with carbapenem-resistant *Klebsiella pneumoniae* after liver transplantation: the importance of pre- and posttransplant colonization. Am J Transplant. 2015;15:1708–15.
176. Lübbert C, Becker-Rux D, Rodloff AC, et al. Colonization of liver transplant recipients with KPC-producing *Klebsiella pneumoniae* is associated with high infection rates and excess mortality: a case-control analysis. Infection. 2014;42:309–16.
177. Barchiesi F, Montalti R, Castelli P, et al. Carbapenem-resistant *Klebsiella pneumoniae* influences the outcome of early infections in liver transplant recipients. BMC Infect Dis. 2016;16(1):538.
178. Mills JP, Wilck MB, Weikert BC, et al. Successful treatment of a disseminated infection with extensively drug-resistant *Klebsiella pneumoniae* in a liver transplant recipient with a fosfomycin-based multidrug regimen. Transpl Infect Dis. 2016;18(5):777–81.
179. Ziakas PD, Pliakos EE, Zervou FN, et al. MRSA and VRE colonization in solid organ transplantation: a meta-analysis of published studies. Am J Transplant. 2014;14:1887–94.
180. de Gouvea EF, Castelo Branco R, Monteiro RC, et al. Surveillance for vancomycin-resistant enterococci colonization among patients of a liver transplant program. Transpl Int. 2005;18:1218–20.
181. Hagen EA, Lautenbach E, Olthoff K, et al. Low prevalence of colonization with vancomycin-resistant Enterococcus in patients awaiting liver transplantation. Am J Transplant. 2003;3:902–5.
182. Bakir M, Bova JL, Newell KA, et al. Epidemiology and clinical consequences of vancomycin-resistant enterococci in liver transplant patients. Transplantation. 2001;72:1032–7.
183. McNeil SA, Malani PN, Chenoweth CE, et al. Vancomycin-resistant enterococcal colonization and infection in liver transplant candidates and recipients: a prospective surveillance study. Clin Infect Dis. 2006;42:195–203.
184. Orloff SL, Busch AM, Olyaei AJ, et al. Vancomycin-resistant Enterococcus in liver transplant patients. Am J Surg. 1999;177:418–22.
185. El-Khoury J, Fishman JA. Linezolid in the treatment of vancomycin-resistant enterococcus faecium in solid organ transplant recipients: report of a multicenter compassionate-use trial. Transpl Infect Dis. 2003;5:121–5.
186. Calfee DP, Salgado CD, Milstone AM, et al. Strategies to prevent methicillin-resistant *Staphylococcus aureus* transmission and infection in acute care hospitals: 2014 update. Infect Control Hosp Epidemiol. 2014;35(suppl 2):S108–32.

187. Singh N, Paterson DL, Chang FY, Gayowski T, Squier C, Wagener MM, Marino IR. Methicillin-resistant *Staphylococcus aureus*: the other emerging resistant gram-positive coccus among liver transplant recipients. Clin Infect Dis. 2000;30:322–7.
188. Hand J, Patel G. Multidrug-resistant organisms in liver transplant: mitigating risk and managing infections. Liver Transpl. 2016;22(8):1143–53.
189. Frenette C, Sperlea D, Leharova Y, et al. Impact of an infection control and antimicrobial stewardship program on solid organ transplantation and hepatobiliary surgical site infections. Infect Control Hosp Epidemiol. 2016;37(12):1468–74.
190. Ramos A, Ortiz J, Asensio Á, et al. Risk factors for Clostridium difficile diarrhea in patients with solid organ transplantation. Prog Transplant. 2016;26(3):231–7.
191. Albright JB, Bonatti H, Mendez J, et al. Early and late onset Clostridium difficile-associated colitis following liver transplantation. Transpl Int. 2007;20(10):856–66.
192. Sullivan T, Weinberg A, Rana M, et al. The epidemiology and clinical features of Clostridium difficile infection in liver transplant recipients. Transplantation. 2016;100(9):1939–43.
193. Andes DR, Safdar N, Baddley JW, et al. The epidemiology and outcomes of invasive Candida infections among organ transplant recipients in the United States: results of the transplant-associated infection surveillance network (TRANSNET). Transpl Infect Dis. 2016;18(6):921–31.
194. Silveira FP, Kusne S, the AST Infectious Diseases Community of Practice. Candida infections in solid organ transplantation. Am J Transplant. 2013;13(Suppl 4):220–7.
195. Husain S, Tollemar J, Dominguez EA, et al. Changes in the spectrum and risk factors for invasive candidiasis in liver transplant recipients: prospective, multicenter, case-controlled study. Transplantation. 2003;75(12):2023–9.
196. Singh N, Winston DJ, Limaye AP, et al. Performance characteristics of galactomannan and b-d-Glucan in high-risk liver transplant recipients. Transplantation. 2015;99(12):2543–50.
197. Pappas PJ, Kauffman CA, Andes DR. Clinical practice guideline for the management of candidiasis: 2016 update by the Infectious Diseases Society of America. Clin Infect Dis. 2016;62(4):e1–50.
198. Winston DJ, Pakrasi A, Busuttil RW. Prophylactic fluconazole in liver transplant recipients. A randomized, double-blind, placebo-controlled trial. Ann Intern Med. 1999;131(10):729–3.
199. Kusne S, Tobin D, Pasculle AW, et al. Candida carriage in the alimentary tract of liver transplant candidates. Transplantation. 1994;57(3):398–402.
200. Giannella M, Bartoletti M, Morelli M, et al. Antifungal prophylaxis in liver transplant recipients: one size does not fit all. Transpl Infect Dis. 2016;18(4):538–44.
201. Wajszczuk CP, Dummer JS, Ho M, et al. Fungal infections in liver transplant recipients. Transplantation. 1985;40(4):347–53.
202. Sganga G, Bianco G, Frongillo F, et al. Fungal infections after liver transplantation: incidence and outcome. Transplant Proc. 2014;46(7):2314–8.
203. Morgan J, Wannemuehler KA, Marr KA, et al. Incidence of invasive aspergillosis following hematopoietic stem cell and solid organ transplantation: interim results of a prospective multicenter surveillance program. Med Mycol. 2005;43(Suppl 1):S49–58.
204. Pappas PA, Alexander BD, Andes AR, et al. Invasive fungal infections among organ transplant recipients: results of the Transplant-Associated Infection Surveillance Network (TRANSNET). Clin Infect Dis. 2010;50(8):1101–11.
205. Fortún J, Martín-Dávila P, Moreno S, et al. Risk factors for invasive aspergillosis in liver transplant recipients. Liver Transpl. 2002;8(11):1065–70.
206. Paterson DL, Singh N. Invasive aspergillosis in transplant recipients. Medicine (Baltimore). 1999;78(2):123–38.
207. Singh N, Arnow P, Bonham A, et al. Invasive aspergillosis in liver transplant recipients in the 1990s. Transplantation. 1997;64(5):716–20.
208. Gavalda J, Len O, San Juan R, et al. Risk factors for invasive aspergillosis in solid-organ transplant recipients: a case-control study. Clin Infect Dis. 2005;41:52–9.
209. Singh N, Avery RK, Munoz P, et al. Trends in risk profiles for and mortality associated with invasive aspergillosis among liver transplant recipients. Clin Infect Dis. 2003;36:46–52.
210. Singh N, Husain S, the AST Infectious Diseases Community of Practice. Aspergillosis in solid organ transplantation. Am J Transplant. 2013;13(Suppl 4):228–41.
211. Husain S, Paterson DL, Studer SM, et al. Aspergillus galactomannan antigen in the bronchoalveolar lavage fluid for the diagnosis of invasive aspergillosis in lung transplant recipients. Transplantation. 2007;83(10):1330–6.
212. Patterson TF, Thompson GR, Denning DW, et al. Practice guidelines for the diagnosis and management of Aspergillosis: 2016 update by the Infectious Diseases Society of America. Clin Infect Dis. 2016;63(4):433–42.
213. Balogh J, Gordon Burroughs S, Boktour M, et al. Efficacy and cost-effectiveness of voriconazole prophylaxis for prevention of invasive aspergillosis in high-risk liver transplant recipients. Liver Transpl. 2016;22(2):163–70.
214. Winston DJ, Limaye AP, Pelletier S, et al. Randomized, double-blind trial of anidulafungin versus fluconazole for prophylaxis of invasive fungal infections in high-risk liver transplant recipients. Am J Transplant. 2014;14(12):2758–64.
215. Perrella A, Esposito C, Amato G, et al. Antifungal prophylaxis with liposomal amphotericin B and caspofungin in high-risk patients after liver transplantation: impact on fungal infections and immune system. Infect Dis (Lond). 2016;48(2):161–6.
216. Fortún J, Muriel A, Martín-Dávila P, et al. Caspofungin versus fluconazole as prophylaxis of invasive fungal infection in high-risk liver transplantation recipients: a propensity score analysis. Liver Transpl. 2016;22(4):427–35.
217. Echenique IA, Ison MG. Update on donor derived infections in liver transplantation. Liver Transpl. 2013;19(6):575–85.
218. Collins GM, Dubernard JM, Land W, et al. Procurement, preservation and allocation of vascularized organs. London: Kluwer Academic Publishers; 1997.
219. Doucette KE, Al-Saif M, Kneteman N, et al. Donor-derived bacteremia in liver transplant recipients despite antibiotic prophylaxis. Am J Transplant. 2013;13(4):1080–3.
220. Miceli MH, Gonulalan M, Perri MB, et al. Transmission of infection to liver transplant recipients from donors with infective endocarditis: lessons learned. Transpl Infect Dis. 2015;17(1):140–6.
221. Caballero F, Lopez-Navidad A, Domingo P, et al. Successful transplantation of organs retrieved from a donor with enterococcal endocarditis. Transpl Int. 1998;11:387–9.
222. Ison MG, Nalesnik MA. An update on donor-derived disease transmission in organ transplantation. Am J Transplant. 2011;11:1123–30.
223. Ison MG, Grossi P, AST Infectious Diseases Community of Practice. Donor-derived infections in solid organ transplantation. Am J Transplant. 2013;13:22–30.
224. Ison MG, Hager J, Blumberg E, et al. Donor-derived disease transmission events in the United States: data reviewed by the OPTN/UNOS Disease Transmission Advisory Committee. Am J Transplant. 2009;9(8):1929–35.
225. Singh N, Huprikar S, Burdette SD, for American Society of Transplantation, Infectious Diseases Community of Practice, Donor-Derived Fungal Infection Working Group, et al. Donor-derived fungal infections in organ transplant recipients: guidelines of the American Society of Transplantation, Infectious Diseases Community of Practice. Am J Transplant. 2012;12:2414–28.

226. Morris MI, Daly JS, Blumberg E, et al. Diagnosis and management of tuberculosis in transplant donors: a donor-derived infections consensus conference report. Am J Transplant. 2012;12:2288–300.
227. Wakelin SJ, Casey J, Robertson A, et al. The incidence and importance of bacterial contaminants of cadaveric renal perfusion fluid. Transpl Int. 2005;17:680–6.
228. Ruiz P, Gastaca M, Gonzalez J, et al. Incidence and clinical relevance of bacterial contamination in preservation solution for liver transplantation. Transplant Proc. 2009;41:2169–71.
229. Janny S, Bert F, Dondero F, et al. Microbiological findings of culture-positive preservation fluid in liver transplantation. Transpl Infect Dis. 2011;13:9–14.
230. Baddley JW, Schain DC, Gupte AA, et al. Transmission of *Cryptococcus neoformans* by organ transplantation. Clin Infect Dis. 2011;52:e94–8.
231. Kanj SS, Welty-Wolf K, Madden J, et al. Fungal infections in lung and heart-lung transplant recipients. Report of 9 cases and review of the literature. Medicine (Baltimore). 1996;75:142–56.
232. Ooi BS, Chen BT, Lim CH, et al. Survival of a patient transplanted with a kidney infected with *Cryptococcus neoformans*. Transplantation. 1971;11:428–9.
233. Centers for Disease Control and Prevention (CDC). Transplantation-transmitted tuberculosis – Oklahoma and Texas, 2007. MMWR Morb Mortal Wkly Rep. 2008;57:333–6.
234. Kotton CN, Lattes R, for AST Infectious Diseases Community of Practice. Parasitic infections in solid organ transplant recipients. Am J Transplant. 2009;9(suppl 4):S234–51.
235. Hamilton KW, Abt PL, Rosenbach MA, et al. Donor-derived Strongyloides stercoralis infections in renal transplant recipients. Transplantation. 2011;91:1019–24.
236. Chin-Hong PV, Schwartz BS, Bern C, et al. Screening and treatment of Chagas disease in organ transplant recipients in the United States: recommendations from the Chagas in Transplant Working Group. Am J Transplant. 2011;11:672–80.
237. Altclas JD, Barcan L, Nagel C, et al. Organ transplantation and Chagas disease. JAMA. 2008;299:1134.
238. Ljungman P, Griffiths P, Paya C. Definitions of cytomegalovirus infection and disease in transplant recipients. Clin Infect Dis. 2002;34:1094–7.
239. Paya CV, Hermans PE, Wiesner RH, et al. Cytomegalovirus hepatitis in liver transplantation: prospective analysis of 93 consecutive orthotopic liver transplantations. J Infect Dis. 1989;160:752–8.
240. Gane E, Saliba F, Valdecasas GJ, et al. Randomised trial of efficacy and safety of oral ganciclovir in the prevention of cytomegalovirus disease in liver-transplant recipients. The Oral Ganciclovir International Transplantation Study Group [corrected]. Lancet. 1997;350:1729–33.
241. Paya C, Humar A, Dominguez E, et al. Efficacy and safety of valganciclovir vs. oral ganciclovir for prevention of cytomegalovirus disease in solid organ transplant recipients. Am J Transplant. 2004;4:611–20.
242. Razonable RR, van Cruijsen H, Brown RA, et al. Dynamics of cytomegalovirus replication during preemptive therapy with oral ganciclovir. J Infect Dis. 2003;187:1801–8.
243. Singh N, Wannstedt C, Keyes L, et al. Who among cytomegalovirus-seropositive liver transplant recipients is at risk for cytomegalovirus infection? Liver Transpl. 2005;11:700–4.
244. Arthurs SK, Eid AJ, Pedersen RA, et al. Delayed-onset primary cytomegalovirus disease after liver transplantation. Liver Transpl. 2007;13:1703–9.
245. Razonable RR. Epidemiology of cytomegalovirus disease in solid organ and hematopoietic stem cell transplant recipients. Am J Health Syst Pharm. 2005;62:S7–S13.
246. Razonable RR, Rivero A, Rodriguez A, et al. Allograft rejection predicts the occurrence of late-onset cytomegalovirus (CMV) disease among CMV-mismatched solid organ transplant patients receiving prophylaxis with oral ganciclovir. J Infect Dis. 2001;184:1461–4.
247. Singh N. Late-onset cytomegalovirus disease as a significant complication in solid organ transplant recipients receiving antiviral prophylaxis: a call to heed the mounting evidence. Clin Infect Dis. 2005;40(5):704–8.
248. Kim JM, Kim SJ, Joh JW, et al. Early and delayed onset cytomegalovirus infection of liver transplant recipients in endemic areas. Transplant Proc. 2010;42:884–9.
249. Razonable RR, Paya CV. Infections and allograft rejection – intertwined complications of organ transplantation. Swiss Med Wkly. 2005;135:571–3.
250. O'Grady JG, Alexander GJ, Sutherland S, et al. Cytomegalovirus infection and donor/recipient HLA antigens: interdependent cofactors in pathogenesis of vanishing bile-duct syndrome after liver transplantation. Lancet. 1988;2:302–5.
251. Noack KB, Wiesner RH, Batts K, et al. Severe ductopenic rejection with features of vanishing bile duct syndrome: clinical, biochemical, and histologic evidence for spontaneous resolution. Transplant Proc. 1991;23:1448–51.
252. Ludwig J, Wiesner RH, Batts KP, et al. The acute vanishing bile duct syndrome (acute irreversible rejection) after orthotopic liver transplantation. Hepatology. 1987;7:476–83.
253. Gao LH, Zheng SS. Cytomegalovirus and chronic allograft rejection in liver transplantation. World J Gastroenterol. 2004;10(13):1857–61.
254. Pastacaldi S, Teixeira R, Montalto P, et al. Hepatic artery thrombosis after orthotopic liver transplantation: a review of nonsurgical causes. Liver Transpl. 2001;7:75–81.
255. Madalosso C, de Souza NF Jr, Ilstrup DM, et al. Cytomegalovirus and its association with hepatic artery thrombosis after liver transplantation. Transplantation. 1998;66:294–7.
256. Munoz-Price LS, Slifkin M, Ruthazer R, et al. The clinical impact of ganciclovir prophylaxis on the occurrence of bacteremia in orthotopic liver transplant recipients. Clin Infect Dis. 2004;39(9):1293–9.
257. George MJ, Snydman DR, Werner BG, et al. The independent role of cytomegalovirus as a risk factor for invasive fungal disease in orthotopic liver transplant recipients. Boston center for liver transplantation cmvig-study group. Cytogam, Medimmune, Inc. Gaithersburg, Maryland. Am J Med. 1997;103(2):106–13.
258. Walker RC, Marshall WF, Strickler JG, et al. Pretransplantation assessment of the risk of lymphoproliferative disorder. Clin Infect Dis. 1995;20(5):1346–53.
259. Stratta RJ, Shaefer MS, Markin RS, et al. Clinical patterns of cytomegalovirus disease after liver transplantation. Arch Surg. 1989;124(12):1443–50.
260. Razonable RR. Cytomegalovirus infection after liver transplantation: current concepts and challenges. World J Gastroenterol. 2008;14(31):4849–60. Epub 2008/08/30.
261. Singh N, Dummer JS, Kusne S, et al. Infections with cytomegalovirus and other herpesviruses in 121 liver transplant recipients: transmission by donated organ and the effect of OKT3 antibodies. J Infect Dis. 1988;158(1):124–31.
262. Razonable RR, Humar A, AST Infectious Diseases Community of Practice. Cytomegalovirus in solid organ transplantation. Am J Transplant. 2013;13(Suppl 4):93–106.
263. Mumtaz K, Faisal N, Husain S, et al. Universal prophylaxis or preemptive strategy for cytomegalovirus disease after liver transplantation: a systematic review and meta-analysis. Am J Transplant. 2015;15(2):472–81.
264. Marcelin JA, Beam E, Razonable RR. Cytomegalovirus infection in liver transplant recipients: updates on clinical management. World J Gastroenterol. 2014;20(31):10658–67.

265. Kostakis ID, Sotiropoulos GC, Kouraklis G. Pneumocystis jirovecii pneumonia in liver transplant recipients: a systematic review. Transplant Proc. 2014;46(9):3206–8.
266. Panel on Opportunistic Infections in HIV-Infected Adults and Adolescents. Guidelines for the prevention and treatment of opportunistic infections in HIV-infected adults and adolescents: recommendations from the Centers for Disease Control and Prevention, the National Institutes of Health, and the HIV Medicine Association of the Infectious Diseases Society of America. Available at http://aidsinfo.nih.gov/contentfiles/lvguidelines/adult_oi.pdf. Accessed 2/2018.
267. Martina SI, Fishman JA, the AST Infectious Diseases Community of Practice. Pneumocystis pneumonia in solid organ transplantation. Am J Transplant. 2013;13(Suppl 4):272–9.
268. Baddley JW, Forrest GN, the AST Infectious Diseases Community of Practice (2013). Cryptococcosis in solid organ transplantation. Am J Transplant. 2013;13(Suppl 4):242–9.
269. Singh N, Dromer F, Perfect JR, et al. Cryptococcosis in solid organ transplant recipients: current state of the science. Clin Infect Dis. 2008;47:1321–7.
270. Husain S, Wagener MM, Singh N. *Cryptococcus neoformans* infection in organ transplant recipients: variables influencing clinical characteristics and outcome. Emerg Infect Dis. 2001;7:375–81.
271. Singh N, Alexander BD, Lortholary O, et al. *Cryptococcus neoformans* in organ transplant recipients: impact of calcineurin-inhibitor agents on mortality. J Infect Dis. 2007;195:756–64.
272. Vilchez RA, Fung J, Kusne S. Cryptococcosis in organ transplant recipients: an overview. Am J Transplant. 2002;2:575–80.
273. Jabbour N, Reyes J, Kusne S, et al. Cryptococcal meningitis after liver transplantation. Transplantation. 1996;61:146–9.
274. Perfect JR, Dismukes WE, Dromer F, et al. Clinical practice guidelines for the management of cryptococcal disease: 2010 update by the Infectious Diseases Society of America. Clin Infect Dis. 2010;50:291–322.
275. Freifeld A, Iwen PC, Lesiak BL, et al. Histoplasmosis in solid organ transplant recipients at a large Midwestern university transplant center. Transpl Infect Dis. 2005;7:109–15.
276. Grim S, Proia L, Miller R, et al. A multicenter study of histoplasmosis and blastomycosis after solid organ transplantation. Transpl Infect Dis. 2012;14:17–23.
277. Batista M, Pierrotti LC, Abdala E, et al. Endemic and opportunistic infections in Brazilian solid organ transplant recipients. Tropical Med Int Health. 2011;16:1134–42.
278. Cuellar-Rodriguez J, Avery RK, Lard M, et al. Histoplasmosis in solid organ transplant recipients: 10 years of experience at a large transplant center in an endemic area. Clin Infect Dis. 2009;49:710–6.
279. Miller R, Assi M, AST Infectious Diseases Community of Practice. Endemic fungal infections in solid organ transplantation. Am J Transplant. 2013;13:250–61.
280. Vucicevic D, Carey EJ, Blair JE. Coccidioidomycosis in liver transplant recipients in an endemic area. Am J Transplant. 2011;11:111–9.
281. Blair J. Coccidioidomycosis in patients who have undergone transplantation. Ann N Y Acad Sci. 2007;1111:365–76.
282. Holt C, Winston DJ, Kubak B, et al. Coccidioidomycosis in liver transplant patients. Clin Infect Dis. 1997;24:216–21.
283. Blair J, Logan JL. Coccidioidomycosis in solid organ transplantation. Clin Infect Dis. 2001;33:1536–44.
284. Gauthier GM, Safdar N, Klein BS, Andes DR. Blastomycosis in solid organ transplant recipients. Transpl Infect Dis. 2007;9:310–7.
285. Pedersen M, Seetharam A. Infections after orthotopic liver transplantation. J Clin Exp Hepatol. 2014;4(4):347–60.
286. Hamandi B, Husain S, Grootendorst P, et al. Clinical and microbiological epidemiology of early and late infectious complications among solid-organ transplant recipients requiring hospitalization. Transpl Int. 2016;29(9):1029–38.
287. Kumar D, Prasad GV, Zaltzman J, et al. Community-acquired West Nile virus infection in solid-organ transplant recipients. Transplantation. 2004;77(3):399.
288. Clark NM, Reid GE. ATS infectious, disease community, of practice Nocardia infections in solid organ transplantation. Am J Transplant. 2013;13:83–92.
289. Husain S, McCurry K, Dauber J, et al. Nocardia infection in lung transplant recipients. J Heart Lung Transplant. 2002;21:354–9.
290. Peleg AY, Husain S, Qureshi ZA, et al. Risk factors, clinical characteristics, and outcome of Nocardia infection in organ transplant recipients: a matched case–control study. Clin Infect Dis. 2007;44:1307–14.
291. Coussement J, Lebeaux D, van Delden C, et al. Nocardia infection in solid organ transplant recipients: a multicenter European case-control study. Clin Infect Dis. 2016;63:338–45.
292. Park BJ, Pappas PG, Wannemuehler KA, et al. Invasive non-aspergillus mold infections in transplant recipients, United States, 2001–2006. Emerg Infect Dis. 2011;17(10):1855–64.
293. Silveira FP, Husain S. Fungal infections in solid organ transplantation. Med Mycol. 2007;45:305–20.
294. Singh N, Chang FY, Gayowski T, et al. Infections due to dematiaceous fungi in organ transplant recipients: case report and review. Clin Infect Dis. 1997;24:369–74.
295. Eshraghian A, Imanieh MH, Dehghani SM, et al. Post-transplant lymphoproliferative disorder after liver transplantation: incidence, long-term survival and impact of serum tacrolimus level. World J Gastroenterol. 2017;23:1224–32.
296. Penn I. Posttransplantation de novo tumors in liver allograft recipients. Liver Transpl Surg. 1996;2:52–9.
297. Green M, Michaels MG. Epstein-Barr virus infection and post-transplant lymphoproliferative disorder. Am J Transplant. 2013;13(Suppl 3):41–54.
298. Singh N, Paterson DL. Mycobacterium tuberculosis infection in solid-organ transplant recipients: impact and implications for management. Clin Infect Dis. 1998;27(5):1266–77.
299. Nahid P, Dorman SE, Alipanah N, et al. Official American Thoracic Society/Centers for Disease Control and Prevention/Infectious Diseases Society of America Clinical Practice Guidelines: treatment of drug susceptible tuberculosis. Clin Infect Dis. 2016;63(7):e147–95.
300. Weltermann B, Herwig A, Dehnen D, et al. Vaccination status of pneumococcal and other vaccines in 444 liver transplant patients compared to a representative population sample. Ann Transplant. 2016;21:200–7.
301. Roni DA, Pathapati RM, Kumar AS, et al. Safety and efficacy of hepatitis B vaccination in cirrhosis of liver. Adv Virol. 2013;2013:196704. Epub 2013 Jun 6.
302. Danziger-Isakov L, Kumar D, the AST Infectious Diseases Community of Practice. Vaccination in solid organ transplantation. Am J Transplant. 2013;13(Suppl 4):311–7.
303. Bratzler DW, Dellinger EP, Olsen KM, et al. Clinical practice guidelines for antimicrobial prophylaxis in surgery. Am J Health-Syst Pharm. 2013;70:195–283.
304. Todo S, Demetris AJ, Van Thiel D, et al. Orthotopic liver transplantation for patients with hepatitis B virus-related liver disease. Hepatology. 1991;13(4):619–26.
305. Lau JY, Bain VG, Davies SE, et al. High-level expression of hepatitis B viral antigens in fibrosing cholestatic hepatitis. Gastroenterology. 1992;102(3):956–62.
306. Marzano A, Gaia S, Ghisetti V, et al. Viral load at the time of liver transplantation and risk of hepatitis B virus recurrence. Liver Transpl. 2005;11(4):402–9.

307. Abdelmalek MF, Pasha TM, Zein NN, et al. Subclinical reactivation of hepatitis B virus in liver transplant recipients with past exposure. Liver Transpl. 2003;9(12):1253–7.
308. Wright TL, Donegan E, Hsu HH, et al. Recurrent and acquired hepatitis C viral infection in liver transplant recipients. Gastroenterology. 1992;103(1):317–22.
309. Lake JR, Shorr JS, Steffen BJ, et al. Differential effects of donor age in liver transplant recipients infected with hepatitis B, hepatitis C and without viral hepatitis. Am J Transplant. 2005;5(3):549–57.
310. Freeman RB, Tran S, Lee YM, et al. Serum hepatitis C RNA titers after liver transplantation are not correlated with immunosuppression or hepatitis. Transplantation. 1996;61(4):542–6.
311. Berenguer M. Natural history of recurrent hepatitis C. Liver Transpl. 2002;8(10 Suppl 1):S14–8.
312. Verna EC, Abdelmessih R, Samomao MA, et al. Cholestatic hepatitis C following liver transplantation: an outcome-based histological definition, clinical predictors, and prognosis. Liver Transpl. 2013;19(1):78–88.
313. McGory RW, Ishitani MB, Oliveira WM, et al. Improved outcome of orthotopic liver transplantation for chronic hepatitis B cirrhosis with aggressive passive immunization. Transplantation. 1996;61(9):1358–64.
314. Charlton M, Everson GT, Flamm SL, et al. Ledipasvir and sofosbuvir plus ribavirin for treatment of HCV infection in patients with advanced liver disease. Gastroenterology. 2015;149(3):649–59.
315. O'Leary JG, Brown K, Burton J, et al. Efficacy and safety of simeprevir and sofosbuvir with and without ribavirin for 12 weeks in subjects with recurrent genotype 1 hepatitis C post-orthotopic liver transplant: the GALAXY study. Transpl Int. 2017;30(2):196–208.
316. Brown RS, O'Leary J, Redy KR, et al. Interferon-free therapy for genotype 1 hepatitis C in liver transplant recipients: real world experience from the hepatitis C therapeutic registry and research network. Liver Transpl. 2016;22(1):24–33.
317. Fontana RJ, Brown RS, Moreno-Zamora A, et al. Daclatasvir combined with sofosbuvir or simeprevir in liver transplant recipients with severe recurrent hepatitis C infection. Liver Transpl. 2016;22:446–58.
318. Kwo PY, Mantry PS, Coakley E, et al. An interferon-free antiviral regimen for HCV after liver transplantation. N Engl J Med. 2014;371(25):2375–82.
319. Kemmer NM, Miskovsky EP. Hepatitis A. Infect Dis Clin N Am. 2000;14(3):605–15.
320. Arslan M, Wiesner RH, Poterucha JJ, et al. Hepatitis A antibodies in liver transplant recipients: evidence for loss of immunity post-transplantation. Liver Transpl. 2000;6(2):191–5.
321. Arslan M, Wiesner RH, Poterucha JJ, et al. Safety and efficacy of hepatitis A vaccination in liver transplantation recipients. Transplantation. 2001;72(2):272–6.
322. Askling HH, Rombo L, van Vollenhoven R, et al. Hepatitis A vaccine for immunosuppressed patients with rheumatoid arthritis: a prospective, open-label, multi-centre study. Travel Med Infect Dis. 2014;12(2):134–42.
323. Garcia Garrido HM, Wieten RW, Grobusch MP, et al. Response to hepatitis A vaccination in immunocompromised travelers. J Infect Dis. 2015;212(3):378–85.
324. Patra S, Kumar A, Trivedi SS, et al. Maternal and fetal outcomes in pregnant women with acute hepatitis E virus infection. Ann Intern Med. 2007;147(1):28–33.
325. Hamid SS, Atiq F, Shehzad A, et al. Hepatitis E virus superinfection in patients with chronic liver disease. Hepatology. 2002;36(2):474–8.
326. Ramachandran J, Eapen C, Kang G, et al. Hepatitis E superinfection produces severe decompensation in patients with chronic liver disease. J Gastroenterol Hepatol. 2004;19(2):134–8.
327. Coilly A, Haim-Boukobza B, Roche TM, Antonini A, et al. Post-transplantation hepatitis E: transfusion-transmitted hepatitis rising from the ashes. Transplantation. 2013;96(2):e4–6.
328. Schlosser B, Stein A, Neuhaus R, et al. Liver transplant from a donor with occult HEV infection induced chronic hepatitis and cirrhosis in the recipient. J Hepatol. 2012;56(2):500–2.
329. Haagsma EB, van den Berg AP, Porte RJ, et al. Chronic hepatitis E virus infection in liver transplant recipients. Liver Transpl. 2008;14(4):547–53.
330. Kamar N, Garrouste C, Haagsma EB, et al. Factors associated with chronic hepatitis in patients with hepatitis E virus infection who have received solid organ transplants. Gastroenterology. 2011;140(5):1481–9.
331. Pischke S, Suneetha PV, Baechlein C, et al. Hepatitis E virus infection as a cause of graft hepatitis in liver transplant recipients. Liver Transpl. 2010;16(1):74–82.
332. Pischke S, Behrendt P, Manns MP, et al. HEV-associated cryoglobulinaemia and extrahepatic manifestations of hepatitis E. Lancet Infect Dis. 2014;14(8):678–9.
333. Legrand-Abravanel F, Kamar N, Sandres-Saune K, et al. Hepatitis E virus infection without reactivation in solid-organ transplant recipients, France. Emerg Infect Dis. 2011;17(1):30–7.
334. Buffaz C, Scholtes C, Dron AG, et al. Hepatitis E in liver transplant recipients in the Rhone-Alps region in France. Eur J Clin Microbiol Infect Dis. 2014;33(6):1037–43.
335. Aggarwal R. Hepatitis E: clinical presentation in disease-endemic areas and diagnosis. Semin Liver Dis. 2013;33(1):30–40.
336. Wang Y, Zhou X, Debing Y, et al. Calcineurin inhibitors stimulate and mycophenolic acid inhibits replication of hepatitis E virus. Gastroenterology. 2014;146(7):1775–83.
337. Zhou X, Wang Y, Metselaar HJ, et al. Rapamycin and everolimus facilitate hepatitis E virus replication: revealing a basal defense mechanism of PI3K-PKB-mTOR pathway. J Hepatol. 2014;61(4):746–54.
338. Pischke S, Stiefel P, Franz B, et al. Chronic hepatitis E in heart transplant recipients. Am J Transplant. 2012;12(11):3128–33.
339. Kamar N, Izopet J, Tripon S, et al. Ribavirin for chronic hepatitis E virus infection in transplant recipients. N Engl J Med. 2014;370(12):1111–20.
340. Kamar N, Rostaing L, Abravanel F, et al. Ribavirin therapy inhibits viral replication on patients with chronic hepatitis E virus infection. Gastroenterology. 2010;139(5):1612–8.
341. Mallet V, Nicand E, Sultanik P, et al. Brief communication: case reports of ribavirin treatment for chronic hepatitis E. Ann Intern Med. 2010;153(2):85–9.

Infections in Kidney and Pancreas Transplantation

4

Megan K. Morales, Matthew Cooper, Peter Abrams, and Joseph G. Timpone Jr.

Abbreviations

AB	Asymptomatic bacteriuria
ATG	Antithymocyte globulin
BKPyV	BK polyomavirus
CDI	Clostridium difficile infection
CMV	Cytomegalovirus
CNI	Calcineurin inhibitors
CRAB	Carbapenem-resistant *Acinetobacter baumannii*
DAA	Direct-acting agent
EBV	Epstein-Barr virus
eGFR	Estimated glomerular filtration rate
EIA	Enzyme immunoassay
FDA	Food and Drug Administration
FQ	Fluoroquinolone
HBV	Hepatitis B virus
HCV	Hepatitis C virus
HIV	Human immunodeficiency virus
HLA	Human leukocyte antigen
HRD	High infectious risk donor
HSV	Herpes simplex virus
ICU	Intensive care unit
IGRA	Interferon-gamma release assay
INH	Isoniazid
IPA	Invasive pulmonary aspergillosis
IVIG	Intravenous immunoglobulin
KDIGO	Kidney disease: improving global outcomes (clinical practice guidelines sponsored by the National Kidney Foundation)
KPC	Klebsiella pneumoniae carbapenemase
KS	Kaposi sarcoma
MDR	Multidrug resistant
MDRO	Multidrug-resistant organism
mTOR	Mammalian target of rapamycin
NAT	Nucleic acid testing
OI	Opportunistic infection
OKT3	Muromonab-CD3
OPO	Organ procurement organization
OPTN	Organ Procurement and Transplantation Network
PAK	Pancreas after kidney
PCP	Pneumocystis pneumonia
PCR	Polymerase chain reaction
PEP	Postexposure prophylaxis
PF	Perfusion fluid
PPFC	Peripancreatic fluid collection
PTA	Pancreas transplant alone (i.e., not combined with renal transplantation)
PTLD	Posttransplant lymphoproliferative disorder
QALY	Quality-adjusted life year
RNA	Ribonucleic acid
SOT	Solid organ transplant
SPK	Simultaneous pancreas-kidney transplant
SRTR	Scientific Registry of Transplant Recipients
SVR	Sustained virologic response
TB	Tuberculosis
TMP-SMX	Trimethoprim-sulfamethoxazole
UNOS	United Network for Organ Sharing
UTI	Urinary tract infection
VZV	Varicella-zoster virus
WNV	West Nile virus

M. K. Morales (✉)
University of Maryland School of Medicine, Institute of Human Virology/Department of Infectious Diseases, Baltimore, MD, USA
e-mail: mmorales@ihv.umaryland.edu

M. Cooper
MedStar Georgetown Transplant Institute, Washington, DC, USA
e-mail: matthew.cooper@gunet.georgetown.edu

P. Abrams
MedStar Georgetown University Hospital, MedStar Georgetown Transplant Institute, Washington, DC, USA
e-mail: peter.l.abrams@gunet.georgetown.edu

J. G. Timpone Jr.
MedStar Georgetown University Hospital, Division of Infectious Diseases and Travel Medicine, Washington, DC, USA
e-mail: timponej@gunet.georgetown.edu

A. Safdar (ed.), *Principles and Practice of Transplant Infectious Diseases*, https://doi.org/10.1007/978-1-4939-9034-4_4

Introduction

The primary indication for kidney transplantation is end-stage renal disease (ESRD) severe enough to require renal replacement therapy (RRT; e.g., dialysis) to sustain an individual's life. Kidney transplantation results in improved patient survival and improved quality of life when compared to patients who remain on renal replacement therapy. Unfortunately, the demand for organs greatly outweighs kidney availability, a trend which has persisted over the past several decades. In 2015, the national Organ Procurement and Transplantation Network/Scientific Registry of Transplant Recipients (OPTN/SRTR) reported that 97,680 patients were on the waiting list, of which 61,234 were active [1]. The SRTR estimates that approximately 50% of listed patients have been on dialysis for at least 4 years [1]. Briefly, there are three types of kidney transplants which include (1) deceased donor kidney transplant, (2) living-related donor kidney transplant, and (3) living-unrelated donor kidney transplant. A total of 18,597 adult and pediatric kidney transplants including multi-organ transplantation occurred in 2015, of which 5626 were living donor transplants [1]. Regardless of the kidney transplant type, kidney transplantation offers a survival benefit as compared to patients on either hemodialysis or peritoneal dialysis. This survival advantage is likely due to the incorporation of better immunosuppressive regimens, improved management of the medical comorbidities in the posttransplantation period, and improved preventive and treatment strategies for infectious complications during the posttransplantation period. Renal allograft and patient survival statistics can be found at https://optn.transplant.hrsa.gov/data/view-data-reports/national-data/#. In general, renal allograft and patient survival rates are better for living-related donor type versus deceased donor type renal allograft. Deceased donor 5-year renal allograft and patient survival are 74.3% and 82.9%, respectively, while living donor 5-year renal allograft and patient survival are 85.5% and 91.9%, respectively.

More than 40% of ESRD in the United States is secondary to diabetes mellitus (DM)-related nephropathy, for which select patients are candidates for pancreas transplantation. The three forms of pancreas transplantation include simultaneous pancreas kidney (SPK), pancreas after kidney (PAK), and pancreas transplant alone (PTA); all achieve similar endpoints of curing an individual's insulin-deficient DM, preventing diabetic nephropathy and halting and often reversing the secondary complications of DM including retinopathy, neuropathy, gastroparesis, ketoacidosis, and hypoglycemic unawareness. Most candidates for pancreas transplantation suffer from long-standing type 1 diabetes with risk for severe secondary complications. Select patients with type 2 DM who are insulin-deficient and demonstrate phenotypic features of type 1 DM can also benefit from pancreas transplantation.

A large number of patients whose progressive chronic kidney disease (CKD) eventually meets criteria for kidney transplantation will experience many years of medical decline. This clinical deterioration includes constitutional symptoms such as increasing fatigue and malaise associated with CKD-related anemia. Other comorbidities of CKD include progressive cardiovascular disease, peripheral and autonomic neuropathy, bone disease, and sexual dysfunction. The social and emotional toll of CKD is extensive and profound, affecting not just patients but also their dependents and extended family. The transplant center assessment, therefore, focuses on the spectrum of morbidity associated with CKD, including the medical, surgical, immunologic, nutritional, and psychosocial condition of each candidate for the purpose of discerning the risks of surgery and the introduction of immunosuppression versus the potential benefit that may be achieved through transplantation.

Transplantation Options

It is increasingly appreciated that an individual's overall state of health prior to transplantation is an important factor in determining their subsequent clinical outcome. Accordingly, understanding transplant surgical complications resulting in infection often requires a consideration of the underlying medical condition of the kidney or kidney/pancreas transplant recipient prior to surgery. The same risk factors for surgical site infection (SSI) that have been well enumerated by organizations such as the National Healthcare Safety Network (NHSN) similarly apply to kidney and kidney/pancreas transplant patients. These risk factors include age, obesity, malnutrition, prolonged preoperative hospitalization, infection at distal sites, cancer, hyperglycemia, immunosuppression, and duration of surgery [2]. Beyond these general risk factors, the immediate period after transplantation is critical in determining surgical risk of infection as the allograft organ(s) is recovering from perioperative ischemia-reperfusion injury and the recipient is receiving peak level immunosuppression therapy. Furthermore, the details of the surgical technique itself used in the transplant operation are highly relevant to surgical infectious complications.

The multidisciplinary team will determine which of the kidney transplant categories is most appropriate for a potential recipient and may include deceased donation from brain-dead deceased donor, donation after cardiac death, or high kidney donor profile index kidney or living donation from a related or unrelated donor. Based on projections of survival benefit following transplantation, an individual candidate may be suited for one or more of these transplant options. Of the three types of pancreas transplants noted above, SPK is performed most commonly to address the multiple morbidities of the diabetic transplant candidate and shows superior survival compared to kidney transplant alone in this population [3].

Surgical Approaches and Complications

Except for one critical difference, the surgical approach is similar between kidney transplant and kidney/pancreas transplant. Both operations involve either midline or curvilinear incisions in the lower abdomen, with dissection and ligation of the inferior epigastric vessels, mobilization of the ipsilateral rectus muscle and gonadal structures, ligation of proximal and distal lymphatics in the ipsilateral iliac fossa, and mobilization of the ipsilateral common, external, and occasionally internal iliac arteries and veins. Both kidney and pancreas are connected to the iliac vessels for perfusion and venous drainage. The kidney transplant ureter is usually connected to the extraperitoneal portion of the bladder; rarely, the transplant ureter is insufficient in length to reach the bladder and is therefore connected to the recipient's native ureter. It is important to note that a standard kidney transplant does not involve opening the peritoneum and avoids contact with the bowel or other intraperitoneal organs. The kidney allograft is transplanted into the retroperitoneal space in either the right or left lower abdominal quadrants. There is preference to transplanting the kidney allograft on the left side in patients receiving an SPK or in anticipation of a PAK transplant. Conversely, in pancreas transplantation, the duodenal segment surrounding the head of the pancreas allograft is commonly connected intra-abdominally to the recipient's jejunum in a side-to-side configuration to accomplish enteric exocrine drainage. A minority of transplant surgeons prefer to connect the transplant duodenum to the recipient bladder.

When evaluating or risk-stratifying pancreas transplant recipients for surgical infectious complications, it is critical to know whether the pancreas transplant involves bladder or enteric exocrine drainage. The incidence of urinary tract infections (UTIs) is significantly higher with bladder drainage [4]. It is thought that the highly alkaline, bicarbonate-rich exocrine drainage of the pancreas leads to injury to the mucosal lining of the recipient bladder and the alterations in acid-base balance of the urine combine to cause higher rates of UTIs. The incidence of peritonitis is higher with bowel drainage, as leakage of pancreatic enzymes into the abdomen together with enteric leakage can lead to peritonitis and intra-abdominal abscess [5]. It is likewise critical to ascertain whether the pancreas transplant has encountered any technical complications. A high-volume pancreas transplant group reported a much higher incidence of bacterial and fungal complications in the cohort of patients who experienced any significant surgical complication [6]. For example, complications including hematuria and urethral stricture following bladder drainage may lead to UTIs, prostatitis, epididymitis, and pyelonephritis [7]. Furthermore, the readmission rate for pancreas transplant recipients is well-known to be much higher than for kidney recipients. This increased incidence results from higher rates of dehydration, increased rates of rejection, and increased rates of infection. Higher rates of hospitalization in the pancreas transplant population place these patients at higher risk for healthcare-associated infections (HAI).

Similar to pancreas transplant, recipients of kidney transplants with postoperative complications are at an increased risk of infectious complications. Well-described complications of kidney transplant include lymphocele, subcutaneous hematoma, peri-allograft hematoma, urine leak, and ureteral stricture. If not addressed in a timely fashion, all of these surgical complications can lead to allograft kidney dysfunction, and also secondary systemic infection in recipients can be life-threatening. An important factor that may affect initial allograft function is the cold ischemic time in deceased donor kidney allografts. After surgical removal of a kidney from a donor, it is placed in cold preservation fluid, prior to transplantation into the recipient; this period of time is known as the cold ischemic time (CIT). Prolonged CIT has been associated with delayed graft function and allograft failure. There is a proportional increase in allograft failure for each additional hour of CIT. There is a low rate of allograft failure of 4% within first year after transplantation with CIT of <36 h [8, 9]. While a threshold CIT has not been established, a typical cutoff time is 24 h but may be extended up to 48 h at the discretion of the transplant center.

An important factor that could contribute to early risk of infection, specifically UTI or allograft pyelonephritis, is the placement of a ureteral stent. Ureteral stents may be selectively placed at the time of surgery to prevent a ureteral stricture occurring from a prolonged CIT in a deceased donor kidney allograft. Ureteral stents in the absence of persistent urinary leak are typically removed via cystoscopy 3–4 weeks following transplantation procedure.

Prompt diagnosis and intervention to correct the complications noted above is critically important, requiring ongoing close collaboration between the medical and surgical teams.

Immunosuppressive Regimens

A primary reason for the improved allograft survival of kidney and pancreas transplants in the modern era is the broad adoption of induction therapy at the time of transplantation of either organ. Compared to conventional immunosuppressive agent therapy alone, a large number of controlled-randomized trials demonstrate that induction therapy involving biologic antibodies in addition to conventional immunosuppression is superior in decreasing kidney and pancreas transplant rejection and allograft failure rates

[10]. An exception to this general rule is made for genetically identical donor-recipient transplants due to the significantly reduced immunologic risk for graft rejection in this relatively small cohort of patients. Induction agents can be classified as either depleting or nondepleting antilymphocyte agents. The optimal prophylactic induction therapy for kidney and kidney/pancreas transplantation remains controversial. In general, transplant centers in the United States use alemtuzumab or rabbit antithymocyte globulin (rATG) as first-line induction, both of which are lymphocyte-depleting agents but have very different mechanisms and side-effect profiles. Patients who cannot tolerate, or have mitigating circumstances that preclude, first-line induction will generally receive basiliximab induction, a nondepleting interleukin-2 receptor antagonist.

In addition to induction therapy, all recipients of kidney and kidney/pancreas transplants receive maintenance immunosuppressive therapy with a combination of agents including corticosteroids such as prednisone; calcineurin inhibitors like cyclosporine A, tacrolimus; mTOR inhibitors, everolimus, sirolimus; antiproliferative agents such as mycophenolate mofetil, mycophenolate sodium, or belatacept, a costimulation inhibitor. Although the optimal maintenance regimen remains unclear, well over 90% of solid organ transplant recipients in the modern era are discharged home on a regimen including tacrolimus as the primary maintenance drug. Tacrolimus is a calcineurin-inhibitor (CNI) drug that decreases organ rejection rates by inhibiting production of interleukin-2, a molecule that promotes development and proliferation of T cells in response to the detection of a foreign antigen. Maintenance immunotherapy is required in kidney and kidney/pancreas transplant recipients to prevent acute rejection and the loss of the allografts over the long term. The first year following transplantation is generally the period of highest immunosuppression levels. The overall level of immunosuppression is slowly reduced overtime, with many factors influencing this gradual taper including allograft function as well as history of rejection or infection.

Pretransplantation Issues Concerning End-Stage Renal Disease and Dialysis Patients

Of the approximately 120,000 people awaiting transplantation in the United States, the vast majority, over 99,000, await kidney transplants [11]. The majority of patients who undergo renal transplantation will have been on dialysis prior to transplantation, leaving them vulnerable to infection in the pretransplant setting that may impact their eligibility for transplantation or the course of the transplant itself. In 2014, 4761 patients died while waiting for a kidney transplant, and another 3668 people became too sick to receive a transplant [11, 12]. The median wait time for an individual's first renal transplant was 3.6 years and may be longer in certain regions of the country [12, 13]. Wait time continues to accrue if a patient is inactivated, as may happen while being treated for infection or completing pretransplantation evaluation; inactive patients now make up approximately 40% of those listed for transplant [14].

Infectious Complications of Hemodialysis and Peritoneal Dialysis

The major bacterial infections in patients on hemodialysis include catheter-related bloodstream infections and respiratory tract infections; infection is the second leading cause of death after cardiovascular causes in patients undergoing maintenance hemodialysis [15]. The rates of bloodstream infections vary, depending upon the type of hemodialysis catheter used, with arteriovenous fistulas having the lowest rates of infection. Catheter-related bloodstream infections have been reported to occur in 0.3/100 patient-months for native arteriovenous fistula, 0.7/100 patient-months for arteriovenous grafts, 4.6/100 patient-months for cuffed hemodialysis catheters, and 7.3/100 patient-months for non-cuffed hemodialysis catheters [16]. In the HEMO study, the authors noted that 21% of the first infection-related hospital admission was due to a vascular access infection [17]. The authors also noted that while only 7.6% of the study population had hemodialysis catheters for vascular access, these catheters accounted for a disproportionate amount of vascular access infections (32%), as compared to arteriovenous fistulas/grafts [17]. It has been estimated that there is a tenfold increase in the relative risk of bloodstream infections with tunneled hemodialysis catheters as compared to arteriovenous fistulas [18]. One prospective study of 472 patients who had a recently placed hemodialysis catheter reported that 35% of patients experienced a catheter-related bloodstream infection at 3 months, and 54% experienced a catheter-related bloodstream infection at 6 months [19]. Despite these increased rates of infection associated with tunneled hemodialysis catheters, the prolonged maturation time for arteriovenous fistulas necessitates temporary use of such catheters for most patients initiating hemodialysis. The most common causative organisms for bloodstream infections in hemodialysis patients are due to staphylococcal species, specifically *Staphylococcus aureus*, and coagulase-negative staphylococci such as *Staphylococcus epidermidis* [15]. Bloodstream infections due to *S. aureus* occur as a result of infection with a person's own endogenous strain, as >50% of patients on hemodialysis are carriers of *S. aureus* [20, 21]. The high rate of *S. aureus* carriage and colonization, or both, the presence of indwelling vascular access catheters, and uremia-related neutrophil dysfunction, contribute greatly to the high rates of *S. aureus* infections in this patient population [20]. It has been estimated that in patients on hemodialysis who are colonized with *S. aureus*, 65% of these isolates were resistant to methicillin [22]. Methicillin-resistant *Staphylococcus aureus* (MRSA) is common among hemodialysis patients, and therefore empiric treatment with vancomycin is warranted in patients with suspected bloodstream infections [23]. Infections due to enterococci and Gram-negative rods can occur, although such infections are less common [15]. In addition to bloodstream infections, metastatic foci of infection may be seen, most typically with bloodstream infections due to *S. aureus*. The common types of infections associated with metastatic foci from bloodstream infection include endocarditis, osteomyelitis especially involving the vertebral column, epidural abscesses, septic arthritis, and septic pulmonary emboli [15, 22]. Persons receiving hemodialysis are 17.8 times more likely to develop endocarditis than the general population, *S. aureus* accounting for 57.9% of cases [24, 25]. Furthermore, the rates of metastatic foci of infection were noted to be more common with *S. aureus* and have been reported to occur in 10–40% of patients with *S. aureus* bacteremia [26, 27].

Patients on hemodialysis are also at increased risk for respiratory tract infections [15] due to community-acquired pathogens such as *Streptococcus pneumonia*, as well as healthcare-associated pathogens, given their frequent exposure to the healthcare setting. Seasonal influenza is also common among persons on hemodialysis; therefore, annual influenza vaccine is indicated for this high-risk population. It is extremely important that patients on hemodialysis be vaccinated for both influenza and pneumococcus, because pneumonia-associated death rates are 14–16 times higher as compared to the general population [28]. *Mycobacterium tuberculosis* is another important pulmonary pathogen in the hemodialysis population, and screening for latent tuberculosis infection is routinely preformed during pretransplant evaluation of potential renal allograft recipients.

The most common infectious complication of chronic peritoneal dialysis is peritonitis. It is estimated that the rate of peritonitis in patients initiating peritoneal dialysis is 42 per 100 patient-years [29]. Another study observed that 37% of patients on peritoneal dialysis developed peritonitis with an annual rate of 0.37 episodes of peritonitis per year at risk [30]. Infections at the exit site of peritoneal dialysis catheters have also been reported. Several large observational studies have reported that Gram-positive cocci account for 50–60%, Gram-negative rods accounted for approximately 15%, and fungi accounted for approximately 2% of cases of peritonitis due to peritoneal dialysis [31, 32]. The majority of Gram-positive cocci infections are due to coagulase-negative staphylococci and *S. aureus* [32], although *Enterococcus* species including vancomycin-resistant *Enterococcus* (VRE) have been reported. Gram-negative enterics and *Pseudomonas aeruginosa* are also associated with peritonitis in peritoneal dialysis patients. It has been reported that non-pseudomonal Gram-negative rods have a worse outcome than peritonitis due to coagulase-negative staphylococcus or *S. aureus* [33]. Peritonitis due to *Pseudomonas aeruginosa* can result in significant morbidity and is often associated with catheter exit-site infections [34]. Fungi are a relatively rare cause of peritonitis in this setting; however, the most common cause is *Candida* species – most often due to *Candida albicans*, *Candida parapsilosis*, and *Candida glabrata* [35]. Other unusual fungal pathogens have been reported and include *Aspergillus* species, *Paecilomyces*, *Penicillium*, *Zygomycetes*, and *Rhodotorula* [35, 36]. Overall, fungal peritonitis is associated with high mortality rates of 20–30% as well as marked inflammation of the peritoneal membrane resulting in dropout from peritoneal dialysis [35]. In patients on peritoneal dialysis who undergo kidney transplantation, there appears to be an ongoing risk for the development of peritonitis, and therefore many authors recommend the immediate removal of the peritoneal dialysis catheter as opposed to waiting for the establishment of renal allograft function [37]. While good outcomes for kidney transplantation in patients on peritoneal dialysis have been reported, Martins et al. found less favorable results among patients undergoing simultaneous pancreas-kidney transplants who utilized peritoneal dialysis, as compared to those on hemodialysis at the time of transplantation, including higher rates of thrombosis-driven relaparotomy, pancreatic loss due to infection, thrombosis-related kidney loss, and inferior survival with infection as the leading cause of death [38].

The management of bloodstream infections due to hemodialysis vascular access catheters and peritonitis associated with peritoneal dialysis is beyond the scope of this chapter. Treatment guidelines are available at: http://cid.oxfordjournals.org/content/49/1/1.full and http://www.pdiconnect.com/content/30/4/393.full.pdf, respectively [23, 39].

Viral Infections in Hemodialysis Patients and Considerations for Kidney Transplantation

Blood-borne pathogens due to viruses are important clinical aspects in the management of patients receiving hemodialysis. The most important viruses include hepatitis B virus (HBV), hepatitis C virus (HCV), and human immunodeficiency virus (HIV). HBV and HCV transmission have also been documented in peritoneal dialysis patients, albeit at a significantly lower rate [40]. The prevention and management of these viruses are crucial in patients being considered for kidney and kidney-pancreas transplantation.

The transmission of viral hepatitis is a real concern for hemodialysis patients and staff. As recently as 2013, a patient acquired novel hepatitis B virus (HBV) infection through contamination in her dialysis center from a source patient who had failed renal transplantation and reactivated quiescent HBV infection [41]. Guidelines target both prevention of infection via available vaccinations as well as routine testing and infection prevention measures to prevent nosocomial transmission and can be fully reviewed at the CDC website for Dialysis Safety – http://www.cdc.gov/dialysis/guidelines/index.html [42].

A national surveillance study of US dialysis centers in 2002 showed a 1% prevalence of dialysis patients who were seropositive for hepatitis B surface antigen (HBsAg) and an annual infection incidence of 0.12% [43]. Although most HD patients who acquire HBV infection will not develop severe or fulminant hepatitis, only a minority will clear the infection converting to HBsAg negative. These patients are more likely then patients without kidney disease to have persistent antigenemia and chronic elevation of liver enzymes [44]. Once additionally immunosuppressed after transplantation, even those who seemingly cleared infection previously may reactivate, particularly if they never developed surface antibodies (HBsAb) [45].

Hepatitis B vaccination is recommended for susceptible dialysis and CKD patients as well as healthcare workers, including those at dialysis centers [46]. In the same 2002 survey, approximately half of hemodialysis patients and 90% of staff received vaccination, and both groups had increasing vaccination rates over the 5-year period [43]. Ideally, HBV vaccination, which occurs at intervals of 0, 1, and 6 months, is administered prior to the initiation of dialysis, as well as for peritoneal and home dialysis patients who may require in-center hemodialysis in the future. Vaccination prior to dialysis has been shown to result in higher immunogenicity or antibody titers [47]. Hemodialysis and immunocompromised patients require a "double dose" (40 μg) of HBV vaccine and should have follow-up serologic testing to confirm vaccine response. If titer response 1–2 months following completion of the vaccine series is not ≥10 mIU/mL, a second vaccination series should be administered. Hemodialysis patients should undergo yearly HBsAb testing with administration of a booster dose if titers subsequently decline to <10 mIU/mL [48]. The list of recommended vaccines for patients on dialysis being considered for kidney transplantation is outlined in Table 4.1.

Table 4.1 Recommended vaccinations for adults with renal disease – 2016 CDC Guidelines [49]

[a]Yearly influenza (inactivated only for renal transplant recipients)
Tdap (once in adulthood, then Td booster every 10 years)
Pneumococcal (PCV13, then PPSV23 at least 8 weeks later)
Hepatitis B (higher 40 μg dose)
[a]Zoster (Shingrix, age >50 or taking/anticipating immunosuppressive therapy)
Human papilloma virus (females up to age 26, males up to age 21)
[a]MMR (born after 1957 if not already vaccinated or having immunity)
[a]Varicella (born after 1980 not already vaccinated or having immunity)

[a]Live virus vaccinations are not recommended for transplant recipients

Risk factors for HBV infection among hemodialysis patients in non-endemic regions include [43, 50, 51]:

- Lack of a protocol for HBV-infected patients
- Patients in the same center positive for HBsAg
- Lack of separate space and dialysis machines for HBsAg-positive patients
- Low (<50%) HBV vaccination rates within a dialysis unit
- Preparation of injectable medications outside of a dedicated medication room, such as on a cart or in a treatment area
- Longer duration on hemodialysis, with 4% higher odds ratio of HBV prevalence per year

Those patients known to be chronically infected with HBV should be treated, with the goal of maintaining undetectable viral loads and normal transaminases. Patients both with and without cirrhosis are at risk for hepatocellular carcinoma so should undergo regular liver cancer screening. Entecavir (Baraclude®, Bristol-Myers Squibb, Princeton, NJ) and tenofovir (Viread®, Gilead Sciences, Foster City, CA) are the most commonly used agents and have a high barrier to resistance in HBV. For patients on hemodialysis, either agent should be administered once every 7 days after dialysis. Lamivudine (Epivir®, ViiV Healthcare, Quebec, Canada) is an alternative option administered at a decreased daily dose but has a lower barrier to resistance. After transplantation, doses must be adjusted with improvement of renal function. Of note, due to the recognized potential nephrotoxicity of tenofovir, alternative agents may be considered in some cases. Tenofovir alafenamide (TAF, Gilead Sciences, Foster City, CA) was approved as a part of combination antiretroviral therapy in HIV patients and provides a more favorable toxicity profile with regard to renal and bone laboratory measurements. Early studies using TAF show promise for the treatment of chronic HBV and may be another option during post-kidney transplantation period [52, 53]. It is important to confirm HIV negativity when treating for HBV to avoid development of HIV resistance as these agents are active against both viruses, and treatment of HIV would require at least two additional antiretroviral agents.

Reported hepatitis C virus (HCV) prevalence of US and European dialysis centers ranges from 2.6% to 22.9%, with a mean of 13.5% [54]. HCV infection is associated with an increased relative risk for all-cause and cardiovascular mortality in dialysis patients [55]. Nosocomial HCV transmission may be influenced by prevalence of HCV within a dialysis unit, low personnel-to-patient ratio, or dialysis in close proximity to HCV-infected patients [56, 57] although this may largely be avoided with strict adherence to infection control practices. Increased HCV prevalence was associated with longer duration on hemodialysis, male gender, Black race, diabetes, coinfection with HBV, prior renal transplant, or alcohol or substance abuse in the preceding 12 months. Whereas, HCV seroconversion was associated with longer time on dialysis, HIV/AIDS or HBV infection, and recurrent cellulitis or gangrene, at the patient level and an increase in facility HCV prevalence, at the center level [54]. Approximately half of centers reported a seroconversion during the 2–4-year study period. An increase in highly trained staff was associated with both lower HCV prevalence and risk of seroconversion.

HCV infection has been identified as an independent risk factor for graft loss and mortality in renal transplant patients [58–60]. It should be noted that these studies were conducted before the widespread use of direct-acting agents (DAAs) against HCV infection. While combinations of DAAs such as sofosbuvir (Sovaldi®, Gilead Sciences, Foster City, CA)/ simeprevir (Olysio®, Janssen Therapeutics, Titusville, NJ) and ombitasvir/paritaprevir/ritonavir/dasabuvir (Viekira Pak®, AbbVie Inc., North Chicago, IL) have revolutionized the treatment of chronic HCV infection, data on the use of these agents in patients with chronic kidney disease is still evolving. The approval of fixed dose elbasvir and grazoprevir combination Zepatier (Merck & Co. Inc., Whitehouse Station, New Jersey) in January 2016 marked the first DAA therapy approved for patients with HCV genotypes 1, the most common in the United States and genotype 4 infections in patients on hemodialysis [61]. In the C-SURFER study, genotype 1 patients with eGFR less than 30 mL/min per 1.73 m^2, (76% of whom were on hemodialysis, 20% treatment experienced and 6% with hepatic cirrhosis) experienced 94% sustained virologic response (SVR) after 12 weeks of therapy [62]. Genotypes 2, 3, 5, and 6 still require the use of sofosbuvir-based regimens which is renally excreted and has limited data in patients on hemodialysis. A small series including 11 hemodialysis patients and 1 peritoneal dialysis patient found lower SVR rates in the dialysis group but reported only minor adverse events including fatigue, rash/ itching, anemia, diarrhea, and decreased appetite with a regimen of half-dose sofosbuvir plus simeprevir [63]. Another study involving pre- and post-kidney or kidney/liver transplant recipients included ten patients on dialysis who were treated with daily sofosbuvir with good tolerability and SVR rates [64]. In the United States, use of sofosbuvir is currently approved for patients with eGFR >30 mL/min. The 2008 Kidney Disease Improving Global Outcomes (KDIGO) guidelines, sponsored by the National Kidney Foundation, recommend treatment prior to renal transplantation as sustained virologic response (SVR) before transplant reduces the risk of hepatic and extrahepatic complications after transplantation [65]. In certain regions with very high organ demand, however, transplantation of a HCV-positive donor kidney will drastically shorten wait times, and therefore many providers may choose to delay treatment until after transplantation. Data supports the use of renal graft from HCV-positive kidney donors showing improved survival in recipients of such grafts versus remaining on the transplant waitlist and continued dialysis [66].

Lee et al. published a multicenter cohort study comparing HBV-mono-infected or HCV-mono-infected to seronegative kidney transplant recipients and found that patients with HBV had worse survival but no difference in graft function as compared to HBV-negative patients [67]. Hepatic complications constituted the primary cause of increased mortality. There was improved patient survival on entecavir compared to lamivudine. While HCV infection did not lower patient survival, it was associated with an increased incidence of renal allograft failure and acute rejection.

As a result of the widespread use of effective combination antiretroviral therapy for the treatment of HIV infection, morbidity and mortality due to opportunistic infections and neoplasms has declined dramatically. Therefore, the major morbidity and mortality has now shifted to other causes such as cardiovascular etiologies, chronic kidney disease, end-stage liver disease, and non-opportunistic malignant neoplasms [68]. Chronic kidney disease and the need for renal replacement therapy in HIV-infected patients are multifactorial; the common causes include HIV-associated nephropathy, immune complex disease, coinfection with HBV and HCV, HIV-associated thrombotic microangiopathy, drug toxicity, and medical comorbidities such as hypertension and diabetes that are often encountered in patients receiving antiretroviral medications. Several HIV cohort studies have observed that 3.1–6% of HIV-infected patients have chronic kidney disease and 1.7% of patients have end-stage renal disease [69, 70]. HIV prevalence in the hemodialysis population varies between 0.67% and 20%, which reflects the overall prevalence of HIV within that region [71, 72].

Stock et al. led a multicenter prospective study of renal transplantation in HIV-infected persons which found 3-year patient and graft survival rates of 88% and 74%, respectively, which fell between national rates for recipients 65 years and older and all comers [73]. Additionally, there was no evidence of accelerated HIV disease progression or virologic failure in the posttransplantation period [73]. However, there were surprisingly higher rates of allograft rejection, up to 33% [73]. Risk factors for acute allograft rejection in the multivariate model included transplant from a deceased donor and cyclosporine use, whereas a higher posttransplantation CD4+ T-cell count was marginally protective. More recently, using the Scientific Registry of Transplant Recipients (SRTR) data of 510 HIV-positive adult kidney recipients, Locke et al. found that HIV-negative and HIV mono-infected kidney transplant recipients had similar graft survival and patient survival, whereas HIV/HCV coinfected patients had worse outcomes [74]. They identified several risk factors to predict higher rates of graft loss among HIV-positive kidney transplants that should be taken into account

Table 4.2 Common infections in the prerenal transplant (dialysis-dependent) period

System	Infection	Organisms
Bloodstream (hemodialysis)	Catheter-related bloodstream infection	*Staphylococcus aureus*, coagulase-negative staphylococci
		Less commonly enterococcus species, Gram-negative bacteria
	Metastatic foci of bloodstream infection: endocarditis, osteomyelitis (especially vertebral), epidural abscess, septic arthritis, septic pulmonary emboli	Same as that causing bloodstream infection
Respiratory tract	Pneumonia, upper respiratory tract infection	Community acquired pathogens, especially *Streptococcus pneumoniae*
		Healthcare acquired pathogens
		Seasonal influenza
	Tuberculosis	*Mycobacterium tuberculosis*
Intra-abdominal (peritoneal dialysis)	Peritonitis	Gram-positive cocci, especially coagulase negative staphylococci and *Staphylococcus aureus* (50–60%)
		Gram-negative bacilli, including *Pseudomonas aeruginosa* (15%)
		Fungi, especially *Candida albicans*, *C. parapsilosis*, *C. glabrata*; also reported *Aspergillus* species, *Paecilomyces*, *Penicillium*, *Zygomycetes*, and *Rhodotorula* (2%)
	Catheter exit site infection	Gram-positive cocci, especially *S. aureus* and Streptococcus spp.
Hepatic	Viral hepatitis	Hepatitis B virus, Hepatitis C virus

in the pretransplantation process: HCV coinfection increased risk by 2.72-fold; >3 human leukocyte antigen (HLA) mismatches increased risk by 1.80-fold in coinfected recipients plus 3 HLA mismatches having an amplified 3.86-fold risk of graft loss [59]. These very encouraging findings support the role of kidney transplantation as a viable option for HIV-infected persons with chronic kidney disease on dialysis.

As for all solid organ transplant recipients, potential candidates for kidney or kidney-pancreas transplant should have HIV virologic control before proceeding to transplantation. While transplant protocols may vary by hospital, generally recipient criteria for potential HIV-positive recipients include a CD4+ T-cell count of 200 cells per cubic millimeter or greater, undetectable HIV plasma RNA level, a stable antiretroviral regimen, and no active opportunistic infection, which were the selection criteria for the prospective multicenter HIV kidney transplant study [73].

Dr. Elmi Muller was the first surgeon to transplant HIV-positive recipients with kidneys from aviremic HIV-positive donors at the Groote Schuur Hospital in Cape Town, South Africa in 2008 [75]. The results of this case series of 27 HIV recipients who received kidneys from deceased HIV-infected donors noted 5-year posttransplant patient and allograft survival rate of 74% and 84%, respectively, among individuals with well-controlled HIV disease [75]. Beginning in 2016, select centers in the United States have begun performing HIV-positive to HIV-positive renal transplants in addition to positive-to-positive liver transplants as part of a multicenter research trial (ClinicalTrials.gov identifier number: NCT02602262).

Mittal et al. reported the first pancreas transplant alone in an HIV-positive recipient with good outcomes [76]. Reported outcomes of SPK transplants in HIV-positive patients have been mixed with two of four patients in a review series experiencing graft failure including one death [77].

Common infections in the pretransplantation period are summarized in Table 4.2.

Pharmacologic Considerations in Patients with Chronic Kidney Disease Undergoing Kidney Transplantation

Patients on hemodialysis also require careful titration of renal-dosed medications before and after transplant. In the pretransplant setting, this may translate to limited HCV treatment options or difficulty optimizing a pretransplant HIV regimen. In the posttransplant setting, this may lead to resistance or failure of virologic suppression if antiretrovirals are underdosed, for instance, or breakthrough opportunistic infections if prophylactic antimicrobials are underdosed. Specifically, antiretroviral agents which require dose modification in patients with chronic kidney disease include reverse transcriptase inhibitors emtricitabine, lamivudine, and tenofovir. In general, the protease inhibitors, non-nucleoside reverse transcriptase inhibitors, and integrase inhibitors do not warrant dose adjustment in the setting of chronic kidney disease [78]. However, in managing HIV-infected patients in the pretransplant period, consideration should be given to selecting a regimen that avoids drug interactions with anticipated immunosuppressives introduced after transplantation. Specifically, protease inhibitors are potent inhibitors of CYP3A4 isoenzymes and can result in increased drug exposure of the calcineurin inhibitors [78]. Conversely, the NNRTIs can result in decreased drug exposure of the calcineurin inhibitors [78]. Regimens that include integrase inhibitors such as raltegravir lack drug interactions with the CYP450 system and may be a preferred regimen for appropriate patients [79]. More recently, cobicistat, a potent inhibitor of CYP3A4 isoenzyme, has been complexed to several antiretrovirals in order to improve drug exposure. It can be anticipated that cobicistat will also interact with the antirejection immunosuppressive regimen, and therefore avoidance of these agents should be considered when constructing an antiretroviral regimen for an HIV-infected kidney transplant candidate. Maraviroc, which is an HIV CCR5 entry inhibitor, may show promise in the posttransplantation setting, as this may provide the added benefit of improved allograft survival, as loss or blockade of the CCR5 receptor has been associated with reduced allograft rejection rates [80].

Conversely, overdosing of certain antimicrobials or antiretrovirals in the setting of pretransplant declining renal function or posttransplant acute or chronic allograft rejection may negatively impact graft function, as may be seen with the use of tenofovir or trimethoprim-sulfamethoxazole (Table 4.3). Other important anti-infective agents that could result in significant drug interactions with the immunosuppressive regimen due to CYP 450 isoenzyme inhibition include the triazole antifungal agents such as fluconazole and voriconazole (Table 4.4). These agents can cause increased drug exposure of immunosuppressives such as the calcineurin inhibitors.

Table 4.3 Commonly used anti-infectives in the renal transplant recipient requiring dose adjustment for renal function

Medication	Indication/use
Acyclovir/valacyclovir	HSV prevention and treatment
Aminoglycosides (amikacin, tobramycin, gentamicin)	Gram-negative bacterial infection
Amphotericin B	Fungal infection, especially *Aspergillus* spp. and *Zygomycetes*
β-lactam and cephalosporin classes	Bacterial infection
Ciprofloxacin, levofloxacin	Treatment of bacterial infections, treatment of Polyoma BK Virus (PyBKV) infection
Colistin	Gram-negative bacterial infection
Daptomycin	Gram-positive bacterial infection
Emtricitabine, lamivudine, tenofovir	HIV therapy
Ertapenem, meropenem, imipenem	Resistant Gram-negative bacterial infection
Fluconazole	Candida prevention and treatment
Foscarnet	Resistant CMV and HSV infection
Ganciclovir/valganciclovir	CMV prevention and treatment
Trimethoprim-sulfamethoxazole	Urinary tract infection and *Pneumocystis* prevention and treatment
Vancomycin, intravenous	Resistant Gram-positive bacterial infections

Table 4.4 Anti-infectives modulating cytochrome P450 drug metabolism (anti-infectives and immunosuppressants metabolized via CYP450 isoenzyme)

Inducers	Inhibitors	
Will accelerate substrate metabolism and decrease drug effect	Will slow substrate metabolism and increase drug effect	Post-transplant maintenance immunosuppressants that are CYP450 substrates
Nevaripine (CYP3A4, CYP2B6)	Ciprofloxacin (CYP1A2)	Cyclosporine (CYP3A4)
Efavirenz (CYP3A4)	Clarithromycin (CYP3A4)	Everolimus (CYP3A4)
Etravirine (CYP3A4)	Cobicistat[a] (CYP3A4, CYP2D6)	Prednisone (CYP3A4)
Rifampin, Rifabutin (CYP1A2, CYP2C9, CYP2C19, CYP3A4)	Erythromycin (CYP3A4)	Sirolimus (CYP3A4)
	Etravirine (CYP2C9, CYP2C19)	Tacrolimus (CYP3A4)
	Fluconazole (CYP2C9, CYP2C19, CYP3A4)	
	Isavuconazole (CYP3A4)	
	Isoniazid (CYP2C19)	
	Itraconazole (CYP3A4)	
	Ketoconazole (CYP3A4)	
	Metronidazole (CYP2C9)	
	Posaconazole (CYP3A4)	
	Ritonavir (as part of a boosted protease inhibitor regimen)[b] (CYP2C9, CYP2C19, CYP2D6, CYP3A4)	
	Terbinafine (CYP2D6)	
	Trimethoprim-sulfamethoxazole (CYP2C9)	
	Voriconazole (CYP3A4, CYP2C19, CYP2C9)	

[a]As part of a boosted HIV regimen with atazanavir, darunavir, elvitegravir

[b]Boosted protease inhibitor regimens: Atazanavir, darunavir, or lopinavir with ritonavir

Pretransplantation Screening for Potential Recipients

Routine screening testing to be done for renal transplant candidates mirrors that of other solid organ transplant candidates and includes serologic testing for immunity to vari-

Table 4.5 Infectious screening for the pre-renal transplant recipient

Laboratory testing
HIV Ag/Ab (4th generation) assay and Nucleic Acid Test (NAT)
Hepatitis serologies:
Hepatitis A antibody
Hepatitis B surface antigen, surface antibody, core antibody, and NAT
Hepatitis C antibody and NAT
Vaccination titers: measles, mumps, rubella, varicella
Syphilis screen – either treponemal or nontreponemal test
Latent TB screen – generally interferon gamma release assay preferred over tuberculin skin test
CMV IgG antibody
EBV antibodies
Based on regions of endemicity
Strongyloides antibody
Coccidioides serology
T. cruzi serology
Imaging
Chest radiography
Should be performed for any patient with a positive TB screening test
May warrant further evaluation if pulmonary nodules suggest infectious etiology, such as fungal or mycobacterial infection

cella, measles, mumps and rubella, serologic and nucleic acid testing (NAT) for HIV, HBV, and HCV, and screens for syphilis and latent tuberculosis. Patients from endemic regions may additionally undergo screening for latent strongyloidiasis, coccidioidomycosis, and, rarely, histoplasmosis, HTLV, or trypanosomiasis. The recipient's CMV and EBV serostatus should be established by serology [81]. Patients may remain listed for years awaiting deceased donor renal allograft transplantation, and screening for viral infections such as HBV and HCV should be kept up to date. Serologic screening tests and recommended imaging are summarized in Table 4.5.

As with other solid organ transplant recipients, renal transplantation places recipients at an increased risk of developing tuberculosis (TB), estimated at 20–74 times higher risk among solid organ transplant recipients, so testing for latent tuberculosis should be included as part of routine pretransplantation screening [82]. It has been well established that patients on hemodialysis are 6–25 times more likely to develop tuberculosis as compared to the general population [83]. Moreover, latent tuberculous infection (LTBI) has been reported to be as high as 20–70% in the hemodialysis population [83]. Therefore, screening for LTBI, and treatment of LTBI, is warranted in all patients on hemodialysis and of particular importance for those who are being considered for listing for kidney transplantation. Most dialysis centers routinely perform annual tuberculin skin testing (TST). Presence of uremia in patients with chronic kidney disease undergoing HD alters macrophage and T-cell functions; the resulted anergy has been noted in as many as 44% of such patients compared with 16% anergy in the general population, making TST less optimal screening tool for this population [83]. A retrospective study of dialysis patients found the two-step, or boosted, TST to have a sensitivity of 14% and specificity of 88% among dialysis patients using an abnormal chest X-ray as a proxy [84]. Two studies demonstrated that a single-step TST had a sensitivity of 11.3% and 14.7%, and an additional 12.1% and 13.1% of the hemodialysis patients, respectively, had a positive TST using the two-step method [83]. Given concerns for poor sensitivity of TST in the dialysis population, most transplant centers now rely on serum interferon-gamma release assays (IGRA) using QuantiFERON-TB Gold in tube (Qiagen, Victoria, Australia) or T-SPOT.TB (Oxford Immunotec, Oxfordshire, England). In hemodialysis patients, the sensitivities of IGRAs for the diagnosis of LTBI have ranged from 22% to 71.4%, and the specificity was noted to be as low as 41.9% and as high as 100% [83]. In renal transplant patients, TST and IGRA results may have only fair agreement, but TST induration size may correlate with positive IGRA [85]. In a prospective study following potential kidney transplant recipients after TST or IGRA testing, Kim et al. found that 13% of 312 patients had positive TST or clinical risk factors requiring pretransplant isoniazid (INH) therapy and none of these patients developed active tuberculosis. In the remaining 272 patients, 71 had a positive T-Spot alone and a negative TST; these patients did not receive INH, and four patients went on to develop active tuberculosis infection after undergoing kidney transplantation. This study demonstrates that T-spot is a more effective method for screening latent tuberculosis in patients being evaluated for kidney transplantation [86]. Based on the high rates and heightened risk of active tuberculosis disease in patients with chronic kidney disease on dialysis, screening for latent and active TB is an essential part of the pretransplant evaluation. While it appears that IGRAs may be the preferred screening modality for LTBI, if TST is the only available modality, then a two-step TST should be performed. Active TB needs to also be ruled out based on a careful assessment of signs and symptoms, and a chest X-ray should be performed as part of the pretransplant evaluation. In high-risk patients, or patients with indeterminate results, high-resolution CT imaging of the thorax may be warranted. Recommendations for the screening, diagnosis, and management of TB in solid organ transplant recipients are available and should be implemented as part of the pretransplant evaluation [87].

Though not a routine part of pretransplant screening, an abnormal pretransplant urodynamic assessment is associated with more frequent urinary complications [88]. Other screenings have been proposed to estimate the risk for bacterial and opportunistic infections (OIs) during posttransplant setting require further validation studies. It was interesting to note that a measured immune risk phenotype prior to transplantation defined as +CMV serology plus CD4/CD8 ratio <1 and/or CD8 T cell count >90th percentile was associated with higher risk for severe bacterial infections and OIs after transplantation [89].

Living Donor and Deceased Donor Screening for Occult Infection

In 2014, 5537 of 17,107 kidney transplants came from living donors [12], and an increasing number are donated via paired exchange in which potential recipients with willing donors may be matched in a larger pool to those with more compatible kidneys. Five hundred forty-four such unrelated paired donations were performed in 2014 [11]. Any potential living kidney donor must undergo their own screening evaluation for occult infection prior to transplantation including clinical history and laboratory evaluation for HIV, HBV, HCV, CMV, and Epstein-Barr virus (EBV) serostatus, syphilis screen, and TB screening. At-risk live donors, defined by regional and seasonal infection-risk variation, may additionally require screening for coccidioidomycosis, strongyloidiasis, West Nile virus, and latent or subclinical *Trypanosoma cruzi* infection [90]. Although there is currently no data regarding Zika virus screening among solid organ graft donors, living kidney donors from Zika virus endemic areas may have prior infection. The Organ Procurement and Transplantation Network (OPTN)/United Network for Organ Sharing (UNOS) Ad Hoc Disease Transmission Advisory Committee does not recommend prior Zika virus infection as a strict exclusion criteria from organ donation; however, the risk of donor-derived infection should be balanced with benefits of transplantation [91]. As the Zika virus outbreak continues in Central and South America, the Caribbean, Mexico, and now parts of Florida and Texas, this will likely be an evolving area of research and guidelines as Zika-infected donors are assessed for organ donation and renal or other transplant recipients travel to the evolving endemic regions and develop new Zika virus infection after undergoing transplantation.

There is an increasing number of deceased donor renal allografts coming from high infection-risk donors (HRD), in part driven by an ongoing epidemic of recreational drug use and overdose deaths. The US Public Health Service currently defines 12 criteria for being at increased risk of recent HIV, HBV, and/or HCV infection, with concern of transferring infection via allograft during a "window" period where recently acquired viremia is not yet detectable by antibody or nucleic acid testing [92] (see Tables 4.6 and 4.7). Actual risk of HIV acquisition during the window period has been estimated between 0.04 and 4.9 per 10,000 donors based on NAT testing. The window for highest HIV infection risk exists in injection drug users (4.9 per 10,000 donors), men who have sex with men (4.2 per 10,000), commercial sex workers (2.7 per 10,000), incarcerated donors (0.9 per 10,000), donors exposed to HIV through blood (0.6 per 10,000), donors engaging in high-risk sexual activities (0.3 per 10,000), and hemophiliacs (0.035 per 10,000) [93]. Pooled risk of window period HCV transmission from

Table 4.6 Special situation donor criteria

High-risk donor criteria	Extended criteria donor
People who have had sex with a person known or suspected to have HIV, HBV, or HCV infection in the preceding 12 months	Donor aged >60 years Donor aged >50 years, plus two of the following:
Men who have had sex with men (MSM) in the preceding 12 months	History of hypertension Serum creatinine ≥1.5
Women who have had sex with a man with a history of MSM behavior in the preceding 12 months	Death resulting from a stroke
People who have had sex in exchange for money or drugs in the preceding 12 months	
People who have had sex with a person who had sex in exchange for money or drugs in the preceding 12 months	
People who have had sex with a person who injected drugs by intravenous, intramuscular or subcutaneous route for nonmedical reasons the preceding 12 months	
A child who is ≤18 months of age and born to a mother known to be infected with, or at an increased risk for, HIV, HBV or HCV infection	
A child who has been breastfed within the preceding 12 months and the mother is known to be infected with, or at increased risk for, HIV infection	
People who have injected drugs by intravenous, intramuscular, or subcutaneous routes for nonmedical reasons in the preceding 12 months	
People who have been in lockup, jail, prison, or a juvenile correctional facility for more than 72 consecutive hours in the preceding 12 months	
People who have been newly diagnosed with, or have been treated for, syphilis, gonorrhea, *Chlamydia*, or genital ulcers in the preceding 12 months	
People who have been on hemodialysis in the preceding 12 months – *at increased risk for recent HCV infection only*	

Table 4.7 Window period lengths

	Serology	Nucleic acid test (NAT)
HIV	Third-generation/standard serology: 19–20 days	5–6 days
	Fourth-generation/combined Ag/Ab serology 7–15 days	
HCV	58–65 days	3–5 days
HBV	36–44 days	20–25 days

HRDs ranges from 0.027 to 32.4 per 10,000 donors, with the highest risk categories being injection drug users (32.4 per 10,000), commercial sex workers and donors exhibiting high-risk behavior (12.3 per 10,000), men who have sex with men (3.5 per 10,000), incarcerated donors (0.8 per 10,000), donors exposed to HIV-infected blood (0.4 per 10,000), and hemophiliacs (0.027 per 10,000) [93].

As of 2010, approximately 9% of deceased kidney donors were classified as HRD [94]. A decision analytic Markov model of renal failure treatment modalities estimated that use of HRD kidneys as compared to discarding these organs would result in higher patient survival, a greater number of quality-adjusted life years (QALY) (5.6 vs. 5.1 years per patient), more kidney transplants, and lower cost of care ($60,000 vs. $71,000 per QALY). They estimated a lower total number of infections, 13.1 vs. 14.8 infections per 1000 patients over 20 years occurring in recipients of HRD organs because of the increased time on hemodialysis if HRD organs are discarded, which in turn carries higher HCV incidence [95]. Because HRDs tend to be younger with less medial comorbidities, recipients of HRD renal transplants have a significantly improved 5-year graft survival compared with non-HRD expanded criteria donor kidney recipients of 84% vs. 78%, respectively ($p < 0.001$) [96].

Infectious Diseases Considerations for Incompatible Kidney Transplant Recipients

Some potential kidney transplant recipients may have otherwise acceptable donors except for the presence of preformed human leukocyte antigen (HLA) antibodies or ABO blood group incompatibility. Similarly, some patients on the wait list for a deceased donor may be highly sensitized, often due to previous blood product transfusion, pregnancy or prior transplantation, and subsequently have longer wait times and decreased likelihood of finding a suitable donor. These patients may be candidates for HLA or ABO-incompatible kidney transplant. Recipients of incompatible kidney transplants have a survival benefit over patients who do not undergo transplantation or wait for a deceased donor allograft, with an 8-year survival benefit significant across all levels of donor-specific antibody [97]. To prevent antibody-mediated rejection and graft loss in these cases, patients undergo pretransplantation desensitization with rituximab, intravenous immunoglobulin (IVIG), and/or plasmapheresis, although specific protocols vary by center. Rituximab is associated with numerous potential adverse events, including cytopenias/hypogammaglobulinemia and increased infectious risks (see Table 4.8). In the United States, rituximab carries a boxed warning for HBV reactivation which may lead to fulminant hepatitis, liver failure, or death [98]. Patients should be screened for HBV typically as part of routine pretransplant screening; see the section above entitled Pretransplantation Screening for Potential Recipients prior to treatment. Those with positive surface antigen should start treatment, and patients with negative HBsAg and a positive core antibody (HBcAb) should have ongoing monitoring for reactivation [98, 99]. HBV reactivation has been reported greater than a year after rituximab therapy [98, 100]. Other newly acquired or reactivated viral infections at increased risk following rituximab use include CMV, herpes simplex virus (HSV), parvovirus B19, varicella zoster virus (VZV), West Nile virus, and HCV [98]. Rituximab also carries a boxed warning against progressive multifocal leukoencephalopathy (PML) due to JC polyomavirus [98]. Data has been mixed as to increased risk of infection after incompatible kidney transplant but generally shows at least a trend toward increased viral infection and surgical complications [101–103]. However, actual increased risk may be impacted by immunosuppressive regimen, splenectomy, or preconditioning regimen all of which may vary between centers, making it difficult to standardize risks across the population as a whole [103]. Overall patient and allograft survival and acute rejection are comparable to HLA and ABO compatible kidney transplants [101, 102].

Table 4.8 Infectious risks associated with rituximab use [98, 104]

Bacterial/mycobacterial	Sepsis, sinusitis, nasopharyngitis, bronchitis, pneumonia, cellulitis, urinary tract infection, colitis
	Mycobacterium avium, *Mycobacterium kansasii*
Viral	Hepatitis B reactivation
	Cytomegalovirus (CMV)
	Herpes simplex virus (HSV)
	Parvovirus B19
	Varicella zoster virus (VZV)
	West Nile virus (WNV)
	Hepatitis C
	Progressive multifocal leukoencephalopathy (PML) caused by JC virus
	BK virus
Fungal	Pneumocystis pneumonia
Parasitic	Babesiosis
Non-infectious	Infusion reaction (fever, rigors, nausea, pruritus, angioedema, hypotension, headache, vomiting, rash, and other symptoms) may mimic acute infection

Infections in the Posttransplantation Period: An Overview

Infections contribute significantly to the morbidity and mortality that is experienced in the solid organ transplant recipient. It is estimated that infections account for 15–20% of the causes of mortality in kidney transplant recipients, although this has been declining over the past several years due to improvements in anti-infective prophylaxis strategies [105]. Candidates for kidney and kidney-pancreas transplantations carry with them their own "baggage" that places them at risk for infectious complications, specifically uremia which is associated with depressed T-cell functions, as well as diabetes mellitus which contributes to hosts' suppressed immune response, and the potential hyperglycemia that places patients at risk for infection after surgery. Several factors contribute to infections following transplantation and include (1) environmental and external factors such as pathogens acquired from the healthcare environment including Gram-negative enteric bacteria or the external environment like endemic mycoses or molds; (2) reactivation of prior infections in the recipient such as HSV, VZV, and CMV; (3) donor-derived infections; (4) iatrogenic complications associated with surgery or hospitalization; and (5) overall state of immunosuppression due to antirejection regimen and infection with immunomodulatory viruses such as CMV, EBV, HBV, HCV, or HIV or both [106, 107]. Another factor that is unique to kidney transplant recipients is the type of renal replacement therapy that precedes transplantation. Postoperative infection rates are notably higher in patients on peritoneal vs. hemodialysis prior to undergoing transplantation (67.5% vs. 25.9%; $p < 0.00001$) [108]. A timeline has been proposed by several authors [107] to categorize the types of infections that are encountered in the posttransplantation period and will be addressed here.

Early Infections Following Kidney and Kidney-Pancreas Transplants

The immediate posttransplantation period has been defined as <30 days from the time of transplantation and is most typically due to healthcare-acquired pathogens, although donor-derived infections can also occur in rare situations.

Early Infections: Risk Factors

There are numerous risk factors associated with the development of infectious complications in the initial posttransplantation period. The majority of these early infections are healthcare acquired, and are related to the risk of exposure to the healthcare setting, and risk of complications of the actual surgical procedure. Other unique factors also contribute to infection risk and are reviewed below.

A Cochrane analysis found insufficient evidence to link early (<14 days) or late (>14 days) steroid withdrawal or steroid avoidance to risk of infection in the postoperative period [109]. They identified only one trial in which significantly more urinary tract infections (UTIs) were reported in the late withdrawal group compared to steroid avoidance, with a relative risk of 0.41 [110].

Markers reported to be independent predictors of infection in the kidney transplant population include elevated ferritin, magnesium deficiency, and vitamin D deficiency, although they may be altered by other illness or physiologic stressors, therefore warranting further study [111–113].

Hypogammaglobulinemia, defined as IgG level <350 mg/dL, has also been identified as a risk factor for severe opportunistic infection and higher number of infections in the first 3 months after transplantation compared to patients with normal serum immunoglobulin levels and may be modifiable with immunoglobulin infusions and monitoring of levels [114, 115].

Approximately one in three renal transplant recipients will have an early readmission occurring within the first 30 days after renal transplantation [116]. Infectious complications appear to be an important cause for early readmission. A large retrospective review identified surgical site problems as the primary cause of early readmission, which may include superficial wound infection or symptomatic perinephric fluid collection. The second most common reason for readmission was UTI with or without bloodstream infection, followed by pneumonia and fever of unknown origin. Other nonsurgical complications leading to readmission included colitis, epididymitis, neutropenia, leukocytosis, pancreatitis, cholangitis, lower extremity cellulitis, and PD catheter infection. Discharge-level factors associated with readmission included electrolyte abnormalities and delayed graft function. Previously published data has also cited older age, black race, low educational level, and medical comorbidities such as hypertension, obesity, diabetes mellitus, cardiovascular disease, HCV, stroke, chronic obstructive pulmonary disease, prior transplant, and frailty as risk factors for early readmission. Donor risk factors associated with recipient readmission include age, expanded criteria donor status, donation after circulatory death, and cold ischemic time. Transplant risk factors include HLA mismatch, length of stay, lack of induction therapy, waitlist time, delayed graft function, and, in one study, weekend discharge [117–120].

Early Infections: Surgical Complications

Renal transplant recipients are at risk for the typical postoperative complications and infections of immunocompetent surgical patients. The most common infections include surgical site infections, urinary tract infections, hospital-acquired pneumonia, and central line-associated bloodstream infections (CLABSI) [106]. The typical causative bacterial organisms are those that are most commonly associated with the particular site of infection. Therefore, it can be anticipated that surgical site infections are predominantly due to Gram-positive cocci, in particular *Staphylococcus aureus*, whereas UTIs are commonly due to enteric Gram-negative bacilli.

UTIs are the most common infection in renal transplant recipients, with US Renal Data System reporting a cumulative incidence of 17% within the first 6 months following transplantation [121]. Ureteral stents placed at the time of renal allograft transplantation confer increased risk for UTI within the first month following transplant (11.4% vs. 0.3% of non-stented allograft recipients; $P < 0.001$) [122].

In addition to the typical postsurgical infectious complications, there are risks unique to the kidney transplantation procedure. Perfusion fluid (PF) used following deceased donor nephrectomy, if contaminated, may lead to serious infection in the recipient [123]. Use of empiric antifungal agents in the perioperative period is routinely given in case of yeast contamination of PF [123]. Ranghino et al. analyzed recipients with bacterial contamination of PF and found an overall incidence of 38.4%, with half being staphylococci and 9.9% *Candida albicans*. Targeted preemptive therapy of PF contamination did not reduce the rate of PF-related allograft infection, which were low despite high frequency of such contamination. The authors suggest a reasonable reduction in the use of antibiotic therapy can be considered along with close monitoring.

As many as 10–34% of pancreas transplant recipients experience complications requiring relaparotomy [124–126], most commonly due to vascular graft thrombosis and intra-abdominal infection but also pancreatitis, bleeding, and stump and anastomotic leaks [125, 126]. Approximately half of those undergoing relaparotomy require graft pancreatectomy [126], but this may be performed in as many as 70% of patients when done for leaks or abscesses [125, 126]. Risk factors for early relaparotomy include donor age >40 years and recipient obesity [125] as well as bladder drainage versus enteric drainage (18.2% vs. 5.8%; $p < 0.05$). Relaparotomy did not significantly affect patient survival consistently between studies, but relaparotomy is consistently associated with significantly lower graft survival [125–127].

Clinically significant peripancreatic fluid collections (PPFC) were found in 16% of pancreas-kidney transplant recipients in a study by Singh et al. [128]. The majority of PPFCs occurred within the first month and may occur up to 3 months after undergoing transplantation. Most patients required relaparotomy except for two in this series who underwent drainage by interventional radiology. Over half (56%) of PPFC were infected; all had bacterial infection with the most common organisms being *Enterococcus faecalis*, coliform/enteric pathogens, *Staphylococcus* spp., and lactobacillus, and 10% of these patients' cultures additionally isolated *Candida*. Multidrug-resistant (MDR) bacteria were isolated in 11%. Similar patient and kidney graft survival was seen in patients with and without PPFC; however, significantly lower total pancreas graft survival resulted (68% vs. 85%), and a greater incidence of infection was also observed (75% vs. 46%; $P < 0.05$) during 5 years following transplantation. Patients with PPFCs had significantly greater incidence of recurrent UTI (58% vs. 36%), bacteremia (31% vs. 3%), and fungal (28% vs. 1%) and viral infection (28% vs. 14%) compared to patients without the evidence of PPFC ($p < 0.001$) [128].

Early Infections: Healthcare-Acquired Infections

As noted above, kidney and pancreas-kidney recipients are at risk of typical postoperative and nosocomial infectious complications in the early posttransplantation period, as well as unique infectious risks related to their transplantation.

In addition to the healthcare-acquired pathogens noted above, a growing problem in hospitals is the increased incidence of *Clostridium difficile* infection (CDI) colitis. Higher CDI incidence has been reported in the solid organ transplant population [129]. Unique CDI risk factors in the kidney and kidney-pancreas transplant population include male gender (82% vs. 48%; $p = 0.003$), deceased donor recipients (84% vs. 64%; $p = 0.045$), leukopenia (18% vs. 4%; $p = 0.038$), recent gastrointestinal procedure within the preceding 3 months (18% vs. 4%; $p = 0.038$), and more days of cumulative and restrictive antimicrobial exposure and more cephalosporin use (43% vs. 16%; $p = 0.008$).

Infection with MDR and extensive drug-resistant organisms is also of increasing concern worldwide and in patients undergoing allograft transplantation. In transplant recipients, exposure to prolonged stays in intensive care units, extensive preemptive and empiric use of broad-spectrum antibiotics and immunosuppressive antirejection therapy, and systemic corticosteroids may be the harbingers of these severe infections. Extended-spectrum beta-lactamase (ESBL)-producing *Enterobacteriaceae* such as *Escherichia coli* and *Klebsiella pneumoniae* have become increasingly prevalent. In SOT recipients with *Klebsiella pneumoniae* infection, over half may be ESBL producers [130]. ESBL-producing *Enterobacteriaceae* have been isolated in up to 11% of urinary cultures in one hospitalized kidney transplant cohort [131]. The urinary tract is the most commonly infected site in renal transplant recipients with MDR infection [132–134], and MDROs accounted for 69% of isolates in symptomatic renal transplant recipients with UTI [132]. Comparison of bacterial species and susceptibilities in a renal transplant population over 10 years has shown a significant increased presence of *Klebsiella pneumoniae* (9.5% vs. 15.6%), *Pseudomonas aeruginosa* (1.8% vs. 7.9%), and *Enterobacter cloacae* (0.6% vs. 3.1%) as well as higher drug non-susceptibility rates for all antibiotic classes with the exception of fosfomycin [132]. Routine perioperative antimicrobial prophylaxis may be ineffective against resistant bacteria or yeast that may have been present in the donor allograft or bloodstream at the time of procurement [135]. In deceased liver donors, risk of donor allograft infection with any bacterial organism is increased if the donor received vasopressors ($p = 0.22$) or cardiopulmonary resuscitation ($p = 0.036$) or had a prolonged intensive care unit stay of 7 days or more ($p \leq 0.0001$) [136], although as little as 2 days may be sufficient for the donor to acquire an MDR organism (MDRO) [137]. Transmission of resistant pathogens leads to high morbidity and mortality. In a tertiary care hospital outbreak with *Klebsiella pneumoniae* carbapenemase (KPC)-producing *K. pneumoniae*, the incidence of KPC infection in renal transplant recipients was 26.3%, and overall 30-day mortality among the SOT recipients was 42% [133]. A prolonged outbreak of carbapenem-resistant *Enterobacter gergoviae* involving renal transplant recipients identified flaws in infection prevention practices of cleaning and handling urinary devices as a contributing factor for the infection risk [134]. Recipient risk factors for acquisition included advanced age, ureteral stent use, retransplantation, and male gender. A kidney-pancreas recipient with donor-derived carbapenem-resistant *Acinetobacter baumannii* (CRAB) with blaOXA-23 carbapenemase gene who died less than 1 week following transplant had developed widespread and deep-seated infection including acute mitral valve endocarditis with splenic and renal septic emboli, myocarditis, peritonitis, and pneumonia which were confirmed on postmortem examination [138].

The above data demonstrates that MDR organisms such as ESBL producing *Enterobacteriaceae*, carbapenem-resistant *Enterobacteriaceae* (CRE), *Pseudomonas*, and *Acinetobacter* spp. substantially contribute to morbidity and mortality in recipients of solid allograft transplant. Therefore, clinicians caring for these patients will need to be aware of their local hospital antibiograms when making empiric antibiotic selection for suspected infection in this high-risk patient population.

Early Infections: Donor-Derived Infection

Huaman et al. analyzed UNOS data on all primary, single organ deceased donor kidney transplants from 2008 to 2013 and found an incidence of donor blood culture positivity in 8.1% of cases [139]. Donor blood culture positivity was associated with delayed graft function but did not impact graft or patient survival. Although bacterial colonization at a distant site, such as the respiratory tract, in a renal allograft recipient does not warrant uniform use of antibacterial therapy, it may rarely signify unrecognized bacteremia [135]. Return of positive donor blood cultures after transplantation may warrant treatment in the recipient. The most common pathogens include coagulase-negative staphylococci and *Staphylococcus aureus*, although Gram-negative infections are being seen in increasing numbers. The exact duration is unknown, but it is recommended to treat the recipient with targeted antibiotics for a minimum of 7–10 days [140, 141]. Use of a kidney allograft from a donor with respiratory colonization of KPC or CRAB may still be considered with close follow-up, but urine culture positivity with these resistant organisms should be considered a contraindication to use of that kidney unless infection is eradicated prior to transplantation [135]. Donor bacteremia with an MDRO should likewise be avoided if recognized prior to transplantation [135].

The risk of donor-derived viral hepatitis and HIV is low, but donor-derived transmissions have been documented. A quantitative review of the literature including 9 studies with 1385 kidney recipients found only 45 had seroconversion of hepatitis B markers [142]. Hepatitis B core antibody accounted for the majority of those who tested positive after receiving a core antibody positive graft. Only 0.28% of recipients converted to surface antigen positivity, and there was no symptomatic hepatitis nor were patient or graft outcomes worse with seroconversion [135, 142]. Both HCV and HIV have been inadvertently transmitted when donors had unrecognized infection. The first known transmission of HIV and HCV to four recipients- two kidneys, liver, and heart- resulted in two deaths and allograft failure in the other two recipients [143]. Human error has been a factor in other instances of transplantation of HIV-positive organs into negative recipients. In Taiwan, miscommunication by phone between a transplant coordinator and laboratory technician with regard to an HIV test resulted in five recipients being transplanted with HIV-positive organs, including heart, liver, lungs, and two kidneys [144]. Patients were started on postexposure prophylaxis (PEP) within 36 h after transplant, and reportedly, follow-up testing of the recipients was negative for HIV; the duration and exact PEP regimen as well as interval to follow-up testing were not defined. Three Italian patients also received HIV-positive organs as the result of an error in documentation after misreading of a computer printout [145]. Further testing from a tissue bank laboratory was faxed on a weekend without verbal communication and resulted in a delay of 5 days until the donor's status was recognized by the transplanting institution. These patients also received HIV medication and have had negative HIV NAT testing and functioning grafts reported at 7 years after transplantation [135]. In both situations, neither donor's family was aware of their HIV status. Transmission and accidental use of HIV-positive renal allografts has not been limited to deceased donors. In 2009, an adult male potential donor tested negative for HIV 79 days before transplant but had unprotected sex with a male with unknown HIV status in the interval before transplantation [146]. The kidney recipient had a posttransplantation course complicated by hospitalizations for febrile illness, renal insufficiency and possible rejection and then tested positive for HIV and had a CD4 cell count <100 cells/μL when hospitalized with refractory oral and esophageal candidiasis.

Human T-cell lymphotropic virus type 1 (HTLV-1) is another retrovirus that has had documented transmission via organ transplantation [147]. HTLV-1 has pockets of endemicity worldwide, but seroprevalence is extremely low in the United States, accounting for 0.0034% among blood donors [148]. It is largely asymptomatic, but in a minority of patients (2–5%), it may cause adult T-cell leukemia- lymphoma or, even more rarely, HTLV-1-associated myelopathy, also known as tropical spastic paraparesis [149]. Twelve published cases of HTLV-1-associated myelopathy from Spain and Japan, including nine kidney recipients, reviewed by Ramanan et al., have resulted from reactivation, primary infection, and donor-derived infection [147]. The first donor-derived case in the United States, reported in 2014, occurred after deceased donor renal transplantation from a donor who emigrated from the Dominican Republic in childhood and resulted in recipient myelopathy at 5 months after transplant [147]. The low seroprevalence in the United States led to a high degree of organ wastage due to false-positive results as well as a lack of FDA-licensed testing in many organ procurement organization (OPO) labs, so in 2009 the OPTN ceased to recommend universal donor screening [149].

In the early posttransplantation period, clinicians should be aware of the rare possibility of donor-derived neurotropic viruses. Transmission of West Nile virus (WNV) has also occurred as a donor-derived infection after transplantation [135]. The kidney may be the site of prolonged WNV replication and shedding, and testing of urine instead of blood has been proposed [135]. The first two clusters of rabies transmission via SOT to non-vaccinated recipients reported development of symptoms and death within 6 weeks of transplantation [135, 150]. Recently a renal allograft recipient developed delayed donor-derived rabies at 18 months after transplantation; however, three other recipients from the same donor survived [151]. Clusters of donor-derived lymphocytic choriomeningitis virus (LCMV) have been reported with poor survival outcomes in the recipients [152].

Donor-derived infections due to other miscellaneous causes have occurred. Immunosuppression is a risk factor for dissemination of latent *Strongyloides* infection, which may persist for decades after leaving an endemic area, typically subtropical climates but also portions of the Southeastern United States. Hyperinfection syndrome from massive larval proliferation and autoinfection after SOT immune suppression carries a mortality rate of greater than 50% [153]. Kidney recipients may reactivate in the setting of profound immunosuppression, but donor-derived infection has also occurred, with the majority of reported cases in the United States occurring in renal transplant recipients [154]. While Chagas disease due to *Trypanosoma cruzi* is endemic in Central and South America, it is estimated that 300,000 persons living in the United States are infected with *T. cruzi* [155]. Transfusion-related and donor-derived infections have occurred predominantly in heart transplant recipients. In 2001, donor-derived Chagas disease from a cadaveric donor from Central America occurred in three recipients: one kidney transplant, one kidney-pancreas, and one recipient of hepatic allograft. The recipient of kidney-pancreas transplant was febrile and diagnosed after a finding of trypomastigotes on a peripheral blood smear; the other recipients were later found to have positive culture for Chagas disease parasite. Despite treatment with nifurtimox, the kidney-pancreas and liver recipients died of myocarditis and hepatic and renal failure, respectively [156]. Primary infection and reactivation have also been documented, most typically in cardiac transplant recipients, however rarely a cause for renal allograft failure [157].

Common infections in the early postoperative period are summarized in Table 4.9.

Opportunistic Infections in Kidney and Pancreas-Kidney Transplant Recipients, First 6 Months Following Transplantation

Opportunistic Bacterial Infections

Solid organ transplant recipients as a whole are at greatly increased risk of TB infection, usually reactivation of latent infection, and carry a 20- to 74-fold higher rates than the general population [82, 158]. The cumulative incidence in renal transplant recipients is 5%, with approximately 40% of cases occurring in the first year [159]. Pulmonary TB represented 78% of cases, including disseminated disease. Predictably, active tuberculosis infection has an unfavorable impact on graft and patient survival, particularly in patients with disseminated disease [158, 159]. Therefore, IGRA testing for latent TB infection should prompt treatment for latent TB in renal transplant recipients and has shown to reduce the risk for serious TB active infection in this group (RR 0.31) [158]. Those treated with isoniazid (INH) have no significant difference in the incidence of hepatitis. Most centers elect to treat with INH to avoid the drug-drug interactions between rifampin and steroids, as well as its effect on decreased CNI drug exposure and serum levels. However, there is data to support the use of rifampin-based regimens; they were well tolerated, without untoward effect on allograft function or increased risk for rejection [160].

Nontuberculous mycobacterial (NTM) infections are rare in renal transplant patients. A single-center study over a 7-year period identified 34 cases of NTM disease in SOT recipients, with only three episodes noted in kidney or kidney-pancreas recipients [161]. *Mycobacterium abscessus* and *Mycobacterium avium intracellulare* were the most

Table 4.9 Common infections in the early (≤30 day) post-kidney or kidney-pancreas transplantation period

Route of acquisition	Infection	Organisms	Risk factors
Surgical	Urinary tract infection	Gram-negative bacilli (especially *Enterobacteriaceae* and *Pseudomonas aeruginosa*), *Enterococcus* spp.	Placement of ureteral stents (kidney recipients), bladder drainage method (pancreas recipients) Candiduria: contamination of perfusion fluid
	Surgical site infection	Gram-positive cocci, less commonly Gram-negative bacilli	Obesity, older age, impaired glycemic control
	Pyelonephritis due to contamination of perfusion fluid	Staphylococci (50%), *Candida* species (10%)	
	Anastomotic leaks and peripancreatic fluid collections (pancreas recipients)	Enteric Gram-negative bacilli *Enterococcus* spp., *Staphylococcus* spp., *Lactobacillus*, *Candida* spp.; multidrug-resistant organisms (11%)	Enteric drainage method
Healthcare acquired	Urinary tract infection	*Enterococcus* spp., enteric Gram-negative bacilli especially *E. coli*	Presence of urinary catheter
	Pneumonia	Gram-negative bacilli, *S. aureus*	Mechanical ventilation especially if prolonged, aspiration, chronic lung disease
	Central line-associated bloodstream infection (CLABSI)	*Staphylococcus* spp., *Enterococcus* spp. Gram-negative bacilli	Indwelling central vascular catheter
	Colitis	*Clostridium difficile*	Deceased donor, leukopenia, recent gastrointestinal procedure in the preceding 3 months, more days of cumulative and restrictive antimicrobial exposure, more cephalosporin use
	Multidrug resistant organism (MDRO) infection, most commonly in the urinary tract	ESBL-producing *Enterobacteriaceae* (especially *E. coli* and *Klebsiella pneumoniae*), *P. aeruginosa* and *Enterobacter cloacae*; carbapenemase-producing *K. pneumoniae* (KPC); carbapenem resistant *Acinetobacter baumannii* (CRAB); vancomycin-resistant enterococci (VRE)	Prolonged intensive care/hospital stays, extensive antibiotic exposure
Donor-derived	Urinary tract infection (donor bacteriuria)	Enteric Gram-negative bacilli	
	Bloodstream infection (donor bacteremia)	Coagulase-negative staphylococci, *Staphylococcus aureus*, less commonly Gram-negative bacilli	
	Viral hepatitis	Hepatitis B virus, hepatitis C virus	High-risk donor Human error (such as in testing or reporting donor serologies)
	Retrovirus infection	HIV, HTLV	HTLV: Donor from endemic region HIV: High-risk donor Human error (such as in testing or reporting donor serologies)
	Neurotropic virus	West Nile virus, rabies virus, LCMV	
	Parasitic infection	Strongyloides stercoralis, Trypanosoma cruzi	Donor from endemic region

common pathogens, and the lung was the most common site of disease. Lung transplant recipients had the highest risk of infection. Infections due to *Nocardia* species are a relatively uncommon cause of infection in kidney and pancreas allograft recipients.

Fungal Infections

The risk of reactivation of endemic dimorphic fungal infections depends on individuals' exposure to the specific geographic locations. *Histoplasma capsulatum* is the most widely prevalent endemic dimorphic fungi causing human illness (see Fig. 4.1). Assi et al. reviewed over 150 histoplasmosis cases occurring in solid organ transplant recipients over a 7-year period, 67% of which occurred in kidney, kidney-pancreas, and pancreas recipients [162]. The median time to diagnosis was 27 months after transplantation; however, one-third of cases were diagnosed in the first year. Disseminated disease was present in 81% of the cases, and approximately one-third had severe disease requiring care in ICU. A 10% attributable mortality was observed with *Histoplasma* infec-

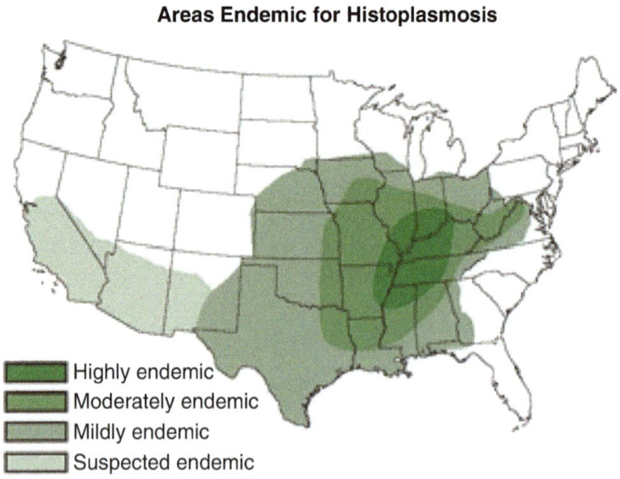

Fig. 4.1 Areas endemic for histoplasmosis [163]. (Reprinted from National Center for Emerging and Zoonotic Infectious Diseases, Centers for Disease Control and Prevention (CDC). 21 Nov 2015. http://www.cdc.gov/fungal/pdf/histoplasmosis-lifecycle508c.pdf)

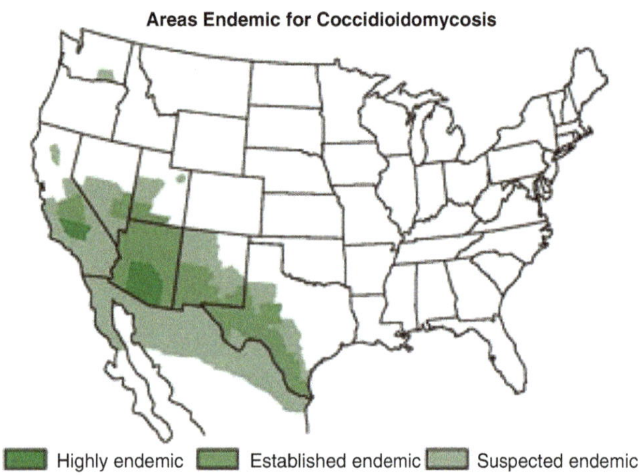

Fig. 4.2 Areas endemic to coccidioidomycosis. Known and suspected areas where the fungus that causes Valley fever lives in the United States [165]. (Reprinted from National Center for Emerging and Zoonotic Infectious Diseases, Centers for Disease Control and Prevention (CDC). Aug 2016. http://www.cdc.gov/features/valleyfever/)

tion and most deaths occurring within 1 month of infection diagnosis. Older age and severity of fungal disease were risk factors for death in these high-risk patients with histoplasmosis. Urinary histoplasma antigen was the most sensitive diagnostic test and was positive in 93% of the cases.

Coccidioidomycosis, caused by the dimorphic fungi *Coccidioides immitis* and *Coccidioides posadasii*, is endemic to the Southwestern United States, particularly Arizona and Southern California, as well as Northern Mexico and Central America [164] (Fig. 4.2). Coccidioidomycosis typically causes a self-limiting febrile illness with respiratory features; however, dissemination with multi-organ involvement may occur in immunocompromised patients and carries a substantial morbidity and mortality [164, 166, 167]. Dissemination rates in dialysis and renal transplant recipients are high between 25% and 75%; the spleen, kidneys, skin, pancreas, bone marrow, thyroid, lymph nodes, and CNS are the common extrapulmonary sites involved [166, 167]. The median time between transplantation and infection was 6 months, although infections have been seen 4 years after transplantation. Prophylaxis against coccidioidomycosis may be targeted in renal transplant recipients with recent infection or positive serology at the time of transplantation.

Cryptococcus neoformans is an encapsulated yeast found in soil, frequently associated with contamination by bird feces, and may be inhaled by a human host. It is the third most common invasive fungal infection in SOT recipients, following *Candida* and *Aspergillus* [168]. Cryptococcosis may manifest as meningitis, pulmonary infection, skin disease, or dissemination infection. Cryptococcosis may present with greater delay than other fungal infections; the median time to onset was 575 days in a large surveillance study of invasive fungal infection in SOT recipients [168]. Kidney transplant recipients may present with cryptococcal disease even later than liver or lung recipients [169]. A recent single-center survey found 1.2% incidence of cryptococcosis, which included disseminated, meningeal, and cutaneous disease [170]. Half of their cases occurred within the first 6 months following transplantation. Additional immunosuppression risk factors were noted in half of these patients including concurrent CMV infection with leukopenia or increased drug-induced immunosuppression preceding the cryptococcal infection. Blood cultures were positive in only half of cases. Cryptococcal immune reconstitution inflammatory syndrome (IRIS) is an increasingly recognized complication in SOT recipients, and clinical presentation may not be too dissimilar to what has been extensively reported in patients with AIDS receiving highly active antiretroviral therapy [169].

The incidence rate of invasive aspergillosis (IA) is lower in renal allograft recipients compared with other solid organs transplantation. Since renal transplants are the most frequently performed transplants, the overall burden is highest [171]. The estimated incidence of IA in renal transplant recipients is <0.5% [172, 173]. Approximately half of episodes occur in the first 3–6 months after transplantation although late IA 6 months after undergoing transplantation procedures occurs more commonly in renal than other SOT recipients [171, 173]. Risk factors for early IA seen within 3 months of transplant procedure include a longer duration of renal replacement therapy pretransplant and the presence of leukopenia [174] as well as acute rejection and the need for dialysis in the first weeks [171]. Risk of late IA is associated with donor CMV seropositivity [174]. Underlying lung disease and chronic heart failure also increase the risk for IA [171, 173]. The patients with IA were also more likely to have had a bloodstream infection, CMV disease, HCV, or low lymphocyte counts in the immediate postoperative period, although these may be surrogate markers of overall profound immunosuppression or healthcare exposures [171]. Mortality ranges from 40% to 60%, most of which is attributable to IA [171, 174]. Positivity of serum galactomannan correlates with increased mortality [173, 174]. Of survivors, 25% experienced graft loss. Renal allograft aspergilloma has been reported occurring late after transplantation. Graft aspergilloma typically requires a surgical approach in addition to systemic mold-active antifungal drug therapy although successful medical treatment alone has been reported [175]. Treatment of aspergillosis in any SOT recipient requires careful adjustment of CNI dosage in conjunction with azole use, typically voriconazole. Intravenous voriconazole contains cyclodextrin for solubility and may accumulate in the setting of renal dysfunction and dialysis, although it does not cause profound toxic effects. The liposomal formulation of amphotericin B (AmBisome®, Gilead, Foster City, CA) does not achieve adequate penetration for fungal pyelonephritis, and the nonliposomal formulation (amphotericin B deoxycholate) must be used, which carries higher risk of renal dysfunction, electrolyte abnormalities, as well as infusion-related reactions and discomfort.

Prophylaxis against *Pneumocystis jiroveci*, formerly *P. carinii*, pneumonia (PCP) is universally recommended in solid organ transplant recipients. The incidence of PCP in renal transplant recipients ranges from 0.6% to 14%, and the period of greatest risk occurs between 2 and 6 months after transplantation [176, 177]. PCP is the most common opportunistic infection leading to ICU admission in renal transplant recipients, and approximately one-half require mechanical ventilation [178]. Trimethoprim-sulfamethoxazole (TMP-SMX) is the prophylactic agent of choice as it is the most effective and also prophylaxes against additional pathogens, including *Toxoplasma gondii*, *Listeria monocytogenes*, *Nocardia* spp., and urinary pathogens. TMP-SMX may also prevent infection with *Nocardia*, although breakthroughs have been reported while on PCP drug prophylaxis. Concerns specific to renal transplant recipients include the need for dose adjustment in the setting of delayed graft function or fluctuating renal function. Hyperkalemia and a mild increase in serum creatinine level, though not truly reflective of an actual decrease in renal dysfunction, may occur during TMP-SMX therapy, which may be difficult to manage in some renal allograft recipients. For patients with sulfa allergy or an inability to tolerate TMP-SMX, dapsone, inhaled pentamidine, or atovaquone are alternative therapies that are less effective and do not provide additional prophylaxis against the aforementioned pathogens. PCP coinfection with CMV is common, and definitive diagnosis should be pursued to ensure treatment of all active pathogens [176]. Any late allograft dysfunction and subsequent use of T-cell depleting immunosuppression and corticosteroids should prompt resumption of PCP prophylaxis.

Outbreaks of pneumocystis pneumonia have also occurred among renal transplant recipients in Europe, Japan, and Canada [179–181]. The Canadian outbreak represented the first such in North America in recent decades [179]. All patients had received 1 year of TMP-SMX prophylaxis after transplantation. The median time between transplant and PCP infection was over 10 years. Affected patients had lower eGFR (29.3 mL/min vs 66.3 mL/min, $p = 0.028$) and lymphopenia (0.51×10^9/L vs 1.25×10^9/l, $p = 0.002$). Four patients who had genotyping done had an identical fungal strain. Overlapping ambulatory care visits were identified as the potential source of transmission. Genotyping done in the Canadian and other cohorts has identified a predominant strain being responsible for outbreaks, presumably from a common human or environmental source [179, 180]. After an outbreak, the entire renal transplant population should resume prophylaxis for 6–12 months [179–181].

Viral Infections

BK Polyomavirus Virus

BK polyomavirus (BKV) is a small double-stranded DNA virus in the polyomavirus family with four serologic groups and genotypes, each of which may elicit specific, non-cross-reactive antibody responses [182]. It was discovered in 1971 and named for the index patient's initials [183]. Infection is thought to be acquired in childhood via oral and respiratory secretions, and initial infection is generally mild in patients with intact immune function [183]. Among the general population, seroprevalence is estimated between 60% and 80% with highest seroprevalence of 91% between the ages of 5 and 9 years [184, 185]. Age and BKV titers have a significant association with linearly declining titers at a rate of 8.7% per 10 years [184, 185]. BKV infects proximal tubule epithelial cells, where it persists and, when reactivated by immune suppression, replicates and produces infectious virus particles within the cells [186]. While immunosuppression likely plays a role in reactivation of the virus, mouse models also show mechanical and chemical injury contributing to newly acquired infection or BKV infection reactivation [187].

BKV infection is an important cause of renal allograft dysfunction and graft loss. The most common presentations include asymptomatic rise in creatinine, nephropathy, and ureteral stenosis. Hemorrhagic cystitis is an uncommon manifestation in renal transplant recipients but is the most common presentation of BKV infection in hematopoietic stem cell transplant recipients [183]. In kidney transplant recipients who develop an unexplained rise in creatinine, BKV PCR in urine and serum should be obtained as part of the evaluation.

Incidence has been increasing since the mid-1990s, thought to be due to the use of more intensive immunosuppression regimens [188]. Incidence of BKV infection peaks around 1 and 3 months following transplantation; infections do occur later within the first year after transplantation [189–192]. Asymptomatic BKV shedding may be found in up to 10% of the general population and approximately 20–32% of renal transplant candidates [184, 185, 191–194].

Because the BKV seroprevalence is so high in the general population, it is not considered an exclusion criterion for donors, although seronegative recipients may acquire donor-derived BKV infection. In a study of 20 donor-recipient pairs, sequencing was consistent with donor derivation of BK infection [195]. Measurable presence of BKV pretransplant is considered a risk factor for posttransplant BK virus replication, higher rates of graft dysfunction, and higher serum creatinine levels [192–194], although no association was found between pretransplant BK viruria and posttransplant BK viruria or viremia in a 2016 prospective study by Bicalho et al. [191].

Fluoroquinolone (FQ) prophylaxis against BKV showed promise in in vitro and observational studies and was proposed to inhibit host topoisomerase used by the virus for replication but failed to prevent infection in prospective and randomized controlled trials [182, 196–198]. Lebreton et al. completed a 3-month prospective study of ciprofloxacin prophylaxis in patients who had additional pretransplantation immune suppression and found that neither rates of BKV infection nor bacterial infection differed [197]. Knoll et al. performed a double-blinded placebo controlled trial with 3 months of levofloxacin prophylaxis, which did not prevent BK viruria [196]. The levofloxacin prophylaxis was associated with an increased risk of adverse events such as bacterial resistance and nonsignificant increased risk of suspected tendonitis. A systematic review concluded that FQ prophylaxis is ineffective in preventing BKV infection and found no significant differences in FQ-resistant infection [198]. Brennan et al. found that randomized use of tacrolimus versus cyclosporine A did not impact the incidence of future BK viruria or viremia, although in patients who did develop viruria, levels were highest in tacrolimus and lowest in cyclosporine A treated patients [199].

BKV infection progresses to nephropathy in 1–10% of kidney transplant recipients [190]. Preemptive PCR monitoring of viral DNA in urine or blood is recommended, usually at least monthly immediately after transplant, and then at 3 months' interval (Fig. 4.3). Elevated BKV DNA levels in blood should trigger further evaluation and an early reduction in drug-induced immunosuppression to prevent progression to nephropathy [190]. BKV viruria typically precedes viremia by 6–12 weeks and may be present in 10–40% of renal transplant recipients without any clinical or histological evidence of BK nephropathy [183, 190, 199, 200]. Persistent high-level viruria for more than 2 months or viremia PCR ≥10,000 copies/mL in the setting of renal dysfunction have an increased positive predictive value for BKV nephropathy [190, 200]. Because of the frequency of viral shedding in the urine, some centers use viremia as a screening methodology, which may be more predictive and identify a narrower group of patients for closer monitoring. The advantages of screening for viruria or urine decoy cells include a high negative predictive value and less invasive testing [190]. Renal biopsy remains the gold standard for diagnosis and should be pursued if viruria or viremia is present in high sustained levels or is seen in conjunction with elevated creatinine or persistent urine cytologic changes, although some centers will elect to make changes in immunosuppression and treat based on high sustained viremia alone.

"Decoy cells" are epithelial cells with typical cytopathic effects including enlarged nuclei and basophilic nuclear inclusions and are characteristic for BKV infection that can be seen in urine cytology. JC virus is another human polyomavirus that may cause the presence of decoy cells in urine. However, infection with JC virus is more likely to be asymptomatic and less likely to result in polyomavirus nephropathy [200]. Risk factors for graft loss in recipients with BKV infection include serum creatinine >2 mg/dL, early BK virus nephropathy within the first 6 months following transplant, and presence of microvascular inflammation including glomerulitis and peritubular capillaritis [201]. Other identified risk factors can be further classified as donor-related, recipient-related, and transplant-related, although there is some discordance between studies, such as preceding CMV infection as a potential risk factor, indicating an area of evolving understanding [183, 190, 202–210]. (Table 4.10) Protective factors include centers with higher transplant volume and living kidney donation [203].

Standard of care involves reduction of immunosuppression which is typically sufficient to clear viremia and viruria plus decoy cells or both. Reduction of immunosuppression is less likely to clear decoy cells due to JC virus infection, with <50% clearance versus 93% clearance in patients with BKV-associated decoy cells; this being said, the observed risk of graft loss is minimal even in those who fail to clear decoy cells in the urine following reduced antirejection-associated immune suppression [200]. The mTOR (mammalian target of rapamycin) inhibitors have in vitro antiviral activity, therefore replacing CNIs with these agents have been suggested for select patients with immunological risk for BK nephropathy [188, 189]. Use of cyclosporine A in place of tacrolimus has also been suggested in patients with persistent BK viremia [190]. The proposed adjuvant therapies include fluoroquinolones, leflunomide, cidofovir, and intravenous immunoglobulin (IVIG) [183, 190].

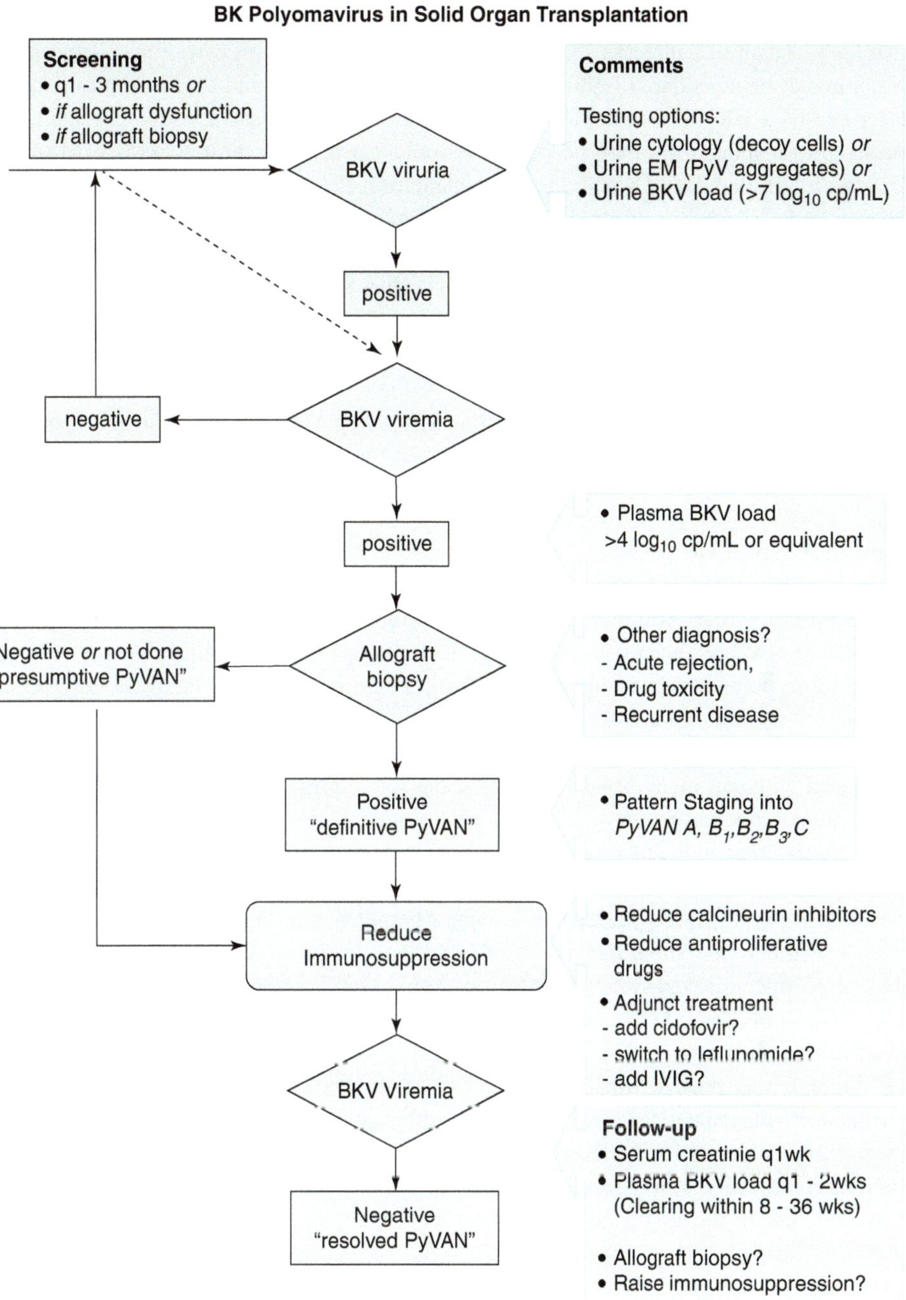

Fig. 4.3 BK polyomavirus screen. Screening and management of kidney transplant patients for BKV replication and polyomavirus-associated nephropathy (PyVAN) [190]. (Reprinted with permission from Hirsch and Randhawa [190] with permission from John Wiley and Sons)

Table 4.10 Risk factors for BK polyomavirus nephropathy

Donor-related risk factors	Recipient-related risk factors	Transplant-related risk factors
HLA-mismatch Deceased donor High BK virus-specific antibody titers (suggesting more recent exposure and possibly higher burden in the kidney) Female gender Ischemia-reperfusion injury Advanced donor age	Pediatric recipients or older age Male gender Low or absent BK virus-specific antibody titers White or African American ethnicity	Ureteral stents or trauma Delayed graft function Acute rejection Antirejection treatment Steroid exposure Lymphocyte-depleting induction Higher immunosuppressive drug levels Tacrolimus-based suppression regimen Diabetes mellitus Cytomegalovirus infection

After clearing plasma BKV DNA and nephropathy by histology, a cautious increase in maintenance immunosuppression can be considered [190]. Cases of IRIS have been described with BKV infection [190, 211]. With close monitoring, re-transplantation may be considered and carries a 93% graft survival rate 3 years after transplantation [212]. Dharnidharka et al. found that 17.5% would require intervention for recurrent infection [212].

Brincidofovir is an oral form of cidofovir that shows promise as a future therapeutic option [182]. Research focused on ELISPOT assay may also help to better define the immune response to BKV in individualized treatment decisions [213]. Rare but increasing reports of long-standing PV nephropathy and renourinary neoplasms also warrant ongoing evaluation [214].

Human Adenovirus

Human adenoviruses (AdV) are non-enveloped double-stranded DNA viruses within the *Adenoviridae* family [215] which have also been seen with increasing frequency due to use of more potent immunosuppression [215]. There are 7 species (A–G) which are further subdivided into serotypes, of which 52 have been identified [215]. Certain serotypes are associated with particular disease manifestations [215, 216]. In immunocompetent patients, it causes self-limited respiratory, gastrointestinal, and conjunctival disease year-round and is most commonly seen in children or military recruits [215]. In renal transplant recipients, it causes hemorrhagic cystitis or tubulointerstitial nephritis [216] and may lead to acute graft rejection and systemic dissemination [217–221]. Species B serotypes 7, 11, 34, and 35 are particularly associated with hemorrhagic cystitis. In addition to gross hematuria, patients may present with dysuria and fever as well as coinfection with bacterial UTI, BK virus infection, or concurrent AdV viremia [217]. Time to onset following transplantation may vary widely from days to a year or more, but most will fall in the first 1–3 months after transplantation [215, 217, 220].

Humar et al. detected plasma adenovirus DNA in 6.5% of kidney recipients over a 1-year study period [222]. Among all SOT recipients, over half (58%) were asymptomatic, while another 21% had vague or nonspecific symptoms. The remaining patients experienced gastrointestinal or respiratory symptoms at equal rates of 10.5% each. No effect on acute graft rejection was observed; however, subsequent CMV infection rates were higher in kidney transplant recipients with adenovirus viremia.

Unlike preemptive CMV and BK screening following renal transplantation, adenovirus screening is not routinely performed. If disease is suspected, the diagnosis can be established with PCR or with rapid antigen tests such as immunofluorescence assays in respiratory samples or by enzyme immunoassay, immunochromatography, or latex agglutination in stool samples [216]. While most serotypes grow well in cell cultures, with the exception of serotypes 40 and 41, viral culture may take up to 28 days for viral growth and ex vivo cytopathic changes to appear in the cell line cultures [215, 216]. Typical cytopathic effects seen in tissue include nuclear enlargement, peripheral condensed chromatin, and basophilic nuclear inclusions representing viral particles [216, 218], and renal biopsy may additionally show tubular cell necrosis. Many patients may continue to shed virus for a prolonged period of time after recovery from an infection or in asymptomatic patients without the evidence of viral disease.

The U.S. Food & Drug Administration (FDA) has not approved any agent for the treatment for AdV infection. Cidofovir is active against all AdV serotypes and widely used for treatment of AdV disease in the immunosuppressed population [215]. Cidofovir undergoes intracellular conversion to become the preferred substrate for the AdV DNA polymerase, leading to viral DNA chain termination [223]. For mild cases a reduction in drug-induced immune suppression alone may be sufficient, although no standardized algorithm exists. Cidofovir carries a significant risk of nephrotoxicity, which can be seen in up to half of patients, and neutropenia and uveitis may occur [216]. It requires renal dose adjustment and should be given with probenecid and intravenous hydration to mitigate the risk of nephrotoxicity. Thrice-weekly dosing may be less nephrotoxic however may result in breakthrough of CMV or HSV infections [216]. CMX001, or brincidofovir, the lipid conjugate of cidofovir, achieves higher intracellular levels compared with cidofovir, does not carry the same nephrotoxicity risk and shows promise as a potentially safe and effective treatment for AdV infection [223].

Serial quantitative PCRs are useful in monitoring the course of disease and defining the end of therapy [220]. Median duration of AdV infection in the urinary tract is 15 days [217]. Use of IVIG for patients with hypogammaglobulinemia may also be helpful as an adjunctive therapy [114, 216].

Cytomegalovirus (CMV)

Like BKV, CMV seroprevalence is common in the general population, typically following a primary infection in childhood that then establishes lifelong latency. Human CMV is a β herpes virus and the largest virus to infect humans [224]. Seroprevalence rates in the United States reach 60–70% and rates are near 100% in parts of Africa [224, 225]. In healthy adults, infection may be asymptomatic or present with features of acute infectious mononucleosis. Similar to HSCT, in solid organ transplant recipients CMV is associated with serious and potentially life-threatening illness. The virus itself additionally encodes genes that downregulate the host immune system [224].

CMV infection in renal transplant recipients may present as asymptomatic viremia, CMV syndrome typically consisting of fever, malaise, leukopenia and thrombocytopenia, or end-organ, tissue-invasive disease. The most common site of CMV organ disease in renal transplant recipients involves the upper or lower gastrointestinal tract presenting as esophagitis, enteritis, and/or colitis [226, 227]. CMV disease involving the lungs, retina, pancreas, and liver is less common in these patients. In general, tissue-invasive CMV disease has a predilection to involve the allograft of solid organ transplant recipients [228]. The renal allograft may be the site of subclinical or latent CMV disease, viruria being not uncommon in renal transplant recipients [229]. However, among viremic renal transplant recipients, viral inclusions are found in <1% of biopsies performed for increasing serum creatinine levels [230]. In an observational study, the majority of these biopsies showed interstitial nephritis with tubulitis, although a wide spectrum of histopathology has been associated with CMV in the renal allograft [230]. In this select subgroup of patients with CMV viral inclusions, treatment with ganciclovir and documented clearance of virus had not resulted in normalization of serum creatinine levels. In patients receiving a pancreas or pancreas-kidney transplant, gastrointestinal disease is the most common manifestation of tissue-invasive CMV disease [231].

Donor and recipient CMV serostatus is an important determinant in prevention strategies for CMV infection following transplantation. In early prophylaxis trials using valacyclovir, between 48% and 67% of patients in the control group developed CMV disease within the first year after transplant [232, 233]. CMV seronegative recipients (R−) had a far higher incidence of CMV disease than their seropositive counterparts (48% vs. 6%) [232]. Biopsy-confirmed acute graft rejection 6 months after transplantation occurred in more than half of patients in whom antiviral prophylaxis was not given [232, 233]. A large prospective study of 609 kidney and kidney-pancreas recipients, who received standardized universal CMV prophylaxis, found 17.7% developed CMV viremia over a 4-year period of which 88% were asymptomatic [210]. Those with symptomatic CMV disease presented with either CMV syndrome or tissue-invasive disease [210]. Infection occurred at a median of 5.6 months after transplant. Multivariate analysis identified D+/R− serostatus ($p \leq 0.0001$), donor age >50 years ($p = 0.013$), higher mean tacrolimus dose ($p = 0.0009$), and higher mean mycophenolic acid blood level ($p = 0.01$) to be risk factors for CMV infection. D−/R− status is the lowest risk for CMV infection. Authors found symptomatic CMV infection, when compared with asymptomatic viremia or no viremia, to have a significantly negative impact on graft survival, conferring a 3.5 times higher risk for graft loss ($p = 0.04$) [210]. A pooled analysis of randomized controlled trials found patients receiving mTOR inhibitors were significantly less likely to have CMV viremia, infection, or end-organ disease as compared to those receiving mycophenolate [234].

Disease rates are similar among pancreas transplant recipients. A study of 130 simultaneous pancreas-kidney (SPK) or pancreas after kidney (PAK), all of whom received antiviral prophylaxis for a median duration of 49 days, had an overall CMV infection rate of 24%, which diverged when classified by recipient serostatus to 44% in D+/R− and 8.2% in R+ group [235]. Another large retrospective study of pancreas and pancreas-kidney recipients found CMV infection in 17.1%; asymptomatic viremia was noted in 4.8%, and CMV disease including CMV syndrome or tissue-invasive disease was present in 10.2% of patients [231]. The cumulative incidence of CMV infection was 20% within 10 years after transplantation [231]. Risk factors for the total cohort included D+/R− status (OR = 16.075), preceding non-CMV infections such as bacterial, fungal, or other viral infections (OR = 6.362), and duration of antiviral prophylaxis (OR = 0.984) [235]. Among the D+/R− group, only non-CMV infection was identified as a risk factor for CMV disease (OR = 10.7). In another large group of 407 pancreas recipients, the incidence of CMV infection was 20.2% in D+/R−, 16.5% in D+/R+, 5.0% in D−/R+, and 2.8% in D−/R−; most of these infections occurred 3 months and beyond after transplantation [236]. Infection was less common in SPK. Immune suppression was not reduced in 72%, and no CMV-related deaths or graft loss were noted.

Valganciclovir prophylaxis after renal transplantation is protective against CMV, HSV, and varicella zoster virus (VZV). Nevertheless, routine monitoring should be done with pp65 antigen or quantitative CMV PCR at regular intervals or if there is clinical suspicion of CMV disease. The longest duration of prophylaxis is recommended for those at highest risk of CMV infection – those with D+/R− status. The American Society of Transplantation (AST) Infectious Diseases Community of Practice regularly updates CMV guidelines, including recommendations for prophylaxis [228] (Table 4.11). Universal prophylaxis may be more

Table 4.11 Risk, recommended prophylaxis, and duration by donor/recipient CMV serostatus

Donor/recipient CMV status	Degree of relative risk	Prophylaxis agents and dosing, assuming normal renal function	Minimum duration of prophylaxis
D+/R−	Highest risk	Valganciclovir[a] 900 mg oral daily	6 months
D+/R+, D−/R+	Moderate risk	Valganciclovir[a] 900 mg oral daily	3–6 months
D−/R−	Lowest risk	Acyclovir 400 mg oral twice daily or valacyclovir 500 mg oral twice daily[b]	3 months

[a]Oral ganciclovir 1gram three times daily may be substituted
[b]D−/R− prophylactic approach may vary by transplant center

cost-effective than a preemptive monitoring strategy, which employs regularly scheduled CMV PCR monitoring [234]. In the setting of acute rejection and treatment with lymphocyte-depleting agents or high-dose corticosteroids, resumption of valganciclovir prophylaxis for 1–3 months is warranted. A preemptive strategy may alternatively be considered [228].

Treatment is twofold, including reduction of immunosuppression and targeted inhibition of the viral DNA polymerase with intravenous ganciclovir or oral valganciclovir. Oral valganciclovir can be used in patients with mild to moderate disease, whereas intravenous ganciclovir is indicated for patients with severe or life-threatening disease and high CMV viral loads or in patients with unpredictable enteric drug absorption [228]. Induction treatment should be maintained for a minimum of 2 weeks but should be extended until resolution of symptoms and virologic suppression has been documented using antigenemia or PCR [228].

Treatment options for drug-resistant CMV include high-dose intravenous ganciclovir (7.5–10 mg/kg every 12 h), foscarnet, and cidofovir. Both ganciclovir and valganciclovir require intracellular phosphorylation into ganciclovir monophosphate via phosphotransferase, a product of the UL97 gene of CMV. Monophosphate is then phosphorylated by cellular enzymes to ganciclovir triphosphate [224]. Mutation in the UL97 gene results in ganciclovir-resistant virus and may be seen in patients requiring repeated treatment courses and following long-standing low drug level exposure. Viral resistance to ganciclovir may vary depending on the site of mutation [228]. In this setting, high-dose ganciclovir or foscarnet may be considered, based on individual genotypic assays. The addition of the UL54 gene mutation can confer cross-resistance to ganciclovir, foscarnet, and cidofovir [228].

Potential toxicities from CMV treatment in renal transplant recipients are considerable. Myelosuppression may be seen with ganciclovir and valganciclovir, compounded by concurrent use of trimethoprim-sulfamethoxazole prophylaxis in many cases. Additionally, as renal function may improve or fluctuate in the posttransplantation setting, dose adjustments of valganciclovir prophylaxis may lag, leading to inadequate intracellular levels and breakthrough infection or development of de novo drug-resistant viral isolates. Use of either foscarnet or cidofovir carries risk for significant nephrotoxicity, making management of resistant virus in the renal transplant recipient additionally challenging. Foscarnet therapy requires close electrolyte monitoring as hypocalcemia, hypomagnesemia, and hypophosphatemia may also result [224]. Cidofovir undergoes uptake by the proximal convoluted renal tubular cells, leading to cell degeneration and necrosis which may be irreversible and require patients to receive renal replacement therapy [237]. Adequate intravenous hydration should be maintained, and coadministration of probenecid reduces cidofovir reuptake by renal tubular cells.

Epstein-Barr Virus

Epstein-Barr virus (EBV), another of the human herpes viruses, causes acute infectious mononucleosis among immunocompetent individuals and lymphoma in HIV-infected individuals. It is transmitted through saliva, body fluids such as with sexual contact, blood transfusion, or via organ transplantation. Within the SOT population, EBV infection may cause posttransplant lymphoproliferative disorder (PTLD). PTLD incidence varies by type of SOT and occurs at the lowest rates in renal transplant recipients, with an approximate incidence of 0.46% in the first year and then 1.1–1.4% cumulative incidence by 5 years after undergoing transplantation [238–240]. However, as renal transplants are by far the most commonly performed among the solid organs, kidney transplant recipients make up the highest absolute number of PTLD cases [238]. Using the UNOS database, the PTLD rate among pancreas transplant recipients was estimated at 1% with a mean follow-up time of 5 years [241]. Risk factors for development of PTLD in the pancreas allograft recipients were similar to those identified in renal allograft patients.

Identified risk factors for development of PTLD in renal transplant recipients include history of pretransplant malignancy, fewer HLA matches, or treatment with antithymocyte globulin (ATG) or muromonab-CD3 (OKT3) [239]. A 10-year single-center prospective trial, however, found no significant association between induction or maintenance immunosuppression regimens and occurrence of PTLD [238]. Recipient age has had conflicting impact on development of PTLD between American and French registry data [239, 240]. Recipient EBV serostatus is considered to be the most important factor in development of PTLD. Use of mycophenolate and azathioprine are associated with a lower risk of PTLD, whereas IL2-receptor inhibitors and sirolimus use do not appear to impact the risk for PTLD [239]. Monthly EBV PCR testing has a low positive predictive value of 16.7%, although a 95.2% negative predictive value is appealing [238]. Nevertheless, regular monitoring is standard of care in most centers, and KDIGO guidelines suggest monitoring high-risk (EBV D+/R−) kidney transplant recipients for EBV with NAT testing, and that any patients with increasing EBV load have a reduction in immunosuppression [242] (Table 4.12).

Table 4.12 Epstein-Barr virus monitoring in high-risk* renal transplant recipients [242]

Time after transplantation	Recommended frequency of monitoring
First week	Once
3–6 months	At least monthly
6–12 months	Every 3 months

Additional monitoring is recommended after treatment for acute rejection

High risk is considered EBV seropositive donor and seronegative recipient (D+/R−)

The role of prophylaxis in preventing PTLD remains ill-defined. Although antiviral prophylaxis is not generally given to target EBV or prevent the development of PTLD specifically, when routine antiviral prophylaxis became widespread both acyclovir prophylaxis for HSV and ganciclovir or valganciclovir for CMV prophylaxis demonstrated a decline in PTLD rates [243–245]. This was first observed in a cohort of pancreas-kidney recipients receiving different anti-CMV prophylactic regimens including oral acyclovir or intravenous ganciclovir followed by oral acyclovir [244]. A multicenter, case-control study of renal transplant recipients assessed the impact of immunosuppressive and antiviral therapy on PTLD in this population and found that prophylactic antiviral use was associated with up to 83% PTLD risk reduction [246]. For every 30 days of ganciclovir use, risk of PTLD during the first year was 38% lower, with an odds ratio of 0.62. Acyclovir was less effective but still resulted in reduced risk for PTLD (odds ratio 0.83). Results were strongest within the first year following transplantation. A retrospective registry study of over 44,000 deceased-donor kidney transplants found nearly identical rates of lymphoma during the first year after transplant among patients who did and did not receive ani-CMV prophylaxis [247]. They did, however, find a complete absence of lymphomas in patients who had received anti-CMV immunoglobulin in the first year following transplantation. This protection did not extend beyond 1 year, and all three groups developed lymphoma at similar rates in the subsequent 5 years. A prospective randomized trial with EBV D+/R−solid organ recipients found no difference in (1) incidence of detectable EBV viral load within the first year posttransplant, (2) time to first detectable viral load, or (3) time to high-level viral load between patients given ganciclovir for 3 months or ganciclovir plus immune globulin therapy [248]. Three of these 34 patients developed PTLD, all of whom were in the immune globulin treatment group.

The treatment of PTLD is complicated and involves reduction in iatrogenic antirejection drug-mediated immune suppression, antiviral therapy, and rituximab-based chemotherapy regimens. Five-year survival of renal transplant recipients with PTLD is just over 60% [239, 240]. Graft PTLD has an improved 5-year survival rate of approximately 80% [240]. Older age, pretransplant malignancy, OKT3 use, HBV or HCV infection, late-onset PTLD, and multiple site involvement or high Ann Arbor staging have been identified as risk factors for death [239]. Good prognostic markers include mycophenolic acid use which was associated with improved survival [239, 240]. Among pancreas allograft recipients with PTLD, 1-, 3-, and 5-year survival rates were 91%, 76%, and 70%, compared to 97%, 93%, and 88% in patients without PTLD [241].

Community-Acquired/Late Infectious Complications in Kidney and Pancreas-Kidney Transplant Recipients

As renal transplant recipients approach 1 year and beyond after transplantation, they are more likely to acquire community-based infections. Up to 6% of renal recipients will have a life-threatening complication requiring ICU admission, most at or beyond the 6-month posttransplant mark [178]. The most common ICU diagnoses for these admissions are cardiac pulmonary edema, bacterial pneumonia, acute graft pyelonephritis, and bloodstream infection. The most common opportunistic infection is PCP, with approximately half needing mechanical ventilation. The most common immune suppression-associated systemic toxicities include drug-related neutropenia, sirolimus-related pneumonitis, and posterior reversible encephalopathy syndrome (PRES). Acute kidney injury is common with 40% requiring renal replacement therapy. Hospital mortality ranges up to 30%, while half of patients are discharged free from dialysis.

In a matched, case-control propensity-adjusted study of SOT and non-SOT controls with blood culture proven sepsis, of which approximately 40% of the SOT were kidney or pancreas-kidney transplants, those with SOT were more likely to have:

- A higher number of comorbidities [OR 8.2]
- Higher sepsis-related organ failure assessment scores [OR 1.2]
- Presence of nosocomial infection [OR 36.3]
- Appropriate initial antibiotics [OR 0.04]
- Lower white blood cell count [OR 0.93] [249]

Interestingly, after adjustment for clinical presentation, severity of illness, and types of infection, SOT recipients with sepsis had a significantly lower risk of death at 28 days and 90 days when compared with non-SOT patients [249]. The authors suggest that immune suppression for transplantation may account for this survival benefit due to modulation of the inflammatory response. These patients were also, however, more likely to receive initial appropriate antibiotics, and it was not reported if these patients received earlier or more infectious disease consultations to assist with treatment of sepsis although presumably most SOT recipients are well-linked to care and counseled to call their center early on for any sign or symptom of possible infection [250]. A large retrospective study using University Health System Consortium ICD coding data found SOT recipients hospitalized with sepsis or severe sepsis were more likely to be younger and insured by Medicare and found a similar lower in-hospital mortality compared to non-SOT patients for those with kidney, liver, and kidney-pancreas transplants but not those with heart or lung transplant who in fact had higher mortality rates [251].

For patients with pancreas or pancreas-kidney transplants, urinary tract infections are the most common urological complications, followed by hematuria, bladder calculi, reflux pancreatitis, and urine leaks related to the pancreatic graft [252]. The urinary bladder drainage method in pancreas transplantation is associated with a higher frequency of urologic complications and rarely requires conversion to enteric diversion [252–254]. Flow issues should be considered in any kidney or pancreas-kidney recipient as abnormal or blocked flow may increase risk for infection and may complicate success in achieving cure or preventing recurrence.

Asymptomatic bacteriuria is common and may account for approximately half of diagnosed UTIs in renal transplant recipients [255]. The bulk of asymptomatic bacteriuria occurs in the early posttransplantation period – particularly the first month – with enteric pathogens such as *Enterococcus faecalis* and *Escherichia coli* [255, 256]. Identified risk factors for asymptomatic bacteriuria include female gender, induction with ATG, presence of comorbidities, acute rejection, and CMV infection. Treatment in renal transplant recipients has ranged from 30% to 100% in series, but evolution to symptomatic UTI is similar between treated and untreated patients, and in both groups, it is typically not the same bacterial pathogen to cause the asymptomatic bacteriuria and the UTI [255, 256]. El Amari et al. found persistent bacteriuria in nearly half of treated episodes with selection of a resistant pathogen in 78% [256]. Conversely, more than half of untreated patients (59%) may have spontaneous bacterial clearance in the urine, particularly if they have low-grade bacteriuria without pyuria. Traditionally, however, asymptomatic bacteriuria was treated in the posttransplantation period with the intent of preventing future UTI or development of graft pyelonephritis; this approach continues to be controversial. In a randomized controlled trial, kidney transplant recipients underwent systematic screening for asymptomatic bacteriuria beyond the second month after transplant and found no differences in the frequency of pyelonephritis, lower UTI, acute rejection, graft function, and all-cause mortality up to 24 months among the antibiotic treatment group vs. patients randomized to no antibiotic control group [257]. There were no additional complications of antibiotic use including *Clostridium difficile* colitis or colonization or infection with drug-resistant organisms in the antibiotic treatment group.

Pyelonephritis in the renal transplant recipient has distinct clinical characteristics. It is defined as the presence of fever plus urinary culture growth with greater than 10^5 CFU/mL and/or bacteremia along with at least one of the following symptoms: pain over the allograft site, chills, cystitis with dysuria, increased urinary frequency, or urgency [258, 259]. The incidence rate of acute graft pyelonephritis is 4.4 episodes per 100 patient-years [258]. In this study, risk factors for the development of acute graft pyelonephritis included the presence of glomerulonephritis as the underlying disease and the previous occurrence of at least two episodes of asymptomatic bacteriuria, and odds ratio was higher with increasing number of episodes of asymptomatic bacteriuria. As mentioned above, the relationship between asymptomatic bacteriuria and the development of acute graft pyelonephritis remains unsettled. In the 3-year follow-up, there was no significant difference in levels of serum creatinine, creatinine clearance, or 24-h proteinuria between patients with and without acute graft pyelonephritis.

Candiduria may represent asymptomatic colonization or, less commonly, true infection. Generally, it does not warrant treatment in adults unless they are neutropenic or will be undergoing urinary tract instrumentation. Ureteral stents remaining in place after transplantation may become colonized and make candiduria difficult to clear. Echinocandins do not achieve adequate levels in the urine to be used for treatment, whereas fluconazole and nonliposomal amphotericin B may be used. In challenging cases of azole-resistant candiduria or fungal pyelonephritis, flucytosine may be added but is generally not used alone due to a low barrier for development of resistance during or following monotherapy. Surgical evaluation may be needed in some cases of pyelonephritis, particularly due to *Aspergillus* spp. [175].

Rejection often mimics infection and should be included in the differential diagnosis of patients presenting with renal allograft dysfunction and fever. Nearly half of patients with allograft failure are hospitalized with fever within 6 months of failure [260]. Patients weaned off immunosuppression after failure have less documented infection than those patients maintained on immunosuppression (38% vs. 88%, $p < 0.001$), although they are at risk for increased alloimmunization. In both groups, the most common infection is dialysis catheter-related bloodstream infection. Hospitalized patients with documented infection are less likely to have allograft nephrectomy performed (30% vs. 81%; $p < 0.001$). Mortality was higher in simultaneous pancreas-kidney recipients and those hospitalized with documented infection.

Emerging fungal pathogens in the renal transplant population tend to occur late after 18 months following transplantation [261]. Relevant pathogens include *Scedosporium*, *Pseudallescheria* spp. and *Fusarium* spp., Zygomycetes such as *Rhizopus*, *Mucor*, and dermatiaceous molds like *Ochroconis, Verruconis, Cladophialophora, Bipolaris, Rhinocladiella,* and *Fonsecaea* species. The most common sites of infection include respiratory tract and paranasal sinuses, skin, and central nervous system.

Dermatophytosis is common in renal transplant recipients, occurring in 42% of patients in one screening study [262]. Infection was chronic lasting more than a year in 40% of the patients. Tinea cruris and tinea corporis were the most common infections observed, with *Trichophyton rubrum* being a common pathogen.

Post-kidney or kidney-pancreas transplant recipients are at risk for malignancies which occur later posttransplantation and are associated with the use of chronic immunosuppressive therapy. A malignancy of infectious origin is Kaposi Sarcoma (KS), due to reactivation or donor-derived acquisition of human herpes virus 8 (HHV-8) [263]. Incidence ranges from 0.5% in Western and Northern countries to approximately 5%

in Mediterranean regions, the Middle East, and South Africa. The skin is the primary site of KS, but visceral organ involvement can occur as well; involvement of the allograft is rare. An approach to treatment may involve reduction of immune suppression, change of regimen to include an mTOR inhibitor such as sirolimus, which has an antiviral effect, local treatments including laser, surgery, cryotherapy or radiotherapy, or systemic chemotherapy in severe cases.

As patients get farther out from transplant, they may engage in more outdoor activities or travel with the potential for exposure to infection, and the risk of acquiring severe travel-related illness is higher in immunocompromised persons [264]. An increasing number of parasitic infections are reported in SOT recipients, including intestinal giardiasis in a SPK recipient [265] and strongyloidiasis, of which kidney recipients constitute the majority of donor-derived infections [154]. Travel-related Chikungunya has been reported in an HIV-positive renal transplant as well [264]. West Nile virus is another mosquito-borne illness but endemic to parts of the United States. Transplant recipients have a higher risk of neurological complications from WNV [135, 266], as seen in three kidney and pancreas-kidney recipients in the 2012 epidemic, two of whom survived after treatment with IVIG [266]. Transmission of WNV has also occurred as a donor-derived infection after transplantation [135]. The kidney may be the site of prolonged WNV replication and shedding, and testing of urine instead of blood has been proposed [135].

Common infections beyond the first month posttransplantation are summarized in Table 4.13.

Table 4.13 Common infections in the intermediate and late (community phase) post-kidney or kidney-pancreas transplantation period

Category	Infection	Organisms	Route of acquisition	Risk factors
Bacteria and mycobacteria	Asymptomatic bacteriuria (AB), urinary tract infection, acute graft pyelonephritis	Enteric Gram-negative bacilli (especially *E. coli*), *Enterococcus* spp.	Community acquired, healthcare associated	For AB: female gender, induction with antithymocyte globulin, presence of comorbidities, acute rejection, CMV infection Acute graft pyelonephritis: ± recurrent asymptomatic bacteriuria In pancreas-kidney transplant: vesicular drainage method
	Bacterial pneumonia	*S. pneumoniae*, *S. aureus*, Gram-negative bacilli, atypical bacteria	Community acquired, healthcare associated	
	Bloodstream infection	*S. aureus*, coagulase-negative staphylococci	Community acquired, healthcare associated	Graft failure with resumption of hemodialysis, particularly via temporary catheter
	Tuberculosis, most commonly pulmonary and disseminated	*Mycobacterium tuberculosis*	Primary: Reactivation Secondary: Donor-derived, community acquired	Positive IGRA test, from an endemic region, increased immunosuppression
Fungus	Endemic mycoses	*Histoplasma capsulatum*, *Coccidioides immitis*, *C. posadasii*, less commonly *Blastomyces dermatitidis*	Reactivation, primary community acquisition	Living in region of endemicity
	Cryptococcosis (meningitis, pulmonary infection, cutaneous disease, dissemination)	*Cryptococcus neoformans*, *Cryptococcus gattii*	Environmental (inhalation)	
	Pneumocystis pneumonia	*Pneumocystis jiroveci*, formerly P. carinii	Primary: Environmental (inhalation) Secondary: Healthcare-associated outbreak	Use of T-cell depleting immunosuppression including steroids
	Aspergillosis	*A. fumigatus*, *A. niger*, other species	Environmental (inhalation)	Renal replacement therapy, leukopenia, allograft rejection, comorbid lung disease or heart failure, CMV
	Other mold infection (respiratory tract infection, sinusitis, skin/dermatophytosis or central nervous system infection)	*Zygomycetes*, dematiaceous molds, *Scedosporium/Pseudallescheria*, Fusarium species Dermatophytosi: *Trichophyton rubrum*	Environmental	
	Urinary tract infection, pyelonephritis	Candida species, Aspergillus species	Endogenous, environmental, healthcare associated	Candiduria: presence of ureteral stents

(continued)

Table 4.13 (continued)

Category	Infection	Organisms	Route of acquisition	Risk factors
Viral	Polyomavirus nephropathy	BK virus, JC virus (rare)	Primary: Reactivation Secondary: Donor-derived in a seronegative recipient	HLA mismatches, deceased donor, high donor BK virus-specific Ab titers, low or absent recipient BK virus-specific Ab titers, higher overall immunosuppressed state, allograft injury (delayed graft function, ischemia-reperfusion injury), ureteral stents, CMV infection
	Asymptomatic viremia, CMV syndrome (fever, malaise, cytopenias), tissue-invasive disease (esophagitis, enteritis/colitis, pneumonitis, hepatitis, viruria, or rarely renal allograft involvement)	Cytomegalovirus	Primary: Reactivation Secondary: Donor-derived in a seronegative recipient, transfusion related with non-leukoreduced blood products, or rarely new community acquisition	Donor positive/recipient negative serostatus, allograft rejection
	Adenovirus hemorrhagic cystitis, allograft rejection, respiratory tract disease, gastroenteritis, hepatitis, myocarditis, dissemination	Adenovirus	Reactivation, primary community acquisition	
	Posttransplant lymphoproliferative disorder (PTLD)	Epstein-Barr virus	Primary: Donor-derived Secondary: Reactivation	Recipient EBV-negative serostatus, history of pretransplant malignancy, fewer HLA matches, overall higher immunosuppressed state
	Hepatitis	Hepatitis B virus, hepatitis C virus	Reactivation, donor derived	Chronic HBV or HCV infection in recipient, high-risk donor
	Progressive multifocal leukoencephalopathy (PML)	JC virus	Reactivation	
	Kaposi sarcoma (KS) of skin or viscera	Human herpes virus 8 (HHV8)	Primary: Reactivation Secondary: Donor-derived in a seronegative recipient	Regionality (Mediterranean, Middle East, South Africa)
Parasitic	Disseminated strongyloidiasis	Strongyloides stercoralis	Reactivation, primary community acquisition	History of residence in or travel to an endemic region

Use of Antimicrobial Prophylaxis in the Kidney and Pancreas-Kidney Transplant Recipient

The use of antimicrobial prophylaxis is a vital tool in preventing infection and complications in kidney and pancreas-kidney transplant recipients. Infection rates have improved with the introduction of standardized antimicrobial prophylaxis after transplant [267]. The ideal prophylaxis targets diseases that are either common or carry significant morbidity and mortality and confers little toxicity. Cost-effectiveness may be a consideration when comparing prophylactic modalities as well. If a patient has significant allergies to antibiotics that are known before transplant, consultation with an allergist may be considered for allergy testing to better delineate options for treatment in the event of infection after transplant.

Trimethoprim-sulfamethoxazole (TMP-SMX) is the cornerstone of antimicrobial prophylaxis in renal transplant recipients, with the aim at preventing urinary tract infections, pyelonephritis, urosepsis, and pneumocystis pneumonia. Prior to its routine use in renal transplant recipients, 30–40% of recipients developed UTIs within the first 4 months following transplantation, and they were often associated with Gram-negative bacteremia, significant graft dysfunction, and relapse [267]. KDIGO guidelines recommend its use for at least 6 months after transplantation with the indication of preventing urinary tract infections and pneumocystis; prophylaxis should be extended or reinstituted for at least 6 weeks after treatment for acute rejection [242]. TMP-SMX carries potential added benefits as it also confers protection against additional pathogens, such as *Toxoplasma gondii*, *Listeria monocytogenes*, and *Nocardia* spp., among others [268, 269]. TMP-SMX is inexpensive and easily accessible but may cause significant adverse reactions in some patients, including cytopenias, hepatic necrosis, and drug rashes ranging from urticaria to Stevens-Johnson syndrome (SJS) and toxic epidermal necrolysis (TEN) [269]. While the sulfamethoxazole may be nephrotoxic at high doses, the trimethoprim may cause a minor, generally $\leq$0.4 mg/dL increase in serum creatinine without truly impacting glomerular filtration rate as it inhibits tubular creatinine secretion [270, 271]. This effect is more pronounced in patients with chronic kidney disease or higher serum creatinine prior to use [270]. It must be dose adjusted in the setting of renal allograft dysfunction if creatinine clearance falls below 30 mL/min [269]. Hyperkalemia and GI upset may also be dose-limiting side effects in some patients. Other options for pneumocystis prophylaxis include dapsone, which may have cross-allergenicity with TMP-SMX and may rarely cause life-threatening hemolysis in patients with or without glucose-6-phosphate dehydrogenase (G6PD) deficiency or methemoglobinemia. Atovaquone is administered as an oral solution and may cause gastrointestinal upset. Inhaled pentamidine should be used with caution in patients prone to bronchospasm and is the least effective agent against PCP as it may not prevent upper lobe pneumocystis or the rare extrapulmonary pneumocystis infection. These alternative agents do not confer protection against the broader range of pathogens covered by TMP-SMX.

Despite TMP-SMX broader antimicrobial coverage, however, retrospective data is conflicted as to its effectiveness in preventing asymptomatic bacteriuria or UTI and trends toward increased amoxicillin and TMP-SMX resistance within 30 days of use [272, 273]. Conversely, it has been shown to reduce the incidence of sepsis in renal transplant recipients as compared to those without prophylaxis [274]. Randomized controlled trials, however, have shown efficacy of TMP-SMX prophylaxis. Renal transplant recipients randomized to receive TMP-SMX had fewer hospital days with fever and bloodstream infections when receiving high-dose prophylaxis (320/1600 mg daily, compared to 160/800 mg daily). Both doses, however, were effective in preventing urinary tract infection after, but not before, catheter removal. TMP-SMX use did not result in colonization or infection with TMP-SMX-resistant Gram-negative bacilli, and patients were less likely to be colonized with *Candida*, possibly due to less antibiotic treatment for infection; however, their infections were more likely to be caused by resistant bacteria than the placebo group. TMP-SMX prophylaxis was found to be cost-beneficial and to have minimal effect on the hosts' microflora [275]. Another randomized, controlled trial using various doses of TMP-SMX found that prophylaxis with high dose (320/1600 mg daily) reduced UTI in the first month after transplant as compared with patients given low or moderate dose prophylaxis [276]. For patients intolerant of TMP-SMX, ciprofloxacin has been studied as an alternative for UTI prophylaxis. Low-dose ciprofloxacin (250 mg daily) as compared to single strength (80/400 mg daily) TMP-SMX daily for 6 months showed ciprofloxacin to be at least as effective as TMP-SMX in preventing urinary tract infection and had better tolerability [277]. Pneumocystis pneumonia occurred in 14% of the ciprofloxacin group; no cases were observed in the TMP-SXM group; however, a follow-up uncontrolled study found ciprofloxacin prophylaxis combined with monthly aerosolized pentamidine was effective in preventing both UTI and pneumocystis pneumonia.

The use of routine perioperative surgical prophylaxis, typically directed at preventing wound infections, will vary by center protocol. Among a retrospective study of 349 renal transplant recipients who received TMP-SMX but not additional perioperative antibiotic prophylaxis, wound infections developed in only 7 patients (2%) and were more common in obese and older patients [122]. All wound infections in the study period were superficial and responded well to wound drainage and outpatient antibiotic therapy. Without additional perioperative antibiotic prophylaxis, the incidence of UTI in the first postoperative month was still low, occurring in 1.7% of patients overall, although this was notably higher in patients who had ureteral stents (11.4% vs 0.3%, $P < 0.001$). The authors suggest that, given the rarity of perioperative bacterial infection in the renal transplant population on TMP-SMX prophylaxis, routine perioperative antibiotic prophylaxis be restricted to patients older than 60, with a body mass index greater than 35, or complicated transplants requiring ureteral stents in order to reduce emergence of drug resistance, costs, and adverse events. However, most centers still opt to give at least short-term prophylaxis with cefazolin or similar agents, and this remains an area for ongoing study.

Oral and esophageal *Candida* prophylaxis with clotrimazole lozenges, nystatin, or fluconazole is recommended for 1–3 months after transplantation and for 1 month after treatment with antilymphocyte antibody [242]. This is also effective against contamination of perfusion fluid with *Candida* species. Use of fluconazole requires concurrent adjustment and monitoring of immunosuppressant levels.

Prophylaxis for tuberculosis should be given for renal transplant recipients diagnosed with latent TB infection or those meeting criteria for non-transplant patients such as a known active TB exposure. Screening and diagnosis of latent TB in the renal transplant recipient is discussed further in the Pretransplantation Screening for Potential Recipients section. In the case of renal or pancreas-renal transplant recipients where bridging therapy with dialysis is an option, there is generally sufficient time in the pretransplant evaluation for patients to undergo TB screening, have imaging done to rule out active disease, discuss prophylaxis options, and begin – or possibly even complete – treatment prior to transplantation. However, latent TB should never be a barrier to proceeding to urgent or life-saving transplantation, but treatment should be started as soon as possible after transplant, ideally within 1 month. A notable exception is patients undergoing simultaneous liver -kidney transplant who may not tolerate the hepatotoxic side effects of TB prophylaxis until after transplant. The most frequently used prophylactic regimens include daily INH for 9 months or rifampin daily for 4 months, although use of rifampin in the posttransplant period has greater potential

Table 4.14 Antimicrobial prophylaxis in the kidney and kidney-pancreas transplant recipient

Agent	Indication	Duration posttransplantation
Acyclovir	Prevention of recurrent HSV outbreaks	Varies
	Prevention of herpes viruses infection in CMV D−/R− patients (vs. a preemptive monitoring strategy which may be used in some centers)	At least 3 months Extend or reinstitute for 6 weeks after treatment with a T-cell depleting antibody
	Postexposure prophylaxis in a susceptible patient after varicella exposure if varicella Ig and IVIG are not available or if greater than 96 h have elapsed between exposure and initiation of care	7 days
Antifungal (clotrimazole, nystatin, fluconazole)	Prevention of oral or esophageal candidiasis, prevention of Candida UTI/pyelonephritis in the setting of perfusion fluid contamination	1–3 months after transplant Extend or reinstitute for 1 month after treatment with antilymphocyte antibody
Entecavir	Treatment of patients with positive HBsAg or detectable serum HBV DNA	Lifelong
	Prevention of reactivation of latent HBV in a core-Ab positive recipient	Low risk for reactivation Consider prophylaxis or preemptive monitoring strategy with ALT and HBV DNA NAT
	Prevention of transmission from a core-Ab positive donor	
Ganciclovir/ valganciclovir	Prevention of CMV viremia/infection in D+/R−, D−/R+, and D+/R+ patients	3–6 months Extend for 1–3 months after treatment for acute rejection
Isoniazid (INH) Co-administered with vitamin B6	Latent tuberculosis	9 months If started prior to transplantation, no need for extension as long as there are no significant interruptions in therapy
Trimethoprim-sulfamethoxazole (TMP-SMX)	Prevention of urinary tract infection and pneumocystis	At least 6 months Extend or reinstitute for at least 6 weeks after treatment for acute rejection
Varicella Ig	Postexposure prophylaxis in a susceptible patient after varicella exposure if presenting within the first 96 h after exposure	Single dose, may be repeated

for interaction with a number of commonly used antirejection medications. Substitution of rifabutin may have less profound drug-drug interactions [242] but is not recommended among the first-line latent TB regimens by the CDC [278]. Use of either isoniazid or rifampin should prompt a discussion with the patient regarding hepatotoxicity side effects and symptoms of acute liver failure; regular liver function testing is advised. Patients with diabetes, renal failure, HIV, alcoholism, and malnutrition are at increased risk of developing neuropathy from INH use and should take concurrent pyridoxine for prevention of drug-induced neurotoxicity [279]; in most clinical practices, all patients on INH will receive pyridoxine as it has little adverse effect.

CMV prophylaxis with oral ganciclovir or valganciclovir should be administered to all kidney transplant recipients who do not fall into the donor-negative/recipient-negative CMV serostatus group for at least 3 months after transplantation and for 6 weeks after treatment with a T-cell depleting antibody [242]. For the highest risk serogroup (D+/R−), prophylaxis should be extended to 6 months [228]. CMV prophylaxis also confers a protective effect against other herpes viruses, including HSV, VZV, and EBV.

For kidney transplant recipients who experience frequent HSV outbreaks, prophylactic antiviral medication may be considered [242]. If a known varicella exposure occurs in a susceptible recipient, varicella zoster immunoglobulin or intravenous immunoglobulin (IVIG) can be administered within 96 hours of exposure; if neither varicella Ig or IVIG is available or greater than 96 hours have elapsed since exposure, a 7-day course of oral acyclovir can be started within 7–10 days following exposure [242].

A general summary of antimicrobial prophylaxis use is outlined in Table 4.14.

References

1. Hart A, Smith JM, Skeans MA, et al. OPTN/SRTR 2015 annual data report: kidney. Am J Transplant. 2017;17:21–116.
2. Centers for Disease Control and Prevention (CDC). Surveillance for surgical site infection (SSI) events. https://www.cdc.gov/nhsn/acute-care-hospital/ssi/. Updated 2016. Accessed 2 Jan 2017.
3. Wai PY, Sollinger HW. Long-term outcomes after simultaneous pancreas-kidney transplant. Curr Opin Organ Transplant. 2011;16(1):128–34.
4. Sollinger HW, Geffner SR. Pancreas transplantation. Surg Clin N Am. 1994;74(5):1183–95.
5. Hesse UJ, Sutherland DE, Simmons RL, Najarian JS. Intra-abdominal infections in pancreas transplant recipients. Ann Surg. 1986;203(2):153–62.
6. Pancreatic transplantation. Informa Healthcare USA; 2007.
7. Baktavatsalam R, Little DM, Connolly EM, Farrell JG, Hickey DP. Complications relating to the urinary tract associated with bladder-drained pancreatic transplantation. Br J Urol. 1998;81(2):219–23.

8. Ponticelli CE. The impact of cold ischemia time on renal transplant outcome. Kidney Int. 2015;87(2):272–5.
9. Debout A, Foucher Y, Trebern-Launay K, et al. Each additional hour of cold ischemia time significantly increases the risk of graft failure and mortality following renal transplantation. Kidney Int. 2015;87(2):343–9.
10. Cai J, Terasaki PI. Induction immunosuppression improves long-term graft and patient outcome in organ transplantation: an analysis of united network for organ sharing registry data. Transplantation. 2010;90(12):1511–5.
11. Organ procurement and transplantation network. http://optn.transplant.hrsa.gov/. Accessed Aug 2016.
12. National kidney foundation: organ donation and transplantation statistics. https://www.kidney.org/news/newsroom/factsheets/Organ-Donation-and-Transplantation-Stats. Updated 2016. Accessed Aug 2016.
13. United states renal data system. Chapter 7: transplantation. https://www.usrds.org/2015/view/v2_07.aspx. Updated 2013. Accessed Aug 2016.
14. Matas AJ, Smith JM, Skeans MA, et al. OPTN/SRTR 2013 annual data report: kidney. Am J Transplant. 2015;15(Suppl 2):1–34.
15. Eleftheriadis T, Liakopoulos V, Leivaditis K, Antoniadi G, Stefanidis I. Infections in hemodialysis: a concise review – part 1: bacteremia and respiratory infections. Hippokratia. 2011;15(1):12–7.
16. Klevens RM, Tokars JI, Andrus M. Electronic reporting of infections associated with hemodialysis. Nephrol News Issues. 2005;19(7):37–8. 43
17. Allon M, Depner TA, Radeva M, et al. Impact of dialysis dose and membrane on infection-related hospitalization and death: results of the HEMO study. J Am Soc Nephrol. 2003;14(7):1863–70.
18. Taylor G, Gravel D, Johnston L, et al. Incidence of bloodstream infection in multicenter inception cohorts of hemodialysis patients. Am J Infect Control. 2004;32(3):155–60.
19. Shingarev R, Barker-Finkel J, Allon M. Natural history of tunneled dialysis catheters placed for hemodialysis initiation. J Vasc Interv Radiol. 2013;24(9):1289–94.
20. Vandecasteele SJ, Boelaert JR, De Vriese AS. Staphylococcus aureus infections in hemodialysis: what a nephrologist should know. Clin J Am Soc Nephrol. 2009;4(8):1388–400.
21. Lederer SR, Riedelsdorf G, Schiffl H. Nasal carriage of meticillin resistant staphylococcus aureus: the prevalence, patients at risk and the effect of elimination on outcomes among outclinic haemodialysis patients. Eur J Med Res. 2007;12(7):284–8.
22. Johnson LB, Jose J, Yousif F, Pawlak J, Saravolatz LD. Prevalence of colonization with community-associated methicillin-resistant staphylococcus aureus among end-stage renal disease patients and healthcare workers. Infect Control Hosp Epidemiol. 2009;30(1):4–8.
23. Allon M. Treatment guidelines for dialysis catheter-related bacteremia: an update. Am J Kidney Dis. 2009;54(1):13–7.
24. Abbott KC, Agodoa LY. Hospitalizations for bacterial endocarditis after initiation of chronic dialysis in the United States. Nephron. 2002;91(2):203–9.
25. Kamalakannan D, Pai RM, Johnson LB, Gardin JM, Saravolatz LD. Epidemiology and clinical outcomes of infective endocarditis in hemodialysis patients. Ann Thorac Surg. 2007;83(6):2081–6.
26. Marr KA, Sexton DJ, Conlon PJ, Corey GR, Schwab SJ, Kirkland KB. Catheter-related bacteremia and outcome of attempted catheter salvage in patients undergoing hemodialysis. Ann Intern Med. 1997;127(4):275–80.
27. Maya ID, Carlton D, Estrada E, Allon M. Treatment of dialysis catheter-related staphylococcus aureus bacteremia with an antibiotic lock: a quality improvement report. Am J Kidney Dis. 2007;50(2):289–95.
28. Sarnak MJ, Jaber BL. Pulmonary infectious mortality among patients with end-stage renal disease. Chest. 2001;120(6):1883–7.
29. Pulliam J, Li NC, Maddux F, Hakim R, Finkelstein FO, Lacson E Jr. First-year outcomes of incident peritoneal dialysis patients in the United States. Am J Kidney Dis. 2014;64(5):761–9.
30. Mujais S. Microbiology and outcomes of peritonitis in North America. Kidney Int Suppl. 2006;103(103):S55–62.
31. Port FK, Held PJ, Nolph KD, Turenne MN, Wolfe RA. Risk of peritonitis and technique failure by CAPD connection technique: a national study. Kidney Int. 1992;42(4):967–74.
32. Kim DK, Yoo TH, Ryu DR, et al. Changes in causative organisms and their antimicrobial susceptibilities in CAPD peritonitis: a single center's experience over one decade. Perit Dial Int. 2004;24(5):424–32.
33. Bunke CM, Brier ME, Golper TA. Outcomes of single organism peritonitis in peritoneal dialysis: gram negatives versus gram positives in the network 9 peritonitis study. Kidney Int. 1997;52(2):524–9.
34. Piraino B, Bernardini J, Florio T, Fried L. Staphylococcus aureus prophylaxis and trends in gram-negative infections in peritoneal dialysis patients. Perit Dial Int. 2003;23(5):456–9.
35. Matuszkiewicz-Rowinska J. Update on fungal peritonitis and its treatment. Perit Dial Int. 2009;29(Suppl 2):S161–5.
36. Unal A, Koc AN, Sipahioglu MH, et al. CAPD-related peritonitis caused by rhodotorula mucilaginosa. Perit Dial Int. 2009;29(5):581–2.
37. Warren J, Jones E, Sener A, et al. Should peritoneal dialysis catheters be removed at the time of kidney transplantation? Can Urol Assoc J. 2012;6(5):376–8.
38. Martins LS, Malheiro J, Pedroso S, et al. Pancreas-kidney transplantation: impact of dialysis modality on the outcome. Transpl Int. 2015;28(8):972–9.
39. Li PKT, Szeto CC, Piraino B, et al. ISPD guidelines recommendations: peritoneal dialysis-related infections recommendations: 2010 update. Dial Int. 2010;30:393–423.
40. Cendoroglo Neto M, Draibe SA, Silva AE, et al. Incidence of and risk factors for hepatitis B virus and hepatitis C virus infection among haemodialysis and CAPD patients: evidence for environmental transmission. Nephrol Dial Transplant. 1995;10(2):240–6.
41. Rhea S, Moorman A, Pace R, et al. Hepatitis B reverse seroconversion and transmission in a hemodialysis center: a public health investigation and case report. Am J Kidney Dis. 2016;68(2):292–5. https://doi.org/10.1053/j.ajkd.2016.03.424.
42. CDC dialysis safety: guidelines and recommendations. http://www.cdc.gov/dialysis/guidelines/index.html. Updated 2016. 2016.
43. Finelli L, Miller JT, Tokars JI, Alter MJ, Arduino MJ. National surveillance of dialysis-associated diseases in the United States, 2002. Semin Dial. 2005;18(1):52–61.
44. Harnett JD, Parfrey PS, Kennedy M, Zeldis JB, Steinman TI, Guttmann RD. The long-term outcome of hepatitis B infection in hemodialysis patients. Am J Kidney Dis. 1988;11(3):210–3.
45. Kanaan N, Kabamba B, Marechal C, et al. Significant rate of hepatitis B reactivation following kidney transplantation in patients with resolved infection. J Clin Virol. 2012;55(3):233–8.
46. Chi C, Patel P, Pilishvili T, Moore M, Murphy T, Strikas R. Guidelines for vaccinating kidney dialysis patients and patients with chronic kidney disease: summarized from recommendations of the advisory committee on immunization practices (ACIP). http://www.cdc.gov/vaccines/pubs/downloads/dialysis-guide-2012.pdf. Updated July, 2015. 2016.
47. Recommendations of the advisory committee on immunization practices (ACIP): use of vaccines and immune globulins for persons with altered immunocompetence. MMWR Recomm Rep. 1993;42(RR-4):1–18.
48. Mast EE, Weinbaum CM, Fiore AE, et al. A comprehensive immunization strategy to eliminate transmission of hepatitis B virus infection in the United States: recommendations of the advisory committee on immunization practices (ACIP) part II: immunization of adults. MMWR Recomm Rep. 2006;55(RR-16):1–33; quiz CE1–4.

49. CDC adult immunization schedule. http://www.cdc.gov/vaccines/schedules/hcp/adult.html. Updated 2016. Accessed 2016.
50. Tokars JI, Alter MJ, Miller E, Moyer LA, Favero MS. National surveillance of dialysis associated diseases in the United States – 1994. ASAIO J. 1997;43(1):108–19.
51. Burdick RA, Bragg-Gresham JL, Woods JD, et al. Patterns of hepatitis B prevalence and seroconversion in hemodialysis units from three continents: the DOPPS. Kidney Int. 2003;63(6):2222–9.
52. Buti M, Gane E, Seto WK, et al. A phase 3 study of tenofovir alafenamide compared with tenofovir disoproxil fumarate in patients with HBeAg-negative, chronic hepatitis B: week 48 efficacy and safety results. Int Liver Congr. 2016. https://www.journal-of-hepatology.eu/article/S0168-8278(16)01637-8/abstract
53. Chan H, Fung S, Seto WK, Chuang W-L, et al. A phase 3 study of tenofovir alafenamide compared with tenofovir disoproxil fumarate in patients with HBeAg-positive chronic HBV: week 48 efficacy and safety results. Barcelona: The International Liver Congress™, EASL – European Association for the Study of the Liver; 2016.
54. Fissell RB, Bragg-Gresham JL, Woods JD, et al. Patterns of hepatitis C prevalence and seroconversion in hemodialysis units from three continents: the DOPPS. Kidney Int. 2004;65(6):2335–42.
55. Cacoub P, Desbois AC, Isnard-Bagnis C, Rocatello D, Ferri C. Hepatitis C virus infection and chronic kidney disease: time for reappraisal. J Hepatol. 2016;65(1 Suppl):S82–94.
56. dos Santos JP, Loureiro A, Cendoroglo Neto M, Pereira BJ. Impact of dialysis room and reuse strategies on the incidence of hepatitis C virus infection in haemodialysis units. Nephrol Dial Transplant. 1996;11(10):2017–22.
57. Petrosillo N, Gilli P, Serraino D, et al. Prevalence of infected patients and understaffing have a role in hepatitis C virus transmission in dialysis. Am J Kidney Dis. 2001;37(5):1004–10.
58. Belga S, Doucette KE. Hepatitis C in non-hepatic solid organ transplant candidates and recipients: a new horizon. World J Gastroenterol. 2016;22(4):1650–63.
59. Locke JE, Shelton BA, Reed RD, et al. Identification of optimal donor-recipient combinations among human immunodeficiency virus (HIV)-positive kidney transplant recipients. Am J Transplant. 2016;16(8):2377–83.
60. Carpio R, Pamugas GE, Danguilan R, Que E. Outcomes of renal allograft recipients with hepatitis C. Transplant Proc. 2016;48(3):836–9.
61. FDA news release: FDA approves zepatier for treatment of chronic hepatitis C genotypes 1 and 4. http://www.fda.gov/NewsEvents/Newsroom/PressAnnouncements/ucm483828.htm. Updated 2016. 2016.
62. Roth D, Nelson DR, Bruchfeld A, et al. Grazoprevir plus elbasvir in treatment-naive and treatment-experienced patients with hepatitis C virus genotype 1 infection and stage 4–5 chronic kidney disease (the C-SURFER study): a combination phase 3 study. Lancet. 2015;386(10003):1537–45.
63. Bhamidimarri KR, Czul F, Peyton A, et al. Safety, efficacy and tolerability of half-dose sofosbuvir plus simeprevir in treatment of hepatitis C in patients with end stage renal disease. J Hepatol. 2015;63(3):763–5.
64. Beinhardt S, Al Zoairy R, Ferenci P, et al. DAA-based antiviral treatment of patients with chronic hepatitis C in the pre- and post-kidney transplantation setting. Transpl Int. 2016;29(9):999–1007.
65. Kidney Disease: Improving Global Outcomes. KDIGO clinical practice guideline for the prevention, diagnosis, evaluation, and treatment of hepatitis C in chronic kidney disease. Kidney Int. 2008;73(Supplement 109):S1–S99.
66. Abbott KC, Lentine KL, Bucci JR, Agodoa LY, Peters TG, Schnitzler MA. The impact of transplantation with deceased donor hepatitis c-positive kidneys on survival in wait-listed long-term dialysis patients. Am J Transplant. 2004;4(12):2032–7.
67. Lee J, Cho JH, Lee JS, et al. Pretransplant hepatitis B viral infection increases risk of death after kidney transplantation: a multicenter cohort study in Korea. Medicine (Baltimore). 2016;95(21):e3671.
68. Palella FJ Jr, Baker RK, Moorman AC, et al. Mortality in the highly active antiretroviral therapy era: changing causes of death and disease in the HIV outpatient study. J Acquir Immune Defic Syndr. 2006;43(1):27–34.
69. Jotwani V, Li Y, Grunfeld C, Choi AI, Shlipak MG. Risk factors for ESRD in HIV-infected individuals: traditional and HIV-related factors. Am J Kidney Dis. 2012;59(5):628–35.
70. Peters L, Grint D, Lundgren JD, et al. Hepatitis C virus viremia increases the incidence of chronic kidney disease in HIV-infected patients. AIDS. 2012;26(15):1917–26.
71. Perez G, Ortiz-Interian C, Lee H, et al. Human immunodeficiency virus and human T-cell leukemia virus type I in patients undergoing maintenance hemodialysis in Miami. Am J Kidney Dis. 1989;14(1):39–43.
72. Vigneau C, Guiard-Schmid JB, Tourret J, et al. The clinical characteristics of HIV-infected patients receiving dialysis in France between 1997 and 2002. Kidney Int. 2005;67(4):1509–14.
73. Stock PG, Barin B, Murphy B, et al. Outcomes of kidney transplantation in HIV-infected recipients. N Engl J Med. 2010;363(21):2004–14.
74. Locke JE, Mehta S, Reed RD, et al. A national study of outcomes among HIV-infected kidney transplant recipients. J Am Soc Nephrol. 2015;26(9):2222–9.
75. Muller E, Barday Z, Mendelson M, Kahn D. HIV-positive-to-HIV-positive kidney transplantation – results at 3 to 5 years. N Engl J Med. 2015;372(7):613–20.
76. Mittal S, Choudhary P, Callaghan C, Hilton R, Drage M. First case of pancreas transplant alone in patient with diabetes and HIV infection. Int J STD AIDS. 2016;27:1350–3.
77. Miro JM, Ricart MJ, Trullas JC, et al. Simultaneous pancreas-kidney transplantation in HIV-infected patients: a case report and literature review. Transplant Proc. 2010;42(9):3887–91.
78. Primeggia J, Timpone JG Jr, Kumar PN. Pharmacologic issues of antiretroviral agents and immunosuppressive regimens in HIV-infected solid organ transplant recipients. Infect Dis Clin N Am. 2013;27(2):473–86.
79. Tricot L, Teicher E, Peytavin G, et al. Safety and efficacy of raltegravir in HIV-infected transplant patients cotreated with immunosuppressive drugs. Am J Transplant. 2009;9(8):1946–52.
80. Latinovic O, Kuruppu J, Davis C, Le N, Heredia A. Pharmacotherapy of HIV-1 infection: focus on CCR5 antagonist maraviroc. Clin Med Ther. 2009;1:1497–510.
81. Fischer SA, Avery RK, AST Infectious Disease Community of Practice. Screening of donor and recipient prior to solid organ transplantation. Am J Transplant. 2009;9(Suppl 4):S7–18.
82. Bumbacea D, Arend SM, Eyuboglu F, et al. The risk of tuberculosis in transplant candidates and recipients: a TBNET consensus statement. Eur Respir J. 2012;40(4):990–1013.
83. Segall L, Covic A. Diagnosis of tuberculosis in dialysis patients: current strategy. Clin J Am Soc Nephrol. 2010;5(6):1114–22.
84. Foster R, Ferguson TW, Rigatto C, Lerner B, Tangri N, Komenda P. A retrospective review of the two-step tuberculin skin test in dialysis patients. Can J Kidney Health Dis. 2016;3:28. -016-0119-4. eCollection 2016.
85. Kim SY, Jung GS, Kim SK, et al. Comparison of the tuberculin skin test and interferon-gamma release assay for the diagnosis of latent tuberculosis infection before kidney transplantation. Infection. 2013;41(1):103–10.
86. Kim SH, Lee SO, Park JB, et al. A prospective longitudinal study evaluating the usefulness of a T-cell-based assay for latent tuberculosis infection in kidney transplant recipients. Am J Transplant. 2011;11(9):1927–35.

87. Subramanian AK, Morris MI, AST Infectious Diseases Community of Practice. Mycobacterium tuberculosis infections in solid organ transplantation. Am J Transplant. 2013;13(Suppl 4):68–76.
88. Blanchet P, Droupy S, Eschwege P, et al. Urodynamic testing predicts long-term urological complications following simultaneous pancreas-kidney transplantation. Clin Transplant. 2003;17(1):26–31.
89. Crepin T, Gaiffe E, Courivaud C, et al. Pre-transplant end-stage renal disease-related immune risk profile in kidney transplant recipients predicts post-transplant infections. Transpl Infect Dis. 2016;18(3):415–22.
90. Levi ME, Kumar D, Green M, et al. Considerations for screening live kidney donors for endemic infections: a viewpoint on the UNOS policy. Am J Transplant. 2014;14(5):1003–11.
91. Organ procurement and transplantation network: Guidance on Zika virus. https://optn.transplant.hrsa.gov. Updated 2016. Accessed Aug 2016.
92. Seem DL, Lee I, Umscheid CA, Kuehnert MJ, United States Public Health Service. PHS guideline for reducing human immunodeficiency virus, hepatitis B virus, and hepatitis C virus transmission through organ transplantation. Public Health Rep. 2013;128(4):247–343.
93. Kucirka LM, Sarathy H, Govindan P, et al. Risk of window period HIV infection in high infectious risk donors: systematic review and meta-analysis. Am J Transplant. 2011;11(6):1176–87.
94. Kucirka LM, Dagher NN, Montgomery RA, Segev DL, Singer AL. High infectious risk organ donors in kidney transplantation: risks, benefits, and current practices. Dial Transplant. 2010;39(5):186–9.
95. Schweitzer EJ, Perencevich EN, Philosophe B, Bartlett ST. Estimated benefits of transplantation of kidneys from donors at increased risk for HIV or hepatitis C infection. Am J Transplant. 2007;7(6):1515–25.
96. Limkemann AJ, Wolfe L, Sharma A, et al. Outcomes of kidney transplants and risk of infection transmission from increased infectious risk donors. Clin Transpl. 2016;30(8):886–93.
97. Orandi BJ, Luo X, Massie AB, et al. Survival benefit with kidney transplants from HLA-incompatible live donors. N Engl J Med. 2016;374(10):940–50.
98. Rituxan (rituximab): package insert. http://www.accessdata.fda.gov/drugsatfda_docs/label/2010/103705s5311lbl.pdf. Accessed 30 Nov 2016.
99. Hwang JP, Somerfield MR, Alston-Johnson DE, et al. Hepatitis B virus screening for patients with cancer before therapy: American society of clinical oncology provisional clinical opinion update. J Clin Oncol. 2015;33(19):2212–20.
100. Huang YH, Hsiao LT, Hong YC, et al. Randomized controlled trial of entecavir prophylaxis for rituximab-associated hepatitis B virus reactivation in patients with lymphoma and resolved hepatitis B. J Clin Oncol. 2013;31(22):2765–72.
101. Habicht A, Broker V, Blume C, et al. Increase of infectious complications in ABO-incompatible kidney transplant recipients – a single centre experience. Nephrol Dial Transplant. 2011;26(12):4124–31.
102. Kahwaji J, Sinha A, Toyoda M, et al. Infectious complications in kidney-transplant recipients desensitized with rituximab and intravenous immunoglobulin. Clin J Am Soc Nephrol. 2011;6(12):2894–900.
103. Choi BH, Han DJ. Ongoing higher infection rate in ABO-incompatible kidney transplant recipient: is it a serious problem? A single-center experience. Ann Surg Treat Res. 2016;91(1):37–44.
104. Gea-Banacloche JC. Rituximab-associated infections. Semin Hematol. 2010;47(2):187–98.
105. Briggs JD. Causes of death after renal transplantation. Nephrol Dial Transplant. 2001;16(8):1545–9.
106. Rubin RH. Infectious disease complications of renal transplantation. Kidney Int. 1993;44(1):221–36.
107. Fishman JA. Infection in solid-organ transplant recipients. N Engl J Med. 2007;357(25):2601–14.
108. Passalacqua JA, Wiland AM, Fink JC, Bartlett ST, Evans DA, Keay S. Increased incidence of postoperative infections associated with peritoneal dialysis in renal transplant recipients. Transplantation. 1999;68(4):535–40.
109. Montero N, Webster AC, Royuela A, Zamora J, Crespo Barrio M, Pascual J. Steroid avoidance or withdrawal for pancreas and pancreas with kidney transplant recipients. Cochrane Database Syst Rev. 2014;(9):CD007669.
110. Cantarovich D, Karam G, Hourmant M, et al. Steroid avoidance versus steroid withdrawal after simultaneous pancreas-kidney transplantation. Am J Transplant. 2005;5(6):1332–8.
111. Fernandez-Ruiz M, Lopez-Medrano F, Andres A, et al. Serum iron parameters in the early post-transplant period and infection risk in kidney transplant recipients. Transpl Infect Dis. 2013;15(6):600–11.
112. Van Laecke S, Vermeiren P, Nagler EV, et al. Magnesium and infection risk after kidney transplantation: an observational cohort study. J Infect. 2016;73(1):8–17.
113. Park YJ, Kim SU, Lee KH, et al. Vitamin D deficiency is associated with increased risk of bacterial infections after kidney transplantation. Korean J Intern Med. 2017; 32:505-513.
114. Mawhorter S, Yamani MH. Hypogammaglobulinemia and infection risk in solid organ transplant recipients. Curr Opin Organ Transplant. 2008;13(6):581–5.
115. Broeders EN, Wissing KM, Hazzan M, et al. Evolution of immunoglobulin and mannose binding protein levels after renal transplantation: association with infectious complications. Transpl Int. 2008;21(1):57–64.
116. Lubetzky M, Yaffe H, Chen C, Ali H, Kayler LK. Early readmission after kidney transplantation: examination of discharge-level factors. Transplantation. 2016;100(5):1079–85.
117. McAdams-Demarco MA, Grams ME, Hall EC, Coresh J, Segev DL. Early hospital readmission after kidney transplantation: patient and center-level associations. Am J Transplant. 2012;12(12):3283–8.
118. McAdams-DeMarco MA, Law A, Salter ML, et al. Frailty and early hospital readmission after kidney transplantation. Am J Transplant. 2013;13(8):2091–5.
119. Taber DJ, Palanisamy AP, Srinivas TR, et al. Inclusion of dynamic clinical data improves the predictive performance of a 30-day readmission risk model in kidney transplantation. Transplantation. 2015;99(2):324–30.
120. Harhay M, Lin E, Pai A, et al. Early rehospitalization after kidney transplantation: assessing preventability and prognosis. Am J Transplant. 2013;13(12):3164–72.
121. Abbott KC, Swanson SJ, Richter ER, et al. Late urinary tract infection after renal transplantation in the United States. Am J Kidney Dis. 2004;44(2):353–62.
122. Laftavi MR, Rostami R, Feng L, et al. The role of antibiotic prophylaxis in the new era of immunosuppression. Transplant Proc. 2011;43(2):533–5.
123. Ranghino A, Diena D, Simonato F, et al. Clinical impact of bacterial contamination of perfusion fluid in kidney transplantation. Springerplus. 2016;5:7. -015-1658-3. eCollection 2016.
124. Meirelles Junior RF, Salvalaggio P, Pacheco-Silva A. Pancreas transplantation: review. Einstein (Sao Paulo). 2015;13(2):305–9.
125. Humar A, Kandaswamy R, Granger D, Gruessner RW, Gruessner AC, Sutherland DE. Decreased surgical risks of pancreas transplantation in the modern era. Ann Surg. 2000;231(2):269–75.
126. Manrique A, Jimenez C, Lopez RM, et al. Relaparotomy after pancreas transplantation: causes and outcomes. Transplant Proc. 2009;41(6):2472–4.

127. Gruessner RW, Sutherland DE, Troppmann C, et al. The surgical risk of pancreas transplantation in the cyclosporine era: an overview. J Am Coll Surg. 1997;185(2):128–44.
128. Singh RP, Vrakas G, Hayek S, et al. Clinically significant peripancreatic fluid collections after simultaneous pancreas-kidney transplantation. Transplantation. 2013;95(10):1263–9.
129. Shah SA, Tsapepas DS, Kubin CJ, et al. Risk factors associated with clostridium difficile infection after kidney and pancreas transplantation. Transpl Infect Dis. 2013;15(5):502–9.
130. Linares L, Cervera C, Hoyo I, et al. Klebsiella pneumoniae infection in solid organ transplant recipients: epidemiology and antibiotic resistance. Transplant Proc. 2010;42(8):2941–3.
131. Pilmis B, Scemla A, Join-Lambert O, et al. ESBL-producing enterobacteriaceae-related urinary tract infections in kidney transplant recipients: incidence and risk factors for recurrence. Infect Dis (Lond). 2015;47(10):714–8.
132. Origuen J, Fernandez-Ruiz M, Lopez-Medrano F, et al. Progressive increase of resistance in enterobacteriaceae urinary isolates from kidney transplant recipients over the past decade: narrowing of the therapeutic options. Transpl Infect Dis. 2016;18(4):575–84.
133. Bergamasco MD, Barroso Barbosa M, de Oliveira Garcia D, et al. Infection with klebsiella pneumoniae carbapenemase (KPC)-producing K. pneumoniae in solid organ transplantation. Transpl Infect Dis. 2012;14(2):198–205.
134. Freire MP, de Oliveira Garcia D, Cury AP, et al. Outbreak of IMP-producing carbapenem-resistant enterobacter gergoviae among kidney transplant recipients. J Antimicrob Chemother. 2016;71(9):2577–85.
135. Fishman JA, Grossi PA. Donor-derived infection – the challenge for transplant safety. Nat Rev Nephrol. 2014;10(11):663–72.
136. Wu TJ, Lee CF, Chou HS, Yu MC, Lee WC. Suspect the donor with potential infection in the adult deceased donor liver transplantation. Transplant Proc. 2008;40(8):2486–8.
137. Martins N, Martins IS, de Freitas WV, et al. Severe infection in a lung transplant recipient caused by donor-transmitted carbapenem-resistant acinetobacter baumannii. Transpl Infect Dis. 2012;14(3):316–20.
138. Patel G, Perez F, Hujer AM, et al. Fulminant endocarditis and disseminated infection caused by carbapenem-resistant acinetobacter baumannii in a renal-pancreas transplant recipient. Transpl Infect Dis. 2015;17(2):289–96.
139. Huaman MA, Vilchez V, Mei X, Davenport D, Gedaly R. Donor positive blood culture is associated with delayed graft function in kidney transplant recipients: a propensity score analysis of the UNOS database. Clin Transplant. 2016;30(4):415–20.
140. Lumbreras C, Sanz F, Gonzalez A, et al. Clinical significance of donor-unrecognized bacteremia in the outcome of solid-organ transplant recipients. Clin Infect Dis. 2001;33(5):722–6.
141. Chong PP, Razonable RR. Diagnostic and management strategies for donor-derived infections. Infect Dis Clin N Am. 2013;27(2):253–70.
142. Mahboobi N, Tabatabaei SV, Blum HE, Alavian SM. Renal grafts from anti-hepatitis B core-positive donors: a quantitative review of the literature. Transpl Infect Dis. 2012;14(5):445–51.
143. Ison MG, Llata E, Conover CS, et al. Transmission of human immunodeficiency virus and hepatitis C virus from an organ donor to four transplant recipients. Am J Transplant. 2011;11(6):1218–25.
144. Parry J. Taiwan transplant team blamed for HIV positive organ blunder. BMJ. 2011;343:d6523.
145. Villa E, Nanni Costa A. HIV-positive organs used for transplant in Italy due to human error. Euro Surveill. 2007;12(3):E070308.1.
146. Centers for Disease Control and Prevention (CDC). HIV transmitted from a living organ donor – New York city, 2009. MMWR Morb Mortal Wkly Rep. 2011;60(10):297–301.
147. Ramanan P, Deziel PJ, Norby SM, Yao JD, Garza I, Razonable RR. Donor-transmitted HTLV-1-associated myelopathy in a kidney transplant recipient – case report and literature review. Am J Transplant. 2014;14(10):2417–21.
148. Dodd RY, Notari EP, Nelson D, et al. Development of a multi-system surveillance database for transfusion-transmitted infections among blood donors in the United States. Transfusion. 2016;56:2781–9.
149. Organ Procurement and Transplantation Network. Guidance for HTLV-1 screening and confirmation in potential donors and reporting potential HTLV-1 infection. https://optn.transplant.hrsa.gov/resources/guidance/guidance-for-htlv-1-screening-and-confirmation-in-potential-donors-and-reporting-potential-htlv-1-infection. Updated 2014. Accessed 24 Sept 2016.
150. Srinivasan A, Burton EC, Kuehnert MJ, et al. Transmission of rabies virus from an organ donor to four transplant recipients. N Engl J Med. 2005;352(11):1103–11.
151. Vora NM, Basavaraju SV, Feldman KA, et al. Raccoon rabies virus variant transmission through solid organ transplantation. JAMA. 2013;310(4):398–407.
152. Macneil A, Stroher U, Farnon E, et al. Solid organ transplant-associated lymphocytic choriomeningitis, United States, 2011. Emerg Infect Dis. 2012;18(8):1256–62.
153. Roxby AC, Gottlieb GS, Limaye AP. Strongyloidiasis in transplant patients. Clin Infect Dis. 2009;49(9):1411–23.
154. Abanyie FA, Gray EB, Delli Carpini KW, et al. Donor-derived strongyloides stercoralis infection in solid organ transplant recipients in the United States, 2009–2013. Am J Transplant. 2015;15(5):1369–75.
155. Bern C. Antitrypanosomal therapy for chronic Chagas' disease. N Engl J Med. 2011;364(26):2527–34.
156. Centers for Disease Control and Prevention (CDC). Chagas disease after organ transplantation – United States, 2001. MMWR Morb Mortal Wkly Rep. 2002;51(10):210–2.
157. Arias LF, Duque E, Ocampo C, et al. Detection of amastigotes of trypanosoma cruzi in a kidney graft with acute dysfunction. Transplant Proc. 2006;38(3):885–7.
158. Currie AC, Knight SR, Morris PJ. Tuberculosis in renal transplant recipients: the evidence for prophylaxis. Transplantation. 2010;90(7):695–704.
159. Meinerz G, da Silva CK, Goldani JC, Garcia VD, Keitel E. Epidemiology of tuberculosis after kidney transplantation in a developing country. Transpl Infect Dis. 2016;18(2):176–82.
160. Sun HY. Treating tuberculosis in solid organ transplant recipients. Curr Opin Infect Dis. 2014;27(6):501–5.
161. Longworth SA, Vinnard C, Lee I, Sims KD, Barton TD, Blumberg EA. Risk factors for nontuberculous mycobacterial infections in solid organ transplant recipients: a case-control study. Transpl Infect Dis. 2014;16(1):76–83.
162. Assi M, Martin S, Wheat LJ, et al. Histoplasmosis after solid organ transplant. Clin Infect Dis. 2013;57(11):1542–9.
163. CDC. Areas endemic for histoplasmosis. Centers for Disease Control and Prevention; 2015. http://www.cdc.gov/fungal/pdf/histoplasmosis-lifecycle508c.pdf.
164. Blair JE, Logan JL. Coccidioidomycosis in solid organ transplantation. Clin Infect Dis. 2001;33(9):1536–44.
165. CDC. Areas endemic to coccidioidomycosis. Centers for Disease Control and Prevention; 2016. http://www.cdc.gov/features/valleyfever/.
166. Antony SJ, Dummer SJ, McNeil KK, Salas I. Coccidioidomycosis in renal transplant recipients. Infect Dis Clin Pract. 2005;13(5):250–4.
167. Cohen IM, Galgiani JN, Potter D, Ogden DA. Coccidioidomycosis in renal replacement therapy. Arch Intern Med. 1982;142(3):489–94.
168. Pappas PG, Alexander BD, Andes DR, et al. Invasive fungal infections among organ transplant recipients: results of the transplant-associated infection surveillance network (TRANSNET). Clin Infect Dis. 2010;50(8):1101–11.

169. Singh N, Dromer F, Perfect JR, Lortholary O. Cryptococcosis in solid organ transplant recipients: current state of the science. Clin Infect Dis. 2008;47(10):1321–7.
170. Marques S, Carmo R, Ferreira I, Bustorff M, Sampaio S, Pestana M. Cryptococcosis in renal transplant recipients: a single-center experience. Transplant Proc. 2016;48(7):2289–93.
171. Lopez-Medrano F, Silva JT, Fernandez-Ruiz M, et al. Risk factors associated with early invasive pulmonary aspergillosis in kidney transplant recipients: results from a multinational matched case-control study. Am J Transplant. 2016;16(7):2148–57.
172. Cornet M, Fleury L, Maslo C, Bernard JF, Brucker G, Invasive Aspergillosis Surveillance Network of the Assistance Publique-Hopitaux de Paris. Epidemiology of invasive aspergillosis in France: a six-year multicentric survey in the greater Paris area. J Hosp Infect. 2002;51(4):288–96.
173. Hoyo I, Sanclemente G, de la Bellacasa JP, et al. Epidemiology, clinical characteristics, and outcome of invasive aspergillosis in renal transplant patients. Transpl Infect Dis. 2014;16(6):951–7.
174. Heylen L, Maertens J, Naesens M, et al. Invasive aspergillosis after kidney transplant: case-control study. Clin Infect Dis. 2015;60(10):1505–11.
175. Shannon EM, Reid MJ, Chin-Hong P. Late aspergilloma of a renal allograft without need for operative management: a case report and review of the literature. Transpl Infect Dis. 2016;18(2):261–5.
176. Rodriguez M, Fishman JA. Prevention of infection due to pneumocystis spp. in human immunodeficiency virus-negative immunocompromised patients. Clin Microbiol Rev. 2004;17(4):770–82, table of contents.
177. Lufft V, Kliem V, Behrend M, Pichlmayr R, Koch KM, Brunkhorst R. Incidence of pneumocystis carinii pneumonia after renal transplantation. Impact of immunosuppression. Transplantation. 1996;62(3):421–3.
178. Canet E, Zafrani L, Azoulay E. The critically ill kidney transplant recipient: a narrative review. Chest. 2016;149(6):1546–55.
179. Mulpuru S, Knoll G, Weir C, et al. Pneumocystis pneumonia outbreak among renal transplant recipients at a North American transplant center: risk factors and implications for infection control. Am J Infect Control. 2016;44(4):425–31.
180. de Boer MGJ, de Fijter JW, Kroon FP. Outbreaks and clustering of *Pneumocystis* pneumonia in kidney transplant recipients: a systematic review. Med Mycol. 2011;49(7):673–80.
181. Gianella S, Haeberli L, Joos B, et al. Molecular evidence of interhuman transmission in an outbreak of pneumocystis jirovecii pneumonia among renal transplant recipients. Transpl Infect Dis. 2010;12(1):1–10.
182. Wright AJ, Gill JS. Strategies to prevent BK virus infection in kidney transplant recipients. Curr Opin Infect Dis. 2016;29(4):353–8.
183. Balba GP, Javaid B, Timpone JG Jr. BK polyomavirus infection in the renal transplant recipient. Infect Dis Clin N Am. 2013;27(2):271–83.
184. Knowles WA, Pipkin P, Andrews N, et al. Population-based study of antibody to the human polyomaviruses BKV and JCV and the simian polyomavirus SV40. J Med Virol. 2003;71(1):115–23.
185. Egli A, Infanti L, Dumoulin A, et al. Prevalence of polyomavirus BK and JC infection and replication in 400 healthy blood donors. J Infect Dis. 2009;199(6):837–46.
186. Low J, Humes HD, Szczypka M, Imperiale M. BKV and SV40 infection of human kidney tubular epithelial cells in vitro. Virology. 2004;323(2):182–8.
187. Atencio IA, Shadan FF, Zhou XJ, Vaziri ND, Villarreal LP. Adult mouse kidneys become permissive to acute polyomavirus infection and reactivate persistent infections in response to cellular damage and regeneration. J Virol. 1993;67(3):1424–32.
188. Jouve T, Rostaing L, Malvezzi P. Place of mTOR inhibitors in management of BKV infection after kidney transplantation. J Nephropathol. 2016;5(1):1–7.
189. El Ansary M, Abd Elhamid S, Saadi G, et al. Prevalence of polyoma BK virus infection among living-donor renal transplant recipients. Transpl Infect Dis. 2016;18(4):529–37.
190. Hirsch HH, Randhawa P, AST Infectious Diseases Community of Practice. BK polyomavirus in solid organ transplantation. Am J Transplant. 2013;13(Suppl 4):179–88.
191. Bicalho CS, Oliveira RR, Pierrotti LC, et al. Pre-transplant shedding of BK virus in urine is unrelated to post-transplant viruria and viremia in kidney transplant recipients. Clin Transpl. 2016;30(7):796–801.
192. Thakur R, Arora S, Nada R, Minz M, Joshi K. Prospective monitoring of BK virus reactivation in renal transplant recipients in North India. Transpl Infect Dis. 2011;13(6):575–83.
193. Hayat A, Mukhopadhyay R, Radhika S, et al. Adverse impact of pretransplant polyoma virus infection on renal allograft function. Nephrology (Carlton). 2008;13(2):157–63.
194. Mitterhofer AP, Tinti F, Pietropaolo V, et al. Role of BK virus infection in end-stage renal disease patients waiting for kidney transplantation – viral replication dynamics from pre- to post-transplant. Clin Transpl. 2014;28(3):299–306.
195. Schmitt C, Raggub L, Linnenweber-Held S, Adams O, Schwarz A, Heim A. Donor origin of BKV replication after kidney transplantation. J Clin Virol. 2014;59(2):120–5.
196. Knoll GA, Humar A, Fergusson D, et al. Levofloxacin for BK virus prophylaxis following kidney transplantation: a randomized clinical trial. JAMA. 2014;312(20):2106–14.
197. Lebreton M, Esposito L, Mengelle C, et al. A 3-month course of ciprofloxacin does not prevent BK virus replication in heavily immunosuppressed kidney-transplant patients. J Clin Virol. 2016;79:61–7.
198. Song TR, Rao ZS, Qiu Y, et al. Fluoroquinolone prophylaxis in preventing BK polyomavirus infection after renal transplant: a systematic review and meta-analysis. Kaohsiung J Med Sci. 2016;32(3):152–9.
199. Brennan DC, Agha I, Bohl DL, et al. Incidence of BK with tacrolimus versus cyclosporine and impact of preemptive immunosuppression reduction. Am J Transplant. 2005;5(3):582–94.
200. Drachenberg CB, Hirsch HH, Papadimitriou JC, et al. Polyomavirus BK versus JC replication and nephropathy in renal transplant recipients: a prospective evaluation. Transplantation. 2007;84(3):323–30.
201. Mohamed M, Parajuli S, Muth B, et al. In kidney transplant recipients with BK polyomavirus infection, early BK nephropathy, microvascular inflammation, and serum creatinine are risk factors for graft loss. Transpl Infect Dis. 2016;18(3):361–71.
202. Hirsch HH, Knowles W, Dickenmann M, et al. Prospective study of polyomavirus type BK replication and nephropathy in renal-transplant recipients. N Engl J Med. 2002;347(7):488–96.
203. Dharnidharka VR, Cherikh WS, Abbott KC. An OPTN analysis of national registry data on treatment of BK virus allograft nephropathy in the United States. Transplantation. 2009;87(7):1019–26.
204. Schold JD, Rehman S, Kayle LK, Magliocca J, Srinivas TR, Meier-Kriesche HU. Treatment for BK virus: incidence, risk factors and outcomes for kidney transplant recipients in the United States. Transpl Int. 2009;22(6):626–34.
205. Hirsch HH, Vincenti F, Friman S, et al. Polyomavirus BK replication in de novo kidney transplant patients receiving tacrolimus or cyclosporine: a prospective, randomized, multicenter study. Am J Transplant. 2013;13(1):136–45.
206. Manitpisitkul W, Drachenberg C, Ramos E, et al. Maintenance immunosuppressive agents as risk factors for BK virus nephropathy: a case-control study. Transplantation. 2009;88(1):83–8.
207. Prince O, Savic S, Dickenmann M, Steiger J, Bubendorf L, Mihatsch MJ. Risk factors for polyoma virus nephropathy. Nephrol Dial Transplant. 2009;24(3):1024–33.

208. Bohl DL, Storch GA, Ryschkewitsch C, et al. Donor origin of BK virus in renal transplantation and role of HLA C7 in susceptibility to sustained BK viremia. Am J Transplant. 2005;5(9):2213–21.
209. Thomas A, Dropulic LK, Rahman MH, Geetha D. Ureteral stents: a novel risk factor for polyomavirus nephropathy. Transplantation. 2007;84(3):433–6.
210. Elfadawy N, Flechner SM, Liu X, et al. CMV viremia is associated with a decreased incidence of BKV reactivation after kidney and kidney-pancreas transplantation. Transplantation. 2013;96(12):1097–103.
211. Schaub S, Mayr M, Egli A, et al. Transient allograft dysfunction from immune reconstitution in a patient with polyoma BK-virus-associated nephropathy. Nephrol Dial Transplant. 2007;22(8):2386–90.
212. Dharnidharka VR, Cherikh WS, Neff R, Cheng Y, Abbott KC. Retransplantation after BK virus nephropathy in prior kidney transplant: an OPTN database analysis. Am J Transplant. 2010;10(5):1312–5.
213. Sawinski D, Goral S. BK virus infection: an update on diagnosis and treatment. Nephrol Dial Transplant. 2015;30(2):209–17.
214. Papadimitriou JC, Randhawa P, Rinaldo CH, Drachenberg CB, Alexiev B, Hirsch HH. BK polyomavirus infection and renourinary tumorigenesis. Am J Transplant. 2016;16(2):398–406.
215. Echavarria M. Adenoviruses in immunocompromised hosts. Clin Microbiol Rev. 2008;21(4):704–15.
216. Florescu MC, Miles CD, Florescu DF. What do we know about adenovirus in renal transplantation? Nephrol Dial Transplant. 2013;28(8):2003–10.
217. Nanmoku K, Ishikawa N, Kurosawa A, et al. Clinical characteristics and outcomes of adenovirus infection of the urinary tract after renal transplantation. Transpl Infect Dis. 2016;18(2):234–9.
218. Sujeet K, Vasudev B, Desai P, et al. Acute kidney injury requiring dialysis secondary to adenovirus nephritis in renal transplant recipient. Transpl Infect Dis. 2011;13(2):174–7.
219. Komiya T, Goto N, Takeda A, et al. A case of acute rejection with adenovirus infection after ABO-incompatible kidney transplantation. Clin Transplant. 2009;23(Suppl 20):27–30.
220. Watcharananan SP, Avery R, Ingsathit A, et al. Adenovirus disease after kidney transplantation: course of infection and outcome in relation to blood viral load and immune recovery. Am J Transplant. 2011;11(6):1308–14.
221. Kozlowski T, Nickeleit V, Andreoni K. Donor-transmitted adenovirus infection causing kidney allograft nephritis and graft loss. Transpl Infect Dis. 2011;13(2):168–73.
222. Humar A, Kumar D, Mazzulli T, et al. A surveillance study of adenovirus infection in adult solid organ transplant recipients. Am J Transplant. 2005;5(10):2555–9.
223. Wold WS, Toth K. New drug on the horizon for treating adenovirus. Expert Opin Pharmacother. 2015;16(14):2095–9.
224. Crumpacker CS II, Zhang JL. Cytomegalovirus. In: Mandell GL, Bennett JE, Dolin R, editors. Principles and practices of infectious diseases. Philadelphia: Churchill Livingstone; 2010. p. 1971–87.
225. Zhang LJ, Hanff P, Rutherford C, Churchill WH, Crumpacker CS. Detection of human cytomegalovirus DNA, RNA, and antibody in normal donor blood. J Infect Dis. 1995;171(4):1002–6.
226. Arthurs SK, Eid AJ, Pedersen RA, et al. Delayed-onset primary cytomegalovirus disease and the risk of allograft failure and mortality after kidney transplantation. Clin Infect Dis. 2008;46(6):840–6.
227. Eid AJ, Arthurs SK, Deziel PJ, Wilhelm MP, Razonable RR. Clinical predictors of relapse after treatment of primary gastrointestinal cytomegalovirus disease in solid organ transplant recipients. Am J Transplant. 2010;10(1):157–61.
228. Razonable RR, Humar A, AST Infectious Diseases Community of Practice. Cytomegalovirus in solid organ transplantation. Am J Transplant. 2013;13(Suppl 4):93–106.
229. Naraqi S, Jackson GG, Jonasson O, Rubenis M. Search for latent cytomegalovirus in renal allografts. Infect Immun. 1978;19(2):699–703.
230. Kashyap R, Shapiro R, Jordan M, Randhawa PS. The clinical significance of cytomegaloviral inclusions in the allograft kidney. Transplantation. 1999;67(1):98–103.
231. Parsaik AK, Bhalla T, Dong M, et al. Epidemiology of cytomegalovirus infection after pancreas transplantation. Transplantation. 2011;92(9):1044–50.
232. Lowance D, Neumayer HH, Legendre CM, et al. Valacyclovir for the prevention of cytomegalovirus disease after renal transplantation. International valacyclovir cytomegalovirus prophylaxis transplantation study group. N Engl J Med. 1999;340(19):1462–70.
233. Reischig T, Jindra P, Mares J, et al. Valacyclovir for cytomegalovirus prophylaxis reduces the risk of acute renal allograft rejection. Transplantation. 2005;79(3):317–24.
234. Malvezzi P, Jouve T, Rostaing L. Use of everolimus-based immunosuppression to decrease cytomegalovirus infection after kidney transplant. Exp Clin Transplant. 2016;14(4):361–6.
235. Fallatah SM, Marquez MA, Bazerbachi F, et al. Cytomegalovirus infection post-pancreas-kidney transplantation – results of antiviral prophylaxis in high-risk patients. Clin Transplant. 2013;27(4):503–9.
236. Shah AP, Chen JM, Fridell JA. Incidence and outcomes of cytomegalovirus in pancreas transplantation with steroid-free immunosuppression. Clin Transplant. 2015;29(12):1221–9.
237. Lalezari JP, Stagg RJ, Kuppermann BD, et al. Intravenous cidofovir for peripheral cytomegalovirus retinitis in patients with AIDS. A randomized, controlled trial. Ann Intern Med. 1997;126(4):257–63.
238. Hosseini-Moghaddam SM, Alhomayeed B, Soliman N, Weir MA, House AA. Primary Epstein-Barr virus infection, seroconversion, and post-transplant lymphoproliferative disorder in seronegative renal allograft recipients: a prospective cohort study. Transpl Infect Dis. 2016;18(3):423–30.
239. Caillard S, Dharnidharka V, Agodoa L, Bohen E, Abbott K. Posttransplant lymphoproliferative disorders after renal transplantation in the United States in era of modern immunosuppression. Transplantation. 2005;80(9):1233–43.
240. Caillard S, Lelong C, Pessione F, Moulin B, French PTLD Working Group. Post-transplant lymphoproliferative disorders occurring after renal transplantation in adults: report of 230 cases from the French registry. Am J Transplant. 2006;6(11):2735–42.
241. Jackson K, Ruppert K, Shapiro R. Post-transplant lymphoproliferative disorder after pancreas transplantation: a united network for organ sharing database analysis. Clin Transplant. 2013;27(6):888–94.
242. Kasiske BL, Zeier MG, Chapman JR, et al. KDIGO clinical practice guideline for the care of kidney transplant recipients: a summary. Kidney Int. 2010;77(4):299–311.
243. Malouf MA, Chhajed PN, Hopkins P, Plit M, Turner J, Glanville AR. Anti-viral prophylaxis reduces the incidence of lymphoproliferative disease in lung transplant recipients. J Heart Lung Transplant. 2002;21(5):547–54.
244. Stratta RJ, Taylor RJ, Bynon JS, et al. Viral prophylaxis in combined pancreas-kidney transplant recipients. Transplantation. 1994;57(4):506–12.
245. Davis CL, Harrison KL, McVicar JP, Forg PJ, Bronner MP, Marsh CL. Antiviral prophylaxis and the Epstein Barr virus related post-transplant lymphoproliferative disorder. Clin Transplant. 1995;9(1):53–9.
246. Funch DP, Walker AM, Schneider G, Ziyadeh NJ, Pescovitz MD. Ganciclovir and acyclovir reduce the risk of post-transplant lymphoproliferative disorder in renal transplant recipients. Am J Transplant. 2005;5(12):2894–900.

247. Opelz G, Daniel V, Naujokat C, Fickenscher H, Dohler B. Effect of cytomegalovirus prophylaxis with immunoglobulin or with antiviral drugs on post-transplant non-Hodgkin lymphoma: a multicentre retrospective analysis. Lancet Oncol. 2007;8(3):212–8.
248. Humar A, Hebert D, Davies HD, et al. A randomized trial of ganciclovir versus ganciclovir plus immune globulin for prophylaxis against Epstein-Barr virus related posttransplant lymphoproliferative disorder. Transplantation. 2006;81(6):856–61.
249. Kalil AC, Syed A, Rupp ME, et al. Is bacteremic sepsis associated with higher mortality in transplant recipients than in nontransplant patients? A matched case-control propensity-adjusted study. Clin Infect Dis. 2015;60(2):216–22.
250. Bahr NC, Beaudoin A, Drekonja D. Rapid access to comprehensive care may explain better outcomes in persons with sepsis with solid organ transplant versus those without solid organ transplant. Clin Infect Dis. 2015;60(12):1869–70.
251. Donnelly JP, Locke JE, MacLennan PA, et al. Inpatient mortality among solid organ transplant recipients hospitalized for sepsis and severe sepsis. Clin Infect Dis. 2016;63(2):186–94.
252. Medina Polo J, Morales JM, Blanco M, et al. Urological complications after simultaneous pancreas-kidney transplantation. Transplant Proc. 2009;41(6):2457–9.
253. Hickey DP, Bakthavatsalam R, Bannon CA, O'Malley K, Corr J, Little DM. Urological complications of pancreatic transplantation. J Urol. 1997;157(6):2042–8.
254. Regueiro Lopez JC, Padillo Ruiz FJ, Requena Tapia MJ, Alvarez Kindelan J, Carmona Campos E, Anglada Curado J. Urologic complications of pancreas-kidney simultaneous transplantation. Actas Urol Esp. 1998;22(3):193–203.
255. Golebiewska JE, Debska-Slizien A, Rutkowski B. Treated asymptomatic bacteriuria during first year after renal transplantation. Transpl Infect Dis. 2014;16(4):605–15.
256. El Amari EB, Hadaya K, Buhler L, et al. Outcome of treated and untreated asymptomatic bacteriuria in renal transplant recipients. Nephrol Dial Transplant. 2011;26(12):4109–14.
257. Origuen J, Lopez-Medrano F, Fernandez-Ruiz M, et al. Should asymptomatic bacteriuria be systematically treated in kidney transplant recipients? Results from a randomized controlled trial. Am J Transplant. 2016;16(10):2943–53.
258. Fiorante S, Fernandez-Ruiz M, Lopez-Medrano F, et al. Acute graft pyelonephritis in renal transplant recipients: incidence, risk factors and long-term outcome. Nephrol Dial Transplant. 2011;26(3):1065–73.
259. Rubin RH. Infection in the organ transplant recipient. In: Rubin RH, Young LS, Russel P, editors. Clinical approach to infection in the compromised host. 3rd ed. New York: Plenum Publishing Corporation; 1981. p. 629–705.
260. Woodside KJ, Schirm ZW, Noon KA, et al. Fever, infection, and rejection after kidney transplant failure. Transplantation. 2014;97(6):648–53.
261. Shoham S. Emerging fungal infections in solid organ transplant recipients. Infect Dis Clin N Am. 2013;27(2):305–16. Epub 2013 Apr 17.
262. Sentamil Selvi G, Kamalam A, Ajithados K, Janaki C, Thambiah AS. Clinical and mycological features of dermatophytosis in renal transplant recipients. Mycoses. 1999;42(1–2):75–8.
263. Hosseini-Moghaddam SM, Soleimanirahbar A, Mazzulli T, Rotstein C, Husain S. Post renal transplantation Kaposi's sarcoma: a review of its epidemiology, pathogenesis, diagnosis, clinical aspects, and therapy. Transpl Infect Dis. 2012;14(4):338–45.
264. Dalla Gasperina D, Balsamo ML, Garavaglia SD, Rovida F, Baldanti F, Grossi PA. Chikungunya infection in a human immunodeficiency virus-infected kidney transplant recipient returning to Italy from the Dominican Republic. Transpl Infect Dis. 2015;17(6):876–9.
265. Kristensen AA, Horneland R, Birn H, Svensson M. Giardia lamblia infection after pancreas-kidney transplantation. BMJ Case Rep. 2016; https://doi.org/10.1136/bcr-2015-211515.
266. Yango AF, Fischbach BV, Levy M, et al. West Nile virus infection in kidney and pancreas transplant recipients in the Dallas-Fort worth metroplex during the 2012 Texas epidemic. Transplantation. 2014;97(9):953–7.
267. Tolkoff-Rubin NE, Cosimi AB, Russell PS, Rubin RH. A controlled study of trimethoprim-sulfamethoxazole prophylaxis of urinary tract infection in renal transplant recipients. Rev Infect Dis. 1982;4(2):614–8.
268. Rubin RH, Swartz MN. Trimethoprim-sulfamethoxazole. N Engl J Med. 1980;303(8):426–32.
269. Bactrim [package insert]. https://accessdata.fda.gov/drugsatfda_docs/label.2014.017377s074lbl.pdf. Updated 01 Nov 2013. Accessed 05 Dec 2016.
270. Delanaye P, Mariat C, Cavalier E, Maillard N, Krzesinski JM, White CA. Trimethoprim, creatinine and creatinine-based equations. Nephron Clin Pract. 2011;119(3):c187–93; discussion c193–4.
271. Berglund F, Killander J, Pompeius R. Effect of trimethoprim-sulfamethoxazole on the renal excretion of creatinine in man. J Urol. 1975;114(6):802–8.
272. Singh R, Bemelman FJ, Hodiamont CJ, Idu MM, Ten Berge IJ, Geerlings SE. The impact of trimethoprim-sulfamethoxazole as pneumocystis jiroveci pneumonia prophylaxis on the occurrence of asymptomatic bacteriuria and urinary tract infections among renal allograft recipients: a retrospective before-after study. BMC Infect Dis. 2016;16:90. -016-1432-3.
273. Ariza-Heredia EJ, Beam EN, Lesnick TG, Kremers WK, Cosio FG, Razonable RR. Urinary tract infections in kidney transplant recipients: role of gender, urologic abnormalities, and antimicrobial prophylaxis. Ann Transplant. 2013;18:195–204.
274. Horwedel TA, Bowman LJ, Saab G, Brennan DC. Benefits of sulfamethoxazole-trimethoprim prophylaxis on rates of sepsis after kidney transplant. Transpl Infect Dis. 2014;16(2):261–9.
275. Fox BC, Sollinger HW, Belzer FO, Maki DG. A prospective, randomized, double-blind study of trimethoprim-sulfamethoxazole for prophylaxis of infection in renal transplantation: clinical efficacy, absorption of trimethoprim-sulfamethoxazole, effects on the microflora, and the cost-benefit of prophylaxis. Am J Med. 1990;89(3):255–74.
276. Khosroshahi HT, Mogaddam AN, Shoja MM. Efficacy of high-dose trimethoprim-sulfamethoxazol prophylaxis on early urinary tract infection after renal transplantation. Transplant Proc. 2006;38(7):2062–4.
277. Hibberd PL, Tolkoff-Rubin NE, Doran M, et al. Trimethoprim-sulfamethoxazole compared with ciprofloxacin for the prevention of urinary tract infection in renal transplant recipients. A double-blind, randomized controlled trial. Online J Curr Clin Trials. 1992. Doc No 15:[4083 words; 46 paragraphs]. https://www.ncbi.nlm.nih.gov/pubmed/1343609.
278. Centers for Disease Control and Prevention (CDC). Treatment regimens for latent TB infections. http://cdc.gov/tb/topic/treatment/ltbi.htm. Accessed 5 Dec 2016.
279. Steichen O, Martinez-Almoyna L, De Broucker T. Isoniazid induced neuropathy: consider prevention. Rev Mal Respir. 2006;23(2 Pt 1):157–60.

Infections in Intestinal and Multivisceral Transplantation

5

Raffaele Girlanda, Joseph G. Timpone Jr, Kevin M. Soriano, and Thomas M. Fishbein

Introduction

Intestinal and multivisceral transplantation (IMVTx) has evolved from being an experimental procedure to become an effective treatment for patients with irreversible intestinal failure (IF) and life-threatening complications from parenteral nutrition (PN) [1]. The availability of more potent immunosuppression compared to the early era, especially the use of tacrolimus and of induction therapy, resulted in decreased incidence of acute rejection and improved patient survival up to 90% at 1-year post-transplant in experienced centers, comparable to the survival of patients on home PN. However, IMVTx poses a greater immunological and infectious challenge compared to other solid organs. Unlike the liver or kidney transplant, the intestinal and multivisceral grafts contain a large number of immune cells, and their lumen is heavily colonized by microbes that are transferred to the recipient. As a consequence, on the one hand, the intestine is a highly immunogenic graft being so heavily populated by immune cells; on the other hand, it carries a high risk of infections given the rich composition of microbes. In fact, severe acute rejection remains the main cause of graft loss and death, and infectious complications cause major morbidity pre- and post-transplant. Furthermore, sepsis with multi-organ failure is a major cause of death after treatment of severe rejection. Therefore, the balance between effective immunosuppression and prophylaxis of infections is a major challenge in the management of IMVTx recipients. In addition, IF in itself presents a combination of risk factors for severe infections in the IMVTx candidate, including short gut, bacterial overgrowth, prolonged central venous access for PN, and others. Furthermore, the transplant candidate often carries the sequelae of prior complex abdominal surgery, resulting in defects of the abdominal wall, enterocutaneous fistulae, chronic obstruction, and abscesses. The complexity of scenarios presented by patients with IF and by IMVTx recipients makes them among the highest risk among transplant recipients. Over the last decade there has been significant progress in the management of IMVTx patients including a better understanding of the immunologic mechanisms at play in the gut and improved treatment of infections. At the same time, increasing interest has been focused on the role of the gut microbiome (see below) in the pathogenesis of intestinal and extraintestinal disease. These recent discoveries are likely to translate in improved outcomes of IMVTx recipients. In this chapter, after a brief presentation of current indications and outcomes of IMVTx, we outline recent advances in intestinal immunology and describe specific risk factors for infections associated with IF and IMVTx. We also discuss the current management of common infections after IMVTx.

R. Girlanda (✉) · J. G. Timpone Jr · K. M. Soriano · T. M. Fishbein
Georgetown University Hospital, Washington, DC, USA
e-mail: Raffaele.Girlanda@gunet.georgetown.edu; timponej@gunet.georgetown.edu; kms383@georgetown.edu; Thomas.M.Fishbein@medstar.net

Indications for Intestinal and Multivisceral Transplantation and Types of Graft

According to the 2009 Intestinal Transplant Registry report, more than 2200 IMVTx have been performed worldwide since 1985 [2]. However, the number of transplants performed so far has only recently increased, reaching 200 transplants/year only in the last 4 years. Therefore, IMVTx represents the most recent development in abdominal organ transplantation. In addition, unlike liver or kidney transplants that are performed in virtually every transplant program, IMVTx is performed in very few specialized centers: as of 2009, only 8 centers worldwide have performed 100 IMVTx or more; therefore current experience remains concentrated in very few transplant programs.

The indication for IMVTx as recognized by the Centers for Medicare and Medicaid Services [3] is irreversible IF defined as the loss of nutritional autonomy of the gut associated with life-threatening complications of PN including liver failure, loss of central venous access secondary to thrombosis,

A. Safdar (ed.), *Principles and Practice of Transplant Infectious Diseases*, https://doi.org/10.1007/978-1-4939-9034-4_5

systemic sepsis from line infection requiring hospitalization, and frequent episodes of dehydration [4–6]. The most common cause of IF is short bowel syndrome secondary to a number of different etiologies in adults and children (Table 5.1).

Table 5.1 Causes of short bowel syndrome in adults and children

Adult	Pediatric (congenital)
Mesenteric vein thrombosis and/or bowel ischemia	Gastroschisis
Crohn's disease requiring multiple small bowel resections	Intestinal atresia
Abdominal trauma due to gunshot wounds	Intestinal volvulus
Radiation enteritis	Congenital short small bowel
Recurrent small bowel obstruction	Necrotizing enterocolitis
Motility disorders	
Neoplasm's of the mesentery (e.g., GIST[a])	
Iatrogenic complications of multiple abdominal surgeries	

[a]Gastrointestinal stromal tumor

Other causes of IF include motility disorders, malabsorption (mucosal defects), and neoplasms of the mesentery.

The intestine is transplanted either as isolated small intestine or combined with the liver in patients with parenteral nutrition-associated liver failure (PNALD). Alternatively, patients with disease involving the foregut and/or the entire colon receive a multivisceral graft that, in addition to the small intestine, includes the stomach and/or the colon (Fig. 5.1).

The donor colon (usually the cecum, right and transverse colon) is included in the graft in selected recipients with absent native colon in order to improve water reabsorption and prevent severe dehydration episodes and renal failure. Since the colon carries a higher microbial load than the small intestine, in the initial experiences of IMVTx, the colon was excluded from the graft to reduce the risk of sepsis post-transplant [7]. However, more recent reports demonstrated that the infection risk and graft survival associated with inclusion of the colon are comparable to non-colon grafts [8, 9].

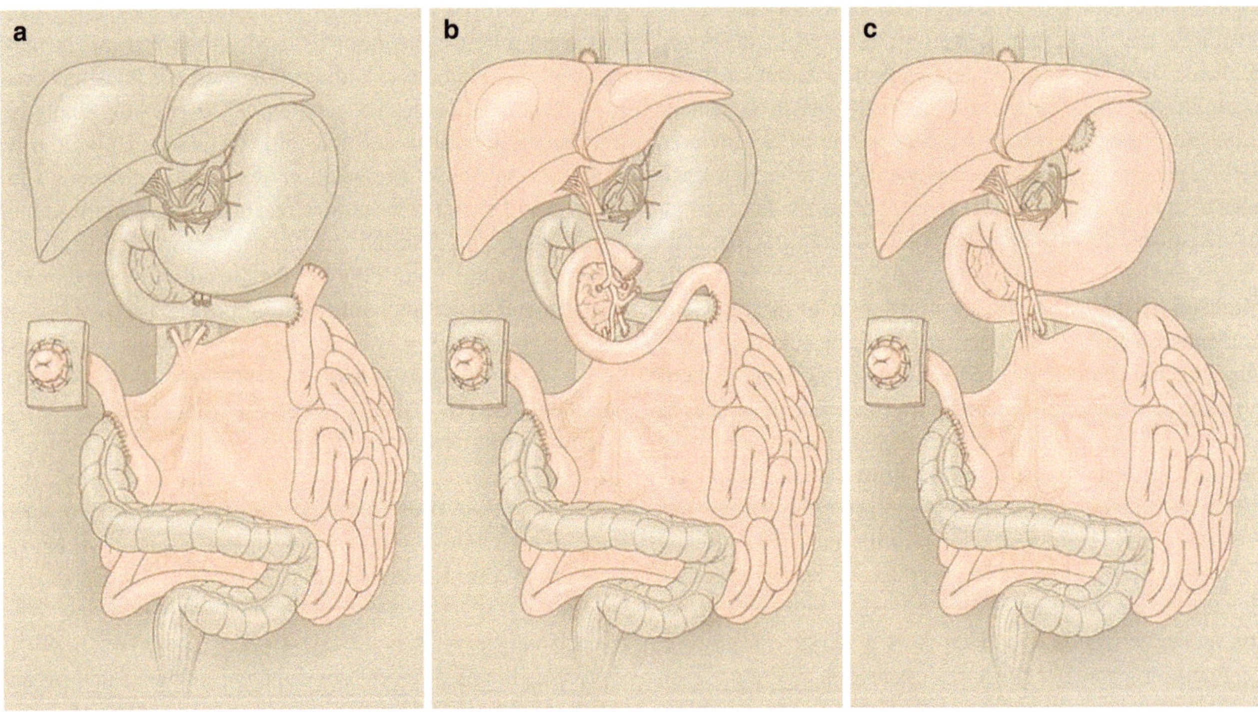

Fig. 5.1 Three types of transplants in intestinal failure. When the small intestine (jejunoileum) is transplanted alone, it is referred to as an isolated intestinal transplant (Panel a), with systemic drainage to the vena cava. A composite liver and intestinal transplant usually includes the duodenum and an intact biliary system and portal circulation, with the native foregut preserved (Panel b). In a multivisceral transplant, which involves the liver, stomach, duodenum, pancreas, and small intestine, the foregut is removed, and a new stomach is transplanted (Panel c). This type of transplant sometimes includes the colon, kidney, or both. The transplanted organs are shown in pink, and the native organs or structures are shown in light brown. (From Fishbein [1]. http://www.nejm.org/doi/full/10.1056/NEJMra0804605. Copyright © (2009) Massachusetts Medical Society. Reprinted with permission)

Immunosuppression

Given the higher immunogenicity of the intestinal graft and higher incidence of acute rejection compared to other solid organ transplants, IMVTx recipients receive heavier immunosuppression compared to other organ recipients. Although protocols vary between centers, generally immunosuppression regimens for IMVTx include induction with T cell-depleting agents such as thymoglobulin or alemtuzumab or the non-T cell-depleting anti-CD25 interleukin-2 receptor blockers (basiliximab, daclizumab). Alemtuzumab (Campath) is a monoclonal antibody targeting CD52 used in some conditioning regimens for bone marrow transplantation, kidney transplantation, and islet cell transplantation. Maintenance immunosuppressive treatment is usually with a combination of tacrolimus, sirolimus, mycophenolate mofetil, and corticosteroids. The introduction of the calcineurin inhibitor tacrolimus in 1990 made a significant impact in reducing the incidence of rejection and improving survival compared to the cyclosporine era [10]. Recently, with the use of the newer induction regimens, acute cellular rejection rates within the first 90 days have been reported to decrease to 30–50% [1]. Target tacrolimus trough levels are typically higher than levels maintained in other abdominal organ transplants: 20–25 ng/ml for the first month with gradual de crease to the 12–20 range for the first 6 months and then 5–8 indefinitely. Monitoring for rejection includes frequent surveillance endoscopy and biopsy. Episodes of rejection are graded as mild, moderate, or severe according to established parameters based on crypt apoptosis and distortion of the epithelial architecture [11, 12]. Treatment of rejection mandates increased immunosuppression based on the severity of the rejection episode: mild and moderate rejection is generally treated with pulse corticosteroids and increased tacrolimus levels, whereas severe rejection is usually treated with T cell-depleting antibodies (thymoglobulin or alemtuzumab). Traditionally the target of immune therapy against rejection has focused on T cell-mediated mechanisms. Recently, antibody-mediated mechanisms responsible for acute and chronic allograft damage are being investigated and targeted by novel therapies, especially in kidney and heart transplantation. Although donor-specific antibodies have been implicated in worsening episodes of IMVTx rejection [13], a definite entity of antibody-mediated rejection has not been established in IMVTx [14].

Antibacterial agents against intraluminal-colonizing organisms such as aerobic Gram-negative bacilli and anaerobes (e.g., ciprofloxacin and metronidazole) are often added to the treatment of severe rejection given the high risk of bacterial translocation and sepsis associated with exfoliation of the intestinal mucosa. Prophylaxis of opportunistic infections post-transplant generally follows established guidelines adopted for other solid organ transplants. However, due to the high rates of rejection, prophylaxis is often intensified or extended beyond the standard duration and is usually resumed during treatment of rejection episodes and will be described in more detail below.

Immunology of the Intestine

The gut has the largest mucosal surface in the body, estimated to extend up to 200 m^2, making it a very efficient absorptive surface for nutrients. At the same time, the intestinal mucosa is a protective barrier against invasion of pathogens. The barrier is constituted of a single layer of columnar epithelial cells (enterocytes) linked at the apico-lateral membranes by intercellular tight junctions to prevent the paracellular diffusion of luminal contents. As discovered in recent studies, the intestinal epithelium functions not only as a mechanical barrier but also as an immune barrier. In case of B cell deficiency, for example, the enterocyte takes on immune functions at the expenses of metabolic function by upregulating INF pathways and reducing the expression of genes of fat uptake and metabolism, as evidenced by the occurrence of lipid malabsorption in HIV [15]. In addition, enterocytes actively participate to defense mechanisms by interacting with immune cells: goblet cells, for example, which are typically producing mucous for the mucosal barrier, are also able to deliver luminal antigens to dendritic cells of the *lamina propria*, and goblet cell deficiency or dysfunction in mice and humans has been linked to the development of intestinal inflammation [16]. The impact of immune functions of the intestinal epithelium on the barrier function of the graft during posttransplant immune depletion is still incompletely understood and may have implications on the risk of rejection post-transplant.

In addition to the intestinal epithelium, other barrier structures limit the invasion of pathogens: a layer of mucins (membrane-bound glycoproteins or glycocalyx) produced by the goblet cells, secretory IgA, and antimicrobial peptides (defensins) secreted by Paneth cells. Within the epithelium and underneath it, a large number of immune cells (lymphocytes, macrophages, and dendritic cells) populate the intestinal mucosa and the mesenteric lymph nodes. These immune cells are constantly exposed to foreign antigens and to resident bacterial flora. In normal conditions, a delicate balance is maintained between immune protection from infection and tolerance to harmless antigens of commensal microbes and nutrients. Special mechanisms regulate this balance in the intestinal wall, and the interplay between different cell populations of the intestinal wall is only beginning to being discovered. Alterations of the immune homeostasis of the gut are increasingly being recognized and implicated in the pathogenesis of inflammatory bowel disease and of extraintestinal autoimmune disorders [17]. Also, breach to the intestinal barrier predisposes to bacterial translocation (see below) and sepsis. The complex equilibrium between tolerance to nutrients and rejection of potential pathogens is maintained by special characteristics of the immune cells of the intestine, different from immune cells of the rest of the body. Intestinal macrophages, for example, unlike macrophages present in other organs, have the ability to clear antigens from the *lamina propria* without mounting an inflammatory response. Indeed, intestinal macrophages do not express the LPS coreceptor (CD14), the Fc receptors (CD89, CD16, CD32, and CD64), or receptors for IL-2 (CD25) and IL-3 (CD123). In addition, intestinal macrophages do not produce pro-inflammatory cytokines IL-1 and TNF after stimulation with LPS [18]. This role of intestinal macrophages is critically important to maintain a noninflammatory state within the *lamina propria* of the gastrointestinal tract. In fact, despite close proximity with immunostimulatory bacteria, intestinal macrophages acquire profound "inflammatory anergy" while retaining avid scavenger and host defense functions. A second important component of mononuclear phagocytes of the intestinal mucosa is constituted by dendritic cells (DC). Several subsets of DC have been characterized at multiple levels: in the *lamina propria*, in isolated lymph follicles, in Peyer's patches, and in mesenteric lymph nodes. DC are characterized by very high plasticity, their phenotype and function being driven by local tissue factors. DC in the intestine can both drive or suppress effector responses: in the *lamina propria*, DC extend dendrites between enterocytes, penetrate epithelial tight junctions, and sample luminal contents and microbiota [19, 20], thus priming naïve T cells for an immune response. Other sub-types of DC (CD103+ DC) promote the conversion of naïve T cells into regulatory T cell via TGF-β and retinoic acid [21]. Therefore, under normal circumstances the aggregate function of DC of the intestine contributes to maintain intestinal immune homeostasis. Mutations in genes coding for bacterial sensing receptors such as NOD2 in DC have recently been described [22] and are likely to impact on the risk of infections and/or rejection after IMVTx. Finally, several studies have recently highlighted the features of multiple subsets of T cells in the gut (T-helper 17 cells, γδ T cells, natural killer (NK) cells, and NK T cells). These cells contribute to the mucosal response to pathogens by secreting cytokines which in turn induce the secretion of chemokines and antimicrobial peptides, thereby orchestrating the response of the mucosal barrier against pathogens. In particular, Th17 cells [23], a subset of T-helper cell distinct from Th1 and Th2, have recently been shown to play multiple roles in the gut defense including recruitment of neutrophils to areas of bacterial infection, induction of proliferation of enterocytes, and production of defensins [24–26].

Microbes

Unlike other transplants that are sterile, the intestine is transplanted with a large content of intraluminal commensal microbes. In the past, the intestinal graft used to be "decontaminated" at the time of procurement by flushing the lumen with antimicrobial decontamination solution. The chemical damage of such solutions to the graft mucosa and the recognition of the important role of the intraluminal flora have made this decontamination now obsolete.

The intestinal lumen is populated by a tremendous number of commensal microorganisms, estimated to reach 10^{14} bacteria belonging to over 1000 species, predominantly comprised of the heterogeneous, Gram-positive phylum *Firmicutes* (which includes organisms such as *Bacillus sp.*, *Lactobacillus, and Clostridia sp.*) and the Gram-negative anaerobic bacilli, *Bacteroides*. Importantly, the cumulative genetic material carried by intestinal microbes (microbiome) is 100× the size of the human genome. Microbes play multiple roles in host metabolism, including energy recovery from nutrients, generation of digestible carbohydrates and short-chain fatty acids from otherwise nondigestible fibers, and synthesis of amino acids and vitamins. In addition, intraluminal microbes exert immune functions advantageous to the host including competition with pathogens and maintenance of the trophism of the colonic epithelium by synthesis of short-chain fatty acids, like butyrate, an essential growth factor for colonic enterocytes [27]. An increasing interest has recently focused on the role of gut microbiota in health and disease and on the mechanisms regulating this symbiotic relationship between microbes and human intestine [28, 29]. Both beneficial and deleterious effects are being discovered as a consequence of alterations or manipulations of this equilibrium (i.e., alteration of the gastrointestinal microbiome also known as dysbiosis). In fact, germ-free animals are more susceptible to infections; on the other hand, colonization of germ-free mice with a single bacterial species is sufficient to enhance the mucosal immune system, including increased numbers of intraepithelial lymphocytes and increased activity of local antigen-presenting cells (APCs) [30]. Intestinal bacterial commensals communicate via innate detection systems (nucleotide oligomerization domain [NOD] and other Toll-like receptors [TLRs]) to generate adaptive lymphoid tissue and maintain intestinal homeostasis: the peptidoglycan of Gram-negative bacteria induces the generation of isolated lymphoid follicles in the intestinal wall which later mature into large B cell clusters [31]. In IMVTx intraluminal pathogens can be the source of sepsis following damage to the mucosal barrier secondary to rejection or preservation injury (translocation; see below). Finally, although the exact cause-effect relationship remains to be clarified, alterations of the intraluminal flora of the graft have been recently associated with increased risk of rejection [32].

Bacterial Translocation

Damage to protective barriers of the intestinal mucosa results in bacterial translocation, the passage of viable bacteria or their products, such as lipopolysaccharide and bacterial DNA, from the gut lumen to extraintestinal sites [27]. Under normal circumstances, a low-grade portal vein endotoxemia of gut origin is rapidly cleared by the reticuloendothelial system of the liver. The diseased gut, however, can translocate endotoxin in large amounts such that systemic endotoxemia can be present in patients with acute inflammatory bowel disease [33] and in children with necrotizing enterocolitis, even in absence of bacteremia [34]. A recent study documented increased bacterial DNA in the intestinal wall of children with NEC [35]. The systemic consequences of bacterial translocation (endotoxemia) include damage to the vascular endothelium with induction of intravascular coagulation, increased muscle protein degradation, suppression of cellular immunity, cholestasis, and septic shock. The mechanisms leading to translocation include direct transmucosal migration across the bowel wall toward the mesenteric lymph nodes or migration into the peritoneal cavity. Pretransplant intestinal stasis and bacterial overgrowth increase the risk of translocation. Posttransplant immunosuppression and damage to the bowel wall secondary to ischemia-reperfusion, infection, (especially viral) or rejection result in altered permeability of the graft mucosa and increased risk of bacterial translocation. Episodes of graft dysfunction requiring resumption of parenteral nutrition result in protein depletion and increased mucosa permeability [36]. Cicalese et al. [37] found 44% incidence of bacterial translocation in human IMVTx with an average of 1.9 episodes per patient (defined as simultaneous positivity of stool and blood culture); a third of all episodes of bacterial translocation occurred within the first month post-transplant, and risk factors included prolonged cold ischemia time (>9 hours), inclusion of the colon in the graft, and rejection.

High Infection Risk in Intestinal Transplantation

As compared to other types of solid organ transplantation, IMVTx recipients present a unique clinical situation that predisposes them to an exceedingly high risk for infectious complications. Rates of infection have been reported to be as high as 90% [38] and are likely related to the high density of microbes within the donor intestinal allograft and the potential for bacterial translocation associated with damaged intestinal mucosa in the setting of acute rejection. This coupled with the need for higher levels of immunosuppression necessary to treat and prevent rejection can result in a "perfect storm" for the development of infection. This high risk of infection begins during the pretransplant period and persists throughout the perioperative and postoperative periods and remains an important threat in the years of follow-up in patients who have undergone successful IMVTx. Table 5.2 demonstrates the major risk factors for infection in persons with intestinal failure and small intestinal transplantation.

Table 5.2 Risk factors for infection in patients with intestinal failure and small intestinal transplantation

Pre-transplant risk factors	Post-transplant risk factors
Intra-abdominal anatomic abnormalities resulting in:	Technically complicated surgery
Recurrent enterocutaneous fistulas	Intestinal allograft with dense microbial burden
Recurrent intra-abdominal abscesses/peritonitis	Intensive immunosuppression
Bacterial translocation	Rejection
Total parenteral nutrition	High rates of acute rejection
Recurrent CLABSIs[a]	Mucosal injury with rejection
Fungemia	
Immunosuppression secondary to malnutrition	Bacterial translocation
Frequent hospitalizations	Bloodstream infections/sepsis
Increased risk for HCAIs[b]	Possible decreased absorption of anti-infective prophylactic medication
Colonization/infection with MDROs[c]	Recurrent hospitalizations
	Increased risk for HCAIs[b]
	Colonization/infection MDROs[c]

[a]Central line-associated bloodstream infections
[b]Healthcare-associated infections
[c]Multidrug-resistant organisms

Risk of Infection in the Pretransplantation Period in Patients with Short Bowel Syndrome

Intestinal failure in both adult and pediatric patient populations is associated with multiple medical comorbidities that can result in multiple hospital admissions and prolonged lengths of stay which increases the exposure to and infection with healthcare-associated pathogens. Patients with IF and short gut syndrome are at particular risk for infection due to (1) anatomical alterations as a result of their underlying disease and/or surgical interventions, (2) the relative immunosuppression associated with protein-calorie malnutrition, and (3) the presence of intravascular catheters and gastrojejunostomy tubes for nutritional support.

The underlying diseases experienced by patients with IF often result in multiple surgical procedures such as the resection of ischemic bowel (as in the setting of mesenteric thrombosis) or the resection and repair of multiple intra-abdominal fistulae (as experienced in Crohn's disease). Additionally, these patients also develop spontaneous intra-abdominal abscesses from perforations associated with diseased bowel. Enterocutaneous fistula formation is another common complication in this patient group and may serve as a source of abdominal sepsis and colonization with enteric bacteria as well as streptococcal and staphylococcal species. It is estimated that 80% of deaths associated with enterocutaneous fistulas are due to abdominal sepsis [39–41]. Enterocutaneous fistulas can be associated with peritonitis and discrete intra-abdominal abscesses. Approximately 50% of patients with enterocutaneous fistulas will have an intra-abdominal abscess present on abdominal imaging [42]. Therefore it is important for clinicians caring for patients with IF and enterocutaneous fistulas to have a high index of suspicion for intra-abdominal infections. Although the indications for a surgical approach in this setting is beyond the scope of this chapter, successful management of intra-abdominal abscesses associated with enterocutaneous fistulas using computed tomographic percutaneous drainage has been successful at our center, as well as being reported by others [43]. Patients with enterocutaneous fistulas complicated by intra-abdominal infection also require appropriate antibiotic therapy – which often times is of an extended duration, due to either recurrences or failure to adequately drain the abscess cavity. The need for prolonged antibiotic treatment in this patient population as well as a prolonged hospital length of stay can place them at risk for colonization and infection with multidrug-resistant organisms [44–46].

Intestinal failure is associated with malnutrition. Protein-calorie malnutrition can contribute to a patient's net state of immunosuppression and results in an increased risk of infection. Malnutrition is associated with T lymphocyte depletion and their response to mitogens, failure of B cells to respond appropriately to antigen presentation, and decreased function of neutrophils [47]. Savendahl and colleagues demonstrated that in the setting of a 7-day fast, there can be a decrease in circulating CD3 lymphocytes, as well as CD4 T-helper lymphocytes. In that same study, there was an attenuated IL-2 response to mitogen stimulation [48]. Neonates with necrotizing enterocolitis and congenital abnormalities resulting in short gut syndrome may be in a more precarious situation than adults with short bowel syndrome as a result of their immunologic immaturity. Therefore it is imperative that patients with short bowel syndrome are cared for by physicians with expertise in hyperalimentation and nutritional supplementation. Unfortunately, the chronic use of PN places patients at risk for catheter-related bloodstream infections and liver disease. It is estimated that 50% of patients on chronic PN will develop liver disease within 5–7 years [49]. Chronic liver disease can also contribute to the level of immunosuppression in this patient population, being associated with defects in humoral immunity and neutrophil dysfunction. These patients often have decreased capacity for the opsonization of foreign antigens due to hypocomplementemia [50]. Neutrophil chemotaxis and adherence is also depressed in patients with liver disease [51]. Finally, it has been noted that in cirrhotic patients, the sinusoidal macrophages (Kupffer cells), which play an important role in the clearance of bacteria and foreign antigens, may be bypassed due to portosystemic shunting [52]. Overall, patients with short bowel syndrome who are being considered for small intestinal transplantation may experience secondary immunodeficiency either due to their nutritional state or PN-induced chronic liver disease.

Parenteral nutrition is an important treatment for patients with short bowel syndrome but carries with it a risk for central line-associated bloodstream infections (CLABSIs). In a prospective study evaluating home infusion therapy in 827 outpatients, the rate of infection was 0.99 infections/1000 days. The use of PN was an independent risk factor for the development of infection [53]. Other risk factors are micronutrient deficiency and immune dysfunction. Central line-associated bloodstream infections are important causes of hospitalization and may contribute to both morbidity and mortality in this patient group during the pretransplant period. In one study, PN was identified as the most important risk factor for the development of CLABSI [54]. In addition to isolated bacteremia, chronic central vascular catheter use is associated with endovascular infections such as endocarditis and suppurative thrombophlebitis.

In the neonatal population with short bowel syndrome, CLABSIs are quite common and in one study occurred in 66% of children on home PN within the first 6 months of hospital discharge [55]. In that same study, the highest incidence occurred within the first month, and the most common infections were due to polymicrobial causes followed by Gram-positive, Gram-negative, and fungal causes, respectively [55]. Moreover, the use of PN in the neonatal patient population with short bowel syndrome has been associated with the relatively rapid development of cholestasis, and this has been observed as a complication of infection and sepsis [56, 57].

In one observational study, the risk of CLABSIs in patients receiving chronic PN (mean duration of follow-up was 4.5 years) was noted to be 80.9% [58]. Additionally, 78.9% of these patients had more than one CLABSI, and 23.8% of these episodes were polymicrobial [58]. Although the majority of patients with CLABSIs present with either fevers or a clinical syndrome consistent with sepsis, in one study, 33% of patients with SBS and liver disease on PN had occult bacteremia just prior to their intestinal transplantation.

This patient group had more postoperative days of mechanical ventilation and a more prolonged length of stay as compared to patients who did not have occult bacteremia at the time of transplantation [59].

Microbiology of CLABSIs

Although patients with SBS are a clinically unique population, it is reasonable to assume that the microbiology of CLABSIs is similar to other patient populations. There are no large studies on the causes of CLABSIs in persons on chronic PN who are awaiting IMVTx. It has been our experience that these patients have CLABSIs due to similar pathogens such as staphylococci, enterococci, *Candida* species, and Gram-negative bacilli. The SCOPE (Surveillance and Control OF Pathogens of Epidemiological Importance) study reported on a total of 24,179 cases of CLABSIs in hospitalized patients over a 7-year period and noted a rate of 60 cases/10,000 patient admissions. In this study, Gram-positive organisms accounted for 65%, Gram-negative bacilli accounted for 25%, and fungi accounted for 9.5% of CLABSIs. The most common isolates were coagulase-negative staphylococci (31%), *Staphylococcus aureus* (22%), *Enterococcus* (9%), *Candida* species (9%), *Escherichia coli* (6%), *Klebsiella* species (5%), *Pseudomonas* species (4%), *Enterobacter* species (4%), *Serratia* species (2%), and *Acinetobacter baumannii* (1%) [60].

In general, patients with SBS often require frequent hospitalizations and are likely to have similar microbiological causes of CLABSIs. However, there are several factors that distinguish this patient group and warrant further consideration when assessing these patients for a presumed CLABSI. Although colonization by skin flora (staphylococci and streptococci) is the most likely source of CLABSIs, due to alterations in the integrity of the gastrointestinal tract, they may be at increased risk for enteric pathogens such as Gram-negative bacilli, enterococci and vancomycin-resistant enterococci. As these patients are on PN, the role of contaminated infusates as a source needs to also be considered. Gram-negative organisms such as *Serratia* and *Pseudomonas* species have been associated with infusate contamination [61, 62]. *Candida parapsilosis* fungemia has been associated with contaminated TPN infusate [63–65].

In addition to the risk of contaminated infusate, patients with SBS have numerous risk factors that are associated with invasive candidiasis and candidemia. Specifically, these include the chronic use of central vascular catheters, the use of broad-spectrum antibiotics, the use of PN, and multiple intra-abdominal surgical procedures [66–68]. Candidemia has been associated with mortality rates as high as 47% in adults and 29% in children [67]. While *C. albicans* remains the most common isolate, non-*albicans* species such as *C. glabrata* have been reported more recently [68, 69]. Furthermore, PN appears to place these patients at increased risk for fungemia due to all *Candida* species and has also been associated with *Candida* chorioretinitis and endophthalmitis in other patient populations receiving PN [70–72].

Practice guidelines for the treatment and management of CLABSIs have been established [73]. In addition to appropriately targeted antibiotic therapy, catheter removal is warranted for CLABSIs due to *Staphylococcus aureus*, *Candida* species, and multidrug-resistant Gram-negative bacilli. Catheter removal is also warranted in the setting of sepsis and the presence of or evidence of metastatic foci of infection [73]. Unfortunately, this patient population is also at risk for catheter-associated thrombosis which may often limit vascular access options and in select situations may result in the need for line salvage in the setting of a bloodstream infection. Antibiotic lock therapy and ethanol lock therapy have been employed to supplement systemic antibiotic therapy when considering line salvage [73–75].

Additionally, in a small study of pediatric patients with either small intestinal transplantation or SBS on PN who had frequent CLABSIs, the use of tobramycin lock therapy was effective in reducing CLABSIs and decreasing the number of hospital admissions due to CLABSIs [76]. Practice guidelines for the treatment of catheter-related bloodstream infections have been published and report additional information on this important management issue [73]. In summary, patients with SBS, who are being considered for IMVTx, have both anatomical and immunological alterations that predispose them to bacterial and fungal infections. Bloodstream infections and intra-abdominal infections are the most common infectious complications that these patients experience prior to transplantation. The routine use of PN, as well as the frequent need for hospitalization, places them at increased risk for healthcare-associated infections due to multidrug-resistant pathogens and *Candida* species prior to the time of their transplantation. Therefore this unique patient group carries a risk of antimicrobial selection pressure that may need to be considered when choosing for a surgical antibiotic prophylactic regimen at the time of transplantation.

Pretransplant Evaluation

The pretransplant evaluation includes not only a comprehensive assessment of the patient's clinical status to rule out contraindications for transplant but also optimization of the nutritional status, patient's compliance, and adequate support system post-transplant. This is essential for IMVTx patients because the hospital stay is often more prolonged than other transplants and the posttransplant recovery period may be slow and complicated by infections or need for repeat surgery. Since virtually every IMVTx candidate presents with a significant infection history (catheter-related bacteremia, previous multiple operations), the optimization of nutrition and compliance and support system are important to reduce the infection risk post-transplant. The panel of pretransplant laboratory tests in the evaluation of the IMVTx candidate is comparable to the panel of other organ recipients and includes viral serology (*hepatitis A, hepatitis B, hepatitis C, herpes simplex virus, CMV, EBV, human immunodeficiency virus, varicella-zoster virus, measles, rubella*) and toxoplasmosis. Patients with a positive tuberculin skin test (PPD) pre-transplant or a history of prior tuberculosis undergo additional screening to rule out active disease. The use of interferon-gamma release assays has not yet been studied in this patient population but may offer some benefit in screening patients for latent tuberculous infection, based on some data from its use in liver transplant candidates [77, 78]. Imaging studies (Doppler survey of central veins, echocardiogram, and computed tomography imaging of the thorax, abdomen, and pelvis) assess the patency of central vessels and rule out occult or known foci of untreated/unresolved infections such as bacterial endocarditis due to frequent episodes of pretransplant bacteremia or fungemia or intra-abdominal abscess as a complication of an enterocutaneous fistula. Aggressive management of pretransplant infections in order to reduce the infection risk post-transplant includes repair of enterocutaneous fistulae and of abdominal wall defects when feasible, drainage of abscesses, and management of bacterial overgrowth. The identification of pretransplant colonizing flora may assist in decisions regarding an individualized peri-transplant prophylactic antimicrobial regimen, although in one study, pretransplant stool surveillance cultures were not predictive of the types of bacteria that were isolated in the setting of a documented infection in the post-transplant setting [79]. Pretransplant vaccination is recommended as for other solid organ transplant recipients (see guidelines of AST Infectious Disease Community of Practice, AJT) [80]. Inactivated vaccines are recommended for post-transplant immunization. Although theoretically the administration of foreign antigen for the purpose of vaccination can cross-reactivate clones of immune cells, there has been no definite documentation of increased risk of rejection related to vaccination.

Approach to Common Post-intestinal Transplant Infections

Timeline of Infections

The timeline of post-transplant infections in solid organ transplant recipients has traditionally been classified into (1) perioperative (first 4 weeks) post-transplantation often due to healthcare-associated infections and due to underlying disease/chronic condition; (2) early post-transplantation (1–6 months), often due to opportunistic pathogens due to higher levels of immunosuppression; and (3) late post-transplantation (>6 months) often due to community-acquired pathogens, molds, as well as manifestations of later viral infections and infection-related neoplasms such as post-transplant lymphoproliferative disorders [PTLD] associated with prolonged enhanced immune suppression [81]. In IMVTx recipients this timeline is not well delineated and is often altered by several factors which include (1) prolonged hospital stay in the post-transplantation period as a result of the complications, (2) the relatively higher rates of repeat surgery, (3) the need for recurrent hospitalizations due to other complications, (4) a more intensive immunosuppressive regimen and maintaining tacrolimus at higher levels for more prolonged durations as compared to other types of solid organ transplant recipients, (5) higher rates and often numerous rejection episodes, and (6) the risk of bacterial translocation that can be associated with mucosal damage that is seen with rejection. As a result, these patients appear to always be at risk for the bacterial and fungal infections that are typically seen within the first month post-transplantation and are often encountered months and even years after transplantation – depending upon the number of readmissions that a patient experiences. Additionally, there is a persistence of the risk of hospital-acquired infections well beyond the first month as these patients often have prolonged initial lengths of stay post-transplantation. Therefore healthcare-associated bacterial infections and fungal infections (due primarily to *Candida* species and *Aspergillus*) remain a persistent or reemergent threat throughout the lifetime of IMVTx recipient. While it is expected that the risk of opportunistic pathogens is highest from 1 month through 6 months post-transplantation, given the relatively high rates of rejection, the clinician caring for these patients needs to "reset" this timeline after each rejection episode, and appropriate prophylaxis should be continued or resumed. These rejection episodes can theoretically contribute to the risk of bacterial or fungal infections as the damaged mucosa allows a portal of entry for colonizing intestinal bacteria and *Candida* species. Finally, the bioavailability and drug exposure of prophylactic agents such as trimethoprim-sulfamethoxazole, valganciclovir, and the azole antifungal agents may demonstrate wide variability in the setting of acute and chronic intestinal allograft rejection; therefore, opportunistic infections could potentially occur despite the use of these prophylactic agents.

There is only one published prospective study that defines a timeline for the development of various types of infections. In a small cohort of IMVTx recipients, it was noted that the median time from the day of transplant to the development of bacterial infections was 11 days, viral infections (CMV and EBV) was 91 days, and fungal infections was 181 days [38].

Based on our own clinical experience and the limited reports in the medical literature, IMVTx recipients may always be at risk for bacterial and fungal infections – especially if they have been recently hospitalized. Although viral infections can typically occur within 1–6 months from transplantation, the numerous rejection episodes may extend this risk to the late post-transplantation period (i.e., >6 months). Therefore we will divide our discussion of infections in IMVTx recipients as follows: (1) the "immediate" post-transplant period (<6 weeks) and (2) the "later" post-transplant period (>6 weeks). Bacterial infections will be addressed in the "immediate" posttransplantation period section, whereas viral, fungal, and parasitic infections will be presented in the "later" posttransplantation section. A proposed timeline and the most common infections in IMVTx are depicted in Table 5.3.

Perioperative Infections

Overview, Incidence, and Risk Factors

Infection continues to be an important cause of morbidity and mortality in patients receiving IMVTx [1, 82, 83]. In one series, infection was the attributable cause of mortality in 17.8% of intestinal transplant recipients and was present in 76.2% of the patients who had died [83]. Furthermore, in one large retrospective series, infection was the second most common cause associated with allograft loss after rejection [82]. It is estimated that nearly 90% of patients who have undergone IMVTx develop a bacterial infection by their follow-up at 6 months [83], and approximately 61% develop a bloodstream infection during their first 6 months post shown to occur in 58–80% of patients who have undergone IMVTx [38, 83, 84]. As most of the studies are small and there is no uniformity in the type of induction and maintenance immunosuppressive regimens, it is difficult to establish clear risk factors that predispose this patient group to such high rates of infection. For example, in one study, there were similar rates of bacterial infections within the first month of transplantation (approximately 60%) when induction therapy with daclizumab (humanized monoclonal antibody to the alpha subunit of the IL-2 T cell receptor) was compared to alemtuzumab [85]. It has been postulated that these high rates of infection are related to bacterial translocation of intraluminal enteric gut flora from the intestinal allograft to sterile sites such as the peritoneum and the bloodstream. It is conceivable that the presence of bacterial flora within the small bowel allograft could gain access to the lymphatics and bloodstream in the immediate postoperative setting as a result of microscopic gastrointestinal mucosal trauma which could occur during

Table 5.3 Common infections in small intestinal and multivisceral transplant recipients

Pre-ITx[a]	"Immediate" post-ITx	"Later" post-ITx
Bacterial/fungal infections • Intra-abdominal abscess • Peritonitis • CLABSIs – Enteric Gm(-) rods – Staphylococci – Enterococci – Candida • Health care associated infections	Bacterial/fungal infections • Intra-abdominal infections (abscess, peritonitis) • CLABSIs • HCAP • Surgical site infection • UTI Etiologies • lGm(-) enterics • Enterococci/VRE • Staphylococci • Candida species • Aspergillus	• Bacterial/fungal infections (health care associated infections) • CLABSIs • Sepsis • Fungal infections – Candida – Aspergillus • Viral infections of the intestinal allograft – CMV – EBV associated PTLD – Adenovirus – Rotavirus – Norovirus • Miscellaneous – PCP – Nocardia – Invasive molds – GI protozoa (isospora, cryptosporidia – Strongyloides stercoralis
Months – Years Pre-ITx	0 Date of ITx	6 Weeks post-ITx / Months – Years Post-ITx

[a]Intestinal transplant

cold ischemia time. Additionally, there are animal models that have demonstrated that bacterial translocation has been associated with antibiotic use, bacterial overgrowth and gastrointestinal dysmotility, malnutrition, use of TPN, and ischemic injury and subsequent bowel reperfusion [37, 86, 87]. All of the above factors are seen in this patient group and can be further compounded by the high level of immunosuppression that is necessary to prevent rejection of this allograft which is rich in lymphoid tissue. In the setting of small bowel allograft rejection, the mucosal injury could facilitate bacterial translocation, and this has been reported in approximately 10% of patients who had undergone IMVTx [37]. In that same study, by obtaining simultaneous stool samples, it was estimated that 44% of the patients who had developed infections (approximately 2.0 episodes/patient) had experienced bacterial translocation that resulted in a documented infection. Bacterial translocation was most commonly documented during the first postoperative month at an incidence of 31%. The organisms that were most commonly associated with bacterial translocation were coagulase-negative staphylococci, *Klebsiella pneumoniae, Enterococcus faecalis, Enterococcus faecium, and Enterobacter cloacae* [37]. A prolonged ischemic time (>9 hours) and the inclusion of a colon as part of the allograft were associated with bacterial translocation [37]. More recently, it has been noted that colonic inclusion was not associated with an increased risk of bacteremia [88], and colonic inclusion as part of the small bowel allograft is considered to be an appropriate option in the management of IF in patients with SBS [8]. The role of bacterial translocation as a contributory cause may be further supported by the predominance of enteric pathogens that are noted as a cause of infection in this patient population [84]. It has also been reported that the microbial environment of the small intestinal allograft shifts from a population of predominantly anaerobic bacteria to a population of *Enterobacteriaceae* and lactobacilli [89].

The role of donor-derived and recipient-derived infections has contributed to the infectious disease-associated morbidity in solid organ transplant recipients during the immediate postoperative period [90]. The role of donor-derived infections may be increasingly important in the setting of small intestinal transplantation as the small bowel allograft (with or without the colon) has a high density of bacterial flora [37]. It is also possible that these donors, while hospitalized, can develop intestinal colonization by drug-resistant enteric bacteria. Concern over the risk of transmission of bacterial and fungal infections from the donor allograft has resulted in the use of gut decontamination protocols at many centers [39, 82, 83]. In a rat model of orthotopic small intestinal transplantation, rats were given polymyxin E and tobramycin by orogastric gavage postoperatively. There was a significant reduction in the amount of enteric bacteria in the ileum and cecum and marked reduction in bacterial translocation to the mesenteric lymph nodes of the group that received the postoperative gut decontamination as compared to the group that did not receive gut decontamination [91]. Selective gut decontamination protocols are employed postoperatively and given as an oral suspension via a gastrostomy or jejunostomy tube into the intestinal allograft. These gut decontamination suspensions target predominantly enteric Gram-negative organisms and fungi and have included various combinations of polymyxin, tobramycin, gentamicin, clindamycin, nystatin, and amphotericin B [38, 83, 84]. The routine use of selective gut decontamination in the intestinal allograft is no longer being employed at our center due to concerns that this practice may result in a "less favorable" intraluminal microbial environment.

Recipient-derived infections have also contributed to the postoperative infectious complications in solid organ transplant recipients, including the transmission of resistant organisms [90, 92]. One study has demonstrated the high prevalence of extended-spectrum B-lactamase (ESBL)-producing *Klebsiella pneumoniae* in stool surveillance cultures of pediatric patients who were undergoing or have received liver or small intestinal transplantation [92]. Bacteremia due to ESBL-producing *Klebsiella pneumoniae* was also noted in this patient population, which supports the hypothesis that colonization of the recipient with multidrug-resistant organisms can result in infections post-transplantation [92]. It is interesting to note that in another study, there was no concordance between the types of organisms isolated from stool surveillance cultures preoperatively and the types of organisms associated with documented infections in the post-intestinal transplant period [79]. Although there is no definitive data, donor-derived and recipient-derived infections likely play an important contributory role in the immediate posttransplantation period, and clinicians may consider altering the perioperative antimicrobial regimen based on prior microbiological history.

Infections in the "Immediate" Posttransplantation Period (<6 Weeks)

The complicated nature of the surgical procedures used in small intestinal and multivisceral transplantation places this patient population at increased risk for healthcare-associated infections in the immediate postoperative period. These patients tend to have prolonged postoperative lengths of stay which expose them to the microbial environment of the hospital. Therefore the predominant initial infectious diseases threat to these patients is bacterial and fungal infections which are characteristic of the types of infections that accompany any critically ill patient who has undergone extensive intra-abdominal surgery. Based on our observations and previous discussion, the "immediate" posttransplantation period will be defined as <6 weeks from the time of transplantation. This is a somewhat arbitrary cutoff, as these patients can experience these types of infections any time post transplantation, given their need for hospital readmission due to various complications such as rejection, surgical complications, acute kidney injury, etc.

Sites of Infections in the "Immediate" Posttransplantation Period

As in other critically ill postoperative patients, healthcare-associated infections predominate at this time and most commonly involve the bloodstream, surgical site, abdomen, respiratory tract, and urinary tract. It has been our experience that the mean length of stay for adult patients who have undergone IMVTx is 24 days; this increases to 42 days in patients who develop one or more infections. In patients who develop multiple infections (>2), the length of stay increases to 71 days [84]. Based on our observations and those of others, bacterial infections occur in at least 58% of patients within the first 4 weeks post-transplantation and then increase to approximately 80% by 8 weeks post transplantation [83, 84]. The incidence of bacterial infections decreases to 3% per month after 6 months from the time of transplantation [83]. Initial bacterial infections occur very early in the post-operative period with a mean or median time to first infection of 9–11 days [38, 83, 84].

Bloodstream infections and sepsis are an important cause of bacterial infection and represent 26–59% of all bacterial sites of infection during the early postoperative period [38, 83, 84]. In one study, 1.6 episodes of bacteremia occurred per patient, with 2.1 episodes occurring in patients with this type of infection [83]. The 6-month cumulative incidence in adults and pediatric patients who had undergone IMVTx at our center was noted to be 61% and was more common in patients who had also received a liver as part of their transplantation [88]. Pediatric transplant recipients were also more likely to develop a bloodstream infection than the adult patients. This same study did not find an association between the inclusion of a colon or acute rejection with regard to the development of a bloodstream infection, which may call into question the role of bacterial translocation in the setting of rejection [88]. Interestingly, we have observed that bacterial infections preceded episodes of rejection by 15 days in the majority of patients who developed allograft rejection within the first month [84].

The predominant causative organisms associated with bloodstream infections were Gram-positive cocci – accounting for 59–66% of the isolates – followed by Gram-negative enterics accounting for 34–41% of the isolates, and *Candida* species accounting for approximately 3% of the isolates [83, 88]. Of note, *Enterococcus* species (including vancomycin-resistant *Enterococcus faecium)* were noted to be the most common Gram-positive isolate identified which supports the intestinal tract as a source [88].

The management of bloodstream infections is beyond the scope of this chapter but clearly includes source control (i.e., central vascular catheter removal or drainage of an intra-abdominal abscess), along with appropriate targeted antimicrobial treatment.

Intra-abdominal infections including intra-abdominal abscesses, infected intra-abdominal fluid collections, and peritonitis are quite common and account for approximately 13–37% of bacterial infections within the immediate postoperative period (Fig. 5.2) [38, 83, 84].

It was noted in one study that the presence of an intra-abdominal abscess and a positive peritoneal culture was associated with a high mortality within the first month of

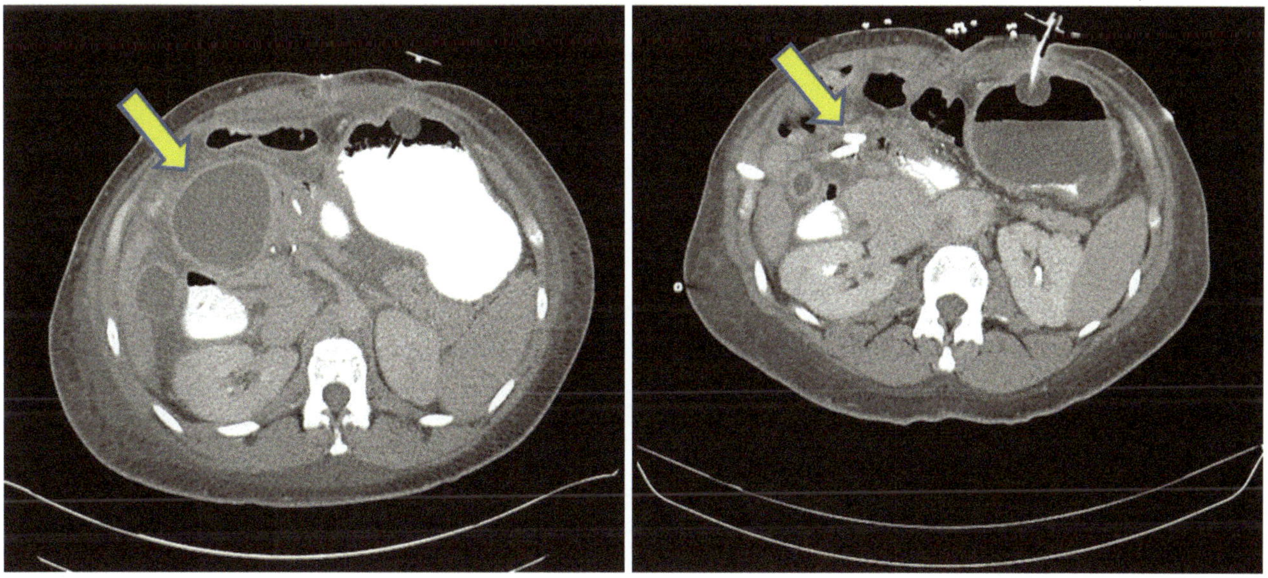

Fig. 5.2 CT scan of abdominal fluid collection post-Tx pre- and post-percutaneous drainage. (Fluid culture: *E. faecium*)

diagnosis (approximately 30%) in small intestinal transplant recipients [83]. Collectively, enteric pathogens including *pseudomonas aeruginosa*, *Enterococcus* species (including vancomycin-resistant *Enterococcus*), *Enterobacter cloacae*, *E. coli*, and *Candida* species have been most commonly reported [83, 84]. Given the reportedly high mortality rate, it is imperative to establish a diagnosis in an effort to improve patient outcomes. The use of computed tomography (CT) to identify intra-abdominal fluid collections and/or abscesses should be employed if there is a high index of clinical suspicion. Management options can include CT-guided percutaneous drainage of intra-abdominal fluid collections as well as exploratory laparotomy and intra-abdominal washout along with appropriate targeted antimicrobial agents.

Respiratory tract infections including healthcare-associated pneumonia (HCAP) account for 14–17% of bacterial infections in small intestinal recipients [38, 83, 84]. It has been reported that 39.5% of HCAPs occur within the first 2 months post-transplantation, with a median onset of 36.5 days. The microbiology of HCAPs in this patient population does not differ from other patient populations and includes *Pseudomonas aeruginosa, Klebsiella pneumoniae, Escherichia coli, Acinetobacter baumannii,* and *Staphylococcus aureus* [83, 84],. The clinician caring for these patients should refer to the practice guidelines for the diagnostic and management of HCAP (Practice Guidelines for HCAP, IDSA). Other atypical bacterial respiratory pathogens have not been reported in this patient population. Although tuberculous and non-tuberculous *Mycobacteria* can cause disease in solid organ transplant recipients (often between months 1–6 post-transplantation), to date, no cases have been reported in IMVTx recipients. We have seen a case of pulmonary infection with *Nocardia* asteroids that disseminated to the central nervous system in a multivisceral transplant recipient – occurring many months after transplantation.

Surgical site infections account for 9–17% of bacterial infections in small intestinal transplant recipients, with a higher percentage due to Gram-negative enterics as the causative pathogens [83, 84]. Urinary tract infections accounted for 15–17% of the bacterial infections in small intestinal or multivisceral transplant recipients [38, 84]. There have also been other types of bacterial infections reported at other miscellaneous sites which include empyema, cholangitis, sinusitis, otitis media, and septic arthritis [83].

As discussed previously, multidrug-resistant organisms may be a common occurrence in small intestinal and multivisceral transplant recipients. It has been our experience that drug-resistant organisms account for 47% of all bacterial infections within the immediate postoperative period, with 71% of Gram-positive cocci demonstrating significant resistance and 39% of Gram-negative enterics exhibiting significant resistance. Vancomycin-resistant *Enterococci* accounted for 75% of all enterococcal isolates, and 100% of *Staphylococcus aureus* isolates were methicillin resistant. Thirty-one percent of *Klebsiella* and *E. coli* isolates were ESBL-producing, and 39% of *Pseudomonas aeruginosa* isolates were multidrug-resistant [84]. The predominance of these multidrug-resistant organisms in the immediate postoperative period raises the possibility to consider empiric coverage for multidrug-resistant organisms based on local antimicrobial resistance patterns when an infection is suspected.

Antimicrobial Prophylaxis in the Peri- and Postoperative Transplant Periods

Although protocols are often center-specific, antimicrobial prophylaxis against bacterial, fungal, viral, and protozoal pathogens follows many of the same principles as in other solid organ transplantations. Perioperative prophylaxis for bacterial infections includes agents such as ampicillin/sulbactam, as well as piperacillin/tazobactam. The duration of surgical prophylaxis varies from 3 days to approximately 7 days and is often center-specific. At our center, ampicillin/sulbactam has been the preferred agent of choice and is maintained for at least 3 days postoperatively or until biopsy confirms mucosal integrity of the allograft. Some centers also employ the use of selective gut decontamination in the donor allograft and recipient (see above).

Antifungal prophylaxis with azole therapy such as fluconazole, as well as a lipid preparation of amphotericin B, has been used by most centers. It has been our practice to discontinue fluconazole once the first allograft biopsy was noted to be normal. Some centers maintain antifungal prophylaxis until the time of hospital discharge [38]. Significant drug interactions exist between the azole antifungals, fluconazole, and voriconazole, with tacrolimus due to inhibition of cytochrome P450 isoenzymes [93]. Therefore, the initiation or discontinuation of azole antifungal agents needs to be coordinated with the close monitoring of tacrolimus levels.

All IMVTx recipients receive intravenous ganciclovir at a dosage of 5 mg/kg every 12 hours to prevent infection with cytomegalovirus (CMV) and other herpes viruses. At our center, patients are usually maintained at this induction dose for at least 2 weeks and then are switched to maintenance dosing with oral valganciclovir. Most centers also employ the use of CMV hyperimmune globulin for CMV prophylaxis. We routinely use CMV hyperimmune globulin at a dosage of 150 mg/kg weekly until postoperative day 30.

Prophylaxis for *Pneumocystis jiroveci* with trimethoprim-sulfamethoxazole is also initiated postoperatively and maintained for at least 6 months after transplantation. It is not unreasonable to consider lifelong prophylaxis due to the high level of immunosuppression that these patients undergo. Trimethoprim-sulfamethoxazole may also provide prophylaxis against *Toxoplasma gondii*, *Listeria monocytogenes*, and some *Nocardia* species.

Infections in the "Late" Post-transplant Period (>6 Weeks)

Viral Infections

Cytomegalovirus (CMV)

CMV, a double-stranded DNA herpesvirus, is among the most common viral infections post-transplantation and causes significant morbidity. Here we discuss aspects of CMV infection pertinent to IMVTx and refer to published guidelines for issues related to aspects common to other solid organ transplantations [94–96].

Historically, CMV has been a major cause of morbidity since the early era of intestinal transplantation. In the first report on 38 patients, an incidence of 39% of CMV disease was found, most commonly during the second month post-transplantation and affecting the intestinal graft in 81%. Factors associated with disease were donor +/recipient serostatus, isolated intestinal transplantation, and the amount of immunosuppression (tacrolimus levels and cumulative corticosteroid dose) [97]. In early reports there was no significant impact on survival at 1 and 2 years [97, 98]. Importantly, undetectable CMV plasma viremia by PCR was reported in 48% of patients with clinical and histopathological invasive CMV disease [97, 99]. In pediatric recipients CMV disease was reported with a lower incidence than in adult recipients (24%), at a median of 53 days post-transplantation, and affecting the intestinal allograft in 90%. Importantly, no CMV disease occurred in the subgroup of D−/R− patients [98]. Resolution of CMV occurred in >90% cases after 2–4 weeks of antiviral therapy, but recurrence rates as high as 50% were documented, similar to adult intestinal allograft recipients and to other solid organ transplant recipients [94]. The cumulative doses of corticosteroid boluses and steroid recycles were associated with a higher incidence of CMV in children [98]. More recent experience in pediatric intestinal transplant recipients reported an 18% incidence of CMV infection post-transplantation and a decreased incidence of invasive CMV disease (7%) [100] compared to earlier experience. At our center, we observed an 18.2% incidence of CMV infection/disease among 88 adult and pediatric IMVTx recipients over a 5-year period [101]. The majority of invasive CMV disease involves the intestinal allograft, and recurrences are reported between 50% and 86% [98, 100]. Furthermore, CMV disease significantly shortened survival with an 11-fold increase in mortality risk when not only the direct cytopathic effects of CMV were considered but also the indirect immunomodulatory effects and the associated increase risk of other infections including EBV and subsequent PTLD [100].

The donor and recipient CMV serologic status is an important predictor of post-transplant CMV infection [5, 99]. The highest risk for development of invasive CMV, recurrent CMV, and ganciclovir-resistant CMV is in CMV-seronegative recipients of a CMV-seropositive donor (D+/R–). While not an absolute contraindication to transplantation, D+/R– status is an indication for more intensive monitoring and more stringent preventive strategies post-transplantation than in donor/recipient pairs with a lower risk of CMV. However, the seropositive recipient, regardless of donor status, is at risk for CMV reactivation and usually receives either prophylaxis or preemptive monitoring and therapy. Irrespective of donor/recipient serostatus, intestinal transplant recipients are at high risk for CMV disease, given the heavy immunosuppressive regimens (including high tacrolimus levels) used in these patients. Although practices remain center-specific, some programs (including ours) now exclude CMV-seropositive donor intestinal allografts for CMV-seronegative recipients who are awaiting isolated small intestinal transplantation. In fact, CMV disease in D+/R– takes much longer to resolve histologically (up to 7 months) and, in addition to involving the graft, also more frequently involves the native gastrointestinal tract [98]. It is also an established practice that seronegative recipients receive CMV-negative blood products during the transplant and postoperatively.

Manifestations of CMV infection and disease post-intestinal transplantation include asymptomatic detectable CMV DNA, a viral syndrome (fever, myalgia, leukopenia, elevated transaminases), and end-organ involvement. CMV enteritis post-transplantation, in addition to systemic symptoms, manifests with increased ileostomy output or diarrhea and gastrointestinal bleeding and affects the intestinal allograft more than the native gastrointestinal tract [98, 100]. Endoscopic findings of CMV allograft enteritis vary between mild (superficial ulceration) (Fig. 5.3) and severe mucosal

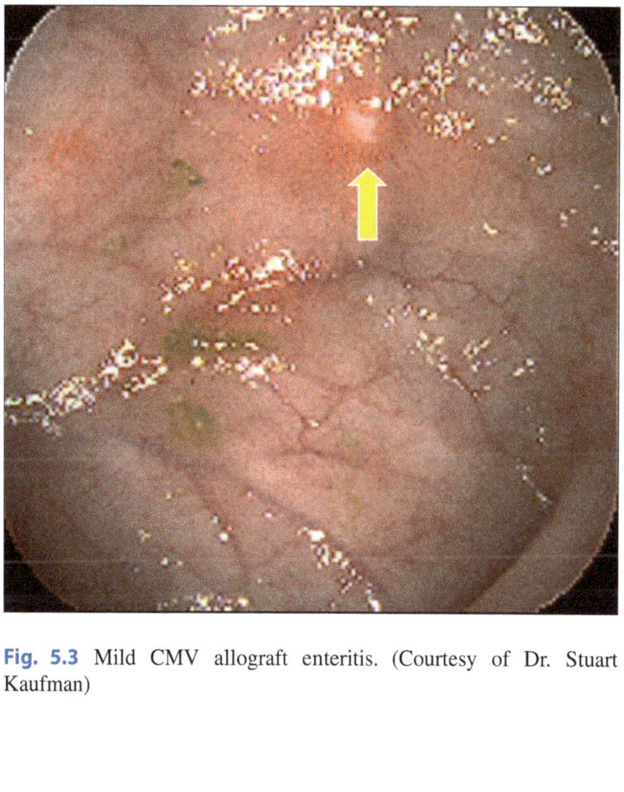

Fig. 5.3 Mild CMV allograft enteritis. (Courtesy of Dr. Stuart Kaufman)

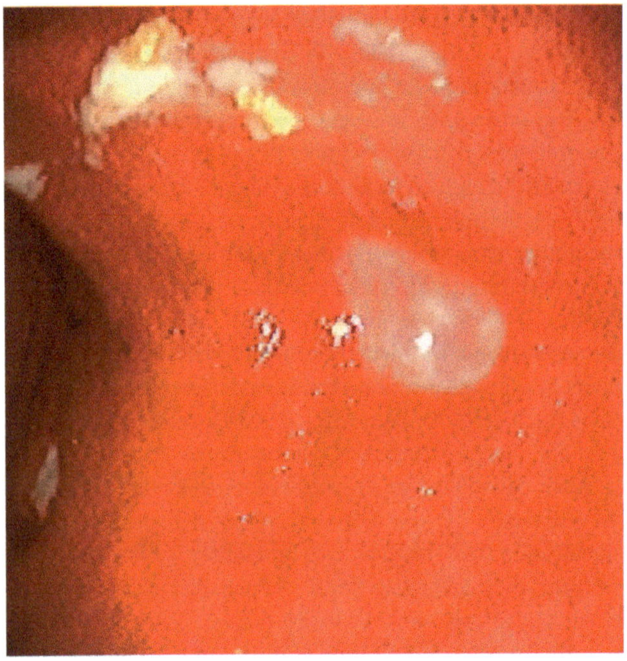

Fig. 5.4 Severe CMV allograft enteritis. (Courtesy of Dr. Stuart Kaufman)

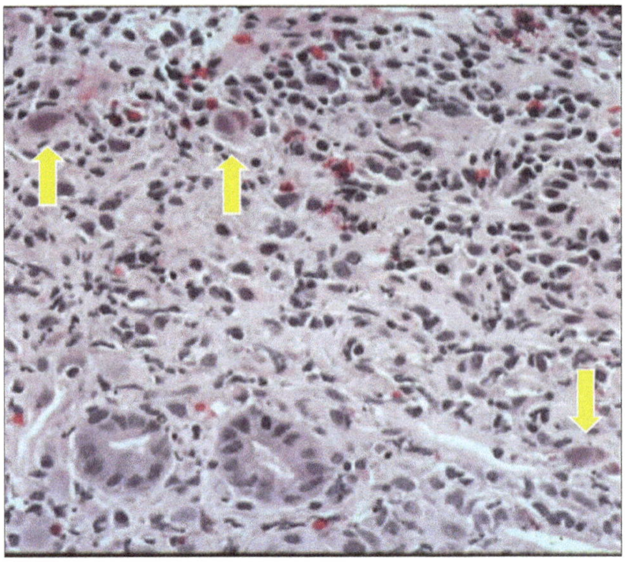

Fig. 5.5 CMV enteritis with inclusion bodies and inflammatory infiltrate

damage (Fig. 5.4) with the potential for bowel perforation, especially following T cell depletion therapy (e.g., thymoglobulin) for acute rejection.

Histologic features suggestive of CMV allograft enteritis include mucosal damage (crypt and villous loss), plasma cell and lymphocyte infiltrate with few eosinophils, and CMV inclusion bodies (Fig. 5.5) with positive CMV immunostaining [102].

In IMVTx recipients, other organs are less frequently involved and include the lungs [98], liver, and kidneys. One patient at our center developed a CMV polyradiculitis that resulted in a severe sensory-motor deficit of the lower extremities.

Generally early prophylaxis is recommended for all intestinal transplant recipients with intravenous ganciclovir for 14–100 days post-transplant in association with CMV immune globulin followed by oral valganciclovir. The optimal duration of antiviral prophylaxis is not uniformly established, and options vary between 3 and 6 months to indefinitely. After completion of prophylaxis, CMV DNA PCR is monitored indefinitely for preemptive resumption of therapy, and intravenous ganciclovir is usually resumed during treatment of acute rejection episodes. Prophylaxis in the form of valganciclovir and CMV immunoglobulin is costly, but it lowers the risk in such a high-risk population like intestinal transplant recipients. As in other solid organ transplants, late-onset CMV disease is a potential problem with prophylaxis, occurring in 15–30% of cases after discontinuation of prophylaxis, whereas CMV resistance has been observed with both prophylaxis and preemptive therapy [94]. The efficacy of prophylaxis with either CMV immune globulin (CMVIG) or intravenous immune globulin (IVIG) in combination with ganciclovir/valganciclovir in high-risk transplant recipients has been investigated in few studies [103, 104], but in intestinal transplantation, practices remain center-based.

The treatment of CMV disease follows guidelines established for other solid organ transplant recipients and usually includes intravenous ganciclovir at a dose of 5 mg/kg every 12 hours for 2–4 weeks or until negative viral replication [105, 106]. Oral valganciclovir 900 mg twice daily may be considered as long as the intestinal allograft is functioning. In most other patient populations, oral valganciclovir may achieve similar drug exposure as intravenous ganciclovir given its good bioavailability (approximately 60%). The pharmacokinetics of valganciclovir in small intestinal transplant recipients has not been extensively studied, although one case report noted a bioavailability of 64.7% when used for CMV prophylaxis in a small intestinal recipient [107]. However in the setting of the small intestinal transplant recipient, intravenous ganciclovir may be preferred over valganciclovir, as valganciclovir may provide sub-optimal drug exposure when allograft function is questionable (as in the setting of acute or chronic rejection). In the setting of CMV allograft enteritis, it is our preference to treat with intravenous ganciclovir to ensure adequate drug exposure. Many centers including ours employ the use of CMV hyperimmune globulin in addition to intravenous ganciclovir for the treatment of invasive CMV disease.

Ganciclovir-resistant CMV has been reported in 1–2% of solid organ transplant recipients, and risk factors include prolonged oral prophylaxis, D+/R– serostatus, and heavy immunosuppression [94, 96]. At our center we noted a rate of nearly 6% for ganciclovir-resistant CMV among all of our IMVTx recipients. However, in those patients with either CMV viremia or invasive disease, we documented a rate of 31% of ganciclovir resistance, which appears to be the highest rate among all types of solid organ transplantations [101]. In our series, all patients with ganciclovir resistance were D+/R– serostatus, and 80% (4/5) of these patients had invasive CMV allograft enteritis. Two of the 5 patients with ganciclovir resistance had both the UL 97 and UL 54 mutation [101]. The diagnosis of CMV resistance is confirmed by genotypic testing, and treatment options include lowering baseline immunosuppression level, intravenous foscarnet adjusted for renal function, cidofovir, or leflunomide. Recently a case has been reported of multidrug-resistant cytomegalovirus in a modified multivisceral transplant recipient [108].

Although it is established that intensified immunosuppression to treat rejection increases the risk of subsequent CMV infection, it is also commonly recognized that CMV increases the risk of rejection at least in kidney transplant recipients. The mechanism is attributed to an immunostimulatory effect of both CMV infection and CMV disease [98, 109], but to date a definite link between CMV and rejection has yet to be established in IMVTx [98].

Epstein-Barr Virus (EBV)

Epstein-Barr Virus (EBV) is another double-stranded herpesvirus. EBV-related posttransplant lymphoproliferative disorders (PTLD) are feared complications among all solid organ transplants. EBV infects, transforms, and immortalizes B lymphocytes and in transplant recipients may progress to PTLD due to inadequate anti-EBV cytotoxic T cells. It can also progress from EBV-driven proliferation to EBV-independent lymphoma. Guidelines have been published on the diagnosis and management of EBV-related disease in solid organ transplant [110]. Among organ transplant recipients, IMVTx are at the highest risk for development of PTLD (up to 32%) compared to other solid organ transplant recipients (1–12%) [110]. However, the incidence of PTLD in IMVTx recipients has recently decreased to 5–10% compared to the early era (30%) secondary to routine quantitative EBV DNA PCR monitoring [111]. In fact, patients with undetectable or low viral loads for the first 6 months after IMVTx are unlikely to develop PTLD regardless of their pretransplant EBV serological status [112]. The decreased incidence of acute rejection after IMVTx (and its treatment) has also contributed to reduce the incidence of EBV-related disease [111].

EBV-seronegative recipients of a graft from an EBV-seropositive donor are at greatest risk of post-transplant infection, although EBV-seropositive recipients remain at significant risk [111]. Usually PTLD follows primary EBV infection in seronegative recipient (most commonly pediatric recipients) of an EBV-seropositive graft, although PTLD can also develop in the seropositive recipient secondary to EBV reactivation under the influence of augmented immunosuppression. Protocols for the surveillance of EBV, diagnosis, and management of PTLD in solid organ transplant patients have been published elsewhere [110, 113].

The timing of development of PTLD is most commonly within the first year post-transplant, but cases have been described as late as 10 years post-transplant, especially EBV-negative PTLD or the rare T cell PTLD [114].

Main risk factors for PTLD are primary EBV infection post-transplantation and the net state of immunosuppression, especially the use of high dose or repeated courses of antilymphocyte globulins which impact on the cytotoxic activity of EBV-specific T cells [110, 115]. Cytomegalovirus infection may also contribute to the net state of immunosuppression and is known to be a risk factor for PTLD [110].

Clinical manifestations of EBV infection post-transplantation include infectious mononucleosis (fever, malaise, exudative pharyngitis, lymphadenopathy, hepatosplenomegaly, and atypical lymphocytosis), specific organ diseases such as hepatitis, pneumonitis, gastrointestinal symptoms, and hematological manifestations such as leucopenia, thrombocytopenia, hemolytic anemia, and hemophagocytosis. Manifestations of PTLD are multiple and include subcutaneous hard and immobile nodules, generalized lymphadenopathy, snoring in children due to adenoidal hypertrophy, mouth breathing with ulcerating palatine tonsils, pneumonia with lung and/or mediastinal masses, diarrhea secondary to diffuse small bowel mucosal infiltration, gastrointestinal bleeding in case of multiple ulcerating lesions, and abdominal pain with or without bowel obstruction [111, 116]. PTLD of the intestinal graft can be discovered incidentally during routine surveillance endoscopy for rejection or following symptoms of mass, abdominal pain, partial obstruction, feeding intolerance in children, fever, and gastrointestinal bleeding [111].

Endoscopically PTLD of the graft may present as a protruding intramural mass with central umbilication (Fig. 5.6) which histologically appears as a lymphocytic mass without follicular organization (Fig. 5.7) and positive on CD20 immunostaining (Fig. 5.8).

Histological diagnosis of PTLD is confirmed by in situ hybridization of EBV DNA and the more sensitive RNA in situ hybridization targeting EBV-encoded small nuclear RNA (EBER) [117].

Prophylaxis with antivirals (ganciclovir) does not impact on EBV-driven B cell proliferation but may reduce the number of EBV-infected cells, thus reducing the risk of PTLD especially in EBV D+/R– mismatch [114].

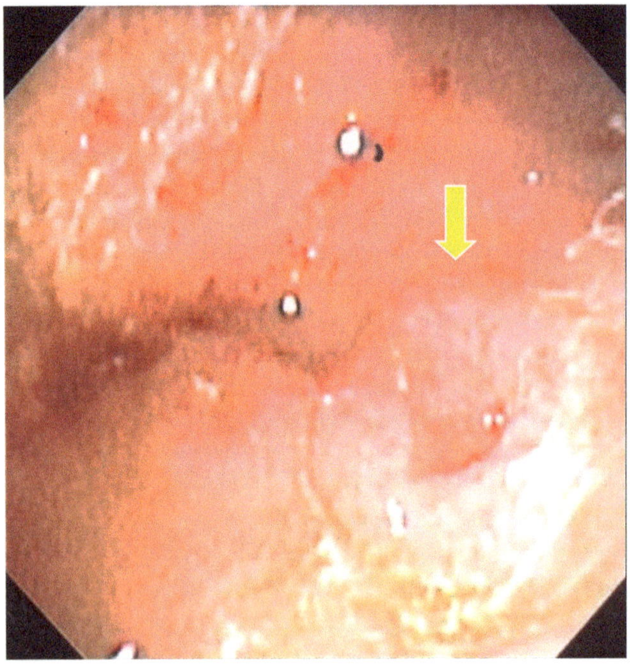

Fig. 5.6 PTLD: endoscopically protruding intramural mass with central umbilication. (Courtesy of Dr. Stuart Kaufman)

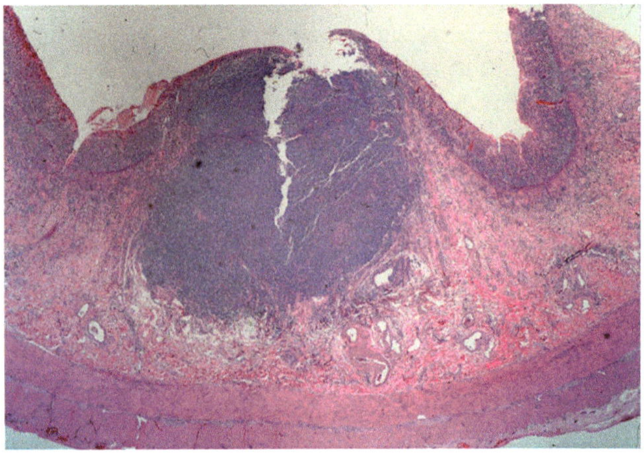

Fig. 5.7 PTLD: intramural lymphoid mass with absent follicular organization

The treatment of PTLD includes reduction of immunosuppression in combination with intravenous ganciclovir, CMV immune globulin, and rituximab (anti-CD20 monoclonal antibody) [118]. The response to reduction of immunosuppression is variable (between 20% and 80%) based on different weaning protocols and on the heterogeneity of disease (localized/diffuse, monomorphic/polymorphic). Aggressive reduction of immunosuppression requires frequent endoscopy and biopsy to monitor the graft for rejection.

Although used off-label, the anti B cell antibody (rituximab) has been used with success in the treatment of PTLD,

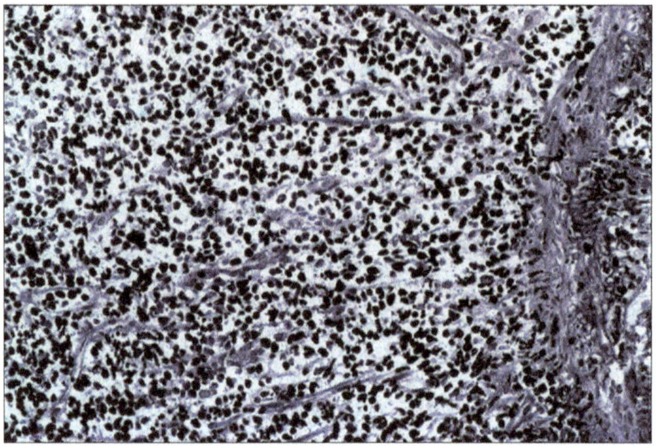

Fig. 5.8 PTLD: CD-20 [B-cell marker] stain

with response rates reported between 50% and 60%, and a low incidence of relapses are also reported [119–121].

Localized PTLD involvement of the graft represents the only situation potentially cured with limited resection and preservation of the graft, whereas diffuse involvement of the graft and/or poor response to therapy often mandates allograft enterectomy.

Most resistant cases of PTLD are considered for chemotherapy (based on cyclophosphamide and corticosteroids), with remission rates of 60% but with significant 2-year mortality of 30–50% often related to toxicity of chemotherapy [122, 123].

Intestinal Allograft Viral Enteritis

Overall, bacterial and viral infections target the intestinal graft with an incidence up to 39% after IMVTx [124], especially in infants and children. Two thirds of allograft infections are secondary to viral enteritis which, in addition to systemic DNA viruses CMV, EBV, and adenovirus, include enterotropic RNA viruses norovirus and rotavirus. The morbidity and mortality associated with systemic DNA viruses are significant, whereas infections with enterotropic viruses are usually associated with a lower mortality risk. Viral enteritis may be clinically indistinguishable from rejection, but it is critical to differentiate between these entities because treatment of rejection could result in viral dissemination. Conversely, decreasing immunosuppressive therapy for presumed viral enteritis may promote graft rejection. Furthermore, it is important to identify the correct pathogen because antiviral treatment may improve CMV infection, whereas no standard treatment is established for adenoviral or other viral infections.

Adenovirus

Adenovirus is a systemic DNA virus with tropism for multiple cell lines, including enterocytes. Like EBV, adenovirus may remain latent in lymphoid tissue thus exposing the

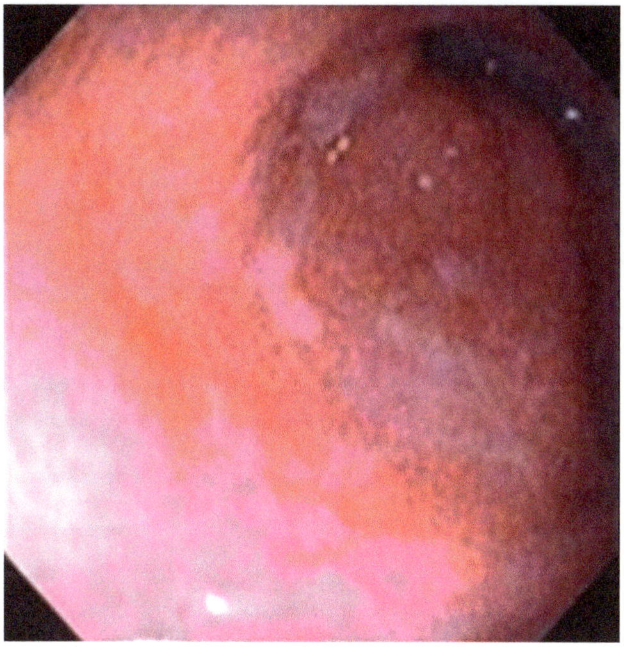

Fig. 5.9 Adenovirus allograft enteritis. (Courtesy of Dr. Stuart Kaufman)

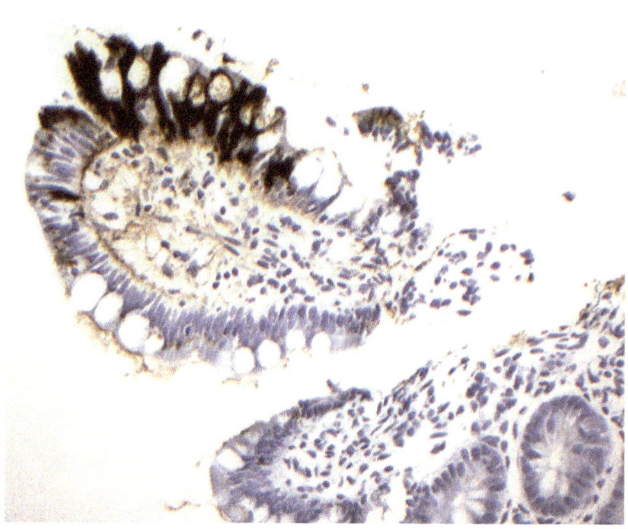

Fig. 5.10 Adenovirus allograft enteritis: enlarged and atypical nuclei with positive immunohistochemical stain for antibody to adenovirus (H&E-stained and immunohistochemical-stained sections, 200×)

recipient to the risk of reactivation post-transplantation. Adenovirus infection is more common in infants than in young children and adults with an incidence reported between 20 and 50% in pediatric intestinal transplant series [125–127], and in 80% of the cases, it occurs within the first 6 months post-transplantation. In a recent study, 36% of the cases were diagnosed in the first month, 32% in the following 5 months, 16% of the cases between 6 and 12 months after transplantation, and 16% after 1 year [100].

The intestinal allograft is more susceptible to adenoviral infection than other target organs, with an incidence of up to 80% of infections involving the intestinal graft [128]. The spectrum of manifestations of adenoviral infection varies between early asymptomatic viral replication, usually of donor origin, to adenoviral enteritis which is usually related to level of immunosuppression within the first 6–12 months post-transplant (Fig. 5.9).

Cases of late infection are sporadic. The main manifestation of adenoviral enteritis is usually osmotic diarrhea, infrequently accompanied by fever and rarely by gastrointestinal bleeding. Endoscopic appearances also vary and include erythema, edema, and increased mucous production, often not limited to the transplanted intestine but also involving the native bowel. Histologically the main features of adenoviral enteritis are apoptosis (like in rejection), villous injury (usually more prominent than in rejection), and cytopathic nuclear inclusions, the latter being a key component to differentiate adenoviral infection from rejection [129, 130].

The diagnosis is confirmed by serum and tissue DNA PCR and by immunohistochemistry (Fig. 5.10).

Usually mild adenoviral infection is limited to the graft in the setting of low immunosuppression, involves more the ileum than the jejunum, (unlike norovirus and rotavirus that affect more the jejunum than the ileum; see below), persists usually for 1–2 weeks, and only rarely produces extra GI manifestations. On the contrary, a more severe disease is usually associated with heavy immunosuppression like after treatment for rejection and causes multi-system involvement (the lungs, liver, pancreas) with significant mortality up to 20% [126]. Routine monitoring in the peripheral blood is not recommended in solid organ transplant recipients [131]. We monitor adenovirus DNA PCR in small children with suspicious viral illness or episodes of graft dysfunction. The management of adenoviral infection includes supportive treatment, reduction of immunosuppression levels, and cidofovir [131]. Although there is no established antiviral treatment for adenovirus infection, cidofovir is considered the standard of care. However, data are lacking to evaluate the efficacy and the response rate of adenovirus enteritis to cidofovir in IMVTx.

Rotavirus

Rotavirus enteritis presents with sudden watery osmotic diarrhea causing significant dehydration requiring intravenous fluid resuscitation and often temporary parenteral nutrition. Like other causes of viral enteritis, it usually affects the pediatric population, although adult recipients are not excluded from infection [132]. The severity and duration of infection are related to the intensity of immunosuppression and are typically worse during the first months after transplant. Endoscopically the infection appears with mild erythema, villous atrophy, and edema (Fig. 5.11) or normal mucosa.

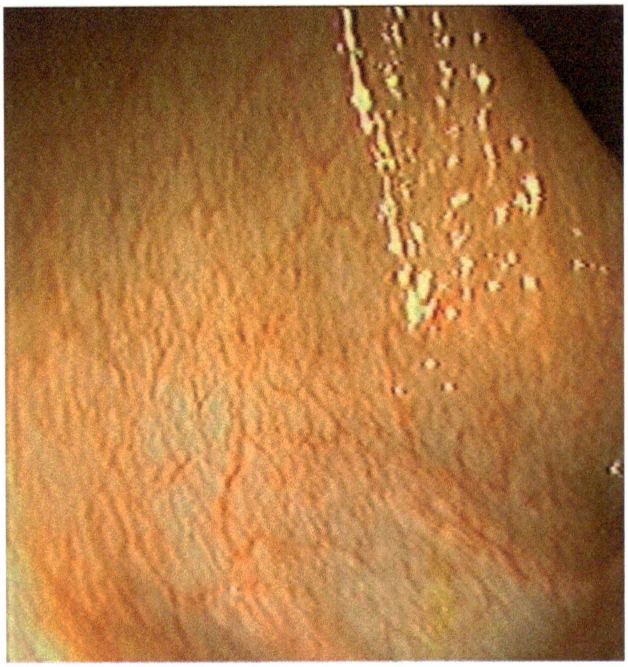

Fig. 5.11 Rotavirus allograft enteritis. (Courtesy of Dr. Stuart Kaufman)

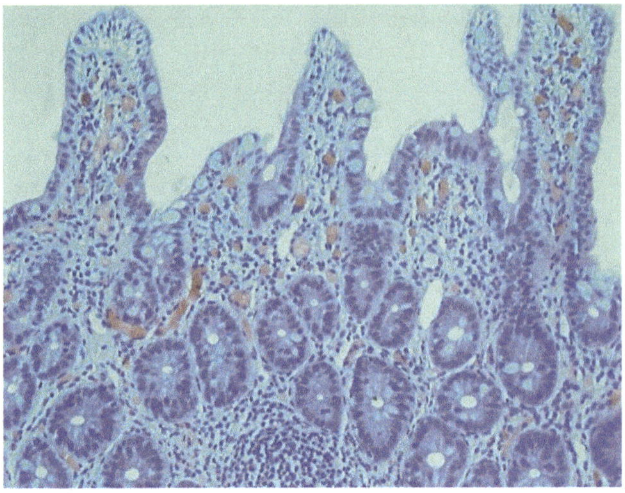

Fig. 5.12 Rotavirus allograft enteritis

The endoscopic jejunal changes are often more visible than the ileal. The differentiation between viral enteritis and acute rejection is not endoscopically or histologically immediate: key endoscopic features of rejection include a coarse mucosal surface with focal erosions. On biopsy, rejection is characterized by single/multiple crypt apoptosis with nuclear fragmentation, but usually, unlike in viral infections, the surface epithelium is preserved.

Other histological characteristics of rotavirus enteritis are villus blunting, mixed inflammatory infiltrate, superficial epithelial disarray, and goblet cell depletion (Fig. 5.12).

The diagnosis is confirmed by culture and immunostaining. The treatment for patients with rotaviral infection includes supportive care and endoscopic surveillance of the graft with biopsy while the patient is recovering. Although most cases are self-limited, rejection can be associated with or follow rotavirus infection in up to 69% of patients with rotaviral enteritis [132] and requires prompt diagnosis and treatment. Mechanisms implicated in rejection during or after infection include diarrhea-related poor drug absorption resulting in sub-therapeutic tacrolimus levels and immune activation secondary to viral infection.

Norovirus

Norovirus, a single-stranded RNA virus, is a common cause of acute self-limited enteritis in healthy persons but can cause protracted diarrhea and severe dehydration especially in pediatric IMVTx recipients [133, 134]. In the immunocompetent host, epidemics caused by this virus are particularly common among persons confined to institutions and other enclosed areas and often spread by contaminated foods. In the immunosuppressed population and after IMVTx, the incidence of norovirus infection is not known given the absence of established monitoring strategies. The timing of infection varies between 17 days and 1 year post-transplant in the limited published series [134].

Typically norovirus enteritis is characterized by protracted excretion of viruses (up to 80 days) [134] and by persistent osmotic diarrhea worsened by enteral feeding. Prolonged excretion of norovirus into ileostomy fluid from immunosuppressed infants may be a risk factor for nosocomial spread. Although antibodies produced in response to acute infection may be long-lasting, there is the potential for recurrent disease with the same or heterotypic strain. Histologically norovirus enteritis shows apoptosis involving both villous enterocytes and crypts, making it more challenging to differentiate from rejection based solely on biopsy. The diagnosis is confirmed by RT-PCR of biopsy material and of intestinal fluid [133]. Management of norovirus enteritis includes supportive care with intravenous fluids, nutritional supplementation, and reduction of maintenance immunosuppression levels (target trough tacrolimus levels <10 ng/ml, discontinuation of sirolimus, and reduction of steroid dose). Although often protracted, the infection is usually self-limited with restoration of normal graft function and limited morbidity unless superimposed to other infections (adenovirus, CMV).

Fungal Infections

The increased availability of diverse and potent immunosuppressive drugs has improved the outcomes of IMVTx but at the same time has increased the risk of opportunistic infections, including fungal infections. As in other solid organ transplant recipients, fungal infections pose major challenges in the management of small intestinal transplant recipients.

Usually fungal infections are healthcare-acquired infections due predominantly to *Candida* species and *Aspergillus*. Risk factors for fungal infections in the IMVTx recipients include the use of central venous catheters, PN, broad-spectrum antibiotics, intra-abdominal surgery requiring reoperation, and intensive immunosuppressive regimens. *Candida* and *Aspergillosis* are the two major fungal pathogens in small intestinal transplant recipients, with a reported incidence of approximately 25% [128, 135] and will be discussed here. While a number of other fungal infections have been reported in other types of solid organ transplant recipients [136], the endemic mycoses, as well as emerging molds, have rarely been reported in the small intestinal and multivisceral transplant recipient and are covered in the section entitled "Miscellaneous Infections" [137].

Candida

Candida spp. are the most common invasive fungal infections after solid organ transplantation, and this trend is also seen in IMVTx recipients [66, 138]. While *Candida* is usually a healthcare-associated infection occurring during the first 3 months post-transplantation in other solid organ recipients, in intestinal transplantation it can also occur later as it may be associated with intensification of immunosuppression (i.e., corticosteroids) for the treatment of rejection episodes. In a study of pediatric small bowel recipients, it was noted that nearly 80% of candidemia episodes occurred greater than 6 months from the time of transplantation, with a median time of 163 days post-transplantation [128]. At that same center, it was noted that approximately 70% of pediatric small intestinal transplant recipients developed fungemia within 1 year of transplantation and was associated with TPN and antibiotic use [100]. The incidence of invasive candidiasis is reported to be up to 28% of intestinal transplant recipients [38, 139].

The main risk factors for *Candida* infection in small intestinal transplant recipients are the presence of central vascular catheters, use of PN, exposure to broad-spectrum antibiotics, use of immunosuppression for induction and rejection episodes, anastomotic leaks or intra-abdominal collections, the need for multiple abdominal surgical procedures, and the presence of a multivisceral graft. Additional risk factors common to other transplants are renal failure and recent CMV infection.

The clinical manifestations of *Candida* infection in this patient population post-transplantation predominantly involve the bloodstream and the abdominal cavity. In one series, candidemia accounted for 66%, and *Candida* intra-abdominal infections accounted for 29% of all yeast infections [128]. Other sites of infection include the urinary tract and respiratory tract. We have observed an endovascular infection at a mesenteric anastomotic site due to *Candida albicans* in a small intestinal transplant recipient.

In general, *C. albicans* accounts for approximately 50% of all infections, and non-*albicans Candida* species collectively account for the other 50%. However in the small intestinal transplant recipient, 63% of *Candida* infections are due to non-*albicans Candida*, and *C. albicans* account for only 37% [128]. The diagnosis of invasive candidiasis depends on the demonstration of candida in sterile body sites, although culture methods, especially blood cultures, often have limited sensitivity (70%) [66].

Many centers employ the use of antifungal prophylaxis (usually with fluconazole) in the immediate postoperative period. The duration of fluconazole prophylaxis for *Candida* infection is variable and may be up to 4 weeks post-transplantation, but it is prolonged further in the presence of ongoing intestinal mucosal injury or in the setting of rejection episodes.

Candidemia has been associated with a mortality risk up to 40% [140] especially if empiric antifungal treatment is delayed until positive blood cultures are documented [141]. The management of candidemia follows the same guidelines as used for other patient populations [66]. Empiric treatment of candidemia may include the triazole agents such as fluconazole and voriconazole, the echinocandins such as caspofungin and micafungin, and the lipid preparations of amphotericin B. Based on limited data from one series [128], as well as our own observations [84], empiric antifungal therapy targeted at non-*albicans Candida* species such as *Candida glabrata* should be considered in the setting of fungemia. As fluconazole prophylaxis is used at our center, echinocandins are used initially for the management of candidemia until final species identification is available. In addition, it is recommended to remove infected central venous catheters, to obtain ophthalmologic exam to rule out candida chorioretinitis/endophthalmitis and maintain intravenous antifungal treatment for at least 2 weeks after there is documented clearance of blood cultures [66]. As stated previously, there are significant drug interactions between the azole antifungal agents and tacrolimus; therefore, close monitoring of tacrolimus levels should be performed when these agents are used and then discontinued [93].

Aspergillosis

Aspergillus spp. is a common filamentous mold in the environment that usually does not cause significant disease in the immunocompetent population. In the immunosuppressed patient, it may invade the lungs (invasive aspergillosis; see Fig. 5.13) and spread to other organs, including the sinuses, brain (Fig. 5.14), gastrointestinal tract, skin, and very rarely the bones.

Invasive aspergillosis represents only 1–3% of invasive fungal infections in small intestinal transplant recipients but is associated with significant morbidity and mortality up to 60–90% [142–144]. The most important risk factor for the development of aspergillosis in solid organ transplant recipients is the net state of immunosuppression associated with the intensity of the immunosuppressive therapies, as well as coinfection with immunomodulatory viruses such as CMV. As there are no case-controlled studies in the IMVTx population that determine risk factors for invasive aspergillosis, probably the most appropriate comparison can be made with liver transplant recipients (as many small intestinal transplant recipients include a liver). Factors that are associated with an increased risk of invasive aspergillosis in liver transplant recipients include re-transplantation, kidney injury requiring renal replacement therapy, CMV infection, and prolonged stay in an ICU [145–150].

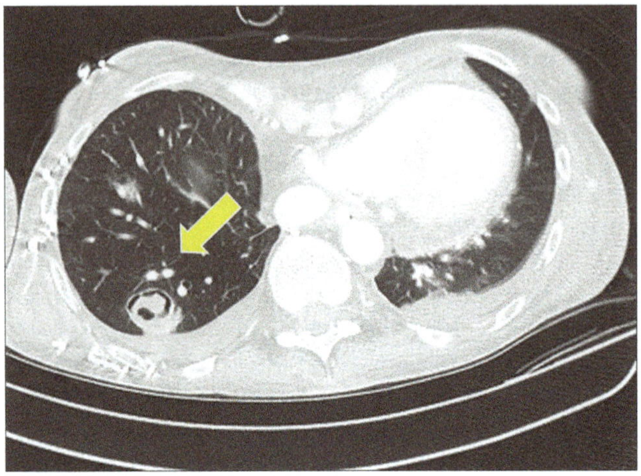

Fig. 5.13 Invasive lung aspergilloma

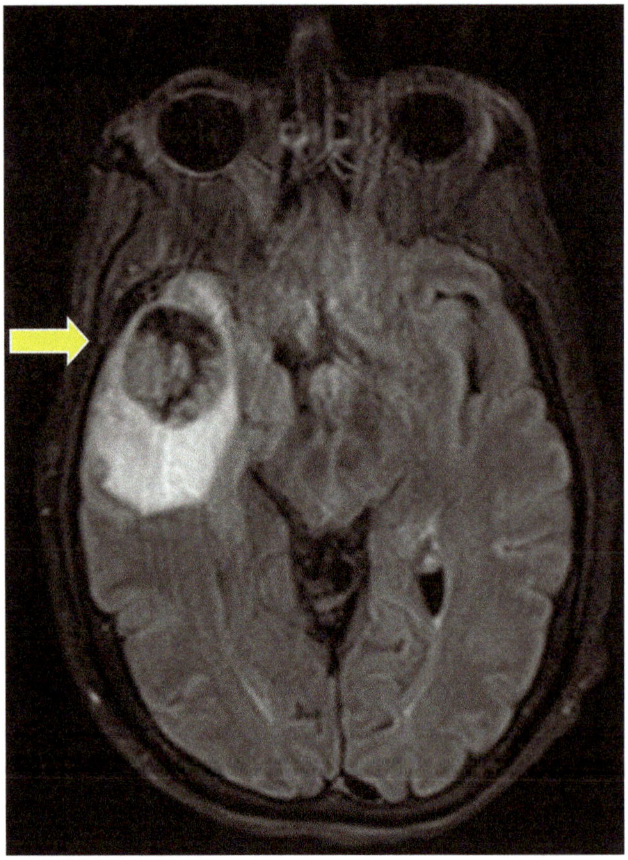

Fig. 5.14 Intracranial post-transplant aspergilloma

Notably, acute kidney injury, CMV infection, and prolonged ICU stays are important postoperative complications in the small intestinal transplant recipient and potentially could increase the risk of aspergillosis in this patient population as well.

The most common site of infection due to *Aspergillus* are the lungs, and patients may present with fever, cough, chest pain, and shortness of breath. Angioinvasion results in necrosis of tissue, which may ultimately lead to cavitation (Fig. 5.13) and/or hemoptysis. In the few cases reported in the literature, as well as our own observations, dissemination to the central nervous system appears to be common [143]. A definitive diagnosis of invasive aspergillosis can be difficult to make without confirmed histopathology demonstrating tissue invasion of the mold. As there are no large case series in the small intestinal transplant patient population, clinicians should use guidelines that are established for other solid organ transplant recipients [142].

There are no established guidelines for the prophylaxis of invasive aspergillosis in IMVTx recipients. The treatment of invasive aspergillosis includes voriconazole as the first-line agent. Alternatives may include liposomal amphotericin B, caspofungin, micafungin, and posaconazole. The surgical excision or debridement of single lung lesions may be indicated for persistent or life-threatening hemoptysis or for lesions invading the pericardium or lesions not responding to maximal antifungal therapy. Depending on location, access, and potential neurological sequelae, surgical resection is also considered in selected cases of intracranial aspergillosis (Fig. 5.14). Due to the lack of data in the small intestinal transplant patient population, optimal management should be based on established guidelines [142].

Miscellaneous Infections

Although bacteria, fungi, and viruses are the predominant causes of infection in the IMVTx recipient, this section will address the isolated and unusual case reports that have been reported in the literature in this specific patient population.

Pneumocystis jiroveci is an important cause of pneumonia in solid organ transplant recipients as well as other immunocompromised hosts but has only rarely been seen in IMVTx recipients. We have seen one case in an adult with an isolated small intestinal transplant recipient. There are two case reports of *Pneumocystis* pneumonia in pediatric patients. One case occurred in an 8-month-old who had intestinal failure and a congenital immunodeficiency with abnormal lymphocyte function who underwent a small intestinal and liver transplantation. The postoperative course was complicated by *Pneumocystis* pneumonia and graft versus host disease, and the child expired on the 23rd postoperative day [151]. The other case of *Pneumocystis* pneumonia occurred in a 2.5-year-old who underwent a living-related small intestinal transplantation that was complicated by four episodes of rejection and CMV infection and ultimately succumbed to *Pneumocystis* pneumonia 16 months after transplantation [152]. Donor-derived disseminated toxoplasmosis has been reported in a pediatric patient who had received a small intestinal transplantation [153].

Several intestinal parasites have been identified as causes of infection in small intestinal transplant recipients. In one case series of cryptosporidioses among pediatric solid organ transplant recipients, one case of cryptosporidioses was diagnosed in a small intestinal transplant recipient which did resolve with treatment [154]. There is also a single case report of *Isospora belli* infection that was diagnosed 3 months after a successful small intestinal transplantation which resolved with treatment with trimethoprim-sulfamethoxazole [155]. There have been two case reports of infection due to *Strongyloides stercoralis* in isolated intestinal transplant recipients, one of which was complicated by *Strongyloides* hyperinfection syndrome and associated with polymicrobial bacteremia and meningitis [156, 157]. We have also recently observed a case of *Strongyloides* infection in a multivisceral transplant recipient (personal communication, J. Timpone). What is interesting to note about all three of these patients is that the source of the *Strongyloides* was donor derived [156, 157]. All three cases were treated with (and responded to) ivermectin, although one case also received thiabendazole [156, 157].

Isolated cases of endemic mycoses have not been reported in the small intestinal and multivisceral transplant population; however, cryptococcosis has been identified. In one retrospective review of solid organ transplant recipients at a single center, one case of cryptococcal meningitis was reported in a small intestinal transplant recipient [158]. Molds other than aspergillus have been rarely reported in small intestinal and multivisceral transplant recipients. There is an isolated case report of an invasive sinusitis due to *Trichoderma longibrachiatum* in an adult patient on tacrolimus and prednisone who had received a combined small intestinal and liver transplantation. The patient was treated with surgical debridement, amphotericin B, and itraconazole with resolution of the infection [159]. There was also a case report of an invasive esophagitis due to the dematiaceous fungus *Cladophialophora bantiana* in a small intestinal transplant recipient [160].

There have been two cases of mucormycosis reported: one case of *Cunninghamella bertholletiae* cutaneous infection which occurred in the setting of treatment of acute rejection 1 year after multivisceral transplantation [161] and one case of *Lichtheimia ramosa* (formerly *Absidia* species) infection presenting as gastrointestinal hemorrhage occurring 5 days postoperatively in the stomach allograft of a modified multivisceral transplant recipient [162]. Given the intensity of immunosuppression seen in this patient population, infections due to unusual molds should be anticipated by the clinicians caring for these patients.

Infections due to *Mycobacterium tuberculosis* have not been reported in small intestinal and multivisceral transplant recipients, although this population may be at increased risk. There has only been one case report of nontuberculous mycobacteria, and this was a surgical site infection due to *Mycobacterium abscessus*, occurring 8 months post-transplantation [163]. Disseminated infections due to *Nocardia* species have been reported. In an adult patient with an isolated small intestinal transplant, prostatitis and bacteremia due to *Nocardia asteroides* complex were reported [164]. The patient was successfully treated with ceftriaxone and trimethoprim-sulfamethoxazole [164]. We have observed another patient at our center who had undergone a multivisceral transplantation and then developed disseminated infection due to *Nocardia asteroides* involving the lungs and the central nervous system. This patient was successfully treated with a prolonged course of meropenem and trimethoprim-sulfamethoxazole.

The most common viral infections have already been discussed previously. Notably, in one small case series (n = 11), infections due to human herpesvirus 6 have not been reported in a patient population that was not receiving valganciclovir prophylaxis [165]. However in another case series (n = 27), two cases of HHV-6 have been reported in two pediatric small intestinal transplant recipients presenting with pancytopenia and encephalitis which responded to ganciclovir [163]. In that same case series, there was one case of BK polyoma virus infection that presented with hemorrhagic cystitis and viremia occurring 5 months after small intestinal transplantation [163].

Conclusion

Intestinal and multivisceral transplantation have become effective treatment options for patients with irreversible intestinal failure although the immunological and infectious challenges remain significant. Effective antiviral, antibacterial, and antifungal agents are now available and significantly reduce the morbidity risk in intestinal transplant recipients. Advances in understanding the immunological homeostasis of the gut will likely result in improved immunosuppressive regimens to manage intestinal allograft rejection and ultimately decrease the rates of infection in this population.

Acknowledgment Dr. Stuart S Kaufman, MD for endoscopic pictures, Dr. Therese Cermak, MD for histology slides, and Michele Malloy for editorial assistance.

References

1. Fishbein TM. Intestinal transplantation. N Engl J Med. 2009;361(10):998–1008. http://0-ovidsp.ovid.com.library.lausys.georgetown.edu/ovidweb.cgi?T=JS&CSC=Y&NEWS=N&PAGE=fulltext&D=medl&AN=19726774; http://catalog.library.georgetown.edu:4550/resserv?sid=OVID:medline&id=pmid:19726774&id=doi:&issn=0028-4793&isbn=&volume=361&issue=10&spage=998&pages=998-1008&date=2009&title=New+England+Journal+of+Medicine&atitle=Intestinal+transplantation.&aulast=Fishbein&pid=%3Cauthor%3EFishbein+TM%3C%2Fauthor%3E%3CAN%3E19726774%3C%2FAN%3E%3CDT%3EJournal+Article%3C%2FDT%3E.
2. Intestinal Transplant Association. Intestinal transplant registry report. 2009.
3. Centers for Medicare & Medicaid Services. Centers for medicare & medicaid services. http://www.cms.gov/. Updated 2012. Accessed 8/16/2012, 2012.
4. Harper SJF, Jamieson NV. Intestinal and multivisceral transplantation. Surgery. 2014;32(7):377–83.
5. Blackwell V, Holdaway L, Reddy S, et al. Careful donor selection reduces the risk of cytomegalovirus viraemia following intestinal transplant: the oxford experience. Transplantation. 2015;99(6):S75.
6. Martinez Rivera A, Wales PW. Intestinal transplantation in children: Current status. Pediatr Surg Int. 2016;32(6):529–40. https://doi.org/10.1007/s00383-016-3885-2.
7. Todo S, Tzakis A, Reyes J, et al. Small intestinal transplantation in humans with or without the colon. Transplantation. 1994;57(6):840–8.
8. Matsumoto CS, Kaufman SS, Fishbein TM. Inclusion of the colon in intestinal transplantation. Curr Opin Organ Transplant. 2011;16(3):312–5. http://0-ovidsp.ovid.com.library.lausys.georgetown.edu/ovidweb.cgi?T=JS&CSC=Y&NEWS=N&PAGE=fulltext&D=medl&AN=21467934; http://catalog.library.georgetown.edu:4550/resserv?sid=OVID:medline&id=pmid:21467934&id=doi:&issn=1087-2418&isbn=&volume=16&issue=3&spage=312&pages=312-5&date=2011&title=Current+Opinion+in+Organ+Transplantation&atitle=Inclusion+of+the+colon+in+intestinal+transplantation.&aulast=Matsumoto&pid=%3Cauthor%3EMatsumoto+CS%2CKaufman+SS%2CFishbein+TM%3C%2Fauthor%3E%3CAN%3E21467934%3C%2FAN%3E%3CDT%3EJournal+Article%3C%2FDT%3E.
9. Kato T, Selvaggi G, Gaynor JJ, et al. Inclusion of donor colon and ileocecal valve in intestinal transplantation. Transplantation. 2008;86(2):293–7. http://0-ovidsp.ovid.com.library.lausys.georgetown.edu/ovidweb.cgi?T=JS&CSC=Y&NEWS=N&PAGE=fulltext&D=medl&AN=18645493.
10. Todo S, Reyes J, Furukawa H, et al. Outcome analysis of 71 clinical intestinal transplantations. Ann Surg. 1995;222(3):270–80. http://0-ovidsp.ovid.com.library.lausys.georgetown.edu/ovidweb.cgi?T=JS&CSC=Y&NEWS=N&PAGE=fulltext&D=med3&AN=7677458.
11. Lee RG, Nakamura K, Tsamandas AC, et al. Pathology of human intestinal transplantation. Gastroenterology. 1996;110(6):1820–34. http://0-ovidsp.ovid.com.library.lausys.georgetown.edu/ovidweb.cgi?T=JS&CSC=Y&NEWS=N&PAGE=fulltext&D=med4&AN=8964408.
12. Wu T, Abu-Elmagd K, Bond G, Nalesnik MA, Randhawa P, Demetris AJ. A schema for histologic grading of small intestine allograft acute rejection. Transplantation. 2003;75(8):1241–8. http://0-ovidsp.ovid.com.library.lausys.georgetown.edu/ovidweb.cgi?T=JS&CSC=Y&NEWS=N&PAGE=fulltext&D=med4&AN=12717210.
13. Tsai HL, Island ER, Chang JW, et al. Association between donor-specific antibodies and acute rejection and resolution in small bowel and multivisceral transplantation. Transplantation. 2011;92(6):709–15. http://0-ovidsp.ovid.com.library.lausys.georgetown.edu/ovidweb.cgi?T=JS&CSC=Y&NEWS=N&PAGE=fulltext&D=medl&AN=21804443.
14. Dick AA, Horslen S. Antibody-mediated rejection after intestinal transplantation. Curr Opin Organ Transplant. 2012;17(3):250–7. https://doi.org/10.1097/MOT.0b013e3283533847.
15. Shulzhenko N, Morgun A, Hsiao W, et al. Crosstalk between B lymphocytes, microbiota and the intestinal epithelium governs immunity versus metabolism in the gut. Nat Med. 2011;17(12):1585–93. http://0-ovidsp.ovid.com.library.lausys.georgetown.edu/ovidweb.cgi?T=JS&CSC=Y&NEWS=N&PAGE=fulltext&D=medc&AN=22101768.
16. McDole JR, Wheeler LW, McDonald KG, et al. Goblet cells deliver luminal antigen to CD103+ dendritic cells in the small intestine. Nature. 2012;483(7389):345–9. http://0-ovidsp.ovid.com.library.lausys.georgetown.edu/ovidweb.cgi?T=JS&CSC=Y&NEWS=N&PAGE=fulltext&D=medl&AN=22422267.
17. Xavier RJ, Podolsky DK. Unravelling the pathogenesis of inflammatory bowel disease. Nature. 2007;448(7152):427–34. http://0-ovidsp.ovid.com.library.lausys.georgetown.edu/ovidweb.cgi?T=JS&CSC=Y&NEWS=N&PAGE=fulltext&D=med4&AN=17653185.
18. Smythies LE, Sellers M, Clements RH, et al. Human intestinal macrophages display profound inflammatory anergy despite avid phagocytic and bacteriocidal activity. J Clin Invest. 2005;115(1):66–75. http://0-ovidsp.ovid.com.library.lausys.georgetown.edu/ovidweb.cgi?T=JS&CSC=Y&NEWS=N&PAGE=fulltext&D=med4&AN=15630445; http://catalog.library.georgetown.edu:4550/resserv?sid=OVID:medline&id=pmid:15630445&id=doi:&issn=0021-9738&isbn=&volume=115&issue=1&spage=66&pages=66-75&date=2005&title=Journal+of+Clinical+Investigation&atitle=Human+intestinal+macrophages+display+profound+inflammatory+anergy+despite+avid+phagocytic+and+bacteriocidal+activity.&aulast=Smythies&pid=%3Cauthor%3ESmythies+LE%2CSellers+M%2CClements+RH%2CMosteller-Barnum+M%2CMeng+G%2CBenjamin+WH%2COrenstein+JM%2CSmith+PD%3C%2Fauthor%3E%3CAN%3E15630445%3C%2FAN%3E%3CDT%3EJournal+Article%3C%2FDT%3E.
19. Rescigno M, Rotta G, Valzasina B, Ricciardi-Castagnoli P. Dendritic cells shuttle microbes across gut epithelial monolayers. Immunobiology. 2001;204(5):572–81. http://0-ovidsp.ovid.com.library.lausys.georgetown.edu/ovidweb.cgi?T=JS&CSC=Y&NEWS=N&PAGE=fulltext&D=med4&AN=11846220.
20. Niess JH, Brand S, Gu X, et al. CX3CR1-mediated dendritic cell access to the intestinal lumen and bacterial clearance. Science. 2005;307(5707):254–8. http://0-ovidsp.ovid.com.library.lausys.georgetown.edu/ovidweb.cgi?T=JS&CSC=Y&NEWS=N&PAGE=fulltext&D=med4&AN=15653504.
21. Coombes JL, Siddiqui KR, Arancibia-Carcamo CV, et al. A functionally specialized population of mucosal CD103+ DCs induces Foxp3+ regulatory T cells via a TGF-beta and retinoic acid-dependent mechanism. J Exp Med. 2007;204(8):1757–64. https://doi.org/10.1084/jem.20070590.
22. Lough D, Abdo J, Guerra-Castro JF, et al. Abnormal CX3CR1+ lamina propria myeloid cells from intestinal transplant recipients with NOD2 mutations. Am J Transplant. 2012;12(4):992–1003. http://0-ovidsp.ovid.com.library.lausys.georgetown.edu/ovidweb.cgi?T=JS&CSC=Y&NEWS=N&PAGE=fulltext&D=medl&AN=22233287.
23. Tesmer LA, Lundy SK, Sarkar S, Fox DA. Th17 cells in human disease. Immunol Rev. 2008;223:87–113. http://0-ovidsp.ovid.com.library.lausys.georgetown.edu/ovidweb.cgi?T=JS&CSC=Y&NEWS=N&PAGE=fulltext&D=medl&AN=18613831.
24. Liang SC, Tan XY, Luxenberg DP, et al. Interleukin (IL)-22 and IL-17 are coexpressed by Th17 cells and cooperatively

enhance expression of antimicrobial peptides. J Exp Med. 2006;203(10):2271–9. http://0-ovidsp.ovid.com.library.lausys.georgetown.edu/ovidweb.cgi?T=JS&CSC=Y&NEWS=N&PAGE=fulltext&D=med4&AN=16982811; http://catalog.library.georgetown.edu:4550/resserv?sid=OVID:medline&id=pmid:16982811&id=doi:&issn=0022-1007&isbn=&volume=203&issue=10&spage=2271&pages=2271-9&date=2006&title=Journal+of+Experimental+Medicine&atitle=Interleukin+%28IL%29-22+and+IL-17+are+coexpressed+by+Th17+cells+and+cooperatively+enhance+expression+of+antimicrobial+peptides.&aulast=Liang&pid=%3Cauthor%3ELiang+SC%2CTan+XY%2CLuxenberg+DP%2CKarim+R%2CDunussi-Joannopoulos+K%2CCollins+M%2CFouser+LA%3C%2Fauthor%3E%3CAN%3E16982811%3C%2FAN%3E%3CDT%3EComparative+Study%3C%2FDT%3E.

25. Korn T, Oukka M, Kuchroo V, Bettelli E. Th17 cells: effector T cells with inflammatory properties. Semin Immunol. 2007;19(6):362–71. https://doi.org/10.1016/j.smim.2007.10.007.
26. Rubino SJ, Geddes K, Girardin SE. Innate IL-17 and IL-22 responses to enteric bacterial pathogens. Trends Immunol. 2012;33(3):112–8. http://0-ovidsp.ovid.com.library.lausys.georgetown.edu/ovidweb.cgi?T=JS&CSC=Y&NEWS=N&PAGE=fulltext&D=medl&AN=22342740; http://catalog.library.georgetown.edu:4550/resserv?sid=OVID:medline&id=pmid:22342740&id=doi:&issn=1471-4906&isbn=&volume=33&issue=3&spage=112&pages=112-8&date=2012&title=Trends+in+Immunology&atitle=Innate+IL-17+and+IL-22+responses+to+enteric+bacterial+pathogens.&aulast=Rubino&pid=%3Cauthor%3ERubino+SJ%2CGeddes+K%2CGirardin+SE%3C%2Fauthor%3E%3CAN%3E22342740%3C%2FAN%3E%3CDT%3EJournal+Article%3C%2FDT%3E.
27. Brenchley JM, Douek DC. Microbial translocation across the GI tract. Annu Rev Immunol. 2012;30:149–73. https://doi.org/10.1146/annurev-immunol-020711-075001.
28. Molloy MJ, Bouladoux N, Belkaid Y. Intestinal microbiota: shaping local and systemic immune responses. Semin Immunol. 2012;24(1):58–66. https://doi.org/10.1016/j.smim.2011.11.008.
29. Shanahan F. The host-microbe interface within the gut. Best Pract Res Clin Gastroenterol. 2002;16(6):915–31. http://0-ovidsp.ovid.com.library.lausys.georgetown.edu/ovidweb.cgi?T=JS&CSC=Y&NEWS=N&PAGE=fulltext&D=med4&AN=12473298.
30. Umesaki Y, Okada Y, Matsumoto S, Imaoka A, Setoyama H. Segmented filamentous bacteria are indigenous intestinal bacteria that activate intraepithelial lymphocytes and induce MHC class II molecules and fucosyl asialo GM1 glycolipids on the small intestinal epithelial cells in the ex-germ-free mouse. Microbiol Immunol. 1995;39(8):555–62. http://0-ovidsp.ovid.com.library.lausys.georgetown.edu/ovidweb.cgi?T=JS&CSC=Y&NEWS=N&PAGE=fulltext&D=med3&AN=7494493.
31. Bouskra D, Brezillon C, Berard M, et al. Lymphoid tissue genesis induced by commensals through NOD1 regulates intestinal homeostasis. Nature. 2008;456(7221):507–10. http://0-ovidsp.ovid.com.library.lausys.georgetown.edu/ovidweb.cgi?T=JS&CSC=Y&NEWS=N&PAGE=fulltext&D=medl&AN=18987631.
32. Oh PL, Martinez I, Sun Y, Walter J, Peterson DA, Mercer DF. Characterization of the ileal microbiota in rejecting and nonrejecting recipients of small bowel transplants. Am J Transplant. 2012;12(3):753–62. http://0-ovidsp.ovid.com.library.lausys.georgetown.edu/ovidweb.cgi?T=JS&CSC=Y&NEWS=N&PAGE=fulltext&D=medl&AN=22152019.
33. Palmer KR, Duerden BI, Holdsworth CD. Bacteriological and endotoxin studies in cases of ulcerative colitis submitted to surgery. Gut. 1980;21(10):851–4. http://0-ovidsp.ovid.com.library.lausys.georgetown.edu/ovidweb.cgi?T=JS&CSC=Y&NEWS=N&PAGE=fulltext&D=med2&AN=7439804; http://catalog.library.georgetown.edu:4550/resserv?sid=OVID:medline&id=pmid:7439804&id=doi:&issn=0017-5749&isbn=&volume=21&issue=10&spage=851&pages=851-4&date=1980&title=Gut&atitle=Bacteriological+and+endotoxin+studies+in+cases+of+ulcerative+colitis+submitted+to+surgery.&aulast=Palmer&pid=%3Cauthor%3EPalmer+KR%2CDuerden+BI%2CHoldsworth+CD%3C%2Fauthor%3E%3CAN%3E7439804%3C%2FAN%3E%3CDT%3EJournal+Article%3C%2FDT%3E.
34. Scheifele DW, Olsen EM, Pendray MR. Endotoxinemia and thrombocytopenia during neonatal necrotizing enterocolitis. Am J Clin Pathol. 1985;83(2):227–9.
35. Bucher BT, McDuffie LA, Shaikh N, et al. Bacterial DNA content in the intestinal wall from infants with necrotizing enterocolitis. J Pediatr Surg. 2011;46(6):1029–33. https://doi.org/10.1016/j.jpedsurg.2011.03.026.
36. Rothman D, Latham MC, Walker WA. Transport of macromolecules in malnourished animals:: I. evidence for increased uptake of intestinal antigens. Nutr Res. 1982;2(4):467–73.
37. Cicalese L, Sileri P, Green M, Abu-Elmagd K, Kocoshis S, Reyes J. Bacterial translocation in clinical intestinal transplantation. Transplantation. 2001;71(10):1414–7. http://0-ovidsp.ovid.com.library.lausys.georgetown.edu/ovidweb.cgi?T=JS&CSC=Y&NEWS=N&PAGE=fulltext&D=med4&AN=11391228; http://catalog.library.georgetown.edu:4550/resserv?sid=OVID:medline&id=pmid:11391228&id=doi:&issn=0041-1337&isbn=&volume=71&issue=10&spage=1414&pages=1414-7&date=2001&title=Transplantation&atitle=Bacterial+translocation+in+clinical+intestinal+transplantation.&aulast=Cicalese&pid=%3Cauthor%3ECicalese+L%2CSileri+P%2CGreen+M%2CAbu-Elmagd+K%2CKocoshis+S%2CReyes+J%3C%2Fauthor%3E%3CAN%3E11391228%3C%2FAN%3E%3CDT%3EJournal+Article%3C%2FDT%3E.
38. Guaraldi G, Cocchi S, Codeluppi M, et al. Outcome, incidence, and timing of infectious complications in small bowel and multivisceral organ transplantation patients. Transplantation. 2005;80(12):1742–8. http://0-ovidsp.ovid.com.library.lausys.georgetown.edu/ovidweb.cgi?T=JS&CSC=Y&NEWS=N&PAGE=fulltext&D=med4&AN=16378070; http://catalog.library.georgetown.edu:4550/resserv?sid=OVID:medline&id=pmid:16378070&id=doi:&issn=0041-1337&isbn=&volume=80&issue=12&spage=1742&pages=1742-8&date=2005&title=Transplantation&atitle=Outcome%2C+incidence%2C+and+timing+of+infectious+complications+in+small+bowel+and+multivisceral+organ+transplantation+patients.&aulast=Guaraldi&pid=%3Cauthor%3EGuaraldi+G%2CCocchi+S%2CCodeluppi+M%2CDi+Benedetto+F%2CDe+Ruvo+N%2CMasetti+M%2CVenturelli+C%2CPecorari+M%2CPinna+AD%2CEsposito+R%3C%2Fauthor%3E%3CAN%3E16378070%3C%2FAN%3E%3CDT%3EJournal+Article%3C%2FDT%3E.
39. Kaushal M, Carlson GL. Management of enterocutaneous fistulas. Clin Colon Rectal Surg. 2004;17(2):79–88. https://doi.org/10.1055/s-2004-828654.
40. Soeters PB, Ebeid AM, Fischer JE. Review of 404 patients with gastrointestinal fistulas. Impact of parenteral nutrition. Ann Surg. 1979;190(2):189–202. http://0-ovidsp.ovid.com.library.lausys.georgetown.edu/ovidweb.cgi?T=JS&CSC=Y&NEWS=N&PAGE=fulltext&D=med1&AN=111638.
41. McLauchlan GJ, Anderson ID, Grant IS, Fearon KC. Outcome of patients with abdominal sepsis treated in an intensive care unit. Br J Surg. 1995;82(4):524–9. http://0-ovidsp.ovid.com.library.lausys.georgetown.edu/ovidweb.cgi?T=JS&CSC=Y&NEWS=N&PAGE=fulltext&D=med3&AN=7613902.
42. Thomas HA. Radiologic investigation and treatment of gastrointestinal fistulas. Surg Clin North Am. 1996;76(5):1081–94.
43. Kwon SH, Oh JH, Kim HJ, Park SJ, Park HC. Interventional management of gastrointestinal fistulas. Korean J Radiol. 2008;9(6):541–9. http://0-ovidsp.ovid.com.library.lausys.georgetown.edu/ovidweb.

cgi?T=JS&CSC=Y&NEWS=N&PAGE=fulltext&D=medl&AN=19039271.
44. Paterson DL. The epidemiological profile of infections with multidrug-resistant pseudomonas aeruginosa and acinetobacter species. Clin Infect Dis. 2006;43(Suppl 2):S43–8. http://0-ovidsp.ovid.com.library.lausys.georgetown.edu/ovidweb.cgi?T=JS&CSC=Y&NEWS=N&PAGE=fulltext&D=med4&AN=16894514.
45. Jacobson KL, Cohen SH, Inciardi JF, et al. The relationship between antecedent antibiotic use and resistance to extended-spectrum cephalosporins in group I beta-lactamase-producing organisms. Clin Infect Dis. 1995;21(5):1107–13.
46. Fraimow HS, Tsigrelis C. Antimicrobial resistance in the intensive care unit: mechanisms, epidemiology, and management of specific resistant pathogens. Crit Care Clin. 2011;27(1):163–205. https://doi.org/10.1016/j.ccc.2010.11.002.
47. Santos JI. Nutrition, infection, and immunocompetence. Infect Dis Clin N Am. 1994;8(1):243–67.
48. Savendahl L, Underwood LE. Decreased interleukin-2 production from cultured peripheral blood mononuclear cells in human acute starvation. J Clin Endocrinol Metab. 1997;82(4):1177–80.
49. Garg M, Jones RM, Vaughan RB, Testro AG. Intestinal transplantation: Current status and future directions. J Gastroenterol Hepatol. 2011;26(8):1221–8. http://0-ovidsp.ovid.com.library.lausys.georgetown.edu/ovidweb.cgi?T=JS&CSC=Y&NEWS=N&PAGE=fulltext&D=medl&AN=21595748; http://catalog.library.georgetown.edu:4550/resserv?sid=OVID:medline&id=pmid:21595748&id=doi:10.1111%2Fj.1440-1746.2011.06783.x&issn=0815-9319&isbn=&volume=26&issue=8&spage=1221&pages=1221-8&date=2011&title=Journal+of+Gastroenterology+%26+Hepatology&atitle=Intestinal+transplantation%3A+current+status+and+future+directions.&aulast=Garg&pid=%3Cauthor%3EGarg+M%2CJones+RM%2CVaughan+RB%2CTestro+AG%3C%2Fauthor%3E%3CAN%3E21595748%3C%2FAN%3E%3CDT%3EJournal+Article%3C%2FDT%3E.
50. Carbone J, Micheloud D, Salcedo M, et al. Humoral and cellular immune monitoring might be useful to identify liver transplant recipients at risk for development of infection. Transpl Infect Dis. 2008;10(6):396–402. https://doi.org/10.1111/j.1399-3062.2008.00329.x.
51. Altin M, Rajkovic IA, Hughes RD, Williams R. Neutrophil adherence in chronic liver disease and fulminant hepatic failure. Gut. 1983;24(8):746–50. http://0-ovidsp.ovid.com.library.lausys.georgetown.edu/ovidweb.cgi?T=JS&CSC=Y&NEWS=N&PAGE=fulltext&D=med2&AN=6873736.
52. Seki S, Habu Y, Kawamura T, et al. The liver as a crucial organ in the first line of host defense: the roles of kupffer cells, natural killer (NK) cells and NK1.1 ag+ T cells in T helper 1 immune responses. Immunol Rev. 2000;174:35–46. http://0-ovidsp.ovid.com.library.lausys.georgetown.edu/ovidweb.cgi?T=JS&CSC=Y&NEWS=N&PAGE=fulltext&D=med4&AN=10807505.
53. Tokars JI, Cookson ST, McArthur MA, Boyer CL, McGeer AJ, Jarvis WR. Prospective evaluation of risk factors for bloodstream infection in patients receiving home infusion therapy. Ann Intern Med. 1999;131(5):340–7. http://0-ovidsp.ovid.com.library.lausys.georgetown.edu/ovidweb.cgi?T=JS&CSC=Y&NEWS=N&PAGE=fulltext&D=med4&AN=10475886.
54. Ishizuka M, Nagata H, Takagi K, Kubota K. Total parenteral nutrition is a major risk factor for central venous catheter-related bloodstream infection in colorectal cancer patients receiving post-operative chemotherapy. Eur Surg Res. 2008;41(4):341–5. http://0-ovidsp.ovid.com.library.lausys.georgetown.edu/ovidweb.cgi?T=JS&CSC=Y&NEWS=N&PAGE=fulltext&D=medl&AN=18841020.
55. Mohammed A, Grant FK, Zhao VM, Shane AL, Ziegler TR, Cole CR. Characterization of posthospital bloodstream infections in children requiring home parenteral nutrition. J Parenter Enter Nutr. 2011;35(5):581–7. http://0-ovidsp.ovid.com.library.lausys.georgetown.edu/ovidweb.cgi?T=JS&CSC=Y&NEWS=N&PAGE=fulltext&D=medl&AN=21799191.
56. Sondheimer JM, Asturias E, Cadnapaphornchai M. Infection and cholestasis in neonates with intestinal resection and long-term parenteral nutrition. J Pediatr Gastroenterol Nutr. 1998;27(2):131–7. http://0-ovidsp.ovid.com.library.lausys.georgetown.edu/ovidweb.cgi?T=JS&CSC=Y&NEWS=N&PAGE=fulltext&D=med4&AN=9702641.
57. Beath SV, Davies P, Papadopoulou A, et al. Parenteral nutrition-related cholestasis in postsurgical neonates: multivariate analysis of risk factors. J Pediatr Surg. 1996;31(4):604–6. http://0-ovidsp.ovid.com.library.lausys.georgetown.edu/ovidweb.cgi?T=JS&CSC=Y&NEWS=N&PAGE=fulltext&D=med4&AN=8801324.
58. Marra AR, Opilla M, Edmond MB, Kirby DF. Epidemiology of bloodstream infections in patients receiving long-term total parenteral nutrition. J Clin Gastroenterol. 2007;41(1):19–28. http://0-ovidsp.ovid.com.library.lausys.georgetown.edu/ovidweb.cgi?T=JS&CSC=Y&NEWS=N&PAGE=fulltext&D=med4&AN=17198060.
59. Matsumoto C, Kaufman S, Fennelly E, Davis J, Gupta P, Fishbein TM. Impact of positive preoperative surveillance blood cultures from chronic indwelling catheters in cadaveric intestinal transplant recipients. Transplant Proc. 2006;38(6):1676–7. http://0-ovidsp.ovid.com.library.lausys.georgetown.edu/ovidweb.cgi?T=JS&CSC=Y&NEWS=N&PAGE=fulltext&D=med4&AN=16908244.
60. Wisplinghoff H, Bischoff T, Tallent SM, Seifert H, Wenzel RP, Edmond MB. Nosocomial bloodstream infections in US hospitals: analysis of 24,179 cases from a prospective nationwide surveillance study. Clin Infect Dis. 2004;39(3):309–17. http://0-ovidsp.ovid.com.library.lausys.georgetown.edu/ovidweb.cgi?T=JS&CSC=Y&NEWS=N&PAGE=fulltext&D=med4&AN=15306996.
61. Ostrowsky BE, Whitener C, Bredenberg HK, et al. Serratia marcescens bacteremia traced to an infused narcotic. N Engl J Med. 2002;346(20):1529–37. http://0-ovidsp.ovid.com.library.lausys.georgetown.edu/ovidweb.cgi?T=JS&CSC=Y&NEWS=N&PAGE=fulltext&D=med4&AN=12015392.
62. Centers for Disease Control and Prevention (CDC): Morbidity and Mortality Weekly Report. *Pseudomonas* bloodstream infections associated with a heparin/saline flush --- missouri, new york, texas, and michigan, 2004--2005 http://www.cdc.gov/mmwr/preview/mmwrhtml/mm5411a1.htm. Updated 2005. Accessed 8/3/2012, 2012.
63. Maki DG. Infections due to infusion therapy. In: Jarvis WR, editor. Bennett and brachman's hospital infections. 5th ed. Philadelphia: Lippincott Williams & Wilkins; 2007.
64. Plouffe JF, Brown DG, Silva J Jr, Eck T, Stricof RL, Fekety FR Jr. Nosocomial outbreak of *candida parapsilosis* fungemia related to intravenous infusions. Arch Intern Med. 1977;137(12):1686–9. http://0-ovidsp.ovid.com.library.lausys.georgetown.edu/ovidweb.cgi?T=JS&CSC=Y&NEWS=N&PAGE=fulltext&D=med1&AN=412474.
65. Solomon SL, Khabbaz RF, Parker RH, et al. An outbreak of *candida parapsilosis* bloodstream infections in patients receiving parenteral nutrition. J Infect Dis. 1984;149(1):98–102. http://0-ovidsp.ovid.com.library.lausys.georgetown.edu/ovidweb.cgi?T=JS&CSC=Y&NEWS=N&PAGE=fulltext&D=med2&AN=6420478.
66. Pappas PG, Kauffman CA, Andes D, et al. Clinical practice guidelines for the management of candidiasis: 2009 update by the infectious diseases society of america. Clin Infect Dis. 2009;48(5):503–35.
67. Pappas PG, Rex JH, Lee J, et al. A prospective observational study of candidemia: epidemiology, therapy, and influences on mortality in hospitalized adult and pediatric patients. Clin Infect Dis. 2003;37(5):634–43. http://0-ovidsp.ovid.com.library.lausys.georgetown.edu/ovidweb.cgi?T=JS&CSC=Y&NEWS=N&PAGE=fulltext&D=med4&AN=12942393.

68. Tortorano AM, Peman J, Bernhardt H, et al. Epidemiology of candidaemia in europe: results of 28-month european confederation of medical mycology (ECMM) hospital-based surveillance study. Eur J Clin Microbiol Infect Dis. 2004;23(4):317–22. http://0-ovidsp.ovid.com.library.lausys.georgetown.edu/ovidweb.cgi?T=JS&CSC=Y&NEWS=N&PAGE=fulltext&D=med4&AN=15029512.
69. Trick WE, Fridkin SK, Edwards JR, Hajjeh RA, Gaynes RP, National Nosocomial Infections Surveillance System Hospitals. Secular trend of hospital-acquired candidemia among intensive care unit patients in the united states during 1989–1999. Clin Infect Dis. 2002;35(5):627–30. http://0-ovidsp.ovid.com.library.lausys.georgetown.edu/ovidweb.cgi?T=JS&CSC=Y&NEWS=N&PAGE=fulltext&D=med4&AN=12173140.
70. Curry CR, Quie PG. Fungal septicemia in patients receiving parenteral hyperalimentation. N Engl J Med. 1971;285(22):1221–5. http://0-ovidsp.ovid.com.library.lausys.georgetown.edu/ovidweb.cgi?T=JS&CSC=Y&NEWS=N&PAGE=fulltext&D=med1&AN=5000319.
71. Henderson DK, Edwards JE Jr, Montgomerie JZ. Hematogenous candida endophthalmitis in patients receiving parenteral hyperalimentation fluids. J Infect Dis. 1981;143(5):655–61. http://0-ovidsp.ovid.com.library.lausys.georgetown.edu/ovidweb.cgi?T=JS&CSC=Y&NEWS=N&PAGE=fulltext&D=med2&AN=6787141.
72. Montgomerie JZ, Edwards JE Jr. Association of infection due to *candida albicans* with intravenous hyperalimentation. J Infect Dis. 1978;137(2):197–201. http://0-ovidsp.ovid.com.library.lausys.georgetown.edu/ovidweb.cgi?T=JS&CSC=Y&NEWS=N&PAGE=fulltext&D=med1&AN=415098.
73. Mermel LA, Allon M, Bouza E, et al. Clinical practice guidelines for the diagnosis and management of intravascular catheter-related infection: 2009 update by the infectious diseases society of america. Clin Infect Dis. 2009;49(1):1–45. http://0-ovidsp.ovid.com.library.lausys.georgetown.edu/ovidweb.cgi?T=JS&CSC=Y&NEWS=N&PAGE=fulltext&D=medl&AN=19489710.
74. Fortun J, Grill F, Martin-Davila P, et al. Treatment of long-term intravascular catheter-related bacteraemia with antibiotic-lock therapy. J Antimicrob Chemother. 2006;58(4):816–21. http://0-ovidsp.ovid.com.library.lausys.georgetown.edu/ovidweb.cgi?T=JS&CSC=Y&NEWS=N&PAGE=fulltext&D=med4&AN=16899468.
75. Rijnders BJ, Van Wijngaerden E, Vandecasteele SJ, Stas M, Peetermans WE. Treatment of long-term intravascular catheter related bacteraemia with antibiotic lock: randomized, placebo-controlled trial. J Antimicrob Chemother. 2005;55(1):90–4. https://doi.org/10.1093/jac/dkh488.
76. Onder AM, Kato T, Simon N, et al. Prevention of catheter-related bacteremia in pediatric intestinal transplantation/short gut syndrome children with long-term central venous catheters. Pediatr Transplant. 2007;11(1):87–93. https://doi.org/10.1111/j.1399-3046.2006.00634.x.
77. Casas S, Munoz L, Moure R, et al. Comparison of the 2-step tuberculin skin test and the quantiFERON-TB gold in-tube test for the screening of tuberculosis infection before liver transplantation. Liver Transpl. 2011;17(10):1205–11. http://0-ovidsp.ovid.com.library.lausys.georgetown.edu/ovidweb.cgi?T=JS&CSC=Y&NEWS=N&PAGE=fulltext&D=medl&AN=22279622.
78. Theodoropoulos N, Lanternier F, Rassiwala J, et al. Use of the QuantiFERON-TB gold interferon-gamma release assay for screening transplant candidates: a single-center retrospective study. Transpl Infect Dis. 2012;14(1):1–8. http://0-ovidsp.ovid.com.library.lausys.georgetown.edu/ovidweb.cgi?T=JS&CSC=Y&NEWS=N&PAGE=fulltext&D=medl&AN=21883759.
79. John M, Gondolesi G, Herold BC, Kaufman S, Fishbein T, Posada R. Impact of surveillance stool culture guided selection of antibiotics in the management of pediatric small bowel transplant recipients. Pediatr Transplant. 2006;10(2):198–204. http://0-ovidsp.ovid.com.library.lausys.georgetown.edu/ovidweb.cgi?T=JS&CSC=Y&NEWS=N&PAGE=fulltext&D=med4&AN=16573607.
80. Danzinger-Isakov L, Kumar D, AST Infectious Diseases Community of Practice. Guidelines for vaccination of solid organ transplant candidates and recipients. Am J Transplant. 2009;9(Suppl 4):S258–62. http://0-ovidsp.ovid.com.library.lausys.georgetown.edu/ovidweb.cgi?T=JS&CSC=Y&NEWS=N&PAGE=fulltext&D=medl&AN=20070687.
81. Fishman JA. Infection in solid-organ transplant recipients. N Engl J Med. 2007;357(25):2601–14. http://0-ovidsp.ovid.com.library.lausys.georgetown.edu/ovidweb.cgi?T=JS&CSC=Y&NEWS=N&PAGE=fulltext&D=med4&AN=18094380.
82. Abu-Elmagd KM, Costa G, Bond GJ, et al. Evolution of the immunosuppressive strategies for the intestinal and multivisceral recipients with special reference to allograft immunity and achievement of partial tolerance. Transplant Int. 2009;22(1):96–109. http://0-ovidsp.ovid.com.library.lausys.georgetown.edu/ovidweb.cgi?T=JS&CSC=Y&NEWS=N&PAGE=fulltext&D=medl&AN=18954362; http://catalog.library.georgetown.edu:4550/resserv?sid=OVID:medline&id=pmid:18954362&id=doi:&issn=0934-0874&isbn=&volume=22&issue=1&spage=96&pages=96-109&date=2009&title=Transplant+International&atitle=Evolution+of+the+immunosuppressive+strategies+for+the+intestinal+and+multivisceral+recipients+with+special+reference+to+allograft+immunity+and+achievement+of+partial+tolerance.&aulast=Abu-Elmagd&pid=%3Cauthor%3EAbu-Elmagd+KM%2CCosta+G%2CBond+GJ%2CWu+T%2CMurase+N%2CZeevi+A%2CSimmons+R%2CSoltys+K%2CSindhi+R%2CStein+W%2CDemetris+A%2CMazariegos+G%3C%2Fauthor%3E%3CAN%3E18954362%3C%2FAN%3E%3CDT%3EJournal+Article%3C%2FDT%3E.
83. Loinaz C, Kato T, Nishida S, et al. Bacterial infections after intestine and multivisceral transplantation. the experience of the university of miami (1994–2001). Hepatogastroenterology. 2006;53(68):234–42. http://0-ovidsp.ovid.com.library.lausys.georgetown.edu/ovidweb.cgi?T=JS&CSC=Y&NEWS=N&PAGE=fulltext&D=med4&AN=16608031; http://catalog.library.georgetown.edu:4550/resserv?sid=OVID:medline&id=pmid:16608031&id=doi:&issn=0172-6390&isbn=&volume=53&issue=68&spage=234&pages=234-42&date=2006&title=Hepato-Gastroenterology&atitle=Bacterial+infections+after+intestine+and+multivisceral+transplantation.+The+experience+of+the+University+of+Miami+%281994-2001%29.&aulast=Loinaz&pid=%3Cauthor%3ELoinaz+C%2CKato+T%2CNishida+S%2CWeppler+D%2CLevi+D%2CDowdy+L%2CNery+JR%2CMittal+N%2CVianna+R%2CFortun+J%2CDe+la+Cruz+J%2CMadariaga+J%2CTzakis+A%3C%2Fauthor%3E%3CAN%3E16608031%3C%2FAN%3E%3CDT%3EJournal+Article%3C%2FDT%3E.
84. Primeggia J, Matsumoto CS, Fishbein TM, Karacki PS, Fredette TM, Timpone JG. Infection among adult small bowel and multivisceral transplant recipients in the 30-day postoperative period. Transpl Infect Dis. 2013;15(5):441–8.
85. Kimura T, Lauro A, Cescon M, et al. Impact of induction therapy on bacterial infections and long-term outcome in adult intestinal and multivisceral transplantation: a comparison of two different induction protocols: Daclizumab vs. alemtuzumab. Clin Transpl. 2009;23(3):420–5. http://0-ovidsp.ovid.com.library.lausys.georgetown.edu/ovidweb.cgi?T=JS&CSC=Y&NEWS=N&PAGE=fulltext&D=medl&AN=19537304.
86. Berg RD. Promotion of the translocation of enteric bacteria from the gastrointestinal tracts of mice by oral treatment with penicillin, clindamycin, or metronidazole. Infect Immun. 1981;33(3):854–61. http://0-ovidsp.ovid.com.library.lausys.georgetown.edu/ovidweb.cgi?T=JS&CSC=Y&NEWS=N&PAGE=fulltext&D=med2&AN=6456996.
87. Mainous M, Xu DZ, Lu Q, Berg RD, Deitch EA. Oral-TPN-induced bacterial translocation and impaired immune defenses are reversed

by refeeding. Surgery. 1991;110(2):277–83. http://0-ovidsp.ovid.com.library.lausys.georgetown.edu/ovidweb.cgi?T=JS&CSC=Y&NEWS=N&PAGE=fulltext&D=med3&AN=1907032.
88. Akhter K, Timpone J, Matsumoto C, Fishbein T, Kaufman S, Kumar P. Six-month incidence of bloodstream infections in intestinal transplant patients. Transpl Infect Dis. 2012;14(3):242–7. https://doi.org/10.1111/j.1399-3062.2011.00683.x.
89. Hartman AL, Lough DM, Barupal DK, et al. Human gut microbiome adopts an alternative state following small bowel transplantation. Proc Natl Acad Sci U S A. 2009;106(40):17187–92. http://0-ovidsp.ovid.com.library.lausys.georgetown.edu/ovidweb.cgi?T=JS&CSC=Y&NEWS=N&PAGE=fulltext&D=medl&AN=19805153.
90. Fishman JA, Issa NC. Infection in organ transplantation: Risk factors and evolving patterns of infection. Infect Dis Clin North Am. 2010;24(2):273–83. http://0-ovidsp.ovid.com.library.lausys.georgetown.edu/ovidweb.cgi?T=JS&CSC=Y&NEWS=N&PAGE=fulltext&D=medl&AN=20466270; http://catalog.library.georgetown.edu:4550/resserv?sid=OVID:medline&id=pmid:20466270&id=doi:&issn=0891-5520&isbn=&volume=24&issue=2&spage=273&pages=273-83&date=2010&title=Infectious+Disease+Clinics+of+North+America&atitle=Infection+in+organ+transplantation%3A+risk+factors+and+evolving+patterns+of+infection.&aulast=Fishman&pid=%3Cauthor%3EFishman+JA%2CIssa+NC%3C%2Fauthor%3E%3CAN%3E20466270%3C%2FAN%3E%3CDT%3EJournal+Article%3C%2FDT%3E.
91. Lee TK, Heeckt P, Smith SD, Lee KK, Rowe MI, Schraut WH. Postoperative selective bowel decontamination prevents gram-negative bacterial translocation in small-bowel graft recipients. J Surg Res. 1995;58(5):496–502. http://0-ovidsp.ovid.com.library.lausys.georgetown.edu/ovidweb.cgi?T=JS&CSC=Y&NEWS=N&PAGE=fulltext&D=med3&AN=7538186.
92. Green M, Barbadora K. Recovery of ceftazidime-resistant *klebsiella pneumoniae* from pediatric liver and intestinal transplant recipients. Pediatr Transplant. 1998;2(3):224–30. http://0-ovidsp.ovid.com.library.lausys.georgetown.edu/ovidweb.cgi?T=JS&CSC=Y&NEWS=N&PAGE=fulltext&D=med4&AN=10084747.
93. Dodds-Ashley E. Management of drug and food interactions with azole antifungal agents in transplant recipients. Pharmacotherapy. 2010;30(8):842–54. http://0-ovidsp.ovid.com.library.lausys.georgetown.edu/ovidweb.cgi?T=JS&CSC=Y&NEWS=N&PAGE=fulltext&D=medl&AN=20653361.
94. Kotton CN, Kumar D, Caliendo AM, et al. International consensus guidelines on the management of cytomegalovirus in solid organ transplantation. Transplantation. 2010;89(7):779–95. http://0-ovidsp.ovid.com.library.lausys.georgetown.edu/ovidweb.cgi?T=JS&CSC=Y&NEWS=N&PAGE=fulltext&D=medl&AN=20224515; http://catalog.library.georgetown.edu:4550/resserv?sid=OVID:medline&id=pmid:20224515&id=doi:&issn=0041-1337&isbn=&volume=89&issue=7&spage=779&pages=779-95&date=2010&title=Transplantation&atitle=International+consensus+guidelines+on+the+management+of+cytomegalovirus+in+solid+organ+transplantation.&aulast=Kotton&pid=%3Cauthor%3EKotton+CN%2CKumar+D%2CCaliendo+AM%2CAsberg+A%2CChou+S%2CSnydman+DR%2CAllen+U%2CHumar+A%2CTransplantation+Society+International+CMV+Consensus+Group%3C%2Fauthor%3E%3CAN%3E20224515%3C%2FAN%3E%3CDT%3EJournal+Article%3C%2FDT%3E.
95. Humar A, Snydman D, AST Infectious Diseases Community of Practice. Cytomegalovirus in solid organ transplant recipients. Am J Transplant. 2009;9(Suppl 4):S78–86. https://doi.org/10.1111/j.1600-6143.2009.02897.x.
96. Eid AJ, Razonable RR. New developments in the management of cytomegalovirus infection after solid organ transplantation. Drugs. 2010;70(8):965–81. https://doi.org/10.2165/10898540-000000000-00000.
97. Manez R, Kusne S, Green M, et al. Incidence and risk factors associated with the development of cytomegalovirus disease after intestinal transplantation. Transplantation. 1995;59(7):1010–4.
98. Bueno J, Green M, Kocoshis S, et al. Cytomegalovirus infection after intestinal transplantation in children. Clin Infect Dis. 1997;25(5):1078–83. http://0-ovidsp.ovid.com.library.lausys.georgetown.edu/ovidweb.cgi?T=JS&CSC=Y&NEWS=N&PAGE=fulltext&D=medc&AN=9402361.
99. Avsar Y, Cicinnati V, Kabar I, et al. Allograft failure in an intestinal graft recipient after cytomegalovirus disease without dnaemia. Transpl Int. 2013;26(Suppl 1):28–32.
100. Florescu DF, Langnas AN, Grant W, et al. Incidence, risk factors, and outcomes associated with cytomegalovirus disease in small bowel transplant recipients. Pediatr Transplant. 2012;16(3):294–301. https://doi.org/10.1111/j.1399-3046.2011.01628.x.
101. Timpone JG, Yimen M, Cox S, et al. Resistant cytomegalovirus in intestinal and multivisceral transplant recipients. Transpl Infect Dis. 2016;18(2):202–9. https://doi.org/10.1111/tid.12507.
102. Talmon GA. Histologic features of cytomegalovirus enteritis in small bowel allografts. Transplant Proc. 2010;42(7):2671–5. http://0-ovidsp.ovid.com.library.lausys.georgetown.edu/ovidweb.cgi?T=JS&CSC=Y&NEWS=N&PAGE=fulltext&D=medl&AN=20832567.
103. Ichihara H, Nakamae H, Hirose A, et al. Immunoglobulin prophylaxis against cytomegalovirus infection in patients at high risk of infection following allogeneic hematopoietic cell transplantation. Transplant Proc. 2011;43(10):3927–32. https://doi.org/10.1016/j.transproceed.2011.08.104.
104. Mor E, Meyers BR, Yagmur O, et al. High-dose acyclovir and intravenous immune globulin reduce the incidence of CMV disease after liver transplantation. Transplant Int. 1995;8(2):152–6. http://0-ovidsp.ovid.com.library.lausys.georgetown.edu/ovidweb.cgi?T=JS&CSC=Y&NEWS=N&PAGE=fulltext&D=med3&AN=7766298.
105. Florescu DF, Abu-Elmagd K, Mercer DF, Qiu F, Kalil AC. An international survey of cytomegalovirus prevention and treatment practices in intestinal transplantation. Transplantation. 2014;97(1):78–82. https://doi.org/10.1097/TP.0b013e3182a6baa2.
106. Nagai S, Mangus RS, Anderson E, et al. Cytomegalovirus infection after intestinal/multivisceral transplantation: a single-center experience with 210 cases. Transplantation. 2016;100(2):451–60. https://doi.org/10.1097/TP.0000000000000832.
107. Fortun Abete J, Martin-Davila P, Moreno S, Quijano Y, de Vicente E, Pou L. Pharmacokinetics of oral valganciclovir and intravenous ganciclovir administered to prevent cytomegalovirus disease in an adult patient receiving small-intestine transplantation. Antimicrob Agents Chemother. 2004;48(7):2782–3. http://0-ovidsp.ovid.com.library.lausys.georgetown.edu/ovidweb.cgi?T=JS&CSC=Y&NEWS=N&PAGE=fulltext&D=med4&AN=15215150.
108. Goldsmith PM, Husain MM, Carmichael A, Zhang H, Middleton SJ. Case report: multidrug-resistant cytomegalovirus in a modified multivisceral transplant recipient. Transplantation. 2012;93(7):e30–2. https://doi.org/10.1097/TP.0b013e318249b163.
109. Sagedal S, Nordal KP, Hartmann A, et al. The impact of cytomegalovirus infection and disease on rejection episodes in renal allograft recipients. Am J Transplant. 2002;2(9):850–6. http://0-ovidsp.ovid.com.library.lausys.georgetown.edu/ovidweb.cgi?T=JS&CSC=Y&NEWS=N&PAGE=fulltext&D=med4&AN=12392291.
110. Allen U, Preiksaitis J, AST Infectious Diseases Community of Practice. Epstein-barr virus and posttransplant lymphoproliferative disorder in solid organ transplant recipients. Am J Transplant. 2009;9(Suppl 4):S87–96. http://0-ovidsp.ovid.com.library.lausys.georgetown.edu/ovidweb.cgi?T=JS&CSC=Y&NEWS=N&PAGE=fulltext&D=medl&AN=20070701.

111. Kaufman S. Small intestinal transplantation. In: Kleinman RE, Walker WA, editors. Walker's pediatric gastrointestinal disease: physiology, diagnosis, management. Hamilton/Lewiston: BC Decker; 2008. p. 621.
112. Green M, Bueno J, Rowe D, et al. Predictive negative value of persistent low epstein-barr virus viral load after intestinal transplantation in children. Transplantation. 2000;70(4):593–6. http://0-ovidsp.ovid.com.library.lausys.georgetown.edu/ovidweb.cgi?T=JS&CSC=Y&NEWS=N&PAGE=fulltext&D=med4&AN=10972215.
113. Vrakas G, Arantes R, Day N, Reddy S, Friend P, Vaidya A. Post transplantation lymphoproliferative disorder after intestinal transplantation. Transplantation. 2014;98(Suppl 1):244
114. Gross TG. Management of posttransplant lymphoproliferative disease. In: Langnas AN, editor. Intestinal failure : diagnosis, management and transplantation. Malden: Blackwell Pub; 2008.
115. Opelz G, Dohler B. Lymphomas after solid organ transplantation: a collaborative transplant study report. Am J Transplant. 2004;4(2):222–30.http://0-ovidsp.ovid.com.library.lausys.georgetown.edu/ovidweb.cgi?T=JS&CSC=Y&NEWS=N&PAGE=fulltext&D=med4&AN=14974943.
116. Hryhorczuk AL, Kim HB, Harris MH, Vargas SO, Zurakowski D, Lee EY. Imaging findings in children with proliferative disorders following multivisceral transplantation. Pediatr Radiol. 2015;45(8):1138–45. https://doi.org/10.1007/s00247-015-3303-2.
117. Plant AS, Venick RS, Farmer DG, Upadhyay S, Said J, Kempert P. Plasmacytoma-like post-transplant lymphoproliferative disorder seen in pediatric combined liver and intestinal transplant recipients. Pediatr Blood Cancer. 2013;60(11):E137–9. https://doi.org/10.1002/pbc.24632.
118. Lauro A, Arpinati M, Pinna AD. Managing the challenge of PTLD in liver and bowel transplant recipients. Br J Haematol. 2015;169(2):157–72. https://doi.org/10.1111/bjh.13213.
119. Oertel SH, Verschuuren E, Reinke P, et al. Effect of anti-CD 20 antibody rituximab in patients with post-transplant lymphoproliferative disorder (PTLD). Am J Transplant. 2005;5(12):2901–6. http://0-ovidsp.ovid.com.library.lausys.georgetown.edu/ovidweb.cgi?T=JS&CSC=Y&NEWS=N&PAGE=fulltext&D=med4&AN=16303003.
120. Pescovitz MD. The use of rituximab, anti-CD20 monoclonal antibody, in pediatric transplantation. Pediatr Transplant. 2004;8(1):9–21. http://0-ovidsp.ovid.com.library.lausys.georgetown.edu/ovidweb.cgi?T=JS&CSC=Y&NEWS=N&PAGE=fulltext&D=med4&AN=15009836.
121. Pescovitz MD. Rituximab, an anti-cd20 monoclonal antibody: history and mechanism of action. Am J Transplant. 2006;6(5 Pt 1):859–66. http://0-ovidsp.ovid.com.library.lausys.georgetown.edu/ovidweb.cgi?T=JS&CSC=Y&NEWS=N&PAGE=fulltext&D=med4&AN=16611321.
122. Buell JF, Gross TG, Hanaway MJ, et al. Chemotherapy for post-transplant lymphoproliferative disorder: the Israel penn international transplant tumor registry experience. Transplant Proc. 2005;37(2):956–7. http://0-ovidsp.ovid.com.library.lausys.georgetown.edu/ovidweb.cgi?T=JS&CSC=Y&NEWS=N&PAGE=fulltext&D=med4&AN=15848588.
123. Gross TG, Bucuvalas JC, Park JR, et al. Low-dose chemotherapy for epstein-barr virus-positive post-transplantation lymphoproliferative disease in children after solid organ transplantation. J Clin Oncol. 2005;23(27):6481–8. http://0-ovidsp.ovid.com.library.lausys.georgetown.edu/ovidweb.cgi?T=JS&CSC=Y&NEWS=N&PAGE=fulltext&D=med4&AN=16170157.
124. Ziring D, Tran R, Edelstein S, et al. Infectious enteritis after intestinal transplantation: incidence, timing, and outcome. Transplantation. 2005;79(6):702–9. http://0-ovidsp.ovid.com.library.lausys.georgetown.edu/ovidweb.cgi?T=JS&CSC=Y&NEWS=N&PAGE=fulltext&D=med4&AN=15785377; http://catalog.library.georgetown.edu:4550/resserv?sid=OVID:medline&id=pmid:15785377&id=doi:&issn=0041-1337&isbn=&volume=79&issue=6&spage=702&pages=702-9&date=2005&title=Transplantation&atitle=Infectious+enteritis+after+intestinal+transplantation%3A+incidence%2C+timing%2C+and+outcome.&aulast=Ziring&pid=%3Cauthor%3EZiring+D%2CTran+R%2CEdelstein+S%2CMcDiarmid+SV%2CGajjar+N%2CCortina+G%2CVargas+J%2CRenz+JF%2CCherry+JD%2CKrogstad+P%2CMiller+M%2CBusuttil+RW%2CFarmer+DG%3C%2Fauthor%3E%3CAN%3E15785377%3C%2FAN%3E%3CDT%3EJournal+Article%3C%2FDT%3E.
125. McLaughlin GE, Delis S, Kashimawo L, et al. Adenovirus infection in pediatric liver and intestinal transplant recipients: utility of DNA detection by PCR. Am J Transplant. 2003;3(2):224–8. http://0-ovidsp.ovid.com.library.lausys.georgetown.edu/ovidweb.cgi?T=JS&CSC=Y&NEWS=N&PAGE=fulltext&D=med4&AN=12603217.
126. Pinchoff RJ, Kaufman SS, Magid MS, et al. Adenovirus infection in pediatric small bowel transplantation recipients. Transplantation. 2003;76(1):183–9. http://0-ovidsp.ovid.com.library.lausys.georgetown.edu/ovidweb.cgi?T=JS&CSC=Y&NEWS=N&PAGE=fulltext&D=med4&AN=12865807.
127. Berho M, Torroella M, Viciana A, et al. Adenovirus enterocolitis in human small bowel transplants. Pediatr Transplant. 1998;2(4):277–82. http://0-ovidsp.ovid.com.library.lausys.georgetown.edu/ovidweb.cgi?T=JS&CSC=Y&NEWS=N&PAGE=fulltext&D=med4&AN=10084729.
128. Florescu DF, Islam MK, Mercer DF, et al. Adenovirus infections in pediatric small bowel transplant recipients. Transplantation. 2010;90(2):198–204. http://0-ovidsp.ovid.com.library.lausys.georgetown.edu/ovidweb.cgi?T=JS&CSC=Y&NEWS=N&PAGE=fulltext&D=medl&AN=20467354.
129. Adeyi OA, Randhawa PA, Nalesnik MA, et al. Posttransplant adenoviral enteropathy in patients with small bowel transplantation. Arch Pathol Lab Med. 2008;132(4):703–5. http://0-ovidsp.ovid.com.library.lausys.georgetown.edu/ovidweb.cgi?T=JS&CSC=Y&NEWS=N&PAGE=fulltext&D=medl&AN=18384224.
130. Kaufman SS, Magid MS, Tschernia A, LeLeiko NS, Fishbein TM. Discrimination between acute rejection and adenoviral enteritis in intestinal transplant recipients. Transplant Proc. 2002;34(3):943–5. http://0-ovidsp.ovid.com.library.lausys.georgetown.edu/ovidweb.cgi?T=JS&CSC=Y&NEWS=N&PAGE=fulltext&D=med4&AN=12034252.
131. Ison MG, Green M, AST Infectious Diseases Community of Practice. Adenovirus in solid organ transplant recipients. Am J Transplant. 2009;9(Suppl 4):S161–5. http://0-ovidsp.ovid.com.library.lausys.georgetown.edu/ovidweb.cgi?T=JS&CSC=Y&NEWS=N&PAGE=fulltext&D=medl&AN=20070676.
132. Adeyi OA, Costa G, Abu-Elmagd KM, Wu T. Rotavirus infection in adult small intestine allografts: A clinicopathological study of a cohort of 23 patients. American Journal of Transplantation. 2010;10(12):2683–9. http://0-ovidsp.ovid.com.library.lausys.georgetown.edu/ovidweb.cgi?T=JS&CSC=Y&NEWS=N&PAGE=fulltext&D=medl&AN=21114645; http://catalog.library.georgetown.edu:4550/resserv?sid=OVID:medline&id=pmid:21114645&id=doi:10.1111%2Fj.1600-6143.2010.03311.x&issn=1600-6135&isbn=&volume=10&issue=12&spage=2683&pages=2683-9&date=2010&title=American+Journal+of+Transplantation&atitle=Rotavirus+infection+in+adult+small+intestine+allografts%3A+a+clinicopathological+study+of+a+cohort+of+23+patients.&aulast=Adeyi&pid=%3Cauthor%3EAdeyi+OA%2CCosta+G%2CAbu-Elmagd+KM%2CWu+T%3C%2Fauthor%3E%3CAN%3E21114645%3C%2FAN%3E%3CDT%3EJournal+Article%3C%2FDT%3E.
133. Kaufman SS, Chatterjee NK, Fuschino ME, et al. Calicivirus enteritis in an intestinal transplant recipient. Am J Transplant. 2003;3(6):764–8.

134. Kaufman SS, Chatterjee NK, Fuschino ME, et al. Characteristics of human calicivirus enteritis in intestinal transplant recipients. J Pediatr Gastroenterol Nutr. 2005;40(3):328–33. http://0-ovidsp.ovid.com.library.lausys.georgetown.edu/ovidweb.cgi?T=JS&CSC=Y&NEWS=N&PAGE=fulltext&D=med4&AN=15735487; http://catalog.library.georgetown.edu:4550/resserv?sid=OVID:medline&id=pmid:15735487&id=doi:&issn=0277-2116&isbn=&volume=40&issue=3&spage=328&pages=328-33&date=2005&title=Journal+of+Pediatric+Gastroenterology+%26+Nutrition&atitle=Characteristics+of+human+calicivirus+enteritis+in+intestinal+transplant+recipients.&aulast=Kaufman&pid=%3Cauthor%3EKaufman+SS%2CChatterjee+NK%2CFuschino+ME%2CMorse+DL%2CMorotti+RA%2CMagid+MS%2CGondolesi+GE%2CFlorman+SS%2CFishbein+TM%3C%2Fauthor%3E%3CAN%3E15735487%3C%2FAN%3E%3CDT%3ECase+Reports%3C%2FDT%3E.

135. Singh N. Antifungal prophylaxis for solid organ transplant recipients: seeking clarity amidst controversy. Clin Infect Dis. 2000;31(2):545–53. http://0-ovidsp.ovid.com.library.lausys.georgetown.edu/ovidweb.cgi?T=JS&CSC=Y&NEWS=N&PAGE=fulltext&D=med4&AN=10987719.

136. Kubak BM, Huprikar SS, AST Infectious Diseases Community of Practice. Emerging & rare fungal infections in solid organ transplant recipients. Am J Transplant. 2009;9(Suppl 4):S208–26. http://0-ovidsp.ovid.com.library.lausys.georgetown.edu/ovidweb.cgi?T=JS&CSC=Y&NEWS=N&PAGE=fulltext&D=medl&AN=20070683.

137. Brizendine KD, Vishin S, Baddley JW. Antifungal prophylaxis in solid organ transplant recipients. Expert Rev Antiinfect Ther. 2011;9(5):571–81. http://0-ovidsp.ovid.com.library.lausys.georgetown.edu/ovidweb.cgi?T=JS&CSC=Y&NEWS=N&PAGE=fulltext&D=medl&AN=21609268.

138. Pappas PG, Alexander BD, Andes DR, et al. Invasive fungal infections among organ transplant recipients: results of the transplant-associated infection surveillance network (TRANSNET). Clin Infect Dis. 2010;50(8):1101–11. http://0-ovidsp.ovid.com.library.lausys.georgetown.edu/ovidweb.cgi?T=JS&CSC=Y&NEWS=N&PAGE=fulltext&D=medl&AN=20218876.

139. Kusne S, Furukawa H, Abu-Elmagd K, et al. Infectious complications after small bowel transplantation in adults: an update. Transplant Proc. 1996;28(5):2761–2. http://0-ovidsp.ovid.com.library.lausys.georgetown.edu/ovidweb.cgi?T=JS&CSC=Y&NEWS=N&PAGE=fulltext&D=medc&AN=8908045.

140. Sauvat F, Dupic L, Caldari D, et al. Factors influencing outcome after intestinal transplantation in children. Transplant Proc. 2006;38(6):1689–91. http://0-ovidsp.ovid.com.library.lausys.georgetown.edu/ovidweb.cgi?T=JS&CSC=Y&NEWS=N&PAGE=fulltext&D=med4&AN=16908249.

141. Morrell M, Fraser VJ, Kollef MH. Delaying the empiric treatment of candida bloodstream infection until positive blood culture results are obtained: a potential risk factor for hospital mortality. Antimicrob Agents Chemother. 2005;49(9):3640–5. http://0-ovidsp.ovid.com.library.lausys.georgetown.edu/ovidweb.cgi?T=JS&CSC=Y&NEWS=N&PAGE=fulltext&D=med4&AN=16127033.

142. Singh N, Husain S, AST Infectious Diseases Community of Practice. Invasive aspergillosis in solid organ transplant recipients. Am J Transplant. 2009;9(Suppl 4):S180–91. http://0-ovidsp.ovid.com.library.lausys.georgetown.edu/ovidweb.cgi?T=JS&CSC=Y&NEWS=N&PAGE=fulltext&D=medl&AN=20070679.

143. Kohler S, Gerlach U, Guckelberger O, et al. Successful treatment of invasive sphenoidal, pulmonary and intracerebral aspergillosis after multivisceral transplantation. Transplant Int. 2009;22(5):589–91. http://0-ovidsp.ovid.com.library.lausys.georgetown.edu/ovidweb.cgi?T=JS&CSC=Y&NEWS=N&PAGE=fulltext&D=medl&AN=19175558.

144. Vianna R, Misra V, Fridell JA, Goldman M, Mangus RS, Tector J. Survival after disseminated invasive aspergillosis in a multivisceral transplant recipient. Transplant Proc. 2007;39(1):305–7. http://0-ovidsp.ovid.com.library.lausys.georgetown.edu/ovidweb.cgi?T=JS&CSC=Y&NEWS=N&PAGE=fulltext&D=med4&AN=17275530.

145. Singh N, Avery RK, Munoz P, et al. Trends in risk profiles for and mortality associated with invasive aspergillosis among liver transplant recipients. Clin Infect Dis. 2003;36(1):46–52. http://proxy.library.georgetown.edu/login?url=http://ovidsp.ovid.com/ovidweb.cgi?T=JS&CSC=Y&NEWS=N&PAGE=fulltext&D=med4&AN=12491201.

146. Gavalda J, Len O, San Juan R, Aguado JM, Fortun J, Lumbreras C, Moreno A, Munoz P, Blanes M, Ramos A, Rufi G, Gurgui M, Torre-Cisneros J, Montejo M, Cuenca-Estrella M, Rodriguez-Tudela JL, Pahissa A. RESITRA (Spanish Network for Research on Infection in Transplantation). Risk factors for invasive aspergillosis in solid-organ transplant recipients: a case-control study. Clin Infect Dis. 2005;41(1):52–9. http://proxy.library.georgetown.edu/login?url=http://ovidsp.ovid.com/ovidweb.cgi?T=JS&CSC=Y&NEWS=N&PAGE=fulltext&D=med4&AN=15937763.

147. Kusne S, Torre-Cisneros J, Manez R, et al. Factors associated with invasive lung aspergillosis and the significance of positive aspergillus culture after liver transplantation. J Infect Dis. 1992;166(6):1379–83. http://proxy.library.georgetown.edu/login?url=http://ovidsp.ovid.com/ovidweb.cgi?T=JS&CSC=Y&NEWS=N&PAGE=fulltext&D=med3&AN=1431256.

148. Osawa M, Ito Y, Hirai T, et al. Risk factors for invasive aspergillosis in living donor liver transplant recipients. Liver Transpl. 2007;13(4):566–70. http://proxy.library.georgetown.edu/login?url=http://ovidsp.ovid.com/ovidweb.cgi?T=JS&CSC=Y&NEWS=N&PAGE=fulltext&D=med4&AN=17394155.

149. George MJ, Snydman DR, Werner BG, et al. The independent role of cytomegalovirus as a risk factor for invasive fungal disease in orthotopic liver transplant recipients. Boston center for liver transplantation CMVIG-study group. Cytogam, MedImmune, Inc. Gaithersburg, Maryland. Am J Med. 1997;103(2):106–13. http://proxy.library.georgetown.edu/login?url=http://ovidsp.ovid.com/ovidweb.cgi?T=JS&CSC=Y&NEWS=N&PAGE=fulltext&D=med4&AN=9274893.

150. Collins LA, Samore MH, Roberts MS, et al. Risk factors for invasive fungal infections complicating orthotopic liver transplantation. J Infect Dis. 1994;170(3):644–52. http://proxy.library.georgetown.edu/login?url=http://ovidsp.ovid.com/ovidweb.cgi?T=JS&CSC=Y&NEWS=N&PAGE=fulltext&D=med3&AN=8077723.

151. Reyes J, Todo S, Green M, et al. Graft-versus-host disease after liver and small bowel transplantation in a child. Clin Transpl. 1997;11(5 Pt 1):345–8. http://0-ovidsp.ovid.com.library.lausys.georgetown.edu/ovidweb.cgi?T=JS&CSC=Y&NEWS=N&PAGE=fulltext&D=medc&AN=9361921.

152. Uemoto S, Fujimoto Y, Inomata Y, et al. Living-related small bowel transplantation: the first case in Japan. Pediatr Transplant. 1998;2(1):40–4. http://0-ovidsp.ovid.com.library.lausys.georgetown.edu/ovidweb.cgi?T=JS&CSC=Y&NEWS=N&PAGE=fulltext&D=med4&AN=10084759.

153. Campbell AL, Goldberg CL, Magid MS, Gondolesi G, Rumbo C, Herold BC. First case of toxoplasmosis following small bowel transplantation and systematic review of tissue-invasive toxoplasmosis following noncardiac solid organ transplantation. Transplantation. 2006;81(3):408–17. http://0-ovidsp.ovid.com.library.lausys.georgetown.edu/ovidweb.cgi?T=JS&CSC=Y&NEWS=N&PAGE=fulltext&D=med4&AN=16477228.

154. Gerber DA, Green M, Jaffe R, Greenberg D, Mazariegos G, Reyes J. Cryptosporidial infections after solid organ transplantation in children. Pediatr Transplant. 2000;4(1):50–5. http://0-ovidsp.

ovid.com.library.lausys.georgetown.edu/ovidweb.cgi?T=JS&CSC=Y&NEWS=N&PAGE=fulltext&D=med4&AN=10731059.

155. Gruz F, Fuxman C, Errea A, et al. Isospora belli infection after isolated intestinal transplant. Transpl Infect Dis. 2010;12(1):69–72. http://0-ovidsp.ovid.com.library.lausys.georgetown.edu/ovidweb.cgi?T=JS&CSC=Y&NEWS=N&PAGE=fulltext&D=medl&AN=19708892; http://catalog.library.georgetown.edu:4550/resserv?sid=OVID:medline&id=pmid:19708892&id=doi:&issn=1398-2273&isbn=&volume=12&issue=1&spage=69&pages=69-72&date=2010&title=Transplant+Infectious+Disease&atitle=Isospora+belli+infection+after+isolated+intestinal+transplant.&aulast=Gruz&pid=%3Cauthor%3EGruz+F%2CFuxman+C%2CErrea+A%2CTokumoto+M%2CFernandez+A%2CVelasquez+J%2CNagel+C%2CRuf+A%2CMaurino+E%2CNachman+F%2CRumbo+M%2CGondolesi+G%3C%2Fauthor%3E%3CAN%3E19708892%3C%2FAN%3E%3CDT%3ECase+Reports%3C%2FDT%3E.

156. Hsu CN, Tseng SH, Chang SW, Chen Y. *Strongyloides stercoralis* infection in an intestinal transplant recipient. Transpl Infect Dis. 2013;15(4):E139–43. https://doi.org/10.1111/tid.12104.

157. Patel G, Arvelakis A, Sauter BV, Gondolesi GE, Caplivski D, Huprikar S. Strongyloides hyperinfection syndrome after intestinal transplantation. Transpl Infect Dis. 2008;10(2):137–41. http://0-ovidsp.ovid.com.library.lausys.georgetown.edu/ovidweb.cgi?T=JS&CSC=Y&NEWS=N&PAGE=fulltext&D=medl&AN=17605735; http://catalog.library.georgetown.edu:4550/resserv?sid=OVID:medline&id=pmid:17605735&id=doi:-&issn=1398-2273&isbn=&volume=10&issue=2&spage=137&pages=137-41&date=2008&title=Transplant+Infectious+Disease&atitle=Strongyloides+hyperinfection+syndrome+after+intestinal+transplantation.&aulast=Patel&pid=%3Cauthor%3EPatel+G%2CArvelakis+A%2CSauter+BV%2CGondolesi+GE%2CCaplivski+D%2CHuprikar+S%3C%2Fauthor%3E%3CAN%3E17605735%3C%2FAN%3E%3CDT%3ECase+Reports%3C%2FDT%3E.

158. Wu G, Selvaggi G, Nishida S, et al. Graft-versus-host disease after intestinal and multivisceral transplantation. Transplantation. 2011;91(2):219–24. http://0-ovidsp.ovid.com.library.lausys.georgetown.edu/ovidweb.cgi?T=JS&CSC=Y&NEWS=N&PAGE=fulltext&D=medl&AN=21076376; http://catalog.library.georgetown.edu:4550/resserv?sid=OVID:medline&id=pmid:21076376&id=doi:&issn=0041-1337&isbn=&volume=91&issue=2&spage=219&pages=219-24&date=2011&title=Transplantation&atitle=Graft-versus-host+disease+after+intestinal+and+multivisceral+transplantation.&aulast=Wu&pid=%3Cauthor%3EWu+G%2CSelvaggi+G%2CNishida+S%2CMoon+J%2CIsland+E%2CRuiz+P%2CTzakis+AG%3C%2Fauthor%3E%3CAN%3E21076376%3C%2FAN%3E%3CDT%3EJournal+Article%3C%2FDT%3E.

159. Furukawa H, Kusne S, Sutton DA, et al. Acute invasive sinusitis due to trichoderma longibrachiatum in a liver and small bowel transplant recipient. Clin Infect Dis. 1998;26(2):487–9. http://proxy.library.georgetown.edu/login?url=http://ovidsp.ovid.com/ovidweb.cgi?T=JS&CSC=Y&NEWS=N&PAGE=fulltext&D=med4&AN=9502475.

160. Singh N, Chang FY, Gayowski T, Marino IR. Infections due to dematiaceous fungi in organ transplant recipients: case report and review. Clin Infect Dis. 1997;24(3):369–74. http://proxy.library.georgetown.edu/login?url=http://ovidsp.ovid.com/ovidweb.cgi?T=JS&CSC=Y&NEWS=N&PAGE=fulltext&D=med4&AN=9114187.

161. Ashkenazi-Hoffnung L, Bilavsky E, Avitzur Y, Amir J. Successful treatment of cutaneous zygomycosis with intravenous amphotericin B followed by oral posaconazole in a multivisceral transplant recipient. Transplantation. 2010;90(10):1133–5. https://doi.org/10.1097/TP.0b013e3181f86916.

162. Irtan S, Lamerain M, Lesage F, et al. Mucormycosis as a rare cause of severe gastrointestinal bleeding after multivisceral transplantation. Transpl Infect Dis. 2013;15(6):E235–8. https://doi.org/10.1111/tid.12147.

163. Rege A, Chaubal G, Reddy J, Vikraman D, Kadiyala R, Sudan D. Unusual rare infections following intestinal transplantation. Transplantation. 2015;99(6):S73.

164. Qu L, Strollo DC, Bond G, Kusne S. Nocardia prostatitis in a small intestine transplant recipient. Transpl Infect Dis. 2003;5(2):94–7. http://proxy.library.georgetown.edu/login?url=http://ovidsp.ovid.com/ovidweb.cgi?T=JS&CSC=Y&NEWS=N&PAGE=fulltext&D=med4&AN=12974790.

165. Pascher A, Klupp J, Schulz RJ, Dignass A, Neuhaus P. CMV, EBV, HHV6, and HHV7 infections after intestinal transplantation without specific antiviral prophylaxis. Transplant Proc. 2004;36(2):381–2. http://proxy.library.georgetown.edu/login?url=http://ovidsp.ovid.com/ovidweb.cgi?T=JS&CSC=Y&NEWS=N&PAGE=fulltext&D=med4&AN=15050166.

Infections in Limbs, Integuments, and Face Transplantation

6

Justin M. Broyles and Chad R. Gordon

Introduction

Solid organ transplantation poses a unique problem in the prophylaxis, treatment, and prevention of microbial colonization and infection. Early infection remains one of the most important causes of morbidity and mortality in patients undergoing solid organ transplantation. By nature of the immunosuppressive regimen, the patient is continually at risk for developing infections which threaten the survivability of the transplanted allograft. A myriad of factors dictates the solid organ transplant recipient's risk of infection, including time from transplant procedure, antimicrobial prophylaxis, environmental exposure, and immunosuppressive regimen given to prevent and treat graft rejection. The net sum of all of these factors dictates that patient's overall risk for developing infectious complications would provide direction in how to develop and implement strategies for prevention and effective management of such complications.

Infections in solid organ transplant recipients can be classified into three broad categories based upon the length of time from transplantation [1, 2]. In the 1st month after surgery, infections that occur are similar to those of other solid organ transplants or surgeries involving that region of the body. These include superficial and deep surgical site infections, catheter-related infections, ventilator-associated pneumonia, and urinary tract infections [1]. The risk factors which appear to contribute to these infections include (1) prolonged mechanical ventilation, (2) prolonged indwelling intravascular catheter placement, (3) prolonged ICU stay, and (4) the development of hematomas or seromas at the surgical site [3–6]. Upon recognition of these problems, immediate action should be taken to remove the suspected potential source for infection. Additionally, judicious culture-directed antibiotics should be initiated in an effort to eradicate the suspected organism(s). Some of the more virulent organisms that can be associated within this 1st month following transplant surgery include methicillin-resistant *Staphylococcus aureus* (MRSA), vancomycin-resistant *Enterococcus* (VRE), and Gram-negative organisms including *Klebsiella* and *Pseudomonas* spp. Rarely, the allograft may be contaminated or procured from a donor with active systemic infection, which virtually ensures the recipient will become colonized or infected due to graft-transmitted pathogen.

The second category in the posttransplant infection timetable ranges from the 2nd to 6th month after initial transplantation. This period is dominated by opportunistic infections that result from the immunosuppressive actions of the various posttransplant medications given to the patient. These infectious can be either derived from the environment, recrudescence of remotely acquired latent infections, or worsening of subclinical infections acquired from the donor allograft [2]. Common infections which occur during this initial phase are oral candidiasis and the reactivation of herpes simplex virus (HSV), type I or II. Common guidelines dictate prophylaxis against these pathogens with either nystatin or clotrimazole for thrush prevention or acyclovir or valacyclovir for HSV suppression [7–10]. Other more serious viral infections that occur during this timeframe include cytomegalovirus (CMV), Epstein-Barr virus (EBV), parvovirus, polyomaviruses, hepatitis B virus (HBV), and hepatitis C virus (HCV). Fungal colonization and subsequent invasive disease can also occur during this window, and common culprits are *Aspergillus* spp., *Pneumocystis jirovecii*, and *Cryptococcus* spp. Six months after the transplant, the patient enter the third and final timeframe for infection risk [11, 12]. From this point on the patient will fall into one of three distinct populations. The first group is comprised of patients who have done well up to this point and are candidates to have their immunosuppression gradually reduced. These patients will slowly approach the infection risk of the general population that resides in patients proximity, albeit, these individuals will

J. M. Broyles · C. R. Gordon (✉)
Department of Plastic and Reconstructive Surgery, The Johns Hopkins Hospital, Baltimore, MD, USA
e-mail: cgordon@jhmi.edu

A. Safdar (ed.), *Principles and Practice of Transplant Infectious Diseases*, https://doi.org/10.1007/978-1-4939-9034-4_6

harbor some degree of increased susceptibility for the community-acquired infections. Therefore, annual influenza vaccinations and updated new-generation pneumococcal vaccinations are especially important in transplant recipients [13, 14]. The second group of patients is characterized by patients who have had difficulties with rejection and have to have their immunosuppressive regimen intensified. Because of this, these patients will maintain an infection risk identical to those seen in the patients during the second period following transplantation. Finally, a third group of patients is comprised of patients who have done well but will develop effects of long-term viral infections such as BK polyomavirus, CMV, HBV, HCV, and human papillomavirus infection (HPV) [2] (Table 6.1).

Comprehension of this timetable is essential and provides guidance to healthcare providers in effective prevention, anticipating, and treating infections that may be encountered in individuals undergoing composite tissue allotransplantation. While this may not be an absolute timetable, it should however serve as a guide in evaluation of each individual patient to better refine protocols and treatment interventions.

Treatment Modalities in Solid Organ Transplantation

There are three ways to prevent and treat infections in solid organ transplant patients. The most obvious way to eradicate an active infection is with the most effective antimicrobial regimen. Prophylaxis is the administration of antimicrobial agents to a susceptible population of patients in order to prevent expected or anticipated infections during various posttransplant periods. Preemptive therapy is the administration of antimicrobial agents to a subgroup of patients defined by certain clinical characteristics that predicts a heightened risk for a specific infectious disease.

Table 6.1 Timing of infectious complications in solid organ transplants

<1 month	1–6 months	>6 months
Aspergillus	*Aspergillus*	*Aspergillus*, atypical molds
Candida	Adenovirus	Community-acquired pneumonia
Aspiration	CMV	CMV
Catheter-related infectious	*Cryptococcus neoformans*	EBV
Clostridium difficile colitis	EBV	HSV
HSV	HSV	HSV encephalitis
Wound infectious	*Pneumocystis carinii*	JC polyomavirus infection
(*Staphylococcus aureus*)	VZV	

Unique Considerations in Composite Tissue Allotransplantation

Each solid organ transplant hosts its own unique properties which make perioperative care unique. Facial and hand composite tissue allotransplants can consist of many different types of tissue such as skin, fat, muscle, bone, nerves, lymphatics, and mucosal services, all of which have a variety of antigenic properties [15, 16]. Therefore, such patients demand a higher degree of drug-induced immune suppression comparable to recipients of other interval visceral transplants. Anatomic and physiologic features of a particular transplant can dictate unique treatment considerations. For example, the alveolar lining in a lung transplant recipient is exposed to the outside environment leading to infections resulting from environmental colonization of the mucosal surfaces due to specific community- and hospital-acquired pathogens. Composite tissue transplant recipients, such as face and limb allografts, also share direct contact with the external environment. Therefore, these transplants can be prone to unique infections not routinely seen in patients undergoing other internal visceral transplantations.

Composite facial transplantation, depending upon the extent of the anatomy of the transplanted graft, may contain many unique mucosal surfaces. These include oral mucosa, nasal mucosa, sinus mucosa, and the mucosa of the upper airways. The oral mucosa can be a source of many pathogenic microorganisms including *Streptococcus* spp., *Capnocytophaga* spp., *Candida* spp., and various microaerophilic and facultative anaerobic bacteria. The sinuses, nasal mucosa, and upper airways can harbor fungal spores including *Aspergillus* and *Rhizopus*, among other rare filamentous molds that can result in serious invasive disease during the posttransplant periods of iatrogenic drug-induced immune suppression [17–19]. Additionally, the patients, both donor and recipient, may become colonized by any variety of drug-resistant potential pathogens prior to undergoing transplantation procedure. These organisms may become clinically relevant after transplantation resulting in soft tissue infections, pneumonia, and various other difficult-to-treat systemic infections [20–24].

Both facial and hand allotransplantation grafts contain large amounts of donor-derived external skin. While native skin is normally colonized by a host of innocuous microorganisms, it is possible that allograft skin may be colonized with certain pathogens such as *Staphylococcus aureus*, *Propionibacterium* spp., diphtheroids, *Corynebacterium*, and other various Gram-negative organisms. This should be kept in mind when devising strategies for prevention and treatment protocols for possible surgical site infections in these high-risk patients. Additionally, these risks can be potentiated by an extended stay in intensive care units or prolonged hospitalization [25–28].

Bacterial Infections

The exposed oral surfaces of a composite facial allotransplant expose the recipient to donor-derived pathogens as well as continuous exposure of the environmental microflora. Immediate oral antimicrobial prophylaxis should concentrate on organisms such as Streptococci, *Capnocytophaga* spp., anaerobic bacteria, and *Candida* spp. Ampicillin-sulbactam provides adequate bacterial prophylaxis for these patients and should be implemented immediately [29]. Nystatin or clotrimazole can provide treatment as well as prophylaxis for *Candida* spp. during this period. If the patient develops an oral infection despite prophylactic measures, the source should be immediately assessed, and culture-directed antibiotic therapy should be promptly given. If there is any concern for methicillin-resistant *Staphylococcus aureus* (MRSA) or Gram-negative bacterial infection, empiric therapy with vancomycin and piperacillin-tazobactam should be started. The duration of prophylaxis is dependent upon a myriad of factors including physician judgment, duration of ICU stay(s), healing of intraoral suture lines, and intensity of antirejection drug-induced immune suppression.

The face transplant recipient is at a heightened risk for bacterial infection involving the paranasal sinuses. Close attention must be directed toward fevers or leukocytosis in the absence of any obvious clinical sign of infection. Serial imaging of the sinuses can be performed, and endoscopic cultures may be obtained if sinusitis is suspected [30]. The common bacterial pathogens include *Streptococcus pneumoniae*, *Moraxella catarrhalis*, *Staphylococcus aureus*, and other streptococci species. However, care must be taken to exclude fungal etiology.

Patients who receive hand or face transplants have similar risks of acquiring pneumonia as recipients of other solid organ transplants. Risk factors for the development of pneumonia in transplant patients include mechanical ventilation, prolonged ICU stay, sedation, history of smoking cigarettes, and patients with underlying asthma or COPD [31, 32]. Face or hand transplant patients who develop pneumonia within the 1st month following transplantation are often susceptible to pathogens associated during ICU stay such as *Pseudomonas aeruginosa*, *Klebsiella pneumonia*, *Acinetobacter* spp., and MRSA. These infections can be either healthcare-associated pneumonia (HAP), ventilator-associated pneumonia (VAP), or community-acquired pneumonia (CAP).

Antimicrobial prevention of pneumonia in the immunosuppressed solid organ transplant recipients has been advocated by many. One of the more effective prophylactic therapies in solid organ transplant recipients is the use of trimethoprim-sulfamethoxazole for the first 6 months following transplantation [33–36]. At many transplant centers, the incidence of *Pneumocystis jirovecii* pneumonia in patients who do not receive prophylaxis is greater than 10%. Prophylaxis with trimethoprim-sulfamethoxazole may also reduce the risk of other important opportunistic pathogens such as *Listeria monocytogenes*, *Toxoplasma gondii*, and *Nocardia asteroides*.

Patient undergoing composite tissue allotransplants are also at higher risk for catheter-related infections. The use of indwelling intravascular devices is nearly universal in this population due to the need for accessible vascular access for medications, transfusion of blood and blood products, monitoring of physiologic parameters, blood draws, and parenteral nutritional supplementation. Bloodstream infection due to microorganisms other than coagulase-negative staphylococcus thought to be related to an infected intravascular devise; it is prudent to remove such infected devices, especially in the severely immunocompromised transplant recipients. Finally, all lines should be discontinued when no longer needed.

Diarrhea is a common problem in solid organ transplant recipients [37–39]. *Clostridium difficile* is the most common cause of healthcare-associated diarrhea. In the hospitalized population, *Clostridium difficile* is responsible for 10–25% of cases of antibiotic-associated diarrhea [40–42]. The risk of becoming colonized with toxigenic *Clostridium difficile* in hospitalized patients is proportional to the length of stay, and most colonization occur within 3 weeks after hospitalization [43, 44]. The incidence of *Clostridium difficile* infection (CDI) in solid organ transplant recipients is highest within the first 3 months due to the immunosuppressive regimen and frequent antimicrobial exposures [45]. Face and hand transplant patients are likely to receive multiple antimicrobial agents for prevention and treatment of bacterial infection and are at an elevated risk for *Clostridium difficile* infection. Diagnosis is confirmed by stool assay identifying the virulent *Clostridium difficile* or one or more if its toxins. Patients with CDI commonly present with copious, malodorous diarrhea, elevated white blood cell count, persistent fever, and abdominal pain. This may progress to abdominal distention, ileus, toxic megacolon, bowel perforation, complicated peritonitis, and sepsis requiring emergent colectomy. Treatment options include cessation of the offending antibiotic drug when possible, treatment with oral vancomycin, and intravenous metronidazole in combination with oral vancomycin for patients with serious illness [46].

CMV Infection and End-Organ Disease

CMV infection has traditionally been one of the more devastating infectious complications following solid organ transplantation. Seroprevalence of CMV in the general population approaches 60–80% depending upon the region. Therefore, most organ donors and recipients have prior exposure to CMV infection [47, 48]. Accordingly, CMV infection occurs in 50% of solid organ transplant recipients within the first 3 months if no antiviral prophylaxis is given.

CMV is a beta herpesvirus that retains a lifelong latency following the primary exposure/infection. It is an immunomodulatory virus that can cause many secondary immunologic phenomenon in addition to the primary infection [49, 50]. Posttransplant infection occurs either as a reactivation of latent remotely acquired infection or via acquisition of the virus from the donor tissue or unscreened blood or blood products. Individuals who are CMV seronegative prior to transplantation and acquire the virus from the donor tissue are at the highest risk for invasive CMV disease, which in most cases result in a devastating complication due to the immunologic novelty of the newly acquired viral infection compounded by the severity of drug-induced immune suppression given in the early posttransplant period.

CMV infection can manifest itself in one of three clinical scenarios. Asymptomatic viremia refers to detectable levels of CMV in a peripheral blood assay in the absence of clinical symptoms. CMV syndrome describes the signs and symptoms of acute CMV infection. This includes fevers, chills, myalgias, leukopenia, thrombocytopenia, and elevation of liver function tests. Finally, end-organ CMV disease refers to specific tissue damage caused by mostly uninterrupted intracellular CMV replication. Histopathology of the affected tissue demonstrates CMV inclusion bodies. Various forms of CMV tissue invasive disease include CMV pneumonitis, hepatitis, esophagitis, gastritis, enteritis, retinitis, colitis, and encephalitis [51].

The two major prevention strategies against CMV infections in face and hand transplantation are prophylaxis and preemptive therapy. Prophylaxis refers to providing antiviral drug for infection prevention given to at risk patients who undergo transplantation. Preemptive therapy refers to providing antiviral therapy to individuals with evidence of high risk for CMV end-organ disease such as those with asymptomatic CMV viremia. When universal prophylaxis was compared with preemptive therapy, results indicated that both strategies were comparable in preventing CMV disease and reducing the incidence allograft rejection in solid organ transplantation [52–54]. Although the strategies appeared to equally prevent CMV disease, patients who received universal anti-CMV prophylaxis were less likely to experience potentially life-threatening bacterial and fungal infections due to probably immune-modulating effect of CMV reactivation or acute infection, especially in the severely immunocompromised transplant recipients [55]. Both preemptive and universal prophylactic strategies have reduced the rate of symptomatic CMV infection to <10%. The most commonly used drug for CMV prophylaxis is valganciclovir, and at most transplant center, it is continued for 3 months following transplantation. In the face transplant performed at the Cleveland Clinic, intravenous ganciclovir followed by oral valganciclovir is given for 5 months.

Prophylaxis and preemptive CMV treatment is not without consequence. Both ganciclovir and valganciclovir have the potential for causing drug-induced multi-lineage myelosuppression resulting in profound neutropenia, anemia, and severe thrombocytopenia. Additionally, these drugs can produce renal dysfunction, gastrointestinal toxicities, and mental status changes. Ganciclovir and valganciclovir are both potentially teratogenic, and this should be kept in mind if the patient undergoing transplantation is of childbearing age. Due to their potential for promoting adverse reactions, ganciclovir and valganciclovir should not be administered together.

The effects of acute CMV infection can be devastating in the presence of a face or hand transplant. This has been illustrated most notably in the second French face transplant that was performed in 2007. This patient developed ganciclovir-resistant CMV infection with an episode of acute rejection. This episode required 8 weeks of therapy with foscarnet to prevent continuing rejection and declining CMV viremia [56]. Foscarnet therapy can result in renal failure requiring renal replacement therapy. Therefore, great care must be practiced when starting the patients on high-dose foscarnet induction therapy.

The impact of CMV infection in the setting of composite tissue allotransplantation has been clearly illustrated in its brief history [57, 58]. In a cohort of hand transplants form Pittsburg, PA, five of nine patients had clinically relevant CMV infection. Two of these patients had high viral loads; several had relapsing or remitting courses of treatment with combination of foscarnet and cidofovir. The face transplant patient from the Cleveland Clinic developed refractory CMV viremia. Her treatment was further complicated by recurrent neutropenia associated with ganciclovir and valganciclovir usage despite supportive care with recombinant myeloid growth factor use such as granulocyte colony-stimulating factor. Other antiviral medications have been considered; however, the risk posed by these medications was deemed too high in an already tenuous situation. Foscarnet is nephrotoxic and in the absence of adequate precautions can lead to urogenital contact ulceration. Cidofovir can lead to nephrotoxicity, cytopenias, and ocular problems. After consultation with multiple specialty services, she received the investigational drug CMX001 (combines Chimerix's Lipid-Antiviral-Conjugate Technology with cidofovir) under emergency IND from the FDA. The implementation of this regimen resulted in reduced CMV viral load, which after 6 weeks of therapy became undetectable in the peripheral blood [59].

CMV infection remains an important pathogen in solid organ transplantation; it appears as if this association may be particularly strong in patients undergoing composite tissue allotransplantation [56–58]. Indeed, CMV infection has been a major complication in two of the first four face transplants as well as five of nine hand transplant recipients. While most would advocate not performing seropositive transplants to a seronegative recipient, however, the high CMV seroprevalence in the general population makes this approach impractical by severely limiting the donor graft pool. Future research in safe and effective new antiviral drugs, standardizing CMV prevention and preemptive treatment strategies, will ensure the greatest benefit for patients undergoing composite tissue allotransplantation.

Other Viral Infections

Viruses other than CMV can contribute to morbidity and mortality after solid organ transplantation. These agents commonly display temporal patterns of infection, with the 1st month displaying HSV seropositive recipients at heightened risk of HSV-1 and HSV-2 infection [60]. The 2nd to 6th months following transplantation are characterized by lowered cell-mediated immunity due to the intensifying effects of immunosuppression. CMV is the most serious infection during this period. Six months after transplantation, varicella-zoster virus (VZV) reactivation resulting single or multiple dermatomal herpes zoster or disseminated disease may occur. Human papillomavirus (HPV), adenoviruses, respiratory syncytial virus (RSV), influenza, and parainfluenza can occur at any time, although severe disease is witnessed in the first 3 months following transplantation [61, 62] (Figs. 6.1 and 6.2). A thorough understanding of the various infectious presentations and their treatments will prepare the team to deal with these problems as they arise.

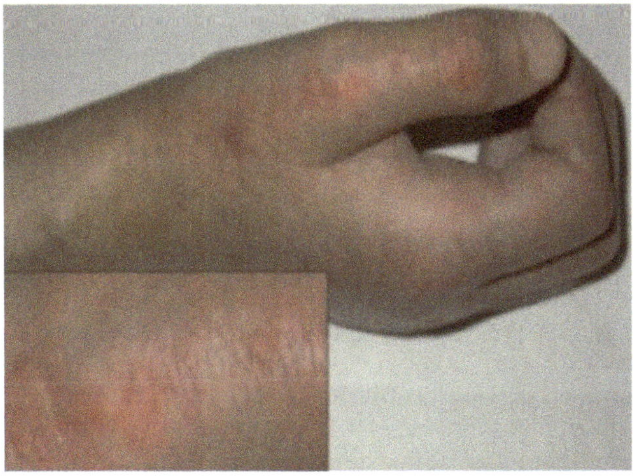

Fig. 6.1 Hand transplant displaying papillomavirus-associated warts at the back of both hands at 9 months after double forearm transplantation [63]. (Reprinted from Schneeberger et al. [63], with permission from Springer)

HSV1 is a ubiquitous virus and reaches a prevalence of 80% among people over the age of 60. This virus may reactivate as cutaneous and mucosal eruptions presenting as painful vesicular lesions. HSV2 is less common with a prevalence of 30% among adults in the general population. The clinical presentation can be genital, perianal, or generalized mucocutaneous vesicular lesions. Additionally, there is a potential for disseminated visceral disease involving the lungs, gastrointestinal tract, and central nervous system. Because the incidence of clinically significant disease in HSV seropositive recipients' approaches 70%, antiviral prophylaxis with acyclovir is recommended during the first 4 weeks after transplantation [64]. The first face transplant recipient in France received HSV prophylaxis; however, she developed orolabial HSV on day 185 posttransplant, which responded to a combination of oral valacyclovir and topical acyclovir cream [26].

The VZV is a highly transmissible virus that causes chickenpox and varicella zoster. After primary infection, the virus remains dormant in the dorsal root ganglia. Approximately 90% of adults are either varicella-seropositive or have immunity from prior immunization. Majority of VZV infections in transplant recipients are as a result of reactivation of dormant remotely acquired virus. In seronegative patients, vaccination should be given at least 4 weeks prior to the anticipated transplantation procedure. Additionally, the live-attenuated virus should be avoided after the patient has undergone transplantation.

Epstein-Barr virus may cause clinically symptomatic disease any period after organ transplantation. Posttransplant lymphoproliferative disorder (PTLD) is a life-threatening complication due to EBV reactivation and may present with a variety of features ranging from reactive lymphadenopathy to malignant treatment-refractory lymphoma. Risk factors include (1) recent EBV infection, (2) coinfection with CMV, and (3) profound drug-induced immune suppression [65, 66]. Prescreening of transplant recipients may identify a patient who is seropositive and help guide therapy. However, there is no clear established role for antiviral prophylaxis. If patients are found to have PTLD, the mainstay of treatment is reduction in immunosuppression. However, new strategies in treating PTLD in solid organ transplants include anti-CD20 monoclonal antibodies given in an effort to limit the proliferation of EBV-infected immortalized cells.

Various other herpesviruses such as herpesvirus 6 (HHV-6) can cause infection in transplant patients. Seropositivity in the general population is high, and reactivation following transplantation may occur resulting in pancytopenia, pneumonitis, hepatitis, and meningoencephalitis. To date, there has been no clear antiviral prophylaxis established. Herpesvirus 8 (HHV-8) is the primary agent of Kaposi sarcoma, Castleman's disease, and body cavity or primary effusion lymphoma. There is no clear role for antiviral

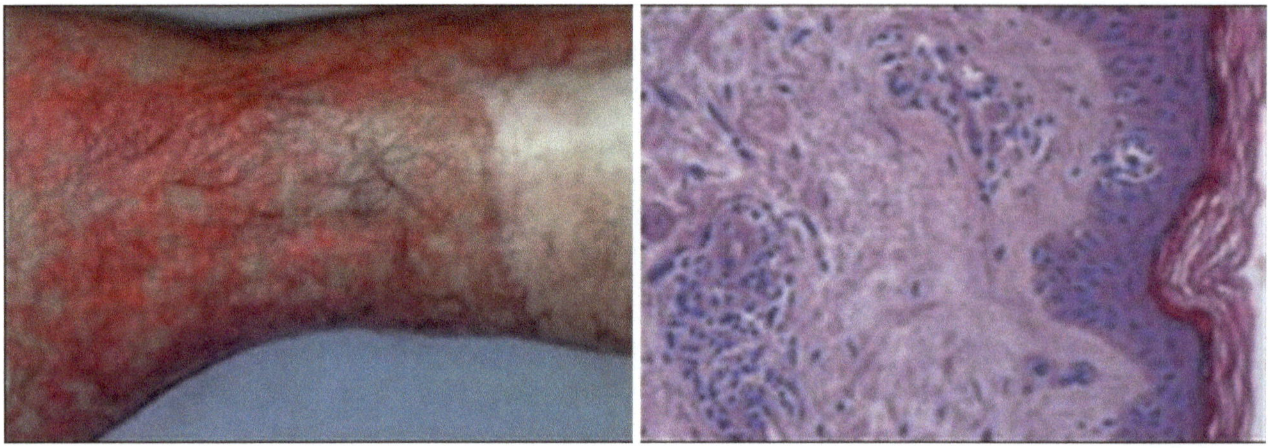

Fig. 6.2 Hand transplant displaying disseminated erythema and papulous lesions as signs of rejection at 55 days after hand transplantation. Histology demonstrated perivascular and interstitial mononuclear cell infiltrates [63]. (Reprinted from Schneeberger et al. [63], with permission from Springer)

prophylaxis for this pathogen, and reduction in drug-induced immune suppression remains the cornerstone for treating patients with HHV 8-related disease.

Both HBV and HCV have been exhaustively studied within the solid organ transplant population. Many studies have been performed identifying the virus' role in predicting, performing, and recovering from liver failure and liver transplantation. To date, there have been no hand or face transplant donors or recipients who have been seropositive for HBV or HCV. However, vaccination against HBV is universally recommended in the preoperative setting.

The clinical manifestations of respiratory viral diseases are often typical, and solid organ transplant recipients are at risk to develop more severe and prolonged illness. Symptoms include congestion and rhinorrhea to an increasingly severe lower respiratory tract infection. Because there is no pathognomonic symptom for a specific virus, judicious culturing or preferably nested PCR respiratory pathogen panels should be performed for any transplant patient suspected respiratory viral disease. Influenza, parainfluenza, RSV, and adenoviruses may result in severe lower respiratory tract infections, and every effort must be made to deter progression to lower respiratory disease. Prevention is the most important strategy for respiratory viruses. Infection control measures are critical and should be strictly implemented in the transplant units. Accordingly, patients with suspected influenza or other respiratory viruses should be isolated using standard and droplet precautions. Additionally, the patients and healthcare workers should receive mandatory annual influenza vaccination. If the patient is found to have influenza, treatment should be implemented according to seasonal viral drug-resistance profile; common agents used in prevention and treatment of influenza viral infections include M2 inhibitors and neuraminidase inhibitor. By implementing policies such as strict adherence to handwashing, contact and droplet precautions as part of hospital infection control strategies, and unwavering compliance with annual influenza vaccination recommendations, infection rates can be reduced in these highly susceptible patients with the potential for devastating respiratory viral disease.

Fungal Infections

Universal antifungal prophylaxis in solid organ transplantation is not accepted based on available data. However, targeted prophylaxis according to risk criteria is generally more evidence based. Additionally, one can start antifungal therapy based upon a positive diagnostic test prior to clinically evident disease. This allows for appropriate dosing of antifungal agents at an early stage of infection and the reduction of unnecessary treatment and toxicity. *Candida*, *Aspergillus*, and *Cryptococcus* species are the most frequent causes of infection in patients undergoing solid organ transplantation. *Histoplasma capsulatum* and *Coccidioides immitis* can cause serious disease, albeit, such infections are only prevalent in certain geographic regions and are less common.

Invasive fungal infections can be broadly categorized into one of two groups, geographically endemic fungi and opportunistic fungal infections. Geographically endemic fungi are endemic to a particular region and present as reactivation of a remotely acquired latent infection or a newly acquired primary infection in a person visiting these specific regions. Opportunistic infections rarely cause clinically relevant invasive disease in immunocompetent patients and have no geographical restriction. Examples of opportunistic fungi include *Candida*, *Aspergillus*, and *Cryptococcus neoformans*.

Candida yeast is the most common opportunistic fungal infection in organ allograft recipients. *Candida* is part of the normal microflora of skin and orointestinal tract; it also frequently colonizes lower genitourinary mucosa in women. Oral candidiasis is common in the early posttransplant period. Other forms of infection include catheter-related candidemia and deep surgical site infections. The treatment for topical and mucosal candidiasis is nystatin or clotrimazole and frequently suggested for oral prophylaxis. The first full-face transplant recipient in France developed oral candidiasis on postoperative day 18. The initial presentation of "diffuse erythema and edema" appeared indistinguishable from acute graft rejection and illustrated the importance of recognizing and treating these infections when they occur. The patient's symptoms resolved with systemic antifungal therapy.

Cryptococcus is an encapsulated yeast found in the soil and has the potential for severe invasive systemic disease in the immunocompromised patients. Most cases of cryptococcal disease occur during 1st year after transplantation [67]. Fungal meningitis, cellulitis, and pneumonia are common diseases. An increased intracranial pressure in patients with cryptococcal meningitis mandate neurosurgical decompression along with combination antifungal drugs and other aspects of medical management.

Coccidioidomycosis and histoplasmosis are both endemic to certain geographic regions in the United States. Coccidioidomycosis is found predominantly in the southwestern United States. Fungal spores are acquired through inhalation. Infections are mostly seen within the 1st year following transplantation and often present as reactivation of remotely acquired infection [68, 69]. The infection presents clinically with acute respiratory infection. Generally, the disease will resolve rapidly, but a small percentage of patients may go on to develop chronic pulmonary disease. A smaller number of patients will progress to develop disseminated disease involving skin, joints, and central nervous system. Histoplasmosis is the most prevalent fungus in the Americas. It is geographically centered in the Midwest region of the United States. Most infections are asymptomatic; however, disseminated pulmonary disease can occur in the immunocompromised individuals.

Aspergillus is ubiquitous filamentous mold commonly isolated from soil and water. Transmission of the fungus is via inhalation of infectious germinating microconidia. Infection in immunocompetent patients is rare, and this fungus typically only becomes invasive in individuals who are severely immunocompromised. The principal manifestation of invasive fungal disease involves the lower respiratory tract resulting in bronchitis, fungal lung nodules that may progress to necrotizing pneumonia and systemic dissemination. Lung transplant recipients are at a higher risk than other solid organ recipients, in part, due to the exposure of allograft to the external environment and prolonged respiratory tract fungal colonization prior to undergoing transplantation procedure.

Risk factors for the development of invasive fungal infections include prolonged ICU stay, extensive exposure to broad-spectrum antibiotics, diabetes mellitus, exposure to agricultural or horticultural products, and marijuana smoking [70]. Preventative strategies include avoidance of exposures in the hospital and limitation of environmental exposure once discharged from the hospital. The face transplant patient at Cleveland Clinic received prophylaxis with voriconazole, which had to be discontinued due to an elevation in liver enzymes and derangement of tacrolimus serum levels. This difficulty is seen with several commonly used triazole antifungal drugs. Additionally, the patient was monitored for histoplasmosis with the urinary *Histoplasma* antigen for approximately 4 months due to exposure to chickens early in life. Fortunately, this patient never developed invasive fungal disease and did well without antifungal prophylaxis.

Other Infections in Face and Hand Transplantation

Because of the intense immunosuppression required in composite tissue allotransplantation, the patients are at risks for a myriad of infectious agents. In addition to traditional bacterial and viral pathogens, these patients are at risk for mycobacterial and parasitic infections. Because these pathogens can be difficult to detect and devastating if they become disseminated, a thorough preoperative screening for *Mycobacterium tuberculous*, *Strongyloides stercoralis*, *Leishmania* spp., and *Trypanosoma cruzi* should be performed. Patients with a history of exposure to *Mycobacterium* should be screened using new-generation gamma interferon release assays and offered isoniazid prophylaxis for untreated latent tuberculosis infection. Positive *Strongyloides* serology should prompt the consideration of preoperative ivermectin therapy.

Immunization Strategies in Composite Tissue Allotransplantation

Face and hand transplants are entirely elective operations; therefore, care must be taken to ensure that the patients have exhaustive evaluation for prevention and prophylaxis prior to becoming a candidate for transplantation. Several infections are associated with an increased risk of solid organ graft rejection and dysfunction. Infections are a major determinant of the patient's overall prognosis. Interventions to prevent infection include vaccination, antimicrobial prophylaxis, and preemptive therapy. A thorough evaluation of vaccination and immunization status prior to transplantation includes a thorough history and physical examination, a complete vaccination history, and standard measurement of titers for HBV, HCV, VZV, varicella, measles, mumps, and rubella.

To further optimize the patient's status prior transplantation, they should undergo further serologic evaluation for CMV, HSV I and II, VZV, EBV, human immunodeficiency virus, HBV, HCV, *Treponema pallidum*, *C. neoformans*, and *Toxoplasma gondii*. Additionally, if the patient lives in an endemic area or there is suspicion for infection, additional serologic titers should be sent for *S. stercoralis*, *Leishmania* spp., *T. cruzi*, *Histoplasma capsulatum*, and *Coccidioides immitis*. One should keep in mind that the patient risks losing immunity with higher degree of immunosuppression; there needs to be a well thought-out delicate balance between risk assessment for certain infections and prevention and treatment for such infections.

The patient should receive appropriate vaccinations prior to transplantation and initiation of immunosuppressive therapy. Pneumococcal vaccine should be administered if not given in the prior 5 years [71]. Tetanus-diphtheria-acellular pertussis (Tdap) should be given if the last tetanus immunization was greater than 10 years before transplantation [72]. HBA and HBV vaccines should be given to seronegative or patients with low titers. Seasonal influenza vaccination, including H1N1 when recommended by the Centers for Disease Control and Prevention, should be administered according to existing guidelines. Poliovirus and *Haemophilus influenza* vaccines should also be given if the vaccination status is questionable [71]. Finally, women aged 9–26 years of age should receive the HPV vaccination. The indications for recombinant HPV vaccination may possibly extend in the future. To these authors' knowledge, there have been no studies to assess long-term efficacy of pretransplant vaccination in this patient population. Due to an increased risk of infection, patients who have started immunotherapy should not receive live-attenuated vaccines.

Lifestyle Adaptations in Composite Tissue Allotransplantation

Once the patient's immediate surgical needs have been met, the face or hand transplant patient enters the recovery period. Here, the patient has been discharge from the inpatient hospital setting, and they begin intensive physical and occupational therapy as well as psychosocial rehabilitation. In this period, it is imperative that the patient is educated for potential environmental exposure risks and how to avoid them. Recipients of face and hand transplants can enjoy many of the activities of everyday life; however, there are certain precautions regarding water, food, animals, and travel-related exposure that should be addressed and periodically reinforced. For instance, the face transplant patient at Cleveland Clinic suffered from transient diarrheal illness. Further investigation revealed *Aeromonas* in her stool and drew attention to the issues surrounding well water as a potential source for the infection.

Patient should try and consciously limit their exposure to pets and other animals, including farm animals. Face and hand transplant patients can be owners of dogs, cats, and other pets, and their emotional attachment to these animals is often strong due to the fact that many of the patients have had difficulty integrating into the society prior to transplantation. The patient should be screened and educated that further exposure to the animals is not without significant risk. For example, exposure to cat feces can lead to *T. gondii* infection. Birds and parrots can transmit fungal infections as well as *Chlamydia psittaci*. Finally, reptiles and amphibians can transmit *Salmonella typhi*. With meticulous education, screening, and prevention, these patients can minimize their infectious risk.

Concomitant Facial and Upper Extremity Transplantation

The combination of facial and upper extremity transplantation appears to provide a solution to one of the most challenging problems in reconstructive surgery. This large surgical undertaking puts an increased stress on the already strained immune system. Undoubtedly, the most puzzling aspect of this proposed solution is unquestionably how the immunosuppressive regimen will change.

It is evident that larger composite tissue allografts contain more donor-derived epidermis. The skin, the largest organ in the human body, contains a variety of immune cells including Langerhans cells and keratinocytes making it the most antigenic tissue component in the allograft. It is not clear as to whether this type of increased antigenic load directly equates to the need for increased levels of immunosuppression and whether this would equate with negative outcomes. To date, there has been no difference in rejection between wrist-level hand versus more extensive higher levels transplantation with more allograft donor skin involved although there are several conflicting studies indicating amplified immunologic responses with an increased antigenic quantity of donor skin transplanted [73, 74].

Additionally, it is unclear if a larger transplant will increase the infection risk. Although intuitive, it is unclear if any additional precautions should be taken and if perioperative topical skin care has any role in preventing these infections. What is clear is that as composite tissue allotransplantation becomes more commonplace and these operations become more aggressive, our understanding in the spectrum of infectious complications will improve.

Conclusions

All patients undergoing long-term immunosuppression for solid organ transplantation are at risk for the development of infectious complications that could not only threaten the viability of the transplanted graft, but this may also threaten their life. As we enter the era of reconstructive transplantation, these risks cannot be understated. It is important that the medical and surgical teams, the patient, and the patient's family are aware of the risk and benefits of this life improving intervention as well as the signs and symptoms of secondary complication such as infections, graft rejection, and drug toxicities. While face and extremity transplants appear to have much in common with solid organ transplants, it is clear that certain subtleties do exist. Namely, the apparent unique microflora in facial transplant and the seemingly increased risk of CMV infection and rejection appear to provide new avenues for investigation. Future work should provide greater insight into the novel strategies for safe effective CMV prevention and treatment of end-organ disease.

References

1. Rubin RH, Wolfson JS, Cosimi AB, Tolkoff-Rubin NE. Infection in the renal transplant patient. Am J Med. 1981;70:405–11.
2. Fishman JA, Rubin RH. Infection in organ-transplant recipients. N Engl J Med. 1998;338:1741–51.
3. Guideline for prevention of nosocomial pneumonia: Centers for Disease Control and Prevention. Respir Care. 1994;39: 1191–236.
4. Cook D, Randolph A, Kernerman P. Central venous catheter replacement strategies: a systematic review of the literature. Crit Care Med. 1997;25:1417–24.
5. Garibaldi RA, Burke JP, Britt MR, Miller MA, Smith CB. Meatal colonization and catheter-associated bacteriuria. N Engl J Med. 1980;303:316–8.
6. Garibaldi RA, Burke JP, Dickman ML, Smith CB. Factors predisposing to bacteriuria during indwelling urethral catheterization. N Engl J Med. 1974;291:215–9.
7. Gluckman E, Lotsberg J, Devergie A, Zhao XM, Melo R, Gomez-Morales M, et al. Prophylaxis of herpes infections after bone-marrow transplantation by oral acyclovir. Lancet. 1983;2: 706–8.
8. Ljungman P. Prophylaxis against herpesvirus infections in transplant recipients. Drugs. 2001;61:187–96.
9. Meyers JD, Wade JC, Mitchell CD, Saral R, Lietman PS, Durack DT, et al. Multicenter collaborative trial of intravenous acyclovir for treatment of mucocutaneous herpes simplex virus infection in the immunocompromised host. Am J Med. 1982;73:229–35.
10. Quintiliani R, Owens NJ, Quercia RA, Klimek JJ, Nightingale CH. Treatment and prevention of oropharyngeal candidiasis. Am J Med. 1984;77:44–8.
11. San Juan R, Aguado JM, Lumbreras C, Díaz-Pedroche C, López-Medrano F, Lizasoain M, RESITRA Network, et al. Incidence, clinical characteristics and risk factors of late infection in solid organ transplant recipients: data from the RESITRA study group. Am J Transplant. 2007;7:964–71.
12. Kirkman RL, Strom TB, Weir MR, Tilney NL. Late mortality and morbidity in recipients. Transplantation. 1982;34:347–51.
13. Prevention of pneumococcal disease: recommendations of the Advisory Committee on Immunization Practices (ACIP) Centers for Disease Control. Recomm Rep. 1997;46(RR-8):1–24.
14. Danzinger-Isakov L, Kumar D. Guidelines for vaccination of solid organ transplant candidates and recipients. Am J Transplant. 2009;9(Suppl 4):S258.
15. Gordon CR. Composite tissue allografts: should we reconsider the terminology? Plast Reconstr Surg. 2009;124:464e–5e.
16. Gordon CR, Siemionow M, Zins J. Composite tissue allotransplantation: a proposed classification system based upon relative complexity. Transplant Proc. 2009;41:481–4.
17. Cuellar-Rodriguez J, Avery RK, Lard M, Budev M, Gordon SM, Shrestha NK, et al. Histoplasmosis in solid organ transplant recipients: 10 years of experience at a large transplant center in an endemic area. Clin Infect Dis. 2009;49:710–6.
18. Singh N, Lortholary O, Alexander BD, Gupta KL, John GT, Pursell K, Cryptococcal Collaborative Transplant Study Group, et al. Allograft loss in renal transplant recipients with *Cryptococcus neoformans* associated immune reconstitution syndrome. Transplantation. 2005;80:1131–3.
19. Husain S, Alexander BD, Munoz P, Avery RK, Houston S, Pruett T, et al. Opportunistic mycelial fungal infections in organ transplant recipients: emerging importance of non-Aspergillus mycelial fungi. Clin Infect Dis. 2003;37:221–9.
20. Herrero IA, Issa NC, Patel R. Nosocomial spread of linezolid-resistant, vancomycin-resistant Enterococcus faecium. N Engl J Med. 2002;346:867–9.
21. Fishman JA. Vancomycin-resistant Enterococcus in liver transplantation: what have we left behind? Transpl Infect Dis. 2003;5:109–11.
22. Lo Presti F, Riffard S, Vandenesch F, Reyrolle M, Ronco E, Ichai P, Etienne J. The first clinical isolate of Legionella parisiensis, from a liver transplant patient with pneumonia. J Clin Microbiol. 1997;35:1706–9.
23. Harbarth S, Pittet D, Romand J. Fatal concomitant nosocomial Legionnaires' disease and cytomegalovirus pneumonitis after cardiac transplantation. Intensive Care Med. 1996;22:1133–4.
24. Bert F, Bellier C, Lassel L, Lefranc V, Durand F, Belghiti J, et al. Risk factors for *Staphylococcus aureus* infection in liver transplant recipients. Liver Transpl. 2005;11:1093–9.
25. Devauchelle B, Badet L, Lengelé B, Morelon E, Testelin S, Michallet M, et al. First human face allograft: early report. Lancet. 2006;368:203–9.
26. Dubernard JM, Lengelé B, Morelon E, Testelin S, Badet L, Moure C, et al. Outcomes 18 months after the first human partial face transplantation. N Engl J Med. 2007;357:2451–60.
27. Guo S, Han Y, Zhang X, Lu B, Yi C, Zhang H, et al. Human facial allotransplantation: a 2-year follow-up study. Lancet. 2008;372:631–8.
28. Meningaud JP, Benjoar MD, Hivelin M, Hermeziu O, Toure G, Lantieri L. The procurement of total human face graft for allotransplantation: a preclinical study and the first clinical case. Plast Reconstr Surg. 2010;126:1181–90.
29. Gordon CR, Avery RK, Abouhassan W, Siemionow M. Cytomegalovirus and other infectious issues related to face transplantation: specific considerations, lessons learned, and future recommendations. Plast Reconstr Surg. 2011;127(4):1515–23.
30. Siemionow MZ, Papay F, Djohan R, Bernard S, Gordon CR, Alam D, et al. First U.S. near-total human face transplantation: a paradigm shift for massive complex injuries. Plast Reconstr Surg. 2010;125:111–22.
31. National Nosocomial Infections (NNIS) system: data summary from Jan 1992–June 2001. Am J Infect Control. 2001;29:408–21.
32. Cook DJ, Walter SD, Cook RJ, Griffith LE, Guyatt GH, Leasa D, et al. Incidence of and risk factors for ventilator-associated pneumonia in critically ill patients. Ann Intern Med. 1988;129: 433–40.

33. Fishman JA. Prevention of infection caused by Pneumocystis carinii in transplant recipients. Clin Infect Dis. 2001;33(8):1397.
34. Nathan SD, Ross DJ, Zakowski P, Kass RM, Koerner SK. Utility of inhaled pentamidine prophylaxis in lung transplant recipients. Chest. 1994;105:417–20.
35. Olsen SL, Renlund DG, O'Connell JB, Taylor DO, Lassetter JE, Eastburn J. Prevention of Pneumocystis carinii in cardiac transplantation recipients by trimethoprim-sulfamethoxazole. Transplantation. 1993;56:359–62.
36. Torre Cisneros J, de la Mata M, Lopez Cillero P, Sanchez Guijo P, Mino P. Effectiveness of daily low-dose cotrimoxazole prophylaxis for Pneumocystis carinii pneumonia in liver transplantation—an open clinical trial. Transplantation. 1996;62:1519–21.
37. Altiparmak MR, Trablus S, Pamuk ON, Apaydin S, Sariyar M, Oztürk R, et al. Diarrhoea following renal transplantation. Clin Transpl. 2002;16:212–6.
38. Bunnapradist S, Neri L, Wong W, Lentine KL, Burroughs TE, Pinsky BW, et al. Incidence and risk factors for diarrhea following kidney transplantation and association with graft loss and mortality. Am J Kidney Dis. 2008;51:478–86.
39. Wong NA, Bathgate AJ, Bellamy CO. Colorectal disease in liver allograft recipients: a clinicopathological study with follow-up. Eur J Gastroenterol Hepatol. 2002;14:231–6.
40. Barbut F, Corthier G, Charpak Y, Cerf M, Monteil H, Fosse T. Prevalence and pathogenicity of Clostridium difficile in hospitalized patients. A French multicenter study. Arch Intern Med. 1996;156:1449–54.
41. Johnson S, Gerding DN. Clostridium difficile-associated diarrhea. Clin Infect Dis. 1998;26(5):1027–34, quiz 1035–1036.
42. Riley TV. Clostridium difficile: a pathogen of the nineties. Eur J Clin Microbiol Infect Dis. 1998;17:137–41.
43. Clabots CR, Johnson S, Olson MM, Peterson LR, Gerding DN. Acquisition of Clostridium difficile by hospitalized patients: evidence for colonized new admissions as a source of infection. J Infect Dis. 1992;166:561–7.
44. McFarland LV, Mulligan ME, Kwok RY, Stamm WE. Nosocomial acquisition of Clostridium difficile infection. N Engl J Med. 1989;320:204–10.
45. Munksgaard B. Clostridium difficile. Am J Transplant. 2004;4:28–30.
46. Aslam S, Musher DM. An update on diagnosis, treatment, and prevention of Clostridium difficile-associated disease. Gastroenterol Clin N Am. 2006;35:315–35.
47. Singh N, Wannstedt C, Keyes L, Gayowski T, Wagener MN, Cacciarelli TV. Efficacy of valganciclovir administered as preemptive therapy for cytomegalovirus disease in liver transplant recipients: impact on viral load and late-onset cytomegalovirus disease. Transplantation. 2005;79:85–90.
48. Singh N. Antiviral drugs for cytomegalovirus in transplant recipients: advantages of preemptive therapy. Rev Med Virol. 2006;16:281–7.
49. Rubin RH, Cosimi AB, Tolkoff-Rubin NE, Russell PS, Hirsch MS. Infectious disease syndromes attributable to cytomegalovirus and their significance among renal transplant recipients. Transplantation. 1977;24:458–64.
50. Rubin RH. The indirect effects of cytomegalovirus infection on the outcome of organ transplantation. JAMA. 1989;261:3607–9.
51. Ljungman P, Griffiths P, Paya C. Definitions of cytomegalovirus infection and disease in transplant recipients. Clin Infect Dis. 2002;34:1094–7.
52. Kalil AC, Levitsky J, Lyden E, Stoner J, Freifeld AG. Meta-analysis: the efficacy of strategies to prevent organ disease by cytomegalovirus in solid organ transplant recipients. Ann Intern Med. 2005;143:870–80.
53. Strippoli GF, Hodson EM, Jones CJ, Craig JC. Pre-emptive treatment for cytomegalovirus viraemia to prevent cytomegalovirus disease in solid organ transplant recipients. Cochrane Database Syst Rev. 2006;1:CD005133.
54. Hodson EM, Jones CA, Webster AC, Strippoli GF, Barclay PG, Kable K. Antiviral medications to prevent cytomegalovirus disease and early death in recipients of solid-organ transplants: a systematic review of randomised controlled trials. Lancet. 2005;365:2105–15.
55. Munoz-Price LS, Slifkin M, Ruthazer R, Poutsiaka DD, Hadley S, Freeman R, et al. The clinical impact of ganciclovir prophylaxis on the occurrence of bacteremia in orthotopic liver transplant recipients. Clin Infect Dis. 2004;39:1293–9.
56. Lantieri L, Meningaud J-P, Grimbert P, Bellivier F, Lefaucheur JP, Ortonne N, et al. Repair of the lower and middle parts of the face by composite tissue allotransplantation in a patient with massive plexiform neurofibroma: a 1-year follow-up study. Lancet. 2008;372:639–45.
57. Gordon C, Siemionow M, Papay F, Pryor L, Gatherwright J, Kodish E, et al. The world's experience with facial transplantation: what have we learned thus far? Ann Plast Surg. 2009;63:572–8.
58. Schneeberger S, Lucchina S, Lanzetta M, Brandacher G, Bösmüller C, Steurer W, et al. Cytomegalovirus-related complications in human hand transplantation. Transplantation. 2005;80:441–7.
59. Painter W, Mossad S, Siemionow M. First use of CMX001, a novel antiviral drug, for the suppression of cytomegalovirus infection in solid organ transplant patients: a case series. American Transplant Congress 2010, oral late-breaking abstract presentation, San Diego, CA.
60. Razonable RR, Eid AJ. Viral infections in transplant recipients. Minerva Med. 2009;100:479–501.
61. Englund JA, Boeckh M, Kuypers J, Nichols WG, Hackman RC, Morrow RA, et al. Brief communication: fatal human metapneumovirus infection in stem-cell transplant recipients. Ann Intern Med. 2006;144:344–9.
62. Kim YJ, Boeckh M, Englund JA. Community respiratory virus infections in immunocompromised patients: hematopoietic stem cell and solid organ transplant recipients, and individuals with human immunodeficiency virus infection. Semin Respir Crit Care Med. 2007;28:222–42.
63. Schneeberger S, Ninkovic M, Margreiter R. Hand transplantation: the Innsbruck experience, Ch 17. In: Transplantation of composite tissue allographs. Springer, Boston; 2008. p. 234–250. https://link.springer.com/chapter/10.1007%2F978-0-387-74682-1_17. Epub accessed 2016.
64. Zuckerman R, Wald A. Herpes simplex virus infections in solid organ transplant recipients. Am J Transplant. 2009;4:104–7.
65. Walker RC, Marshall WF, Strickler JG, Wiesner RH, Velosa JA, Habermann TM, et al. Pretransplantation assessment of the risk of lymphoproliferative disorder. Clin Infect Dis. 1995;20:1346–53.
66. Walker RC, Paya CV, Marshall WF, Strickler JG, Wiesner RH, Velosa JA, et al. Pretransplantation seronegative Epstein–Barr virus status is the primary risk factor for posttransplantation lymphoproliferative disorder in adult heart, lung, and other solid organ transplantations. J Heart Lung Transplant. 1995;14:214–21.
67. Husain S, Wagener MM, Singh N. *Cryptococcus neoformans* infection in organ transplant recipients: variables influencing clinical characteristics and outcome. Emerg Infect Dis. 2001;7:375–81.
68. Blair JE, Logan JL. Coccidioidomycosis in solid organ transplantation. Clin Infect Dis. 2001;33:1536–44.
69. Cohen IM, Galgiani JN, Potter D, Ogden DA. Coccidioidomycosis in renal replacement therapy. Arch Intern Med. 1982;142:489–94.
70. Hadley S, Karchmer AW. Fungal infections in solid organ transplant recipients. Infect Dis Clin N Am. 1995;9:1045–74.
71. Centers for Disease Control and Prevention. Recommended adult immunization schedule—United States, October 2007–September 2008. 56th ed. Atlanta: Centers for Disease Control and Prevention; 2007. p. Q1–4.

72. Kretsinger K, Broder KR, Cortese MM, Joyce MP, Ortega-Sanchez I, Lee GM, Centers for Disease Control and Prevention, Advisory Committee on Immunization Practices, Healthcare Infection Control Practices Advisory Committee. Preventing tetanus, diphtheria, and pertussis among adults: use of tetanus toxoid, reduced diphtheria toxoid, and acellular pertussis vaccine. Recommendations of the Advisory Committee on Immunization Practices (ACIP) and recommendation of ACIP, supported by the Healthcare Infection Control Practices Advisory Committee (HICPAC), for use of TDaP among health-care personnel. MMWR Recomm Rep. 2006;55(RR-17):1–37.
73. Gordon CR, Zor F, Siemionow M. Skin area quantification in preparation for concomitant upper extremity and face transplantation: a cadaver study and literature review. Transplantation. 2011;91(9):1050–6.
74. Gordon CR, Zor F, Cetrulo C, Brandacher G, Sachs J, Lee WP. Concomitant face and hand transplantation: perfect solution or perfect storm? Ann Plast Surg. 2011;67(3):309–14.

Principles of Hematopoietic Stem Cell Transplantation

7

Michelle Limei Poon, Richard E. Champlin, and Partow Kebriaei

Introduction

Hematopoietic stem cell transplantation (HSCT) refers to the process of intravenous infusion of self-renewing hematopoietic stem and progenitor cells to restore normal hematopoiesis and/or treat malignancy. The term "hematopoietic stem cell transplantation" has replaced the term bone marrow transplantation because the current advances in the field of transplantation have allowed these self-renewing progenitor and stem cells to be derived not just from bone marrow but also from peripheral blood and umbilical cord blood. In addition, HSCT can be further characterized according to whether they are obtained from the patients themselves (referred to as autologous transplantation), a genetically identical twin (referred to as syngeneic transplantation), or from another individual (referred to as allogeneic transplantation). After decades of refinement, transplantation of both autologous and allogeneic hematopoietic stem cells has become increasingly safe and effective. HSCT now forms an integral part of the curative treatment of hematological malignancies, metabolic disorders, and benign hematological disorders including hemoglobinopathies, immune deficiency syndromes, as well as inherited and acquired marrow failure syndromes. Thus, not surprisingly, the NMDP reports more than 50,000 autologous and allogeneic transplants being done worldwide annually for the treatment of various disorders [1].

The initial concept of the curative potential of HSCT was through allowing increased, myeloablative doses of chemotherapy to be given while avoiding the risk of permanent marrow aplasia. While this may be true for autologous HSCT, the basis for allogeneic HSCT is engraftment of donor-derived hematopoietic stem cells into the recipient. These cells reconstitute hematopoiesis and immunity. Following successful transplantation, recipients are considered chimeras with hematopoietic and immune cells derived from the donor, while mesenchymal and epithelial tissues remain predominantly host derived. Importantly, there is an additional component of an immunotherapeutic graft-versus-leukemia effect, mediated by immunologically competent lymphocytes within the donor graft, which helps improve chances for a cure. The evidence for this graft-versus-tumor effect (GVT) has been clearly demonstrated by studies which show (1) an inverse correlation between relapse and severity of graft-versus-host disease (GVHD) and a comparatively higher rate of relapse following syngeneic or autologous HSCT using the same myeloablative conditioning regimen [2], (2) a higher incidence of relapse rates in T-cell-depleted grafts, and, most significantly, (3) the observations that donor lymphocyte infusions (DLIs) given at a time distant from the original conditioning regimen can treat leukemia relapse successfully. In addition, the potency of the GVT effect varies among the various diseases [3–6]. Indolent lymphoid and myeloid malignancies are most responsive to GVT effects, with durable remissions noted after modulation of immunosuppression or DLI in patients with chronic myeloid leukemia, chronic lymphoid leukemia, and follicular lymphoma [7]. In contrast, diseases such as high-grade lymphoma and acute lymphoblastic leukemia appear less susceptible to the GVT effect, although patients with GVHD do have a reduced risk for relapse [8]. The rapid rate of proliferation of these malignancies may also outpace a developing immune response leading to a generally poor response to DLI. Reduced-intensity conditioning (RIC) regimens were developed based on the potency of the GVT effect rather than the intensity of the conditioning regimen. The advent of RIC regimens has made HSCT accessible to older and more medically infirm patients.

Other progresses in the field of HSCT have included the increasing use of alternative donor sources such as umbilical cord blood transplants and haploidentical transplantations

M. L. Poon
National University Hospital, Department of Hematology Oncology, Singapore, Singapore

R. E. Champlin · P. Kebriaei (✉)
MD Anderson Cancer Center, Department of Stem Cell Transplantation and Cellular Therapy, Houston, TX, USA
e-mail: rchampli@mdanderson.org; pkebriae@mdanderson.org

A. Safdar (ed.), *Principles and Practice of Transplant Infectious Diseases*, https://doi.org/10.1007/978-1-4939-9034-4_7

again allowing HSCT to be made accessible to patients who have no matched donors and who previously would have been precluded from a HSCT. These transplantations however are associated with higher risks of morbidity and mortality, including higher risks of infective complications, due to delayed immune reconstitution.

In this chapter, we aim to look at some important principles of HSCT including the immunobiology of stem cell transplantation, as well as the impact of HSCT on the host immune system, and discuss the principles of immune reconstitution following HSCT. In addition, we will also discuss the choice of preparative regimens, stem cell sources, the importance of post-transplant immunosuppressive therapy, as well as the indications for HSCT. The complications related to HSCT will be briefly touched upon, but these will be covered in greater detail in the relevant chapters.

Historical Perspectives of HSCT

There has been increased interest in the use of marrow cells to facilitate hematopoietic reconstitution since the late nineteenth and early twentieth century, with reports of the use of oral, intramuscular, and intramedullary injections of marrow infusions to facilitate hematopoietic recovery in patients with leukemia or marrow aplasia. In 1939, Osgood et al. reported the first unsuccessful attempt to treat a patient with aplastic anemia using intravenous infusion of viable marrow cells [9]. These early attempts, however, were carried out in isolation, and it was not until the clinical observations of the severe myelosuppressive effects of radiation among nuclear bomb survivors at Hiroshima and Nagasaki that concerted research efforts were started to develop methods to reverse the myelosuppressive effects of radiation, including the use of marrow infusion. Early pivotal work by Jacobson et al. in 1948 demonstrated that mice who had splenic shielding could survive otherwise lethal doses of irradiation with marrow recovery [10]. He further showed that bone marrow failure following otherwise lethal doses of irradiation could also be prevented by infusing either spleen cells or bone marrow cells from a litter mate into the animal [11]. The mechanisms of these findings were initially poorly understood and attributed to either a hormone or growth factor contained in the infusion. Further studies however in the 1950s and 1960s debunked the "hormonal theory" and confirmed that it was the living cells within the marrow infusion that were responsible for hematopoietic recovery. These studies formed the initial basis for the development of stem cell infusion as a treatment for leukemia and bone marrow failure. Further advances in the field of HSCT came with the understanding of the concept of histocompatibility, as a result of the canine studies done by E. Donnall Thomas and colleagues in Seattle in the 1960s. They noted that in lethally irradiated dogs, marrow grafts from mismatched littermates always failed, while grafts between dog lymphocyte antigen (DLA)-matched donors and recipients showed improved survival. They also demonstrated that the administration of a short course of MTX for immunosuppression after grafting improved the long-term survival of matched recipients [12–14]. This understanding of the major histocompatibility complex (MHC) and human leucocyte antigens (HLA) as the major determinants of graft rejection further advanced laboratory studies and clinical applications of allogeneic HSCT. This led to the first successful reports of clinical HSCT for patients with immunodeficiency disorders, aplastic anemias, and advanced leukemias in the late 1960s and early 1970s [7, 15–17].

The initial transplants were associated with significant morbidity and mortality as a result of complications from infections and graft-versus-host disease (GVHD). In the last 10–20 years, however, the outcomes of HSCT have improved dramatically due to refinements in the transplant approach, as well as better supportive care/infectious disease management. Better tissue typing of donors and recipients using molecular methods and improved understanding of the pathogenesis of GVHD and improved GVHD prophylactic measures have led to reduced rates of both acute and chronic GVHD. Improved and novel, reduced-intensity conditioning regimens, together with the increased numbers of matched unrelated donor (MUD) registries and development of alternative stem cell sources including cord blood and haploidentical sources, have made HSCT more accessible to a larger patient population, who would have been ineligible for transplant previously. In addition, improvements in supportive care, and especially in the field of infectious diseases, have further reduced infection-related morbidity and mortality. The summation of these exciting developments has led to HSCT being a standard treatment option not just for many hematological malignancies but also for benign disorders including immunodeficiency syndromes, metabolic disorders, and defective hematopoietic states. Rarely, allogeneic HSCT may also have a role in situations of nuclear accidents, where it may be used to treat victims who receive exposure to marrow-ablative doses of radiation, such as following the Chernobyl nuclear disaster in 1986 [18]. While such situations are rare, this concept has been brought to the forefront again with the recent Japanese Fukushima nuclear disaster, and with the increasing use of nuclear resources as a source of energy, as well as the constant threat of nuclear warfare worldwide.

Basic Principles of HSCT

Immunobiology of HSCT

The fundamental principles underlying the development of stem cell transplantation are the use of a combination of drugs and/or radiotherapy (conditioning regimen) to eradicate the underlying disease process and to create space within the bone marrow niches for the incoming marrow cells. The conditioning regimen also has the role of immunosuppressing the host in order to prevent a host-versus-graft reaction. Hematopoietic stem cells (HSCs) with the capacity for self-renewal and differentiation into the various lineages are collected either from the patient (autologous transplants) or from the donor (allogeneic transplant). Following the conditioning regimen, HSC are then introduced. These cells then migrate through the blood and across endothelial vasculature to various organs, and eventually to the marrow niches, a process termed homing. Homing is a coordinated multistep process, which usually occurs rapidly within 24 h, and is the first and most essential step in clinical stem cell transplantation. The understanding of the details of this complex process remains the work of much ongoing research.

Durable engraftment of allogeneic HSC is subsequently dependent on the donor CD8+ T cells which are needed to overcome any residual host-versus-graft response created by the donor-specific host T cells (that remain following the conditioning). Donor CD8 and CD4 T cells interact with peptide antigens complexed with MHC class I and II molecules, respectively, on antigen-presenting cells (APCs) of the recipient. This leads to subsequent donor T-cell proliferation and a successful allo-response against residual recipient T cells, causing the elimination of the recipient immune system. Donor T-cell engraftment is important in establishing long-term hematopoiesis. CD34 stem cells and their progeny within the graft also help in engraftment by blocking residual host T-cell function through a "veto" effect, as well as by further differentiating into natural killer (NK) cells which favor engraftment through their recognition and killing of residual recipient lymphocytes. Once engrafted, donor HSCs continue to maintain hematopoiesis as well as aid in immune reconstitution within the host.

Reconstitution of Immunity Following Allogeneic HSCT

Reconstitution of immunity post HSCT involves the reconstitution of different immune cell subsets, including NK cells, the T and B cells, APCs, and the production of antibodies.

Recovery of Innate Immunity

NK cells, derived from the infused CD34 progenitor cells, and driven by lymphocyte growth factors and cytokines, are the first immune cells to reach normal levels and are crucial components of the innate immune system. Donor-derived antigen-presenting cells (APC) including monocyte-macrophages, dendritic cells (myeloid and plasmacytoid), and Langerhans cells also develop from CD34 cells within weeks after the transplant and return to normal levels within 6 weeks following the transplant.

Recovery of Adaptive Immunity

The initial T-cell recovery in the first 3 months following HSCT is dependent on peripheral expansion of post-thymic donor T lymphocytes that were transfused within the graft. These T cells consist predominantly of central and effector memory cells with a smaller population of naive T cells and end-stage effector cells. These memory T cells are driven by cytokines and the presence of alloreactive antigens, as well as reactivating viruses, and expand and mature into an expanded memory pool but with decreased diversity in both naive and memory lymphocytes. The TCR repertoire resulting from these early expansions is typically skewed and oligoclonal. These post-thymic cells are largely responsible for the success or failure of the transplant through their impact on engraftment, GVHD, GVT, and reactivating viruses.

While early post-transplant T-cell reconstitution is dependent upon peripheral T-cell expansion, an optimal cellular immunity, with a diverse T-cell receptor (TCR) repertoire, is only achieved following thymopoiesis, which normally starts about 120 days post-transplant. CD4-positive T cells rely more on thymic production of naive T cells after HSCT and hence reconstitute later than CD8 + T cells, leading to an inversion of the CD4/CD8 ratio prior to thymopoiesis. Naive T cells are formed by the CD34 precursors within the marrow and processed by the recipient thymus to form a new immune repertoire. In children and young adults where the thymus function is normal, a new T-cell repertoire develops within 1–2 years. In contrast, in older patients with limited thymic activity, naive T cells and total CD4+ T-cell reconstitution may be impaired indefinitely leading to higher risks of opportunistic infections, leukemia relapse, and chronic GVHD.

B-cell reconstitution post HSCT recapitulates the normal B-cell development. However, this process is commonly impaired due to prolonged low levels of circulating B cells, a relative deficit of mature B cells due to impaired immunoglobulin class switching, and a diminished ability to undergo somatic hypermutation. The reconstitution of the B-cell compartment representing humoral immunity may take up to 2 years after HSCT and may result in patients being at high risks of infection by encapsulated organisms and may also result in diminished vaccine responses to infectious antigens even after normal B-cell numbers have been achieved.

1. The pattern of reconstitution of immunity explains the pattern of infective complications seen post-transplantation. Re-engraftment (D1-30): Bacterial infections are commonest during this period followed by fungal infections especially candidemia and invasive aspergillosis, due to the significant neutropenia while awaiting engraftment of HSCs.
2. Post-engraftment (D30-100): Viral and fungal infections (especially mold infections) may develop as a result of the defective cellular and humoral immunity, as well as defective phagocytic function.
3. Late post-engraftment (days >100): Risks for viral and fungal infections persist until eventual recovery of cellular and humoral immunity.

Importantly, there are a number of factors that affect immune reconstitution post-transplant. These include the age of the patient, the transplant preparative regimen, and whether anti-T-cell therapy such as antithymocyte globulin (ATG) or alemtuzumab was included, the graft source, and the development of GVHD. These will be discussed in the subsequent relevant sections below.

Technical Aspects of HSCT

Tissue Typing and Donor Selection

The major histocompatibility complex (MHC) is the term given to genes clustered on the short arm of chromosome six that form the human leukocyte antigen (HLA) system. The most important HLAs include HLA A, B, and C (found on the class 1 loci) and HLA DR, DQ (found on the class 2 loci). A single set of MHC alleles described as a haplotype are inherited from each parent, resulting in HLA pairs. As a result of this inheritance, parents are half matched with their children, while the probability that two siblings would share the same haplotypes would be one in four. In allogeneic HSCT, donor and recipient are matched for HLA in order to reduce GVHD (where immunologically active cells from the graft attack body tissues in the transplant recipient/host) or, less commonly, graft rejection (where immunologically active cells from the recipient/host reject the donor cells). While histocompatibility was previously defined by serologic assays (also called low-resolution HLA typing), the development of molecular assays has resulted in the serologic groups being further subdivided into specific alleles (high-resolution typing). Studies have shown that HLA matching of donors and recipients at a high-resolution level (using molecular methods of typing) especially for unrelated transplants have been associated with reduced GVHD rates and improved overall survival. Currently, a "matched" donor is defined on the basis of HLA high-resolution matching at four loci, HLA A, B, C, and DRB1, ("8/8" match) or five loci, HLA A, B, C, DRB1, and DQB1 ("10/10" match).

Sibling donors are the preferred donor source, because of the least risks of GVHD and graft rejection. For patients without a fully HLA-matched sibling donor, alternatives include an unrelated HLA fully matched donor or partially matched cord blood units or a partially HLA-matched family member [19–21].

MUD Donors

Depending on the ethnic background of the patient, the possibility of identifying a HLA-matched unrelated (MUD) donor is between 50% and 80%. As a result of better HLA matching with improved molecular typing techniques, the current results of matched unrelated donor transplants for malignancy are not significantly different compared with HSCT from matched sibling donor transplants [22, 23]. This has led to the use of MUD HSCTs for patients at an earlier stage in their disease, and these transplants now account for almost 15% of all allogeneic transplants performed worldwide. Problems with using MUD donors however include the longer time (up to 2–3 months or longer) needed to identify and procure cells from an unrelated donor, which may not be fast enough for patients with rapidly progressive malignancies.

Umbilical Cord Blood Donors

Umbilical cord blood transplantation was first performed successfully by Gluckman et al. in a patient with Fanconi's anemia in 1988 [24]. Since then, the field has expanded rapidly, with over 25,000 cord blood transplants performed worldwide and over 500,000 cord bloods being collected for public use. The umbilical cord contains fetal blood collected following the delivery of the placenta and separation from the fetus and is rich in hematopoietic and progenitor cells [25]. Normally up to 50–100 cc of cord blood can be collected from each delivery. The small volumes of cord blood available usually results in much lower stem cell dose as compared to that collected from peripheral blood or bone marrow, for the adult patient. The advantages of umbilical cord blood transplant over an unrelated donor include the rapidity at which the product can be obtained (usually less than 4 weeks). In addition, because of the high percentage of naive T cells present within the cord blood, HLA mismatches in up to two of six HLAs are acceptable in cord blood transplant, allowing for a higher likelihood of finding a donor for a patient with rarer HLA genotypes. The rates of aGVHD with UCBTs also appear lower compared with normal unrelated BM transplants, and this is again attributed to the high naive T-cell population present within the cord blood graft [26]. The low stem cell dose and possibly the smaller number of lineage committed late progenitor cells within cord blood grafts however, especially for adult patients, lead to higher risks of graft rejection, slower engraftment and immune reconstitution, and higher infective complications and treatment-related mortality (TRM) compared with unrelated HSCTs. In addition, no remaining product is left after infusion in the event of disease relapse or graft rejection. While there has been no randomized controlled trials comparing the outcomes of UCBT to other graft sources, there have been a number of retrospective studies in the literature which has explored this issue. In one of the largest studies, a review of registry data from the CIBMTR, comparing the outcomes of 165 myeloablative single UCBT with 888 MUD peripheral blood stem cell (PBSC) recipients and 472 MUD bone marrow (BM) recipients, it was found that UCBT was associated with higher TRM, but overall DFS and OS were similar among all three groups [27]. In an attempt to overcome the poor outcomes associated with the low cell doses in the cord blood grafts, there has been a shift toward using double rather than single cord blood units [28], as well as studies looking at ex vivo expansion of one of the cord blood units [29, 30] or the use of CD34 cells from haploidentical donors for temporary support while awaiting cord blood engraftment [31]. Brunstein et al. reported data from Seattle and Minnesota, comparing double UCBT with related, matched, or 1-antigen-mismatched MUD and found TRM was higher [dUCB (34%, 95% CI, 25%–42%), MRD (24%, 95% CI, 17%–39%), and MUD (14%, 95% CI, 9%–20%), but relapse rates were lower in the UCBT group (15%, 95% CI, 9%–22%) compared with MRD (43%, 95% CI, 35%–52%) or MUD (37%, 95% CI, 29%–46%), leading to comparable overall survival among the different groups [32].

Haploidentical Donors

Haploidentical transplantation is another alternative for patients with no unrelated donors. It involves alloHSCT using a partially HLA-matched family member among first-degree relatives, who share at least one haplotype with the potential recipient. The advantage of haploidentical transplantation includes donor availability, since virtually all patients should have a haploidentical donor. The initial experiences with haploidentical HSCT using unmanipulated bone marrow grafts with standard immunosuppressive therapy post-transplant were associated with dismal outcomes with high rates of graft rejection, GVHD and TRM, especially in the setting of two or more HLA mismatches [33–35]. This led to work by several groups to overcome the immunological barrier through novel graft manipulation techniques, improved GVHD prophylaxis, and the development of new conditioning regimens. Most strategies have involved T-cell depletion pre-transplant, using either in vivo techniques (using monoclonal antibodies or antithymocyte globulin) or ex vivo techniques using T-cell depletion with agglutination and E-rosetting methods and CD34+-selected cells, a technique pioneered by the Perugia group in Italy [19, 36, 37]. While these techniques have been associated with marked reduction in graft failure and GVHD rates, delayed immune reconstitution and high TRM due to infections remain a significant deterrence. In addition long-term disease control with haploidentical HSCT is limited in patients with active disease at time of transplant. Another novel approach in the field of haploidentical transplant has been the use of post-transplantation cyclophosphamide to overcome the HLA barrier [38–40]. It has been shown in animal models that both graft rejection and GVHD after histoincompatible BMT can be mitigated by the post-transplant administration of high-dose cyclophosphamide, which is known to be highly toxic to proliferating alloreactive lymphocytes, though high relapse rates remain an issue.

Given the differences between the various stem cell sources, generally sibling donors are preferred, followed by MUD donors. For patients with no MUD donors, the selection of cord blood versus haploidentical family member donor remains largely dependent on institutional expertise, in the absence of comparative studies.

HSC Acquisition

Following identification of a donor, procurement of hematopoietic progenitor cells is necessary before proceeding with a HSCT. Collection of sufficient numbers of hematopoietic stem cells is required for reconstitution of hematopoiesis and immunity post-transplantation. These stem cells primarily reside in the bone marrow, and in the past, all hematopoietic transplantation utilized unfractionated bone marrow cells harvested via repeated aspirations from the posterior iliac crest. However, HSCs also circulate in low frequency in the peripheral blood, and since the 1980s, hematopoietic growth factors, primarily granulocyte colony-stimulating factor (GCSF), have been used to mobilize higher numbers of HSC into the peripheral blood pool, and HSCs are then collected via an aphaeresis procedure from the donor [41, 42]. Importantly, there are many significant differences in the composition of peripheral blood HSC as compared with marrow grafts. GCSF-stimulated peripheral blood grafts have an approximately two to five times higher HSC concentration than in bone marrow, as well as one log more T cells than marrow grafts [43]. In contrast, bone marrow grafts contain mesenchymal stromal cells, as well as reticular endothelial cells, macrophages, fibroblasts, endothelial progenitor cells, adipocytes, and osteogenic progenitor cells, which provide various cell-to-cell interactions essential for hematopoiesis and progenitor cell differentiation. Some consistent differences in outcomes identified from comparative studies include faster engraftment of all cell lineages, faster immune recovery (see section on Immune reconstitution post-transplant), and a trend toward more overall and extensive chronic GVHD rates in PB transplants [44–51]. In addition, an individual patient meta-analysis using data from the nine randomized trials also found an improved overall survival and disease-free survival in patients with late-stage hematologic malignancies disease who received a PBHC transplant compared to a bone marrow transplant [52]. The results of these studies, as well as the ease of PBHC collection as compared to BM harvests, have led to increased use of PBHC grafts, and currently, about 70% of all allogeneic transplants in Europe and worldwide are performed with PBHC instead of BM grafts. What is important to realize however is that these prospective randomized studies comparing PBHC vs. BM transplants have been done in matched sibling transplants and mainly included patients with leukemias and other hematologic malignancies. For other patients with benign disorders such as aplastic anemia, where a graft-versus-tumor effect is not needed, retrospective registry data has suggested that BM grafts are the preferred option over PBHC grafts because of their lower risks for chronic GVHD [53]. In the matched unrelated setting, a large Phase III, randomized, multicenter, trial looking at the issue of PBHC versus BM graft has been recently reported in abstract form [54]. In this large study involving 278 subjects from 50 centers in the United States and Canada, PBHC grafts appear to be associated with higher rates of chronic GVHD and BM associated with increased rate of graft failure, with similar rates of acute GVHD, relapse, non-relapse mortality and overall survival.

Currently, selection of the optimal source of stem cells depends on the underlying disease subtype, as well as the donor and transplant type. In patients undergoing autologous transplantation, PBHCs are now almost universally used in preference to BM grafts since chronic GVHD is not an issue of concern. For allogeneic matched-related donor transplants, the use of PBHCs will be preferable in patients being allografted for advanced leukemias, whereas for transplants done for benign disorders such as aplastic anemia, BM grafts are preferable. In the unrelated donor setting, the optimal graft choice remains unclear, though given the recent intriguing data from the BMT-CTN studies; the choice for BM versus PB HSC depends on individuals' concerns for chronic GVHD versus graft failure.

Preparative Regimens

Myeloablative Versus Reduced-Intensity Conditioning

Following the selection of the appropriate donor and stem cell source, patients are then put on conditioning regimens prior to the infusion of the hematopoietic stem cells. For autologous transplant, where the hematopoietic cells come from the patient themselves, the only role of the conditioning regimen is tumor eradication. In contrast, in myeloablative allogeneic transplant, the conditioning regimens have three main roles:

1. First, reduction of the disease burden to a minimal level
2. Second, creation of "space" within the marrow microenvironment to allow engraftment of HSC
3. Third, to provide sufficient host immunosuppression to prevent graft rejection and allow donor cells engraftment

Until recently, all patients received myeloablative conditioning regimens, defined as a regimen which contained a combination of agents expected to produce profound and irreversible pancytopenia and myeloablation within 1–3 weeks from administration and which needed hematopoietic stem cell infusion to restore hematopoiesis. When given with stem cell rescue, the ability to escalate doses of agents used in myeloablative regimens is limited by their toxicity to organs and tissues other than the bone marrow.

The discovery of the curative potential of the immune-mediated GVT effect has led to increasing use of reduced-intensity conditioning (RIC) regimens [55, 56]. These reduced-intensity conditioning regimens have been designed not to eradicate malignancy but rather to provide sufficient immunosuppression and immunoablation to achieve engraftment and allow induction of a GVT effect. They are associated with lower toxicities and hence can be safely performed in many patients in whom HSCT would have been previously contraindicated. Although all these low-dose nonablative preparative conditioning regimens devised are broadly classified as "reduced-intensity" transplants, there are significant differences in the relative degree of immunosuppression and myelosuppression involved, and they can be further divided into the truly nonmyeloablative regimens (NMA) and RIC regimens [57]. Nonmyeloablative regimens are defined as regimens associated with minimal cytopenia that do not require stem cell support. In nonmyeloablative regimens, the conditioning regimen is mainly for immunosuppression to allow stem cell engraftment and depends mainly on the GVT effect for disease control. The lack of neutropenia with such regimens reduces risks of bacterial sepsis, and hence such treatments are very tolerable and may even be performed in the outpatient setting. In contrast, RIC regimens are a category of regimens which are intermediate in intensity between myeloablative and NMA regimens. These regimens have an element of antitumor effect in addition to their immunosuppressive effect. They are associated with observable aplasia and have greater toxicities compared to NMA regimens but have the advantage of greater debulking of residual disease. With RIC regimens, cytopenias may be prolonged, and stem cell support required, and although unlike myeloablative regimens, autologous recovery would eventually occur, the pancytopenia would be of such duration to cause significant morbidity and mortality.

GVHD and Its Prophylaxis

GVHD is a major cause of morbidity and mortality in allogeneic HSCT patients. Acute GVHD typically occurs within the first 100 days post-transplant and is due to the reactivity of the mature donor T lymphocytes present in the graft directed against disparate major or minor histocompatibility of the host. In contrast, chronic GVHD is a syndrome of disordered immune dysregulation with features similar to that of a number of autoimmune disorders and generally develop between 100 days and 2 years post-transplant. These cutoffs however are not absolute, and patients can present with symptoms typical of chronic GVHD in the early weeks after transplant and with symptoms typical of acute GVHD at times beyond day 100.

The pathophysiology of acute GVHD involves three phases [58]. The first phase involves conditioning regimen-related tissue injury, which results in cytokine release, upregulation of HLA molecules as well as activation of macrophages, and generation of a pro-inflammatory state. In the second phase, alloreactive T cells recognize allogeneic antigens presented on host dendritic cells and become activated and expand. In the third phase, there is generation of effector cells and cytokines that are responsible for tissue injury. The skin, GI tract, and liver are the primary target tissues of acute GVHD. In contrast, chronic GVHD is a syndrome of immune dysregulation with generation of autoreactive T cells directed against shared MHC determinants and production of autoantibodies. Chronic GVHD is related to thymic dysfunction and failure of the thymus to delete autoreactive cells and induce tolerance, and may be associated with significant immunosuppression, and a higher risk for opportunistic infections.

Pharmacological immunosuppression is generally administered for the first 6 months post-transplant to reduce the incidence and severity of GVHD, and the current standard of care combines either cyclosporine or tacrolimus with a short course of methotrexate [59, 60]. Cyclosporine and tacrolimus prevent activation of T cells, whereas methotrexate targets proliferating T cells that were activated in the early post-transplant phase by host antigens. Addition of corticosteroids is the first line of therapy in patients who develop acute GVHD [61], and approximately half of patients have a sustained response with steroid dose being able to be tapered off. Steroid-resistant GVHD has an unfavorable prognosis. With current immunosuppressive prophylaxis, the incidence of acute GVHD is about 25–50% of patients after transplants from an HLA identical sibling, and up to 60–90% has been reported following transplants from mismatched and unrelated donors, while chronic GVHD affects 25–60% of recipients of allogeneic transplantation who survive more than 6 months after transplant.

Table 7.1 Complications after hematopoietic transplantation

Complications
Immune complications
Graft rejection
Acute graft-vs-host disease
Chronic graft-vs-host disease
Regimen-related toxicity of the preparative regimen
Mucositis
Hemorrhagic cystitis
Veno-occlusive disease of the liver
Diffuse alveolar hemorrhage and interstitial pneumonitis
Hematologic complications
Cytopenias
Hemolytic anemia
Thrombotic thrombocytopenic purpura and hemolytic disorders
Infections and immunodeficiency
EBV-associated lymphoproliferative disease
Late complications:
Growth disturbances
Endocrine-related issues: e.g., hypothyroidism, hypogonadism, and sterility
Cataracts
Avascular necrosis
Secondary malignancies
Cognitive deficits (with TBI-based regimens)

Treatment-Related Complications

Hematopoietic transplantation has been associated with a number of serious complications including immune-mediated processes such as graft failure and graft-versus-host disease, toxicities from the pre-transplant conditioning regimen, as well as infections related to neutropenia and post-transplant immune deficiency. Supportive care post-transplantation including hydration, close monitoring, appropriate use of growth factors to hasten WBC recovery, appropriate use of antimicrobial prophylaxis, and good nutritional support are important in preventing these complications. Table 7.1 summarizes the complications associated with HSCT.

Indications for HSCT

Malignant Disorders

Both autologous and allogeneic HSCT are now well established as important treatments for hematological malignancies. Selection of the type of transplantation (autologous or allogeneic) depends on the type of malignancy, age, availability of a suitable donor, the ability to collect a tumor free graft, the stage of disease, as well as disease susceptibility to the GVT effect.

Autologous transplants do not require HLA-matched donors, as the stem cells come from the patients themselves, hence making this process readily available.

Autologous transplants are also associated with lower TRM than allogeneic transplants, because of various factors, including faster immune reconstitution and lower opportunistic infections, lower risk of life-threatening complications, and no GVHD issues and only rare graft failure issues. The process is hence well tolerated and can be offered to older patients.

However, autologous transplants have several drawbacks including potential contamination of the autograft by clonogenic tumor cells that can contribute to relapse, as well as the lack of an immune-mediated graft-versus-malignancy effect, hence leading to higher relapse rates as compared to allogeneic transplants. In addition, the use of high-dose chemotherapy, especially in patients with extensive prior therapy, may be associated with risks of developing therapy-related myelodysplastic syndrome and secondary leukemias.

Benign Disorders

In addition to their benefits in patients with hematological malignancies, allogeneic transplantation is also indicated in nonmalignant disorders including immunodeficiency disease, metabolic diseases, hemoglobinopathies, and aplastic anemia as well as other marrow failure syndromes.

Table 7.2 provides recommendations on the appropriate timing for transplantation consultation, based on the 2012 guidelines were developed jointly by the National Marrow Donor Program® (NMDP) and the American Society for Blood and Marrow Transplantation (ASBMT) [1].

Table 7.2 Indications for stem cell transplantation

Hematologic malignancies
(i) Acute myeloid leukemia (AML)
High-risk AML including antecedent hematological disease (e.g., myelodysplasia (MDS)), therapy-related AML, or induction failure
CR1 with intermediate- or poor-risk cytogenetics or molecular markers
Relapsed AML
(ii) Acute lymphoblastic leukemia (ALL)
CR1 standard risk or
CR1 high risk including persistent minimal residual disease, poor-risk cytogenetics (e.g., Philadelphia chromosome (t(9;22)) or 11q23 rearrangements), high WBC (>30,000–50,000) at diagnosis, no CR within 4 weeks of initial treatment, and induction failure, persistent minimal residual disease
ALL after relapse
(iii) Myelodysplastic syndromes (MDS)
Intermediate-1 or -2(INT-1 or INT-2) or high IPSS score
Any MDS with poor prognostic features, including older age, refractory cytopenias, adverse cytogenetics, transfusion dependent
(iv) Chronic myeloid leukemia
No hematologic response post-tyrosine kinase inhibitor (TKI) initiation
No complete cytogenetic response post-TKI initiation
Disease progression
Intolerance to TKI
Accelerated phase or blast crisis (myeloid or lymphoid)
(v) Chronic lymphocytic leukemia (CLL)
High-risk cytogenetics or molecular features (e.g., 11q or 17p deletions, unmutated Ig V_H mutational status)
Short initial remission
Poor initial response
Fludarabine-resistant
(vi) Non-Hodgkin lymphoma
Follicular
Poor response to initial treatment
Initial remission duration <12 months
Second relapse
Transformation to diffuse large B-cell lymphoma
Diffuse large B-cell or high-grade lymphoma
At first or subsequent relapse
CR1 for patients with high or high-intermediate IPI risk
No CR with initial treatment
(vii) Hodgkin lymphoma
No initial CR
First or subsequent relapse
(viii) Multiple myeloma
After initiation of therapy
At first progression
Other malignant diseases
(i) Germ cell tumors if
Short initial remission
Poor initial response
(ii) Neuroblastoma if
Short initial remission
Poor initial response or at progression
Nonmalignant disorders
(i) Immune deficiency disease (including severe combined immunodeficiency syndromes, Wiskott-Aldrich syndrome, Omenn syndrome, X-linked lymphoproliferative syndrome, Kostmann syndrome): at the time of diagnosis
(ii) Inherited metabolic disorders (including Hurler's syndrome, adrenoleukodystrophy, and others): at diagnosis
(iii) Hemoglobinopathies
Thalassemia major: at the time of diagnosis
Sickle cell disease with aggressive course (CNS or lung complications, frequent pain crises)
(iv) Hemophagocytic lymphohistiocytosis (HLH): at diagnosis
(v) Severe aplastic anemia and other marrow failure syndromes (including Fanconi anemia, Diamond-Blackfan anemia, and others): at diagnosis

Adapted from the 2012 guidelines developed by the National Donor Marrow Program and the American Society for Blood And Marrow Transplantation [1]

Future Directions

Over the last two decades, the increased understanding of the various aspects of HSCT has led to significant improved safety of this procedure and increased applicability of this treatment to a larger patient population and provided a means of delivering potentially curative treatment in many situations where it was not previously possible. Areas under current development include the improvement preparative regimens through the use of molecularly targeted anticancer therapies, the broadened use of alternative donors, and continuous improvement in supportive care for patients. In addition, promising work has been done with the use of adoptive cellular therapy such as the use of T cells with chimeric receptor antigens, tumor vaccines, as well as the use of expanded NK cells to augment the GVT effects. Major challenges ahead remain the development of strategies to enhance the immune antitumor effect with both autologous and allogeneic transplants, as well as strategies to separate the GVT effect from the GVHD effect so as to improve upon TRM. Carefully planned prospective clinical trials and collaborative efforts from the various research groups will be necessary to attain these goals.

References

1. National marrow donor program website https://www.bethematch.org.
2. Horowitz MM, Gale RP, Sondel PM, Goldman JM, Kersey J, Kolb HJ, et al. Graft-versus-leukemia reactions after bone marrow transplantation. Blood. 1990;75(3):555–62.
3. Collins RH Jr, Shpilberg O, Drobyski WR, Porter DL, Giralt S, Champlin R, et al. Donor leukocyte infusions in 140 patients with relapsed malignancy after allogeneic bone marrow transplantation. J Clin Oncol. 1997;15(2):433–44.
4. Kolb HJ, Mittermüller J, Clemm C, Holler E, Ledderose G, Brehm G, et al. Donor leukocyte transfusions for treatment of recurrent chronic myelogenous leukemia in marrow transplant patients. Blood. 1990;76(12):2462–5.
5. Kolb HJ, Schattenberg A, Goldman JM, Hertenstein B, Jacobsen N, Arcese W, et al. Graft-versus-leukemia effect of donor lymphocyte transfusions in marrow grafted patients. Blood. 1995;86(5):2041–50.
6. Porter DL, Roth MS, McGarigle C, Ferrara JL, Antin JH. Induction of graft-versus-host disease as immunotherapy for relapsed chronic myeloid leukemia. N Engl J Med. 1994;330(2):100–6.
7. van Besien KW, de Lima M, Giralt SA, Moore DF Jr, Khouri IF, Rondón G, et al. Management of lymphoma recurrence after allogeneic transplantation: the relevance of graft-versus-lymphoma effect. Bone Marrow Transplant. 1997;19(10):977–82.
8. Collins RH Jr, Goldstein S, Giralt S, Levine J, Porter D, Drobyski W, et al. Donor leukocyte infusions in acute lymphocytic leukemia. Bone Marrow Transplant. 2000;26(5):511–6.
9. Osgood E. Aplastic anemia treated with daily transfusions and intravenous marrow: case report. Ann Intern Med. 1939;13:357–67.
10. Jacobson LO, Simmons EL, Marks EK, Robson MJ, Bethard WF, Gaston EO. The role of the spleen in radiation injury and recovery. J Lab Clin Med. 1950;35(5):746–70.
11. Jacobson LO, Simmons EL, Bethard WF. Studies on hematopoietic recovery from radiation injury. J Clin Invest. 1950;29(6):825.
12. Storb R, Epstein RB, Bryant J, Ragde H, Thomas ED. Marrow grafts by combined marrow and leukocyte infusions in unrelated dogs selected by histocompatibility typing. Transplantation. 1968;6(4):587–93.
13. Storb R, Epstein RB, Graham TC, Thomas ED. Methotrexate regimens for control of graft-versus-host disease in dogs with allogeneic marrow grafts. Transplantation. 1970;9(3):240–6.
14. Storb R, Rudolph RH, Thomas ED. Marrow grafts between canine siblings matched by serotyping and mixed leukocyte culture. J Clin Invest. 1971;50(6):1272–5.
15. Bach FH, Albertini RJ, Joo P, Anderson JL, Bortin MM. Bone-marrow transplantation in a patient with the Wiskott-Aldrich syndrome. Lancet. 1968;2(7583):1364–6.
16. Gatti RA, Meuwissen HJ, Allen HD, Hong R, Good RA. Immunological reconstitution of sex-linked lymphopenic immunological deficiency. Lancet. 1968;2(7583):1366–9.
17. Mathe G, Amiel JL, Schwarzenberg L, Cattan A, Schneider M, Devries MJ, et al. Successful allogenic bone marrow transplantation in man: chimerism, induced specific tolerance and possible anti-leukemic effects. Blood. 1965;25:179–96.
18. Champlin RE, Kastenberg WE, Gale RP. Radiation accidents and nuclear energy: medical consequences and therapy. Ann Intern Med. 1988;109(9):730–44.
19. Aversa F, Tabilio A, Velardi A, Cunningham I, Terenzi A, Falzetti F, et al. Treatment of high-risk acute leukemia with T-cell-depleted stem cells from related donors with one fully mismatched HLA haplotype. N Engl J Med. 1998;339(17):1186–93.
20. Kernan NA, Bartsch G, Ash RC, Beatty PG, Champlin R, Filipovich A, et al. Analysis of 462 transplantations from unrelated donors facilitated by the National Marrow Donor Program. N Engl J Med. 1993;328(9):593–602.
21. Rubinstein P, Carrier C, Scaradavou A, Kurtzberg J, Adamson J, Migliaccio AR, et al. Outcomes among 562 recipients of placental-blood transplants from unrelated donors. N Engl J Med. 1998;339(22):1565–77.
22. Flomenberg N, Baxter-Lowe LA, Confer D, Fernandez-Vina M, Filipovich A, Horowitz M, et al. Impact of HLA class I and class II high-resolution matching on outcomes of unrelated donor bone marrow transplantation: HLA-C mismatching is associated with a strong adverse effect on transplantation outcome. Blood. 2004;104(7):1923–30.
23. Yakoub-Agha I, Mesnil F, Kuentz M, Boiron JM, Ifrah N, Milpied N, et al. Allogeneic marrow stem-cell transplantation from human leukocyte antigen-identical siblings versus human leukocyte antigen-allelic-matched unrelated donors (10/10) in patients with standard-risk hematologic malignancy: a prospective study from the French Society of Bone Marrow Transplantation and Cell Therapy. J Clin Oncol. 2006;24(36):5695–702.
24. Gluckman E, Broxmeyer HA, Auerbach AD, Friedman HS, Douglas GW, Devergie A, et al. Hematopoietic reconstitution in a patient with Fanconi's anemia by means of umbilical-cord blood from an HLA-identical sibling. N Engl J Med. 1989;321(17):1174–8.
25. Cairo MS, Wagner JE. Placental and/or umbilical cord blood: an alternative source of hematopoietic stem cells for transplantation. Blood. 1997;90(12):4665–78.
26. Rocha V, Wagner JE Jr, Sobocinski KA, Klein JP, Zhang MJ, Horowitz MM, Gluckman E. Graft-versus-host disease in children who have received a cord-blood or bone marrow transplant from an HLA-identical sibling. Eurocord and International Bone Marrow Transplant Registry Working Committee on Alternative Donor and Stem Cell Sources. N Engl J Med. 2000;342(25):1846–54.
27. Eapen M, Rocha V, Sanz G, Scaradavou A, Zhang M-J, Arcese W, et al. Effect of graft source on unrelated donor haemopoietic stem-cell transplantation in adults with acute leukaemia: a retrospective analysis. Lancet Oncol. 2010;11(7):653–60.
28. Barker JN, Weisdorf DJ, DeFor TE, Blazar BR, McGlave PB, Miller JS, et al. Transplantation of 2 partially HLA-matched umbilical cord blood units to enhance engraftment in adults with hematologic malignancy. Blood. 2005;105(3):1343–7.
29. Shpall EJ, Quinones R, Giller R, Zeng C, Baron AE, Jones RB, et al. Transplantation of ex vivo expanded cord blood. Biol Blood Marrow Transplant. 2002;8(7):368–76.

30. Robinson SN, Simmons PJ, Yang H, Alousi AM, Marcos de Lima J, Shpall EJ. Mesenchymal stem cells in ex vivo cord blood expansion. Best Pract Res Clin Haematol. 2011;24(1): 83–92.
31. Liu H, Rich ES, Godley L, Odenike O, Joseph L, Marino S, et al. Reduced-intensity conditioning with combined haploidentical and cord blood transplantation results in rapid engraftment, low GVHD, and durable remissions. Blood. 2011;118(24):6438–45.
32. Brunstein CG, Gutman JA, Weisdorf DJ, Woolfrey AE, Defor TE, Gooley TA, et al. Allogeneic hematopoietic cell transplantation for hematologic malignancy: relative risks and benefits of double umbilical cord blood. Blood. 2010;116(22):4693–9.
33. Anasetti C, Amos D, Beatty PG, Appelbaum FR, Bensinger W, Buckner CD, et al. Effect of HLA compatibility on engraftment of bone marrow transplants in patients with leukemia or lymphoma. N Engl J Med. 1989;320(4):197–204.
34. Anasetti C, Beatty PG, Storb R, Martin PJ, Mori M, Sanders JE, et al. Effect of HLA incompatibility on graft-versus-host disease, relapse, and survival after marrow transplantation for patients with leukemia or lymphoma. Hum Immunol. 1990;29(2): 79–91.
35. Beatty PG, Clift RA, Mickelson EM, Nisperos BB, Flournoy N, Martin PJ, et al. Marrow transplantation from related donors other than HLA-identical siblings. N Engl J Med. 1985;313(13): 765–71.
36. Aversa F, Tabilio A, Terenzi A, Velardi A, Falzetti F, Giannoni C, et al. Successful engraftment of T-cell-depleted haploidentical "three-loci" incompatible transplants in leukemia patients by addition of recombinant human granulocyte colony-stimulating factor-mobilized peripheral blood progenitor cells to bone marrow inoculum. Blood. 1994;84(11):3948–55.
37. Aversa F, Terenzi A, Tabilio A, Falzetti F, Carotti A, Ballanti S, et al. Full haplotype-mismatched hematopoietic stem-cell transplantation: a phase II study in patients with acute leukemia at high risk of relapse. J Clin Oncol. 2005;23(15):3447–54.
38. Luznik L, Jalla S, Engstrom LW, Iannone R, Fuchs EJ. Durable engraftment of major histocompatibility complex-incompatible cells after nonmyeloablative conditioning with fludarabine, low-dose total body irradiation, and posttransplantation cyclophosphamide. Blood. 2001;98(12):3456–64.
39. Luznik L, O'Donnell PV, Symons HJ, Chen AR, Leffell MS, Zahurak M, et al. HLA-haploidentical bone marrow transplantation for hematologic malignancies using nonmyeloablative conditioning and high-dose, posttransplantation cyclophosphamide. Biol Blood Marrow Transplant. 2008;14(6):641–50.
40. O'Donnell PV, Luznik L, Jones RJ, Vogelsang GB, Leffell MS, Phelps M, et al. Nonmyeloablative bone marrow transplantation from partially HLA-mismatched related donors using posttransplantation cyclophosphamide. Biol Blood Marrow Transplant. 2002;8(7):377–86.
41. Champlin RE. Peripheral blood progenitor cells: a replacement for marrow transplantation? Semin Oncol. 1996;23(2 Suppl 4): 15–21.
42. Anderlini P, Korbling M. The use of mobilized peripheral blood stem cells from normal donors for allografting. Stem Cells. 1997;15(1):9–17.
43. Körbling M, Huh YO, Durett A, Mirza N, Miller P, Engel H, et al. Allogeneic blood stem cell transplantation: peripheralization and yield of donor-derived primitive hematopoietic progenitor cells (CD34+ Thy-1dim) and lymphoid subsets, and possible predictors of engraftment and graft-versus-host disease. Blood. 1995;86(7):2842–8.
44. Bensinger WI, Martin PJ, Storer B, Clift R, Forman SJ, Negrin R, et al. Transplantation of bone marrow as compared with peripheral-blood cells from HLA-identical relatives in patients with hematologic cancers. N Engl J Med. 2001;344(3): 175–81.
45. Blaise D, Kuentz M, Fortanier C, Bourhis JH, Milpied N, Sutton L, et al. Randomized trial of bone marrow versus lenograstim-primed blood cell allogeneic transplantation in patients with early-stage leukemia: a report from the Societe Francaise de Greffe de Moelle. J Clin Oncol. 2000;18(3):537–46.
46. Couban S, Simpson DR, Barnett MJ, Bredeson C, Hubesch L, Howson-Jan K, et al. A randomized multicenter comparison of bone marrow and peripheral blood in recipients of matched sibling allogeneic transplants for myeloid malignancies. Blood. 2002;100(5):1525–31.
47. Heldal D, Tjønnfjord G, Brinch L, Albrechtsen D, Egeland T, Steen R, et al. A randomised study of allogeneic transplantation with stem cells from blood or bone marrow. Bone Marrow Transplant. 2000;25(11):1129–36.
48. Mahmoud F, Abul H, al-Seleh Q, Morgan G, Haines D, al-Ramly M, et al. Differential expression of interferon gamma by mitogen-stimulated peripheral blood mononuclear cells among Kuwaiti psoriasis patients. J Dermatol. 1999;26(1):23–8.
49. Powles R, Mehta J, Kulkarni S, Treleaven J, Millar B, Marsden J, et al. Allogeneic blood and bone-marrow stem-cell transplantation in haematological malignant diseases: a randomised trial. Lancet. 2000;355(9211):1231–7.
50. Schmitz N, Beksar M, Hasenclever D, Bacigalupo A, Ruutu T, Nagler A, et al. Transplantation of mobilized peripheral blood cells to HLA-identical siblings with standard-risk leukemia. Blood. 2002;100(3):761–7.
51. Vigorito AC, Azevedo WM, Marques JF, Azevedo AM, Eid KA, Aranha FJ, et al. A randomised, prospective comparison of allogeneic bone marrow and peripheral blood progenitor cell transplantation in the treatment of haematological malignancies. Bone Marrow Transplant. 1998;22(12):1145–51.
52. Stem Cell Trialists' Collaborative Group. Allogeneic peripheral blood stem-cell compared with bone marrow transplantation in the management of hematologic malignancies: an individual patient data meta-analysis of nine randomized trials. J Clin Oncol. 2005;23(22):5074–87.
53. Schrezenmeier H, Passweg JR, Marsh JC, Bacigalupo A, Bredeson CN, Bullorsky E, et al. Worse outcome and more chronic GVHD with peripheral blood progenitor cells than bone marrow in HLA-matched sibling donor transplants for young patients with severe acquired aplastic anemia. Blood. 2007;110(4): 1397–400.
54. Anasetti C, Logan BR, Lee SJ, Waller EK, Weisdorf DJ, Wingard JR, et al. Increased incidence of chronic graft-versus-host disease (GVHD) and no survival advantage with filgrastim-mobilized peripheral blood stem cells (PBSC) compared to bone marrow (BM) transplants from unrelated donors: results of Blood and Marrow Transplant Clinical Trials Network (BMT CTN) protocol 0201, a phase III, prospective, randomized trial. ASH Ann Meet Abstr. 2011;118(21):1.
55. Giralt S, Estey E, Albitar M, van Besien K, Rondón G, Anderlini P, et al. Engraftment of allogeneic hematopoietic progenitor cells with purine analog-containing chemotherapy: harnessing graft-versus-leukemia without myeloablative therapy. Blood. 1997;89(12):4531–6.
56. Slavin S, Nagler A, Naparstek E, Kapelushnik Y, Aker M, Cividalli G, et al. Nonmyeloablative stem cell transplantation and cell therapy as an alternative to conventional bone marrow transplantation with lethal cytoreduction for the treatment of malignant and nonmalignant hematologic diseases. Blood. 1998;91(3): 756–63.

57. Bacigalupo A, Ballen K, Rizzo D, Giralt S, Lazarus H, Ho V, et al. Defining the intensity of conditioning regimens: working definitions. Biol Blood Marrow Transplant. 2009;15(12):1628–33.
58. Ferrara JL, Deeg HJ. Graft-versus-host disease. N Engl J Med. 1991;324(10):667–74.
59. Przepiorka D, Ippoliti C, Khouri I, Woo M, Mehra R, Le Bherz D, et al. Tacrolimus and minidose methotrexate for prevention of acute graft-versus-host disease after matched unrelated donor marrow transplantation. Blood. 1996;88(11):4383–9.
60. Storb R, Deeg HJ, Pepe M, Appelbaum F, Anasetti C, Beatty P, et al. Long-term follow-up of a controlled trial comparing a combination of methotrexate plus cyclosporine with cyclosporine alone for prophylaxis of graft-versus-host disease in patients administered HLA-identical marrow grafts for leukemia. Blood. 1992;80(2):560–1.
61. Martin PJ, Schoch G, Fisher L, Byers V, Anasetti C, Appelbaum FR, et al. A retrospective analysis of therapy for acute graft-versus-host disease: initial treatment. Blood. 1990;76(8):1464–72.

Infections in Pediatric Transplant Recipients

8

Aspasia Katragkou, Lucy O'Connor, Emmanuel Roilides, and Thomas J. Walsh

Introduction

Infections are major causes of morbidity and mortality in pediatric patients undergoing hematopoietic stem cell and solid organ transplantation (HSCT, SOT, respectively). They also represent the most significant barrier to short- and long-term survival of the implant allograft. Advances in pediatric infectious diseases supportive care have resulted in the ability of patients to undergo intensive immunosuppression and aggressive invasive procedures. The achievements during the past 30 years have resulted in remarkably improved outcome for pediatric transplant recipients. These advances of pediatric infectious disease supportive care have contributed substantially to the improved survival, outcome, and reduction of suffering and pain due to infectious complications.

This chapter reviews the epidemiology, clinical manifestations, and strategies for managing infectious diseases in pediatric transplant recipients. Because the immune defects and the possible etiologic agents for infection vary with the time elapsed since transplantation, the chapter is organized in such a manner. Timetables of infection after hematopoietic stem and solid organ transplantation are useful as they help differential diagnosis, infection control, and, eventually, treatment (Figs. 8.1 and 8.2).

Pediatric Versus Adult Patients

Pediatric transplant patients are different from their adult counterparts in several ways. These include the spectrum of underlying diseases requiring transplantation, the intensity of chemotherapeutic regimens, and the incidence and severity of comorbid medical conditions preceding the transplantation. Additionally, the percentage of patients with indwelling central venous catheters, the community exposures to infectious pathogens, and maturation of the immune system may be different in different ages. Therapeutic and diagnostic issues are also different between adults and children. Many antimicrobial agents lack pediatric approval or rigorous pediatric dose identifying, while important surrogate markers for infection have not been validated in chil-

A. Katragkou
Transplantation-Oncology Infectious Diseases Program, New York-Presbyterian/Weill Cornell Medical Center, New York, NY, USA

3rd Department of Pediatrics, Aristotle University, Hippokration Hospital, Thessaloniki, Greece

Nationwide Children's Hospital, Department of Pediatric Infectious Diseases, Columbus, OH, USA

L. O'Connor
Transplantation-Oncology Infectious Diseases Program, New York-Presbyterian/Weill Cornell Medical Center, New York, NY, USA

University of Manchester School of Medicine, Manchester, UK

E. Roilides
3rd Department of Pediatrics, Hippokration Hospital, School of Health Sciences, Aristotle University of Thessaloniki, Thessaloniki, Greece
e-mail: roilides@med.auth.gr

T. J. Walsh (✉)
Transplantation-Oncology Infectious Diseases Program, New York-Presbyterian/Weill Cornell Medical Center, New York, NY, USA

Department of Pediatrics, New York-Presbyterian/Weill Cornell Medical Center, New York, NY, USA

Department of Microbiology and Immunology, New York-Presbyterian/Weill Cornell Medical Center, New York, NY, USA

Transplant Infectious Diseases Program, Division of Infectious Diseases, Icahn School of Medicine at Mount Sinai, New York, NY, USA
e-mail: thw2003@med.cornell.edu

A. Safdar (ed.), *Principles and Practice of Transplant Infectious Diseases*, https://doi.org/10.1007/978-1-4939-9034-4_8

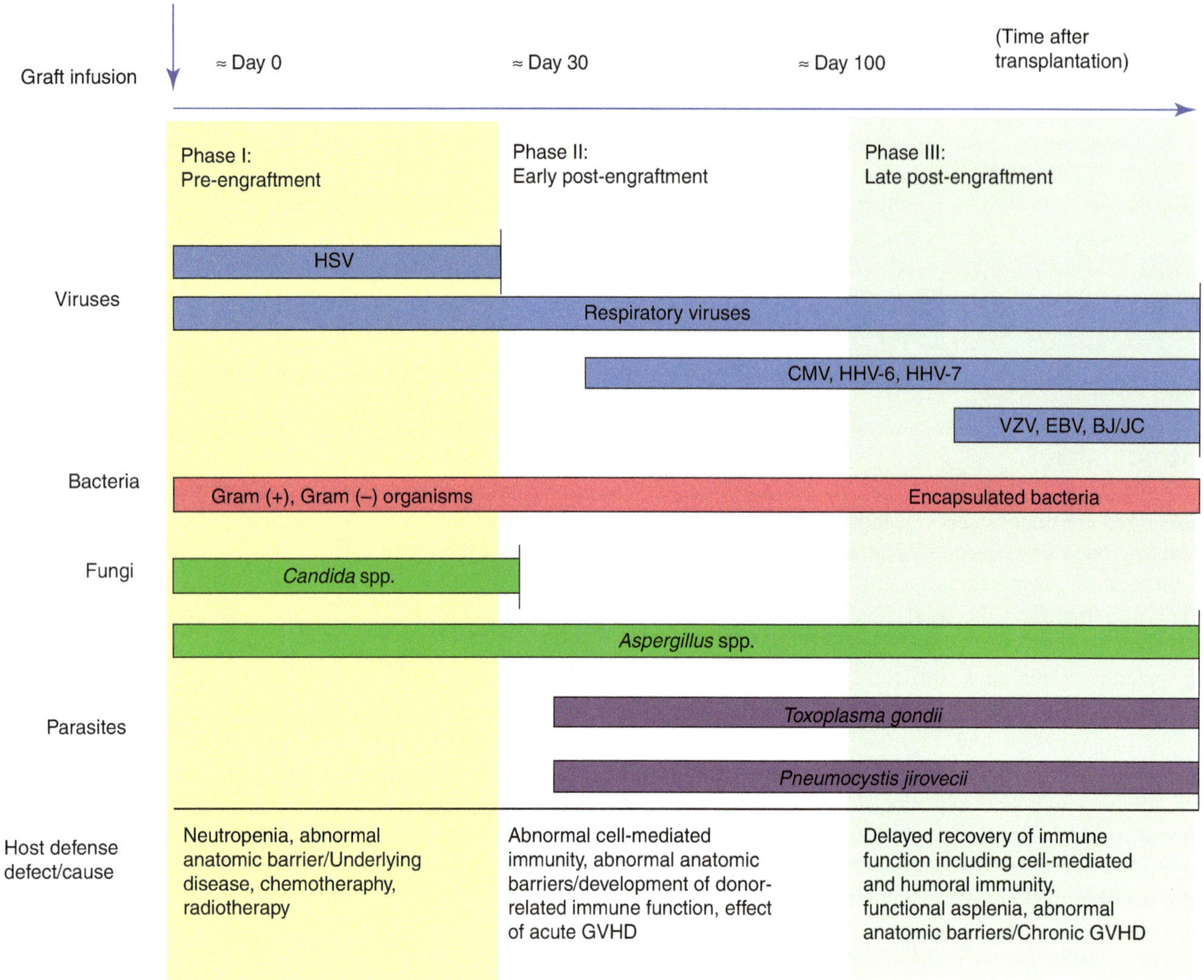

Fig. 8.1 Timing of infections after hematopoietic stem cell transplantation [1]. (Adapted from Tomblyn et al. [1])

dren. Notably, a risk stratification system widely evaluated or clinically adopted in pediatrics is missing. Lastly, a number of psychosocial issues including family dynamics are remarkably different between adults and children [3, 4].

These differences between adult and pediatric patients affect the frequency and nature of episodes of fever and neutropenia. A review of results from four EORTC studies highlighted some of these differences [5]. They reported that the sites of infection and spectrum of infecting organisms are different in children and adults. Children more often do not have a clinically apparent site of infection and consequently have a higher rate of fever without a source. When a defined site is present, children were more likely than their adult counterparts to have upper respiratory tract findings. The overall incidence of bacteremia is similar; however, the rate of death during fever and neutropenia was 1% in children compared to 4% in adults [5].

Infections in Pediatric Hematopoietic Stem Cell Transplantation

Hematopoietic stem cell transplantation involves the intravenous infusion of syngeneic, autologous, or allogeneic stem cells obtained from bone marrow, umbilical cord blood, and peripheral blood. HSCT has become standard of therapy for patients with malignant and nonmalignant hematologic diseases, neuroblastoma, and a variety of genetic conditions. Infections occurring after HSCT are dependent on the underlying primary disease and the suppression of host defenses that occur after transplantation. The severity and type of infections that develop during HSCT depend on a number of factors including the type of transplant, intensity of the preparative regimen, the presence of donor T cells, histocompatibility mismatch, preventive therapy against graft-versus-host disease (GVHD), serologic status

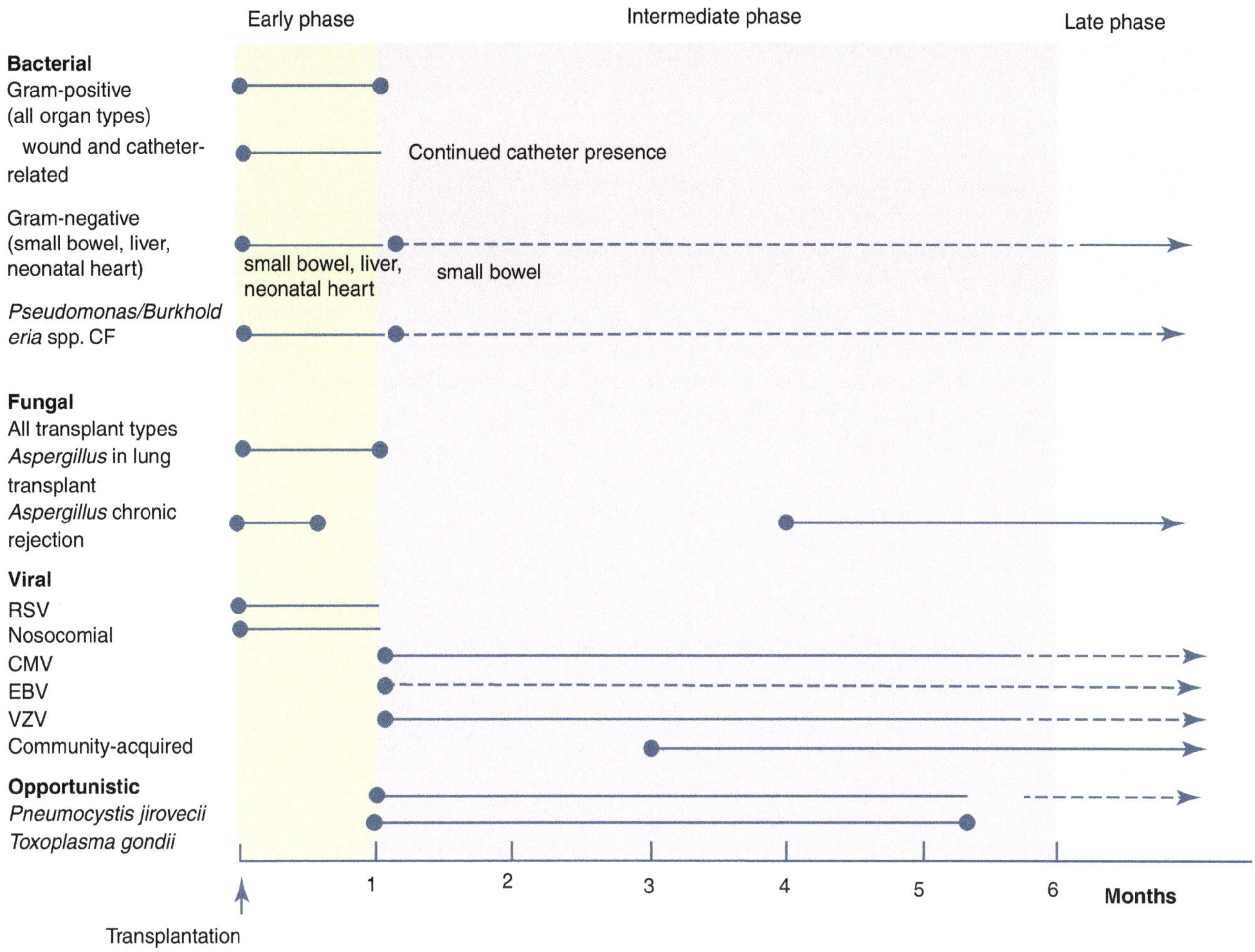

Fig. 8.2 Timing of infections after solid organ transplantation [2]. (Adapted from Fishman [2])

of the donor and recipient, previous antibiotic exposure, and the presence of indwelling medical devices.

Infections During the Pre-engraftment Phase (Phase I)

The pre-engraftment phase begins with the time of the conditioning regimen, usually 5–10 days before stem cell infusion, and continues until engraftment, about 30 days after transplantation. The major host defense defects in this period are aplasia with severe neutropenia and disruptions of the mucocutaneous integrity caused primarily by the myeloablative effects of the conditioning regimens and the use of vascular catheters. Pre-engraftment period is similar to that of patients with hematologic malignancies with neutropenia after chemotherapy. The most common causes of infection in this period are bacteria, fungi, and viruses [6, 7].

Bacterial Infections

Primary bacteremia accounts for approximately one-third of all infections in the pre-engraftment period. The spectrum of etiologic agents is similar to that in other chemotherapy-induced neutropenic patients. Epidemiologic data show a predominance of infections caused by Gram-positive cocci, especially coagulase-negative staphylococci, while, more recently, other organisms like viridans streptococci, *Enterococcus* spp., and *Streptococcus pneumoniae* have become important causes of bacteremia. The rise in staphylococcal and streptococcal infections was related to the use of indwelling intravascular catheters and antibiotic prophylaxis with fluoroquinolones. Gram-negative organisms, such as *Escherichia coli*, *Klebsiella* spp., and *Enterobacter* spp., are isolated in 30–40% of bloodstream infections following transplantation procedure. Methicillin-resistant *S. aureus* (MRSA), vancomycin-resistant *Enterococcus* (VRE), and extended-spectrum beta-lactamase (ESBL)-producing *Enterobacteriaceae* reflect some of the ongoing challenges being particularly worrisome as they display high rates of resistance to many frontline antibiotics [6].

The frequency of catheter-associated bacteremia may vary depending on the institution. The spectrum of etiologic agents includes most frequently staphylococcal and streptococcal spp., while other organisms like *Corynebacterium* spp. and *Stomatococcus* spp. have been implicated.

Pulmonary infections may occur during prolonged neutropenia or later in the course of HSCT with reduced intensity preparatory regimens. During this phase of transplantation, most commonly a number of noninfectious pulmonary complications may also occur (Table 8.1). A less common but potentially lethal infection reported in this period is neutropenic enterocolitis or typhlitis. This is a fulminant necrotizing process of the gastrointestinal tract defined by neutropenia, abdominal pain, and fever. Clinical and imaging findings are non-specific. The etiologic agents responsible for typhlitis include anaerobes and Gram-negative bacilli, especially *P. aeruginosa*. *Clostridium difficile* is recognized increasingly as an important cause of typhlitis. Most patients respond to conservative management without surgical resection of the involved segment of colon [6].

Table 8.1 Differential diagnosis of pneumonia in pediatric transplant recipients [8]

Localized infiltrates	Diffuse infiltrates
Non-neutropenic patients	
Bacteria: *Streptococcus pneumoniae*, *Moraxella* spp., *Legionella* spp., mycobacteria, *Nocardia* spp.	**Fungi**: *Pneumocystis jirovecii*, *Cryptococcus neoformans*, *Histoplasma capsulatum*
Fungi: *Cryptococcus neoformans*, *Histoplasma capsulatum*, *Coccidioides immitis*, *Aspergillus* spp. (the latter especially in HSCT recipients post-engraftment)	**Bacteria**: mycobacteria, *Mycoplasma pneumoniae*, *Chlamydophila pneumoniae*, less commonly *Legionella* spp. and *Nocardia* spp.
Viruses: RSV, adenovirus, influenza, CMV	**Viruses**: RSV, adenovirus, HSV, VZV, CMV, influenza
	Protozoa: *Toxoplasma gondii*
	Drugs: bleomycin, busulfan, cyclophosphamide, methotrexate, cytosine arabinoside
	Radiation
Neutropenic patients	
Bacteria: any Gram-positive or Gram-negative; mycobacteria, *Legionella* spp., *Nocardia* spp.	**Bacteria**: any Gram-positive or Gram-negative; mycobacteria, *Mycoplasma pneumoniae*, *Chlamydophila pneumonia*, less commonly *Legionella* spp. and *Nocardia* spp.
Fungi: *Aspergillus* spp., Zygomycetes, *Fusarium* spp., *Scedosporium* spp., other filamentous fungi (see text)	**Fungi**: *Pneumocystis jirovecii*, *Cryptococcus neoformans*, *Histoplasma capsulatum*
Viruses. RSV, adenovirus, influenza	**Viruses**: RSV, adenovirus, HSV, VZV, CMV, influenza
	Protozoa: *T. gondii*
	Radiation

Adapted from Pizzo and Poplack [8]

Fungal Infections

Candida infections typically occur during the second or following weeks of neutropenia, and *Aspergillus* infections typically occur later during the third and subsequent weeks of neutropenia. A number of clinical and imaging findings may differentiate these common fungal infections [9]. Prolonged severe neutropenia, heavy colonization with *Candida* spp., severe acute and extensive chronic GVHD, and high-dose systemic corticosteroid therapy are factors associated with invasive fungal infections in pediatric HSCT patients [10–12].

The last few decades have witnessed an epidemiologic shift in invasive fungal infections toward a higher prevalence of non-*albicans Candida* spp. and non-*fumigatus Aspergillus* species. Infections due to *Candida tropicalis*, *Candida krusei* or *Aspergillus terreus*, and other molds such as Zygomycetes, *Fusarium*, and *Scedosporium* are on the rise. Most of the filamentous fungi use the respiratory tract as their portal of entry and cause sinopulmonary disease. They have the capacity for hematogenous dissemination to other remote body sites, and due to neurotropism, fungal brain involvement is a dreaded complication for such infections [13–15].

Viral Infections

The most common viral infection is usually due to herpes simplex virus (HSV). It usually occurs within the first 4 weeks after transplantation coinciding with the maximum suppression of the lymphocyte response. Reactivation of latent virus is the primary mechanism of infection, while donor immunity does not prevent reactivation of disease. HSV-seropositive patients before transplantation have 70–80% risk of developing clinical disease regardless of the autologous or allogeneic source of stem cells. Among the common disease manifestations are stomatitis, esophagitis, pneumonitis, and bacterial or fungal superinfection of the skin lesions. HSV-1 accounts for 85% of all HSV-related infections, while HSV-2 is relatively unusual. HSV-2 infection presents with genital ulcers or extragenital vesicles [6, 16].

Enteric viruses such as rotavirus, coxsackie, adenovirus, and respiratory viruses like RSV, influenza, and parainfluenza are usually seasonal or may also occur in epidemics [17]. Among the viruses causing significant morbidity and mortality in this population are adenoviruses, which may lead to disseminated disease with multiple manifestations including hemorrhagic cystitis, pneumonia, nephritis, hepatitis, colitis, and pancreatitis [18–20].

Infections During Early Post-Engraftment Phase (Phase II)

The post-engraftment phase begins with resolution of the neutropenia heralding engraftment, about 30 days after transplantation, and continues approximately 100 days after transplantation. During this period the risk of infection is decreased as major immune defects have resolved. However, there are still abnormalities as recovery of the immune function is asynchronous with different components normalizing at varying times and rates. Infections in this period occur predominantly due to defects in cell-mediated immunity. Other factors that influence the immune response are the presence of acute GVHD and deficits in cellular, humoral, and reticuloendothelial functions [7, 21].

Bacterial Infections

Typically, the bacterial infections in this phase are less common. Gram-positive cocci and less often Gram-negative bacteria are the usual bacterial pathogens associated with the presence of indwelling vascular catheters and complications and consequences from GVHD and anti-GVHD therapy, respectively.

Fungal Infections

Candida spp. and *Aspergillus* spp. are the predominant fungal pathogens during this phase with *Candida* preceding invasive aspergillosis chronologically. Hepatosplenic candidiasis or chronic disseminated candidiasis usually appears during this phase. It is manifested as fever with abdominal symptoms and rising alkaline phosphatase in a patient who has recently recovered from, often prolonged period of, severe neutropenia. Imaging reveals multiple lesions called "bull's eye" in the liver and spleen, blood cultures are usually negative, and definitive diagnosis requires liver biopsy. Brain abscesses are a common manifestation of fungal infections during the period.

Pneumonia due to *Pneumocystis jirovecii* commonly presents with hypoxemia and dyspnea on minor exertion, cough, fever, and bilateral interstitial lung infiltrates. After the introduction of trimethoprim-sulfamethoxazole prophylaxis, the incidence of pneumocystis pneumonia has been decreased to less than 5%.

Protozoan Infections

Toxoplasmosis following HSCT is an infrequent infection usually occurring 2–6 months after transplantation as reactivation of latent disease. Cerebral toxoplasmosis is the usual manifestation associated with high mortality [22–25].

Viral Infections

Prior to routine prophylaxis, CMV pneumonitis was a common cause of viral pneumonia in this phase after HSCT [26]. The most frequent causes of CMV infection and subsequent disease are reactivation of latent virus in seropositive patients and acquisition of CMV from donor marrow in seronegative patients [27]. Among CMV-seronegative recipients of HSCT from seropositive donors, there is a high risk of death due to bacterial infections and invasive mycoses likely due to the indirect immunosuppressive effects of CMV infection on host innate and adaptive immune function [28]. CMV pneumonitis most often occurs between 30 and 100 days after allogeneic bone marrow transplantation, coinciding with the period of highest risk for the development of acute GVHD [29]. CMV pneumonitis is characterized radiographically by diffuse bilateral linear or nodular infiltrates. However, CMV pneumonitis occasionally may present as a lobar or segmental consolidation or as a solitary nodule. The diagnosis of CMV pneumonia can be made by isolation of CMV from BAL fluid, demonstration of either CMV antigen or nucleic acid in pulmonary alveolar macrophages, or characteristic histopathology. Until recently, CMV pneumonitis was associated with an extremely high mortality of greater than 85% despite the use of a variety of antiviral and immunotherapeutic agents. Combined therapy with ganciclovir and intravenous immune globulin either pooled or enriched anti-CMV immunoglobulins has improved survival to more than 50% in allogeneic HSCT recipients with CMV pneumonitis [30, 31]. Despite the limited enrollment and uncontrolled nature of these trials, the dramatic results have led to an acceptance of ganciclovir and immune globulin combination therapy as a standard of care for transplant recipients with CMV pneumonitis.

Although CMV infections predominate in the early post-engraftment period, other viral infections may occur. Among these adenovirus is increasingly recognized as a significant pathogen [32]. The timing of adenovirus infection following HSCT is highly variable, and the median time to onset is 54 days after HSCT [18]. The most severe manifestations of adenovirus disease are due to respiratory and hepatic involvement [33]; however adenovirus may cause disease in other sites such as the urinary and gastrointestinal tract or occasionally in the central nervous system [32]. Reported mortality is as high as 60% in patients with disseminated disease since there are few proven therapeutic options [18, 33, 34]. None of the approved antiviral agents has proven efficacy for the treatment of severe adenovirus infection [32]. Cidofovir is the most widely used antiviral therapy against adenovirus; however, no controlled clinical trials have been performed. When used preemptively, cidofovir can reduce adenovirus viral load. Adenovirus-specific T-cell therapy is in development [35].

Infections During Late Post-Engraftment Phase (Phase III)

The late phase of HSCT occurs around 100 days after transplantation and is characterized by a declining risk of infection. The defects in immune function usually resolve by 1 year after transplantation; however, they are persistent in the presence of chronic GVHD or inadequate stem cell engraftment. Further, up to 90% of patients with extensive GVHD may demonstrate functional asplenia. At the beginning of this stage, the immune defects concern the cellular and humoral arms, which have not fully recovered [21].

Bacterial and Fungal Infections

At this stage encapsulated bacteria such as *Haemophilus influenzae*, *Neisseria meningitidis*, and *Streptococcus pneumoniae* are the predominant causes of bacterial infections. Usually the infections are localized to the skin, upper respiratory tract, and lungs. Invasive fungal infections are rare in this phase, and oropharyngeal candidiasis most frequently occurs [6].

Viral Infections

The usual viral infections in this period are due to VZV, which occur up to 60% of pediatric HSCT recipients. Most infections represent reactivation of VZV. Predisposing factors to VZV infection are acute and chronic GVHD, allogeneic transplant, and lymphoma as underlying disease [6, 36, 37].

Infections in Solid Organ Transplantation

Solid organ transplantation is a major therapeutic option for many children with end-stage organ failure. For a successful SOT, a careful balance between prevention of allograft rejection and immunosuppression-associated infection plays a central role. The risk of infection in the recipients of SOT is determined by the interaction of multitude of factors related to the recipient, the transplantation procedure, and the net state of immunosuppression occurring from the pretransplantation until posttransplantation period (Table 8.2) [3, 38].

Infections in SOT recipients follow a temporal trend and tend to be predictable. While it would be oversimplistic to suggest that specific infections occur only at specific time points, it is, nevertheless, helpful to divide the period following transplantation into specific phases. In each phase specific organisms predominate; however, infectious disease syndromes such as pneumonia can occur at any time during the posttransplant period; however, the etiology changes at different points in time. The timing of infections can be divided into three intervals: early, 0–30 days after transplantation; intermediate, 30–180 days after transplantation; and late, >180 days after transplantation (Fig. 8.2) [39]. However, polymicrobial infections are not uncommon and may occur simultaneously or sequentially. The prototype of this interaction is the immunomodulatory effect of CMV infection,

Table 8.2 Risk factors determining the risk of infections in solid organ transplant recipients [3]

Pretransplantation factors	Peri-transplantation factors	Posttransplantation factors
Young age	Type of organ transplanted	Net state of immunosuppression
Underlying disease	Transplant procedure (injury, prolonged time, technical problems)	Dose, duration, and temporal sequence of immunosuppressive agents (steroids, calcineurin inhibitors, sirolimus)
Duration and frequency of hospitalizations	Indwelling medical devices	Rejection and its treatment (antithymocyte globulin, alemtuzumab, palivizumab)
Palliative surgery before transplantation		
Complications of end-stage organ disease		Host defense defects due to underlying disease
Malnutrition		
Environmental exposures (community, hospitals)		Technical/anatomic abnormalities that compromise the integrity of mucocutaneous barriers
Travel		Neutropenia
		Metabolic abnormalities (protein-calorie malnutrition, uremia, hyperglycemia)
		Viral infections with immunomodulating effect (CMV, EBV, HBV, HCV, HIV)
		Environmental exposure (community, hospital)
		Indwelling medical devices

Adapted from Fonseca-Aten and Michaels [3]

which results in immunosuppression and, thereby, promotes hosts' susceptibility for other opportunistic viral, bacterial, and invasive fungal disease(s) [40, 41].

Early Phase Infections During 0–30 Days After Transplantation

The net state of immunosuppression at this phase is not great despite the high doses of immunosuppressive therapy. Therefore, opportunistic infections that are caused by pathogens such as *Aspergillus*, *Listeria*, and *Nocardia* are rare. There are three main types of infections during this period: (1) infections present in the recipient before undergoing transplantation, which are exacerbated after the transplantation due to transplant surgery and immunosuppressive drug therapy; (2) donor-derived infections which are usually due to critical or terminal illness, organ harvesting procedure and transport, and donor's undiagnosed infections such as West Nile virus, HIV, rabies, and among others [42–44] as well as undiagnosed critical care-related bacterial infections such as pneumonia including HAP/VAP, bacteremia, and endovascular infections; and finally (3) infections transmitted perioperatively that could also occur in an immunocompetent patient. The majority of the infections during the early phase after transplantation is of this last variety and determined by the technical integrity of the operation and the post-surgery use of indwelling medical devices. Early graft injuries resulting from tissue ischemia (bile ducts) or reperfusion injury (lungs) may later become foci of liver or lung abscesses [45].

Intermediate Phase Infections (30–180 Days After Transplantation)

The infections occurring in this phase are the result of immunosuppression and the immunomodulatory effects of coinfecting viruses. There are three types of infections during this period: (1) continuation of infections acquired during the previous phase; (2) opportunistic viral infections such as CMV, Epstein-Barr virus (EBV), herpesvirus-6, and other pathogenic viruses like hepatitis B virus and hepatitis C virus and HIV. However, other rare viral pathogens such as polyomavirus BK and adenovirus have also emerged and (3) opportunistic fungal infections due to *Pneumocystis jirovecii* and *Aspergillus fumigatus* which usually suggest an environmental source. Additionally, infections due to non-endemic and endemic dimorphic fungi like *Cryptococcus* spp., *Histoplasma*, *Coccidioides*, and *Blastomyces* are noted during this period. *Trypanosoma cruzi* and *Strongyloides stercoralis* may cause potentially devastating disease in SOT recipients during this period; a thorough travel and potential exposure history is crucial for evaluating patients being considered for organ transplantation [3, 46].

Late-Phase Infections After 6 Months Following Transplantation

There are three types of infections during this period: (1) patients with good transplantation outcome requiring minimal immune suppression and good allograft function, in which no opportunistic viral infections are at risk from community-acquired respiratory viruses such as influenza, parainfluenza, and respiratory syncytial virus; (2) patients with chronic viral infections that may cause allograft injury such as recipients HCV infection of hepatic allograft, bronchiolitis obliterans in lung transplant recipients, accelerated vasculopathy in heart transplant recipients with CMV infection, or a malignant condition such as posttransplantation lymphoproliferative disorder (PTLD) or skin or anogenital cancer; and (3) patients with poor result from transplantation like repeated episodes of acute and chronic allograft injury, excessive immunosuppression, and chronic viral infections. These patients are at risk for opportunistic infections with *Listeria monocytogenes* or *Nocardia* species, invasive fungal infections such as zygomycetes and dematiaceous molds, and unusual organisms like *Rhodococcus* species [3, 45–47].

Diagnosis and Laboratory Findings

A careful history and physical examination directed toward identifying possible foci of infection is important as a guide to further management. As surrogate markers able to accurately evaluate the relative risk for each patient for infection do not exist, it is essential that these patients be monitored carefully and receive early intervention for signs or symptoms of an infectious disease.

Fever in immunocompromised patients may be the first and only sign of infection [5, 48]. However, one should keep in mind that noninfectious causes such as pyrogenic medications, transfusions of blood products, and drug reactions may also be responsible for a febrile episode. The absence of fever in immunocompromised patients with localizing signs does not exclude the possibility of an ongoing infection. Further, clinical signs and symptoms frequently indicative of an infectious process such as pain, warmth, erythema, and tissue swelling may be blunted or lacking. Patients should be questioned about the presence of any localizing pain or discomfort. Attention on history and physical examination should be focused on areas such as the oropharynx, respiratory tract, perianal area, central venous catheter sites, and any site of recent invasive procedures, as well as the skin and soft tissues.

According to the specific phase after transplantation, the diagnostic approach should be guided toward the most frequent pathogens (Figs. 8.1 and 8.2). Blood cultures should be obtained from all lumens of central venous catheters, when present. Volume of blood cultures is the most important factor for detection of circulating bacteria and fungi. Urine cultures should be routinely submitted where feasible. Other cultures should be obtained based on clinical suspicion including stool, cerebrospinal fluid, central line site, or surgical wound. A routine complete blood count and serum chemistry profile could provide evidence of disease from an infectious agent or indicate noninfectious causes of hepatic or renal disease such as GVHD.

The diagnosis of a catheter-related versus non-catheter-related bacteremia is difficult. Evidence of catheter-related infection as opposed to bacteremia from other sources includes a greater number of colony-forming units per milliliter of blood from cultures of the central line compared with simultaneous peripheral cultures and positive catheter tip cultures. Another approach is to use differential time to positive blood culture. However, as peripheral blood cultures in pediatric patients are inconvenient and contribute little to increasing the diagnostic yield of bacteremia, their utility is questionable. The volume of blood drawn is the critical determinant for recovery of bacteria during bloodstream infections. Thus, two or three blood cultures through the central venous catheter, one set per each lumen will provide a yield similar to that of central cultures plus peripheral cultures but without the patients' discomfort and the potential for contamination from cutaneous flora.

Nasopharyngeal washes for viral pathogens, including respiratory RSV, parainfluenza, influenza, and adenovirus, are important in patients with concomitant upper respiratory tract infection-like symptoms. Nucleic acid detection assays, such as PCR, are useful for detecting and follow-up of the response to therapy of certain pathogens like herpesviruses and parvovirus B19. The impact of PCR on diagnosis of HSV encephalitis is especially apparent [49–53]. Recent advances in PCR may assist in noninvasive diagnosis of CNS toxoplasmosis and detect *Mycoplasma* and *Chlamydia* DNA in BAL samples [54, 55].

Serologic testing is useful for diagnosing toxoplasmosis, bartonellosis, histoplasmosis, and blastomycosis. However, serology tests in transplant recipients are of limited value as these patients are immunosuppressed and a good number of them may have received pooled immunoglobulin therapy. Nevertheless, when PCR is not available, acute and convalescent serum antibody titers against herpesviruses, echoviruses, and the less common arboviruses should be measured. Specific cerebrospinal fluid antibody may be detected in cases of mumps, HSV, or VZV.

A chest radiograph should be obtained in all patients with fever and neutropenia. Routine chest radiographs in asymptomatic neutropenic patients may provide an important baseline for future reference. The presence of a pulmonary infiltrate should also prompt consideration for subsequent evaluation by bronchoscopy for a more definitive microbiological diagnosis. Computed tomography scans of the brain, paranasal sinuses, chest, and the abdomen are useful when evaluating patients with invasive fungal disease. Radiologic examination of the sinuses is useful for diagnosis of sinusitis in children older than 1 year of age. Radiographic evaluation with a CT scan is more sensitive than conventional chest radiography and may provide more information regarding the pattern and extent of disease [56]. Specific findings of a "halo" sign, crescent sign, nodular infiltrate, peripheral pleural-based lung lesions, or wedge-shaped infiltrate are indicative of a possible angioinvasive filamentous fungal disease, including, but not limited to, *Aspergillus* spp. [57–59]. Flexible fiber-optic bronchoscopy can provide evidence for a specific diagnosis in immunocompromised patients with pneumonia. The yield of bronchoscopy depends on the clinical situation and the extent of prior therapy [60]. Bronchoalveolar lavage (BAL) can yield a specific diagnosis in approximately 80% on cases of PCP, whereas it is significantly less sensitive for detection of invasive fungal infections or bacterial infections in patients who have received prior antibiotic therapy. Ultrasound can be used to diagnose abdominal problems such as typhlitis.

The double sandwich ELISA system for detection of galactomannan antigenemia is an important advance in the non-culture diagnosis of invasive aspergillosis among HSCT recipients. Depending upon the patient population, several studies have demonstrated a sensitivity ranging from 50% to 95% and specificity ranging from 87% to 99% for diagnosis of invasive aspergillosis. Additional studies indicate that serial serum galactomannan antigen levels permit therapeutic monitoring and have prognostic implications [61–64]. Coupled with a CT scan that is radiographically compatible with invasive pulmonary aspergillosis in the appropriate host population, a positive serum galactomannan assay establishes a reasonable diagnosis of probable invasive aspergillosis HSCT recipients [65].

Management and Therapy

The initial management of patients with fever and neutropenia after transplantation is similar to that of cancer patients with chemotherapy-induced fever and neutropenia. It is well recognized that bacteremia in the neutropenic host can progress rapidly to septic shock and death making, thus, empirical therapy a therapeutic consensus [66, 67]. Empiric antibiotic therapy should be started after obtaining appropriate samples for culture [68]. When considering a particular empiric antibacterial regimen, the choice should be dictated by the local epidemiology of bacterial infections, antibiotic susceptibility profiles, cost, toxicity, as well as the patient's surveillance isolates. Hence, an empiric antibiotic regimen must cover a broad-spectrum of bacteria, provide high serum bactericidal drug levels, be stable against the emergence of resistant bacteria, and be nontoxic and simple to administer. Several regimens, usually consisting of a cephalosporin, an aminoglycoside, and extended-spectrum penicillin, have been employed [69–71]. A combination that provides broad coverage to Gram-negative bacteria and Gram-positive cocci would be ceftazidime or cefepime with or without vancomycin. If *Pseudomonas aeruginosa* is suspected, an aminoglycoside should be added. Once antibiotics have been initiated empirically, a meticulous investigation of the cause of fever is warranted.

Other clinical findings indicating the addition of other agents as empirical therapy are described in Table 8.3.

Table 8.3 Indications for the addition of specific agents in the empirical therapy of the febrile neutropenic child with transplantation [8]

Head, eyes, ears, nose, throat	
Necrotizing or marginal gingivitis	Add specific anti-anaerobic agent (clindamycin or metronidazole) to empirical therapy
Vesicular or ulcerative lesions	Suspect HSV infection. Culture and begin acyclovir therapy
Sinus congestion, tenderness or nasal ulcerative lesions	Suspect invasive fungal infection with Aspergillus or Zygomycete; obtain imaging studies and ENT consultation. Adjust antifungal therapy according to organism recovered
Gastrointestinal tract	
Retrosternal burning pain	Suspect candida or herpetic esophagitis, or both. Add antifungal therapy and, if no response, acyclovir. Bacterial esophagitis also is a possibility. For patients not responding within 48 h, endoscopy should be considered
Acute abdominal pain	Suspect typhlitis, as well as appendicitis, if pain in right lower quadrant, even in the absence of fever. Add specific anti-anaerobic coverage (e.g., metronidazole to ceftazidime; or substitution of imipenem for ceftazidime) to empirical regimen and monitor closely for need for surgical intervention
Perianal tenderness	Evaluate for anal fissures, perianal cellulitis, perianal fistulas, or perirectal abscesses. Add specific anti-anaerobic drug to empirical regimen, as indicated, and monitor need for surgical intervention, especially when patient is recovering from neutropenia
Respiratory tract	
New focal lesion(s) in patient recovering from neutropenia	Observe carefully, as such lesions may be a consequence of inflammatory response to previously occult pneumonic process detected in concert with neutrophil recovery
New focal lesion(s) in patient with continuing neutropenia	Invasive pulmonary aspergillosis is the chief concern. Rule out other causes of fungal pneumonia. Perform BAL or transthoracic needle aspirate with appropriate direct exams and cultures. Add voriconazole or lipid formulation of amphotericin B, depending upon findings (do not administer voriconazole and amphotericin B simultaneously)
New interstitial pneumonitis	Attempt diagnosis by examination of induced sputum or BAL. If patient is symptomatic, begin empirical treatment with trimethoprim-sulfamethoxazole, pending procedure. Consider noninfectious causes and need for open-lung biopsy if diagnosis is not established

Adapted from Pizzo and Poplack [8]

Guidelines for the management of fever and neutropenia specifically for children with HSCT have recently been published by the International Pediatric Fever and Neutropenia Guideline Panel [68].

Empiric antifungal therapy is recommended for patients who remain persistently granulocytopenic and febrile after 5–7 days of antibiotic therapy without identification of a bacterial cause. Conventional amphotericin B, liposomal amphotericin B, voriconazole, caspofungin, and itraconazole have been well characterized for empirical antifungal therapy for persistent fever in high-risk neutropenic patients. Selection of an agent for empirical antifungal therapy will depend upon the patterns of infection in one's institution, cost, and the risk for end-organ toxicity (e.g., renal or hepatic dysfunction) [72–76].

For patients who remain neutropenic, antifungal therapy should be continued until the resolution of neutropenia. Persistence or recrudescence of fever should prompt a meticulous investigation for non-fungal infections such as bacterial or viral superinfections or for a fungus that is resistant to initial empirical antifungal coverage like *Aspergillus* spp., *Trichosporon*, *Fusarium* spp., *Pseudallescheria boydii*, *Scedosporium* spp., and agents of mucormycosis. Patients who develop a documented fungal infection should be treated with the appropriate antifungal agent (Table 8.4). The indications, dosages, and activity spectrum of the most commonly used antibacterial, antifungal, antiviral, and anti-pneumocystis agents in pediatric patients are shown in Tables 8.4, 8.5, and 8.6.

Catheter-Associated Bacteremia

Removal of chronic indwelling central venous catheters is best determined by the type of organism recovered, the hemodynamic stability of the patient, and the presence of persistent bacteremia, rather than by differences in colony counts suggesting evidence of direct involvement of the catheter (Table 8.7). Removal and replacement of chronic indwelling catheters carry the risk of general anesthesia, pneumothorax, and hemorrhage, particularly in thrombocytopenic patients.

Prevention of Infections

The most efficacious and practical intervention to prevent or reduce infections in the immunocompromised host is adherence to strict handwashing practices [77].

Another measure to decrease the acquisition of new organisms is to maintain a cooked diet during periods of granulocytopenia, with avoidance of fresh fruits and vegetables and non-processed dairy products, because these foods are naturally contaminated with Gram-negative bacteria, especially *E. coli*, *K. pneumoniae*, and *P. aeruginosa* [78, 79].

Environmental sources can contribute to fungal especially *Aspergillus* spp., *Fusarium* spp., and *Zygomycetes* and bacterial such as *Legionella* spp., *Pseudomonas* spp., and *Acinetobacter* spp. colonization and infection. In medical cen-

Table 8.4 Antifungal agents used in children for infections after transplantation

Class	Agent	Route	Spectrum	Daily dose (maximum)			Comments
				Neonates (0–30 days)	Infants (31 days–1 year)	Children (>1–17 years)	
Polyenes	Deoxycholate amphotericin B	IV	Very broad antifungal activity including *Candida* spp., *Aspergillus* spp., Zygomycetes, *Cryptococcus neoformans*, *Histoplasma capsulatum*	Empirical therapy: 0.5–1.5 mg/kg Q24h Documented fungal infections: 1.0–1.5 mg/kg	Empirical therapy: 0.5–1.5 mg/kg Q24h Documented fungal infections: 1.0–1.5 mg/kg Q24h		Children can generally tolerate higher doses than adults
	Lipid formulations (amphotericin B lipid complex, amphotericin B colloidal dispersion, and liposomal amphotericin B)	IV	Same spectrum as deoxycholate formulation	5 mg/kg Q24h	Empirical therapy: 3 mg/kg Q24h Documented fungal infections: 5 mg/kg Q24h (max. dose 10 mg/kg, but no evidence for improved efficacy)		Significantly less nephrotoxicity with efficacy at least equal to that of deoxycholate amphotericin B
Triazoles	Fluconazole	PO, IV	*Candida* spp., (not *C. krusei* and not some strains of *C. glabrata*); *C. neoformans*, *Trichosporon* spp. and *Coccidioides immitis*	Treatment: 12 mg/kg Q24h Prophylaxis: 3 mg/kg twice weekly	12 mg/kg Q24h	3–12 mg/kg Q24h Life threatening infections: 12 mg/kg/day Q12h (max 600 mg/day)	Excellent bioavailability, independent of gastric acidity. Higher dose required in children and infants due to shorter half-life
	Itraconazole	PO, IV	*Aspergillus* spp., *Candida* spp., *H. capsulatum*, *Blastomyces dermatitidis*, and *C. immitis*	Unknown	Unknown	Load with 6 mg/kg/day Q12h × 1 day; maintain with 2.5–5 mg/kg/day Q12h[a] (max 10 mg/kg/day)	Absorption erratic but increased with taking drug with meals or by using cyclodextrin formulation. Dosing Q12h preferred in children. TDM recommended
	Voriconazole	PO, IV	*Candida* spp., *Aspergillus* spp., *Trichosporon* spp. and some strains of *Scedosporium* spp., and *Fusarium* spp.	8–16 mg/kg/day Q12h (IV, PO)		Loading dose 6 mg/kg Q12h day 1, then 4 mg/kg Q12h IV for invasive aspergillus and serious mold infections; 3 mg/kg Q12h for serious candida infections PO, <40 Kg: 200 mg Q12h then 100 mg Q12h 40 Kg: 400 mg Q12h then 200 mg Q12h	Linear pharmacokinetics in children. Higher dosages may be necessary in pediatric patients to achieve comparable adult drug exposures. Pediatric suspension is available; bioavailability is reliable and is enhanced with empty stomach. TDM recommended
	Posaconazole	PO	Zygomycetes, *Candida* spp., and *Aspergillus* spp.	Unknown	Unknown	Prophylaxis: 600 mg/day Q8h For oropharyngeal candidiasis (OPC): Load with 100 mg Q12h × 1 day, maintain with 100 mg/day Q24h For refractory OPC: 800 mg/day Q6-12h	TDM recommended

Table 8.4 (continued)

Class	Agent	Route	Spectrum	Daily dose (maximum) Neonates (0–30 days)	Infants (31 days–1 year)	Children (>1–17 years)	Comments
Echinocandins	Caspofungin	IV	*Candida* spp. and *Aspergillus* spp.	25 mg/m^2 Q24h	50 mg/m^2 Q24h	Load with 70 mg/m^2/day for 1 day; maintain with 50 mg/m^2/day Q24h (max 70 mg)	Dosing should be adjusted for hepatic insufficiency to 35 mg/m^2 Q24h

Adapted from Michelow and McCracken [106]
Abbreviation: TDM therapeutic drug monitoring
[a]IV formulation for itraconazole is available, but dosage and pharmacokinetics have not been defined in pediatric patients

Table 8.5 Antibacterial agents used in children for infections after transplantation

Class	Generic agent name (trade names)	Route	Spectrum[a]	Daily dose (maximum) Neonates (0–30 days)	Infants (31 days–1 years)	Children (>1–17 years)	Comments
Third-generation cephalosporin	Ceftazidime	IV, IM	Enteric bacteria, some Gram-positive aerobes, no anaerobic coverage	0–7 days: 50 mg/kg Q12h 8–30 days: 50 mg/kg Q8h	Inappropriate for mild infections Moderate infections: 90–150 mg/kg/day Q8h (max 6 g/day)		Only ceftazidime covers *Pseudomonas aeruginosa*: 200–300 mg/kg/day recommended for serious pseudomonas infection
Fourth generation cephalosporin	Cefepime	IV, IM	Enteric bacteria, Gram-positive aerobes	0–7 days: 50 mg/kg Q12h 8–30 days: 50 mg/kg Q8h	Inappropriate for mild infections Moderate infections: 100–150 mg/kg/day Q8h or Q12h (max 6 g/day)		Active against some *P. aeruginosa*, *Enterobacter* spp., and *Serratia* spp. resistant to ceftazidime; broader Gram-positive spectrum
Carbapenems	Imipenem-cilastatin	IV, IM	Most Gram-negative including those producing beta-lactamases and *P. aeruginosa*; Gram-positive aerobes, including enterococci; excellent anaerobic coverage	Inappropriate	Inappropriate for mild infections Moderate infections: 60–100 mg/kg/day Q6h (max 4 g/day)		*Stenotrophomonas maltophilia* and *Burkholderia cepacia* not covered. IM form not approved for <12 years of age
	Meropenem	IV	Similar to imipenem	Sepsis: 60 mg/kg/day Q8h Meningitis: 120 mg/kg/day Q8h	Inappropriate for mild infections Moderate infections: 60–120 mg/kg/day Q8h (max 3 g/day)		Less likely than imipenem to cause seizures
Extended-spectrum penicillins	Piperacillin, azlocillin, mezlocillin	IV	Enteric aerobes, including some *P. aeruginosa*, *Enterobacter* spp., *Serratia* spp.; anaerobes	Unknown	Inappropriate for mild infections Moderate infections: 200–300 mg/kg/day Q6h or Q8h (max 21 g/day)		Must be paired with an aminoglycoside for coverage of *P. aeruginosa*
	Piperacillin-tazobactam	IV	Similar to piperacillin, increased activity versus some beta-lactamase-producing Gram-positive cocci, Gram-negative bacilli, and anaerobes	0–7 days: 100 mg/kg Q12h 8–30 days: 100 mg/kg Q8h	Inappropriate for mild infections Moderate infections: 240–300 mg/kg/day of piperacillin Q6h or Q8h (max 12 g/day)		Not adequate as monotherapy for *P. aeruginosa*; aminoglycoside should be added

(continued)

Table 8.5 (continued)

Class	Generic agent name (trade names)	Route	Spectrum[a]	Daily dose (maximum)			Comments
				Neonates (0–30 days)	Infants (31 days–1 years)	Children (>1–17 years)	
Monobactams	Aztreonam	IV	Exclusively aerobic Gram-negative aerobes including *P. aeruginosa*	0–7 days: 30 mg/kg Q12h 8–30 days: 30 mg/kg Q8h	Mild infections: 90 mg/kg/day Q8h (max 4 g/day) Moderate infections: 120 mg/kg/day Q6h (max 4 g/day)		Limited spectrum requires pairing with Gram-positive agent, not cross-reactive with beta lactams so can be used in penicillin or cephalosporin allergic patients
Glycopeptide	Vancomycin	PO, IV	Exclusively Gram-positive	Inappropriate	Inappropriate for mild infections Moderate infections: 40–60 mg/kg Q6h or Q12h (max 3 g/day)		No need to add vancomycin routinely for empirical coverage for fever and neutropenia
Lipopeptide	Daptomycin	IV	Exclusively Gram-positive, including ORSA and susceptible strains of VRE	6 mg/kg Q12h	2–5 years 10 mg/kg/day Q24h 6–11 years 7 mg/kg/day Q24h	4 mg/kg/day Q24h (based on total body weight)	Data in pediatrics are limited at this time
Oxazolidinone	Linezolid	PO, IV	Exclusively Gram-positive, including MRSA, susceptible strains of VRE, and penicillin and cephalosporin resistant *S. pneumoniae*	0–7 days (unless TBW >2 kg): 10 mg/kg Q12h 8–30 days or TBW >2 kg: 10 mg/kg Q8h	30 mg/kg/day Q8h	30 mg/kg/day Q8h >12 years, 1200 mg/day Q12h	Excellent oral bioavailability
Streptogramin	Quinupristin/dalfopristin	IV	Exclusively Gram-positive, similar to linezolid but spectrum does not include *E. faecalis*	Inappropriate	22.5 mg/kg/day Q8h		Venous irritation should be given via central venous catheter

Adapted from Michelow and McCracken [106]

ters where *Aspergillus* spp. and *Fusarium* spp. are a significant problem, special air filtration systems, such as high-efficiency particulate air filters (HEPA filters) and close attention cleaning bathroom facilities, may be helpful [80, 81].

Total protective isolation is a comprehensive regimen designed to reduce patients' endogenous microbial burden while preventing the acquisition of new organisms. A sterile environment is created in a clean-air room with constant positive-pressure airflow. It is maintained by an aggressive program of surface decontamination and sterilization of all objects that enter the room and by an intensive regimen to disinfect the patient, including oral nonabsorbable antibiotics, skin antiseptics, antibiotic sprays and ointments, and a low-microbial diet. The total protective environment reduces the number of infections in profoundly granulocytopenic patients. However, a total protective environment is expensive, and because of the improvement in treating established infections, it does not offer a survival advantage to patients. Total protective isolation is not necessary for the routine care of immunosuppressed patients. Modifications of the approach are used, on occasion, for patients undergoing allogeneic bone marrow transplantation and for patients who are likely to experience periods of 30 or more days of profound neutropenia [82].

In recipients of SOT, the organ donor is frequently the source of various pathogens. To prevent transmissible pathogens from the solid organ donor, the current requirements for donor and recipient screening are provided in Table 8.8 [46, 83].

Antibacterial Prophylaxis

The fluoroquinolone antibiotics are attractive for oral prophylaxis because of their bioavailability, tolerability, and broad-spectrum. These agents have been widely used in

Table 8.6 Antiviral and anti-pneumocystis agents used in children for infections after transplantation

				Daily dose (maximum)			
Class	Agent	Route	Spectrum[a]	Neonates (0–30 days)	Infants (31 days–1 years)	Children (>1–17 years)	Comments
Anti-herpetic agents	Acyclovir	PO, IV	HSV, VZV	0–7 days (unless TBW >2 kg): 40 mg/kg/day Q12h 8–30 days or TBW >2 kg: 60 mg/kg/day Q8h	Empirical therapy: 15–60 mg/kg/day Q8h (IV) 60–80 mg/kg/day Q6-8 h (PO) HSV: 750 mg/m²/day Q8h or 5 mg/kg Q8h VZV: 1500 mg/m²/day Q8h or 10 mg/kg Q8h		IV dose for VZV is twice that for HSV Hydration should be ensured when administering high doses
	Ganciclovir	PO, IV	CMV, HSV, VZV, EBV, HHV-6	CMV: 12 mg/kg/day Q12h	CMV: 10–15 mg/kg/day Q12h for 14 days induction, then 5 mg/kg/day for maintenance/suppression (IV) VZV, HSV: 10 mg/kg/day Q8h (IV) 90 mg/kg/day (PO)		Neutropenia is the major dose-limiting toxicity; not routinely used for HSV, VZV but dose used for CMV is effective for the other herpesviruses
	Foscarnet	PO, IV	HSV, VZV, CMV (including most acyclovir and ganciclovir resistant strains)	Inappropriate	CMV treatment: 180 mg/kg/day Q8h for 14 days then 90–120 mg/kg/day for maintenance/suppression VZV, HSV: 120 mg/kg/day Q8h		Nephrotoxicity is dose-limiting effect; renal function and electrolytes require close monitoring
Anti-pneumocystis agents	Trimethoprim-sulfamethoxazole	PO, IV	*Pneumocystis jirovecii* (formerly, *P. carinii*) also is active against many Gram-positive and Gram-negative bacteria, including *S. maltophilia* and *B. cepacia*	Inappropriate	Empirical therapy: 8–10 mg of TMP/kg/day UTI prophylaxis: 2 mg of TMP/kg/day PCP treatment: 15–20 mg of TMP/kg/day Q12h (IV) PCP prophylaxis: 150 mg of TMP/m²/day Q12h 3×/week		May cause bone marrow suppression in high doses
	Pentamidine	IV, IM	*P. jirovecii*	Inappropriate	4 mg/kg/day Q24h (IV) for treatment		Adverse effects include pancreatitis, hypoglycemia, hypocalcemia, infusional hypotension
	Dapsone	PO	*P. jirovecii*		Prophylaxis: 2 mg/kg/day Q24h (max. 100 mg/day)		High incidence of hemolytic reactions can also cause methemoglobinemia
	Atovaquone	PO	*P. jirovecii*	30 mg/kg/day	45 mg/kg/day	30 mg/kg/day Q12h for treatment, Q24h for prophylaxis (max. 1500 mg/day)	Suspension formulation has better bioavailability

Adapted from Michelow and McCracken [106]

adult oncology patients but are not generally used for prophylaxis in children because of concern of cartilage toxicity with long-term exposure. In adults, comparative studies have shown no advantage of the oral quinolones over more traditional regimens of infection prophylaxis, such as trimethoprim-sulfamethoxazole, for prevention of infection. Moreover, none of the studies of antibacterial prophylaxis has demonstrated a reduction in mortality caused by infection [84, 85].

Antifungal Prophylaxis

Fluconazole is FDA-approved for prevention of deeply invasive fungal infections in neutropenic patients and HSCT recipients when the risk of aspergillosis is not high. Randomized, placebo-controlled studies demonstrated that the prophylactic administration of fluconazole to allogeneic HSCT recipients reduced the incidence of both disseminated and mucosal candidiasis [86, 87]. However the shift in the

Table 8.7 Management of central venous catheters in patients with bacteremia [8]

Criteria for central venous line removal
1. Evidence of a local tunnel infection
2. Persistently positive blood cultures
3. Recurrently positive blood cultures with the same pathogen
4. Positive blood cultures for:
Staphylococcus aureus
Candida spp.
Polymicrobial infections
Atypical mycobacteria (e.g., *M. fortuitum*, *M. chelonae*, *M. abscessus*)
Bacillus spp.

Adapted from Pizzo and Poplack [8]

Table 8.8 Screening requirements for solid organ donors and recipients [46, 83]

Pathogen	Donor	Recipient	Action required
HIV-1 and 2	+	–	Reject donor
	–	+	Accept donor if HIV well controlled
HTLV-1 and 2	+		Exclude donor (may be used in life-threatening conditions)
Hepatitis B virus	HBsAb+	+ or –	Accept donor
	HBsAg+	HBsAb – or +	Reject donor
	HBcAb IgM+	HBsAb – or +	Reject donor
Hepatitis C virus	+	+	Accept (by some centers)
	+	–	Decision depends on urgency
CMV	+ or –	+	Accept
	+	–	Accept (high risk for CMV infection)
EBV	+ or –	+	Accept
	+	–	Accept (higher risk for primary EBV infection and PTLD)
Toxoplasma gondii	+ or –	+	Accept
	+	–	Accept
Treponema pallidum	+	+ or –	Accept
CNS viral pathogens (LCMV, rabies, WNV)	Clinical suspicion of infection		Reject

Modified from Allen and Green [46] and Hayes-Lattin et al. [82]
Abbreviations: PTLD posttransplant lymphoproliferative disease, *LCMV* lymphocytic choriomeningitis virus, *WNV* West Nile virus

colonization pattern toward more resistant species, including *C. glabrata*, *Candida krusei*, *Candida parapsilosis*, *Aspergillus*, and other filamentous spp. fungi, is of concern [88]. More recent studies involving pediatric patients demonstrated that micafungin is superior to fluconazole in prevention of proven and suspected invasive fungal infections in neutropenic HSCT patients [89].

Antiviral Prophylaxis

Acyclovir, given orally or intravenously, is effective prophylaxis against reactivation of HSV in seropositive HSCT recipients [90–92]. Intravenous doses ranging from 250 mg/m^2 every 8 h to 5 mg/kg every 12 h, and oral doses of 400 mg given three times daily, are effective in preventing reactivation of HSV in seropositive individuals. Although acyclovir is therapeutically less active against VZV or CMV, prophylactic acyclovir given to HSCT recipients may nonetheless decrease the occurrence of zoster and invasive CMV disease during the posttransplant period [93, 94]. Refractory lesions may respond to foscarnet [95].

Ganciclovir prophylaxis can reduce the frequency of invasive CMV disease in HSCT recipients. However, myelosuppressive effects of ganciclovir are problematic for most patients, making it undesirable for routine anti-CMV prophylaxis. Targeting transplant recipients at highest risk for severe CMV disease has yielded the practice of "pre-emptive" ganciclovir therapy, that is, treatment of patients who have evidence of CMV reactivation in surveillance assays such as CMV antigenemia, or quantitative CMV PCR. This approach has been shown to effectively suppress CMV viremia, when present and, accordingly, appropriate selection of patients reduces universal need for prophylaxis and dramatically reduces the risk for end-organ CMV disease [96, 97].

Pneumocystis Prophylaxis

There are several effective regimens for *Pneumocystis jirovecii* pneumonia prophylaxis. The choice among them often depends on the patient's tolerance of their various side effects. TMP-SMX, given twice a day for 3 days a week, is considered the first-line regimen [98]. For patients who can tolerate this regimen, protection against PCP is virtually complete [99]. In a number of individuals, presence of skin rash, neutropenia, and gastrointestinal symptoms may limit the routine use of TMP-SMX. Alternative compounds for prevention of PCP in patients who are intolerant of or refractory to TMP/SMX include dapsone, atovaquone, and aerosolized pentamidine.

Immunization

There are no universally accepted recommendations for immunizing children undergoing transplantation. The American Academy of Pediatrics and the CDC regularly publish updated guidelines regarding immunization practices in healthy and transplant pediatric recipients [100, 101] (Table 8.9).

Table 8.9 Immunizations in patients after hematopoietic stem cell transplantation (HSCT) [102]

Vaccine	Recommended time after HSCT
Pneumococcal[a]	12 and 24 months
Haemophilus influenzae type b	12, 14, and 24 months
Tetanus-diphtheria toxoid[a]	12, 14, and 24 months
Inactivated polio	12, 14, and 24 months
Hepatitis B	12, 14, and 24 months
Hepatitis A	Routine administration not recommended
Measles, mumps, rubella (MMR)[a]	24 months
Meningococcal	Routine administration not recommended
Varicella zoster virus[a]	Contraindicated
Influenza	6 months (yearly lifelong)

Modified from Centers for Disease Control and Prevention, Infectious Disease Society of America, American Society of Blood and Marrow Transplantation [102]
[a]See text

Children and adolescents before undergoing HSCT or SOT should receive immunizations recommended for their age at least 4 or 2 weeks before the transplantation, respectively.

Immunizations can be started 6–12 months after HSCT as long as the patient has no persistent complications (GVHD) and is not receiving immunosuppressive therapy.

If the patient is <7 years old, three doses of diphtheria, tetanus toxoids, and acellular pertussis (DTaP) vaccine should be administered starting 6 months after HSCT. If the patient is >7 years old, three doses of tetanus and diphtheria toxoid-containing vaccine [including two doses of tetanus and diphtheria (TD) and one dose of adolescent tetanus toxoid, reduced diphtheria toxoid, and acellular pertussis (Tdap)] should be used [100].

For HSCT recipients who are seronegative to measles and without GVHD or immunosuppression, one dose of MMR vaccine should be given to adolescents and adults and two doses to children at least 24 months after transplantation [100].

Varicella vaccine is contraindicated for HSCT recipients less than 24 months after transplantation. Given the lack of access of immunocompromised patients to the live attenuated varicella vaccine, passive immunoprophylaxis either with varicella zoster immune globulin (VZIG) within 96 h of exposure or regular infusions of gamma globulin is indicated in the high-risk children with no reliable history of varicella. If inadvertent contact occurs between an immunocompromised child and a recent varicella vaccine recipient, administration of VZIG is not recommended as the transmission rate is low and varicella from the Oka strain, albeit unlikely, would be mild and self-limiting. Finally, one should be aware that the varicella vaccine may not be fully protective against varicella, particularly in an outbreak setting.

The 13-valent pneumococcal conjugate vaccine (PCV13) shows good immunogenicity after three doses starting 3–6 months after HSCT. At 12 months after HSCT in children ≥2 years is recommended a dose of pneumococcal polysaccharide vaccine to broaden the serotype coverage given that the patient does not have chronic GVHD. For patients with chronic GVHD, a fourth dose of PCV13 can be given at 12 months after HSCT [100].

After SOT, DTaP, HIB, hepatitis A, hepatitis B, inactivated influenza and pneumococcal and meningococcal conjugate and polysaccharide vaccines can be administered if indicated. Immunization schedules vary between centers, but most experts recommend waiting at least 6 months after transplantation. Administration of live-virus vaccines such as MMR and varicella is advised in patients who are stable at least 6 months after SOT, who are receiving minimal immunosuppressive agents, and who have not had recent episodes of organ rejection.

Household and health-care contacts of HSCT and solid organ transplant recipients should have immunity or be immunized against poliovirus, measles, mumps, varicella, influenza, and hepatitis A [100, 101].

Use of CSFs in Stem Cell Transplantation

Recombinant human cytokines and colony-stimulating factors (CSFs) for adjunctive therapy in immunocompromised patients have been an important assistance in attenuating the myelotoxic effects of HSCT. Granulocyte-CSF (G-CSF; filgrastim) and granulocyte-macrophage-CSF (GM-CSF; sargramostim) have undergone extensive evaluation for their potential role in reducing infectious morbidity during periods of severe immunosuppression. However, they should be used judiciously in order to maximize medical benefit, limit potential toxicity, and be cost-effective. The effects of G-CSF and GM-CSF in prevention of infections in neutropenic patients are perhaps best illustrated in the impact of these agents on stem cell mobilization in HSCT donors. Transfusion of peripheral mobilized stem cells has led to a substantial reduction in depth and duration of neutropenia [103–106]. G-CSF and GM-CSF also are used in HSCT recipients as part of most immediate posttransplant regimens for their impact on shortening the duration of neutropenia. The effects on the incidence of fever or documented infections, antibiotic usage, or duration of hospitalization have been more variable and dependent on clinical trial design. Notably, as these cytokines do not augment platelet recovery, thrombocytopenia remains a challenging problem for HSCT recipients.

References

1. Tomblyn M, Chiller T, Einsele H, Gress R, Sepkowitz K, Storek J, European Blood and Marrow Transplant Group, American Society of Blood and Marrow Transplantation; Canadian Blood and Marrow Transplant Group, Infectious Diseases Society of America, Society for Healthcare Epidemiology of America, Association of Medical Microbiology and Infectious Disease Canada, Centers for Disease Control and Prevention, et al. Guidelines for preventing infectious complications among hematopoietic cell transplantation recipients: a global perspective. Biol Blood Marrow Transplant. 2009;15(10):1143–238.
2. Fishman JA. Infection in organ transplantation. Am J Transplant. 2017;17:856–79.
3. Fonseca-Aten M, Michaels MG. Infections in pediatric solid organ transplant recipients. Semin Pediatr Surg. 2006;15:153–61.
4. Sung L, Phillips R, Lehrnbecher T. Time for paediatric febrile neutropenia guidelines – children are not little adults. Eur J Cancer. 2011;47:811–3.
5. Hann I, Viscoli C, Paesmans M, Gaya H, Glauser M. A comparison of outcome from febrile neutropenic episodes in children compared with adults: results from four EORTC studies. International Antimicrobial Therapy Cooperative Group (IATCG) of the European Organization for Research and Treatment of Cancer (EORTC). Br J Haematol. 1997;99:580–8.
6. Sable CA, Donowitz GR. Infections in bone marrow transplant recipients. Clin Infect Dis. 1994;18:273–81; quiz 282–274.
7. Parkman R, Weinberg KI. Immunological reconstitution following bone marrow transplantation. Immunol Rev. 1997;157:73–8.
8. Infectious complications in pediatric cancer patients. In: Pizzo A, Poplack DG, editors. Principles and practice of pediatric oncology. 5th ed. Philadelphia: Lippincott Williams & Wilkins; 2015.
9. Wingard JR. Empirical antifungal therapy in treating febrile neutropenic patients. Clin Infect Dis. 2004;39(Suppl 1):S38–43.
10. Hovi L, Saarinen-Pihkala UM, Vettenranta K, Saxen H. Invasive fungal infections in pediatric bone marrow transplant recipients: single center experience of 10 years. Bone Marrow Transplant. 2000;26:999–1004.
11. Jantunen E, Ruutu P, Niskanen L, Volin L, Parkkali T, et al. Incidence and risk factors for invasive fungal infections in allogeneic BMT recipients. Bone Marrow Transplant. 1997;19:801–8.
12. O'Donnell MR, Schmidt GM, Tegtmeier BR, Faucett C, Fahey JL, et al. Prediction of systemic fungal infection in allogeneic marrow recipients: impact of amphotericin prophylaxis in high-risk patients. J Clin Oncol. 1994;12:827–34.
13. Nucci M, Marr KA, Queiroz-Telles F, Martins CA, Trabasso P, et al. Fusarium infection in hematopoietic stem cell transplant recipients. Clin Infect Dis. 2004;38:1237–42.
14. Zaoutis TE, Heydon K, Chu JH, Walsh TJ, Steinbach WJ. Epidemiology, outcomes, and costs of invasive aspergillosis in immunocompromised children in the United States, 2000. Pediatrics. 2006;117:e711–6.
15. Morrison VA, Haake RJ, Weisdorf DJ. The spectrum of non-Candida fungal infections following bone marrow transplantation. Medicine (Baltimore). 1993;72:78–89.
16. Fisher BT, Alexander S, Dvorak CC, Zaoutis TE, Zerr DM, et al. Epidemiology and potential preventative measures for viral infections in children with malignancy and those undergoing hematopoietic cell transplantation. Pediatr Blood Cancer. 2012;59:11–5.
17. Wasserman R, August CS, Plotkin SA. Viral infections in pediatric bone marrow transplant patients. Pediatr Infect Dis J. 1988;7:109–15.
18. Hale GA, Heslop HE, Krance RA, Brenner MA, Jayawardene D, et al. Adenovirus infection after pediatric bone marrow transplantation. Bone Marrow Transplant. 1999;23:277–82.
19. Shields AF, Hackman RC, Fife KH, Corey L, Meyers JD. Adenovirus infections in patients undergoing bone-marrow transplantation. N Engl J Med. 1985;312:529–33.
20. van Tol MJ, Claas EC, Heemskerk B, Veltrop-Duits LA, de Brouwer CS, et al. Adenovirus infection in children after allogeneic stem cell transplantation: diagnosis, treatment and immunity. Bone Marrow Transplant. 2005;35(Suppl 1):S73–6.
21. Storek J. Immunological reconstitution after hematopoietic cell transplantation – its relation to the contents of the graft. Expert Opin Biol Ther. 2008;8:583–97.
22. Weber C, Schaper J, Tibussek D, Adams O, Mackenzie CR, et al. Diagnostic and therapeutic implications of neurological complications following paediatric haematopoietic stem cell transplantation. Bone Marrow Transplant. 2008;41:253–9.
23. Slavin MA, Meyers JD, Remington JS, Hackman RC. Toxoplasma gondii infection in marrow transplant recipients: a 20 year experience. Bone Marrow Transplant. 1994;13:549–57.
24. Mele A, Paterson PJ, Prentice HG, Leoni P, Kibbler CC. Toxoplasmosis in bone marrow transplantation: a report of two cases and systematic review of the literature. Bone Marrow Transplant. 2002;29:691–8.
25. Walker M, Zunt JR. Parasitic central nervous system infections in immunocompromised hosts. Clin Infect Dis. 2005;40:1005–15.
26. Wingard JR, Piantadosi S, Burns WH, Zahurak ML, Santos GW, et al. Cytomegalovirus infections in bone marrow transplant recipients given intensive cytoreductive therapy. Rev Infect Dis. 1990;12(Suppl 7):S793–804.
27. Ljungman P, Brand R, Einsele H, Frassoni F, Niederwieser D, et al. Donor CMV serologic status and outcome of CMV-seropositive recipients after unrelated donor stem cell transplantation: an EBMT megafile analysis. Blood. 2003;102:4255–60.
28. Nichols WG, Corey L, Gooley T, Davis C, Boeckh M. High risk of death due to bacterial and fungal infection among cytomegalovirus (CMV)-seronegative recipients of stem cell transplants from seropositive donors: evidence for indirect effects of primary CMV infection. J Infect Dis. 2002;185:273–82.
29. Castagnola E, Cappelli B, Erba D, Rabagliati A, Lanino E, et al. Cytomegalovirus infection after bone marrow transplantation in children. Hum Immunol. 2004;65:416–22.
30. Emanuel D, Cunningham I, Jules-Elysee K, Brochstein JA, Kernan NA, et al. Cytomegalovirus pneumonia after bone marrow transplantation successfully treated with the combination of ganciclovir and high-dose intravenous immune globulin. Ann Intern Med. 1988;109:777–82.
31. Reed EC, Bowden RA, Dandliker PS, Lilleby KE, Meyers JD. Treatment of cytomegalovirus pneumonia with ganciclovir and intravenous cytomegalovirus immunoglobulin in patients with bone marrow transplants. Ann Intern Med. 1988;109:783–8.
32. Walls T, Shankar AG, Shingadia D. Adenovirus: an increasingly important pathogen in paediatric bone marrow transplant patients. Lancet Infect Dis. 2003;3:79–86.
33. Hierholzer JC. Adenoviruses in the immunocompromised host. Clin Microbiol Rev. 1992;5:262–74.
34. Runde V, Ross S, Trenschel R, Lagemann E, Basu O, et al. Adenoviral infection after allogeneic stem cell transplantation (SCT): report on 130 patients from a single SCT unit involved in a prospective multi center surveillance study. Bone Marrow Transplant. 2001;28:51–7.
35. Matthes-Martin S, Feuchtinger T, Shaw PJ, Engelhard D, Hirsch HH, et al. European guidelines for diagnosis and treatment of adenovirus infection in leukemia and stem cell transplantation: summary of ECIL-4 (2011). Transpl Infect Dis. 2012;14:555–63.
36. Leung TF, Chik KW, Li CK, Lai H, Shing MM, et al. Incidence, risk factors and outcome of varicella-zoster virus infection in children after haematopoietic stem cell transplantation. Bone Marrow Transplant. 2000;25:167–72.

37. Maltezou HC, Kafetzis DA, Abisaid D, Mantzouranis EC, Chan KW, et al. Viral infections in children undergoing hematopoietic stem cell transplant. Pediatr Infect Dis J. 2000;19:307–12.
38. Rubin RH, Ikonen T, Gummert JF, Morris RE. The therapeutic prescription for the organ transplant recipient: the linkage of immunosuppression and antimicrobial strategies. Transpl Infect Dis. 1999;1:29–39.
39. Marty FM, Rubin RH. The prevention of infection post-transplant: the role of prophylaxis, preemptive and empiric therapy. Transpl Int. 2006;19:2–11.
40. Rubin RH, Marty FM. Principles of antimicrobial therapy in the transplant patient. Transpl Infect Dis. 2004;6:97–100.
41. Rubin RH. Importance of CMV in the transplant population. Transpl Infect Dis. 1999;1(Suppl 1):3–7.
42. Gottesdiener KM. Transplanted infections: donor-to-host transmission with the allograft. Ann Intern Med. 1989;110:1001–16.
43. Iwamoto M, Jernigan DB, Guasch A, Trepka MJ, Blackmore CG, et al. Transmission of West Nile virus from an organ donor to four transplant recipients. N Engl J Med. 2003;348:2196–203.
44. Srinivasan A, Burton EC, Kuehnert MJ, Rupprecht C, Sutker WL, et al. Transmission of rabies virus from an organ donor to four transplant recipients. N Engl J Med. 2005;352:1103–11.
45. Fishman JA. Infection in solid-organ transplant recipients. N Engl J Med. 2007;357:2601–14.
46. Allen U, Green M. Prevention and treatment of infectious complications after solid organ transplantation in children. Pediatr Clin N Am. 2010;57:459–79.
47. Keough WL, Michaels MG. Infectious complications in pediatric solid organ transplantation. Pediatr Clin N Am. 2003;50:1451–69.
48. Pizzo PA. Management of fever in patients with cancer and treatment-induced neutropenia. N Engl J Med. 1993;328:1323–32.
49. Shi J, Wu Y, Cai M, Shang S. Rapid diagnosis of herpetic encephalitis in children by PCR-microarray technology for simultaneous detection of seven human herpes viruses. Eur J Pediatr. 2010;169:421–5.
50. Schloss L, Falk KI, Skoog E, Brytting M, Linde A, et al. Monitoring of herpes simplex virus DNA types 1 and 2 viral load in cerebrospinal fluid by real-time PCR in patients with herpes simplex encephalitis. J Med Virol. 2009;81:1432–7.
51. Wada K, Mizoguchi S, Ito Y, Kawada J, Yamauchi Y, et al. Multiplex real-time PCR for the simultaneous detection of herpes simplex virus, human herpesvirus 6, and human herpesvirus 7. Microbiol Immunol. 2009;53:22–9.
52. Strick LB, Wald A. Diagnostics for herpes simplex virus: is PCR the new gold standard? Mol Diagn Ther. 2006;10:17–28.
53. Schiff D, Rosenblum MK. Herpes simplex encephalitis (HSE) and the immunocompromised: a clinical and autopsy study of HSE in the settings of cancer and human immunodeficiency virus-type 1 infection. Hum Pathol. 1998;29:215–22.
54. Miyashita N, Saito A, Kohno S, Yamaguchi K, Watanabe A, et al. Multiplex PCR for the simultaneous detection of Chlamydia pneumoniae, Mycoplasma pneumoniae and Legionella pneumophila in community-acquired pneumonia. Respir Med. 2004;98:542–50.
55. Maltezou HC, La-Scola B, Astra H, Constantopoulou I, Vlahou V, et al. Mycoplasma pneumoniae and Legionella pneumophila in community-acquired lower respiratory tract infections among hospitalized children: diagnosis by real time PCR. Scand J Infect Dis. 2004;36:639–42.
56. Heussel CP, Kauczor HU, Heussel GE, Fischer B, Begrich M, et al. Pneumonia in febrile neutropenic patients and in bone marrow and blood stem-cell transplant recipients: use of high-resolution computed tomography. J Clin Oncol. 1999;17:796–805.
57. Kim MJ, Lee KS, Kim J, Jung KJ, Lee HG, et al. Crescent sign in invasive pulmonary aspergillosis: frequency and related CT and clinical factors. J Comput Assist Tomogr. 2001;25:305–10.
58. Milito MA, Kontoyiannis DP, Lewis RE, Liu P, Mawlawi OR, et al. Influence of host immunosuppression on CT findings in invasive pulmonary aspergillosis. Med Mycol. 2010;48:817–23.
59. Greene RE, Schlamm HT, Oestmann JW, Stark P, Durand C, et al. Imaging findings in acute invasive pulmonary aspergillosis: clinical significance of the halo sign. Clin Infect Dis. 2007;44:373–9.
60. Bergen GA, Shelhamer JH. Pulmonary infiltrates in the cancer patient. New approaches to an old problem. Infect Dis Clin N Am. 1996;10:297–325.
61. Baker C. Serial Aspergillus antigen monitoring in pediatric bone marrow transplant patients. J Pediatr Oncol Nurs. 2006;23:300–4.
62. Marr KA, Balajee SA, McLaughlin L, Tabouret M, Bentsen C, et al. Detection of galactomannan antigenemia by enzyme immunoassay for the diagnosis of invasive aspergillosis: variables that affect performance. J Infect Dis. 2004;190:641–9.
63. Boutboul F, Alberti C, Leblanc T, Sulahian A, Gluckman E, et al. Invasive aspergillosis in allogeneic stem cell transplant recipients: increasing antigenemia is associated with progressive disease. Clin Infect Dis. 2002;34:939–43.
64. Maertens J, Van Eldere J, Verhaegen J, Verbeken E, Verschakelen J, et al. Use of circulating galactomannan screening for early diagnosis of invasive aspergillosis in allogeneic stem cell transplant recipients. J Infect Dis. 2002;186:1297–306.
65. Ascioglu S, Rex JH, de Pauw B, Bennett JE, Bille J, et al. Defining opportunistic invasive fungal infections in immunocompromised patients with cancer and hematopoietic stem cell transplants: an international consensus. Clin Infect Dis. 2002;34:7–14.
66. Giamarellou H, Antoniadou A. Infectious complications of febrile leukopenia. Infect Dis Clin N Am. 2001;15:457–82.
67. Klastersky J. Empirical antibiotic therapy in neutropenic cancer patients. Eur J Cancer. 1993;29A(Suppl 1):S6–10.
68. Lehrnbecher T, Phillips R, Alexander S, Alvaro F, Carlesse F, et al. Guideline for the management of fever and neutropenia in children with cancer and/or undergoing hematopoietic stem-cell transplantation. J Clin Oncol. 2012;30:4427–38.
69. Schimpff S, Satterlee W, Young VM, Serpick A. Empiric therapy with carbenicillin and gentamicin for febrile patients with cancer and granulocytopenia. N Engl J Med. 1971;284:1061–5.
70. Schimpff SC, Gaya H, Klastersky J, Tattersall MH, Zinner SH. Three antibiotic regimens in the treatment of infection in febrile granulocytopenic patients with cancer. The EORTC international antimicrobial therapy project group. J Infect Dis. 1978;137:14–29.
71. Walsh TJ, Schimpff SC. Antibiotic combinations for the empiric treatment of the febrile neutropenic patient. Schweiz Med Wochenschr. 1983;14:58–63.
72. Pizzo PA, Robichaud KJ, Gill FA, Witebsky FG. Empiric antibiotic and antifungal therapy for cancer patients with prolonged fever and granulocytopenia. Am J Med. 1982;72:101–11.
73. Walsh TJ, Lee J, Lecciones J, Rubin M, Butler K, et al. Empiric therapy with amphotericin B in febrile granulocytopenic patients. Rev Infect Dis. 1991;13:496–503.
74. Walsh TJ, Finberg RW, Arndt C, Hiemenz J, Schwartz C, et al. Liposomal amphotericin B for empirical therapy in patients with persistent fever and neutropenia. National Institute of Allergy and Infectious Diseases Mycoses Study Group. N Engl J Med. 1999;340:764–71.
75. Walsh TJ, Teppler H, Donowitz GR, Maertens JA, Baden LR, et al. Caspofungin versus liposomal amphotericin B for empirical antifungal therapy in patients with persistent fever and neutropenia. N Engl J Med. 2004;351:1391–402.
76. Boogaerts M, Winston DJ, Bow EJ, Garber G, Reboli AC, et al. Intravenous and oral itraconazole versus intravenous amphotericin B deoxycholate as empirical antifungal therapy for persistent fever in neutropenic patients with cancer who are receiving broad-spectrum antibacterial therapy. A randomized, controlled trial. Ann Intern Med. 2001;135:412–22.

77. Doebbeling BN, Stanley GL, Sheetz CT, Pfaller MA, Houston AK, et al. Comparative efficacy of alternative hand-washing agents in reducing nosocomial infections in intensive care units. N Engl J Med. 1992;327:88–93.
78. Remington JS, Schimpff SC. Occasional notes. Please don't eat the salads. N Engl J Med. 1981;304:433–5.
79. Pizzo PA, Purvis DS, Waters C. Microbiological evaluation of food items. For patients undergoing gastrointestinal decontamination and protected isolation. J Am Diet Assoc. 1982;81:272–9.
80. Anaissie EJ, Stratton SL, Dignani MC, Lee CK, Mahfouz TH, et al. Cleaning patient shower facilities: a novel approach to reducing patient exposure to aerosolized Aspergillus species and other opportunistic molds. Clin Infect Dis. 2002;35:E86–8.
81. Walsh TJ, Dixon DM. Nosocomial aspergillosis: environmental microbiology, hospital epidemiology, diagnosis and treatment. Eur J Epidemiol. 1989;5:131–42.
82. Hayes-Lattin B, Leis JF, Maziarz RT. Isolation in the allogeneic transplant environment: how protective is it? Bone Marrow Transplant. 2005;36:373–81.
83. Fischer SA, Lu K. Screening of donor and recipient in solid organ transplantation. Am J Transplant. 2013;13(Suppl 4):9–21.
84. Dekker AW, Rozenberg-Arska M, Verhoef J. Infection prophylaxis in acute leukemia: a comparison of ciprofloxacin with trimethoprim-sulfamethoxazole and colistin. Ann Intern Med. 1987; 106:7–11.
85. Schmeiser T, Kurrle E, Arnold R, Wiesneth M, Bunjes D, et al. Norfloxacin for prevention of bacterial infections during severe granulocytopenia after bone marrow transplantation. Scand J Infect Dis. 1988;20:625–31.
86. Goodman JL, Winston DJ, Greenfield RA, Chandrasekar PH, Fox B, et al. A controlled trial of fluconazole to prevent fungal infections in patients undergoing bone marrow transplantation. N Engl J Med. 1992;326:845–51.
87. Slavin MA, Osborne B, Adams R, Levenstein MJ, Schoch HG, et al. Efficacy and safety of fluconazole prophylaxis for fungal infections after marrow transplantation – a prospective, randomized, double-blind study. J Infect Dis. 1995;171:1545–52.
88. Walsh TJ, Hiemenz J, Pizzo PA. Evolving risk factors for invasive fungal infections – all neutropenic patients are not the same. Clin Infect Dis. 1994;18:793–8.
89. van Burik JA, Ratanatharathorn V, Stepan DE, Miller CB, Lipton JH, et al. Micafungin versus fluconazole for prophylaxis against invasive fungal infections during neutropenia in patients undergoing hematopoietic stem cell transplantation. Clin Infect Dis. 2004;39:1407–16.
90. Saral R, Ambinder RF, Burns WH, Angelopulos CM, Griffin DE, et al. Acyclovir prophylaxis against herpes simplex virus infection in patients with leukemia. A randomized, double-blind, placebo-controlled study. Ann Intern Med. 1983;99:773–6.
91. Meyers JD, Wade JC, Mitchell CD, Saral R, Lietman PS, et al. Multicenter collaborative trial of intravenous acyclovir for treatment of mucocutaneous herpes simplex virus infection in the immunocompromised host. Am J Med. 1982;73:229–35.
92. Wade JC, Newton B, Flournoy N, Meyers JD. Oral acyclovir for prevention of herpes simplex virus reactivation after marrow transplantation. Ann Intern Med. 1984;100:823–8.
93. Meyers JD, Reed EC, Shepp DH, Thornquist M, Dandliker PS, et al. Acyclovir for prevention of cytomegalovirus infection and disease after allogeneic marrow transplantation. N Engl J Med. 1988;318:70–5.
94. Perren TJ, Powles RL, Easton D, Stolle K, Selby PJ. Prevention of herpes zoster in patients by long-term oral acyclovir after allogeneic bone marrow transplantation. Am J Med. 1988;85:99–101.
95. Erlich KS, Jacobson MA, Koehler JE, Follansbee SE, Drennan DP, et al. Foscarnet therapy for severe acyclovir-resistant herpes simplex virus type-2 infections in patients with the acquired immunodeficiency syndrome (AIDS). An uncontrolled trial. Ann Intern Med. 1989;110:710–3.
96. Schmidt GM, Horak DA, Niland JC, Duncan SR, Forman SJ, et al. A randomized, controlled trial of prophylactic ganciclovir for cytomegalovirus pulmonary infection in recipients of allogeneic bone marrow transplants; The City of Hope-Stanford-Syntex CMV Study Group. N Engl J Med. 1991;324:1005–11.
97. Goodrich JM, Mori M, Gleaves CA, Du Mond C, Cays M, et al. Early treatment with ganciclovir to prevent cytomegalovirus disease after allogeneic bone marrow transplantation. N Engl J Med. 1991;325:1601–7.
98. Hughes WT, Rivera GK, Schell MJ, Thornton D, Lott L. Successful intermittent chemoprophylaxis for Pneumocystis carinii pneumonitis. N Engl J Med. 1987;316:1627–32.
99. Ioannidis JP, Cappelleri JC, Skolnik PR, Lau J, Sacks HS. A meta-analysis of the relative efficacy and toxicity of Pneumocystis carinii prophylactic regimens. Arch Intern Med. 1996;156:177–88.
100. American Academy of Pediatrics. Active immunizations. In: Pickering LK, editor. Red book: 2003 report of the committee on infectious diseases. 29th ed. Elk Grove Village: American Academy of Pediatrics; 2012. p. 83–6.
101. Sullivan KM, Dykewicz CA, Longworth DL, Boeckh M, Baden LR, et al. Preventing opportunistic infections after hematopoietic stem cell transplantation: the Centers for Disease Control and Prevention, Infectious Diseases Society of America, and American Society for Blood and Marrow Transplantation Practice Guidelines and beyond. Hematol Am Soc Hematol Educ Program. 2001;1:392–421.
102. Centers for Disease Control and Prevention; Infectious Disease Society of America; American Society of Blood and Marrow Transplantation. Guidelines for preventing opportunistic infections among hematopoietic stem cell transplant recipients. MMWR Recomm Rep. 2000;49(RR-10):1–125, CE1–7. https://www.cdc.gov/mmwr/preview/mmwrhtml/rr4910a1.htm; Beyer J, Schwella N, Zingsem J, Strohscheer I, Schwaner I, et al. Hematopoietic rescue after high-dose chemotherapy using autologous peripheral-blood progenitor cells or bone marrow: a randomized comparison. J Clin Oncol. 1995;13:1328–35.
103. Schmitz N, Linch DC, Dreger P, Goldstone AH, Boogaerts MA, et al. Randomised trial of filgrastim-mobilised peripheral blood progenitor cell transplantation versus autologous bone-marrow transplantation in lymphoma patients. Lancet. 1996;347:353–7.
104. Klumpp TR, Mangan KF, Goldberg SL, Pearlman ES, Macdonald JS. Granulocyte colony-stimulating factor accelerates neutrophil engraftment following peripheral-blood stem-cell transplantation: a prospective, randomized trial. J Clin Oncol. 1995;13:1323–7.
105. Nemunaitis J, Rosenfeld CS, Ash R, Freedman MH, Deeg HJ, et al. Phase III randomized, double-blind placebo-controlled trial of rhGM-CSF following allogeneic bone marrow transplantation. Bone Marrow Transplant. 1995;15:949–54.
106. Michelow IC, McCracken GH. Antibacterial therapeutic agents. In: Feigin RD, Cherry JD, Demmler-Harrison GJ, Kaplan SL, editors. Feigin and Cherry's textbook of pediatric infectious diseases, vol. 2. Philadelphia: Saunders Elsevier; 2009. p. 3178–227.

Part II

Clinical Disorders in Transplant Recipients

9 Febrile Neutropenia in Transplant Recipients

Lior Nesher and Kenneth V. I. Rolston

Introduction

Hematopoietic transplantation has been used to treat many disorders including neoplastic, hematologic, immunologic, and metabolic diseases. Currently, most hematopoietic transplants are performed for the treatment of hematologic malignancies [1]. Hematopoietic cells for transplantation can be collected from various sources including bone marrow, peripheral blood, and umbilical cord blood. Autologous transplants utilize the patient's own cells, whereas allogeneic transplants utilize cells obtained from a different individual. Syngeneic transplants are between genetically identical twins. Conditioning therapy given prior to hematopoietic transplantation can be myeloablative or non-myeloablative (i.e., reduced intensity) and produces significant neutropenia (absolute neutrophil count [ANC] ≤500 cells/mm^3), which is the most common predisposing factor for the development of bacterial and fungal infections during the pre-engraftment phase. Neutropenia is more prolonged in recipients of myeloablative allogeneic transplants than in recipients of non-myeloablative or autologous transplants. Thus, the frequency and severity of infection in allogeneic transplant recipients are greater than in other transplant subgroups [2–6]. Some patients with hematologic malignancies may have normal or even elevated ANCs but may be at increased risk for infection due to defects in neutrophil function (qualitative neutropenia). These defects include significant reduction in phagocytosis, decreased bactericidal and fungicidal activity, decreased production of superoxide anions, and defects in granulocyte locomotion. Myeloablative conditioning regimens also inflict substantial damage to mucosal barriers causing mucositis of the mouth and gastrointestinal tract, resulting in increased risk of infections arising from these sites [7, 8]. Early recognition and aggressive management of infection is critical for the overall survival of hematopoietic transplant recipients, and delays in the administration of appropriate anti-infective therapy are associated with poorer outcomes [9]. Unfortunately, signs and symptoms commonly associated with infection may be blunted in these highly immunosuppressed patients. Often the only manifestation of infection during an episode of neutropenia is fever. This condition is commonly referred to as "febrile neutropenia." The widely accepted definition of febrile neutropenia is an oral temperature of ≥38.3 °C, or two consecutive readings of >38 °C during a 2 h period, and an absolute neutrophil count of <500/mm^3 [10]. It has been estimated that approximately 80% of allogeneic transplant recipients and a smaller but substantial proportion of allogeneic transplant recipients will develop febrile neutropenia. It is important to keep in mind that some neutropenic patients, especially those receiving corticosteroids, may not mount an adequate inflammatory response and may be afebrile or even hypothermic while developing or harboring a significant infection. A high index of suspicion and close monitoring during periods of increased risk is essential in such patients.

The administration of prompt, broad-spectrum, empiric, antimicrobial therapy has become the standard of care for most febrile neutropenic patients including transplant recipients [10]. The general principles of such therapy for both adult and pediatric patients have been published in guidelines issued by various learned societies [10–13]. Specific treatment regimens for individual patients generally take into consideration local epidemiologic trends and local susceptibility/resistance patterns since geographic and institutional differences do occur. Periodic surveillance studied to monitor changes in the epidemiology of infections and in susceptibility and resistance patterns are important especially in

L. Nesher
Infectious Disease Institute, Faculty of Health Sciences, Ben-Gurion University of the Negev, Beer Sheba, Israel

Soroka University Medical Center affiliated with Faculty of Health Sciences Ben-Gurion University of the Negev, Infectious Disease Institute, Beer Sheba, Israel
e-mail: nesherke@bgu.ac.il

K. V. I. Rolston (✉)
Department of Infectious Diseases, Infection Control & Employee Health, The University of Texas MD Anderson Cancer Center, Houston, TX, USA
e-mail: krolston@mdanderson.org

A. Safdar (ed.), *Principles and Practice of Transplant Infectious Diseases*, https://doi.org/10.1007/978-1-4939-9034-4_9

institutions that perform large numbers of hematopoietic transplants.

Types of Febrile Episodes

Although fever is the most frequent and occasionally the only manifestation of infection in neutropenic patients, a substantial number of patients remain febrile without a specific infection being documented. A specific causative pathogen, most often bacterial or fungal, is identified in only 20–25% of febrile neutropenic episodes, referred to as episodes of microbiologically documented infection [14]. An additional 20–25% of patients will have an identifiable site of infection (e.g., pneumonia, cellulitis, enterocolitis) but will have negative cultures (Fig. 9.1). This may be due to various reasons such as the use of antimicrobial prophylaxis which may render cultures negative or substantially delay the time to positivity or a blunted inflammatory response which can result in paucity of specimens (e.g., sputum) to culture. These episodes are referred to as clinically documented infections. Approximately 40–50% of febrile neutropenic patients have neither clinical evidence of infection nor positive microbiological documentation of one, which are referred to as episodes of unexplained fever. The majority of these episode are probably caused by undetected infections as most of them respond to empiric antimicrobial therapy. A small proportion of patients with fever and neutropenia have noninfectious causes of fever such as drug fever or tumor fever. This is not surprising since fever is induced by cytokine release which is not limited to infections. All febrile neutropenic patients should undergo a thorough evaluation to detect infection before the possibility of a noninfectious etiology is entertained. Most microbiologically documented infections are monomicrobial (i.e., caused by one organism) with Gram-positive bacteria being predominant [10, 15]. However, polymicrobial infections are being documented with increasing frequency at many transplant centers and may account for up to 25% of bacterial infections [16]. Recent data show that ~10–15% of bacteremias in neutropenic patients are polymicrobial [17]. Infections involving deep tissue sites such as pneumonia, enterocolitis, and perirectal infections are often polymicrobial [16, 18]. Most polymicrobial infections are caused by multiple bacterial species although bacterial and fungal, bacterial and viral, or fungal and viral infections may be present at the same time. These infections are generally associated with greater morbidity and mortality than monomicrobial infections.

Sites of Infection

The most common sites of infection documented in neutropenic hematopoietic transplant recipients are listed in Table 9.1. Infections of the respiratory tract occur most often followed by bloodstream infections (including central line-associated bloodstream infection, CLABSI), urinary tract infections, skin and skin structure infections (SSSIs), and infections originating from the oropharynx, the gastrointestinal tract, and the biliary tract [14]. Less frequent but clinically important sites include the central nervous system, the musculoskeletal system, and the end organs such as the spleen and liver. The frequency of bloodstream infection (BSI) varies from center to center and also on the type of transplant, generally being more frequent in allogeneic transplant recipients [19, 20]. Recent data indicate that the incidence of at least one episode of BSI is around 21% with an attributable mortality of ~3% [21]. Approximately 25% of patients with profound neutropenia lasting >10–12 days will develop lung infiltrates. These often do not respond to broad-spectrum antimicrobial therapy and establishing a specific diagnosis in such patients remains a significant challenge [22]. Data regarding other sites of infection are not as robust as those describing BSIs.

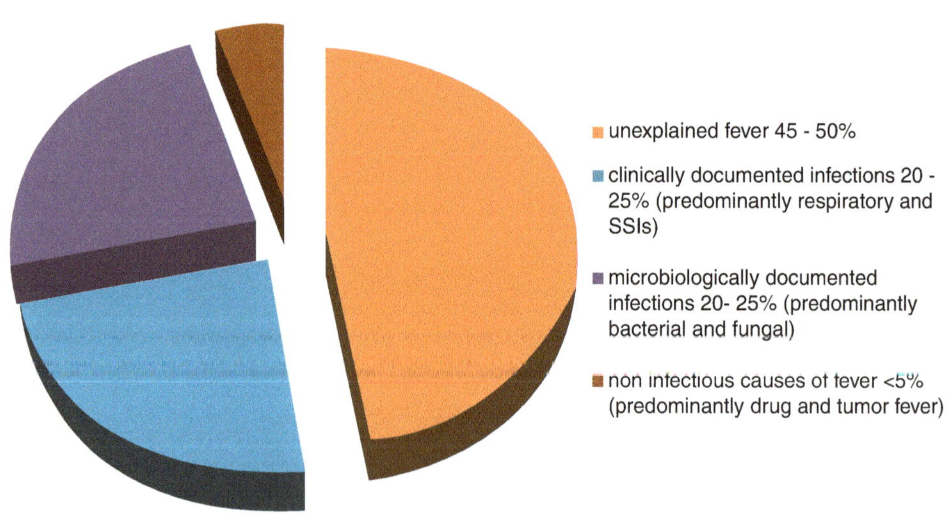

Fig. 9.1 Types and distribution of febrile episodes in neutropenic patients

Table 9.1 Common sites of infection in febrile neutropenic patients

Site of infection[a]	Frequency range
Respiratory tract[b]	35–40%
Bloodstream[c]	15–35%
Urinary tract	5–15%
Skin and skin structure[d]	5–10%
Gastrointestinal tract[e]	5–10%
Other sites[f]	5–10%

These data were extracted from various epidemiologic surveys conducted at the University of Texas MD Anderson Cancer Center between 2004 and 2014

[a]Approximately 15–20 % of patients will have multiple sites of infection (i.e., bacteremia + pneumonia). These are not always caused by the same organisms

[b]Includes the para nasal sinuses, the upper respiratory tract, the lungs, and infections such as empyema

[c]Includes primary and catheter-related bacteremia

[d]Includes infections at surgical sites, bone marrow biopsy sites, and radiation fields

[e]Includes infections arising from the oral cavity, esophagitis, appendicitis, neutropenic enterocolitis, cholangitis, and perirectal infections

[f]Central nervous system, bone, joint, etc.

Most microbiologically documented infections arise from the patient's endogenous microflora, with only a small proportion being acquired from exogenous sources and/or environmental exposure. It is therefore often possible to anticipate the potential etiology of an infection and provide appropriate empiric coverage based on the site where the infection originated. For example, most infections with a cutaneous origin are caused by *Staphylococcus* species and other organisms that colonize the skin (*Bacillus* spp., *Corynebacterium* spp., *Candida* spp.) [23]. Patients with severe oral mucositis and/or poor periodontal status are more likely to have infections caused by viridans group streptococci (VGS) and *Stomatococcus mucilaginosus* [24–26]. In patients with significant lower intestinal mucositis, enterococcal and Gram-negative bacillary infections occur more often. Bacterial infections generally occur during the initial stages of a neutropenic episode, while fungal infections arise more frequently in patients with prolonged (≥7 days) neutropenia. The widespread use of long-term central venous catheters in transplant recipients has had an impact on the frequency and spectrum of infection. The ability of certain organisms (notably coagulase-negative staphylococci (CoNS), *Staphylococcus aureus*, and *Candida* spp.) to produce and get embedded in biofilm, and the poor penetration of many antimicrobial agents into biofilm, makes catheter-related infections difficult to eradicate without removal of the offending catheter [27]. Consequently many transplant centers perform routine weekly blood cultures from central venous catheters in an attempt to detect colonization/infection early [28, 29]. This practice, however, has not been shown to accurately predict the development of CLABSI and may lead to unnecessary interventions [30]. The most common organisms isolated from CLABSI are CoNS. Other organisms include S. *aureus*, *Bacillus* spp., *Corynebacterium* spp., *Pseudomonas aeruginosa*, *Enterobacteriaceae*, *Enterococcus* spp., *Acinetobacter* spp., *Stenotrophomonas maltophilia*, and *Candida* spp. Despite the widespread use of catheters, the infection rate seldom exceeds 15% or more than two episodes per 1000 catheter days [31].

Bacterial Infections

Several recent epidemiologic surveys conducted in pediatric and adult hematopoietic transplant recipients have documented the predominance of Gram-positive organisms over Gram-negative bacilli [32–34]. Some of the reasons for this predominance include (1) the widespread use of central venous catheters, (2) the frequent use of intensive chemotherapeutic regimens that produce significant oral mucositis, and (3) the use of antibacterial prophylaxis (generally with a fluoroquinolone) directed primarily against enteric Gram-negative bacilli. Fluoroquinolone prophylaxis has in fact been show to increase the frequency of Gram-positive infections especially with organisms such as VGS that are often resistant to them [35]. The proportion of Gram-positive infections has been reported to be as high as 70–80% at some centers. Many reports, however, include data only on BSI caused by single organisms (monomicrobial BSI) and either exclude or provide very little details regarding infections at other sites and on polymicrobial infections [36]. These reports provide an overestimate of Gram-positive infections since the majority of bacteremias, particularly CLABSI, are indeed caused by Gram-positive organisms that inhabit the skin. As mentioned previously, BSIs account for only 20–25% of microbiologically documented infections. Infections at most other sites such as lungs, intestinal tract, urinary tract, and biliary tract have a predominance of Gram-negative pathogens. Additionally, ~60–80% of polymicrobial infections have a Gram-negative component, and ~30–35% are caused exclusively by multiple Gram-negative species [16, 18]. Therefore, when all sites of infection, not just BSI and monomicrobial as well as polymicrobial infections are pooled together, the apparent predominance of Gram-positive organisms seems less striking, with Gram-negative organisms being isolated almost as frequently [37]. Indeed, some institutions are beginning to report a resurgence in the frequency of Gram-negative pathogens even in patients with BSI [32]. The main reason for this appears to be the discontinuation of fluoroquinolone prophylaxis at some institutions since this practice has resulted in the emergence of fluoroquinolone-resistant and even multidrug-resistant organisms [32]. For reasons that remain unclear anaerobes are seldom isolated from neutropenic patients, although it is customary to provide anaerobic coverage especially for infections arising from or involving the intestinal tract. Real-time knowledge of local epidemiological patterns is critical, and empiric regimens need to be based on such information. Consequently, transplant centers are encouraged to perform periodic surveillance studies in order to keep abreast of epidemiologic changes. The organisms causing the majority if bacterial infections in neutropenic hematopoietic transplant recipients are listed in Tables 9.2 and 9.3.

Table 9.2 The spectrum of Gram-positive organisms isolated from febrile neutropenic patients

Organism	% Frequency
CoNS[a]	20–50
Staphylococcus aureus[a]	10–30
Enterococcus species[b]	10–20
VGS[c]	5–25
Micrococcus species	2–8
Corynebacterium species	2–5
β hemolytic streptococci[d]	4–6
Bacillus species	4–6
Aerococcus species	<3, respectively
Streptococcus pneumoniae	
Stomatococcus mucilaginosus	
Lactobacillus species	
Leuconostoc species	
Pediococcus species	

These data were extracted from various epidemiologic surveys conducted at the University of Texas MD Anderson Cancer Center between 2004 and 2014

[a]CoNS – coagulase-negative staphylococci – approximately 7% of CoNS were *S. lugdunensis*. >95% of CoNS and >65% of *S. aureus* isolates were methicillin-resistant

[b]Approximately 18% of *Enterococcus species* were vancomycin-resistant enterococci (VRE)

[c]VGS – viridans group streptococci – the most common species were *S. mitis*, *S. sanguis*, and *S. salivarius*

[d]Included groups A, B, C, G, and F

Table 9.3 Spectrum of Gram-negative organisms isolated from febrile neutropenic patients

Organism	% Frequency
Escherichia coli[a]	20–45
Klebsiella species[b]	10–20
Other *Enterobacteriaceae*[c]	15–20
Pseudomonas aeruginosa[d]	18–24
Stenotrophomonas maltophilia[d]	2–5
Acinetobacter species[d]	<3
Other NFGNB[e]	<3

These data were extracted from various epidemiologic surveys conducted at the University of Texas MD Anderson Cancer Center between 2004 and 2014

[a]Approximately 40% of isolates were fluoroquinolone-resistant, approximately 9% produced ESBLS and 4% were multidrug resistant

[b]*K. pneumoniae* 78% and *K. oxytoca* 22%. Increasing rates of ESBL and carbapenemase-producing organisms are being reported

[c]Primarily *Enterobacter* species, *Serratia* species, and *Citrobacter* species

[d]Increasing frequency of multidrug resistant (MDR) isolates (i.e., resistant to at least three classes of antimicrobial agents)

[e]NFGNB – non-fermentative Gram-negative bacilli

Gram-Positive Organisms

Coagulase-negative staphylococci are isolated most often with the most common species being *Staphylococcus epidermidis*, *S. hominis*, and *S. haemolyticus*. These organisms are of low virulence and seldom cause life-threatening infections even in severely neutropenic patients. CLABSI are the most common infections caused by CoNS. These can often be treated with antimicrobial agents alone, although catheter removal may be required if the infection recurs [38]. The one exception is *S. lugdunensis*, which more closely resembles *S. aureus* in virulence [39–41]. Many experts recommend that these organisms should not be considered to be harmless commensals and infections caused by them should be managed like those caused by *S. aureus*. Other Gram-positive organisms that colonize the human skin and cause infections in neutropenic patients include *Bacillus* spp., *Corynebacterium* spp., and *Micrococcus* spp. Like CoNS, these organisms cause CLABSI most often, although serious infections such as endophthalmitis, endocarditis, septic arthritis, and pneumonia develop occasionally. As mentioned, *S. aureus* are more virulent than other staphylococci and are associated with substantial morbidity and mortality. Patients with *S. aureus* bacteremia should be evaluated with infections such as endocarditis and deep-seated abscesses [42]. Unlike CoNS catheter removal is almost always necessary in *S. aureus* CLABSI [43]. Of concern are the increasing rates of methicillin resistance among *S. aureus* (MRSA) isolates worldwide. Although MRSA rates as low as 10% are still reported occasionally, many institutions are reporting MRSA rates in the range of 55–60%, making them more common than methicillin-susceptible isolates. Some MRSA isolates have developed tolerance (MBC ≥32 times the MIC) or reduced susceptibility to vancomycin (referred to as the MIC creep), thereby reducing the therapeutic impact of this agent, which until recently has been considered to be the agent of choice for the treatment of Gram-positive infections in neutropenic patients [44, 45]. Alternative agents are being recommended for infections caused by such organisms [46].

Alpha-hemolytic streptococci or VGS are major components of the human oral microflora. Patients particularly prone to VGS infections are recipients of high-intensity chemotherapy with agents such as cytosine arabinoside which induces severe mucosal damage and facilitates translocation of these organisms into the bloodstream. Other predisposing factors include the use of fluoroquinolone prophylaxis and the use of antacids and histamine type-2 (H2) antagonists. Although not recommended by most authorities, vancomycin-based prophylaxis in the peri-transplant period has been used by some, in order to reduce the frequency of VGS bacteremia [47]. This practice requires close monitoring of patients for the development of resistant organisms such as VRE and/or staphylococcal isolates with reduced susceptibility or resistance to vancomycin. It should only be considered in institutions where the frequency of infections caused by VGS is very high. Also of concern is the possibility that this practice might lead to the development of reduced susceptibility to other agents (daptomycin, dalbavancin). Some investigators believe that mucositis, which generally occurs at the nadir of neutropenia, is the primary predisposing factor for the development of infection in this setting, and have coined the phrase "febrile mucositis." Additionally, periodontal inflammation including gingivitis, periodontitis increases the possibility of VGS bacteremia [24, 48]. The most common manifestation of VGS infection is bacteremia. Approximately 5–10% of patients may develop disseminated infection, the so-called streptococcal toxic shock syndrome in which the mortality rate is in the range of 40–50% despite appropriate therapy [49]. *Streptococcus mitis*, *S. sanguis*, and *S. salivarius* are the species isolated most often from patients with VGS bacteremia. Of increasing concern are reports that up to 20–60% of VGS isolates are non-susceptible or overtly resistant to penicillin [50]. All isolates are currently susceptible to vancomycin, although occasional tolerance to this agent has been described [45]. They are also susceptible to newer-generation quinolones such as moxifloxacin and agents such as linezolid, daptomycin, telavancin, and dalbavancin, although clinical experience with these agents is limited [51–53]. The use of antibiotic combinations may be warranted, especially against organisms with high MICs or tolerance to vancomycin.

The enterococci reside mainly in the lower intestinal tract. They are seldom primary pathogens but are isolated most often following prolonged therapy with broad-spectrum agents such as the carbapenems. The most common manifestations include BSI and urinary tract infections. Enterococci are also often isolated from polymicrobial infections such as neutropenic enterocolitis and perirectal infections. The increased and prolonged use of vancomycin in neutropenic patients was in part responsible for the emergence of vancomycin-resistant enterococci (VRE) globally, and currently, 15–20% of all enterococcal isolates in the United States are VRE. Fecal colonization with VRE in hematopoietic transplant recipients is not uncommon, and approximately 15–40% of colonized patients will develop BSI or other serious infections [54–58]. Consequently, some experts recommend the preemptive use of agents with activity against VRE when patients with fecal colonization develop febrile neutropenia. Fecal decolonization has been attempted, but most attempts have been unsuccessful. Therefore, antimicrobial stewardship and infection control measures to limit the emergence and spread of VRE are extremely important.

Gram-Negative Organisms

The gastrointestinal tract serves as an important source of infection in neutropenic patients, with the predominant pathogens being enteric Gram-negative bacilli. The use of antimicrobial prophylaxis in high-risk neutropenic patients including hematopoietic transplant recipients led to a decline in the frequency and, to some extent, the morbidity and mortality associated with documented Gram-negative infections. This practice also led to the emergence of resistance among *Escherichia coli* and other Gram-negative species [59–61]. Therefore, many institutions are re-evaluating this practice, and some institutions have even discontinued fluoroquinolone prophylaxis in neutropenic patients [32]. Many institutions conduct surveillance studies in high-risk patients looking for fecal colonization with VRE, *Pseudomonas aeruginosa*, and other resistant organisms such as extended-spectrum beta-lactamase (ESBL) producers and carbapenem-resistant *Enterobacteriaceae* (CRE), since positive surveillance cultures often predict the development of infections during subsequent episodes of neutropenia [55, 62, 63]. This information is useful in picking appropriate empiric regimens when colonized patients develop febrile neutropenia, as well as in antimicrobial stewardship efforts if surveillance cultures are negative. ESBL-producing organisms are being reported with increasing frequency [64]. Carbapenemase-producing Gram-negative bacteria (*Klebsiella pneumonia* carbapenemase, KPC; New Delhi metallo-beta-lactamase 1, NDM-1; non-metallo-beta-lactamase producers) have emerged over the past few years and are spreading across the globe [65, 66]. Gram-negative infections are usually associated with greater morbidity and mortality than Gram-positive infections. Many epidemiological studies have shown that *E. coli*, *Klebsiella* species (*K. pneumoniae* and *K. oxytoca*), and *P. aeruginosa* remain the three primary Gram-negative pathogens in neutropenic patients causing 45–60% of such infections [36, 37]. Other *Enterobacteriaceae* (*Citrobacter* spp., *Enterobacter* spp., *Proteus* spp., *Serratia* spp.) are less common, although institutional differences do exist [67, 68]. Nationwide outbreaks of *Serratia marcescens* bacteremia due to contaminated prefilled heparin and saline syringes have been reported [69, 70]. Despite the overall decline in the frequency of Gram-negative infections, the proportion of infections caused by non-fermentative Gram-negative bacilli (NFGNB) such as *P. aeruginosa*, non-aeruginosa pseudomonads, *Stenotrophomonas maltophilia*, and *Acinetobacter* species has increased [67, 71]. Collectively, NFGNB now cause ~40% of all Gram-negative infections, a proportion that has steadily increased over the past two decades. *P. aeruginosa* is the most important and most frequently isolated NFGNB and causes between 15% and 20% of Gram-negative infections [72]. Bacteremia and pneumonia are the two most common manifestations, although infections at various other sites are not uncommon. It is also the most common Gram-negative organism isolated from polymicrobial infections [16]. These organisms develop resistance to antimicrobial agents using multiple mechanisms and often acquire resistance to several classes of agents (multidrug resistance, MDR) and are difficult to treat and eradicate. Combination therapy is often necessary. Prolonged use of fluoroquinolones and carbapenems has been identified as risk factor for the development of resistance [73–75]. Consequently, many antimicrobial stewardship efforts focus on curtailing or minimizing the use of these agents. Colonization/infection with *S. maltophilia* is also being reported more often especially in patients with hematologic malignancies and hematopoietic transplant recipients [76, 77]. The shift from trimethoprim/sulfamethoxazole (which has potent activity against *S. maltophilia*) to fluoroquinolones (which do not) as the preferred agents for antimicrobial prophylaxis in neutropenic patients may account for this increase. These organisms are almost always multidrug resistant, and as is the case with *P. aeruginosa*, combination therapy (trimethoprim/sulfamethoxazole + minocycline or tigecycline) is frequently necessary [77, 78]. Other infrequent but important NFGNB include *Acinetobacter* spp., *Achromobacter* and *Alcaligenes* spp., and non-aeruginosa *Pseudomonas* species such as *P. putida* and *P. fluorescens*. Many outbreaks caused by these organisms have been traced to contaminated dialysis fluid, de-ionized water, mechanical ventilators, and chlorhexidine solution. Many of these organisms are also multidrug resistant.

Anaerobic Infections

Anaerobic infections are seldom documented in febrile neutropenic patients, with the overall range of positive blood cultures being 0–5% [79]. The most common sites of infection are the intestinal tract (neutropenic enterocolitis, perirectal infections, abdominal/pelvic abscesses), complicated skin and skin structure infections, biliary tract infections, and respiratory infections [14, 80]. It is customary to provide anaerobic coverage to treat these infections even if anaerobes have not been isolated. The presence of significant oral or intestinal mucositis increases the risk of anaerobic infections. Purulence, which is the hallmark of anaerobic infections in immunocompetent patients, is often absent in patients with neutropenia. The organisms isolated most often include *Peptostreptococcus* spp., *Fusobacterium nucleatum*, *Bacteroides* spp., *Prevotella* spp., and *Clostridium* spp. Due to the frequent and prolonged use of broad-spectrum antimicrobial agents, *Clostridium difficile*-associated diarrhea is not infrequent in patients with neutropenia [81]. Approximately 13% of hematopoietic transplant recipients develop *C. difficile* infection mainly in the 1st month post-transplantation [82]. Colonization with toxigenic strains of *C. difficile* has been shown to be predictive for the development of *C. difficile*-associated diarrhea in hematopoietic transplant recipients [83, 84]. Response to treatment may be lower and relapses or recurrent infections may be higher in this setting.

The spectrum of bacterial infection in neutropenic patients continues to change with significant geographic and institutional differences being commonplace. In institutions wherein fluoroquinolone prophylaxis is still in use, Gram-positive pathogens predominate, whereas in institutions that have suspended or discontinued the use of fluoroquinolone prophylaxis, Gram-negative pathogens are more common. Resistance patterns also vary from region to region and, indeed, sometimes within the same region or institution. Resistant organisms are uncommon in Scandinavian countries. VRE appears to be more common in the United States than in Europe. The frequency of ESBL-producing, carbapenemase-producing, and MDR Gram-negative organisms appears to be increasing worldwide. Consequently, generating real-time local epidemiologic and susceptibility/resistance data is important.

Fungal Infections

Bacterial infections predominate during the initial 7–10 days of neutropenia. With more prolonged neutropenia, fungal infections begin to develop. Infections caused by *Candida* spp. and *Aspergillus* spp. are documented most often although many opportunistic fungi are pathogenic in this setting (Table 9.4). Invasive candidiasis was the most common fungal infection in neutropenic patients prior to the development of agents such as fluconazole, with *C. albicans* being the predominant species. With the routine usage of antifungal prophylaxis in high-risk patients including hematopoietic transplant recipients, the frequency of invasive candidiasis has been substantially reduced with manifestations like esophagitis and chronic systemic or hepatosplenic candidiasis becoming almost of historic interest. Currently candidemia, most often catheter-related, is the most common manifestation of invasive candidiasis. There has also been a shift in the epidemiology of candidiasis, in part related to the usage of agents such as fluconazole, with the emergence of *Candida* species other than *C. albicans such as C. glabrata*, *C. tropicalis*, *C. parapsilosis*, *C. krusei*, *C. auris* as frequent pathogens in this setting [85, 86]. Regional differences have been documented with a preponderance of different species in different institutions. These differences may be due to divergent use of antifungal prophylaxis and/or geographic diversity. As with bacterial infections, local epidemiologic and susceptibility/resistance data should be used to guide empiric

Table 9.4 The spectrum of fungal and viral infections in neutropenic patients

Fungal pathogens (yeast) – 8–24% of blood stream infections in patients with hematological malignancy
Candida albicans
Other candida species[a]
Trichosporon beigelii
Geotrichum capitatum
Malassezia furfur
Hansenula anomala
Streptomyces cerevisiae
Fungal pathogens (molds) – 2–28% of patients with hematological malignancy
Aspergillus fumigatus
Other Aspergillus species[b]
The Zygomycetes[c]
Fusarium species
Scedosporium species
Viral pathogens
Herpes simplex viruses (reactivation)
Community respiratory viruses[d]

These data were extracted from various epidemiologic surveys conducted at the University of Texas MD Anderson Cancer Center between 2004 and 2014

[a]Includes *C. glabrata, C. tropicalis, C. krusei, C. auris,* and *C. parapsilosis*

[b]Includes *A. flavus, A. niger, A. terreus, and A. oryzae*

[c]*Rhizopus, Mucor, Rhizomucor, Absidia, and Cunninghamella* are the most common human pathogens

[d]Includes influenza A and B, parainfluenza viruses, respiratory syncytial virus (RSV), human metapneumovirus, corona viruses, rhinoviruses, and bocavirus. Infection may not necessarily be more common in neutropenic patients but tends to be more severe

and targeted antifungal therapy. Other yeasts occasionally encountered in this setting include *Trichosporon beigelii, Hansenula anomala,* Geotrichum capitatum, *Malassezia furfur, and Streptomyces cerevisiae.*

Invasive mold infections are the most common life-threatening infections in patients with neutropenia that last longer than 2 weeks [87]. The vast majority of these infections are caused by *Aspergillus* species with *A. fumigatus* being the predominant species. Other species of Aspergillus have emerged as significant pathogens as well, including *A. flavus, A. terreus, A. niger,* and *A. oryzae* (Table 9.4). The most common site of involvement is the lung, resulting in invasive pulmonary aspergillosis (IPA). Other frequent sites of involvement include the paranasal sinuses and the central nervous system. Fungemia is rarely documented. Although still relatively uncommon, mucormycosis has emerged as an increasingly important infection in neutropenic patients in the last 15–20 years [88]. The most common organisms causing this infection are *Mucor* spp., *Rhizopus* spp., *Rhizomucor* spp., *Cunninghamella* spp., and *Absidia* spp. The increasing frequency of mucormycosis has in part been attributed to the use of voriconazole, due to its lack of activity against these organisms [89–91]. Like aspergillosis, common sites of infection include the paranasal sinuses, the rhino-orbital area, the lungs, and the central nervous system [92]. Other uncommon but important molds that cause infection in this setting include *Fusarium* spp. and *Scedosporium* spp. Unlike most other molds, fungemia is a common manifestation of fusariosis and may occur in up to 50% of patients [93]. Necrotic cutaneous lesions are also relatively common. The incidence of *Scedosporium* infection appears to be increasing in recent years. This increase may also be related to the fact that these organisms are resistant to many commonly used antifungal agents [94].

Viral Infections

Viral infections, especially those caused by human herpes viruses, are common in high-risk patients with neutropenia including hematopoietic cell transplant recipients. Most are effectively prevented with antiviral prophylaxis and/or pre-emptive therapy. Most herpes simplex virus (HSV 1 and HSV 2) infections in adults are due to reactivation of latent infections in seropositive patients. The likelihood of viral reactivation depends on the intensity of the chemotherapeutic/conditioning regimen. Reactivation occurs in two-thirds of patients undergoing induction chemotherapy for acute myelogenous leukemia and in recipients of hematopoietic transplants in the absence of antiviral prophylaxis [95, 96]. Ulcerations of the oral and esophageal mucosa, ulcers, or vesicles on the lips, genitalia, skin, or perianal areas are the most common manifestations. The HSVs can cause numerous syndromes including encephalitis, meningitis, myelitis, esophagitis, hepatitis, ocular disease, pneumonia, and erythema multiforme. Reactivation, or less commonly, primary acquisition of other human herpes viruses such as Cytomegalovirus, Epstein-Barr virus, and human herpes virus 6 can also occur, albeit, seen mostly during late transplant period [97–100].

Infections caused by respiratory viruses may not necessarily occur more frequently in neutropenic patients, but their manifestations tend to be more severe in this setting [101]. This may even impact the decision to proceed with hematopoietic cell transplantation, and several guidelines recommend delaying transplantation in patients with pre-transplant upper respiratory tract infections [101–103]. These pathogens include the influenza viruses (influenza A and B), respiratory syncytial virus (RSV), parainfluenza viruses, adenovirus, and metapneumovirus [104]. The risk for infection by these organisms tends to coincide with respiratory virus outbreaks in the general population. The severity of infection and specifically the rate of progression from upper respiratory tract disease to lower respiratory tract disease such as pneumonia depend on the level, duration, and type of immunosuppression [104–107].

Polymicrobial Infections

As previously mentioned, approximately 25–30% of microbiologically documented infections are polymicrobial. In the past polymicrobial infections have been ignored or underappreciated and underreported [16]. Of late, greater attention is being paid to such infections. In general, they are associated with greater morbidity and mortality than monomicrobial infections. This may be because polymicrobial infections frequently involve deep tissues (pneumonia, empyema, neutropenic enterocolitis, perirectal infections) where penetration of antimicrobial agents might be subtherapeutic and large areas of under perfused or necrotic tissue may be present. Recent studies also show that ~15% of bacteremic infections including CLABSI are polymicrobial [17]. Gram-positive organisms, predominantly staphylococci and enterococci, are isolated from up to 40% to 50% of polymicrobial infections, whereas Gram-negative organisms are isolated from ~80% of polymicrobial infections with *P. aeruginosa* and *E. coli* being isolated most often. Approximately one-third are caused by multiple Gram-negative species e.g., *E. coli & P. aeruginosa* [18]. Occasionally bacterial and fungal, bacterial and viral, fungal and viral, or multiple fungal infections may coexist.

It is important to remember that neutropenia is often superimposed on other immunological defects such as impaired cellular or humoral immunity both as a result of the underlying malignancy and/or its treatment prior to transplantation. If such deficits are present in addition to neutropenia, the spectrum of infection widens considerably as these deficits are associated with their own unique set of pathogens.

Management of Febrile Neutropenia

The principles of managing episodes of febrile neutropenia have been developed and refined over several decades [10, 108–110]. Many societies including the Infectious Diseases Society of America (IDSA), the National Comprehensive Cancer Network (NCCN), the American Society of Clinical Oncology (ASCO), and the European Society of Medical Oncology (ESMO) have published evidence-based guidelines that provide current information regarding the management (including prevention) of these episodes [10, 11, 13, 111, 112]. All febrile neutropenic patients should undergo a quick but thorough initial evaluation and should receive prompt, broad-spectrum, empiric, antibiotic therapy based on current local epidemiologic and susceptibility/resistance patterns. Several options are available for initial empiric therapy including (1) monotherapy with a broad-spectrum antipseudomonal agent or (2) various combination regimens. Depending on the patients' risk group, such therapy may be administered in the hospital or in an outpatient setting and may be parenteral or oral. Close monitoring for response or progression of infection, the development of complications or drug-related adverse effects, and the development of superinfections is critical. Modification of the initial regimen may be required in up to 30% of patients depending on the risk group, nature and site of infection, and the development of a superinfection (including a suspected or documented fungal infection). Removal of infected catheters and other medical hardware may be necessary. Surgical intervention may be indicated in specific settings (e.g., perirectal infection/abscess). The overall duration of therapy depends on several factors such as the patients risk group, nature and site of infection, and resolution or persistence of neutropenia. These principles are discussed below.

Initial Evaluation

A detailed history should be taken including the nature and intensity of chemotherapy, prior antibiotic usage (prophylactic and therapeutic), use of corticosteroids or other immunosuppressive agents, recent surgical procedures including placement of medical hardware, allergies, and recent travel or potential exposure to sick contacts. A history of past infection and/or colonization with resistant organisms will also have an impact on the selection of an appropriate empiric antimicrobial regimen. A thorough physical examination is mandatory and often reveals important sites of infection including cutaneous lesions such as ecthyma gangrenosum, cellulitis, and perirectal infection/abscesses. The examination of catheter insertion sites, external auditory meatus, nares and nasal septum, and the oropharynx may also often reveal foci of infection. Additionally, it is important to remember that some neutropenic patients, especially those receiving corticosteroids, may be afebrile. Others may just feel unwell and may even hypothermic. Such patients may harbor serious infections such as Gram-negative septicemia.

Laboratory evaluation should include a complete blood count (CBC) with differential leucocyte count and platelet count, measurement of serum creatinine blood urea nitrogen (BUN) to assess renal function, and measurement of serum electrolytes, total bilirubin, and hepatic transaminase enzymes. At least two sets of blood cultures should be obtained (one from a peripheral vein and the other from a central venous catheter, if present). Each lumen of multi-lumen catheters should be cultured separately [113]. Culture specimens from other sites (urine, wounds, sputum if available) should be obtained as indicated. Chest radiographs are not recommended routinely but should be obtained in patients with respiratory symptoms or signs [114].

The initial evaluation of a febrile neutropenic patient should also include risk assessment as this guides the choice of the empiric antibiotic regimen (combination vs monotherapy), the route of administration (parenteral vs oral), the setting in which therapy is administered (hospital vs outpatient), and the duration of therapy. The most commonly used risk assessment system in adults is the MASCC risk index [115]. High-risk patients have a MASCC risk score of <21 and should be admitted to the hospital for empiric therapy and close monitoring. Low-risk patients have a MASCC risk score of ≥21 and may be candidates for outpatient (oral or parenteral) therapy. Separate risk assessment tools are available for pediatric febrile neutropenic patients [116, 117].

Empiric Therapy

An algorithm for the management of febrile neutropenic patients is provided in Fig. 9.2. Once the initial evaluation and risk assessment have been completed, empiric antibiotic therapy should be administered without undue delay [10]. Low-risk patients can be treated with oral or parenteral regimens (Table 9.5). These can be administered during a short period of hospitalization followed by outpatient therapy or treatment of the entire episode in the outpatient setting. Most oral regimens are fluoroquinolone-based combinations although fluoroquinolone monotherapy has also been shown to be safe and effective [118, 119]. It is important to point out that hematopoietic cell transplant recipients (even those receiving non-myeloablative and/or autologous transplants) seldom fall into the low-risk category. Most hematopoietic transplant recipients with febrile neutropenia will either already be in the hospital or will require hospitalization for the administration of parenteral antibiotic therapy. Monotherapy with an antipseudomonal beta-lactam agent such as cefepime, a carbapenem such as meropenem or imipenem-cilastatin (but not ertapenem, as it is not active against *P. aeruginosa*), or piperacillin-tazobactam is recommended (Table 9.5). Other agents (aminoglycosides, fluoroquinolones, tigecycline, polymyxin-colistin, metronidazole) may be needed if antimicrobial resistance is suspected or documented or a specific pathogen such as an ESBL-producing or carbapenemase-producing Gram-negative bacillus or an anaerobe is isolated. The initial use of agents such as vancomycin, daptomycin, or linezolid is discouraged except when prior colonization or infection with a resistant Gram-positive organism (MRSA, VRE) has been documented or a catheter-related infection is strongly suspected [10, 120]. The empiric use of vancomycin has not been shown to reduce the overall mortality in patients with Gram-positive infections with the possible exception of infections caused by VGS. Additionally, one recent study has demonstrated that the empiric use of linezolid in febrile neu-

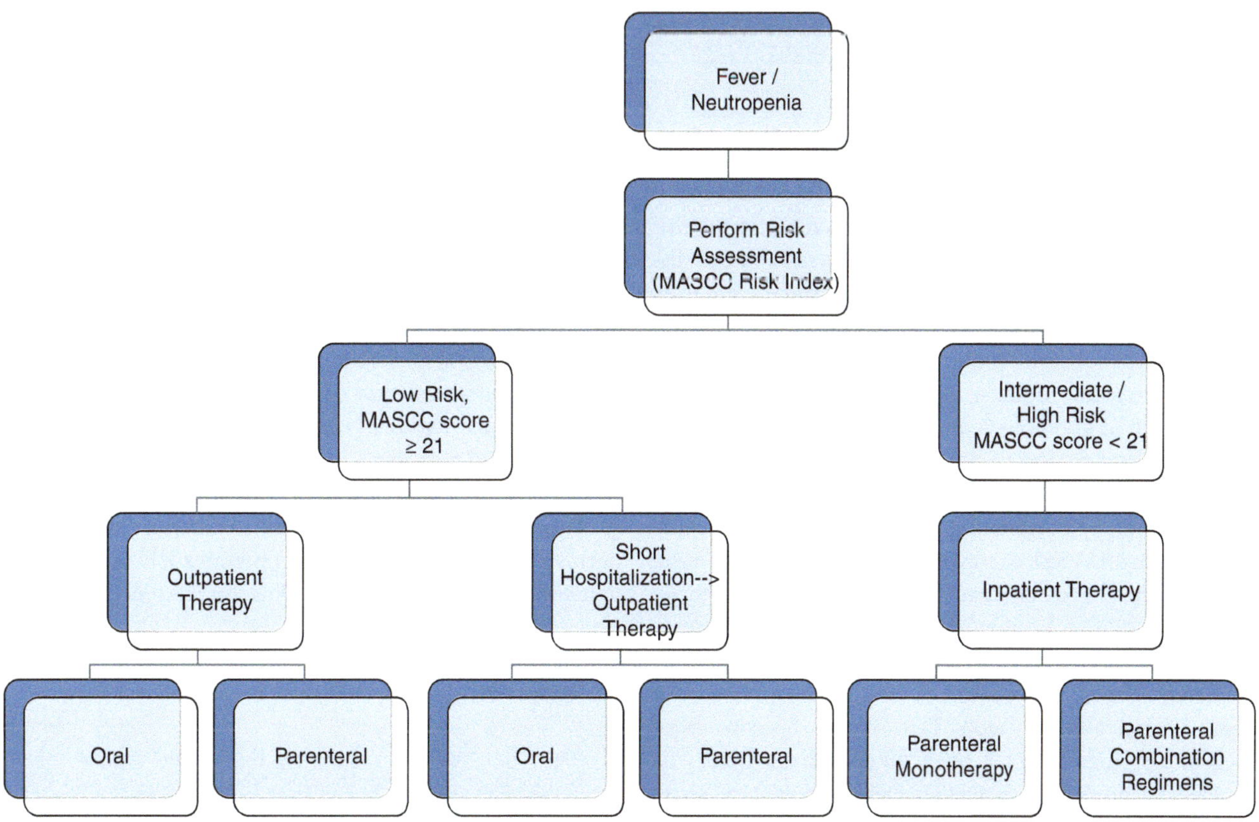

Fig. 9.2 Treatment algorithm for febrile neutropenic patients. Specific agents/regimens are listed in Table 9.5

Table 9.5 Common antibiotic regimens used in febrile neutropenic patients

Regimens
Regimens in low-risk patients
Parenteral regimens
Ceftriaxone or Ertapenem +/− an aminoglycoside
Aztreonam plus clindamycin or azithromycin
Quinolone plus clindamycin or azithromycin
Cefepime
Oral regimens
Quinolone plus amoxicillin/clavulanate
Quinolone plus clindamycin or azithromycin
Quinolone monotherapy
Regimens in intermediate to high-risk patients
Monotherapy
Cefepime
Piperacillin/tazobactam
Carbapenem (meropenem or imipenem/cilastatin)
Combination therapy
Agents used for monotherapy + an aminoglycoside
Agents used for monotherapy + vancomycin[a]

[a]Alternative agents such as daptomycin and linezolid are being used with increasing frequency although clinical data are limited

Table 9.6 Strategies for Antimicrobial stewardship program

Strategies
General strategies
Determine and monitor local epidemiology and resistance patterns
Develop multidisciplinary antimicrobial stewardship team (MAST)
Antimicrobial usage strategies
Limit antibacterial prophylaxis
Encourage targeted/specific therapy
Consider formulary restriction and/or pre-authorization
Create local guidelines and clinical pathways
Consider antimicrobial heterogeneity
Consider de-escalation (streamlining) of empiric regimen
Dose optimization
Parenteral to oral transition
Optimize duration of therapy
Other strategies
Prospective audits of antimicrobial usage with feedback to prescribers
Educational activities (grand rounds, in-services)
Strict adherence to infection control policies

Adapted from [123, 125–127]

tropenic patients colonized with VRE had no impact on mortality as well [121]. Concern has also been raised about the development of linezolid resistance, which has already been reported with increased usage of this agent [122]. Empiric antifungal coverage should be instituted if patients remain febrile after 4–7 days.

Duration of Therapy

The duration of therapy continues to be vigorously debated. In patients with episodes of unexplained fever, therapy is generally continued until marrow recovery (ANC >500 cells/mm^3 for 2 consecutive days). Some experts recommend discontinuation of therapy if the patient has defervesced, even though marrow recovery as defined above has not yet occurred. It is recommended to place these patients on their initial prophylactic regimen until neutropenia resolves. In patients with microbiologically or clinically documented infections, the duration of therapy usually depends on the site of infection (cellulitis or UTI requiring a shorter duration than bacteremia or pneumonia) and the organism isolated. In patients with CLABSI caused by *S. aureus*, *P. aeruginosa*, *Candida* spp. or other fungi, or mycobacteria, catheter removal in addition to appropriate antimicrobial therapy is recommended [43].

Therapy is generally continued until marrow recovery or longer if clinically indicated. The ultimate decision as to when to stop therapy often needs to be individualized and may depend on numerous factors such as the patient's risk group, the presence of a documented infection, and/or the persistence of neutropenia.

Infection Control and Antimicrobial Stewardship

Hand hygiene, cutaneous antisepsis, and maximum sterile barrier precautions are recommended for all procedures such as CVC insertions and bone marrow biopsies. Strict adherence to infection control practices and policies is essential in minimizing the spread of infections and controlling outbreaks, especially those caused by resistant organisms in the hospital and in other healthcare settings. Antimicrobial stewardship is essential especially since the frequent use of antimicrobial therapy in these high-risk patients creates selection pressures leading to the development of resistance. The various strategies for antimicrobial stewardship are listed in Table 9.6 and include a multidisciplinary antibiotic stewardship team (MAST), institutional pathways/guidelines, formulary restrictions or pre-approval requirements for certain agents, and de-escalation or streamlining of therapy when appropriate and feasible [123, 124]. Antimicrobial stewardship programs have been successfully instituted at several institutions [125–127]. Although currently the primary focus of these programs has been stewardship of antibacterial agents, it is anticipated that these programs will soon expand to include antifungal and antiviral agents as well.

References

1. Jones R, Shpall E, Champlin R. In Holland-Frei editor. Hematopoietic cell transplantation. 9th ed. Hoboken: John Wiley and sons. 2017, p 831–41.
2. Almyroudis NG, Fuller A, Jakubowski A, et al. Pre- and post-engraftment bloodstream infection rates and associated mortality

in allogeneic hematopoietic stem cell transplant recipients. Transpl Infect Dis. 2005;7(1):11–7.

3. Sorror ML, Storer BE, Maloney DG, Sandmaier BM, Martin PJ, Storb R. Outcomes after allogeneic hematopoietic cell transplantation with nonmyeloablative or myeloablative conditioning regimens for treatment of lymphoma and chronic lymphocytic leukemia. Blood. 2008;111(1):446–52.
4. Celebi H, Akan H, Akçağlayan E, Ustün C, Arat M. Febrile neutropenia in allogeneic and autologous peripheral blood stem cell transplantation and conventional chemotherapy for malignancies. Bone Marrow Transplant. 2000;26(2):211–4.
5. Gil L, Styczynski J, Komarnicki M. Infectious complication in 314 patients after high-dose therapy and autologous hematopoietic stem cell transplantation: risk factors analysis and outcome. Infection. 2007;35(6):421–7.
6. Zhang WX, Zhao QY, Huang HQ. Febrile neutropenic infection occurred in cancer patients undergoing autologous peripheral blood stem cell transplantation. Transplant Proc. 2015;47(2):523–7.
7. van der Velden WJ, Herbers AH, Netea MG, Blijlevens NM. Mucosal barrier injury, fever and infection in neutropenic patients with cancer: introducing the paradigm febrile mucositis. Br J Haematol. 2014;167(4):441–52.
8. Vera-Llonch M, Oster G, Ford CM, Lu J, Sonis S. Oral mucositis and outcomes of allogeneic hematopoietic stem-cell transplantation in patients with hematologic malignancies. Support Care Cancer. 2007;15(5):491–6.
9. Safdar A, Armstrong D. Infections in patients with hematologic neoplasms and hematopoietic stem cell transplantation: neutropenia, humoral, and splenic defects. Clin Infect Dis. 2011;53(8):798–806.
10. Freifeld AG, Bow EJ, Sepkowitz KA, et al. Clinical practice guideline for the use of antimicrobial agents in neutropenic patients with cancer: 2010 update by the infectious diseases society of America. Clin Infect Dis. 2011;52(4):e56–93.
11. Baden LR, Bensinger W, Angarone M, et al. Prevention and treatment of cancer-related infections. J Natl Compr Cancer Netw. 2012;10(11):1412–45.
12. Lehrnbecher T, Phillips R, Alexander S, et al. Guideline for the management of fever and neutropenia in children with cancer and/or undergoing hematopoietic stem-cell transplantation. J Clin Oncol. 2012;30(35):4427–38.
13. de Naurois J, Novitzky-Basso I, Gill MJ, et al. Management of febrile neutropenia: ESMO clinical practice guidelines. Ann Oncol. 2010;21(Suppl 5):v252–6.
14. Nesher L, Rolston KVI. The current spectrum of infection in cancer patients with chemotherapy related neutropenia. Infection. 2014;42(1):5–13.
15. Nesher L, Rolston KVI, Shah DP, et al. Fecal colonization and infection with Pseudomonas aeruginosa in recipients of allogeneic hematopoietic stem cell transplantation. Transpl Infect Dis. 2015;17(1):33–8.
16. Rolston KV, Bodey GP, Safdar A. Polymicrobial infection in patients with cancer: an underappreciated and underreported entity. Clin Infect Dis. 2007;45(2):228–33.
17. Klastersky J, Ameye L, Maertens J, et al. Bacteraemia in febrile neutropenic cancer patients. Int J Antimicrob Agents. 2007;30(Suppl 1):S51–9.
18. Elting LS, Bodey GP, Fainstein V. Polymicrobial septicemia in the cancer patient. Medicine (Baltimore). 1986;65(4):218–25.
19. Gudiol C, Garcia-Vidal C, Arnan M, et al. Etiology, clinical features and outcomes of pre-engraftment and post-engraftment bloodstream infection in hematopoietic SCT recipients. Bone Marrow Transplant. 2014;49(6):824–30.
20. Piñana JL, Montesinos P, Martino R, et al. Incidence, risk factors, and outcome of bacteremia following autologous hematopoietic stem cell transplantation in 720 adult patients. Ann Hematol. 2014;93(2):299–307.
21. Blennow O, Ljungman P, Sparrelid E, Mattsson J, Remberger M. Incidence, risk factors, and outcome of bloodstream infections during the pre-engraftment phase in 521 allogeneic hematopoietic stem cell transplantations. Transpl Infect Dis. 2014;16(1):106–14.
22. Maschmeyer G, Carratalà J, Buchheidt D, et al. Diagnosis and antimicrobial therapy of lung infiltrates in febrile neutropenic patients (allogeneic SCT excluded): updated guidelines of the Infectious Diseases Working Party (AGIHO) of the German Society of Hematology and Medical Oncology (DGHO). Ann Oncol. 2015;26(1):21–33.
23. Rolston KV, Nesher L, Tarrand JT. Current microbiology of surgical site infections in patients with cancer: a retrospective review. Infect Dis Ther. 2014;3(2):245–56.
24. Raber-Durlacher JE, Laheij AM, Epstein JB, et al. Periodontal status and bacteremia with oral viridans streptococci and coagulase negative staphylococci in allogeneic hematopoietic stem cell transplantation recipients: a prospective observational study. Support Care Cancer. 2013;21(6):1621–7.
25. Blijlevens NM, Donnelly JP, de Pauw BE. Empirical therapy of febrile neutropenic patients with mucositis: challenge of risk-based therapy. Clin Microbiol Infect. 2001;7(Suppl 4):47–52.
26. Fanourgiakis P, Georgala A, Vekemans M, Daneau D, Heymans C, Aoun M. Bacteremia due to Stomatococcus mucilaginosus in neutropenic patients in the setting of a cancer institute. Clin Microbiol Infect. 2003;9(10):1068–72.
27. Singh R, Ray P, Das A, Sharma M. Penetration of antibiotics through Staphylococcus aureus and *Staphylococcus epidermidis* biofilms. J Antimicrob Chemother. 2010;65(9):1955–8.
28. Kanathezhath B, Shah A, Secola R, Hudes M, Feusner JH. The utility of routine surveillance blood cultures in asymptomatic hematopoietic stem cell transplant patients. J Pediatr Hematol Oncol. 2010;32(4):327–31.
29. Rigby H, Fernandez CV, Langley J, Mailman T, Crooks B, Higgins A. Routine surveillance for bloodstream infections in a pediatric hematopoietic stem cell transplant cohort: do patients benefit? Can J Infect Dis Med Microbiol. 2007;18(4):253–6.
30. Nesher L, Chemaly RF, Shah DP, Mulanovich VE, Hosing C, Rolston KVI. Utility of routine surveillance blood cultures in asymptomatic allogeneic hematopoietic stem cell transplant recipients with indwelling central venous catheters at a comprehensive cancer center. Am J Infect Control. 2014;42(10):1084–8.
31. Cecinati V, Brescia L, Tagliaferri L, Giordano P, Esposito S. Catheter-related infections in pediatric patients with cancer. Eur J Clin Microbiol Infect Dis. 2012;31(11):2869–77.
32. Montassier E, Batard E, Gastinne T, Potel G, de La Cochetière MF. Recent changes in bacteremia in patients with cancer: a systematic review of epidemiology and antibiotic resistance. Eur J Clin Microbiol Infect Dis. 2013;32(7):841–50.
33. Macesic N, Morrissey CO, Cheng AC, Spencer A, Peleg AY. Changing microbial epidemiology in hematopoietic stem cell transplant recipients: increasing resistance over a 9-year period. Transpl Infect Dis. 2014;16(6):887–96.
34. Miedema KG, Winter RH, Ammann RA, et al. Bacteria causing bacteremia in pediatric cancer patients presenting with febrile neutropenia – species distribution and susceptibility patterns. Support Care Cancer. 2013;21(9):2417–26.
35. Razonable RR, Litzow MR, Khaliq Y, Piper KE, Rouse MS, Patel R. Bacteremia due to viridans group Streptococci with diminished susceptibility to Levofloxacin among neutropenic patients receiving levofloxacin prophylaxis. Clin Infect Dis. 2002;34(11):1469–74.
36. Wisplinghoff H, Seifert H, Wenzel RP, Edmond MB. Current trends in the epidemiology of nosocomial bloodstream infections in patients with hematological malignancies and solid neoplasms in hospitals in the United States. Clin Infect Dis. 2003;36(9):1103–10. Epub 2003 Apr 14.

37. Yadegarynia D, Tarrand J, Raad I, Rolston K. Current spectrum of bacterial infections in patients with cancer. Clin Infect Dis. 2003;37(8):1144–5.
38. Raad I, Chaftari AM. Advances in prevention and management of central line-associated bloodstream infections in patients with cancer. Clin Infect Dis. 2014;59(Suppl 5):S340–3.
39. Giormezis N, Kolonitsiou F, Makri A, et al. Virulence factors among Staphylococcus lugdunensis are associated with infection sites and clonal spread. Eur J Clin Microbiol Infect Dis. 2015;34(4):773–8.
40. Kleiner E, Monk AB, Archer GL, Forbes BA. Clinical significance of Staphylococcus lugdunensis isolated from routine cultures. Clin Infect Dis. 2010;51(7):801–3.
41. Fadel HJ, Patel R, Vetter EA, Baddour LM. Clinical significance of a single Staphylococcus lugdunensis-positive blood culture. J Clin Microbiol. 2011;49(4):1697–9.
42. Mihu CN, Schaub J, Kesh S, et al. Risk factors for late *Staphylococcus aureus* bacteremia after allogeneic hematopoietic stem cell transplantation: a single-institution, nested case-controlled study. Biol Blood Marrow Transplant. 2008;14(12):1429–33.
43. O'Grady NP, Alexander M, Burns LA, et al. Guidelines for the prevention of intravascular catheter-related infections. Clin Infect Dis. 2011;52(9):e162–93.
44. Sakoulas G, Moise-Broder PA, Schentag J, Forrest A, Moellering RC, Eliopoulos GM. Relationship of MIC and bactericidal activity to efficacy of vancomycin for treatment of methicillin-resistant *Staphylococcus aureus* bacteremia. J Clin Microbiol. 2004;42(6):2398–402.
45. Safdar A, Rolston KV. Vancomycin tolerance, a potential mechanism for refractory gram-positive bacteremia observational study in patients with cancer. Cancer. 2006;106(8):1815–20.
46. Liu C, Bayer A, Cosgrove SE, et al. Clinical practice guidelines by the infectious diseases society of America for the treatment of methicillin-resistant *Staphylococcus aureus* infections in adults and children. Clin Infect Dis. 2011;52(3):e18–55.
47. Seo SK, Xiao K, Huang YT, et al. Impact of peri-transplant vancomycin and fluoroquinolone administration on rates of bacteremia in allogeneic hematopoietic stem cell transplant (HSCT) recipients: a 12-year single institution study. J Infect. 2014;69(4):341–51.
48. Graber CJ, de Almeida KN, Atkinson JC, et al. Dental health and viridans streptococcal bacteremia in allogeneic hematopoietic stem cell transplant recipients. Bone Marrow Transplant. 2001;27(5):537–42.
49. Elting LS, Bodey GP, Keefe BH. Septicemia and shock syndrome due to viridans streptococci: a case-control study of predisposing factors. Clin Infect Dis. 1992;14(6):1201–7.
50. Han XY, Kamana M, Rolston KV. Viridans streptococci isolated by culture from blood of cancer patients: clinical and microbiologic analysis of 50 cases. J Clin Microbiol. 2006;44(1):160–5.
51. Rolston KV, Besece D, Lamp KC, Yoon M, McConnell SA, White P. Daptomycin use in neutropenic patients with documented gram-positive infections. Support Care Cancer. 2014;22(1):7–14.
52. Rolston KVI, Wang W, Nesher L, Coyle E, Shelburne S, Prince RA. In vitro activity of telavancin compared with vancomycin and linezolid against gram-positive organisms isolated from cancer patients. J Antibiot. 2014;67(7):505–9.
53. Rolston KV, Frisbee-Hume S, LeBlanc B, Streeter H, Ho DH. In vitro antimicrobial activity of moxifloxacin compared to other quinolones against recent clinical bacterial isolates from hospitalized and community-based cancer patients. Diagn Microbiol Infect Dis. 2003;47(2):441–9.
54. Matar MJ, Tarrand J, Raad I, Rolston KV. Colonization and infection with vancomycin-resistant enterococcus among patients with cancer. Am J Infect Control. 2006;34(8):534–6.
55. Liss BJ, Vehreschild JJ, Cornely OA, et al. Intestinal colonisation and blood stream infections due to vancomycin-resistant enterococci (VRE) and extended-spectrum beta-lactamase-producing Enterobacteriaceae (ESBLE) in patients with haematological and oncological malignancies. Infection. 2012;40(6):613–9.
56. Bossaer JB, Hall PD, Garrett-Mayer E. Incidence of vancomycin-resistant enterococci (VRE) infection in high-risk febrile neutropenic patients colonized with VRE. Support Care Cancer. 2010;19(2):231–7.
57. Kang M, Xie Y, He C, et al. Molecular characteristics of vancomycin-resistant Enterococcus faecium from a tertiary care hospital in Chengdu, China: molecular characteristics of VRE in China. Eur J Clin Microbiol Infect Dis. 2014;33(6):933–9.
58. Kang Y, Vicente M, Parsad S, et al. Evaluation of risk factors for vancomycin-resistant enterococcus bacteremia among previously colonized hematopoietic stem cell transplant patients. Transpl Infect Dis. 2013;15(5):466–73.
59. Mihu CN, Rhomberg PR, Jones RN, Coyle E, Prince RA, Rolston KV. *Escherichia coli* resistance to quinolones at a comprehensive cancer center. Diagn Microbiol Infect Dis. 2010;67(3):266–9.
60. Bhusal Y, Mihu CN, Tarrand JJ, Rolston KV. Incidence of fluoroquinolone-resistant and extended-spectrum β-lactamase-producing *Escherichia coli* at a comprehensive cancer center in the United States. Chemotherapy. 2011;57(4):335–8.
61. Kern WV, Klose K, Jellen-Ritter AS, et al. Fluoroquinolone resistance of *Escherichia coli* at a cancer center: epidemiologic evolution and effects of discontinuing prophylactic fluoroquinolone use in neutropenic patients with leukemia. Eur J Clin Microbiol Infect Dis. 2005;24(2):111–8.
62. Rolston KV, Nesher L, Mulanovich V, Chemaly R. Intestinal colonisation and blood stream infections due to vancomycin-resistant enterococci (VRE) and extended-spectrum beta-lactamase-producing enterobacteriaceae (ESBLE) in patients with haematological and oncological malignancies. Infection. 2013;41(5):1039–40.
63. Biehl LM, Schmidt-Hieber M, Liss B, Cornely OA, Vehreschild MJ. Colonization and infection with extended spectrum beta-lactamase producing Enterobacteriaceae in high-risk patients – review of the literature from a clinical perspective. Crit Rev Microbiol. 2016;42(1):1–16.
64. Kim SH, Kwon JC, Choi SM, et al. Escherichia coli and *Klebsiella pneumoniae* bacteremia in patients with neutropenic fever: factors associated with extended-spectrum β-lactamase production and its impact on outcome. Ann Hematol. 2013;92(4):533–41.
65. Patel G, Bonomo RA. "Stormy waters ahead": global emergence of carbapenemases. Front Microbiol. 2013;4:48.
66. Pillai DR, McGeer A, Low DE. New Delhi metallo-β-lactamase-1 in Enterobacteriaceae: emerging resistance. CMAJ. 2011;183(1):59–64.
67. Rolston KV, Tarrand JJ. Pseudomonas aeruginosa – still a frequent pathogen in patients with cancer: 11-year experience at a comprehensive cancer center. Clin Infect Dis. 1999;29(2):463–4.
68. Safdar A, Rodriguez GH, Balakrishnan M, Tarrand JJ, Rolston KV. Changing trends in etiology of bacteremia in patients with cancer. Eur J Clin Microbiol Infect Dis. 2006;25(8):522–6.
69. Chemaly RF, Rathod DB, Sikka MK, et al. Serratia marcescens bacteremia because of contaminated prefilled heparin and saline syringes: a multi-state report. Am J Infect Control. 2011;39(6):521–4.
70. Chemaly RF, Rathod DB, Raad II. A tertiary care cancer center experience of the 2007 outbreak of Serratia marcescens bloodstream infection due to prefilled syringes. Infect Control Hosp Epidemiol. 2009;30(12):1237–8.
71. Rolston KV, Kontoyiannis DP, Yadegarynia D, Raad II. Nonfermentative gram-negative bacilli in cancer patients: increasing frequency of infection and antimicrobial susceptibility of clinical isolates to fluoroquinolones. Diagn Microbiol Infect Dis. 2005;51(3):215–8.

72. Hakki M, Limaye AP, Kim HW, Kirby KA, Corey L, Boeckh M. Invasive Pseudomonas aeruginosa infections: high rate of recurrence and mortality after hematopoietic cell transplantation. Bone Marrow Transplant. 2007;39(11):687–93.
73. Ohmagari N, Hanna H, Graviss L, et al. Risk factors for infections with multidrug-resistant Pseudomonas aeruginosa in patients with cancer. Cancer. 2005;104(1):205–12.
74. Aboufaycal H, Sader HS, Rolston K, et al. blaVIM-2 and blaVIM-7 carbapenemase-producing Pseudomonas aeruginosa isolates detected in a tertiary care medical center in the United States: report from the MYSTIC program. J Clin Microbiol. 2007;45(2):614–5.
75. Toleman MA, Rolston K, Jones RN, Walsh TR. blaVIM-7, an evolutionarily distinct metallo-beta-lactamase gene in a Pseudomonas aeruginosa isolate from the United States. Antimicrob Agents Chemother. 2004;48(1):329–32.
76. Demiraslan H, Sevim M, Pala Ç, et al. Risk factors influencing mortality related to Stenotrophomonas maltophilia infection in hematology-oncology patients. Int J Hematol. 2013;97(3):414–20.
77. Safdar A, Rolston KV. Stenotrophomonas maltophilia: changing spectrum of a serious bacterial pathogen in patients with cancer. Clin Infect Dis. 2007;45(12):1602–9.
78. Al-Anazi KA, Al-Jasser AM. Infections caused by Stenotrophomonas maltophilia in recipients of hematopoietic stem cell transplantation. Front Oncol. 2014;4:232.
79. Brook I, Frazier EH. Aerobic and anaerobic infection associated with malignancy. Support Care Cancer. 1998;6(2):125–31.
80. Nesher L, Rolston KV. Neutropenic enterocolitis, a growing concern in the era of widespread use of aggressive chemotherapy. Clin Infect Dis. 2013;56(5):711–7.
81. Huang AM, Marini BL, Frame D, Aronoff DM, Nagel JL. Risk factors for recurrent Clostridium difficile infection in hematopoietic stem cell transplant recipients. Transpl Infect Dis. 2014;16(5):744–50.
82. Willems L, Porcher R, Lafaurie M, et al. Clostridium difficile infection after allogeneic hematopoietic stem cell transplantation: incidence, risk factors, and outcome. Biol Blood Marrow Transplant. 2012;18(8):1295–301.
83. Jain T, Croswell C, Urday-Cornejo V, et al. Clostridium difficile colonization in hematopoietic stem cell transplant recipients: a prospective study of the epidemiology and outcomes involving toxigenic and nontoxigenic strains. Biol Blood Marrow Transplant. 2016;22(1):157–63.
84. Kinnebrew MA, Lee YJ, Jenq RR, et al. Early Clostridium difficile infection during allogeneic hematopoietic stem cell transplantation. PLoS One. 2014;9(3):e90158.
85. Hachem R, Hanna H, Kontoyiannis D, Jiang Y, Raad I. The changing epidemiology of invasive candidiasis: Candida glabrata and *Candida krusei* as the leading causes of candidemia in hematologic malignancy. Cancer. 2008;112(11):2493–9.
86. Maschmeyer G. The changing epidemiology of invasive fungal infections: new threats. Int J Antimicrob Agents. 2006;27(Suppl 1):3–6.
87. Steinbach WJ, Marr KA, Anaissie EJ, et al. Clinical epidemiology of 960 patients with invasive aspergillosis from the PATH Alliance registry. J Infect. 2012;65(5):453–64.
88. Kontoyiannis DP, Wessel VC, Bodey GP, Rolston KV. Zygomycosis in the 1990s in a tertiary-care cancer center. Clin Infect Dis. 2000;30(6):851–6.
89. Marty FM, Cosimi LA, Baden LR. Breakthrough zygomycosis after voriconazole treatment in recipients of hematopoietic stem-cell transplants. N Engl J Med. 2004;350(9):950–2.
90. Kontoyiannis DP, Lionakis MS, Lewis RE, et al. Zygomycosis in a tertiary-care cancer center in the era of Aspergillus-active antifungal therapy: a case-control observational study of 27 recent cases. J Infect Dis. 2005;191(8):1350–60.
91. Pongas GN, Lewis RE, Samonis G, Kontoyiannis DP. Voriconazole-associated zygomycosis: a significant consequence of evolving antifungal prophylaxis and immunosuppression practices? Clin Microbiol Infect. 2009;15(Suppl 5):93–7.
92. Lewis RE, Cahyame-Zuniga L, Leventakos K, et al. Epidemiology and sites of involvement of invasive fungal infections in patients with haematological malignancies: a 20-year autopsy study. Mycoses. 2013;56(6):638–45.
93. Campo M, Lewis RE, Kontoyiannis DP. Invasive fusariosis in patients with hematologic malignancies at a cancer center: 1998–2009. J Infect. 2010;60(5):331–7.
94. Lamaris GA, Chamilos G, Lewis RE, Safdar A, Raad II, Kontoyiannis DP. Scedosporium infection in a tertiary care cancer center: a review of 25 cases from 1989–2006. Clin Infect Dis. 2006;43(12):1580–4.
95. Saral R, Ambinder RF, Burns WH, et al. Acyclovir prophylaxis against herpes simplex virus infection in patients with leukemia. A randomized, double-blind, placebo-controlled study. Ann Intern Med. 1983;99(6):773–6.
96. Saral R, Burns WH, Laskin OL, Santos GW, Lietman PS. Acyclovir prophylaxis of herpes-simplex-virus infections. N Engl J Med. 1981;305(2):63–7.
97. Yoshikawa T, Asano Y, Ihira M, et al. Human herpesvirus 6 viremia in bone marrow transplant recipients: clinical features and risk factors. J Infect Dis. 2002;185(7):847–53.
98. Zerr DM, Boeckh M, Delaney C, et al. HHV-6 reactivation and associated sequelae after hematopoietic cell transplantation. Biol Blood Marrow Transplant. 2012;18(11):1700–8.
99. Mori T, Kato J. Cytomegalovirus infection/disease after hematopoietic stem cell transplantation. Int J Hematol. 2010;91(4):588–95.
100. Cohen L, Yeshurun M, Shpilberg O, Ram R. Risk factors and prognostic scale for cytomegalovirus (CMV) infection in CMV-seropositive patients after allogeneic hematopoietic cell transplantation. Transpl Infect Dis. 2015;17(4):510–7.
101. Campbell AP, Guthrie KA, Englund JA, et al. Clinical outcomes associated with respiratory virus detection before allogeneic hematopoietic stem cell transplant. Clin Infect Dis. 2015;61(2):192–202.
102. Tomblyn M, Chiller T, Einsele H, et al. Guidelines for preventing infectious complications among hematopoietic cell transplant recipients: a global perspective. Preface. Bone Marrow Transplant. 2009;44(8):453–5.
103. Hirsch HH, Martino R, Ward KN, Boeckh M, Einsele H, Ljungman P. Fourth European conference on infections in Leukaemia (ECIL-4): guidelines for diagnosis and treatment of human respiratory syncytial virus, parainfluenza virus, metapneumovirus, rhinovirus, and coronavirus. Clin Infect Dis. 2013;56(2):258–66.
104. Hutspardol S, Essa M, Richardson S, et al. Significant transplantation-related mortality from respiratory virus infections within the first one hundred days in children after hematopoietic stem cell transplantation. Biol Blood Marrow Transplant. 2015;21(10):1802–7.
105. Renaud C, Xie H, Seo S, et al. Mortality rates of human metapneumovirus and respiratory syncytial virus lower respiratory tract infections in hematopoietic cell transplantation recipients. Biol Blood Marrow Transplant. 2013;19(8):1220–6.
106. Shah DP, Ghantoji SS, Mulanovich VE, Ariza-Heredia EJ, Chemaly RF. Management of respiratory viral infections in hematopoietic cell transplant recipients. Am J Blood Res. 2012;2(4):203–18.
107. Egli A, Bucher C, Dumoulin A, et al. Human metapneumovirus infection after allogeneic hematopoietic stem cell transplantation. Infection. 2012;40(6):677–84.
108. Hughes WT, Armstrong D, Bodey GP, et al. 2002 guidelines for the use of antimicrobial agents in neutropenic patients with cancer. Clin Infect Dis. 2002;34(6):730–51.

109. Hughes WT, Armstrong D, Bodey GP, et al. 1997 guidelines for the use of antimicrobial agents in neutropenic patients with unexplained fever. Infectious Diseases Society of America. Clin Infect Dis. 1997;25(3):551–73.
110. Hughes WT, Armstrong D, Bodey GP, et al. From the Infectious Diseases Society of America. Guidelines for the use of antimicrobial agents in neutropenic patients with unexplained fever. J Infect Dis. 1990;161(3):381–96.
111. Flowers CR, Seidenfeld J, Bow EJ, et al. Antimicrobial prophylaxis and outpatient management of fever and neutropenia in adults treated for malignancy: American Society of Clinical Oncology clinical practice guideline. J Clin Oncol. 2013;31(6):794–810.
112. Weissinger F, Auner HW, Bertz H, et al. Antimicrobial therapy of febrile complications after high-dose chemotherapy and autologous hematopoietic stem cell transplantation – guidelines of the Infectious Diseases Working Party (AGIHO) of the German Society of Hematology and Oncology (DGHO). Ann Hematol. 2012;91(8):1161–74.
113. Krause R, Valentin T, Salzer H, et al. Which lumen is the source of catheter-related bloodstream infection in patients with multilumen central venous catheters? Infection. 2013;41(1):49–52.
114. Yolin-Raley DS, Dagogo-Jack I, Niell HB, et al. The utility of routine chest radiography in the initial evaluation of adult patients with febrile neutropenia patients undergoing HSCT. J Natl Compr Cancer Netw. 2015;13(2):184–9.
115. Klastersky J, Paesmans M, Rubenstein EB, et al. The multinational association for supportive care in cancer risk index: a multinational scoring system for identifying low-risk febrile neutropenic cancer patients. J Clin Oncol. 2000;18(16):3038–51.
116. Phillips B, Wade R, Stewart LA, Sutton AJ. Systematic review and meta-analysis of the discriminatory performance of risk prediction rules in febrile neutropaenic episodes in children and young people. Eur J Cancer. 2010;46(16):2950–64.
117. Santolaya ME, Alvarez AM, Avilés CL, et al. Prospective validation of a risk prediction model for severe sepsis in children with cancer and high-risk febrile neutropenia. Pediatr Infect Dis J. 2013;32(12):1318–23.
118. Kern WV, Marchetti O, Drgona L, et al. Oral antibiotics for fever in low-risk neutropenic patients with cancer: a double-blind, randomized, multicenter trial comparing single daily moxifloxacin with twice daily ciprofloxacin plus amoxicillin/clavulanic acid combination therapy – EORTC infectious diseases group trial XV. J Clin Oncol. 2013;31(9):1149–56.
119. Rolston KV, Frisbee-Hume SE, Patel S, Manzullo EF, Benjamin RS. Oral moxifloxacin for outpatient treatment of low-risk, febrile neutropenic patients. Support Care Cancer. 2010;18(1):89–94.
120. Jaksic B, Martinelli G, Perez-Oteyza J, Hartman CS, Leonard LB, Tack KJ. Efficacy and safety of linezolid compared with vancomycin in a randomized, double-blind study of febrile neutropenic patients with cancer. Clin Infect Dis. 2006;42(5):597–607.
121. Lisboa LF, Miranda BG, Vieira MB, et al. Empiric use of linezolid in febrile hematology and hematopoietic stem cell transplantation patients colonized with vancomycin-resistant Enterococcus spp. Int J Infect Dis. 2015;33:171–6.
122. Scheetz MH, Knechtel SA, Malczynski M, Postelnick MJ, Qi C. Increasing incidence of linezolid-intermediate or -resistant, vancomycin-resistant Enterococcus faecium strains parallels increasing linezolid consumption. Antimicrob Agents Chemother. 2008;52(6):2256–9.
123. Dellit TH, Owens RC, McGowan JE, et al. Infectious Diseases Society of America and the Society for Healthcare Epidemiology of America guidelines for developing an institutional program to enhance antimicrobial stewardship. Clin Infect Dis. 2007;44(2):159–77.
124. Nesher L, Tverdek FP, Mahajan SN, Chemaly RF, Rolston KV. Ertapenem usage in cancer patients with and without neutropenia: a report on 97 cases from a comprehensive cancer center. Infection. 2015;43(5):545–50.
125. Tverdek FP, Rolston KV, Chemaly RF. Antimicrobial stewardship in patients with cancer. Pharmacotherapy. 2012;32(8):722–34.
126. Cosgrove SE, Seo SK, Bolon MK, et al. Evaluation of postprescription review and feedback as a method of promoting rational antimicrobial use: a multicenter intervention. Infect Control Hosp Epidemiol. 2012;33(4):374–80.
127. Paskovaty A, Pflomm JM, Myke N, Seo SK. A multidisciplinary approach to antimicrobial stewardship: evolution into the 21st century. Int J Antimicrob Agents. 2005;25(1):1–10.

10 Cytopenias in Transplant Patients

Maura Barry, Sunandana Chandra, and Kenneth B. Hymes

Anemia in Solid Organ Transplants

Anemia is commonly seen after solid organ transplant (SOT). It can result from a number of different etiologies including bleeding or hemorrhage, iron deficiency, hemolysis, drug related, lack of erythropoietin, marrow suppression, and congenital etiologies. The frequency and severity of anemia is dependent on the type of solid organ transplant and the duration of time that has passed since the transplant. Much of the data for the causes of anemia following SOT is from renal transplant and cardiac transplant populations. In these renal transplant patients, the prevalence of anemia is about 40% 1-year posttransplant. Severe anemia, defined as Hb <11 g/dL in males and 10 g/dL in females, is seen in 8.5% of patients 6–60 months post-kidney transplant [1]. Anemia to a hematocrit of less than 33% can persist for greater than 5 years in 25% patients and can result in worsened renal graft function and graft loss [2, 3]. Pre-transplant anemia often seen in dialysis can often improve posttransplant, but then may recur if there is graft failure. About 40% of cardiac transplant patients also experience posttransplant anemia [4]. Pre-transplant anemia that is seen in 25% of this population negatively affects 1-year survival posttransplant [5].

M. Barry (✉)
Division of Hematology and Oncology, Larner College of Medicine at the University of Vermont, University of Vermont Medical Center, Burlington, VT, USA
e-mail: maura.barry@uvmhealth.org

S. Chandra
Division of Hematology and Oncology, Northwestern University Feinberg School of Medicine, Chicago, IL, USA
e-mail: sunandana.chandra@northwestern.edu

K. B. Hymes
Hematology, Coagulation, and Medical Oncology, Laura and Isaac Perlmutter Cancer Center, NYU Langone Health, New York, NY, USA

Hemolysis

Mismatched ABO solid organ transplantation is often employed due to the shortage of transplantable organs. Three different groups of ABO incompatibility can be found in transplantation: minor, major, and bidirectional. Complications arising from minor ABO-mismatched solid organ transplants include the passenger lymphocyte syndrome (PLS) [6]. Recipients of minor ABO-incompatible transplantation express ABO antigens that are not expressed in the donor and may result in a graft-versus-host (GvH) reaction, including delayed hemolysis of recipient red blood cells [7]. Passenger lymphocyte syndrome occurs when antibodies that are produced by the donor B-lymphocytes result in a primary or secondary immune response against the recipient's ABO and Rh antigens. The severity of hemolysis depends on the level of red cell isoagglutinins in the donor tissue that are passively transferred with the organ and the subsequent rise in antibodies in the transplant recipient that occurs 1–3 weeks posttransplant and usually resolves within 3 months posttransplant [7]. In rare instances, PLS can occur due to non-ABO/Rh antibodies if the organ had been previously sensitized to other red cell antigens in the setting of pregnancy or transfusion [8–11]. PLS occurs more frequently in the heart and lung transplants and less frequently in liver and kidney transplants [7].

Drugs

There are numerous drugs that are often used in the solid organ transplant setting that can cause myelosuppression, including anemia, through a variety of pathophysiologic mechanisms. A number of immunosuppressants with various pharmacologic mechanisms of action are used to prolong graft and recipient survival. The immunosuppressants mycophenolate mofetil and tacrolimus have been shown to cause anemia in renal transplant recipients [12]. One-year posttransplant, renal transplant patients with anemia who are on

A. Safdar (ed.), *Principles and Practice of Transplant Infectious Diseases*, https://doi.org/10.1007/978-1-4939-9034-4_10

mycophenolate mofetil have a lower rates of survival and higher rates of cardiovascular death [13]. Sirolimus, another immunosuppressant, may result in greater myelosuppression compared to mycophenolate mofetil [14]. Sirolimus and calcineurin inhibitors such as tacrolimus and cyclosporine have been shown in renal and lung transplant recipients to cause hemolytic anemia, thrombotic thrombocytopenic purpura, and atypical hemolytic uremic syndrome [15–17]. The calcineurin inhibitors have been shown to cause anemia ranging from 1% to 5% in European trials to 38–47% in US trial [18]. The antimetabolite azathioprine, a purine-analog drug, can also cause cytopenias. Mycophenolate mofetil, tacrolimus, azathioprine, and anti-thymocyte globulin have all shown to cause pure red cell aplasia [19, 20].

Primaquine and dapsone are used for PCP treatment, and both can result in hemolysis in glucose-6-phosphate-dehydrogenase-deficient patients, which is not restricted to solid organ transplant settings. In patients with low body weight or renal failure, dapsone may induce a hemolytic anemia and produce methemoglobinemia even if the G6PD levels are normal [21–23].

Ribavirin and interferon can cause bone marrow suppression in liver transplant recipients who are being treated with recurrent hepatitis C virus [24]. Ribavirin is used in treating respiratory syncytial virus after transplant in both the oral and inhaled formulations, both of which can cause bone marrow suppression [25]. In patients who are co-infected with human deficiency virus (HIV) and hepatitis C virus, myelosuppression can be seen with the anti-retroviral medication, AZT, and the anemia can be exacerbated with the co-administration of ribavirin. The antibiotic trimethoprim-sulfamethoxazole can also cause myelosuppression including anemia. Valganciclovir has been reported to cause bone marrow failure in renal transplant patients who received this antiviral as prophylaxis [26].

Newer immunosuppressants have been developed which allow for the sparing of steroids and calcineurin inhibitors, the latter of which can cause chronic nephropathy. These newer agents include alemtuzumab, a human anti-CD52 antibody that depletes T- and B-cells, daclizumab, a human anti-CD25 antibody that targets the IL-2 alpha subunit, and anti-thymocyte globulin (ATG). Alemtuzumab has been reported to be associated with red cell aplasia, autoimmune hemolytic anemia, and idiopathic thrombocytopenia purpura in pancreas transplant patients [27].

Iron Deficiency

Iron deficiency is often overlooked in transplant patients. In renal transplant patients, those with a hematocrit of less than 30% have iron studies checked only 40% of the time [28]. Perioperative bleeding and frequent phlebotomies for laboratory studies can contribute to iron deficiency anemia. Anemia of chronic disease is also frequently seen in the transplant population due to chronic inflammation, abnormal erythropoietin production due to allograft nephropathy after renal transplant. Drugs such as ACE inhibitors that are often used in chronic kidney disease are also associated post-kidney transplant anemia [1].

Infections

Numerous infectious etiologies that can occur during the posttransplant immunosuppressed period have been shown to cause myelosuppression including anemia. Parvovirus B19, a single-stranded DNA virus, has been known to cause red cell aplasia with anemia, reticulocytopenia, and erythroid maturation arrest [29]. Elevated parvoviral B19 titers have been found by PCR in lung transplant recipients who had anemia with other etiologies that were ruled out [30–32]. Cytomegalovirus (CMV) infection as well as its first-line therapies, ganciclovir and valganciclovir, can be associated with bone marrow suppression. Also tuberculosis, histoplasmosis, Epstein-Barr virus (EBV), human herpes virus-6, and human herpes virus-8 infections can be associated with bone marrow suppression and pancytopenia [33]. Posttransplant lymphoproliferative disorder that can be seen with immunosuppressive therapy can also be associated with pancytopenia.

Posttransplant Lymphoproliferative Disorder

Posttransplant lymphoproliferative disorder (PTLD) which includes the spectrum of infectious mononucleosis, EBV-driven polyclonal lymphocyte proliferation, and non-Hodgkin's lymphoma can be seen with solid organ transplantation [29]. PTLD is due to the impaired EBV-specific cytotoxic T-cell activity that allows for recipient B cells that have latent EBV infection to expand. PTLD can result in bone marrow infiltration and pancytopenia, as well as cause autoimmune hemolytic anemia. The severity of PTLD depends on the level of immunosuppression and usually occurs within the 1st year after transplant.

Graft-Versus-Host Disease

Graft-versus-host disease (GVHD) is rarely seen after SOT and is due to the engraftment and proliferation of allograft-associated lymphocytes in the immunosuppressed transplant recipient causing an immune-mediated response toward HLA-unmatched host tissue. Risk factors for the development of GVHD includes the volume of lymphoid tissue that is transplanted and therefore is seen more with small bowel and liver transplants, in those over 65 years of age and with HLA mismatch between donor and recipient [34, 35]. GVHD, in contrast to the development of PTLD, occurs early after SOT, on the order of weeks to months depending on the type of solid organ transplant. The clinical presentation usually includes fever, rash, diarrhea, and cytopenias, and diagnosis is made by histologic confirmation of affected tissue.

Hemophagocytic Syndrome

Hemophagocytic syndrome is a systemic inflammatory disease that can include the symptoms of fever, hepatosplenomegaly, lymphadenopathy, pancytopenia, rash, jaundice, cough, dyspnea, cachexia, and neurologic dysfunction and can often occur in response to a precipitant, such as infection [29]. This syndrome is a result of aberrant immune response of abnormal T-cell activation leading to hemophagocytosis by activated, nonmalignant macrophages that secrete numerous cytokines including interleukin (IL)-1, IL-6, IL-12, and tumor necrosis factor-alpha in the bone marrow, liver, lymph nodes, and spleen, resulting in a "cytokine storm" [29]. Acquired hemophagocytic syndrome has been documented in the renal, liver, heart, and pancreas-kidney solid organ transplants. There have been cases of hemophagocytic syndrome due to disseminated histoplasmosis in renal transplant recipients which were diagnosed by bone marrow biopsy [36].

Leukopenia in Solid Organ Transplants

Leukopenia can be defined as having a white blood cell (WBC) count of less than 3000–4000 cells/μL, with neutropenia defined as an absolute neutrophil count (ANC) <500/mm^3 by the Infectious Diseases Society of America [37]. Leukopenia is commonly seen after solid organ transplantation and can be caused by noninfectious and infectious etiologies. It can signal an underlying infection or disease process, such as posttransplant lymphoproliferative disorder (PTLD). It also increases the risk of developing further complications such as opportunistic infection and can require reduction of immunosuppression, increasing the risk of graft rejection. While there is no data to suggest a clear independent relationship between leukopenia and graft rejection, the complications of leukopenia mentioned above provide ample reason to investigate the etiology of the decreased white cell count. Solid organ transplant recipients are at risk for developing infections due to their medically induced immunodeficiency following transplant, required to prevent rejection of the transplanted organ.

Noninfectious Etiologies

Noninfectious causes of leukopenia include drugs that are often used in transplant settings. Numerous immunosuppressants can cause leukopenia, but given their use in combination, it is difficult to elucidate each agent's individual role in incidence and management. In one retrospective study of adult kidney and pancreas transplantations, the incidence of either leukopenia or neutropenia was 58%, with the first episode occurring at a mean of 91 days posttransplant [38].

One of the most common immunosuppressants, azathioprine, is a purine analog that causes an antimetabolite effect. Azathioprine may result in leukopenia in a dose-dependent manner, as well as based on the duration of treatment. The leukopenia that results from azathioprine is usually reversible upon dose-reduction or drug discontinuation. The leukopenia, often occurring late in the course of therapy, can be related to low or absent levels of S-methyl-transferase (TPMT) activity, which metabolizes 6-mercaptopurine, and can result in increased myelotoxicity [39].

Drugs that result in the depletion of T cells, such as thymoglobulin and alemtuzumab, can also lead to leukopenia in 10–14% of patients [40]. The immunosuppressant, mycophenolate mofetil (MMF), reversibly and noncompetitively inhibits the enzyme, inosine monophosphate dehydrogenase, the rate-limiting enzyme for de novo purine synthesis during lymphocyte proliferation [29]. MMF can result in leukopenia in 13–35% of patients. The myelosuppression of MMF is dose-dependent and is related to the trough level of the active metabolite, mycophenolic acid; however, brief discontinuations of the drug can lead to organ rejection, especially in the era of steroid-sparing regimens [41, 42]. The calcineurin inhibitors such as cyclosporine, tacrolimus, and sirolimus can also lead to cytopenias, including leukopenia.

Infections

Some of these agents can cause leukopenia as one of many symptoms of infection. For example, leukopenia (and often thrombocytopenia as well) have been observed as a sign/symptoms of infection with pathogens such as adenovirus, coronavirus, lymphocytic choriomeningitis virus (LCMV), parainfluenza, ehrlichiosis, and measles [43–45]. In areas endemic for the disease, dengue infection also causes both leukopenia and thrombocytopenia in patients after solid organ transplant [46]. Fungal infections such as histoplasmosis can cause disseminated organ infiltration, with the bone marrow being a common area of involvement, resulting in decreased hematopoiesis and cytopenias [33]. Parvovirus B19, much better known for its role in causing both acute and chronic anemia in solid organ transplants, is also reported to cause acute and chronic leukopenia in approximately 37.5% of solid organ as well as hematopoietic stem cell transplant recipients who develop the infection [32, 47]. An acute infection with HHV-8 can present with fever, splenomegaly, and leukopenia (as part of a pancytopenia), with bone marrow biopsy revealing hypocellularity, plasma cell infiltration, and evidence of viral infection by immunohistochemical staining [33].

A retrospective analysis of liver and kidney transplant recipients was performed to assess the relationship between leukopenia and positive hepatitis B and C serologies. The investigators found that there was no significant correlation between leukopenia and hepatitis C infection, but that the incidence of leukopenia in those with active hepatitis B infection was 7.4%. They posited that, similar to other viruses, infection with hepatitis B virus could lead to "decreased or ineffective leukocyte production in the bone marrow…shifts of cells from the circulation to the marginal blood pools…[and] also produce peripheral destruction of white blood cells due to immune and nonimmune processes" [48].

Cytomegalovirus infection is the most well-known transplant-related infection to cause cytopenias, with leukopenia found in approximately 20% of infected transplant recipients and with most of the data and research conducted in kidney transplant populations [49]. Infection with CMV has direct effects on the bone marrow, inhibiting hematopoiesis by affecting both the bone marrow stroma and the stem cells and hematopoietic precursors [33, 50]. CMV disease (acute symptomatic infection) is most often seen in the first 6 months, particularly during the first 3 months posttransplant, and presents with constitutional complaints such as fever, abdominal pain, diarrhea, and respiratory symptoms along with cytopenias [33, 49, 51]. However, in heart transplant patients, a subclinical infection during the 1st year where infected individuals are asymptomatic has also been associated with leukopenia, with the most significant reductions occurring in the neutrophil and monocyte populations and preservation of the lymphocyte counts [52].

An added challenge when addressing CMV infection and leukopenia results from the frequent finding that the treatments for the disease can result in further leukopenia (discussed in "Noninfectious Etiologies of Leukopenia" section).

Additional diagnoses to consider when assessing the etiologies of leukopenia, as well as pancytopenia, with regard to infection are hemophagocytic syndrome (HPS) which is associated with CMV, EBV, HHV-6, HHV-8, and histoplasmosis, as well as EBV-associated PTLD [29, 33].

Thrombocytopenia and Solid Organ Transplant

As in all cases of thrombocytopenia, when evaluating a finding of low platelets in a patient after SOT, it must be determined whether the primary problem is one of impaired production in the bone marrow or if it is a matter of consumption or sequestration outside the marrow. Infections and drugs are known to suppress megakaryocyte production in the marrow, such as cytomegalovirus and trimethoprim-sulfamethoxazole (TMP-SMX). Additionally, both infections and medications as well as auto- and alloimmune processes can lead to destruction of platelets despite adequate production of megakaryocytes in the bone marrow.

Infectious Etiologies of Thrombocytopenia

Solid organ transplant recipients are at risk for developing infections due to their immunosuppression, and viral infections in particular are a potential contributor to the development of thrombocytopenia following solid organ transplant. Detailed discussions of these infections are found in other chapters of this book, but their involvement in thrombocytopenia is discussed below. In addition to the viral infections that contribute to thrombocytopenia, it is important to remember that thrombocytopenia can be a sign of bacterial infection and sepsis most often in the context of disseminated intravascular coagulation (DIC). Appropriate workup to rule out infection is among the first steps in examining thrombocytopenia in a solid organ recipient.

Cytomegalovirus

The virus of particular concern in regard to platelet count in transplant patients specifically is cytomegalovirus, though thrombocytopenia due to other viruses has also been described, often among a constellation of systemic symptoms.

Cytomegalovirus can cause thrombocytopenia both by decreasing production of and through destruction of platelets. Studies have shown that CMV can impair megakaryocyte production in its early stages by infection of stromal cells, which interferes with growth factor production, as well as by directly infecting myeloid cells [50], similar to CMV-related leukopenia.

The other reported etiology of thrombocytopenia from CMV is due to intravascular destruction of platelets by CMV-associated thrombotic microangiopathy (TMA), with a clinical picture resembling that of thrombotic thrombocytopenic purpura (TTP)/atypical hemolytic uremic syndrome (aHUS), consisting of varying degrees of Coombs-negative hemolytic anemia, thrombocytopenia, acute kidney injury, fever, and neurological findings. While this etiology is more often identified as a drug-related phenomenon, particularly due to the immunosuppressants required to prevent organ rejection (see next section), there have been multiple case reports associating CMV infection as a trigger of TMA in the posttransplant setting [53, 54]. This has been noted with particular frequency in the renal transplant literature, where both de novo and recurrent forms of aHUS were associated with CMV infection in renal transplant recipients. However, particularly in the patients with "de novo" disease, it is possible that CMV may be directly driving the thrombotic microangiopathy, rather than solely by the complement-mediated events of aHUS. Mechanisms thought to be underlying CMV's endothelial effects include activation of CMV-specific cytotoxic immune responses and induction of primitive endothelial dysfunction as well as direct infection of endothelial cells by CMV [55, 56].

However, some investigators question how significant a contributor CMV actually is to thrombotic microangiopathy in transplant patients. In a review of TMA among lung transplant recipients by Hachem and colleagues, an analysis of 24 patients who were diagnosed with TMA following lung transplantation revealed that only 4 patients had evidence of CMV infection, and additionally that there were 229 incidences of CMV viremia among the 237 lung transplant patients who did not develop TMA. Additionally, in their univariate and multivariate analyses, neither CMV viremia nor serologic status was identified as a risk factor for TMA in the study population [57].

Epstein-Barr Virus

Infection with Epstein-Barr virus often results in conditions associated with pancytopenia, such as PTLD and hemophagocytic syndrome, both of which are described in greater detail in previous sections of this chapter (see "Leukopenia and Anemia" sections). EBV should be considered as a possible infectious etiology during the workup of thrombocytopenia, particularly if other systemic signs or symptoms are present.

Other Infectious Etiologies

Other infectious etiologies that have thrombocytopenia among the constellation of presenting symptoms that have been described in organ transplant recipients include coronavirus, particularly SARS, lymphocytic choriomeningitis virus (LCMV), and HHV-6, though the thrombocytopenia is unlikely to be the primary issue at presentation [58]. Parvovirus B-19 and polyoma BK virus infection have also been associated with development of aHUS [55, 59].

It is also important to note that chronic infection with hepatitis C can be an etiology for thrombocytopenia both in and outside the context of solid organ transplantation. The etiology of thrombocytopenia in the setting of hepatitis C infection can be due to hepatocellular damage including fibrosis and/or cirrhosis affecting thrombopoietin (TPO) production, hypersplenism due to portal hypertension, bone marrow suppression, immune dysfunction, and development of platelet autoantibodies [60]. Additionally, treatment for hepatitis C with interferon is known to cause thrombocytopenia.

Noninfectious Etiologies of Thrombocytopenia

There are numerous noninfectious etiologies of thrombocytopenia that have been identified in SOT patients. Many pharmacologic agents have been implicated in the development of thrombocytopenia following SOT through varying mechanisms, such as TMA, decreased megakaryocyte production, and auto- and allo-immune mechanisms of platelet destruction.

Pharmacologic Agents

Calcineurin Inhibitors

The drugs most strongly associated with decreased platelet counts due to thrombotic microangiopathy are the calcineurin inhibitors (CI) cyclosporine and tacrolimus. Calcineurin inhibitor induced TMA often occurs within weeks following SOT, and the CIs are thought to cause direct endothelial injury and platelet aggregation, although the specific mechanism has not been identified. When this is identified, numerous case studies in multiple different organ systems (lung, liver, kidney solid organ transplant) have reported that changing from one CI to another (tacrolimus to cyclosporine or vice versa) or to another class of medication such as sirolimus or mycophenolate mofetil can prevent further episodes of TMA from occurring [61–64]. However, the addition of the mTOR inhibitor sirolimus to a calcineurin inhibitor also increases the chance of developing TMA [57, 65].

Antivirals and Antibiotics

Ganciclovir and valganciclovir are used in prophylaxis and treatment of CMV. Both are known to have myelosuppressive effects, particularly on granulocytes and platelets, but generally there is rapid recovery of counts following withdrawal of the medication.

One of linezolid's most well-known adverse effects is thrombocytopenia, with the package insert reporting a rate of 3% in adults. Other studies have reported rates of grades III–IV thrombocytopenia of approximately 5.2% [66]. No mechanism has been identified for linezolid-related thrombocytopenia, though some evidence suggests that it is an immune-mediated phenomenon [67]. The medication is frequently used in the treatment of vancomycin-resistant enterococcus (VRE), which has been an infection seen in transplant patients, as well as non-transplant patients, with increasing frequency. A multicenter compassionate use trial published in 2003 showed that it was an effective drug in treating VRE, which was identified as having a mortality rate of up to 83%, with the authors reporting a 62% survival rate after treatment with linezolid. Thrombocytopenia was the main adverse effect of treatment, seen in 4.7%, but did not necessitate the cessation of therapy [68]. A second study in liver transplant patients treated with linezolid for VRE infection showed a similar treatment efficacy and again reported no cases (0/46 patients) requiring cessation of therapy due to severe thrombocytopenia, and furthermore found no correlation between treatment duration and platelet counts [69] though other articles advise caution when using linezolid for extended time periods [70]. Thus, while it may or may not require any intervention or change in treatment plan, it should be considered as part of the differential diagnosis when assessing thrombocytopenia.

Heparin

Heparin-induced thrombocytopenia is an additional drug-related event that can occur in the setting of solid organ transplant. Assessment of this as a possible etiology for thrombocytopenia follows the same algorithm as it would for any patient receiving heparin. The probability of the thrombocytopenia being related to heparin use would be based on the 4Ts whether the timing (>10 days following start of heparin use or sooner if heparin was used previously), degree of fall (>50% decrease from baseline), presence of thrombosis, and lack of alternate explanations for the thrombocytopenia suggest that heparin could be the causative agent [71]. Studies reveal that HIT is an uncommon occurrence in liver transplant recipients, and that thrombotic events and HIT antibody positivity were not well correlated [72, 73]. Case studies in renal transplant patients have reported some incidences of HIT posttransplant and graft-failure related to HIT, in part related to previous exposure to heparin in hemodialysis [74, 75].

HIT antibody immunoassays are often sent if a patient develops thrombocytopenia and has received heparin at any time during the hospitalization. However, the high sensitivity but low specificity of the test results in overdiagnosis of heparin-induced thrombocytopenia exposes patients to unnecessary risks associated with therapeutic anticoagulation. Chaturvedi and colleagues examined this phenomenon at Cleveland Clinic and found that utilizing the 4Ts algorithm to first rule out patients at low risk for HIT was a safe, reliable, and cost-effective [76]. Therefore, we recommend that immunoassays for HIT antibodies be utilized only in those patients whose 4T scores suggest intermediate or high probability of heparin-induced thrombocytopenia.

If a HIT antibody immunoassay is sent once a patient is determined to be of intermediate/high risk for HIT, it is important to understand how this test is interpreted. The immunoassay detects the presence of antiplatelet factor 4 (PF4) antibodies in patient serum and is interpreted by optical density (OD). A higher reported OD correlates to a higher titer of the antibody and is more strongly suggestive of a diagnosis of HIT. As mentioned previously, ELISAs for HIT have a high sensitivity (meaning a negative test can rule out the diagnosis) but a low specificity, underscoring the need to first confirm a high pretest probability.

Immune Etiologies

Immune Thrombocytopenic Purpura

Immune thrombocytopenic purpura (ITP) is characterized by very low platelet counts, petechiae and bruising, as well as mucosal bleeding, due to opsonization of platelets in the circulation. Occurrence of ITP following solid organ transplant has been documented particularly in the liver transplant literature, with the cases attributed to either autoimmune ITP, at times precipitated by an identified infectious etiology such as tuberculosis [77] or alloimmune etiologies. The literature reports that chronic renal disease and renal transplant in patients with ITP are noted to be very rare [78], and thus most of our knowledge of ITP as an etiology following transplant is from the liver transplant literature.

One study reported a case series of eight patients who developed ITP following orthotopic liver transplantation (OLT), with a mean time of presentation of ITP since OLT of 5.4 years [79]. These cases were all felt to be autoimmune cases, as there was no history of ITP in the donors. This case series also presented a review of the previous literature on ITP after OLT, and they noted two distinct time patterns of ITP presentation, early (within 3 months) or late (>3 months). The authors note that it has been proposed that the early-onset presentation may be due to passive transfer of antibodies from the donor to the recipient. Those that developed late-onset ITP were felt to have developed the antibodies independently of their donors [79].

Additionally, studies have reported on development of alloimmune thrombocytopenic purpura, with antibodies introduced from donors with a history of ITP [79, 80]. One case study described a case where a donor liver was obtained from a donor who had died after a cerebral hemorrhage secondary to ITP. The recipient developed ITP within 3 days of transplant and subsequently expired after developing portal vein thrombosis. The authors attributed the death to ITP in that they were unable to anticoagulate but were providing blood products that may have resulted in increased likelihood of thrombosis. It is also possible, however, that the donor was producing procoagulant antibodies, as approximately 20–25% of patients with ITP also have antiphospholipid antibodies [81, 82]. Based on this event, the authors recommended excluding cadaveric transplants from donors whose death is attributed to ITP [80].

Other Etiologies

Particularly in liver transplant patients, thrombocytopenia is often seen prior to transplant, and generally approximately 50% of transplant recipients develop worsening thrombocytopenia within 2 weeks following transplant. This acute decrease generally resolves within the 1st month after transplant, and if thrombocytopenia persists, another etiology should be sought [79, 83, 84]. Thrombocytopenia following liver transplant can also be attributed to residual portal hypertension or hypersplenism, if either of these conditions persist following transplant. However, it is important to remain vigilant to other causes particularly drug-related and infectious etiologies that could cause a drop in the platelet count.

Additionally, while case reports exist of TMA with low ADAMTS13 levels attributed to inhibitors present in the blood [85], this is not a common phenomenon, and etiologies of TMA mentioned previously (infectious and drug-related) would be much more likely.

Treatment

In most cases, treatment of the underlying etiology of the thrombocytopenia will result in improvement in platelet counts. That may require antivirals, adjustment of the immunosuppressant regimen, withdrawal of other pharmacologic agents such as heparin, or supportive care. Platelet transfusions may be necessary if bleeding events occur or if additional procedures are necessary, but we do not recommend prophylactic transfusions for maintenance of the platelet count above a specific threshold.

TPO receptor agonists, romiplostim and eltrombopag, have been used in management of chronic thrombocytopenia due to ITP and liver disease and are being studied as a supportive medication in stem cell transplantation [86]. There is a case report in the pediatric transplant literature where romiplostim was used in the peri-transplant setting, which resulted in a platelet-transfusion-free liver transplant [87]. However at this time, there is no data to support use of TPO agonists outside of their approved indications following solid organ transplant.

References

1. Vanrenterghem Y, Ponticelli C, Morales JM, et al. Prevalence and management of anemia in renal transplant recipients: a European survey. Am J Transplant. 2003;3:835–45.
2. Yorgin PD, Scandling JD, Belson A, Sanchez J, Alexander SR, Andreoni KA. Late post-transplant anemia in adult renal transplant recipients. Am J Transplant. 2002;2:429–35.
3. Kolonko A, Pinocy-Mandok J, Kocierz M, et al. Anemia and erythrocytosis after kidney transplantation: a 5 year graft function and survival analysis. Transplant Proc. 2009;8:3046–51.
4. Przybylowski P, Malyszko J, Malyszko J. Anemia is a predictor of outcome in heart transplant recipients. Transplant Proc. 2009;41:322–3231.
5. Taegtmeyer AB, Rogers P, Breen JB, Barton PJ, Banner NR, Yacoub MH. The effects of pre- and post-transplant anemia on 1-year survival after cardiac transplantation. J Heart Lung Transplant. 2008;27:394–9.
6. Yazer MH, Triulzi DJ. Immune hemolysis following ABO-mismatched stem cell or solid organ transplantation. Curr Opin Hematol. 2007;14:664–70.
7. Audet M, Panaro F, Piardi T, et al. Passenger lymphocyte syndrome and liver transplantation. Clin Dev Immunol. 2009;2008:715769.
8. Shortt J, Westall GP, Roxby D. A 'dangerous' group O donor: severe hemolysis in all recipients of organs from a donor with multiple red cell alloantibodies. Am J Transplant. 2008;8:711–4.
9. Seltsam A, Hell A, Heymann G, Salama A. Donor derived alloantibodies and passenger lymphocyte syndrome in two of four patients who received different organs from the same donor. Transfusion. 2001;41:365–70.
10. Salerno CT, Burdine J, Perry EH, Kshettry VR, Hertz MI, Bolman IIIR. Donor-derived antibodies and hemolysis after ABO-compatible but nonidentical heart-lung and lung transplantation. Transplantation. 1998;65:261–4.
11. Panaro F, DeChristopher PJ, Rondelli D. Severe hemolytic anemia due to passenger lymphocytes after living related bowel transplant. Clin Transpl. 2004;18:332–5.
12. Winkelmayer WC, Kewalramani R, Rutstein M, Gabardi S, Vonvisger T, Chandraker A. Pharmacoepidemiology of anemia in kidney transplant recipients. J Am Soc Nephrol. 2004;15:1347–52.
13. Imoagene-Oyedeji AE, Rosas SE, Doyle AM, Goral S, Bloom RD. Posttransplantation anemia at 12 months in kidney recipients treated with mycophenolate mofetil: risk factors and implications for mortality. J Am Soc Nephrol. 2006;17:3240–7.
14. Augustine JJ, Knauss TC, Schulak JA, Bodziak KA, Siegel C, Hricik DE. Comparative effects of sirolimus and mycophenolate mofetil on erythropoiesis in kidney transplant patients. Am J Transplant. 2004;4:2001–6.
15. Pratap B, Abraham G, Srinivas CN, Bhaskar S. Post-renal transplant hemolytic uremic syndrome following combination therapy with tacrolimus and everolimus. Saudi J Kidney Dis Transpl. 2007;18:609–12.
16. Go O, Naqvi A, Tan A, Amzuta I, Lenox R. The spectrum of thrombotic thrombocytopenic purpura: a clinicopathologic demonstration of tacrolimus-induced thrombotic thrombocytopenic purpura in a lung transplant patient. South Med J. 2008;101:744–7.
17. Saito M, Satoh S, Kagaya H, et al. Thrombotic microangiopathy developing in early stage after renal transplantation with a high trough level of tacrolimus. Clin Exp Nephrol. 2008;12:312–5.
18. Maheshwari A, Mishra R, Thuluvath PJ. Post-liver transplant anemia: etiology and management. Liver Transpl. 2004;10:165–73.
19. Nosari A, Marbello L, De Carlis LG, et al. Bone marrow hypoplasia complicating tacrolimus (FK506) therapy. Int J Hematol. 2004;79:130–2.
20. Engelen W, Verpooten GA, Van der Planken M, Helbert MF, Bosmans JL, De Broe ME. Four cases of red blood cell aplasia in association with the use of mycophenolate mofetil in renal transplant patients. Clin Nephrol. 2003;60:119–24.
21. Naik PM, Lyon GM 3rd, Ramirez A, et al. Dapsone-induced hemolytic anemia in lung allograft recipients. J Heart Lung Transplant. 2008;27:1198–202.
22. Ash-Bernal R, Wise R, Wright SM. Acquired methemoglobinemia: a retrospective series of 138 cases at 2 teaching hospitals. Medicine. 2004;83:265–73.
23. Dunford LM, Roy DM, Hahn TE, et al. Dapsone-induced methemoglobinemia after hematopoietic stem cell transplantation. Biol Blood Marrow Transplant. 2006;12:241–2.
24. Balbi E, Leal CR, Pacheco-Moreira LF, et al. Treatment for recurrent hepatitis C virus infection after liver transplantation. Transplant Proc. 2009;41:891–4.
25. Glanville AR, Scott AI, Morton JM, et al. Intravenous ribavirin is a safe and cost-effective treatment for respiratory syncytial virus infection after lung transplantation. J Heart Lung Transplant. 2005;24:2114–9.

26. Ar MC, Ozbalak M, Tuzuner N, et al. Severe bone marrow failure due to valganciclovir overdose after renal transplantation from cadaveric donors: four consecutive cases. Transplant Proc. 2009;41:1648–53.
27. Elimelakh M, Dayton V, Park KS, et al. Red cell aplasia and autoimmune hemolytic anemia following immunosuppression with alemtuzumab, mycophenolate, and daclizumab pancreas transplant recipients. Haematologica. 2007;92:1029–36.
28. Mix TC, Kazmi W, Khan S, et al. Anemia: a continuing problem following kidney transplantation. Am J Transplant. 2003;3:1426–33.
29. Smith EP. Hematologic disorders after solid organ transplantation. Am Soc Hematol Am Soc Hematol Educ Program. 2010;2010:281–6.
30. Park JB, Kim DJ, Woo SY, et al. Clinical implications of quantitative real time-polymerase chain reaction of parvovirus B19 in kidney transplant recipients – a prospective study. Transpl Int. 2009;22:455–62.
31. Florea AV, Ionescu DN, Melhem MF. Parvovirus B19 infection in the immunocompromised host. Arch Pathol Lab Med. 2007;131:799–804.
32. Shekar K, Hopkins PM, Kermeen FD, Dunning JJ, McNeil KD. Unexplained chronic anemia and leukopenia in lung transplant recipients secondary to parvovirus B19 infection. J Heart Lung Transplant. 2008;27:808–11.
33. Marinella MA. Hematologic abnormalities following renal transplantation. Int Urol Nephrol. 2010;42:151–64.
34. Parker A, Bowles K, Bradley JA, et al. Management of post-transplant lymphoproliferative disorder in adult solid organ transplant recipients – BCSH and BTS guidelines. Br J Haematol. 2010;149:693–705.
35. Kato T, Yazawa K, Madono K, Saito J, Hosomi M, Itoh K. Acute graft-vs-host disease in kidney transplantation: case report and review of literature. Transplant Proc. 2009;41:3949–52.
36. Lo MM, Mo JQ, Dixon BP, Czech KA. Disseminated histoplasmosis associated with hemophagocytic lymphohistiocytosis in kidney transplant recipients. Am J Transplant. 2010;10:687–91.
37. Hughes WT, Armstrong D, Bodey GP, et al. Guidelines for the use of antimicrobial agents in neutropenic patients with cancer. Clin Infect Dis. 2002;34:730–51.
38. Hartmann EL, Gatesman M, Roskopf-Somerville J, Stratta R, Farney A, Sundberg A. Management of leukopenia in kidney and pancreas transplant recipients. Clin Transpl. 2008;22:822–8.
39. Dewit O, Moreels T, Baert F, et al. Limitations of extensive TPMT genotyping in the management of azathioprine-induced myelosuppression in IBD patients. Clin Biochem. 2011;44:1062–6.
40. Danesi R, Del Tacca M. Hematologic toxicity of immunosuppressive treatment. Transplant Proc. 2004;36:703–4.
41. The Tricontinental Mycophenolate Mofetil Renal Transplantation Study Group. A blinded, randomized clinical trial of mycophenolate mofetil for the prevention of acute rejection in cadaveric renal transplantation. Transplantation. 1996;61:1029–37.
42. Knoll GA, MacDonald I, Khan A, Van Walraven C. Mycophenolate mofetil dose reduction and the risk of acute rejection after renal transplantation. J Am Soc Nephrol. 2003;14:2381–6.
43. Fischer SA. Emerging viruses in transplantation: there is more to infection after transplant then CMV and EBV. Transplantation. 2008;86:1327–39.
44. Thomas LD, Hongo I, Bloch KC, Tang YW, Dummer S. Human ehrlichiosis in transplant patients. Am J Transplant. 2007;7:1641–7.
45. Arakawa Y, Matsui A, Sasaki N, Nakayama T. Agranulocytosis and thrombocytopenic purpura following measles infection in a living-related orthotopic liver transplantation recipient. Acta Paediatr Jpn. 1997;39:226–9.
46. Wiwanitkit V. Dengue infection in kidney transplant patients: an appraisal on clinical manifestation. Iran J Kidney Dis. 2010;4:168.
47. Eid AJ, Brown RA, Patel R, Razonable RR. Parvovirus B19 infection after transplantation: a review of 98 cases. Clin Infect Dis. 2006;43:40–8.
48. Karakus S, Arin BE, Arat Z, Karakayali H, Haberal M. Impact of hepatitis serology on development of leukopenia after solid organ transplantation. Transplant Proc. 2008;40:199–201.
49. Razeghi E, Hadadi A, Mansor-Kiaei M, Molavi M, Khashayar P, Pourmand G. Clinical manifestation, laboratory findings, and the response of treatment in kidney transplant recipients with CMV infection. Transplant Proc. 2007;39:993–6.
50. Simmons P, Kaushansky K, Torok-Storb B. Mechanisms of cytomegalovirus-mediated myelosuppression: perturbation of stromal cell function versus direct infection of myeloid cells. Proc Natl Acad Sci U S A. 1990;87:1386–90.
51. Kute VB, Vanikar AV, Shah PR, et al. Post-renal transplant cytomegalovirus infection: study of risk factors. Transplant Proc. 2012;44:706–9.
52. Cooke ME, Potena L, Luikart H, Valantine HA. Peripheral blood leukocyte counts in cytomegalovirus infected heart transplant patients: impact of acute disease versus subclinical infection. Transplantation. 2006;82:1419–24.
53. Rane S, Nada R, Minz M, Sakhuja V, Joshi K. Spectrum of cytomegalovirus-induced renal pathology in renal allograft recipients. Transplant Proc. 2012;44:713–6.
54. De Keyzer K, Van Laecke S, Peeters P, Vanholder R. De novo thrombotic microangiopathy induced by cytomegalovirus infection leading to renal allograft loss. Am J Nephrol. 2010;32:491–6.
55. Zuber J, Le Quintrec M, Sberro-Soussan R, Loirat C, Fremeaux-Bacchi V, Legendre C. New insights into postrenal transplant hemolytic uremic syndrome. Nat Rev Nephrol. 2011;7:23–35.
56. Ramasubbu K, Mullick T, Koo A, et al. Thrombotic microangiopathy and cytomegalovirus in liver transplant recipients: a case-based review. Transpl Infect Dis. 2003;5:98–103.
57. Hachem RR, Yusen RD, Chakinala MM, Aloush AA, Patterson GA, Trulock EP. Thrombotic microangiopathy after lung transplantation. Transplantation. 2006;81:57–63.
58. Fischer SA. Emerging viruses in transplantation: there is more to infection after transplant than CMV and EBV. Transplantation. 2008;86:1327–39.
59. Caires RA, Marques IDB, Repizo LP, et al. De novo thrombotic microangiopathy after kidney transplantation: clinical features, treatment, and long-term patient and graft survival. Transplant Proc. 2012;44:2388–90.
60. Fouad YM. Chronic hepatitis C-associated thrombocytopenia: aetiology and management. Trop Gastroenterol. 2013;34:58–67.
61. Smith EP. Hematologic disorders after solid organ transplantation. ASH Educ Program Book. 2010;2010:281–6.
62. Devadoss CW, Vijaya VM, Mahesh E, Venkataramana SR, Girish MS. Tacrolimus associated localized thrombotic microangiopathy developing in early stage after renal transplantation. J Clin Diagn Res. 2012;6:1786–8.
63. Boyer NL, Niven A, Edelman J. Tacrolimus-associated thrombotic microangiopathy in a lung transplant recipient. BMJ Case Rep. 2013;2013:bcr2012007351.
64. Nwaba A, MacQuillan G, Adams LA, et al. Tacrolimus-induced thrombotic microangiopathy in orthotopic liver transplant patients: case series of four patients. Intern Med J. 2013;43:328–33.
65. Fortin MC, Raymond MA, Madore F, et al. Increased risk of thrombotic microangiopathy in patients receiving a cyclosporin-sirolimus combination. Am J Transplant. 2004;4:946–52.
66. Minson Q, Gentry CA. Analysis of linezolid-associated hematologic toxicities in a large veterans affairs medical center. Pharmacotherapy. 2010;30:895–903.
67. Bernstein WB, Trotta RF, Rector JT, Tjaden JA, Barile AJ. Mechanisms for linezolid-induced anemia and thrombocytopenia. Ann Pharmacother. 2003;37:517–20.

68. El-Khoury J, Fishman JA. Linezolid in the treatment of vancomycin-resistant enterococcus faecium in solid organ transplant recipients: report of a multicenter compassionate-use trial. Transpl Infect Dis. 2003;5:121–5.
69. Radunz S, Juntermanns B, Kaiser GM, et al. Efficacy and safety of linezolid in liver transplant patients. Transpl Infect Dis. 2011;13:353–8.
70. Attassi K, Hershberger E, Alam R, Zervos MJ. Thrombocytopenia associated with linezolid therapy. Clin Infect Dis. 2002;34:695–8.
71. Lo GK, Juhl D, Warkentin TE, Sigouin CS, Eichler P, Greinacher A. Evaluation of pretest clinical score (4 T's) for the diagnosis of heparin-induced thrombocytopenia in two clinical settings. J Thromb Haemost. 2006;4:7.
72. Bachmann R, Bachmann J, Lange J, Nadalin S, Konigsrainer A, Ladurner R. Incidence of heparin-induced thrombocytopenia type II and postoperative recovery of platelet count in liver graft recipients: a retrospective cohort analysis. J Surg Res. 2014;186:429–35.
73. Kaneko J, Sugawara Y, Tamura S, Togashi J, Matsui Y, Makuuchi M. Heparin-induced thrombocytopenia after liver transplantation. Transplant Proc. 2008;40:1518–21.
74. Dracopoulos S, Vougas V, Kassimatis TI, Theodoridis T, Ali ME, Apostolou T. Heparin-induced thrombocytopenia type II: a serious hazard in preemptive renal transplantation: a case report. Transplant Proc. 2007;39:3481–4.
75. Muzaffar M, Li X, Ratnam S. Successful preemptive renal retransplantation in a patient with previous acute graft loss secondary to HIT type II: a case report and review of literature. Int Urol Nephrol. 2012;44:991–4.
76. Chaturvedi S, Kohli R, McCrae K. Over-testing for heparin induced thrombocytopenia in hospitalized patients. J Thromb Thrombolysis. 2015;40(1):12–6.
77. Lugao Rdos S, Motta MP, de Azevedo MF, et al. Immune thrombocytopenic purpura induced by intestinal tuberculosis in a liver transplant recipient. World J Gastroenterol. 2014;20:8304–8.
78. Einollahi B. Renal transplantation and idiopathic thrombocytopenic purpura: two case reports. Transplant Proc. 2009;41:2923.
79. Taylor RM, Bockenstedt P, Su GL, Marrero JA, Pellitier SM, Fontana RJ. Immune thrombocytopenic Purpura following liver transplantation: a case series and review of the literature. Liver Tranplant. 2006;12:11.
80. Pereboom IT, de Boer MT, Haagsma EB, van der Heide F, Porcelijn L, Lisman T, Porte RJ. Transmission of idiopathic thrombocytopenic purpura during orthotopic liver transplantation. Transplant Int. 2010;23:3.
81. Kim KJ, Baek IW, Yoon CH, Kim WU, Cho CS. Thrombotic risk in patients with immune thrombocytopenia and its association with antiphospholipid antibodies. Br J Haematol. 2013;161: 706–14.
82. Yang YJ, Yun GW, Song IC, et al. Clinical implications of elevated antiphospholipid antibodies in adult patients with primary immune thrombocytopenia. Korean J Intern Med. 2011;26:449–54.
83. Chatzipetrou MA, Tsaroucha AK, Weppler D, et al. Thrombocytopenia after liver transplantation. Transplantation. 1999;67:702–6.
84. Plevak DJ, Halma GA, Forstrom LA, et al. Thrombocytopenia after liver transplantation. Transplant Proc. 1988;20:630–3.
85. Pham PT, Danovitch GM, Wilkinson AH, et al. Inhibitors of ADAMTS13: a potential factor in the cause of thrombotic microangiopathy in a renal allograft recipient. Transplantation. 2002;74:1077–80.
86. Liesveld JL, Phillips GL 2nd, Becker M, et al. A phase 1 trial of eltrombopag in patients undergoing stem cell transplantation after total body irradiation. Biol Blood Marrow Transplant. 2013;19:1745–52.
87. Minowa K, Arai K, Kasahara M, et al. Romiplostim treatment allows for platelet transfusion-free liver transplantation in pediatric thrombocytopenic patient with primary sclerosing cholangitis. Pediatr Transplant. 2014;18:E212–5.

Infections in Allogeneic Stem Cell Transplantation

11

Marcus R. Pereira, Stephanie M. Pouch, and Brian Scully

Introduction

Allogeneic hematopoietic stem cell transplantation (allo-HSCT) has become a widely used modality of therapy for a variety of malignant and nonmalignant diseases. While many advances have been made in the field, infection remains one of the most severe and frequently encountered complications of HSCT. In this chapter we review the defects in host defenses and important risk factors predisposing allo-HSCT recipients to infection, the major categories of infection and their time courses following transplantation, and preventive strategies.

Risk Factors for Infection Following Allo-HSCT

The severity of defects in host defenses and the subsequent risk of infection are influenced by a complex interaction between several factors. Particularly salient are (1) the underlying illness of the patient, (2) the conditioning regimen, (3) the graft and the closeness of the match, (4) the type of transplant, and (5) the presence of graft-versus-host disease (GVHD). Immediate local and remote epidemiological factors are also important. The timing of impaired host defenses and infectious risk in allo-HSCT recipients are outlined in Fig. 11.1.

M. R. Pereira (✉) · B. Scully
Department of Medicine – Infectious Diseases, Columbia University Medical Center, New York, NY, USA
e-mail: mp2323@cumc.columbia.edu; bs4@cumc.columbia.edu

S. M. Pouch
Division of Infectious Diseases, Emory University, Atlanta, GA, USA
e-mail: spouch@emory.edu

Underlying Host Disease

Infection risk is very much impacted by the disease for which the patient is being transplanted and also by the presence of preceding infections. Acute leukemia, for example, predisposes to neutropenia and other defects of innate immunity. Profound neutropenia (<500 cells/mm^3) of greater than 10-day duration is considered a strong risk factor for bacterial and invasive fungal infection [1]. In addition to neutropenia, other factors that increase risk for invasive aspergillosis include advanced or refractory acute myelogenous leukemia, high-risk myelodysplastic syndrome, chronic neutropenia prior to chemotherapy, iron overload secondary to repeated peripheral blood transfusions, and prior fungal infection [2–6]. Further, antileukemic agents have been shown to diminish antibody response to primary antigens, thereby increasing susceptibility to bacterial pathogens even in the absence of neutropenia [7]. Other underlying diseases such as primary immunodeficiency, for example, may predispose to progression or reactivation of antecedent infections, and individuals with myelodysplastic syndrome who are neutropenic at the time of transplant are at an increased risk of infection and mortality. In addition to innate immune defects, increasing age, waning cellular immunity, organ dysfunction, fragile skin, and prior antibiotic exposure may all contribute to the progression of preexisting infection, including aspergillosis, as well as to the risk for new infections during the posttransplant period [8–11].

The presence of infection immediately preceding allo-HSCT also impacts infectious risk during the posttransplant period. In individuals scheduled to undergo allo-HSCT, active infections should be treated prior to transplantation whenever possible. The timing of allo-HSCT following the initiation of antibiotics for active infection should be made on a case by case basis by an experienced practitioner.

A. Safdar (ed.), *Principles and Practice of Transplant Infectious Diseases*, https://doi.org/10.1007/978-1-4939-9034-4_11

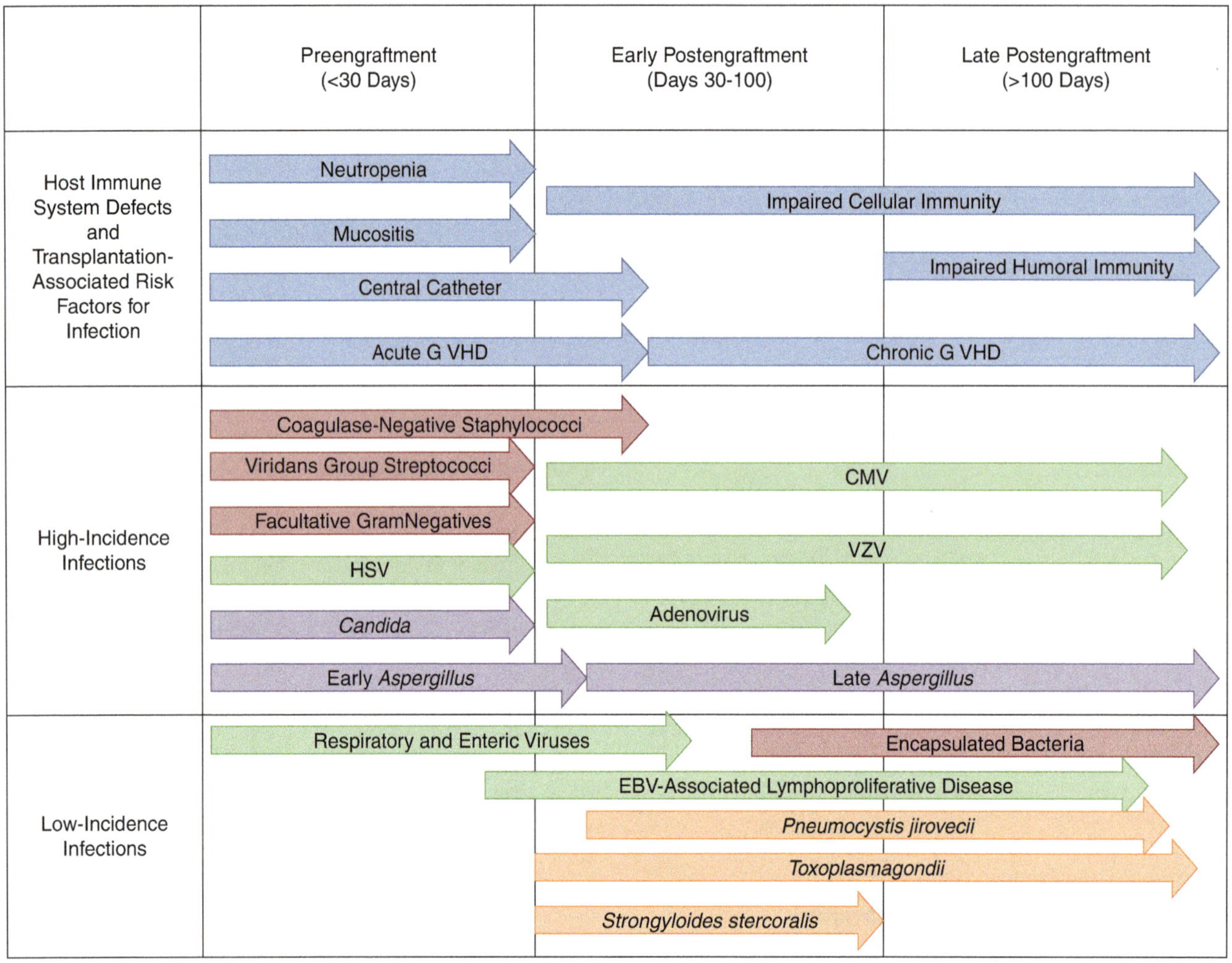

Fig. 11.1 Timeline of host immune defects and infections in Allo-HSCT recipients. Predictable opportunistic infections encountered following allo-HSCT. Immune defects and transplant-associated risk factors are shaded in blue, bacterial infections in pink, viral infections in green, fungal infections in purple, and parasitic infections in orange

The Conditioning Regimen

Prior to transplantation, the prospective recipient must be conditioned so as to allow engraftment of the transplant. The goals of conditioning are twofold: (1) to suppress the recipient's immune system, particularly the T-cell arm, in order to prevent rejection of the graft, and (2) to eliminate the tumor. Many regimens are myeloablative, employing total body irradiation and cytotoxic chemotherapy, with resultant profound and prolonged neutropenia, mucositis, and potential organ toxicities. Recipients of such conditioning are highly susceptible to early infection and sepsis. Less intense regimens increasingly used in some of the more vulnerable older patients may result in minimal neutropenia and mucositis and a correspondingly lower risk of infection [12]. However, recipients of reduced-intensity conditioning regimens may experience prolonged neutropenia should engraftment fail.

The Graft

The closeness of the human leukocyte antigen (HLA) match dictates the likelihood and severity of GVHD as well as the intensity of the immunosuppressive regimen. The various degrees of match include the following: the donor may be an HLA-matched sibling or twin, HLA-matched but unrelated, haploidentical such that donor and recipient share one complete haplotype, or partially matched. The latter two categories often necessitate more intense immunosuppressive regimens to prevent GVHD.

The source of the stem cells also impacts the risk of infection. Bone marrow transplant recipients have more prolonged periods of neutropenia and a higher risk for early infection, but lower risk of GVHD than peripheral stem cells mobilized by granulocyte colony-stimulating factor [13, 14]. Cord blood cells, in contrast, are typically obtained from unrelated donors and confer a much lower stem cell dose than in the other transplants. Cord blood stem cell transplant recipients have delayed engraftment, such that neutropenia may extend for 6 weeks or longer and T-cell immune dysfunction may persist for months to years [15].

Graft-Versus-Host Disease

GVHD occurs when donor T-cells attack the recipient's tissues as a consequence of either T-cell ablation of the graft prior to transplant or by the administration of immunosuppressive drugs after transplantation. When unmanipulated bone marrow or peripheral stem cells are used, $24–300 \times 10^6$/kg CD3 cells are administered. Ex vivo pretreatment of the graft may produce up to a 3-log reduction in cells transplanted and decrease the potential risk and severity of GVHD. However, there is a resultant prolonged T-cell immunodeficiency, and the patient must then walk an immunological-infection tightrope for many months. If an untreated graft is transplanted, then any one of a variety of immunosuppressive regimens may be given. Examples are sirolimus and a calcineurin inhibitor, such as tacrolimus. It appears that these regimens pose a lower infection risk than pretransplant T-cell ablation [16]. Sirolimus therapy has also been associated with a reduced risk of cytomegalovirus (CMV) infection [17, 18].

GVHD is classified as acute when the onset is prior to posttransplant day 100 and chronic when the onset is after day 100. Acute disease may persist into the chronic period, in which case it is termed progressive. While GVHD may respond to treatment and go into remission, it may also reactivate at a later date.

Acute disease, characterized by secretory diarrhea, hepatitis, and skin rash, is categorized according to severity with grades 3 and 4 posing an increased risk of mortality. Corticosteroids are the mainstay of therapy. The intense immunosuppression associated with the condition itself and enhanced by its treatment, combined with disrupted barrier defenses, especially in the intestine, place patients at great risk of infection. CMV infection is common as are other viral, bacterial, and fungal infections such as aspergillosis [19].

In chronic GVHD, humoral defects and functional hyposplenism markedly suppress cellular immunity. Severe pneumococcal, disseminated fungal, and CMV infections are frequently seen in this context [20, 21]. Infections are even more problematic when steroid-refractory disease necessitates the use of potent immunosuppressive regimens such as cyclophosphamide, alemtuzumab, or anti-thymocyte globulin. In this situation, human herpesvirus-6 (HHV6), adenovirus, disseminated fungal and nocardial infections, as well as posttransplant lymphoproliferative disease (PTLD) may occur [22].

Timing of Opportunistic Infections in Allo-HSCT Recipients

Three periods of immunodeficiency occur following hematopoietic stem cell transplantation: pre-engraftment (days 0–30), early post-engraftment (days 30–100), and late post-engraftment (until day 100). The immune suppression that takes place during each of the periods conveys a particular risk for infection and drives the use of standard prophylaxis following transplantation (Figs. 11.1) [23, 24].

Pre-engraftment

The pre-engraftment period is associated with three major risk factors for infection: (1) prolonged neutropenia, (2) disruption of the mucosal barrier related to preparative chemotherapeutic regimens, and (3) the presence and frequent utilization of central venous access [24, 25]. The combined effect of neutropenia and mucositis contributes to high risk of reactivation of HSV in seropositive patients, prompting standard use of acyclovir during this period [26, 27]. These factors also predispose to candidemia and early-onset aspergillosis [24]. While prophylactic antifungals are used in the pre-engraftment period, fluconazole prophylaxis has been linked to an increased risk of non-albicans candidal infections, particularly due to *C. glabrata* and *C. krusei* [28–30]. Voriconazole prophylaxis has also been associated with an increased risk of zygomycosis in this setting [31–34]. Additionally, mechanical disruption of the skin and the use of prophylactic antibiotics targeted toward gut flora increase the risk for bloodstream infections with Gram-positive flora, particularly viridians group streptococci and coagulase-negative staphylococci [25, 35].

Early Post-engraftment

The early post-engraftment period extends from the time of neutrophil recovery (approximately day 30 posttransplantation) until day 100 and is notable for B- and T-lymphocyte dysfunction. In the setting of allo-HSCT recipients, the impact of this immunodeficiency is further mediated by GVHD and CMV infection, as well as their treatments. Such cell-mediated immune dysfunction contributes to increased risk for viral infections, including CMV, adenovirus, varicella zoster virus (VZV), and Epstein-Barr virus (EBV)-related PTLD, as well as late-onset aspergillosis and *Pneumocystis jirovecii* [24].

Late Post-engraftment

The late post-engraftment period extends from day 100 until normal immune function is regained. While immune function generally returns within 18–36 months of transplant, the duration of the late post-engraftment period may be extended in allo-HSCT recipients owing to chronic GVHD and its management. During this time, ongoing humeral and cell-mediated immune dysfunction contributes to the risk for infections with VZV, CMV, late-onset aspergillosis, and infections with encapsulated bacteria [24, 36, 37].

Bacterial Infections

The microbiology of bacterial infections in allo-HSCT patients has evolved over time. In the past decade or so, it has been greatly influenced by the widespread use of fluoroquinolone prophylaxis, the increased prevalence of *Clostridium difficile* infection, and the evolution of conditioning regimens. Once transplanted, patients are at increased risk for bacterial infections for the remainder of their lifetime.

Infection During the Pre-engraftment Period

During the pre-engraftment period, bacteremia occurs in up to 20% of patients [38]. Table 11.1 lists some common infecting pathogens, their particular risks, and their clinical manifestations. The main sources for bacteremia are the oral or gastrointestinal mucositis, the respiratory tract, and the presence of central venous catheters. Infecting organisms are commonly Gram-positive cocci such as *Streptococcus viridans* and enterococci or a variety of fermenting and non-fermenting Gram-negative rods. Enterococci are increasingly resistant to vancomycin, and these strains have been associated with a worse prognosis than vancomycin-sensitive strains [39]. Some recent studies also report an increase in infections due to multidrug resistant (MDR) Gram-negative rods such as *Pseudomonas aeruginosa and* carbapenemase-producing *Klebsiella pneumoniae* [40–43]. The isolation of such resistant bacteria has been associated with the use of fluoroquinolone prophylaxis and third-generation cephalosporins in several reports. These infections carry a high mortality and often relapse.

Gastrointestinal infections are prominent during this period. Necrotizing enterocolitis and typhlitis may occur in any severely neutropenic patient and can serve as a source of bacteremia and sepsis. *Clostridium difficile* colitis is very common, occurring in about 12% of allogeneic transplant patients versus 9% of autologous patients during the pre-engraftment period [44–46]. Extensive antibiotic exposures, mucosal damage from intense chemotherapy, and multiple prior hospitalizations are all contributory [47]. *Clostridium difficile* has been linked to levofloxacin, which is frequently given for bacterial prophylaxis in these patients [48]. Hypervirulent strains of *Clostridium difficile*, including the epidemic North American pulse-field gel electrophoresis type 1 (NAP1) and ribotype 027/toxinotype III strains, have specifically been associated with moxifloxacin and other members of the fluoroquinolone class [49, 50]. An association between *Clostridium difficile* colitis and subsequent GVHD has also been reported [46]. The colitis may be severe, often relapses, and may also serve as a source for secondary bloodstream infections.

Table 11.1 Bacterial infections following allo-HSCT

Bacterial pathogens	Predisposing risks	Clinical manifestations
Streptococcus viridans	Neutropenia, oral mucositis	Bacteremia
Streptococcus pneumoniae	Graft-versus-host disease (GVHD), lack of immunization	Pneumonia, meningitis, sepsis
Enterococcus species	Cephalosporin use, *C. difficile* infection	Bacteremia
Staphylococcus aureus	Central venous lines (CVL), colonization	Bacteremia, pneumonia, soft tissue infection
Coagulase-negative staphylococcus	CVL	Bacteremia
Escherichia coli	Neutropenia, mucositis	Bacteremia, pneumonia
Klebsiella pneumoniae	Neutropenia, mucositis	Bacteremia, pneumonia
Pseudomonas aeruginosa	Neutropenia, mucositis	Bacteremia, pneumonia, ecthyma
Stenotrophomonas maltophilia	CVL, prior broad-spectrum antibiotic exposure	Bacteremia
Acinetobacter species	CVL, prior broad-spectrum antibiotic exposure	Bacteremia, pneumonia
Achromobacter species	CVL, prior broad-spectrum antibiotic exposure	Bacteremia
Anaerobic bacteria (e.g., *Clostridium septicum*, *Bacteroides* species)	Neutropenia, mucositis	Bacteremia, necrotizing enterocolitis, typhlitis
Clostridium difficile	Antibiotic exposure, GVHD, local epidemiology, previous *C. difficile* infection	Colitis, megacolon, secondary bacteremia

The risk of infection and bacteremia during this neutropenic pre-engraftment period is reduced by the use of prophylactic antibiotics. In general fluoroquinolones, usually levofloxacin, are the preferred agents [51]. Prophylaxis should start with the stem cell infusion and should continue until the resolution of the neutropenia or the initiation of antibiotic therapy for neutropenic fever. Several meta-analyses have demonstrated decreased infection-associated morbidity, mortality, as well as cost benefit, with the use of prophylactic antibacterials [52–54]. These agents do, however, increase the risk for selection of resistant bacteria and *Clostridium difficile*-associated disease [55].

Infection During the Early Post-engraftment Period

During the early period after engraftment, the risk of bacterial infections and bacteremia is reduced but ongoing. Risk is increased by general debility, by the presence of renal or hepatic dysfunction, and by the presence of GVHD. Central venous lines are often the source. Most of the patients by this time will have received antibiotic courses making them more likely to be infected with resistant pathogens. Staphylococci, enterococci (often vancomycin resistant), and non-fermenting Gram-negatives such as *Stenotrophomonas maltophilia* and *Acinetobacter* are frequent pathogens [38]. By virtue of their T-cell immunosuppression, these patients are also particularly susceptible to *Listeria* and *Legionella* if exposed [56, 57].

Infection During the Late Post-engraftment Period

During the late period following engraftment, the main predisposing factor for infection is the presence of GVHD. Many patients have B-cell dysfunction and are functionally asplenic [58, 59]. They are thus vulnerable to serious infections with encapsulated bacteria, most notably *Streptococcus pneumoniae,* with pneumonia as the usual source [36, 60, 61]. Some patients are hypogammaglobulinemic, further increasing their risk. Less common are infections due to mycobacteria and *Nocardia.* Case reports suggest a global incidence of nontuberculous mycobacterial infections in allo-HSCT recipients ranging from 0.4% to 4.9% [37, 62–66]. Tuberculosis in this patient population, however, ranges from 0.0014% to 3% in the United States to as high as 8.5% in Taiwan [67–70]. Systemic nocardiosis is rare, and one center reported a cumulative incidence of 1.75%; cases were all observed in patients with extensive chronic GVHD [71].

Preventive strategies include vaccination with the heptavalent conjugate pneumococcal vaccine at 3–6 months post-engraftment for all patients [51]. Immunogenicity of this vaccine, however, appears to be related to immune reconstitution, particularly in allo-HSCT recipients aged 50 and over. In this population, improved vaccine response has been associated with CD4 >200 cells/μL, IgG >500 mg/dL, and phytohemagglutinin within 60% of the lower limit of normal [72]. Patients with active GVHD should also receive antibiotic prophylaxis aimed at pneumococcus. Penicillin V usually suffices, but trimethoprim/sulfamethoxazole or doxycycline may also be considered depending on local resistance patterns. For patients who are severely hypogammaglobulinemic (<400 mg IgG), regular infusions of intravenous immunoglobulin (IVIG) can be considered. Meticulous care of central venous catheters is mandatory [51, 73].

Clostridium Difficile

Clostridium difficile can occur at any time, though the risk is greatest during periods of hospitalization. Risk is increased in proportion to antibiotic exposure, especially perhaps to fluoroquinolones, by the presence of GVHD and of course by nosocomial risks, e.g., during an outbreak. Relapses are common after treatment.

Viral Infections

Viral pathogens are a significant source of morbidity and mortality after allo-HSCT [74]. Allo-HSCT recipients are affected by a wide range of viruses, either through primary infection, donor-derived infection, or reactivation of latent virus.

Cytomegalovirus

CMV continues to be one of the most important pathogens in this group. It is estimated that about 50% of the population in the United States is latently infected with CMV [75]. In other places in the world, including developing nations, the prevalence is even higher [76, 77].

Prior to widespread use of anti-CMV prophylaxis, approximately 80% of seropositive allo-HSCT recipients developed CMV reactivation, usually in the first 3 months after transplantation [78]. Despite prophylaxis with either ganciclovir or valganciclovir, the incidence of CMV reactivation ranges between 20% and 50%, with episodes increasingly occurring after prophylaxis is finished (late CMV) [79–83]. Approximately 6–18% of allo-HSCT recipients with CMV reactivation develop disease [79, 80, 83]. Clinical manifestations of CMV disease are variable and include interstitial pneumonia, enteritis, hepatitis, retinitis, encephalitis, and a CMV syndrome that includes cytopenia and fevers. CMV-related mortality is on average 40–50%, but can be as high as 86% in cases of severe pneumonia [83]. In addition to its direct end-organ effects, CMV disease is also associated with increased bacterial, fungal, and other viral infections [84].

The classic and most important risk factor for CMV reactivation is the serostatus of the recipient and donor, with a CMV-infected (seropositive) patient receiving a graft from a CMV-naïve (seronegative) donor considered the highest risk.

Additional risk factors include total body radiation in the conditioning phase, development of acute and chronic GVHD, T-cell-depleting therapies, steroids at doses greater than 1 mg/kg per day, and the use of mismatched or unrelated donors [78, 79].

Diagnosis of CMV disease remains clinically challenging given the varied and nonspecific presentations. Although PCR analysis of CMV DNA in the serum has become the mainstay of diagnosis, no absolute cutoff in viremia exists for differentiation between infection and disease. The presence of viremia does not automatically indicate disease although studies have shown that the likelihood of disease is high when levels above 10,000 copies/mL are found [85]. Conversely, disease does not always correlate with viremia, especially in cases of gastrointestinal involvement. With the introduction of international units, better studies to correlate disease and viremia will be possible in the future.

Intravenous ganciclovir is first-line therapy for CMV disease in allo-HSCT recipients. In non-severe cases, including asymptomatic viremia, oral valganciclovir can be used. Due to toxicities, foscarnet and cidofovir are considered second-line drugs and reserved for treatment failure due to GCV resistance or in situations where GCV is not tolerated. It is recommended that continuing treatment for 14–21 days after CMV DNA is no longer detectable in serum, followed by 1–3 months of maintenance therapy [86]. CMV immunoglobulins have been studied and in general are reserved for severe cases, especially pneumonia, or lack of response to antiviral therapy [87]. Recent studies have suggested that CMV-specific T-cell administration can be effective in the prophylaxis and treatment of CMV [88].

Although risk-stratified prophylaxis with oral valganciclovir can be effective, problems with toxicity, especially bone marrow suppression, preclude it from being a standard approach. An alternative approach involves frequent serum CMV PCR monitoring and initiation of treatment if viremia is detected. This preemptive approach is usually more logistically difficult and leads to higher rates of CMV reactivation [51]. An elusive goal for many decades, the search for a vaccine has recently shown promising results around glycoprotein B and phosphoprotein 65 epitopes [89, 90].

Epstein-Barr Virus (EBV)

In the United States and worldwide, it is estimated that almost 95% of adults demonstrate past infection with EBV. The spectrum of EBV-related diseases includes asymptomatic viremia, a viral syndrome with fevers and neutropenia, oral hairy leukoplakia, and rarely meningoencephalitis. More importantly, EBV is also associated with 50–70% of cases of PTLD in allo-HSCT recipients [91].

PTLD usually occurs in the first year after transplant and arises when EBV-specific T-lymphocytes are depleted, allowing for unchecked proliferation of donor-derived monoclonal or polyclonal B cells [92]. The spectrum of PTLD includes extranodal lymphocyte infiltration to high-grade B-cell lymphoma and varies from an indolent to fulminant presentation. Although the overall incidence of EBV-related PTLD in this population is approximately 1% (up to 2.8% in children), mortality can be as high as 50–90% [93]. Risk factors include age >50; recipients of mismatched, matched unrelated, or T-cell-depleted transplants; acute and chronic GVHD; and use of T-cell-depleting agents such as thymoglobulin and alemtuzumab [92].

Treatment options range from reduced immunosuppression to chemotherapeutic agents such as rituximab or CHOP. Antiviral agents have a limited role in the treatment or prevention of EBV-PTLD. Given that persistent or increasing EBV viremia usually precedes PTLD, preemptive treatment with rituximab may reduce the risk of progression to PTLD [94, 95].

Herpes Simplex Virus (HSV)

More than 50% of US adults are latently infected with HSV-1 [96]. In allo-HSCT recipients who do not received antiviral prophylaxis, the rate of reactivation can be as high as 80% and often occurs earlier, 2–3 weeks post-engraftment, than other herpesviruses [97, 98]. Clinical manifestations most commonly include oral-labial lesions and esophagitis, but can be varied and cause bone marrow suppression, keratitis, pneumonia, hepatitis, as well as meningoencephalitis [99–104]. HSV-2, on the other hand, is less frequent and is usually involved with perineal lesions only. Recurrent episodes of either HSV-1 or 2 infections may warrant suppressive therapy [51].

Varicella Zoster Virus (VZV)

Similar to HSV, reactivation is the most common cause of VZV-related disease after allo-HSCT, occurring in about 16% of patients in the first year after transplant [105]. Since anti-HSV or CMV prophylaxis is effective against VZV, reactivation usually occurs after prophylaxis has stopped, although breakthrough can also occur [105, 106]. GVHD is a major risk factor for VZV reactivation [107]. Clinical manifestations include either classic or multi-dermatomal shingles with lesions usually taking longer to heal that in immunocompetent patients. Disseminated VZV is a rare but severe occurrence, which can involve the lungs, liver, and CNS [108].

Human Herpesvirus (HHV) 6, 7, and 8

HHV-6 reactivation is common early post allo-HSCT, ranging from 36% to 47% of patients in the first month [109, 110]. The vast majority of cases range from asymptomatic viremia to fevers and transient marrow suppression, but patients can infrequently develop severe disease, including encephalitis, hepatitis, and pneumonitis. Posttransplant acute limbic encephalitis [111] is a form of CNS disease in allo-HSCT recipients that is related to HHV-6 reactivation [112]. In addition to its direct effects, HHV-6 viremia has been found to increase delayed engraftment and GVHD as well as predispose patients to CMV and EBV reactivation [109]. Risk factors for HHV-6 reactivation include cord blood transplantation as well HLA mismatch [113]. Ganciclovir has activity against HHV-6 and is used for treatment [114]. Screening and preventative measures have not been developed.

HHV-7 viremia is also a common occurrence, but its association with post-HSCT disease is not well documented at this time. Reports of CNS disease associated with this virus have been reported [115].

HHV-8 can be transmitted to seronegative recipients, but clinical manifestations of viremia are also not well documented at this time, although it may possibly be related to fever, rash, mild hepatitis, and bone marrow aplasia. Unlike solid organ transplantation, cases of Kaposi's sarcoma are very rare [116].

Adenovirus (ADV)

Besides reactivation of latent infection, allo-HSCT recipients are susceptible to transmission of ADV via the stem cell graft as well as primary acquisition of any of the other >50 serotypes. About 12% of allo-HSCT recipients are affected by ADV reactivation, most of which are children under 5 years of age [117]. Reactivation usually occurs between 30 and 90 days posttransplant. Besides young age, risk factors for reactivation include severe GVHD, high-dose steroids, as well as use of unrelated cord blood [74]. In recipients with ADV viremia, approximately 40–50% develop disease, which ranges from a viral syndrome (fever, elevated liver enzymes, and pancytopenia) to pneumonitis, nephropathy, hemorrhagic cystitis, colitis, myocarditis, and CNS disease. Mortality in the setting of ADV disease is estimated to be around 22% [117].

Diagnosis is usually a combination of high clinical suspicion, serum ADV quantitative PCR, and histology. Treatment is not well defined but usually consists of reduced immunosuppression and cidofovir, which has a high incidence of nephrotoxicity [118]. Preventative measures are also not well defined.

Respiratory Viruses

With continuously improving detection techniques, respiratory viral pathogens have been increasingly recognized as significant sources of morbidity and mortality among recipients of allo-HSCT. These include, among others, influenza [119], parainfluenza [120], RSV [121], human metapneumovirus [122], as well as multiple strains of rhinoviruses, coronaviruses, and bocaviruses [123, 124]. Both community and nosocomial outbreaks are responsible for majority of infections, and rates of respiratory viral infections among allo-HSCT recipients undergo seasonal variation, much like the general population [125]. Estimates vary, but studies have shown that influenza (both A and B), parainfluenza, and RSV are the most common causes of viral respiratory infections [125]. Risk factors include GVHD, lymphopenia, and the presence of children younger than 12 years of age at home. Diagnosis involves clinical suspicion and RT-PCR. Mortality is variable and is usually associated with complications such as respiratory failure and bacterial or fungal superinfection. Preventative measures include vaccination, hand washing, and isolation measures in the setting of outbreaks. Besides anti-influenza drugs, antiviral therapy for most other respiratory viruses remains largely unproven [119, 120].

Hepatitis B Virus

The main risk with hepatitis B virus is reactivation of previously resolved infection, which can occur in up to 20% of cases if prophylaxis is not instituted [126]. Among those who reactivate, liver failure can be a rare complication. It is recommended that both recipients and donors be checked for hepatitis B serologies prior to HSCT and appropriate therapeutic or prophylactic measures taken [127].

Polyoma Viruses (BK and JC)

Although more commonly affecting renal transplant recipients, BK virus reactivation has also been described to cause both hemorrhagic cystitis and nephropathy in allo-HSCT recipients [128–131]. JCV-related progressive multifocal leukoencephalopathy (PML) is a rare but well-described complication in allo-HSCT recipients with dismal prognosis [132].

Fungal Infections

Invasive fungal infections (IFIs) are a major cause of morbidity and mortality among HSCT recipients. Individuals undergoing allo-HSCT are at higher risk for developing IFIs compared to recipients of autologous grafts, largely owing to delayed engraftment and GVHD. The epidemiology of IFIs in HSCT recipients remains dynamic. Since the 1990s, there has been a decrease in the incidence of invasive candidiasis among HSCT recipients due to the more widespread use of fluconazole prophylaxis; however, IFIs due to *Aspergillus* and other filamentous molds remain a significant concern.

Candida

Candida species commonly inhabit the skin and mucosa of the gastrointestinal tract, and disruption of the integrity of either mucosal barrier can lead to invasive candidiasis. In the setting of allo-HSCT, invasive candidiasis typically results from mucositis of the gastrointestinal tract incurred during conditioning. Additional risk factors for invasive candidiasis include HLA mismatch, recipient age, prolonged neutropenia, GVHD, gastrointestinal tract colonization, and CMV disease [133, 134].

In the early 1990s, two large trials demonstrated a significant decrease in candidiasis with the use of fluconazole prophylaxis, and its administration through 75 days posttransplant was later shown to significantly reduce mortality among allo-HSCT recipients [135–137]. This prompted the widespread use of fluconazole prophylaxis in the early posttransplant period. More recent data from the Prospective Antifungal Therapy (PATH) Alliance registry, however, reported a 28% and 23% incidence of invasive candidiasis in allo-HSCT recipients from matched-related and matched-unrelated donors, respectively [138]. While *Candida albicans* accounted for over half of all episodes of invasive candidiasis in HSCT recipients in the 1980s, invasive candidiasis caused by azole-resistant *Candida* species such as *C. glabrata* and *C. krusei* has increased since the 1990s, which may reflect the routine use of fluconazole prophylaxis [28–30, 137, 138].

Invasive candidiasis in allo-HSCT recipients most commonly presents as fungemia or hepatosplenic candidiasis. Candidemia occurs in approximately 3% of HSCT recipients and may be accompanied by sepsis, a discreet palpable vasculitic rash, and/or end-organ involvement including but not limited to meningitis, endophthalmitis, and endocarditis [139]. In contrast, hepatosplenic candidiasis, or chronic disseminated candidiasis, results from invasion of *Candida* species into the portal vasculature with subsequent seeding of the liver and/or spleen during periods of neutropenia. While the exact incidence of hepatosplenic candidiasis remains unknown, one autopsy study identified hepatic candidal infection in 9% of HSCT recipients [140]. Patients typically present with fever and an elevated alkaline phosphatase level following neutrophil recovery. Blood cultures tend to be negative in this setting, but computed tomography of the abdomen demonstrates multiple lesions in the liver and spleen; such lesions decrease in size with recurrent neutropenia, indicating that hepatosplenic candidiasis results from a systemic inflammatory response. Biopsy is required for definitive diagnosis, especially because other IFIs and malignancy can result in a similar clinical syndrome.

The diagnosis of invasive candidiasis remains challenging, particularly because conventional blood cultures may only have a sensitivity of 50% in those with deep fungal infection [141]. Newer diagnostic assays, including the beta-D-glucan test, which detects beta-glucans in the cell wall of molds and yeasts except zygomycetes and cryptococci, may be valuable in the diagnosis of invasive candidiasis. One recent study demonstrated a sensitivity and specificity of 87.5% and 85.5%, respectively, of this assay. The mannan antigen and antibody and the Cand-Tec *Candida* antigen assays have demonstrated lower sensitivities than the beta-D-glucan assay (58.9%, 62.5%, and 13%, respectively) [142].

Given the prevalence of azole-resistant *Candida* species in neutropenic patients, particularly *C. glabrata* and *C. krusei*, management of invasive candidiasis in allo-HSCT recipients should include amphotericin B or an echinocandin such as caspofungin, micafungin, or anidulafungin. Several studies have demonstrated comparable efficacy between both antifungal classes; however, echinocandins have been associated with a more favorable toxicity profile [143, 144]. Voriconazole may be used in situations where additional mold coverage is desired; however, since voriconazole resistance has been seen in 3% of Candida infections in solid organ and HSCT recipients, this agent should not be used unless susceptibility of the isolate is confirmed [145, 146]. As the majority of cases of hepatosplenic candidiasis are caused by *C. albicans*, clinically stable patients may receive fluconazole. Those who are acutely ill or who have relapsed disease should receive 1–2 weeks of induction with liposomal amphotericin B or an echinocandin followed by fluconazole. Duration of therapy for hepatosplenic candidiasis is dependent upon resolution of visceral lesions, typically 3–6 months. Chronic suppressive therapy may be used in individuals at high risk for recurrence, including those with GVHD [146].

Invasive Mold Infections

Aspergillus and other molds are ubiquitous environmental pathogens. HSCT recipients are at high risk of infection with these organisms, which are largely acquired via inhalation of conidia that are inadequately cleared in the setting of immunosuppression. Less common routes of infection include invasion of the gastrointestinal tract or cutaneous inoculation.

Aspergillus

Invasive aspergillosis is the most frequent IFI encountered among allo-HSCT recipients. Data from the PATH Alliance demonstrated an incidence of invasive aspergillosis of 53.5% and 59.8% in recipients of matched-related donor and matched-unrelated donor transplants, respectively [138]. While both autologous and allo-HSCT recipients are at risk for the development of invasive aspergillosis, prolonged neutropenia, as well as GVHD, and its treatment contribute to higher incidences of invasive aspergillosis among allo-HSCT recipients [147, 148].

The onset of invasive aspergillosis following HSCT occurs in a bimodal fashion, with the first peak noted within the first 40 days of transplantation [149] and corresponding to the period of neutropenia. The second peak occurs post-engraftment ("late period"), typically defined as 41+ days following transplant, and tends to arise in the setting of acute or chronic GVHD [147, 148, 150]. Age >40 has been associated with the development of invasive aspergillosis at any time following transplantation, as have donor and recipient polymorphisms in various Toll-like receptors and genes regulating interleukin-1, interleukin-10 promoter, and plasminogen [147, 151–155]. Specifically, donor haplotype 1363T/1063G, which contains two cosegregated single nucleotide polymorphisms in the Toll-like receptor 4 gene, has been associated with the development of invasive aspergillosis [151]. Single nucleotide polymorphisms in the chemokine ligand 10 (CXCL-10) gene have also been demonstrated to reduce dendritic cell CXCL-10 expression when exposed to *Aspergillus* germlings; these polymorphisms have also been associated with invasive aspergillosis following allo-HSCT [154]. Hematologic malignancies other than chronic myelogenous leukemia in the chronic phase, as well as aplastic anemia, myelodysplastic syndrome, mismatched donor, the use of cord blood, summer season, lack of laminar air flow, and local building construction, have been identified as risk factors for invasive aspergillosis in the early posttransplant period. The risk of invasive aspergillosis in the late posttransplant period increases in the setting of underlying multiple myeloma, use of T-cell-depleted or CD34-selected stem cell products, neutropenia, lymphopenia, use of corticosteroids, CMV disease, respiratory virus infection, and GVHD [147, 148]. GVHD and CMV disease are the major risk factors for the development of invasive aspergillosis >6 months after transplantation [148]. The contribution of GVHD to the risk of invasive aspergillosis is highlighted by the fact that conditioning regimens do not appear to impact the incidence of this invasive fungal infection. While the period of neutropenia is shorter and the incidence of early invasive aspergillosis is less in non-myeloablative HSCT recipients, this group remains at highest risk in the late posttransplant period in conjunction with GVHD [12, 156–158].

Aspergillus fumigatus is the most commonly isolated species associated with invasive aspergillosis in allogeneic HSCT recipients; infections with *A. niger*, *A. flavus*, and *A. terreus* are less frequently encountered [147, 159]. The lungs represent the most commonly involved site of infection, though patients may develop sinusitis, CNS disease, and tracheobronchitis. Clinical presentation may be variable, but frequently includes fever, cough, chest pain, hemoptysis, and/or respiratory failure, and the presence of these symptoms should prompt CT of the chest. Lung lesions, with surrounding ground-glass halos, nodular infiltrates, and cavitations, are highly suggestive of pulmonary aspergillosis; however, radiographic findings can be variable in allo-HSCT recipients with concomitant GVHD and include focal infiltrates and/or bronchopneumonia [160]. Given the lack of specificity of symptoms and radiographic findings, prompt microbiologic diagnosis via bronchoscopy should be pursued. Diagnosis of invasive aspergillosis may also be facilitated with use of the *Aspergillus* galactomannan assay, which employs a double-sandwich enzyme immunoassay to detect the galactomannan component of the *Aspergillus* cell wall. While the sensitivity of the serum galactomannan assay has varied between studies, it has proven clinically useful for the diagnosis of invasive aspergillosis and monitoring of clinical response during therapy [161, 162]. The galactomannan assay on bronchoalveolar lavage fluid in patients with hematologic malignancies and HSCT recipients has demonstrated higher sensitivity than bronchoalveolar lavage culture, cytology, and the serum galactomannan assay [163]. Important caveats for the use of galactomannan testing include false negative results in individuals receiving concomitant antifungals, false positive results in children and patients receiving beta-lactams, particularly piperacillin-tazobactam, and cross-reactivity with plasmalyte [164–166]. The beta-D-glucan test, which detects beta-glucans in the cell wall of molds and yeasts except zygomycetes and cryptococci, may also be a valuable adjunctive screening test for invasive aspergillosis particularly in conjunction with the galactomannan assay, though the performance characteristics of the beta-D-glucan assay in the HSCT population have not yet been evaluated.

Empiric therapy for suspected invasive aspergillosis should include a mold-active azole or amphotericin B. The use of an echinocandin can also be entertained, though these agents are fungistatic, rather than fungicidal. Once the diagnosis of invasive aspergillosis has been confirmed, primary therapy should include voriconazole in most patients, as this agent has been associated with improved clinical outcomes and survival rates and less toxicity compared with amphotericin B [167, 168]. Voriconazole is also the preferred therapy for *Aspergillus* tracheobronchitis [168]. Combination therapy with an echinocandin and either amphotericin B or a mold-active azole may be more efficacious than voriconazole alone, however, particularly for salvage therapy [169, 170]. The duration of therapy in allogeneic HSCT recipients should be prolonged and continue at least until immunosuppressives, particularly corticosteroids, are completed.

Prevention of invasive aspergillosis in allogeneic HSCT recipients should include the use of high-efficiency particulate air (HEPA) filtration and/or laminar flow rooms during the pre-engraftment period. In addition, two recent studies have suggested that voriconazole may be appropriate secondary prophylaxis prior to HSCT in patients with previous IA [171, 172].

Other Molds

Mucor and *Rhizopus* species are the most commonly encountered zygomycetes in clinical practice, with an incidence of 8.5% and 5.9% in recipients of matched-related and matched-unrelated allo-HSCT, respectively [138]. Infection with these organisms results in mucormycosis, which can occur in the late posttransplant period and causes devastating sino-orbital, CNS, and gastrointestinal disease, as well as cutaneous lesions and fasciitis. Among HSCT recipients, risk factors for zygomycosis include HLA mismatch, prolonged neutropenia, corticosteroid use, iron overload, and GVHD [173, 174]. Additionally, several studies have noted increasing numbers of zygomycosis cases among patients receiving voriconazole as either prophylaxis or treatment of invasive aspergillosis [32, 111, 175]. Whether this reflects azole-related selective pressure remains unknown.

Fusarium species are environmental organisms, which cause infrequent but severe invasive fungal infection in HSCT recipients. Cases of fusariosis among HSCT recipients have been linked to contamination of central venous catheters and hospital water supply [176, 177]. Risk factors for fusariosis include underlying multiple myeloma and HLA mismatch. As with invasive aspergillosis, the onset of fusariosis occurs in a bimodal fashion; infection in the early posttransplant period is associated with prolonged neutropenia, and late infection is associated with T-cell depletion, corticosteroid use, and GVHD. Infection with *Fusarium* species can mimic invasive aspergillosis; however, patients with fusariosis are more likely to have positive blood cultures and multiple papular or ulcerated skin lesions compared to patients with invasive aspergillosis [176, 178].

Scedosporium apiospermum and *Scedosporium prolificans* have also been isolated in HSCT recipients; their disease spectrum is similar to invasive aspergillosis. Risk factors for *Scedosporium* infection include prolonged neutropenia and GVHD [159, 179, 180].

Miscellaneous Infections

Pneumocystis Jirovecii (PJP)

Due to effective prophylaxis, PCP has become a rare event among allo-HSCT recipients with retrospective studies showing incidence rates from 1.3% to 2.5% [181, 182]. PCP is usually a late occurrence, and risk factors include treatment for GVHD or cessation of PCP prophylaxis [183]. Despite effective treatment, mortality can be high if infection occurs early after transplant [184].

Toxoplasmosis

The majority of cases of toxoplasmosis in allo-HSCT recipients are due to reactivation of latent infection. In the United States, the incidence of toxoplasmosis has been reported to be as low as 0.25% [185], reflecting a low seroprevalence in the population [186]. In regions of the world with a higher seroprevalence, incidence rates of toxoplasmosis are predictably higher [187]. Disease usually occurs in the first 6 months after transplantation [185, 186]. Besides seropositivity, the main risk factor for reactivation is intensification of immunosuppression due to GVHD [186]. The most common clinical presentation is encephalitis, which usually presents with focal neurological deficits. Extra-CNS forms of toxoplasmosis include pneumonitis, chorioretinitis, and myocarditis. Diagnosis of toxoplasmosis in any of the above manifestations requires a high clinical suspicion. A toxoplasma PCR can be obtained in serum and tissue such as CSF and vitreous fluid [188, 189]. First-line treatment includes extensive treatment with pyrimethamine and sulfadiazine. Despite best efforts mortality in allo-HSCT recipients remains high [185, 190]. Prophylaxis is usually accomplished with trimethoprim/sulfamethoxazole [191].

Strongyloides

Strongyloides stercoralis can latently infect auto-HSCT recipients who previously lived or visited endemic areas (tropical and subtropical region worldwide), even many decades earlier. In the setting of immunosuppression, the parasite's life cycle is accelerated and cause hyperinfection and disseminated disease [192]. Clinical manifestations include intestinal obstruction, respiratory failure including alveolar hemorrhage, bacterial sepsis, or meningitis [193]. Because of delays in diagnosis, infections can be devastating and carry high mortality. Patients from endemic areas should be serologically screened and treated with ivermectin prior transplant [193].

Preventative Strategies

Like solid organ transplant recipients, allo-HSCT recipients can benefit from measures aimed to prevent infectious complications in the posttransplant period. These can include infection control practices in hospitals and outpatient clinics as well as guidelines for the prevention of opportunistic infections.

The CDC/IDSA and ASBMT have published extensive evidence-based infection control guidelines that include specific practices regarding room ventilation, isolation and barrier precautions, cleaning, hand hygiene, equipment disinfection, plants, patient skin and oral care, prevention of intravascular catheter-related infections, construction and renovations, as well as healthcare workers [194].

In terms of specific infections, guidelines from the CDC were published in 2000. Because many of these organisms not only involve reactivation of latent infection in the recipient but can also be donor-derived, both donors and recipients should be universally tested for CMV, EBV, HIV I/II, HTLV I/II (although this is not done in all centers), hepatitis B and C, syphilis, and *M. tuberculosis* (in donor only if from endemic country). Additionally, all recipients should be tested for HSV I/II, VZV, and *Toxoplasma*. Potential donors and recipients

Table 11.2 Pretransplant screening in candidate allo-HSCT donors and recipients

Donor screening	Recipient screening
Standard	
CMV IgG	CMV IgG
EBV VCA IgG	EBV VCA IgG
VZV IgG	HSV I/II IgG
HIV Ab and NAT	VZV IgG
HTLV I//II Ab	HIV Ab and NAT
Hepatitis B surface Ag and core Ab	HTLV I/II Ab
Hepatitis C Ab, NAT	Hepatitis B surface Ag and core Ab
Syphilis screening (RPR)	Hepatitis C Ab, NAT
	Syphilis screening (RPR)
	Latent Tb screening (PPD or IGRA)
Optional (if risk factors are present)	
Hepatitis B NAT	Hepatitis B NAT
West Nile virus Ab	West Nile virus Ab
Toxoplasma Ab	*Toxoplasma* Ab
Strongyloides Ab	*Strongyloides* Ab
Trypanosoma cruzi	*Trypanosoma cruzi*
Leishmania Ab/PCR	*Coccidioides* Ab
Babesia Ab	*Histoplasma* Ab
Rickettsia Ab	*Brucella* Ab
Coxiella burnetii Ab	

Table 11.3 Recommended and optional vaccination of allo-HSCT recipients [195]

Vaccine	Comments on use after allo-HSCT	Time post-HSCT to initiate vaccine
Recommended		
Pneumococcal conjugate (PCV)	3–4 doses, a fourth dose with PPSV23[a] may be beneficial	3–6 months
Tetanus, diphtheria, acellular pertussis	3 doses, DTaP preferred over Tdap	6–12 months
Haemophilus influenzae conjugate	3 doses	6–12 months
Meningococcal conjugate	1 dose, follow country recommendations for general population	6–12 months
Inactivated polio	3 doses	6–12 months
Recombinant hepatitis B	3 doses, follow country recommendations for general population	6–12 months
Inactivated influenza	Yearly	4–6 months
Measles, mumps, rubella (live)	1–2 doses, all children and measles seronegative adults, not recommended if active GVHD or on immunosuppression	>24 months
Optional		
Hepatitis A	Follow country recommendations for general population	12 months
Varicella (Varivax, live)	Limited data regarding safety and efficacy. Not recommended if active GVHD or on immunosuppression	>24 months
Human papillomavirus	Follow country recommendations for general population	No data
Yellow fever (live)	Limited data regarding safety and efficacy. The risk-benefit balance may favor use of the vaccine in patients residing in or traveling to endemic areas	>24 months
Rabies	Appropriate for use in HCT recipients with potential occupational exposures to rabies. Postexposure administration of rabies vaccine with human rabies Ig can be administered any time after HCT, as indicated	12–24 months
Tick-borne encephalitis	According to local policy in endemic areas	No data
Japanese B encephalitis	According to local policy when residing in or travelling to endemic areas	No data

Adapted and printed by permission from Macmillan Publishers Ltd.: Nature Publishing Group, Bone Marrow Transplantation, Vaccination of hematopoietic cell transplant recipients, Ljungman P, Cordonnier C, Einsele H, Englund J, Machado CM, et al.; Center for International Blood and Marrow Transplant Research; National Marrow Donor Program; European Blood and Marrow Transplant Group; American Society of Blood and Marrow Transplantation; Canadian Blood and Marrow Transplant Group; Infectious Disease Society of America; Society for Healthcare Epidemiology of America; Association of Medical Microbiology and Infectious Diseases Canada; Centers for Disease Control and Prevention Vol. 44/No. 8, pages 521–526, © 2009

Contraindicated vaccines: BCG (live), oral polio (live), intranasal live influenza, cholera (live), typhoid (live and IM), *Rotavirus*, zoster vaccine (Zostavax, live)

[a]PPV23: 23-valent pneumococcal vaccine

should also be tested for *Strongyloides* and *Trypanosoma cruzi* if they have epidemiologic risks. Patients with evidence of syphilis, *Strongyloides*, or latent tuberculosis infection should be treated in the pretransplant period (see Table 11.2).

Vaccinations are an important component of disease prevention. Because of predictable decline in antibody titers posttransplant, it is recommended that recipients be revaccinated in the post-engraftment at the appropriate time (see Table 11.3) [195].

Prophylaxis in the posttransplant period is usually aimed at the most common and predictable organisms. A discussion of strategies to prevent CMV is beyond the scope of this chapter but includes either preemptive treatment in cases of CMV viremia or universal prophylaxis for those at risk for CMV reactivation. Recipients not at risk for CMV should receive acyclovir for HSV prophylaxis. PCP and *Toxoplasma* prophylaxis is accomplished with sulfamethoxazole/trimethoprim for 6–13 months, although this practice varies when taking into consideration the myelosuppressive effects of this drug combination. Dapsone, atovaquone, and pentamidine are alternatives for PCP prophylaxis. Of those, only atovaquone has activity against *Toxoplasma* as well. Many centers also institute bacterial and fungal prophylaxis in the peri-transplant period until neutropenia resolves.

References

1. Bodey GP, Buckley M, Sathe YS, Freireich EJ. Quantitative relationships between circulating leukocytes and infection in patients with acute leukemia. Ann Intern Med. 1966;64(2):328–40.
2. Wingard JR, Leather HL. Empiric antifungal therapy for the neutropenic patient. Oncology (Williston Park). 2001;15(3):351–63. discussion 363–4, 367–9
3. Cornely OA, Maertens J, Winston DJ, Perfect J, Ullmann AJ, Walsh TJ, et al. Posaconazole vs. fluconazole or itraconazole prophylaxis in patients with neutropenia. N Engl J Med. 2007;356(4):348–59.
4. Lortholary O, Gangneux JP, Sitbon K, Lebeau B, de Monbrison F, Le Strat Y, et al. Epidemiological trends in invasive aspergillosis in France: the SAIF network (2005–2007). Clin Microbiol Infect. 2011;17(12):1882–9.
5. Kontoyiannis DP, Chamilos G, Lewis RE, Giralt S, Cortes J, Raad II, et al. Increased bone marrow iron stores is an independent risk factor for invasive aspergillosis in patients with high-risk hematologic malignancies and recipients of allogeneic hematopoietic stem cell transplantation. Cancer. 2007;110(6):1303–6.
6. Pagano L, Akova M, Dimopoulos G, Herbrecht R, Drgona L, Blijlevens N. Risk assessment and prognostic factors for mould-related diseases in immunocompromised patients. J Antimicrob Chemother. 2011;66(Suppl 1):i5–14.
7. Hersh EM, Carbone PP, Wong VG, Freireich EJ. Inhibition of the primary immune response in man by anti-metabolites. Cancer Res. 1965;25(7):997–1001.
8. Filipovich A. Hematopoietic cell transplantation for correction of primary immunodeficiencies. Bone Marrow Transplant. 2008;42(Suppl 1):S49–52.
9. Smith AR, Gross TG, Baker KS. Transplant outcomes for primary immunodeficiency disease. Semin Hematol. 2010;47(1):79–85.
10. Scott BL, Park JY, Deeg HJ, Marr KA, Boeckh M, Chauncey TR, et al. Pretransplant neutropenia is associated with poor-risk cytogenetic features and increased infection-related mortality in patients with myelodysplastic syndromes. Biol Blood Marrow Transplant. 2008;14(7):799–806.
11. Verschraegen CF, van Besien KW, Dignani C, Hester JP, Andersson BS, Anaissie E. Invasive Aspergillus sinusitis during bone marrow transplantation. Scand J Infect Dis. 1997;29(4):436–8.
12. Junghanss C, Marr KA, Carter RA, Sandmaier BM, Maris MB, Maloney DG, et al. Incidence and outcome of bacterial and fungal infections following nonmyeloablative compared with myeloablative allogeneic hematopoietic stem cell transplantation: a matched control study. Biol Blood Marrow Transplant. 2002;8(9):512–20.
13. Nucci M, Andrade F, Vigorito A, Trabasso P, Aranha JF, Maiolino A, De Souza CA. Infectious complications in patients randomized to receive allogeneic bone marrow or peripheral blood transplantation. Transpl Infect Dis. 2003;5(4):167–73.
14. Eyrich M, Lang P, Lal S, Bader P, Handgretinger R, Klingebiel T, et al. A prospective analysis of the pattern of immune reconstitution in a paediatric cohort following transplantation of positively selected human leucocyte antigen-disparate haematopoietic stem cells from parental donors. Br J Haematol. 2001;114(2):422–32.
15. Safdar A, Rodriguez GH, De Lima MJ, Petropoulos D, Chemaly RF, Worth LL, et al. Infections in 100 cord blood transplantations: spectrum of early and late posttransplant infections in adult and pediatric patients 1996–2005. Medicine (Baltimore). 2007;86(6):324–33.
16. van Burik JA, Carter SL, Freifeld AG, High KP, Godder KT, Papanicolaou GA, et al. Higher risk of cytomegalovirus and aspergillus infections in recipients of T cell-depleted unrelated bone marrow: analysis of infectious complications in patients treated with T cell depletion versus immunosuppressive therapy to prevent graft-versus-host disease. Biol Blood Marrow Transplant. 2007;13(12):1487–98.
17. Marty FM, Bryar J, Browne SK, Schwarzberg T, Ho VT, Bassett IV, et al. Sirolimus-based graft-versus-host disease prophylaxis protects against cytomegalovirus reactivation after allogeneic hematopoietic stem cell transplantation: a cohort analysis. Blood. 2007;110(2):490–500.
18. Demopoulos L, Polinsky M, Steele G, Mines D, Blum M, Caulfield M, et al. Reduced risk of cytomegalovirus infection in solid organ transplant recipients treated with sirolimus: a pooled analysis of clinical trials. Transplant Proc. 2008;40(5):1407–10.
19. Wingard JR, Hsu J, Hiemenz JW. Hematopoietic stem cell transplantation: an overview of infection risks and epidemiology. Infect Dis Clin N Am. 2010;24(2):257–72.
20. Bjorklund A, Aschan J, Labopin M, Remberger M, Ringden O, Winiarski J, Ljungman P. Risk factors for fatal infectious complications developing late after allogeneic stem cell transplantation. Bone Marrow Transplant. 2007;40(11):1055–62.
21. Yamasaki S, Heike Y, Mori S, Fukuda T, Maruyama D, Kato R, et al. Infectious complications in chronic graft-versus-host disease: a retrospective study of 145 recipients of allogeneic hematopoietic stem cell transplantation with reduced- and conventional-intensity conditioning regimens. Transpl Infect Dis. 2008;10(4):252–9.
22. Fuji S, Kapp M, Einsele H. Challenges to preventing infectious complications, decreasing re-hospitalizations, and reducing cost burden in long-term survivors after allogeneic hematopoietic stem cell transplantation. Semin Hematol. 2012;49(1):10–4.
23. Guidelines for preventing opportunistic infections among hematopoietic stem cell transplant recipients. MMWR Recomm Rep. 2000;49(RR-10):1–125, CE1–7.
24. Dykewicz CA. Summary of the guidelines for preventing opportunistic infections among hematopoietic stem cell transplant recipients. Clin Infect Dis. 2001;33(2):139–44.
25. Marena C, Zecca M, Carenini ML, Bruschi A, Bassi ML, Olivieri P, et al. Incidence of, and risk factors for, nosocomial infections among hematopoietic stem cell transplantation recipients, with impact on procedure-related mortality. Infect Control Hosp Epidemiol. 2001;22(8):510–7.
26. Gluckman E, Lotsberg J, Devergie A, Zhao XM, Melo R, Gomez-Morales M, et al. Prophylaxis of herpes infections after bone-marrow transplantation by oral acyclovir. Lancet. 1983;2(8352):706–8.
27. Wade JC, Newton B, Flournoy N, Meyers JD. Oral acyclovir for prevention of herpes simplex virus reactivation after marrow transplantation. Ann Intern Med. 1984;100(6):823–8.
28. Wingard JR, Merz WG, Rinaldi MG, Johnson TR, Karp JE, Saral R. Increase in *Candida krusei* infection among patients with bone marrow transplantation and neutropenia treated prophylactically with fluconazole. N Engl J Med. 1991;325(18):1274–7.
29. Persons DA, Laughlin M, Tanner D, Perfect J, Gockerman JP, Hathorn JW. Fluconazole and *Candida krusei* fungemia. N Engl J Med. 1991;325(18):1315.
30. Wingard JR, Merz WG, Rinaldi MG, Miller CB, Karp JE, Saral R. Association of *Torulopsis glabrata* infections with fluconazole prophylaxis in neutropenic bone marrow transplant patients. Antimicrob Agents Chemother. 1993;37(9):1847–9.

31. Siwek GT, Dodgson KJ, de Magalhaes-Silverman M, Bartelt LA, Kilborn SB, Hoth PL, et al. Invasive zygomycosis in hematopoietic stem cell transplant recipients receiving voriconazole prophylaxis. Clin Infect Dis. 2004;39(4):584–7.
32. Kontoyiannis DP, Lionakis MS, Lewis RE, Chamilos G, Healy M, Perego C. Zygomycosis in a tertiary-care cancer center in the era of Aspergillus-active antifungal therapy: a case-control observational study of 27 recent cases. J Infect Dis. 2005;191(8):1350–60.
33. Lionakis MS, Kontoyiannis DP. Sinus zygomycosis in a patient receiving voriconazole prophylaxis. Br J Haematol. 2005;129(1):2.
34. van Well GT, van Groeningen I, Debets-Ossenkopp YJ, van Furth AM, Zwaan CM. Zygomycete infection following voriconazole prophylaxis. Lancet Infect Dis. 2005;5(9):594.
35. Collin BA, Leather HL, Wingard JR, Ramphal R. Evolution, incidence, and susceptibility of bacterial bloodstream isolates from 519 bone marrow transplant patients. Clin Infect Dis. 2001;33(7):947–53.
36. Ochs L, Shu XO, Miller J, Enright H, Wagner J, Filipovich A. Late infections after allogeneic bone marrow transplantations: comparison of incidence in related and unrelated donor transplant recipients. Blood. 1995;86(10):3979–86.
37. Roy V, Weisdorf D. Mycobacterial infections following bone marrow transplantation: a 20 year retrospective review. Bone Marrow Transplant. 1997;19(5):467–70.
38. Almyroudis NG, Fuller A, Jakubowski A, Sepkowitz K, Jaffe D, Small TN, et al. Pre- and post-engraftment bloodstream infection rates and associated mortality in allogeneic hematopoietic stem cell transplant recipients. Transpl Infect Dis. 2005;7(1):11–7.
39. Avery R, Kalaycio M, Pohlman B, Sobecks R, Kuczkowski E, Andresen S, et al. Early vancomycin-resistant enterococcus (VRE) bacteremia after allogeneic bone marrow transplantation is associated with a rapidly deteriorating clinical course. Bone Marrow Transplant. 2005;35(5):497–9.
40. Mikulska M, Del Bono V, Raiola AM, Bruno B, Gualandi F, Occhini D, et al. Blood stream infections in allogeneic hematopoietic stem cell transplant recipients: reemergence of Gram-negative rods and increasing antibiotic resistance. Biol Blood Marrow Transplant. 2009;15(1):47–53.
41. Trecarichi EM, Tumbarello M, Caira M, Candoni A, Cattaneo C, Pastore D, et al. Multidrug resistant Pseudomonas aeruginosa bloodstream infection in adult patients with hematologic malignancies. Haematologica. 2011;96(1):e1–3. author reply e4
42. Mikulska M, Del Bono V, Bruzzi P, Raiola AM, Gualandi F, Van Lint MT, et al. Mortality after bloodstream infections in allogeneic haematopoietic stem cell transplant (HSCT) recipients. Infection. 2012;40(3):271–8.
43. Garnica M, Maiolino A, Nucci M. Factors associated with bacteremia due to multidrug-resistant Gram-negative bacilli in hematopoietic stem cell transplant recipients. Braz J Med Biol Res. 2009;42(3):289–93.
44. Arango JI, Restrepo A, Schneider DL, Callander NS, Ochoa-Bayona JL, Restrepo MI, et al. Incidence of Clostridium difficile-associated diarrhea before and after autologous peripheral blood stem cell transplantation for lymphoma and multiple myeloma. Bone Marrow Transplant. 2006;37(5):517–21.
45. Bobak D, Arfons LM, Creger RJ, Lazarus HM. Clostridium difficile-associated disease in human stem cell transplant recipients: coming epidemic or false alarm? Bone Marrow Transplant. 2008;42(11):705–13.
46. Alonso CD, Treadway SB, Hanna DB, Huff CA, Neofytos D, Carroll KC, Marr KA. Epidemiology and outcomes of Clostridium difficile infections in hematopoietic stem cell transplant recipients. Clin Infect Dis. 2012;54(8):1053–63.
47. Anand A, Glatt AE. Clostridium difficile infection associated with antineoplastic chemotherapy: a review. Clin Infect Dis. 1993;17(1):109–13.
48. Loo VG, Poirier L, Miller MA, Oughton M, Libman MD, Michaud S, et al. A predominantly clonal multi-institutional outbreak of Clostridium difficile-associated diarrhea with high morbidity and mortality. N Engl J Med. 2005;353(23):2442–9.
49. Biller P, Shank B, Lind L, Brennan M, Tkatch L, Killgore G, et al. Moxifloxacin therapy as a risk factor for Clostridium difficile-associated disease during an outbreak: attempts to control a new epidemic strain. Infect Control Hosp Epidemiol. 2007;28(2):198–201.
50. Goorhuis A, Van der Kooi T, Vaessen N, Dekker FW, Van den Berg R, Harmanus C, et al. Spread and epidemiology of Clostridium difficile polymerase chain reaction ribotype 027/toxinotype III in The Netherlands. Clin Infect Dis. 2007;45(6):695–703.
51. Tomblyn M, Chiller T, Einsele H, Gress R, Sepkowitz K, Storek J, Center for International Blood and Marrow Research, National Marrow Donor program, European Blood and MarrowTransplant Group, American Society of Blood and Marrow Transplantation, Canadian Blood and Marrow Transplant Group, Infectious Diseases Society of America, Society for Healthcare Epidemiology of America, Association of Medical Microbiology and Infectious Disease Canada, Centers for Disease Control and Prevention, et al. Guidelines for preventing infectious complications among hematopoietic cell transplantation recipients: a global perspective. Biol Blood Marrow Transplant. 2009;15(10):1143–238.
52. Gafter-Gvili A, Fraser A, Paul M, Leibovici L. Meta-analysis: antibiotic prophylaxis reduces mortality in neutropenic patients. Ann Intern Med. 2005;142(12 Pt 1):979–95.
53. van de Wetering MD, de Witte MA, Kremer LC, Offringa M, Scholten RJ, Caron HN. Efficacy of oral prophylactic antibiotics in neutropenic afebrile oncology patients: a systematic review of randomised controlled trials. Eur J Cancer. 2005;41(10):1372–82.
54. Cruciani M, Rampazzo R, Malena M, Lazzarini L, Todeschini G, Messori A, Concia E. Prophylaxis with fluoroquinolones for bacterial infections in neutropenic patients: a meta-analysis. Clin Infect Dis. 1996;23(4):795–805.
55. Bow EJ. Fluoroquinolones, antimicrobial resistance and neutropenic cancer patients. Curr Opin Infect Dis. 2011;24(6):545–53.
56. Chang J, Powles R, Mehta J, Paton N, Treleaven J, Jameson B. Listeriosis in bone marrow transplant recipients: incidence, clinical features, and treatment. Clin Infect Dis. 1995;21(5):1289–90.
57. Harrington RD, Woolfrey AE, Bowden R, McDowell MG, Hackman RC. Legionellosis in a bone marrow transplant center. Bone Marrow Transplant. 1996;18(2):361–8.
58. Storek J, Witherspoon RP, Webb D, Storb R. Lack of B cells precursors in marrow transplant recipients with chronic graft-versus-host disease. Am J Hematol. 1996;52(2):82–9.
59. Kalhs P, Panzer S, Kletter K, Minar E, Stain-Kos M, Walter R, et al. Functional asplenia after bone marrow transplantation. A late complication related to extensive chronic graft-versus-host disease. Ann Intern Med. 1988;109(6):461–4.
60. Youssef S, Rodriguez G, Rolston KV, Champlin RE, Raad II, Safdar A. Streptococcus pneumoniae infections in 47 hematopoietic stem cell transplantation recipients: clinical characteristics of infections and vaccine-breakthrough infections, 1989–2005. Medicine (Baltimore). 2007;86(2):69–77.
61. Engelhard D, Cordonnier C, Shaw PJ, Parkalli T, Guenther C, Martino R, Infectious Disease Working Party of the European Bone Marrow Transplantation (IDWP-EBMT), et al. Early and late invasive pneumococcal infection following stem cell transplantation: a European Bone Marrow Transplantation survey. Br J Haematol. 2002;117(2):444–50.
62. Cordonnier C, Martino R, Trabasso P, Held TK, Akan H, Ward MS, European Blood and Marrow Transplant Group Infectious Diseases Working Party, et al. Mycobacterial infection: a difficult and late diagnosis in stem cell transplant recipients. Clin Infect Dis. 2004;38(9):1229–36.

63. Unal E, Yen C, Saiman L, George D, Della-Latta P, van de Ven C, et al. A low incidence of nontuberculous mycobacterial infections in pediatric hematopoietic stem cell transplantation recipients. Biol Blood Marrow Transplant. 2006;12(11):1188–97.
64. Doucette K, Fishman JA. Nontuberculous mycobacterial infection in hematopoietic stem cell and solid organ transplant recipients. Clin Infect Dis. 2004;38(10):1428–39.
65. Au WY, Cheng VC, Ho PL, Yuen KY, Hung I, Ma SY, et al. Nontuberculous mycobacterial infections in Chinese hematopoietic stem cell transplantation recipients. Bone Marrow Transplant. 2003;32(7):709–14.
66. Gaviria JM, Garcia PJ, Garrido SM, Corey L, Boeckh M. Nontuberculous mycobacterial infections in hematopoietic stem cell transplant recipients: characteristics of respiratory and catheter-related infections. Biol Blood Marrow Transplant. 2000;6(4):361–9.
67. Russo RL, Dulley FL, Suganuma L, França IL, Yasuda MA, Costa SF. Tuberculosis in hematopoietic stem cell transplant patients: case report and review of the literature. Int J Infect Dis. 2010;14(Suppl 3):e187–91.
68. Navari RM, Sullivan KM, Springmeyer SC, Siegel MS, Meyers JD, Buckner CD, et al. Mycobacterial infections in marrow transplant patients. Transplantation. 1983;36(5):509–13.
69. Kurzrock R, Zander A, Vellekoop L, Kanojia M, Luna M, Dicke K. Mycobacterial pulmonary infections after allogeneic bone marrow transplantation. Am J Med. 1984;77(1):35–40.
70. Wang JY, Chang YL, Lee LN, Chen JH, Tang JL, Yang PC, Lee YC. Diffuse pulmonary infiltrates after bone marrow transplantation: the role of open lung biopsy. Ann Thorac Surg. 2004;78(1):267–72.
71. Daly AS, McGeer A, Lipton JH. Systemic nocardiosis following allogeneic bone marrow transplantation. Transpl Infect Dis. 2003;5(1):16–20.
72. Pao M, Papadopoulos EB, Chou J, Glenn H, Castro-Malaspina H, Jakubowski AA, et al. Response to pneumococcal (PNCRM7) and haemophilus influenzae conjugate vaccines (HIB) in pediatric and adult recipients of an allogeneic hematopoietic cell transplantation (alloHCT). Biol Blood Marrow Transplant. 2008;14(9):1022–30.
73. Toscano CM, Bell M, Zukerman C, Shelton W, Novicki TJ, Nichols WG, et al. Gram-negative bloodstream infections in hematopoietic stem cell transplant patients: the roles of needleless device use, bathing practices, and catheter care. Am J Infect Control. 2009;37(4):327–34.
74. Benjamin D, Miller WC, Bayliff S, Martel L, Alexander K, Martin PL. Infections diagnosed in the first year after pediatric stem cell transplantation. Pediatr Infect Dis J. 2002;21(3):227–34.
75. Bate SL, Dollard SC, Cannon MJ. Cytomegalovirus seroprevalence in the United States: the national health and nutrition examination surveys, 1988–2004. Clin Infect Dis. 2010;50(11):1439–47.
76. Urwijitaroon Y, Teawpatanataworn S, Kitjareontarm A. Prevalence of cytomegalovirus antibody in Thai-northeastern blood donors. Southeast Asian J Trop Med Public Health. 1993;24(Suppl 1):180–2.
77. Souza MA, Passos AM, Treitinger A, Spada C. Seroprevalence of cytomegalovirus antibodies in blood donors in southern, Brazil. Rev Soc Bras Med Trop. 2010;43(4):359–61.
78. Miller W, Flynn P, McCullough J, Balfour HH Jr, Goldman A, Haake R, et al. Cytomegalovirus infection after bone marrow transplantation: an association with acute graft-v-host disease. Blood. 1986;67(4):1162–7.
79. Montesinos P, Sanz J, Cantero S, Lorenzo I, Martín G, Saavedra S, et al. Incidence, risk factors, and outcome of cytomegalovirus infection and disease in patients receiving prophylaxis with oral valganciclovir or intravenous ganciclovir after umbilical cord blood transplantation. Biol Blood Marrow Transplant. 2009;15(6):730–40.
80. Goodrich JM, Bowden RA, Fisher L, Keller C, Schoch G, Meyers JD. Ganciclovir prophylaxis to prevent cytomegalovirus disease after allogeneic marrow transplant. Ann Intern Med. 1993;118(3):173–8.
81. Winston DJ, Ho WG, Bartoni K, Du Mond C, Ebeling DF, Buhles WC, Champlin RE. Ganciclovir prophylaxis of cytomegalovirus infection and disease in allogeneic bone marrow transplant recipients. Results of a placebo-controlled, double-blind trial. Ann Intern Med. 1993;118(3):179–84.
82. Ayala E, Greene J, Sandin R, Perkins J, Field T, Tate C, et al. Valganciclovir is safe and effective as pre-emptive therapy for CMV infection in allogeneic hematopoietic stem cell transplantation. Bone Marrow Transplant. 2006;37(9):851–6.
83. Boeckh M, Leisenring W, Riddell SR, Bowden RA, Huang ML, Myerson D, et al. Late cytomegalovirus disease and mortality in recipients of allogeneic hematopoietic stem cell transplants: importance of viral load and T-cell immunity. Blood. 2003;101(2):407–14.
84. Nichols WG, Corey L, Gooley T, Davis C, Boeckh M. High risk of death due to bacterial and fungal infection among cytomegalovirus (CMV)-seronegative recipients of stem cell transplants from seropositive donors: evidence for indirect effects of primary CMV infection. J Infect Dis. 2002;185(3):273–82.
85. Boeckh M, Nichols WG, Papanicolaou G, Rubin R, Wingard JR, Zaia J. Cytomegalovirus in hematopoietic stem cell transplant recipients: current status, known challenges, and future strategies. Biol Blood Marrow Transplant. 2003;9(9):543–58.
86. Boeckh M, Ljungman P. How we treat cytomegalovirus in hematopoietic cell transplant recipients. Blood. 2009;113(23):5711–9.
87. Alexander BT, Hladnik LM, Augustin KM, Casabar E, McKinnon PS, Reichley RM, et al. Use of cytomegalovirus intravenous immune globulin for the adjunctive treatment of cytomegalovirus in hematopoietic stem cell transplant recipients. Pharmacotherapy. 2010;30(6):554–61.
88. Mui TS, Kapp M, Einsele H, Grigoleit GU. T-cell therapy for cytomegalovirus infection. Curr Opin Organ Transplant. 2010;15(6):744–50.
89. Bernstein DI. Vaccines for cytomegalovirus. Infect Disord Drug Targets. 2011;11(5):514–25.
90. Kharfan-Dabaja MA, Boeckh M, Wilck MB, Langston AA, Chu AH, Wloch MK, et al. A novel therapeutic cytomegalovirus DNA vaccine in allogeneic haemopoietic stem-cell transplantation: a randomised, double-blind, placebo-controlled, phase 2 trial. Lancet Infect Dis. 2012;12(4):290–9.
91. Jagadeesh D, Woda BA, Draper J, Evens AM. Post transplant lymphoproliferative disorders: risk, classification, and therapeutic recommendations. Curr Treat Options in Oncol. 2012;13(1):122–36.
92. Landgren O, Gilbert ES, Rizzo JD, Socié G, Banks PM, Sobocinski KA, et al. Risk factors for lymphoproliferative disorders after allogeneic hematopoietic cell transplantation. Blood. 2009;113(20):4992–5001.
93. Ocheni S, Kroeger N, Zabelina T, Sobottka I, Ayuk F, Wolschke C, et al. EBV reactivation and post transplant lymphoproliferative disorders following allogeneic SCT. Bone Marrow Transplant. 2008;42(3):181–6.
94. Blaes AH, Cao Q, Wagner JE, Young JA, Weisdorf DJ, Brunstein CG. Monitoring and preemptive rituximab therapy for Epstein-Barr virus reactivation after antithymocyte globulin containing nonmyeloablative conditioning for umbilical cord blood transplantation. Biol Blood Marrow Transplant. 2010;16(2):287–91.
95. Styczynski J, Einsele H, Gil L, Ljungman P. Outcome of treatment of Epstein-Barr virus-related post-transplant lymphop-

roliferative disorder in hematopoietic stem cell recipients: a comprehensive review of reported cases. Transpl Infect Dis. 2009;11(5):383–92.
96. Xu F, Sternberg MR, Kottiri BJ, McQuillan GM, Lee FK, Nahmias AJ, et al. Trends in herpes simplex virus type 1 and type 2 seroprevalence in the United States. JAMA. 2006;296(8):964–73.
97. Meyers JD, Flournoy N, Thomas ED. Infection with herpes simplex virus and cell-mediated immunity after marrow transplant. J Infect Dis. 1980;142(3):338–46.
98. Wade JC, Day LM, Crowley JJ, Meyers JD. Recurrent infection with herpes simplex virus after marrow transplantation: role of the specific immune response and acyclovir treatment. J Infect Dis. 1984;149(5):750–6.
99. Gasparetto EL, Escuissato DL, Inoue C, Marchiori E, Müller NL. Herpes simplex virus type 2 pneumonia after bone marrow transplantation: high-resolution CT findings in 3 patients. J Thorac Imaging. 2005;20(2):71–3.
100. Ramsey PG, Fife KH, Hackman RC, Meyers JD, Corey L. Herpes simplex virus pneumonia: clinical, virologic, and pathologic features in 20 patients. Ann Intern Med. 1982;97(6):813–20.
101. Kaufman B, Gandhi SA, Louie E, Rizzi R, Illei P. Herpes simplex virus hepatitis: case report and review. Clin Infect Dis. 1997;24(3):334–8.
102. Momméja-Marin H, Lafaurie M, Scieux C, Galicier L, Oksenhendler E, Molina JM. Herpes simplex virus type 2 as a cause of severe meningitis in immunocompromised adults. Clin Infect Dis. 2003;37(11):1527–33.
103. Robinson MJ, Newton C. Bilateral herpes simplex keratitis in a patient with graft-vs-host disease. Am J Ophthalmol. 1991;112(4):468–9.
104. Ballen KK, Donadio D, Bouloux C, McCarthy P, Weinstein H, Antin JH. Herpes simplex virus and neutropenia following bone marrow transplantation. Transplantation. 1992;54(3):553–5.
105. Rogers JE, Cumpston A, Newton M, Craig M. Onset and complications of varicella zoster reactivation in the autologous hematopoietic cell transplant population. Transpl Infect Dis. 2011;13(5):480–4.
106. Oshima K, Takahashi T, Mori T, Matsuyama T, Usuki K, Asano-Mori Y, et al. One-year low-dose valacyclovir as prophylaxis for varicella zoster virus disease after allogeneic hematopoietic stem cell transplantation. A prospective study of the Japan Hematology and Oncology Clinical Study Group. Transpl Infect Dis. 2010;12(5):421–7.
107. Steer CB, Szer J, Sasadeusz J, Matthews JP, Beresford JA, Grigg A. Varicella-zoster infection after allogeneic bone marrow transplantation: incidence, risk factors and prevention with low-dose aciclovir and ganciclovir. Bone Marrow Transplant. 2000;25(6):657–64.
108. Kim DH, Messner H, Minden M, Gupta V, Kuruvilla J, Wright J, Lipton J. Factors influencing varicella zoster virus infection after allogeneic peripheral blood stem cell transplantation: low-dose acyclovir prophylaxis and pre-transplant diagnosis of lymphoproliferative disorders. Transpl Infect Dis. 2008;10(2):90–8.
109. Zerr DM, Boeckh M, Delaney C, Martin PJ, Xie H, Adler AL, et al. HHV-6 reactivation and associated sequelae after hematopoietic cell transplant. Biol Blood Marrow Transplant. 2012;18(11):1700–8.
110. Zerr DM, Corey L, Kim HW, Huang ML, Nguy L, Boeckh M. Clinical outcomes of human herpesvirus 6 reactivation after hematopoietic stem cell transplantation. Clin Infect Dis. 2005;40(7):932–40.
111. Trifilio SM, Bennett CL, Yarnold PR, McKoy JM, Parada J, Mehta J, et al. Breakthrough zygomycosis after voriconazole administration among patients with hematologic malignancies who receive hematopoietic stem-cell transplants or intensive chemotherapy. Bone Marrow Transplant. 2007;39(7):425–9.
112. Hill JA, Koo S, Guzman Suarez BB, Ho VT, Cutler C, Koreth J, et al. Cord-blood hematopoietic stem cell transplant confers an increased risk for human herpesvirus-6-associated acute limbic encephalitis: a cohort analysis. Biol Blood Marrow Transplant. 2012;18(11):1638–48.
113. Yamane A, Mori T, Suzuki S, Mihara A, Yamazaki R, Aisa Y, et al. Risk factors for developing human herpesvirus 6 (HHV-6) reactivation after allogeneic hematopoietic stem cell transplantation and its association with central nervous system disorders. Biol Blood Marrow Transplant. 2007;13(1):100–6.
114. Olli-Lähdesmäki T, Haataja L, Parkkola R, Waris M, Bleyzac N, Ruuskanen O. High-dose ganciclovir in HHV-6 encephalitis of an immunocompetent child. Pediatr Neurol. 2010;43(1):53–6.
115. Yoshikawa T, Yoshida J, Hamaguchi M, Kubota T, Akimoto S, Ihira M, et al. Human herpesvirus 7-associated meningitis and optic neuritis in a patient after allogeneic stem cell transplantation. J Med Virol. 2003;70(3):440–3.
116. de Medeiros BC, Rezuke WN, Ricci A Jr, Tsongalis G, Shen PU, Bona RD, et al. Kaposi's sarcoma following allogeneic hematopoietic stem cell transplantation for chronic myelogenous leukemia. Acta Haematol. 2000;104(2–3):115–8.
117. van Tol MJD, Kroes ACM, Schinkel J, Dinkelaar W, Claas ECJ, et al. Adenovirus infection in paediatric stem cell transplant recipients: increased risk in young children with a delayed immune recovery. Bone Marrow Transplant. 2005;36(1):39–50.
118. Taniguchi K, Yoshihara S, Tamaki H, Fujimoto T, Ikegame K, Kaida K, et al. Incidence and treatment strategy for disseminated adenovirus disease after haploidentical stem cell transplantation. Ann Hematol. 2012;91(8):1305–12.
119. Nichols WG, Guthrie KA, Corey L, Boeckh M. Influenza infections after hematopoietic stem cell transplantation: risk factors, mortality, and the effect of antiviral therapy. Clin Infect Dis. 2004;39(9):1300–6.
120. Nichols WG, Corey L, Gooley T, Davis C, Boeckh M. Parainfluenza virus infections after hematopoietic stem cell transplantation: risk factors, response to antiviral therapy, and effect on transplant outcome. Blood. 2001;98(3):573–8.
121. Avetisyan G, Mattsson J, Sparrelid E, Ljungman P. Respiratory syncytial virus infection in recipients of allogeneic stem-cell transplantation: a retrospective study of the incidence, clinical features, and outcome. Transplantation. 2009;88(10):1222–6.
122. Debur MC, Vidal LR, Stroparo E, Nogueira MB, Almeida SM, Takahashi GA, et al. Human metapneumovirus infection in hematopoietic stem cell transplant recipients. Transpl Infect Dis. 2010;12(2):173–9.
123. Milano F, Campbell AP, Guthrie KA, Kuypers J, Englund JA, et al. Human rhinovirus and coronavirus detection among allogeneic hematopoietic stem cell transplantation recipients. Blood. 2010;115(10):2088–94.
124. Weigt SS, Gregson AL, Deng JC, Lynch JP 3rd, Belperio JA. Respiratory viral infections in hematopoietic stem cell and solid organ transplant recipients. Semin Respir Crit Care Med. 2011;32(4):471–93.
125. Chemaly RF, Ghosh S, Bodey GP, Rohatgi N, Safdar A, Keating MJ, et al. Respiratory viral infections in adults with hematologic malignancies and human stem cell transplantation recipients: a retrospective study at a major cancer center. Medicine (Baltimore). 2006;85(5):278–87.
126. Hammond SP, Borchelt AM, Ukomadu C, Ho VT, Baden LR, Marty FM. Hepatitis B virus reactivation following allogeneic hematopoietic stem cell transplantation. Biol Blood Marrow Transplant. 2009;15(9):1049–59.
127. Giaccone L, Festuccia M, Marengo A, Resta I, Sorasio R, Pittaluga F, et al. Hepatitis B virus reactivation and efficacy of prophylaxis with lamivudine in patients undergoing allogeneic stem cell transplantation. Biol Blood Marrow Transplant. 2010;16(6):809–17.

128. Sanchez-Pinto LN, Laskin BL, Jodele S, Hummel TR, Yin HJ, Goebel J. BK virus nephropathy in a pediatric autologous stem-cell transplant recipient. Pediatr Blood Cancer. 2011;56(3):495–7.
129. Lekakis LJ, Macrinici V, Baraboutis IG, Mitchell B, Howard DS. BK virus nephropathy after allogeneic stem cell transplantation: a case report and literature review. Am J Hematol. 2009;84(4):243–6.
130. O'Donnell PH, Swanson K, Josephson MA, Artz AS, Parsad SD, Ramaprasad C, et al. BK virus infection is associated with hematuria and renal impairment in recipients of allogeneic hematopoietic stem cell transplants. Biol Blood Marrow Transplant. 2009;15(9):1038–1048 e1.
131. Dropulic LK, Jones RJ. Polyomavirus BK infection in blood and marrow transplant recipients. Bone Marrow Transplant. 2008;41(1):11–8.
132. Steurer M, Clausen J, Gotwald T, Gunsilius E, Stockhammer G, Gastl G, Nachbaur D. Progressive multifocal leukoencephalopathy after allogeneic stem cell transplantation and posttransplantation rituximab. Transplantation. 2003;76(2):435–6.
133. Goodrich JM, Reed EC, Mori M, Fisher LD, Skerrett S, Dandliker PS, et al. Clinical features and analysis of risk factors for invasive candidal infection after marrow transplantation. J Infect Dis. 1991;164(4):731–40.
134. Marr KA, Seidel K, White TC, Bowden RA. Candidemia in allogeneic blood and marrow transplant recipients: evolution of risk factors after the adoption of prophylactic fluconazole. J Infect Dis. 2000;181(1):309–16.
135. Goodman JL, Winston DJ, Greenfield RA, Chandrasekar PH, Fox B, Kaizer H, et al. A controlled trial of fluconazole to prevent fungal infections in patients undergoing bone marrow transplantation. N Engl J Med. 1992;326(13):845–51.
136. Slavin MA, Osborne B, Adams R, Levenstein MJ, Schoch HG, Feldman AR, et al. Efficacy and safety of fluconazole prophylaxis for fungal infections after marrow transplantation – a prospective, randomized, double-blind study. J Infect Dis. 1995;171(6):1545–52.
137. Marr KA, Seidel K, Slavin MA, Bowden RA, Schoch HG, Flowers ME, et al. Prolonged fluconazole prophylaxis is associated with persistent protection against candidiasis-related death in allogeneic marrow transplant recipients: long-term follow-up of a randomized, placebo-controlled trial. Blood. 2000;96(6):2055–61.
138. Neofytos D, Horn D, Anaissie E, Steinbach W, Olyaei A, Fishman J, et al. Epidemiology and outcome of invasive fungal infection in adult hematopoietic stem cell transplant recipients: analysis of Multicenter Prospective Antifungal Therapy (PATH) Alliance registry. Clin Infect Dis. 2009;48(3):265–73.
139. Horn DL, Neofytos D, Anaissie EJ, Fishman JA, Steinbach WJ, Olyaei AJ, et al. Epidemiology and outcomes of candidemia in 2019 patients: data from the prospective antifungal therapy alliance registry. Clin Infect Dis. 2009;48(12):1695–703.
140. Rossetti F, Brawner DL, Bowden R, Meyer WG, Schoch HG, Fisher L, et al. Fungal liver infection in marrow transplant recipients: prevalence at autopsy, predisposing factors, and clinical features. Clin Infect Dis. 1995;20(4):801–11.
141. Hart PD, Russell E Jr, Remington JS. The compromised host and infection. II. Deep fungal infection. J Infect Dis. 1969;120(2):169–91.
142. Held J, Kohlberger I, Rappold E, Busse Grawitz A, Häcker G. Comparison of (1->3)-beta-D-glucan, mannan/anti-mannan antibodies, and Cand-Tec Candida antigen as serum biomarkers for candidemia. J Clin Microbiol. 2013;51(4):1158–64.
143. Mora-Duarte J, Betts R, Rotstein C, Colombo AL, Thompson-Moya L, Smietana J, Caspofungin Invasive Candidiasis Study Group, et al. Comparison of caspofungin and amphotericin B for invasive candidiasis. N Engl J Med. 2002;347(25):2020–9.
144. Kuse ER, Chetchotisakd P, da Cunha CA, Ruhnke M, Barrios C, Raghunadharao D, Micafungin Invasive Candidiasis Working Group, et al. Micafungin versus liposomal amphotericin B for candidaemia and invasive candidosis: a phase III randomised double-blind trial. Lancet. 2007;369(9572):1519–27.
145. Lockhart SR, Wagner D, Iqbal N, Pappas PG, Andes DR, Kauffman CA, et al. Comparison of in vitro susceptibility characteristics of Candida species from cases of invasive candidiasis in solid organ and stem cell transplant recipients: Transplant-Associated Infections Surveillance Network (TRANSNET), 2001 to 2006. J Clin Microbiol. 2011;49(7):2404–10.
146. Pappas PG, Kauffman CA, Andes D, Benjamin DK Jr, Calandra TF, Edwards JE Jr, Infectious Diseases Society of America, et al. Clinical practice guidelines for the management of candidiasis: 2009 update by the Infectious Diseases Society of America. Clin Infect Dis. 2009;48(5):503–35.
147. Wald A, Leisenring W, van Burik JA, Bowden RA. Epidemiology of Aspergillus infections in a large cohort of patients undergoing bone marrow transplantation. J Infect Dis. 1997;175(6):1459–66.
148. Marr KA, Carter RA, Boeckh M, Martin P, Corey L. Invasive aspergillosis in allogeneic stem cell transplant recipients: changes in epidemiology and risk factors. Blood. 2002;100(13):4358–66.
149. Seo KW, Kim DH, Sohn SK, Lee NY, Chang HH, Kim SW, et al. Protective role of interleukin-10 promoter gene polymorphism in the pathogenesis of invasive pulmonary aspergillosis after allogeneic stem cell transplantation. Bone Marrow Transplant. 2005;36(12):1089–95.
150. Garcia-Vidal C, Upton A, Kirby KA, Marr KA. Epidemiology of invasive mold infections in allogeneic stem cell transplant recipients: biological risk factors for infection according to time after transplantation. Clin Infect Dis. 2008;47(8):1041–50.
151. Bochud PY, Chien JW, Marr KA, Leisenring WM, Upton A, Janer M, et al. Toll-like receptor 4 polymorphisms and aspergillosis in stem-cell transplantation. N Engl J Med. 2008;359(17):1766–77.
152. Kesh S, Mensah NY, Peterlongo P, Jaffe D, Hsu K, VAN DEN Brink M, et al. TLR1 and TLR6 polymorphisms are associated with susceptibility to invasive aspergillosis after allogeneic stem cell transplantation. Ann N Y Acad Sci. 2005;1062:95–103.
153. Zaas AK, Liao G, Chien JW, Weinberg C, Shore D, Giles SS, et al. Plasminogen alleles influence susceptibility to invasive aspergillosis. PLoS Genet. 2008;4(6):e1000101.
154. Mezger M, Steffens M, Beyer M, Manger C, Eberle J, et al. Polymorphisms in the chemokine (C-X-C motif) ligand 10 are associated with invasive aspergillosis after allogeneic stem-cell transplantation and influence CXCL10 expression in monocyte-derived dendritic cells. Blood. 2008;111(2):534–6.
155. Sainz J, Pérez E, Gómez-Lopera S, Jurado M. IL1 gene cluster polymorphisms and its haplotypes may predict the risk to develop invasive pulmonary aspergillosis and modulate C-reactive protein level. J Clin Immunol. 2008;28(5):473–85.
156. Martino R, Caballero MD, Canals C, San Miguel J, Sierra J, Rovira M, alloPBSCT and Infectious/nonifectious Complications Subcommittees of the Grupo Español de Transplante Hematopoyético (GETH), et al. Reduced-intensity conditioning reduces the risk of severe infections after allogeneic peripheral blood stem cell transplantation. Bone Marrow Transplant. 2001;28(4):341–7.
157. Fukuda T, Boeckh M, Carter RA, Sandmaier BM, Maris MB, Maloney DG, et al. Risks and outcomes of invasive fungal infections in recipients of allogeneic hematopoietic stem cell transplants after nonmyeloablative conditioning. Blood. 2003;102(3):827–33.
158. Labbé AC, Su SH, Laverdière M, Pépin J, Patiño C, Cohen S, et al. High incidence of invasive aspergillosis associated with intestinal graft-versus-host disease following nonmyeloablative transplantation. Biol Blood Marrow Transplant. 2007;13(10):1192–200.

159. Marr KA, Carter RA, Crippa F, Wald A, Corey L. Epidemiology and outcome of mould infections in hematopoietic stem cell transplant recipients. Clin Infect Dis. 2002;34(7):909–17.
160. Kojima R, Tateishi U, Kami M, Murashige N, Nannya Y, Kusumi E, et al. Chest computed tomography of late invasive aspergillosis after allogeneic hematopoietic stem cell transplantation. Biol Blood Marrow Transplant. 2005;11(7):506–11.
161. Marr KA, Balajee SA, McLaughlin L, Tabouret M, Bentsen C, Walsh TJ. Detection of galactomannan antigenemia by enzyme immunoassay for the diagnosis of invasive aspergillosis: variables that affect performance. J Infect Dis. 2004;190(3):641–9.
162. Boutboul F, Alberti C, Leblanc T, Sulahian A, Gluckman E, Derouin F, Ribaud P. Invasive aspergillosis in allogeneic stem cell transplant recipients: increasing antigenemia is associated with progressive disease. Clin Infect Dis. 2002;34(7):939–43.
163. Nguyen MH, Leather H, Clancy CJ, Cline C, Jantz MA, Kulkarni V, et al. Galactomannan testing in bronchoalveolar lavage fluid facilitates the diagnosis of invasive pulmonary aspergillosis in patients with hematologic malignancies and stem cell transplant recipients. Biol Blood Marrow Transplant. 2011;17(7):1043–50.
164. Marr KA, Laverdiere M, Gugel A, Leisenring W. Antifungal therapy decreases sensitivity of the Aspergillus galactomannan enzyme immunoassay. Clin Infect Dis. 2005;40(12):1762–9.
165. Machetti M, Furfaro E, Viscoli C. Galactomannan in piperacillin-tazobactam: how much and to what extent? Antimicrob Agents Chemother. 2005;49(9):3984–5.
166. Hage CA, Reynolds JM, Durkin M, Wheat J, Knox KS. Plasmalyte as a cause of false-positive results for Aspergillus galactomannan in bronchoalveolar lavage fluid. J Clin Microbiol. 2007;45(2):676–7.
167. Herbrecht R, Denning DW, Patterson TF, Bennett JE, Greene RE, Oestmann JW, Invasive Fungal Infections Group of the European Organisation for Research and Treatment of Cancer and the Global Aspergillus Study Group, et al. Voriconazole versus amphotericin B for primary therapy of invasive aspergillosis. N Engl J Med. 2002;347(6):408–15.
168. Walsh TJ, Anaissie EJ, Denning DW, Herbrecht R, Kontoyiannis DP, Marr KA, Infectious Diseases Society of America, et al. Treatment of aspergillosis: clinical practice guidelines of the Infectious Diseases Society of America. Clin Infect Dis. 2008;46(3):327–60.
169. Kontoyiannis DP, Hachem R, Lewis RE, Rivero GA, Torres HA, Thornby J, et al. Efficacy and toxicity of caspofungin in combination with liposomal amphotericin B as primary or salvage treatment of invasive aspergillosis in patients with hematologic malignancies. Cancer. 2003;98(2):292–9.
170. Marr KA, Schlamm HT, Herbrecht R, Rottinghaus ST, Bow EJ, Cornely OA, et al. Combination antifungal therapy for invasive aspergillosis. Clin Infect Dis. 2004;39(6):797–802.
171. Cordonnier C, Rovira M, Maertens J, Olavarria E, Faucher C, Bilger K, Voriconazole for Secondary Prophylaxis of Invasive Fungal Infections in Patients With Allogeneic Stem Cell Transplants (VOSIFI) study group, Infectious Diseases Working Party, European Group for Blood and Marrow Transplantation, et al. Voriconazole for secondary prophylaxis of invasive fungal infections in allogeneic stem cell transplant recipients: results of the VOSIFI study. Haematologica. 2010;95(10):1762–8.
172. El-Cheikh J, Castagna L, Wang L, Esterni B, Faucher C, Fürst S, et al. Impact of prior invasive aspergillosis on outcome in patients receiving reduced-intensity conditioning allogeneic hematopoietic stem cell transplant. Leuk Lymphoma. 2010;51(9):1705–10.
173. Gaziev D, Baronciani D, Galimberti M, Polchi P, Angelucci E, Giardini C, et al. Mucormycosis after bone marrow transplantation: report of four cases in thalassemia and review of the literature. Bone Marrow Transplant. 1996;17(3):409–14.
174. Roden MM, Zaoutis TE, Buchanan WL, Knudsen TA, Sarkisova TA, Schaufele RL, et al. Epidemiology and outcome of zygomycosis: a review of 929 reported cases. Clin Infect Dis. 2005;41(5):634–53.
175. Imhof A, Balajee SA, Fredricks DN, Englund JA, Marr KA. Breakthrough fungal infections in stem cell transplant recipients receiving voriconazole. Clin Infect Dis. 2004;39(5):743–6.
176. Nucci M, Marr KA, Queiroz-Telles F, Martins CA, Trabasso P, Costa S, et al. Fusarium infection in hematopoietic stem cell transplant recipients. Clin Infect Dis. 2004;38(9):1237–42.
177. Anaissie EJ, Kuchar RT, Rex JH, Francesconi A, Kasai M, Müller FM, et al. Fusariosis associated with pathogenic fusarium species colonization of a hospital water system: a new paradigm for the epidemiology of opportunistic mold infections. Clin Infect Dis. 2001;33(11):1871–8.
178. Boutati EI, Anaissie EJ. Fusarium, a significant emerging pathogen in patients with hematologic malignancy: ten years' experience at a cancer center and implications for management. Blood. 1997;90(3):999–1008.
179. Husain S, Muñoz P, Forrest G, Alexander BD, Somani J, Brennan K, et al. Infections due to Scedosporium apiospermum and Scedosporium prolificans in transplant recipients: clinical characteristics and impact of antifungal agent therapy on outcome. Clin Infect Dis. 2005;40(1):89–99.
180. Bhatti Z, Shaukat A, Almyroudis NG, Segal BH. Review of epidemiology, diagnosis, and treatment of invasive mould infections in allogeneic hematopoietic stem cell transplant recipients. Mycopathologia. 2006;162(1):1–15.
181. De Castro N, Neuville S, Sarfati C, Ribaud P, Derouin F, Gluckman E, et al. Occurrence of Pneumocystis jiroveci pneumonia after allogeneic stem cell transplantation: a 6-year retrospective study. Bone Marrow Transplant. 2005;36(10):879–83.
182. Torres HA, Chemaly RF, Storey R, Aguilera EA, Nogueras GM, Safdar A, et al. Influence of type of cancer and hematopoietic stem cell transplantation on clinical presentation of Pneumocystis jiroveci pneumonia in cancer patients. Eur J Clin Microbiol Infect Dis. 2006;25(6):382–8.
183. Lyytikäinen O, Ruutu T, Volin L, Lautenschlager I, Jokipii L, et al. Late onset Pneumocystis carinii pneumonia following allogeneic bone marrow transplantation. Bone Marrow Transplant. 1996;17(6):1057–9.
184. Tuan IZ, Dennison D, Weisdorf DJ. Pneumocystis carinii pneumonitis following bone marrow transplantation. Bone Marrow Transplant. 1992;10(3):267–72.
185. Mulanovich VE, Ahmed SI, Öztürk T, Khokhar FA, Kontoyiannis DP, de Lima M. Toxoplasmosis in allo-SCT patients: risk factors and outcomes at a transplantation center with a low incidence. Bone Marrow Transplant. 2011;46(2):273–7.
186. Slavin MA, Meyers JD, Remington JS, Hackman RC. Toxoplasma gondii infection in marrow transplant recipients: a 20 year experience. Bone Marrow Transplant. 1994;13(5):549–57.
187. Derouin F, Devergie A, Auber P, Gluckman E, Beauvais B, Garin YJ, Lariviere M. Toxoplasmosis in bone marrow-transplant recipients: report of seven cases and review. Clin Infect Dis. 1992;15(2):267–70.
188. Cavattoni I, Ayuk F, Zander AR, Zabelina T, Bacher A, Cayroglu E, et al. Diagnosis of Toxoplasma gondii infection after allogeneic stem cell transplant can be difficult and requires intensive scrutiny. Leuk Lymphoma. 2010;51(8):1530–5.
189. Edvinsson B, Lundquist J, Ljungman P, Ringdén O, Evengård B. A prospective study of diagnosis of Toxoplasma gondii infection after bone marrow transplantation. APMIS. 2008;116(5):345–51.
190. Bautista G, Ramos A, Forés R, Regidor C, Ruiz E, de Laiglesia A, et al. Toxoplasmosis in cord blood transplantation recipients. Transpl Infect Dis. 2012;14(5):496–501.

191. Derouin F, Pelloux H. Prevention of toxoplasmosis in transplant patients. Clin Microbiol Infect. 2008;14(12):1089–101.
192. Wirk B, Wingard JR. Strongyloides stercoralis hyperinfection in hematopoietic stem cell transplantation. Transpl Infect Dis. 2009;11(2):143–8.
193. Gupta S, Jain A, Fanning TV, Couriel DR, Jimenez CA, Eapen GA. An unusual cause of alveolar hemorrhage post hematopoietic stem cell transplantation: a case report. BMC Cancer. 2006;6:87.
194. Recommendations of the Center for International Blood and Marrow Transplant Research (CIBMTR®), the National Marrow Donor Program (NMDP), the European Blood and Marrow Transplant Group (EBMT), the American Society of Blood and Marrow Transplantation (ASBMT), the Canadian Blood and Marrow Transplant Group (CBMTG), the Infectious Disease Society of America (IDSA), the Society for Healthcare Epidemiology of America (SHEA), the Association of Medical Microbiology and Infectious Diseases Canada (AMMI), the Centers for Disease Control and Prevention (CDC), Tomblyn M, Chiller T, Einsele H, Gress R, Sepkowitz K, et al. Guidelines for preventing infectious complications among hematopoietic cell transplant recipients: a global perspective. Bone Marrow Transplant. 2009;44(8):453–558.
195. Ljungman P, Cordonnier C, Einsele H, Englund J, Machado CM, Center for International Blood and Marrow Transplant Research, National Marrow Donor Program, European Blood and Marrow Transplant Group, American Society of Blood and Marrow Transplantation, Canadian Blood and Marrow Transplant Group, Infectious Disease Society of America, Society for Healthcare Epidemiology of America, Association of Medical Microbiology and Infectious Diseases Canada, Centers for Disease Control and Prevention, et al. Vaccination of hematopoietic cell transplant recipients. Bone Marrow Transplant. 2009;44(8):521–6.

Complications Arising from Preparatory Conditioning Regimens for Stem Cell Transplantation

12

Jasmine Zain, Merav Bar, and Amar Safdar

Introduction

Hematopoietic stem cell transplantation (HSCT) is performed to provide long-term cures for patients with advanced hematological malignancies and other nonmalignant disorders. However, transplantation procedures can result in complications that can affect any organ system in the body. Many factors may contribute toward these complications including direct effects of old and newer modalities in transplant conditioning, severe and prolong pancytopenia, immunosuppressive antineoplastic drugs, graft-versus-host disease (GVHD), and infections, especially opportunistic viral, bacterial, and fungal infections. Factors that may help elucidate complications related to pretransplant conditioning include the following: (1) the incidence of complications appears to be similar between autologous and allogeneic stem cell transplants, (2) complication occurs less frequently in the setting of reduced intensity conditioning (RIC), and (3) complications associated with radiation therapy (XRT) and total body irradiation (TBI) are mostly abrogated when nonradiation-based preparatory regimen is administered. The differences between the risk for various complications among autologous and allogeneic stem cell graft recipients may not only represent toxicity from the conditioning regimen; patients undergoing allograft transplantation are also given immunosuppressive drugs for prevention and treatment of acute and/or chronic GVHD. Introduction of RIC may further assist in elucidating complications arising from drugs used for prevention and treatment of GVHD during the post-transplant period. Adults undergoing cord blood stem cell transplantation experience prolonged periods of pancytopenia, thereby placing such patients at an increased risk for infection and hemorrhagic complications. In this chapter a focused discussion includes systemic toxicities related with various preparatory regimens among adult patients undergoing stem cell transplantation based on aforementioned principles is presented [1, 2]. Where possible, the authors intend to identify effects of GVHD and/or underlying immune suppression that may have contributed toward various systemic complications.

J. Zain
Department of Hematology/Hematopoietic Cell Transplantation, City of Hope National Medical Center, Duarte, CA, USA
e-mail: jazain@coh.org

M. Bar
Clinical Research Division, Fred Hutchinson Cancer Research Center, Seattle, WA, USA
e-mail: mbar@fhcrc.org

A. Safdar (✉)
Clinical Associate Professor of Medicine, Texas Tech University Health Sciences Center El Paso, Paul L. Foster School of Medicine, El Paso, TX, USA
e-mail: amar.safdar@cidimmunology.com

Conditioning Regimens

Preparatory conditioning regimens given prior to HSCT have two main functions: (1) to provide tumor cytoreduction and (2), in allogeneic HSCT, to suppress hosts' immune response against the allograft and to prevent early graft rejection. Traditionally, preparatory regimens consist of high-dose chemotherapy and/or chemotherapy plus total body irradiation (TBI) with the objective for near-total eradication of cancer. However, high-dose, myeloablative conditioning regimens are associated with significant systemic toxicity including pancytopenia, injury to internal organs and skin. The regimen-related toxicity (RRT) poses a major obstacle in achieving successful transplant outcome. Modifications in traditional myeloablative conditioning include reduced-intensity conditioning regimens (RIC). Patients undergoing RIC are given lower doses of chemotherapy, and containment of cancer in the recipients mainly relies upon the donor graft-mediated anticancer cellular immune response known as "graft-versus-tumor" (GVT) or "graft-versus-leukemia" effect. RIC transplants are better tolerated and may be offered to older patients, patients with medical comorbidities, or "heavily pretreated patients" in whom multiple courses of

A. Safdar (ed.), *Principles and Practice of Transplant Infectious Diseases*, https://doi.org/10.1007/978-1-4939-9034-4_12

Table 12.1 Toxicities of common agents used in HSCT conditioning regimens

Agent	Known MTD	Acute DLT	Chronic DLT	Mechanism of injury	Treatment
Cyclophosphamide	200 mg/kg	Nausea, hemorrhagic myocarditis, acute CHF, SIADH, Cardiac arrhythmias, hemorrhagic cystitis resulting from secretion of active drug metabolites into the bladder	CHF	Direct myocardial toxicity due to leakage of drug from damaged endothelium; and renal tubular injury	Supportive care, use of Mesna to prevent hemorrhagic cystitis, and bladder irrigation
Melphalan	200 mg/m^2	Mucositis, GI toxicity, SOS, diffuse pulmonary alveolitis, and SIADH			
Busulfan	20 mg/kg given over 4 days, steady-state PKs over 4 days more predictable of toxicity than actual dose	SOS, neurotoxicity characterized by seizure; mucositis, radiation recall and pulmonary fibrosis, and gonadal toxicity	Ovarian failure, infertility, and azoospermia		
Thiotepa	1135 mg/m^2	CNS toxicity including somnolence, confusion and coma; oral and esophageal mucositis, enterocolitis, liver toxicity and SOS, acute dermatitis manifested as desquamating dermatitis; interstitial pneumonitis and cardiac toxicity			
1,3-bis (2-chloroethyl)-1-nitrosourea (BCNU)	900–1200 mg/m^2	Pulmonary toxicity, SOS, hypotension, myocardial ischemia, renal toxicity, and encephalopathy		Depletion of pulmonary glutathione reductase	
Cisplatin	300 mg/m^2	Renal dysfunction including electrolyte wasting; ototoxicity and high-frequency hearing loss; peripheral neuropathy; nausea and vomiting			
Carboplatin	1600–2400 mg/m^2	Liver toxicity, mucositis, peripheral neuropathy, ototoxicity, nephrotoxicity			
Etoposide	25–60 mg/kg or 2400 mg/m^2	Mucositis, GI toxicity	Secondary leukemias		
Doxorubicin	150–165 mg/m^2 delivered over 96 h as a CI	Cardiac toxicity (cumulative for doses above 350–400 mg/m^2, this may be lower in patients with existing cardiac risk factors), orointestional mucositis resulting in stomatitis, diarrhea, and typhlitis	Secondary malignancies		
Paclitaxel	725–750 mg/m^2	Peripheral neuropathy, and mucositis	Secondary malignancies		
Bortezomib		Peripheral neuropathy			
Bendamustine					
Fludarabine		Neurologic toxicity			
Clofarabine					
Ifosfamide	18–20 mg/m^2	Renal, and urinary bladder toxicity; neurotoxicity may present as somnolence, lethargy, confusion, and seizures			Mesna infusion
Cytarabine	36 gm/m^2 for 4–12 doses at 12 h intervals	Neurotoxicity, particularly cerebellar			
TBI	10–16 Gy	GI toxicity includes severe mucositis; hepatic and pulmonary toxicity	Growth retardation, chronic pulmonary insufficiency, secondary malignancies, and cataracts		Shielding of internal organs; targeted delivery of radiation like total marrow irradiation or total lymphoid irradiation

antineoplastic therapy have been given for the treatment of recurring or relapsed cancer; in the past such patients were considered high risk for traditional myeloablative HSCT. Recent advances in targeted antineoplastic drugs like radioimmunotherapy, proteasome inhibitor, and monoclonal antibodies are being incoorporated in preparatory regimens with the intent to minimize systemic toxicity. Table 12.1 provides an outline of adverse events associated with commonly used modalities for conditioning given in preparation for stem cell transplantation.

Orointestinal Complications

Damage to the mucosa of orointestinal tract is common in patients undergoing HSCT. The ensuing mucositis may be severe after myeloablative stem cell allograft transplantation. It is important to note that mucosal damage resulting from conditioning regimens can overlap with orointestinal acute GVHD and enterocolitis due to opportunistic cytomegalovirus or adenovirus infection. Therefore, it is essential to thoroughly evaluate the patients, especially if symptoms appear more than 2 weeks post-transplantation. Following are the common presentations of orointestinal toxicities among patients undergoing HSCT.

Emesis and Anorexia

Most conditioning regimens are associated with emesis and anorexia [3, 4]. The pathogenesis of chemotherapy-induced emesis includes direct drug-induced stimulation of central vomiting center and local injury to cell lining of the orointestinal tract. Nausea and vomiting in such cases can last for up to 3 weeks after transplant procedure [5]. The main process during days 1-10 following transplantion is damage to the mucosal lining, resulting in systemic translocation of bacteria and bacterial endotoxins, triggering various aspects of innate immune response that includes acute-phase protein, and local release of proinflammatory cytokines. Cytokines such as interleukin-1, interleukin- 6, and tumor necrosis factor alpha via systemic circulation penetrate the blood-brain barrier suppressed brain regulation of appetite may result in devestating anorexia. Conditioning-induced anorexia is prominent during the first 3 weeks after transplantation.

Mucositis

Oral mucositis is a common transplant-related complication, usually seen during the first 2–3 weeks after HSCT. Mucositis may affect up to 80% of transplant recipients and frequently associated with myeloablative regimens that include radiation [6]. Mucositis occurs in phases starting with erythema and atrophy progressing to ulceration and the final, healing phase. Mucositis is common with cytarabine, etoposide, high-dose melphalan, and treatement with multiple alkylating agents [7, 8]. Preexisting periodontal disease and prior radiation to the head and neck area increase the risk for mucositis. Chemotherapy-induced symptomatic mucositis usually starts 5–10 days after initiation of the conditioning and may take up to 3 weeks to heal. The healing phase can be delayed if additional factors like methotrexate used as GVHD prophylaxis, bacterial and fungal infections, and in patients with recrudescence of oral HSV infection. Morbidity and risk of death due to mucositis include severe oral pain and dysphagia with marked decline in oral calorie intake, recurrent bleeding, superimposed viral (HSV), bacterial and fungal (*Candida*) infections, edema of the upper airway, and airway obstruction. The extent and severity of oral mucositis correlates with the risk for infection, prolonged hospital stay, and hospital mortality [9]. Treatment is usually supportive and includes analgesia, oral rinsing solutions, and parenteral nutrition. Severe mucosal swelling and upper airway edema may require endotracheal intubation to secure patients' airway. Prevention strategies are developed to minimize the risk for mucositis. Palifermin, a recombinant human keratinocyte growth factor, it was approved by FDA for prevention of mucositis in patients undergoing autologous and allogeneic HSCT. Preclinical data in mice showed protective effects of palifermin against chemotherapy and radiation-induced mucositis [10–12] and led to clinical trials [13, 14]. Phase III study in patients following autologous transplants after TBI conditioning demonstrated a decreased incidence and duration of grade III–IV mucositis. Goldberg et al. conducted a retrospective study in 251 patients undergoing allogeneic HSCT, 154 of whom received palifermin during peritransplant period. In all patients, treatment with palifermin significantly reduced the number of days needed for (1) total parenteral nutrition (TPN; 13 vs. 16 days; $P = 0.006$), (2) patient-controlled analgesia (PCA; 6 vs. 10 days; $P = 0.023$), and length of hospitalization (32 vs. 37 days; $P = 0.014$). However, the effect of palifermin was only significant in patients who received TBI; this benefit was not evident in patients given busulfan-based conditioning [15].

Injury to mucosal barrier may also result in diarrhea, gastrointestinal bleeding, susceptibility to infections, and risk of death [16, 17]. Typhilitis is a particularly serious complication. Cecal edema, mucosal friability, and mucosal ulceration, accompanied with fever, abdomonal pain, and diarrhea are salient features; polymicrobial infections may reasult in severe sepsis [3]. The pathophysiology of neutropenic typhlitis is not fully understood; it is hypothesized that an acute mucosal injury caused by cytotoxic drugs serves as a trigger, followed by secondary infection of the bowel wall, progressing to systemic infection and sepsis with increased risk for bowel perforation [18]. Typhlitis may progress rapidly and mortality rate of up to 20% may be seen in high-risk patients. High index of suspicion, early diagnosis and timely institution of aggressive medical therapy that includes complete bowel rest, broad-spectrum antimicrobials, elecrolyte, mineral, and intravascular homeostasis among other supportive measures is essential for improve outcome [19].

Diarrhea

Diarrhea is seen in nearly half of patients receiving high-dose chemotherapy and radiation-based conditioning as a result of mucosal damage, which usually resolves within 3 weeks after transplantation [4, 20]. Patients with other complications such as superimposed infections or GVHD involving the orointestinal tract, the duration of diarrhea my be prolonged. Preparatory regimen with radiation, alkylating agents, cytarabine, high-dose melphalan, or busulfan frequently result in diarrheal illness. Radiation- or chemotherapy-induced diarrhea is classified as osmotic or secretory diarrhea [21, 22]. The underlying processes include (1) damage to the intestinal mucosa and crypts resulting in reduced chloride absorption causing an osmotic load, (2) alteration in gut motility with reduced transit time due to direct effect of chemotherapy, and (3) mucositis resulting in decreased water absorption. Additionally, chemotherapy and radiation change the composition of the native intestinal microbiota, which may also contributes to diarrhea following HSCT; intestinal yeast overgrowth may play a role in some patients. Organisms that may cause diarrhea in stem cell transplant recipients include infection due to exotoxin producing *Clostridium difficile* and, less commonly, tissue-invasive disease due to *C. perfringens*, and *C. septicum.* It is important to recognize that enterocolitis due to opportunistic viral infections such as CMV, and adenovirus are difficult to distinguish clinically from other causes of diarrheal illness in such patients.

Conditioning-Induced Liver Complications

Hepatic complications are a major cause of morbidity and mortality following HSCT. The frequency and severity of liver complications however, have declined in the recent years [23]. Hepatotoxicity due to pre-transplant conditioning is usually seen within the first 3 weeks after transplants [24]. Sinusoidal obstruction syndrome (SOS) or veno-occlusive disease (VOD) is the main complication. Treatment-induced damage to the endothelial cells in the hepatic sinusoids clinically presents as tender hepatomegaly, fluid retention, weight gain, and elevated serum bilirubin level [25–27]. SOS is a direct manifestation of conditioning-related hepatotoxicity. The major risk factors are radiation and specific chemotherapy agents used in high doses particularly cytoxan (Cy) and busulfan (Bu). Combination regimens with chemotherapy and TBI has shown a correlation between cytoxan and TBI dose. The incidence of SOS after conditioning regimens that include cyclophosphamide at a dose of 120 mg/kg plus TBI greater than 14 Gy can be as high as 50% [24]; however, the incidence of SOS can be minimized with reduced-intensity regimens [28]. In the past, gemtuzumab ozogamicin exposure was associated with the risk of SOS in patients undergoing myeloablative allogeneic HSCT [29]. Additional risk factors for SOS include: (1) variations in the metabolism of cyclophosphamide and other chemotherapy drugs [30, 31]; (2) underlying fibroinflammatory liver diseases [32], and (3) concomitant use of drugs during and after conditioning therapy that either affect the metabolism of cytotoxic drugs such as triazole-based antifungals, or cause concomitant liver injury like sirolimus (Table 12.1). During the 1990s, the overall incidence of SOS at Fred Hutchinson Cancer Research Center was 38% with 7% of the patients having severe disease after cyclophosphamide and TBI preparatory regimen. A favorable reduction (12% with 2% severe disease) was noted after oral busulfan plus cyclophosphamide combination was introduced [31, 33]. There has been an appreciable decline in the frequency and severity of SOS during the past decade and probably represent (1) lower doses of TBI being used, (2) replacement of cyclophosphamide with fludarabine, (3) conditioning regimens that do not contain either cyclophosphamide or high-dose TBI, and (4) therapeutic drug monitoring that allows individualized dosing of chemotherapeutic drugs adjusted for variability of drug metabolism [24]. Prevention of severe sinusoidal liver injury begins with an assessment of patients risk due to underlying liver disease (Table 12.2) and tailoring appropriate conditioning regimen for select group of at-risk patients [25, 31, 34]. There are no satisfactory treatments for SOS; however complete recovery from SOS occurs in more than 70% of patients with supportive care, that include management of sodium and water balance, preservation of renal blood flow, and paracenteses, as needed. Patients with poor prognosis are recognized by a steep rise in total serum bilirubin level, increase body weight, serum ALT level of greater than 750 U/L, portal pressure greater than 20 mm Hg, development of portal vein thrombosis, and development of multi-organ failure [24]. However, liver failure is an uncommon cause of death in patients with SOS; most patients die from secondary renal and cardiopulmonary failure, or both [26, 35]. Treatment with defibrotide, a compound porcine oligodeoxyribonucleotides with procoagulant and fibrinolytic properties may ameliorate SOS disease in select group of patients [36, 37]. Recent observation that octerotide prophylaxis may reduce the incidence of SOS after HSCT was interesting and needs further evaluation [38].

Table 12.2 Risk factors for SOS in patients undergoing HSCT [24]

Liver diseases at baseline	Specific conditioning regimens	Concomitant drugs during conditioning therapy
Inflammatory diseases	Cyclophosphamide-based	Itraconazole
Chronic hepatitis B or C	CY 120 mg/kg plus TBI (greater risk with higher TBI dosing)	Sirolimus (rapamycin)
Nonalcoholic steatohepatitis	BCV (BCNU + CY + VP-16)	Norethisterone
Alcoholic hepatitis	BU + CY (greater risk without therapeutic drug monitoring of BU)	
Fibrotic diseases	Melphalan-based	
Cirrhosis	BU + MEL + thiotepa	
Lobular fibrosis	BU + MEL	
Extramedullary hematopoiesis with sinusoidal fibrosis		
Cholestatic disorders	Other regimens	
Jaundice caused by intrahepatic cholestasis	BU + TBI (greater risk with higher TBI dosing)	
Past history		
Prior SOS from conventional chemotherapy	Gemtuzumab ozogamicin-containing myeloablative regimens	
Recent exposure to gemtuzumab ozogamicin	High-dose radiolabeled antibody myeloablative regimens	
Prior liver irradiation		
Prior myeloablative hematopoietic cell transplant		

Reprinted and adapted from McDonald [24], with permission from John Wiley and Sons

Conditioning-Induced Renal Complications

Acute Renal Failure

Acute kidney injury (AKI) is a common complication in patients undergoing HSCT, and usually seen within the first 3 months after transplantation [39]. The incidence, timing and severity is different among patients following myeloablative versus RIC preparatory regimen, thereby emphasizing differential nephrotoxic potential of conditioning regimens. In 1989 Zager et al. reported that 53% of patients who underwent myeloablative HSCT developed AKI after a mean 14 days post-transplantation [40]. Since then several studies have evaluated renal injury in patients undergoing myeloablative transplantation [35, 41–48]. First 3 months after transplantation is when most episodes of AKI are observed; the incidence range between 21% and 73% after myeloablative allogeneic transplants; it is 12–19% for patients undergoing autologous stem cell graft transplantation. The cause of AKI include: (1) direct renal toxicity from cytotoxic drugs; (2) indirect damage sustained from intense conditioning regimens, i.e., patients with SOS; (3) GVHD via cytokine- and immune-related kidney injury; (4) nephrotoxicity from calcineurin inhibitors such as cyclosporine and tacrolimus; (5) dehydration and other conditions with depletion of intravascular volume; and (6) opportunistic CMV, or adenovirus infections that may involve the kidneys. Myeloablative conditioning is an independent risk factor for the development of AKI [43]. Severe AKI was shown to be more frequent in patients undergoing myeloablative HSCT compared with those treated with RIC [41, 43, 44, 46, 49, 50]. Several studies have evaluated the incidence and time of occurrence of AKI in patients given RIC and ranges from 29% to 56%; most cases are observed during the 2nd month after transplantation [42, 43, 46, 49–55]. Factors shown to increase the risk of AKI in RIC transplant recipients include, requirement for mechanical ventilation [50], previous autologous SCT, preexisting chronic kidney disease (CKD) [56, 57], acute GVHD, CMV reactivation [49], incomplete HLA-matched stem cell allograft transplantation, presence of sepsis [55], methotrexate given for GVHD prophylaxis, three or more antineoplastic treatments before transplantation, and patients with preexisting diabetes mellitus [54].

Chronic Renal Failure

AKI in the early post-transplant period is a risk factor for CKD. In a retrospective study, 158 adults received myeloablative allogeneic HSCT [58], proteinuria was noted in 23% of patients; prevalence of stage 3 or stage 4 CKD was 17%. Initiation of chronic renal replacement therapy or kidney transplantation for end-stage kidney disease was performed in 4% after an average 11 years following transplantation. In this study, presence of AKI after transplant was significantly associated with the risk for severe CKD (≥ stage 3). Another large study included 1,635 adult and pediatric patients who underwent myeloablative or RIC HSCT at the Fred Hutchinson Cancer Research Center between 1991 and 2002 [59]. A total of 23% developed CKD at a median of 191 (range, 131–516) days after transplantation. Presence of AKI was a prominent risk for CKD in the late transplant period [59]. Lack of resolution of structural and functional renal abnormalities back to the baseline after AKI episode and persistence of reduced renal reserves predicted the risk for CKD [60, 61]. AKI after transplant was associated with a higher risk for hypertension, which further increased the risk for CKD [62]. RIC regimen did not reduce the incidence of CKD. In an another retrospective study, the risk for CKD was 55% at 6 months, 50% at 9 months, and 45% at 12 months after RIC transplants [63]. Overall, 66%

of the patients developed CKD within 1 year following RIC transplantation. AKI during the first 3 months following transplantation was associated with the risk for CKD. Hingorani et al. reported albuminuria (ACR >30 mg/gm and proteinuria as >300 mg per day) on day 100 was associated with greater risk of CKD 1 year after HSCT; they also found that overt albuminuria was associated with an increase risk of non-cancer relapse death, and reduced 1 year post-transplant survival [64].

Immune System Complications and Immune Reconstitution

Conditioning regimens are designed to suppress hosts' immune response in order to allow the donor hematopoietic stem cells to establish stable engraftment. After HSCT, there is a prolonged period of immune deficiency affecting both the innate and the adaptive component of immune system thereby enhancing hosts' vulnerability to a variety of infections and other complications. Several factors contribute to immune deficiency state after HSCT, including: advance age, preparative regimen like myeloablative vs RIC; source of stem cell graft such as bone marrow, vs. G-CSF-mobilized peripheral blood stem cells, or stem cells derived from umbilical cord blood; graft manipulation, donor-recipient human leukocyte antigen (HLA) and non-HLA (minor) antigen mismatch; drug-induced immune suppression, and presence of acute or chronic GVHD [65].

Innate Immunity

Epithelial barriers are an important component of innate immune defense that are compromised on account of chemotherapy and/or radiation-induced mucositis or mucosal disruption resulting from acute or chronic GVHD. Direct injury to epithelial cells and cell-cell junctions or desmosomes facilitate systemic translocation of pathogens and microbial byproducts through the skin intergumentary system, respiratory, orointestinal, and genitourinary tracts. The epithelial barriers often recover quickly after transplant, however, presence of secretory acellular antimicrobial components such as cationic peptides, lyzosome, secretory immunoglobulins may remain subnormal for a potentially extended duration, especially in patients with GVHD [66, 67]. Cells of the innate immunity, including neutrophils, natural killer (NK) cells, monocytes, macrophages, and dendritic cells including antigen-presenting cells (APCs), are destroyed by the conditioning regimen in patients undergoing autologous and allogeneic HSCT. Various classes of immune cells originating from the hematopoietic progenitor cells start the process of recovery within weeks after transplantation [68–70]. However, despite recovery of the innate cell counts, some of the cell functions may not recover fully for months after transplantation [65]. NK cells reach normal levels within 3 months after transplantation and regain their ability to destroy malignant cells early in the post-transplant period [71, 72]. Additional events like GVHD, opportunistic viral infections such as CMV, and medications particularly high-dose systemic corticosteroids may further dampen prospects of immune recovery.

Adaptive Immunity

Myeloablative preparatory conditioning regimens comprises of agents that have myeloablative capacity resulting in destruction of hosts' adaptive immune system. Restitution and recovery of adaptive immune response in recipients after allogeneic stem cell grafts transplantoriginates from mature lymphoid cells from the donor derived effecter immune cells. The newly engrafted stem cells differentiate into common lymphoid progenitors (CLP) a common precursor to both T and B lymphocytes. If T-cell depletion methods are not used, the graft also contains antigen-specific T cells and naïve T cells that undergo peripheral expansion outside the thymus; lacking capacity for self-recognition. The proliferation, maturation, and differentiation of the donor-derived T cells into a diverse immune repertoire are dependent on adequate thymic function in recipients and controlled by the expression of surface molecules on thymic stromal cells and cytokines secreted by these important regulatory cells [73]. Immune regulatroy thymic activity is a complex process; dependent upon the patient age and prior treatments at the time of transplantation. Chemotherapy and radiation before HSCT and as preparatory conditioning regimen results in thymic dysfunction causing delayed T-cell immune reconstitution [74]. B cells derived from the common lymphoid progenitors undergo differentiation in the bone marrow, and the number of B cells usually returns to normal levels within 1–2 months after HSCT; however, serum immunoglobulin levels may remain subnormal for several months after transplantation [75]. The maturation process of B cells is dependent on the interactions with antigen-specific T lymphocytes. Therefore, defects in T-cell maturation due to inadequate thymic function or ongoing iatrogenic immunosuppression may also adversely affects B-cell maturation and B-cell function. Plasma cells are relatively resistant to chemotherapy and irradiation; studies have shown that persistence of antibody producing residual plasma cells of hosts origin may linger for a year after HSCT [76, 77]. However, a durable source of antibody production requires both antigen-specific donor T cells and mature B donor-derived lymphocytes. RIC regimens are immunosuppressive rather than immunoablative, and the immunological outcome in RIC transplant recipients' depends upon the degree of elimination of the residual recipients' immune system following donor-derived T lymphocytes repopulation and functional recovery. The immune reconstitution after RIC HSCT is not significantly different from the immune reconstitution after myeloablative HSCT, although this occurs early after RIC transplants compared with patients undergoing myeloablative HSCT [78]. In most cases, T lymphocytes are all from donor origin within 3–4 months after RIC transplantation [79]. In patients following autologous HSCT, the number and function of NK cells return to normal as early as day 14 after transplantation; the quantitative and functional B-cell recovery may be delayed up to 18 months after HSCT, and T-cell subsets' (CD3, CD4, and CD8) recovery does not return to normal for a year or in some cases longer after transplant procedure [80].

The prolonged immunodeficiency state after allogeneic HSCT results in significant morbidity due to potentially life-threatening bacterial, viral, fungal and protozoal infections, this may also have a negative influence on the much desired graft-versus-tumor effect [81]. Since the immune reconstitution process after autologous HSCT is more rapid, opportunistic infections are not as common in patients undergoing these procedures [78].

Neurologic Complications

Conditioning regimens can lead to both short- and long-term neurologic complications in patients undergoing HSCT. In addition, patient may experience neurological symptoms due to neurotoxicity from immunosuppressive drugs or infections that directly or indirectly affect the nervous system. Up to 3% of patients will have neurological complications after autologous transplants; whereas 44% after allogeneic transplants may experience these complications [82, 83].

Neurologic Toxicity

Direct neurotoxic effects of specific chemotherapeutic agent and radiation can result in acute encephalopathy, and new-onset seizures, as well as long-term complications such as peripheral neuropathy and cognitive impairment may adversly impact patients' quality of life. Among the common chemotherapeutic agents used in conditioning, busulfan and carmustine (BCNU) are most likely to cause seizures as they readily cross the blood-brain barrier. About 10% of patients receiving high-dose busulfan, defined as 4 mg/kg for 4 days, will experience generalized seizures [84]. BCNU typically used in conditioning regimens for lymphoma and Hodgkin's disease may result in seizures at doses of 300 mg/m^2. Anticonvulsant prophylaxis is recommended when these medications are being administered. Oral phenytoin and levetiracetam are commonly used for this purpose, and it is imperative that a therapeutic level of the anticonvulsant be achieved before chemotherapy is commenced. Other agents associated with acute CNS toxicity include ifosfamide as part of high-dose ICE regimens that may result in seizures, confusion, mutism, disordered sensorium, and even comma. Ifosfamide neurotoxicity results due to the accumulation of chloroacetaldehyde, a chloral hydrate-like compound which is an important metabolite of the drug. There is no prophylaxis, but methylene blue has been used to treat neurological toxicity in select cases [85]. High-dose mechlorethamine used with TBI and fludarabine is also associated with encephalopathy; fludarabine-associated encephalopathy may present late in some patients. High-dose cytarabine used in BEAM and other conditioning regimens given for lymphoproliferative disorders is associated with cerebellar symptoms in over 10% of cases; permanent Purkinje fiber damage observed in nearly 3% of cases [86]. This can also result in seizures and transient encephalopathy. High-dose Ara-C can cause peripheral neuropathy and demyelinating polyneuropathy similar to Guillain-Barre syndrome [87]. Cisplatin and VP-16 are associated with a delayed axonal neuropathy that develops approximately 2 months after the administration of these drugs, and recovery is gradual and protracted [88]. Cisplatin neurotoxicity involves large sensory fibers resulting in a deficit in proprioception with preserved tactile and pain sensations without motor deficits. It correlates with cumulative toxicity with symptoms usually occurring at doses of 300–600 mg/m^2. Other problems include ototoxicity that involves high-frequency hearing loss, and ultimately speech frequency hearing loss may occur with continued drug exposure. Cisplatin has also been reported to result in CNS toxicity including Lhermitte phenomenon, which is presented as cortical blindness and seizures [89]. By contrast VP-16 and paclitaxel neuropathies affect all sensory fibers. Manifestations can include paresthesia and sensory disturbances of the distal extremities; cases of motor and autonomic neuropathy have also been described. Prior exposure to other neurotoxic agents like vincristine can exacerbate such symptoms. High-dose paclitaxel at a minimum dose of 625 mg/m^2 used in some conditioning regimens for solid tumors is associated with a high incidence of peripheral sensory neuropathy within 5 days after the drug is given [90]. High-dose methotrexate (5 gm/m^2) may be associated with transient leukoencephalopathy [91], while the use of intrathecal methotrexate can rarely result in hemiparesis. A delayed onset chronic leukoencephalopathy may result in patients after intrathecal MTX and whole brain radiation [92]. Neurologic signs develop within 4–5 months after transplantation and progress to dysarthria, ataxia, dysphasia, spasticity, upper motor neuron weakness, spasticity, seizures, confusion, and eventually death. The combination of TBI and amphotericin B has also been reported to lead to a similar leukoencephalopathy. Intrathecal cytarabine and the depot version are associated with a predictable aseptic meningitis due to meningeal irritation. Concomitant use of steroids either given intrathecally or systemically may ameliorate symptoms [86]. Some of the newer agents that are being used in conditioning regimens like bortezomib may cause peripheral neuropathy [93]. This is usually reversible with dose modification or discontinuation of the drug.

Central Nervous System Infections

Conditioning regimens lead to a period of pancytopenia and immune suppression that increases the risk for infections involving the CNS. Most of these present in the immediate post-transplant period, and late infections can also occur in patients with prolonged immunosuppression due to GVHD or graft dysfunction. The incidence of CNS infections is 5% in allogeneic transplants and as high as 8–15% in autopsy series [94]. The presenting symptoms are altered mental status, delirium, and altered sensorium. Meningeal signs or focal neurologic deficits are less common. Workup should include imaging studies and spinal fluid examination once intracranial mass lesion(s) with potential for herniation is ruled out. Aspergillosis was the most common infection accounting for 30–50% of CNS infections [94]. The newer mold-active triazole drugs like voriconazole have better CNS penetration as compared to other antifungals and currently recommended for the treatment of CNS aspergillosis. Systemic candidiasis in patients with fungemia can result in CNS involvements in nearly 3% of cases; seen in up to 15% in autopsy series [95]. Protozoal infections that include *Toxoplasmosis gondii* CNS disease mostly noted in the early post-transplant period, especially if patients, in whom prophylaxis with trimethoprim-sulfamethoxazole was deferred [94].

Bacterial infections are less common in the era of aggressive antibacterial prophylaxis and routine antimicrobial therapy for suscepted or porven infections. However, cases of meningitis due to *Listeria monocytogenes*, penicillin-nonsusceptible *Streptococcus pneumoniae*, and *Stomatococcus mucilaginous* have been reported in patients after allogeneic and autologous stem cell transplants; these infections are usually seen during the early post-transplant period. However, in patients with chronic GVHD, such infections may present late after HSCT. CNS mycobacterial infections are rare in patients undergoing HSCT [94].

CMV reactivation is a common and serious complication after allograft transplants. Unlike patients with HIV/AIDS, CMV chorioretinitis is seldom seen in patients following HSCT for reasons still not well understood [96]. Similarly, herpes simplex encephalitis is rare in post-transplant setting despite up to 80% of seropositive patients may experience high-level viral reactivation after undergoing stem cell transplantation. There are few reports in literature; the presentation and findings in HSCT recipients are mostly diffuse brain involvement that is not limited to the temporal lobe. EEG shows periodic lateralized epileptiform discharges characteristic of herpetic encephalitis and may precede before radiolographic changes become evident [96]. Activation of VZV mainly as mucocutaneous disease is seen 4–5 months after transplantation; viral encephalitis may seldom occur. Postherpetic neuralgias can develop in up to 25% of patients despite antiviral therapy and secondary prophylaxis. Cranial nerves can be involved resulting in symptoms of facial palsy, hearing loss, and unusual features like arm weakness from cervical neuralgia or a neurogenic bladder from the involvement of lumbosacral plexus [97]. Adenovirus and other herpes viruses like Epstein-Barr virus or human herpesvirus 6 can cause fatal meningoencephalitis during the periods of pancytopenia and severe cellular immunosuppression. Progressive multifocal leukoencephalopathy (PML) caused by JC virus is a rare complication that may present late after allogeneic transplantation and even rare among patients in whom autologous stem cell transplantation was performed years prior to PML presentation [98, 99].

Vascular Complications

In the early post-transplant period following myeloablative conditioning, patients are typically pancytopenic for nearly 2 weeks and are at risk for intracranial bleeding due to severe thrombocytopenia. Subdural hematoma may occur, whereas intracerebral hemorrhage is often fatal. Subdural hematomas are the most common form of intracranial hemorrhage in this group of patients; clinical presentation includes mental status changes without acute localizing neurologic signs [100, 101]. Treatment requires maintenance of platelet count of greater than 75,000/mm^3, correction of any coagulation abnormalities, and surgical treatment, as necessary [102]. The clinical presentation for intracerebral hemorrhage reported in up to 3% of allogeneic transplant recipients may present with an acute localizing neurologic event accompanied by decreased sensorium. Fatal transtentorial herniation may occur if not recognized and treated promptly with surgical decompression. Cerebellar bleeds may present with more subtle signs of gait abnormalities and nystagmus, which can progress to changes in sensorium.

Ischemic strokes can also occur in the early post-transplant period. These can arise from thrombotic emboli in patients with infectious and noninfectious endocarditis or a hypercoagulable state resulting from disseminated intravascular coagulation in patients with multi-organ failure (MOF) or severe sepsis [103, 104]. Rare cases of vasospasm associated with the infusion of cryopreserved stem cells have been reported [105]. Intracranial infections and meningitis can lead to endarteritis, resulting in an ischemic events; a compication occasionally seen in patients with CNS aspergillosis. Sinusoidal infections either bacterial or fungal may extend into the carotid artery and the venous cavernous sinus causing vascular compromise and stroke. Conditioning chemotherapy can lead to endothelial damage, which may be exacerbated by calcineurin inhibitors. The hypercoagulable state and non-bacterial thrombotic endocarditis carries a high risk for stroke. Thrombotic microangiopathy seen in 5–15% of stem cell transplant patients can also cause acute mental status changes. The presence of fragmented RBCs, elevated LDH, and renal insufficiency are the classic features. Treatment consists of discontinuation of calcineurin inhibitors, infusion of cryoprecipitate poor plasma, or plasmapheresis [104].

Metabolic Encephalopathy

Acute metabolic complications after conditioning regimens can lead to acute mental status changes that present as altered sensorium. The leading causes include sepsis, use of sedatives and other neurotrophic medications, hypoxia from various respiratory complications; uremia and liver failure [106]. Multi-organ failure (MOF) is a significant cause of mortality in patients undergoing transplantation. Severe CNS dysfunction is a salient feature of this syndrome, which is thought to reflect an excessive systemic inflammatory response. Prolonged critical care unit stay in transplant patients may result in critical care polyneuropathy that is thought to occur due to impaired blood flow to the peripheral nerves [107]. Vasogenic edema with characteristic radiologic findings has been associated with the use of calcineurin inhibitors. Radiation-based conditioning regimens and the use of high-dose chemotherapy may contribute to the breakdown of blood-brain barrier resulting in the release of endothelin and other vasoactive peptides that may trigger vascular and neurological changes well documented with calcineurin inhibitors [108].

Delayed Neurologic Complications

Intensive chemotherapy and radiation are well-recognized cause for chronic neurologic sequelae. Ongoing immunosuppression, GVHD, and infections may beother contributing factors. Both the central and peripheral nervous system may be involved; In general, the neurologic complications are less frequent among recipients of autologous stem cell graft compared with those undergoing allogeneic transplants. Leukoencephalopathy can arise in the setting of aggressive intrathecal chemotherapy in combination with cranial irradiation with TBI dose of 1800–2400 cGY or higher. This is an irreversible complication and can leave a patient in a permanent vegetative state. Adequate shielding of cranium and judicious use of intrathecal chemotherapy has reduced the risk for this devastating complication [109]. Vasculitic changes in the CNS as well as peripheral neuropathy have been described in the setting of GVHD. Cognitive impairment, memory dysfunction, and shortened attention span are reported in patients, particularly children after stem cell transplantation; these CNS complications may or may not be directly attributed to preparatory pre-transplant conditioning particularly patients receiving cranial irradiation [110, 111]. Radiation-induced neurocognitive impairment due to brain irradiation in patients with CNS lymphoma or leukemia, presents as a biphasic illness; a subacute transient decline that peaks around 4 months and a late irreversible neurocognitive dysfunction that becomes evident several months to years after brain irradiation was given [112].

Cardiovascular System

Cardiac complications occur at a rate of 2–28% despite aggressive pre-transplant screening and implementation of reduced-intensity conditioning regimens. They are an increasing problem as stem cell transplants are being offered to older patients. Congestive heart failure, and arrhythmias are common; pericardial effusions, and rarely, infectious or noninfectious endocarditis may be seen [113].

Acute Cardiac Complications

High-dose cyclophosphamide, prior history of anthracycline use, chest and mediastinal radiation are risk factors for CHF. This is exacerbated in patients with pancytopenias, particularly severe anemia, fluid overload, and renal dysfunction. Cyclophosphamide can result in cardiac toxicity within 3 weeks following administration. This occurs at doses above 150 mg/kg. Besides CHF, it can also cause pericardial effusion and cardiac tamponade. Pathophysiology of cyclophosphamide-related cardiac injury is related to endothelial damage resulting in extravasation of active drug metabolites into the myocardium causing direct cellular injury by severe depletion of cardiac thiol stores. Fractionated cyclophosphamide can reduce the incidence of cardiac injury. The risk of cardiac toxicity is increased by concomitant administration of cytarabine or mitoxantrone [114]. Melphalan and fludarabine, commonly used for reduced-intensity conditioning, are associated with a 2–14% incidence of cardiac toxicity in the acute setting [115]. Pancytopenia, particularly severe neutropenia following pre-transplant conditioning can lead to infections, which may present as pericarditis with pericardial effusions, and less commonly, endocarditis with or without valvular dysfunction. Cardiac arrhythmias can also be a manifestation of acute cardiac injury associated with conditioning regimens. Rituximab, cyclophosphamide, and melphalan are the most common agents associated with cardiac arrhythmias [116].

Delayed Cardiac Complications

Several antineoplastic agents that are part of pre-transplant conditioning can result in long-term cardiac complications. Late effects consist of arrhythmias, congestive heart failure, myocardial infarction, hypertension, angina, pericarditis, and valvular heart disease. In a study of 248 patients with chronic myeloid leukemia, the incidence of delayed cardiac complications was 33% compared with age-controlled general population, and the degree of cardiac impairment was greater after unrelated donor stem cell transplants (48%) as compared with 29% in related donor HSCT and 18% in patients following autologous transplants [117]. Other than direct cardiotoxicity from chemotherapeutic agents, GVHD appears to be a major factor associated with cardiovascular complications. There is an increased incidence of coronary artery disease in survivors of stem cell transplantation due to the delayed effects of chest radiation, hyperlipidemia associated with calcineurin inhibitor therapy, corticosteroid use, endocrine dysfunctions, physical inactivity, and overall physical deconditioning. Vascular sequelae of the seldom seen infective and non-infective endocarditis can lead to permanent valvular dysfunction; it is important ot note that sudden, severe aortic valve regurgitation is a life-threatneing cardiac emergency [118].

Pulmonary Complications

In nearly 60% of transplant recipients, pulmonary complications are expected and may result in 30% of deaths attributed to non-(cancer) relapse mortality (NRM) [119]. Pulmonary complications after transplant may have various causes such as infections, direct effects of the drugs or radition used in pre-transplant conditioning, non-cardiogenic pulmonary edema, fluid overload states, diffuse alveolar hemorrhage, and idiopathic pneumonia syndrome, as well as late obstructive and restrictive lung disease each with unique clinical and diagnostic features. GVHD also affects the respiratory tract [120, 121].

Infections

Severe neutropenia following high-dose conditioning regimens substantially increases the risk for acute pulmonary infections. Pneumonia is the leading cause of death after HSCT. In the first 30 days, patients are most susceptible to bacterial pneumonia with an incidence up to 15%. Myeloablative conditioning regimens are more likely to cause bacterial pneumonia compared with reduced-intensity regimens. Atypical clinical presentation and absence of consolidation on CXR is not uncommon in neutropenic patients with penumonia. Bacterial pneumonia can be a rapidly progressive illness resulting in acute respiratory failure and death. Therefore, high-index of suspicion is of paramount importance in managing patients during pre-engraftment neutropenia, in particular those with fever without localizing sign(s) of infection.

Respiratory viral infections due to respiratory syncytial virus, influenza, parainfluenza, and adenovirus can lead to debilitating acute illness in the early post-transplant period and in patients with GVHD-related prolonge immunosuppression [122, 123]. CMV reactivation and viral pneumonitis among other CMV manifestations of systemic disease are usually seen after engraftment, herald by recovery in peripheral blood cell count usually between day 30 and day 100 after transplantation. This is related to the ongoing immunosuppression in the post-transplant period rather than conditioning regimen-associated complication; furthermore, CMV end-organ disease is rarely seen in patients following autologous stem cell transplants [124].

Prolonged neutropenia, and continued immunosuppression increases the risk for invasive fungal disease (IFD); aspergillosis mostly involve lungs and less frequently paranasal sinuses with the risk for intraorbital and intracranial extension. These neurotropic filamentous fungi may cause intracranial infection via hemtogenous seeding. In recipients of cord blood stem cells, the incidence of invasive fungal infections is highest among adults undergoing allogenic HSCT; which in most part is a reflection of delayed hematopoietic engraftment and therefore, extended duration of neutropenia [125]. Chronic GVHD and drug-induced cellular immune suppression also places the patient at risk for invasive fungal disease. Dyspnea and cough are usually present. CT scan of chest should be obtained early and findings such as pulmonary nodules with the classic "Halo sign" indicating hemorrhage in the adjoining lung tissue that tends to disapper after first week of infection; dense areas of consolidation in peripheral lung, near pleura, or thick wall cavitation with seldom seen “air crescent sign” are highly suggestive of pulmonary IFD. Hyphae seen in bronchoalveolar lavage samples have a positive predictive value of 80%; however it has low sensitivity. Voriconazole and other mold-active triazole drugs such as posaconazole and isavuconazonium sulfate have replaced amphotericin B as the gold standard of therapy for most cases of pulmonary fungal disease. Echinocandins and lipid formulations of amphotericin B may still be used in select cases. The incidence of *Pneumocystis jirovecii* pneumonia was up to 15% in patients undergoing transplantation. Routine prophylaxis with trimethoprim-sulfamethoxazole has almost eliminated this serious fungal lung disease in the susceptible population. BAL is the diagnostic procedure of choice, with a yield of nearly 90%. Treatment consists of high-dose trimethoprim-sulfamethoxazole; corticosteroids are reserved for patients with severe hypoxemia.

Idiopathic Pneumonia Syndrome

Also known as interstitial pneumonia, is an acute pulmonary syndrome with widespread alveolar injury, with multilobar infiltrates, increased alveolar to arterial oxygen gradient, and restrictive pulmonary dys function in the absence of infection or cardiogenic lung disease. The histopathologic findings consist of interstitial pneumonitis; diffuse alveolar damage; cryptogenic organizing pneumonia (COP), formerly bronchiolitis obliterans organizing pneumonia (BOOP); and lymphocytic bronchitis. The incidence is 3–15% and associated with high-dose conditioning regimens compared to RIC; suggesting toxicity from pre-transplant preparatory regimen as a contributing factor. The incidence is also higher in patients who undergo allogeneic transplantation compared with patients given autologous stem cell grafts [126]. Symptoms occur early in the post-transplant period, usually within the first 100 days and are fairly typical for pneumonia such as dyspnea, fever, hypoxemia, and mostly non-productive cough. Infections need to be ruled out, and treatment consists of high-dose corticosteroids. This condition may rapidly progress to respiratory failure requiring assisted mechanical ventilation [121, 127]. COP is usually seen as a complication of GVHD within the first 1–3 months after HSCT. Pathologically it consists of small airway injury and interstitial inflammation with granulation plugs in the small airways. Patients with COP respond to high-dose steroids; however, long-term respiratory complications in such patients are not uncommon.

Diffuse alveolar hemorrhage (DAH) is seen in 5% of HSCT recipients. The characteristic features include fever, cough, and respiratory compromise during the early post-transplant period usually within the first 30 days. Diffuse ground-glass infiltrates are suggestive, by no means diagnostic. Diagnosis requires progressively bloodier return of BAL aliquots and 20% or more blood-laden macrophages. Patients may need mechanical ventilation, and treatment consists of corticosteroids given in high doses such as 125 or 250 mg of methylprednisolone every 6 h for 4–5 days followed by a gradual tapering steriod dose schedule. Mortality is high, up to 60% at 6 months. Risk factors for DAH include high-dose conditioning regimen, total body irradiation, renal insufficiency, older age, and previous history of GVHD [128–130].

Late-Onset Pulmonary Complications

Late complications affecting the airways and lungs are seen in 7–26% of patients undergoing HSCT; common causes are lung infections, TBI-based conditioning regimen, and GVHD [131, 132]. Mucositis due to aggressive preparatory conditioning reduces mucociliary clearance and mucous retention in the respiratory tract. Chronic inflammation ensues, alveoli and pulmonary interstitium are both affected, recurring or perisstent hemorrhage, and edema promotes fibrosis resulting in chronic obstructive and/or restrictive lung disease. High-dose regimens containing carmustine are known to cause delayed pulmonary syndrome seen approximately 10 weeks after transplantation. Symptoms consist of dyspnea, nonproductive cough, and fever. PFT show a mild restrictive defect although severe defect in lung diffusion capacity becomes evident. Radiographic presentation comprises of scattered diffuse ground-glass infiltrates. Patients respond to corticosteroids; however, progressive respiratory failure and death may occur in nearly 8% of patients [133, 134].

Bronchiolitis obliterans is seen as a late complication and often associated with chronic GVHD. Methotrexate and respiratory viral infections within first 100 days after transplants increases the risk of bronchiolitis obliterans. Some patients may progress to obstructive lung disease and respiratory failure [135].

Late idiopathic pulmonary syndrome (IPS) defined as a noninfectious interstitial pneumonitis may occur in 6–18% of HSCT recipients between 3 and 24 months after transplantation. It is characterized by thickening of the interstitial space with a cellular infiltrate, accumulation of fluid, and fibrotic tissue. Radiographic studies show diffuse pulmonary infiltrates, and the symptoms consist of progressive dyspnea, hypoxemia, and fevers. High-dose radiotherapy and GVHD are the risk factors associated with this complication. Treatment includes high-dose corticosteroid therapy [136–138].

Patients undergoing HSCT are at increased risk for secondary malignancies including lung cancer, head and neck cancers that are usually seen 2 years after transplantation. Total body irradiation during preparatory conditioning is a well-described risk factor.

Hematologic Complications

Myeloablative conditioning regimens are designed to erode marrow function completely; recovery of the resultant pancytopenia requires successful engraftment, which is an amalgam of variables such as stem cell graft source i.e., autologous vs. allogeneic; dose of nucleated stem cells; marrow-derived vs. PBSC vs. cord blood-derved; donor factors i.e., related vs. unrelated; ABO blood type, major, and minor HLA antigen compatibility. RIC is designed to creat a hosts' milieu of immune suppression rather than myelosuppression. Therefore, as expected RIC is associated with low systemic and myelotoxicity. The duration of pancytopenia is shorter and conceivably less infectious, and non-infections complications, including the need for transfusions.

Conditioning regimens are associated with hemolytic complications secondary to thrombotic microangiopathy (TM); a Coombs' negative hemolysis associated with RBC fragmentation, thrombocytopenia; renal and neurologic abnormalities [139, 140]. The incidence varies from 1% in autologous transplants and up to 70% in small series of patients following allogeneic transplants particularly where tacrolimus and sirolimus was used for GVHD prophylaxis [141, 142]. RIC is associated with 15–23% incidence of TM, with the highest risk in patients with prior myeloablative transplant (<6 months), suggesting a potential role of cytotoxic conditioning therapy for this syndrome [104, 143]. The majority of TM cases occur within the first 3 months after transplants. Unlike thrombotic thrombocytopenic purpura, ADAMTS13 deficiency or a decrease in the von Willebrand multimers cannot be demonstrated in the transplant-related TM. Mortality can be as high as 50–90% [144–146]. Pathophysiology of transplant-related TM consist of injury to the vascular endothelium from irradiation, dose-intense chemotherapy, as well as injury due to calcineurin inhibitors. Certain viral infections such as HHV6, parvovirus B19, CMV, or adenovirus; possibly aspergillosis may act as a trigger for post-HSCT TM. Treatment consists of supportive care, removal of offending agents, and potential role of the compliment inhibitor such as eculizumab [147–149]. Among long-term hematologic complications also include increased risk of MDS and acute leukemia during the late transpant period.

Endocrine Complications

The effect of pre-transplant conditioning on endocrine dysruption involves growth and skeletal development, metabolic function, gonadal and sexual function, and fertility. Radiation-based conditioning exposes the hypothalamic-pituitary axis to the effects of radiation at doses of 10–14 Gy [150]. The degree of damage is directly proportional to the cumulative radiation dose received with hypopituitarism observed with > or equale to 20 Gy. At the standard doses of 12 Gy used in TBI, the damage to the hypopituitary axis is minimal, however, concomitant or prior use of systemic and intrathecal chemotherapy may lower this threshold particularly in patients given high-dose methotrexate [151].

Growth Hormone Dysfunction

Children undergoing HSCT are highly susceptible; the incidence of short stature may range from 4–60% and correlates with young age at the time of transplantation. TBI and cranial irradiation are the strongest predictors for growth retardation due to: skeletal dysplasia of the spine by direct effects of chemotherapy and irradiation, radiation-induced hypopituitarism, hypothyroidism, and possibly precocious puberty resulting in early closure of bone epiphysis. In addition, use of glucocorticoids can blunt the secretion of growth hormone (GH), and direct effects of Bu and Cy on the epiphyseal growth plate may also contribute to growth retardation in children given radiation sparing preparatory regimen [152, 153]. In adults, there are no clearly recognizable syndromes associated with GH deficiency. However, GH deficiency may be associated with lean body mass and muscule wasting and increased body fat; cardiovascular adverse events and reduced bone mineral density [154].

Bone Metabolism and Osteoporosis

Patients undergoing HSCT exhibit bone loss particularly within the first 6 months [155, 156]. Typically, 5–15% bone loss is expected in lumbar spine and femoral neck within the 1st year after HSCT; osteopenia is noted in 50–60% and osteoporosis in 20% of stem cell transplant recipients [157]. The pathogenesis of bone loss in is multifactorial. Prolonged use of glucocorticoids, alterations in calcium and magnesium homeostasis in patients given calcineurin inhibitors contribute to bone loss [158, 159]. It is prudent to be aware of this complication, assess bone density by DEXA scans at regular intervals, and replenish calcium, vitamin D; and bisphosphonate therapy as indicated.

Thyroid Dysfunction

Thyroid dysfunction is seen 2–56%, and effects both autologous and allogeneic stem cell graft recipients [160, 161]. Conditioning regimen is thought to play a role, as expected, radiation-based conditioning would elicit direct damage to the thyroid tissue and to the hypothalamus and pituitary gland. The incidence of thyroid dysfunction after single dose irradiation is higher (23–73%) compared with 10–28% seen with fractionated dose therapy [162]. Similarly, patients undergoing allogeneic vs. autologous HSCT have higer risk for thyroid dysfunction as a result of immunosuppressive drugs [163, 164]. In the post-transplant period, thyroid dysfunction presents as euthyroid sick syndrome (ETS), hypothyroidism, autoimmune disease, or a thyroid nodule.

ETS is the most common thyroid dysfunction observed during first 3 months following HSCT. It is characterized by low free T3 and free T4 and a normal or low TSH; and regarded as an indicator for poor overall prognosis. Hypothyroidism is a common long-term thyroid complication after transplantation, with a cumulative incidence of 48% after 5 years and 67% after 8 years; however, median time to diagnosis is 4 years post-HSCT. Single-dose TBI carries higher risk for hypothyroidism (50%) compared with fractionated TBI (15%). The incidence of hypothyroidism is lower (11%) in patients given non-radiation conditioning. In this case the mechanism appears to be related to the effects of chemotherapy on the cytokines that control thyroid function; in addition GVHD may elicit thyroid dysfunction via immune/inflammatory pathway [163, 165, 166]. The incidence of thyroid nodules is higher in patients undergoing HSCT (27%) compared with the general population (4%) [162]. Although most patients with thyroid nodules have no symptoms, although 5–10% may be malignant, therefore, rigorous evaluation should be performed at the time of initial diagnosis and follow up. Patients, particularly children undergoing HSCT, have an increased risk for thyroid cancers compared with the general population, with an overall incidence of 0.2%. Radiation (TBI)-associated relative risk for nodules and thyroid malignancies is estimated between 0.6–14.9 and 3.6, respectively [167, 168].

Secondary Malignancies After HCT

Secondary malignancies are a rare and usually late complication; total body irradiation and chronic GVHD appears to be the strongest risk factors [169].

Solid Tumors

Secondary solid cancer following HSCT was performed by the Center for International Blood and Marrow Transplant Research (CIBMTR) [170]. Risk factors for solid cancers in a multi-institutional cohort of 28,874 allogeneic transplant recipients, who underwent myeloablative transplantation was assessed. Approximately 70% had received TBI-based conditioning. New solid tumors were reported in 153 transplant recipients, with a cumulative incidence of 1% after 10 years, 2.2% after 15 years, and 3.3% 20 years after transplantation. In this study, transplant recipients developed solid organ malignancies twice the rate of age- and gender-matched general population. Risk for tumors involving the oral cavity, liver, thyroid, bone, soft tissue, melanoma, brain and CNS were prominent. Risk for invasive solid tumor cancers was strongly related with age at time of transplant, exposure to radiation as part of the conditioning regimen, and development of moderate-to-severe chronic GVHD. However, risk factors for solid tumors differed by the type of tumor. Radiation was found to be a major factor for non-squamous cell carcinoma (SCC), especially among patients who had survived 5 years or longer after transplant. Whereas, chronic GVHD was associated with an increased risk for SCC, during both early and late post-transplant period [170]. The overall risk for secondary solid tumor was twofold higher in patients in whom radiation was a part of pre-transplant conditioning compared with patients given radiation sparing prepartory regimen. The increased solid tumor risk with radiation was most significant for patients younger than 10 years of age at the time of transplantation and remained high up to the age of 30 years. Patients 30 years and older at the time of transplant did not display higher risk for secondary solid organ malignancies despite receiving TBI conditioning.

The risks of secondary solid organ malignancies in nonradiation-based HSCT conditioning, with busulfan-cyclophosphamide was evlauted in 4,318 patients [171]. The cumulative incidence of solid cancers was 0.8% after 5 years and 2% after 10 years following transplantation. HSCT recipients had 1.4× higher rate of solid organ cancer compared with age- and gender-matched general population. Lung cancer was common, followed by breast cancer; significantly elevated risk was also observed for tumors involving the oral cavity, esophagus, soft tissue, and brain. On multivariate analysis, old age, lower performance status at time of transplantation, and chronic GVHD were important predictors for such cancers [171]. It is hypothesized that busulfan can cause pulmonary injury and fibrosis [172]; exposure to alkylator chemotherapy and particularly in patients with history of smoking increases the risk for lung cancer [173]. There might have been a synergistic carcinogenic effect of smoking and busulfan-cyclophosphamide lung cancer in non-TBI HSCT study [170, 171, 174–177].

The pathophysiology of secondary solid organ malignancies after allogeneic HSCT is not well understood and most likely a culmination of number of factors. Differences in type of malignancies related with TBI exposure versus busulfan-cyclophosphamide preparatory therapy or chronic GVHD suggest divergent carcinogensis pathways. Radiation may increase the risk of post-transplant malignancies by inhibiting DNA repair mechanisms resulting in gene translocation and gene instability due to breaks in double-strand DNA. Chronic GVHD and prolong exposure to immunosuppressive drugs likely increase the risk for secondary malignancies by inhibiting cancer-protecting immunologic defense mechanisms; for example, increased incidence of SCC involving female genital tract or head and neck cancer due to infection with human papilloma virus is related with chronic GVHD and prolonged immunosuppressive therapy [170, 171, 177–179].

Post-Transplant Lymphoproliferative Disorder

Post-transplant lymphoproliferative disorder (PTLD) is a serious complication in patients undergoing solid organ transplants (SOT) and allogeneic HSCT. PTLD is a heterogeneous group of lymphoproliferative diseases with a wide-spectrum of underlying pathology and clinical manifestations that range from benign lymphoid hyperplasia to aggressive lymphoma [180]. The incidence of PTLD is 1–10% after SOT and 0.5–1% after HSCT [181–185]. Most SOT-related PTLD is of host origin [186], whereas PTLD in allogeneic HSCT recipients is predominately of donor origin [187]. The highest risk for PTLD is in patients with drug-induced severe immune suppression for prevention and treatment of solid organ allograft rejection; rate between 10% and 25% are observed in SOT subgroup that require high doses of antirejection therapy that is commonly given for a prolong duration after heart, lung, and multivisceral transplants [181, 182, 188]. The incidence rates are lower (1% and 5%) after kidney and liver transplantation, as these patients in most cases, do not require intense drug-induced immunosuppressive state [184, 188]. An estimated 50–70% of all PLTD cases are associated with EBV infection [189–191], the risk is higher in EBV-negative recipient given allograft from EBV-positive donor [190, 192].

In HSCT recipients, the main risk factors for PTLD are T-cell depletion (TCD), and HLA mismatch, unrelated donor graft transplants. Severity of GVHD, and transplantation for primary immune deficiency disorders are additional contributing factors [185, 187, 193]. The median time from transplantation for PTLD in SOT patients varies from 30 to 72 months [183, 189, 194–197]. Among HSCT recipients, PTLD has a more rapid onset with a median time between 4 and 6 months after transplantation [185, 187, 198].

The incidence of EBV-negative PTLD is 10–20%; it usually occurs late and responds poorly to treatment [169, 196, 197]. PTLD have a diverse clinical presentation based on location and the degree an organ is involved. Presenting symptoms include fever, lymphadenopathy, weight loss, anorexia, fatigue, sepsis-like syndrome, and multi-organ dysfunction. Extra-nodal involvement is relatively common; sites such as the gastrointestinal tract, lung, skin, bone marrow, and central nervous system are frequently affected [183, 189, 194, 197, 199, 200]. PTLD in patients after HSCT usually has an aggressive course with extensive disseminated disease, involving multiple organs [201]. Prognostic factors associated with poor survival include older age, elevated LDH, presence of B symptoms, multi-organ involvement, decreased performance status, advanced stage of the disease, involvement of the allograft in solid organ recipients, >1 extra-nodal sites, and CNS or bone marrow involvement [202, 203]. At present there is no consensus on standard treatment for PTLD; reduction in immune suppression, when possible is the main treatment strategy. Additional therapeutic options include rituximab, chemotherapy, antiviral therapy, cytokine therapy, adoptive immunotherapy, surgery, and radiation [202, 204]. Given the heterogeneity of PTLD, survival is variable with an overall median survival range between ~1.5 and 8 years [180]. Mortality rate may be high (70–90%) in patients following high-risk allogeneic HSCT [185].

Secondary Myelodysplastic Syndrome and Leukemia

Recipient-Derived Myelodysplastic Syndrome and Acute Myelogenous Leukemia

Treatment-related myelodysplastic syndrome (MDS) and acute myelogenous leukemia (AML) may occur after autologous HSCT. Up to 10% of patients with lymphoma treated with either conventional or high-dose antineoplastic therapy, and those after autologous stem cell transplants may develop treatment-related MDS or AML within 10 years after the primary therapy [205, 206]. Main risk factors are prior exposure to alkylating agents and the purine nucleotide analog like fludarabine, and TBI as part of the preparatory regimen [205, 206]. Cases of treatment-related MDS/AML have been reported in patients who were treated with radioimmunotherapy; however the possible contribution of radioimmunotherapy to the risk for secondary malignancies is still unclear since most patients had been previously treated with alkylating agents [207]. The pathogenesis of alkylating drug and TBI-induced MDS/AML is a result of chromosomal damage of hematopoietic precursors; possibly other yet unknown tumor promoting external elements and unrecognized hosts' genetic haecceity may also play a role. The neoplastic transformation of the hematopoietic stem cells is a multiple step process, which is most likely initiated by prior exposure to cytotoxic drugs and accelerated by high-dose chemo- and radiation therapy used in transplant conditioning. Therefore, patients undergoing autologous HSCT should be carefully evaluated for pre-transplantation risk(s) for secondary MDS/AML, and selection of conditioning regimen must be tailored accordingly.

Donor-Derived MDS and AML

In the allogeneic setting, secondary MDS and AML after HSCT are thought to occur as a result of oncogenic transformation of the apparently normal donor hematopoietic stem cells exposed to a foreign environment [208]. Donor-derived MDS/AML is a rare complication after HSCT, and its incidence has been reported between 0.12% and 5% [208–210]. Alteration of the bone marrow microenvironment following allogeneic stem cell transplantation resulting from high -doses cytotoxic and immunosuppressive drugs may influence normal hematopoietic progenitor cells to undergo leukemic transformation via a complex mechanism(s) that may involve interaction between donor hematopoietic progenitor cells, and recipients' unique stromal cells and signalling milieu, influence of growth factors, selective impact via cytokines and chemokine dysregulation, among others [208]. In large survey conducted by European Group for Blood and Marrow Transplantation (EBMT), 14 donor-derived leukemia were reported among 10,489 allogeneic HSCT recipients. The median time to onset was 17 months, with a range of 4–164 months after transplantation. No specific risk factors, such as type of conditioning regimen, donor graft manipulation, or type and degree of recipients' immune suppression were identified [209]. It is important to differentiate secondary leukemia after allogenic transplant from relapse of the original disease, which is an important cause of death in patients undergoing allogeneic stem cell transplantation [211].

The current understanding of secondary malignancies after HSCT is based on studies that evaluated mainly patients who have received myeloablative conditioning. Less is known about the repertoire and risks for secondary malignancies after reduced-intensity HSCT recipients; long-term follow up studies are needed to assess post-transplant cancer risk this population.

Conclusion

HSCT is an effective life-saving treatment modality for many hematologic malignancies and a growing number of nonmalignant hematologic and autoimmune disorders. However, as discussed in the aforementioned text, there are a number of short- and long-term complications associated with preparatory regimens given prior to transplantation. In this chapter, we have enumerated common and less frequently noted complications attributed to various conditioning regimens used to achieve cytoreduction, antitumor effect, myeloablation, and immunosuppression. Additional complications and toxicities may occur as a result of GVHD, opportunistic infections, and disruption in various aspects of hosts' immune response. Whenever the transplant procedure is performed, a life is at risk, and the question of risk vs. benefit needs to be discussed in great detail with the patient along with quality of life issues and reasonable expectations in near and far post-transplant period. The goal always is to minimize transplant-related risks, which can be achieved with better understanding of such complications. As we move forward into the era of targeted and molecular biologics, it remains imperative that feasiability of new agents with better therapeutic index and safety profiles be incorporated in next generation preparatory regimens with the aim to reduce the burden of complications and achieve sustained cancer remission following hematopoietic stem cell transplantation.

References

1. Zain J, O'Connor O. Pralatrexate: basic understanding and clinical development. Expert Opin Pharmacother. 2010;11(10):1705–14.
2. O'Connor OA, Pro B, Pinter-Brown L, Bartlett N, Popplewell L, Coiffier B, et al. Pralatrexate in patients with relapsed or refractory peripheral T-cell lymphoma: results from the pivotal PROPEL study. J Clin Oncol. 2011;29(9):1182–9.
3. Strater SI, McDonald GB. In: Appelbaum FR, Forman SJ, Negrin RS, Blume KG, editors. Thomas' hematopoietic cell transplantation. Wiley-Blackwell, Hoboken, NJ; 2009. p. 1434–55.
4. Tuncer HH, Rana N, Milani C, Darko A, Al-Homsi SA. Gastrointestinal and hepatic complications of hematopoietic stem cell transplantation. World J Gastroenterol. 2012;18(16):1851–60.
5. Malone FR, Leisenring WM, Storer BE, Lawler R, Stern JM, Aker SN, et al. Prolonged anorexia and elevated plasma cytokine levels following myeloablative allogeneic hematopoietic cell transplant. Bone Marrow Transplant. 2007;40(8):765–72.
6. Vera-Llonch M, Oster G, Ford CM, Lu J, Sonis S. Oral mucositis and outcomes of allogeneic hematopoietic stem-cell transplantation in patients with hematologic malignancies. Support Care Cancer. 2007;15(5):491–6.
7. Sonis ST, Elting LS, Keefe D, Peterson DE, Schubert M, Hauer-Jensen M, et al. Perspectives on cancer therapy-induced mucosal injury: pathogenesis, measurement, epidemiology, and consequences for patients. Cancer. 2004;100(9 Suppl):1995–2025.
8. Wardley AM, Jayson GC, Swindell R, Morgenstern GR, Chang J, Bloor R, et al. Prospective evaluation of oral mucositis in patients receiving myeloablative conditioning regimens and haemopoietic progenitor rescue. Br J Haematol. 2000;110(2):292–9.
9. Sonis ST, Oster G, Fuchs H, Bellm L, Bradford WZ, Edelsberg J, et al. Oral mucositis and the clinical and economic outcomes of hematopoietic stem-cell transplantation. J Clin Oncol. 2001;19(8):2201–5.
10. Dorr W, Noack R, Spekl K, Farrell CL. Modification of oral mucositis by keratinocyte growth factor: single radiation exposure. Int J Radiat Biol. 2001;77(3):341–7.
11. Farrell CL, Bready JV, Rex KL, Chen JN, DiPalma CR, Whitcomb KL, et al. Keratinocyte growth factor protects mice from chemotherapy and radiation-induced gastrointestinal injury and mortality. Cancer Res. 1998;58(5):933–9.
12. Farrell CL, Rex KL, Kaufman SA, Dipalma CR, Chen JN, Scully S, Lacey DL. Effects of keratinocyte growth factor in the squamous epithelium of the upper aerodigestive tract of normal and irradiated mice. Int J Radiat Biol. 1999;75(5):609–20.
13. Meropol NJ, Somer RA, Gutheil J, Pelley RJ, Modiano MR, Rowinsky EK, et al. Randomized phase I trial of recombinant human keratinocyte growth factor plus chemotherapy: potential role as mucosal protectant. J Clin Oncol. 2003;21(8):1452–8.
14. Spielberger R, Stiff P, Bensinger W, Gentile T, Weisdorf D, Kewalramani T, et al. Palifermin for oral mucositis after intensive therapy for hematologic cancers. N Engl J Med. 2004;351(25):2590–8.
15. Goldberg JD, Zheng J, Castro-Malaspina H, Jakubowski AA, Heller G, van den Brink MR, Perales MA. Palifermin is efficacious in recipients of TBI-based but not chemotherapy-based allogeneic hematopoietic stem cell transplants. Bone Marrow Transplant. 2013;48(1):99–104. Epub 2012 Jul 2

16. Rapoport AP, Miller Watelet LF, Linder T, Eberly S, Raubertas RF, Lipp J, et al. Analysis of factors that correlate with mucositis in recipients of autologous and allogeneic stem-cell transplants. J Clin Oncol. 1999;17(8):2446–53.
17. Blijlevens NM, Donnelly JP, de Pauw BE. Prospective evaluation of gut mucosal barrier injury following various myeloablative regimens for haematopoietic stem cell transplant. Bone Marrow Transplant. 2005;35(7):707–11.
18. Morgan C, Tillett T, Braybrooke J, Ajithkumar T. Management of uncommon chemotherapy-induced emergencies. Lancet Oncol. 2011;12(8):806–14.
19. Altinel E, Yarali N, Isik P, Bay A, Kara A, Tunc B. Typhlitis in acute childhood leukemia. Med Princ Pract. 2012;21(1):36–9.
20. Epstein RJ, McDonald GB, Sale GE, Shulman HM, Thomas ED. The diagnostic accuracy of the rectal biopsy in acute graft-versus-host disease: a prospective study of thirteen patients. Gastroenterology. 1980;78(4):764–71.
21. Gibson RJ, Keefe DM. Cancer chemotherapy-induced diarrhoea and constipation: mechanisms of damage and prevention strategies. Support Care Cancer. 2006;14(9):890–900.
22. Stringer AM, Gibson RJ, Bowen JM, Logan RM, Yeoh AS, Keefe DM. Chemotherapy-induced mucositis: the role of gastrointestinal microflora and mucins in the luminal environment. J Supp Oncol. 2007;5(6):259–67.
23. Gooley TA, Chien JW, Pergam SA, Hingorani S, Sorror ML, Boeckh M, et al. Reduced mortality after allogeneic hematopoietic-cell transplantation. N Engl J Med. 2010;363(22):2091–101.
24. McDonald GB. Hepatobiliary complications of hematopoietic cell transplantation, 40 years on. Hepatology. 2010;51(4):1450–60.
25. DeLeve LD, Shulman HM, McDonald GB. Toxic injury to hepatic sinusoids: sinusoidal obstruction syndrome (veno-occlusive disease). Semin Liver Dis. 2002;22(1):27–42.
26. Coppell JA, Richardson PG, Soiffer R, Martin PL, Kernan NA, Chen A, et al. Hepatic veno-occlusive disease following stem cell transplantation: incidence, clinical course, and outcome. Biol Blood Marrow Transplant. 2010;16(2):157–68.
27. Howard M, Shulman LBF, Gary Schoch H, Henne KW, McDonald GB. Venoocclusive disease of the liver after marrow transplantation: histological correlates of clinical signs and symptoms. Hepatology. 1994;19(5):1171–81.
28. Hogan WJ, Maris M, Storer B, Sandmaier BM, Maloney DG, Schoch HG, Woolfrey AE, Shulman HM, Storb R, McDonald GB. Hepatic injury after nonmyeloablative conditioning followed by allogeneic hematopoietic cell transplantation: a study of 193 patients. Blood. 2004;103(1):78–84.
29. Wadleigh M, Richardson PG, Zahrieh D, Lee SJ, Cutler C, Ho V, et al. Prior gemtuzumab ozogamicin exposure significantly increases the risk of veno-occlusive disease in patients who undergo myeloablative allogeneic stem cell transplantation. Blood. 2003;102(5):1578–82.
30. McCune JS, Batchelder A, Guthrie KA, Witherspoon R, Appelbaum FR, Phillips B, et al. Personalized dosing of cyclophosphamide in the total body irradiation-cyclophosphamide conditioning regimen: a phase II trial in patients with hematologic malignancy. Clin Pharmacol Ther. 2009;85(6):615–22.
31. McDonald GB, Slattery JT, Bouvier ME, Ren S, Batchelder AL, Kalhorn TF, et al. Cyclophosphamide metabolism, liver toxicity, and mortality following hematopoietic stem cell transplantation. Blood. 2003;101(5):2043–8.
32. Strasser SI, Myerson D, Spurgeon CL, Sullivan KM, Storer B, Schoch HG, et al. Hepatitis C virus infection and bone marrow transplantation: a cohort study with 10-year follow-up. Hepatology. 1999;29(6):1893–9.
33. McCune JS, Batchelder A, Deeg HJ, Gooley T, Cole S, Phillips B, et al. Cyclophosphamide following targeted oral busulfan as conditioning for hematopoietic cell transplantation: pharmacokinetics, liver toxicity, and mortality. Biol Blood Marrow Transplant. 2007;13(7):853–62.
34. McDonald GB, Frieze D. A problem-oriented approach to liver disease in oncology patients. Gut. 2008;57(7):987–1003.
35. Hingorani SR, Guthrie K, Batchelder A, Schoch G, Aboulhosn N, Manchion J, McDonald GB. Acute renal failure after myeloablative hematopoietic cell transplant: incidence and risk factors. Kidney Int. 2005;67(1):272–7.
36. Chopra R, Eaton JD, Grassi A, Potter M, Shaw B, Salat C, et al. Defibrotide for the treatment of hepatic veno-occlusive disease: results of the European compassionate-use study. Br J Haematol. 2000;111(4):1122–9.
37. Richardson P, Linden E, Revta C, Ho V. Use of defibrotide in the treatment and prevention of veno-occlusive disease. Expert Rev Hematol. 2009;2(4):365–76.
38. Corbacioglu S, Cesaro S, Faraci M, Valteau-Couanet D, Gruhn B, Rovelli A, et al. Defibrotide for prophylaxis of hepatic veno-occlusive disease in paediatric haemopoietic stem-cell transplantation: an open-label, phase 3, randomised controlled trial. Lancet. 2012;379(9823):1301–9.
39. Lopes JA, Jorge S. Acute kidney injury following HCT: incidence, risk factors and outcome. Bone Marrow Transplant. 2011;46(11):1399–408.
40. Zager RA, O'Quigley J, Zager BK, Alpers CE, Shulman HM, Gamelin LM, et al. Acute renal failure following bone marrow transplantation: a retrospective study of 272 patients. Am J Kidney Dis. 1989;13(3):210–6.
41. Parikh CR, McSweeney PA, Korular D, Ecder T, Merouani A, Taylor J, et al. Renal dysfunction in allogeneic hematopoietic cell transplantation. Kidney Int. 2002;62:566–73.
42. Hahn T, Rondeau C, Shaukat A, Jupudy V, Miller A, Alam AR, et al. Acute renal failure requiring dialysis after allogeneic blood and marrow transplantation identifies very poor prognosis patients. Bone Marrow Transplant. 2003;32(4):405–10.
43. Parikh CR, Schrier RW, Storer B, Diaconescu R, Sorror ML, Maris MB, et al. Comparison of ARF after myeloablative and nonmyeloablative hematopoietic cell transplantation. Am J Kidney Dis. 2005;45(3):502–9.
44. Kersting S, Koomans HA, Hene RJ, Verdonck LF. Acute renal failure after allogeneic myeloablative stem cell transplantation: retrospective analysis of incidence, risk factors and survival. Bone Marrow Transplant. 2007;39(6):359–65.
45. Lopes JA, Jorge S, Silva S, de Almeida E, Abreu F, Martins C, et al. An assessment of the RIFLE criteria for acute renal failure following myeloablative autologous and allogeneic haematopoietic cell transplantation. Bone Marrow Transplant. 2006;38(5):395.
46. Ando M, Mori J, Ohashi K, Akiyama H, Morito T, Tsuchiya K, et al. A comparative assessment of the RIFLE, AKIN and conventional criteria for acute kidney injury after hematopoietic SCT. Bone Marrow Transplant. 2010;45(9):1427–34.
47. Hosing C, Nash R, McSweeney P, Mineishi S, Seibold J, Griffith LM, et al. Acute kidney injury in patients with systemic sclerosis participating in hematopoietic cell transplantation trials in the United States. Biol Blood Marrow Transplant. 2011;17(5):674–81.
48. Fadia A, Casserly LF, Sanchorawala V, Seldin DC, Wright DG, Skinner M, Dember LM. Incidence and outcome of acute renal failure complicating autologous stem cell transplantation for AL amyloidosis. Kidney Int. 2003;63(5):1868–73.
49. Kersting S, Dorp SV, Theobald M, Verdonck LF. Acute renal failure after nonmyeloablative stem cell transplantation in adults. Biol Blood Marrow Transplant. 2008;14(1):125–31.
50. Parikh CR, Sandmaier BM, Storb RF, Blume KG, Sahebi F, Maloney DG, et al. Acute renal failure after nonmyeloablative hematopoietic cell transplantation. J Am Soc Nephrol. 2004;15(7):1868–76.

51. Lopes JA, Goncalves S, Jorge S, Raimundo M, Resende L, Lourenco F, et al. Contemporary analysis of the influence of acute kidney injury after reduced intensity conditioning haematopoietic cell transplantation on long-term survival. Bone Marrow Transplant. 2008;42(9):619–26.
52. Liu H, Ding JH, Liu BC, Zhao G, Chen BA. Early renal injury after nonmyeloablative allogeneic peripheral blood stem cell transplantation in patients with chronic myelocytic leukemia. Am J Nephrol. 2007;27(4):336–41.
53. Parikh CR, Yarlagadda SG, Storer B, Sorror M, Storb R, Sandmaier B. Impact of acute kidney injury on long-term mortality after nonmyeloablative hematopoietic cell transplantation. Biol Blood Marrow Transplant. 2008;14(3):309–15.
54. Pinana JL, Valcarcel D, Martino R, Barba P, Moreno E, Sureda A, et al. Study of kidney function impairment after reduced-intensity conditioning allogeneic hematopoietic stem cell transplantation. A single-center experience. Biol Blood Marrow Transplant. 2009;15(1):21–9.
55. Liu H, Li YF, Liu BC, Ding JH, Chen BA, Xu WL, Qian J. A multicenter, retrospective study of acute kidney injury in adult patients with nonmyeloablative hematopoietic SCT. Bone Marrow Transplant. 2010;45(1):153–8.
56. Chertow GM, Burdick E, Honour M, Bonventre JV, Bates DW. Acute kidney injury, mortality, length of stay, and costs in hospitalized patients. J Am Soc Nephrol. 2005;16(11):3365–70.
57. Uchino S, Kellum JA, Bellomo R, Doig GS, Morimatsu H, Morgera S, et al. Acute renal failure in critically ill patients: a multinational, multicenter study. JAMA. 2005;294(7):813–8.
58. Ando M, Ohashi K, Akiyama H, Sakamaki H, Morito T, Tsuchiya K, Nitta K. Chronic kidney disease in long-term survivors of myeloablative allogeneic haematopoietic cell transplantation: prevalence and risk factors. Nephrol Dial Transplant. 2010;25(1):278–82.
59. Hingorani S, Guthrie KA, Schoch G, Weiss NS, McDonald GB. Chronic kidney disease in long-term survivors of hematopoietic cell transplant. Bone Marrow Transplant. 2007;39(4):223–9.
60. Ishani A, Xue JL, Himmelfarb J, Eggers PW, Kimmel PL, Molitoris BA, Collins AJ. Acute kidney injury increases risk of ESRD among elderly. J Am Soc Nephrol. 2009;20(1):223–8.
61. Lo LJ, Go AS, Chertow GM, McCulloch CE, Fan D, Ordonez JD, Hsu CY. Dialysis-requiring acute renal failure increases the risk of progressive chronic kidney disease. Kidney Int. 2009;76(8):893–9.
62. Hoffmeister PA, Hingorani SR, Storer BE, Baker KS, Sanders JE. Hypertension in long-term survivors of pediatric hematopoietic cell transplantation. Biol Blood Marrow Transplant. 2010;16(4):515–24.
63. Weiss AS, Sandmaier BM, Storer B, Storb R, McSweeney PA, Parikh CR. Chronic kidney disease following non-myeloablative hematopoietic cell transplantation. Am J Transplant. 2006;6(1):89–94.
64. Hingorani SR, Seidel K, Lindner A, Aneja T, Schoch G, McDonald G. Albuminuria in hematopoietic cell transplantation patients: prevalence, clinical associations, and impact on survival. Biol Blood Marrow Transplant. 2008;14(12):1365–72.
65. Bosch M, Khan FM, Storek J. Immune reconstitution after hematopoietic cell transplantation. Curr Opin Hematol. 2012;19(4):324–35.
66. Chaushu G, Itzkovitz-Chaushu S, Yefenof E, Slavin S, Or R, Garfunkel AA. A longitudinal follow-up of salivary secretion in bone marrow transplant patients. Oral Surg Oral Med Oral Pathol Oral Radiol Endod. 1995;79(2):164–9.
67. D'Orsogna LJ, Wright MP, Krueger RG, McKinnon EJ, Buffery SI, Witt CS, et al. Allogeneic hematopoietic stem cell transplantation recipients have defects of both switched and igm memory B cells. Biol Blood Marrow Transplant. 2009;15(7):795–803.
68. Hashimoto D, Merad M. Harnessing dendritic cells to improve allogeneic hematopoietic cell transplantation outcome. Semin Immunol. 2011;23(1):50–7.
69. Bensinger WI, Clift R, Martin P, Appelbaum FR, Demirer T, Gooley T, et al. Allogeneic peripheral blood stem cell transplantation in patients with advanced hematologic malignancies: a retrospective comparison with marrow transplantation. Blood. 1996;88(7):2794–800.
70. Storek J, Dawson MA, Storer B, Stevens-Ayers T, Maloney DG, Marr KA, et al. Immune reconstitution after allogeneic marrow transplantation compared with blood stem cell transplantation. Blood. 2001;97(11):3380–9.
71. De Angelis C, Mancusi A, Ruggeri L, Capanni M, Urbani E, Velardi A, Stern M. Expansion of CD56-negative, CD16-positive, KIR-expressing natural killer cells after T cell-depleted haploidentical hematopoietic stem cell transplantation. Acta Haematol. 2011;126(1):13–20.
72. Marcenaro E, Carlomagno S, Pesce S, Moretta A, Sivori S. Bridging innate NK cell functions with adaptive immunity. Adv Exp Med Biol. 2011;780:45–55.
73. Koch U, Radtke F. Mechanisms of T cell development and transformation. Annu Rev Cell Dev Biol. 2011;27:539–62.
74. Toubert A, Glauzy S, Douay C, Clave E. Thymus and immune reconstitution after allogeneic hematopoietic stem cell transplantation in humans: never say never again. Tissue Antigens. 2012;79(2):83–9.
75. Witherspoon RP, Storb R, Ochs HD, Fluornoy N, Kopecky KJ, Sullivan KM, et al. Recovery of antibody production in human allogeneic marrow graft recipients: influence of time posttransplantation, the presence or absence of chronic graft-versus-host disease, and antithymocyte globulin treatment. Blood. 1981;58(2):360–8.
76. Lum LG, Seigneuret MC, Storb R. The transfer of antigen-specific humoral immunity from marrow donors to marrow recipients. J Clin Immunol. 1986;6(5):389–96.
77. Wimperis JZ, Brenner MK, Prentice HG, Reittie JE, Karayiannis P, Griffiths PD, Hoffbrand AV. Transfer of a functioning humoral immune system in transplantation of T-lymphocyte-depleted bone marrow. Lancet. 1986;1(8477):339–43.
78. Packman R, Weinberg KI. In: Appelbaum FR, Forman SJ, Negrin RS, Blume KG, editors. Thomas' hematopoietic cell transplantation. Wiley-Blackwell, Hoboken, NJ; 2009. p. 222–31.
79. Niederwieser D, Maris M, Shizuru JA, Petersdorf E, Hegenbart U, Sandmaier BM, et al. Low-dose total body irradiation (TBI) and fludarabine followed by hematopoietic cell transplantation (HCT) from HLA-matched or mismatched unrelated donors and postgrafting immunosuppression with cyclosporine and mycophenolate mofetil (MMF) can induce durable complete chimerism and sustained remissions in patients with hematological diseases. Blood. 2003;101(4):1620–9.
80. Porrata LF, Litzow MR, Markovic SN. Immune reconstitution after autologous hematopoietic stem cell transplantation. Mayo Clinic Proc Mayo Clinic. 2001;76(4):407–12.
81. Peggs KS, Mackinnon S. Immune reconstitution following haematopoietic stem cell transplantation. Br J Haemol. 2004;124(4):407–20.
82. Guerrero A, Perez-Simon JA, Gutierrez N, Caballero D, Ortin F, Gomez-Sanchez JC, et al. Neurological complications after autologous stem cell transplantation. Eur Neurol. 1999;41(1):48–50.
83. de Brabander C, Cornelissen J, Smitt PA, Vecht CJ, van den Bent MJ. Increased incidence of neurological complications in patients receiving an allogenic bone marrow transplantation from alternative donors. J Neurol Neurosurg Psychiatry. 2000;68(1):36–40.

84. De La Camara R, Tomas JF, Figuera A, Berberana M, Fernandez-Ranada JM. High dose busulfan and seizures. Bone Marrow Transplant. 1991;7(5):363–4.
85. Pallotta MG, Velazco A, Sadler A. Ifosfamide extrapyramidal neurotoxicity. Cancer. 1992;70(11):2743–5.
86. Glantz MJ, Jaeckle KA, Chamberlain MC, Phuphanich S, Recht L, Swinnen LJ, et al. A randomized controlled trial comparing intrathecal sustained-release cytarabine (DepoCyt) to intrathecal methotrexate in patients with neoplastic meningitis from solid tumors. Clin Cancer Res. 1999;5(11):3394–402.
87. Baker WJ, Royer GL Jr, Weiss RB. Cytarabine and neurologic toxicity. J Clin Oncol. 1991;9(4):679–93.
88. Imrie KR, Couture F, Turner CC, Sutcliffe SB, Keating A. Peripheral neuropathy following high-dose etoposide and autologous bone marrow transplantation. Bone Marrow Transplant. 1994;13(1):77–9.
89. Mollman JE. Cisplatin neurotoxicity. N Engl J Med. 1990;322(2):126–7.
90. Rowinsky EK, Donehower RC. Paclitaxel (taxol). N Engl J Med. 1995;332(15):1004–14.
91. Ebner F, Ranner G, Slavc I, Urban C, Kleinert R, Radner H, et al. MR findings in methotrexate-induced CNS abnormalities. AJR Am J Roentgenol. 1989;153(6):1283–8.
92. Bleyer WA. Neurologic sequelae of methotrexate and ionizing radiation: a new classification. Cancer Treat Rep. 1981;65(Suppl 1):89–98.
93. Dimopoulos MA, Mateos MV, Richardson PG, Schlag R, Khuageva NK, Shpilberg O, et al. Risk factors for, and reversibility of, peripheral neuropathy associated with bortezomib-melphalan-prednisone in newly diagnosed patients with multiple myeloma: subanalysis of the phase 3 VISTA study. Eur J Haematol. 2011;86(1):23–31.
94. Bleggi-Torres LF, de Medeiros BC, Werner B, Neto JZ, Loddo G, Pasquini R, de Medeiros CR. Neuropathological findings after bone marrow transplantation: an autopsy study of 180 cases. Bone Marrow Transplant. 2000;25(3):301–7.
95. Verfaillie C, Weisdorf D, Haake R, Hostetter M, Ramsay NK, McGlave P. Candida infections in bone marrow transplant recipients. Bone Marrow Transplant. 1991;8(3):177–84.
96. Patchell RA, White CL 3rd, Clark AW, Beschorner WE, Santos GW. Neurologic complications of bone marrow transplantation. Neurology. 1985;35(3):300–6.
97. Meyers JD. Treatment of herpesvirus infections in the immunocompromised host. Scand J Infect Dis Suppl. 1985;47:128–36.
98. Vu T, Carrum G, Hutton G, Heslop HE, Brenner MK, Kamble R. Human herpesvirus-6 encephalitis following allogeneic hematopoietic stem cell transplantation. Bone Marrow Transplant. 2007;39(11):705–9.
99. Re D, Bamborschke S, Feiden W, Schroder R, Lehrke R, Diehl V, Tesch H. Progressive multifocal leukoencephalopathy after autologous bone marrow transplantation and alpha-interferon immunotherapy. Bone Marrow Transplant. 1999;23(3):295–8.
100. Graus F, Saiz A, Sierra J, Arbaiza D, Rovira M, Carreras E, Tolosa E, Rozman C. Neurologic complications of autologous and allogeneic bone marrow transplantation in patients with leukemia: a comparative study. Neurology. 1996;46(4):1004–9.
101. Pomeranz S, Naparstek E, Ashkenazi E, Nagler A, Lossos A, Slavin S, Or R. Intracranial haematomas following bone marrow transplantation. J Neurol. 1994;241(4):252–6.
102. Kannan K, Koh LP, Linn YC. Subdural hematoma in two hematopoietic stem cell transplant patients with post-dural puncture headache and initially normal CT brain scan. Ann Hematol. 2002;81(9):540–2.
103. Patchell RA, White CL 3rd, Clark AW, Beschorner WE, Santos GW. Nonbacterial thrombotic endocarditis in bone marrow transplant patients. Cancer. 1985;55(3):631–5.
104. Shimoni A, Yeshurun M, Hardan I, Avigdor A, Ben-Bassat I, Nagler A. Thrombotic microangiopathy after allogeneic stem cell transplantation in the era of reduced-intensity conditioning: the incidence is not reduced. Biol Blood Marrow Transplant. 2004;10(7):484–93.
105. Hoyt R, Szer J, Grigg A. Neurological events associated with the infusion of cryopreserved bone marrow and/or peripheral blood progenitor cells. Bone Marrow Transplant. 2000;25(12):1285–7.
106. Gordon B, Lyden E, Lynch J, Tarantolo S, Pavletic ZS, Bishop M, et al. Central nervous system dysfunction as the first manifestation of multiple organ dysfunction syndrome in stem cell transplant patients. Bone Marrow Transplant. 2000;25(1):79–83.
107. Haire WD, Ruby EI, Gordon BG, Patil KD, Stephens LC, Kotulak GD, et al. Multiple organ dysfunction syndrome in bone marrow transplantation. JAMA. 1995;274(16):1289–95.
108. Zoja C, Furci L, Ghilardi F, Zilio P, Benigni A, Remuzzi G. Cyclosporin-induced endothelial cell injury. Lab Investig. 1986;55(4):455–62.
109. Thompson CB, Sanders JE, Flournoy N, Buckner CD, Thomas ED. The risks of central nervous system relapse and leukoencephalopathy in patients receiving marrow transplants for acute leukemia. Blood. 1986;67(1):195–9.
110. Bush NE, Haberman M, Donaldson G, Sullivan KM. Quality of life of 125 adults surviving 6–18 years after bone marrow transplantation. Soc Sci Med. 1995;40(4):479–90.
111. Solaro C, Murialdo A, Giunti D, Mancardi G, Uccelli A. Central and peripheral nervous system complications following allogeneic bone marrow transplantation. Eur J Neurol. 2001;8(1):77–80.
112. Tallet AV, Azria D, Barlesi F, Spano JP, Carpentier AF, Goncalves A, Metellus P. Neurocognitive function impairment after whole brain radiotherapy for brain metastases: actual assessment. Radiat Oncol. 2012;7:77.
113. Cazin B, Gorin NC, Laporte JP, Gallet B, Douay L, Lopez M, Najman A, Duhamel G. Cardiac complications after bone marrow transplantation. A report on a series of 63 consecutive transplantations. Cancer. 1986;57(10):2061–9.
114. Gottdiener JS, Appelbaum FR, Ferrans VJ, Deisseroth A, Ziegler J. Cardiotoxicity associated with high-dose cyclophosphamide therapy. Arch Intern Med. 1981;141(6):758–63.
115. Ritchie DS, Seymour JF, Roberts AW, Szer J, Grigg AP. Acute left ventricular failure following melphalan and fludarabine conditioning. Bone Marrow Transplant. 2001;28(1):101–3.
116. Hidalgo JD, Krone R, Rich MW, Blum K, Adkins D, Fan MY, et al. Supraventricular tachyarrhythmias after hematopoietic stem cell transplantation: incidence, risk factors and outcomes. Bone Marrow Transplant. 2004;34(7):615–9.
117. Baker KS, Gurney JG, Ness KK, Bhatia R, Forman SJ, Francisco L, et al. Late effects in survivors of chronic myeloid leukemia treated with hematopoietic cell transplantation: results from the Bone Marrow Transplant Survivor Study. Blood. 2004;104(6):1898–906.
118. Murdych T, Weisdorf DJ. Serious cardiac complications during bone marrow transplantation at the University of Minnesota, 1977–1997. Bone Marrow Transplant. 2001;28(3):283–7.
119. Quabeck K. The lung as a critical organ in marrow transplantation. Bone Marrow Transplant. 1994;14(Suppl 4):S19–28.
120. Kantrow SP, Hackman RC, Boeckh M, Myerson D, Crawford SW. Idiopathic pneumonia syndrome: changing spectrum of lung injury after marrow transplantation. Transplantation. 1997;63(8):1079–86.
121. Clark JG, Madtes DK, Martin TR, Hackman RC, Farrand AL, Crawford SW. Idiopathic pneumonia after bone marrow transplantation: cytokine activation and lipopolysaccharide amplification in the bronchoalveolar compartment. Crit Care Med. 1999;27(9):1800–6.

122. Ebbert JO, Limper AH. Respiratory syncytial virus pneumonitis in immunocompromised adults: clinical features and outcome. Respiration. 2005;72(3):263–9.
123. Boeckh M, Englund J, Li Y, Miller C, Cross A, Fernandez H, Kuypers J, et al. Randomized controlled multicenter trial of aerosolized ribavirin for respiratory syncytial virus upper respiratory tract infection in hematopoietic cell transplant recipients. Clin Infect Dis. 2007;44(2):245–9.
124. Osarogiagbon RU, Defor TE, Weisdorf MA, Erice A, Weisdorf DJ. CMV antigenemia following bone marrow transplantation: risk factors and outcomes. Biol Blood Marrow Transplant. 2000;6(3):280–8.
125. Ruggeri A, Peffault de Latour R, Carmagnat M, Clave E, Douay C, Larghero J, et al. Outcomes, infections, and immune reconstitution after double cord blood transplantation in patients with high-risk hematological diseases. Transpl Infect Dis. 2011;13(5):456–65.
126. Clark JG, Hansen JA, Hertz MI, Parkman R, Jensen L, Peavy HH. NHLBI workshop summary. Idiopathic pneumonia syndrome after bone marrow transplantation. Am Rev Respir Dis. 1993;147(6 Pt 1):1601–6.
127. Weiner RS, Bortin MM, Gale RP, Gluckman E, Kay HE, Kolb HJ, et al. Interstitial pneumonitis after bone marrow transplantation. Assessment of risk factors. Ann Intern Med. 1986;104(2): 168–75.
128. Robbins RA, Linder J, Stahl MG, Thompson AB 3rd, Haire W, Kessinger A, Armitage JO, et al. Diffuse alveolar hemorrhage in autologous bone marrow transplant recipients. Am J Med. 1989;87(5):511–8.
129. Lewis ID, DeFor T, Weisdorf DJ. Increasing incidence of diffuse alveolar hemorrhage following allogeneic bone marrow transplantation: cryptic etiology and uncertain therapy. Bone Marrow Transplant. 2000;26(5):539–43.
130. Metcalf JP, Rennard SI, Reed EC, Haire WD, Sisson JH, Walter T, Robbins RA. Corticosteroids as adjunctive therapy for diffuse alveolar hemorrhage associated with bone marrow transplantation. University of Nebraska Medical Center Bone Marrow Transplant Group. Am J Med. 1994;96(4):327–34.
131. Soubani AO, Miller KB, Hassoun PM. Pulmonary complications of bone marrow transplantation. Chest. 1996;109(4):1066–77.
132. Palmas A, Tefferi A, Myers JL, Scott JP, Swensen SJ, Chen MG, et al. Late-onset noninfectious pulmonary complications after allogeneic bone marrow transplantation. Br J Haematol. 1998;100(4):680–7.
133. Aronin PA, Mahaley MS Jr, Rudnick SA, Dudka L, Donohue JF, Selker RG, Moore P. Prediction of BCNU pulmonary toxicity in patients with malignant gliomas: an assessment of risk factors. N Engl J Med. 1980;303(4):183–8.
134. Shen YC, Chiu CF, Chow KC, Chen CL, Liaw YC, Yeh SP. Fatal pulmonary fibrosis associated with BCNU: the relative role of platelet-derived growth factor-B, insulin-like growth factor I, transforming growth factor-beta1 and cyclooxygenase-2. Bone Marrow Transplant. 2004;34(7):609–14.
135. Yoshihara S, Yanik G, Cooke KR, Mineishi S. Bronchiolitis obliterans syndrome (BOS), bronchiolitis obliterans organizing pneumonia (BOOP), and other late-onset noninfectious pulmonary complications following allogeneic hematopoietic stem cell transplantation. Biol Blood Marrow Transplant. 2007;13(7): 749–59.
136. Yanik G, Cooke KR. The lung as a target organ of graft-versus-host disease. Semin Hematol. 2006;43(1):42–52.
137. Down JD, Mauch P, Warhol M, Neben S, Ferrara JL. The effect of donor T lymphocytes and total-body irradiation on hemopoietic engraftment and pulmonary toxicity following experimental allogeneic bone marrow transplantation. Transplantation. 1992;54(5):802–8.
138. Shankar G, Cohen DA. Idiopathic pneumonia syndrome after bone marrow transplantation: the role of pre-transplant radiation conditioning and local cytokine dysregulation in promoting lung inflammation and fibrosis. Int J Exp Pathol. 2001;82(2):101–13.
139. Ho VT, Cutler C, Carter S, Martin P, Adams R, Horowitz M, et al. Blood and marrow transplant clinical trials network toxicity committee consensus summary: thrombotic microangiopathy after hematopoietic stem cell transplantation. Biol Blood Marrow Transplant. 2005;11(8):571–5.
140. Ruutu T, Barosi G, Benjamin RJ, Clark RE, George JN, Gratwohl A, et al. Diagnostic criteria for hematopoietic stem cell transplant-associated microangiopathy: results of a consensus process by an International Working Group. Haematologica. 2007;92(1):95–100.
141. Cutler C, Henry NL, Magee C, Li S, Kim HT, Alyea E, et al. Sirolimus and thrombotic microangiopathy after allogeneic hematopoietic stem cell transplantation. Biol Blood Marrow Transplant. 2005;11(7):551–7.
142. Pettitt AR, Clark RE. Thrombotic microangiopathy following bone marrow transplantation. Bone Marrow Transplant. 1994;14(4):495–504.
143. Nakamae H, Yamane T, Hasegawa T, Nakamae M, Terada Y, Hagihara K, et al. Risk factor analysis for thrombotic microangiopathy after reduced-intensity or myeloablative allogeneic hematopoietic stem cell transplantation. Am J Hematol. 2006;81(7):525–31.
144. Bernardo A, Ball C, Nolasco L, Moake JF, Dong JF. Effects of inflammatory cytokines on the release and cleavage of the endothelial cell-derived ultralarge von Willebrand factor multimers under flow. Blood. 2004;104(1):100–6.
145. Rabinowe SN, Soiffer RJ, Tarbell NJ, Neuberg D, Freedman AS, Seifter J, et al. Hemolytic-uremic syndrome following bone marrow transplantation in adults for hematologic malignancies. Blood. 1991;77(8):1837–44.
146. van der Plas RM, Schiphorst ME, Huizinga EG, Hene RJ, Verdonck LF, Sixma JJ, Fijnheer R. von Willebrand factor proteolysis is deficient in classic, but not in bone marrow transplantation-associated, thrombotic thrombocytopenic purpura. Blood. 1999;93(11):3798–802.
147. Llamas P, Romero R, Cabrera R, Sanjuan I, Fores R, Fernandez MN. Management of thrombotic microangiopathy following allogeneic transplantation: what is the role of plasma exchange? Bone Marrow Transplant. 1997;20(4):305–6.
148. Ruutu T, Hermans J, Niederwieser D, Gratwohl A, Kiehl M, Volin L, B, et al. Thrombotic thrombocytopenic purpura after allogeneic stem cell transplantation: a survey of the European Group for Blood and Marrow Transplantation (EBMT). Br J Haematol. 2002;118(4):1112–9.
149. de Fontbrune FS, Galambrun C, Sirvent A, Huynh A, Faguer S, Nguyen S, et al. Use of eculizumab in patients with allogeneic stem cell transplant-associated thrombotic microangiopathy: a study from the SFGM-TC. Transplantation. 2015;99(9):1953–9.
150. Shalet SM. Radiation and pituitary dysfunction. N Engl J Med. 1993;328(2):131–3.
151. Kauppila M, Koskinen P, Irjala K, Remes K, Viikari J. Long-term effects of allogeneic bone marrow transplantation (BMT) on pituitary, gonad, thyroid and adrenal function in adults. Bone Marrow Transplant. 1998;22(4):331–7.
152. Shalitin S, Phillip M, Stein J, Goshen Y, Carmi D, Yaniv I. Endocrine dysfunction and parameters of the metabolic syndrome after bone marrow transplantation during childhood and adolescence. Bone Marrow Transplant. 2006;37(12):1109–17.
153. Holm K, Nysom K, Rasmussen MH, Hertz H, Jacobsen N, Skakkebaek NE, et al. Growth, growth hormone and final height after BMT. Possible recovery of irradiation-induced growth hormone insufficiency. Bone Marrow Transplant. 1996;18(1):163–70.

154. Carroll PV, Christ ER, Bengtsson BA, Carlsson L, Christiansen JS, Clemmons D, et al. Growth hormone deficiency in adulthood and the effects of growth hormone replacement: a review. Growth Hormone Research Society Scientific Committee. J Clin Endocrinol Metab. 1998;83(2):382–95.
155. Schulte CM, Beelen DW. Bone loss following hematopoietic stem cell transplantation: a long-term follow-up. Blood. 2004;103(10):3635–43.
156. Valimaki MJ, Kinnunen K, Volin L, Tahtela R, Loyttyniemi E, Laitinen K, et al. A prospective study of bone loss and turnover after allogeneic bone marrow transplantation: effect of calcium supplementation with or without calcitonin. Bone Marrow Transplant. 1999;23(4):355–61.
157. Weilbaecher KN. Mechanisms of osteoporosis after hematopoietic cell transplantation. Biol Blood Marrow Transplant. 2000;6(2A):165–74.
158. Ebeling PR, Thomas DM, Erbas B, Hopper JL, Szer J, Grigg AP. Mechanisms of bone loss following allogeneic and autologous hemopoietic stem cell transplantation. J Bone Miner Res. 1999;14(3):342–50.
159. Stern JM, Sullivan KM, Ott SM, Seidel K, Fink JC, Longton G, Sherrard DJ. Bone density loss after allogeneic hematopoietic stem cell transplantation: a prospective study. Biol Blood Marrow Transplant. 2001;7(5):257–64.
160. Boulad F, Bromley M, Black P, Heller G, Sarafoglou K, Gillio A, et al. Thyroid dysfunction following bone marrow transplantation using hyperfractionated radiation. Bone Marrow Transplant. 1995;15(1):71–6.
161. Sanders JE. Endocrine complications of high-dose therapy with stem cell transplantation. Pediatr Transplant. 2004;8(Suppl 5):39–50.
162. Michel G, Socie G, Gebhard F, Bernaudin F, Thuret I, Vannier JP, et al. Late effects of allogeneic bone marrow transplantation for children with acute myeloblastic leukemia in first complete remission: the impact of conditioning regimen without total-body irradiation – a report from the Societe Francaise de Greffe de Moelle. J Clin Oncol. 1997;15(6):2238–46.
163. Toubert ME, Socie G, Gluckman E, Aractingi S, Esperou H, Devergie A, et al. Short- and long-term follow-up of thyroid dysfunction after allogeneic bone marrow transplantation without the use of preparative total body irradiation. Br J Haematol. 1997;98(2):453–7.
164. Afify Z, Shaw PJ, Clavano-Harding A, Cowell CT. Growth and endocrine function in children with acute myeloid leukaemia after bone marrow transplantation using busulfan/cyclophosphamide. Bone Marrow Transplant. 2000;25(10):1087–92.
165. Tauchmanova L, Selleri C, Rosa GD, Pagano L, Orio F, Lombardi G, et al. High prevalence of endocrine dysfunction in long-term survivors after allogeneic bone marrow transplantation for hematologic diseases. Cancer. 2002;95(5):1076–84.
166. Berger C, Le-Gallo B, Donadieu J, Richard O, Devergie A, Galambrun C, et al. Late thyroid toxicity in 153 long-term survivors of allogeneic bone marrow transplantation for acute lymphoblastic leukaemia. Bone Marrow Transplant. 2005;35(10):991–5.
167. Kaplan MM, Garnick MB, Gelber R, Li FP, Cassady JR, Sallan SE, et al. Risk factors for thyroid abnormalities after neck irradiation for childhood cancer. The Am J Med. 1983;74(2):272–80.
168. Cohen A, Rovelli A, van Lint MT, Merlo F, Gaiero A, Mulas R, et al. Secondary thyroid carcinoma after allogeneic bone marrow transplantation during childhood. Bone Marrow Transplant. 2001;28(12):1125–8.
169. Majhail NS. Secondary cancers following allogeneic haematopoietic cell transplantation in adults. Br J Haematol. 2011;154(3):301–10.
170. Rizzo JD, Curtis RE, Socie G, Sobocinski KA, Gilbert E, Landgren O, et al. Solid cancers after allogeneic hematopoietic cell transplantation. Blood. 2009;113(5):1175–83.
171. Majhail NS, Brazauskas R, Rizzo JD, Sobecks RM, Wang Z, Horowitz MM, et al. Secondary solid cancers after allogeneic hematopoietic cell transplantation using busulfan-cyclophosphamide conditioning. Blood. 2011;117(1):316–22.
172. Ginsberg SJ, Comis RL. The pulmonary toxicity of antineoplastic agents. Semin Oncol. 1982;9(1):34–51.
173. Travis LB, Gospodarowicz M, Curtis RE, Clarke EA, Andersson M, Glimelius B, et al. Lung cancer following chemotherapy and radiotherapy for Hodgkin's disease. J Natl Cancer Inst. 2002;94(3):182–92.
174. Cohen A, Rovelli A, Merlo DF, van Lint MT, Lanino E, Bresters D, et al. Risk for secondary thyroid carcinoma after hematopoietic stem-cell transplantation: an EBMT Late Effects Working Party Study. J Clin Oncol. 2007;25(17):2449–54.
175. Friedman DL, Rovo A, Leisenring W, Locasciulli A, Flowers ME, Tichelli A, et al. Increased risk of breast cancer among survivors of allogeneic hematopoietic cell transplantation: a report from the FHCRC and the EBMT-Late Effect Working Party. Blood. 2008;111(2):939–44.
176. Leisenring W, Friedman DL, Flowers ME, Schwartz JL, Deeg HJ. Nonmelanoma skin and mucosal cancers after hematopoietic cell transplantation. J Clin Oncol. 2006;24(7):1119–26.
177. Schwartz JL, Kopecky KJ, Mathes RW, Leisenring WM, Friedman DL, Deeg HJ. Basal cell skin cancer after total-body irradiation and hematopoietic cell transplantation. Radiat Res. 2009;171(2):155–63.
178. Savani BN, Stratton P, Shenoy A, Kozanas E, Goodman S, Barrett AJ. Increased risk of cervical dysplasia in long-term survivors of allogeneic stem cell transplantation – implications for screening and HPV vaccination. Biol Blood Marrow Transplant. 2008;14(9):1072–5.
179. Savani BN, Goodman S, Barrett AJ. Can routine posttransplant HPV vaccination prevent commonly occurring epithelial cancers after allogeneic stem cell transplantation? Clin Cancer Res. 2009;15(7):2219–21.
180. Jagadeesh D, Woda BA, Draper J, Evens AM. Post transplant lymphoproliferative disorders: risk, classification, and therapeutic recommendations. Curr Treat Options in Oncol. 2012;13(1):122–36.
181. Cockfield SM. Identifying the patient at risk for post-transplant lymphoproliferative disorder. Transpl Infect Dis. 2001;3(2):70–8.
182. Opelz G, Dohler B. Lymphomas after solid organ transplantation: a collaborative transplant study report. Am J Transplant. 2004;4(2):222–30.
183. Caillard S, Lelong C, Pessione F, Moulin B. Post-transplant lymphoproliferative disorders occurring after renal transplantation in adults: report of 230 cases from the French registry. Am J Transplant. 2006;6(11):2735–42.
184. Hartmann C, Schuchmann M, Zimmermann T. Posttransplant lymphoproliferative disease in liver transplant patients. Curr Infect Dis Rep. 2011;13(1):53–9.
185. Bhatia S, Ramsay NK, Steinbuch M, Dusenbery KE, Shapiro RS, Weisdorf DJ, et al. Malignant neoplasms following bone marrow transplantation. Blood. 1996;87(9):3633–9.
186. Weissmann DJ, Ferry JA, Harris NL, Louis DN, Delmonico F, Spiro I. Posttransplantation lymphoproliferative disorders in solid organ recipients are predominantly aggressive tumors of host origin. Am J Clin Pathol. 1995;103(6):748–55.
187. Shapiro RS, McClain K, Frizzera G, Gajl-Peczalska KJ, Kersey JH, Blazar BR, et al. Epstein-Barr virus associated B cell lymphoproliferative disorders following bone marrow transplantation. Blood. 1988;71(5):1234–43.

188. Opelz G, Henderson R. Incidence of non-Hodgkin lymphoma in kidney and heart transplant recipients. Lancet. 1993;342(8886–8887):1514–6.
189. Oton AB, Wang H, Leleu X, Melhem MF, George D, Lacasce A, et al. Clinical and pathological prognostic markers for survival in adult patients with post-transplant lymphoproliferative disorders in solid transplant. Leuk Lymphoma. 2008;49(9):1738–44.
190. Paya CV, Fung JJ, Nalesnik MA, Kieff E, Green M, Gores G, et al. Epstein-Barr virus-induced posttransplant lymphoproliferative disorders. ASTS/ASTP EBV-PTLD Task Force and The Mayo Clinic Organized International Consensus Development Meeting. Transplantation. 1999;68(10):1517–25.
191. Nourse JP, Jones K, Gandhi MK. Epstein-Barr virus-related post-transplant lymphoproliferative disorders: pathogenetic insights for targeted therapy. Am J Transplant. 2011;11(5):888–95.
192. McDonald RA, Smith JM, Ho M, Lindblad R, Ikle D, Grimm P, et al. Incidence of PTLD in pediatric renal transplant recipients receiving basiliximab, calcineurin inhibitor, sirolimus and steroids. Am J Transplant. 2008;8(5):984–9.
193. Zutter MM, Martin PJ, Sale GE, Shulman HM, Fisher L, Thomas ED, Durnam DM. Epstein-Barr virus lymphoproliferation after bone marrow transplantation. Blood. 1988;72(2):520–9.
194. Leblond V, Dhedin N, Mamzer Bruneel MF, Choquet S, Hermine O, Porcher R, et al. Identification of prognostic factors in 61 patients with posttransplantation lymphoproliferative disorders. J Clin Oncol. 2001;19(3):772–8.
195. Johnson LR, Nalesnik MA, Swerdlow SH. Impact of Epstein-Barr virus in monomorphic B-cell posttransplant lymphoproliferative disorders: a histogenetic study. Am J Surg Pathol. 2006;30(12):1604–12.
196. Nelson BP, Nalesnik MA, Bahler DW, Locker J, Fung JJ, Swerdlow SH. Epstein-Barr virus-negative post-transplant lymphoproliferative disorders: a distinct entity? Am J Surg Pathol. 2000;24(3):375–85.
197. Leblond V, Davi F, Charlotte F, Dorent R, Bitker MO, Sutton L, et al. Posttransplant lymphoproliferative disorders not associated with Epstein-Barr virus: a distinct entity? J Clin Oncol. 1998;16(6):2052–9.
198. Novoa-Takara L, Perkins SL, Qi D, Shidham VB, Vesole DH, Hariharan S, et al. Histogenetic phenotypes of B cells in posttransplant lymphoproliferative disorders by immunohistochemical analysis correlate with transplant type: solid organ vs hematopoietic stem cell transplantation. Am J Clin Pathol. 2005;123(1):104–12.
199. Buell JF, Gross TG, Hanaway MJ, Trofe J, Roy-Chaudhury P, First MR, Woodle ES. Posttransplant lymphoproliferative disorder: significance of central nervous system involvement. Transplant Proc. 2005;37(2):954–5.
200. Cavaliere R, Petroni G, Lopes MB, Schiff D. Primary central nervous system post-transplantation lymphoproliferative disorder: an International Primary Central Nervous System Lymphoma Collaborative Group Report. Cancer. 2010;116(4):863–70.
201. Tsao L, Hsi ED. The clinicopathologic spectrum of posttransplantation lymphoproliferative disorders. Arch Pathol Lab Med. 2007;131(8):1209–18.
202. Evens AM, David KA, Helenowski I, Nelson B, Kaufman D, Kircher SM, et al. Multicenter analysis of 80 solid organ transplantation recipients with post-transplantation lymphoproliferative disease: outcomes and prognostic factors in the modern era. J Clin Oncol. 2010;28(6):1038–46.
203. Knight JS, Tsodikov A, Cibrik DM, Ross CW, Kaminski MS, Blayney DW. Lymphoma after solid organ transplantation: risk, response to therapy, and survival at a transplantation center. J Clin Oncol. 2009;27(20):3354–62.
204. Trappe R, Oertel S, Leblond V, Mollee P, Sender M, Reinke P, et al. Sequential treatment with rituximab followed by CHOP chemotherapy in adult B-cell post-transplant lymphoproliferative disorder (PTLD): the prospective international multicentre phase 2 PTLD-1 trial. Lancet Oncol. 2012;13(2):196–206.
205. Armitage JO, Carbone PP, Connors JM, Levine A, Bennett JM, Kroll S. Treatment-related myelodysplasia and acute leukemia in non-Hodgkin's lymphoma patients. J Clin Oncol. 2003;21(5):897–906.
206. Kalaycio M, Rybicki L, Pohlman B, Sobecks R, Andresen S, Kuczkowski E, Bolwell B. Risk factors before autologous stem-cell transplantation for lymphoma predict for secondary myelodysplasia and acute myelogenous leukemia. J Clin Oncol. 2006;24(22):3604–10.
207. Focosi D, Cecconi N, Boni G, Orciuolo E, Galimberti S, Petrini M. Acute myeloid leukaemia after treatment with (90) Y-ibritumomab tiuxetan for follicular lymphoma. Hematol Oncol. 2008;26(3):179–81.
208. Flynn CM, Kaufman DS. Donor cell leukemia: insight into cancer stem cells and the stem cell niche. Blood. 2007;109(7):2688–92.
209. Hertenstein B, Hambach L, Bacigalupo A, Schmitz N, McCann S, Slavin S, et al. Development of leukemia in donor cells after allogeneic stem cell transplantation – a survey of the European Group for Blood and Marrow Transplantation (EBMT). Haematologica. 2005;90(7):969–75.
210. Pulsipher MA, Chitphakdithai P, Miller JP, Logan BR, King RJ, et al. Adverse events among 2408 unrelated donors of peripheral blood stem cells: results of a prospective trial from the National Marrow Donor Program. Blood. 2009;113(15):3604–11.
211. Barrett AJ, Battiwalla M. Relapse after allogeneic stem cell transplantation. Expert Rev Hematol. 2010;3(4):429–41.

Intravascular Catheter and Implantable Device Infections in Transplant Patients

13

Nasia Safdar, Cybele Lara R. Abad, and Dennis G. Maki

Introduction

The use of intravascular devices for administration of drugs, fluids, blood products, and nutritional support is essential to medical care. Unfortunately, these intravascular devices have a significant potential to produce iatrogenic disease, especially bloodstream infection originating from colonization of the device used for access or from contamination of the infusate administered through the device [1–4]. Over two-thirds of all healthcare-associated bacteremia originate from devices used for vascular access [5]. Patients with hematologic malignancies undergoing stem cell transplantation (SCT), who have inherently compromised immune function because of their malignancy and are further incapacitated due to the preparative regimen or graft-versus-host disease (GVHD), are particularly prone to device-related infections [6].

Every year more than five million central venous catheters (CVC) are inserted in the United States [7]. More than 250,000 intravascular catheter-related bloodstream infections (IVDR BSI) occur annually with an associated mortality of 12–25% [7]. A recent meta-analysis found mortality to be significantly increased in intensive care unit (ICU) patients who had IVDR BSI compared with those without IVDR BSI (odds ratio [OR], 1.96; 95% confidence interval [CI], 1.25–3.09) (Fig. 13.1) [8]. Each episode of IVDR BSI significantly increases hospital length of stay, and the added healthcare costs range from $4,000 to $56,000 per episode [9–11].

Probably more than any other healthcare-associated infection, IVDR BSI is preventable [5, 12–15].

N. Safdar (✉) · D. G. Maki
Section of Infectious Diseases, Department of Medicine, University of Wisconsin-Madison, School of Medicine and Public Health, and the William S. Middleton Memorial Veterans Hospital, Madison, WI, USA
e-mail: ns2@medicine.wisc.edu; dgmaki@medicine.wisc.edu

C. L. R. Abad
Section of Infectious Diseases, Department of Medicine, University of the Philippines Manila, Philippine General Hospital, Manila, Philippines

This chapter focuses on the epidemiology and prevention of IVDR BSI in transplant patients. Given the paucity of data specific to the transplant population, we extrapolate from studies in other populations, particularly the critically ill and patients with cancer.

The first step to preserve vascular access is a highly effective institutional program for prevention of IVDR BSI. In recent years, a large volume of high-quality research studies have delineated key measures for prevention, and IVDR BSI rates in the ICU have declined markedly in most institutions [13, 16–27]. However, despite adherence to best practices, IVDR BSI continues to pose formidable challenges, especially in solid organ and stem cell transplant patients [28].

Pathogenesis of IVDR BSI

There are two major sources of IVDR BSI: (1) colonization of the IVD, or device-related infection, and (2) contamination of the fluid administered through the device, or infusate-related infection [29]. Contaminated infusate is the cause of most epidemic intravascular device-related BSI [4, 30]; in contrast, catheter-related infections are responsible for most *endemic* device-related BSI. A major route of BSI in transplant patients may be translocation of gut and oral flora into the bloodstream as a result of mucositis, called mucosal barrier injury-related BSI. These infections may be mistakenly classified as IVDR BSI if the patient has an IVD in place at the time of positive blood culture.

Understanding the pathogenesis of IVDR BSI is fundamental to devising effective strategies for prevention and treatment of these infections; however, relatively few published studies have determined the mechanism of IVDR colonization and infection using sophisticated molecular techniques to prove or disprove potential routes of infection [31–37].

In order for microorganisms to cause catheter-related infection, they must first gain access to the extraluminal or intraluminal surface of the device where they can adhere

A. Safdar (ed.), *Principles and Practice of Transplant Infectious Diseases*, https://doi.org/10.1007/978-1-4939-9034-4_13

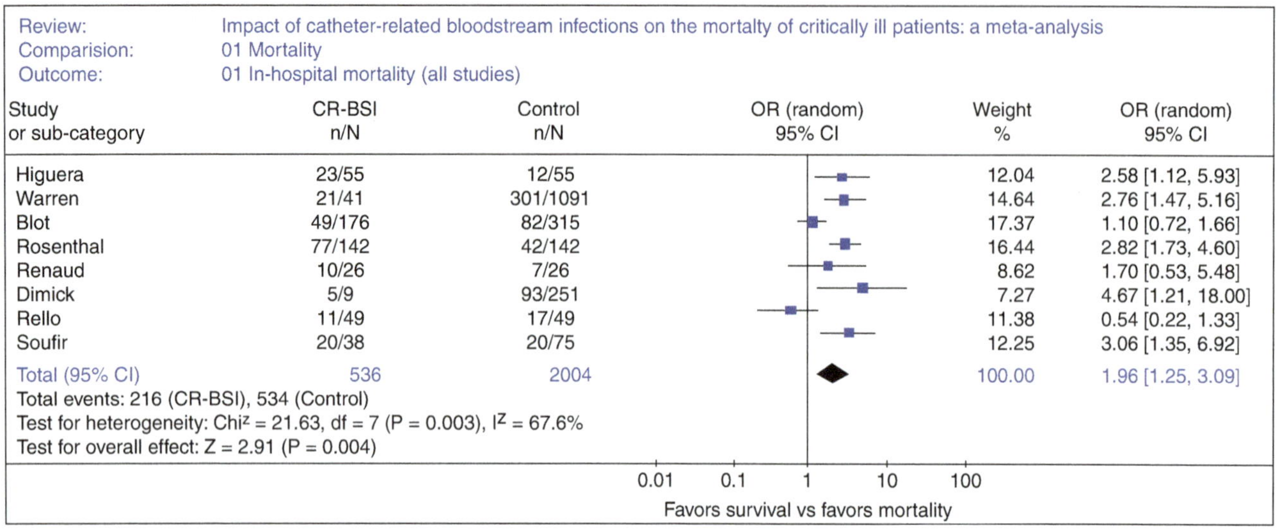

Fig. 13.1 Attributable mortality of IVDR BSI in critically ill patients [8]. (Reprinted from Siempos et al. [8], © 2009, http://journals.lww.com/ccmjournal/Abstract/2009/07000/Impact_of_catheter_related_bloodstream_infections.22.aspx, with permission from Wolters Kluwer Health, Inc.)

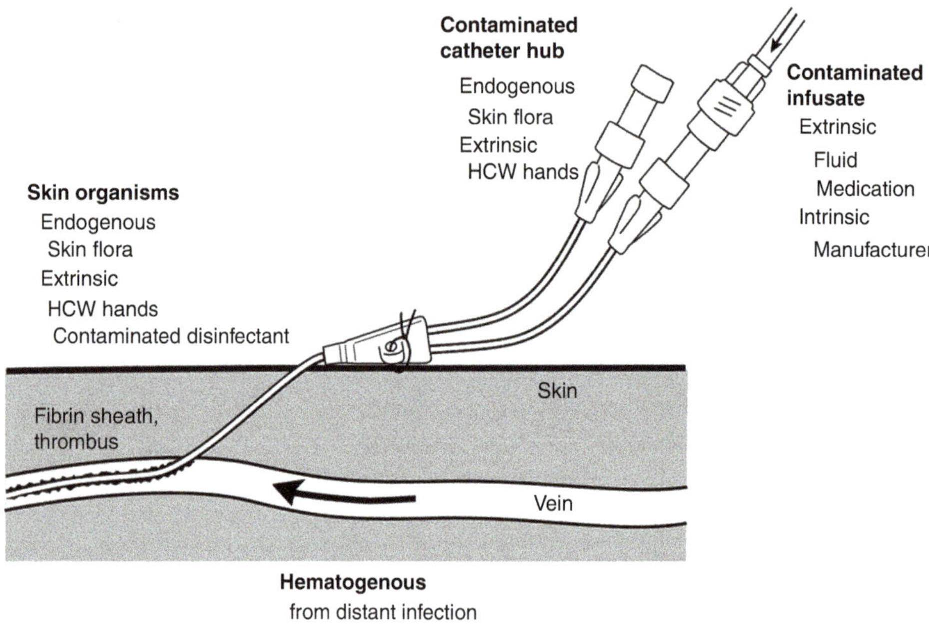

Fig. 13.2 Potential sources of infection of a percutaneous IVD: the contiguous skin flora, contamination of the catheter hub and lumen, contamination of infusate, and hematogenous colonization of the IVD from distant, unrelated sites of infection [42]. (Reprinted from Crnich and Maki [42], by permission of Oxford University Press)

and become incorporated into a biofilm that allows sustained colonization and ultimately hematogenous dissemination [38]. Microorganisms gain access to the implanted IVD by one of three mechanisms: (1) skin organisms invade the percutaneous tract, probably facilitated by capillary action [39], at the time of insertion or in the days following; (2) microorganisms contaminate the catheter hub and lumen when the catheter is inserted over a percutaneous guidewire or later manipulated [40]; or (3) organisms are carried hematogenously to the implanted IVD from remote sources of local infection, such as a pneumonia [41] or from gut or mouth translocation due to inflammation or mucositis (Fig. 13.2) [42].

With short-term IVDs that are in place <14 days, such as peripheral IV catheters, arterial catheters, and non-cuffed, non-tunneled CVCs, most catheter-related BSIs are of cutaneous origin, from the insertion site, and gain access extraluminally or occasionally intraluminally [37, 43, 44]. For long-term catheters, such as tunneled, cuffed CVCs, totally implantable ports, and peripherally inserted central catheters (PICCs), luminal colonization has been shown to be the major mechanism leading to BSI [45, 46]. A characteristic pulsed-field gel electrophoresis image obtained from a short-term non-cuffed CVC causing BSI is shown in Fig. 13.3 and from a long-term catheter (PICC) in Fig. 13.4.

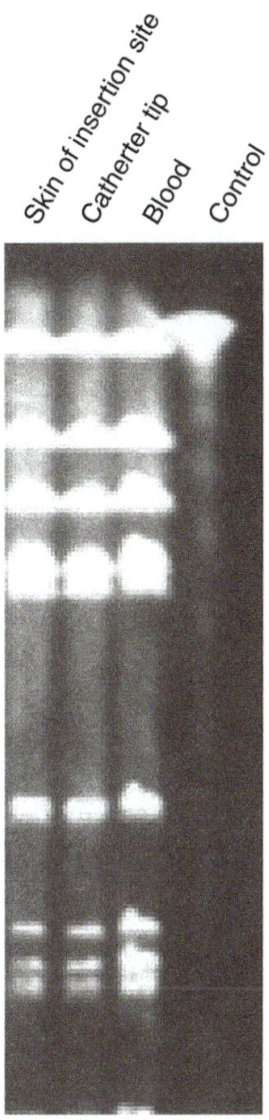

Fig. 13.3 Pulsed-field gel electrophoresis image showing the probable pathogenesis of a CVC-related bacteremia with coagulase-negative Staphylococcus. The isolates from the skin of the insertion site, catheter tip, and blood and were concordant, indicating an extraluminal route of infection [37]. (Reprinted from Safdar and Maki [37], with permission of Springer)

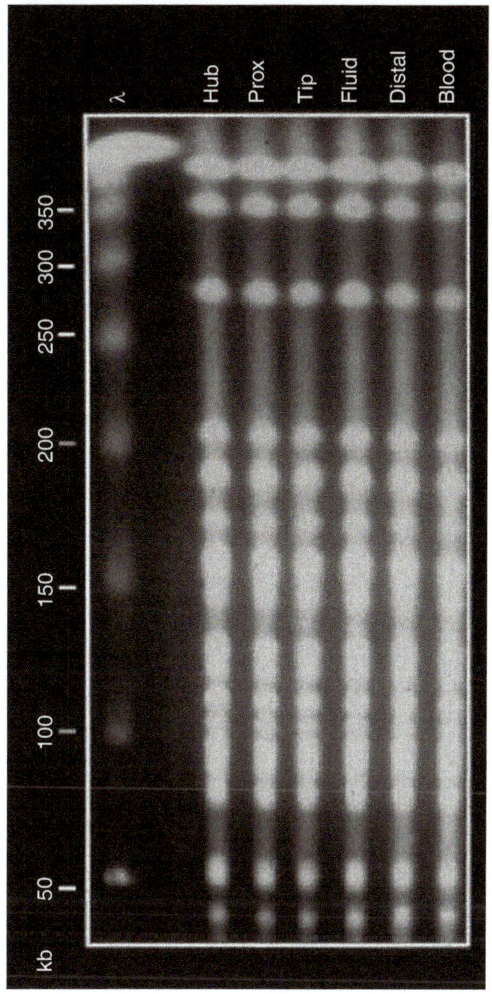

Fig. 13.4 Pulsed-field gel electrophoresis image showing the probable pathogenesis of a PICC-related bacteremia with *Serratia marcescens*. The isolates from the catheter tip, blood, hub, and fluid were all concordant, indicating an intraluminal route of infection

Microbiology

Antimicrobial resistance, now considered to be at global-crisis levels, continues to loom large, and the organisms implicated in IVDR BSI are no exception. In the past two decades, the proportion of IVDR BSI caused by multidrug-resistant (MDR) organisms, such as methicillin-resistant *Staphylococcus aureus* (MRSA) and fluconazole-resistant *Candida* species, has risen inexorably [7, 47–49]. Overall, the organisms encountered most frequently in IVDR BSI are coagulase-negative staphylococci (CoNS) (31%), *Staphylococcus aureus* (20%), enterococci (9%), and *Candida* species (9%) [25–27, 47, 50].

In one large prospective surveillance study using data from SCOPE (Surveillance and Control of Pathogens of Epidemiological Importance), comprising 24,179 cases of nosocomial BSI reported over a 7-year period from 49 hospitals, the rates of MRSA infection increased from 22% of all *S. aureus* BSI in 1995 to 75% in 2001 ($p < 0.001$), and resistance to vancomycin was found in 60% of *Enterococcus faecium* isolates [47].

There is a paucity of data on the epidemiology and microbiology of IVDR BSI in the transplant population. However, a large multicenter study among 38 acute care hospitals, the majority of which were oncology and bone marrow transplant-capable centers, recently implemented the National Healthcare Safety Network (NHSN) surveillance definition of mucosal barrier injury laboratory-confirmed bloodstream infection (MBI-LCBI). In a study by See et al. [51], among 168 central line-associated bloodstream infections (CLABSI) from patients who met one of the two patient criteria of the MBI-LCBI definition, *E. faecium*, *E. coli*, and CoNS (16.0%, 12.6%, 12% of organisms, respectively) were the organisms most commonly reported. In comparison, among 121 cases of CLABSI from patients who did not meet the MBI-LCBI definition's patient criteria, CoNS and *S. aureus* were the top organisms isolated, and both *E. faecium* and *E. coli* organisms were less commonly reported, with a joint rank of sixth (7.2% of organisms). This difference in the underlying etiologic organism favors the addition of mucosal barrier injury-related BSI as a separate entity from CLABSI particularly for the neutropenic transplant population, as the pathogenesis of bacteremia in this group of patients can arise from a wholly different mechanism.

Diagnosis

Accurate and early diagnosis of IVDR BSI is essential in guiding management decisions, and a variety of diagnostic tests have been developed to help guide therapy. These tests are broadly categorized as methods that require removal of the IVD and those that do not. In general, those that require removal involve quantitative or qualitative cultures of the catheter segment, and those that do not require removal involve paired blood cultures or cytospin examination (Table 13.1) [52].

A meta-analysis by Safdar et al. examined the eight most common diagnostic methods used to evaluate catheter-related bloodstream infection, including qualitative catheter segment culture, semiquantitative catheter segment culture, or quantitative catheter segment culture, each in concordance with results of concomitant blood cultures; qualitative blood culture drawn through an IVD; quantitative blood culture drawn through an IVD, paired quantitative peripheral, and IVD-drawn blood cultures; acridine orange leukocyte cytospin testing; and differential time to positivity. Overall sensitivity was highest for the qualitative catheter segment culture (0.9), followed by IVD-drawn qualitative blood culture and paired quantitative blood cultures (both 0.87). The acridine orange cytospin test had the lowest sensitivity (0.72). Among all the tests, the paired quantitative cultures had the highest specificity (0.98), whereas the qualitative segment culture had the lowest (0.72). However, most methods had acceptable sensitivity and specificity, and the commonly used differential time to positivity test is the preferred method [52].

Notably, in this meta-analysis, only a few studies included immune-compromised patients [53–60], and none exclusively studied the transplant population. Since, there have been only a few additional studies involving the transplant population [61–63]. All these studies evaluated the use of a catheter removal sparing method, the acridine orange leukocyte cytospin (AOLC) test. In a study by Abdelkefi et al., among 26 of 245 hematopoietic stem cell transplant recipients who had a positive differential time to positivity test, the cytospin test was only positive in two of the 26 patients and had a very low sensitivity of 7% [63]. A study by Farina et al. showed similar results, with AOLC testing negative despite positive culture results [62]. In contrast, a smaller study by Krause et al. involving 16/51 hematopoietic stem cell transplant patients showed conflicting results, with much higher sensitivity at 70% and a 100% positive predictive value and a 88% negative predictive value [61]. Certainly, more information regarding the applicability of these and other methods of diagnoses in this particular population is needed.

Table 13.1 Major diagnostic methods for IVDR BSI [52]

Diagnostic method	Description	Criteria for positivity
Methods requiring device removal		
Qualitative catheter segment culture	A segment from the removed catheter is immersed in broth media and incubated for 24–72 h	Any growth
Semiquantitative catheter segment culture	A 5-cm segment of the catheter is rolled four times across a blood agar plate and incubated	≥15 CFU
Quantitative catheter segment culture	A segment from the removed catheter is flushed with broth or sonicated in broth, followed by serial dilutions, surface plating on blood agar, and incubation	≥1000 CFU
Methods not requiring device removal		
Qualitative blood culture through the device	One or more conventional blood cultures are drawn through the device	Any growth
Quantitative blood culture through the device	A blood culture drawn through the device and processed by pour-plate methods or a lysis-centrifugation technique (Isolator, Wampole Laboratories, Cranbury, New Jersey)	≥100 CFU/mL
Paired quantitative blood cultures	Concomitant quantitative blood cultures are drawn through the device and percutaneously and are monitored continuously	Cultures are positive from both sites and the concentration of microorganisms in the culture from the device is 3- to 5-fold greater than in the peripherally drawn culture
Differential time to positivity	Concomitant conventional blood cultures are drawn through the device and percutaneously and are monitored continuously	Both blood cultures are positive and the catheter-drawn blood culture turns positive ≥2 h earlier than the peripherally drawn culture
Acridine orange leukocyte cytospin	Approximately 1 mL of blood is aspirated from the catheter; the cells are lysed with sterile water; and the specimen is centrifuged, stained with acridine orange, and examined microscopically	Visualization of any microorganisms

Abbreviation: CFU colony-forming units

Table 13.2 Recommendations for prevention of IVDR BSI, 2011 CDC HICPAC Guideline [7, 64, 65]

Recommendation	Rating[a]
Education, training, staffing	
Educate all relevant healthcare personnel regarding indications for IVC use, proper procedures for insertion and maintenance, and infection-control measures	IA
Ensure appropriate nursing staff levels in ICUs	IB
Surveillance	
Conduct institutional surveillance for rates of IVDR BSI, monitor trends, identifying lapses in infection-control practices	IA
Express ICU data as number of IVDR BSIs per 1000 catheter days	IB
Antisepsis	
Maximal sterile barrier precautions during catheter insertion: cap, mask, sterile gown, sterile gloves, and large sterile sheet	IB
Hand hygiene: wash hands with antiseptic-containing soap and water or waterless alcohol-based product: before insertion or any manipulation of any IVC	IB
Gloves: required for any manipulation of any IVC	IB
Sterile gloves required for arterial and central catheters	
Clean gloves acceptable for peripheral IVCs if site not touched after application of skin antiseptics	
Cutaneous antisepsis: use before insertion and during dressing changes: 2% chlorhexidine is preferred, an iodophor or 70% alcohol are acceptable	IA
Insertion	
When possible, use subclavian site when using a non-tunneled CVC	IB
Use ultrasound guidance and designated personnel for insertion and maintenance of IVCs	IB
Use sterile gauze or sterile, transparent semipermeable dressing	IA
Do not give prophylactic antibiotics to prevent catheter colonization or BSI	IA
Maintenance	
Change dressing at least weekly	IIII
Monitor site visually or by palpation through intact dressing on regular basis and remove dressing for full exam if tender, fever without obvious source, or other manifestations suggesting local or BSI	
Do not routinely culture catheter tips	IB
Do not use topical antibiotic ointments or creams (except with dialysis catheters)	IB
Remove IVCs as soon as not necessary	IB
Do not routinely replace CVCs, PICCs, HD catheters or pulmonary artery catheters to prevent IVDR BSI	
Replace peripheral venous catheters at least every 72–96 h in adults	IB
Replace administration sets no more frequently than at 72 h unless infection or unless infusing blood products or lipid emulsions	
If after implementing a comprehensive strategy to reduce rates of IVDR BSI and rates remain high, use antimicrobial or antiseptic-impregnated CVC in adults if CVC is expected to remain >5 days	IB
Other strategies recently addressed in current guidelines	
Consider antimicrobial lock solutions for use in all long-term devices	II
Chlorhexidine-impregnated dressings (Biopatch®) should be used with all short-term catheters	IA
A sutureless catheter securement device (StatLock®) is preferred to sutures	II
Adhere to the IHI bundle for CVCs	IA
Chlorhexidine bathing in the ICU	II

Abbreviations: IVDR BSI intravascular catheter-related bloodstream infection, *CVC* central venous catheter, *HD* hemodialysis, *IVC* intravenous catheter, *PICC* peripherally inserted central venous catheter, *IHI* Institute for Healthcare Improvement

[a]CDC categories of evidence: IA: Strongly recommended for implementation and strongly supported by well-designed experimental, clinical, or epidemiologic studies, IB: Strongly recommended for implementation and supported by some experimental, clinical or epidemiologic studies, and a strong theoretical rationale, IC: Required by state or federal regulations, rules, or standards, II: Suggested for implementation and supported by suggestive clinical or epidemiologic studies or a theoretical rationale [7]

Prevention of IVDR BSI

In 2002, the Healthcare Infection Control Practices Advisory Committee (HICPAC) of the CDC published a comprehensive guideline for the prevention of IVDR BSI [7]. This guideline was recently updated in 2011 [64] and provides recommendations for: all healthcare workers on best practices for catheter insertion and care; the surveillance of infection rates; practicing maximal antisepsis, including hand hygiene and barrier precautions; choosing the optimal insertion site and dedicated insertion personnel; and removing the device as soon as it is deemed unnecessary [64]. Table 13.2 summarizes the recommendations of the guideline [7, 64, 65]. Highlighted below are topics of importance in prevention as well as other strategies recently addressed in the guideline (Table 13.3) [66–78]. The recommendations are rated based on the strength of evidence supporting them as follows: IA, strongly recommended for implementation and strongly supported by well-designed experimental, clinical, or epidemiologic studies; IB, strongly recommended for implementation and supported by some

Table 13.3 Novel strategies for the prevention of catheter-related bloodstream infections [66–78]

Strategy	Study	Design	Technology	Outcome
Antimicrobial lock solutions				
	Safdar et al. (2006) [67]	Meta-analysis	Vancomycin-containing locks versus heparin	50% risk reduction (RR, 0.49; 95% CI, 0.26–0.95)
	Yahav et al. (2008) [68]	Systematic review and meta-analysis	Various antibiotics[a]	*Antibiotic solutions:*
			Antibiotic plus antiseptic[b]	RR, 0.44 (95% CI, 0.38–0.5)
			Antiseptic[c]	*Non-antibiotic antiseptic solutions alone*:
				RR, 0.9 (95% CI, 0.48–1.69)
				Non-antibiotic antiseptic solutions + other prevention methods[d]*:*
				RR, 0.25 (95% CI, 0.13–0.5)
	Sanders et al. (2008) [69]	Double-blind randomized trial	Ethanol-containing locks versus heparin	OR, 0.18 (95% CI, 0.05–0.65)
Antimicrobial catheters				
	Veenstra et al. (1999) [70]	Meta-analysis	Antiseptic-impregnated CVCs[e]	OR, 0.56 (95% CI, 0.37–0.84)
	Ramritu et al. (2008) [71]	Systematic review	Antibiotic-impregnated CVCs[f]	RR, 0.39 (95% CI, 0.17–0.92)
	Crnich et al. (2002) [66]	Meta-analysis	Silver-impregnated CVCs	RR, 0.40 (95% CI, 0.24–0.68)
	Ramritu et al. (2008) [71]	Systematic review	Antibiotic versus first-generation antiseptic-impregnated CVCs	RR, 0.12 (95% CI 0.02–0.67)[g]
	Hockenhull et al. (2009) [72]	Meta-analysis	Anti-infective CVCs (all types)	OR, 0.49 (95% CI 0.37–0.64)[h]
Chlorhexidine dressings				
	Maki et al. (2000) [73]	Randomized, controlled trial	Chlorhexidine-impregnated sponge dressing	IVDR BSI: RR 0.37 (0.17–0.80)
	Ho et al. (2006) [74]	Meta-analysis	Chlorhexidine-impregnated dressing versus placebo or povidine-iodine dressing	Catheter or exit site colonization: 14.3% vs 27.2%; OR, 0.4 (95% CI, 0.26–0.61)
				IVDR BSI: 2.2% vs 3.8%; OR, 0.58 (95% CI, 0.29–1.14, $p = 0.11$)
	Timsit et al. (2009) [75]	Randomized, controlled trial	Chlorhexidine-impregnated dressing versus standard dressing	IVDR BSI: 0.4 vs 1.3 per 1000 catheter days; HR, 0.024 (95% CI, 0.09–0.65; $p = 0.005$)
Cutaneous antisepsis				
	Chaiyakunapruk et al. (2002) [76]	Meta-analysis	Chlorhexidine versus povidone-iodine	RR, 0.49 (95% CI, 0.28–0.88)[i]
	Maki et al. (1991) [77]	RCT	Chlorhexidine vs alcohol versus povidone-iodine	IVDR BSI RR 0.16, $p = 0.04$
Mupirocin prophylaxis				
	Tacconelli et al. (2003) [78]	Meta-analysis	Mupirocin prophylaxis in dialysis patients[j]	Decrease in *S. aureus* bacteremia in hemodialysis patients by 78%; RR 0.22 (95% CI, 0.11–0.42)

Abbreviations: CI confidence interval, *EDTA* ethylenediamine tetraacetic acid, *HR* hazard ratio, *IVDR BSI* intravascular catheter-related bloodstream infection, *OR* odds ratio, *RR* relative risk

[a]Gentamicin; gentamicin + citrate; gentamicin + vancomycin; gentamicin + cefazolin; cefotaxime

[b]Minocycline with EDTA

[c]Citrate; citrate with taurolidine

[d]Nasal mupirocin and exit-site iodine dressing

[e]Chlorhexidine-silver sulfadiazine

[f]Minocycline and rifampin

[g]Reduced risk with antibiotic catheters

[h]Reduced risk with anti-infective catheters: all types combined, see text for subgroup analysis

[i]Reduced with chlorhexidine

[j]Six studies used intranasal mupirocin two to three times daily for 5–14 days with various maintenance schedules; four studies used mupirocin applied to catheter exit site

experimental, clinical, or epidemiologic studies and a strong theoretical rationale; IC, required by state or federal regulations, rules, or standards; and II, suggested for implementation and supported by suggestive clinical or epidemiologic studies or a theoretical rationale [7].

Cutaneous Antisepsis

Iodophors, such as 10% povidone-iodine, or 70% alcohol were historically the most widely used agents for cutaneous antisepsis of the insertion site in US centers [79, 80].

However, several studies, including a meta-analysis, have shown that 2% chlorhexidine (CHG) is unequivocally superior for preventing IVDR BSI [76, 77] and is now recommended by the HICPAC Guideline as the agent of first choice (rating IA) [7, 64, 77, 79].

Topical Antimicrobials

The HICPAC Guideline specifically recommends against the application of topical antimicrobial ointments or creams to the IVD insertion site, except in the case of hemodialysis catheters [7] to avoid promotion of fungal infection and antimicrobial resistance (rating IA). The Guideline also discourages the use of intranasal mupirocin for staphylococcal decolonization before IVD insertion or during the use of an IVD as a means to prevent colonization or IVDR BSI (rating IA) [7]. A meta-analysis of mupirocin prophylaxis to prevent *S. aureus* infections in patients undergoing dialysis showed a 63% reduction (95% CI, 50–73%) in the rate of overall *S. aureus* infections [78]. The study population included both hemodialysis and peritoneal dialysis patients. Of the ten studies, six used intranasal mupirocin two to three times daily for 5–14 days, with various maintenance schedules, and four used mupirocin applied to the catheter exit site. In patients undergoing hemodialysis, *S. aureus* bacteremias were reduced by 78% (relative risk [RR], 0.22; 95% CI, 0.11–0.42). However, the differences in site, frequency, and duration of mupirocin treatment in these studies and the resulting clinical heterogeneity make it difficult to offer robust recommendations [78].

A randomized, double-blind, placebo-controlled trial evaluating mupirocin prophylaxis for nosocomial *S. aureus* infections in nonsurgical patients found that restricting the use of intranasal mupirocin to patients shown to be carriers on admission did not prevent nosocomial *S. aureus* infections [81]. Increasing reports of mupirocin resistance [82–87] has called decolonization with mupirocin into question as a strategy to prevent IVDR BSI, even in hemodialysis centers, and we do not recommend topical or intranasal mupirocin for prevention of IVDR BSI.

The early promise of mupirocin has suggested that other topical approaches to preventing IVDR BSI bear study. One such agent is honey, which has long been known to have antibacterial properties. In a randomized, controlled trial (RCT) to compare the effect of thrice-weekly application of Medihoney (commercially available; pooled antibacterial honeys including *Leptospermum* species honey; Medihoney Pty Ltd., Brisbane, Australia) to the IVD exit site versus mupirocin in 101 patients receiving hemodialysis through tunneled and cuffed CVCs, catheter-associated bacteremia rates in the two arms were similar (0.97 versus 0.85 episodes per 1000 catheter days; $p > 0.05$) [88]. Although these results are promising, a larger trial powered to show equivalence or superiority is needed to establish the utility of Medihoney for the prevention of IVDR BSI in patients receiving hemodialysis through cuffed and tunneled CVCs.

Maximal Barrier Precautions

The use of maximal barrier precautions, including cap, sterile gown, mask, large sterile drape, and sterile gloves, significantly reduces the rate of IVDR BSI when used during catheter insertion [7, 89, 90]. In an RCT, Raad et al. compared maximal barrier precautions with minimal precautions such as sterile gloves and a small fenestrated drape, and found the CVC-related BSI rate to be 6.3 times higher in the control group ($p = 0.06$) [89]. The HICPAC Guideline recommends that maximal barrier precautions be used for all central IVD insertions, including PICCs (rating IB) [64].

Insertion Site

According to the HICPAC Guideline, the preferred site for insertion of non-tunneled CVCs in adult patients is the subclavian vein (rating 1B) [7]. However, the subclavian site is typically avoided in hemodialysis patients and patients with advanced kidney disease to avoid stenosis (1A). The femoral site has been reported to be associated with higher rates of catheter colonization as well as an increased risk of deep vein thrombosis compared to cephalad sites in adults [7, 43, 91–93]. In an RCT with uncuffed CVCs comparing femoral with subclavian sites, catheters inserted in a femoral site were associated with a higher incidence of infectious complications (19.8% vs 4.5%; $p < 0.001$) [93].

The internal jugular vein site has also been associated with higher rates of IVDR BSI than the femoral or subclavian sites in several studies [7, 43, 94]. However, a recent RCT comparing the jugular and femoral sites found no difference in the risk of infection between the two sites (2.3 vs 1.5, $p = 0.42$) [95]. A prospective, observational study comparing the subclavian, internal jugular, and femoral insertion sites found colonization lowest at the subclavian site but no difference in rates of infection between sites [95, 96].

Using real-time ultrasound guidance for catheter insertion significantly reduces mechanical complications deriving from catheter insertion and catheter infection [7, 97, 98]. In a randomized study, real-time ultrasound guidance versus the landmark technique for catheter placement in the internal jugular vein resulted in significantly fewer complications, including fewer IVDR BSI ($p < 0.001$) [98]. A meta-analysis found that the use of ultrasound for insertion at internal jugular and subclavian vein sites reduced cannulation failure (RR, 0.32; 95% CI, 0.18–0.55), the need for multiple placement attempts (RR, 0.60; 95% CI, 0.45–0.79), and complications during catheter placement (RR, 0.22; 95% CI,

0.10–0.45) in comparison with insertions using anatomic landmarks [97].

Although no RCT to date has compared the three insertion sites, based on the available data we recommend the subclavian site as the first preferred site for CVC insertion and routinely employing real-time ultrasound to minimize mechanical complications.

Simulation-Based Training

A recent observational study, completed in an urban teaching hospital, evaluated the impact of a simulation-based educational intervention on the rates of IVDR BSI in a medical ICU [99]. As part of this study, 92 second- and third-year internal medicine and emergency medicine residents completed the educational program, which included a pretest, an informational video demonstrating proper CVC insertion technique, training with ultrasound and hands-on practice using a simulator device, and a posttest with a required minimum score [99]. There were 3.2 infections per 1000 catheter days in the 16 months prior to the educational intervention in this medical ICU, and 4.9 infections per 1000 catheter days in a comparator unit in the same hospital, the surgical ICU, during the pre-intervention period. The rate of IVDR BSIs in the medical ICU during the 16-month intervention period, when all of the second- and third-year residents had completed the training, decreased to 0.5 per 1000 catheter days. The rate in the surgical ICU, where no rotating residents completed the simulation training, remained stable at 5.3 per 1000 catheter days during the same 16-month interval [99]. This study highlights the value of cutting-edge programs for training healthcare personnel in proper CVC insertion techniques, addressing a priority recommendation in the CDC HICPAC Guideline for the Prevention of IVDR BSI [7].

Chlorhexidine-Impregnated Insertion Site Dressings

The application of a chlorhexidine (CHG)-impregnated sponge dressing (BioPatch®, Johnson & Johnson Gateway) over the CVC insertion site has been shown to greatly reduce the incidence of IVDR BSI in several randomized trials [5, 73, 75, 79, 100, 101]. A large, randomized, open, controlled trial compared this dressing to standard sterile dressings in 601 chemotherapy patients, with 9,731 catheterization days, and showed a significant reduction in IVDR BSI in the intervention group (6.4%, 19 of 300) compared to the control group (11.3%, 34 of 301; $p = 0.016$, RR, 0.54; 95% CI, 0.31–0.94) [101]. In ICU patients, the use of CHG-impregnated dressings led to significantly fewer IVDR BSIs when compared with standard sterile dressings, in a large, multicenter RCT ($p = 0.005$, HR, 0.024; 95% CI, 0.09–0.65) [75, 100].

The latest 2011 guideline recommends the use of CHG-impregnated dressings for short-term catheters in patients older than two months of age if the CLABSI rate is not decreasing despite adherence to basic multimodal prevention measures (IB). However, there is considerable emerging data indicating that CHG-impregnated dressings are effective in reducing IVDR BSI, and we recommend their use as part of standard care [73, 75, 79, 100, 101].

Chlorhexidine Bathing

Daily bathing with liquid CHG or the use of CHG-impregnated washcloths has been studied extensively in the past few years [102–104] for its impact on reducing healthcare-associated infections. A meta-analysis by O'Horo et al. which included 12 studies examined the efficacy of daily bathing with CHG, focusing mainly on healthcare-associated BSIs, including CLABSI [102]. Ten of the 12 studies were carried out in the ICU setting, and none included the transplant population. The results showed that 291 patients in the CHG arm developed BSI over 67,775 days compared to 557 patients in the control arm who developed BSI over 69,617 days (OR, 0.44; 95% CI, 0.33–0.59; $p < 0.0001$).

Data regarding the use of CHG bathing among transplant recipients is lacking. The study by Climo et al., a multicenter cluster-randomized, crossover trial, involved a total of nine units, of which one was exclusively bone marrow transplant patients [105]. However, results specific to the bone marrow population were not provided. Overall, the risk of acquiring primary BSI was significantly lower among patients bathed with CHG than among those bathed with non-antimicrobial cloths. In addition, the longer the length of stay in the unit, the lower the risk for a primary BSI among those bathed with CHG; for example, RR at day 7 was 0.69 compared to 0.51 at 14 days.

Anti-infective-Impregnated Catheters

The HICPAC Guideline recommends the use of anti-infective-coated CVCs if the catheter is expected to remain longer than five days and is used in combination with a comprehensive IVDR BSI reduction strategy (rating IB) [7]. However, the majority of studies have focused on the use of antimicrobial-coated CVCs used as short-term devices, and few data have been published on their use as long-term devices [71, 79]. Several types of catheters are available: catheters coated either externally, the first generation, or externally and internally, the second generation, with chlorhexidine and sulfadiazine silver (CSS); catheters coated with minocycline or rifampin; and silver-impregnated catheters [5]. Silver-coated catheters include silver-, platinum-, and carbon-coated catheters and silver ion/alloy catheters.

A recent comprehensive meta-analysis of anti-infective-coated catheters included clinical trials comparing antimicrobial-coated CVCs with either a standard CVC or another antimicrobial-coated CVC [106]. The main outcomes were catheter colonization and catheter-related BSI. The first-generation CSS CVCs were shown to reduce colonization (OR, 0.51; 95% CI, 0.42–0.60) and catheter-related BSI (OR, 0.68; 95% CI, 0.47–0.98). Minocycline-rifampin-coated CVCs also reduced catheter colonization (OR, 0.39; 95% CI, 0.27–0.55) and catheter-related BSI (OR, 0.29; 95% CI 0.16–0.52) and performed better than the CSS CVCs for reducing catheter colonization and BSI (OR, 0.18; 95% CI, 0.07–0.51). A small retrospective study among kidney transplant patients also showed that silver ion (AgION)-coated polyurethane catheters were less likely to be colonized with bacteria (58% vs 6.6%), compared to plain polyurethane catheters [107].

The choice of which catheter to use is governed by many factors including efficacy, cost, cost-effectiveness, and risk of promoting drug resistance. A recent analysis (2008) found an estimated cost savings of £138.20, approximately $227, for every anti-infective catheter inserted [11]. Antibiotic resistance is a particular concern with antibiotic-impregnated catheters, although trials assessing the efficacy of minocycline-rifampin-coated catheters have not found evidence of emergence of drug resistance to date [71].

Anti-infective Lock Solutions

The major mechanism of IVDR BSI in long-term IVDs is intraluminal colonization. For this reason, antimicrobial lock solutions have been a logical step to prevent colonization of the intraluminal surfaces of long-term IVDs to prevent IVDR BSI. A small volume of the antimicrobial solution is instilled into the lumen of the IVD and allowed to dwell for a prescribed period, after which it is either removed or flushed into the patient's bloodstream.

A meta-analysis of seven RCTs, involving mostly cancer patients, comparing a vancomycin-containing lock solution with sterile saline showed a significantly reduced risk of IVDR BSI (RR, 0.49; 95% CI, 0.26–0.95) [67]. Ethanol has also recently been shown to be safe and effective as an antimicrobial lock solution [69, 79, 107]. A recently published prospective, double-blind RCT comparing ethanol with heparinized saline in granulocytopenic hematology patients showed a four-fold reduction in IVDR BSI in the ethanol group compared to controls (OR, 0.18; 95% CI, 0.05–0.65) [69]. In contrast, a similar study comparing heparinized saline with 70% ethanol locks in patients with hematologic malignancies and tunneled CVCs did not show a reduction in device-associated infection with the use of ethanol locks [108].

A recent meta-analysis of 23 studies [109] published in 2014 reported data on a variety of lock solutions and involved a total of 2,896 patients, including patients on hemodialysis, adult and pediatric oncology patients, critically ill neonates, and patients receiving total parenteral nutrition. The use of antimicrobial lock solutions led to a 69% reduction in CLABSI rate (RR, 0.31; 95% CI, 0.24–0.40) and a 32% reduction in the rate of exit site infections (RR, 0.68; 95% CI, 0.49–0.95) compared with heparin, without significantly affecting catheter failure due to noninfectious complications (RR, 0.83; 95% CI, 0.65–1.06).

While a number of new antibiotics show promise as lock solutions based on in vitro studies [110], further research of their efficacy in clinical trials is mandatory.

Given the promising data, we recommend the use of anti-infective lock solutions for prevention of IVDR BSI with long-term IVDs in patients at high risk for IVDR BSI, such as those receiving hemodialysis. In general, antiseptic lock solutions are preferable to antibiotic lock solutions because of their greater spectrum of activity and lower risk of promoting antibiotic resistance.

Anti-infective Luer-Activated Devices

In addition to the above novel technology-based strategies for prevention of IVDR BSI, an emerging role of needleless connectors in the pathogenesis of IVDR BSI must be mentioned, with conjecture of possible preventive strategies.

Needleless connectors were developed in response to demands for enhanced safety for healthcare workers, to prevent needlestick injuries universally, and are an integral component of infusion systems in use across North America. Although needleless connectors, when properly used, clearly reduce the risk for needlestick injuries during access of an IVD or injection port [111–115], some reports published over the past decade have raised concerns about a potential increased risk of iatrogenic IVDR BSI associated with the use of luer-activated, valved connectors [43, 116–120]. Most of these studies have been retrospective and uncontrolled, and suboptimal manipulation of the device, rather than the device itself, may have been responsible for some of the increased incidence of BSI in some settings. However, many hospitals experienced sharp increases in primary BSI following introduction of a new connector, and intensified infection control practices had no impact; only after removing the new connector from the hospital did rates of CVC-associated BSI return to baseline levels [121]. Most notably, multiple commercial valved connectors have been implicated, indicating that these devices can become contaminated and result in iatrogenic BSI.

Typically, healthcare personnel disinfect the connector before accessing with 70% (v/v) isopropyl alcohol. Although needleless connectors appeared to reduce contamination in comparison with standard caps [122], a recent study by Menyhay and Maki found that conventional methods of disinfection of the membranous septum may not prevent microbial entry if the membrane of the luer-activated device (LAD) is heavily contaminated, which may account for the increased risk for CVC-associated BSI seen in some centers [123].

This issue has been addressed with the development of a new technology. The V-Link with VitaShield (Baxter Healthcare) is a LAD protected with interior and exterior antimicrobial coating and was recently approved by the FDA. The V-Link with VitaShield is effective against 99.9% of pathogens known to cause IVDR BSI in in vitro testing and was recently shown in a simulation study to prevent internal contamination, even with heavy contamination of the membranous septum [124].

Saralex-cl (Menyhay Healthcare Systems), another promising device, is an antimicrobial barrier cap that threads onto the end of a needleless LAD system. A recent prospective in vitro study compared standard disinfection of common LADs using 70% isopropyl alcohol with the new antiseptic barrier cap [125]. This new antiseptic cap which bathes the connector septum with 0.25 mL of 2% CHG in 70% isopropyl alcohol is almost totally effective in preventing transmission of pathogens across the membranes of pre-contaminated LADs when compared to standard techniques (positive control, 100% transmission; standard disinfection with 70% alcohol, 20 transmissions in 30 trials, 67% transmission; Saralex-cl, 1 transmission in 60 trials, 1.6% transmission; $p<0.001$) [120]. Data on the clinical efficacy of antimicrobial-coated LADs and antimicrobial barrier caps based on RCTs is needed.

Catheter Securement

Choices for securement of a percutaneous uncuffed CVC or PICC include sutures, tape, or novel catheter securement devices, such as StatLock® (Venetec International, a subsidiary of CR Bard). Sutures are often painful for the patient, pose the risk of needlestick injury to the provider placing them, and foster infection at the catheter insertion site, increasing the risk of catheter-related BSI. StatLock®, a sutureless catheter securement device, reduces catheter-related complications including IVDR BSI [126–128]. A randomized trial comparing suture securement to the StatLock® with peripherally inserted central catheters showed a significant reduction in the number of catheter-related BSIs in the StatLock® group (2 vs 10; $p = 0.032$) [127]. We recommend the use of a sutureless securement device for peripheral IV and extended dwell catheters, such as non-cuffed CVCs and PICCs.

Intensive Insulin Therapy

Glycemic control in critically ill ICU patients is essential for prevention of IVDR BSI. However, the optimum level of glycemic control is controversial. A large, RCT in 1,548 critically ill patients in a surgical ICU, the majority of whom had undergone surgical procedures, compared intensive insulin therapy for the maintenance of blood glucose level between 80 and 110 mg/dL by using continuous insulin infusions with conventional subcutaneous insulin therapy given only if blood glucose levels exceeded 215 mg/dL, striving to maintain levels between 180 and 200 mg/dL [129]. The study found a markedly reduced ICU and hospital mortality with intensive glycemic control [8% with conventional treatment vs 4.6% with intensive treatment ($p < 0.04$)]. The greatest reduction in mortality was seen in patients with multi-organ failure due to a septic focus [129]. Most noteworthy, the incidence of nosocomial BSI was cut in half from 8% to 4%. A similar study in medical ICU patients found no reduction in mortality or difference in bacteremia rates with intensive control [130].

A meta-analysis which included 29 RCTs and 8,432 patients found no difference in hospital mortality with tight glucose control versus moderate control (21.6% vs 23.3%; RR, 0.93; 95% CI, 0.85–1.03), and the results did not change when patients were stratified by type of ICU: surgical, medical, or medical-surgical. However, tight glucose control was associated with a reduced risk of septicemia of 10.9% vs 13.4% in the moderate control group (RR, 0.76; 95% CI, 0.59–0.97) [130].

In the NICE SUGAR study, a large RCT of 6,104 adult ICU patients, intensive glycemic control (goal 81–108 mg/dL) was associated with increased mortality compared to conventional control (goal ≤180 mg/dL) (OR, 1.14; 95% CI, 1.02–1.28; $p = 0.02$) [131]. The study population included more medical than surgical ICU patients. The intensive group had 36.9% surgical and 63.1% medical patients, whereas the conventional group included 37.2% surgical and 62.8% medical ICU patients. Severe hypoglycemia, defined as ≤40 mg/dL was significantly more common in the intensive control group (6.8% vs 0.5%; $p < 0.001$) [131].

A recent meta-analysis of 26 trials involving a total of 13,567 patients, including the data from the NICE SUGAR trial, found no mortality benefit to intensive insulin therapy in critically ill patients; the pooled RR of death with intensive therapy using insulin drip as compared with moderate control using subcutaneous insulin was 0.93 (95% CI, 0.83–1.04) [132]. However, when analyzed separately, surgical ICU patients experienced significant benefit (RR, 0.63; 95% CI, 0.44–0.91), while patients in nonsurgical ICUs did not.

Based on these studies, all hospitalized patients are likely to benefit from moderate glycemic control, and we recommend the use of intensive glycemic control with an insulin drip in surgical ICU patients to reduce the risk of healthcare-associated infections, particularly BSI. However, stringent monitoring to avoid severe hypoglycemia is critical, and a glycemic target that can be achieved safely should be chosen, generally 120–130 mg/dL.

Achieving High-Level Compliance with Essential Control Measures Through Institutional Systems

A multifaceted approach with near-100% compliance is essential to consistently and maximally reduce the risk of IVDR BSI. The Institute for Healthcare Improvement (IHI) has developed the concept of "bundles" to aid in risk reduction. A bundle, according to the IHI, is a structured way of improving the processes of care and patient outcomes using a set of practices, generally three to five, which when performed collectively and reliably have been shown to improve patient outcomes [133]. The IHI-recommended evidence-based bundle for CVC care includes the following: (1) hand hygiene before IVD insertion; (2) maximal barrier precautions during the insertion procedure; (3) cutaneous antisepsis with CHG; (4) optimal catheter insertion site selection, with the subclavian vein the preferred site for CVCs; and (5) daily review of continued need for the catheter, with immediate removal when no longer needed [133]. In a pre-post trial in 100 Michigan hospitals, Pronovost et al. showed that development of effective systems within the hospitals which assured a very high level of compliance with the bundle for every CVC insertion resulted in a striking reduction in IVDR BSI in the individual hospitals over 18 months, with a reduction from pre-study baseline at 0–3 months of 0.62 (95% CI, 0.47–0.81) and at 16–18 months of 0.34 (95% CI, 0.23–0.5) [13]. These numbers represented an overall 66% reduction in rates of IVDR BSI, which was maintained for several months [15].

Bhutta et al. undertook a prospective quasi-experimental study in a children's hospital which included the stepwise introduction of interventions over a 5-year period [134]. The interventions included maximal barrier precautions, a transition to antibiotic-impregnated CVCs, annual hand washing campaigns, and the use of CHG in lieu of povidone-iodine. Significant decreases in rates of infection occurred over the intervention period and were sustained over a 3-year follow-up. Annual rates of CVC-associated BSI decreased from 9.7 per 1000 days in 1997 to 3.0 per 1000 days in 2005 (RR, 0.75; 95% CI, 0.35–1.26). The investigators found that multifaceted interventions of this nature and development of systems to achieve uniformly high compliance reduce IVDR BSI but require strong institutional support.

The recent implementation of a multifaceted approach in a pediatric cardiac ICU, which included CVC insertion and maintenance bundles, CHG-impregnated dressings, nurse and physician education, and the addition of a unit-based infection control nurse, resulted in a reduction in the rate of IVDR BSI from 7.8 to 2.3 infections per 1000 catheter days over a period of less than 2 years [135]. Pronovost et al. have outlined the essential steps to establishing an effective institutional system to achieve these recommended results [14].

A recent meta-analysis by Blot et al. also investigated the efficacy of quality improvement interventions, including personnel education, catheter care bundles, and checklists in decreasing CLABSI. Results among the 41 studies showed an infection rate decrease (OR, 0.39; 95% CI, 0.33–0.46; $p < 0.001$), which was more pronounced for trials implementing a bundle or checklist approach ($p = 0.03$) [136]. These results suggest that quality improvement interventions contribute to the prevention of CLABSI.

Summary

The use of intravascular devices is now standard of care for many patients, including transplant recipients. Unfortunately, these devices, especially when used in the long term, increase the risk of bloodstream infections through external or internal colonization of the lumen. The key to preventing device-related bloodstream infection is establishment of, and strict compliance with, a multifaceted approach to consistently and maximally reduce the risk of IVDR BSI. This approach has largely been streamlined into a few steps called the bundle of care and consists of hand hygiene, use of maximal barrier precautions, antisepsis, and removal of the line when it is no longer necessary.

In critically ill transplant patients where access is crucial and yet difficult to obtain, removal of the infected device may not be a feasible option, and catheter salvage is a viable alternative. Fortunately, there are now evidence-based recommendations from guidelines and several recent studies that have evaluated the use of salvage therapy, both for prevention and treatment of device-related bacteremia. Among the options, the use of antibiotic or antiseptic lock solutions in combination with systemic therapy appears to be the most promising. Data among the transplant population remains scant at this time, and more prospective, randomized controlled trials are needed in the future to evaluate whether current recommendations for the general population are applicable to this population.

References

1. Raad I, Hachem R, Hanna H, et al. Sources and outcome of bloodstream infections in cancer patients: the role of central venous catheters. Eur J Clin Microbiol Infect Dis. 2007;26(8):549–56.
2. Hachem R, Raad I. Prevention and management of long-term catheter related infections in cancer patients. Cancer Investig. 2002;20(7–8):1105–13.
3. Longuet P, Douard MC, Arlet G, Molina JM, Benoit C, Leport C. Venous access port – related bacteremia in patients with acquired immunodeficiency syndrome or cancer: the reservoir as a diagnostic and therapeutic tool. Clin Infect Dis. 2001;32(12):1776–83.
4. Safdar N, Maki DG. Antibiotic resistance and prevention of CVC-associated BSIs, catheter-associated urinary tract infection and Clostridium difficile. In: Jarvis W, editor. Bennett and Brachman's hospital infections. Philadelphia: Williams and Wilkins; 2007. p. 395–416.
5. Raad I, Hanna H, Maki D. Intravascular catheter-related infections: advances in diagnosis, prevention, and management. Lancet Infect Dis. 2007;7(10):645–57.
6. Lukenbill J, Rybicki L, Sekeres MA, et al. Defining incidence, risk factors, and impact on survival of central line-associated blood stream infections following hematopoietic cell transplantation in acute myeloid leukemia and myelodysplastic syndrome. Biol Blood Marrow Transplant. 2013;19(5):720–4.
7. O'Grady NP, Alexander M, Dellinger EP, et al. Guidelines for the prevention of intravascular catheter-related infections. Infect Control Hosp Epidemiol. 2002;23(12):759–69.
8. Siempos II, Kopterides P, Tsangaris I, Dimopoulou I, Armaganidis AE. Impact of catheter-related bloodstream infections on the mortality of critically ill patients: a meta-analysis. Crit Care Med. 2009;37(7):2283–9.
9. Pittet D, Tarara D, Wenzel RP. Nosocomial bloodstream infection in critically ill patients. Excess length of stay, extra costs, and attributable mortality. JAMA. 1994;271(20):1598–601.
10. Maki DG, Kluger DM, Crnich CJ. The risk of bloodstream infection in adults with different intravascular devices: a systematic review of 200 published prospective studies. Mayo Clin Proc. 2006;81(9):1159–71.
11. Hockenhull JC, Dwan K, Boland A, et al. The clinical effectiveness and cost-effectiveness of central venous catheters treated with anti-infective agents in preventing bloodstream infections: a systematic review and economic evaluation. Health Technol Assess. 2008;12(12):iii–v, xi–xii, 1–154.
12. Raad II. Commentary: zero tolerance for catheter-related bloodstream infections: the unnegotiable objective. Infect Control Hosp Epidemiol. 2008;29(10):951–3.
13. Pronovost P, Needham D, Berenholtz S, et al. An intervention to decrease catheter-related bloodstream infections in the ICU. N Engl J Med. 2006;355(26):2725–32.
14. Pronovost PJ, Berenholtz SM, Needham DM. Translating evidence into practice: a model for large scale knowledge translation. BMJ. 2008;337:a1714.
15. Pronovost PJ, Goeschel CA, Colantuoni E, et al. Sustaining reductions in catheter related bloodstream infections in Michigan intensive care units: observational study. BMJ. 2010;340:c309.
16. Reduction in central line-associated bloodstream infections among patients in intensive care units – Pennsylvania, April 2001–March 2005. MMWR Morb Mortal Wkly Rep. 2005;54(40):1013–6.
17. Frankel HL, Crede WB, Topal JE, Roumanis SA, Devlin MW, Foley AB. Use of corporate Six Sigma performance-improvement strategies to reduce incidence of catheter-related bloodstream infections in a surgical ICU. J Am Coll Surg. 2005;201(3):349–58.
18. Gastmeier P, Geffers C. Prevention of catheter-related bloodstream infections: analysis of studies published between 2002 and 2005. J Hosp Infect. 2006;64(4):326–35.
19. Jeffries HE, Mason W, Brewer M, et al. Prevention of central venous catheter-associated bloodstream infections in pediatric intensive care units: a performance improvement collaborative. Infect Control Hosp Epidemiol. 2009;30(7):645–51.
20. Lobo RD, Levin AS, Oliveira MS, et al. Evaluation of interventions to reduce catheter-associated bloodstream infection: continuous tailored education versus one basic lecture. Am J Infect Control. 2010;38(6):440–8.
21. Miller RS, Norris PR, Jenkins JM, et al. Systems initiatives reduce healthcare-associated infections: a study of 22,928 device days in a single trauma unit. J Trauma. 2010;68(1):23–31.
22. Render ML, Brungs S, Kotagal U, et al. Evidence-based practice to reduce central line infections. Jt Comm J Qual Patient Saf. 2006;32(5):253–60.
23. Rosenthal VD, Guzman S, Pezzotto SM, Crnich CJ. Effect of an infection control program using education and performance feedback on rates of intravascular device-associated bloodstream infections in intensive care units in Argentina. Am J Infect Control. 2003;31(7):405–9.
24. Zuschneid I, Schwab F, Geffers C, Ruden H, Gastmeier P. Reducing central venous catheter-associated primary bloodstream infections in intensive care units is possible: data from the German nosocomial infection surveillance system. Infect Control Hosp Epidemiol. 2003;24(7):501–5.
25. Edwards JR, Peterson KD, Andrus ML, Dudeck MA, Pollock DA, Horan TC. National Healthcare Safety Network (NHSN) report, data summary for 2006 through 2007, issued November 2008. Am J Infect Control. 2008;36(9):609–26.
26. Edwards JR, Peterson KD, Andrus ML, et al. National Healthcare Safety Network (NHSN) report, data summary for 2006, issued June 2007. Am J Infect Control. 2007;35(5):290–301.
27. Edwards JR, Peterson KD, Mu Y, et al. National Healthcare Safety Network (NHSN) report: data summary for 2006 through 2008, issued December 2009. Am J Infect Control. 2009;37(10):783–805.
28. Digiorgio MJ, Fatica C, Oden M, et al. Development of a modified surveillance definition of central line-associated bloodstream infections for patients with hematologic malignancies. Infect Control Hosp Epidemiol. 2012;33(9):865–8.
29. Maki DG, Goldman DA, Rhame FS. Infection control in intravenous therapy. Ann Intern Med. 1973;79(6):867–87.
30. Maki D, Mermel L. Infections due to infusion therapy. CINAAGINCOURT. 1999;15:71–95. http://doctorlib.info/medical/infections/39.html
31. Douard MC, Clementi E, Arlet G, et al. Negative catheter-tip culture and diagnosis of catheter-related bacteremia. Nutrition. 1994;10(5):397–404.
32. Nouwen JL, Wielenga JJ, van Overhagen H, et al. Hickman catheter-related infections in neutropenic patients: insertion in the operating theater versus insertion in the radiology suite. J Clin Oncol. 1999;17(4):1304.
33. Livesley MA, Tebbs SE, Moss HA, Faroqui MH, Lambert PA, Elliott TS. Use of pulsed field gel electrophoresis to determine the source of microbial contamination of central venous catheters. Eur J Clin Microbiol Infect Dis. 1998;17(2):108–12.
34. Darouiche RO, Raad II, Heard SO, et al. A comparison of two antimicrobial-impregnated central venous catheters. Catheter Study Group. N Engl J Med. 1999;340(1):1–8.
35. Maki DG, Stolz SM, Wheeler S, Mermel LA. Prevention of central venous catheter-related bloodstream infection by use of an antiseptic-impregnated catheter. A randomized, controlled trial. Ann Intern Med. 1997;127(4):257–66.
36. Garland JS, Alex CP, Sevallius JM, et al. Cohort study of the pathogenesis and molecular epidemiology of catheter-related bloodstream infection in neonates with peripherally inserted central venous catheters. Infect Control Hosp Epidemiol. 2008;29(3):243–9.

37. Safdar N, Maki DG. The pathogenesis of catheter-related bloodstream infection with noncuffed short-term central venous catheters. Intensive Care Med. 2004;30(1):62–7.
38. Marrie TJ, Costerton JW. Scanning and transmission electron microscopy of in situ bacterial colonization of intravenous and intraarterial catheters. J Clin Microbiol. 1984;19(5):687–93.
39. Cooper GL, Schiller AL, Hopkins CC. Possible role of capillary action in pathogenesis of experimental catheter-associated dermal tunnel infections. J Clin Microbiol. 1988;26(1):8–12.
40. Sitges-Serra A, Linares J, Garau J. Catheter sepsis: the clue is the hub. Surgery. 1985;97(3):355–7.
41. Maki DG, Jarrett F, Sarafin HW. A semiquantitative culture method for identification of catheter-related infection in the burn patient. J Surg Res. 1977;22(5):513–20.
42. Crnich CJ, Maki DG. The promise of novel technology for the prevention of intravascular device-related bloodstream infection. I. Pathogenesis and short-term devices. Clin Infect Dis. 2002;34(9):1232–42.
43. Yokoe DS, Mermel LA, Anderson DJ, et al. A compendium of strategies to prevent healthcare-associated infections in acute care hospitals. Infect Control Hosp Epidemiol. 2008;29(Suppl 1):S12–21.
44. Bjornson HS, Colley R, Bower RH, Duty VP, Schwartz-Fulton JT, Fischer JE. Association between microorganism growth at the catheter insertion site and colonization of the catheter in patients receiving total parenteral nutrition. Surgery. 1982;92(4):720 7.
45. Sitges-Serra A, Puig P, Linares J, et al. Hub colonization as the initial step in an outbreak of catheter-related sepsis due to coagulase negative staphylococci during parenteral nutrition. JPEN J Parenter Enteral Nutr. 1984;8(6):668–72.
46. Raad I, Costerton W, Sabharwal U, Sacilowski M, Anaissie E, Bodey GP. Ultrastructural analysis of indwelling vascular catheters: a quantitative relationship between luminal colonization and duration of placement. J Infect Dis. 1993;168(2):400–7.
47. Wisplinghoff H, Bischoff T, Tallent SM, Seifert H, Wenzel RP, Edmond MB. Nosocomial bloodstream infections in US hospitals: analysis of 24,179 cases from a prospective nationwide surveillance study. Clin Infect Dis. 2004;39(3):309–17.
48. Trick WE, Fridkin SK, Edwards JR, Hajjeh RA, Gaynes RP. Secular trend of hospital-acquired candidemia among intensive care unit patients in the United States during 1989–1999. Clin Infect Dis. 2002;35(5):627–30.
49. Lorente L, Jimenez A, Santana M, et al. Microorganisms responsible for intravascular catheter-related bloodstream infection according to the catheter site. Crit Care Med. 2007;35(10):2424–7.
50. Sipsas NV, Lewis RE, Tarrand J, et al. Candidemia in patients with hematologic malignancies in the era of new antifungal agents (2001–2007): stable incidence but changing epidemiology of a still frequently lethal infection. Cancer. 2009;115(20):4745–52.
51. See I, Iwamoto M, Allen-Bridson K, Horan T, Magill SS, Thompson ND. Mucosal barrier injury laboratory-confirmed bloodstream infection: results from a field test of a new National Healthcare Safety Network definition. Infect Control Hosp Epidemiol. 2013;34(8):769–76.
52. Safdar N, Fine JP, Maki DG. Meta-analysis: methods for diagnosing intravascular device-related bloodstream infection. Ann Intern Med. 2005;142(6):451–66.
53. Raad I, Hanna H, Boktour M, et al. Management of central venous catheters in patients with cancer and candidemia. Clin Infect Dis. 2004;38(8):1119–27.
54. Jones PG, Hopfer RL, Elting L, Jackson JA, Fainstein V, Bodey GP. Semiquantitative cultures of intravascular catheters from cancer patients. Diagn Microbiol Infect Dis. 1986;4(4):299–306.
55. Douard MC, Arlet G, Leverger G, et al. Quantitative blood cultures for diagnosis and management of catheter-related sepsis in pediatric hematology and oncology patients. Intensive Care Med. 1991;17(1):30–5.
56. Douard MC, Arlet G, Longuet P, et al. Diagnosis of venous access port-related infections. Clin Infect Dis. 1999;29(5):1197–202.
57. Franklin JA, Gaur AH, Shenep JL, Hu XJ, Flynn PM. In situ diagnosis of central venous catheter-related bloodstream infection without peripheral blood culture. Pediatr Infect Dis J. 2004;23(7):614–8.
58. Malgrange VB, Escande MC, Theobald S. Validity of earlier positivity of central venous blood cultures in comparison with peripheral blood cultures for diagnosing catheter-related bacteremia in cancer patients. J Clin Microbiol. 2001;39(1):274–8.
59. Gaur AH, Flynn PM, Giannini MA, Shenep JL, Hayden RT. Difference in time to detection: a simple method to differentiate catheter-related from non-catheter-related bloodstream infection in immunocompromised pediatric patients. Clin Infect Dis. 2003;37(4):469–75.
60. Seifert H, Cornely O, Seggewiss K, et al. Bloodstream infection in neutropenic cancer patients related to short-term nontunnelled catheters determined by quantitative blood cultures, differential time to positivity, and molecular epidemiological typing with pulsed-field gel electrophoresis. J Clin Microbiol. 2003;41(1):118–23.
61. Krause R, Auner HW, Gorkiewicz G, et al. Detection of catheter-related bloodstream infections by the differential-time-to-positivity method and gram stain-acridine orange leukocyte cytospin test in neutropenic patients after hematopoietic stem cell transplantation. J Clin Microbiol. 2004;42(10):4835–7.
62. Farina C, Bonanomi E, Benetti G, Fumagalli R, Goglio A. Acridine orange leukocyte cytospin test for central venous catheter – related bloodstream infection: a pediatric experience. Diagn Microbiol Infect Dis. 2005;52(4):337–9.
63. Abdelkefi A, Achour W, Torjman L, et al. Detection of catheter-related bloodstream infections by the Gram stain-acridine orange leukocyte cytospin test in hematopoietic stem cell transplant recipients. Bone Marrow Transplant. 2006;37(6):595–9.
64. O'Grady NP, Alexander M, Burns LA, et al. Guidelines for the prevention of intravascular catheter-related infections. Clin Infect Dis. 2011;52(9):e162–93.
65. O'Grady NP, Alexander M, Dellinger EP, Gerberding JL, Heard SO, Maki DG, et al. Guidelines for the prevention of intravascular catheter-related infections. Centers for Disease Control and Prevention. MMWR Recomm Rep. 2002;51(RR-10):1–29.
66. Crnich CJ, Maki DG. The promise of novel technology for the prevention of intravascular device related bloodstream infection. II. Long-term devices. Clin Infect Dis. 2002;34(10):1362–8.
67. Safdar N, Maki DG. Use of vancomycin-containing lock or flush solutions for prevention of bloodstream infection associated with central venous access devices: a meta-analysis of prospective, randomized trials. Clin Infect Dis. 2006;43(4):474–84.
68. Yahav D, Rozen-Zvi B, Gafter-Gvili A, Leibovici L, Gafter U, Paul M. Antimicrobial lock solutions for the prevention of infections associated with intravascular catheters in patients undergoing hemodialysis: systematic review and meta-analysis of randomized, controlled trials. Clin Infect Dis. 2008;47(1):83–93.
69. Sanders J, Pithie A, Ganly P, et al. A prospective double-blind randomized trial comparing intraluminal ethanol with heparinized saline for the prevention of catheter-associated bloodstream infection in immunosuppressed haematology patients. J Antimicrob Chemother. 2008;62(4):809–15.
70. Veenstra DL, Saint S, Saha S, Lumley T, Sullivan SD. Efficacy of antiseptic-impregnated central venous catheters in preventing catheter-related bloodstream infection: a meta-analysis. JAMA. 1999;281(3):261–7.
71. Ramritu P, Halton K, Collignon P, et al. A systematic review comparing the relative effectiveness of antimicrobial-coated catheters in intensive care units. Am J Infect Control. 2008;36(2):104–17.
72. Hockenhull JC, Dwan KM, Smith GW, et al. The clinical effectiveness of central venous catheters treated with anti-infective

agents in preventing catheter-related bloodstream infections: a systematic review. Crit Care Med. 2009;37(2):702–12.
73. Maki D, Mermel L, Kluger D, et al. The efficacy of a chlorhexidine impregnated sponge (Biopatch) for the prevention of intravascular catheter-related infection-a prospective randomized controlled multicenter study. Abstr Intersci Conf Antimicrob Agents Chemother. 2000;40:422–4. (abstr 1430).
74. Ho KM, Litton E. Use of chlorhexidine-impregnated dressing to prevent vascular and epidural catheter colonization and infection: a meta-analysis. J Antimicrob Chemother. 2006;58(2):281–7.
75. Timsit JF, Schwebel C, Bouadma L, Geffroy A, Garrouste-Orgeas M, Pease S, et al. Chlorhexidine-impregnated sponges and less frequent dressing changes for prevention of catheter-related infections in critically ill adults: a randomized controlled trial. JAMA. 2009;301(12):1231–41.
76. Chaiyakunapruk N, Veenstra DL, Lipsky BA, Saint S. Chlorhexidine compared with povidone-iodine solution for vascular catheter-site care: a meta-analysis. Ann Intern Med. 2002;136(11):792–801.
77. Maki DG, Ringer M, Alvarado CJ. Prospective randomised trial of povidone-iodine, alcohol, and chlorhexidine for prevention of infection associated with central venous and arterial catheters. Lancet. 1991;338(8763):339–43.
78. Tacconelli E, Carmeli Y, Aizer A, Ferreira G, Foreman MG, D'Agata EM. Mupirocin prophylaxis to prevent *Staphylococcus aureus* infection in patients undergoing dialysis: a meta-analysis. Clin Infect Dis. 2003;37(12):1629–38.
79. Safdar N, Crnich CJ, Maki DG. The pathogenesis of ventilator-associated pneumonia: its relevance to developing effective strategies for prevention. Respir Care. 2005;50(6):725–39; discussion 739–741.
80. Clemence MA, Walker D, Farr BM. Central venous catheter practices: results of a survey. Am J Infect Control. 1995;23(1):5–12.
81. Wertheim HF, Vos MC, Ott A, et al. Mupirocin prophylaxis against nosocomial *Staphylococcus aureus* infections in nonsurgical patients: a randomized study. Ann Intern Med. 2004;140(6):419–25.
82. Babu T, Rekasius V, Parada JP, Schreckenberger P, Challapalli M. Mupirocin resistance among methicillin-resistant *Staphylococcus aureus*-colonized patients at admission to a tertiary care medical center. J Clin Microbiol. 2009;47(7):2279–80.
83. Orrett FA. The emergence of mupirocin resistance among clinical isolates of methicillin-resistant *Staphylococcus aureus* in Trinidad: a first report. Jpn J Infect Dis. 2008;61(2):107–10.
84. Perkins D, Hogue JS, Fairchok M, Braun L, Viscount HB. Mupirocin resistance screening of methicillin-resistant *Staphylococcus aureus* isolates at Madigan Army Medical Center. Mil Med. 2008;173(6):604–8.
85. Rossney A, O'Connell S. Emerging high-level mupirocin resistance among MRSA isolates in Ireland. Euro Surveill. 2008;13(14). pii=8084. Available online: http://www.eurosurveillance.org/ViewArticle.aspx?ArticleId=8084.
86. Graber CJ, Schwartz BS. Failure of decolonization in patients with infections due to mupirocin-resistant strains of community-associated methicillin-resistant *Staphylococcus aureus*. Infect Control Hosp Epidemiol. 2008;29(3):284; author reply 284–285
87. Cavdar C, Saglam F, Sifil A, et al. Effect of once-a-week vs thrice-a-week application of mupirocin on methicillin and mupirocin resistance in peritoneal dialysis patients: three years of experience. Ren Fail. 2008;30(4):417–22.
88. Johnson DW, van Eps C, Mudge DW, Wiggins KJ, Armstrong K, Hawley CM, et al. Randomized, controlled trial of topical exit-site application of honey (Medihoney) versus mupirocin for the prevention of catheter-associated infections in hemodialysis patients. J Am Soc Nephrol. 2005;16(5):1456–62.
89. Raad II, Hohn DC, Gilbreath BJ, et al. Prevention of central venous catheter-related infections by using maximal sterile barrier precautions during insertion. Infect Control Hosp Epidemiol. 1994;15(4 Pt 1):231–8.
90. Mermel LA, McCormick RD, Springman SR, Maki DG. The pathogenesis and epidemiology of catheter-related infection with pulmonary artery Swan-Ganz catheters: a prospective study utilizing molecular subtyping. Am J Med. 1991;91(3B):197S–205S.
91. Goetz AM, Wagener MM, Miller JM, Muder RR. Risk of infection due to central venous catheters: effect of site of placement and catheter type. Infect Control Hosp Epidemiol. 1998;19(11):842–5.
92. Joynt GM, Kew J, Gomersall CD, Leung VY, Liu EK. Deep venous thrombosis caused by femoral venous catheters in critically ill adult patients. Chest. 2000;117(1):178–83.
93. Merrer J, De Jonghe B, Golliot F, et al. Complications of femoral and subclavian venous catheterization in critically ill patients: a randomized controlled trial. JAMA. 2001;286(6):700–7.
94. Richet H, Hubert B, Nitemberg G, et al. Prospective multicenter study of vascular-catheter-related complications and risk factors for positive central-catheter cultures in intensive care unit patients. J Clin Microbiol. 1990;28(11):2520–5.
95. Parienti JJ, Thirion M, Megarbane B, et al. Femoral vs jugular venous catheterization and risk of nosocomial events in adults requiring acute renal replacement therapy: a randomized controlled trial. JAMA. 2008;299(20):2413–22.
96. Gowardman JR, Robertson IK, Parkes S, Rickard CM. Influence of insertion site on central venous catheter colonization and bloodstream infection rates. Intensive Care Med. 2008;34(6):1038–45.
97. Randolph AG, Cook DJ, Gonzales CA, Pribble CG. Ultrasound guidance for placement of central venous catheters: a meta-analysis of the literature. Crit Care Med. 1996;24(12):2053–8.
98. Karakitsos D, Labropoulos N, De Groot E, et al. Real-time ultrasound-guided catheterisation of the internal jugular vein: a prospective comparison with the landmark technique in critical care patients. Crit Care. 2006;10(6):R162.
99. Barsuk JH, Cohen ER, Feinglass J, McGaghie WC, Wayne DB. Use of simulation-based education to reduce catheter-related bloodstream infections. Arch Intern Med. 2009;169(15):1420–3.
100. Timsit JF, Cheval C, Gachot B, et al. Usefulness of a strategy based on bronchoscopy with direct examination of bronchoalveolar lavage fluid in the initial antibiotic therapy of suspected ventilator-associated pneumonia. Intensive Care Med. 2001;27(4):640–7.
101. Ruschulte H, Franke M, Gastmeier P, et al. Prevention of central venous catheter related infections with chlorhexidine gluconate impregnated wound dressings: a randomized controlled trial. Ann Hematol. 2009;88(3):267–72.
102. O'Horo JC, Silva GL, Munoz-Price LS, Safdar N. The efficacy of daily bathing with chlorhexidine for reducing healthcare-associated bloodstream infections: a meta-analysis. Infect Control Hosp Epidemiol. 2012;33(3):257–67.
103. Climo MW, Wong ES. Effect of daily chlorhexidine bathing on hospital-acquired infection. N Engl J Med. 2013;368(6):533–42.
104. Lowe CF, Lloyd-Smith E, Sidhu, Ritchie G, Sharma A, Jang W, et al. Reduction in hospital-associated methicillin-resistant Staphylococcus aureus and vancomycin-resistant Enterococcus with daily chlorhexidine gluconate bathing for medical inpatients. Am J Infect Control. 2017;45(3):255–9.
105. Climo MW, Wong ES. Daily chlorhexidine bathing and hospital-acquired infection. N Engl J Med. 2013;368(24):2332.
106. Casey AL, Mermel LA, Nightingale P, Elliott TS. Antimicrobial central venous catheters in adults: a systematic review and meta-analysis. Lancet Infect Dis. 2008;8(12):763–76.
107. Loertzer H, Soukup J, Hamza A, et al. Use of catheters with the AgION antimicrobial system in kidney transplant recipients to reduce infection risk. Transplant Proc. 2006;38(3):707–10.

108. Worth LJ, Slavin MA, Heath S, Szer J, Grigg AP. Ethanol versus heparin locks for the prevention of central venous catheter-associated bloodstream infections: a randomized trial in adult haematology patients with Hickman devices. J Hosp Infect. 2014;88(1):48–51.
109. Zacharioudakis IM, Zervou FN, Arvanitis M, Ziakas PD, Mermel LA, Mylonakis E. Antimicrobial lock solutions as a method to prevent central line-associated bloodstream infections: a meta-analysis of randomized controlled trials. Clin Infect Dis. 2014;59(12):1741–9.
110. Bookstaver PB, Williamson JC, Tucker BK, Raad II, Sherertz RJ. Activity of novel antibiotic lock solutions in a model against isolates of catheter-related bloodstream infections. Ann Pharmacother. 2009;43(2):210–9.
111. Mendelson MH, Short LJ, Schechter CB, et al. Study of a needleless intermittent intravenous-access system for peripheral infusions: analysis of staff, patient, and institutional outcomes. Infect Control Hosp Epidemiol. 1998;19(6):401–6.
112. Skolnick R, LaRocca J, Barba D, Paicius L. Evaluation and implementation of a needleless intravenous system: making needlesticks a needless problem. Am J Infect Control. 1993;21(1):39–41.
113. Gartner K. Impact of a needleless intravenous system in a university hospital. J Healthc Mater Manag. 1993;11(8):44–6, 48–49.
114. Lawrence D. HAI – a high visibility problem: recent studies show that hospitals with low HAI rates rely heavily on IT, but the jury is still out on where a CIO should begin. Healthc Inform. 2008;25(12):22, 24.
115. Jarvis WR, Murphy C, Hall KK, et al. Health care-associated bloodstream infections associated with negative- or positive-pressure or displacement mechanical valve needleless connectors. Clin Infect Dis. 2009;49(12):1821–7.
116. Do AN, Ray BJ, Banerjee SN, Illian AF, Barnett BJ, Pham MH, et al. Bloodstream infection associated with needleless device use and the importance of infection-control practices in the home health care setting. J Infect Dis. 1999;179(2):442–8.
117. Cookson ST, Ihrig M, O'Mara EM, et al. Increased bloodstream infection rates in surgical patients associated with variation from recommended use and care following implementation of a needleless device. Infect Control Hosp Epidemiol. 1998;19(1):23–7.
118. McDonald LC, Banerjee SN, Jarvis WR. Line-associated bloodstream infections in pediatric intensive-care-unit patients associated with a needleless device and intermittent intravenous therapy. Infect Control Hosp Epidemiol. 1998;19(10):772–7.
119. Kellerman S, Shay DK, Howard J, et al. Bloodstream infections in home infusion patients: the influence of race and needleless intravascular access devices. J Pediatr. 1996;129(5):711–7.
120. Rupp ME, Sholtz LA, Jourdan DR, et al. Outbreak of bloodstream infection temporally associated with the use of an intravascular needleless valve. Clin Infect Dis. 2007;44(11):1408–14.
121. Maragakis LL, Bradley KL, Song X, et al. Increased catheter-related bloodstream infection rates after the introduction of a new mechanical valve intravenous access port. Infect Control Hosp Epidemiol. 2006;27(1):67–70.
122. Casey AL, Worthington T, Lambert PA, Quinn D, Faroqui MH, Elliott TS. A randomized, prospective clinical trial to assess the potential infection risk associated with the PosiFlow needleless connector. J Hosp Infect. 2003;54(4):288–93.
123. Menyhay SZ, Maki DG. Disinfection of needleless catheter connectors and access ports with alcohol may not prevent microbial entry: the promise of a novel antiseptic-barrier cap. Infect Control Hosp Epidemiol. 2006;27(1):23–7.
124. Maki DG. In vitro studies of a novel antimicrobial luer-activated needleless connector for prevention of catheter-related bloodstream infection. Clin Infect Dis. 2010;50(12):1580–7.
125. Menyhay SZ, Maki DG. Preventing central venous catheter-associated bloodstream infections: development of an antiseptic barrier cap for needleless connectors. Am J Infect Control. 2008;36(10):S174 e15.
126. Schears GJ. Summary of product trials for 10,164 patients: comparing an intravenous stabilizing device to tape. J Infus Nurs. 2006;29(4):225–31.
127. Yamamoto AJ, Solomon JA, Soulen MC, et al. Sutureless securement device reduces complications of peripherally inserted central venous catheters. J Vasc Interv Radiol. 2002;13(1):77–81.
128. Frey AM, Schears GJ. Why are we stuck on tape and suture? A review of catheter securement devices. J Infus Nurs. 2006;29(1):34–8.
129. van den Berghe G, Wouters P, Weekers F, et al. Intensive insulin therapy in the critically ill patients. N Engl J Med. 2001;345(19):1359–67.
130. Van den Berghe G, Wilmer A, Hermans G, et al. Intensive insulin therapy in the medical ICU. N Engl J Med. 2006;354(5):449–61.
131. Finfer S, Chittock DR, Su SY, et al. Intensive versus conventional glucose control in critically ill patients. N Engl J Med. 2009;360(13):1283–97.
132. Griesdale DE, de Souza RJ, van Dam RM, et al. Intensive insulin therapy and mortality among critically ill patients: a meta-analysis including NICE-SUGAR study data. CMAJ. 2009;180(8):821–7.
133. Haraden C. What is a bundle? 2006. 09/07/2006. Available from: http://www.ihi.org/IHI/Topics/CriticalCare/IntensiveCare/ImprovementStories/WhatIsaBundle.htm.
134. Bhutta A, Gilliam C, Honeycutt M, et al. Reduction of bloodstream infections associated with catheters in paediatric intensive care unit: stepwise approach. BMJ. 2007;334(7589):362–5.
135. Costello JM, Morrow DF, Graham DA, Potter-Bynoe G, Sandora TJ, Laussen PC. Systematic intervention to reduce central line-associated bloodstream infection rates in a pediatric cardiac intensive care unit. Pediatrics. 2008;121(5):915–23.
136. Blot K, Bergs J, Vogelaers D, Blot S, Vandijck D. Prevention of central line-associated bloodstream infections through quality improvement interventions: a systematic review and meta-analysis. Clin Infect Dis. 2014;59(1):96–105.

Surgical Site Infections: Wound and Stump Infections

14

Nasia Safdar, Sara A. M. Zerbel, and Elizabeth Ann Misch

Background and Prevalence

Surgical site infections (SSI) following transplantation have been linked to increased mortality, graft rejection, increased length of stay, and increased resource utilization [1, 2]. SSIs can be categorized by the anatomical depth at which the infection occurs. Superficial SSIs involve the skin and subcutaneous tissue of the surgical incision only. Deep SSIs involve the deep soft tissues (e.g., fascia and muscle). Organ/space infections involve tissue beyond the fascia and muscle including the intra-abdominal cavity, solid organs, bone, mediastinum, and spinal tissue (see Fig. 14.1). The Centers for Disease Control and Prevention's (CDC) National Healthcare Safety Network (NHSN) defines the time frame for superficial, deep and organ/space SSIs as occurring within the 30 days after surgery for select procedures such as if no implant is present. For other procedures, such as if an implant is present, deep and organ/space infections can be linked back to a surgical procedure for up to 90 days after surgery. See Table 14.1 for detailed NHSN definitions of SSI. Rates of SSI vary and can reach as high as 37% for some transplant procedures [3]. The risk of infection depends greatly on type of surgery and patient-specific factors. A number of factors predispose transplant patients to SSI including immunosuppression, reoperation, diabetes, and obesity [4–13]. The route of infection is dependent on the type of transplant surgery and may be both endogenous and exogenous sources. Microorganisms in posttransplant SSIs are primarily bacterial; however, fungal infections may also play a role [14–16]. Multidrug-resistant organisms are an increasingly common culprit in SSI [9–11] in this population due to a heavy exposure to the healthcare system, use of prophylactic antibiotics, and immunosuppression. There are few guidelines to direct therapy. In general, management with debridement alone is not sufficient in the transplant population, due to impaired host defenses. Culture or PCR of tissues is critical to diagnose resistant or unexpected pathogens. Depending upon local epidemiology and site of infection, antibiotics to target resistant Gram-positive and Gram-negative organisms (including *Pseudomonas*), *Candida*, and, on occasion, *Aspergillus*, may be necessary. Measures to prevent SSI during the preoperative, intraoperative, and postop-

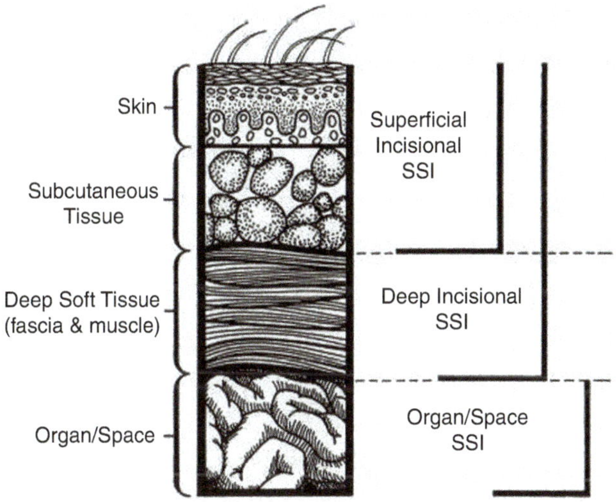

Fig. 14.1 Cross-section of abdominal wall depicting CDC classifications of SSI [17]. (Reprinted from Mangram et al. [17], © 1999, with permission from Elsevier)

N. Safdar (✉)
Section of Infectious Diseases, Department of Medicine, University of Wisconsin-Madison, School of Medicine and Public Health, and the William S. Middleton Memorial Veterans Hospital, Madison, WI, USA
e-mail: ns2@medicine.wisc.edu

S. A. M. Zerbel
UnityPoint Health-Meriter, Department of Performance Improvement, Madison, WI, USA
e-mail: sara.zerbel@unitypoint.org

E. A. Misch
Division of Infectious Diseases, Department of Medicine, University of Wisconsin-Madison, School of Medicine and Public Health, Madison, WI, USA
e-mail: eamisch@medicine.wisc.edu

A. Safdar (ed.), *Principles and Practice of Transplant Infectious Diseases*, https://doi.org/10.1007/978-1-4939-9034-4_14

Table 14.1 CDC's NHSN definition of SSI [17]

A *superficial incisional SSI* must meet each of the following criteria:
1. Infection occurs within 30 days after operative procedure
2. Involves only skin and subcutaneous tissue of the incision
3. Patient has at least one of the following:
a. Purulent drainage from the superficial incision
b. Organisms isolated from an aseptically obtained culture of fluid or tissue from the superficial incision
c. At least one of the following signs or symptoms of infection: pain or tenderness, localized swelling, redness, or heat, and superficial incision are deliberately opened by surgeon and are culture-positive or not cultured. A culture-negative finding does not meet this criterion
d. Diagnosis of superficial incisional SSI by the surgeon or attending physician
A *deep incisional SSI* must meet each of the following criteria:
1. Infection occurs within 30 days after the operative procedure for select procedures or within 90 days for others (such as if an implant is in place) and the infection appears to be related to the operative procedure
2. Involves deep soft tissues (e.g., fascial and muscle layers) of the incision
3. Patient has at least one of the following:
a. Purulent drainage from the deep incision but not from the organ/space component of the surgical site
b. A deep incision spontaneously dehisces or is deliberately opened by a surgeon and is culture-positive or not cultured, and the patient has at least one of the following signs or symptoms: fever (>38 °C), or localized pain or tenderness. A culture-negative finding does not meet this criterion
c. An abscess or other evidence of infection involving the deep incision is found on direct examination, during reoperation, or by histopathologic or radiographic examination
d. Diagnosis of a deep incisional SSI by a surgeon or attending physician
An *organ/space SSI* must meet each of the following criteria:
1. Infection occurs within 30 days after the operative procedure for select procedures e or within 90 days for others (such as if an implant is in place) and the infection appears to be related to the operative procedure
2. Infection involves any part of the body, excluding the skin incision, fascia, or muscle layers, that is opened or manipulated during the operative procedure
3. Patient has at least one of the following:
a. Purulent drainage from a drain that is placed through a stab wound into the organ/space
b. Organisms isolated from an aseptically obtained culture of fluid or tissue in the organ/space
c. An abscess or other evidence of infection involving the organ/space that is found on direct examination, during reoperation, or by histopathologic or radiologic examination
d. Diagnosis of an organ/space SSI by a surgeon or attending physician

erative period should be evidence-based and incorporated into hospital quality control initiatives.

The incidence of SSI as published by NHSN is 3.28% in patients undergoing heart transplant, 3.67–6.57% for kidney transplant, and 11.61–20.10% for liver transplant [18]

Table 14.2 Posttransplant SSI rates [3, 18]

Organ transplanted	Published SSI range	Source
Living-donor liver transplant	37%	Iinuma et al. [3]
Liver transplant	11.61–20.10%	NHSN [18]
Heart transplant	3.28%	NHSN [18]
Kidney transplant	3.67–6.57%	NHSN [18]

(Table 14.2). A prospective study of 113 living-donor liver transplant recipients showed an SSI rate of 37%, with intra-abdominal abscess and peritonitis as the most common infections [3].

Major Risk Factors for SSI

Patients undergoing solid organ transplant are at an increased risk for development of SSI. A number of factors are known to increase the risk for infection in the transplant population including immunosuppression, recurrent rejection, reoperation, diabetes mellitus, and obesity [3, 8–11, 19–21]. The CDC uses the following equation to estimate risk for SSI:

$$\frac{\text{Dose of bacterial contamination} \times \text{virulence}}{\text{Resistance of the host patient}} = \text{Risk of SSI}$$

Immunosuppression

The last two decades have witnessed tremendous advances in transplantation including the development of drugs that suppress the body's immune system to aid the transplant and long-term acceptance of allogeneic tissue. However, these drugs simultaneously create an environment within the body that allows invasion by opportunistic pathogens [4, 22]. Environmental and skin organisms that offer little risk to patients with intact immune systems may colonize and infect immunosuppressed patients. In addition, due to immunosuppression, symptoms and signs of SSI may be attenuated in transplant patients. With a suboptimal immune response, redness, heat, and swelling may not be present as they would be in a patient with an intact immune system. With a lack of early symptoms, SSIs in immunosuppressed transplant patients are at risk for staying undetected until they become more severe. Patients undergoing transplant of cadaveric allografts are additionally at an increased risk for infection due to the elevated level of immunosuppression required for acceptance of the transplanted organ. Because of the high risk of infection in immunosuppressed patients, it is advisable to complete a comprehensive preoperative physical to evaluate for sources of potential current or previous infection and successfully treat any infections prior to surgery.

Repeat Surgery

Each time a surgical incision is made, there is a risk for contamination with endogenous organisms which consequently increases the risk for infection. Reoperation at the allograft site presents a unique risk for SSI [10, 23]. Patients undergoing reoperation for transplantation are more likely to be highly immunosuppressed in an effort to save the transplanted organ. They are also very likely to have a number of comorbidities that will impact wound healing. In addition, rejection of a transplanted organ often leads to tissue necrosis which can fuel an organ/space infection at the site of the transplant. Anastomotic leaks followed by repeat surgery have also been shown to greatly increase the risk of infection in liver transplant patients [1].

Diabetes Mellitus

Diabetes mellitus adds to the risk of SSI, and with a high incidence in renal and pancreas transplant patients, it can be a common factor in many transplant patients. In a retrospective study of 680 liver transplant patients, Park et al. found that severe hyperglycemia was independently associated with SSI following liver transplantation [24]. Additionally, a prospective study of 1400 kidney transplant patients showed that diabetic patients were at increased risk of developing incisional SSIs after surgery [20]. Although diabetes mellitus is an immutable patient factor, perioperative blood glucose levels can be monitored and strictly controlled, which may reduce SSI and improve outcomes.

Obesity

Many studies have linked obesity with a number of comorbidities, including heart disease, diabetes, cancer, vascular disease, hypertension, and, with these, an increased risk of postoperative wound infection. In addition to the comorbidities that often coexist with obesity, there is an increased risk of suboptimal or underdosing of preoperative antibiotic prophylaxis, as well as concerns regarding postoperative wound care. A review by Holley et al. showed that the most frequently reported postrenal transplant complication in obese patients (BMI ≥30) was wound infection and wound disruption [13]. In another review by Johnson et al., obese patients (BMI >30) were more likely to experience postrenal transplant superficial wound breakdown and wound dehiscence [19]. Due to the increased risk for postoperative wound infection in obese patients, an attempt at significant weight reduction prior to surgery may be indicated for optimal outcomes.

Mechanism of Surgical Site Infection

Type of Transplant

Risks for SSI vary greatly depending on the type of transplant procedure (Table 14.2). Surgery at a sterile body site as in heart transplant is generally lower risk for a SSI than surgery at body sites that can be more easily contaminated by the endogenous bacteria of the gastrointestinal tract, respiratory tract, or genitourinary tract. The CDC describes four types of wound classifications: (1) clean, (2) clean contaminated, (3) contaminated, and (4) dirty/infected (see Table 14.3) [17]. Heart and pancreas transplants are generally considered clean wounds. However, lung, kidney, intestine, and liver transplants are generally considered clean contaminated. If bile or urine is infected, then a liver or kidney transplant, respectively, is considered contaminated. This risk for infection is lowest for clean wounds and highest for dirty wounds.

Endogenous Sources

As described previously, the risk for SSI is directly related to the level of microorganism contamination at the wound site.

Table 14.3 Surgical wound classification [17]

Wound class	Definition
Class I/clean	An uninfected operative wound in which no inflammation is encountered and the respiratory, alimentary, genital, or uninfected urinary tract is not entered. In addition, clean wounds are primarily closed and, if necessary, drained with closed drainage. Operative incisional wounds that follow non-penetrating (blunt) trauma should be included in this category if they meet the criteria
Class II/ clean-contaminated	An operative wound in which the respiratory, alimentary, genital, or urinary tracts are entered under controlled conditions and without unusual contamination. Specifically, operations involving the biliary tract, appendix, vagina, and oropharynx are included in this category, provided no evidence of infection or major break in technique is encountered
Class III/ contaminated	Open, fresh, accidental wounds. In addition, operations with major breaks in sterile technique (e.g., open cardiac massage) or gross spillage from the GI tract, and incisions in which acute, non-purulent inflammation is encountered are included in this category
Class IV/ dirty-infected	Old traumatic wounds with retained devitalized tissue and those that involve existing clinical infection or perforated viscera. This definition suggests that the organisms causing postoperative infection were present in the operative field before the operation

When a SSI does develop after a clean wound procedure, the infecting organism is much more likely to be endogenous normal skin flora. In particular, Gram-positive bacteria and especially *Staphylococcus species* dominate as the causative agent of infections after clean procedures. Alternatively, with clean-contaminated procedures, the causative agent is much more likely to be endogenous flora of the respiratory, gastrointestinal, or genitourinary tract depending on the type of surgery. The antibiotic chosen for surgical prophylaxis must take into consideration the wound class as well as the type and location of surgery.

Exogenous Sources

Most sources of SSI originate from endogenous normal flora and asymptomatic and symptomatic infections that are present at the time of surgery. However, lapses in surgical technique, hand hygiene compliance, postoperative wound care procedures, and postoperative infections from invasive devices are also contributing factors to the risk of SSI. Given the depressed immune status of the transplant patient, any number of exogenous sources could lead to a postoperative wound infection.

Early Onset

In general, infections that occur within the first week of surgery and are organ/space infections are a result of anastomotic leaks or other contamination of the open surgical site during surgery by endogenous or exogenous sources. These types of infections generally require, at minimum, drainage of fluid collections and possibly repeat surgery. Since the symptoms of SSI can be obscured by immunosuppression, there should be a high level of suspicion for SSI if a patient develops even a slightly elevated white blood cell count or fever.

Late Onset

SSIs that develop after the first two postoperative weeks can have a variety of sources. Postoperative wound care in combination with immunosuppression therapy can play an important role in these late-onset infections. Late-onset organ/space infections in posttransplant patients could be related to rejection of the transplanted organ. In addition, for surgery that involves an implant, deep and organ/space infections may develop as far out as several weeks after surgery. An example of late onset SSI might be a deep sternal wound infection and mediastinitis after heart and lung transplant, since sternal wires are considered implants by the CDC definition.

Diagnosis

The clinical presentation of SSI in immune-compromised (IC) patients may be attenuated in comparison to the normal host. In heart transplant patients, for example, sternal dehiscence, fever (approximately 25–30% of patients), or pain out of proportion to that expected following a sternotomy incision may be the only indicator of an infection at the operative site [9, 25, 26]. In a series of liver transplant recipients, leukocytosis and fever were seen in only 53% and 34%, respectively, of patients [12]. Clinicians should be aware that the differential diagnosis of skin and soft tissue infection in IC patients includes routine (*Staphylococcus*, *Streptococcus*, Gram-negative organisms, *Clostridium*) as well as atypical pathogens (yeasts, mold, mycobacteria) [27–32] and systemic, noninfectious syndromes (drug eruption, pyoderma gangrenosum, and Sweet's syndrome, among others) [33–35]. Thus, patients who fail to respond to empiric antibiotics may require biopsy of the involved tissue to direct therapy toward a proven pathogen or establish an alternate diagnosis. Material can be obtained during debridement or through a separate procedure (punch biopsy) and should be sent for bacterial Gram stain and stains for fungal, acid-fast, and modified acid-fast organisms. Tissue should be submitted separately to the microbiology laboratory, for bacterial, fungal, and mycobacterial culture, and to pathology (fresh frozen section and fixed sections). Immunohistochemistry, PCR, and special stains can be added onto fresh or fixed tissues and may permit more rapid diagnosis of pathogens (e.g., cytomegalovirus, fungi, mycobacteria). Histological evidence of inflammation may be scant even in cases of proven infection.

Microbiology

Recent case series of SSIs in liver transplant recipients emphasize a shift toward a predominance of Gram-negative pathogens, *Enterococcus* (often vancomycin-resistant), and drug-resistant Gram-positive and Gram-negative bacteria. *Candida* species are also reported [36–39]. In patients who received either small bowel or multivisceral transplant, 57% experienced an SSI within 30 days of surgery, with Gram-negative and Gram-positive organisms and *Candida* represented [40]. SSIs in kidney transplant recipients frequently involve Gram-positive bacteria, specifically, *Staphylococci* and *Enterococci* [8, 23, 41]. Frequent rates of Gram-positive organisms and *Candida* are reported in some series of postoperative wound infections in kidney pancreas transplant patients [21, 42], while a predominance of Gram-negative organisms has been reported in others [20]. Heart transplant patients have high rates of SSIs, with incidences of 8–15% [38, 43]. *Staphylococci*, methicillin-resistant *Staphylococcus aureus*, and *Candida* species are commonly isolated, but Gram-negative organisms are also encountered [9, 25, 44–46]. Microbiological data on SSIs in the lung transplant population is particularly lacking. In a single study of 31 "deep" SSIs occurring after lung transplantation [47], MSSA, MRSA, *Enterococcus*, *Pseudomonas*, and other Gram-negative bacteria, mycobacteria, and molds were identified.

Treatment

Most of the studies cited above are retrospective and offer few insights as to the comparative effectiveness of different antibiotic regimens for prophylaxis or treatment of SSIs. Treatment of SSIs in transplant patients is not standardized, in part because the microbiology is different than for non-transplant surgery and has not been as systematically surveyed. Existing guidelines for the treatment of SSIs in general surgical patients [48] may not be fully applicable to the transplant setting, where methicillin-resistant *Staphylococci*, vancomycin-resistant *Enterococci* SSIs, and multidrug-resistant pathogens are frequently encountered and mortality rates can be as high as 30% [44]. For immunocompetent patients, opening and draining the wound is the cornerstone of management. Antibiotics are then added if there is evidence of a "significant systemic response," such as redness, tissue induration, fever, tachycardia, or leukocytosis [48]. By contrast, in transplant patients the inflammatory response is markedly blunted in the first 30 days after transplant. Since systemic signs may be masked in this population, antibiotics are considered mandatory for the treatment of SSI. In general, tissue should be promptly sampled and treatment should be guided by organisms recovered on culture. When empiric, antibiotic selection should be broad and informed by the available epidemiology. For example, given that Gram-positive bacteria, including MRSA, *Candida*, and Gram-negative bacteria are reported in SSI series of heart transplant patients, an empiric antibiotic regimen could reasonably include vancomycin, linezolid, daptomycin, telavancin, or ceftaroline, an antifungal agent (an echinocandin or fluconazole), and an extended-spectrum beta-lactam, third- or fourth-generation cephalosporin, or antipseudomonal carbapenem for Gram-negative pathogens. If institution-specific epidemiology suggests high rates of MDROs, antibiotic coverage of Gram-negative organisms should be designed using local antibiograms.

Other critical aspects of management include drainage of associated collections (by catheter, needle aspiration, or surgery), repair of anastomotic leaks, and the debridement of necrotic or unviable tissue. Infrequently, the dose of immunosuppressive medications may need to be reduced, raising the prospect of graft loss.

Prevention

Despite the increased risk for SSI associated with transplant surgery, there are measures that can be taken to reduce the incidence of SSI in this patient population. Dosing and choice of preoperative antibiotic, careful surgical technique to minimize tissue damage, nutritional support, surgical site antisepsis, and postoperative wound care are among the key areas for SSI prevention.

Preoperative

Screening for Infection and Colonization

A thorough preoperative history and physical should be completed to inspect for active infections at surgical or remote body sites. If possible, surgery should be delayed until infections are treated. Transplant centers should routinely evaluate transplant candidates for potential colonization with multidrug resistant organisms. Individuals who have had recent lengthy hospitalizations, live in a long term care environment, have been on multiple courses of antibiotic treatment, or have been incarcerated are all at higher risk for colonization with drug-resistant organisms. A patient with a history of MRSA could undergo a decolonization protocol prior to surgery to reduce the risk of infection with the colonizing organism [49]. Active screening for MDROs may be indicated when protocols for decolonization of known carriers are in place. Type of surgery and sources for potential infection should be considered when developing such protocols. Generally MRSA decolonization protocols are more effective when used for clean procedures in which *Staphylococcal* species are more likely to cause infection.

Antiseptic Preoperative Bath or Shower

Some studies have shown a benefit of preoperative skin bathing with the antiseptic agent chlorhexidine gluconate (CHG). Bathing with CHG the night before and the morning of surgery has been shown to decrease risk of bacterial colonization at the site, but studies have not consistently found a major effect on SSI [50]. Additionally, some studies support the use of a CHG-impregnated cloth, which is used to apply CHG to the skin where it is then left to dry. Leaving the CHG on the skin may have an increased benefit as compared to washing it away, especially in clean procedures where normal skin flora is often the etiological agent of SSI.

Preoperative Hair Removal

A number of studies confirm that hair removal should not be performed unless the hair at the surgical site will interfere with the operative procedure. If the hair must be removed, it should not be shaved. Shaving produces small nicks and cuts in the skin that can serve as a portal of entry for microorganisms. Clipping the hair or using depilatory creams has been shown to lower the risk of SSI as compared to shaving. Furthermore, the Association for Perioperative Registered Nurses (AORN) guidelines state that preoperative hair removal should take place outside the operating suite to prevent contamination of the sterile field.

Tobacco Cessation

A link has been shown between the use of nicotine and an increased risk of SSI through delayed wound healing. Tobacco cessation should be encouraged preoperatively. The CDC recommends that patients be instructed to abstain from products containing nicotine for at least 30 days before elective operation.

Wash and Prep the Incision Site

In an effort to reduce bacterial load on the skin prior to surgery, the patient's skin should be washed and cleaned around the incision site. This should be followed with the application of a surgical prep that is allowed to dry on the skin. The use of products containing alcohol in addition to CHG or povidone iodine has shown superior results in prevention of SSI in comparison to aqueous povidone iodine alone [51].

Prophylactic Antibiotic Choice and Timing

The most effective time for antibiotic administration is within 30 min prior to incision. Between 1 and 2 h prior to incision is effective for vancomycin and fluoroquinolones. Prophylactic antibiotic choice depends primarily on the sight of infection and likely bacterial contaminants. For clean procedures, it is important to cover for Gram-positive organisms, whereas clean-contaminated procedures that could involve gastrointestinal flora should cover for Gram-negative anaerobes. Antibiotic dosing will depend on patient's weight and creatinine clearance [52].

Intraoperative

Antibiotic Re-dosing

Antibiotic re-dosing should be completed as appropriate for long surgeries. Generally re-dosing is indicated when the half-life of the given prophylactic antibiotic is reached. Antibiotic re-dosing is also indicated when there is a high volume of blood loss (>1500 mL) and should also take into account patient renal function [52].

Temperature Management

Research has shown that the incidence of SSI is significantly increased in hypothermic patients undergoing surgery [53]. Hypothermia, even when mild, results in subcutaneous vasoconstriction which causes tissues hypoxia. When the cells of the immune system cannot reach the tissue, the risk for infection is elevated. All efforts should be made to maintain a minimum body temperature of 36 °C. This can be achieved through advanced technology in active warming devices such as a Bair Hugger or similar device.

Technique

In a retrospective review of 166 liver transplant patients who developed SSI at a single hospital from 2003 to 2008, Hellinger et al. found an association between SSI rate and surgeon that was independent of all other risk factors evaluated [54]. Wound closure technique can play a role in risk for SSI. Tissue damage can also impact the rate of SSI. Excessive tissue injury, which can be caused by overuse of electrocautery, has been shown to elevate the risk for SSI. Surgical techniques such as multilayered wound closure that prevent the occurrence of dead spaces have also been shown to decrease the risk of wound infection.

Postoperative

Control of Serum Blood Glucose

A number of studies have linked diabetes mellitus to poor wound healing and an increased risk for postoperative wound infection [5]. Taking this one step further, research in diabetic patients showed that controlled serum blood glucose levels after open heart surgery are linked to a reduction in SSI [7]. Efforts should be made to control blood glucose perioperatively at a level less than 200 mg/dl.

Wound Care

Protecting the surgical wound from contamination leads to a decreased risk of SSI. Surgical wounds that have been closed primarily should be covered with a sterile dressing for 24–48 h. Hand hygiene should be performed before and after dressing changes. Sterile technique should be used when changing surgical incision dressings. The patient and family should be educated regarding proper wound care and symptoms of SSI prior to discharge from the hospital.

The Role of the Environment

The preoperative, intraoperative, and postoperative environment should be a particular focus for transplant patients due to their diminished immune response. Preoperatively, patients with suppressed immune systems should be roomed in a protective environment with HEPA-filtered positive pressure airflow whenever possible to prevent opportunistic infections prior to surgery. In the OR suite, as with any surgical procedure, the air should be HEPA-filtered and air flow should be positive to the hall, with minimal traffic into the

OR during the case. After surgery, the patient should ideally return to a protective environment where environmental contamination can be kept to a minimum. Protective precautions policies for immunosuppressed patients should incorporate HVAC controls and the use of personal protective equipment for the patient and staff, and prohibit plants and flowers from the patient's environment.

Summary

Advances in immunosuppressive therapies have led to success in transplantation outcomes. However, infections remain a challenge for this population. SSIs are a common complication of transplantation and can range from superficial skin and subcutaneous tissue infections to deep and organ/space infections. Multiple factors play a role in the increased risk of SSI among transplant patients, including immunosuppression, repeat surgeries, diabetes mellitus, and obesity. The mechanism of post-transplant SSI can vary depending on the organ, with the possibility of both endogenous and exogenous sources for bacterial and fungal contamination. SSIs generally present within the first 30 days after transplant and can be related to contamination with normal body flora during incision or leaks at the site of anastomosis. Organisms involved in SSIs are generally bacterial, but fungal organisms also play a role. Multidrug-resistant organisms are increasingly common in the transplant population. Guidelines for antibiotic therapy are lacking. We believe tissue sampling is essential to direct antibiotic selection. Empiric regimens should be broad and cover resistant Gram-positive (MRSA, VRE), resistant Gram-negative organisms and, depending upon the site of infection, fungal pathogens. Prevention of SSIs should focus on preoperative, intraoperative, and postoperative periods and use evidence-based practices, including preoperative assessments for infection and colonization with pathogenic organisms, surgical site preparation, tobacco cessation, antibiotic prophylaxis, surgical technique, and wound care.

References

1. Hollenbeak CS, Alfrey EJ, Souba WW. The effect of surgical site infections on outcomes and resource utilization after liver transplantation. Surgery. 2001;130:388–95.
2. Hollenbeak CS, Alfrey EJ, Sheridan K, Burger TL, Dillon PW. Surgical site infections following pediatric liver transplantation: risks and costs. Transplant Infect Dis. 2003;5:72–8.
3. Iinuma Y, Senda K, Fujihara N, et al. Surgical site infection in living-donor liver transplant recipients: a prospective study. Transplantation. 2004;78:704–9.
4. Dunn DL. Problems related to immunosuppression. Infection and malignancy occurring after solid organ transplantation. Crit Care Clin. 1990;6:955–77.
5. Terranova A. The effects of diabetes mellitus on wound healing. Plast Surg Nurs. 1991;11:20–5.
6. Saleem TF, Cunningham KE, Hollenbeak CS, Alfrey EJ, Gabbay RA. Development of diabetes mellitus post-renal transplantation is associated with poor short-term clinical outcomes. Transplant Proc. 2003;35:2916–8.
7. Zerr KJ, Furnary AP, Grunkemeier GL, Bookin S, Kanhere V, Starr A. Glucose control lowers the risk of wound infection in diabetics after open heart operations. Ann Thorac Surg. 1997;63:356–61.
8. Wszola M, Kwiatkowski A, Ostaszewska A, et al. Surgical site infections after kidney transplantation – where do we stand now? Transplantation. 2013;95:878–82.
9. Zuckermann A, Barten MJ. Surgical wound complications after heart transplantation. Transplant Int. 2011;24:627–36.
10. Shah H, Hellinger WC, Heckman MG, et al. Surgical site infections after liver retransplantation: incidence and risk factors. Liver Transplant. 2014;20:930–6.
11. Said A, Safdar N, Lucey MR, et al. Infected bilomas in liver transplant recipients, incidence, risk factors and implications for prevention. Am J Transplant. 2004;4:574–82.
12. Reid GE, Grim SA, Sankary H, Benedetti E, Oberholzer J, Clark NM. Early intra-abdominal infections associated with orthotopic liver transplantation. Transplantation. 2009;87:1706–11.
13. Holley JL, Shapiro R, Lopatin WB, Tzakis AG, Hakala TR, Starzl TE. Obesity as a risk factor following cadaveric renal transplantation. Transplantation. 1990;49:387–9.
14. Blair JE, Kusne S. Bacterial, mycobacterial, and protozoal infections after liver transplantation – part I. Liver Transplant. 2005;11:1452–9.
15. Singh N, Paterson DL, Chang FY, et al. Methicillin-resistant *Staphylococcus aureus*: the other emerging resistant gram-positive coccus among liver transplant recipients. Clin Infect Dis. 2000;30:322–7.
16. Chang FY, Singh N, Gayowski T, Drenning SD, Wagener MM, Marino IR. *Staphylococcus aureus* nasal colonization and association with infections in liver transplant recipients. Transplantation. 1998;65:1169–72.
17. Berríos-Torres SI, Umscheid CA, Bratzler DW, et al. Centers for Disease Control and Prevention guideline for the prevention of surgical site infection. JAMA Surg. 2017;152(8):784–91.
18. Edwards JR, Peterson KD, Mu Y, et al. National Healthcare Safety Network (NHSN) report: data summary for 2006 through 2008, issued December 2009. Am J Infect Control. 2009;37:783–805.
19. Johnson DW, Isbel NM, Brown AM, et al. The effect of obesity on renal transplant outcomes. Transplantation. 2002;74:675–81.
20. Ramos A, Asensio A, Munez E, et al. Incisional surgical site infection in kidney transplantation. Urology. 2008;72:119–23.
21. Perdiz LB, Furtado GHC, Linhares MM, Gonzalez AM, Pestana JOM, Medeiros EAS. Incidence and risk factors for surgical site infection after simultaneous pancreas–kidney transplantation. J Hosp Infect. 2009;72:326–31.
22. Esposito S. Immune system and surgical site infection. J Chemother. 2001;13 Spec No 1:12–6.
23. Menezes FG, Wey S, Xe, et al. Risk factors for surgical site infection in kidney transplant recipients. Infect Control Hosp Epidemiol. 2008;29:771–3.
24. Park C, Hsu C, Neelakanta G, et al. Severe intraoperative hyperglycemia is independently associated with surgical site infection after liver transplantation. Transplantation. 2009;87:1031–6.
25. Ramos A, Asensio A, Muñez E, et al. Incisional surgical infection in heart transplantation. Transplant Infect Dis. 2008;10:298–302.
26. Sénéchal M, LePrince P, Tezenas du Montcel S, et al. Bacterial mediastinitis after heart transplantation: clinical presentation, risk factors and treatment. J Heart Lung Transplant. 2004;23:165–70.
27. Albano L, Bretagne S, Mamzer-Bruneel M-F, et al. Evidence that graft-site candidiasis after kidney transplantation is acquired dur-

ing organ recovery: a multicenter study in France. Clin Infect Dis. 2009;48:194–202.
28. Talbot TR, Hatcher J, Davis SF, Pierson RN 3rd, Barton R, Dummer S. Scedosporium apiospermum pneumonia and sternal wound infection in a heart transplant recipient. Transplantation. 2002;74:1645–7.
29. Vallabhaneni S, Purfield AE, Benedict K, et al. Cardiothoracic surgical site phaeohyphomycosis caused by Bipolaris mould, multiple US states, 2008–2013: a clinical description. Med Mycol. 2016;54:318–21.
30. El-Sayed Ahmed MM, Almanfi A, Aftab M, Singh SK, Mallidi HR, Frazier OH. Aspergillus mediastinitis after orthotopic heart transplantation: a case report. Tex Heart Inst J. 2015;42:468–70.
31. Gandhi V, Nagral A, Nagral S, Das S, Rodrigues C. An unusual surgical site infection in a liver transplant recipient. BMJ Case Rep. 2010;2010:bcr0220102702.
32. Unai S, Miessau J, Karbowski P, Bajwa G, Hirose H. Sternal wound infection caused by Mycobacterium chelonae. J Card Surg. 2013;28:687–92.
33. Ogata K, Takamori H, Ikuta Y, et al. Pyoderma gangrenosum in an abdominal surgical site: a case report. Surg Case Rep. 2015;1:122.
34. Faghihi G, Abtahi-Naeini B, Nikyar Z, Jamshidi K, Bahrami A. Postoperative pyoderma gangrenosum: a rare complication after appendectomy. J Postgrad Med. 2015;61:42–3.
35. Minocha R, Sebaratnam DF, Choi JYJ. Sweet's syndrome following surgery: cutaneous trauma as a possible aetiological co-factor in neutrophilic dermatoses. Australas J Dermatol. 2015;56:e74–e6.
36. Avkan-Oguz V, Unek T, Firuzan E, et al. Bacterial pathogens isolated in liver transplant recipients with surgical site infection and antibiotic treatment. Transplant Proc. 2015;47:1495–8.
37. Karapanagiotou A, Kydona C, Papadopoulos S, et al. Infections after orthotopic liver transplantation in the intensive care unit. Transplant Proc. 2012;44:2748–50.
38. Dorschner P, McElroy LM, Ison MG. Nosocomial infections within the first month of solid organ transplantation. Transplant Infect Dis. 2014;16:171–87.
39. Yeganegi M, Watson CS, Martins A, et al. Effect of Lactobacillus rhamnosus GR-1 supernatant and fetal sex on lipopolysaccharide-induced cytokine and prostaglandin-regulating enzymes in human placental trophoblast cells: implications for treatment of bacterial vaginosis and prevention of preterm labor. Am J Obstet Gynecol. 2009;200:532 e1–8.
40. Primeggia J, Matsumoto CS, Fishbein TM, Karacki PS, Fredette TM, Timpone JG. Infection among adult small bowel and multivisceral transplant recipients in the 30-day postoperative period. Transplant Infect Dis. 2013;15:441–8.
41. Harris AD, Fleming B, Bromberg JS, et al. Surgical site infection after renal transplantation. Infect Control Hosp Epidemiol. 2015;36:417–23.
42. Steurer W, Bonatti H, Obrist P, et al. Incidence of intraabdominal infection in a consecutive series of 40 enteric-drained pancreas transplants with FK506 and MMF immunosuppression. Transplant Int. 2000;13(Suppl 1):S195–8.
43. Centofanti P, Savia F, La Torre M, et al. A prospective study of prevalence of 60-days postoperative wound infections after cardiac surgery. An updated risk factor analysis. J Cardiovasc Surg. 2007;48:641–6.
44. Filsoufi F, Rahmanian PB, Castillo JG, Pinney S, Broumand SR, Adams DH. Incidence, treatment strategies and outcome of deep sternal wound infection after orthotopic heart transplantation. J Heart Lung Transplant. 2007;26:1084–90.
45. Lepelletier D, Perron S, Bizouarn P, et al. Surgical-site infection after cardiac surgery: incidence, microbiology, and risk factors. Infect Control Hosp Epidemiol. 2005;26:466–72.
46. Sánchez-Lázaro IJ, Almenar L, Blanes M, et al. Timing, etiology, and location of first infection in first year after heart transplantation. Transplant Proc. 2010;42:3017–9.
47. Shields RK, Clancy CJ, Minces LR, et al. Epidemiology and outcomes of deep surgical site infections following lung transplantation. Am J Transplant. 2013;13:2137–45.
48. Stevens DL, Bisno AL, Chambers HF, et al. Practice guidelines for the diagnosis and management of skin and soft tissue infections: 2014 update by the Infectious Diseases Society of America. Clin Infect Dis. 2014;59:e10–52.
49. Bode LG, Kluytmans JA, Wertheim HF, et al. Preventing surgical-site infections in nasal carriers of *Staphylococcus aureus*. N Engl J Med. 2010;362:9–17.
50. Chlebicki MP, Safdar N, O'Horo JC, Maki DG. Preoperative chlorhexidine shower or bath for prevention of surgical site infection: a meta-analysis. Am J Infect Control. 2013;41:167–73.
51. Darouiche RO, Wall MJ Jr, Itani KM, et al. Chlorhexidine-alcohol versus povidone-iodine for surgical-site antisepsis. N Engl J Med. 2010;362:18–26.
52. Alexander JW, Solomkin JS, Edwards MJ. Updated recommendations for control of surgical site infections. Ann Surg. 2011;253:1082–93.
53. Mangram AJ, Horan TC, Pearson ML, Silver LC, Jarvis WR. Guideline for prevention of surgical site infection, 1999. Hospital Infection Control Practices Advisory Committee. Infect Control Hosp Epidemiol. 1999;20:250–78; quiz 79–80.
54. Hellinger WC, Heckman MG, Crook JE, et al. Association of surgeon with surgical site infection after liver transplantation. Am J Transplant. 2011;11:1877–84.

Endovascular Infections and Endocarditis

15

Walter Zingg and Didier Pittet

Introduction

Acute bloodstream infection (BSI) is one of the most severe forms of infection. BSI may be primary or secondary and community-acquired or healthcare-associated. BSI is frequently observed among immunocompromised and critically ill patients, but is rarely asymptomatic and may be associated with multiple organ failure [1–3]. Infective endocarditis (IE) is either acute or subacute, the latter being more common with underlying vascular disease.

The term "bloodstream infection" includes all forms of microbiologically confirmed or non-confirmed bacteremia and fungemia. Acute BSI should be distinguished from *septicemia, clinical sepsis,* and *sepsis,* which refer to clinical syndromes. Definitions are summarized in Table 15.1 [8]. Strictly speaking, IE is a BSI variant, but for practical reasons, it is often considered a separate entity. Diagnosis of IE follows the modified Duke criteria as outlined in Table 15.2 [9].

Epidemiology

Severe sepsis is not rare (3/1000 population; 2.3/100 hospital discharges), and particularly frequent in the elderly with an incidence increasing by >100-fold with age (0.2/1000 in children compared to 26.2/1000 in persons >85 years old) [10]. It is an expensive (US$ 22,100/case) and potentially fatal condition (28.6%). Laboratory-confirmed BSI accounts for 30–40% of all cases of severe sepsis and septic shock. In the healthcare setting, BSI contributes to 12–15% of all healthcare-associated infections (HAI) as reported in the European Prevalence of Infection in Intensive Care (EPIC) studies [11–13]. Almost half of all positive blood cultures in the hospital setting are due to healthcare-associated BSI [14]. Of these, most are primary and associated with central catheter use [15].

Most surveillance systems today, such as the United States National Healthcare Safety Network (NHSN), the German Krankenhaus Infektions Surveillance System (KISS), or the International Nosocomial Infection Control Consortium (INICC), focus on catheter-associated, laboratory-confirmed, primary BSI (CLABSI), with rates

Table 15.1 Definitions of bloodstream infections [4–6]

Type	Criteria
Positive blood culture	Pathogens identified from one or more blood cultures
Laboratory-confirmed BSI	One or more positive blood cultures with a recognized pathogen; or common skin contaminant (diphteroids, *Bacillus* spp., *Propionibacterium* spp., coagulase-negative staphylococci, or micrococci) cultured from two or more blood cultures obtained on separate occasions, and at least one of the following signs or symptoms: fever (>100.4 °F [38 °C]) or hypothermia (<98.6 °F [37 °C]); chills; low blood pressure (systolic blood pressure ≤90 mm Hg or a decrease >40 mm Hg from baseline)
Primary BSI	Laboratory-confirmed BSI occurring without a documented distal source of infection, but including those associated or related with an intravascular device
Secondary BSI	Laboratory-confirmed BSI occurring in the presence of a documented distal source of infection
Catheter-associated BSI	Primary BSI and presence (>2 calendar days) of an intravascular device
Catheter-related BSI	Primary BSI and at least one of the following: positive semiquantitative culture of the catheter (>15 CFU/catheter segment) with the same organism; [4] positive quantitative culture of the catheter (>10^3 CFU/catheter segment) with the same organism; [7] quantitative blood cultures obtained from the catheter and a peripheral vein with a ≥5: 1 ratio (catheter versus peripheral vein); [5] or differential time to positivity >2h of blood cultures simultaneously obtained from the catheter and a peripheral vein [6]

BSI bloodstream infection, *CFU* colony-forming unit

W. Zingg · D. Pittet (✉)
Infection Control Programme and WHO Collaborating Centre on Patient Safety, University of Geneva Hospitals and Faculty of Medicine, Geneva, Switzerland
e-mail: walter.zingg@hcuge.ch; didier.pittet@hcuge.ch

A. Safdar (ed.), *Principles and Practice of Transplant Infectious Diseases*, https://doi.org/10.1007/978-1-4939-9034-4_15

Table 15.2 Infective endocarditis: modified Duke criteria

Major criteria
Blood culture positive for IE
Typical microorganisms consistent with IE from 2 separate blood cultures:
Viridans streptococci, *Streptococcus bovis*, HACEK group, *Staphylococcus aureus*
Community-acquired enterococci in the absence of a primary focus
Microorganisms consistent with IE from persistently positive blood cultures, defined as follows:
At least 2 positive cultures of blood samples obtained >12 h apart
All of 3 or a majority of >4 separate cultures of blood (with first and last sample obtained at least 1 h apart)
Single positive blood culture for *Coxiella burnetii* or IgG antibody titer >1: 800
Evidence of endocardial involvement
Echocardiogram positive for IE (TEE recommended in patients with prosthetic valves, rated at least "possible IE" by clinical criteria, or complicated IE [paravalvular abscess]; TTE as first test in other patients), defined as follows:
Oscillating intracardiac mass on valve or supporting structures in the path of regurgitant jets or on implanted material in the absence of an alternative anatomic explanation
Abscess
New partial dehiscence of prosthetic valve
New valvular regurgitation (worsening or changing of pre-existing murmur not sufficient)
Minor criteria
Predisposition, predisposing heart condition, or injection drug use
Fever (temperature >38 °C)
Vascular phenomena, major arterial emboli, septic pulmonary infarcts, mycotic aneurysm, intracranial hemorrhage, conjunctival hemorrhages, and Janeway lesions
Immunologic phenomena: glomerulonephritis, Osler's nodes, Roth's spots, and rheumatoid factor
Microbiological evidence: positive blood culture, but does not meet a major criterion as noted above[a] or serological evidence of active infection with an organism consistent with IE
Echocardiographic minor criteria eliminated
Definite infective endocarditis
Pathologic criteria
1. Microorganisms demonstrated by culture or histologic examination of a vegetation, a vegetation that has embolized or an intracardiac abscess specimen
2. Pathologic lesions; vegetation or intracardiac abscess confirmed by histologic examination showing active endocarditis
Clinical criteria
1. 2 major criteria
2. 1 major criterion and 3 minor criteria
3. 5 minor criteria
Possible infective endocarditis
1. 1 major criterion and 1 minor criterion
2. 3 minor criteria
Rejected
1. Firm alternate diagnosis explaining evidence of infective endocarditis
2. Resolution of infective endocarditis syndrome with antibiotic therapy for <4 days
3. No pathologic evidence of infective endocarditis at surgery or autopsy, with antibiotic therapy for <4 days
4. Does not meet the criteria for possible infective endocarditis as detailed above

[a]Excludes single positive cultures for coagulase-negative staphylococci and organisms that do not cause endocarditis HACEK Haemo philus parainfluenzae, H. aphrophilus, Actinobacillus actinomycetemcomitans, Cardiobacterium homi nis, Eikenella corrodens, and Kingella kingae, *IE* infective endocarditis, *TEE* trans-esophageal echoca rdiography, *TTE* trans-thoracic echocardiography

reported as episodes per 1000 device-days. CLABSI incidence density rates are known to be high in the intensive care unit (ICU), but non-ICU settings may have similar rates (Table 15.3) [16–29, 31–35]. The large differences among studies reporting on CLABSI are due to variable definitions and reporting systems. Thus, comparison and benchmarking should be performed with caution [36, 37].

Severe sepsis and septic shock are associated with increased morbidity, end-organ dysfunction, and risk of death [38]. Clinical sepsis has been reported to represent up to two-thirds of CLABSI, and focusing on microbiologically documented BSI may underestimate true CLABSI rates [15]. However, surveillance of clinical sepsis has been mostly abandoned because the definition of this infection leaves too much room for interpretation and is resource demanding [15]. The exception to this rule is BSI-surveillance in the neonatal intensive care unit (NICU) because blood cultures from neonates are often unreliable [39]. In adults, false-negative blood cultures are most likely due to previous antibiotic treatment.

Table 15.3 Incidence of healthcare-associated bloodstream infections in various healthcare settings [16–30]

Report	No. of hospitals	Type of hospital	Per 1000 admissions or discharges	Per 1000 patient-days	Per 1000 device-days
Hospital-wide series					
Brun-Buisson[a] [16]	24	Any	4.4	–	–
Banerjee [19]	124	Community	1.3	–	–
Banerjee [19]	124	University	6.5	–	–
Pittet [30]	1	University	13.2	1.5	–
Marschall [27]	1	Teaching	–	1.3	5.7
Zingg [28]	1	University	–	0.2	4.2
ICU series					
Richards [25]	205 mixed	Any	7.5	2.4	–
Legras [26]	5 mixed	Any	48	3.8	–
Renaud [17]	15 mixed	Any	33.8	4.5	–
Richards [20]	112 medical	Any	16.3	4.1	–
Richards [21]	61 pediatric	Any	14.6	3.7	–
Raymond [22]	20 pediatric	Any	8.9	3.4	–
Gastmeier [23]	72 pediatric	Any	–	2.1	–
Gilio [24]	1 pediatric	University	6	1.5	–
Richards [18]	93 coronary	Any	4.8	1.7	6.3
Zingg [29]	1 mixed	University	–	4.7	2.3

[a]Both community-acquired and healthcare-associated infections were reported together

Patients with BSI have higher mortality compared to those without BSI [17, 40]. Attributable mortality from CLABSI is between 2% and 35% [41]. Healthcare-associated BSI, particularly CLABSI, is associated with morbidity, prolonged length of hospital stay, and increased resource utilization in almost all groups of patients [1, 16, 17, 31–33, 41–51]. Interestingly, mortality from secondary BSI is higher compared to primary BSI (29–45% vs. 18–29%, respectively). Furthermore, mortality from CLABSI is lower than mortality from other primary BSI (15–26% vs. 18–29%, respectively) [17, 40]. Although the reason for this remains unclear, delayed antibiotic therapy for community-acquired BSI and serious comorbidities in the context of secondary BSI may partially explain such trends. Microbiological factors have been found to be important in the context of mortality among patients with healthcare-associated BSI, even after adjustment for major confounders such as patients' underlying conditions [40]. Pathogens independently associated with mortality include *Candida* spp. and *Pseudomonas aeruginosa*. Coagulase-negative staphylococci (CoNS) are less associated with mortality compared to other pathogens, although they are the most frequently isolated [40].

BSI is the most frequent type of infection in patients after hematopoietic stem cell transplantation (HSCT) with rates of approximately 11–19 per 1000 neutropenic days [52, 53]. Most BSI occur within the first 30 days after transplantation. In this period, there is no difference in BSI between allogeneic and autologous transplants, most likely due to neutropenia, which is similar in both groups [54]. Prolonged neutropenia is the most important risk factor for BSI and attributable mortality [54–56]. In the long term, BSI occurs almost exclusively in allogeneic transplant patients because of the prevention and treatment of graft-versus-host disease with immunosuppressive drugs [57].

IE accounts for about 1% of all cases of severe sepsis [10]. The estimated incidence is 3–10/100,000 patient-years with a low incidence in childhood and a peak incidence up to 15/100,000 patient-years in the elderly [58–66]. The incidence among children has been estimated at around 0.2–1.25/1000 hospital admissions, with an average age of 5–13 years [67–70]. Historically, the most important reason for IE was rheumatic heart disease. However, it has been estimated that the proportion of IE patients with this disease has decreased by 12% per decade, while the proportion of IE patients after valve surgery has increased by 9% in the same period [71]. Mortality from IE is approximately 20–25% during hospitalization, and up to one-third in the 1st year [10, 59, 63–65, 72]. Immunosuppressed and hemodialysis patients are particularly at risk [64]. In general, IE is a rather rare event after solid organ transplantation (SOT), but the overall incidence is still higher compared to the general population [73–75]. By contrast, IE is frequent (1.5%) after heart transplantation with an exceptionally high mortality of up to 80% and a dramatic reduction of the survival rate from 9.3 to 1.4 years [76]. The annual incidence of IE among prosthetic valve recipients is 1–4% [77]. Patients with prosthetic valves and a history of past IE have the highest risk for recurrent IE. Other risk factors for IE include congenital malformations, rheumatic fever, degenerative valve lesions, and even mitral valve prolapse [78]. Although the individual risk of IE from mitral valve prolapse is small, the high prevalence of this heart condition in the general population makes it relevant. Among congenital malformations, the ventricular septal defect is particularly of risk due to high blood flow and pressure gradients [81]. In recent years, intravenous drug use and healthcare-associated bacteremia have been recognized as emerging risk factors for IE [79, 80].

Pathogenesis

Microorganisms are not likely to attach to the vascular endothelium. However, host factors and cofactors such as fibrinogen, fibronectin, calcium, magnesium, and iron facilitate bacteria attachment on foreign material, such as intravascular catheters [82–92]. Streptococci possess fibronectin-binding proteins, platelet-aggregating factors and glucans, which facilitate adherence to endocardial lesions and vegetations [93]. *Staphylococcus aureus* adheres to host-tissue ligands, such as fibrinogen, via genetically defined microbial surface proteins, commonly referred to as "microbial surface components recognizing adhesive matrix molecules" (MSCRAMM) [94–96]. After adherence, the attachment becomes irreversible, and the microorganisms start to produce an extracellular matrix. This matrix protects microorganisms from host defense mechanisms and antibiotics, and allows them to proliferate in a protected environment. This process is called biofilm formation [97]. Thrombus formation around the catheter is thought to further increase the risk of catheter-related BSI, [98] although clinical evidence on this topic is controversial [99–101]. Main risk factors for catheter-related BSI include catheter dwell time [102], femoral rather than the subclavian access site [103, 104], parenteral nutrition [105–107], guidewire exchange [108, 109], multi-lumen catheters [110], and previous HSCT [111, 112].

The pathogenesis of IE is initiated by turbulent flow and pressure gradients creating stress on endocardial tissue. Such stress is maximal on the atrial surface of the atrioventricular valves and the ventricular surface of the semilunar valves. In valve insufficiency, flow jets damage structures, such as the mitral chordae (aortic insufficiency), the atrial wall (mitral regurgitation), or the septal leaflet of the tricuspid valve (ventricular septal defect) [113, 114]. Defects in the endocardium provoke the deposition of fibrin and platelets [115], an ongoing process resulting in thrombus formation. At any time, such a thrombus may become colonized by microorganisms due to transient bacteremia or fungemia. Once attached, microorganisms are covered by further deposition of fibrin and platelets and proliferate in a protected environment. This cycle of fibrin and platelet deposition, together with the proliferation of microorganisms in the presence of pressure gradients and sheering forces, results in the formation of the typical IE vegetations. Gradually, the process triggers an inflammatory response that is exemplified by elevated levels of inflammatory markers, such as C-reactive protein, tumor necrosis factor alpha, immune complexes, the rheumatoid factor, and increased the erythrocyte sedimentation rate [116]. The deposition of immune complexes can result in kidney amyloidosis.

Microbiology

The distribution of microorganisms causing intravascular infections varies according to source, age (neonates, children, adults), and resources [16, 17, 20–22, 25, 30–33, 117–126]. Healthcare-associated BSI are mainly due to Gram-positive organisms in high-income countries (Table 15.4) [25, 30, 128, 129]. In countries with limited resources, Gram-negative pathogens and among these, non-fermentative organisms such as *Pseudomonas* spp. and *Acinetobacter* spp., are predominant (Table 15.4) [119–123]. This may be the result of breaches in basic infection control procedures, such as the multiple use of infusates or handling of catheteres without complying with aseptic procedures [120, 130]. The shift toward Gram-positive cocci in high-income countries is mainly due to coagulase-negative staphylococci (CoNS), and is a consequence of the abundant use of central catheters and the fact that the proportion of patients with risk factors, such as neutropenia, SOT, HSCT, prematurity, or the use of immunosuppressive agents, has increased in the past years [131]. The mean interval between admission and infection depends on the microorganism and is shortest (13 days) for *Escherichia coli*, followed by *S. aureus* (16 days), *Candida* spp. and *Klebsiella* spp. (22 days), enterococci (23 days), and *Acinetobacter* spp. (26 days) [129].

The proportion of *Candida* spp. has increased over the years due to the use of broad-spectrum antibiotics, intravascular devices, total parenteral nutrition, and prolonged neutropenia in patients with chemotherapy [132–139]. But only recently, first reports suggested no further increase and even trends toward a reduction of *Candida* infections, at least in North America [140, 141]. By contrast, an important shift in the epidemiology of *Candida* BSI has occurred over the past decades with decreasing infections due to *C. albicans*, but increasing infections due to non-albicans species, in particular *C. glabrata* [142]. The emergence of this species is a problem because it is often resistant to fluconazole [143]. BSI due to *Candida* spp. has a poor prognosis. Mortality from BSI with this microorganism ranges between 15% and 55%, particularly when antifungal treatment is delayed or intravascular catheters are left in place [132, 144].

CoNS are the most common pathogens isolated from blood cultures, particularly in primary BSI [14]. They are mostly contaminants, but the detection of CoNS may not always be harmless, and mortality up to 12% has been reported, particularly in neutropenic patients [14, 145]. By contrast, mortality from *S. aureus* BSI ranges between 13% and 25% with higher proportions in healthcare-associated compared to community-acquired infections [146, 147]. Detection of *S. aureus* on a catheter tip is a predictor for subsequent bacteremia, even in the absence of clinical signs and negative blood cultures at the time of catheter removal [148–150].

Table 15.4 Microbiology of healthcare-associated bloodstream infections [2, 17, 20, 21, 25, 30, 33, 117, 119–122, 125, 127]

Author	Year of publication	No. of organisms	CoNS (%)	*S. aureus* (%)	*S. pneumoniae* (%)	Enterococci (%)	Other GPC (%)	*E. coli* (%)	*Enterobacter* (%)	*P. aeruginosa* (%)	Other GNB (%)	Yeasts (%)
High-income countries												
Pittet [30]	1995	3464	26	16	NR	4	12	12	6	9	8	7
Valles [33]	1997	511	28	20	NR	6	3	6	10	9	15	5
Edmond [2]	1999	10,617	32	16	NR	11	1	6	7	4	16	8
Richards [20]	1999	2971	36	15	NR	16	NR	3	6	3	11	12
Richards [21]	1999	1887	40	9	6	NR	1	3	5	5	21	10
Renaud [17]	2001	111	18	14	NR	7	5	NR	25	NR	15	7
Luzzaro [117]	2002	1478	13	23	1	9	12	15	8	9	11	9
Richards [25]	2000	4394	40	12	11	NR	7	2	7	4	5	12
Low- and middle-income countries												
Pawar [125]	2004	17	6	12	NR	NR	NR	47	6	NR	18	12
Almuneef [127]	2006	73	14	7	NR	10	1	4	10	11	35	8
Moreno [122]	2006	126	10	37	NR	NR	NR	NR	NR	6	45	2
Girao [121]	2008	1286	12	27	NR	8	NR	NR	7	9	30	6
Macias [120]	2010	108	10	14	NR	4	1	NR	8	23	35	5
Rosenthal [119]	2010	5433	NR	14	NR	2	NR	11	NR	46	26	NR

CoNS, coagulase-negative staphylococci, *GNB* Gram-negative bacilli, *GPC* Gram-positive cocci, *NR* not reported

Table 15.5 Most common microorganisms in healthcare-associated vascular infections, large series 1995–2012 [2, 20, 21, 30, 32, 52, 117, 129, 151–163]

All-cause		HSCT transplants		Solid organ transplants	
Gram-positive bacteria					
CoNS	31.8%	CoNS	41.0%	*Enterococcus* spp.	16.9%
Staphylococcus aureus[c]	16.6%	*Streptococcus* spp.	12.3%	CoNS[b]	14.0%
Enterococcus spp.	10.4%	*Enterococcus* spp.	10.1%	*Staphylococcus aureus*[a]	10.3%
Streptococcus spp.	2.4%	*Staphylococcus aureus*[a]	2.9%	*Streptococcus* spp.	2.7%
		Listeria spp.	0.2%	*Listeria* spp.	0.7%
Gram-negative bacteria					
Escherichia coli	8.2%	*Escherichia coli*	8.9%	*Pseudomonas* spp.	11.4%
Pseudomonas spp.	5.7%	*Pseudomonas* spp.	4.5%	*Klebsiella* spp.	6.7%
Klebsiella spp.	5.6%	*Klebsiella* spp.	2.7%	*Escherichia coli*	5.6%
Enterobacter spp.	4.7%	*Stenotrophomonas maltophilia*	1.9%	*Acinetobacter* spp.	4.2%
Serratia spp.	1.5%	*Enterobacter* spp.	1.6%	*Enterobacter* spp.	4.0%
Acinetobacter spp.	0.7%	*Acinetobacter* spp.	1.0%	*Stenotrophomonas maltophilia*	3.7%
		Serratia spp.	0.3%	*Serratia* spp.	1.1%
Fungi/other microorganisms					
Candida spp.	8.8%	*Candida* spp.	5.3%	*Candida* spp.	5.2%
Anaerobes	0.5%	Anaerobes	1.4%	Anaerobes	1.3%
Other microorganisms	3.1%	Other microorganisms	5.9%	Other microorganisms	12.2%
Authors					
Pittet [30]		Dettenkofer [152]		Rodriguez [156]	
Edmond [2]		Wisplinghoff [129]		Shi [157]	
Richards [20]		Danziger-Isakov [153]		Iida [158]	
Richards [21]		Dettenkofer [154]		Mikulska [159]	
Palmer [151]		Ortega [155]		Hsu [160]	
Luzzaro [117]		Laws [52]		Karvellas [161]	
Lyytikäinen [32]				Lee [162]	
				Busca [163]	

CoNS coagulase-negative staphylococci, HSCT Hematopoietic stem cell transplantation
[a]Including methicillin-resistant *Staphylococcus aureus* (MRSA)

The distribution of pathogens in SOT demonstrates a predominance of Gram-positive bacteria similar to healthcare-associated BSI in HSCT (Table 15.5). Emerging BSI in SOT due to *Candida* spp. are the result of antifungal prophylaxis [164]. In addition, rare causes such as *Mycobacterium avium intracellulare*, and *Listeria* spp. have been reported [165, 166]. Vascular infections due to donor organs are not frequent, although donor organs may be contaminated with CoNS, *S. aureus*, *Streptococcus pyogenes*, *Enterobacteriaceae*, *Enterococcus*, *Pseudomonas*, *Candida* spp., and *Aspergillus* [167, 168]. Recently however, infections including BSI due to donor organs colonized with carbapenem-resistant Gram-negative organisms such as *K. pneumoniae* or *A. baumannii* after lung, liver, kidney, or heart transplantation have been described [169–171]. Independent from donor organ contamination, patients after SOT and HSCT are at increased risk for BSI.

In bone marrow transplant patients, time from transplantation to first positive blood culture is between 5 and 10 days [172]. Most pathogens are Gram-positive bacteria with a large proportion of viridians streptococci and enterococci [159, 173]. Mucositis is a risk condition for BSI due to enterococci and anaerobes such as *Fusobacterium* and *Clostridium* spp. [159, 174]. The incidence of pre- and post-engraftment BSI is similar in allogeneic HSCT recipients (22% and 19.5%, respectively). Pre-engraftment rates are highest for viridans streptococci (58), *Enterobacteriaceae* (39), and *E. faecium* (34) [173]. Attributable mortality from BSI is low except for infections due to *P. aeruginosa, Enterobacter* spp., *Serratia*, and *Citrobacter* spp. [172]. No significant difference in the distribution of pathogens was identified in neutropenic and non-neutropenic patients with hematological malignancies or solid neoplasms and BSI [175].

IE is largely due to Gram-positive bacteria, mostly *S. aureus* and streptococci, predominantly from the viridians group; however, enterococci or *S. pneumoniae* have been described as well. CoNS rarely cause IE, particularly on native valves [176]. Overall, a third of native valve IE are due to *S. aureus* [177]. Mortality from *S. aureus* IE is 20% [178], and patients are more likely to experience an embolic event (61%) or to have a central nervous system complication. More than half of the cases occur in patients with intravascular devices. IE due to other Gram-positive bacilli such as *Corynebacterium* spp., *L. monocytogenes,* or *Lactobacillus* are very rare. Gram-negative bacteria only cause few IE (4–5%) with a predominance of bacteria from the HACEK group (*Haemophilus* spp., *Actinobacillus actinomycetemcomitans*, *Cardiobacterium hominis*, *Eikenella corrodens*, *Kingella kingae*). In a large study of 2761 patients with definite IE according to the Duke criteria, only 49 (1.8%) had endocarditis (20 native valve, 29 prosthetic valve or device) due to non-HACEK Gram-negative bacilli, with *E. coli* and *P. aeruginosa* being the most common pathogens [179]. Most IE due to non-HACEK Gram-negative bacilli were healthcare-associated and in patients with implanted intravascular devices.

IE after SOT is infrequent but the microorganisms differ from non-transplant patients. *S. aureus*, *Candida*, and *Aspergillus* spp. are predominant, but viridians streptococci remain rather rare (4%) [75]. Other pathogens found in this group include *Coxiella burnetii*, *Nocardia*, *Listeria* spp., *Pseudomonas* spp., *Enterococcus* spp., *Oerskovia xanthineolytica*, and *Weissella confusa* [74, 180–184]. Most fungal IE are due to *Candida* spp. with *C. albicans* being the most common microorganism, but other *Candida* spp. such as *C. krusei*, *C. parapsilosis*, *C. tropicalis*, or *C. guillermondii* have been reported as well. *Aspergillus* spp., including *A. fumigatus*, *A. flavus*, *A. terreus*, and *A. niger*, are isolated particularly in lung transplant recipients after cystic fibrosis, and IE due to these pathogens are associated with a poor prognosis [75, 76, 185, 186]. Fungal infections predominate in the first 30 days after transplantation (20%), while bacteria are responsible for most infections (80%) after this period [75].

The most common organism in "culture-negative" IE is *Coxiella burnetii*. Other pathogens such as *Bartonella* spp., *Brucella* spp., *Chlamydia* spp., *Mycoplasma hominis*, *Legionella pneumophila*, rickettsiae, and *Tropheryma whipplei* have been rarely described [187].

Clinical Signs

Fever is the hallmark of all vascular infections. Fever in the absence of other symptoms and, in particular, in the presence of an intravascular device must be considered a BSI until proven otherwise. Sepsis is characterized additionally by hemodynamic abnormalities. The symptoms of IE relate to systemic infection, (septic) emboli, metastatic infective foci, congestive heart failure, or immune complex-associated lesions [188]. Acute IE is characterized by fever, new or changed heart murmurs, and skin manifestations such as splinter hemorrhages, Osler nodes, Roth spots, or Janeway lesions. Subacute IE may present less typically without or with moderate fever only, but with malaise, anorexia/weight loss, heart failure, arthralgia, splenomegaly, or glomerulonephritis.

Diagnosis

Blood cultures should be obtained from patients with clinical signs suggestive for BSI. Severe sepsis and septic shock are associated with increased morbidity, mortality, and end-organ dysfunction [38]. Accordingly, when sepsis is suspected, it is not possible to wait until the results of blood cultures are available, and empirical antimicrobial treatment is initiated as soon as possible. Positive blood culture results with a recognized pathogen are sufficient to diagnose BSI, particularly when clinical signs such as fever, hypothermia, chills, or low blood pressure are present. BSI due to skin contaminants need confirmation with additional blood cultures and the presence of clinical signs. The classification into primary or secondary, and catheter-associated or catheter-related BSI, can be done based on additional clinical signs and laboratory findings, and whether a catheter is in place (Table 15.1). Inappropriate blood culture sampling may produce false-positive results, particularly when skin contaminants are identified [189]. If CLABSI is suspected and the catheter is removed, the tip should be cultured either by using the Maki roll-plate technique or the Brun-Buisson vortex method [4, 190, 191]. Alternatively, if the catheter is left in place, two blood culture samples – from the catheter and from a peripheral vein – should be obtained simultaneously to measure the differential time to positivity [192]. To avoid missing infections, all lumens of a multi-lumen catheter should be tested [193].

The diagnosis of IE follows the modified major and minor Duke criteria distinguishing definite, possible, and rejected IE (Table 15.2). Prior antibiotic use may result in culture-negative IE, less likely to be classified as definite IE by the Duke criteria [194]. Clinical signs, such as fever, embolic complications, new or changed heart murmurs, and predisposing factors (e.g., rheumatic heart disease, congenital heart disease, mitral valve prolapse, or previous cardiac surgery) should raise suspicion for IE, even in the absence of positive blood cultures.

Laboratory Findings

Overall, only 10–15% of performed blood cultures turn positive. Even in the presence of a systemic inflammatory response syndrome, blood cultures are negative in 40–60% of cases [31]. Due to challenges of blood culture sampling in terms of technique, volume and availability of adequate blood culture bottles, the situation in neonates is even more pronounced [39]. The quality of blood cultures is better among older children but is not optimal either when compared to adults [189]. Prophylactic or preemptive antibiotic treatment at the time of sampling makes the interpretation of negative blood culture results difficult [195–197]. This can be bypassed by using nucleic acid testing with a multiplex polymerase chain reaction (PCR) identifying a wide range of microorganisms [198, 199]. However, most negative test results are true negative. After SOT and HSCT, blood cultures should be obtained generously from febrile patients in the first 30 days after transplantation. BSI is less frequent in autologous HSCT recipients after engraftment, and in SOT recipients once immunosuppressive therapy is less intensive.

Most patients with IE have positive blood cultures, but they may remain negative for a long time in subacute IE due to non-common pathogens such as *Candida* spp. or microorganisms of the HACEK group. However, blood cultures in IE are negative only in 10–15% of cases, although rates up to 31% have been described [200–204]. Potential reasons for blood culture-negative IE are (1) right-sided IE, (2) previous administration of antibiotics, (3) fungi, (4) viruses, and (5) pathogens that do not grow in regular culture conditions such as *Bartonella* spp., *Brucella* spp., *Chlamydia* spp., *Mycoplasma hominis*, *Legionella pneumophila*, rickettsiae, *Coxiella burnetii*, and *Tropheryma whipplei* [203, 205]. Pathogens of blood culture-negative IE can still be identified by serological tests and by PCR in valve tissue obtained by surgery [205, 208–214]. In particular, fungi are be detected more readily in biopsies [215]. Microbiological culturing of heart valves on the other hand, has a low sensitivity [206, 207]. By applying a range of methods (microbiology, serology, molecular techniques), a pathogen can be identified in up to 63% of culture-negative IE cases [187].

Upon IE suspicion, two blood culture bottles for aerobic and anaerobic cultures and a serum vial should be obtained immediately, the latter to search for rheumatoid factor and antibodies directed against *Coxiella burnetii*, *Bartonella* spp., *Brucella* spp., *Chlamydia* spp., *Mycoplasma pneumonia*, *Legionella pneumophila*, and *Aspergillus* spp. [204, 210]. Two additional samplings of blood culture bottles for aerobic and anaerobic cultures are obtained after 2 and 4 h.

Inflammatory markers such as C-reactive protein, procalcitonin, erythrocyte sedimentation rate, and tumor necrosis factor alpha are elevated in vascular infections. Presence or absence of rheumatoid factor can distinguish between patients with definite and rejected IE based on the modified Duke criteria [116]. Autoantibodies, such as antinuclear antibodies and anticardiolipin, can be present in IE, but they are less specific than the rheumatoid factor [216].

General Principles of Management

The management of BSI combines early antimicrobial treatment and the active search for a source of infection that might require specific therapeutic interventions. Either delayed or inappropriate antibiotic treatment is associated with higher mortality [34, 128, 217–219]. Similar results were observed for candidemia where mortality was significantly higher when antifungal therapy was delayed [144, 220, 221]. Conversely, inappropriate antibiotic treatment was not found to be a risk for developing septic shock in patients with positive blood cultures in one study, [31] but mortality of those requiring inotropic drugs was significantly higher – 85% vs. 75% and 58% vs. 24%, respectively.

The choice of antibiotics to start empiric therapy should be based on knowledge of the local epidemiology and susceptibility of pathogens, and the source of infection. A multidisciplinary approach, allowing close collaboration between the physician in charge of the patient, the infectious disease specialist, and the microbiology laboratory, improves the accuracy of empiric therapy. Once susceptibility testing of the microorganisms is available, antimicrobial treatment should be adjusted accordingly. In some conditions, pathogens identified from other body sites may also need to be taken into account for selecting the appropriate antimicrobials. In addition, specific measures such as abscess drainage , adequate surgical management of peritonitis, or removal of infected prosthetic material are necessary to control the infection. Follow-up of inflammatory markers can help to shorten antimicrobial treatment. Procalcitonin-based de-escalation of antimicrobial therapy can reduce exposure to antibiotics by almost 30% [222–224].

In the case of primary BSI or sepsis, central lines should be removed if in place at the time of infection. Catheter retention may result in a severalfold increase in risk for recurrence of BSI. However, recent data suggest that antibiotic locks in addition to systemic antibiotic therapy can be used as a salvage strategy if CLABSI involves long-term catheters, signs of exit site or tunnel infection are absent, and blood cultures reveal the presence of CoNS or enterococci [225, 226]. Removal of the catheter is mandatory in severe or complicated infections, in the presence of shock, in case of recurrent BSI, and when microorganisms such as *S. aureus*, Gram-negative bacilli, or *Candida* spp. are isolated [227]. Relapse, continuous fever, or bacteremia despite catheter removal requires an active search for complications, such as metastatic abscesses, septic thrombophlebitis, or endocarditis. Following the completion of antimicrobial therapy, careful follow-up is mandatory owing to the frequent occurrence of late complications [228, 229]. Recovery of *S. aureus* on a catheter tip may suggest the initiation of therapy, even in the absence of clinical signs and negative blood cultures [148].

Antibiotic therapy is the cornerstone in the treatment of IE, with the addition of an aminoglycoside to an antibiotic regimen with activity against Gram-positive bacteria [210, 230, 231]. Although the addition of an aminoglycoside in the 1st weeks of treatment is recommended by international guidelines, clinical trials did not show that such combination therapies decrease mortality or bacteriological failure, or reduce the need for surgery [210, 232–235]. For IE due to methicillin-resistant staphylococci, vancomycin remains the therapy of choice. Other antibiotics such as linezolid or daptomycin have been shown to be effective, but have not been proven to be superior to vancomycin [236, 237]. Furthermore, linezolid alone is bacteriostatic, but in the treatment of IE, a bacteriocidal substance is encouraged. Appropriate antibiotics must be initiated as early as possible in the treatment of IE because a delay in antibiotic therapy worsens the clinical outcome [210, 238, 239] e.g. IE-related stroke [240].

Heart surgery is necessary in 25–42% of patients with IE [62, 73, 241]. The two primary objectives of surgery are the total removal of infected tissue and reconstruction of the cardiac morphology [210]. Surgery can improve long-term survival, in particular for left-sided IE [242, 243]. However, a significant proportion of patients with a recommended indication does not receive cardiac surgery [244]. Because IE is a multifactorial event, a standardized management by a skilled multidisciplinary team is required for best outcome [245, 246].

Prevention

As for any other healthcare-associated infection, the prevention of BSI in the hospital relies on the basic principles of hygiene, particularly hand hygiene practices [247–249]. It has been shown that improved hand hygiene and good work organization prevents the transmission of pathogens [250]. For the prevention of device-associated infections, there is good evidence that multimodal strategies combining procedural and technical interventions are effective [29, 251–254]. "Procedural" interventions include the introduction of standardized, written procedures for catheter insertion and catheter care. "Technical" interventions include the use of alcohol-based chlorhexidine for skin antisepsis, devices (catheters, connectors, sponges, dressings) impregnated with chlorhexidine, chlorhexidine-silver sulfadiazine, silver and antibiotics, and the use of lock solutions with agents such as taurolidine, citrate, or EDTA. Alcohol based, chlorhexidine-containing skin antiseptics have now become standard of care. The use of a chlorhexidine-impregnated sponge was found effective in two randomized controlled trials [255, 256]. Daily bathing with a chlorhexidine-containing solution in the ICU reduced bacteremia due to vancomycin-resistant enterococci (VRE), as well as VRE-colonization and methicillin-resistant *S. aureus* (MRSA) acquisition. This allowed to reduce colonization pressure and shows the importance of microorganism transmission in the pathogenesis of BSI with multidrug-resistant pathogens [257]. Two meta-analyses demonstrated that chlorhexidine-silver sulfadiazine-impregnated catheters are effective in reducing catheter colonization, but not CLABSI, while rifampicin-minocycline-coated catheters are effective in reducing both catheter colonization and CLABSI [258, 259]. Most studies with central venous catheters are conducted in the ICU, including catheters with relatively short dwell times. No data on the efficacy of antibiotic-coated devices are available for long dwell-times, and there is evidence that chlorhexidine-silver sulfadiazine impregnation is not effective in the long run [260]. The efficacy of lock solutions as a prevention strategy remains undetermined at present, although some studies show promising results [261–263]. A recent study among children reported that a taurolidine citrate lock solution was associated with a significant BSI reduction in immunocompromised pediatric patients [264]. Ethanol locks in CLABSI prevention on the other hand remain controversial. Although the substance worked well in vitro [265, 266] and among patients with long-term catheters, [267–269] three recent randomized controlled trials did not find any significant efficacy [270–272].

Educational programs or global preventive strategies based on the strict application of specific preventive measures and careful control of all factors associated with infection have been shown to be effective in reducing infection rates. Such programs must be multidisciplinary in preparation and multimodal in implementation in order to be effective [29, 251, 253, 273–277]. Education and training should use different modes such as bedside teaching, workshops, or simulator training [278–283]. Ex cathedra teaching or disseminating guidelines alone are not sufficient to change behavior of healthcare workers [284].

IE prophylaxis has produced contradictory results [285, 286] and has never been shown effective in clinical studies [113, 287, 288]. This is most likely due to the fact that IE is a rare event, even in the absence of prophylaxis. The procedure-related risk for IE due to dental procedures can be estimated as 1:14,000,000 for the general population and 1:95,000 for patients with previous IE [78, 289]. No potential index procedure can be associated with IE [63]. The existing evidence does not support the extensive use of antibiotic prophylaxis recommended in previous guidelines. Prophylaxis should be limited to patients at highest risk for IE or at high risk for adverse outcome from IE [231]. Compared to previous recommendations, all recent guidelines limit prophylaxis to clearly defined patients at risk and to dental procedures (Table 15.6) [231, 290] or do not recom-

Table 15.6 Patients at risk for infective endocarditis

1. Patients with a prosthetic valve or prosthetic material used for cardiac valve repair
2. Patients with previous infective endocarditis
3. Patients with congenital heart disease:
Cyanotic congenital heart disease, without surgical repair, or with residual defects, palliative shunts, or conduits
Congenital heart disease with complete repair with prosthetic material whether placed by surgery or by percutaneous technique, up to 6 months after the procedure
When a residual defect persists at the site of implantation of a prosthetic material or device by cardiac surgery or percutaneous technique

mend antibiotic prophylaxis at all [291]. However, all guidelines emphasize the importance of good oral hygiene in IE prevention [231, 290–293]. This is reasonable because it has been shown that transient bacteremia is associated most likely with tooth brushing, flossing, or chewing [294, 295]. IE prophylaxis is recommended only for dental procedures requiring manipulation of the gingival or periapical region or the teeth or perforation or the oral mucosa [231]. It is not recommended for any procedure of the respiratory, gastrointestinal, or urogenital tract, or for skin or soft tissue interventions. Prophylaxis is administered as a single dose 30–60 min before the dental procedure either with penicillin or ampicillin, or clindamycin in case of penicillin allergy.

References

1. Pittet D, Tarara D, Wenzel RP. Nosocomial bloodstream infection in critically ill patients. Excess length of stay, extra costs, and attributable mortality. JAMA. 1994;271(20):1598–601.
2. Edmond MB, Wallace SE, McClish DK, Pfaller MA, Jones RN, Wenzel RP. Nosocomial bloodstream infections in United States hospitals: a three-year analysis. Clin Infect Dis. 1999;29(2):239–44.
3. Marshall JC, Vincent JL, Fink MP, Cook DJ, Rubenfeld G, Foster D, et al. Measures, markers, and mediators: toward a staging system for clinical sepsis. A report of the Fifth Toronto Sepsis Roundtable, Toronto, Ontario, Canada, October 25-26, 2000. Crit Care Med. 2003;31(5):1560–7.
4. Brun-Buisson C, Abrouk F, Legrand P, Huet Y, Larabi S, Rapin M. Diagnosis of central venous catheter-related sepsis. Critical level of quantitative tip cultures. Arch Intern Med. 1987;147(5):873–7.
5. Kite P, Dobbins BM, Wilcox MH, McMahon MJ. Rapid diagnosis of central-venous-catheter-related bloodstream infection without catheter removal. Lancet. 1999;354(9189):1504–7.
6. Blot F, Nitenberg G, Chachaty E, Raynard B, Germann N, Antoun S, et al. Diagnosis of catheter-related bacteraemia: a prospective comparison of the time to positivity of hub-blood versus peripheral-blood cultures. Lancet. 1999;354(9184):1071–7.
7. Sherertz RJ, Raad II, Belani A, Koo LC, Rand KH, Pickett DL, et al. Three-year experience with sonicated vascular catheter cultures in a clinical microbiology laboratory. J Clin Microbiol. 1990;28(1):76–82.
8. Zingg W, Eggimann P, Pittet D. Acute bloodstream infection. In: Vincent JL, Abraham E, Moore FA, Kochanek P, Fink MP, editors. Textbook of critical care. Philadelphia: Saunders; 2011. p. 1004–9.
9. Li JS, Sexton DJ, Mick N, Nettles R, Fowler VG Jr, Ryan T, et al. Proposed modifications to the Duke criteria for the diagnosis of infective endocarditis. Clin Infect Dis. 2000;30(4):633–8.
10. Angus DC, Linde-Zwirble WT, Lidicker J, Clermont G, Carcillo J, Pinsky MR. Epidemiology of severe sepsis in the United States: analysis of incidence, outcome, and associated costs of care. Crit Care Med. 2001;29(7):1303–10.
11. Vincent JL, Bihari DJ, Suter PM, Bruining HA, White J, Nicolas-Chanoin MH, et al. The prevalence of nosocomial infection in intensive care units in Europe. Results of the European Prevalence of Infection in Intensive Care (EPIC) study. EPIC International Advisory Committee. JAMA. 1995;274(8):639–44.
12. Lyytikäinen O, Kanerva M, Agthe N, Möttönen T, Ruutu P, Finnish Prevalence Survey Study Group. Healthcare-associated infections in Finnish acute care hospitals: a national prevalence survey, 2005. J Hosp Infect. 2008;69(3):288–94.
13. Vincent JL, Rello J, Marshall J, Silva E, Anzueto A, Martin CD, EPIC II Group of Investigators, et al. International study of the prevalence and outcomes of infection in intensive care units. JAMA. 2009;302(21):2323–9.
14. Favre B, Hugonnet S, Correa L, Sax H, Rohner P, Pittet D. Nosocomial bacteremia: clinical significance of a single blood culture positive for coagulase-negative staphylococci. Infect Control Hosp Epidemiol. 2005;26(8):697–702.
15. Hugonnet S, Sax H, Eggimann P, Chevrolet J-C, Pittet D. Nosocomial bloodstream infection and clinical sepsis. Emerg Infect Dis. 2004;10(1):76–81.
16. Brun-Buisson C, Doyon F, Carlet J. Bacteremia and severe sepsis in adults: a multicenter prospective survey in ICUs and wards of 24 hospitals. French Bacteremia-Sepsis Study Group. Am J Respir Crit Care Med. 1996;154(3 Pt 1):617–24.
17. Renaud B, Brun-Buisson C. Outcomes of primary and catheter-related bacteremia. A cohort and case-control study in critically ill patients. Am J Respir Crit Care Med. 2001;163(7):1584–90.
18. Richards MJ, Edwards JR, Culver DH, Gaynes RP. Nosocomial infections in coronary care units in the United States. National Nosocomial Infections Surveillance System. Am J Cardiol. 1998;82(6):789–93.
19. Banerjee SN, Emori TG, Culver DH, Gaynes RP, Jarvis WR, Horan T, et al. Secular trends in nosocomial primary bloodstream infections in the United States, 1980–1989. National Nosocomial Infections Surveillance System. Am J Med. 1991;91(3B):86S–9S.
20. Richards MJ, Edwards JR, Culver DH, Gaynes RP. Nosocomial infections in medical intensive care units in the United States. National Nosocomial Infections Surveillance System. Crit Care Med. 1999;27(5):887–92.
21. Richards MJ, Edwards JR, Culver DH, Gaynes RP. Nosocomial infections in pediatric intensive care units in the United States. National Nosocomial Infections Surveillance System. Pediatrics. 1999;103(4):e39.
22. Raymond J, Aujard Y. Nosocomial infections in pediatric patients: a European, multicenter prospective study. European Study Group. Infect Control Hosp Epidemiol. 2000;21(4):260–3.
23. Gastmeier P, Hentschel J, de Veer I, Obladen M, Rüden H. Device-associated nosocomial infection surveillance in neonatal intensive care using specified criteria for neonates. J Hosp Infect. 1998;38(1):51–60.
24. Gilio AE, Stape A, Pereira CR, Cardoso MF, Silva CV, Troster EJ. Risk factors for nosocomial infections in a critically ill pediatric population: a 25-month prospective cohort study. Infect Control Hosp Epidemiol. 2000;21(5):340–2.
25. Richards MJ, Edwards JR, Culver DH, Gaynes RP. Nosocomial infections in combined medical-surgical intensive care units in the United States. Infect Control Hosp Epidemiol. 2000;21(8):510–5.
26. Legras A, Malvy D, Quinioux AI, Villers D, Bouachour G, et al. Nosocomial infections: prospective survey of incidence in five French intensive care units. Intensive Care Med. 1998;24(10):1040–6.
27. Marschall J, Leone C, Jones M, Nihill D, Fraser VJ, Warren DK. Catheter-associated bloodstream infections in general medical patients outside the intensive care unit: a surveillance study. Infect Control Hosp Epidemiol. 2007;28(8):905–9.
28. Zingg W, Sax H, Inan C, Cartier V, Diby M, Clergue F, et al. Hospital-wide surveillance of catheter-related bloodstream infection: from the expected to the unexpected. J Hosp Infect. 2009;73(1):41–6.
29. Zingg W, Imhof A, Maggiorini M, Stocker R, Keller E, Ruef C. Impact of a prevention strategy targeting hand hygiene and catheter care on the incidence of catheter-related bloodstream infections. Crit Care Med. 2009;37(7):2167–73; quiz 2180.

30. Pittet D, Wenzel RP. Nosocomial bloodstream infections. Secular trends in rates, mortality, and contribution to total hospital deaths. Arch Intern Med. 1995;155(11):1177–84.
31. Vallés J, Rello J, Ochagavía A, Garnacho J, Alcalá MA. Community-acquired bloodstream infection in critically ill adult patients: impact of shock and inappropriate antibiotic therapy on survival. Chest. 2003;123(5):1615–24.
32. Lyytikäinen O, Lumio J, Sarkkinen H, Kolho E, Kostiala A, Ruutu P, Hospital Infection Surveillance Team. Nosocomial bloodstream infections in Finnish hospitals during 1999–2000. Clin Infect Dis. 2002;35(2):e14–9.
33. Valles J, Leon C, Alvarez-Lerma F. Nosocomial bacteremia in critically ill patients: a multicenter study evaluating epidemiology and prognosis. Spanish Collaborative Group for Infections in Intensive Care Units of Sociedad Espanola de Medicina Intensiva y Unidades Coronarias (SEMIUC). Clin Infect Dis. 1997;24(3):387–95.
34. Kollef MH, Sherman G, Ward S, Fraser VJ. Inadequate antimicrobial treatment of infections: a risk factor for hospital mortality among critically ill patients. Chest. 1999;115(2):462–74.
35. Elhanan G, Raz R, Pitlik SD, Sharir R, Konisberger H, Samra Z, et al. Bacteraemia in a community and a university hospital. J Antimicrob Chemother. 1995;36(4):681–95.
36. Eggimann P, Hugonnet S, Sax H, Touveneau S, Chevrolet JC, Pittet D. Ventilator-associated pneumonia: caveats for benchmarking. Intensive Care Med. 2003;29(11):2086–9.
37. Richards C, Emori TG, Edwards J, Fridkin S, Tolson J, Gaynes R. Characteristics of hospitals and infection control professionals participating in the National Nosocomial Infections Surveillance System 1999. Am J Infect Control. 2001;29(6):400–3.
38. Rangel-Frausto MS, Pittet D, Hwang T, Woolson RF, Wenzel RP. The dynamics of disease progression in sepsis: Markov modeling describing the natural history and the likely impact of effective antisepsis agents. Clin Infect Dis. 1998;27(1):185–90.
39. Connell TG, Rele M, Cowley D, Buttery JP, Curtis N. How reliable is a negative blood culture result? Volume of blood submitted for culture in routine practice in a children's hospital. Pediatrics. 2007;119(5):891–6.
40. Pittet D, Li N, Woolson RF, Wenzel RP. Microbiological factors influencing the outcome of nosocomial bloodstream infections: a 6 year validated, population based model. Clin Infect Dis. 1997;24(6):1068–78.
41. Siempos II, Kopterides P, Tsangaris I, Dimopoulou I, Armaganidis AE. Impact of catheter-related bloodstream infections on the mortality of critically ill patients: a meta-analysis. Crit Care Med. 2009;37(7):2283–9.
42. Pittet D, Thiévent B, Wenzel RP, Li N, Auckenthaler R, Suter PM. Bedside prediction of mortality from bacteremic sepsis. A dynamic analysis of ICU patients. Am J Respir Crit Care Med. 1996;153(2):684–93.
43. Soufir L, Timsit JF, Mahe C, Carlet J, Regnier B, Chevret S. Attributable morbidity and mortality of catheter-related septicemia in critically ill patients: a matched, risk-adjusted, cohort study. Infect Control Hosp Epidemiol. 1999;20(6):396–401.
44. Leibovici L, Drucker M, Konigsberger H, Samra Z, Harrari S, Ashkenazi S, Pitlik SD. Septic shock in bacteremic patients: risk factors, features and prognosis. Scand J Infect Dis. 1997;29(1):71–5.
45. Forgacs IC, Eykyn SJ, Bradley RD. Serious infection in the intensive therapy unit: a 15-year study of bacteraemia. Q J Med. 1986;60(232):773–9.
46. Smith RL, Meixler SM, Simberkoff MS. Excess mortality in critically ill patients with nosocomial bloodstream infections. Chest. 1991;100(1):164–7.
47. Rello J, Ricart M, Mirelis B, Quintana E, Gurgui M, Net A, Prats G. Nosocomial bacteremia in a medical-surgical intensive care unit: epidemiologic characteristics and factors influencing mortality in 111 episodes. Intensive Care Med. 1994;20(2):94–8.
48. Pittet D, Wenzel RP. Nosocomial bloodstream infection in the critically ill. JAMA. 1994;272:1819–20.
49. Digiovine B, Chenoweth C, Watts C, Higgins M. The attributable mortality and costs of primary nosocomial bloodstream infections in the intensive care unit. Am J Respir Crit Care Med. 1999;160(3):976–81.
50. Rello J, Ochagavia A, Sabanes E, Roque M, Mariscal D, Reynaga E, Valles J. Evaluation of outcome of intravenous catheter-related infections in critically ill patients. Am J Respir Crit Care Med. 2000;162(3 Pt 1):1027–30.
51. Dimick JB, Pelz RK, Consunji R, Swoboda SM, Hendrix CW, Lipsett PA. Increased resource use associated with catheter-related bloodstream infection in the surgical intensive care unit. Arch Surg. 2001;136(2):229–34.
52. Laws HJ, Kobbe G, Dilloo D, Dettenkofer M, Meisel R, Geisel R, et al. Surveillance of nosocomial infections in paediatric recipients of bone marrow or peripheral blood stem cell transplantation during neutropenia, compared with adult recipients. J Hosp Infect. 2006;62(1):80–8.
53. Mendes ET, Dulley F, Basso M, Batista MV, Coracin F, Guimarães T, et al. Healthcare-associated infection in hematopoietic stem cell transplantation patients: risk factors and impact on outcome. Int J Infect Dis. 2012;16(6):e424–8.
54. Benjamin DK Jr, Miller WC, Bayliff S, Martel L, Alexander K, Martin PL. Infections diagnosed in the first year after pediatric stem cell transplantation. Pediatr Infect Dis J. 2002;21(3):227–34.
55. Tomonari A, Takahashi S, Ooi J, Tsukada N, Konuma T, Kobayashi T, et al. Bacterial bloodstream infection in neutropenic adult patients after myeloablative cord blood transplantation: experience of a single institution in Japan. Int J Hematol. 2007;85(3):238–41.
56. Wisplinghoff H, Cornely OA, Moser S, Bethe U, Stützer H, Salzberger B, et al. Outcomes of nosocomial bloodstream infections in adult neutropenic patients: a prospective cohort and matched case-control study. Infect Control Hosp Epidemiol. 2003;24(12):905–11.
57. Goker H, Haznedaroglu IC, Chao NJ. Acute graft-vs-host disease: pathobiology and management. Exp Hematol. 2001;29(3):259–77.
58. Hoen B, Alla F, Selton-Suty C, Béguinot I, Bouvet A, Briançon S, Association pour l'Etude et la Prévention de l'Endocardite Infectieuse (AEPEI) Study Group, et al. Changing profile of infective endocarditis: results of a 1-year survey in France. JAMA. 2002;288(1):75–81.
59. Hoen B, Chirouze C, Cabell CH, Selton-Suty C, Duchêne F, Olaison L, International Collaboration on Endocarditis Study Group, et al. Emergence of endocarditis due to group D streptococci: findings derived from the merged database of the International Collaboration on Endocarditis. Eur J Clin Microbiol Infect Dis. 2005;24(1):12–6.
60. Hogevik H, Olaison L, Andersson R, Lindberg J, Alestig K. Epidemiologic aspects of infective endocarditis in an urban population. A 5-year prospective study. Medicine (Baltimore). 1995;74(6):324–39.
61. Berlin JA, Abrutyn E, Strom BL, Kinman JL, Levison ME, Korzeniowski OM, et al. Incidence of infective endocarditis in the Delaware Valley, 1988–1990. Am J Cardiol. 1995;76(12):933–6.
62. Bouza E, Menasalvas A, Muñoz P, Vasallo FJ, del Mar Moreno M, García Fernández MA. Infective endocarditis – a prospective study at the end of the twentieth century: new predisposing conditions, new etiologic agents, and still a high mortality. Medicine (Baltimore). 2001;80(5):298–307.
63. van der Meer JT, Thompson J, Valkenburg HA, Michel MF. Epidemiology of bacterial endocarditis in The Netherlands. I. Patient characteristics. Arch Intern Med. 1992;152(9):1863–8.

64. Cabell CH, Jollis JG, Peterson GE, Corey GR, Anderson DJ, Sexton DJ, et al. Changing patient characteristics and the effect on mortality in endocarditis. Arch Intern Med. 2002;162(1):90–4.
65. Thuny F, Di Salvo G, Belliard O, Avierinos JF, Pergola V, Rosenberg V, et al. Risk of embolism and death in infective endocarditis: prognostic value of echocardiography: a prospective multicenter study. Circulation. 2005;112(1):69–75.
66. Sy RW, Kritharides L. Health care exposure and age in infective endocarditis: results of a contemporary population-based profile of 1536 patients in Australia. Eur Heart J. 2010;31(15):1890–7.
67. Zakrzewski T, Keith JD. Bacterial endocarditis in infants and children. J Pediatr. 1965;67:1179–93.
68. Johnson DH, Rosenthal A, Nadas AS. A forty-year review of bacterial endocarditis in infancy and childhood. Circulation. 1975;51(4):581–8.
69. Sholler GF, Hawker RE, Celermajer JM. Infective endocarditis in childhood. Pediatr Cardiol. 1986;6(4):183–6.
70. Fukushige J, Igarashi H, Ueda K. Spectrum of infective endocarditis during infancy and childhood: 20-year review. Pediatr Cardiol. 1994;15(3):127–31.
71. Tleyjeh IM, Abdel-Latif A, Rahbi H, Scott CG, Bailey KR, Steckelberg JM, et al. A systematic review of population-based studies of infective endocarditis. Chest. 2007;132(3):1025–35.
72. Wallace SM, Walton BI, Kharbanda RK, Hardy R, Wilson AP, Swanton RH. Mortality from infective endocarditis: clinical predictors of outcome. Heart. 2002;88(1):53–60.
73. Ruttmann E, Bonatti H, Legit C, Ulmer H, Stelzmueller I, Antretter H, et al. Severe endocarditis in transplant recipients – an epidemiologic study. Transpl Int. 2005;18(6):690–6.
74. Bishara J, Robenshtok E, Weinberger M, Yeshurun M, Sagie A, Pitlik S. Infective endocarditis in renal transplant recipients. Transpl Infect Dis. 1999;1(2):138–43.
75. Paterson DL, Dominguez EA, Chang FY, Snydman DR, Singh N. Infective endocarditis in solid organ transplant recipients. Clin Infect Dis. 1998;26(3):689–94.
76. Sherman-Weber S, Axelrod P, Suh B, Rubin S, Beltramo D, Manacchio J, et al. Infective endocarditis following orthotopic heart transplantation: 10 cases and a review of the literature. Transpl Infect Dis. 2004;6(4):165–70.
77. Bayer AS, Nelson RJ, Slama TG. Current concepts in prevention of prosthetic valve endocarditis. Chest. 1990;97(5):1203–7.
78. Steckelberg JM, Wilson WR. Risk factors for infective endocarditis. Infect Dis Clin N Am. 1993;7(1):9–19.
79. Wilson LE, Thomas DL, Astemborski J, Freedman TL, Vlahov D. Prospective study of infective endocarditis among injection drug users. J Infect Dis. 2002;185(12):1761–6.
80. Mathew J, Addai T, Anand A, Morrobel A, Maheshwari P, Freels S. Clinical features, site of involvement, bacteriologic findings, and outcome of infective endocarditis in intravenous drug users. Arch Intern Med. 1995;155(15):1641–8.
81. Gersony WM, Hayes CJ. Bacterial endocarditis in patients with pulmonary stenosis, aortic stenosis, or ventricular septal defect. Circulation. 1977;56(1 Suppl):I84–7.
82. Raad I, Costerton W, Sabharwal U, Sacilowski M, Anaissie E, Bodey GP. Ultrastructural analysis of indwelling vascular catheters: a quantitative relationship between luminal colonization and duration of placement. J Infect Dis. 1993;168(2):400–7.
83. Banin E, Brady KM, Greenberg EP. Chelator-induced dispersal and killing of Pseudomonas aeruginosa cells in a biofilm. Appl Environ Microbiol. 2006;72(3):2064–9.
84. Falcieri E, Vaudaux P, Huggler E, Lew D, Waldvogel F. Role of bacterial exopolymers and host factors on adherence and phagocytosis of Staphylococcus aureus in foreign body infection. J Infect Dis. 1987;155(3):524–31.
85. Hoffman LR, D'Argenio DA, MacCoss MJ, Zhang Z, Jones RA, Miller SI. Aminoglycoside antibiotics induce bacterial biofilm formation. Nature. 2005;436(7054):1171–5.
86. Mehall JR, Kite CA, Saltzman DA, Wallett T, Jackson RJ, Smith SD. Prospective study of the incidence and complications of bacterial contamination of enteral feeding in neonates. J Pediatr Surg. 2002;37(8):1177–82.
87. Mehall JR, Saltzman DA, Jackson RJ, Smith SD. Fibrin sheath enhances central venous catheter infection. Crit Care Med. 2002;30(4):908–12.
88. Qin Z, Ou Y, Yang L, Zhu Y, Tolker-Nielsen T, Molin S, Qu D. Role of autolysin-mediated DNA release in biofilm formation of Staphylococcus epidermidis. Microbiology. 2007;153(Pt 7):2083–92.
89. Rhodes ER, Shoemaker CJ, Menke SM, Edelmann RE, Actis LA. Evaluation of different iron sources and their influence in biofilm formation by the dental pathogen Actinobacillus actinomycetemcomitans. J Med Microbiol. 2007;56(Pt 1):119–28.
90. Sheth NK, Franson TR, Sohnle PG. Influence of bacterial adherence to intravascular catheters on in-vitro antibiotic susceptibility. Lancet. 1985;2(8467):1266–8.
91. Vaudaux P, Pittet D, Haeberli A, Lerch PG, Morgenthaler JJ, Proctor RA, et al. Fibronectin is more active than fibrin or fibrinogen in promoting Staphylococcus aureus adherence to inserted intravascular catheters. J Infect Dis. 1993;167(3):633–41.
92. Lin MH, Shu J-C, Huang H-Y, Chengg Y-C, Fitgerald JR, editors. Involvement of iron in biofilm formation by Staphylococcus aureus. PLoS One. 2012;7(3):e34388.
93. Moreillon P, Que YA, Bayer AS. Pathogenesis of streptococcal and staphylococcal endocarditis. Infect Dis Clin N Am. 2002;16(2):297–318.
94. Greene C, McDevitt D, Francois P, Vaudaux PE, Lew DP, Foster TJ. Adhesion properties of mutants of Staphylococcus aureus defective in fibronectin-binding proteins and studies on the expression of fnb genes. Mol Microbiol. 1995;17(6):1143–52.
95. Darouiche RO. Device-associated infections: a macroproblem that starts with microadherence. Clin Infect Dis. 2001;33(9):1567–72.
96. Darouiche RO, Landon GC, Patti JM, Nguyen LL, Fernau RC, McDevitt D, et al. Role of Staphylococcus aureus surface adhesins in orthopaedic device infections: are results model-dependent? J Med Microbiol. 1997;46(1):75–9.
97. Schachter B. Slimy business – the biotechnology of biofilms. Nat Biotechnol. 2003;21(4):361–5.
98. Timsit JF, Farkas JC, Boyer JM, Martin JB, Misset B, Renaud B, Carlet J. Central vein catheter-related thrombosis in intensive care patients: incidence, risks factors, and relationship with catheter-related sepsis. Chest. 1998;114(1):207–13.
99. Akl EA, Vasireddi SR, Gunukula S, Yosuico VE, Barba M, Sperati F, et al. Anticoagulation for patients with cancer and central venous catheters. Cochrane Database Syst Rev. 2011;(2):CD006468.
100. Abdelkefi A, Achour W, Ben Othman T, Ladeb S, Torjman L, Lakhal A, et al. Use of heparin-coated central venous lines to prevent catheter-related bloodstream infection. J Support Oncol. 2007;5(6):273–8.
101. Abdelkefi A, Ben Othman T, Kammoun L, Chelli M, Romdhane NB, Kriaa A, et al. Prevention of central venous line-related thrombosis by continuous infusion of low-dose unfractionated heparin, in patients with haemato-oncological disease. A randomized controlled trial. Thromb Haemost. 2004;92(3):654–61.
102. Richet H, Hubert B, Nitemberg G, Andremont A, Buu-Hoi A, Ourbak P, et al. Prospective multicenter study of vascular catheter-related complications and risk factors for positive central-catheter cultures in intensive care unit patients. J Clin Microbiol. 1990;28(11):2520–5.
103. Merrer J, De Jonghe B, Golliot F, Lefrant JY, Raffy B, Barre E, French Catheter Study Group in Intensive Care, et al.

Complications of femoral and subclavian venous catheterization in critically ill patients: a randomized controlled trial. JAMA. 2001;286(6):700–7.
104. Goetz AM, Wagener MM, Miller JM, Muder RR. Risk of infection due to central venous catheters: effect of site of placement and catheter type. Infect Control Hosp Epidemiol. 1998;19(11):842–5.
105. Chen HS, Wang FD, Lin M, Lin YC, Huang LJ, Liu CY. Risk factors for central venous catheter-related infections in general surgery. J Microbiol Immunol Infect. 2006;39(3):231–6.
106. Opilla MT, Kirby DF, Edmond MB. Use of ethanol lock therapy to reduce the incidence of catheter-related bloodstream infections in home parenteral nutrition patients. JPEN J Parenter Enteral Nutr. 2007;31(4):302–5.
107. Zingg W, Posfay-Barbe KM, Pfister RE, Touveneau S, Pittet D. Individualized catheter surveillance among neonates: a prospective, 8-year, single-center experience. Infect Control Hosp Epidemiol. 2011;32(1):42–9.
108. Cobb DK, High KP, Sawyer RG, Sable CA, Adams RB, Lindley DA, et al. A controlled trial of scheduled replacement of central venous and pulmonary-artery catheters. N Engl J Med. 1992;327(15):1062–8.
109. Cook D, Randolph A, Kernerman P, Cupido C, King D, Soukup C, Brun-Buisson C. Central venous catheter replacement strategies: a systematic review of the literature. Crit Care Med. 1997;25(8):1417–24.
110. Zurcher M, Tramer MR, Walder B. Colonization and bloodstream infection with single- versus multi-.lumen central venous catheters: a quantitative systematic review. Anesth Analg. 2004;99(1):177–82.
111. Adler A, Yaniv I, Solter E, Freud E, Samra Z, Stein J, et al. Catheter-associated bloodstream infections in pediatric hematology-oncology patients: factors associated with catheter removal and recurrence. J Pediatr Hematol Oncol. 2006;28(1):23–8.
112. Adler A, Yaniv I, Steinberg R, Solter E, Samra Z, Stein J, Levy I. Infectious complications of implantable ports and Hickman catheters in paediatric haematology-oncology patients. J Hosp Infect. 2006;62(3):358–65.
113. Bashore TM, Cabell C, Fowler V Jr. Update on infective endocarditis. Curr Probl Cardiol. 2006;31(4):274–352.
114. Robard S. Blood velocity and endocarditis. Circulation. 1963;27:24.
115. Johnson CM. Adherence events in the pathogenesis of infective endocarditis. Infect Dis Clin N Am. 1993;7(1):21–36.
116. Gouriet F, Bothelo-Nevers E, Coulibaly B, Raoult D, Casalta JP. Evaluation of sedimentation rate, rheumatoid factor, C reactive protein, and tumor necrosis factor for the diagnosis of infective endocarditis. Clin Vaccine Immunol. 2006;13(2):301.
117. Luzzaro F, Viganò EF, Fossati D, Grossi A, Sala A, Sturla C, Saudelli M, et al. Prevalence and drug susceptibility of pathogens causing bloodstream infections in northern Italy: a two-year study in 16 hospitals. Eur J Clin Microbiol Infect Dis. 2002;21(12):849–55.
118. Garden OJ, Sim AJ. A comparison of tunnelled and nontunnelled subclavian vein catheters: a prospective study of complications during parenteral feeding. Clin Nutr. 1983;2(1):51–4.
119. Rosenthal VD, Maki DG, Jamulitrat S, Medeiros EA, Todi SK, Gomez DY, INICC Members, et al. International Nosocomial Infection Control Consortium (INICC) report, data summary for 2003–2008, issued June 2009. Am J Infect Control. 2010;38(2):95–104.e2.
120. Macias AE, Huertas M, de Leon SP, Munoz JM, Chavez AR, Sifuentes-Osornio J, et al. Contamination of intravenous fluids: a continuing cause of hospital bacteremia. Am J Infect Control. 2010;38(3):217–21.
121. Girão E, Levin AS, Basso M, Gobara S, Gomes LB, Medeiros EA, et al. Trends and outcome of 1121 nosocomial bloodstream infections in intensive care units in a Brazilian hospital, 1999–2003. Int J Infect Dis. 2008;12(6):e145–6.
122. Moreno CA, Rosenthal VD, Olarte N, Gomez WV, Sussmann O, Agudelo JG, et al. Device-associated infection rate and mortality in intensive care units of 9 Colombian hospitals: findings of the International Nosocomial Infection Control Consortium. Infect Control Hosp Epidemiol. 2006;27(4):349–56.
123. Agarwal R, Gupta D, Ray P, Aggarwal AN, Jindal SK. Epidemiology, risk factors and outcome of nosocomial infections in a Respiratory Intensive Care Unit in North India. J Infect. 2006;53(2):98–105.
124. de Brito CS, de Brito DV, Abdallah VO, Gontijo Filho PP. Occurrence of bloodstream infection with different types of central vascular catheter in critically neonates. J Infect. 2010;60(2):128–32.
125. Pawar M, Mehta Y, Kapoor P, Sharma J, Gupta A, Trehan N. Central venous catheter-related blood stream infections: incidence, risk factors, outcome, and associated pathogens. J Cardiothorac Vasc Anesth. 2004;18(3):304–8.
126. Su BH, Hsieh HY, Chiu HY, Lin HC, Lin HC. Nosocomial infection in a neonatal intensive care unit: a prospective study in Taiwan. Am J Infect Control. 2007;35(3):190–5.
127. Almuneef MA, Memish ZA, Balkhy HH, Hijazi O, Cunningham G, Francis C. Rate, risk factors and outcomes of catheter-related bloodstream infection in a paediatric intensive care unit in Saudi Arabia. J Hosp Infect. 2006;62(2):207–13.
128. Hugonnet S, Harbarth S, Ferrière K, Ricou B, Suter P, Pittet D. Bacteremic sepsis in intensive care: temporal trends in incidence, organ dysfunction, and prognosis. Crit Care Med. 2003;31(2):390–4.
129. Wisplinghoff H, Bischoff T, Tallent SM, Seifert H, Wenzel RP, Edmond MB. Nosocomial bloodstream infections in US hospitals: analysis of 24,179 cases from a prospective nationwide surveillance study. Clin Infect Dis. 2004;39(3):309–17.
130. Macias AE, de Leon SP, Huertas M, Maravilla E, Romero C, Montoya TG, et al. Endemic infusate contamination and related bacteremia. Am J Infect Control. 2008;36(1):48–53.
131. Bizzarro MJ, Raskind C, Baltimore RS, Gallagher PG. Seventy-five years of neonatal sepsis at Yale: 1928–2003. J Hosp Infect. 2006;62(2):207–13.
132. Bassetti M, Trecarichi EM, Righi E, Sanguinetti M, Bisio F, Posteraro B, et al. Incidence, risk factors, and predictors of outcome of candidemia. Survey in 2 Italian university hospitals. Diagn Microbiol Infect Dis. 2007;58(3):325–31.
133. Boo TW, O'reilly B, O'leary J, Cryan B. Candidaemia in an Irish tertiary referral hospital: epidemiology and prognostic factors. Mycoses. 2005;48(4):251–9.
134. Cheng YR, Lin LC, Young TG, Liu CE, Chen CH, Tsay RW. Risk factors for candidemia-related mortality at a medical center in central Taiwan. J Microbiol Immunol Infect. 2006;39(2):155–61.
135. Dimopoulos G, Ntziora F, Rachiotis G, Armaganidis A, Falagas ME. Candida albicans versus non-albicans intensive care unit-acquired bloodstream infections: differences in risk factors and outcome. Anesth Analg. 2008;106(2):523–9, table of contents.
136. Klevay MJ, Horn DL, Neofytos D, Pfaller MA, Diekema DJ, PATH Alliance. Initial treatment and outcome of Candida glabrata versus Candida albicans bloodstream infection. Diagn Microbiol Infect Dis. 2009;64(2):152–7.
137. Labelle AJ, Micek ST, Roubinian N, Kollef MH. Treatment-related risk factors for hospital mortality in Candida bloodstream infections. Crit Care Med. 2008;36(11):2967–72.
138. Odds FC, Hanson MF, Davidson AD, Jacobsen MD, Wright P, Whyte JA, et al. One year prospective survey of Candida bloodstream infections in Scotland. J Med Microbiol. 2007;56(Pt 8):1066–75.

139. Yapar N, Uysal U, Yucesoy M, Cakir N, Yuce A. Nosocomial bloodstream infections associated with Candida species in a Turkish University Hospital. Mycoses. 2006;49(2):134–8.
140. Fridkin SK, Kaufman D, Edwards JR, Shetty S, Horan T. Changing incidence of Candida bloodstream infections among NICU patients in the United States: 1995–2004. Pediatrics. 2006;117(5):1680–7.
141. Labbe AC, Pepin J, Patino C, Castonguay S, Restien C, Laverdiere M. A single-centre 10-year experience with Candida bloodstream infections. Can J Infect Dis Med Microbiol. 2009;20(2):45–50.
142. Trick WE, Fridkin SK, Edwards JR, Hajjeh RA, Gaynes RP, National Nosocomial Infections Surveillance System Hospitals. Secular trend of hospital-acquired candidemia among intensive care unit patients in the United States during 1989–1999. Clin Infect Dis. 2002;35(5):627–30.
143. Lee I, Zaoutis TE, Fishman NO, Morales KH, Nachamkin I, Lautenbach E. Risk factors for fluconazole resistance in patients with Candida glabrata bloodstream infection: potential impact of control group selection on characterizing the association between previous fluconazole use and fluconazole resistance. Am J Infect Control. 2010;38(6):456–60.
144. Garey KW, Rege M, Pai MP, Mingo DE, Suda KJ, Turpin RS, Bearden DT. Time to initiation of fluconazole therapy impacts mortality in patients with candidemia: a multi-institutional study. Clin Infect Dis. 2006;43(1):25–31.
145. Horasan ES, Ersoz G, Tombak A, Tiftik N, Kaya A. Bloodstream infections and mortality-related factors in febrile neutropenic cancer patients. Med Sci Monit. 2011;17(5):CR304–9.
146. Lyytikäinen O, Ruotsalainen E, Järvinen A, Valtonen V, Ruutu P. Trends and outcome of nosocomial and community-acquired bloodstream infections due to Staphylococcus aureus in Finland, 1995–2001. Eur J Clin Microbiol Infect Dis. 2005;24(6):399–404.
147. Turnidge JD, Kotsanas D, Munckhof W, Roberts S, Bennett CM, Nimmo GR, Australia New Zealand Cooperative on Outcomes in Staphylococcal Sepsis, et al. Staphylococcus aureus bacteraemia: a major cause of mortality in Australia and New Zealand. Med J Aust. 2009;191(7):368–73.
148. Ekkelenkamp MB, van der Bruggen T, van de Vijver DA, Wolfs TF, Bonten MJ. Bacteremic complications of intravascular catheters colonized with Staphylococcus aureus. Clin Infect Dis. 2008;46(1):114–8.
149. Park KH, Kim SH, Song EH, Jang EY, Lee EJ, Chong YP, et al. Development of bacteraemia or fungaemia after removal of colonized central venous catheters in patients with negative concomitant blood cultures. Clin Microbiol Infect. 2010;16(6):742–6.
150. Ruhe JJ, Menon A. Clinical significance of isolated Staphylococcus aureus central venous catheter tip cultures. Clin Microbiol Infect. 2006;12(9):933–6.
151. Palmer SM, Alexander BD, Sanders LL, Edwards LJ, Reller LB, Davis RD, Tapson VF. Significance of blood stream infection after lung transplantation: analysis in 176 consecutive patients. Transplantation. 2000;69(11):2360–6.
152. Dettenkofer M, Ebner W, Bertz H, Babikir R, Finke J, Frank U, et al. Surveillance of nosocomial infections in adult recipients of allogeneic and autologous bone marrow and peripheral blood stem-cell transplantation. Bone Marrow Transplant. 2003;31(9):795–801.
153. Danziger-Isakov LA, Sweet S, Delamorena M, Huddleston CB, Mendeloff E, Debaun MR. Epidemiology of bloodstream infections in the first year after pediatric lung transplantation. Pediatr Infect Dis J. 2005;24(4):324–30.
154. Dettenkofer M, Wenzler-Röttele S, Babikir R, Bertz H, Ebner W, Meyer E, Hospital Infection Surveillance System for Patients with Hematologic/Oncologic Malignancies Study Group, et al. Surveillance of nosocomial sepsis and pneumonia in patients with a bone marrow or peripheral blood stem cell transplant: a multicenter project. Clin Infect Dis. 2005;40(7):926–31.
155. Ortega M, Rovira M, Almela M, Marco F, de la Bellacasa JP, Martínez JA, et al. Bacterial and fungal bloodstream isolates from 796 hematopoietic stem cell transplant recipients between 1991 and 2000. Ann Hematol. 2005;84(1):40–6.
156. Rodríguez C, Muñoz P, Rodríguez-Créixems M, Yañez JF, Palomo J, Bouza E. Bloodstream infections among heart transplant recipients. Transplantation. 2006;81(3):384–91.
157. Shi SH, Kong HS, Xu J, Zhang WJ, Jia CK, Wang WL, et al. Multidrug resistant gram-negative bacilli as predominant bacteremic pathogens in liver transplant recipients. Transpl Infect Dis. 2009;11(5):405–12.
158. Iida T, Kaido T, Yagi S, Yoshizawa A, Hata K, Mizumoto M, et al. Posttransplant bacteremia in adult living donor liver transplant recipients. Liver Transpl. 2010;16(12):1379–85.
159. Mikulska M, Del Bono V, Prinapori R, Boni L, Raiola AM, Gualandi F, et al. Risk factors for enterococcal bacteremia in allogeneic hematopoietic stem cell transplant recipients. Transpl Infect Dis. 2010;12(6):505–12.
160. Hsu RB, Tsai MK, Lee PH, Le CM, Chen MF, Wang SS, et al. Bloodstream infection in heart transplant recipients: 12-year experience at a university hospital in Taiwan. Eur J Cardiothorac Surg. 2011;40(6):1362–7.
161. Karvellas CJ, McPhail M, Pink F, Asthana S, Muiesan P, Heaton N, et al. Bloodstream infection after elective liver transplantation is associated with increased mortality in patients with cirrhosis. J Crit Care. 2011;26(5):468–74.
162. Lee SO, Kang SH, Abdel-Massih RC, Brown RA, Razonable RR. Spectrum of early-onset and late-onset bacteremias after liver transplantation: implications for management. Liver Transpl. 2011;17(6):733–41.
163. Busca A, Cavecchia I, Locatelli F, D'Ardia S, De Rosa FG, Marmont F, et al. Blood stream infections after allogeneic stem cell transplantation: a single-center experience with the use of levofloxacin prophylaxis. Transpl Infect Dis. 2012;14(1):40–8.
164. van Hal SJ, Marriott DJ, Chen SC, Nguyen Q, Sorrell TC, Ellis DH, Slavin MA, Australian Candidaemia Study. Candidemia following solid organ transplantation in the era of antifungal prophylaxis: the Australian experience. Transpl Infect Dis. 2009;11(2):122–7.
165. Nagy GS, Rubin RH. Disseminated Mycobacterium avium-intracellulare in a kidney transplant recipient. Transpl Infect Dis. 2001;3(4):220–30.
166. Rapose A, Lick SD, Ismail N. Listeria grayi bacteremia in a heart transplant recipient. Transpl Infect Dis. 2008;10(6):434–6.
167. Cerutti E, Stratta C, Romagnoli R, Serra R, Lepore M, Fop F, et al. Bacterial- and fungal-positive cultures in organ donors: clinical impact in liver transplantation. Liver Transpl. 2006;12(8):1253–9.
168. Kumar D, Cattral MS, Robicsek A, Gaudreau C, Humar A. Outbreak of pseudomonas aeruginosa by multiple organ transplantation from a common donor. Transplantation. 2003;75(7):1053–5.
169. Goldberg E, Bishara J, Lev S, Singer P, Cohen J. Organ transplantation from a donor colonized with a multidrug-resistant organism: a case report. Transpl Infect Dis. 2012;14(3):296–9.
170. Ariza-Heredia EJ, Patel R, Blumberg EA, Walker RC, Lewis R, Evans J, et al. Outcomes of transplantation using organs from a donor infected with Klebsiella pneumoniae carbapenemase (KPC)-producing K. pneumoniae. Transpl Infect Dis. 2012;14(3):229–36.
171. Martins N, Martins IS, de Freitas WV, de Matos JA, Magalhães AC, Girão VB, et al. Severe infection in a lung transplant recipient caused by donor-transmitted carbapenem-resistant Acinetobacter baumannii. Transpl Infect Dis. 2012;14(3):316–20.
172. Collin BA, Leather HL, Wingard JR, Ramphal R. Evolution, incidence, and susceptibility of bacterial bloodstream isolates

from 519 bone marrow transplant patients. Clin Infect Dis. 2001;33(7):947–53.
173. Almyroudis NG, Fuller A, Jakubowski A, Sepkowitz K, Jaffe D, Small TN, et al. Pre- and post-engraftment bloodstream infection rates and associated mortality in allogeneic hematopoietic stem cell transplant recipients. Transpl Infect Dis. 2005;7(1): 11–7.
174. Lark RL, McNeil SA, VanderHyde K, Noorani Z, Uberti J, Chenoweth C. Risk factors for anaerobic bloodstream infections in bone marrow transplant recipients. Clin Infect Dis. 2001;33(3):338–43.
175. Wisplinghoff H, Seifert H, Wenzel RP, Edmond MB. Current trends in the epidemiology of nosocomial bloodstream infections in patients with hematological malignancies and solid neoplasms in hospitals in the United States. Clin Infect Dis. 2003;36(9):1103–10.
176. Zinkernagel AS, Speck RF, Ruef C, Zingg W, Berger-Bachi B, Springer B. Rapidly destructive Staphylococcus epidermidis endocarditis. Infection. 2005;33(3):148–50.
177. Miro JM, Anguera I, Cabell CH, Chen AY, Stafford JA, Corey GR, International Collaboration on Endocarditis Merged Database Study Group, et al. Staphylococcus aureus native valve infective endocarditis: report of 566 episodes from the International Collaboration on Endocarditis Merged Database. Clin Infect Dis. 2005;41(4):507–14.
178. Fowler VG Jr, Sanders LL, Kong LK, McClelland RS, Gottlieb GS, Li J, et al. Infective endocarditis due to Staphylococcus aureus: 59 prospectively identified cases with follow-up. Clin Infect Dis. 1999;28(1):106–14.
179. Morpeth S, Murdoch D, Cabell CH, Karchmer AW, Pappas P, Levine D, International Collaboration on Endocarditis Prospective Cohort Study (ICE-PCS) Investigators, et al. Non-HACEK gram-negative bacillus endocarditis. Ann Intern Med. 2007;147(12):829–35.
180. Avery RK, Barnes DS, Teran JC, Wiedemann HP, Hall G, Wacker T, et al. Listeria monocytogenes tricuspid valve endocarditis with septic pulmonary emboli in a liver transplant recipient. Transpl Infect Dis. 1999;1(4):284–7.
181. Nasim A, Baqi S, Akhtar SF. Pseudomonas aeruginosa endocarditis in renal transplant recipients. Transpl Infect Dis. 2012;14(2):180–3.
182. Archuleta S, Murphy B, Keller MJ. Successful treatment of vancomycin-resistant Enterococcus faecium endocarditis with linezolid in a renal transplant recipient with human immunodeficiency virus infection. Transpl Infect Dis. 2004;6(3):117–9.
183. Urbina BY, Gohh R, Fischer SA. Oerskovia xanthineolytica endocarditis in a renal transplant patient: case report and review of the literature. Transpl Infect Dis. 2003;5(4):195–8.
184. Harlan NP, Kempker RR, Parekh SM, Burd EM, Kuhar DT. Weissella confusa bacteremia in a liver transplant patient with hepatic artery thrombosis. Transpl Infect Dis. 2011;13(3): 290–3.
185. Philippe B, Grenet D, Honderlick P, Longchampt E, Dupont B, Picard C, Stern M. Severe Aspergillus endocarditis in a lung transplant recipient with a five-year survival. Transpl Infect Dis. 2010;12(3):273–6.
186. Lázaro M, Ramos A, Ussetti P, Asensio A, Laporta R, Muñez E, et al. Aspergillus endocarditis in lung transplant recipients: case report and literature review. Transpl Infect Dis. 2011;13(2):186–91.
187. Fournier PE, Thuny F, Richet H, Lepidi H, Casalta JP, Arzouni JP, et al. Comprehensive diagnostic strategy for blood culture-negative endocarditis: a prospective study of 819 new cases. Clin Infect Dis. 2010;51(2):131–40.
188. Lederman MM. Infections of the heart and vessels. In: Andreoli TE, et al., editors. Essentials of medicine. Philadelphia: W.B. Saunders; 2001.
189. Gonsalves WI, Cornish N, Moore M, Chen A, Varman M. Effects of volume and site of blood draw on blood culture results. J Clin Microbiol. 2009;47(11):3482–5.
190. Bouza E, Alvarado N, Alcalá L, Sánchez-Conde M, Pérez MJ, Muñoz P, et al. A prospective, randomized, and comparative study of 3 different methods for the diagnosis of intravascular catheter colonization. Clin Infect Dis. 2005;40(8):1096–100.
191. Maki DG, Weise CE, Sarafin HW. A semiquantitative culture method for identifying intravenous-catheter-related infection. N Engl J Med. 1977;296(23):1305–9.
192. Raad I, Hanna HA, Alakech B, Chatzinikolaou I, Johnson MM, Tarrand J. Differential time to positivity: a useful method for diagnosing catheter-related bloodstream infections. Ann Intern Med. 2004;140(1):18–25.
193. Guembe M, Rodríguez-Créixems M, Sánchez-Carrillo C, Pérez-Parra A, Martín-Rabadán P, Bouza E. How many lumens should be cultured in the conservative diagnosis of catheter-related https://www.ncbi.nlm.nih.gov/pubmed/15879906bloodstream infections? Clin Infect Dis. 2010;50(12):1575–9.
194. Siddiqui BK, Tariq M, Jadoon A, Alam M, Murtaza G, Abid B, et al. Impact of prior antibiotic use in culture-negative endocarditis: review of 86 cases from southern Pakistan. Int J Infect Dis. 2009;13(5):606–12.
195. Vandecasteele SJ, Van Eldere J, Merckx R, Peetermans WE. The effect of systemic antibiotics on the microbiological diagnosis of experimental foreign body infections caused by Staphylococcus epidermidis. Diagn Microbiol Infect Dis. 2004;48(2):89–95.
196. Kennedy MJ, Jackson MA, Kearns GL. Delayed diagnosis of penicillin-resistant Streptococcus mitis endocarditis following single-dose amoxicillin prophylaxis in a child. Clin Pediatr (Phila). 2004;43(8):773–6.
197. Pazin GJ, Saul S, Thompson ME. Blood culture positivity: suppression by outpatient antibiotic therapy in patients with bacterial endocarditis. Arch Intern Med. 1982;142(2):263–8.
198. Afshari A, Schrenzel J, Ieven M, Harbarth S. Bench-to-bedside review: rapid molecular diagnostics for bloodstream infection – a new frontier? Crit Care. 2012;16(3):222.
199. Yanagihara K, Kitagawa Y, Tomonaga M, Tsukasaki K, Kohno S, Seki M, et al. Evaluation of pathogen detection from clinical samples by real-time polymerase chain reaction using a sepsis pathogen DNA detection kit. Crit Care. 2010;14(4):R159.
200. Tunkel AR, Kaye D. Endocarditis with negative blood cultures. N Engl J Med. 1992;326(18):1215–7.
201. Nakatani S, Mitsutake K, Hozumi T, Yoshikawa J, Akiyama M, Yoshida K, Committee on Guideline for Prevention and Management of Infective Endocarditis, Japanese Circulation Society, et al. Current characteristics of infective endocarditis in Japan: an analysis of 848 cases in 2000 and 2001. Circ J. 2003;67(11):901–5.
202. Lamas CC, Eykyn SJ. Blood culture negative endocarditis: analysis of 63 cases presenting over 25 years. Heart. 2003;89(3):258–62.
203. Houpikian P, Raoult D. Blood culture-negative endocarditis in a reference center: etiologic diagnosis of 348 cases. Medicine (Baltimore). 2005;84(3):162–73.
204. Raoult D, Casalta JP, Richet H, Khan M, Bernit E, Rovery C, et al. Contribution of systematic serological testing in diagnosis of infective endocarditis. J Clin Microbiol. 2005;43(10):5238–42.
205. Marín M, Muñoz P, Sánchez M, del Rosal M, Alcalá L, Rodríguez-Créixems M, Bouza E, Group for the Management of Infective Endocarditis of the Gregorio Marañón Hospital. Molecular diagnosis of infective endocarditis by real-time broad-range polymerase chain reaction (PCR) and sequencing directly from heart valve tissue. Medicine (Baltimore). 2007;86(4):195–202.
206. Miyazato A, Ohkusu K, Tabata M, Uwabe K, Kawamura T, Tachi Y, et al. Comparative molecular and microbiological diagnosis of 19 infective endocarditis cases in which causative microbes were

identified by PCR-based DNA sequencing from the excised heart valves. J Infect Chemother. 2012;18(3):318–23.
207. Muñoz P, Bouza E, Marín M, Alcalá L, Rodríguez Créixems M, Group for the Management of Infective Endocarditis of the Gregorio Marañón Hospital, et al. Heart valves should not be routinely cultured. J Clin Microbiol. 2008;46(9):2897–901.
208. Millar B, Moore J, Mallon P, Xu J, Crowe M, Mcclurg R, et al. Molecular diagnosis of infective endocarditis – a new Duke's criterion. Scand J Infect Dis. 2001;33(9):673–80.
209. Bosshard PP, Kronenberg A, Zbinden R, Ruef C, Böttger EC, Altwegg M. Etiologic diagnosis of infective endocarditis by broad-range polymerase chain reaction: a 3-year experience. Clin Infect Dis. 2003;37(2):167–72.
210. Thuny F, Grisoli D, Collart F, Habib G, Raoult D. Management of infective endocarditis: challenges and perspectives. Lancet. 2012;379(9819):965–75.
211. Breitkopf C, Hammel D, Scheld HH, Peters G, Becker K. Impact of a molecular approach to improve the microbiological diagnosis of infective heart valve endocarditis. Circulation. 2005;111(11):1415–21.
212. Rovery C, Greub G, Lepidi H, Casalta JP, Habib G, Collart F, Raoult D. PCR detection of bacteria on cardiac valves of patients with treated bacterial endocarditis. J Clin Microbiol. 2005;43(1):163–7.
213. Branger S1, Casalta JP, Habib G, Collard F, Raoult D. Streptococcus pneumoniae endocarditis: persistence of DNA on heart valve material 7 years after infectious episode. J Clin Microbiol. 2003;41(9):4435–7.
214. Fenollar F, Raoult D. Molecular diagnosis of bloodstream infections caused by non-cultivable bacteria. Int J Antimicrob Agents. 2007;30(Suppl 1):S7–15.
215. Thuny F, Habib G. When should we operate on patients with acute infective endocarditis? Heart. 2010;96(11):892–7.
216. Bojalil R, Mazón-González B, Carrillo-Córdova JR, Springall R, Amezcua-Guerra LM. Frequency and clinical significance of a variety of autoantibodies in patients with definite infective endocarditis. J Clin Rheumatol. 2012;18(2):67–70.
217. Harbarth S, Garbino J, Pugin J, Romand JA, Lew D, Pittet D. Inappropriate initial antimicrobial therapy and its effect on survival in a clinical trial of immunomodulating therapy for severe sepsis. Am J Med. 2003;115(7):529–35.
218. Ibrahim EH, Sherman G, Ward S, Fraser VJ, Kollef MH. The influence of inadequate antimicrobial treatment of bloodstream infections on patient outcomes in the ICU setting. Chest. 2000;118(1):146–55.
219. Harbarth S, Ferrière K, Hugonnet S, Ricou B, Suter P, Pittet D. Epidemiology and prognostic determinants of bloodstream infections in surgical intensive care. Arch Surg. 2002;137(12):1353–9; discussion 1359.
220. Morrell M, Fraser VJ, Kollef MH. Delaying the empiric treatment of candida bloodstream infection until positive blood culture results are obtained: a potential risk factor for hospital mortality. Antimicrob Agents Chemother. 2005;49(9):3640–5.
221. Parkins MD, Sabuda DM, Elsayed S, Laupland KB. Adequacy of empirical antifungal therapy and effect on outcome among patients with invasive Candida species infections. J Antimicrob Chemother. 2007;60(3):613–8.
222. Bouadma L, Luyt CE, Tubach F, Cracco C, Alvarez A, Schwebel C, et al. Use of procalcitonin to reduce patients' exposure to antibiotics in intensive care units (PRORATA trial): a multicentre randomised controlled trial. Lancet. 2010;375(9713):463–74.
223. Harbarth S, Albrich WC, Muller B. When once is not enough – further evidence of procalcitonin-guided antibiotic stewardship. Crit Care. 2009;13(4):165.
224. Nobre V, Harbarth S, Graf JD, Rohner P, Pugin J. Use of procalcitonin to shorten antibiotic treatment duration in septic patients: a randomized trial. Am J Respir Crit Care Med. 2008;177(5):498–505.
225. Fernandez-Hidalgo N, Almirante B, Calleja R, Ruiz I, Planes AM, Rodriguez D, et al. Antibiotic-lock therapy for long-term intravascular catheter-related bacteraemia: results of an open, non-comparative study. J Antimicrob Chemother. 2006;57(6):1172–80.
226. Fortún J, Grill F, Martín-Dávila P, Blázquez J, Tato M, Sánchez-Corral J, et al. Treatment of long-term intravascular catheter-related bacteraemia with antibiotic-lock therapy. J Antimicrob Chemother. 2006;58(4):816–21.
227. Mermel LA, Allon M, Bouza E, Craven DE, Flynn P, O'Grady NP, et al. Clinical practice guidelines for the diagnosis and management of intravascular catheter-related infection: 2009 update by the Infectious Diseases Society of America. Clin Infect Dis. 2009;49(1):1–45.
228. Maki DG, et al. Hospital infections. 4th ed. Philadelphia: Lippincott-Raven; 1998.
229. Rosen AB, Fowler VG Jr, Corey GR, Downs SM, Biddle AK, Li J, Jollis JG. Cost-effectiveness of transesophageal echocardiography to determine the duration of therapy for intravascular catheter-associated Staphylococcus aureus bacteremia. Ann Intern Med. 1999;130(10):810–20.
230. Baddour LM, Wilson WR, Bayer AS, Fowler VG Jr, Bolger AF, Levison ME, Committee on Rheumatic Fever, Endocarditis, and Kawasaki Disease, Council on Cardiovascular Disease in the Young, Councils on Clinical Cardiology, Stroke, and Cardiovascular Surgery and Anesthesia, American Heart Association, Infectious Diseases Society of America, et al. Infective endocarditis: diagnosis, antimicrobial therapy, and management of complications: a statement for healthcare professionals from the Committee on Rheumatic Fever, Endocarditis, and Kawasaki Disease, Council on Cardiovascular Disease in the Young, and the Councils on Clinical Cardiology, Stroke, and Cardiovascular Surgery and Anesthesia, American Heart Association: endorsed by the Infectious Diseases Society of America. Circulation. 2005;111(23):e394–434.
231. Habib G, Hoen B, Tornos P, Thuny F, Prendergast B, Vilacosta I, ESC Committee for Practice Guidelines, et al. Guidelines on the prevention, diagnosis, and treatment of infective endocarditis (new version 2009): the Task Force on the Prevention, Diagnosis, and Treatment of Infective Endocarditis of the European Society of Cardiology (ESC). Endorsed by the European Society of Clinical Microbiology and Infectious Diseases (ESCMID) and the International Society of Chemotherapy (ISC) for Infection and Cancer. Eur Heart J. 2009;30(19):2369–413.
232. Ribera E, Gómez-Jimenez J, Cortes E, del Valle O, Planes A, Gonzalez-Alujas T, et al. Effectiveness of cloxacillin with and without gentamicin in short-term therapy for right-sided Staphylococcus aureus endocarditis. A randomized, controlled trial. Ann Intern Med. 1996;125(12):969–74.
233. Korzeniowski O, Sande MA. Combination antimicrobial therapy for Staphylococcus aureus endocarditis in patients addicted to parenteral drugs and in nonaddicts: a prospective study. Ann Intern Med. 1982;97(4):496–503.
234. Abrams B, Sklaver A, Hoffman T, Greenman R. Single or combination therapy of staphylococcal endocarditis in intravenous drug abusers. Ann Intern Med. 1979;90(5):789–91.
235. Coppens L, Hanson B, Klastersky J. Therapy of staphylococcal infections with cefamandole or vancomycin alone or with a combination of cefamandole and tobramycin. Antimicrob Agents Chemother. 1983;23(1):36–41.
236. Birmingham MC, Rayner CR, Meagher AK, Flavin SM, Batts DH, Schentag JJ. Linezolid for the treatment of multidrug-resistant, gram-positive infections: experience from a compassionate-use program. Clin Infect Dis. 2003;36(2):159–68.
237. Fowler VG Jr, Boucher HW, Corey GR, Abrutyn E, Karchmer AW, Rupp ME, S. aureus Endocarditis and Bacteremia Study

Group, et al. Daptomycin versus standard therapy for bacteremia and endocarditis caused by Staphylococcus aureus. N Engl J Med. 2006;355(7):653–65.
238. Lodise TP, McKinnon PS, Swiderski L, Rybak MJ. Outcomes analysis of delayed antibiotic treatment for hospital-acquired Staphylococcus aureus bacteremia. Clin Infect Dis. 2003;36(11):1418–23.
239. Fernández-Hidalgo N, Almirante B, Tornos P, González-Alujas MT, Planes AM, Larrosa MN, et al. Prognosis of left-sided infective endocarditis in patients transferred to a tertiary-care hospital – prospective analysis of referral bias and influence of inadequate antimicrobial treatment. Clin Microbiol Infect. 2011;17(5):769–75.
240. Dickerman SA, Abrutyn E, Barsic B, Bouza E, Cecchi E, Moreno A, ICE Investigators, et al. The relationship between the initiation of antimicrobial therapy and the incidence of stroke in infective endocarditis: an analysis from the ICE Prospective Cohort Study (ICE-PCS). Am Heart J. 2007;154(6):1086–94.
241. Shapira N, Merin O, Rosenmann E, Dzigivker I, Bitran D, Yinnon AM, Silberman S. Latent infective endocarditis: epidemiology and clinical characteristics of patients with unsuspected endocarditis detected after elective valve replacement. Ann Thorac Surg. 2004;78(5):1623–9.
242. Bannay A, Hoen B, Duval X, Obadia JF, Selton-Suty C, Le Moing V, AEPEI Study Group, et al. The impact of valve surgery on short- and long-term mortality in left-sided infective endocarditis: do differences in methodological approaches explain previous conflicting results? Eur Heart J. 2011;32(16):2003–15.
243. Lalani T, Cabell CH, Benjamin DK, Lasca O, Naber C, Fowler VG, International Collaboration on Endocarditis-Prospective Cohort Study (ICE-PCS) Investigators, et al. Analysis of the impact of early surgery on in-hospital mortality of native valve endocarditis: use of propensity score and instrumental variable methods to adjust for treatment-selection bias. Circulation. 2010;121(8):1005–13.
244. Delahaye F, Rial MO, de Gevigney G, Ecochard R, Delaye J. A critical appraisal of the quality of the management of infective endocarditis. J Am Coll Cardiol. 1999;33(3):788–93.
245. Botelho-Nevers E, Thuny F, Casalta JP, Richet H, Gouriet F, Collart F, et al. Dramatic reduction in infective endocarditis-related mortality with a management-based approach. Arch Intern Med. 2009;169(14):1290–8.
246. Thuny F, Fournier PE, Casalta JP, Gouriet F, Lepidi H, Riberi A, et al. Investigation of blood culture-negative early prosthetic valve endocarditis reveals high prevalence of fungi. Heart. 2010;96(10):743–7.
247. Pittet D, Hugonnet S, Harbarth S, Mourouga P, Sauvan V, Touveneau S, Perneger TV. Effectiveness of a hospital-wide programme to improve compliance with hand hygiene. Infection Control Programme. Lancet. 2000;356(9238):1307–12.
248. Hugonnet S, Perneger TV, Pittet D. Alcohol-based handrub improves compliance with hand hygiene in intensive care units. Arch Intern Med. 2002;162(9):1037–43.
249. World Health Organization. WHO guidelines for hand hygiene in health care. Geneva: World Health Organization; 2009.
250. Pessoa-Silva CL, Hugonnet S, Pfister R, Touveneau S, Dharan S, Posfay-Barbe K, Pittet D. Reduction of health care associated infection risk in neonates by successful hand hygiene promotion. Pediatrics. 2007;120(2):e382–90.
251. Eggimann P, Harbarth S, Constantin MN, Touveneau S, Chevrolet JC, Pittet D. Impact of a prevention strategy targeted at vascular-access care on incidence of infections acquired in intensive care. Lancet. 2000;355(9218):1864–8.
252. Eggimann P, Hugonnet S, Sax H, Harbarth S, Chevrolet JC, Pittet D. Long-term reduction of vascular access-associated bloodstream infection. Ann Intern Med. 2005;142(10):875–6.
253. Pronovost P, Needham D, Berenholtz S, Sinopoli D, Chu H, Cosgrove S, et al. An intervention to decrease catheter-related bloodstream infections in the ICU. N Engl J Med. 2006;355(26):2725–32.
254. Pronovost PJ, Goeschel CA, Colantuoni E, Watson S, Lubomski LH, Berehnnholtz SM, et al. Sustaining reductions in catheter related bloodstream infections in Michigan intensive care units: observational study. BMJ. 2010;340:c309.
255. Timsit JF, Schwebel C, Bouadma L, Geffroy A, Garrouste-Orgeas M, Pease S, Dressing Study Group, et al. Chlorhexidine-impregnated sponges and less frequent dressing changes for prevention of catheter-related infections in critically ill adults: a randomized controlled trial. JAMA. 2009;301(12):1231–41.
256. Ruschulte H, Franke M, Gastmeier P, Zenz S, Mahr KH, Buchholz S, et al. Prevention of central venous catheter related infections with chlorhexidine gluconate impregnated wound dressings: a randomized controlled trial. Ann Hematol. 2009;88(3):267–72.
257. Climo MW, Sepkowitz KA, Zuccotti G, Fraser VJ, Warren DK, Perl TM, et al. The effect of daily bathing with chlorhexidine on the acquisition of methicillin-resistant Staphylococcus aureus, vancomycin-resistant Enterococcus, and healthcare-associated bloodstream infections: results of a quasi-experimental multicenter trial. Crit Care Med. 2009;37(6):1858–65.
258. Niel-Weise BS, Stijnen T, van den Broek PJ. Anti-infective-treated central venous catheters for total parenteral nutrition or chemotherapy: a systematic review. J Hosp Infect. 2008;69(2):114–23.
259. Ramritu P, Halton K, Collignon P, Cook D, Fraenkel D, Battistutta D, et al. A systematic review comparing the relative effectiveness of antimicrobial-coated catheters in intensive care units. Am J Infect Control. 2008;36(2):104–17.
260. Walder B, Pittet D, Tramer MR. Prevention of bloodstream infections with central venous catheters treated with anti-infective agents depends on catheter type and insertion time: evidence from a meta-analysis. Infect Control Hosp Epidemiol. 2002;23(12):748–56.
261. Maki DG, Ash SR, Winger RK, Lavin P, AZEPTIC Trial Investigators. A novel antimicrobial and antithrombotic lock solution for hemodialysis catheters: a multi-center, controlled, randomized trial. Crit Care Med. 2011;39(4):613–20.
262. Raad II, Fang X, Keutgen XM, Jiang Y, Sherertz R, Hachem R. The role of chelators in preventing biofilm formation and catheter-related bloodstream infections. Curr Opin Infect Dis. 2008;21(4):385–92.
263. Ferreira Chacon JM, Hato de Almeida E, de Lourdes Simões R, Lazzarin C Ozório V, Alves BC, Mello de Andréa ML, et al. Randomized study of minocycline and edetic acid as a locking solution for central line (port-a-cath) in children with cancer. Chemotherapy. 2011;57(4):285–91.
264. Dümichen MJ, Seeger K, Lode HN, Kühl JS, Ebell W, Degenhardt P, et al. Randomized controlled trial of taurolidine citrate versus heparin as catheter lock solution in paediatric patients with haematological malignancies. J Hosp Infect. 2012;80(4):304–9.
265. Sherertz RJ, Boger MS, Collins CA, Mason L, Raad II. Comparative in vitro efficacies of various catheter lock solutions. Antimicrob Agents Chemother. 2006;50(5):1865–8.
266. Takla TA, Zelenitsky SA, Vercaigne LM. Effectiveness of a 30% ethanol/4% trisodium citrate locking solution in preventing biofilm formation by organisms causing haemodialysis catheter-related infections. J Antimicrob Chemother. 2008;62(5):1024–6.
267. Cober MP, Kovacevich DS, Teitelbaum DH. Ethanol-lock therapy for the prevention of central venous access device infections in pediatric patients with intestinal failure. JPEN J Parenter Enteral Nutr. 2010;35(1):67–73.
268. Jones BA, Hull MA, Richardson DS, Zurakowski D, Gura K, Fitzgibbons SC, et al. Efficacy of ethanol locks in reducing central

venous catheter infections in pediatric patients with intestinal failure. J Pediatr Surg. 2010;45(6):1287–93.
269. Oliveira C, Nasr A, Brindle M, Wales PW. Ethanol locks to prevent catheter-related bloodstream infections in parenteral nutrition: a meta-analysis. Pediatrics. 2012;129(2):318–29.
270. Crnich CJ, Duster M, Jones A, Maki DG. Prospective randomized double-blind trial of an ethanol lock for prevention of CLABSI. In: 49th Interscience Conference on Antimicrobial Agents and Chemotherapy [Abstract]. San Francisco; 2009
271. Slobbe L, Doorduijn JK, Lugtenburg PJ, El Barzouhi A, Boersma E, van Leeuwen WB, Rijnders BJ. Prevention of catheter-related bacteremia with a daily ethanol lock in patients with tunnelled catheters: a randomized, placebo-controlled trial. PLoS One. 2010;5(5):e10840.
272. Perez MJ, et al. Ethanol lock therapy in the prevention of catheter-related bloodstream infections after major heart surgery. In: 22nd European Congress of Clinical Microbiology and Infectious Diseases [Abstract]: London; 2012. p. P1355.
273. DePalo VA, McNicoll L, Cornell M, Rocha JM, Adams L, Pronovost PJ. The Rhode Island ICU collaborative: a model for reducing central line-associated bloodstream infection and ventilator-associated pneumonia statewide. Qual Saf Health Care. 2010;19(6):555–61.
274. Marra AR, Cal RG, Durão MS, Correa L, Guastelli LR, Moura DF Jr, et al. Impact of a program to prevent central line-associated bloodstream infection in the zero tolerance era. Am J Infect Control. 2010;38(6):434–9.
275. Miller MR, Griswold M, Harris JM 2nd, Yenokyan G, Huskins WC, Moss M, et al. Decreasing PICU catheter-associated bloodstream infections: NACHRI's quality transformation efforts. Pediatrics. 2010;125(2):206–13.
276. Peredo R, Sabatier C, Villagra A, Gonzalez J, Hernandez C, Perez F, et al. Reduction in catheter-related bloodstream infections in critically ill patients through a multiple system intervention. Eur J Clin Microbiol Infect Dis. 2010;29(9):1173–7.
277. Pérez Parra A, Cruz Menárguez M, Pérez Granda MJ, Tomey MJ, et al. A simple educational intervention to decrease incidence of central line-associated bloodstream infection (CLABSI) in intensive care units with low baseline incidence of CLABSI. Infect Control Hosp Epidemiol. 2010;31(9):964–7.
278. Britt RC, Novosel TJ, Britt LD, Sullivan M. The impact of central line simulation before the ICU experience. Am J Surg. 2009;197(4):533–6.
279. Barsuk JH, Cohen ER, Feinglass J, McGaghie WC, Wayne DB. Use of simulation-based education to reduce catheter-related bloodstream infections. Arch Intern Med. 2009;169(15):1420–3.
280. Barsuk JH, Cohen ER, McGaghie WC, Wayne DB. Long-term retention of central venous catheter insertion skills after simulation-based mastery learning. Acad Med. 2010;85(10 Suppl):S9–12.
281. Barsuk JH, McGaghie WC, Cohen ER, O'Leary KJ, Wayne DB. Simulation-based mastery learning reduces complications during central venous catheter insertion in a medical intensive care unit. Crit Care Med. 2009;37(10):2697–701.
282. Khouli H, Jahnes K, Shapiro J, Rose K, Mathew J, Gohil A, et al. Performance of medical residents in sterile techniques during central vein catheterization: randomized trial of efficacy of simulation-based training. Chest. 2011;139(1):80–7.
283. Sherertz RJ, Ely EW, Westbrook DM, Gledhill KS, Streed SA, Kiger B, et al. Education of physicians-in-training can decrease the risk for vascular catheter infection. Ann Intern Med. 2000;132(8):641–8.
284. Larson EL, Quiros D, Lin SX. Dissemination of the CDC's Hand Hygiene Guideline and impact on infection rates. Am J Infect Control. 2007;35(10):666–75.
285. Hall G, Hedström SA, Heimdahl A, Nord CE. Prophylactic administration of penicillins for endocarditis does not reduce the incidence of postextraction bacteremia. Clin Infect Dis. 1993;17(2):188–94.
286. Lockhart PB, Brennan MT, Sasser HC, Fox PC, Paster BJ, Bahrani-Mougeot FK. Bacteremia associated with toothbrushing and dental extraction. Circulation. 2008;117(24):3118–25.
287. Lacassin F, Hoen B, Leport C, Selton-Suty C, Delahaye F, Goulet V, et al. Procedures associated with infective endocarditis in adults. A case control study. Eur Heart J. 1995;16(12):1968–74.
288. Strom BL, Abrutyn E, Berlin JA, Kinman JL, Feldman RS, Stolley PD, et al. Risk factors for infective endocarditis: oral hygiene and nondental exposures. Circulation. 2000;102(23):2842–8.
289. Pallasch TJ. Antibiotic prophylaxis: problems in paradise. Dent Clin N Am. 2003;47(4):665–79.
290. Wilson W, Taubert KA, Gewitz M, Lockhart PB, Baddour LM, Levison M, American Heart Association Rheumatic Fever, Endocarditis, and Kawasaki Disease Committee, American Heart Association Council on Cardiovascular Disease in the Young, American Heart Association Council on Clinical Cardiology, American Heart Association Council on Cardiovascular Surgery and Anesthesia, Quality of Care and Outcomes Research Interdisciplinary Working Group, et al. Prevention of infective endocarditis: guidelines from the American Heart Association: a guideline from the American Heart Association Rheumatic Fever, Endocarditis, and Kawasaki Disease Committee, Council on Cardiovascular Disease in the Young, and the Council on Clinical Cardiology, Council on Cardiovascular Surgery and Anesthesia, and the Quality of Care and Outcomes Research Interdisciplinary Working Group. Circulation. 2007;116(15):1736–54.
291. Prophylaxis against infective endocarditis: antimicrobial prophylaxis against infective endocarditis in adults and children undergoing interventional procedures [Internet]. 2008.
292. da Silva DB, Souza IP, Cunha MC. Knowledge, attitudes and status of oral health in children at risk for infective endocarditis. Int J Paediatr Dent. 2002;12(2):124–31.
293. Duva X, Leport C. Prophylaxis of infective endocarditis: current tendencies, continuing controversies. Lancet Infect Dis. 2008;8(4):225–32.
294. Forner L, Larsen T, Kilian M, Holmstrup P. Incidence of bacteremia after chewing, tooth brushing and scaling in individuals with periodontal inflammation. J Clin Periodontol. 2006;33(6):401–7.
295. Roberts GJ. Dentists are innocent! "Everyday" bacteremia is the real culprit: a review and assessment of the evidence that dental surgical procedures are a principal cause of bacterial endocarditis in children. Pediatr Cardiol. 1999;20(5):317–25.

Gastrointestinal Infections and *Clostridium difficile* Infection

16

Stephen Harold and Herbert L. DuPont

Introduction

Gastrointestinal infections developing before, during, and after organ transplant is one of the leading causes of treatment failures among transplant recipients. In addition to significant increase in morbidity and mortality, GI complications also escalate the cost of treatment due to prolonged periods of hospitalization [1]. In this chapter, we provide an overview of the gastrointestinal infections with special emphasis on the *Clostridium difficile* (*C. difficile*) infection (CDI) in transplant recipients. In Fig. 16.1 we outline important factors in the development of CDI.

Transplants are broadly classified into hematopoietic stem cell transplant (HSCT), bone marrow transplant (BMT), and solid organ transplant (SOT). Recent changes in transplant immunosuppressant regimes have dramatically reduced the incidence of acute graft rejection. Newer immunosuppressive agents provide profound and sustained immunosuppression that effectively reduces the number of organ dysfunction or rejection and prolongs the survival of transplant recipient. On the contrary, it increases the risk of infection in this patient population due to disruption of the delicate balance between immunosuppression and host defense mechanism [2, 3]. The risk of infection in this subset of patients is due to interplay of multiple predisposing factors such as the type of transplant, conditioning regimens, use of antibiotics and immunosuppressive agents, and time period following transplantation [2]. Knowledge of the impact of immunologic state and therapies administered on the risk of infectious diseases including CDI can be critical to outcome in transplantation.

S. Harold
Baylor College of Medicine, Houston, TX, USA
e-mail: harold@bcm.edu

H. L. DuPont (✉)
Baylor St. Luke's Medical Center, Department of Research, Houston, TX, USA

Center for Infectious Diseases, University of Texas School of Public Health, Houston, TX, USA

Kelsey Research Foundation, Houston, TX, USA

Baylor College of Medicine, Houston, TX, USA

University of Texas McGovern School of Medicine Houston, Houston, TX, USA
e-mail: herbert.l.dupont@uth.tmc.edu

Clostridium difficile Infection (CDI)

CDI rates have tripled in hospitals in the United States (US) since the 1990s. Rates are rising due to changes in organism virulence but more importantly because of changing resistance of the host [4]. This review focuses on the problem of CDI in patients undergoing transplantation.

History

Bacillus difficilis was identified in 1935 by Hall and O'Toole as a common constituent of neonatal bowel flora [5]. The organisms, while now known as *C. difficile*, earned its appellation due to the difficulty experienced in the laboratory in characterizing the organisms' fermentation patterns. In the 1950s, pseudomembranous enterocolitis was thought to occur infrequently in surgical patients and was generally attributed to *Staphylococcus aureus* [6, 7]. The modern era of CDI began in the early 1970s with a prospective study of 200 patients treated with clindamycin, wherein 21% of the patients reported diarrhea and 10% were found to be suffering from pseudomembranous colitis (PMC) [8]. In 1977, a toxin produced by a *Clostridium* species was proposed as the cause of clindamycin-induced ileocecitis in hamsters [9], and in 1978, *C. difficile* was clearly identified as the causal agent of antibiotic-associated colitis in humans [10].

A. Safdar (ed.), *Principles and Practice of Transplant Infectious Diseases*, https://doi.org/10.1007/978-1-4939-9034-4_16

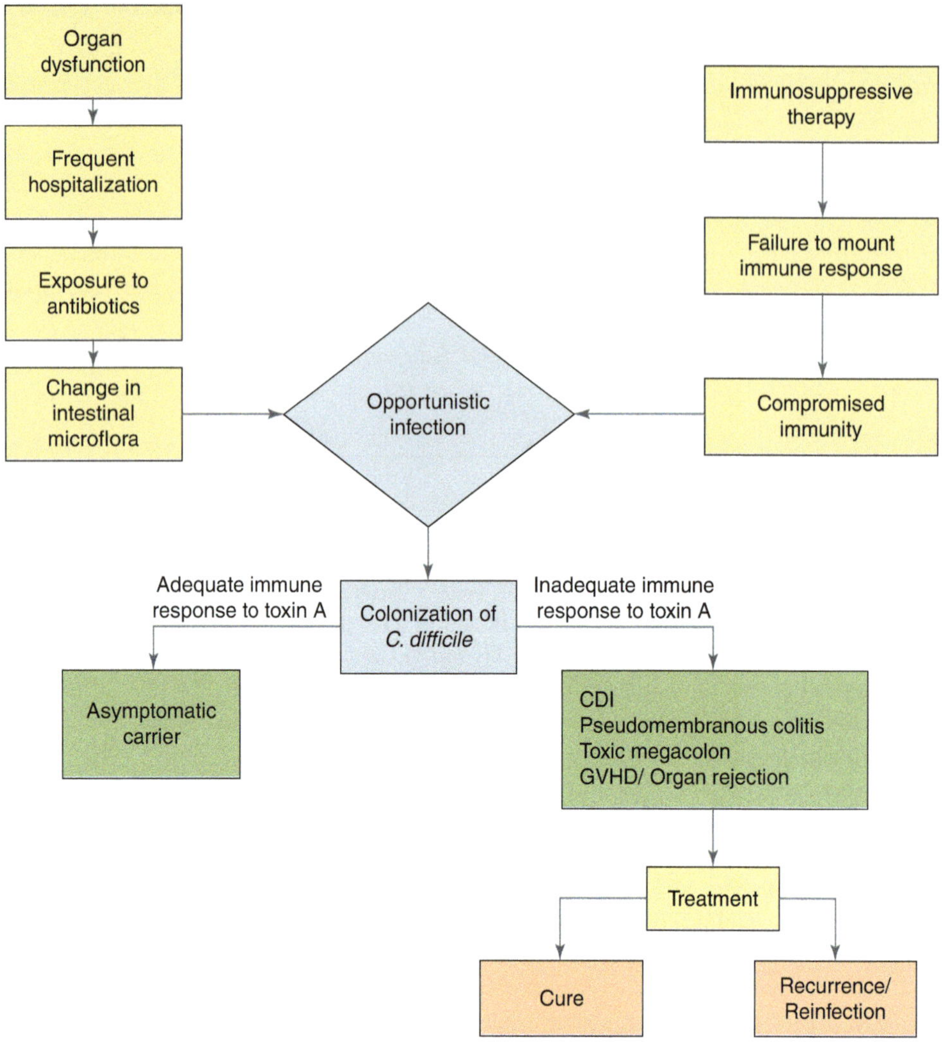

Fig. 16.1 An algorithm identifying risk factors associated with the development of *Clostridium difficile* infection in hospitalized patients including transplant recipients

Epidemiology

CDI is the most commonly identified cause of antibiotic-associated diarrhea found in 15–25% of cases [1, 11–13]. CDI was also reported in 5–7% of autologous BMT and 13–15% of allogeneic BMT patients [14–17]. Lung transplant recipients were shown to be more susceptible to CDI and were more likely to have severe CDI than all other SOT patients [18]. It is also the most common cause of enteric infections among liver transplant recipients [19]. The emergence of a so-called NAP1 hypervirulent strain further increased the incidence of CDI in some places of Canada, the US, and Europe since 2000 and is associated with increased morbidity and mortality where it occurs. The mortality rate due to CDI averages 1–2.5% of cases of infection [12].

Risk Factors

Most patients with CDI develop their infection when three factors are aligned: (1) elderly and infirm host, often immunosuppressed; (2) receipt of an antibiotic that dramatically alters colonic flora; and (3) exposure to *C. difficile* spores, often in a healthcare facility [4]. The specific antibiotic used in patients that leads to a disruption of normal bacterial flora is important [20, 21]. The antibiotics that are mostly associated with CDI are penicillins, cephalosporins, fluoroquinolones, and clindamycin [22–24]. Other predisposing factors for CDI are advanced age (greater than 65 years), severe underlying diseases, enteral feeding, use of proton pump inhibitors and chemotherapeutic agents, surgery, immunosuppression, and prolonged hospital stay leading to exposure to *C. difficile* spores [25, 26]. Most patients acquiring CDI have a combination of these risk factors.

Route of Transmission

C. difficile is a spore-forming gram-positive bacillus. *C. difficile* spores are non-vegetative forms that are acid and heat resistant. Spores of the organism are viable for prolonged period of time and are resistant to commonly used disinfectants and antiseptics. Ten percent Clorox is the preferred disinfectant yet is poorly tolerated as a general hospital disinfectant. The major reservoirs of infection are patients with CDI or asymptomatic carriers of *C. difficile* that contaminate the environment. Transmission of *C. difficile* is through fecal-oral route. Exposure may occur through direct contact with contaminated surfaces or through oral inoculation via contaminated materials like thermometers. When ingested, the spores of *C. difficile* survive gastric acidity, germinate to vegetative forms when exposed to bile salts, and colonize the gut [27]. CDI mostly occurs after antimicrobial therapy that disrupts the normal bacterial flora of the colon, facilitating colonization of the gut by *C. difficile*. Depending on the immune status of the individual, the incubation period of illness varies from few days to 8 weeks, and they clinically manifest with varying degrees of severity [21, 28] (Fig. 16.1).

Pathogenicity of *C. difficile* Infection

Pathogenesis of the disease is due to elaboration of two virulent toxins, toxin A, an enterotoxin, and toxin B, a cytotoxin. These toxins are large antigenic proteins that mediate an acute inflammatory diarrhea, characterized by proteinaceous exudate containing large number of neutrophils. Toxin A, which is a 308-kD cytotoxin and enterotoxin, induces marked intestinal inflammation, fluid secretion, and mucosal injury, while Toxin B, which is a 270-kD cytotoxic protein, stimulates the release of inflammatory cytokines from monocytes. It also activates calcium influx required for actin disassembly during cytotoxicity [29, 30]. A third toxin, named CDT, is a member of the iota family of binary toxins, which comprises the *Clostridium botulinum* C2 toxin and iota toxin subfamilies. CDT comprises two independent unlinked protein chains, CDTa (the enzymic component) and CDTb (the binding component) [31, 32]. The binding component CDTb mediates entry of CDTa into the cell, which potentiates the ADP ribosylation of actin and leads to disorganization of the cytoskeleton [33]. The exact pathogenic role of the binary toxin CDT in *C. difficile* infections is still not fully understood although it is associated with the hypervirulent NAP1 strain. Since they act synergistically with other toxins and depolymerize the actin cytoskeleton by a complementary mechanism, they are considered to be an additional virulence factor that contributes to the increased morbidity and mortality [34, 35]. *C. difficile* toxins inflame and destroy the colonic mucosal lining and form the typical "pseudomembranes" [36, 37].

The surface layer proteins (SLPs) of *C. difficile* also play a significant role in activating the host immune response in CDI. SLPs are the outermost surface components of the bacterium and are responsible for gut colonization and adhesion to the intestinal mucosa. A possible mediation of the SLPs in binding to both the intestinal epithelial cells and some components of their extracellular matrix fibers resulting in further epithelial damage has been proposed. In addition, the pathogenicity of *C. difficile* infection is attributed to the loss of the delicate balance between regulatory and inflammatory cytokines in the immune regulatory cells like monocytes and dendritic cells [38].

Although the *C. difficile* bacteria are noninvasive, their toxins penetrate the mucosal barrier and initiate an immune response in the host [39]. The ability of the host to mount an immune response against toxins is a key factor that accounts for the spectrum of clinical manifestation [29, 40]. Low serum and/or intestinal antibody response to *C. difficile* toxin A is associated with severe, prolonged, and recurrent CDI [41]. Adequate antibody response to toxin A is therefore an important element in clinical recovery from *C. difficile* diarrhea [40]. A genetic polymorphism in the promoter region of interleukin 8 gene has been associated with increased rates of CDI [42] and disease recurrence [43]. Presence of this polymorphism apparently leads to recurrence by prevention of immune response to the toxin(s) of *C. difficile* during a bout of CDI [44]. This genetic marker has not been studied in CDI in patients with transplantation.

Host Immune Response to *C. difficile* Colonization and Infection in Transplant Patients

The therapeutic prescription in transplant recipients includes a delicate balance between immunosuppression to protect the patient from graft-versus-host disease (GVHD)/organ rejection and simultaneous protection from life-threatening bacterial, viral, and fungal infection. With the advent of newer molecules and newer immunosuppressive regimens, the augmented immunosuppression confers protection against GVHD but inhibits the ability to mount a microbial specific cytotoxic T-lymphocyte response [45].

Immunosuppression deactivates immune competence in the transplant recipient through multiple pathways including suppression of anti-inflammatory cytokines and suppression of antibody-mediated response to toxins by immunosuppressive agents, frequent use of antibiotics, and longer and more frequent hospital admissions. These immunosuppressive pathways reduce their ability to mount an aggressive humoral response to the *C. difficile* toxin soon after the infection. Intensified immunosuppressive therapy and pulse steroid therapy that prevent transplant rejection are also major contributors of posttransplant hypogammaglobulinemia (HGG) that is observed in 69.6% of transplant patients [46]. This inhibits immunoglobulin production primarily through an indirect pathway by altering lymphokine production by the T cells which in turn alters the B-cell function. A few newer immunosuppressive agents affect B-cell function through a direct pathway too [47, 48]. Hence these patients are unable to initiate a specific immune response against *C. difficile*'s toxin A and SLP [41, 49]. Besides, HGG is associated with increased incidence of opportunistic infection. Consequently, broad-spectrum antibiotics are used extensively as a prophylactic as well as therapeutic measure resulting in destruction of the normal intestinal flora. In addition, multiple antibiotics are administered to transplant recipients as perioperative prophylaxis or postoperative therapy. These antibiotics alter the intestinal microecology and reduce the resistance to colonization of the bowel by *C. difficile*. This ultimately results in increased incidence of antibiotic-associated diarrhea and CDI [50]. Iatrogenic immunosuppression in transplant recipients thus offsets the fine balance and makes the patient more vulnerable to CDI.

Emergence of a Hypervirulent Strain

A hypervirulent or BI/027/NAP1 toxinotype III strain of *C. difficile* has emerged during the past decade. This strain of bacteria possesses a binary toxin, with an 18-bp deletion in the tcdC gene that demonstrates in vitro resistance to fluoroquinolones [34, 51, 52]. The BI/027 strain produces 3 to 13 times more toxins and sporulates at a higher degree than historical strains [53]. In the US and UK isolates, the NAP1/027 strain produced 16 times more of toxin A and 23 times more of toxin B concentrations than other strains [54]. These factors contribute to hypervirulence, increased severity of the disease, and widespread emergence of this epidemic strain all too often resulting in the development of toxic megacolon requiring colectomy, leukemoid reaction, shock, and death [34]. The importance of this organism in transplantation medicine has not been established.

CDI in BMT Patients

BMT patients appear to be at increased risk of developing infectious gastroenteritis [55] most probably related to prolonged hospitalizations with enhanced exposure to infectious spores, treatment with numerous prophylactic broad-spectrum antibiotics, myeloablative chemotherapy, and altered integrity of the intestinal mucosa [14, 15, 56]. Cytopenias are frequently seen in these patients in spite of submyeloablative doses of chemotherapy. Prolonged neutropenia and placement of indwelling catheters prior to mobilization process predispose them to infections. Prophylactic antibiotics are given due to high risk of infection following intense chemotherapy to enhance stem cell yield. All these factors predispose this population to increased risk of CDI [57]. However, the duration of immunosuppression is shorter in BMT patients than in SOT patients. Nevertheless, neutropenia seldom occurs in patients following SOT, whereas in HSCT recipients severe neutropenia is routinely seen during the pre-engraftment period. CDI accounts for 1.3–20.4% of all diarrheal diseases in BMT patients [58]. The incidence of CDI is 5–7% in autologous transplant patients [15, 55], while Yolken et al. reported 15%, and Chakrabarti et al. reported CDI 13% in allogeneic BMT patients [17, 59]. This may be due to shorter duration of neutropenia in patients undergoing autologous BMT because of increased use of hematopoietic growth factors [14, 60]. In allogeneic BMT patients, donor effector T cell may cause GVHD, and diarrhea is the common clinical presentation of intestinal tract GVHD [16]. High-dose steroids and antibiotics given to suppress the host anti-inflammatory response in patients with GVHD could have attributed to higher incidence of CDI in allogeneic BMT patients [16].

The average time to onset of CDI after autologous BMT is less than a week [16, 61] and after allogeneic BMT is 33–38 days [16, 17]. Mobilization of stem cells is done by administration of cytokines like filgrastim alone, chemotherapy alone, or both. However, the stem cell yield is greater for those patients receiving a combination of cytokines and chemotherapy. This frequently results in prolonged periods of cytopenias including neutropenia [62]. Moreover, these conditioning regimens, which are indispensable for stem cell mobilization, damage the integrity of mucosal barriers [55]. In addition, the placement of indwelling catheters prior to mobilization of stem cells and prophylactic use of antibiotics destroys the ecologic balance of the normal intestinal flora and promotes colonization of the gut by pathogenic organisms such as *C. difficile* in BMT patients [13, 57]. All these factors along with intense immunosuppressive therapy to prevent GVHD in allogeneic hematopoietic graft recipients may predispose BMT patients to earlier onset of CDI [57] than SOT patients. In a study of patients with CDI having previously undergone HSCT, the 1-year incidence of recurrent CDI was 31% with most recurrences seen in within 6 months of the initial infection [63].

CDI in SOT Patients

It was determined in one study that CDI was five times more common in sold organ transplant recipients than among general medicine inpatients and that CDI was associated with increased 30-day readmission for transplanted patients [64]. Reported incidence of CDI in SOT patients ranges from 1% to 31%: 3–7% in liver, 1–16% in kidney, 8–15% in heart, and 7–31% in lung transplant patients [46, 50, 65–67]. In one study the median time from transplantation until development of CDI was 51 days (14–249 days range) with liver recipients having the shortest time to infection, median 36 days, and lung recipients a longer time to infection, median 136 days [68]. Hospitalized children with solid organ transplant recipients are at increased rates of CDI [69].

Poor pretransplant conditions such as end-stage organ failure and long waiting times, longer and more frequent hospital admissions, and prolonged/protracted immune suppression over a period of 12 months in SOT patients increase the risk of CDI [65, 67]. These prolonged periods of immune suppression predispose SOT patients to repeated infections, which exposes them to repeated courses of broad-spectrum antibiotics. The use of antibiotics in this group of patients alters the intestinal flora favoring the colonization of gut by *C. difficile* [50]. Suppression of anti-inflammatory and antibody-mediated immune response reduces their ability to mount an effective humoral response to the *C. difficile* toxin after the infection. In addition, immunosuppressive and steroid therapy in the post-transplant period given to prevent transplant rejection is a major contributor of HGG in a vast majority of transplant patients [46]. This inhibits immunoglobulin production primarily through an indirect pathway by altering lymphokine production by the T cells, which in turn alters the B-cell function. A few newer immunosuppressive agents affect B-cell function through a direct pathway too [47, 48]. Hence, these patients are unable to initiate a specific immune response against *C. difficile*'s toxin A and SLP. Besides, HGG is associated with increased risk of opportunistic infection [46]. Another common risk factor in SOT patients is gastric acid suppression by proton pump inhibitors. Hospitalized patients receiving proton pump inhibitors are two times more likely to develop CDI [70]. Though gastric acid does not have any action on the spores, it destroys the vegetative forms and reduces the ability of the spores to germinate. Proton pump inhibitors also alter the gastrointestinal flora, facilitating colonization of the colon by *C. difficile* [71]. In a study by Dallal et al. [18], it was observed that the risk of developing CDI was 46 times higher in lung transplant recipients and they were 8 times more likely to have severe forms of CDI than all other patients with CDI. This may be due to more intense immunosuppression to prevent rejection and frequent use of antibiotics to treat recurrent pulmonary infection as lung transplant recipients are the only SOT patients in whom the allograft is directly exposed to the environment [18]. Poor pretransplantation condition associated with end-stage liver failure, longer waiting times, operative stress, and the required immune suppression impair the normal defense mechanism and predispose liver transplant recipients to higher incidence of infections. Administration of frequent, more diverse, and prolonged use of antimicrobials favor increased incidence of CDI in liver transplant patients than kidney transplant patients. Further, certain newer immunosuppressive agents may cause severe mucosal damage and increase the incidence of CDI in this population [65, 67]. The incidence of CDI in kidney transplant recipients may be low because of underreporting [72]. Further, induction of immunosuppressive treatment and recent use of antibiotics are risk factors that favor CDI in this population [73]. CDI in adult kidney recipients appeared to represent a different pattern by their presentation at a later age invariably associated with use of antibiotics [72]. HGG has been reported in kidney, lung, heart, and liver transplant patients. Severe HGG was observed in approximately 10% of heart transplant patients, which increases the risk of CDI in this subset of transplant patients [48, 74, 75].

CDI occurs more frequently in the first 3 months after transplantation mostly due to enhanced immunosuppression, increased exposure to healthcare settings due to prolonged hospital stay, frequent use of antibiotics, and debilitated condition prior to transplant [50, 65, 66]. Late-onset CDI correlate with the onset of HGG due to exposure to antimicrobials or intensified immunosuppression to treat graft rejection [66, 72, 76, 77]. The outcome of CDI in recipients of solid organ transplants is good with recurrence the major complication as seen in non-transplant patients [78].

Clinical Features

Depending on the immune response to toxin A of *C. difficile*, infected patients exhibit a wide spectrum of clinical manifestations. Patients with a high titer of IgG to toxin A may remain as asymptomatic carriers of *C. difficile* [29]. Approximately 2–3% of healthy adults are asymptomatic carriers of *C. difficile* [79]. Symptomatic patients present with watery diarrhea, cramping, fever, dehydration, and leukocytosis. Some of the complications of CDI include fulminant colitis, hypoalbuminemia, pseudomembranous colitis, toxic megacolon, and perforation of the colon [37, 80]. Recurrent CDI occurs in 10–25% of CDI and is more often due to relapse than reinfection. Some of the risk factors associated with relapse include age greater than 65 years, prolonged hospitalization, prolonged antibiotic use, diverticulosis, and comorbidities [81]. An increased secretion of IgG to toxin A is associated with decreased risk of recurrence [41].

Diagnosis

Though there is no gold standard test to confirm the diagnosis of CDI, the commonly used tests are enzyme immunoassay (EIA) for toxin A/B, glutamate dehydrogenase (GDH), nucleic acid amplification tests (NAATs), toxigenic culture (TC), and cytotoxin neutralization (CTN) test [82, 83]. Diagnosis of CDI is made following detection of *C. difficile* toxin in stool samples in a patient with new onset diarrhea, often associated with antibiotic use. Stool toxin test is the most specific diagnostic test for CDI with sensitivity of 67–100% depending upon the method of toxin testing employed. EIAs are done to detect toxin A and/or toxin B, but they have low sensitivity. In some institutions, a two-step process is being used to detect CDI [84]. Initially, a cost-effective screening test is done to detect the presence of GDH in stools. As the presence of GDH does not differentiate between toxigenic and non-toxigenic strains of *C. difficile*, patients with stool specimen positive for GDH are subject to further evaluation by assays to confirm the presence of toxigenic *C. difficile*. Stool culture followed by testing the isolate for toxin production is a highly sensitive method (89–100%) with high specificity (84–99%). NAATs such as real-time polymerase chain reaction (RT-PCR) are as sensitive as culture for diagnosing CDI. A stool sample to be tested should be sent to the laboratory as soon as possible as the toxins secreted by *C. difficile* strains undergo degradation within hours [81]. Computed tomography imaging is a useful test that shows colonic thickening, and colonoscopy is also very sensitive showing characteristic white yellow mucosal plaques or pseudomembrane formation [85–87]. False-positive tests commonly occur regardless of test because of *C. difficile* carriage making it difficult to determine if CDI was the diagnosis or diarrhea due to another cause. In a logistic regression model, allogeneic HSCT was identified as a significant risk factor (OR 18.6, $p < 0.01$) compared with other patients for colonization by *C. difficile* [88].

In the absence of above mentioned confirmatory laboratory findings, the following factors may be suggestive of CDI: (1) marked leukocytosis (WBC >15 × 10^9/L), (2) hypoalbuminemia (<30 g/L), and (3) rise in serum creatinine level (133 μM or 1.5 times the premorbid level) [89].

Treatment

General management includes discontinuing of offending antibiotic if possible together with fluid and electrolyte replacement, anti-*C. difficile* antimicrobial therapy and institution of infection control measures. Specific anti-*C. difficile* treatment [85] includes administration of oral vancomycin, oral or intravenous metronidazole, or oral fidaxomicin for 10–14 days [90–92] (Table 16.1). Vancomycin and fidaxomicin are the two FDA-approved drugs for CDI. Response rate to treatment is 86–100%. Oral vancomycin and fidaxomicin are the preferred treatments of CDI [92]. IV metronidazole is helpful for the management of patients with CDI who cannot take oral medications when combined with vancomycin enemas [93]. Though fidaxomicin is associated with lower frequency of recurrence than vancomycin, recurrences are not eliminated, and the drug is much more expensive. See Table 16.1 for summary of treatment options for CDI. Recurrence rate of CDI after appropriate therapy averages 25% [94]. Because of the importance of anti-*C. difficile* antibody development in CDI to ultimate recovery, anti-*C. difficile* toxin vaccines and antibody preparations are in development. A humanized anti-toxin A and B monoclonal antibody preparation reduced the occurrence of CDI recurrence in patients treated with standard anti-CDI therapy [95]. Pooled human immunoglobulin has been used with variable success in treating recurrent CDI [96].

Table 16.1 Specific anti-*C. difficile* treatment

Therapeutic agent	Dose	Comments
Metronidazole	500 mg 3–4 times a day for 10–14 days PO or IV	Not as effective as other drugs when given orally due to high gut absorption; can be given IV if oral route unavailable; give orally when can
Oral vancomycin	125 mg four times a day for 10–14 days	Standard therapy for moderately ill or severely ill patients
Fidaxomicin	200 mg every 12 h for 10 days	Lower recurrence rate than vancomycin but remains the most expensive option

Other drugs with potential value: ramoplanin, rifalazil, rifaximin, tinidazole, nitazoxanide, teicoplanin, and fusidic acid

First recurrent CDI can be managed with a repeat course of the initial antibiotic. Recurrent cases beyond the first recurrence can be treated with pulsed or tapered dose of oral vancomycin over a month or longer [97]. Patients with fulminant CDI may require colectomy for cure [98]. Fecal microbiota transplant (FMT), a process by which feces from a healthy donor is directly transplanted into the duodenum or lower gastrointestinal tract or is administered as frozen FMT capsules to restore normal ecology, has been used increasingly for severe cases of post-antibiotic colitis and more frequently for refractory and recurrent cases of CDI [82, 99–102], the most successful treatment in immunocompetent hosts. However, recommended guidelines suggested avoidance of FMT in SOT recipients due to risk of infection from the organisms in the fecal material [84]. Nevertheless, in a retrospective study of 80 immunocompromised patients, including 19 SOT recipients, who had received FMT for refractory/recurrent/severe CDI, an overall cure rate of 89% was reported [103]. Though there were few severe adverse effects or related adverse effects, infections definitely related to FMT were not reported in this study which fits with another study of FMT for recurrent CDI in HSCT recipients [104]. Though seemingly not appealing, FMT is emerging as an inexpensive, safe, and efficient treatment of refractory and recurrent CDI [105–108]. There are limited centers for this option but the outcome is excellent. More research is needed to understand the positive elements of donor feces studied by metagenomic analyses in the therapy of severe or recurrent CDI.

Recommended Prevention and Control Measures

Preventive measures that effectively reduce the incidence of *C. difficile* infections and cross-infection in hospital settings include a precise and early diagnosis, early initiation of specific treatment, adopting enteric precautions for symptomatic patients, promoting hand hygiene using soap and water, and adopting barrier precautions. Combination of hand hygiene and contact precaution can result in 60–80% reduction in spread of CDI [109, 110]. As a primary preventive step, environmental disinfection with 10% sodium hypochlorite should be routinely employed in hospital rooms confining or having confined patients with CDI [111]. The use of broad-spectrum antibiotics should be limited by adhering to antibiotic policy of the hospital which should be reviewed periodically [112]. *C. difficile* should be systematically investigated in patients with more serious forms of nosocomial diarrhea. Educational programs for clinical and ancillary clinical staff can help prevent transmission of *C. difficile* from patient to patient. Strict antiseptic measures including use of disposable gloves, mask, and gown, frequent washing of hands with soap and water, and use of disposable thermometers and enhanced environmental cleaning must be enforced. Isolation methods such as private rooms or cohorting of infected patients have been effective in reducing the rate of CDI. Surveillance should be instituted in order to detect hospital and community outbreaks [81, 85].

Patients with CDI continue to excrete the organism for long periods. There is no established treatment for the frequent patient in the hospital who becomes colonized by *C. difficile*. It is therefore essential that patients' rooms be thoroughly sanitized to reduce the potential for reinfection of patients, as this is one of the commonest causes for recurrence of symptoms.

Other Gastrointestinal Infections

Other non-*C. difficile* causes of diarrhea may be seen in the first 6 months after transplantation. Though the infections seen in BMT and SOT patients are similar, there is significant difference in the duration and degree of immunosuppression. Infections that occur in the first month following SOT include endogenous pathogens infecting the patient pretransplant such as herpes viruses, those transmitted from the donor as, for example, hepatitis virus, and those related to the procedure itself such as gram-negative sepsis. Opportunistic infections that occur from 1 to 6 months following SOT include viral, fungal, and parasitic infections. Beyond the first 6 months, SOT patients are at a higher risk for community-acquired infections and lymphoproliferative diseases like B- and T-cell lymphoma due to continued intense immunosuppression [2].

Mucositis is common following BMT [113] and mucosal ulcerations which may be due to cytomegalovirus (CMV), herpes simplex virus, fungal agents, or *Entamoeba histolytica* [114, 115]. Diarrhea due to *E. histolytica*, *Giardia lamblia*, *Cryptosporidium* spp., *Strongyloides stercoralis*, CMV, and noroviruses are known to occur during the period of immunosuppression in BMT patients [116]. Abscess in the perianal region mostly due to bacteria is known to occur during neutropenic episodes [117]. Hepatitis B and hepatitis C may be transmitted from the donor, or reactivation of the virus in an infected recipient may occur in the posttransplant period [118, 119]. Fatal fulminant hepatitis B has been reported in hepatitis B-infected recipients in the absence of viral prophylaxis [120]. Fungal infections are less common in BMT patients due to antifungal prophylaxis [121, 122].

CMV infection is the most common infection that occurs within the first year of SOT, with a peak incidence at 4–6 months after transplant [45, 123]. Lung transplant and heart transplant patients are at a higher risk of developing CMV infection than other SOT patients. CMV hepatitis is more severe in orthoptic liver transplant patients than in any other SOT recipients [124]. Kidney and kidney-pancreas transplant patients are at a lower risk of developing CMV infection as the latent viral load is low in the allograft [123]. This is more likely to occur in those patients who receive antilymphocyte antibody in addition to conventional immunosuppression or mycophenolate mofetil (MMF) for maintenance [124–126].

Herpes simplex virus infection is the second most commonly occurring viral infection in SOT patients. It has great predilection for the squamous epithelium of the esophagus; however, it can involve the intestine and liver in the absence of appropriate prophylaxis. It is mostly due to reactivation of latent virus and hence manifests within the first 4 weeks of transplantation [127]. Other herpes virus infections are less common. However, the risk of dissemination of varicella-zoster virus increases with use of MMF immunotherapy.

Fungal infections usually develop after the first month of SOT especially in patients who have discontinued fungal prophylaxis [127]. Liver transplant patients are at a higher risk to develop invasive fungal infection in general and *Candida albicans* in particular than other SOT patients; while infection by *Aspergillus* spp. is highly prevalent in lung transplant and heart-lung transplant patients [128].

Conclusions

The incidence of CDI in the immunosuppressed population is greater than in the general population and is dependent on receipt of antibiotics and other drugs and exposure to *C. difficile*. Recovery from CDI depends upon the patient's ability to mount a quantitative immune response and presence of comorbidities. Disruption of the delicate balance between iatrogenic immunosuppression to prevent organ rejection and the ability to mount an immune response against pathogenic agents results in life-threatening or recurrent infections by *C. difficile* and other pathogens.

Prompt diagnosis and early treatment of CDI, effective infection control measures, and prudent use of antibiotics may help reduce morbidity and mortality due to CDI. Understanding the gravity of the disease and strict implementation of hand hygiene and antiviral and antifungal prophylaxis may help prevent other gastrointestinal infections following transplantation.

References

1. Kyne L, Hamel MB, Polavaram R, Kelly CNP. Health care costs and mortality associated with nosocomial diarrhea due to Clostridium difficile. Clin Infect Dis. 2002;34(3):346–53.
2. Fishman JA. Infection in solid-organ transplant recipients. N Engl J Med. 2007;357(25):2601–14.
3. Meier-Kriesche HU, Li S, Gruessner RW, Fung JJ, Bustami RT, Barr ML, et al. Immunosuppression: evolution in practice and trends, 1994–2004. Am J Transplant. 2006;6(5 Pt 2):1111–31.
4. DuPont HL. The search for effective treatment of Clostridium difficile infection. N Engl J Med. 2011;364(5):473–5.
5. Hall IC, OT E. Intestinal flora in newborn infants with a description of a new pathogenic anaerobe, *Bacillus difficilis*. Am J Dis Child. 1935;49:390–402.
6. Pettet JD, Baggenstoss AH, Dearing WH, Judd ES Jr. Postoperative pseudomembranous enterocolitis. Surg Gynecol Obstet. 1954;98(5):546–52.
7. Altemeier WA, Hummel RP, Hill EO. Staphylococcal enterocolitis following antibiotic therapy. Ann Surg. 1963;157:847–58.
8. Tedesco FJ, Barton RW, Alpers DH. Clindamycin-associated colitis. A prospective study. Ann Intern Med. 1974;81(4):429–33.
9. Bartlett JG, Chang TW, Gurwith M, Gorbach SL, Onderdonk AB. Antibiotic-associated pseudomembranous colitis due to toxin-producing clostridia. N Engl J Med. 1978;298(10):531–4.
10. Bartlett JG, Moon N, Chang TW, Taylor N, Onderdonk AB. Role of Clostridium difficile in antibiotic-associated pseudomembranous colitis. Gastroenterology. 1978;75(5):778–82.
11. Oldfield EC 3rd. Clostridium difficile-associated diarrhea: risk factors, diagnostic methods, and treatment. Rev Gastroenterol Disord. 2004;4(4):186–95.
12. Schroeder MS. Clostridium difficile – associated diarrhea. Am Fam Physician. 2005;71(5):921–8.
13. Bartlett JG. Antibiotic-associated diarrhea. Clin Infect Dis. 1992;15(4):573–81.
14. Avery R, Pohlman B, Adal K, Bolwell B, Goldman M, Kalaycio M, et al. High prevalence of diarrhea but infrequency of documented Clostridium difficile in autologous peripheral blood progenitor cell transplant recipients. Bone Marrow Transplant. 2000;25(1):67–9.
15. Bilgrami S, Feingold JM, Dorsky D, Edwards RL, Bona RD, Khan AM, et al. Incidence and outcome of Clostridium difficile infection following autologous peripheral blood stem cell transplantation. Bone Marrow Transplant. 1999;23(10):1039–42.
16. Alonso CD, Treadway SB, Hanna DB, Huff CA, Neofytos D, Carroll KC, et al. Epidemiology and outcomes of Clostridium difficile infections in hematopoietic stem cell transplant recipients. Clin Infect Dis. 2012;54(8):1053–63.
17. Chakrabarti S, Lees A, Jones SG, Milligan DW. Clostridium difficile infection in allogeneic stem cell transplant recipients is associated with severe graft-versus-host disease and non-relapse mortality. Bone Marrow Transplant. 2000;26(8):871–6.
18. Dallal RM, Harbrecht BG, Boujoukas AJ, Sirio CA, Farkas LM, Lee KK, et al. Fulminant Clostridium difficile: an underappreciated and increasing cause of death and complications. Ann Surg. 2002;235(3):363–72.
19. Stelzmueller I, Biebl M, Graziadei I, Wiesmayr S, Margreiter R, Bonatti H. Regarding diarrhea in liver transplant recipients: etiology and management. Liver Transpl. 2006;12(1):163–4.
20. Kelly CP, LaMont JT. Clostridium difficile infection. Annu Rev Med. 1998;49:375–90.
21. Castagliuolo I, LaMont JT. Pathophysiology, diagnosis and treatment of Clostridium difficile infection. Keio J Med. 1999;48(4):169–74.
22. McFarland LV, Surawicz CM, Stamm WE. Risk factors for Clostridium difficile carriage and *C. difficile*-associated diarrhea in a cohort of hospitalized patients. J Infect Dis. 1990;162(3):678–84.
23. Bignardi GE. Risk factors for Clostridium difficile infection. J Hosp Infect. 1998;40(1):1–15.
24. Bartlett JG, Perl TM. The new Clostridium difficile – what does it mean? N Engl J Med. 2005;353(23):2503–5.
25. Gerding DN, Johnson S, Peterson LR, Mulligan ME, Silva J Jr. Clostridium difficile-associated diarrhea and colitis. Infect Control Hosp Epidemiol. 1995;16(8):459–77.
26. Kee VR. Clostridium difficile infection in older adults: a review and update on its management. Am J Geriatr Pharmacother. 2012;10(1):14–24.
27. Blondeau JM. What have we learned about antimicrobial use and the risks for Clostridium difficile-associated diarrhoea? J Antimicrob Chemother. 2009;63(2):238–42.
28. Theunissen C, Knoop C, Nonhoff C, Byl B, Claus M, Liesnard C, et al. Clostridium difficile colitis in cystic fibrosis patients with and without lung transplantation. Transpl Infect Dis. 2008;10(4):240–4.
29. Kyne L, Warny M, Qamar A, Kelly CP. Asymptomatic carriage of Clostridium difficile and serum levels of IgG antibody against toxin A. N Engl J Med. 2000;342(6):390–7.
30. Carter GP, Rood JI, Lyras D. The role of toxin A and toxin B in the virulence of Clostridium difficile. Trends Microbiol. 2012;20(1):21–9.
31. Gulke I, Pfeifer G, Liese J, Fritz M, Hofmann F, Aktories K, et al. Characterization of the enzymatic component of the ADP-ribosyltransferase toxin CDTa from Clostridium difficile. Infect Immun. 2001;69(10):6004–11.
32. Considine RV, Simpson LL. Cellular and molecular actions of binary toxins possessing ADP-ribosyltransferase activity. Toxicon. 1991;29(8):913–36.
33. Aktories K, Wegner A. Mechanisms of the cytopathic action of actin-ADP-ribosylating toxins. Mol Microbiol. 1992;6(20):2905–8.
34. McDonald LC, Killgore GE, Thompson A, Owens RC Jr, Kazakova SV, Sambol SP, et al. An epidemic, toxin gene-variant strain of Clostridium difficile. N Engl J Med. 2005;353(23):2433–41.
35. Ananthakrishnan AN. Clostridium difficile infection: epidemiology, risk factors and management. Nat Rev Gastroenterol Hepatol. 2011;8(1):17–26.
36. Poxton IR, McCoubrey J, Blair G. The pathogenicity of Clostridium difficile. Clin Microbiol Infect. 2001;7(8):421–7.
37. Poutanen SM, Simor AE. Clostridium difficile-associated diarrhea in adults. Can Med Assoc J. 2004;171(1):51–8.
38. Ausiello CM, Cerquetti M, Fedele G, Spensieri F, Palazzo R, Nasso M, et al. Surface layer proteins from Clostridium difficile induce inflammatory and regulatory cytokines in human monocytes and dendritic cells. Microbes Infect. 2006;8(11):2640–6.
39. Flegel WA, Muller F, Daubener W, Fischer HG, Hadding U, Northoff H. Cytokine response by human monocytes to Clostridium difficile toxin A and toxin B. Infect Immun. 1991;59(10):3659–66.
40. Sanchez-Hurtado K, Corretge M, Mutlu E, McIlhagger R, Starr JM, Poxton IR. Systemic antibody response to Clostridium diffi-

cile in colonized patients with and without symptoms and matched controls. J Med Microbiol. 2008;57(Pt 6):717–24.
41. Kyne L, Warny M, Qamar A, Kelly CP. Association between antibody response to toxin A and protection against recurrent Clostridium difficile diarrhoea. Lancet. 2001;357(9251):189–93.
42. Jiang ZD, DuPont HL, Garey K, Price M, Graham G, Okhuysen P, et al. A common polymorphism in the interleukin 8 gene promoter is associated with Clostridium difficile diarrhea. Am J Gastroenterol. 2006;101(5):1112–6.
43. Garey KW, Jiang ZD, Ghantoji S, Tam VH, Arora V, DuPont HL. A common polymorphism in the interleukin-8 gene promoter is associated with an increased risk for recurrent Clostridium difficile infection. Clin Infect Dis. 2010;51(12):1406–10.
44. Jiang ZD, Garey KW, Price M, Graham G, Okhuysen P, Dao-Tran T, et al. Association of interleukin-8 polymorphism and immunoglobulin G anti-toxin A in patients with Clostridium difficile-associated diarrhea. Clin Gastroenterol Hepatol. 2007;5(8):964–8.
45. Fishman JA, Rubin RH. Infection in organ-transplant recipients. N Engl J Med. 1998;338(24):1741–51.
46. Munoz P, Giannella M, Alcala L, Sarmiento E, Fernandez Yanez J, Palomo J, et al. Clostridium difficile-associated diarrhea in heart transplant recipients: is hypogammaglobulinemia the answer? J Heart Lung Transplant. 2007;26(9):907–14.
47. Carpenter CB. Immunosuppression in organ transplantation. N Engl J Med. 1990;322(17):1224–6.
48. Yamani MH, Avery RK, Mawhorter SD, Young JB, Ratliff NB, Hobbs RE, et al. Hypogammaglobulinemia following cardiac transplantation: a link between rejection and infection. J Heart Lung Transplant. 2001;20(4):425–30.
49. Drudy D, Calabi E, Kyne L, Sougioultzis S, Kelly E, Fairweather N, et al. Human antibody response to surface layer proteins in Clostridium difficile infection. FEMS Immunol Med Microbiol. 2004;41(3):237–42.
50. Gunderson CC, Gupta MR, Lopez F, Lombard GA, LaPlace SG, Taylor DE, et al. Clostridium difficile colitis in lung transplantation. Transpl Infect Dis. 2008;10(4):245–51.
51. Curry SR, Marsh JW, Muto CA, O'Leary MM, Pasculle AW, Harrison LH. tcdC genotypes associated with severe TcdC truncation in an epidemic clone and other strains of Clostridium difficile. J Clin Microbiol. 2007;45(1):215–21.
52. Hubert B, Loo VG, Bourgault AM, Poirier L, Dascal A, Fortin E, et al. A portrait of the geographic dissemination of the Clostridium difficile North American pulsed-field type 1 strain and the epidemiology of *C. difficile*-associated disease in Quebec. Clin Infect Dis. 2007;44(2):238–44.
53. Akerlund T, Persson I, Unemo M, Noren T, Svenungsson B, Wullt M, et al. Increased sporulation rate of epidemic Clostridium difficile Type 027/NAP1. J Clin Microbiol. 2008;46(4):1530–3.
54. Warny M, Pepin J, Fang A, Killgore G, Thompson A, Brazier J, et al. Toxin production by an emerging strain of Clostridium difficile associated with outbreaks of severe disease in North America and Europe. Lancet. 2005;366(9491):1079–84.
55. van Kraaij MG, Dekker AW, Verdonck LF, van Loon AM, Vinje J, Koopmans MP, et al. Infectious gastro-enteritis: an uncommon cause of diarrhoea in adult allogeneic and autologous stem cell transplant recipients. Bone Marrow Transplant. 2000;26(3):299–303.
56. Bobak D, Arfons LM, Creger RJ, Lazarus HM. Clostridium difficile-associated disease in human stem cell transplant recipients: coming epidemic or false alarm? Bone Marrow Transplant. 2008;42(11):705–13.
57. Jillella AP, Ustun C, Robach E, Sertkaya D, DiPiro C, Kallab AM, et al. Infectious complications in patients receiving mobilization chemotherapy for autologous peripheral blood stem cell collection. J Hematother Stem Cell Res. 2003;12(2):155–60.
58. Chopra T, Chandrasekar P, Salimnia H, Heilbrun LK, Smith D, Alangaden GJ. Recent epidemiology of Clostridium difficile infection during hematopoietic stem cell transplantation. Clin Transpl. 2011;25(1):E82–7.
59. Yolken RH, Bishop CA, Townsend TR, Bolyard EA, Bartlett J, Santos GW, et al. Infectious gastroenteritis in bone-marrow-transplant recipients. N Engl J Med. 1982;306(17):1010–2.
60. Mossad SB, Longworth DL, Goormastic M, Serkey JM, Keys TF, Bolwell BJ. Early infectious complications in autologous bone marrow transplantation: a review of 219 patients. Bone Marrow Transplant. 1996;18(2):265–71.
61. Arango JI, Restrepo A, Schneider DL, Callander NS, Ochoa-Bayona JL, Restrepo MI, et al. Incidence of Clostridium difficile-associated diarrhea before and after autologous peripheral blood stem cell transplantation for lymphoma and multiple myeloma. Bone Marrow Transplant. 2006;37(5):517–21.
62. Webb IJ, Eickhoff CE, Elias AD, Ayash LJ, Wheeler CA, Schwartz GN, et al. Kinetics of peripheral blood mononuclear cell mobilization with chemotherapy and/or granulocyte-colony-stimulating factor: implications for yield of hematopoietic progenitor cell collections. Transfusion (Paris). 1996;36(2):160–7.
63. Mani S, Rybicki L, Jagadeesh D, Mossad SB. Risk factors for recurrent Clostridium difficile infection in allogeneic hematopoietic cell transplant recipients. Bone Marrow Transplant. 2016;51(5):713–7.
64. Donnelly JP, Wang HE, Locke JE, Mannon RB, Safford MM, Baddley JW. Hospital-onset Clostridium difficile infection among solid organ transplant recipients. Am J Transplant. 2015;15(11):2970–7.
65. Stelzmueller I, Goegele H, Biebl M, Wiesmayr S, Berger N, Tabarelli W, et al. Clostridium difficile colitis in solid organ transplantation – a single-center experience. Dig Dis Sci. 2007;52(11):3231–6.
66. Albright JB, Bonatti H, Mendez J, Kramer D, Stauffer J, Hinder R, et al. Early and late onset Clostridium difficile-associated colitis following liver transplantation. Transplant Int. 2007;20(10):856–66.
67. Niemczyk M, Leszczyniski P, Wyzgal J, Paczek L, Krawczyk M, Luczak M. Infections caused by clostridium difficile in kidney or liver graft recipients. Ann Transplant. 2005;10(2):70–4.
68. Tsapepas DS, Martin ST, Miao J, Shah SA, Scheffert J, Fester K, et al. Clostridium difficile infection, a descriptive analysis of solid organ transplant recipients at a single center. Diagn Microbiol Infect Dis. 2015;81(4):299–304.
69. Pant C, Deshpande A, Desai M, Jani BS, Sferra TJ, Gilroy R, et al. Outcomes of Clostridium difficile infection in pediatric solid organ transplant recipients. Transplant Infect Dis. 2016;18(1):31–6.
70. Dubberke ER, Reske KA, Yan Y, Olsen MA, McDonald LC, Fraser VJ. Clostridium difficile – associated disease in a setting of endemicity: identification of novel risk factors. Clin Infect Dis. 2007;45(12):1543–9.
71. Jump RL, Pultz MJ, Donskey CJ. Vegetative Clostridium difficile survives in room air on moist surfaces and in gastric contents with reduced acidity: a potential mechanism to explain the association between proton pump inhibitors and *C. difficile*-associated diarrhea? Antimicrob Agents Chemother. 2007;51(8):2883–7.
72. West M, Pirenne J, Chavers B, Gillingham K, Sutherland DE, Dunn DL, et al. Clostridium difficile colitis after kidney and kidney-pancreas transplantation. Clin Transpl. 1999;13(4):318–23.
73. Keven K, Basu A, Re L, Tan H, Marcos A, Fung JJ, et al. Clostridium difficile colitis in patients after kidney and pancreas-kidney transplantation. Transpl Infect Dis. 2004;6(1):10–4.
74. Yamani MH, Avery R, Mawhorter S, Young JB, McNeill A, Cook DJ, et al. Hypogammaglobulinemia after heart transplantation: impact of pre-emptive use of immunoglobulin replacement

(CytoGam) on infection and rejection outcomes. Transpl Infect Dis. 2001;3(Suppl 2):40–3.
75. Doron S, Ruthazer R, Werner BG, Rabson A, Snydman DR. Hypogammaglobulinemia in liver transplant recipients: incidence, timing, risk factors, and outcomes. Transplantation. 2006;81(5):697–703.
76. Mawhorter S, Yamani MH. Hypogammaglobulinemia and infection risk in solid organ transplant recipients. Curr Opin Organ Transplant. 2008;13(6):581–5.
77. Arslan H, Inci EK, Azap OK, Karakayali H, Torgay A, Haberal M. Etiologic agents of diarrhea in solid organ recipients. Transpl Infect Dis. 2007;9(4):270–5.
78. Hsu JL, Enser JJ, McKown T, Leverson GE, Pirsch JD, Hess TM, et al. Outcomes of Clostridium difficile infection in recipients of solid abdominal organ transplants. Clin Transpl. 2014;28(2):267–73.
79. Kawecki D, Chmura A, Pacholczyk M, Lagiewska B, Adadynski L, Wasiak D, et al. Detection of Clostridium difficile in stool samples from patients in the early period after liver transplantation. Transplant Proc. 2007;39(9):2812–5.
80. Kelly CP, Pothoulakis C, LaMont JT. Clostridium difficile colitis. N Engl J Med. 1994;330(4):257–62.
81. Hookman P, Barkin JS. Clostridium difficile associated infection, diarrhea and colitis. World J Gastroenterol. 2009;15(13): 1554–80.
82. Dupont HL. Diagnosis and management of Clostridium difficile infection. Clin Gastroenterol Hepatol. 2013;11(10):1216–23.
83. Avila MB, Avila NP, Dupont AW. Recent advances in the diagnosis and treatment of clostridium difficile infection. F1000Res. 2016;5:F1000 Faculty Rev-118.
84. Dubberke ER, Burdette SD. Practice ASTIDCo. Clostridium difficile infections in solid organ transplantation. Am J Transplant. 2013;13(Suppl 4):42–9.
85. Cohen SH, Gerding DN, Johnson S, Kelly CP, Loo VG, McDonald LC, et al. Clinical practice guidelines for Clostridium difficile infection in adults: 2010 update by the Society for Healthcare Epidemiology of America (SHEA) and the Infectious Diseases Society of America (IDSA). Infect Control Hosp Epidemiol. 2010;31(5):431–55.
86. Bartlett JG. Clinical practice. Antibiotic-associated diarrhea. N Engl J Med. 2002;346(5):334–9.
87. Gerding DN, Olson MM, Peterson LR, Teasley DG, Gebhard RL, Schwartz ML, et al. Clostridium difficile-associated diarrhea and colitis in adults. A prospective case-controlled epidemiologic study. Arch Intern Med. 1986;146(1):95–100.
88. Akahoshi Y, Kimura S, Nakano H, Harada N, Kameda K, Ugai T, et al. Significance of a positive Clostridium difficile toxin test after hematopoietic stem cell transplantation. Clin Transpl. 2016;30(6):703–8.
89. Debast SB, Bauer MP, Kuijper EJ, European Society of Clinical M, Infectious D. European Society of Clinical Microbiology and Infectious Diseases: update of the treatment guidance document for Clostridium difficile infection. Clin Microbiol Infect. 2014;20(Suppl 2):1–26.
90. Johnson S, Louie TJ, Gerding DN, Cornely OA, Chasan-Taber S, Fitts D, et al. Vancomycin, metronidazole, or tolevamer for Clostridium difficile infection: results from two multinational, randomized, controlled trials. Clin Infect Dis. 2014;59(3): 345–54.
91. Zar FA, Bakkanagari SR, Moorthi KM, Davis MB. A comparison of vancomycin and metronidazole for the treatment of Clostridium difficile-associated diarrhea, stratified by disease severity. Clin Infect Dis. 2007;45(3):302–7.
92. Louie TJ, Miller MA, Mullane KM, Weiss K, Lentnek A, Golan Y, et al. Fidaxomicin versus vancomycin for Clostridium difficile infection. N Engl J Med. 2010;364(5):422–31.
93. Dupont HL. Diagnosis and management of Clostridium difficile infection. Clin Gastroenterol Hepatol. 2013;11(10):1216–23; quiz e73.
94. Garey KW, Sethi S, Yadav Y, DuPont HL. Meta-analysis to assess risk factors for recurrent Clostridium difficile infection. J Hosp Infect. 2008;70(4):298–304.
95. Lowy I, Molrine DC, Leav BA, Blair BM, Baxter R, Gerding DN, et al. Treatment with monoclonal antibodies against Clostridium difficile toxins. N Engl J Med. 2010;362(3):197–205.
96. Wilcox MH. Descriptive study of intravenous immunoglobulin for the treatment of recurrent Clostridium difficile diarrhoea. J Antimicrob Chemother. 2004;53(5):882–4.
97. Gerding DN, Muto CA, Owens RC Jr. Treatment of Clostridium difficile infection. Clin Infect Dis. 2008;46(Suppl 1):S32–42.
98. Hall JF, Berger D. Outcome of colectomy for Clostridium difficile colitis: a plea for early surgical management. Am J Surg. 2008;196(3):384–8.
99. Gough E, Shaikh H, Manges AR. Systematic review of intestinal microbiota transplantation (fecal bacteriotherapy) for recurrent Clostridium difficile infection. Clin Infect Dis. 2011;53(10):994–1002.
100. Silverman MS, Davis I, Pillai DR. Success of self-administered home fecal transplantation for chronic Clostridium difficile infection. Clin Gastroenterol Hepatol. 2010;8(5):471–3.
101. O'Horo JC, Jindai K, Kunzer B, Safdar N. Treatment of recurrent Clostridium difficile infection: a systematic review. Infection. 2014;42(1):43–59.
102. Drekonja D, Reich J, Gezahegn S, Greer N, Shaukat A, MacDonald R, et al. Fecal microbiota transplantation for Clostridium difficile infection: a systematic review of the evidence. Fecal microbiota transplantation for Clostridium difficile infection: a systematic review of the evidence. VA evidence-based synthesis program reports. Washington (DC) Ann Intern Med. 2015;162(9):630–8.
103. Kelly CR, Ihunnah C, Fischer M, Khoruts A, Surawicz C, Afzali A, et al. Fecal microbiota transplant for treatment of Clostridium difficile infection in immunocompromised patients. Am J Gastroenterol. 2014;109(7):1065–71.
104. Webb BJ, Brunner A, Ford CD, Gazdik MA, Petersen FB, Hoda D. Fecal microbiota transplantation for recurrent Clostridium difficile infection in hematopoietic stem cell transplant recipients. Transpl Infect Dis. 2016;18(4):628–33.
105. Bilal M, Khehra R, Strahotin C, Mitre R. Long-term follow-up of fecal microbiota transplantation for treatment of recurrent Clostridium difficile infection in a dual solid organ transplant recipient. Case Rep Gastroenterol. 2015;9(2):156–9.
106. Boyle ML, Ruth-Sahd LA, Zhou Z. Fecal microbiota transplant to treat recurrent Clostridium difficile infections. Crit Care Nurse. 2015;35(2):51–64; quiz 5.
107. Borody T, Fischer M, Mitchell S, Campbell J. Fecal microbiota transplantation in gastrointestinal disease: 2015 update and the road ahead. Expert Rev Gastroenterol Hepatol. 2015;9(11):1379–91.
108. Hirsch BE, Saraiya N, Poeth K, Schwartz RM, Epstein ME, Honig G. Effectiveness of fecal-derived microbiota transfer using orally administered capsules for recurrent Clostridium difficile infection. BMC Infect Dis. 2015;17:15.
109. Muto CA, Blank MK, Marsh JW, Vergis EN, O'Leary MM, Shutt KA, et al. Control of an outbreak of infection with the hypervirulent Clostridium difficile BI strain in a university hospital using a comprehensive "bundle" approach. Clin Infect Dis. 2007;45(10):1266–73.
110. Riddle DJ, Dubberke ER. Clostridium difficile infection in solid organ transplant recipients. Curr Opin Organ Transplant. 2008;13(6):592–600.
111. Gerding DN, Muto CA, Owens RC Jr. Measures to control and prevent Clostridium difficile infection. Clin Infect Dis. 2008;46(Suppl 1):S43–9.

112. Davey P, Brown E, Fenelon L, Finch R, Gould I, Hartman G, et al. Interventions to improve antibiotic prescribing practices for hospital inpatients. Cochrane Database Syst Rev. 2005;4:CD003543.
113. Wingard JR, Niehaus CS, Peterson DE, Jones RJ, Piantadosi S, Levin LS, et al. Oral mucositis after bone marrow transplantation. A marker of treatment toxicity and predictor of hepatic veno-occlusive disease. Oral Surg Oral Med Oral Pathol. 1991;72(4):419–24.
114. Fries BC, Riddell SR, Kim HW, Corey L, Dahlgren C, Woolfrey A, et al. Cytomegalovirus disease before hematopoietic cell transplantation as a risk for complications after transplantation. Biol Blood Marrow Transplant. 2005;11(2):136–48.
115. Pico JL, Avila-Garavito A, Naccache P. Mucositis: its occurrence, consequences, and treatment in the oncology setting. Oncologist. 1998;3(6):446–51.
116. Kang G, Srivastava A, Pulimood AB, Dennison D, Chandy M. Etiology of diarrhea in patients undergoing allogeneic bone marrow transplantation in South India. Transplantation. 2002;73(8):1247–51.
117. Salazar R, Sola C, Maroto P, Tabernero JM, Brunet J, Verger G, et al. Infectious complications in 126 patients treated with high-dose chemotherapy and autologous peripheral blood stem cell transplantation. Bone Marrow Transplant. 1999;23(1):27–33.
118. Perez RM, Ferreira AS, Silva IS, Medina-Pestana JO, Lanzoni VP, Silva AE, et al. Hepatitis C virus infection in renal transplant patients: a comparative study with immunocompetent patients. Clin Transpl. 2005;19(6):763–8.
119. Mohanty SR, Cotler SJ. Management of hepatitis B in liver transplant patients. J Clin Gastroenterol. 2005;39(1):58–63.
120. Lin PC, Poh SB, Lee MY, Hsiao LT, Chen PM, Chiou TJ. Fatal fulminant hepatitis B after withdrawal of prophylactic lamivudine in hematopoietic stem cell transplantation patients. Int J Hematol. 2005;81(4):349–51.
121. Ullmann AJ, Lipton JH, Vesole DH, Chandrasekar P, Langston A, Tarantolo SR, et al. Posaconazole or fluconazole for prophylaxis in severe graft-versus-host disease. N Engl J Med. 2007;356(4):335–47.
122. Slavin MA, Osborne B, Adams R, Levenstein MJ, Schoch HG, Feldman AR, et al. Efficacy and safety of fluconazole prophylaxis for fungal infections after marrow transplantation – a prospective, randomized, double-blind study. J Infect Dis. 1995;171(6):1545–52.
123. Weikert BC, Blumberg EA. Viral infection after renal transplantation: surveillance and management. Clin J Am Soc Nephrol. 2008;3(Suppl 2):S76–86.
124. Fishman JA, Emery V, Freeman R, Pascual M, Rostaing L, Schlitt HJ, et al. Cytomegalovirus in transplantation – challenging the status quo. Clin Transpl. 2007;21(2):149–58.
125. Sarmiento JM, Munn SR, Paya CV, Velosa JA, Nguyen JH. Is cytomegalovirus infection related to mycophenolate mofetil after kidney transplantation? A case-control study. Clin Transpl. 1998;12(5):371–4.
126. Keown P, Häyry P, Morris P, Stiller C, Barker C, Carr L, et al. A blinded, randomized clinical trial of mycophenolate mofetil for the prevention of acute rejection in cadaveric renal transplantation. The Tricontinental Mycophenolate Mofetil Renal Transplantation Study Group. Transplant. 1996;61(7):1029–37.
127. Helderman JH, Goral S. Gastrointestinal complications of transplant immunosuppression. J Am Soc Nephrol. 2002;13(1):277–87.
128. Patel R, Paya CV. Infections in solid-organ transplant recipients. Clin Microbiol Rev. 1997;10(1):86–124.

Hepatobiliary Tract Infections

17

Jonathan Merola, Robert M. Mocharla, Alexander Z. Jow, Samuel H. Sigal, and Amar Safdar

Introduction

Patients undergoing solid-organ and hematopoietic stem cell transplantation are at risk for numerous infections involving the hepatobiliary tract. Hepatobiliary tract infections contribute significantly to increased morbidity and mortality among recipients of solid-organ allografts, particularly in patients undergoing liver transplantation. Bacteria and less frequently yeast within the gastrointestinal tract may colonize a dysfunctional biliary system resulting in increased susceptibility for ascending cholangitis. Additionally, opportunistic viral infections such as varicella zoster virus, cytomegalovirus, and Epstein-Barr virus may trigger life-threatening acute illnesses or perpetuate malignancies during the posttransplant period. Fungal and protozoal infections may also find refuge within the biliary tract of immunosuppressed host and requiring multifaceted treatment approach. A thoughtful balance between utilization and adjustment of immunosuppressive medications, which are essential for graft preservation, while limiting the risk for opportunistic bacterial, fungal, viral, and parasitic disease, is pivotal in developing a fastidious approch towards patients undergoing allograft transplantation.

Strategies for infection prevention play an important role in mitigating the risk for infections during the posttransplant period. A thorough pretransplant assessment includes (1) surveillance of active and latent infections, (2) early institution of appropriate antimicrobial drug prophylaxis, and (3) appropriate active and passive immunization. A high level of suspicion for biliary tract and infections involving the liver along with improved new-generation diagnostic tests for early diagnosis, and prompt initiation of effective antimicrobial therapy, as expected, are deemed critical in improved patient outcomes. Lowering drug-induced immune suppression, when possible, remains pivotal in addressing management of infections in this high-risk group. Here were present a comprehensive review of important infections in transplant population involving the hepatobiliary tract.

J. Merola
Department of Surgery, Yale School of Medicine, Yale-New Haven Hospital, New Haven, CT, USA
e-mail: jonathan.merola@yale.edu

R. M. Mocharla
Division of Gastroenterology, NYU School of Medicine, Department of Internal Medicine, New York, NY, USA
e-mail: robert.mocharla@nyumc.org

A. Z. Jow
Division of Gastroenterology, Mid-Atlantic Kaiser Permanente Medical Group, Springfield, VA, USA

S. H. Sigal (✉)
Division of Gastroenterology and Hepatology, Department of Medicine, Albert Einstein College of Medicine, Montefiore Medical Center, Bronx, NY, USA
e-mail: ssigal@montefiore.com

A. Safdar
Clinical Associate Professor of Medicine, Texas Tech University Health Sciences Center El Paso, Paul L. Foster School of Medicine, El Paso, TX, USA
e-mail: amar.safdar@cidimmunology.com

Bacterial Infections

Pretransplant Cholangitis

Acute cholangitis is a common bacterial infection affecting patients undergoing liver transplantation with advanced liver and/or biliary tract disease. The disease process typically involves an ascending bacterial infection originating in the duodenum that migrates into the lower biliary tract. If untreated, the disease can progress resulting in life-threatening systemic dissemination such as bloodstream invasion, sepsis, severe sepsis, multiorgan dysfunction and death. In the pretransplant setting, cholangitis can develop as a complication of cirrhosis due to any etiology as well as be the first manifestation of chronic liver disease. Cirrhotic patients are prone to cholangitis due to altered biliary motility and anatomic aberrancy involving the biliary tract. In patients with chronic liver disease being considered for liver

A. Safdar (ed.), *Principles and Practice of Transplant Infectious Diseases*, https://doi.org/10.1007/978-1-4939-9034-4_17

transplantation, underlying biliary disease increases the risk for cholangitis; these include patients with primary or secondary cholangitis and less commonly, other causes of primary biliary tract disease. Following transplantation, such infections may result from technical complications arising from vascular insufficiency and/or compromised biliary duct anastomoses.

In the normally functioning biliary system, the sphincter of Oddi and the constant forward flow of bile prevents retrograde spread of bacteria from the duodenum into the biliary tract. With the frequent clearing of bacteriostatic bile salts, bacterial multiplication is kept in check. These protective systems, however, are less effective in patients with chronic liver and/or biliary tract disease. Inflammatory damage to the hepatocyte and epithelial cells in the bile ducts distort the normal hepatic architecture and bile flow, predisposing to biliary stasis and gallstone formation. The presence of gallstones in turn serves as a nidus that promotes the risk for ascending cholangitis. Bile aspirated from individuals without gallstone disease is usually sterile. However, nearly 32% of bile cultures taken from cancer patients with gallstones demonstrate bacterial colonization [1].

Primary sclerosing cholangitis (PSC) is characterized by chronic inflammatory damage of the intrahepatic and extrahepatic bile ducts, the resulting fibrosis leads to strictures throughout the biliary tract. Although the precise etiology of this disease is not known, due its co-occurrence with inflammatory bowel disease, especially ulcerative colitis, autoimmune damage is presently the favored hypothesis for this progressive and devastating illness. Chronic inflammation impedes normal excretion of bile due to stricture formation and anatomic distortion of bile duct system, resulting in frequent episodes of cholangitis. Patients with PSC are also at a higher risk for gallstone formation. Endoscopic treatment to dilate or place stents in the region of severe bile duct narrowing is often undertaken to alleviate bile stasis and to reduce the risk for recurrent infections.

Secondary sclerosing cholangitis (SSC) is radiographically and clinically similar to PSC. Recurring injury to the bile ducts seen in patients with chronic gallstone disease, recurrent pancreatitis, surgical trauma to the biliary system, treatment with antineoplastic drugs, eosinophilic cholangitis, recurrent bacterial cholangitis, and HIV cholangiopathy are some of the common causes [2]. Injury to the bile duct results in anatomic damage and aberration in bile excretion predisposing to ascending bacterial colonization and infections. Finally, cholangitis may be associated with congenital diseases such Caroli disease and Caroli syndrome. Caroli disease involves the cystic dilation of intrahepatic bile ducts, and Caroli syndrome involves bile duct dilatation as well as congenital hepatic fibrosis [3]. These patients are prone to recurrent acute cholangitis, which manifest as the presenting sign in nearly two-thirds of the patients [4]. The true incidence of cholangitis is likely underestimated, as biliary strictures likely lead to frequent, and conceivably transient bacterial infection.

Acute cholangitis characteristically presents with jaundice, fever, and right upper quadrant abdominal pain. Because patients with chronic liver or biliary tract disease may be chronically jaundiced and have abdominal pain and fever from other causes such as spontaneous bacterial peritonitis, the diagnosis may not be readily perceived. In addition, intrahepatic fibrosis may prevent the development of intrahepatic biliary dilatation [5]. Among patients with hepatic cirrhosis, the diagnostic approach with ultrasound, CT scan, MRCP, and ERCP is the same as for the non-cirrhotic patient. However, ERCP carries significant risk for complications in patients with cirrhosis due to (1) the adverse effects of sedation in preexisting hepatic encephalopathy, (2) risk of uncontrolled bleeding due to coagulopathy, and (3) procedure-associated pancreatitis. ERCP-associated pancreatitis is a serious complication, especially in patients with end-stage liver disease. However, diagnosis and relief from bile duct obstruction is crucial in preventing future infections and other complications.

The causative organisms of acute cholangitis are of intestinal origin and similar to those associated with cholecystitis. Aerobic Gram-negative bacteria (GNB) such as *Escherichia coli*, *Klebsiella* spp. and *Enterobacter* spp.; occasionally, Gram-positive bacteria (GPB) such as *Enterococcus* spp. are isolated. Anaerobes such as *Bacteroides fragilis* or *Clostridium perfringens* are uncommon pathogens [6]. In patients with PSC, *Candida* species are increasingly isolated from the bile cultures [7]. Concurrent yeast and bacterial polymicrobial infection may result in a more severe form of cholangitis. Systemic antifungals should be considered early in the course of therapy for acute cholangitis, especially in patients with known biliary tract yeast colonization, in whom initial empiric antibacterial therapy has failed.

Effective treatment consists of a multifaceted approach including systemic antimicrobials, biliary tract drainage, and supportive care. Current recommendations are to cover broadly for aerobic GNB, GPB, and anaerobes. More than 50% of cases respond well to conservative antimicrobial treatment alone, given for 7–10 days [8]. If patients' clinical status declines or infection fails to improve within the first 24 h after treatment with antibiotics has commenced, emergent drainage of the biliary tract is recommended. Patient with cirrhosis experience high frequency of complications following ERCP and sphincterotomy. Approximately 3–8% of cirrhotic patients will experience bleeding, and 4–5% may develop acute pancreatitis following sphincterotomy [9, 10]. Other complications such as secondary cholangitis, cholecystitis, stent occlusion, stent migration, and bile leak are also more frequent in patients with cirrhosis of liver [10]. Cholangitis in patients with PSC commonly requires dilation and/or stenting of bile duct strictures. Placement of a foreign object act as an additional nidus, that increases the risk for future infections; recurrent cholangitis was more common after stent placement compared with PSC patients, in whom only balloon dilation was performed [10]. Finally, percutaneous transhepatic cholangiography (PTC) can be employed in cases in which ERCP is not possible due to prior surgery; however, PTC carries an increased risk for bacteremia, hemorrhage, hemobilia, and creation of vascular-biliary fistula. This technique cannot be employed in patients with significant ascites as the ascitic fluid prevents maturation of the cutaneobiliary tract [11].

For patients with frequent, recurrent cholangitis associated with surgical alterations of the biliary tract such as hepaticojejunostomy and sphincteroplasty, the use of long-term antibiotic prophylaxis with rotating antibiotic regimens including amoxicillin-clavulanic acid, trimethoprim-sulfamethoxazole, or ciprofloxacin are proposed to reduce recurrences of cholangitis episodes [12, 13]. As with all long-term antibiotic prophylaxis, colonization and infection due to drug-resistant organisms remain a serious concern.

Finally, potential liver transplant recipients with PSC, during the episodes of recurrent cholangitis, have an increased risk of death; however, it is considerably lower during the intervals without such infection episodes. To account for this additional risk of death, patients who have two or more serious episodes of cholangitis requiring hospitalization and intravenous antibiotic therapy within a 6-month period are eligible to receive MELD exception points to prioritize their prospect for hepatic allograft transplantation [14].

Posttransplantation Cholangitis

Cholangitis that occurs after transplantation procedure can be classified into conditions associated with anatomic alterations in liver transplant recipients and those associated with anti-rejection drug regimen-induced immune suppression. With the first category, bacterial pathogens are most common. In the subsequent category, polymicrobial infections associated with high level of drug-induced, cumulative immune suppression become more prominent. Temporal-relationship, and other associated features such as source of the hepatic allograft, transplantation procedure, and the underlying etiology of end-stage liver disease are important features in assessing patients with cholangitis after transplantation.

Bacterial Cholangitis

Acute cholangitis is the most common infectious complication in liver transplant recipients and may arise at any time after undergoing transplantation. Alterations in the normal biliary anatomy predisposes to infections resulting from choledochojejunostomy anastomosis. Most surgical complications involve the biliary system; 15–30% of transplant recipients will experience a complication involving the biliary tract [15]. Surgical complications such as bile leakage, wound dehiscence, and bile duct strictures are commonly associated with the risk of cholangitis. Recurrence of primary disease in patients with PSC is a well-known risk for acute cholangitis. Finally, viral infections may involve the liver and confer a greater risk of cholangitis by promoting bile stasis.

The causes and risks associated with the infection can roughly be grouped according to two main time periods: within 30 days and after 1st month following transplantation [16]. The incidence of acute cholangitis begins to decrease after the 1st year following transplantation. This is presumably due to a decline in the risk factors for cholangitis that usually manifest early after transplant surgery.

During the first several weeks immediately following liver transplantation, surgical complications are the main cause of acute cholangitis. Acute cholangitis in the first 30 days following transplant is commonly related to biliary anastomotic leaks. Bile leaks usually manifest within the first 30 days after transplant surgery, with a mean time for presentation being 17 days [17]. Subsequently, acute cholangitis as a direct result of surgical complication becomes much less common. Placement of biliary T-tube in the duct-o-duct anastomosis increases the overall risk for complications, including the risk for cholangitis [18].

After the first month, strictures in the biliary tract become the leading cause of cholangitis. Strictures can be classified as either anastomotic or non-anastomotic strictures and typically present around 6 months after transplantation [19]. Anastomotic strictures are short, limited to the surgical anastomosis site, resulting from fibrotic scar tissue formation. Non-anastomotic strictures are typically multiple, long, and proximal to the site of anastomosis involving within the transplanted hepatic allograft. They are divided into three main groups based on causative etiology: macroangiopathic, microangiopathic, and immunogenic. Macroangiopathic strictures are related to vascular events, the most common being hepatic artery thrombosis and hepatic artery stenosis, with an incidence of 1–3% [20]. Non-anastomotic strictures due to microangiopathic complications are related to ischemic events that occur during perioperative period involving donor liver or surgical and postsurgical complications in the recipients such as inadequate tissue perfusion or the need for systemic vasopressor support. Bile duct complications are more frequent in patients undergoing living donor transplantation (LDT) due to the complex biliary and vascular grafting techniques; bile leaks and strictures may occur in up to 12.6 and 5.8% of LDT cases, respectively [21]. Finally, recurrence of primary sclerosing cholangitis can cause immunogenic strictures. Of all the causes of biliary strictures, immunogenic strictures present furthest from the transplant procedure.

The most such complications will present within the first 18 months after transplant; however, they may be encountered years after transplantation [22, 23]. Approximately 10–20% of patients undergoing transplantation for PSC will develop disease recurrence with a median presentation time of 68 months [23, 24]. These cases are associated with HLA subtype, presence of acute cellular rejection, and necessity for chronic systemic corticosteroid therapy for ulcerative colitis [24].

Transplant recipients may or may not present with typical symptoms suggestive of acute cholangitis, and comparable clinical presentation of other conditions may initially obscure the diagnosis. Abdominal pain is not uncommon after liver transplant surgery. Liver biochemistries may be abnormal due for a variety of reasons. As a result, it is often difficult to diagnose an acute episode of cholangitis based on classic physical and laboratory findings. In addition, biliary dilatation is frequently absent in patients with cholangitis due to local edema, blood clots, and sludge in the bile ducts that obscure accurate visualization of the biliary tract. Abdominal ultrasound has low diagnostic sensitivity of 38–68% [25]. As a result, diagnostic MRCP is recommended in all appropriate clinical settings.

Treatment of acute cholangitis in the transplant population is similar to treatment approach for patients with acute cholangitis during pretransplant period; prompt initiation of empiric antibiotic coverage for GNB and GPB is recommended. Concomitant fungal infection may be present in 1–12% among such infections, typically *Candida* spp., rarely *Aspergillus* spp., and it is exceedingly rare to find extrapulmonary *Pneumocystis* as a concurrent fungal pathogen [16, 26]. Antifungal coverage should also be considered in patients receiving intensified antirejection regimen. Invasive fungal disease of the biliary tract is often rapidly fatal unless effective systemic treatment is given empirically and high level of suspicion plays an important role in such decision making [27]. Finally, ERCP-assisted biliary decompression with drainage and placement of stents may be needed.

Cholangitis Associated with Immunosuppression

Immunosuppression used to prevent or treat liver graft rejection predisposes the patients to infection with a variety of viruses and fungi which are normally harmless in individuals with intact immune function. In patients with CMV hepatitis, viral infection may extend to involve the biliary tract; fungal infections primarily *Candida* spp. and less commonly *Aspergillus* spp. may occur, especially in highly susceptible population with (1) documented fungal infection prior to transplantation; (2) advanced renal disease; (3) patients after prolonged transplant operative time; and (4) those with a choledochojejunostomy.

Cholecystitis

Cholelithiasis and cholecystitis are prevalent in the general population, nearly 500,000 cholecystectomies are performed annually in the United States [28]. Detection and treatment of the disease among otherwise healthy individuals is generally successful without significant morbidity and mortality. However, gallbladder disease and surgery in the cirrhotic patient carries significant risk. Development of gallstones and progression to cholecystitis is common in patients with hepatic cirrhosis, this is ascribed to high levels of estrogen, unconjugated bilirubin, and increased risk for hemolysis. In patients with cirrhosis of liver, gallstones may develop at a frequency of 38% higher compared with general population [29, 30]. The prevalence of gallstones increases with disease severity, and recent studies have suggested chronic hepatitis C viral infection as an independent risk factor for gallstone disease in patients with cirrhosis [31, 32].

Clinical presentation of cholecystitis in patients with cirrhosis may be similar to that observed in the general population; however, presence of abdominal distension and abdominal pain from ascites, preexisting liver test abnormalities may obscure the diagnosis. The bacteriology of acute cholecystitis in cirrhosis is similar to that of cholecystitis in otherwise healthy patient, namely, the normal intestinal flora. Gram-negative bacilli such as *E.coli*, *Klebsiella pneumoniae*, *Klebsiella oxytoca*, and *Enterobacter* spp. and anaerobes such as *Bacteroides* and *Fusobacterium* spp. are frequently isolated. Due to higher frequency of exposure to the healcare environment including hospitalization and frequent antibiotic use including antimicrobials given for prevention of spontaneous bacterial peritonitis in patients with end-stage cirrhosis; the probability of infections due to multidrug-resistant organisms (MDROs) is a concern. Colonization of the gastrointestinal tract with MDROs and unusual pathogens resulting from altered hosts' microbiota is regarded as an important contributor in the changing spectrum of the causative agents for acute cholecystitis [33, 34]. Additionally, cirrhotic patients are at increased risk for renal failure due to impairments in normal renal circulation [35]. Predictive factors for renal failure in this population include, higher baseline MELD score of greater than 27 and severity of infection; therefore, administration of albumin with antibiotics has been proposed to improve outcomes in high-risk individuals [36].

Curative therapy for cholecystitis involves surgical removal of the gallbladder, however, patients with cirrhosis are poor surgical candidates. Derangements in fluid dynamics due to portal hypertension, dysregulation in coagulation cascade, and overall poor functional performance status in patients with end-stage liver disease are some of the salient factors contributing to the significant risk associated with surgery. Cirrhosis follows cardiovascular disease such as congestive heart failure in predicting complications during and after surgery. Prior to the advent of laparoscopic cholecystectomy, advanced cirrhosis was considered as a contraindication for cholecystectomy due to high mortality rates approaching 25–83%. Such patients were managed conservatively with systemic antibiotics and supportive care [37, 38]. Surgical complications included intra-abdominal hemorrhage, variceal bleed, development or worsening of ascites, superimposed infection(s), and cardiovascular compromise. With laparoscopy advanced cholecystectomy techniques, favorable outcomes have improved substantially [39] and should be attempted as the initial approach for a select group of patients [40]. Laparoscopic surgery is associated with shorter hospital stay, earlier resumption of enteral feeding, earlier ambulation, less blood loss, and reduced pain during the postoperative period [41]. Additionally, postoperative ascites is less common after laparoscopic procedure; probably a reflection on reduced disruption of hepatic and biliary lymphatic circulation and lower risk of bleeding in the peritoneal cavity [42]. In cases where laparoscopic total cholecystectomy is not possible due to extensive fibrosis and/or severe local inflammation, subtotal cholecystectomy procedure that leaves the posterior wall of the gallbladder intact along the liver allows symptomatic relief and clinical resolution of the infection, while mitigating the aforementioned risk of complications associated with a more invasive surgical dissection needed during total cholecystectomy procedure [42–44].

Operation risk was initially assessed with Child-Turcotte-Pugh classification. Individuals with Child-Pugh A or B score were considered safe to undergo surgical procedure, whereas those with Child-Pugh C were managed with conservative therapy alone [45, 46]. More recently, the MELD (model for end-stage liver disease) scoring system, which also includes serum bilirubin, INR, and serum creatinine levels, has shown to be a more accurate predictor of postoperative survival. In a retrospective study between 1995 and 2009, complications following surgery significantly increased in patients with MELD scores greater than 13 [47]. Postoperative complications including hemorrhage, abdominal fluid collection, wound infection, and pulmonary infection increased from 11.6% in those with a MELD score of <13 to as high as 45.8% in patients with a MELD score higher than 13 [48, 49]. Many of the surgical complications were a result of portal hypertension, which increases the risk for hemorrhage, formation of ascites, and renal failure during and after surgery. Placement of transjugular intrahepatic portosystemic shunt (TIPS) is now routinely used to lower portal circulation pressure in patients with end-stage liver disease with refractory ascites and/or recurrent, or severe varecieal bleed. This procedure has made liver and intra-abdominal surgery possible in patients, in whom such procedures otherwise would have been differed [50–53]. Patients with advanced cirrhosis are still considered high-risk candidates for laparoscopic cholecystectomy, despite best medical optimization efforts. For appropriate patients, liver transplantation is the only feasible approach. As a provisional measure for patients in urgent need for biliary tract decompression, percutaneous drainage via transhepatic route by placement of cholecystostomy tube or immediate gallbladder aspiration may be considered. Numerous studies have examined this technique versus laparoscopic cholecystectomy among high-risk patients such as elderly and those with multiple comorbidities; favorable results accompanied by reduced complication rates make this as a first-line approach for a select group of high-risk individuals. Treatment success rates approach 83–85% with 30-day mortality rates between 12 and 15% among otherwise inoperable patients [54, 55]. Similar studies involving patients with severe cirrhosis have shown similar favorable outcomes [56]. Finally, placement of stents in the cystic duct during ERCP has also been evaluated. A case series involving 13 nonsurgical candidates with advanced cirrhosis and symptomatic gallbladder disease reported successful stent placement from gallbladder into the duodenum with complete resolution of symptoms and absence of major complications with the procedure [57].

Hepatic Abscess

Hepatic abscesses are a rare, albeit a life-threatening complication in patients undergoing allograft transplantation [58]. As with other serious infections, a high index of suspicion, prompt diagnosis, and institution of appropriate therapy are the essential components for better outcome [58]. Risk factors include diabetes mellitus, hepatic artery thrombosis, and strictures involving the bile duct anastomosis site. Most liver abscesses develop within the first 3 months following transplantation surgery; liver ultrasonography remains the quickest and safest diagnostic test [58, 59]. Enteric Gram-negative bacilli are common causative organisms, including enteric organims with hyperproduction of capsular polysaccharide or those exhibiting hypermucoviscosity, such monomicrobial infections can lead to large, multiloculated intrahepatic collections. Polymicrobial infections, mixed aerobic, ananerobic bacteria and less frequently *Candida* spp. infection may occur. Treatment involves surgical or intervention radiology-assisted abscess drainage, and broad-spectrum intravenous antibiotics.

Viral Infections

Cytomegalovirus

Cytomegalovirus (CMV) is a member of the β-herpesvirus group and is endemic around the world with seroprevalence rates ranging from 45 to 100% [60, 61]. In immunocompetent hosts, primary CMV infection most commonly presents without symptoms or as a self-limiting mononucleosis-like syndrome. Infected individuals harbor the virus for life in a latent phase. However, reaction of the virus in immunocompromised individuals following allograft transplantation is common and associated with significant morbidity and death [62].

Primary CMV infection in the general popultion presents as asymptomatic infection, and in 10% as mild self-limiting illness; whereas, life-threatening viral disease may rarely lead to severe cholestatic hepatitis and fulminant hepatic failure (FHH) [63–67]. CMV may involve any internal organ; in abdominal organ transplant recipients, gastrointestinal viral disease is most frequently encountered. In one report, FHH due to CMV infection was successfully treated with an emergency living-donor liver transplantation and ganciclovir therapy continued during the posttransplant period. Following liver transplantation, CMV is the most common viral pathogen that affects the overall outcome after transplantation. The clinical impact of CMV infection can be categorized as direct or an indirect viral effect. Direct effects of CMV can manifest as either CMV syndrome with fever, viral myelosuppression, or tissue-invasive end-organ viral disease [68]. CMV may involve any organ resulting in hepatitis, esophagitis, gastritis, enteritis, colitis, meningioencephalitis, retinitis, and pneumonitis to name a few. Transplanted liver allografts are more susceptible to tissue-invasive CMV disease compared with the risk of viral disease involviong the native organ. Reactivation of latent CMV infection in CMV seropositive recipient or allograft-transmitted primary CMV infection in CMV naive liver transplant recipient are well-established risk factor for poor allograft function and patient survival [62, 69, 70]. CMV has the ability to upregulate alloantigen presentation thereby promoting the risk of both, acute and chronic allograft rejection; CMV-induced immune dysregulation included stunted hosts' cellular immune response increases the risk for infection due to other opportunistic pathogens; and its adverse impact on accelerated HCV recurrence after liver transplantation are all important issues [71]. CMV infection has been linked to the vanishing bile duct syndrome, chronic rejection noticeable by ductopenia, and extrahepatic bile duct strictures resulting in chronic cholestasis and eventual allograft failure [72–74].

Epstein-Barr Virus Infection

Epstein-Barr virus (EBV), a member of the herpes virus family, is a nearly ubiquitous infection in humans. According to the World Health Organization (WHO), nearly 95% of the world's population by the age of 35–40 years has latent EBV infection [75]. The virus is transmitted via oropharyngeal secretions and consists of a linear DNA genome, nucleocapsid, and viral envelope. Infection is usually transmitted in early adolescence, and most primary infections are asymptomatic with only 30% presenting as acute viral illness [75]. Primary clinical EBV infection, known as infectious mononucleosis, causes a flu-like illness, patients may have fever, pharyngitis, generalized lymphadenopathy, splenomegaly, atypical lymphocytosis, and elevations in transaminase levels. Acute infection is usually a self-limiting illness and managed with supportive care; most infections resolve in 4–6 weeks. Less than 5% of patients present with jaundice [76]. In very rare instances, acute EBV infection leads to fulminant hepatic failure with jaundice, aminotransferase levels elevated to 10,000–20,000 international units; hepatic encephalopathy, coagulopathy, and thrombocytopenia are other common features. In some, an alarming progression of disease may result in nearly 90% mortality [77]. Although fulminant hepatic failure is more common in immunocompromised patients [78], this has been reported in individuals with competent immune function, both adults and children are at risk for this rare complication [79, 80]. Serologic testing confirms acute EBV primary infection; blood EBV quantitative PCR is better to assess severity of infection. Low levels of free EBV DNA are usually present in acute infection, whereas high viral DNA levels are noted in severe life-threatening cases; patients with fatal EBV infection tend to have 100× higher EBV DNA level in blood [81]. Liver transplantation is the only curative treatment once disease has progressed to fulminant hepatic failure. Although there is no expert consensus or ongoing trials to assess pharmacotherapy, high-dose steroids, antiviral agents; plasmapheresis is recommended while awaiting liver transplantation. Finally, there is limited information regarding the risk for EBV recurrence after transplantation in patients with EBV-induced liver failure. A single case report noted prevention of EBV recurrence up to 2 years after hepatic allograft transplantation with a regimen of acyclovir, low-dose antirejection immune suppression, and anti-EBV gamma globulin therapy; however, this has not been replicated in other reports [77]. In the posttransplant period, acute EBV infection can either be the result of a primary infection or more commonly reactivation of remotely acquired latent viral infection. EBV has been implicated in a number of diseases that may occur in this population, such as posttransplant lymphoproliferative disorder, lymphoma, nasopharyngeal carcinoma, Burkett's lymphoma, and Hodgkin's disease and are discussed in detail elsewhere [82–86].

Herpes Simplex

Herpes simplex virus (HSV) is a common, double-stranded DNA virus with two subtypes HSV-1 and HSV-2; in the developed world prevalence of HSV-1 is around 80% and HSV-2 nearly 30% [87, 88]. Primary and recurrent HSV infection may rarely result in a disseminated infection that may result in fulminant hepatitis. Less than 1% of acute liver failure and 2% of viral-induced acute liver failure are caused by HSV [87, 89]. HSV hepatitis most commonly affects infants who acquire the virus via vertical transmission and adults with impaired cellular immunity due to malignancy, HIV/AIDS, and treatment with immunosuppressive anti-rejection or anti-GVHD drugs [90–92]. Though commonly associated with immune deficiency, 25% of patients with HSV hepatitis are seen in patients with apparently competent immune function [87]. The development of HSV hepatitis can occur as a result of large inoculums at the time of initial infection that overwhelm natural immune defenses or secondary to dissemination from recrudescent herpetic lesion in the absence of an effective hosts' immune response. Virulence through reactivation of latent virus with superimposed infection due to a new viral strain and infection due to hepatotropic viral strain promote risk for HSV hepatitis [92–94].

Patients with HSV hepatitis most commonly present with fever (98%), coagulopathy (84%), encephalopathy (80%), and leukopenia (71%) [87]. A rise in transaminase levels in the absence of jaundice is a characteristic feature of severe HSV hepatitis [90]. The presence of a herpetic rash can be observed in 40–60% of cases [87, 92]. Diagnosis of HSV hepatitis is challenging, as most cases are diagnosed during postmortem examination [87]. Pelvic examination may be helpful as women may less evident vaginal or cervical herpetic lesions while sparing the vulva or perineum [87, 95]. Tzanck smear, or direct fluorescent antibody staining of skin lesions aid in diagnosis [87, 96]. Serologic testing has limited clinical use [87]. Detection of HSV DNA in blood by PCR and/or demonstration/isolation of the virus in liver biopsy samples is needed for establishing diagnosis [87, 97]. Gross pathologic specimens of HSV hepatitis are characterized by a mottled appearance with multiple red-yellow necrotic lesions. Histologic examination often reveals centrilobular hemorrhagic necrosis, scattered acidophilic bodies, and intranuclear ground-glass inclusions with margination of chromatin. The inflammatory response in these tissue specimens is often minimal [90, 98, 99].

Clinical suspicion alone should prompt initiation of high-dose intravenous acyclovir given as 10 mg/kg dose every 8 h adjusted to renal dysfunction, when present [94, 100]. In a review of 134 patients with HSV hepatitis, 49 were treated with acyclovir within 4 days of the symptoms onset; 51% deaths and progression to liver transplant vs. 81% in the untreated group was a significant difference in outcome [87]. Risk factors for death and liver transplantation include age > 40, male gender, coagulopathy, immunosuppression, encephalopathy, ALT >5000, platelets <75,000 U, and the absence of treatment with acyclovir. A delay in institution of antiviral therapy of 4.7 vs. 3.5 days from the onset of symptoms was significantly related with the risk for death or need for urgent liver transplantation. Three of seven patients who underwent orthotopic liver transplantation for HSV acute liver failure survived [87]. Children have a significantly better 5-year survival (74%) compare with long-term survival of 27% seen in adult liver transplant recipients with fulminant HSV hepatitis [92].

Acyclovir prophylaxis is recommended for all patients undergoing liver transplantation for HSV liver failure [98, 100]. However, several recent reports have noted recurrence of infection due to acyclovir-resistant HSV strains following transplantation, close monitoring is recommneded for possible recurrent infection due to a mutant viral strains [97, 98]. Foscarnet therapy followed by liver retransplantation in such cases demonstrated a 43% survival rate, though the degree of immune suppression in patients with severe sepsis-like syndrome should be deemed carefully [101–103].

Fungal Infections

Aspergillosis

Aspergillus is a ubiquitous, saprophytic fungus that is widely distributed in the natural environment and the second most common cause of invasive fungal disease (IFD) in patients undergoing liver transplantation [104, 105]. Nearly one quarter of all IFD is due to *Aspergillus* spp. and account for 1–8% of infections in the post-liver transplant period [106]. Risk factors of invasive aspergillosis include renal insufficiency, retransplantation, CMV infection, thrombocytopenia, leukocytopenia, recurrent bacterial infections, allograft dysfunction, fulminant hepatic failure, high requirement for blood and blood products, and treatment with anti CD3 monoclonal antibodies [106–113]. Invasive aspergillosis historically manifest within 3 weeks after liver transplantation. However, several recent studies have noted that most cases of invasive aspergillosis are seen 100 days after transplant surgery [108, 114–116]. This late occurrence coincides with CMV infection and prophylaxis with fluconazole, when used does not provide adequate protection against filamentous molds such as *Aspergillus* spp. [106]. Hepatic *Aspergillus* spp. abscesses were described in liver and in renal transplant recipients, especially during treatment with high-dose corticosteroid therapy for acute allograft rejection [117, 118].

Invasive aspergillosis (IA) typically manifest as a sinopulmonary disease in patients undergoing allogeneic hematopoietic stem cell transplantation, and due to neurotropism, fungal brain involvement may also occur, although fungal brain abscesses are not common complications in allograft transplant patients with IA. Given its ability to invade blood vessels, fungus may be disseminated widely and patients may have clinically diverse presentations, including involvement of the eyes, liver, spleen, heart, kidneys, bone, and brain [119]. In patients with seldom seen aspergillosis of the liver, fungal abscesses and mycotic aneurysms are notible presentations [117, 120–123]. Posttransplant mycotic abscesses carry a significant mortality of nearly 60%; it is important to note that ruptured mycotic aneurysm may be the initial presentation of IA in patients undergoing liver allograft transplants [117, 120–123]. Early diagnosis continues to pose a challenge and thought to contribute toward high mortality seen with these infections [124–126]. All liver abscesses require guided aspiration to establish correct diagnosis and early institution of appropriate therapy [117, 120–122]. Fungal stains and culture of fine-needle aspirates samples from intra- or extrahepatic collections should be performed routinely; however, to establish diagnosis of proven IFD, it is important to demonstrate tissue invasion by molds; and tissue biopsy should be pursued when possible in patients suspected for invasive aspergillosis [117, 120–122]. The role of ancillary fungal antigen assays such as beta D glucan and galactomannan for diagnosis of IA involving hepatic allograft remain uncertain.

Amphotericin was effective in the treatment of hepatic mycotic pseudoaneurysms [127]. Mortality rate associated with aspergillus abscesses in allograft transplant recipients was unacceptably high, despite treatment with amphotericin B [117, 120–122]. The addition of broad-spectrum triazole-based drugs such as voriconazole, posaconazole and the recent addition of isavuconazonium sulfate in the current antifungal armamentarium provided a less toxic and more effective treatment option for these life-threatening opportunistic pathogens. Similarly, echinocandins including caspofungin, micafungin, and anidulafungin also considered safe treatment option and with significantly less potential for drug-drug interaction compared with the triazole drugs. Reduced intragenic, drug-induced immune suppression is important in solid allograft transplant patients with an active invasive fungal disease, an option that is not available for patients with IFD following allogeneic HSCT. Surgical drainage, excision of necrotic tissue, or resection of the infected devitalized organ is considered as important as treatment with effective antifungal drugs [117, 119, 121, 128, 129]. However, due to various reasons, patients with IFD during posttransplant period may not be suitable candidate for surgical resection or debridement.

Candidiasis

Candida is a commensal yeast normally found on skin and mucus membranes of upper respiratory, orointestinal, and genitourinary tracts [119]. Particular disease-causing species of *Candida* may lead to tissue invasive infection with a potential for widespread hematogenous systemic dissemination. Yeast colonization involving multiple body-sites, yeast overgrowth in patients with impaired milieu inflicting alterations in hosts' protective microbiota, presences of indwelling foreign devices such as intravascular catheters, and surgical drains increases the risk for invasive candidiasis in severely immunosuppressed patients undergoing transplantation. Individuals treated with extended and often multiple courses of broad-spectrum antibiotics and prolonged exposure to healthcare that includes doctors office visit, repeat hospitalizations among others, are vulnerable to these complications.

Candida infection plays a particularly prominent role in the development of cholangitis. In a recent retrospective study of 171 patients with PSC that were followed for 20 years, the presence of *Candida* in biliary cultures was associated with a significantly poor transplant-free survival compared to patients with sterile bile cultures [130]. Infection with *Candida* and *Enterococcus* is responsible for sclerosing cholangitis in critically ill patients, this entity represents severe biliary disease, which may rapidly progress to liver cirrhosis; distinguished from PSC by a more rapid clinical course and absence of a prior history of liver disease or injury responsible for bile duct obstruction [131].

Early diagnosis of invasive candidiasis presents a challenge as clinical features are not specific and *Candida* colonization is particularly common in such hospitalized patients; furthermore, lack of sensitivity of routine blood cultures makes diagnosis of fungemia difficult. The fungal antigen assasys like beta-D-glucan assay, which detects fungal cell wall complex sugar in blood and bronchoscopy samples, common to most clinically relevant fungi, are increasingly used to diagnose *Candida* spp. invasive disease. Several studies in renal transplant recipients have noted a diagnostic specificity of 80% and a sensitivity of 50% with this assay [132–134]. Dialysis with cellulose membranes, concomitant use of certain antibiotics, perhaps infection due to *S. pneumoniae*, use of albumin products, coagulation factors, and human plasma-derived albumin and globulin may occasionally result in false-positive detection of beta-D-glucan in sterile body fluid samples [135]. Recently, flow cytometry has been used to identify yeast colonization in patients undergoing living-donor liver transplantation [136].

Empiric antifungal therapy is recommended in organ transplant patients with persistent fever, despite treatement with broad-spectrum antibiotics [119]. Historically, amphotericin B was considered the drug of choice at a dose of 0.5–0.7 mg/kg/day [119]. Echinocandins, such as caspofungin, micafungin, or anidulafungin, have shown high degree of efficacy and excellent safety profile compared with amphotericin B in patients undergoing solid-organ and hematopoietic stem cell transplantation [137–141]. A recent case report by Goicoechea et al. has documented biliary excretion of caspofungin at levels above the MIC_{50} for *C. albicans* [142].

Transient elevation of serum transaminases was observed in patients receiving caspofungin 70 mg daily along with cyclosporine; FDA has cautioned against such combination therapy [143, 144]. Fluconazole remains an alternative agent for *C. albicans* infections, although increasing resistance among the *C. glabrata* clinical isolates warrants fluconazole use as first-line agent, especially in transplant patients with invasive candidiasis, which may include anastomosis site abscesses, fungal cholangitis, with or without evidence of fungemia [145–147].

Protozoal Infections

Cryptosporidium

Cryptosporidium is a genus of protozoan parasites that causes an acute, self-limited diarrheal illness in the normal host, whereas in patients with severe immune suppression, *Cryptosporidium* may be responsible for debilitating chronic diarrheal illness. The most common species affecting humans is *Cryptosporidium parvum*, which is ubiquitous in natural water source around the world; transmission occurs via ingestion of water or food contaminated with mature oocysts. Cryptosporidiosis is an uncommon illness among transplant recipients in the United States and Europe; however, such infections are more visible in the immunosuppressed patients residing or visiting *Cryptospridium* endemic regions in the Middle East, India, South America, or Africa.

Extraintestinal manifestations are rare; biliary tract involvement has been noted in patients with advanced HIV/AIDS, those with congenital immunodeficiencies, and in patients undergoing organ allograft transplantation [148–154]. Biliary manifestations observed in patients with AIDS include acalculous cholecystitis, sclerosing cholangitis, and pancreatitis [148, 149]. Diagnosis of cryptosporidiosis is based on microscopic examination of stool with findings of oocysts similar to size and shape of yeasts [154]. Immunofluorescent assays that employ monoclonal antibodies against *Cryptosporidium* oocysts and antigen-detection assays by ELISA and immunochromatographic formats are also available and have higher sensitivity compared with stool studies using acid-fast staine. Initial management should focus on replacement of fluids and electrolytes. Treatment includes reducing the degree of drug-induced immunosuppression; antiparasitic agents active against *C. parvum* are nitazoxanide, paromomycin, or macrolide antibiotics [154]. To date, only five cases of *C. parvum*-associated sclerosing cholangitis have been reported in the transplant population [150–152]. One case was reported in an adult renal transplant recipient with a reversal of cholangiopathy secondary to *C. parvum* after reduction in immunosuppression [152]. Three other cases were in children in a series of 461 pediatric liver transplant recipients who developed diarrhea with a diffuse cholangitis while on immunosuppression with tacrolimus and prednisone [151]. Bile duct anastomosis was revised in all three children, and one required retransplantation procedure. The fifth case was in an adult liver transplant recipient in whom the diagnosis of *C. parvum*-associated sclerosing cholangitis was made after percutaneous core biopsy of the liver showed *C. parvum* lining the bile duct epithelium [150]. In this patient, diarrhea and liver abnormalities resolved after treatment with azithromycin plus paromomycin, and follow-up liver biopsy was negative for the parasite.

Entamoeba Histolytica

Entamoeba histolytica is transmitted via oral-fecal contamination; such infections are common in the developing countries and areas of poor water sanitation. Disease initially involves the intestinal mucosa, the amoeba subsequently penetrates hepatic tissue forming multiple cysts or liver abscesses throughout the organ, although most patients present with a single prominent liver lesion and other smaller cysts scattered throughtout the organ. Patients present with vague abdominal discomfort or pain and a history of prolonged diarrheal illness. Laboratory evaluation may reveal leukocytosis, but liver tests are usually unremarkable. Diagnosis includes a high index of suspicion along with fecal antigen and/or serum antigen tests. Radiographic imaging show multiple cysts in the liver. Paromomycin is recommended for treatment due to limited cyst penetration by metronidazole. Surgical drainage is generally not required.

There is no clear consensus as to increased risk for amebic liver disease in patients with hepatic cirrhosis. A report in the 1980s suggested a reduced prevalence of hepatic amebiasis in patients with cirrhosis; which was hypothesized to reflect reduced number of viable hepatocytes susceptible to amoebic invasion and severely altered hepatic architecture [155]. More recent reports, however, suggest contrary to be the case. A decade-long review of liver abscesses among cirrhotic patients in a high-incidence region of Thailand reported that 36% were due to amoebiasis [156].

Treatment is usually effective against protozoal infections; however, in nearly 7% of successfully treated individuals, residual hepatic lesions may persist on ultrasound; these are vestiges of previously treated infection and do not require further antiparasitic therapy [157]. For unclear reasons, the residual lesions can persist for years at the site of prior infection, and as long as patients are not symptomatic, this does not warrant further therapy. This holds true for individuals being considered for organ transplantation. A recent report described a patient who had residual abscess cavity after receiving treatment for amoebic liver disease; patient underwent successful renal transplantation without infection recurrence during posttransplant follow up [158].

Mycobacterial Infection

Tuberculosis is the most common mycobacterial infection worldwide. In the developed world, incidence of active tuberculosis infection after allograft transplantation is less than 1%. Whereas, in the developing world, active tuberculosis may be encountered in as high as 15% of transplant recipients [159, 160]. Predisposing factors for acute tuberculosis include coinfection with HCV and/or HIV and severe drug-induced cellular immune suppression [161–163]. Most cases are reactivation of latent tuberculosis rather than newly acquired, primary infection. In 63%, infection is confined to the lungs. Extrapulmonary foci of infection may be seen in 12% of the cases with active tuberculosis infection. Disseminated tuberculosis may occur in upto 25% of transplant patients and involves various extrapulmonary sites. Gastrointestinal tract is the most common non-pulmonary infection site; nearly half of such patients (48%) will demonstrate tuberculous hepatitis.

Following transplantation, diagnosis of tuberculous hepatitis may be challenging as common presenting symptoms are non-specific, which may include recurring fever, along with other constitutional symptoms, and a vague right upper quadrant discomfort. Most patients with active tuberculosis will present within first year after transplantation [160, 164]. Common laboratory findings are elevated liver enzymes, including high alkaline phosphatase levels and coagulation abnormalities. Elevated alkaline phosphatase is the most common finding seen in 75–87% of patients, whereas elevated serum transaminase levels are noted in 35–75% of patients [165, 166]. Isolated cases of tuberculous hepatitis may occur, although it is rare to see tuberculosis confined to the liver as most patients will have concurrent pulmonary disease [166, 167].

Demonstration of acid-fast bacilli and/or a positive *M. tuberculosis* cultures in liver biopsy samples confirms the diagnosis of active tuberculosis infection. In contrast to the general population, presence of granuloma in the hepatic parenchyma in itself is not diagnostic for active tuberculosis infection, especially in allograft transplant recipients as granulomas may occur with other conditions such as acute cellular allograft rejection, recurrence of PBC, infections due to nontuberculous mycobacteria; hepatosplenic candidiasis, nocardiosis, and endemic mycoses among others. In a retrospective analysis, in patients after liver transplantation, less than 3% of granulomas were attributed to active *M. tuberculous* infection [168].

The common nontuberculous mycobacterial infections in patients undergoing allogeneic HSCT or SOT, are as follows: *Mycobacterium avium complex*, *Mycobacterium haemophilum*, *Mycobacterium kansasii*, *Mycobacterium abscessus*, and *Mycobacterium chelonae*. These insidious infections may present months to years after transplantation; a variety of organ systems may be involved [169]. It is not uncommon for hepatic *M. kansasii* infection to present with a protracted febrile illness accompanied by abdominal pain; multiple liver abscesses may be seen on imaging [170]. Granulomatous liver disease due to MAC may present as portal hypertension and ascites [171]. Elevated alkaline phosphatase serum levels may be the only finding, transaminase and bilirubin levels are often within the normal range. Treatment of mycobacterial infection is presented in Chapter 56.

Schistosomiasis

Schistosoma is an infection of trematode fluke that affect nearly 200 million people in the endemic regions worldwide [172]. Transmission occurs through infectious cercariae that emerge and released from freshwater snails into the local water reservoirs such as lakes, ponds, and rivers. The cercariae penetrate human skin and transform into immature worms [173]. Worms mature over 6 weeks and hone to target vessels in the mesentery and bladder, producing eggs that erode into the walls of the intestine and urinary bladder [173]. Three major *Schistosoma* species are known to cause disease. *Schistosoma mansoni* is prominent in Africa and South America, whereas *Schistosoma japonicum* intestinal and hepatic schistosomiasis is prevalent in Asia. Hepatic schistosomiasis results from entrapment of eggs lodged in the portal venules, initiating an inflammatory cascade that ultimately leads to portal fibrosis and venous congestion [173]. *Schistosoma haematobium* is associated with urinary bladder infestation; post-obstructive nephropathy is the consequence of chronic bladder and ureteral inflammation among patients in Africa and the Middle East [174, 175].

Acute schistosomiasis infection is asymptomatic although patients may experience fever, headache, myalgia, abdominal pain, or a systemic serum sickness-like reaction known as Katayama fever, which results from immune responses to parasitic invasion and migration [173]. Liver abscesses may occur in persons with early schistosome infections due to the sequestration of encapsulated bacteria in the integument of the adult worms [176]. Chronic schistosomiasis may occur in 60% of infected individuals, leading to extensive liver disease in 4–8% of cases [172, 177]. Patients with hepatic schistosomiasis may present with variceal bleeding and splenomegaly due to portal congestion; synthetic liver function indices are often normal, and histologically, tissue infiltration with inflammatory cells is routinely noted. Advanced fibrosis in patients with long-standing schistosomal infection

Table 17.1 A summary of hepatobiliary tract infections in patients undergoing liver trnasplantation, along with clinical features, diagnosis and treatment

Infection	Pathogens	Clinical features	Diagnosis	Treatment
Cholangitis	*E.coli, Klebsiella, Enterobacter, Enterococcus* (plus fungal following transplantation)	Jaundice, fever, RUQ pain	Ultrasound, CT, MRCP (avoid ERCP in cirrhotics)	7–10 days antimicrobials, emergent drainage if no response within 24 h
Cholecystitis	*E.coli, Klebsiella, Enterobacter, Bacteroides*	RUQ pain	Ultrasound	Cholecystectomy, percutaneous drainage with abx if surgery contraindicated
Viral	CMV	Hepatitis, biliary stasis	Serum PCR, viral ctx, liver biopsy	Ganciclovir, transplant for FHH
	EBV	Jaundice, FHH	Serum PCR	Transplant for FHH (bridge w/ steroids, antivirals, plasmapheresis)
	HSV	Fever, coagulopathy, encephalopathy, leukopenia	Serum PCR, liver biopsy	IV acyclovir
Fungal	*Aspergillus*	Variable, usually always pulmonary involvement	Abscess drainage with culture	Itraconazole, voriconazole, or caspofungin, consider surgical drainage
	Candida	Primarily involves biliary tract (cholangitis), usually within 1st 30d of transplant	Difficult dx; can try beta-D-glucan or flow cytometry if suspicious	Amphotericin B
Protozoal	*Cryptococcus*	Diarrhea with cholangitis and/or cholecystitis	Stool oocysts or antibody oocyst testing	Nitazoxanide, paromomycin, or macrolides
	E. histolytica	Vague abdominal pain with diarrhea	Fecal or serum antigen, radiographic cysts	Paromomycin
Mycobacterial	*M. tuberculosis*	Sweats, weight loss, almost always pulmonary involvement	Biopsy with AFB stain or positive culture	Extrapulmonary TB regimen with close LFT monitoring
Trematode	*Schistosome*	Fever, myalgia, abdominal pain (Katayama fever – serum sickness)	Eggs in stool or on mucosal biopsy	Praziquantel (oxamniquine if *S. mansoni*)

resembles clay pipestems histologically and known as Symmers pipestem fibrosis [178].

Diagnosis is established by demonstrating schistosome eggs in the stool sample. The extent of fecal egg output correlates with the burden of mature worms and the extent of disease in infections due to *S. mansoni* and *S. japonicum* [173]. ELISA assays are useful for population screening, however, a + ELISA test result does not predict the activity of parasite in an individual [173]. Identification of *Schistosoma* eggs on mucosal biopsy remains the most sensitive method of diagnosis, although there are no widely accepted screening guidelines for patients undergoing allograft transplantation. It has been suggested that individuals from endemic areas, particularly the Middle East, Africa, South America, and Asia, should undergo serological and stool screening for ova and parasites during the pretransplant assessment [173, 179–181].

Effective treatment of schistosomiasis is achieved with three doses of 20 mg/kg praziquantel or oxamniquine given every 8 h for *S. mansoni* infection. Early treatment can result in total resolution of fibrosis, particularly in patients with early and mild disease [182]. Response to treatment may be followed by serial stool analysis. Epidemiological studies have demonstrated that high levels of IgE correlate with long-term resistance to schistosomal reinfection in individuals residing in the endemic regions [183].

Schistosoma-HCV coinfection is a leading indication for transplantation in Egypt and Saudi Arabia [184–186]. Mass treatment programs for schistosomiasis prior to 1980 utilized non-disposable syringes and needles, which significantly worsened the spread of HCV and regarded as largely responsible for the high HCV prevalence and transmission rates in the North African countries [187]. Clinical studies have demonstrated that *Schistosoma*-HCV coinfection accelerates liver injury compared with HCV-positive patients without schistosomiasis; co-infection has as been known to increases the risk for hepatocellular carcinoma [184, 187–189]. It has been suggested that TH1 response, critical for containment and resolution of acute HCV infection, is downregulated by a prominent TH2 cellular immune response garnered to tackle the invading parasites [190–192].

Recent evidence has demonstrated that patients with schistosomiasis in the absence of detectable organ damage may be viable liver and kidney donors. A study compared schistosoma-positive 20 living kidney donors with 20 uninfected donors; the investigators found no significant difference in graft survival over an average of 3.5-year follow-up [193]. Several case reports have demonstrated similar findings in recipients of liver allograft from schistosoma-seropositive donors [194–196]. Moreover, a large trial by Mahmoud et al. demonstrated no significant difference in renal allograft function; incidence and frequency of acute vs. chronic graft rejection between patients with schistosoma infection vs. no evidence of schistosoma infection [197]. In this trial, however, immunosuppression in schistosoma-positive patients was challenging due to higher doses of cyclosporine needed to achieve target blood level, which probably reflected poor intestinal drug absorption in the presence of parasitic infestation [198].

Recurrence of schistosomiasis after liver transplant is rare, with only few case reports described in the literature, and all of such cases were successfully treated with praziquantel [179, 186]. Transplant recipients are at increased risk for reinfection particularly in endemic areas where re-exposure to parasite remains high. A study in Egypt by Sobh et al. demonstrated that 23% of allograft recipients were diagnosed with reinfection during posttransplant follow-up [199]. End-stage kidney or end-stage liver disease may be present for many decades after the initial exposure to the parasites, and it is recommended that previously infected patients be treated prophylactically before undergoing allogeneic transplantation, as adult worms can survive for several years after the initial exposure [179, 194]. Table 17.1 provides a summary of hepatobiliary tract infections in patients undergoing liver transplantation.

References

1. Csendes A, Becerra M, Burdiles P, Demian I, Bancalari K, Csendes P. Bacteriological studies of bile from the gallbladder in patients with carcinoma of the gallbladder, cholelithiasis, common bile duct stones and no gallstones disease. Eur J Surg. 1994;160(6–7):363–7.
2. Abdalian R, Heathcote EJ. Sclerosing cholangitis: a focus on secondary causes. Hepatology. 2006;44(5):1063–74.
3. Ananthakrishnan AN, Saeian K. Caroli's disease: identification and treatment strategy. Curr Gastroenterol Rep. 2007;9(2):151–5.
4. Giovanardi RO. Monolobar Caroli's disease in an adult. Case report. Hepato-Gastroenterology. 2003;50(54):2185–7.
5. Brant WE. The core curriculum: ultrasound. 1st ed. Philadelphia: Lippincott Williams & Wilkins; 2001.
6. Lum DF, Leung JW. Bacterial cholangitis. Curr Treat Options Gastroenterol. 2001;4(2):139–46.
7. Kulaksiz H, Rudolph G, Kloeters-plachky P, Sauer P, Geiss H, Stiehl A. Biliary candida infections in primary sclerosing cholangitis. J Hepatol. 2006;45(5):711–6.
8. Boey JH, Way LW. Acute cholangitis. Ann Surg. 1980;191(3):264–70.
9. Artifon EL, Da silveira EB, Aparicio D, et al. Management of common bile duct stones in cirrhotic patients with coagulopathy: a comparison of supra-papillary puncture and standard cannulation technique. Dig Dis Sci. 2011;56(6):1904–11.
10. Alkhatib AA, Hilden K, Adler DG. Comorbidities, sphincterotomy, and balloon dilation predict post-ERCP adverse events in PSC patients: operator experience is protective. Dig Dis Sci. 2011;56(12):3685–8.
11. Classen M, Tytgat GNJ, Lightdale CJ. Gastroenterological endoscopy. 2nd ed. Stuttgart: Thieme; 2010.
12. Van den hazel SJ, Speelman P, Tytgat GN, Van leeuwen DJ. Successful treatment of recurrent cholangitis with antibiotic maintenance therapy. Eur J Clin Microbiol Infect Dis. 1994;13(8):662–5.
13. Bu LN, Chen HL, Chang CJ, et al. Prophylactic oral antibiotics in prevention of recurrent cholangitis after the Kasai portoenterostomy. J Pediatr Surg. 2003;38(4):590–3.
14. Gores GJ, Gish RG, Shrestha R, Wiesner RH. Model for end-stage liver disease (MELD) exception for bacterial cholangitis. Liver Transpl. 2006;12(12 Suppl 3):S91–2.
15. Gonzalez MR, Cascales PA, Abellan I, et al. The evolution of therapeutic strategies for biliary tract complications after liver transplantation over a period of 20 years. Transplant Proc. 2012;44(7):2093–5.
16. Aberg F, Makisalo H, Hockerstedt K, Isoniemi H. Infectious complications more than 1 year after liver transplantation: a 3-decade nationwide experience. Am J Transplant. 2011;11(2):287–95.
17. Gunawansa N, Mccall JL, Holden A, Plank L, Munn SR. Biliary complications following orthotopic liver transplantation: a 10-year audit. HPB (Oxford). 2011;13(6):391–9.
18. Scatton O, Meunier B, Cherqui D, et al. Randomized trial of choledochocholedochostomy with or without a T tube in orthotopic liver transplantation. Ann Surg. 2001;233(3):432–7.
19. Sharma S, Gurakar A, Jabbour N. Biliary strictures following liver transplantation: past, present and preventive strategies. Liver Transpl. 2008;14(6):759–69.
20. Akun E, Yaprak O, Killi R, Balci NC, Tokat Y, Yuzer Y. Vascular complications in hepatic transplantation: single-center experience in 14 years. Transplant Proc. 2012;44(5):1368–72.
21. Wang SF, Huang ZY, Chen XP. Biliary complications after living donor liver transplantation. Liver Transpl. 2011;17(10):1127–36.
22. Verdonk RC, Buis CI, Van der Jagt EJ, et al. Nonanastomotic biliary strictures after liver transplantation, part 2: management, outcome, and risk factors for disease progression. Liver Transpl. 2007;13(5):725–32.
23. Alexander J, Lord JD, Yeh MM, Cuevas C, Bakthavatsalam R, Kowdley KV. Risk factors for recurrence of primary sclerosing cholangitis after liver transplantation. Liver Transpl. 2008;14(2):245–51.
24. Fosby B, Karlsen TH, Melum E. Recurrence and rejection in liver transplantation for primary sclerosing cholangitis. World J Gastroenterol. 2012;18(1):1–15.
25. Ayoub WS, Esquivel CO, Martin P. Biliary complications following liver transplantation. Dig Dis Sci. 2010;55(6):1540–6.
26. Ohkubo T, Sugawara Y, Takayama T, Kokudo N, Makuuchi M. The risk factors of fungal infection in living-donor liver transplantations. J Hepatobiliary Pancreat Sci. 2012;19(4):382–8.
27. Yuchong C, Dingheng Z, Zhizhong Y, Hongyu Y, Jing H, Jianghan C. Aspergillosis of biliary tract after liver transplantation: a case report. Mycopathologia. 2010;170(2):117–21.
28. Schirmer BD, Winters KL, Edlich RF. Cholelithiasis and cholecystitis. J Long-Term Eff Med Implants. 2005;15(3):329–38.
29. Fornari F, Imberti D, Squillante MM, et al. Incidence of gallstones in a population of patients with cirrhosis. J Hepatol. 1994;20(6):797–801.
30. Maggi A, Solenghi D, Panzeri A, et al. Prevalence and incidence of cholelithiasis in patients with liver cirrhosis. Ital J Gastroenterol Hepatol. 1997;29(4):330–5.
31. Acalovschi M, Buzas C, Radu C, Grigorescu M. Hepatitis C virus infection is a risk factor for gallstone disease: a prospective hospital-based study of patients with chronic viral C hepatitis. J Viral Hepat. 2009;16(12):860–6.
32. Bini EJ, Mcgready J. Prevalence of gallbladder disease among persons with hepatitis C virus infection in the United States. Hepatology. 2005;41(5):1029–36.
33. Cardentey-Reyes A, Jacobs F, Struelens MJ, Rodriguez-Villalobos H. First case of bacteremia caused by Moellerella wisconsensis: case report and a review of the literature. Infection. 2009;37(6):544–6.

34. Oteo J, Gomez-Garces JL, Alos JI. Acute cholecystitis and bacteremia caused by Kluyvera ascorbata in a cirrhotic patient. Clin Microbiol Infect. 1998;4(2):113–5.
35. Fasolato S, Angeli P, Dallagnese L, et al. Renal failure and bacterial infections in patients with cirrhosis: epidemiology and clinical features. Hepatology. 2007;45(1):223–9.
36. Guevara M, Terra C, Nazar A, et al. Albumin for bacterial infections other than spontaneous bacterial peritonitis in cirrhosis. A randomized, controlled study. J Hepatol. 2012;57(4):759–65.
37. Cryer HM, Howard DA, Garrison RN. Liver cirrhosis and biliary surgery: assessment of risk. South Med J. 1985;78(2):138–41.
38. Aranha GV, Sontag SJ, Greenlee HB. Cholecystectomy in cirrhotic patients: a formidable operation. Am J Surg. 1982;143(1):55–60.
39. Cappellani A, Cacopardo B, Zanghi A, Cavallaro A, Di Vita M, Alfano G, Lo Menzo E. Retrospective survey on laparoscopic cholecystectomy in the cirrhotic patient. Eur Rev Med Pharmacol Sci. 2008;12(4):257–60.
40. Hamad MA, Thabet M, Badawy A, et al. Laparoscopic versus open cholecystectomy in patients with liver cirrhosis: a prospective, randomized study. J Laparoendosc Adv Surg Tech A. 2010;20(5):405–9.
41. Poggio JL, Rowland CM, Gores GJ, Nagorney DM, Donohue JH. A comparison of laparoscopic and open cholecystectomy in patients with compensated cirrhosis and symptomatic gallstone disease. Surgery. 2000;127(4):405–11.
42. Palanivelu C, Rajan PS, Jani K, et al. Laparoscopic cholecystectomy in cirrhotic patients: the role of subtotal cholecystectomy and its variants. J Am Coll Surg. 2006;203(2):145–51.
43. Cakmak A, Genc V, Orozakunov E, Kepenekci I, Cetinkaya OA, Hazinedaroglu MS. Partial cholecystectomy is a safe and efficient method. Chirurgia (Bucur). 2009;104(6):701–4.
44. Sharp CF, Garza RZ, Mangram AJ, Dunn EL. Partial cholecystectomy in the setting of severe inflammation is an acceptable consideration with few long-term sequelae. Am Surg. 2009;75(3):249–52.
45. Curro G, Baccarani U, Adani G, Cucinotta E. Laparoscopic cholecystectomy in patients with mild cirrhosis and symptomatic cholelithiasis. Transplant Proc. 2007;39(5):1471–3.
46. Curro G, Iapichino G, Melita G, Lorenzini C, Cucinotta E. Laparoscopic cholecystectomy in Child-Pugh class C cirrhotic patients. JSLS. 2005;9(3):311–5.
47. Delis S, Bakoyiannis A, Madariaga J, Bramis J, Tassopoulos N, Dervenis C. Laparoscopic cholecystectomy in cirrhotic patients: the value of MELD score and Child Pugh classification in predicting outcome. Surg Endosc. 2010;24(2):407–12.
48. Arif R, Seppelt P, Schwill S, et al. Predictive risk factors for patients with cirrhosis undergoing heart surgery. Ann Thorac Surg. 2012;94(6):1947–52.
49. Song CS, Yoon MY, Kim HJ, et al. Usefulness of model for end-stage liver disease score for predicting mortality after intra-abdominal surgery in patients with liver cirrhosis in a single hospital. Korean J Gastroenterol. 2011;57(6):340–5.
50. Schlenker C, Johnson S, Trotter JF. Preoperative transjugular intrahepatic portosystemic shunt (TIPS) for cirrhotic patients undergoing abdominal and pelvic surgeries. Surg Endosc. 2009;23(7):1594–8.
51. Azoulay D, Buabse F, Damiano I, et al. Neoadjuvant transjugular intrahepatic portosystemic shunt: a solution for extrahepatic abdominal operation in cirrhotic patients with severe portal hypertension. J Am Coll Surg. 2001;193(1):46–51.
52. Chalret du Rieu M, Carrere N, Bureau C, Lagarde S, Otal P, Pradere B. Transjugular intrahepatic portosystemic shunt before hepatic surgery in a patient with cirrhosis and portal hypertension: case report. J Chir (Paris). 2009;146(2):191–4.
53. Gil A, Martinez-Regueira F, Hernandez-Lizoain JL, et al. The role of transjugular intrahepatic portosystemic shunt prior to abdominal tumoral surgery in cirrhotic patients with portal hypertension. Eur J Surg Oncol. 2004;30(1):46–52.
54. Mckay A, Abulfaraj M, Lipschitz J. Short- and long-term outcomes following percutaneous cholecystectomy for acute cholecystitis in high-risk patients. Surg Endosc. 2012;26(5):1343–51.
55. Saeed SA, Masroor I. Percutaneous cholecystectomy (PC) in the management of acute cholecystitis in high risk patients. J Coll Phys Surg Pak. 2010;20(9):612–5.
56. Aranha GV, Kruss D, Greenlee HB. Therapeutic options for biliary tract disease in advanced cirrhosis. Am J Surg. 1988;155(3):374–7.
57. Shrestha R, Trouillot TE, Everson GT. Endoscopic stenting of the gallbladder for symptomatic gallbladder disease in patients with end-stage liver disease awaiting orthotopic liver transplantation. Liver Transpl Surg. 1999;5(4):275–81.
58. Nikeghbalian S, Salahi R, Salahi H, et al. Hepatic abscesses after liver transplant: 1997–2008. Exp Clin Transplant. 2009;7(4):256–60.
59. Torbenson M, Wang J, Nichols L, Jain A, Fung J, Nalesnik MA. Causes of death in autopsied liver transplantation patients. Mod Pathol. 1998;11(1):37–46.
60. Bate SL, Dollard SC, Cannon MJ. Cytomegalovirus seroprevalence in the United States: the national health and nutrition examination surveys, 1988–2004. Clin Infect Dis. 2010;40:1439–47.
61. Cannon NJ, Schmid DS, Hyde TB. Review of cytomegalovirus seroprevalence and demographic characteristics associated with infection. Rev Med Virol. 2010;20:202–13.
62. Razonable RR, Emery VC. Management of CMV infection and disease in transplant patients. Herpes. 2004;11:77–86.
63. Rafailidis PI, Mourtzoukou EG, Varbobitis IC, Falagas ME. Severe cytomegalovirus infection in apparently immunocompetent patients: a systematic review. Virol J. 2008;5:47.
64. Giroud O, Meier P, San Millán D, Praz G. Severe CMV infection: not only in immunocompromised patients. Rev Med Suisse. 2010;6:1918–21.
65. Yu YD, Park GC, Park PJ, Choi YI, et al. Cytomegalovirus infection-associated fulminant hepatitis in an immunocompetent adult requiring emergency living-donor liver transplantation: report of a case. Surg Today. 2013;43(4):424–8.
66. Fernández-Ruiz M, Muñoz-Codoceo C, López-Medrano F, Faré-Garciá R, et al. Cytomegalovirus myopericarditis and hepatitis in an immunocompetent adult: successful treatment with oral valganciclovir. Intern Med. 2008;47:1963–6.
67. Shusterman NH, Fauenhoffer C, Kinsey MD. Fatal massive hepatic necrosis in cytomegalovirus mononucleosis. Ann Intern Med. 1978;88:810–2
68. Ljungman P, Griffiths P, Paya C. Definition of cytomegalovirus infection and disease in transplant recipients. Clin Infect Dis. 2002;34:1094–7.
69. Arthurs SK, Eid AJ, Pedersen RA, Dierkhising RA, Kremers WK, Patel R, Razonable RR. Delayed-onset primary cytomegalovirus disease after liver transplantation. Liver Transpl. 2007;13:1703–9.
70. Razonable RR, Paya CV. Herpesvirus infection in transplant recipients: current challenges in the clinical management of cytomegalovirus and Epstein-Barr virus infections. Herpes. 2003;10:60–5.
71. Razonable RR, Paya CV. Infections and allograft rejection – intertwined complications of organ transplantation. Swiss Med Wkly. 2005;135:571–3.
72. O'Grady JG, Alexander GJ, Sutherland S, Donaldson PT, Harvey F, Portmann B, Calne RY, Williams R. Cytomegalovirus infection and donor/recipient HLA antigens: interdependent co-factors in pathogenesis of vanishing bile-duct syndrome after transplantation. Lancet. 1988;2:302–5.
73. Noack KB, Wiesner RH, Batts K, van Hoek B, Ludwig J. Severe ductopenic rejection with features of vanishing bile duct syndrome: clinical, biochemical, and histologic evidence for spontaneous resolution. Transplant Proc. 1991;23:1448–145.

74. Kowdley KV, Fawaz KA, Kaplan MM. Extrahepatic biliary stricture associated with cytomegalovirus in a liver transplant recipient. Transpl Int. 1996;9:161–3.
75. World Health Organization. Immunization vaccines and biologicals http://www.who.int/vaccine_research/diseases/viral_cancers/en/index1.html. Accessed 17 Jun 2017.
76. White NJ, Juel-jensen BE. Infectious mononucleosis hepatitis. Semin Liver Dis. 1984;4(4):301–6.
77. Feranchak AP, Tyson RW, Narkewicz MR, Karrer FM, Sokol RJ. Fulminant Epstein-Barr viral hepatitis: orthotopic liver transplantation and review of the literature. Liver Transpl Surg. 1998;4(6):469–76.
78. Papatheodoridis GV, Delladetsima JK, Kavallierou L, Kapranos N, Tassopoulos NC. Fulminant hepatitis due to Epstein-Barr virus infection. J Hepatol. 1995;23(3):348–50.
79. Collin L, Moulin P, Jungers M, Geubel AP. Epstein-Barr virus (EBV)-induced liver failure in the absence of extensive liver-cell necrosis: a case for cytokine-induced liver dysfunction. J Hepatol. 2004;41(1):174–5.
80. Ader F, Chatellier D, Le Berre R, Morand P, Fourrier F. Fulminant Epstein-Barr virus (EBV) hepatitis in a young immunocompetent subject. Med Mal Infect. 2006;36(7):396–8.
81. Yamamoto M, Kimura H, Hironaka T, et al. Detection and quantification of virus DNA in plasma of patients with Epstein-Barr virus-associated diseases. J Clin Microbiol. 1995;33(7):1765–8.
82. Wang D, Liebowitz, Kleff E. An EBV membrane protein expressed in immortalized lymphoctyes transforms established rodent cells. Cell. 1985;43(3 Pt 2):831–40.
83. Birx DL, Redfield RR, Tosato G. Defective regulation of Epstein-Barr virus infection in patients with acquired immunodeficiency syndrome (AIDS) or AIDS-related disorders. N Engl J Med. 1986;314(14):874–9.
84. Baumforth KR, Young LS, Flavell KJ, Constandinou C, Murray PG. The Epstein-Barr virus and its association with human cancers. MP Mol Pathol. 1999;52(6):307–22.
85. Ben-Ari Z, Amlot P, Lachmanan SR, Tur-Kaspa R, Rolles K, Burroughs AK. Posttransplantation lymphoproliferative disorder in liver recipients: characteristics, management, and outcome. Liver Transpl Surg. 1999;5(3):184–91.
86. Taylor AL, Marcus R, Bradley JA. Post-transplant lymphoproliferative disorders (PTLD) after solid organ transplantation. Crit Rev Oncol Hematol. 2005;56(1):155–67.
87. Norvell JP, Blei AT, Javanovic BD, Letisky J. Herpes simplex virus hepatitis: an analysis of the published literature and institutional cases. Liver Transpl. 2007;13:1428–34.
88. Rosenthal SL, Stanberry LR, Biro FM. Seroprevalence of herpes simplex virus types 1 and 2 and cytomegalovirus in adolescents. Clin Infect Dis. 1997;24:135–9.
89. Schiodt DT, Shakil O, McGuire B, Samuel G, Lee W, the Acute Liver Failure Study Group. Viral hepatitis-related acute liver failure. Am J Gastroenterol. 2003;98:448–53.
90. Kaufman B, Gandhi SA, Louie E, Rizzi R, Illei P. Herpes simplex virus hepatitis: vase report and review. Clin Infect Dis. 1997;24:334–8.
91. Halliday J, Lokan J, Angus PW, Gow P. A case of fulminant hepatic failure in pregnancy. Hepatology. 2010;51:341–2.
92. Moldovan B, Mentha G, Manjno P, et al. Demographics and outcomes of severe herpes simplex virus hepatitis: a registry-based study. J Hepatol. 2011;55:1222–6.
93. Graham BB, Kaul DR, Saint S, Janssen WJ. Clinical problem-solving. Kiss of death. N Engl J Med. 2009;360:2564–8.
94. Ichai P, Roque Alfonso AM, Sebagh M, et al. Herpes simplex virus-associated acute liver failure: a difficult diagnosis with a poor prognosis. Liver Transpl. 2005;11:1550–5.
95. Smith PJ, Hunter J. Cervical infection with herpes simplex virus. Lancet. 1981;1:1051.
96. Sharma S, Mosunjac M. Herpes simplex hepatitis in adults: a search for muco-cutaneous clues. J Clin Gastroenterol. 2004;38:697–704.
97. Riedgier C, Sauer P, Matevossian E, Muller MW, Buchler P, Friess H. Herpes simplex virus sepsis and acute liver failure. Clin Transpl. 2009;23(S21):37–41.
98. Longerich T, Christoph E, Penzel R, et al. Recurrent herpes simplex virus hepatitis after liver retransplantation despite acyclovir therapy. Liver Transpl. 2005;11(10):1289–94.
99. Jacques SM, Qureshi F. Herpes simplex virus hepatitis in pregnancy: a clinicopathologic study of three cases. Hum Pathol. 1992;23:183–7.
100. Montalbano M, Slapak-Green GI, Neff GW. Fulminant hepatic failure from herpes simplex virus: post liver transplantation acyclovir therapy and literature review. Transplant Proc. 2005;37:4393–6.
101. Shanley CJ, Braun DK, Brown K. Fulminant hepatic failure secondary to herpes simplex virus hepatitis. Successful outcome after orthotopic liver transplantation. Transplantation. 1995;59:145–9.
102. Rivera-Penera T, Moreno J, Skaff C, McDiarmid S, Vargas J, Ament ME. Delayed encephalopathy in fulminant hepatic failure in the pediatric population and the role of liver transplantation. J Pediatr Gastroenterol Nur. 1997;24:128–34.
103. Devictor D, Desplanques L, Debray D, et al. Emergency liver transplantation for fulminant liver failure in infants and children. Hepatology. 1992;16:1156–62.
104. Paya CV. Prevention of fungal and hepatitis virus infections in liver transplantation. Clin Infect Dis. 2001;33(S1):1813–21.
105. Badiee P, Albozi A, Malekhosseini SA, Nikeghbalian S, Shakiba E. Determining the incidence of aspergillosis after liver transplant. Exp Clin Transplant. 2010;8(3):220–3.
106. Singh N, Peterson DL. Aspergillus infections in transplant recipients. Clin Microbiol Rev. 2005;18:44–69.
107. Singh N, Pruett TL, Houston S, et al. Invasive aspergillosis in the recipients of liver transplantation. Liver Transpl. 2006;12:1205–9.
108. Rosenhagen M, Feldhues R, Schmidt J, Hoppe-Tichy T, Geiss HK. A risk profile for invasive aspergillosis in liver transplant recipients. Infection. 2009;37:313–9.
109. Gavalda J, Len O, San Juan R, et al. Risk factors for invasive aspergillosis in solid organ transplant recipients: a case-control study. Clin Infect Dis. 2005;41:52–9.
110. Patel R, Portela D, Badley AD, et al. Risk factors of invasive Candida and non-Candida fungal infections after liver transplantation. Transplantation. 1996;62:926–34.
111. Kusne S, Torre-Ciseneros J, Manez R, et al. Factors associated with invasive lung aspergillosis and the significant of positive Aspergillus culture after liver transplantation. J Infect Dis. 1992;166:1379–83.
112. Fortun J, Martin-Davila P, Moreno S, et al. Risk factors for invasive aspergillosis in liver transplant recipients. Liver Transpl. 2002;8:1065–70.
113. Gayowski T, Marino IR, Singh N, et al. Orthotopic liver transplantation in high-risk patients: risk factors associated with mortality and infectious morbidity. Transplantation. 1998;65:499–504.
114. Grossi P, Farina C, Fiocchi R, Dalla GD. Prevalence and outcome of invasive fungal infections in 1963 thoracic organ transplant recipients: a multicenter retrospective study. Italian Study Group of Fungal Infections in Thoracic Organ Transplant Recipients. Transplantation. 2000;70:112–6.
115. Montoya JG, Chaparro SV, Celis D, et al. Invasive aspergillosis in the setting of cardiac transplantation. Clin Infect Dis. 2003;37(S3):S281–92.
116. Singh N. The changing face of invasive aspergillosis in liver transplant in liver transplant recipients. Liver Transpl. 2002;8(11):1071–2.
117. Mazza D, Gugenheim J, Toouli J, Moniel J. Survival of a liver graft recipient treated for an aspergillar liver abscess. Clin Infect Dis. 1996;23:831–2.

118. Gupta KL, Rajaram KG, Joshi K, Sakhuja V. Progression of hepatic aspergillosis following second renal transplantation in a patient with recurrent glomerulonephritis. Indian J Pathol Microbiol. 2012;55(4):580–2.
119. Marik P. Fungal infections in solid organ transplantation. Expert Opin Pharmacother. 2006;7(3):297–305.
120. Schroter GP, Hoelscher M, Putnam CW, Porter KA, Starzl TE. Fungus infection after liver transplantation. Ann Surg. 1977;186:115–22.
121. Durand F, Bernuau J, Dupont B, et al. Aspergillus intraabdominal abscess after liver transplantation successfully treated with itraconazole. Transplantation. 1992;54:734–5.
122. Kusne S, Dummer JS, Singh N, et al. Infections after liver transplantation: an analysis of 101 consecutive cases. Medicine (Baltimore). 1988;67:132–43.
123. Zhan HX, Lv Y, Zhang Y, et al. Hepatic and renal artery rupture due to Aspergillus and Mucor mixed infection after combined liver and kidney transplantation: a case report. Transplant Proc. 2008;40:1771–3.
124. Falcone M, Massetti AP, Russo A, Vullo V, Venditti M. Invasive aspergillosis in patients with liver disease. Med Mycol. 2011;49:406–13.
125. Rosen HR. Disease recurrence following liver transplantation. Clin Liver Dis. 2000;4:675–89.
126. Munoz SJ, Rothstein KD, Reich D, Manzabeitia C. Long-term care of the liver transplant recipient. Clin Liver Dis. 2000;4:691–710.
127. Rudich SM, Kinkhabwala MM, Murray NGB, et al. Successful treatment of mycotic hepatic artery pseudoaneurysms with arterial reconstruction and liposomal amphotericin B. Liver Transpl Surg. 1998;4:91–3.
128. Herbrecht R, Denning DW, Patterson TF, et al. Vorticonazole versus amphotericin B for primary therapy of invasive aspergillosis. NEJM. 2002;347:408–15.
129. Thomas A, Korb V, Guillemain R, et al. Clinical outcomes of lung-transplant recipients treated by voriconazole and caspofungin combination in aspergillosis. J Clin Pharm Ther. 2010;35:49–53.
130. Kirchner GI, Scherer MN, Obed A, et al. Outcome of patients with ischemic-like cholangiopathy with secondary sclerosing cholangitis after liver transplantation. Scand J Gastroenterol. 2011;46:471–8.
131. Saito T, Senda K, Takakura S, et al. Biliary bacteria in living related liver transplant recipients: microbiology and rapid detection system using flow cytometry. Clin Chem Lab Med. 2003;41(2):159–63.
132. Sendid B, Poirot JL, Tabouret M, et al. Combined detection of mannanaemia and antimannan antibodies as a strategy for diagnosis of systemic infection caused by pathogenic Candida species. J Med Microbiol. 2002;51(5):433–42.
133. Persat F, Topenot R, Piens MA, THeiebaut A, Dannaoui E, Picot S. Evaluation of different commercial ELISA methods for the serodiagnosis of systemic candidosis. Mycoses. 2002;45(11–12):455–60.
134. Bar W, Hecker H. Diagnosis of systemic Candida infections in patients of the intensive care unit. Significance of serum antigens and antibodies. Mycoses. 2002;45(1–2):22–8.
135. Wingard JR. Have novel serum markers supplanted tissue diagnosis for invasive fungal infections in acute leukemia and transplantation? Best Pract Res Clin Hematol. 2012;25:487–91.
136. Kusne S, Blair JE. Viral and fungal infections after liver transplantation-part II. Liver Transpl. 2006;12:2–11.
137. Mora-Duarte J, Betts R, Rotstein C, et al. Comparison of caspofungin and amphotericin B for invasive candidiasis. N Engl J Med. 2002;347:2020–9.
138. Kartsonis NA, Saah A, Lipka CJ, Talor A, Sable CA. Second-ling therapy with caspofungin for mucosal or invasive candidiasis: results from the caspofungin compassionate-use study. J Antimicrob Chemother. 2004;53:878–81.
139. Colombo AL, Perfect J, Dinubile M, et al. Global distribution and outcomes for Candida species causing invasive candidiasis: results from a n international randomized double-blind study of caspofungin versus amphotericin B for the treatment of invasive candidiasis. Eur J Clin Microbiol Infect Dis. 2003;22:470–4.
140. Walsh TJ, Teppler H, Donowitz GR, et al. A randomized, double-blind, multicenter study of caspofungin versus liposomal amphotericin B for empiric antifungal therapy in pediatric patients with persistent fever and neurtopenia. N Engl J Med. 2004;351:1391–402.
141. Maertens JA, Madero L, Reilly AF, et al. A randomized, double-blind multicenter study of caspofungin versus liposomal amphotericin B for empiric antifungal therapy in pediatric patients with persistent fever and neutropenia. Pediatr Infect Dis J. 2010;29:415–20.
142. Goicoechea M, Fierer J, Johns S. Treatment of candidal cholangitis with caspofungin therapy in a patient with a liver transplant: documentation of biliary excretion of caspofungin. Clin Infect Dis. 2004;38(7):1040–1.
143. Marr KA, Hachem R, Papanicolaou G, et al. Retrospective study of the hepatic safety profile of patients concomitantly treated with caspofungin and cyclosporine A. Transpl Infect Dis. 2004;6:110–6.
144. San-Rodriguez C, Lopez-Duarte M, Jurado M, et al. Safety of the concomitant use of caspofungin and cyclosporine A in patients with invasive fungal infections. Bone Marrow Transplant. 2004;34:13–20.
145. Crucani M, Mengoli C, Malena M, et al. Antifungal prophylaxis in liver transplant patients: a systematic review and meta-analysis. Liver Transpl. 2006;12:850–8.
146. Concia E, Azzini AM, Conti M. Epidemiology, incidence and risk factors for invasive candidiasis in high-risk patients. Drugs. 2009;69(S1):5–14.
147. Fortun J, Lopez-San Roman A, Velasco JJ. Selection of candida glabrata strains with reduced susceptibility to azoles in four liver transplant patients with invasive candidiasis. Eur J Clin Microbiol Infect Dis. 1997;16(4):314–8.
148. Vakil NB, Schwartz SM, Buggy BP, et al. Biliary cryptosporidiosis in HIV-infected people after the waterborne outbreak of cryptosporidiosis in Milwaukee. N Engl J Med. 1996;334:19–23.
149. Bonacini M. Hepatobiliary complications in patients with human immunodeficiency virus infection. Am J Med. 1992;92:404–11.
150. Denkinger CM, Hariquopal P, Ruiz P, Dowdy LM. Cryptosporodium parvum-associated sclerosing cholangitis in a liver transplant patient. Transpl Infect Dis. 2008;10:133–6.
151. Campos M, Jouzdani E, Sempoux C, Buts JP, Reding R, Otte JB, Sokal EM. Sclerosing cholangitis associated to cryptosporidiosis in liver-transplanted children. Eur J Pediatr. 2000;159:113–5.
152. Abdo A, Klassen J, Urbanski S, Raber E, Swain MG. Reversible sclerosing cholangitis secondary to cryptosporidiosis in a renal transplant patient. J Hepatol. 2003;38:688–91.
153. Davis JJ, Heyman MB, Ferrell L, Kerner J, Kerlan R Jr, Thaler MM. Sclerosing cholangitis associated with chronic cryptosporidiosis child with a congenital immunodeficiency disorder. Am J Gastroenterol. 1987;82:1196–202.
154. Huang DB, White AC. An updated review on cryptosporidium and Giardia. Gastroenterol Clin N Am. 2006;35:291–314.
155. Falaiye JM, Okeke GC, Fregene AO. Amoebic abscess in the cirrhotic liver. Gut. 1980;21(2):161–3.
156. Wiwanitkit V, Suwansaksri N, Suwansaksri J. Causative agents of liver abscess in those with liver cirrhosis: a 10-year case review of hospitalized patients in Thailand. Ann Trop Med Parasitol. 2002;96(5):513–6.
157. Blessman J, Khoa ND, Van an L, Tannich E. Ultrasound patterns and frequency of focal liver lesions after successful treatment of amoebic liver abscess. Trop Med Int Health. 2006;11(4):504–8.

158. Choudhrie AV, Kumar S, Gopalakrishnan G. Residual amoebic liver abscess in a prospective renal transplant recipient. Saudi J Kidney Dis Transpl. 2012;23(1):99–101.
159. Aguado JM, Herrero JA, Gavalda J, et al. Clinical presentation and outcome of tuberculosis in kidney, liver, and heart transplant recipients in Spain. Spanish Transplantation Infection Study Group, GESITRA. Transplantation. 1997;63(9):1278–86.
160. Garcia-Goez JF, Linares L, Benito N, et al. Tuberculosis in solid organ transplant recipients at a tertiary hospital in the last 20 years in Barcelona, Spain. Transplant Proc. 2009;41(6):2268–70.
161. Miro JM, Blanes M, Norman F, Martin-Davila P. Infections in solid organ transplantation in special situations: HIV-infection and immigration. Enferm Infecc Microbiol Clin. 2012;30(Suppl 2):76–85.
162. Torres J, Aguado JM, San Juan R, et al. Hepatitis C virus, an important risk factor for tuberculosis in immunocompromised: experience with kidney transplantation. Transpl Int. 2008;21(9):873–8.
163. Bosch W, Poowanawittayakom N, Chaikriangkrai K, et al. Tuberculous hepatitis in renal transplant recipients following alemtuzumab induction therapy. Transpl Infect Dis. 2013;15(1):E33–9.
164. Munoz P, Rodriguez C, Bouza E. Mycobacterium tuberculosis infection in recipients of solid organ transplants. Clin Infect Dis. 2005;40(4):581–7.
165. Essop AR, Posen JA, Hodkinson JH, Segal I. Tuberculosis hepatitis: a clinical review of 96 cases. Q J Med. 1984;53(212):465–77.
166. Alvarez SZ. Hepatobiliary tuberculosis. J Gastroenterol Hepatol. 1998;13(8):833–9.
167. Mat O, Abramowicz D, Peny MO, et al. Tuberculosis presenting as acute hepatitis in a renal transplant recipient. Transpl Int. 1994;7(1):67–9.
168. Ferrell LD, Lee R, Brixko C, Bass NM, Lake JR, Roberts JP, Ascher N, Rabkin J. Hepatic granulomas following liver transplantation. Clinicopathologic features in 42 patients. Transplantation. 1995;60(9):926–33.
169. Nagy GS, Rubin RH. Disseminated Mycobacterium avium-intracellulare in a kidney transplant recipient. Transpl Infect Dis. 2001;3(4):220–30.
170. Kaur P, Fishman JA, Misdraji J, Varma MC, Kotton CN. Disseminated Mycobacterium kansasii infection with hepatic abscesses in a renal transplant recipient. Transpl Infect Dis. 2011;13(5):531–5.
171. Patel R, Roberts GD, Keating MR, Paya CV. Infections due to nontuberculous mycobacteria in kidney, heart, and liver transplant recipients. Clin Infect Dis. 1994;19(2):263–73.
172. Chitsulo L, Engels D, Montresor A, Savioli L. The global status of schistosomiasis and its control. Acta Trop. 2000;77:41–51.
173. Ross AGP, Bartley PB, Sleigh AC, Olds GR, Li Y, Williams GM, McManus DP. Current concepts: schistosomiasis. N Engl J Med. 2002;346:1212–20.
174. Sobh M, Moustafa F, Sally S, Deelder A, Ghoneim M. Characterization of kidney lesion in early schistosomal specific nephropathy. Nephrol Dial Transplant. 1988;3:392–8.
175. Ghoneim MA. Bilharziasis: the lower genitourinary tract. In: Husain I, editor. Tropical urology and renal disease. Chap. 16. Edinburgh: Churchill Livingstone; 1984. p. 261–80.
176. Lambertucci JR, Rayes AA, Serufo JC, Gerspacher-Lara R, Brasileiro Filho G, Teixeira R, Antunes CM, Goes AM, Coelho PM. Schistosomiasis and associated infections. Mem Inst Oswaldo Cruz. 1998;93(Suppl 1):135–9.
177. Andrade ZA. Schistosomiasis and liver fibrosis. Parasite Immunol. 2009;31:656–63.
178. Symmers WSC. Note on a new form of liver cirrhosis due to the presence of ova of Bilharzia haematobium. J Pathol Bacteriol. 1904;9:237–9.
179. Hoare M, Gelson WT, Davies SE, Curran M, Alexander GJ. Hepatic and intestinal schistosomiasis after orthotopic liver transplant. Liver Transpl. 2005;11:1603–7.
180. Pungpapong S, Krishna M, Abraham SC, Keaveny AP, Dickson RD, Nakhleh RE. Clinicopathologic findings and outcomes of liver transplantation using grafts from donors with unrecognized and unusual diseases. Liver Transpl. 2006;12:310–5.
181. Kotton CN, Lattes R. Parasitic infections in solid organ transplant recipients. Am J Transplant. 2009;9(S4):S243–51.
182. Berhe N, Myrvang B, Gundersen SG. Reversibility of schistosomal periportal thickening/fibrosis after praziquantel therapy: a twenty-six month follow-up study in Ethiopia. Am J Trop Med Hyg. 2008;78(2):228–34.
183. Hagan P, Blumenthal UJ, Dunn D, Simpson AJG, Wilkins HA. Human IgE, IgG4 and resistance to reinfection with Schistosoma haematobium. Nature. 1991;349:243–5.
184. Halim AB, Garry RF, Dash S, Gerber MA. Effect of schistosomiasis and hepatitis on liver disease. Am J Top Med Hyg. 1999;60:915–20.
185. Khalaf H, El-Meteini M, El-Sefi T, et al. Evolution of living donor liver transplantation in Egypt. Saudi Med J. 2005;26:1394–7.
186. Ahmed K, Safdar K, Kemmer M, Atiq M, Wang J, Neff GW. Intestinal schistosomiasis following orthotopic liver transplantation: a case report. Transplant Proc. 2007;39:3502–4.
187. Strickland GT. Liver disease in Egypt: hepatitis C superseded schistosomiasis as a result of iatrogenic and biological factors. Hepatology. 2006;43:915–22.
188. Gad A, Tanaka E, Orii K, Rokhara A, Nooman Z, Serwah AH, et al. Relationship between hepatitis C virus infection and schisotomal liver disease: not simply an additive effect. J Gastroenterol. 2001;36:753–8.
189. Bedwani R, El-Khwsky F, El-Shazly M, Seif HA, Zaki A, Renganathan E, et al. Hepatitis viruses, schistosomal infection and liver cancer in Egypt. Int J Cancer. 1996;68:688–9.
190. Kamal SM, Rasensack JW, Biachi L, Al TA, El Sayed KK, Peter T, et al. Acute hepatitis C without and with schistosomiasis: correlation with hepatitis C-specific CD4(+) T-cell and cytokine response. Gastroenterology. 2001;121:646–56.
191. Maizels RM, Bundy DA, Selkirk ME, Smith DF, Anderson RM. Immunological modulation and evasion by helminth parasites in human populations. Nature. 1993;365:797–805.
192. Parana R, Codes L, Andrade Z. Is splenectomy a cause of antiviral treatment failure in hepatitis C virus infection? Hepatology. 2001;33:1340.
193. Sobh MA, El-Sharkawy SE, Shokeir AA, Moustafa FE, El-Sherif AK, Ghoneim MA. Effects of schistosomiasis on living kidney donors. Scand J Urol Nephrol. 1992;26:409–12.
194. Andraus W, Pugliese V, Pecora R, D'Albuquerque LA. Intentional use of *Schistosoma mansoni*-infected grafts in living donor liver transplantation. Liver Transpl. 2012;18(7):867–8.
195. Pungpapong S, Krishna M, Abraham SC, Keaveny AP, Dickson RC, Nakhleh RE. Clinicopathologic findings and outcomes of liver transplantation using grafts from donors with unrecognized and unusual diseases. Liver Transpl. 2006;12:310–5.
196. Pannegeon V, Masini JP, Paye F, Chazouilleres O, Girard PM. *Schistosoma mansoni* infection and liver graft. Transplantation. 2005;80:287.
197. Mahmoud KM, Sobh MA, El-Agroudy AE, Mostafa FE, Baz ME, Shokeir AA, Ghoneim MA. Impact of schistosomiasis on patient and graft outcome after renal transplantation: 10 years' follow-up. Nephrol Dial Transplant. 2001;16(11):2214–21.
198. Shokeir AA. Renal transplantation: the impact of schistosomiasis. BJU Int. 2001;88:915–20.
199. Sobh MA, El-Agroudy AE, Moustafa FE, Shokeir AA, El-Shazly A, Ghoneim MA. Impact of schistosomiasis on patient and graft outcome after kidney transplantation. Nephrol Dial Transplant. 1992;7:858–64.

Ocular Infections in Transplant Patients

18

Ann-Marie Lobo, Lucia Sobrin, and Marlene L. Durand

Abbreviations

AIDS	Acquired immunodeficiency syndrome
ARN	Acute retinal necrosis
BCG	Bacillus Calmette-Guerin vaccine
CMV	Cytomegalovirus
CMVR	Cytomegalovirus retinitis
CNS	Central nervous system
EBV	Epstein-Barr virus
GVHD	Graft versus host disease
HAART	Highly active antiretroviral therapy
HIV	Human immunodeficiency virus
HSCT	Hematopoietic stem cell transplant
HSV	Herpes simplex virus
HZO	Herpes zoster ophthalmicus
IRS	Immune recovery syndrome
PCR	Polymerase chain reaction
PORN	Progressive outer retinal necrosis
TB	Tuberculosis
VZV	Varicella zoster virus

A.-M. Lobo
Department of Ophthalmology and Visual Sciences, Illinois Eye and Ear Infirmary, University of Illinois at Chicago, Chicago, IL, USA
e-mail: alobo2@uic.edu

L. Sobrin
Department of Ophthalmology, Harvard Medical School, Massachusetts Eye and Ear Infirmary, Boston, MA, USA
e-mail: lucia_sobrin@meei.harvard.edu

M. L. Durand (✉)
Department of Medicine, Harvard Medical School, Massachusetts General Hospital, Division of Infectious Diseases, Boston, MA, USA
e-mail: mdurand@mgh.harvard.edu

Introduction

Transplant patients may develop infections in any part of the eye and ocular adnexa. The most common site of ocular infection is in the posterior segment of the eye, which includes the vitreous, retina, choroid, and optic nerve. Posterior segment infections occur most often from either hematogenous spread of systemic infection like endophthalmitis or reactivation of latent infections such as viral retinitis, and ocular toxoplasmosis. The anterior segment of the eye includes the conjunctiva, sclera, cornea, aqueous, iris, and ciliary body. These structures can be infected either through direct inoculation in cases of keratitis or corneal infection or via hematogenous spread resulting in endophthalmitis. Various terms are used to define the location and structures of the eye involved in infectious and inflammatory processes. Endophthalmitis refers to a bacterial or fungal infection involving the vitreous and/or aqueous humors. Uveitis refers to an inflammatory or infectious process involving the uvea, which is comprised of the iris, ciliary body, and choroid. The uvea is highly vascular, so the choroid may be the first structure involved if a bacteremia or fungemia seeds the eye. Retinitis is considered a type of uveitis, even though the retina is not part of the uvea. In many cases of infection involving the retina, there is also underlying choroidal involvement, hence the term chorioretinitis. In treating intraocular infections, the blood-eye barrier must be considered. This is similar to the blood-brain barrier and prevents some antibiotics from achieving therapeutic intraocular levels.

Ocular Complications in Transplant Patients

The most common ocular complications in transplant patients are noninfectious. Cataract is the most common complication in several studies and usually occurs as a complication of corticosteroid therapy or, in allogeneic

A. Safdar (ed.), *Principles and Practice of Transplant Infectious Diseases*, https://doi.org/10.1007/978-1-4939-9034-4_18

hematopoietic stem cell transplant (HSCT) recipients, total body irradiation. In a study of 71 pediatric renal transplant recipients with a mean follow-up of 5.6 years, cataract was the most common ocular complication and occurred in 8% [1]. Similarly, in a study of 46 lung transplant recipients who underwent eye examination, cataract was the most common finding, occurring in 28% of patients [2]. In a prospective study of 115 heart, lung, or heart-lung transplant recipients, cataracts were again the most common finding, occurring in 17%, followed by hypertensive changes (8%), chorioretinal scarring (5%), and diabetic retinopathy (3%) [3]. In bone marrow transplant recipients, a major ocular complication is dry eyes related to chronic graft versus host disease (GVHD). In a prospective study of 101 consecutive patients who received allogenic stem cell transplants between 2004 and 2007, ocular GVHD developed in 54% and consisted mainly of dry eyes and conjunctivitis [4].

The incidence of ocular infections after solid organ or HSCT is low, with studies from around the world reporting an incidence of approximately 2%. In a study of 1198 solid organ or bone marrow transplant recipients examined at an eye clinic in Korea between 1995 and 2005, 33 had retinal complications, including 21 (1.8%) with infectious etiologies (15 viral, 5 fungal, 1 *Toxoplasma*) [5]. Over 80% of these eye infections occurred within the first year posttransplant. Of the viral infections, cytomegalovirus (CMV) retinitis was the most common (11 cases), while acute retinal necrosis (ARN) occurred in 3 and progressive outer retinal necrosis (PORN) in 1. A review of 860 patients who had received heart, lung, or liver transplants in Sydney, Australia, between 1984 and 1997 identified 19 (2%) who had non-cataract ocular complications [6]. Of these, ocular infections occurred in 14 patients (1.6%), with viral infections in 11 (5 ARN, 3 CMV retinitis, 2 herpes simplex virus keratitis, 1 herpes zoster ophthalmicus), fungal chorioretinitis in 2, and bacterial dacryocystitis in 1. These infections occurred from 5 months to 4 years posttransplantation. A study of heart, lung, and heart-lung recipients in London found only 1 of 115 (0.8%) developed an ocular infection (*Aspergillus* endophthalmitis) [3]. A study of 620 patients who underwent allogeneic stem cell transplant from 1997 to 2007 in Riyadh, Saudi Arabia, found ocular infections in 16 (2.6%), with keratitis in 11 patients (bacterial 10, viral 1), CMV retinitis in 4 patients, and mold endophthalmitis in 1 patient [7]. A study of 313 patients who received heart transplants at the Mayo Clinic in Rochester, Minnesota, between 1988 and 2006 found 6 patients (1.9%) with potentially serious eye infections (1 CMV retinitis, 1 *Aspergillus* endophthalmitis, 3 herpes zoster ophthalmicus, 1 preseptal cellulitis), while 2 others had minor infections (conjunctivitis, blepharitis) [8].

Common Eye Infections in Transplant Patients

Viral Retinitis

Acute Retinal Necrosis

The acute retinal necrosis syndrome (ARN) is a rapidly progressive viral retinitis that was first described in 1971 [9]. Although ARN is mainly reported in immunocompetent patients, it is still one of the most common infections seen in transplant patients. The onset of ARN occurred 7 months to 7 years posttransplant in several studies, with the average onset greater than 1 year posttransplant [5, 6, 10]. Most cases have been described in solid organ transplant patients rather than HSCT recipients. ARN is caused by varicella zoster virus (VZV), herpes simplex virus (HSV) types 1 and 2, and less commonly CMV. In non-transplant patients, VZV is the most common etiology, causing 60% of cases, while HSV causes 30–40% and CMV less than 10% of cases [11, 12]. The relative frequency of these etiologies in transplant patients has not been described. In transplant patients, the herpes viruses may be more likely than other infections to present solely in the eye without concomitant extraocular infection or graft rejection [5]. In immunocompetent patients, there is an age distribution for the different viral etiologies with VZV more likely to be the cause of ARN in older patients and HSV type 2 more likely in younger patients [13]. It is unclear whether this distribution also exists in transplant patients.

ARN usually presents with unilateral eye pain, photophobia, and decreased vision. The eye pain may be mild or absent. In up to 30% of cases, ARN occurs in both eyes, although usually one eye is affected before the onset of symptoms in the other. The American Uveitis Society has established the following clinical criteria for diagnosis of ARN: (1) focal well-demarcated areas of retinal necrosis located in the retinal periphery, (2) rapid circumferential progression of necrosis, (3) occlusive vasculopathy, and (4) prominent inflammation (white blood cells) in the vitreous and aqueous [14]. Clinical exam is significant for a panuveitis (which produces symptoms of pain and blurred vision) and peripheral retinal whitening/retinitis (Fig. 18.1a, b).

The differential diagnosis of ARN includes CMV retinitis, *Toxoplasma* chorioretinitis, ocular syphilis, and infectious endophthalmitis. The ocular findings in CMV retinitis differ from CMV-ARN and are discussed below; one major difference is that CMV-ARN has marked intraocular inflammation, while this is not a feature of CMV retinitis. Nearly all patients develop ARN as reactivation of latent infection due to VZV, HSV, or CMV, although rare cases have been described after recent acquisition of virus. Although ARN is primarily a clinical diagnosis, other diag-

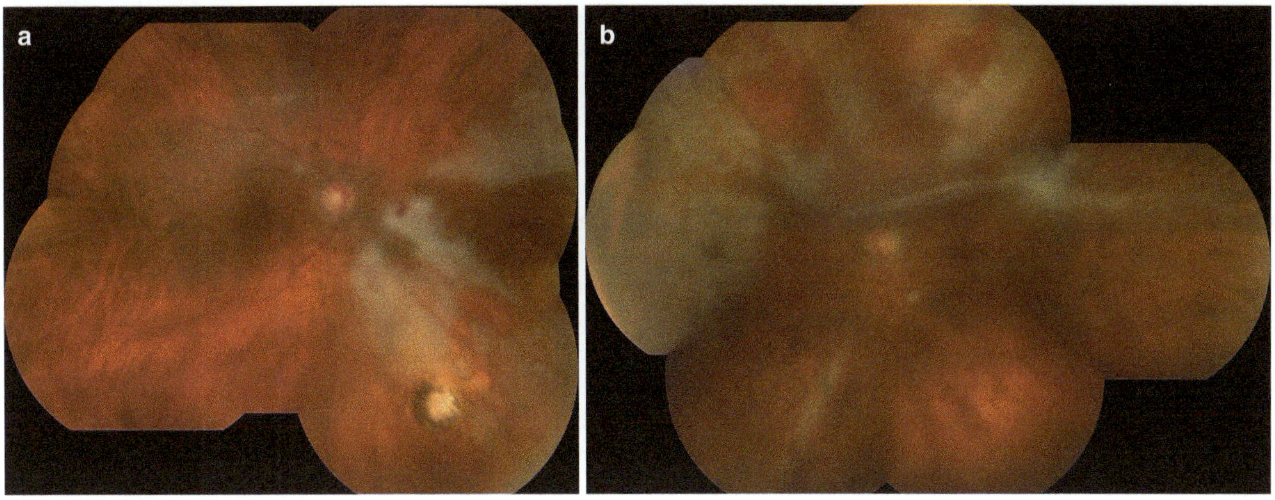

Fig. 18.1 (**a**, **b**) Acute retinal necrosis (ARN): fundus photographs of each eye demonstrating peripheral retinal whitening with hemorrhages and vitritis. Vitreous PCR was positive for CMV. The patient had been CMV seronegative when he received a kidney 14 months earlier from a CMV-seropositive donor. He developed bilateral ARN 2 months after completing a year of valganciclovir prophylaxis

nostic tests may be helpful in distinguishing specific viral etiology and in tailoring treatment. Serum antibody titers are generally not helpful in diagnosis, given the high baseline level of seropositivity in the general population. However, negative serology (IgM and IgG) for a particular virus (e.g., HSV or CMV) usually excludes that pathogen as an etiology of ARN. Molecular diagnostic testing with polymerase chain reaction (PCR) from ocular fluid samples provides a more specific test for identifying viral pathogens in ARN [13]. Aqueous fluid sampling is a relatively safe office procedure and can be used even in cases of primarily posterior segment disease including necrotizing retinitis even though the quantitative yield can be low [15, 16]. A vitreous aspirate has a higher yield and can also be obtained in the office but has more potential for complications, including infection and retinal detachment. A diagnostic vitrectomy can be performed in the operating room to obtain a larger sample of fluid for testing, especially in cases of minimal anterior segment inflammation. Clinicians should have a low threshold for performing molecular diagnostic testing in transplant patients with ARN in whom the viral etiology is unclear. Aqueous and/or vitreous sampling for viral PCR is especially important if initial empiric antiviral therapy does not halt progression of retinitis by funduscopic examination. Quantitative PCR can also be used to monitor response to therapy; if there is no significant decline in viral load from vitreous aspirate signifying potential antiviral resistance, a change in antiviral therapy can be implemented [17, 18]. However, the results of such quantitative PCR testing may not be available in a timely fashion, and decisions must be made day by day based on the ophthalmologist's examination of the eye. Progression of ARN in one eye or new involvement of the other eye while on intravenous antiviral therapy should prompt immediate change in therapy in order to save vision in this potentially blinding infection.

Treatment of ARN in transplant patients always includes intravenous antiviral therapy initially and may also include intravitreal injections of antiviral agents. Intravenous acyclovir is the standard initial therapy for ARN in immunocompetent patients, in whom CMV-ARN is very uncommon [19]. Intravenous acyclovir has also been used successfully in treating transplant patients with VZV and HSV ARN [10]. Valacyclovir has been used in treatment of early ARN in immunocompetent patients, but we do not recommend this, especially in immunosuppressed patients as retinitis may progress rapidly. One question in treating ARN is whether intravenous ganciclovir, rather than intravenous acyclovir, should be used initially in transplant patients and other severely immunosuppressed patients, given the increased likelihood of CMV-ARN in immunosuppressed patients. This question has not been answered. Successful treatment of ARN requires daily communication between the infectious disease specialist and the retina specialist, with the goal of halting retinitis progression as quickly as possible. Failure of intravenous acyclovir to halt progression of retinitis may signify either CMV-ARN or acyclovir-resistant HSV or VZV (e.g., due to thymidine kinase mutation). CMV-ARN requires intravenous ganciclovir (acyclovir is ineffective), but progression despite ganciclovir may occur and may signify ganciclovir-resistant CMV. Such patients would be given intravenous foscarnet or, failing that, intravenous cidofovir, plus intravitreal foscarnet injections. Transplant patients on chronic acyclovir prophylaxis are at increased risk for acyclovir-resistant HSV and VZV, and ganciclovir will not be effective for such patients: intravenous foscarnet should be given. Cidofovir may be necessary in cases that continue to progress despite foscarnet. Intravitreal injections of foscarnet may be used to supplement systemic therapy. Intravitreal injection of ganciclovir (for acyclovir-sensitive HSV or VZV and ganciclovir-sensitive CMV) or foscarnet within 48 h of initiation of systemic therapy may prevent rapid progression of retinitis and improve visual prognosis [11]. Multiple intravitreal antiviral injections may be given to halt the progression of retinal necrosis.

Systemic intravenous antiviral therapy should be given for a minimum of 1–2 weeks and can then be transitioned to an oral antiviral (valacyclovir or valganciclovir, if patients responded to intravenous acyclovir or ganciclovir, respectively). Valacyclovir or valganciclovir is usually given for several months in immunocompetent patients, although the optimal duration of this therapy is unknown. Dosing may then be reduced to provide long-term prophylaxis, which may be necessary indefinitely in the transplant patient. In patients who require intravenous foscarnet for acyclovir-resistant HSV or VZV or for ganciclovir-resistant CMV, an oral equivalent is not currently available, so long-term prophylactic therapy becomes more difficult.

A late complication of ARN is retinal detachment, which occurs 4 weeks to 6 months after the acute infection [20]. Barrier retinal laser photocoagulation can be performed at the edges of retinal necrosis early in the course in an attempt to prevent subsequent retinal detachment, but many patients with extensive necrosis may still develop retinal detachment [21, 22]. The severity of vitreous inflammation in the acute phase of infection may prevent adequate visualization of the retina for laser therapy. Vitrectomy with or without silicone oil tamponade can be performed to repair retinal detachments associated with ARN.

Visual prognosis in ARN is guarded, and more than 50% of patients develop retinal detachment [21]. One retrospective study of 58 patients with unilateral ARN diagnosed between 1981 and 2008 and who had at least 6 months of follow-up reported that significant vision loss (≤20/200) in the affected eye occurred in 50% of patients by 3 months and 75% by 5 years [20]. Patients with worse initial visual acuity or who developed a retinal detachment had worse outcomes in this study. This study found that 19% of ARN patients were immunocompromised, but did not note whether any were transplant recipients. The rate of significant visual loss from ARN is unknown in the transplant population. One study that included three patients treated with intravenous acyclovir found that all three had excellent outcomes [6], while another study of four patients (five eyes infected) found that final visual acuity was <20/200 in 40% [5]. Viral etiology also affects prognosis, and VZV has been associated with worse visual prognosis and more rapid necrosis compared to HSV [11].

Progressive Outer Retinal Necrosis

Progressive outer retinal necrosis (PORN) is a variant of a herpetic necrotizing retinitis that primarily involves the "outer" (deeper) layers of the retina. This rapidly progressive infection is characterized by lack of inflammation and retinal vasculitis. PORN initially was described only in severely immunosuppressed AIDS patients [23, 24]. This syndrome has also been noted in several cases of hematopoietic stem cell transplant (HSCT) and kidney transplant patients [5, 25, 26]. VZV is the most common etiology for PORN, and the majority of transplant patients have an antecedent history of disseminated or localized herpes zoster infection prior to the development of necrotizing outer retinal necrosis. Several reported cases of PORN in HSCT patients occurred in the setting of significant immunosuppression for graft versus host disease [26, 27].

Rather than a blurred vision, patients often present with complaints of painless dimming of vision or constriction of their visual field. Visual complaints may be out of proportion to what is seen on clinical examination in early stages of disease. Clinical exam reveals multifocal circumscribed creamy deep retinal lesions in the periphery of the retina although the central macula can also be involved. These lesions rapidly progress to become confluent areas of retinal whitening with perivascular sparing (Fig. 18.2). Progression to near total vision loss is often very rapid in PORN, and timely and aggressive antiviral therapy is essential. Unlike cases of ARN, there is no inflammation in the anterior chamber or vitreous and no occlusive vasculitis in PORN. The optic nerve can be involved with profound visual loss. Many

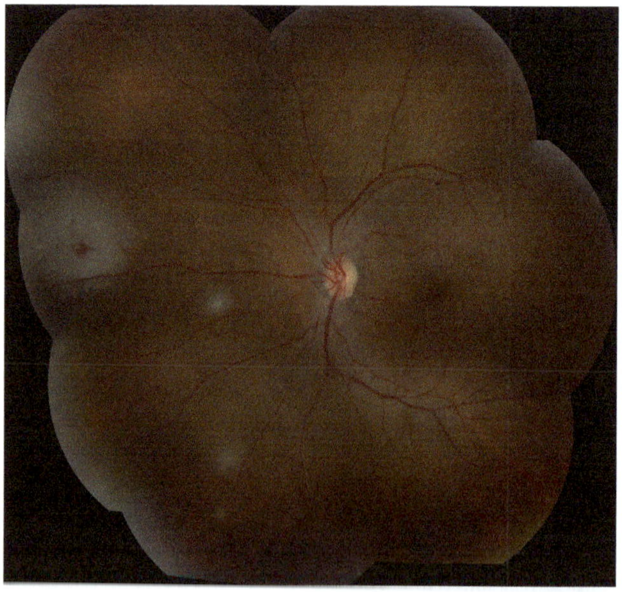

Fig. 18.2 Progressive outer retinal necrosis (PORN): fundus photograph demonstrating areas of retinal whitening and minimal vitritis. The risk factor in this patient was AIDS

patients present with retinal detachments which often occur early in the course of the disease [28].

The differential diagnosis for PORN includes ARN, atypical toxoplasmosis, CMV retinitis, and ocular syphilis. Diagnosis is primarily clinical, but in cases of uncertainty, ocular fluid sampling for PCR can be performed. There have been rare cases of PCR positive for CMV and HSV from vitreous samples of patients with PORN [29].

Treatment for PORN also differs from ARN in that intravenous acyclovir has been found to be ineffective in many cases of PORN. Because many immunosuppressed patients have already been treated with prophylactic acyclovir or valacyclovir, there is concern that acyclovir resistance may be highly prevalent in patients who subsequently develop PORN [24]. Intravenous ganciclovir and foscarnet are the systemic therapies of choice due to the aggressive and rapid course of this disease. Induction doses of ganciclovir can be given for 3 weeks and foscarnet for 2 weeks followed by maintenance therapy until the retinitis has completely regressed [28]. Early treatment with intravitreal antiviral therapy, either foscarnet or ganciclovir, is also recommended; intravitreal therapy can be given as frequently as three injections per week at the outset of disease followed by weekly injections until the retinitis has stabilized. Barrier laser photocoagulation can be performed at the borders of areas of retinal necrosis, although even when performed, many patients still may develop retinal detachments. The absence of vitreous inflammation makes laser treatment more feasible in PORN compared with many cases of ARN.

PORN has the worst visual prognosis of all types of viral retinitis, with reports of greater than 60% of patients losing vision to the level of no light perception [23]. Macula and optic nerve involvement can cause profound vision loss, and 70% of patients develop retinal detachments [28]. The aggressive use of intravenous and intravitreal antiviral therapies has improved visual outcomes, but early diagnosis and treatment are paramount. Transplant patients with history of herpes zoster should be referred immediately for evaluation if they develop any new visual complaints.

CMV Retinitis

CMV retinitis (CMVR) is an opportunistic infection most commonly seen in AIDS patients prior to the era of highly active antiretroviral therapy (HAART). While the overall incidence of CMVR has declined in AIDS patients in association with HAART therapy, this disease process has been reported in both the solid organ transplant and hematopoietic stem cell transplant (HSCT) populations. The incidence of CMVR after solid organ transplantation is reportedly between 2% and 15% compared to 0.19–2.2% for HSCT populations [6, 29–31], but there is some variation by study. A review of 101 studies from 1987 to 2007 involving 12,653 liver transplant patients found CMV retinitis in only 0.1% [32]. The incidence of CMVR may be increasing due to the earlier recognition and treatment of CMV reactivation and decreased likelihood of lethal systemic CMV disease early in the posttransplant course [33]. The source of CMV infection can either be a CMV-antibody-positive donor, reactivation of latent CMV, or primary infection with CMV in the setting of transfusion or immunosuppression [5]. Characteristics associated with the development of CMVR in transplant patients include severe immunosuppression and/or lymphopenia, graft versus host disease, and other systemic infections [5, 33]. Viral retinitis has been reported more commonly in heart transplant patients likely due to the high level of immunosuppression required [5, 6]. In HSCT, risk factors for CMVR include unrelated donors, delayed lymphocyte engraftment, and increased CMV reactivation in the CMV-seropositive graft recipients [31].

Clinical Presentation

Patients often present with complaints of floaters and blurred vision, but many patients may be asymptomatic if lesions are in the peripheral retina. Bilateral involvement is common, occurring in 40% of HSCT patients in one study [29] and 60% of solid organ transplant patients in another [34]. There are two characteristic fundus lesions seen on clinical examination: (1) a wedge-shaped area of hypopigmented retinal infiltrate along a vascular arcade often with associated intraretinal hemorrhages and (2) a peripheral yellow granular retinal lesion with a scarred center and an active border that slowly expands. Other associated clinical signs include satellite lesions adjacent to the main lesion, retinal vascular sheathing, and rarely extensive exudation along retinal blood vessels referred to as "frosted branch angiitis." In contrast to other ocular infections, such as ARN and toxoplasmosis, CMVR has minimal anterior segment and vitreous inflammation.

The differential diagnosis for CMVR includes HSV or VZV retinitis, atypical ocular toxoplasmosis, fungal or bacterial endophthalmitis, and ocular syphilis. CMVR can generally be diagnosed based on clinical examination. In atypical cases, molecular diagnostic tests such as PCR can be performed from aqueous or vitreous fluid samples. In most cases of CMVR, transplant patients may already have known systemic CMV disease and positive CMV antigenemia.

The immune reconstitution syndrome (IRS) (also called immune recovery uveitis) has also been reported in transplant patients who have been treated for CMVR. IRS is thought to be an immune reaction to CMV antigens in patients with active or inactive disease but is more common with larger-sized lesions [35]. This syndrome presents in the eye with vitritis, optic nerve edema, macular edema, and epiretinal membrane formation which can decrease visual acuity.

Treatment

The treatment of CMVR involves systemic induction therapy as well as local intravitreal therapy with ganciclovir or foscarnet. Intravitreal therapy serves as an important adjunct therapy for CMVR, especially in patients who cannot tolerate high-dose systemic therapy due to neutropenia [33]. In severe cases with rapid progression of retinitis, a ganciclovir sustained release implant can be inserted [36]. There have been cases of transplant patients who develop CMVR in spite of CMV prophylaxis with valganciclovir or ganciclovir, with one series reporting that 7 of 11 transplant patients were on ganciclovir for CMV antigenemia prior to the development of CMVR [5]. In patients where retinitis continues to progress despite standard therapy with ganciclovir or valganciclovir, ganciclovir resistance should be suspected, and alternative therapy with foscarnet (intravenous and/or intravitreal) or cidofovir is imperative [32]. Such patients should have samples of plasma tested for ganciclovir resistance (e.g., UL97 and UL54 gene sequencing). Duration of maintenance therapy varies for CMVR in transplant patients and depends on the level of cumulative immune suppression, systemic disease and adverse effects. Treatment of ocular IRS usually includes systemic or periocular corticosteroids in addition to ongoing antiviral therapy.

Prognosis

Visual prognosis for transplant patients with CMVR is guarded. In one large series of CMVR in patients without HIV, the majority of patients had decreased visual acuity within 1 year following diagnosis [35]. Causes of ocular morbidity and limited visual prognosis include retinal scarring and retinal detachment. Retinal necrosis leads to the development of retinal tears and subsequent detachment. Transplant patients with CMVR have a lower likelihood of developing retinal detachment compared to AIDS patients regardless of HAART therapy [35].

Endophthalmitis

Endophthalmitis means bacterial or fungal infection involving the vitreous and/or aqueous. Endophthalmitis may be either exogenous, introduced from outside in, such as after eye surgery or eye trauma, or endogenous, due to hematogenous seeding of bacteria or fungi. The most common type of endophthalmitis in the general population is exogenous and bacterial, while the most common type in the transplant population is endogenous and fungal.

Cataract surgery is the most common type of ocular surgery, with over two million surgeries performed annually in the United States alone. Endophthalmitis develops postoperatively in approximately 0.1% of cases, and 75% of patients develop symptoms (decreased vision, eye discomfort, redness) within the first week after eye surgery. Bacteria cause nearly all cases in western countries, with coagulase-negative staphylococci accounting for 70% of cases. Cataracts (opacities of the lens) are common in the transplant population, occurring in at least 15% of patients as noted above. Both corticosteroid therapy and total body irradiation are risk factors in the transplant population. Many of these patients will eventually require cataract surgery, so post-cataract endophthalmitis is a risk in this population. However, this infection has not been specifically mentioned in reviews of ocular infections in transplant patients, so the incidence may be the same as in the general population.

Endogenous fungal endophthalmitis is the most common type of endophthalmitis in transplant patients and is often associated with disseminated fungal infection or fungal infection at another site. Blood cultures may be negative, however, as fungemia may be transient. It is worth noting a nomenclature issue: in the literature, fungal chorioretinitis (i.e., without significant vitritis) is sometimes distinguished from fungal "endophthalmitis," a term that implies significant vitritis. However, most of the transplant literature does not make this distinction, and we will only note the degree of vitritis here, when relevant.

Fungal endophthalmitis accounts for 20–25% of posterior segment infections in transplant patients, second only to viral retinitis [5–7]. Overall, 0.1–0.4% of transplant patients develop fungal endophthalmitis [5–7]. The onset is within 1 year of transplant in nearly all cases. Because infections are endogenous, the "back" of the eye is usually seeded first – often the highly vascular choroid. This infection may be clinically silent at first, but then the patient develops decrease in vision with or without eye pain. On examination, fluffy white lesions may be seen in the posterior pole with minimal vitritis – this is termed chorioretinitis and is typical of early endogenous *Candida* infections. Patients with more severe eye infection usually have significant vitritis (white blood cells in the vitreous), often coalesced as "fluff balls" or a "string of pearls," as well as inflammation in the aqueous (Fig. 18.3). At this stage, there may be eye pain and a "red eye." On examination, a hypopyon (layer of white blood cells in the aqueous) may be present. There may be so much intraocular inflammation that the view of the retina is obscured. In some cases of mold endophthalmitis in transplant patients, the primary appearance is of a subretinal abscess.

Both yeasts and molds have been described as causes of fungal endophthalmitis in transplant patients. Patients with *Candida* endophthalmitis may have concurrent or antecedent candidemia. *Aspergillus* endophthalmitis is the most common type of mold endophthalmitis in transplant patients and accounts for over half of cases [37]. There is often another

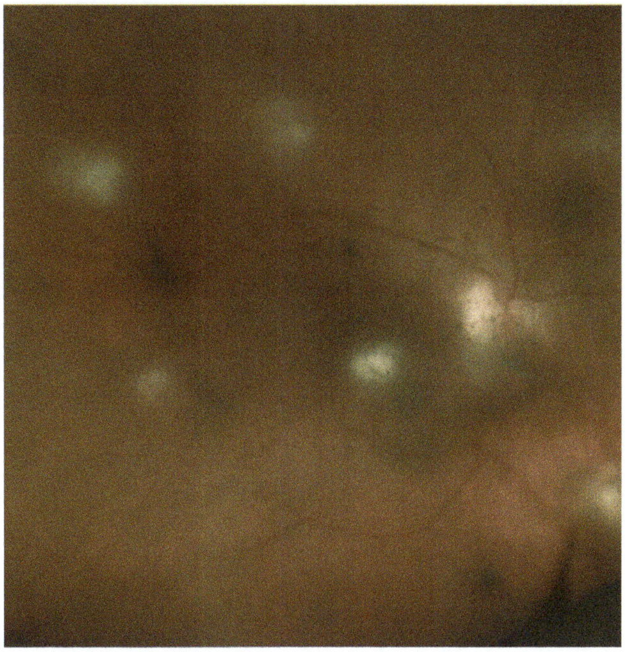

Fig. 18.3 Fungal endophthalmitis: fundus photograph demonstrating several vitreous "fluff balls" typical of fungal endophthalmitis. Gram stain and fungal stain of aqueous humor samples demonstrated yeast, but cultures of the aqueous, vitreous, and blood were negative. The risk factor in this patient was intravenous drug abuse

organ infected concurrently, such as *Aspergillus* endocarditis [8] and pulmonary aspergillosis [6]. Endogenous *Aspergillus* endophthalmitis may be unrecognized during life, especially if patients are too ill to complain of eye symptoms. In an autopsy series of 85 liver transplant patients, 6 patients were found to have *Aspergillus* endophthalmitis, but only 1 was diagnosed before death [38]. The eye was the second most common site of infection, after the lungs.

Scedosporium apiospermum (the asexual form of *Pseudallescheria boydii*) is another common cause of fungal endophthalmitis in transplant patients [39]. It is often associated with disseminated infection, and mortality is at least 50% in transplant patients and nearly 100% in lung transplant recipients. This fungus is resistant to amphotericin but usually responds to voriconazole. Successful treatment using long-term voriconazole has been described in two lung transplant patients with disseminated infection including endophthalmitis [40]. *Fusarium* endophthalmitis is the second most common cause of mold endophthalmitis worldwide, after *Aspergillus*, but in non-immunocompromised patients, this infection usually arises exogenously – either as an extension of *Fusarium* keratitis (corneal infection), after eye trauma, or as a nosocomial complication of eye surgery in tropical countries. In transplant patients, *Fusarium* is usually associated with disseminated infection, as in the case of a HSCT patient with bilateral endophthalmitis who died despite maximal therapy [41].

Bacterial endophthalmitis is rare in transplant patients and nearly always occurs from bacteremic seeding, although blood cultures may be negative at the time of presentation with eye findings. Case reports have described other bacterial etiologies, including a case of bilateral *Pseudomonas* endophthalmitis in a cystic fibrosis patient after lung transplantation [42], *Listeria* endophthalmitis in a renal transplant patient [43], and *Nocardia* endophthalmitis in a cardiac transplant patient [44].

Treatment of fungal endophthalmitis requires systemic antifungal therapy optimized for the fungus involved. In cases of *Candida* chorioretinitis without vitritis, or with minimal vitritis, systemic therapy alone may be sufficient to also treat the eye infection. However, if significant vitritis is present or in cases of mold endophthalmitis, intravitreal injections of antifungal agents must also be given. These are either amphotericin or voriconazole injections and may be repeated more than once. Vitrectomy, if the patient is well enough to undergo eye surgery, is often essential to control intraocular mold infections; in these cases, an injection of antifungal (amphotericin or voriconazole) is given at the end of the case.

The prognosis for endogenous fungal endophthalmitis in transplant patients has been poor, and many die of the systemic fungal disease. However, successful therapy is increasingly common in the era of the new antifungal agents.

Rare Eye Infections in Transplant Patients

Infectious Uveitis

Ocular Toxoplasmosis

Ocular toxoplasmosis is the most common infectious cause of posterior uveitis in the world. In transplant patients, toxoplasmosis can present as encephalitis, pneumonitis, or myocarditis, but it has been reported infrequently in the eye. In one series of 102 non-AIDS immunocompromised patients, 6% of patients developed chorioretinitis, and 70% of these patients had concomitant encephalitis [45]. The overall incidence of reactivation of toxoplasmosis in HSCT patients who have known *Toxoplasma* IgG seropositivity is 2% [46]. The majority of cases of toxoplasmosis in HSCT develop within 6 months after transplant [47]. Ocular toxoplasmosis in transplant patients is most often reactivation of latent disease, although reports of acquired infection from transplantation have been described, particularly in cardiac and liver transplants [48]. Immunocompromised patients with positive antibodies to *Toxoplasma* prior to transplantation may be more likely to have reactivation of disease. Other risk factors for ocular toxoplasmosis in the transplant patient include prior episodes of ocular toxoplasmosis and severe GVHD.

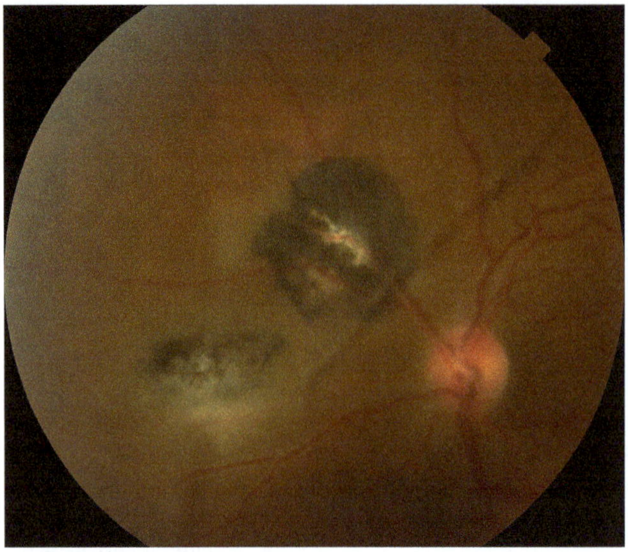

Fig. 18.4 Toxoplasma chorioretinitis: fundus photograph demonstrating pigmented chorioretinal scar with adjacent active area of hypopigmented chorioretinitis

Clinical Presentation

Patients may present with complaints of blurred vision, floaters, eye pain, and scotomata. Clinical examination reveals a mild cellular reaction in the anterior and posterior chambers with areas of white-yellow chorioretinal lesions which may be adjacent to an area of pigmented chorioretinal scarring (Fig. 18.4). These lesions are generally more bright white and have borders with smooth contours compared to CMV retinitis lesions. There can be associated retinal vasculitis. Patients may have multiple lesions and bilateral involvement. In contrast with ocular toxoplasmosis in immunocompetent patients, which is often associated with significant vitritis, transplant patients may have mild inflammation and more extensive chorioretinal necrosis, making it difficult to distinguish from viral retinitis [49].

Diagnostic Tests

Most cases of ocular toxoplasmosis are diagnosed clinically. Serologic testing for *Toxoplasma* antibodies (IgM and IgG) can be helpful, particularly if patients were seronegative prior to transplantation. Molecular diagnostic testing with PCR may be performed on ocular fluid samples in cases of atypical toxoplasmosis, Goldmann-Witmer coefficient testing comparing antibodies in ocular fluids and serum may be inconclusive in severely immunosuppressed patients who may not be able to mount a sufficient antibody response for detection. One case of ocular toxoplasmosis was diagnosed in a HSCT patient based on fine needle aspiration biopsy of the chorioretinal lesion demonstrating *Toxoplasma gondii* tachyzoites and intracytoplasmic cysts; this approach can be reserved for atypical cases where it is unclear if the retinal process is infectious or a recurrence of leukemia [50]. Because of the potential for systemic *Toxoplasma* infection including encephalitis, neuroimaging should be performed in immunocompromised patients with ocular toxoplasmosis.

Treatment

The treatment for ocular toxoplasmosis in the immunocompromised patient is sulfadiazine, plus pyrimethamine, with folinic acid rescue; clindamycin may also be added for "triple therapy." Patients must be monitored closely for adverse effects of medications including additional bone marrow suppression with pyrimethamine and renal failure with sulfadiazine. Trimethoprim-sulfamethoxazole has been used to treat immunocompetent patients. Prophylactic treatment with either trimethoprim-sulfamethoxazole 160 mg/800 mg or combination of pyrimethamine/sulfadiazine has been recommended in transplant patients with known prior episodes of *Toxoplasma* chorioretinitis [47]. This prophylactic therapy is continued for months to years or even lifelong, with the duration depending on factors such as the degree and duration of immune suppression, type of transplantation procedure, and the presence of GVHD or allograft rejection.

Prognosis

The visual prognosis for ocular toxoplasmosis is dependent on the location of chorioretinal lesions. Once treated, lesions involving the macula or adjacent to the optic nerve become fibrotic scars with associated poor visual acuity. Patients with peripheral lesions generally have a good visual prognosis, with full recovery to baseline visual acuity with treatment. Potential complications which may also affect visual prognosis include retinal detachment and reactivation of infection.

Ocular Tuberculosis

Ocular involvement of tuberculosis (TB) is rare. In a large series of patients from the United States during the era of TB sanatoria, only 1.4% of patients with pulmonary TB had ocular involvement [51]. The incidence of TB in solid organ transplant populations was reported to be 25–50 times higher than the general population, according to one recent series from a single center in the United States [52]. The majority of transplant patients present with pulmonary or disseminated TB within the first year after transplantation when the level of immunosuppression is highest. Ocular TB in transplant patients is rare and has been reported in a handful of cases, mainly in renal transplant patients with disseminated or pulmonary involvement [53, 54]. Ocular TB occurs following hematogenous spread from pulmonary or disseminated infection.

Patients may present with complaints of blurred vision, floaters, or eye pain, depending on the location of the ocular involvement. One of the most common manifestations of ocular TB is a choroidal granuloma ("tubercle") which appears as a gray or yellow mass deep to the retina with or without inflammation. Choroidal tubercles can be found in both eyes, range in size from one-fourth to several disc diameters, and are histopathologically similar to tubercles found in other parts of the body, with caseating granulomas containing acid-fast bacilli [55]. Untreated, choroidal granulomas can grow in size and become subretinal abscesses as the choroid is replaced with necrotic tissue. Other types of ocular involvement include multifocal chorioretinitis which can coalesce to form serpiginous choroiditis, retinal vasculitis (mainly periphlebitis), vitritis, panuveitis, granulomatous anterior uveitis, and scleritis. The differential diagnosis of ocular TB includes ocular syphilis, ocular toxoplasmosis, viral retinitis, and noninfectious etiologies such as sarcoidosis and ocular Behcet's disease.

Diagnosis of ocular TB in the absence of pulmonary or disseminated TB can be challenging. Immunosuppressed patients are more likely to have a negative tuberculin skin test even in the presence of active TB. Interferon gamma release assays (IGRA), may be more sensitive in detecting TB in immunosuppressed patients and in patients with prior BCG vaccination [56]. Culture of ocular fluids rarely produces positive results. Ocular fluid sampling can be performed for molecular diagnostic testing, but the sensitivity and diagnostic yield of TB PCR in ocular fluids are low. [57]. Because transplant patients with ocular TB most likely have systemic involvement, it is important to perform a thorough workup for evidence of disseminated TB.

Treatment of ocular TB consists of standard multidrug TB therapy as used for systemic infections. A quinolone antibiotic is sometimes substituted for ethambutol given concern for ethambutol-associated optic neuropathy. In patients with severe intraocular inflammation, where the inflammation alone may be harmful to the retina, local or systemic corticosteroids may be used. However, systemic corticosteroids should be used with caution in transplant patients with disseminated disease.

Visual prognosis depends on the extent and location of ocular involvement. Patients with large choroidal granulomas or subretinal abscesses who present with more advanced disease are at risk for significant vision loss. Early recognition of eye involvement and treatment with antitubercular therapy is important for preventing severe vision loss and for treating systemic infection.

Infectious Keratitis: Herpes Zoster Ophthalmicus, Herpes Simplex

Reactivation of VZV is a common complication in solid organ transplant and HSCT patients. VZV in the distribution of the first branch of the trigeminal nerve, also known as herpes zoster ophthalmicus (HZO), can cause significant morbidity. The incidence of HZO in one series of HSCT in children was 1.2% [58]. Patients present with the vesicular rash in a dermatomal distribution. Herpes simplex keratitis can also occur in transplant patients and can be distinguished from VZV by the absence of the dermatomal rash. There have also been rare instances of bilateral HSV keratitis in patients with graft versus host disease following SCT [59].

Patients often complain of eye pain, redness, tearing, and blurred vision, although there may be eye involvement in the absence of significant symptoms. Clinical examination may reveal a corneal pseudodendrite in HZO (similar to the dermatologic vesicular lesion in zoster) or a corneal epithelial dendrite in HSV. Both HZO and HSV may also present with stromal keratitis, anterior uveitis, scleritis, and conjunctivitis. HZO can cause an optic neuropathy or extraocular muscle palsy. Both entities can cause elevated eye pressure on presentation. Systemic antiviral therapy should be instituted within 72 h of the development of the rash in HZO to decrease disease duration and potential morbidity, including postherpetic neuralgia. Transplant patients are often treated with intravenous acyclovir for HZO, likely due to concerns for more aggressive disease process or risk of disseminated disease in immunosuppressed patients. There have also been cases of severe HSV keratitis in transplant patients requiring the use of intravenous acyclovir [60]. However, there is concern for acyclovir resistance especially in immunocompromised patients with VZV who may have been on antiviral prophylaxis. There was a case of HZO in a HSCT patient that persisted in spite of intravenous acyclovir therapy [61]. Transplant patients should be maintained on oral antiviral prophylaxis with acyclovir, valacyclovir, or famciclovir to prevent recurrence of inflammation, particularly stromal keratitis and anterior uveitis [62]. Topical and local corticosteroids are used for the treatment of associated corneal stromal disease and intraocular inflammation. Visual prognosis is dependent on the location and severity of eye involvement. A small corneal dendrite in HSV may heal with minimal scarring and preservation of visual acuity. Recurrent inflammation, involvement of the corneal stroma with the development of neovascularization and opacification, and any involvement of the optic nerve can significantly limit visual prognosis.

Orbital and Adnexal Infections

Transplant patients are susceptible to common and uncommon bacterial and fungal infections of the orbit and adnexa. As with immunocompetent patients, orbital infections in transplant patients often develop as an extension of sinus disease. The most common orbital infection in transplant patients is orbital zygomycosis (or mucormycosis). Zygomycosis is an invasive fungal infection with a high rate of morbidity and mortality, particularly in the transplant population. Ubiquitous fungi from the genera *Mucor*, *Absidia*, and *Rhizopus* invade the oral and sinus mucosa of immunocompromised patients and can extend into the orbit and intracranial tissues (rhino-orbital-cerebral mucormycosis). In one large series of patients with zygomycosis, 19.5% of patients developed orbital involvement [63]. In one series of solid organ transplant patients with zygomycosis, the average time to infection after transplant was between 60 and 120 days; risk factors included diabetes or hyperglycemia, acidosis, and renal failure [64]. Patients present with complaints of unilateral headache, eye pain, periorbital swelling, double vision, and vision loss. Signs on exam include periorbital edema with erythema, conjunctival edema (chemosis), ophthalmoplegia, proptosis, and diminished visual acuity. There is often hypesthesia of the first and/or second divisions of cranial nerve 5. In late stages of the disease, examination of the nasal mucosa reveals a black eschar which results from tissue necrosis and infarction due to fungal invasion of blood vessels. Neuroimaging is important to ascertain the extent of invasion; solid organ transplant patients are more likely than diabetic patients to have central nervous system involvement [65]. A high index of suspicion is essential, as the clinical findings often precede any radiologic evidence of infection. An intranasal or sinus "black eschar" may not be present, and biopsy of nasal and sinus mucosa should be performed early. Biopsy of normal mucosa may demonstrate the invasive hyphae. Treatment of zygomycosis includes intravenous amphotericin B and surgical debridement of involved tissues. The liposomal formulation of amphotericin B has been associated with better outcomes than amphotericin B deoxycholate or other antifungal therapies [63, 65]. Posaconazole has been used in rare cases of medication toxicity or treatment failure with amphotericin B, but is not recommended as first-line therapy [63, 66]. There have been reports of breakthrough zygomycosis in patients who are on posaconazole prophylaxis, leading to the concern for potential drug resistance [67]. Isavuconazole is a new antifungal agent that may have similar efficacy as amphotericin against mucormycosis, based on results of a single-arm non-randomized trial [68], although it is currently not recommended as first-line treatment. Exenteration may be necessary in some patients with mucormycosis involving the orbit in order to prevent intracranial extension of disease. Overall prognosis is poor, and mortality rates of rhino-orbital-cerebral zygomycosis in transplant patients have been reported between 52% and 100% [64, 65]. CNS invasion is associated with higher mortality [65].

References

1. Krause I, Snir M, Cleper R, et al. Ocular complications in children and adolescents following renal transplantation. Pediatr Transplant. 2010;14:77–81.
2. Tarabishy AB, Khatib OF, Nocero JR, et al. Ocular complications in patients with lung transplants. Br J Ophthalmol. 2011;95:1295–8.
3. Akerele T, Lightman S. Ocular complications in heart, lung and heart-lung recipients. Br J Ophthalmol. 2007;91:310–2.
4. Westeneng AC, Hettinga Y, Lokhorst H, et al. Ocular graft-versus-host disease after allogeneic stem cell transplantation. Cornea. 2010;29:758–63.
5. Chung H, Kim K, Kim J, et al. Retinal complications in patients with solid organ or bone marrow transplantations. Transplantation. 2007;83(6):694–9.
6. Ng P, McCluskey P, McCaughan G, et al. Ocular complications of heart, lung, and liver transplantation. Br J Ophthalmol. 1998;82(4):423–8.
7. Tabbara KF, Al-GHamdi A, Al-Mohareb F, et al. Ocular findings after allogeneic hematopoietic stem cell transplantation. Ophthalmology. 2009;116:1624–9.
8. Del Pozo JL, van de Beek D, Daly RC, et al. Incidence and clinical characteristics of ocular infections after heart transplantation: a retrospective cohort study. Clin Transplant. 2009;23:484–9.
9. Urayama A, Yamad N, Sasakim T, et al. Unilateral acute uveitis with retinal periarteritis and detachment. Jpn J Clin Ophthalmol. 1971;25:607–19.
10. Akova YA, Altan-Yaycioglu R, Yilmaz G, Azap OK, Haberal M. Opportunistic posterior uveal infections in renal transplant patients. Transplant Proc. 2006;38(5):1348–53.
11. Wong R, Pavesio CE, Laidlaw DA, Williamson TH, Graham EM, Stanford MR. Acute retinal necrosis: the effects of intravitreal foscarnet and virus type on outcome. Ophthalmology. 2010;117(3):556–60.
12. Cochrane TF, Silvestri G, McDowell C, et al. Acute retinal necrosis in the United Kingdom: results of a prospective surveillance study. Eye. 2012;26:370–8.
13. Ganatra JB, Chandler D, Santos C, Kuppermann B, Margolis TP. Viral causes of the acute retinal necrosis syndrome. Am J Ophthalmol. 2000;129(2):166–72.
14. Holland GN. Standard diagnostic criteria for the acute retinal necrosis syndrome. Executive Committee of the American Uveitis Society. Am J Ophthalmol. 1994;117(5):663–7.
15. Tran TH, Rozenberg F, Cassoux N, Rao NA, LeHoang P, Bodaghi B. Polymerase chain reaction analysis of aqueous humour samples in necrotising retinitis. Br J Ophthalmol. 2003;87(1):79–83.
16. Harper TW, Miller D, Schiffman JC, Davis JL. Polymerase chain reaction analysis of aqueous and vitreous specimens in the diagnosis of posterior segment infectious uveitis. Am J Ophthalmol. 2009;147(1):140–147 e2.
17. Cottet L, Kaiser L, Hirsch HH, Baglivo E. HSV2 acute retinal necrosis: diagnosis and monitoring with quantitative polymerase chain reaction. Int Ophthalmol. 2009;29(3):199–201.
18. Arimura E, Deai T, Maruyama K, Uno N, Yamamoto H, Matsumoto C, Shimomura Y. Herpes simplex virus-2 quantification by real-time polymerase chain reaction in acute retinal necrosis. Jpn J Ophthalmol. 2005;49(1):64–5.
19. Blumenkranz MS, Culbertson WW, Clarkson JG, Dix R. Treatment of the acute retinal necrosis syndrome with intravenous acyclovir. Ophthalmology. 1986;93(3):296–300.
20. Tibbetts MD, Shah CP, Young LH, et al. Treatment of acute retinal necrosis. Ophthalmology. 2010;117:818–24.

21. Sternberg P Jr, Han DP, Yeo JH, Barr CC, Lewis H, Williams GA, Mieler WF. Photocoagulation to prevent retinal detachment in acute retinal necrosis. Ophthalmology. 1988;95(10):1389–93.
22. Kanoff J, Sobrin L. New diagnosis and treatment paradigms in acute retinal necrosis. Int Ophthalmol Clin. 2011;51(4):25–31.
23. Engstrom RE Jr, Holland GN, Margolis TP, Muccioli C, Lindley JI, Belfort R Jr, et al. The progressive outer retinal necrosis syndrome. A variant of necrotizing herpetic retinopathy in patients with AIDS. Ophthalmology. 1994;101(9):1488–502.
24. Holland GN. The progressive outer retinal necrosis syndrome. Int Ophthalmol. 1994;18(3):163–5.
25. Kalpoe JS, van Dehn CE, Bollemeijer JG, Vaessen N, Claas EC, Barge RM, et al. Varicella zoster virus (VZV)-related progressive outer retinal necrosis (PORN) after allogeneic stem cell transplantation. Bone Marrow Transplant. 2005;36(5):467–9.
26. Khot A, Dignan F, Taylor S, Potter M, Cubitt D, Treleaven JG. Another case of PORN (bilateral progressive outer retinal necrosis) after allogeneic stem cell transplantation. Bone Marrow Transplant. 2006;37(1):113–4.
27. Gill H, Cheung J, Wong I, Lie AK, Kwong YL. Varicella zoster virus progressive outer retinal necrosis after allogeneic haematopoietic stem cell transplantation. Br J Haematol. 2012;157(3):279.
28. Scott IU, Luu KM, Davis JL. Intravitreal antivirals in the management of patients with acquired immunodeficiency syndrome with progressive outer retinal necrosis. Arch Ophthalmol. 2002;120(9):1219–22.
29. Crippa F, Corey L, Chuang EL, Sale G, Boeckh M. Virological, clinical, and ophthalmologic features of cytomegalovirus retinitis after hematopoietic stem cell transplantation. Clin Infect Dis. 2001;32(2):214–9.
30. Fishburne BC, Mitrani AA, Davis JL. Cytomegalovirus retinitis after cardiac transplantation. Am J Ophthalmol. 1998;125(1):104–6.
31. Xhaard A, Robin M, Scieux C, de Latour RP, Deplus S, Mazeron MC, et al. Increased incidence of cytomegalovirus retinitis after allogeneic hematopoietic stem cell transplantation. Transplantation. 2007;83(1):80–3.
32. Egli A, Bergamin O, Müllhaupt B, Seebach JD, Mueller NJ, Hirsch HH. Cytomegalovirus-associated chorioretinitis after liver transplantation: case report and review of the literature. Transpl Infect Dis. 2008;10(1):27–43.
33. Song WK, Min YH, Kim YR, Lee SC. Cytomegalovirus retinitis after hematopoietic stem cell transplantation with alemtuzumab. Ophthalmology. 2008;115(10):1766–70.
34. Wagle AM, Biswas J, Gopal L, et al. Clinical profile and immunological status of cytomegalovirus retinitis in organ transplant recipients. Indian J Ophthalmol. 2002;50:115–21.
35. Kuo IC, Kempen JH, Dunn JP, Vogelsang G, Jabs DA. Clinical characteristics and outcomes of cytomegalovirus retinitis in persons without human immunodeficiency virus infection. Am J Ophthalmol. 2004;138(3):338–46.
36. Ghosh F, Hansson LJ, Bynke G, Békássy AN. Intravitreal sustained-release ganciclovir implants for severe bilateral cytomegalovirus retinitis after stem cell transplantation. Acta Ophthalmol Scand. 2002;80(1):101–4.
37. Vergoulidou M, Krause L, Foerster MH, et al. Endogenous filamentous fungal endophthalmitis – single-centre survey in patients with acute leukaemia or postallogeneic stem cell transplantation and review of the literature. Mycoses. 2011;54:e704–11.
38. Hunt KE, Glasgow BJ. Aspergillus endophthalmitis. An unrecognized endemic disease in orthotopic liver transplantation. Ophthalmology. 1996;103:757–67.
39. Rogasi PG, Zanazzi M, Nocentini J, et al. Disseminated Scedosporium apiospermum infection in renal transplant recipient: long-term successful treatment with voriconazole: a case report. Transplant Proc. 2007;39:2033–5.
40. Musk M, Chambers D, Weng C, et al. Successful treatment of disseminated Scedosporium infection in 2 lung transplant recipients: review of the literature and recommendations for management. J Heart Lung Transplant. 2006;25:1268–72.
41. Kapp M, Schargus M, Deuchert T, et al. Endophthalmitis as primary clinical manifestation of fatal fusariosis in an allogeneic stem cell recipient. Transpl Infect Dis. 2011;13:274–9.
42. Dua S, Chalermskulrat W, Miller MB, et al. Bilateral hematogenous Pseudomonas aeruginosa endophthalmitis after lung transplantation. Am J Transplant. 2006;6:219–24.
43. Algan M, Jonon B, George JL, et al. *Listeria monocytogenes* endophthalmitis in a renal transplant patient receiving cyclosporin. Ophthalmologica. 1990;201:23–7.
44. Scott M, Mehta S, Rahman HT, et al. Nocardia veterana endogenous endophthalmitis in a cardiac transplant patient. J Ophthalmic Inflamm Infect. 2013;3:44.
45. Israelski DM, Remington JS. Toxoplasmosis in the non-AIDS immunocompromised host. Curr Clin Top Infect Dis. 1993;13:322–56.
46. Brinkman K, Debast S, Sauerwein R, Ooyman F, Hiel J, Raemaekers J. Toxoplasma retinitis/encephalitis 9 months after allogeneic bone marrow transplantation. Bone Marrow Transplant. 1998;21(6):635–6.
47. Peacock JE Jr, Greven CM, Cruz JM, Hurd DD. Reactivation toxoplasmic retinochoroiditis in patients undergoing bone marrow transplantation: is there a role for chemoprophylaxis? Bone Marrow Transplant. 1995;15(6):983–7.
48. Conrath J, Mouly-Bandini A, Collart F, Ridings B. Toxoplasma gondii retinochoroiditis after cardiac transplantation. Graefes Arch Clin Exp Ophthalmol. 2003;241(4):334–8.
49. Chung H, Kim JG, Choi SH, Lee SY, Yoon YH. Bilateral toxoplasma retinochoroiditis simulating cytomegalovirus retinitis in an allogeneic bone marrow transplant patient. Korean J Ophthalmol. 2008;22(3):197–200.
50. Palkovacs EM, Correa Z, Augsburger JJ, Eagle RC Jr. Acquired toxoplasmic retinitis in an immunosuppressed patient: diagnosis by transvitreal fine-needle aspiration biopsy. Graefes Arch Clin Exp Ophthalmol. 2008;246(10):1495–7.
51. Donahue HC. Ophthalmologic experience in a tuberculosis sanatorium. Am J Ophthalmol. 1967;64(4):742–8.
52. Lopez de Castilla D, Schluger NW. Tuberculosis following solid organ transplantation. Transpl Infect Dis. 2010;12(2):106–12.
53. Mehta S, Suratkal L. Ophthalmoscopy in the early diagnosis of opportunistic tuberculosis following renal transplant. Indian J Ophthalmol. 2007;55(5):389–91.
54. Mansour AM. Renal allograft tuberculosis. Tubercle. 1990;71(2):147–8.
55. Biswas J, Madhavan HN, Gopal L, Badrinath SS. Intraocular tuberculosis. Clinicopathologic study of five cases. Retina. 1995;15(6):461–8.
56. Cordero-Coma M, Calleja S, Torres HE, del Barrio I, Franco M, Yilmaz T, et al. The value of an immune response to Mycobacterium tuberculosis in patients with chronic posterior uveitis revisited: utility of the new IGRAs. Eye (Lond). 2010;24(1):36–43.
57. Cutrufello NJ, Karakousis PC, Fishler J, Albini TA. Intraocular tuberculosis. Ocul Immunol Inflamm. 2010;18(4):281–91.
58. Walton RC, Reed KL. Herpes zoster ophthalmicus following bone marrow transplantation in children. Bone Marrow Transplant. 1999;23(12):1317–20.
59. Robinson MJ, Newton C. Bilateral herpes simplex keratitis in a patient with graft-vs-host disease. Am J Ophthalmol. 1991;112(4):468–9.

60. Oshry T. Intravenous acyclovir treatment for extensive herpetic keratitis in a liver transplant patient. Int Ophthalmol. 1998;21:265–8.
61. Fujiwara O, Mitamura Y, Ohtsuka K. Herpes zoster panuveitis progression despite acyclovir treatment in a patient following bone marrow transplantation. Jpn J Ophthalmol. 2005;49(6):536–8.
62. Herpetic Eye Disease Study Group. Oral acyclovir for herpes simplex virus eye disease: effect on prevention of epithelial keratitis and stromal keratitis. Arch Ophthalmol. 2000;118(8):1030–6.
63. Rüping MJ, Heinz WJ, Kindo AJ, Rickerts V, Lass-Flörl C, Beisel C, et al. Forty-one recent cases of invasive zygomycosis from a global clinical registry. J Antimicrob Chemother. 2010;65(2):296–302.
64. Almyroudis NG, Sutton DA, Linden P, Rinaldi MG, Fung J, Kusne S. Zygomycosis in solid organ transplant recipients in a tertiary transplant center and review of the literature. Am J Transplant. 2006;6(10):2365–74.
65. Sun HY, Forrest G, Gupta KL, Aguado JM, Lortholary O, Julia MB, et al. Rhino-orbital-cerebral zygomycosis in solid organ transplant recipients. Transplantation. 2010;90(1):85–92.
66. Stark D, Milliken S, Marriott D, Harkness J. Rhizopus microsporus var. rhizopodiformis sinus-orbital zygomycosis in an immunosuppressed patient: successful treatment with posaconazole after a complicated clinical course. J Med Microbiol. 2007;56(Pt 5):699–701.
67. Schlemmer F, Lagrange-Xélot M, Lacroix C, de La Tour R, Socié G, Molina JM. Breakthrough Rhizopus infection on posaconazole prophylaxis following allogeneic stem cell transplantation. Bone Marrow Transplant. 2008;42(8):551–2.
68. Marty FM, Ostrosky-Zeichner L, Cornely OA, et al. Isavuconazole treatment for mucormycosis: a single-arm open label trial and case-control analysis. Lancet Infect Dis. 2016;16:828–37.

Intracranial, Spinal, and Paraspinal Infections in the Transplant Recipient

19

Matthew W. McCarthy, Axel Rosengart, and Thomas J. Walsh

Introduction

Intracranial, spinal, and paraspinal infections contribute significantly to morbidity and mortality in patients receiving solid organ and stem cell transplants [1, 2] and should be considered a medical emergency [3]. The incidence of CNS involvement varies but is estimated to occur in 5–10% of transplant recipients [4] and is influenced by multiple factors, including the organ transplanted [5], the type and degree of immunosuppression, post-transplant adverse events [1], as well as donor characteristics, e.g., autologous vs. allogeneic [6].

Fungal, viral, bacterial, and parasitic infections of the central nervous system are well-documented in transplant recipients [7]. Because post-transplantation immunosuppressive regimens may modify the clinical presentation of CNS infections, special attention should be given to even minor neurologic symptoms and noninfectious causes such as the toxic effects of calcineurin inhibitors, and lymphoma should be included in the differential diagnosis [3]. Here we review the most common intracranial, spinal, and paraspinal infections in the post-transplant patient.

M. W. McCarthy (✉)
Weill Cornell Medicine, Department of General Internal Medicine, New York, NY, USA
e-mail: mwm9004@med.cornell.edu

A. Rosengart
Cedars-Sinai Medical Center, Departments of Neurology, Neurosurgery and Biomedical Sciences, Los Angeles, CA, USA
e-mail: axel.rosengart@cshs.org

T. J. Walsh
Transplantation-Oncology Infectious Diseases Program, New York-Presbyterian/Weill Cornell Medical Center, New York, NY, USA

Department of Pediatrics, New York-Presbyterian/Weill Cornell Medical Center, New York, NY, USA

Department of Microbiology and Immunology, New York-Presbyterian/Weill Cornell Medical Center, New York, NY, USA

Transplant Infectious Diseases Program, Division of Infectious Diseases, Icahn School of Medicine at Mount Sinai, New York, NY, USA
e-mail: thw2003@med.cornell.edu

Part 1: Intracranial Infection in the Transplant Recipient

Some of the more common organisms responsible for intracranial infection in the transplant recipient include species of *Aspergillus*, *Toxoplasma*, *Candida*, *Klebsiella*, *Cryptococcus*, *Coccidioides*, *Listeria*, and *Mucor*. In the late 1980s, three organisms – *Listeria monocytogenes*, *Aspergillus fumigatus*, and *Cryptococcus neoformans* – accounted for the great majority of these infections in transplant recipients [8]. When presenting as meningoencephalitis or abscesses, these lesions were often multiple and deep-seated and were frequently associated with pulmonary or disseminated infection [9]. However, with the development of new immunosuppressive agents, antimicrobial prophylaxis, shifts in nosocomial flora, and improved diagnostic methods, it is now recognized that a broad array of pathogens cause intracranial infection and tend to occur at discrete time points in the post-transplant patient [10, 11].

These infections can be divided into the early post-transplantation period, intermediate period, and late post-transplantation period and are influenced by epidemiologic exposures, net state of immunosuppression, antimicrobial prophylaxis, and the type of transplantation [3, 12]. Below is a review of intracranial infections at each time point.

Early Time Period Intracranial Infection

The early post-transplant period is generally defined as the first month after transplantation. Because the major effects of exogenous immunosuppression are not yet apparent, the causes of intracranial infection in this time period are those derived from either the donor or recipient and infectious complications of the transplant and hospitalization [13].

A. Safdar (ed.), *Principles and Practice of Transplant Infectious Diseases*, https://doi.org/10.1007/978-1-4939-9034-4_19

Recipient-Derived Infections

An important component of the pretransplant evaluation is to identify and treat any infection in the donor and recipient. Cytomegalovirus, Epstein-Barr virus, *Mycobacterium tuberculosis*, and *Toxoplasma gondii* are examples of pathogens that may exist in a latent state in the recipient and may be reactivated after transplantation, causing intracranial lesions. For this reason, they are routinely screened for prior to transplant [14]. Pretransplant vaccination has also become recognized as an important measure to protect patients from reactivation of latent pathogens. Many inactive and conjugate vaccines have been approved for use in the pretransplant patient. Recommendations for vaccinations of adult transplant recipients including special considerations for household contacts have been published [15].

Donor-Derived Infections

Transmission of donor-derived pathogens has been well-documented in the transplant recipient [16]. In 2010, a case was reported in which a 24-year-old patient developed invasive *Aspergillosis* of the brain 9 days after heart transplantation [17]. Five organs from this patient were subsequently used for transplantation into five recipients. Of the five recipients – two kidney, one liver, one islet cell, and one lung recipient – one lost the kidney graft because of invasive *Aspergillosis* of the transplanted organ. The lung recipient died due to primary non-function unrelated to infection. In the remaining recipients, prompt initiation of therapy prevented the outbreak of symptomatic *Aspergillosis*. Severe malaria, including cerebral malaria, has been reported following organ transplantation, but it is not clear that the incidence of cerebral malaria is elevated in this population [4]. Transplant-transmitted viral encephalitis from West Nile virus and Rabies virus has also been reported within 30 days of transplantation [18, 19].

Infectious Complications Related to Surgery

The organisms responsible for postoperative intracranial infections are often the bacteria and fungi that have colonized the recipient or donor prior to transplant. These include antimicrobial-resistant organisms, such as fluconazole-resistant *Candida* species, methicillin-resistant *Staphylococcus aureus*, vancomycin-resistant *Enterococcus*, *Clostridium difficile*, and resistant Gram-negative bacteria [20–26].

Because recipients are immunosuppressed, they are at risk for developing neurologic sequelae from bacteremia, and the risk is further increased with the use of indwelling vascular access catheters, urinary catheters, and surgical drains. Organ transplantation from donors with fever or viral syndromes is controversial. In cases in which the need for transplantation is not critical, we recommend avoiding the use of organs from donors with unexplained fever, encephalitis, or untreated infectious syndromes [3].

Intermediate Time Period Intracranial Infections (1–6 Months After Transplant)

In the period 1–6 months after transplantation, the composition of intracranial pathogens changes. Opportunistic infections prevail although there is geographic variation given the inter-institution variation in immunosuppressive and antimicrobial prophylaxis strategies. Local epidemiology also plays a role, as endemic fungi, e.g., *Histoplasma capsulatum*, *Coccidioides* spp., and *Cryptococcus gattii*, as well as *Mycobacterium tuberculosis* and nontuberculous mycobacteria have been observed to cause infection [27–29].

Although the incidence has decreased with routine use of antimicrobial prophylaxis, transplant recipients are at increased risk for acquiring infection with *Toxoplasma gondii* and *Pneumocystis jirovecii*, although intracranial infection remains rare. In a multicenter, matched case-control study in a 1:2 ratio, 22 cases of toxoplasmosis were identified among 15,800 solid organ transplant recipients performed in 11 Spanish hospitals between 2000 and 2009 [30]. With respect to central nervous system involvement, five manifested as brain abscesses and one had meningitis.

Antiviral prophylaxis with has decreased the incidence of intracranial viral infections, but the disease has not been eliminated. Herpesviruses have frequently been implicated in interim period intracranial infection [31]. A 2011 analysis of 2628 patients after allogeneic stem cell transplantation found that viral encephalitis occurred in 32 patients [32]. Detected viruses included human herpesvirus 6, Epstein-Barr virus, herpes simplex virus, JC virus, varicella zoster virus, cytomegalovirus, and adenovirus. More than one virus was identified in 16% of patients with viral encephalitis. The median onset time was 106 days after allogeneic stem cell transplantation for the total group of 32 patients, but onset times were shortest in those with HHV-6 encephalitis and longest in those with JC virus-associated progressive multifocal leukoencephalopathy [32].

Progressive multifocal leukoencephalopathy (PML) is a rapidly progressive demyelinating disorder of the central nervous system almost exclusively encountered in immunocompromised individuals and is caused by reactivation of the John Cunningham virus (JCV) [32]. In January, 2011, a 59-year-old woman underwent umbilical cord stem cell transplantation for follicular non-Hodgkin lymphoma [33]. On day 35, the patient developed grade 2 acute GVHD reaction of the skin without other organ dysfunction, and 2 mg/kg methylprednisolone was started. On day 51, the patient developed CMV reactivation in the peripheral blood (detected by PCR = 1359 copies); and an antiviral treatment with ganciclovir (Cymevan) 2.5 mg/kg/day was administrated. On day 68, she developed confusion and short-term memory dysfunction, with abnormal Babinski reflexes on the left. Brain MRI (FLAIR sequence) revealed hyper-intensity lesions in the white matter of the frontal lobes. On day 84, the patient's mental status was stable, and a lumbar cerebrospinal fluid (CSF) examination revealed a white blood cell (WBC) count of 1 cells/L, a normal glucose level of 3.89 mmol/L, and a normal protein level of 389 mg/L. Gram staining and culture were negative. A specimen was sent for polymerase chain reaction (PCR) analysis for JC virus was positive in the CSF and the serum which was negative for CMV, VZV, HHV-6, EBV, and herpes simplex virus by PCR. A treatment with 5 mg/kg/week of cidofovir was initiated on day 86 associated with mefloquine and mirtazapine. However, the patient's neurologic condition continued to deteriorate, and she expired on day 110 after umbilical cord blood transplant; post-mortem neuropathologic examination was not performed secondary to the wishes of the family.

Transplant recipients are also at increased risk for acquiring *Mycobacterium tuberculosis*. Solid organ transplant recipients are 20–74 times more likely to acquire *Mycobacterium tuberculosis* than the general population and more frequently presents with extrapulmonary tuberculosis [34]. After solid organ transplant, the median time to development of tuberculosis is 183 days, and intracranial tuberculosis infection appears to follow that pattern [35]. The most common symptoms of intracranial tuberculosis infection are fever, headache, vomiting, and altered level of consciousness. The basilar meninges and cistern are frequently affected and cause cranial nerve dysfunction, especially of the sixth (abducens or abducent) and seventh (facial) cranial nerves [36, 37]. Tuberculous meningitis may have an insidious onset, so physicians should have a high clinical suspicion in transplant recipients with altered level of consciousness in tuberculosis-endemic areas.

Microsporidia are spore-forming, obligate, intracellular parasites that are ubiquitous and infect invertebrates as well as all classes of vertebrates. At least one case of parasitic involvement of the brain parenchyma in the intermediate time period post-transplantation has been reported [38].

Late Time Period Intracranial Infection (More than 6 Months After Transplant)

More than 6 months after transplantation, most patients with good graft function receive stable and reduced levels of immunosuppression while continuing on some form of antimicrobial prophylaxis. The pathogens that cause intracranial infection tend to more closely resemble the community-acquired pathogens responsible for these infections in immunocompetent hosts.

In contrast, patients with concern for rejection or impaired graft function generally require more significant immunosuppressive therapy and remain at highest risk for opportunistic infections. In addition to the opportunistic pathogens mentioned in prior sections, these patients are at risk for developing intracranial nocardiosis [39], which has a special tropism for neural tissue [40]. Central nervous system nocardiosis is a formation of a parenchymal abscess that can occur in any region of the brain. A matched case-control study of 5126 organ transplant recipients between January 1995 and December 2005 revealed 35 cases of *Nocardia* infection [41]. Of the 35 cases, 7 had disseminated disease, including 3 with CNS involvement, all in the form of brain abscess as 1 presented with a solitary abscess and 1 presented with multiple abscesses.

An emerging pathogen in the immunocompromised host, *Rhodococcus equi*, is a Gram-positive coccobacillus that is a well-documented pathogen in veterinary literature causing pneumonia and sepsis in farm animals, especially in horses and cattle. It is an unusual cause of infection in humans but has recently been described as a cause of intracranial infection in the post-transplant patient. In one case report, a 42-year-old woman developed end-stage renal failure because of hemolytic uremic syndrome and malignant hypertension in 2001 and subsequently underwent kidney transplantation in 2003 [42]. Five years later, while on maintenance of immunosuppressive therapy with mycophenolate mofetil 500 mg BID, tacrolimus 1 mg BID, and prednisolone 7.5 mg once a day, she presented with a deep subcutaneous abscess in her right hip. The abscess was treated with surgical drainage and antibiotic therapy, and *R. equi* was identified in cultures from drained material from the subcutaneous abscess. Five weeks after this episode, she presented again with an abscess in her right hip, for which she again underwent surgical drainage. During her stay at the hospital, she developed epileptic seizures, and imaging revealed two brain abscesses that were not accessible to surgery. She subsequently died 14 days after admission from transtentorial brain herniation.

Conclusions

The nature of intracranial infections after solid organ transplantation continues to evolve, and with improved diagnostic tools, new pathogens have been identified in this subset of patients, including many with significant antimicrobial resistance [43]. An emerging issue is that of donor-derived infection, including West Nile virus, rabies, and lymphocytic choriomeningitis virus [44]. As of 2012, four clusters of organ transplant-associated lymphocytic choriomeningitis virus (LCMV) transmissions have been identified in the United States [45]. In immunocompetent patients, the disease can cause a non-specific febrile illness and, in some cases, aseptic meningitis [46]. In the transplant recipient, LCMV may cause multi-organ failure and often death. Of 15 confirmed cases of transplant-associated LCMV in the United States, 12 patients died of complications from the virus [45].

Part 2: Spinal Infection in the Transplant Recipient

Although rare, spinal infection in the post-transplant patient has been documented [47, 48] and has potentially devastating consequences if not identified and treated appropriately. For most patients, the primary route of infection is via hematogenous spread secondary to bacteremia. Septic emboli lodge at the vertebral end plate as it is supplied by end-arterial circulation. This leads to local infarction, and the avascular vertebrae become involved in the infective process [49]. These infections can be classified by the anatomical location involved: the vertebral column, the intervertebral disk space, and the spinal canal as well as by the time frame in which they occur after organ transplantation (i.e., early, intermediate, and late). Infection in adjacent soft tissues will be discussed later in the chapter.

Because of blunted host immune response, signs and symptoms of spinal infection may vary. The overriding symptom, however, is back pain. Radiculopathy, myelopathy, and sensory loss may accompany focal tenderness. CT scan, magnetic resonance, and bone scan play a vital role in the diagnosis of these infections [50]. The cornerstone of treatment is the identification of the responsible pathogen, appropriate medical therapy including possible surgical debridement, immobilization of the affected segment of the spine, and physical therapy to combat physical deconditioning [50].

Early Time Period Spinal Infection

Spinal infection in the first month after organ transplantation is rare, and incidence remains on the level of the case report [51]. As with intracranial infection, spinal infections in this period are usually attributed to nosocomial factors (surgery and hospitalization) or infection derived from the host or donor that spreads to the spine.

Intermediate Time Period Spinal Infection

Between 1 and 6 months after organ transplantation, bacterial and fungal pathogens predominate and tend to occur as a result of hematogenous seeding to the spine. However, viral complications such as progressive multifocal leukoencephalopathy caused by the reactivation of the JC virus have been reported [33]. The incidence of pyogenic spinal infection continues to occur, but its incidence has been decreased by the routine use of antimicrobial prophylaxis. And as result of improvements in transplant surgical methods, the prevalence of invasive fungal infections – primarily *Candida* and *Aspergillus* species, respectively – has declined as a whole over the past two decades [52]. However, a reduction in the number of spinal infections caused by *Candida* species has been accompanied by a rise in infections caused by *Aspergillus*. A 2010 review of *Aspergillus* spinal infection in solid organ transplant recipients identified 15 cases of spondylodiscitis [48]. Most cases (80%) were afebrile on presentation. All patients presented with progressive pain, showing radiographic evidence of lumbar osteomyelitis and discitis. In liver transplant recipients, the median time to onset was 2.125 months; for heart transplant recipients, it was 5.4 months. *Aspergillus fumigatus* and *Aspergillus flavus* were the most common pathogens, occurring in 84.62% and 15.38% of isolates, respectively. In all of the cases reviewed, heart transplant recipients were more inclined to have spinal *Aspergillosis* than renal or liver graft recipients There has been some success treating these patients with surgical debridement and voriconazole although the data is limited [53].

Late Spinal Infection

The majority of spinal infections reported in the literature occur after 6 months. These patients are often on reduced levels of immunosuppression, and the role of lifetime trimethoprim-sulfamethoxazole or antifungal prophylaxis remains controversial. Such long-term prophylaxis carries some risk of the development of microbial resistance to the prophylactic agents and possible future drug interactions [3]. *Staphylococcus aureus* is frequently implicated in cases of vertebral osteomyelitis in immunocompetent hosts and has similarly been reported in cases of post-transplantation vertebral osteomyelitis [49]. In one case of an orthotropic heart transplantation, the patient presented 14 months post-transplantation, with fever, nausea, vomiting, and severe epigastric pain that was unrelated to food but aggravated by movement and lying supine. Examination revealed bilateral tenderness over the lumbar region with localized tenderness over the lower thoracic and lumbar spine. Blood cultures revealed methicillin-sensitive *Staphylococcus* aureus, and MRI revealed findings consistent with infective diskitis and T-10 vertebral body osteomyelitis. The patient was successfully treated with intravenous and oral antibiotics, and the authors speculate that spinal infection may have resulted from hematogenous spread to areas of previously diseased osteoporotic vertebrae or damaged vertebral facet joints from analgesic injections.

Vertebral osteomyelitis by *Aspergillus* remains rare, although vertebrae are the most common site of *Aspergillus* infection in the bone [54]. In 2003, a case of a 46-year-old man with a 30-year history of type I diabetes, complicated by end-stage renal disease, who underwent simultaneous pancreas/kidney transplantation was reported [55]. One year after his transplant, the patient presented with fever, progressive low back pain, and paravertebral tenderness in the lumbar region. The patient was noted to be neutropenic with a white blood cell count of 1600 cells/mL, and imaging revealed L2–L3 osteopenia and diskitis, without compression, fracture, or abscess. Computed tomography (CT)-guided biopsy of L3 vertebra showed hyphae on mycological smears, and culture revealed *Aspergillus fumigatus*. The patient was treated with amphotericin B 1 mg/kg/day and underwent diskectomy, with debridement and drainage.

Some evidence suggests CMV disease or being a CMV-seronegative recipient of a CMV-seropositive donor organ is a predictor for invasive fungal disease following solid organ transplantation [56] and is now routinely included in the pre-transplantation assessment of both donor and recipient.

Conclusions

Spinal infection in the transplant recipient is an uncommon but aggressive disease that may cause spinal instability, neurological insult, and possibly death. Because the host's immune system is often suppressed, the clinical must retain a high level of suspicion to ensure prompt diagnosis and treatment. Aggressive surgical treatment with concurrent pharmacotherapy can successfully treat these infections and prevent neurological injury.

Part 3: Paraspinal Myositis and Other Paraspinal Infections in the Transplant Recipient

Paraspinal infection in the post-transplant patient is a rare event and includes paraspinal myositis and psoas muscle abscesses. It may be caused by a broad range of bacterial, fungal, parasitic, and viral agents and remains uncommon due to the relative resistance of musculature to infection [57]. Modes of transmission include transcutaneous infection of the deep tissue by needles or catheters, surgery, blunt trauma, and hematogenous seeding from remote sites. Signs and symptoms of paraspinal infection include back or flank pain, fever, inguinal mass, limp, anorexia, and weight loss [58]. In cases of psoas abscess formation, CT is the imaging modality of choice. Management consists of drainage and prompt initiation of antibiotics.

Bacterial causes are categorized by organism and anatomic location (i.e., *Staphylococcus aureus* myositis, group A streptococcal necrotizing myositis, group B streptococcal myositis, clostridial gas gangrene, and nonclostridial myositis). In the transplant recipient, however, atypical pathogens have also been implicated in paraspinal infection. In 2004, a case report detailed the course of a 35-year-old man who underwent combined kidney and pancreas transplantation in 2000 [59]. Two years after undergoing transplantation, the patient developed septic arthritis affecting the right knee and sternoclavicular joints and pain in the left iliac fossa. Radiological investigations demonstrated abnormal gallium uptake in these areas and an associated left psoas abscess. Purulent fluid was aspirated from the psoas abscess; however, no microorganisms were noted by microscopic evaluation or culture. Amplification of 16S rRNA gene was performed on psoas abscess material and demonstrated sequence homologies of 99–100% with *Mycoplasma pneumoniae.* Treatment with oral doxycycline 100 mg BID was then introduced, resulting in a rapid and complete clinical improvement within 3 weeks.

Fungal myositis is rare; *Histoplasma capsulatum* necrotizing myofascitis has been identified in a renal transplant patient, but the infection was of the upper extremity, not the paraspinal muscles [60]. Similarly, severe *Coccidioides immitis* myositis of the lower extremity has been seen in an orthotopic cardiac transplant recipient. For this reason, a careful travel history should be obtained in any transplant recipient with an unexplained febrile illness [61]. Parasitic myositis in the immunocompetent host is most commonly a result of trichinosis or cysticercosis, but other protozoa or helminths may be involved and are often suggested by peripheral eosinophilia and/or travel history [57]. To our knowledge, a parasitic cause of paraspinal infection in the transplant recipient has not been reported. Viruses known to cause myositis in the immunocompetent host include influenza virus and coxsackievirus B. Interestingly, one case of influenza vaccine-induced proximal muscle rhabdomyolysis has been described in a renal transplant patient [62]. The diagnosis of paraspinal infection in the transplant recipient may be subtle and is ultimately determined by the clinical presentation, radiologic imaging, and microbiologic or serologic testing. Therapy is based on the clinical presentation and the underlying pathogen.

Summary

Immunosuppression following organ transplantation increases susceptibility to central nervous system infections [4]. Despite ever-improving surgical techniques, diagnostic modalities, and prophylactic and therapeutic antibiotic regimens, intracranial, spinal, and paraspinal infections remain an important source of morbidity and mortality among transplant recipients. Because signs and symptoms may be subtle, the clinician must retain a high index of suspicion with any patient presenting with fever or neurologic symptoms. These infections should be considered a medical emergency, and treatment should be prompt to minimize the risk of neurologic sequelae and death. Table 19.1 shows a summary of antimicrobial therapy for common pathogens causing infection of the central nervous system in transplant recipients.

Table 19.1 Summary of antimicrobial therapy for common pathogens causing infection of the central nervous system in transplant recipients

Organism	First-line therapy	Second-line therapy/comments
Fungi		
Aspergillus spp.	Voriconazole *Loading dose*: 6 mg/kg IV q12hr *Maintenance dose*: 4 mg/kg IV q12h L-AMB (5–7.5 mg/kg/day IV)	ABLC (5 mg/kg/day IV) Caspofungin *Loading dose*: 70 mg day IV *Maintenance dose*: 50 mg/day IV thereafter Posaconazole (200 mg QID initially and then 400 mg PO BID) Itraconazole (dosage depends upon formulation)
Mucorales	L-AMB (3–5 mg/kg/day IV) ABLC (5 mg/kg/day IV)	Posaconazole (200 mg QID initially and then 400 mg PO BID)
Cryptococcus	*Induction therapy*: liposomal AmB (3–4 mg/kg per day) *or* ABLC (5 mg/kg per day) PLUS flucytosine (100 mg/kg per day) For 2 weeks *Consolidation therapy*: fluconazole (400–800 mg per day) For 8 weeks *Maintenance therapy*: fluconazole (200–400 mg per day) For 6–12 months	*Induction therapy*: liposomal AmB (6 mg/kg per day) *or* ABLC (5 mg/kg per day)
Candida spp.	L-AMB (5–7.5 mg/kg/day IV)	Fluconazole (400–800 mg per day) Micafungin 100 mg IV q12hr Caspofungin *Loading dose*: 70 mg day IV *Maintenance dose*: 50 mg/day IV thereafter
Protozoa		
Toxoplasma	Pyrimethamine (100 mg loading dose PO followed by 25–50 mg daily) plus sulfadiazine (2–4 g/day PO q6hrs)	Pyrimethamine (100 mg loading dose PO followed by 25–50 mg daily) plus azithromycin (500 mg daily) or atovaquone 750 mg Po q12hr
Bacteria		
Listeria monocytogenes	Ampicillin 2 g IV q4hr × 21 days	Trimethoprim-sulfamethoxazole (5 mg/kg [based on the trimethoprim component) IV or PO every 6–12 h Meropenem 1 g IV q8hr
Streptococcus pneumoniae	In patients with isolates that are susceptible to penicillin (MIC ≤0.06 mcg/mL), penicillin (4 million units IV every 4 h) can be used	Ceftriaxone 2 g IV q12hr in patients with penicillin (MIC ≤0.06 mcg/mL)
Methicillin-resistant Staphylococcus aureus	Vancomycin 15–20 mg/kg IV every 8–12 h (not to exceed 2 g per dose or a total daily dose of 60 mg/kg); adjust dose to achieve serum trough concentrations of 15–20 mcg/mL)	Daptomycin 8 mg IV q24hr
Viral		
CMV	Valganciclovir *Induction therapy*: 900 mg PO q12hr 14–21 days *Maintenance therapy*: valganciclovir 900 mg PO q12hr	Ganciclovir 5 mg/kg IV every 12 h
VZV	Valacyclovir (1000 mg PO q8hr) for 7 days	Famciclovir (500 mg PO q8hr)
EBV	Supportive care	
HSV	Acyclovir (10 mg/kg IV every 8 h) for 14–21 days	
WNV	Supportive care	The use of alfa interferon is based upon evidence of efficacy against WNV in vitro and in animal models Hyperimmune globulin on protocol

*Surgical resection may be appropriate for focal lesions
**Dosages are written for adults

References

1. Feltracco P, Barbieri S, Furnari M, Milevoj M, Rizzi S, Galligioni H, et al. Central nervous system infectious complications early after liver transplantation. Transplant Proc. 2010;42(4):1216–22.
2. Koh KN, Park M, Kim BE, Im HJ, Seo JJ. Early central nervous system complications after allogeneic hematopoietic stem cell transplantation in children. Kor J Hematol. 2010;45(3):164–70.
3. Fishman JA. Infection in solid-organ transplant recipients. N Engl J Med. 2007;357(25):2601–14.
4. Walker M, Kublin JG, Zunt JR. Parasitic central nervous system infections in immunocompromised hosts: malaria, microsporidiosis, leishmaniasis, and African trypanosomiasis. Clin Infect Dis. 2006;42(1):115–25.
5. Michalak G, Kwiatkowski A, Bieniasz M, Meszaros J, Czerwinski J, Wszola M, et al. Infectious complications after simultaneous pancreas-kidney transplantation. Transplant Proc. 2005;37(8):3560–3.
6. Patchell RA. Neurological complications of organ transplantation. Ann Neurol. 1994;36(5):688–703.
7. Walker M, Zunt JR. Parasitic central nervous system infections in immunocompromised hosts. Clin Infect Dis. 2005;40(7):1005–15.
8. Conti DJ, Rubin RH. Infection of the central nervous system in organ transplant recipients. Neurol Clin. 1988;6(2):241–60.
9. Britt RH, Enzmann DR, Remington JS. Intracranial infection in cardiac transplant recipients. Ann Neurol. 1981;9(2):107–19.
10. Silveira FP, Husain S. Fungal infections in lung transplant recipients. Curr Opin Pulm Med. 2008;14(3):211–8.
11. Husain S, Tollemar J, Dominguez EA, Baumgarten K, Humar A, Paterson DL, et al. Changes in the spectrum and risk factors for invasive candidiasis in liver transplant recipients: prospective, multicenter, case-controlled study. Transplantation. 2003;75(12):2023–9.
12. Pate R, Paya CV. Infections in solid-organ transplant recipients. Clin Microbiol Rev. 1997;10(1):86–124.
13. Greenwald MA, Kuehnert M, Fishman JA. Infectious disease transmission during organ and tissue transplantation. Emerg Infect Dis. 2012;18(8):e1.
14. Avery RK. Recipient screening prior to solid-organ transplantation. Clin Infect Dis. 2002;35(12):1513–9.
15. Sester M, Gärtner BC, Girndt M, Sester U. Vaccination of the solid organ transplant recipient. Transplant Rev. 2008;22(4):274–84.
16. Fishman JA, Greenwald MA, Grossi PA. Transmission of infection with human allografts: essential considerations in donor screening. Clin Infect Dis. 2012;55(5):720–7.
17. Mueller NJ, Weisser M, Fehr T, Wüthrich RP, Müllhaupt B, Lehmann R, et al. Donor-derived aspergillosis from use of a solid organ recipient as a multiorgan donor. Transplant Infect Dis. 2010;12(1):54–9.
18. Iwamoto M, Jernigan DB, Guasch A, Trepka MJ, Blackmore CG, Hellinger WC, et al. Transmission of West Nile virus from an organ donor to four transplant recipients. N Engl J Med. 2003;348(22):2196–203.
19. Srinivasan A, Burton EC, Kuehnert MJ, Rupprecht C, Sutker WL, Ksiazek TG, Rabies in Transplant Recipients Investigation Team, et al. Transmission of rabies virus from an organ donor to four transplant recipients. N Engl J Med. 2005;352(11):1103–11.
20. Herrero IA, Issa NC, Patel R. Nosocomial spread of linezolid-resistant, vancomycin-resistant Enterococcus faecium. N Engl J Med. 2002;346(11):867–9.
21. Patel R, Rouse MS, Piper KE, Steckelberg JM. Linezolid therapy of vancomycin-resistant Enterococcus faecium experimental endocarditis. Antimicrob Agents Chemother. 2001;45(2):621–3.
22. Fishman JA. Vancomycin-resistant Enterococcus in liver transplantation: what have we left behind? Transplant Infect Dis. 2003;5(3):109–11.
23. Keven K, Basu A, Re L, Tan H, Marcos A, Fung JJ, et al. Clostridium difficile colitis in patients after kidney and pancreas-kidney transplantation. Transplant Infect Dis. 2004;6(1):10–4.
24. West M, Pirenne J, Chavers B, Gillingham K, Sutherland D, Dunn DI, Matas AJ. Clostridium difficile colitis after kidney and kidney-pancreas transplantation. Clin Transpl. 1999;13(4):318–23.
25. Harbarth S, Pittet D, Romand J. Fatal concomitant nosocomial Legionnaires' disease and cytomegalovirus pneumonitis after cardiac transplantation. Intensive Care Med. 1996;22(10):1133–4.
26. Bert F, Bellier C, Lassel L, Lefranc V, Durand F, Belghiti J, et al. Risk factors for Staphylococcus aureus infection in liver transplant recipients. Liver Transplant. 2005;11(9):1093–9.
27. Kauffman CA. Endemic mycoses in patients with hematologic malignancies. Semin Respir Infect. 2002;17(2):106–12.
28. Ljungman P, Griffiths P, Paya C. Definitions of cytomegalovirus infection and disease in transplant recipients. Clin Infect Dis. 2002;34(8):1094–7.
29. Doucette K, Fishman JA. Nontuberculous mycobacterial infection in hematopoietic stem cell and solid organ transplant recipients. Clin Infect Dis. 2004;38(10):1428–39.
30. Fernàndez-Sabé N, Cervera C, Fariñas MC, Bodro M, Muñoz P, Gurguí M, et al. Risk factors, clinical features, and outcomes of toxoplasmosis in solid-organ transplant recipients: a matched case-control study. Clin Infect Dis. 2012;54(3):355–61.
31. Ernst J, Sauerbrei A, Krumbholz A, Egerer R, Mentzel H-J, Kurzai M, et al. Multiple viral infections after haploidentical hematopoietic stem cell transplantation in a child with acute lymphoblastic leukemia. Transplant Infect Dis. 2012;14(5):E82–8.
32. Schmidt-Hieber M, Schwender J, Heinz WJ, Zabelina T, Kühl JS, Mousset S, et al. Viral encephalitis after allogeneic stem cell transplantation: a rare complication with distinct characteristics of different causative agents. Haematologica. 2011;96(1):142–9.
33. El-Cheikh J, Fürst S, Casalonga F, Crocchiolo R, Castagna L, Granata A, et al. JC virus leuko-encephalopathy in reduced intensity conditioning cord blood transplant recipient with a review of the literature. Mediterr J Hematol Infect Dis. 2012;4(1):e2012043.
34. Singh N, Paterson DL. Mycobacterium tuberculosis infection in solid-organ transplant recipients: impact and implications for management. Clin Infect Dis. 1998;27(5):1266–77.
35. Torre-Cisneros J, Doblas A, Aguado JM, San Juan R, Blanes M, Montejo M, Spanish Network for Research in Infectious Diseases, et al. Tuberculosis after solid-organ transplant: incidence, risk factors, and clinical characteristics in the RESITRA (Spanish Network of Infection in Transplantation) cohort. Clin Infect Dis. 2009;48(12):1657–65.
36. Garg RK. Tuberculous meningitis. Acta Neurol Scand. 2010;122(2):75–90.
37. Lincoln EM, Sordillo VR, Davies PA. Tuberculous meningitis in children. A review of 167 untreated and 74 treated patients with special reference to early diagnosis. J Pediatr. 1960;57:807–23.
38. Carlson JR, Li L, Helton CL, Munn RJ, Wasson K, Perez RV, et al. Disseminated microsporidiosis in a pancreas/kidney transplant recipient. Arch Pathol Lab Med. 2004;128(3):e41–3.
39. Zaatreh M, Alabulkarim W. Images in clinical medicine. Disseminated central nervous system nocardiosis. N Engl J Med. 2006;354(26):2802.
40. Beaman BL, Beaman L. Nocardia species: host-parasite relationships. Clin Microbiol Rev. 1994;7(2):213–64.
41. Peleg AY, Husain S, Qureshi ZA, Silveira FP, Sarumi M, Shutt KA, et al. Risk factors, clinical characteristics, and outcome of Nocardia infection in organ transplant recipients: a matched case-control study. Clin Infect Dis. 2007;44(10):1307–14.
42. Rahamat-Langendoen JC, van Mers M, Zijlstra JG, Lo-Ten-Foe JR. Disseminated Rhodococcus equi infection in a kidney transplant patient without initial pulmonary involvement. Diagn Microbiol Infect Dis. 2009;65(4):427–30.

43. Fishman JA, Issa NC. Infection in organ transplantation: risk factors and evolving patterns of infection. Infect Dis Clin N Am. 2010;24(2):273–83.
44. Kaul DR. Donor-derived infection: epidemiology and outcomes. Curr Infect Dis Rep. 2012;14(6):676–82.
45. Macneil A, Ströher U, Farnon E, Campbell S, Cannon D, Paddock DC, LCMV Transplant Investigation Team, et al. Solid organ transplant-associated lymphocytic choriomeningitis, United States, 2011. Emerg Infect Dis. 2012;18(8):1256–62.
46. Jahrling PB, Peters CJ. Lymphocytic choriomeningitis virus. A neglected pathogen of man. Arch Path Lab Med. 1992;116(5):486–8.
47. Korres DS, Papagelopoulos PJ, Zahos KA, Kolia MD, Poulakou GG, Falagas ME. Multifocal spinal and extra-spinal Mycobacterium chelonae osteomyelitis in a renal transplant recipient. Transplant Infect Dis. 2007;9(1):62–5.
48. Li XF, Liu ZD, Xia Q, Dai LY. Aspergillus spondylodiscitis in solid organ transplant recipients. Transplant Proc. 2010;42(10):4513–7.
49. Datta S, Hussain IR, Madden B. Spinal osteomyelitis and diskitis: a rare complication following orthotopic heart transplantation. J Heart Lung Transplant. 2001;20(11):1213–6.
50. Broner FA, Garland DE, Zigler JE. Spinal infections in the immunocompromised host. Orthop Clin N Am. 1996;27(1):37–46.
51. Williams RL, Fukui MB, Meltzer CC, Swarnkar A, Johnson DW, Welch W. Fungal spinal osteomyelitis in the immunocompromised patient: MR findings in three cases. AJNR Am J Neuroradiol. 1999;20(3):381–5.
52. Singh N. Fungal infections in the recipients of solid organ transplantation. Infect Dis Clin N Am. 2003;17(1):113–34, viii.
53. Ersoy A, Dizdar OS, Koc AO, Akalin H, Ener B. Aspergillus fumigatus spondylodiskitis in renal transplant patient: voriconazole experience. Exp Clin Transplant. 2011;9(4):265–9.
54. Hummel M, Schüler S, Weber U, Schwertlick G, Hempel S, Theiss D, et al. Aspergillosis with Aspergillus osteomyelitis and diskitis after heart transplantation: surgical and medical management. J Heart Lung Transplant. 1993;12(4):599–603.
55. Salvalaggio PR, Bassetti M, Lorber MI, Micheletto GC, Friedman AL, Andriole VT, Basadonna GP. Aspergillus vertebral osteomyelitis after simultaneous kidney-pancreas transplantation. Transpl Infect Dis. 2003;5(4):187–90.
56. George MJ, Snydman DR, Werner BG, Griffith J, Falagas ME, Dougherty NN, Rubin RH. The independent role of cytomegalovirus as a risk factor for invasive fungal disease in orthotopic liver transplant recipients. Boston Center for Liver Transplantation CMVIG-Study Group. Cytogam, MedImmune, Inc. Gaithersburg, Maryland. Am J Med. 1997;103(2):106–13.
57. Crum-Cianflone NF. Bacterial, fungal, parasitic, and viral myositis. Clin Microbiol Rev. 2008;21(3):473–94.
58. Mückley T, Schütz T, Kirschner M, Potulski M, Hofmann G, Bühren V. Psoas abscess: the spine as a primary source of infection. Spine. 2003;28(6):E106–13.
59. O'Sullivan MV, Isbel NM, Johnson DW, Rencken K, Byrne S, Graham MM, Playford EG. Disseminated pyogenic Mycoplasma pneumoniae infection in a renal transplant recipient, detected by broad-range polymerase chain reaction. Clin Infect Dis. 2004;39(9):e98–9.
60. Wagner JD, Prevel CD, Elluru R. Histoplasma capsulatum necrotizing myofascitis of the upper extremity. Ann Plast Surg. 1996;36(3):330–3.
61. Vartivarian SE, Coudron PE, Markowitz SM. Disseminated coccidioidomycosis. Unusual manifestations in a cardiac transplantation patient. Am J Med. 1987;83(5):949–52.
62. Raman KS, Chandrasekar T, Reeve RS, Roberts ME, Kalra PA. Influenza vaccine-induced rhabdomyolysis leading to acute renal transplant dysfunction. Nephrol Dial Transplant. 2006;21(2):530–1.

Respiratory Tract Infections: Sinusitis, Bronchitis, and Pneumonia

20

Benjamin A. Miko, Marcus R. Pereira, and Amar Safdar

Introduction

Upper and lower respiratory tract infections are among the most common infectious processes among solid organ and hematopoietic stem cell transplant (HSCT) recipients [1]. As with most infectious syndromes outlined in this text, the increased risk of respiratory tract disease encountered in transplant recipients relates in part to defects in innate and adaptive immunity. Within this population, however, the incidence and microbiological etiology of respiratory infections are quite variable. This is due in part to the use of heterogeneous immunosuppressive regimens and differing prophylactic antibiotic strategies. In addition to diminished host immunity, anatomic breaches in upper and lower respiratory tract defenses may increase the susceptibility of immunocompromised hosts to a variety of common and opportunistic pathogens. Such anatomical considerations are especially important in patients who have undergone thoracic surgery for lung and heart transplantation and individuals who have required prolonged mechanical ventilation. Medical devices such as nasogastric and endotracheal tubes hinder coordinated glottic movement and mucociliary function and act as conduits for the introduction of pathogenic organisms to the respiratory tract [2].

Several immune deficits can affect transplant recipients and consequently increase the risk of upper and lower respiratory tract infections. These include:

1. *Neutropenia*: Commonly associated with medication toxicities, chemotherapy, hematological malignancies, and viral infections, deficits in neutrophil count and function can increase the risk of infection with staphylococci, streptococci, Gram-negative bacilli (GNB), and fungi [3, 4].
2. *T lymphocyte deficiency*: Caused by many transplant immunosuppressive medications that include calcineurin inhibitors, mTOR inhibitors, glucocorticoids. T lymphocyte deficiency is also encountered in the setting of HIV infection, lymphoma, leukemia, and infection/reactivation of various herpesviruses, especially *Cytomegalovirus* (CMV). Patients with cellular immune dysfunction are at increased risk of respiratory infection due to intracellular organisms such as *Listeria monocytogenes*, *Salmonella* spp., *Legionella* spp., and *Toxoplasma gondii*, mycobacteria, fungi-like *Cryptococcus* spp., *Histoplasma capsulatum*, and *Pneumocystis jirovecii*, as well as CMV, *Human herpesvirus 6* (HHV-6), varicella-zoster virus (VZV), and respiratory viruses [5–7].
3. *B lymphocyte deficiency*: Associated with various transplant/oncology medications like azathioprine, mycophenolate, rituximab, and glucocorticoids and hematological malignancies such as leukemia, multiple myeloma, and other causes of humoral immune defects increases the risk of infection with encapsulated bacteria including *S. pneumoniae*, *H. influenzae*, and *N. meningitidis*.
4. *Asplenia and hypocomplementemia*: Similarly increase the risk of infection with encapsulated bacteria as well as *Capnocytophaga*.

Because such immune defects are often mixed, careful attention to clinical and radiographic features as well as recognition of nosocomial versus community sources of infection are critical to making a correct diagnosis and initiating empiric antimicrobial therapy [1]. In both solid organ transplant and HSCT recipients, delays in appropriate antimicrobial therapy may increase the risk of secondary complications and infection-associated deaths, especially in those with

B. A. Miko
Columbia University Medical Center, Division of Infectious Diseases, Department of Medicine, New York, NY, USA
e-mail: bm2266@columbia.edu

M. R. Pereira
Department of Medicine – Infectious Diseases, Columbia University Medical Center, New York, NY, USA
e-mail: mp2323@cumc.columbia.edu

A. Safdar (✉)
Clinical Associate Professor of Medicine, Texas Tech University Health Sciences Center El Paso, Paul L. Foster School of Medicine, El Paso, TX, USA
e-mail: amar.safdar@cidimmunology.com

A. Safdar (ed.), *Principles and Practice of Transplant Infectious Diseases*, https://doi.org/10.1007/978-1-4939-9034-4_20

severe immunosuppression. Therefore, it is common practice to initiate empiric or preemptive antimicrobial therapy in patients for whom the suspicion of infection is high.

This chapter reviews the common respiratory tract infections affecting transplant recipients including sinusitis, bronchitis, tracheobronchitis, and pneumonia. Particular attention is directed to epidemiological risk factors including healthcare exposure, clinical presentation, diagnosis, and common microbiological etiologies. Unique causes of opportunistic pneumonias are reviewed in the final section of this chapter.

Sinusitis

Sinus infections are a common occurrence in transplant recipients, affecting between 4% and 31% of HSCT recipients [8, 9] and probably a similar percent of solid organ transplant recipients [10]. Of note, transplant patients with underlying cystic fibrosis (CF) are at extremely high risk for sinusitis with between 90% and 100% of individuals with CF showing pan-sinusitis on imaging by 8 months of age [11]. In HSCT recipients, risk factors for developing severe rhinosinusitis include graft-versus-host disease (GVHD) [12, 13]. The determinants of sinusitis in solid organ transplant recipients are less clearly defined, possibly due to the heterogeneous disease processes prompting transplantation. Unlike non-immunosuppressed individuals, no studies have linked tobacco, allergy, asthma, and low IgG levels to sinusitis in transplant recipients [13].

In general, sinusitis can be classified temporally as acute (<4 weeks), subacute (4–12 weeks), or chronic (>12 weeks) and in terms of severity as invasive or noninvasive. Typical signs and symptoms include nasal congestion, focal sinus pressure or pain, nasal discharge, and reduced sense of smell although, as is generally the case, transplant recipients can often have a muted clinical picture. Among HSCT recipients, nasal congestion and cough are the most common symptoms of acute sinusitis (80% and 61%, respectively) [8]. The nonspecific nature of these symptoms may ultimately lead to delays in diagnosis resulting in poorer clinical outcomes of invasive infections.

The diagnosis of acute sinusitis is often based entirely on clinical presentation in the immunocompetent patients, whereas in transplant recipients, a high degree of suspision due to dampened clinical signs and symptoms should be accompanied by an appropriate diagnostic investigation that often includes CT or MRI scan of the face and paranasal sinuses. In most cases, cultures of nasal discharge are not helpful; a nasal wash for bacterial cultures and a PCR panel that assesses a number of common and uncommon respiratory viruses may considerably improve diagnostic yeild. When imaging is obtained, fluid levels are found in 86% of cases [6]. Although a wide variety of organisms can cause acute sinusitis, the vast majority of infections are due to viral pathogens. These include rhinovirus, respiratory syncytial virus (RSV), adenovirus, coronavirus, influenza, parainfluenza, and even CMV [14–16]. Viral infections can be short-lived but viral shedding can be prolonged among immunocompromised patients. Bacterial sinus infections are much less common and rarely occur with less than 7 days of symptoms [17]. Common bacterial causes of acute bacterial sinusitis include *S. pneumoniae*, *Haemophilus influenzae*, *Moraxella catarrhalis*, *S. aureus*, and anaerobes. *Pseudomonas* can be a prominent sinus pathogen in cystic fibrosis patients both before and after lung transplantation [18, 19]. While most cases of acute bacterial sinusitis are caused by one predominant organism, up to one quarter have two distinct pathogens present in high concentration [20]. It is important to note, however, that in routine clinical practice, the majority of patients with acute sinusitis do not have a bacterial pathogen isolated.

In the immunocompetent patients treatment of acute sinusitis is usually supportive except in cases where symptoms persist for greater than 7 days, at which point empiric antimicrobial therapy may be warranted. In severely immunocompormised transplant patients with or without neutropenia, approach has been to start treatment early when bacterial sinus infection is suspected. Complications of acute sinusitis include facial cellulitis, preseptal periorbital cellulitis, brain abscess, cavernous sinus thrombosis, and orbital invasion that may result in sight and life threatening orbital (post-septal) cellulitis [21]. Intracraneal extension should be suspected if mental status changes occur or if there are focal neurological signs [22]. CT imaging or MRI scan should be urgently obtained, and otolaryngology evaluation with endoscopy should be sought for both diagnosis (cultures and histology) and therapeutic drainage. Empiric antimicrobials should be initiated while this diagnostic evaluation is pending. In lung transplant recipients with underlying cystic fibrosis, sinus surgery can decrease recurrence of *Pseudomonas*-related sinus infections [18].

Invasive fungal sinus infections are associated with increased morbidity and mortality that may range from 50% and may beupto as high as 90% in patients undergoing solid organ allograft and allogenic hematopoietic stem cell transplantation [23]. Bony erosions can be a sign of invasive disease. There is a correlation with chronicity and invasiveness. Invasive sinus disease is often fungal although bacterial causes such as *Pseudomonas* and *S. aureus* are not uncommon. In transplant recipients, *Candida* and *Aspergillus* species remain the most common fungal organisms to cause sinusitis, resulting in invasive and noninvasive sinus disease [24]. *Rhizopus* is also an important organism associated with rapidly progressive infection with high mortality rate [21]. Even rarer fungal etiologies include *Scopulariopsis* [25], *Fusarium* [26, 27], *Trichoderma* [28], *Scedosporium* [29], and *Pseudallescheria* [30]. *Acanthamoeba* is a rare but well-described parasitic cause of invasive rhinosinusitis in immunosuppressed patients with a strong predilection for intracraneal involvement, in such patients brain infection carries high fatality [31, 32].

Bronchitis and Tracheobronchitis

The terms tracheobronchitis and acute bronchitis are frequently used interchangeably, with acute bronchitis having a preferential use in the literature with the exception of aspergillosis and ventilator-associated tracheobronchial infections [33–35]. As such, both are generally defined as a self-limited inflammation of the large airways of the lung, or bronchi, due to an infection. As opposed to pneumonia, the lower airways are not involved, and chest imaging is generally normal. Patients typically present with a cough lasting more than 5 days, an important factor distinguishing it from mild upper respiratory infection (URI) [36]. Symptoms usually persist for 10–20 days but may extend for more than 4 weeks. Most patients report purulent sputum, indicating sloughing of tracheobronchial epithelium and inflammation. As opposed to bronchiolitis, acute bronchitis does not usually present with progressive cough, wheezing, tachypnea, respiratory distress, and hypoxemia. Chronic bronchitis, on the other hand, entails continuing symptoms on most days of the month for at least 3 months of the year during two consecutive years.

Many studies have shown that community-acquired viruses are by far the most common cause of acute bronchitis [37–40]. These include influenza A and B, adenovirus, rhinovirus, coronavirus, parainfluenza, RSV, and human metapneumovirus [37–40]. Bacteria, particularly atypical organisms, can also cause acute bronchitis; commonly implicated pathogens include *Bordetella pertussis*, *Chlamydophila pneumoniae*, and *Mycoplasma pneumonia*. Among immunocompromised patients, the causative agents of acute bronchitis are largely similar to the general population [41–43]. Opportunistic pathogens can also cause tracheobronchial infections, particularly among lung transplant and allogeneic HSCT recipients. The most important of these include invasive fungal infections, especially *Aspergillus* [35, 44, 45].

Acute bronchitis affects about 5% of adults annually, with the majority of infections occurring during the fall and winter [46]. The incidence of upper respiratory tract infections among solid organ transplant and HSCT recipients appears to be similar to that of the general population [43, 47–49]. Despite similar epidemiology, immunocompromised patients often suffer from prolonged periods viral shedding and progress to pneumonia more frequently [50]. Higher rates of airflow obstruction and increased mortality are also key differences [50, 51]. Respiratory viral infections immediately prior to bone marrow transplant are associated with decreased survival [52]. Among lung transplant recipients, respiratory viral infection, particularly RSV, can be associated with progression of chronic rejection and bronchiolitis obliterans syndrome (BOS) on histopathologic examination [41, 47, 48, 53]. Patients undergoing allogeneic hematopietic stem cell transplantation similarly are at risk for BOS that potentially may have been triggered after an episode of respiratory viral infection [54].

The major procedures employed for diagnosis of upper respiratory tract infections include multiplex PCR platforms and sputum cultures. When a fungal etiology is suspected, bronchoscopy is often performed to establish microbiological diagnosis. Among lung transplant recipients, examination of the bronchial anastomosis is essential to ascertain its integrity and the presence of necrosis.

Treatment for acute bronchitis depends on the causative infectious agent [51]. For the viral organisms without an established therapy, supportive care and close monitoring is recommended. Please refer to each specific pathogen for further information on treatment.

Pneumonia

Guidelines put forth by the Infectious Diseases Society of American (IDSA) and American Thoracic Society (ATS) suggest that the diagnosis of pneumonia requires a constellation of suggestive clinical features such as fever, purulent sputum, leukocytosis, and decline in oxygen saturation, and a demonstrable infiltrate on chest radiograph or other imaging technique with or without supporting microbiological data [55, 56]. As the common clinical and radiographic manifestations of pneumonia may be absent or attenuated in immunosuppressed patients due to impaired inflammatory responses [1], the diagnosis of pneumonia may be difficult to establish in solid allograft transplant and both autologous and allogeneic HSCT recipients. Adding to this diagnostic challenge is the frequent colonization of the upper airway with microorganisms that do not contribute to lung disease, rendering the microbiological diagnosis of pneumonia by conventional culture techniques difficult. Conversely, sterile respiratory tract cultures do not exclude an infectious etiology, particularly in the setting of recent exposure to broad-spectrum antibiotics. The common use of prophylactic antimicrobials in transplant recipients may contribute to suppression of culture results while increasing the risk of infections that are resistant to commonly used antimicrobial agents given for infection prophylaxis such as fluoroquinolones, trimethoprim-sulfamethoxazole, triazole-based antifungals, and valacyclovir or valganciclovir [57–59].

As in the general population, pneumonias occurring in transplant recipients are traditionally defined based on the setting in which they are acquired, i.e., community-acquired vs. hospital-acquired. Until 2016, the IDSA and ATS designated a third category, healthcare-associated pneumonia (HCAP), to delineate patients with significant exposure to nursing homes, dialysis centers, and outpatient clinics. While this was intended to highlight this group's increased risk of multi-drug resistant pathogens, several studies have shown HCAP to be caused by organisms similar to those causing community-acquired pneumonia (CAP) [60–62]. Given that, the HCAP designation was removed from the most-recent IDSA/ATS guidelines for the management of hospital-acquired pneumonia (HAP) and ventilator-associated pneumonia (VAP) [56].

Community-Acquired Pneumonia

CAP, as defined by IDSA and ATS, refers to the radiographic and clinical development of pneumonia in the community setting, distinguishing it from HAP, as outlined below [55, 56]. The distinction of CAP from nosocomial pneumonia remains important as it allows for prediction of likely pathogens and permits prognostic estimations based on epidemiologic descriptions of the underlying cause. Consequently, this distinction provides a framework for decisions regarding the appropriate diagnostic evaluation and empiric antimicrobial therapy.

The etiologic spectrum of bacterial pathogens causing CAP among transplant recipients with mild-to-moderate immunosuppression is similar to that of patients without a history of transplantation. However, a clinically insignificant microbial inoculum in the general population may cause severe infection among patients with underlying immunosuppression. *S. pneumoniae* remains the most commonly identified pathogen and the most frequent cause of lethal CAP [63]. *S. aureus*, nontypeable *Haemophilus influenzae*, *Pseudomonas* spp., and other GNB may also cause life-threatening CAP. Recently, other non-lactose fermenting (NF)-GNB such as *Stenotrophomonas*, *Burkholderia*, *Chryseobacterium*, *Achromobacter*, and *Alcaligenes* species have been increasingly recognized as etiologic agents in both CAP and nosocomial infections [64]. *S. pyogenes*, *Neisseria meningitidis*, and *Moraxella catarrhalis* also cause CAP less frequently. The incidence of CAP associated with the atypical pathogens such as *Mycoplasma pneumoniae*, *Chlamydia pneumoniae*, and *Legionella* spp. varies widely with patient age, seasonal variation, and geographic location. Viral pneumonias, most commonly caused by influenza, parainfluenza, and adenovirus, are also sources of CAP, which may be severe in the setting of transplantation. It is important to note that lower respiratory tract infections may be due to a mixed population of viruses, bacteria, and fungi in solid organ transplant and HSCT recipients [65–70].

The microbiological diagnosis of CAP is based upon recovery of a likely pathogen from an otherwise sterile source like blood, urine, pleural fluid, isolation of a noncommensal organism in respiratory secretions, or positive results of selected serological tests. Although the utility of Gram staining and culture of expectorated sputum in the diagnosis of pneumonia has been debated for years, carefully procured sputum specimens with cytologic confirmation of a lower respiratory source appear to be diagnostically useful, particularly if they are obtained before the initiation of antimicrobial therapy. Timely establishment of an accurate diagnosis contributes to a successful outcome, although treatment should not be withheld while diagnostic interventions are underway. Antimicrobial selection should be based upon the probable infecting organism(s), the severity of the patient's pneumonia, the patient's underlying immune status, and the presence or absence of comorbid conditions [71, 72].

Hospital-Acquired Pneumonia

Lower respiratory tract infections that occur more than 48 h after hospital admission in patients without antecedent clinical symptoms or radiographic findings suggestive of pneumonia are referred to as HAP. The etiological spectrum of microbial pathogens causing HAP among low-risk transplant recipients with no recent antibiotic exposure is similar as that seen in the general population. *H. influenzae*, *S. pneumoniae*, *S. aureus*, and *Enterobacteriaceae* are frequently encountered. Methicillin-resistant *S. aureus* (MRSA) may cause severe HAP, especially among patients with prior MRSA colonization, antibiotic exposure, advanced age, and/or prolonged ventilatory support [73]. Protracted mechanical ventilation and recent antibiotic administration are also associated with increased rates of HAP caused by *P. aeruginosa*, *Acinetobacter baumannii* complex, *Enterobacter* spp., and emerging strains of MDR NF-GNB such as *S. maltophilia*, *Burkholderia cepacia* complex, and *Alcaligenes* (*Achromobacter*) species, which may be difficult to treat. Mortality rates associated with HAP due to MRSA or *P. aeruginosa* are disproportionately higher than those caused by other nosocomial bacterial pathogens [74].

Polymicrobial isolates and MDR pathogens are more common among patients with HAP, particularly when it occurs as a late complication during hospitalization. Because of the frequency with which multiple organisms are identified on a single respiratory sample, recent evidence-based guidelines advocate the use of quantitative or semiquantitative lower respiratory tract cultures obtained either bronchoscopically or noninvasively as part of the initial evaluation of the patients with suspected HAP or VAP [75].

Empiric antibiotic selections for HAP that develop within 7 days of admission should target *S. pneumoniae*, *S. aureus* including MRSA, *Streptococcus* spp., *H. influenzae*, and Enterobacteriaceae. Patients with late HAP occurring >1 week after hospitalization should receive empiric antimicrobial therapy that includes coverage for MDR-GNB. The scope of alternative antimicrobial choices in patients with refractory or slow-to-respond HAP or VAP should be based on institution-dependent susceptibility profiles. If an institution's incidence of MRSA pneumonia is low and respiratory cultures are unavailable or unrevealing, screening for MRSA nasal colonization may be useful in guiding therapy [76]. As the absence of MRSA nasal colonization has a high negative predictive value for MRSA pneumonia, coverage for that organism can often be discontinued early in the treatment course if screening swabs are negative [76].

Pneumonias Caused by Aspiration and Bronchial Obstruction

Aspiration of orogastric contents and mechanical obstruction of the airways may create a favorable milieu for pneumonia caused by microaerophilic or anaerobic bacteria like *Peptostreptococcus* spp. A variety of factors, such as abnormal swallow function, altered cough reflex, impaired mucociliary clearance, altered mental status, the use of sedating medications, chemotherapy-induced mucositis, supine positioning, gastroparesis, mechanical ventilation, and nasogastric tube feeding, all contribute to the increased predilection for aspiration in patients with histories of transplantation or malignancy [77–79]. Pneumonia associated with large-volume aspiration of gastric contents typically occurs as a late finding. The acidic gastric contents act as a poor medium for bacterial growth. Thus, the initial clinical syndrome following aspiration of gastric contents arises from the direct caustic effect of the acidic aspirate on the cells of the alveolar-capillary interface, i.e., chemical pneumonitis. A true bacterial pneumonia, if it occurs, is consequently a superimposed process. Aspiration of oral contents, by contrast, results from inhalation of nonsterile oropharyngeal material. The clinical presentation is often insidious, and the diagnosis is commonly inferred based on a compatible patient risk profile coupled with radiographic evidence of pneumonia.

Chest radiographs may show focal abnormalities that correlate with the patient's position at the time of aspiration. For example, aspiration that occurs while the patient is in the upright position typically localizes to the basilar segments of the lower lobes, whereas the superior segments of the lower lobes and posterior segments of the upper lobes are more frequently affected following aspiration that occurs in the supine position. The major pathogens underlying nosocomial versus community-acquired aspiration pneumonias differ although a microbiologic diagnosis may not be established due to the limited yield of conventional anaerobic cultures [78, 80–82]. If necessary, such cultures may be best obtained bronchoscopically using a protected strategy.

The management of patients with significant lung injury associated with the aspiration of gastric contents includes aggressive supportive care. Upper airway suctioning, pulmonary toilet, and, if necessary, positive pressure ventilation comprise the mainstays of therapy. There is no clearly established role for corticosteroids in this setting, though the practice of prescribing moderate- to high-dose prednisolone is not uncommon. Early and aggressive antimicrobial therapy is recommended for patients with pneumonia secondary to aspiration of oropharyngeal contents. Antimicrobial selections should be tailored to the immune status of the patient and setting in which the aspiration occurred, i.e., community vs. healthcare environment but in general should be broad in spectrum and target Gram-negative organisms and oral anaerobes. Anaerobic coverage may be particularly important in patients with periodontal disease, putrid sputum, or evidence of necrotizing pneumonia [78].

Other Sources of Pneumonia

Transplant recipients with altered pulmonary anatomy specifically lung transplant recipients with bronchial anastomotic strictures may be at risk for obstruction of the airways, atelectasis, and postobstructive pneumonia. The associated pneumonias tend to be polymicrobial in nature including GNB, staphylococci, and anaerobes and may require relief of the obstruction to achieve adequate antimicrobial effects, even if appropriate antibiotics are selected. This is often most rapidly achieved through interventional bronchoscopic techniques such as bronchial dilation with or without stent placement.

The lungs may also become infected via septic emboli arising from suppurative endovascular bacterial and, less commonly, fungal infections. Infected intravascular septic deep venous thrombi are increasingly recognized as a potential source of infection in immunosuppressed patients. The radiographic pattern in these patients is distinctive and includes multicentric, pleomorphic lung nodules with asymmetric, relatively small, thick-walled cavities.

Specific Pathogens

Opportunistic organisms commonly implicated in transplant-related respiratory tract infections are outlined below.

Nocardia and Actinomycosis

Over 30 species of *Nocardia* have been associated with human disease [83]. *Nocardia asteroides* complex, including *N. asteroides* sensu stricto and *N. farcinica*, accounts for nearly 90% of *Nocardia* infections, both in cancer patients and the general population. Risk factors for *Nocardia* pneumonia include profound deficiencies in cellular immunity, prolonged use of high-dose systemic corticosteroids, especially in the treatment of chronic lung diseases [84], and the presence of GVHD. Solid organ transplant recipients are also at particular risk for *Nocardia* infections although this varies based upon the organ transplanted. One review demonstrated infection rates of 3.5%, 2.5%, 1.3%, 0.2%, and 0.1% among recipients of the lungs, hearts, intestines, livers, and kidneys, respectively [85]. *Nocardia* infections commonly occur within the 1st year of transplantation although early (<1 month) and late (>2 years) infections have also been reported [85–87]. Infection with the organism should be considered if nodular pulmonary infiltrates are seen, although reticulonodular or diffuse infiltrates are occasionally described. Solitary nodules associated with irregular, thick-walled cavities that mimic invasive pulmonary aspergillosis, histoplasmosis, necrotizing cancer, or chronic bacterial lung abscess have also been associated with *Nocardia* infection.

Indolent *Nocardia* pneumonia may be clinically indistinguishable from other actinomycetes infections and from pneumonias caused by pulmonary eumycetes. Severely immunosuppressed cancer patients with refractory leukemia or prior allogenic HSCT may present with rapidly progressive multifocal nocardiosis. Spontaneous pneumothorax and hemoptysis are also recognized presentations of *Nocardia* infection among immunocompromised patients. Concomitant brain involvement is not uncommon, and preemptive evaluation is recommended to diagnose asymptomatic brain abscess in patients with pulmonary *Nocardia* infection. Trimethoprim-sulfamethoxazole (10–12 mg/kg daily) is effective against many *Nocardia* species. Retrospective studies suggest that clinical outcomes are improved when appropriate therapy is given for an extended period of time (6–12 months) [88]. Despite aggressive antimicrobial therapy, pulmonary nocardiosis carries a high mortality in immunosuppressed individuals [84]. Pulmonary actinomycosis typically presents in a very similar manner to nocardiosis, although it is classically associated with invasion across tissue plans. As such, pulmonary infection may involve the adjoining pleura and subsequently erode through the chest wall. Isolation of Actinomycetes from the respiratory tract should be evaluated critically as their presence may represent oropharyngeal contamination.

Tuberculosis

Mycobacterium tuberculosis is a rare cause of pulmonary infections in the developed world but is important to consider in severely immunosuppressed patients, especially foreign-born individuals or patients undergoing allograft solid organ or stem cell translantation in the developing countries where tuberculosis is regarded as an endemic disease [89]. Solid organ transplant recipients are estimated to have 20–74 times higher incidence of active tuberculosis than that of the general population [90]. Frequency of disease varies based upon the organ transplanted and the time from transplantation, with two-thirds of cases occurring within 1 year of transplantation [91].

A broad range of clinical manifestations may be possible with tuberculosis infection. Pulmonary tuberculosis may present as an insidious pneumonia that is difficult to distinguish from Actinomycetes and eumycetes infection. Patients with impaired T-cell response may develop rapidly progressive tuberculosis that follows the course of a virulent bacterial infection. Systemic corticosteroid therapy is an independent predictor of both tuberculosis reactivation and suboptimal response to combination antimicrobial therapy. Hence, once the diagnosis of tuberculosis is established, every effort should be made to discontinue steroid therapy if not indicated for a specific syndrome [89]. Just as HIV-infected patients may develop clinical worsening of tuberculosis pneumonia when initiating antiretroviral therapy such as immune reconstitution inflammatory syndrome, tuberculosis-related lung disease in solid organ transplant or HSCT recipients may infrequently worsen as immune function recovers following temporary discontinuation or partial withdrawal of antirejection or anti-GVHD therapy. Nonetheless, minimizing immunosuppression may be helpful in clearing such infections.

Nontuberculous Mycobacteria

Nontuberculous mycobacteria (NTM) are ubiquitous in the environment and generally cause infection only in hosts with specific anatomical or immunological defects [92]. Transplant recipients are at particular risk due to their impaired cell-mediated immunity. Among patients with structural lung disease particularly those before and after lung transplantation, this risk is further compounded by anatomical abnormalities. Epidemiological data are somewhat lacking for these pathogens as NTM infections are not reportable infections [92]. Incidence rates for NTM pulmonary infections are estimated at 0.24–2.8% among heart transplant recipients and 0.46–8.0% among lung transplant recipients [93–95].

Pulmonary NTM infections are classically caused by *M. avium-intracellulare* complex and other slow-growing mycobacteria. These opportunistic pathogens are most frequently associated with chronic, indolent pneumonias. In the United States, the rapidly growing mycobacteria particularly *M. abscessus* and *M. fortuitum* have emerged as another important, albeit less frequent cause of NTM lung disease. The diagnosis of pulmonary NTM infections remains a challenge as identification of these organisms in respiratory cultures may result from colonization of the respiratory tract or environmental contamination. Causality is suggested by identification of NTM in sterile lower respiratory tract specimens coupled with corresponding clinical manifestations such as chronic nonproductive cough and exertional dyspnea and a NTM lung disease compatible radiographic presentation. Fever, night sweats, weight loss, pleuritic chest pain, and pleural effusions are also possible but less frequent in the absence of systemic disseminated infection.

Radiographic features of NTM infection include upper lobe predominant nonspecific nodular lesions and small, thin-walled cavities. Chest CT findings demonstrating the characteristic "tree-in-bud" appearance may also be seen in patients with other chronic infections. The so-called Lady Windermere syndrome, characterized by relapsing or refractory pulmonary NTM infection due to slow-growing mycobacteria, may be seen in patients with defects in endogenous interferon-gamma cellular immune response [96]. NTM pulmonary infections are usually insidious, although rapidly progressive disease has been seen in patients with profound defects in helper T-cells. Treatment should include at least two antimicrobial agents to which the *Mycobacterium* is susceptible.

Pneumocystis jirovecii

Similar to NTM, *P. jirovecii* previously known as *P. carinii* is thought to be ubiquitous in the environment and only causes infection in the setting of impaired immunity. Classically described in HIV-positive individuals with pronounced CD4 lymphocytopenia, *Pneumocystis* is an important pathogen in solid organ transplant recipients [97]. In most immunosuppressed patients, *Pneumocystis* pneumonia presents as a slowly progressive infection accompanied by nonproductive cough, exertional dyspnea, and hypoxemia, although an acute, rapidly progressive form has been described. CT evidence of perihilar infiltrates may be mistaken for pneumonitis caused by common acquired viral infections such as RSV, influenza, parainfluenza, or CMV during the early phase of the infection. Bronchoalveolar lavage typically has a high diagnostic yield either through silver staining or through PCR amplification. High-dose trimethoprim-sulfamethoxazole (15–20 mg/kg daily) given for 21 days is the treatment of choice. Adjuvant systemic corticosteroids should be administered to most patients with severe hypoxemia. Oral atovaquone, primaquine plus clindamycin, and parenteral pentamidine may be given to patients who are intolerant of sulfa-containing regimens.

Invasive Fungal Pneumonia

Invasive pulmonary aspergillosis (IPA) is a relatively common cause of pneumonia in patients undergoing allogeneic HSCT and severely immunosuppressed patients following high-risk solid organ allograft transplantation [98]. Among cancer patients, risk factors for invasive pulmonary aspergillosis include prolonged (>1 week) and severe (<100 cells/μL) neutropenia, refractory leukemia, allogeneic HSCT, GVHD, immunosuppressive therapy, and treatment with high dose systemic corticosteroids [99, 100]. Among solid organ transplant recipients, risk factors vary based upon the organ transplanted but often include renal failure, reoperation/retransplantation, and CMV infection [101]. *Aspergillus fumigatus* is most commonly encountered, although non-*fumigatus Aspergillus* species are increasingly recognized. Similarly, a marked increase in pulmonary invasive fungal infections due to non-*Aspergillus* molds including *Fusarium*, *Pseudallescheria boydii*, and *Scedosporium* spp. and the dematiaceous (black) molds has also been noted, making the selection of an effective empiric regimen more challenging. The increased incidence of pulmonary mucormycosis may be related to changes in antifungal utilization with a shift away from amphotericin B compounds in favor of mold-active triazole drugs like voriconazole [102]. The effects of newer triazole agents like posaconazole and isavuconazonium on the overall feasibility, efficacy and safety in magagement of fungal pneumonia in transplant recipients is evolving and appears encouraging.

While the clinical symptoms of fungal pneumonia may be similar to those seen in bacterial pneumonia, CT imaging may reveal a highly suggestive "halo sign" during the early course of infection and/or less often observed "crescent sign" that becomes apparent during the later course of IPA. Despite this, in most cases of pulmonary mycosis, the only radiographic findings at the time of presentation are peripheral, pleural-based lung nodules, sometimes with thick-walled regular or irregular cavities [103]. The definitive diagnosis of pulmonary invasive fungal infection requires demonstration of fungal hyphae within the involved lung tissue. Therefore, the clinical diagnosis is often made by inference as high prevalence of thrombocytopenia and coagulopathies in transplant recipients render lung biopsies unsafe. It is important to note that isolation of fungi in respiratory samples may misrepresent the etiology of underlying pulmonary infiltrates as they may reflect environmental contamination or respiratory tract colonization.

The measurement of fungal antigens such as serum galactomannan, bronchoalveolar lavage galactomannan, and serum beta-D-glucan can aid in the detection of invasive pulmonary mycosis. Newer assays, including sequence-based nucleic acid amplification techniques, may further alter the diagnostic strategies used for invasive fungal infection in the future. Therapeutic strategies for these infections are discussed elsewhere.

Viruses

As previously noted, respiratory viruses including RSV, influenza A and B, parainfluenza, and adenovirus are common causes of upper respiratory tract infections that may have lower respiratory tract manifestations in immunosuppressed patients. Human metapneumovirus (hMPV) is also recognized as a serious pulmonary pathogen in this population. The spectrum of hMPV disease may range from mild upper respiratory tract infection to serious disseminated infection leading to respiratory failure and encephalitis. Herpesviruses, particularly CMV, are also important causes of pneumonitis in transplant recipients. As invasive CMV disease often affects the transplanted allograft, lung transplant recipients are at particularly high risk of CMV pneumonitis [104]. The virus itself is immunomodulatory in nature, and CMV has been associated with bacterial and fungal superinfections as well as lymphoproliferative disorders [105, 106].

Fever and nonproductive cough are prominent but nonspecific features of viral respiratory tract infection. In patients with extensive lung involvement, dyspnea may appear early in the course of infection. Viral nucleic acids in nasal washes, tracheal aspirates, and bronchial specimens are most frequently used in diagnosing viral respiratory infections through multiplex PCR platforms. Despite that, the isolation of CMV especially by PCR amplification from lower respiratory tract secretions may not necessarily indicate CMV lung infection as even in transplant recipients with severe cellular immune defects; intermittent low-level viral replication and shed virus without developing viral lung disease has been well established. Hosts' risk assessment and CMV disease susceptibility evaluation along with radiographic imaging such as non-iv-contrast chest CT scan prove helpful in discerning active viral lung disease versus non-disease associated CMV respiratory tract viral shedding. Of note, chest CT scans may show ground glass opacities even when conventional chest radiographs are unremarkable, improving the sensitivity of diagnosis. Ganciclovir or foscarnet are commonly prescribed for systemic CMV infections. In transplant recipients with CMV pneumonitis, IVIG immune modulation along with effective antiviral drug if recommended. A detailed discussion is provided regarding specific pathogens and approach towards therapeutic management of lung infections in chapters throughout this book.

References

1. Fishman JA. Infection in solid-organ transplant recipients. N Engl J Med. 2007;357:2601–14.
2. Ibrahim EH, Tracy L, Hill C, Fraser VJ, Kollef MH. The occurrence of ventilator-associated pneumonia in a community hospital: risk factors and clinical outcomes. Chest. 2001;120:555–61.
3. Bodey GP, Buckley M, Sathe YS, Freireich EJ. Quantitative relationships between circulating leukocytes and infection in patients with acute leukemia. Ann Intern Med. 1966;64:328–40.
4. Carlisle PS, Gucalp R, Wiernik PH. Nosocomial infections in neutropenic cancer patients. Infect Control Hosp Epidemiol. 1993;14:320–4.
5. Issa NC, Fishman JA. Infectious complications of antilymphocyte therapies in solid organ transplantation. Clin Infect Dis Off Publ Infect Dis Soc Am. 2009;48:772–86.
6. Roemer E, Blau IW, Basara N, Kiehl MG, Bischoff M, Günzelmann S, et al. Toxoplasmosis, a severe complication in allogeneic hematopoietic stem cell transplantation: successful treatment strategies during a 5-year single-center experience. Clin Infect Dis Off Publ Infect Dis Soc Am. 2001;32:E1–8.
7. Safdar A, Armstrong D. Listeriosis in patients at a comprehensive cancer center, 1955–1997. Clin Infect Dis Off Publ Infect Dis Soc Am. 2003;37:359–64.
8. Savage DG, Taylor P, Blackwell J, Chen F, Szydlo RM, Rule SA, Spencer A, et al. Paranasal sinusitis following allogeneic bone marrow transplant. Bone Marrow Transplant. 1997;19(1):55–9.
9. Shibuya TY, Momin F, Abella E, Jacobs JR, Karanes C, Ratanatharathorn V, et al. Sinus disease in the bone marrow transplant population: incidence, risk factors, and complications. Otolaryngol Head Neck Surg. 1995;113(6):705–11.
10. Dhong HJ, Lee JC, Ryu JS, Cho DY. Rhinosinusitis in transplant patients. Clin Otolaryngol Allied Sci. 2001;26:329–33.
11. Yung MW, Gould J, Upton GJG. Nasal polyposis in children with cystic fibrosis: a long-term follow-up study. Ann Otol Rhinol Laryngol. 2002;111:1081–6.
12. Ortiz E, Sakano E, De Souza CA, Vigorito A, Eid KAB, Chronic GVHD. Predictive factor for rhinosinusitis in bone marrow transplantation. Braz J Otorhinolaryngol. 2006;72:328–32.
13. Thompson AM, Couch M, Zahurak ML, Johnson C, Vogelsang GB. Risk factors for post-stem cell transplant sinusitis. Bone Marrow Transplant. 2002;29:257–61.
14. Rayes A, Sahni K, Hanna C, Suryadevara M, Goyal P, Cherrick I. Cytomegalovirus sinusitis in a child with chronic myelogenous leukemia following bone marrow transplantation. Pediatr Blood Cancer. 2011;56:1140–2.
15. Gwaltney JM. Acute community-acquired sinusitis. Clin Infect Dis. 1996;23(6):1209–23; quiz 1224–5.
16. Mogensen C, Tos M. Quantitative histology of the maxillary sinus. Rhinology. 1977;15:129–40.
17. Fokkens W, Lund V, Mullol J, European Position Paper on Rhinosinusitis and Nasal Polyps Group. EP3OS 2007: European position paper on rhinosinusitis and nasal polyps 2007. A summary for otorhinolaryngologists. Rhinology. 2007;45: 97–101.
18. Holzmann D, Speich R, Kaufmann T, Laube I, Russi EW, Simmen D, et al. Effects of sinus surgery in patients with cystic fibrosis after lung transplantation: a 10-year experience. Transplantation. 2004;77:134–6.
19. Murray TS, Egan M, Kazmierczak BI. Pseudomonas aeruginosa chronic colonization in cystic fibrosis patients. Curr Opin Pediatr. 2007;19:83–8.
20. Evans FO, Sydnor JB, Moore WEC, Moore GR, Manwaring JL, Brill AH, et al. Sinusitis of the maxillary antrum. N Engl J Med. 1975;293:735–9.
21. de Medeiros CR, Bleggi-Torres LF, Faoro LN, Reis-Filho JS, Silva LC, de Medeiros BC, et al. Cavernous sinus thrombosis caused by zygomycosis after unrelated bone marrow transplantation. Transpl Infect Dis. 2001;3:231–4.
22. Li JY, Yong TY, Khoo E, Russ GR, Grove DI, Coates PT, McDonald SP. Isolated sphenoid fungal sinusitis in a renal transplant recipient presenting with bilateral abducens nerve palsy. Transpl Int. 2007;20(7):640–2.
23. Berlinger NT. Sinusitis in immunodeficient and immunosuppressed patients. Laryngoscope. 1985;95:29–33.
24. Lee SY, Yeo CL, Lee WH, Kwa AL, Koh LP, Hsu LY. Prevalence of invasive fungal disease in hematological patients at a tertiary university hospital in Singapore. BMC Res Notes. 2011;4:42.
25. Ellison MD, Hung RT, Harris K, Campbell BH. Report of the first case of invasive fungal sinusitis caused by Scopulariopsis acremonium: review of Scopulariopsis infections. Arch Otolaryngol Head Neck Surg. 1998;124:1014–6.
26. Rombaux P, Eloy P, Bertrand B, Delos M, Doyen C. Lethal disseminated Fusarium infection with sinus involvement in the immunocompromised host: case report and review of the literature. Rhinology. 1996;34:237–41.
27. Richardson SE, Bannatyne RM, Summerbell RC, Milliken J, Gold R, Weitzman SS. Disseminated fusarial infection in the immunocompromised host. Rev Infect Dis. 1988;10:1171–81.
28. Furukawa H, Kusne S, Sutton DA, Manez R, Carrau R, Nichols L, et al. Acute invasive sinusitis due to Trichoderma longibrachiatum in a liver and small bowel transplant recipient. Clin Infect Dis. 1998;26:487–9.
29. Machado CM, Martins MA, Heins-Vaccari EM, CdS L, MCA M, Castelli JB, et al. Scedosporium apiospermum sinusitis after bone marrow transplantation: report of a case. Rev Inst Med Trop Sao Paulo. 1998;40:321–3.
30. Castiglioni B, Sutton DA, Rinaldi MG, Fung J, Kusne S. Pseudallescheria boydii (Anamorph Scedosporium apiospermum). Infection in solid organ transplant recipients in a tertiary medical center and review of the literature. Medicine (Baltimore). 2002;81:333–48.
31. Vernon SE, Acar BC, Pham SM, Fertel D. Acanthamoeba infection in lung transplantation: report of a case and review of the literature. Transpl Infect Dis. 2005;7:154–7.

32. Rivera MA, Padhya TA. Acanthamoeba: a rare primary cause of rhinosinusitis. Laryngoscope. 2002;112:1201–3.
33. Craven DE, Hjalmarson KI. Ventilator-associated tracheobronchitis and pneumonia: thinking outside the box. Clin Infect Dis. 2010;51(Suppl 1):S59–66.
34. van Assen S, Bootsma GP, Verweij PE, Donnelly JP, Raemakers JM. Aspergillus tracheobronchitis after allogeneic bone marrow transplantation. Bone Marrow Transplant. 2000;26:1131–2.
35. Fernández-Ruiz M, Silva JT, San-Juan R, de Dios B, García-Luján R, López-Medrano F, et al. Aspergillus tracheobronchitis: report of 8 cases and review of the literature. Medicine (Baltimore). 2012;91:261–73.
36. Wenzel RP, Fowler AA. Clinical practice. Acute bronchitis. N Engl J Med. 2006;355:2125–30.
37. Falsey AR, Erdman D, Anderson LJ, Walsh EE. Human metapneumovirus infections in young and elderly adults. J Infect Dis. 2003;187:785–90.
38. Boldy DA, Skidmore SJ, Ayres JG. Acute bronchitis in the community: clinical features, infective factors, changes in pulmonary function and bronchial reactivity to histamine. Respir Med. 1990;84:377–85.
39. Jonsson JS, Sigurdsson JA, Kristinsson KG, Guthnadóttir M, Magnusson S. Acute bronchitis in adults. How close do we come to its aetiology in general practice? Scand J Prim Health Care. 1997;15:156–60.
40. Louie JK, Hacker JK, Gonzales R, Mark J, Maselli JH, Yagi S, Drew WL. Characterization of viral agents causing acute respiratory infection in a San Francisco University Medical Center Clinic during the influenza season. Clin Infect Dis. 2005;41:822–8.
41. Gottlieb J, Schulz TF, Welte T, Fuehner T, Dierich M, Simon AR, Engelmann I. Community-acquired respiratory viral infections in lung transplant recipients: a single season cohort study. Transplantation. 2009;87:1530–7.
42. Chemaly RF, Ghosh S, Bodey GP, Rohatgi N, Safdar A, Keating MJ, et al. Respiratory viral infections in adults with hematologic malignancies and human stem cell transplantation recipients: a retrospective study at a major cancer center. Medicine (Baltimore). 2006;85:278–87.
43. Renaud C, Campbell AP. Changing epidemiology of respiratory viral infections in hematopoietic cell transplant recipients and solid organ transplant recipients. Curr Opin Infect Dis. 2011;24:333–43.
44. Tang T-C, Chuang W-Y. Aspergillus tracheobronchitis in allogeneic stem cell transplanted recipient. Eur J Haematol. 2012;88:183.
45. Krenke R, Kołkowska-Leśniak A, Pałynyczko G, Prochorec-Sobieszek M, Konopka L. Ulcerative and pseudomembranous Aspergillus tracheobronchitis in a patient with acute myeloid leukemia. Int J Hematol. 2009;89:257–8.
46. Adams PF, Hendershot GE, Marano MA, Centers for Disease Control and Prevention/National Center for Health Statistics. Current estimates from the National Health Interview Survey, 1996. Vital Health Stat. 1999;10:1–203.
47. Ljungman P, Ward KN, Crooks BN, Parker A, Martino R, Shaw PJ, et al. Respiratory virus infections after stem cell transplantation: a prospective study from the Infectious Diseases Working Party of the European Group for Blood and Marrow Transplantation. Bone Marrow Transplant. 2001;28:479–84.
48. Kumar D, Husain S, Chen MH, Moussa G, Himsworth D, Manuel O, et al. A prospective molecular surveillance study evaluating the clinical impact of community-acquired respiratory viruses in lung transplant recipients. Transplantation. 2010;89:1028–33.
49. López-Medrano F, Aguado JM, Lizasoain M, Folgueira D, Juan RS, Díaz-Pedroche C, et al. Clinical implications of respiratory virus infections in solid organ transplant recipients: a prospective study. Transplantation. 2007;84:851–6.
50. Erard V, Chien JW, Kim HW, Nichols WG, Flowers ME, Martin PJ, et al. Airflow decline after myeloablative allogeneic hematopoietic cell transplantation: the role of community respiratory viruses. J Infect Dis. 2006;193:1619–25.
51. Waghmare A, Englund JA, Boeckh M. How I treat respiratory viral infections in the setting of intensive chemotherapy or hematopoietic cell transplantation. Blood. 2016;127:2682–92.
52. Campbell AP, Guthrie KA, Englund JA, Farney RM, Minerich EL, Kuypers J, et al. Clinical outcomes associated with respiratory virus detection before allogeneic hematopoietic stem cell transplant. Clin Infect Dis. 2015;61:192–202.
53. Fisher CE, Preiksaitis CM, Lease ED, Edelman J, Kirby KA, Leisenring WM, et al. Symptomatic respiratory virus infection and chronic lung allograft dysfunction. Clin Infect Dis. 2016;62:313–9.
54. Chien JW, Duncan S, Williams KM, Pavletic SZ. Bronchiolitis obliterans syndrome after allogeneic hematopoietic stem cell transplantation-an increasingly recognized manifestation of chronic graft-versus-host disease. Biol Blood Marrow Transplant. 2010;16:S106–14.
55. Mandell LA, Wunderink RG, Anzueto A, Bartlett JG, Campbell GD, Dean NC, Infectious Diseases Society of America; American Thoracic Society, et al. Infectious Diseases Society of America/American Thoracic Society consensus guidelines on the management of community-acquired pneumonia in adults. Clin Infect Dis. 2007;44:S27–72.
56. Kalil AC, Metersky ML, Klompas M, Muscedere J, Sweeney DA, Palmer LB, et al. Management of adults with hospital-acquired and ventilator-associated pneumonia: 2016 clinical practice guidelines by the Infectious Diseases Society of America and the American Thoracic Society. Clin Infect Dis. 2016;63(5):e61–e111.
57. Costa SF, Alexander BD. Non-Aspergillus fungal pneumonia in transplant recipients. Clin Chest Med. 2005;26:675–90, vii.
58. Marr KA, Carter RA, Crippa F, Wald A, Corey L. Epidemiology and outcome of mould infections in hematopoietic stem cell transplant recipients. Clin Infect Dis. 2002;34:909–17.
59. Kotloff RM, Ahya VN, Crawford SW. Pulmonary complications of solid organ and hematopoietic stem cell transplantation. Am J Respir Crit Care Med. 2004;170:22–48.
60. Chalmers JD, Rother C, Salih W, Ewig S. Healthcare-associated pneumonia does not accurately identify potentially resistant pathogens: a systematic review and meta-analysis. Clin Infect Dis. 2014;58:330–9.
61. Gross AE, Van Schooneveld TC, Olsen KM, Rupp ME, Bui TH, Forsung E, Kalil AC. Epidemiology and predictors of multidrug-resistant community-acquired and health care-associated pneumonia. Antimicrob Agents Chemother. 2014;58:5262–8.
62. Yap V, Datta D, Metersky ML. Is the present definition of health care-associated pneumonia the best way to define risk of infection with antibiotic-resistant pathogens? Infect Dis Clin N Am. 2013;27:1–18.
63. Bartlett JG. Community-acquired pneumonia. Int J Pract Suppl. 2000;115:18–22.
64. Aisenberg G, Rolston KV, Safdar A. Bacteremia caused by Achromobacter and Alcaligenes species in 46 patients with cancer (1989–2003). Cancer. 2004;101:2134–40.
65. Patterson TF, Kirkpatrick WR, White M, Hiemenz JW, Wingard JR, Dupont B, et al. Invasive aspergillosis. Disease spectrum, treatment practices, and outcomes. I3 Aspergillus Study Group. Medicine (Baltimore). 2000;79:250–60.
66. Junghanss C, Marr KA, Carter RA, Sandmaier BM, Maris MB, Maloney DG, et al. Incidence and outcome of bacterial and fungal infections following nonmyeloablative compared with myeloablative allogeneic hematopoietic stem cell transplantation: a matched control study. Biol Blood Marrow Transplant. 2002;8:512–20.

67. Marr KA, Carter RA, Boeckh M, Martin P, Corey L. Invasive aspergillosis in allogeneic stem cell transplant recipients: changes in epidemiology and risk factors. Blood. 2002;100:4358–66.
68. Ison MG, Hayden FG, Kaiser L, Corey L, Boeckh M. Rhinovirus infections in hematopoietic stem cell transplant recipients with pneumonia. Clin Infect Dis. 2003;36:1139–43.
69. Alangaden GJ, Wahiduzzaman M, Chandrasekar PH, Bone Marrow Transplant Group. Aspergillosis: the most common community-acquired pneumonia with gram-negative Bacilli as copathogens in stem cell transplant recipients with graft-versus-host disease. Clin Infect Dis. 2002;35:659–64.
70. Ascioglu S, Rex JH, de Pauw B, Bennett JE, Bille J, Crokaert F, Invasive Fungal Infections Cooperative Group of the European Organization for Research and Treatment of Cancer, Mycoses Study Group of the National Institute of Allergy and Infectious Diseases, et al. Defining opportunistic invasive fungal infections in immunocompromised patients with cancer and hematopoietic stem cell transplants: an international consensus. Clin Infect Dis. 2002;34:7–14.
71. Mandell LA, Bartlett JG, Dowell SF, File TM Jr, Musher DM, Whitney C, Infectious Diseases Society of America. Update of practice guidelines for the management of community-acquired pneumonia in immunocompetent adults. Clin Infect Dis. 2003;37:1405–33.
72. Niederman MS, Mandell LA, Anzueto A, Bass JB, Broughton WA, Campbell GD, American Thoracic Society, et al. Guidelines for the management of adults with community-acquired pneumonia. Diagnosis, assessment of severity, antimicrobial therapy, and prevention. Am J Respir Crit Care Med. 2001;163:1730–54.
73. Rubinstein E, Kollef MH, Nathwani D. Pneumonia caused by methicillin-resistant *Staphylococcus aureus*. Clin Infect Dis. 2008;46:S378–85.
74. Rello J, Ollendorf DA, Oster G, Vera-Llonch M, Bellm L, Redman R, Kollef MH, VAP Outcomes Scientific Advisory Group. Epidemiology and outcomes of ventilator-associated pneumonia in a large US database. Chest. 2002;122:2115–21.
75. American Thoracic Society & Infectious Diseases Society of America. Guidelines for the management of adults with hospital-acquired, ventilator-associated, and healthcare-associated pneumonia. Am J Respir Crit Care Med. 2005;171:388–416.
76. Dangerfield B, Chung A, Webb B, Seville MT. Predictive value of methicillin-resistant *Staphylococcus aureus* (MRSA) nasal swab PCR assay for MRSA pneumonia. Antimicrob Agents Chemother. 2014;58:859–64.
77. Reza Shariatzadeh M, Huang JQ, Marrie TJ. Differences in the features of aspiration pneumonia according to site of acquisition: community or continuing care facility. J Am Geriatr Soc. 2006;54:296–302.
78. Marik PE. Aspiration pneumonitis and aspiration pneumonia. N Engl J Med. 2001;344:665–71.
79. Cabre M, Serra-Prat M, Palomera E, Almirall J, Pallares R, Clavé P. Prevalence and prognostic implications of dysphagia in elderly patients with pneumonia. Age Ageing. 2010;39:39–45.
80. El-Solh AA, Pietrantoni C, Bhat A, Aquilina AT, Okada M, Grover V, Gifford N. Microbiology of severe aspiration pneumonia in institutionalized elderly. Am J Respir Crit Care Med. 2003;167:1650–4.
81. Mier L, Dreyfuss D, Darchy B, Lanore JJ, Djedaïni K, Weber P, et al. Is penicillin G an adequate initial treatment for aspiration pneumonia? A prospective evaluation using a protected specimen brush and quantitative cultures. Intensive Care Med. 1993;19:279–84.
82. Carratalà J, Mykictiuk A, Fernández-Sabé N, Suárez C, Dorca J, Verdaguer R, et al. Health care-associated pneumonia requiring hospital admission: epidemiology, antibiotic therapy, and clinical outcomes. Arch Intern Med. 2007;167:1393–9.
83. Brown-Elliott BA, Brown JM, Conville PS, Wallace RJ. Clinical and laboratory features of the Nocardia spp. based on current molecular taxonomy. Clin Microbiol Rev. 2006;19:259–82.
84. Torres HA, Reddy BT, Raad II, Tarrand J, Bodey GP, Hanna HA, et al. Nocardiosis in cancer patients. Medicine (Baltimore). 2002;81:388–97.
85. Peleg AY, Husain S, Qureshi ZA, Silveira FP, Sarumi M, Shutt KA, et al. Risk factors, clinical characteristics, and outcome of Nocardia infection in organ transplant recipients: a matched case-control study. Clin Infect Dis. 2007;44:1307–14.
86. Santos M, Gil-Brusola A, Morales P. Infection by Nocardia in solid organ transplantation: thirty years of experience. Transplant Proc. 2011;43:2141–4.
87. Yu X, Han F, Wu J, He Q, Peng W, Wang Y, et al. Nocardia infection in kidney transplant recipients: case report and analysis of 66 published cases. Transpl Infect Dis. 2011;13:385–91.
88. Uttamchandani RB, Daikos GL, Reyes RR, Fischl MA, Dickinson GM, et al. Nocardiosis in 30 patients with advanced human immunodeficiency virus infection: clinical features and outcome. Clin Infect Dis. 1994;18:348–53.
89. De La Rosa GR, Jacobson KL, Rolston KV, Raad II, Kontoyiannis DP, Safdar A. Mycobacterium tuberculosis at a comprehensive cancer centre: active disease in patients with underlying malignancy during 1990-2000. Clin Microbiol Infect. 2004;10:749–52.
90. Muñoz P, Rodríguez C, Bouza E. Mycobacterium tuberculosis infection in recipients of solid organ transplants. Clin Infect Dis. 2005;40:581–7.
91. Singh N, Paterson DL. Mycobacterium tuberculosis infection in solid-organ transplant recipients: impact and implications for management. Clin Infect Dis. 1998;27:1266–77.
92. Keating MR, Daly JS, AST Infectious Diseases Community of Practice. Nontuberculous mycobacterial infections in solid organ transplantation. Am J Transplant. 2013;13(Suppl 4):77–82.
93. Patel R, Roberts GD, Keating MR, Paya CV. Infections due to nontuberculous mycobacteria in kidney, heart, and liver transplant recipients. Clin Infect Dis. 1994;19:263–73.
94. Knoll BM, Kappagoda S, Gill RR, Goldberg HJ, Boyle K, Baden LR, et al. Non-tuberculous mycobacterial infection among lung transplant recipients: a 15-year cohort study. Transpl Infect Dis. 2012;14:452–60.
95. Piersimoni C. Nontuberculous mycobacteria infection in solid organ transplant recipients. Eur J Clin Microbiol Infect Dis. 2012;31:397–403.
96. Safdar A, White DA, Stover D, Armstrong D, Murray HW. Profound interferon gamma deficiency in patients with chronic pulmonary nontuberculous mycobacteriosis. Am J Med. 2002;113:756–9.
97. Martin SI, Fishman JA, AST Infectious Diseases Community of Practice. Pneumocystis pneumonia in solid organ transplantation. Am J Transplant. 2013;13(Suppl 4):272–9.
98. Morgan J, Wannemuehler KA, Marr KA, Hadley S, Kontoyiannis DP, Walsh TJ, et al. Incidence of invasive aspergillosis following hematopoietic stem cell and solid organ transplantation: interim results of a prospective multicenter surveillance program. Med Mycol. 2005;43(Suppl 1):S49–58.
99. Marr KA. Empirical antifungal therapy – new options, new tradeoffs. N Engl J Med. 2002;346:278–80.
100. Marr KA, Patterson T, Denning D. Aspergillosis. Pathogenesis, clinical manifestations, and therapy. Infect Dis Clin N Am. 2002;16:875–94, vi.
101. Singh N, Singh NM, Husain S, AST Infectious Diseases Community of Practice. Aspergillosis in solid organ transplantation. Am J Transplant. 2013;13(Suppl 4):228–41.
102. Kontoyiannis DP, Lionakis MS, Lewis RE, Chamilos G, Healy M, Perego C, et al. Zygomycosis in a tertiary-care cancer center in the

era of Aspergillus-active antifungal therapy: a case-control observational study of 27 recent cases. J Infect Dis. 2005;191:1350–60.
103. Heussel CP, Kauczor HU, Heussel GE, Fischer B, Begrich M, Mildenberger P, Thelen M. Pneumonia in febrile neutropenic patients and in bone marrow and blood stem-cell transplant recipients: use of high-resolution computed tomography. J Clin Oncol. 1999;17:796–805.
104. Razonable R. Direct and indirect effects of Cytomegalovirus: can we prevent them? Enferm Infecc Microbiol Clin. 2010;28:1–5.
105. George MJ, Snydman DR, Werner BG, Griffith J, Falagas ME, Dougherty NN, Rubin RH. The independent role of Cytomegalovirus as a risk factor for invasive fungal disease in orthotopic liver transplant recipients. Boston Center for Liver Transplantation CMVIG-Study Group. Cytogam, MedImmune, Inc. Gaithersburg, Maryland. Am J Med. 1997;103:106–13.
106. Walker RC, Marshall WF, Strickler JG, Wiesner RH, Velosa JA, Habermann TM, et al. Pretransplantation assessment of the risk of lymphoproliferative disorder. Clin Infect Dis. 1995;20:1346–53.

Respiratory Tract Diseases That May Be Mistaken for Infection

21

Robert M. Kotloff, Burton F. Dickey, and Nicholas Vander Els

Introduction

The prevention, diagnosis, and treatment of pneumonia are critical to outcomes among transplantation patients. The diagnosis of pneumonia is usually considered when a new radiographic infiltrate is identified. Rarely, pneumonia may present initially without infiltrates in an immunocompromised host. However, even in severely immunosuppressed patients, infectious microbes cause inflammation through innate immune mechanisms that lead to tissue edema which is evident radiographically. The occurrence of pneumonia that is not apparent when a CT scan is included in the assessment is sufficiently rare that it will not be further considered here. Instead, we begin with an abnormal imaging study of the lungs, which is typically obtained during the workup of a symptom or sign such as cough, fever, or chills. The differential diagnosis of a lung infiltrate in a transplantation patient includes several common non-infectious causes. Failure to accurately diagnose non-infectious causes of lung infiltrates can lead to unnecessary treatment with antibiotics, and more importantly to failure to address the under lying pathophysiologic process. This chapter is focused on clinical presentations of pulmonary disorders that mimic infectious pneumonia.

R. M. Kotloff
Department of Pulmonary Medicine, Respiratory Institute, Cleveland Clinic, Cleveland, OH, USA
e-mail: kotlofr@ccf.org

B. F. Dickey
Department of Pulmonary Medicine, University of Texas MD Anderson Cancer Center, Houston, TX, USA
e-mail: bdickey@mdanderson.org

N. Vander Els (✉)
Pulmonary Service, Memorial Sloan- Kettering Cancer Center, New York, NY, USA
e-mail: vanderen@mskcc.org

Hematopoietic Stem Cell Transplantation (HSCT)

Despite advances in treatment regimens and supportive care, pulmonary complications still occur in up to 60% of HSCT recipients [1]. These complications are mostly due to toxicities from conditioning regimens, delayed bone marrow recovery, prolonged immunosuppressive therapy, and graft-versus-host disease (GVHD). As the incidence of infectious pulmonary complications has diminished, largely due to effective prophylactic therapy, non-infectious pulmonary complications have emerged as a major cause of morbidity and mortality [2]. Pulmonary complications have been divided into those that occur "early" (during the first 100 days after transplantation) and those that occur "late," but this is not a rigid division. In particular, some "late" complications such as cryptogenic organizing pneumonia and constrictive bronchiolitis occur with substantial frequency during the first 100 days.

Pulmonary Edema

Cardiogenic (hydrostatic) pulmonary edema occurs with regularity in transplant patients due to the large volumes of fluid administered with chemotherapy and antibiotics, chemotherapy-induced cardiotoxicity, and co-morbidities (e.g., renal insufficiency) [3]. The classic presentation of cardiogenic pulmonary edema, consisting of acute, bilateral, symmetrical, perihilar infiltrates with interstitial thickening, an enlarged heart, and pleural effusions in a patient with pre-existing heart disease and associated findings of peripheral edema and bibasilar rales, is easy to recognize. However, cardiogenic pulmonary edema may also be the cause of asymmetrical infiltrates in a patient with underlying lung disease, such as bullous emphysema, that precludes alveolar filling in localized regions (see Fig. 21.1). An enlarged heart may not be present on the radiograph if cardiac dysfunction is not longstanding, so that the heart has not had time to

A. Safdar (ed.), *Principles and Practice of Transplant Infectious Diseases*, https://doi.org/10.1007/978-1-4939-9034-4_21

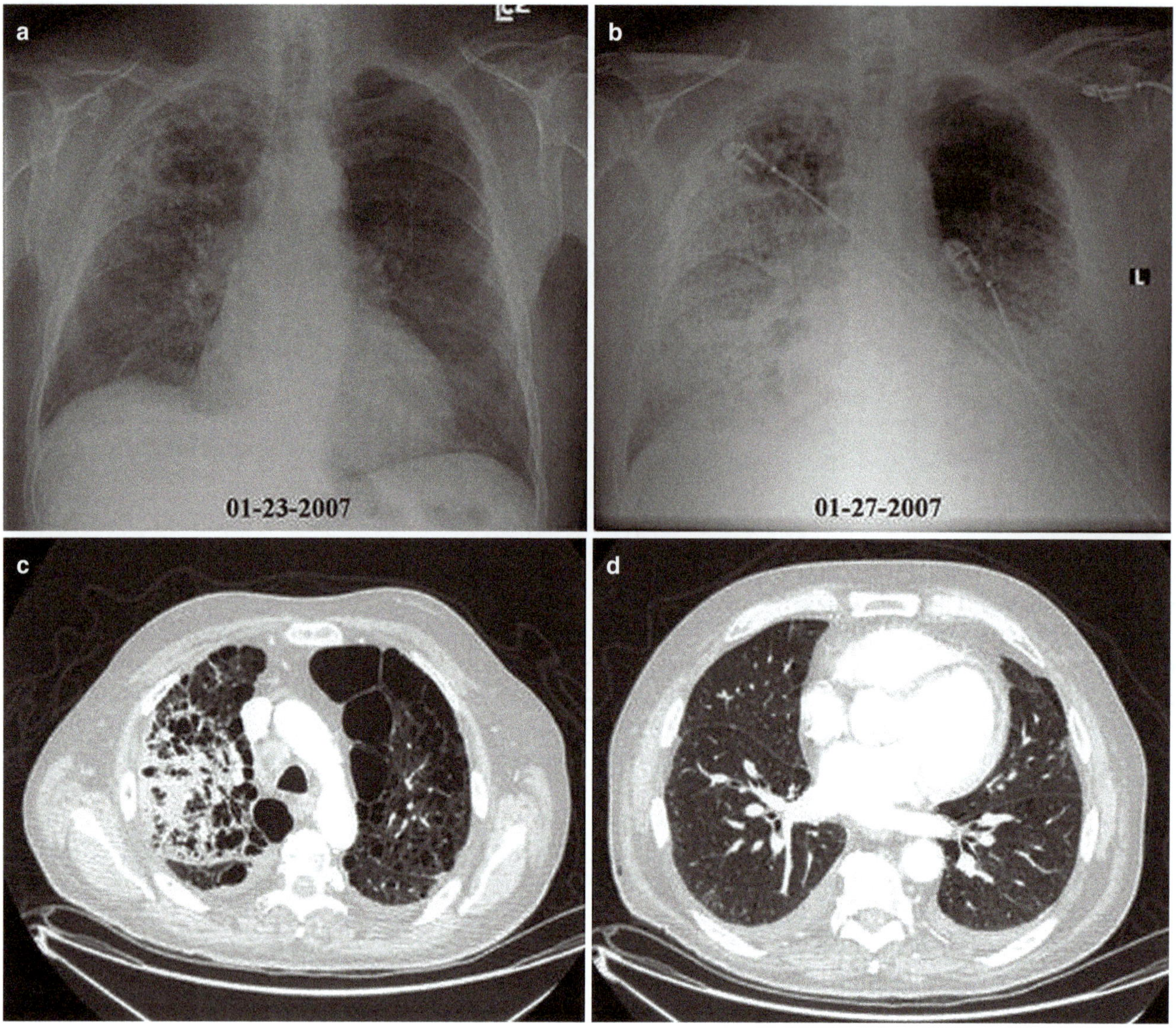

Fig. 21.1 Atypical presentation of congestive heart failure. A 68-year-old male was receiving radiation therapy to a squamous cell carcinoma of the upper lobe of the right lung. He had received 19 of 37 planned fractions, when he was admitted because of increasing dyspnea and cough, presumed to be pneumonia. (**a**) The PA radiograph in the left upper corner shows the right upper lobe with associated radiation pneumonitis. (**b**) The AP radiograph in the right upper corner taken 4 days later shows lung infiltrates that spare the left upper lobe. (**c**) However, the CT angiogram on the lower panel performed on the day of admission 01-24-2007 shows that the left upper chest is mostly occupied by emphysematous bullae, accounting for the sparing of the left upper lung field when pulmonary edema developed. (**d**) The remainder of the lung fields contain ground-glass opacities suggestive of *congestive heart failure*. The diagnosis of congestive heart failure was supported by the patient's history of prior episodes of pulmonary edema, bilateral ankle edema, a depressed left ventricular ejection fraction of 30–35%, moderate mitral regurgitation, elevated BNP of 1043, transudative pleural effusion, and improvement with diuresis [8]. (Reprinted from Kaplan et al. [8], with permission of Springer)

remodel (e.g., acute volume overload or diastolic dysfunction secondary to acute ischemia). In these cases, additional studies can be very helpful in establishing the diagnosis [4–6]. CT of the chest may show the diffuse nature of alveolar infiltrates and pleural effusions that are less apparent on plain films, and may additionally reveal interstitial edema and cardiac chamber enlargement. Review of serial radiographs may show infiltrates that wax and wane in association with variations in patient weight, peripheral edema, or fluid administration. Echocardiography is very supportive when it reveals systolic dysfunction, but it is important to recognize that diastolic dysfunction is an equally prevalent cause of heart failure [7], potentially exacerbated by rhythm disturbances such as atrial fibrillation, valvular dysfunction, or transient ventricular wall stiffening due to ischemia. Brain natriuretic peptide (BNP) levels are quite specific and sensitive but are less elevated in diastolic than in systolic dysfunction [7].

Non-cardiogenic pulmonary edema due to increased permeability of the alveolocapillary membrane (acute lung injury and adult respiratory distress syndrome (ARDS)) can occur as a result of a wide variety of causes in transplant patients. Sepsis is the most common cause of permeability edema of the lungs in general [6, 9, 10] and can cause radiographic infiltrates in transplant patients. In addition, transplant patients are susceptible to lung injury from causes unique to this population, such as from chemotherapy or the effects of acute GVHD. Transplant patients are also frequently exposed to treatments associated with lung injury in the general hospital population, such as transfusion. Transfusion-related acute lung injury (TRALI) is the leading cause of mortality from transfusions [11] and has been associated with all plasma-containing blood products, including immunoglobulins. The incidence of TRALI is not known, but has been estimated at 0.02% per unit transfused and 0.16% per patient transfused [12]. Patients with TRALI commonly present with dyspnea, cough, fever, acute hypoxemia hypotension, and bilateral pulmonary infiltrates within 1–6 h after the transfusion. Transient leukopenia, due to pulmonary sequestration of the circulating pool of leukocytes, may be observed. The mainstay of treatment for TRALI is to discontinue the transfusion, followed by supportive care. Although there has never been a randomized controlled trial of glucocorticoid therapy, they have no effect on the 5–8% mortality. With supportive treatment, infiltrates usually resolve, within 96 h, and survivors have no long-term sequelae [13].

Engraftment Syndrome (ES)

ES is characterized by a constellation of symptoms and signs including fever, erythrodermatous skin rash, diarrhea, and non-cardiogenic pulmonary edema with bilateral pulmonary infiltrates, which generally occur within 5 days of neutrophil engraftment following HSCT. In more severe cases, systemic involvement, i.e., renal failure, hepatic failure, encephalopathy, or seizures, may be observed. Seen most often following autologous HSCT, ES has also been described in those individuals who have undergone allogeneic HSCT with a non-myeloablative preparative therapy. Although the pathophysiology of ES is not well understood, it is thought to result from a combination of endothelial injury due to preconditioning chemotherapy and the production and release of cytokines and products of neutrophil degranulation and oxidative metabolism, leading to capillary leak, with either local injury in the lung or systemic tissue injury [14]. Bronchoalveolar lavage (BAL) may show a neutrophilic alveolitis. Surgical lung biopsies, when obtained, often reveal diffuse alveolar damage. Treatment entails observation and supportive care (i.e., antibiotics, intravenous fluids) in mild cases. High-dose corticosteroid therapy is very effective, often resulting in rapid clinical improvement in those with progressive or symptomatic ES. Respiratory failure requiring mechanical ventilation has been observed, however, in up to one-third of patients [15].

Idiopathic Pneumonia Syndrome (IPS)

In 1993, a panel convened by the NIH proposed a broad working definition of IPS as widespread non-lobar radiographic infiltrates in the absence of congestive heart failure or evidence of lower respiratory tract infection [16]. IPS occurs in 10% of HSCT recipients, usually 14–90 days following transplantation. Mortality rates range from 50% to 70% [17]. Possible etiologies of IPS include direct toxic effects of the chemoradiation conditioning regimen, occult infection, and/or the release of inflammatory cytokines secondary to some as yet unknown inciting stimuli. The association of IPS with the presence of acute GVHD after allogeneic HSCT suggests that alloreactive T cells may be at least one of these stimuli [17, 18].

The clinical presentation is non-specific, with symptoms of dyspnea, cough, and fever associated with diffuse infiltrates on chest radiograph. The diagnosis of IPS largely relies on the exclusion of infection on lower respiratory samples obtained from a diagnostic procedure, e.g., BAL or lung biopsy. Common pathologic findings of non-specific interstitial pneumonitis (NSIP) and/or diffuse alveolar damage (DAD) may be seen. Although no randomized controlled trials of treatment for IPS are available, current standards include high-dose intravenous corticosteroids and supportive care, such as supplemental oxygen and broad-spectrum antibiotics. Recent preclinical and clinical data suggest a potential role for tumor necrosis factor-α (TNF-α) in the pathogenesis of IPS [19 21], and a randomized trial using etanercept, a TNF receptor fusion protein, is being conducted by the Blood and Marrow Transplant Clinical Trials Network.

This same Network has included diffuse alveolar hemorrhage (DAH) within the definition of IPS, and we know of no reason to separate the two. Post-transplantation DAH was initially described in autologous HSCT recipients as widespread lung injury manifested by diffuse radiographic infiltrates that occurred in the absence of identifiable infection. DAH is now known to occur in both allogeneic and autologous transplant recipients and is seen in approximately 5% of all HSCT [22]. The etiology is unclear, but is not clearly related to any specific coagulopathy or to thrombocytopenia [23]. Pre-transplant high-dose chemotherapy, thoracic and/or total body irradiation, and undocumented infections are putative factors which may cause the initial injury, priming the lung for subsequent development of DAH. It can coincide with stem cell engraftment, but late onset (after the first 30 days) has been observed and is associated with a worse prognosis. Hemoptysis occurs in less than 20% of patients.

Bronchoscopic diagnostic criteria include progressively bloodier returns on BAL or the presence of 20% or more hemosiderin-laden macrophages on cytologic inspection of BAL fluid. However, these bronchoscopic criteria may be seen in association with diffuse lung injury from a wide variety of causes, including infections, congestive heart failure, and malignancy. There are no prospective randomized trials addressing the treatment of DAH. Earlier retrospective studies demonstrated reduced need for mechanical ventilation and mortality in a cohort of patients receiving high-dose corticosteroids, but more recent observational studies found no survival benefit [24, 25].

Drug-Induced Lung Injury (DILI)

DILI may present with dyspnea, fever, and pulmonary infiltrates, clinically indistinguishable from a pneumonia [26]. DILI may present at the time of transplantation as a consequence of chemotherapy administered for treatment of an underlying cancer or after transplantation as a consequence of chemotherapy administered as part of the conditioning regimen, or given as prophylaxis of GVHD. Agents of concern are listed in Table 21.1. Symptoms vary with the severity of injury; fever can be absent, and patients may have only dyspnea on exertion or be asymptomatic. In such patients, diffuse infiltrates seen on radiographs or abnormalities on pulmonary function testing may be the only signs of lung injury. There is no pathognomonic finding unique for DILI, and the diagnosis is one of exclusion [27]. Given the severe immune compromise of HSCT patients, bronchoscopy to exclude infection is indicated for most patients with new diffuse infiltrates.

Lung injury may occur either from a drug's cytotoxic mechanism or from its presence as an antigen. The histologic and radiographic patterns produced vary and include Usual Interstitial Pneumonitis (UIP)/fibrosis, hypersensitivity pneumonitis, and acute lung injury (ALI)/ARDS. Bleomycin produces lung injury both by cytotoxic action and as an antigen. It is used primarily to treat Hodgkin's disease and forms a moiety with ferrous ions that induces oxidative injury to tumor cells [28]. Human lungs and skin lack an enzyme, bleomycin hydrolase, which limits injury to other tissues. A UIP/fibrosis pathology is produced, with peripheral and basal infiltrates [29]. (See Fig. 21.2.) Exposure to supplemental oxygen can exacerbate this form of toxicity, by potentiating oxidative injury. As an antibiotic, bleomycin can cause hypersensitivity pneumonitis, with high fevers and acute infiltrates. This presentation tends to be responsive to steroid therapy [28–30]. Methotrexate also produces hypersensitivity pneumonitis. It is used both for the treatment of lymphoma and for prophylaxis against GVHD after HSCT. In contrast to bleomycin, the hypersensitivity from methotrexate can be accompanied by peripheral eosinophilia and thoracic adenopathy [31, 32]. Granulomas are seen on biopsy, and the toxicity is responsive to steroid therapy [31]. The substituted nucleoside fludarabine may also produce granulomatous disease, as well as eosinophilic pneumonia [33, 34]. Etoposide is rarely toxic but can produce a severe hypersensitivity reaction with symptoms of angioedema or ARDS [35, 36]. Etoposide use is common in HSCT, as a component of the ICE

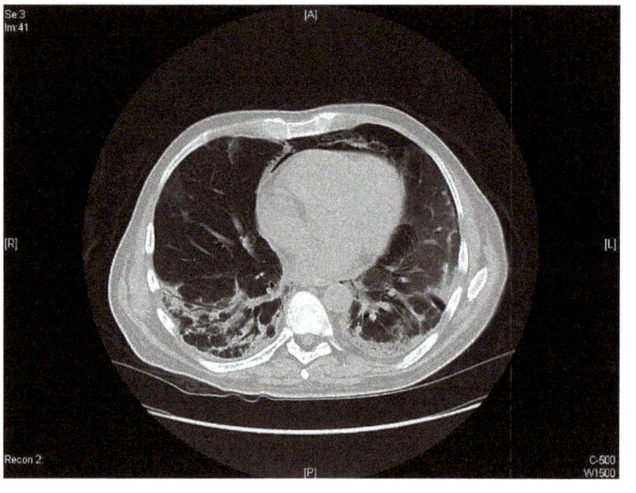

Fig. 21.2 Severe bleomycin toxicity, UIP presentation. Note peripheral and basal pattern of infiltration, as well as spontaneous pneumothorax seen anteriorly

Table 21.1 Chemotherapeutic agents characterized by class, indication, and pulmonary toxicity

Agent	Class	Indication	Pulmonary toxicity
Anti-thymocyte globulin	Monoclonal antibody	Induction agent	ALI/ARDS
Bleomycin	Antibiotic	Lymphoma	IP/H/OP
Busulfan	Alkylating agent	Induction agent	IP/pleural effusion
Carmustine/BCNU	Nitrosourea	Induction agent	IP/fibrosis
Cyclophosphamide	Alkylating agent	Induction/lymphoma	IP/pleuritis
Cytarabine	Substituted nucleoside	AML	Capillary leak
Etoposide	Anti-podophyllotoxin	Induction agent/lymphoma	ALI/ARDS
Fludarabine	Substituted nucleoside	CLL/induction	EP/H
Melphalan	Alkylating agent	Induction agent	IP
Methotrexate	Antimetabolite	Induction/GVHD	H/pleuritis/adenopathy
Sirolimus	mTOR inhibitor	GVHD	IP

Abbreviations: ALI acute lung injury, *EP* eosinophilic pneumonia, *H* hypersensitivity, *IP* interstitial pneumonitis, *OP* organizing pneumonia (ifosfamide, cisplatin, and etoposide) regimen, as a "salvage" regimen for lymphoma, and also as an induction agent [37, 38]. Cytarabine, commonly used to treat acute myeloid leukemia (AML), may cause non-cardiogenic pulmonary edema. This is usually responsive to steroid therapy and is resolved prior to transplant [39]. Dasatinib is a tyrosine kinase inhibitor useful in the treatment of CML. In addition to producing pleural effusions, ground-glass opacities can be seen as well as alveolar septal thickening [40].

HSCT patients receive high-dose chemotherapy as an induction regimen to eliminate marrow cells and prevent rejection of the graft. Following transplantation, immunosuppressive agents to prevent GVHD are prescribed for patients who received allogeneic grafts. Anti-thymocyte globulin is an antibody derived from rabbit or equine serum that can produce interstitial infiltrates and progress to ARDS [41, 42]. The mechanism of lung injury is not clear. As ATG is an anti-leukocyte antibody, the pathogenesis may be similar to that of transfusion-related lung injury (TRALI), or it may stem from its presence as a foreign protein [41, 42]. BCNU may produce DILI within 6 weeks of administration or as late as 20 years after administration to treat pediatric cancers [43, 44]. It presents with diffuse infiltrates and dyspnea, generally without fever, and is irregularly responsive to steroid therapy. The alkylating agents busulfan, melphalan, and cyclophosphamide can all produce a UIP/fibrosing pattern of injury [27]. Busulfan was the first cytotoxic agent described to produce lung injury more than 50 years ago [45]. In one series, the incidence of toxicity was 46% [46]. Today, it is only used as an induction agent for HSCT. Melphalan is well-tolerated at standard doses but given at the high doses used for induction can produce a DIP-like presentation [47]. Cyclophosphamide, used to treat lymphoma and for induction, can produce an early-onset pneumonitis, within 1–6 months of administration, which may be responsive to cessation of the drug or steroid therapy [48]. It can also produce fibrosis and pleural thickening that can chronically progress despite cessation. Rituximab, which is a B-cell-depleting monoclonal antibody, is used to treat lymphomas and rheumatologic ailments. It can be used for induction as well. Symptoms may appear as early as 30 days or as late as 5 months. It rarely causes interstitial lung disease, with only 121 cases reported to date; however, 15% of the cases were fatal [49]. Sirolimus, temsirolimus, and everolimus are mTOR inhibitors used for prevention of GVHD and for treatment of renal and other cancers [50, 51]. The mTOR inhibitors can all cause pneumonitis and are discussed in the subsequent section on solid organ transplantation.

Radiation-Induced Lung Injury

As with DILI, lung injury can be a consequence of radiation administered for control of a tumor prior to transplantation or for radiation administered as part of an induction regimen for HSCT. The symptoms and radiographic findings are a consequence of both radiation injury per se to pulmonary parenchyma and the host immunologic response to the injury. Bilateral lymphocytic alveolitis is seen after radiation is administered to only one lung [52, 53]. Roberts et al. performed bilateral BAL on 17 patients receiving radiation therapy for breast cancer, and bilateral lymphocytic alveolitis was seen even in the 15 asymptomatic patients [52]. This type presentation can be appreciated as part of the natural course of radiation-induced lung injury in the young patient shown in Fig. 21.3. Three months earlier, he had received a hilar "boost" of radiation therapy prior to an HSCT for Hodgkin's disease. Low-grade fevers and increased interstitial markings (Fig. 21.3a, b) evolved over weeks into the dramatic infiltrate seen in Fig. 21.3c. By the time of the final radiograph, fevers had resolved and no steroids were prescribed. In general, radiation lung injury may be treated as a self-limited process, with steroid therapy reserved for patients who are febrile or hypoxic.

Total body irradiation (TBI) administered for induction is associated with acute pulmonary toxicity. Among 101 patients undergoing HSCT with TBI at Duke, one-third developed severe pulmonary toxicity, though the only independent factor correlated with the development of pulmonary toxicity was the number of chemotherapy regimens prior to transplant [54]. Gopal et al. found a similar rate of severe pulmonary toxicity among patients receiving 12 cGy of TBI in 4 once daily fractions (6 of 24 patients, 25%) [55]. There was a lower incidence of severe toxicity among patients treated with 10.2 cGy in 6 twice-daily fractions (7 of 57, 12%); however, the difference was not significant (P-0.19). TBI has also been associated with alveolar hemorrhage in patients undergoing autologous transplantation [23].

Pulmonary Alveolar Proteinosis (PAP)

PAP is a rare complication that may occur within the first 100 days after HSCT [56, 57]. Patients typically present with slowly progressive dyspnea and a non-productive cough. Bilateral diffuse alveolar densities and diffuse ground-glass attenuation with superimposed interlobular septal thickening and intralobular lines in a "crazy-paving" pattern on chest CT are non-specific, but supportive radiographic findings (see Fig. 21.4a). Bronchoscopic examination demonstrates copious, milky BAL effluent, which on cytologic examination contains foamy macrophages engorged with periodic acid-Schiff-positive intracellular inclusions and granular, acellular eosinophilic proteinaceous material (see Fig. 21.4b). Concentrically laminated phospholipid lamellar bodies may be seen on electron microscopy, which is occasionally necessary to confirm the diagnosis. Spontaneous reversal of PAP

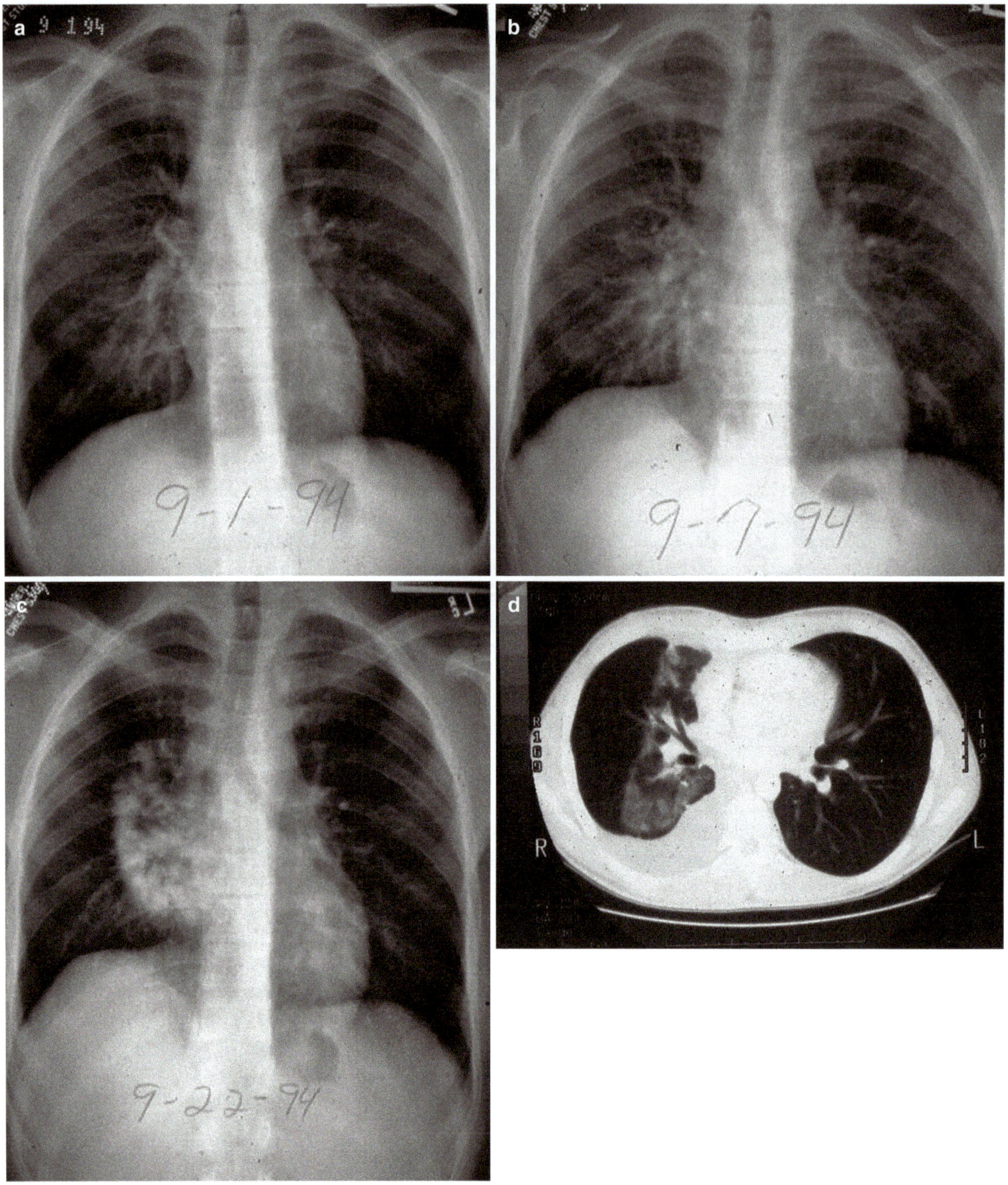

Fig. 21.3 Natural progression of radiation pneumonitis, 3 months after treatment. A young man underwent autologous HSCT for Hodgkin's disease in June of 1994 after receiving a right hilar "boost" to an enlarged lymph node. (**a**) A PA chest radiograph from 09-01-1994 showed increased interstitial markings on the right. (**b**) A PA chest radiograph on 09-07-1994 during a febrile episode attributed to an infected catheter showed an increase in the interstitial infiltrates. (**c**) The pulmonary service was consulted to evaluate this PA chest radiograph on 09-22-1994; however, the patient was asymptomatic. (**d**) A chest CT confirmed the linear border of the infiltrate and revealed an unsuspected small effusion. No treatment was prescribed

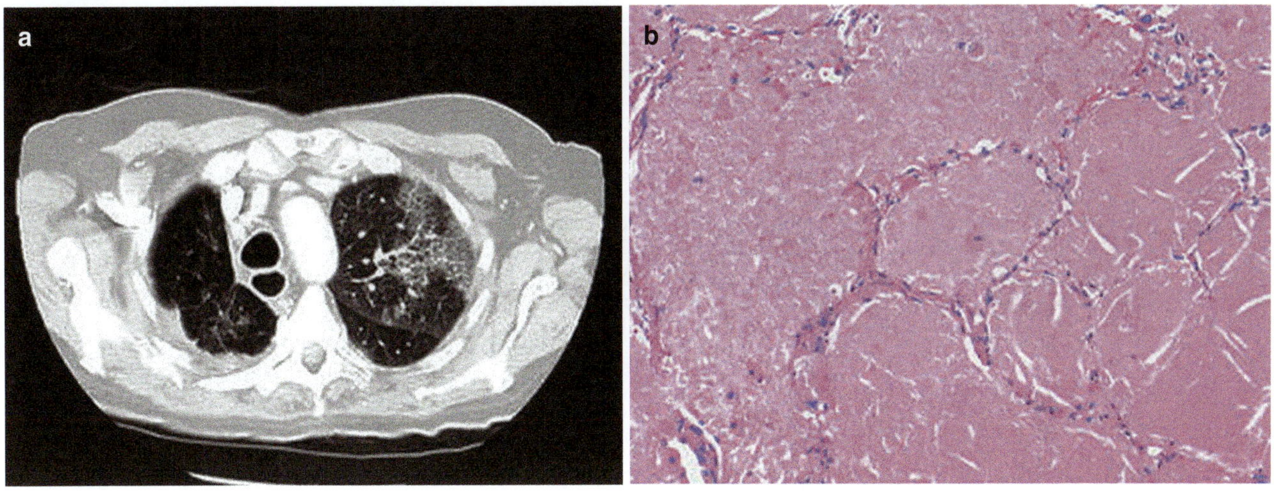

Fig. 21.4 Pulmonary alveolar proteinosis (PAP) in a patient with chronic myeloid leukemia. (**a**) CT chest demonstrates a "crazy-paving" pattern, with a network of smoothly thickened reticular (i.e., septal) lines superimposed on ground-glass opacities. (**b**) Histopathologic findings in PAP include the filling of alveolar spaces with eosinophilic proteinaceous material, which may stain periodic acid-Schiff-positive [8]. (From Kaplan et al. [8], with permission of Springer)

has been described after the resolution of neutropenia or an associated infection. In patients with severe dyspnea and/or significant hypoxemia, whole lung lavage or GM-CSF administered either subcutaneously or via nebulization have been effective in patients with PAP not associated with HSCT [58, 59]. Steroids are not recommended, since they may increase mortality.

Cryptogenic Organizing Pneumonitis (COP)

COP [formerly, Bronchiolitis Obliterans with Organizing Pneumonia (BOOP)] occurs mostly in allogeneic HSCT recipients with GVHD or following CMV pneumonitis [60], with an onset between 1 and 13 months after transplantation. It is less common than post-transplantation constrictive bronchiolitis (PTCB) and should not be confused with it since PTCB is not associated with radiographic infiltrates. Cough and fever are the most common symptoms of COP on presentation; dyspnea, if present, is mild, and, in some cases, patients are asymptomatic [61]. COP usually presents with patchy bilateral alveolar opacities which can be migratory on chest radiograph. The opacities have a lower lobe predominance and are peripheral in location. They may appear as ground-glass opacities or consolidation with air bronchograms on high-resolution CT scans (see Fig. 21.5a). Occasionally, COP can present radiographically as a solitary nodule or mass mimicking a neoplasm or chronic nonresolving pneumonia. In 1 retrospective study of 43 cancer patients, 81% of patients with solid organ tumors had nodular or mass-like radiographic abnormalities, and 19% presented with diffuse infiltrates [62]. In the same study, diffuse infiltrates were seen in the majority of patients with hematologic malignancies, including HSCT, and mimicked infection and drug-induced toxicity.

Pathologically, COP is characterized by the presence of granulation tissue within the lumen of the distal air spaces with or without bronchoalveolar involvement (see Fig. 21.5b). This pathologic picture can be seen with multiple other accompanying diagnoses, such as congestive heart failure, infections, and drug-induced toxicity; hence, in the HSCT recipient, other diagnoses should be excluded before a diagnosis of COP is made. COP is highly responsive to corticosteroids. The minimal effective dose and duration of therapy are unknown; however, a prolonged steroid course with a slow taper is usually necessary due to high relapse rates. Macrolides have been used with success in some cases and might be considered in those individuals who are intolerant to steroid therapy or in whom relapse occurs [63]. Although the specific mechanism of action is not known, macrolides are thought to exert their beneficial effects through anti-inflammatory rather than anti-microbial activities.

Post-transplantation Lymphoproliferative Disorder (PTLD)

PTLD occurs in approximately 1% of HSCT patients, usually within the first 4–12 months after transplantation [1, 64]. The clinical constellation may include fever, lymphadenopathy,

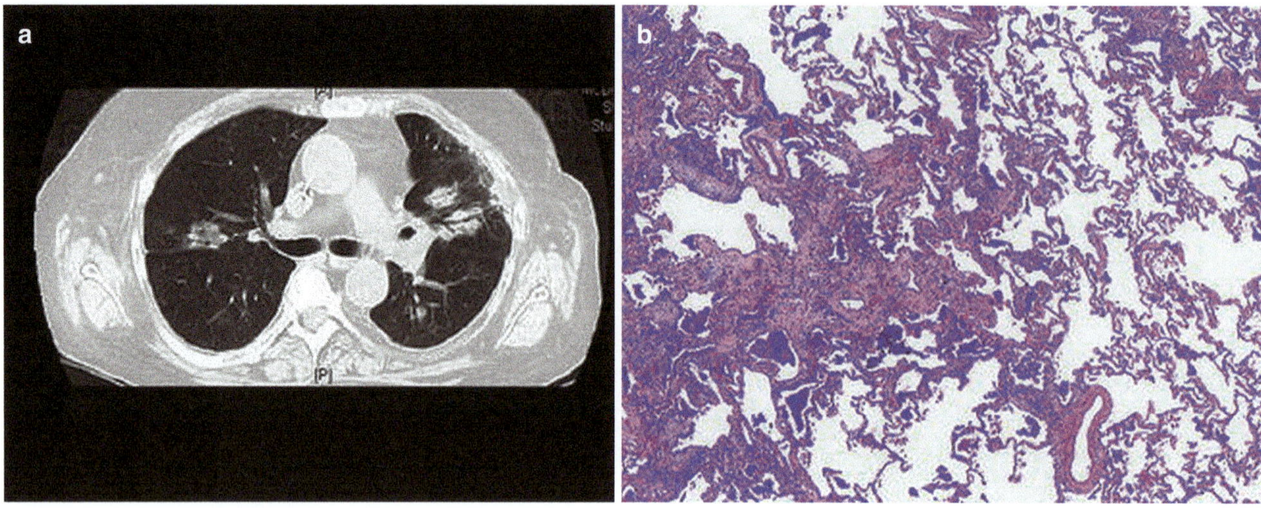

Fig. 21.5 Organizing pneumonia in a patient with a history of chronically waxing and waning pulmonary infiltrates. (**a**) Patchy airspace consolidation with air bronchograms, often in a subpleural location, is a characteristic radiographic presentation for organizing pneumonia. (**b**) On histopathologic examination, granulation tissue can be seen within the lumen of the distal air spaces, swirling into alveoli, associated with chronic inflammation in the surrounding alveoli [8]. (From Kaplan et al. [8], with permission of Springer)

pharyngitis, hepatosplenomegaly, and neurologic symptoms. There appears to be a greater incidence of fulminant, disseminated PTLD in HSCT recipients as compared to solid organ transplant recipients, possibly accounting for the increased mortality associated with PTLD in this population [65]. The lung is involved only 20% of the time, usually as a component of disseminated disease, most commonly with ill-defined nodular infiltrates. It can also present as well-defined nodules, surrounded by a rim of ground-glass density (halo sign), mimicking the features of invasive aspergillosis. Hilar and mediastinal adenopathy and pleural effusions may also be seen. The pathogenesis of PTLD and its treatment are addressed below under Solid Organ Transplantation.

Solid Organ Transplantation

A number of non-infectious pulmonary complications affecting solid organ transplant recipients present with clinical and radiographic features that may mimic infection. These are described in the following sections; complications limited to specific organ recipient populations are noted in the subheadings.

Primary Graft Dysfunction (Lung Transplantation)

Primary graft dysfunction (PGD) represents a form of acute lung injury associated with the development of noncardiogenic pulmonary edema within the first 72 h following lung transplantation [66]. It is presumed to result from ischemia-reperfusion injury to the allograft(s), but inflammatory events triggered by brain death in the donor prior to implantation, as well as surgical trauma and lymphatic disruption, may be contributing factors. In most cases, the process is mild and transient, with fleeting pulmonary infiltrates on chest x-ray. In approximately 10% of cases, however, the presentation and course are similar to the acute respiratory distress syndrome (ARDS) with severe hypoxemia, widespread airspace opacities on chest x-ray, and the need for mechanical ventilator support. In common with ARDS, lung biopsies performed in patients with PGD demonstrate a prevailing pattern of diffuse alveolar damage.

A multitude of factors have been identified as associated with an increased risk of developing PGD, though the causal nature and mechanisms underlying these associations have not been established. Donor-related risk factors include female gender, African-American race, older age, and low donor PaO_2/FiO_2 ratio [67–69]. An elevated level of interleukin-8 in bronchoalveolar lavage fluid recovered from the donor has been associated with the development of severe PGD, supporting the notion that inflammatory events preceding organ harvest may play a role. Recipient risk factors include an underlying diagnosis of idiopathic pulmonary arterial hypertension as well as the presence of elevated pulmonary artery pressures independent of diagnosis. An association between graft ischemic time and PGD has not been consistently demonstrated. A possible explanation for the conflicting data is that ischemic time may become a factor only when it exceeds a certain threshold, suggested by one study as occurring beyond 6 h [70].

PGD should be considered when pulmonary infiltrates appear in the allograft(s) (sparing the native lung in cases of single lung transplantation) within the initial 3 days after lung transplantation. The diagnosis is one of exclusion. Other entities to be considered include volume overload, hyperacute rejection, aspiration pneumonitis, and pulmonary venous outflow obstruction. Pneumonia, transmitted from the donor via the allograft or acquired de novo post-transplantation, is an additional consideration. Evaluation should include assessment of hemodynamics (especially pulmonary capillary wedge pressure if a right heart catheter is in place), bronchoscopy to assess for purulent secretions and to obtain cultures, transesophageal echocardiography to visualize the pulmonary veins, and immunological testing for the presence of donor-specific anti-HLA antibodies.

As with ARDS due to other causes, treatment of severe PGD is supportive. Mechanical ventilation, employing a "low stretch" protocol, is the mainstay of care. Adjunct measures considered when oxygenation is tenuous include use of inhaled nitric oxide or prostacyclin and extracorporeal life support. Results of emergent retransplantation in this setting have been poor [71]. Severe PGD is associated with a mortality rate in the range of 30–40% and represents a leading cause of perioperative death among lung transplant recipients. Recovery among survivors is often protracted, but achievement of normal graft function is possible. Survivors do appear to be at increased risk of developing bronchiolitis obliterans syndrome [72].

Allograft Rejection (Lung Transplantation)

Hyperacute rejection is a rare cause of widespread pulmonary infiltrates in the immediate postoperative period following lung transplantation [73]. This form of rejection is mediated by preformed donor-specific anti-HLA antibodies present in the recipient at the time of transplantation. These antibodies target the pulmonary microvasculature, leading to complement- and neutrophil-mediated damage and widespread deposition of platelet/fibrin thrombi. Hyperacute rejection becomes clinically manifest within minutes to hours of establishing perfusion to the freshly implanted allograft. Intraoperatively, the allograft often appears dusky, mottled, and grossly edematous. Profound hypoxemia, hemodynamic instability, and dense opacification of the allograft(s) on chest x-ray are accompanying features. Four of five patients with this complication reported in the literature died; the one survivor was treated with a combination of plasmapheresis, anti-thymocyte globulin, and cyclophosphamide [74, 75]. Routine screening of all lung transplant candidates for preformed anti-HLA antibodies and either avoidance of donors with the targeted antigens or prospective cross-matching prior to transplantation have proven to be highly effective in minimizing the risk of hyperacute rejection.

Acute cellular rejection is a common alloimmune phenomenon, occurring in up to 75% of lung transplant recipients during the first post-transplant year but diminishing markedly in frequency beyond this time point [76]. It may be clinically and radiographically silent in up to 40% of cases, detected only by surveillance transbronchial lung biopsies. When clinically overt, symptoms include malaise, low-grade fever, dyspnea, and cough. Radiographic features are varied and include consolidation, ground-glass opacities, interstitial opacities, and pleural effusions (Fig. 21.6). A decline in oxygenation and/or spirometry values is often seen. Notably, similar clinical, radiographic, and physiologic features accompany bouts of infection; reliance on these features to make a diagnosis of acute rejection runs the risk of misdiagnosis and needless augmentation of immunosuppression. Rather, transbronchial lung biopsies should be obtained in all suspected cases, unless contraindicated by severe hypoxemia or marginal lung function. The reported sensitivity of transbronchial biopsies in the diagnosis of acute cellular rejection is 61–94% and the specificity exceeds 90% [77]. Diagnosis requires demonstration of perivascular lymphocytic infiltrates that in more severe cases spill over into the adjacent interstitium and alveolar spaces. Lymphocytic bronchiolitis may accompany the parenchymal involvement or may be an independent feature. Standard treatment for acute cellular rejection consists of a 3-day pulse of intravenous methylprednisolone, typically at a dose of 15 mg/kg. In most cases, this leads to clinical and radiographic improvement within several days. Anti-thymocyte globulin is employed in refractory cases.

Antibody-mediated rejection is a more recently recognized but still ill-defined form of acute rejection in lung transplant recipients [78]. In contrast to hyperacute rejection, in which donor-specific anti-HLA alloantibodies are present in the recipient at the time of transplantation, this process is mediated by antibodies that develop de novo after transplantation,

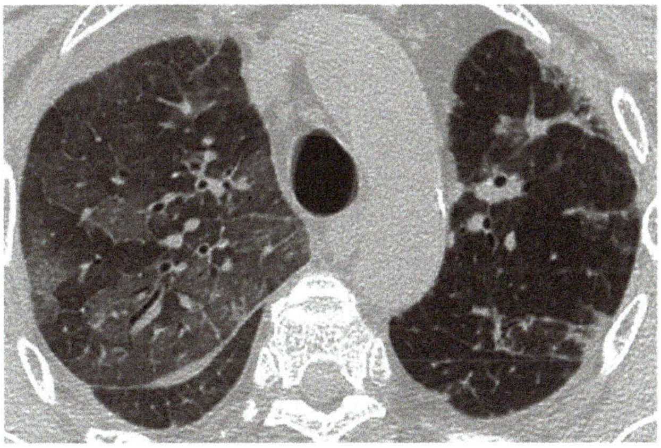

Fig. 21.6 Chest CT demonstrating ground-glass opacities and interlobular septal thickening in the right lung allograft of a single lung transplant recipient. Transbronchial biopsies demonstrated acute cellular rejection

and it is therefore delayed in onset. The clinical presentation can be indistinguishable from acute cellular rejection or infection, with dyspnea, hypoxemia, and diffuse radiographic opacities. Hemoptysis, reflecting the presence of capillaritis, is an important clue but occurs in only 25% of cases [79]. Proposed diagnostic criteria for acute antibody-mediated rejection are (1) presence of circulating donor-specific anti-HLA antibodies, (2) histopathological evidence of capillaritis, and (3) detection of endothelial cell C4d deposition. Treatment with high-dose corticosteroids is effective in less than half of patients; the addition of plasmapheresis is beneficial in the majority of steroid-refractory cases [79]. Intravenous immunoglobulin and anti-CD20 monoclonal antibodies have also been used as adjunctive therapy.

Post-transplantation Lymphoproliferative Disorder (PTLD)

PTLD encompasses a spectrum of abnormal proliferative responses involving B cells in the majority of cases and ranging from benign hyperplasia to frank lymphomas. Epstein-Barr virus is responsible for driving B-cell proliferation in approximately 90% of cases. Proliferation occurs in an unregulated fashion due to absence of the normal cytotoxic T-cell response in the immunosuppressed patient. The proliferating B cells are of recipient origin in most cases. In contrast to B-cell-derived PTLD, the less commonly encountered T-cell neoplasms are predominantly EBV-negative.

The prevalence of PTLD varies considerably among the different solid organ transplant populations. The prevalence is lowest in kidney recipients (1%); intermediate in liver (2–5%), heart (2–5%), and lung (2–8%) transplant recipients; and highest in bowel transplant recipients (up to 30%) [80, 81]. Across all organ types, EBV-naïve recipients who receive organs from EBV-positive donors are at greatest risk for developing PTLD [82]. The net state of immunosuppression and, in particular, the use of anti-lymphocyte antibodies, has also been implicated as a risk factor. A recent study of lung transplant recipients documented a decline in the incidence of PTLD at one large center in recent years; the authors speculate that this may relate to the shift from anti-lymphocyte antibodies to the less immunosuppressive interleukin-2 antagonists for induction [83].

The risk of PTLD is greatest in the first post-transplantation year. The development of this complication may be heralded by constitutional symptoms of fever, malaise, sweats, and weight loss. The particular pattern of organ involvement varies among the different solid organ transplant populations and includes lung, intestine, central nervous system, liver, kidney, and lymph nodes. Intrathoracic involvement occurs in the majority of cases of PTLD in lung and heart-lung transplant recipients. It occurs less commonly in other recipient populations, with reported frequencies of 16–32% in heart transplant recipients, 4.2–24% in liver recipients, and 4.4–15% in kidney recipients [81, 84]. Lung involvement typically manifests as one or multiple nodules or masses (Fig. 21.7). Occasionally, these opacities may have a surrounding halo, mimicking the radiographic appearance of invasive aspergillosis (Fig. 21.8). Airspace consolidation is a less common radiographic

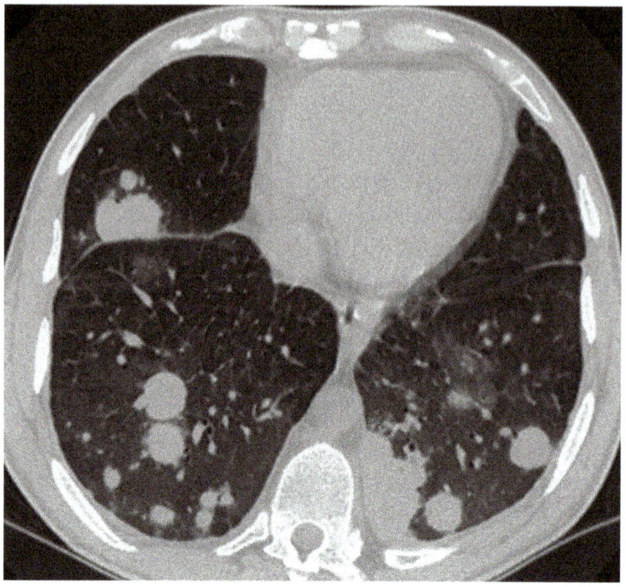

Fig. 21.7 Multiple lung nodules and masses due to PTLD in a bilateral lung transplant recipient

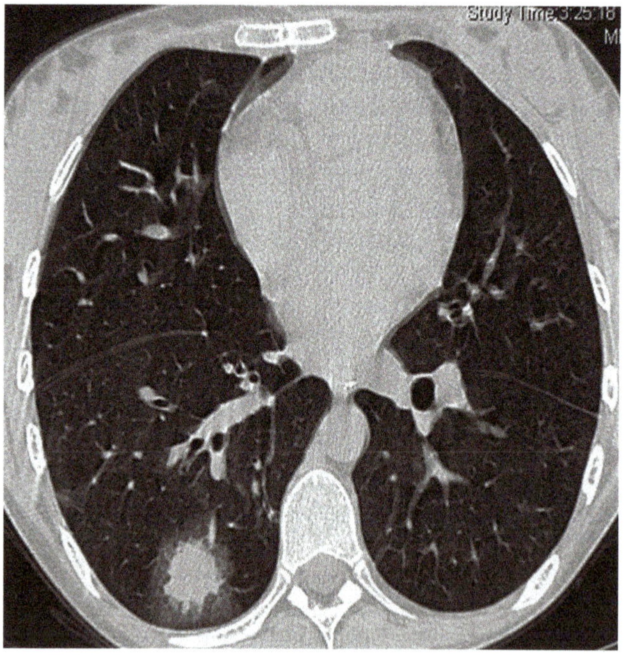

Fig. 21.8 Halo sign (lung nodule with surrounding rim of ground glass) associated with PTLD. This finding is more commonly associated with invasive aspergillosis and invasive lung disease due to other opportunistic mold infections

manifestation, but one that similarly creates diagnostic confusion with infection. Intrathoracic lymphadenopathy may accompany parenchymal abnormalities or may occur in isolation. Pleural effusions are uncommon.

Definitive diagnosis of PTLD requires tissue biopsy; fine needle aspiration rarely yields sufficient material to establish a diagnosis with confidence. Pathological analysis should include flow cytometry to determine clonality, in situ hybridization or immunohistochemical staining to assess for the presence of EBV, and determination of CD-20 expression to assist in planning treatment. Determination of EBV viral load by quantitative polymerase chain reaction assays has been touted as an ancillary diagnostic tool. However, this technique is limited by a lack of consensus on the appropriate specimen source (serum, whole blood, or peripheral mononuclear cells) and by varying threshold value definitions of a positive result. As a consequence of this, performance characteristics of EBV viral load testing in the diagnosis of PTLD vary considerably in the published literature [85, 86].

The initial treatment of PTLD involves reduction in the magnitude of immunosuppression to allow partial reconstitution of host T cellular immunity against EBV. Regression of tumor ensues in up to three-quarters of patients, typically within 2–4 weeks [87]. While often successful, reduction in immunosuppression carries the attendant risk of precipitating acute or chronic allograft rejection, documented in 39% of patients in one series [87]. Factors predictive of failure to respond to reduced immunosuppression include elevated serum lactate dehydrogenase level, severe organ dysfunction (need for hemodialysis, mechanical ventilation, vasopressors (bilirubin >4 mg/dL), and multiple visceral sites of involvement [87].

For patients with CD-20-positive PTLD who fail to respond to reduced immunosuppression alone or have more aggressive tumors, administration of anti-CD20 monoclonal antibodies (rituximab) has emerged as the treatment of choice. This agent is generally well-tolerated and has been associated with remission rates of up to 60% and improved survival [88, 89]. Standard chemotherapy is reserved for patients with CD-20-negative PTLD, for rituximab failures, and for aggressive, life-threatening disease. While effective, chemotherapy is often poorly tolerated and associated with a significant risk of lethal infectious complications [89]. Antiviral therapy is not effective in the treatment of established PTLD, but prophylactic use of antiviral agents for other purposes has been associated with a reduced risk of subsequent development of PTLD.

Lung Cancer (Heart and Lung Transplantation)

The reported incidence of lung cancer is 1.6–4.1% in heart transplant recipients and 2–4% in lung transplant recipients

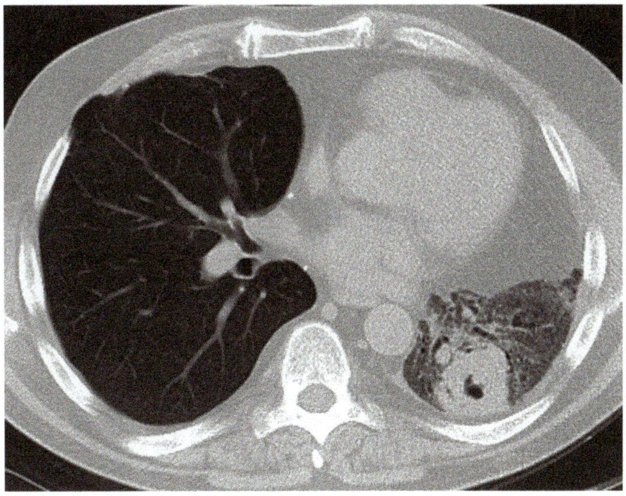

Fig. 21.9 Cavitary squamous cell carcinoma in the fibrotic native lung of a single lung transplant recipient

[90]. These rates are considerably higher than that reported in other solid organ recipient populations and in the general population. It is not clear, however, that these rates truly represent increased risk or simply reflect expected occurrence rates in populations with similar risk factors. Among lung transplant patients, the vast majority of reported cases involve the native lung of single lung transplant recipients with underlying chronic obstructive pulmonary disease or pulmonary fibrosis (Fig. 21.9), the majority of whom were former smokers. In one study that specifically examined the incidence by transplant type, lung cancer developed in 6.9% of single lung transplant recipients compared to none of the bilateral lung recipients [91]. Risk factors other than transplant type that were identified in this study were increasing age and >60 pack-year history of cigarette smoking. Rarely, lung cancer of donor origin has been transmitted to recipients via the allograft. Lung cancer in the transplant recipient often progresses at a rapid pace, potentially leading to initial confusion with an infectious process. Overall prognosis is poor but should not preclude attempts at curative resection in the minority of cases in which early stage disease is encountered.

Sirolimus (mTOR Inhibitor) Pneumonitis

Sirolimus, also known as rapamycin, is used with varying frequency in different solid organ transplant populations as a component of the maintenance immunosuppressive regimen. Since its introduction into clinical practice, there have been numerous reports of interstitial pneumonitis developing in association with sirolimus [92–94]. The incidence of this complication remains poorly defined. Initial reports suggested that interstitial pneumonitis was largely a

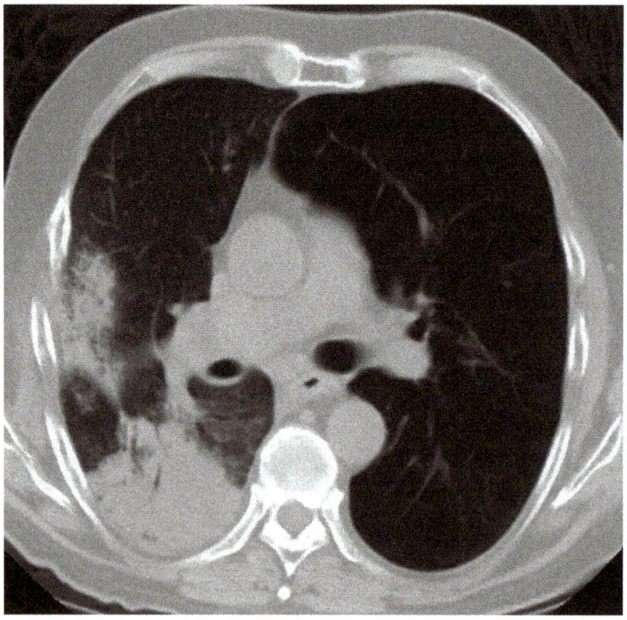

Fig. 21.10 Areas of dense consolidation due to sirolimus pneumonitis in the right lung allograft of a single lung transplant recipient

complication of excessive sirolimus blood concentrations, but more recent reports have documented cases in the setting of therapeutic drug levels. Approximately 50% of cases develop within the first 6 months after initiation of the drug. Onset is usually insidious, but acute and fulminant presentations have been described [95]. Common presenting symptoms include dyspnea, non-productive cough, and fever; hemoptysis is occasionally present. Radiographic abnormalities include bilateral interstitial infiltrates, alveolar consolidation, ground-glass opacities, and nodules (Fig. 21.10). Bronchoalveolar lavage reveals evidence of a lymphocytic alveolitis and, less commonly, of alveolar hemorrhage. Histological findings are diverse and include bronchiolitis obliterans with organizing pneumonia, interstitial lymphocytic infiltrates, alveolar hemorrhage, and non-necrotizing granulomas. Discontinuation of the drug typically leads to prompt clinical improvement while radiographic abnormalities may take several months to fully resolve. In more severe cases, high doses of corticosteroids have been administered, but the true efficacy of these agents remains uncertain.

Conclusion

Multiple common disorders in transplantation patients are associated with radiographic lung infiltrates that can be confused with infectious pneumonia. While pneumonia is a serious complication in transplantation patients, leading to an appropriately high index of suspicion, accurate diagnosis of both infectious and non-infectious etiologies of lung infiltrates is essential to optimal treatment. The identification of non-infectious etiologies of lung infiltrates can usually be made on the basis of clinical findings and imaging studies, but invasive studies are sometimes necessary.

References

1. Kotloff RM, Ahya VN, Crawford SW. Pulmonary complications of solid organ and hematopoietic stem cell transplantation. Am J Respir Crit Care Med. 2004;170(1):22–48.
2. Lim do H, Lee J, Lee HG, Park BB, Peck KR, Oh WS, et al. Pulmonary complications after hematopoietic stem cell transplantation. J Korean Med Sci. 2006;21(3):406–11.
3. Yeh ET, Bickford CL. Cardiovascular complications of cancer therapy: incidence, pathogenesis, diagnosis, and management. J Am Coll Cardiol. 2009;53(24):2231–47.
4. Hunt SA, Abraham WT, Chin MH, Feldman AM, Francis GS, Ganiats TG, et al. 2009 focused update incorporated into the ACC/AHA 2005 guidelines for the diagnosis and management of heart failure in adults: a report of the American College of Cardiology Foundation/American Heart Association Task Force on Practice Guidelines: developed in collaboration with the International Society for Heart and Lung Transplantation. Circulation. 2009;119(14):e391–479.
5. Wilson JF. In the clinic. Heart failure. Ann Intern Med. 2007;147(11):ITC12-1-ITC-6.
6. Ware LB, Matthay MA. Clinical practice. acute pulmonary edema. N Engl J Med. 2005;353(26):2788–96.
7. Maeder MT, Kaye DM. Heart failure with normal left ventricular ejection fraction. J Am Coll Cardiol. 2009;53(11):905–18.
8. Kaplan R, Bashoura L, Shannon VR, Dickey BF, Stover DI. Noninfectious lung infiltrates that may be confused with pneumonia in the cancer patient. In: Safdar A, editor. Principles and practice of cancer infectious disease. New York: Springer; 2011. p. 153–65.
9. Kollef MH, Schuster DP. The acute respiratory distress syndrome. N Engl J Med. 1995;332(1):27–37.
10. Piantadosi CA, Schwartz DA. The acute respiratory distress syndrome. Ann Intern Med. 2004;141(6):460–70.
11. Holness L, Knippen MA, Simmons L, Lachenbruch PA. Fatalities caused by TRALI. Transfus Med Rev. 2004;18(3):184–8.
12. Popovsky MA, Moore SB. Diagnostic and pathogenetic considerations in transfusion-related acute lung injury. Transfusion. 1985;25(6):573–7.
13. Looney MR, Gropper MA, Matthay MA. Transfusion-related acute lung injury: a review. Chest. 2004;126(1):249–58.
14. Spitzer TR. Engraftment syndrome following hematopoietic stem cell transplantation. Bone Marrow Transplant. 2001;27(9):893–8.
15. Capizzi SA, Kumar S, Huneke NE, Gertz MA, Inwards DJ, Litzow MR, et al. Peri-engraftment respiratory distress syndrome during autologous hematopoietic stem cell transplantation. Bone Marrow Transplant. 2001;27(12):1299–303.
16. Clark JG, Hansen JA, Hertz MI, Parkman R, Jensen L, Peavy HH. NHLBI workshop summary. Idiopathic pneumonia syndrome after bone marrow transplantation. Am Rev Respir Dis. 1993;147(6 Pt 1):1601–6.
17. Watkins TR, Chien JW, Crawford SW. Graft versus host-associated pulmonary disease and other idiopathic pulmonary complications after hematopoietic stem cell transplant. Semin Respir Crit Care Med. 2005;26(5):482–9.
18. Yanik G, Hellerstedt B, Custer J, Hutchinson R, Kwon D, Ferrara JL, et al. Etanercept (Enbrel) administration for idiopathic pneumonia syndrome after allogeneic hematopoietic stem cell transplantation. Biol Blood Marrow Transplant. 2002;8(7):395–400.

19. Yanik GA, Ho VT, Levine JE, White ES, Braun T, Antin JH, et al. The impact of soluble tumor necrosis factor receptor etanercept on the treatment of idiopathic pneumonia syndrome after allogeneic hematopoietic stem cell transplantation. Blood. 2008;112(8):3073–81.
20. Tun HW, Wallace KH, Grinton SF, Khoor A, Burger CD. Etanercept therapy for late-onset idiopathic pneumonia syndrome after nonmyeloablative allogeneic hematopoietic stem cell transplantation. Transplant Proc. 2005;37(10):4492–6.
21. Shukla M, Yang S, Milla C, Panoskaltsis-Mortari A, Blazar BR, Haddad IY. Absence of host tumor necrosis factor receptor 1 attenuates manifestations of idiopathic pneumonia syndrome. Am J Physiol Lung Cell Mol Physiol. 2005;288(5):L942–9.
22. Afessa B, Tefferi A, Litzow MR, Krowka MJ, Wylam ME, Peters SG. Diffuse alveolar hemorrhage in hematopoietic stem cell transplant recipients. Am J Respir Crit Care Med. 2002;166(5):641–5.
23. Jules-Elysee K, Stover DE, Yahalom J, White DA, Gulati SC. Pulmonary complications in lymphoma patients treated with high-dose therapy autologous bone marrow transplantation. Am Rev Respir Dis. 1992;146(2):485–91.
24. Majhail NS, Parks K, Defor TE, Weisdorf DJ. Diffuse alveolar hemorrhage and infection-associated alveolar hemorrhage following hematopoietic stem cell transplantation: related and high-risk clinical syndromes. Biol Blood Marrow Transplant. 2006;12(10):1038–46.
25. Lewis ID, DeFor T, Weisdorf DJ. Increasing incidence of diffuse alveolar hemorrhage following allogeneic bone marrow transplantation: cryptic etiology and uncertain therapy. Bone Marrow Transplant. 2000;26(5):539–43.
26. Vahid B, Marik PE. Pulmonary complications of novel antineoplastic agents for solid tumors. Chest. 2008;133(2):528–38.
27. Cooper JA Jr, White DA, Matthay RA. Drug-induced pulmonary disease. Part 1: cytotoxic drugs. Am Rev Respir Dis. 1986;133(2):321–40.
28. Sleijfer S. Bleomycin-induced pneumonitis. Chest. 2001;120(2):617–24.
29. Jules-Elysee K, White DA. Bleomycin-induced pulmonary toxicity. Clin Chest Med. 1990;11(1):1–20.
30. Copper JA Jr. Drug-induced lung disease. Adv Intern Med. 1997;42:231–68.
31. White DA, Orenstein M, Godwin TA, Stover DE. Chemotherapy-associated pulmonary toxic reactions during treatment for breast cancer. Arch Intern Med. 1984;144(5):953–6.
32. White DA, Rankin JA, Stover DE, Gellene RA, Gupta S. Methotrexate pneumonitis. Bronchoalveolar lavage findings suggest an immunologic disorder. Am Rev Respir Dis. 1989;139(1):18–21.
33. Helman DL Jr, Byrd JC, Ales NC, Shorr AF. Fludarabine-related pulmonary toxicity: a distinct clinical entity in chronic lymphoproliferative syndromes. Chest. 2002;122(3):785–90.
34. Trojan A, Meier R, Licht A, Taverna C. Eosinophilic pneumonia after administration of fludarabine for the treatment of non-Hodgkin's lymphoma. Ann Hematol. 2002;81(9):535–7.
35. Siderov J, Prasad P, De Boer R, Desai J. Safe administration of etoposide phosphate after hypersensitivity reaction to intravenous etoposide. Br J Cancer. 2002;86(1):12–3.
36. Gurjal A, An T, Valdivieso M, Kalemkerian GP. Etoposide-induced pulmonary toxicity. Lung Cancer. 1999;26(2):109–12.
37. Moskowitz CH, Bertino JR, Glassman JR, Hedrick EE, Hunte S, Coady-Lyons N, et al. Ifosfamide, carboplatin, and etoposide: a highly effective cytoreduction and peripheral-blood progenitor-cell mobilization regimen for transplant-eligible patients with non-Hodgkin's lymphoma. J Clin Oncol. 1999;17(12):3776–85.
38. Di Ianni M, Ballanti S, Iodice G, Reale A, Falzetti F, Minelli O, et al. High-dose thiotepa, etoposide and carboplatin as conditioning regimen for autologous stem cell transplantation in patients with high-risk Hodgkin's lymphoma. Hematology. 2012;17(1):23–7.
39. Kopterides P, Lignos M, Mentzelopoulos S, Armaganidis A, Pappa V. Cytarabine-induced lung injury: case report. Anticancer Drugs. 2005;16(7):743–5.
40. Bergeron A, Rea D, Levy V, Picard C, Meignin V, Tamburini J, et al. Lung abnormalities after dasatinib treatment for chronic myeloid leukemia: a case series. Am J Respir Crit Care Med. 2007;176(8):814–8.
41. Goligher EC, Cserti-Gazdewich C, Balter M, Gupta V, Brandwein JE. Acute lung injury during antithymocyte globulin therapy for aplastic anemia. Can Respir J. 2009;16(2):e3–5.
42. Sirvent-von Bueltzingsloewen A, Gratecos N, Legros L, Fuzibet JG, Cassuto JP. Antithymocyte-associated reticulonodular pneumonitis during a conditioning regimen of reduced intensity for genoidentical bone marrow transplantation. Bone Marrow Transplant. 2001;27(8):891–2.
43. O'Driscoll BR, Hasleton PS, Taylor PM, Poulter LW, Gattameneni HR, Woodcock AA. Active lung fibrosis up to 17 years after chemotherapy with carmustine (BCNU) in childhood. N Engl J Med. 1990;323(6):378–82.
44. Wilczynski SW, Erasmus JJ, Petros WP, Vredenburgh JJ, Folz RJ. Delayed pulmonary toxicity syndrome following high-dose chemotherapy and bone marrow transplantation for breast cancer. Am J Respir Crit Care Med. 1998;157(2):565–73.
45. Oliner H, Schwartz R, Rubio F, Dameshek W. Interstitial pulmonary fibrosis following busulfan therapy. Am J Med. 1961;31:134–9.
46. Heard BE, Cooke RA. Busulphan lung. Thorax. 1968;23(2):187–93.
47. Akasheh MS, Freytes CO, Vesole DH. Melphalan-associated pulmonary toxicity following high-dose therapy with autologous hematopoietic stem cell transplantation. Bone Marrow Transplant. 2000;26(10):1107–9.
48. Malik SW, Myers JL, DeRemee RA, Specks U. Lung toxicity associated with cyclophosphamide use. Two distinct patterns. Am J Respir Crit Care Med. 1996;154(6 Pt 1):1851–6.
49. Hadjinicolaou AV, Nisar MK, Parfrey H, Chilvers ER, Ostor AJ. Non-infectious pulmonary toxicity of rituximab: a systematic review. Rheumatology (Oxford). 2012;51(4):653–62.
50. White DA, Camus P, Endo M, Escudier B, Calvo E, Akaza H, et al. Noninfectious pneumonitis after everolimus therapy for advanced renal cell carcinoma. Am J Respir Crit Care Med. 2010;182(3):396–403.
51. Johnston L, Florek M, Armstrong R, McCune JS, Arai S, Brown J, et al. Sirolimus and mycophenolate mofetil as GVHD prophylaxis in myeloablative, matched-related donor hematopoietic cell transplantation. Bone Marrow Transplant. 2012;47(4):581–8.
52. Roberts CM, Foulcher E, Zaunders JJ, Bryant DH, Freund J, Cairns D, et al. Radiation pneumonitis: a possible lymphocyte-mediated hypersensitivity reaction. Ann Intern Med. 1993;118(9):696–700.
53. Martin C, Romero S, Sanchez-Paya J, Massuti B, Arriero JM, Hernandez L. Bilateral lymphocytic alveolitis: a common reaction after unilateral thoracic irradiation. Eur Respir J. 1999;13(4):727–32.
54. Wojno KJ, Vogelsang GB, Beschorner WE, Santos GW. Pulmonary hemorrhage as a cause of death in allogeneic bone marrow recipients with severe acute graft-versus-host disease. Transplantation. 1994;57(1):88–92.
55. Gopal R, Ha CS, Tucker SL, Khouri IF, Giralt SA, Gajewski JL, et al. Comparison of two total body irradiation fractionation regimens with respect to acute and late pulmonary toxicity. Cancer. 2001;92(7):1949–58.
56. Cordonnier C, Fleury-Feith J, Escudier E, Atassi K, Bernaudin JF. Secondary alveolar proteinosis is a reversible cause of respiratory failure in leukemic patients. Am J Respir Crit Care Med. 1994;149(3 Pt 1):788–94.

57. Tomonari A, Shirafuji N, Iseki T, Ooi J, Nagayama H, Masunaga A, et al. Acquired pulmonary alveolar proteinosis after umbilical cord blood transplantation for acute myeloid leukemia. Am J Hematol. 2002;70(2):154–7.
58. Beccaria M, Luisetti M, Rodi G, Corsico A, Zoia MC, Colato S, et al. Long-term durable benefit after whole lung lavage in pulmonary alveolar proteinosis. Eur Respir J. 2004;23(4):526–31.
59. Tazawa R, Hamano E, Arai T, Ohta H, Ishimoto O, Uchida K, et al. Granulocyte-macrophage colony-stimulating factor and lung immunity in pulmonary alveolar proteinosis. Am J Respir Crit Care Med. 2005;171(10):1142–9.
60. Afessa B, Litzow MR, Tefferi A. Bronchiolitis obliterans and other late onset non-infectious pulmonary complications in hematopoietic stem cell transplantation. Bone Marrow Transplant. 2001;28(5):425–34.
61. Maldonado F, Daniels CE, Hoffman EA, Yi ES, Ryu JH. Focal organizing pneumonia on surgical lung biopsy: causes, clinicoradiologic features, and outcomes. Chest. 2007;132(5):1579–83.
62. Mokhtari M, Bach PB, Tietjen PA, Stover DE. Bronchiolitis obliterans organizing pneumonia in cancer: a case series. Respir Med. 2002;96(4):280–6.
63. Stover DE, Mangino D. Macrolides: a treatment alternative for bronchiolitis obliterans organizing pneumonia? Chest. 2005;128(5):3611–7.
64. Papadopoulos EB, Ladanyi M, Emanuel D, Mackinnon S, Boulad F, Carabasi MH, et al. Infusions of donor leukocytes to treat Epstein-Barr virus-associated lymphoproliferative disorders after allogeneic bone marrow transplantation. N Engl J Med. 1994;330(17):1185–91.
65. Loren AW, Tsai DE. Post-transplant lymphoproliferative disorder. Clin Chest Med. 2005;26(4):631–45, vii.
66. Christie JD, Bavaria JE, Palevsky HI, Litzky L, Blumenthal NP, Kaiser LR, et al. Primary graft failure following lung transplantation. Chest. 1998;114(1):51–60.
67. Christie JD, Kotloff RM, Pochettino A, Arcasoy SM, Rosengard BR, Landis JR, et al. Clinical risk factors for primary graft failure following lung transplantation. Chest. 2003;124(4):1232–41.
68. Pilcher DV, Snell GI, Scheinkestel CD, Bailey MJ, Williams TJ. High donor age, low donor oxygenation, and high recipient inotrope requirements predict early graft dysfunction in lung transplant recipients. J Heart Lung Transplant. 2005;24(11):1814–20.
69. Whitson BA, Nath DS, Johnson AC, Walker AR, Prekker ME, Radosevich DM, et al. Risk factors for primary graft dysfunction after lung transplantation. J Thorac Cardiovasc Surg. 2006;131(1):73–80.
70. Thabut G, Mal H, Cerrina J, Dartevelle P, Dromer C, Velly JF, et al. Graft ischemic time and outcome of lung transplantation: a multicenter analysis. Am J Respir Crit Care Med. 2005;171(7):786–91.
71. Kawut SM, Lederer DJ, Keshavjee S, Wilt JS, Daly T, D'Ovidio F, et al. Outcomes after lung retransplantation in the modern era. Am J Respir Crit Care Med. 2008;177(1):114–20.
72. Daud SA, Yusen RD, Meyers BF, Chakinala MM, Walter MJ, Aloush AA, et al. Impact of immediate primary lung allograft dysfunction on bronchiolitis obliterans syndrome. Am J Respir Crit Care Med. 2007;175(5):507–13.
73. Choi JK, Kearns J, Palevsky HI, Montone KT, Kaiser LR, Zmijewski CM, et al. Hyperacute rejection of a pulmonary allograft. Immediate clinical and pathologic findings. Am J Respir Crit Care Med. 1999;160(3):1015–8.
74. Bittner HB, Dunitz J, Hertz M, Bolman MR 3rd, Park SJ. Hyperacute rejection in single lung transplantation--case report of successful management by means of plasmapheresis and antithymocyte globulin treatment. Transplantation. 2001;71(5):649–51.
75. Camargo J, Camargo S, Schio SM, Machuca TN, Perin FA. Hyperacute rejection after single lung transplantation: a case report. Transplant Proc. 2008;40:867–9.
76. Hopkins PM, Aboyoun CL, Chhajed PN, Malouf MA, Plit ML, Rainer SP, et al. Prospective analysis of 1,235 transbronchial lung biopsies in lung transplant recipients. J Heart Lung Transplant. 2002;21(10):1062–7.
77. Trulock EP. Lung transplantation. Am J Respir Crit Care Med. 1997;155(3):789–818.
78. Glanville AR. Antibody-mediated rejection in lung transplantation: myth or reality? J Heart Lung Transplant. 2010;29(4):395–400.
79. Astor TL, Weill D, Cool C, Teitelbaum I, Schwarz MI, Zamora MR. Pulmonary capillaritis in lung transplant recipients: treatment and effect on allograft function. J Heart Lung Transplant. 2005;24(12):2091–7.
80. Morgans AK, Reshef R, Tsai DE. Posttransplant lymphoproliferative disorder following kidney transplant. Am J Kidney Dis. 2010;55(1):168–80.
81. Ibrahim HA, Naresh KN. Posttransplant lymphoproliferative disorders. Adv Hematol. 2012;2012:230173.
82. Dharnidharka VR, Lamb KE, Gregg JA, Meier-Kriesche HU. Associations between EBV serostatus and organ transplant type in PTLD risk: an analysis of the SRTR National Registry Data in the United States. Am J Transplant. 2012;12(4):976–83.
83. Kremer BE, Reshef R, Misleh JG, Christie JD, Ahya VN, Blumenthal NP, et al. Post-transplant lymphoproliferative disorder after lung transplantation: a review of 35 cases. J Heart Lung Transplant. 2012;31(3):296–304.
84. Borhani AA, Hosseinzadeh K, Almusa O, Furlan A, Nalesnik M. Imaging of posttransplantation lymphoproliferative disorder after solid organ transplantation. Radiographics. 2009;29(4):981–1000. discussion -2.
85. Allen U, Preiksaitis J, Practice ASTIDCo. Epstein-barr virus and posttransplant lymphoproliferative disorder in solid organ transplant recipients. Am J Transplant. 2009;9(Suppl 4):S87–96.
86. Gulley ML, Tang W. Using Epstein-Barr viral load assays to diagnose, monitor, and prevent posttransplant lymphoproliferative disorder. Clin Microbiol Rev. 2010;23(2):350–66.
87. Tsai DE, Hardy CL, Tomaszewski JE, Kotloff RM, Oltoff KM, Somer BG, et al. Reduction in immunosuppression as initial therapy for posttransplant lymphoproliferative disorder: analysis of prognostic variables and long-term follow-up of 42 adult patients. Transplantation. 2001;71(8):1076–88.
88. Evens AM, David KA, Helenowski I, Nelson B, Kaufman D, Kircher SM, et al. Multicenter analysis of 80 solid organ transplantation recipients with post-transplantation lymphoproliferative disease: outcomes and prognostic factors in the modern era. J Clin Oncol. 2010;28(6):1038–46.
89. Elstrom RL, Andreadis C, Aqui NA, Ahya VN, Bloom RD, Brozena SC, et al. Treatment of PTLD with rituximab or chemotherapy. Am J Transplant. 2006;6(3):569–76.
90. Bellil Y, Edelman MJ. Bronchogenic carcinoma in solid organ transplant recipients. Curr Treat Options Oncol. 2006;7(1):77–81.
91. Dickson RP, Davis RD, Rea JB, Palmer SM. High frequency of bronchogenic carcinoma after single-lung transplantation. J Heart Lung Transplant. 2006;25(11):1297–301.
92. Champion L, Stern M, Israel-Biet D, Mamzer-Bruneel MF, Peraldi MN, Kreis H, et al. Brief communication: sirolimus-associated pneumonitis: 24 cases in renal transplant recipients. Ann Intern Med. 2006;144(7):505–9.
93. Lee HS, Huh KH, Kim YS, Kim MS, Kim HJ, Kim SI, et al. Sirolimus-induced pneumonitis after renal transplantation: a single-center experience. Transplant Proc. 2012;44(1):161–3.
94. Garrean S, Massad MG, Tshibaka M, Hanhan Z, Caines AE, Benedetti E. Sirolimus-associated interstitial pneumonitis in solid organ transplant recipients. Clin Transpl. 2005;19(5):698–703.
95. Chau EM, Chow WH. Sirolimus-induced pneumonitis presenting as acute respiratory distress syndrome. J Heart Lung Transplant. 2006;25(7):867–8.

Skin and Soft Tissue Infection in Transplant Recipients

22

Robert G. Micheletti and Carrie L. Kovarik

Introduction

Transplant patients are vulnerable to a vast array of infectious and noninfectious cutaneous complications related to immunosuppression, chemotherapy and antibiotic exposure, and immunologic interactions between host and donor tissue. The diagnosis and treatment of cutaneous infections are especially challenging due to the vast array of infections—both common and rare—which may occur and the marked variability of appearance, both typical and atypical, with which they may present.

Yet, with this great challenge, comes great opportunity. The skin and mucous membranes form the host's most basic barrier against infection. Visible to the naked eye, their surfaces provide warning of invaders from the outside and, more ominously, dissemination of infections from the inside. Accessible to examination and easily sampled for pathology and culture, the skin can provide a wealth of information on the health of the patient.

In the following chapter, we review common, serious, or otherwise important cutaneous infections and their presentations in the immunocompromised transplant patient. Where possible, we discuss both typical and atypical presentations of these diseases and provide strategies for diagnosis and treatment. In all cases, the clinician must stay alert; maintain appropriate diagnostic suspicion; be aware of relevant history, timing, and systemic symptoms; carry out thorough examinations; and not hesitate to perform appropriate diagnostic studies. Systematic attention to these tenets and the cutaneous exam itself may be lifesaving.

R. G. Micheletti · C. L. Kovarik (✉)
Departments of Medicine and Dermatology, Perelman School of Medicine at the University of Pennsylvania, Philadelphia, PA, USA
e-mail: Robert.micheletti@uphs.upenn.edu; Carrie.kovarik@uphs.upenn.edu

Gram-Positive Bacteria

Staphylococcus

Staphylococci colonize the skin of immunologically intact hosts and are a frequent cause of superficial skin infections. Transplant patients and other immunocompromised patients are no different in this regard. While unusual infections and atypical presentations are seen, common things remain common, and staphylococci often cause skin and soft tissue infections in the transplant population.

Staphylococcal skin colonization is increased in certain populations of patients, including those with pre-existing skin diseases such as atopic dermatitis and cutaneous T-cell lymphoma, as well as those with various types of immunosuppression, such as diabetes, chronic granulomatous disease, hyper IgE syndrome, acquired immunodeficiency syndrome (AIDS), leukopenia, and cancer (particularly hematologic malignancies) [1–3].

Superficial cutaneous staphylococcal infections are common in such patients and increase in incidence with more significant immunodeficiency. Impetigo, with its honey-colored crust, is common in periorificial areas, at sites of injury, or where the normal skin barrier function is otherwise compromised (Fig. 22.1). It may involve weeping skin in a patient with profound lower extremity edema or anasarca, and it can superinfect lesions of herpes simplex or herpes zoster. Patients who develop cutaneous toxicities from chemotherapy or immunotherapy may also develop superinfection of the affected areas. A large number (38%) of those with rash secondary to one of the epidermal growth factor (EGF) receptor inhibitors develop bacterial superinfection of the lesions, most often with *S. aureus* [4].

Folliculitis or furunculosis of hair-bearing areas typically presents with follicular erythematous papules and pustules. It may become quite extensive, causing fever and systemic illness in some patients, but can also be subtle in neutropenic patients whose ability to mount an inflammatory response is

A. Safdar (ed.), *Principles and Practice of Transplant Infectious Diseases*, https://doi.org/10.1007/978-1-4939-9034-4_22

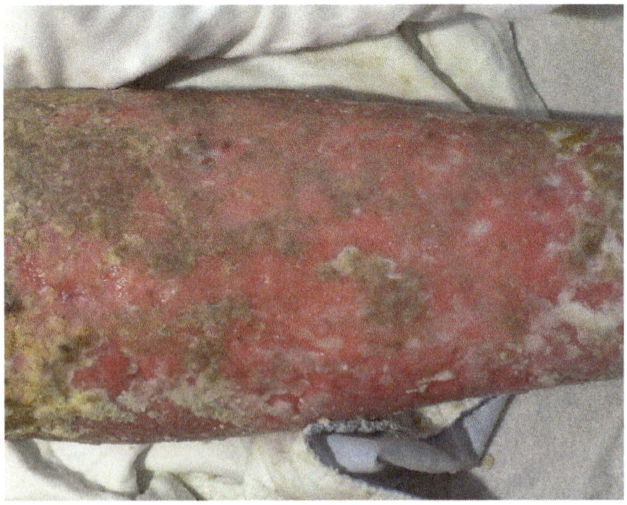

Fig. 22.1 A patient with relapsed cutaneous T-cell lymphoma following stem cell transplantation developed *S. aureus* impetigo superinfection

impaired. Ecthyma typically presents as a shallow ulceration and is most commonly due to staphylococcal or streptococcal species.

Cellulitis in transplant patients generally presents as it does in the general population, with swelling, warmth, and erythema. Special attention to the skin around indwelling lines, which may be covered from view by tape or bulky dressings, is essential to avoid a delay in diagnosis. Irritation or allergy to adhesives or topical cleansers, such as chlorhexidine, may cause some irritation which can be mistaken for cellulitis; clues to a contact dermatitis include linear, geometric, or sharply defined shape, itching, and weeping or scaling of the skin. It is also important to note that atypical presentations of fungal, viral, or other bacterial infections may mimic Gram-positive cellulitis. A high index of suspicion for atypical infections is especially appropriate in cases which do not respond to antibiotic therapy for the usual staphylococcal or streptococcal species.

Staphylococcal scalded skin syndrome (SSSS) is characterized by toxin-mediated generalized erythema and superficial exfoliation caused by local cutaneous infection with *S. aureus* type 71, phage group 2. This bacterium elutes exfoliating toxins A and B, which circulate and cleave the desmosomal protein desmoglein 1 in the superficial epidermis, resulting in widespread peeling. This syndrome is most commonly observed in young children, in whom the prognosis is quite good. Risk factors for adult infection include impaired renal function, which decreases clearance of the toxin, as well as immunosuppression due to systemic steroids, malignancy, or organ transplantation [5]. In adults with these comorbid diseases, the incidence of positive blood cultures and the mortality rate are increased [6].

Unusual presentations of *S. aureus* infection in immunosuppressed patients include blastomycosis-like verrucous plaques with multiple pustules, violaceous plaque-like lesions of folliculitis, monomorphic vesicles or bullae, and chronic suppurative infections with bacterial granules (botryomycosis) [3]. Blistering distal dactylitis, characterized by tender, tense bullae on the fingertips, may also be caused by staphylococcal species [7].

Streptococcus

Like *Staphylococcus*, cutaneous streptococcal infections are quite common. Streptococcal species are responsible for the majority of cellulitis and erysipelas and also cause impetigo and ecthyma.

In immunocompromised patients, all of these more typical manifestations may be seen, but streptococcal infections may be unusually extensive or may appear clinically atypical. *Streptococcus pyogenes* (group A β-hemolytic strep) may cause extensive ecthyma or facial erysipelas that can result in bacteremia [8, 9]. *Streptococcus agalactiae* (group B strep) most commonly causes invasive infection in pregnant women and neonates but is also increased in immunocompromised patients [10]. In addition to erysipelas, cellulitis, and ecthyma, group B strep can cause myositis, necrotizing fasciitis, and toxic shock syndrome, as well as an acute cellulitis-adenitis condition with rapidly enlarging lymph nodes and fever [11].

Streptococcus pneumoniae uncommonly causes skin or soft tissue infection but may result in a facial and neck cellulitis in patients with hematologic malignancies [12]. Pneumococcal cellulitis commonly appears brown or dusky with bulla formation [13]. Necrotizing fasciitis and purpura fulminans/disseminated intravascular coagulation (DIC) are rare but deadly complications of *S. pneumoniae* infection. Transplant patients are at increased risk of such complications as are others who are immunosuppressed, particularly those with functional or anatomical asplenism.

Clostridium

Clostridial myonecrosis (gas gangrene) may be posttraumatic or spontaneous. Underlying immunosuppression, such as that caused by hematologic malignancy or neutrophil dysfunction, increases the risk of spontaneous infection. *Clostridium perfringens* (60%) and *Clostridium septicum* (30%) are the most common isolates from these infections [14], resulting in a 32% and 79% mortality, respectively [15].

Clostridial myonecrosis is characterized by a relatively sudden onset of severe pain in the involved site, rapid extension of infection, and systemic toxicity. The skin may appear pallid or mottled, then a dusky brownish purple. Finally, tense hemorrhagic bullae develop, signaling necrosis of the involved tissue. Crepitus may be detected clinically or on radiographic imaging.

Underlying muscle and soft tissue involvement may be quite extensive, far exceeding what is visible on the skin surface. Rapid progression, sepsis, and death can occur within 1–2 days. Timely diagnosis is essential. Gram staining of the serosanguineous fluid found in the hemorrhagic bullae shows numerous Gram-positive rods. Computed tomography (CT) or other radiographic imaging may help define the extent of infection [15], but surgical debridement and treatment with intravenous antibiotics (high-dose penicillin is the treatment of choice) should not be delayed for imaging studies. Granulocyte colony-stimulating factor (G-CSF) should be considered as adjunctive therapy in neutropenic patients.

Bacillus

Bacillus cereus is best known as a cause of mild food poisoning, but it can also cause life-threatening infection in immunocompromised patients, particularly those with neutropenia following chemotherapy or stem cell transplantation. A single painful vesicle, pustule, or bulla may appear on a digit or extremity at a site of inoculation, followed by necrosis and ulcer or eschar formation, rapidly spreading cellulitis, and high fever [16]. This presentation may mimic that of clostridial myonecrosis, complete with large Gram-positive rods on Gram stain. However, unlike *Clostridium*, *B. cereus* is generally resistant to many beta-lactam antibiotics including most cephalosporins. Vancomycin, aminoglycosides, and carbapenems are acceptable alternatives. Severe infection, with necrotizing fasciitis, endocarditis, and brain abscesses, in immunosuppressed patients has been reported and is frequently fatal [17, 18].

Corynebacterium

Aside from *C. diphtheriae*, corynebacteria are part of the normal skin flora, rarely cause infection, and are susceptible to most antibiotics. *C. jeikeium* most commonly colonizes the perineal, rectal, inguinal, and axillary areas of adult men and postmenopausal women, likely related to increased sebum production, which promotes the growth of lipophilic organisms [19]. Risk factors for colonization are the same as for infection and include indwelling intravenous catheters, neutropenia, prolonged hospitalization, and previous treatment with broad-spectrum antibiotics [20].

Primary cutaneous *C. jeikeium* infection occurs at breaks in the skin barrier due to trauma or nosocomial inoculation, most commonly presenting as a cellulitis. The organism may then enter the bloodstream, leading to septicemia [21]. Secondary skin infection results from hematogenous spread. It may present with nontender subcutaneous nodules, erythematous macules or papules, or nonblanching red papules or pustules with secondary necrosis. *C. jeikeium* is most aggressive in those with hematologic malignancies undergoing chemotherapy or status post stem cell transplantation. This group is most likely to develop *C. jeikeium* sepsis and more commonly develops cutaneous manifestations of the disease. Forty-eight percent of such patients develop skin lesions due to hematogenous spread, making the skin the second most common infected organ [22].

Vancomycin is the agent of choice for the treatment of *C. jeikeium* and should be continued until hematologic recovery. The mortality of *C. jeikeium* sepsis approaches 34% in those with hematologic malignancies but drops to 5% in those with bone marrow recovery [22].

Nocardia

Nocardia is a branching, filamentous aerobic bacteria found in soil and decaying plant matter. It is not part of the normal human flora, so positive cultures should be evaluated carefully [23]. *N. asteroides* is the most common member of the genus to cause human infection. It involves the lungs most frequently, followed by the skin, and the central nervous system (CNS).

Immunocompromised states predispose to nocardial infection. Those with a history of hematologic malignancy, organ transplantation, iatrogenic immunosuppressive therapy, and advanced HIV disease (CD4 < 100) are at greatest risk. *Nocardia* infection is more common following solid organ transplantation than hematopoietic stem cell transplantation. Independent risk factors include high-dose steroid therapy, prior cytomegalovirus infection, and high serum levels of calcineurin inhibitor in the month prior to infection [24].

Cutaneous nocardiosis may be due to primary inoculation or secondary to dissemination. Primary lesions may present with swelling, induration, and purulence of a mycetoma; the beefy red nodules of lymphocutaneous or "sporotrichoid" infection spreading along lymphatics from the site of inoculation; or with the erythema, fluctuance, or ulceration of a more superficial cellulitis, abscess, or crusted nodule (Fig. 22.2) [25–27].

Secondary cutaneous lesions due to hematogenous spread may be indistinguishable from the type of abscesses, nodules, or ulcers seen in primary disease. Therefore, all patients presenting with cutaneous nocardiosis should be screened for systemic involvement with imaging of the lungs and CNS. Cutaneous lesions may be the only sign of otherwise asymptomatic disseminated infection [28]. Dissemination from a primary skin lesion to other organs is rare, but late dissemination from the lungs to the skin or CNS can occur in immunosuppressed patients despite appropriate therapy for pulmonary nocardiosis.

Cutaneous nocardiosis may take on other more atypical forms in immunosuppressed patients. Among the less common presentations described in transplant patients are warm

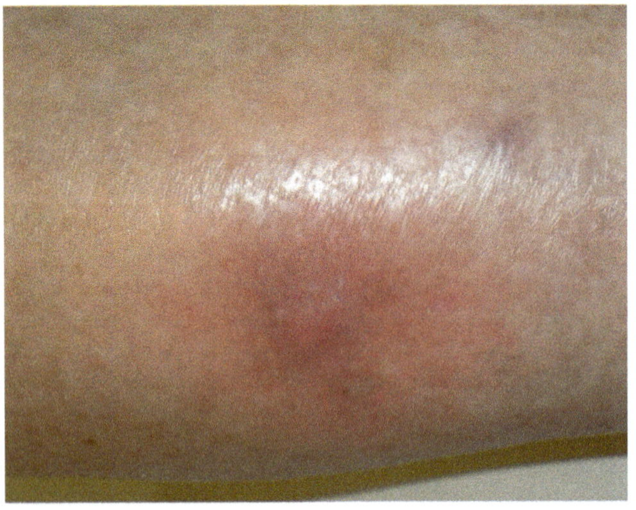

Fig. 22.2 A patient with AML status post stem cell transplantation developed several tender, red, subcutaneous nodules on the legs. Tissue culture grew *Nocardia*

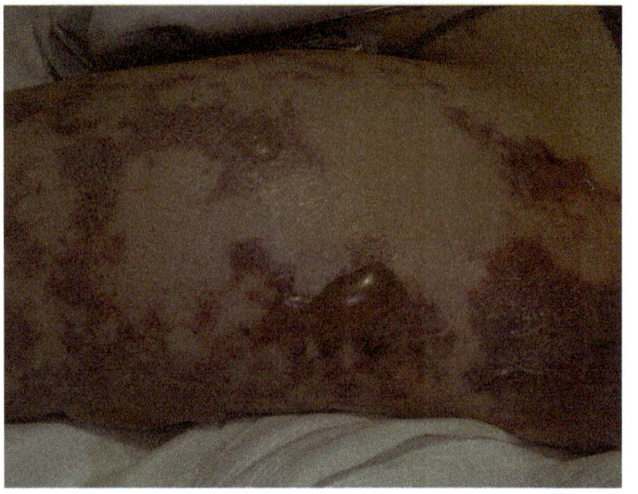

Fig. 22.3 Purpura fulminans and tense bullae in a patient with *E. coli* septicemia. (Image courtesy of Katherine Evans, MD)

and cold subcutaneous nodules [29, 30], pustules, and pyomyositis [31]. Cases of disseminated infection are usually due to *N. asteroides*, but in the organ transplant recipient, *N. nova* is the most frequent cause of disseminated disease.

Cutaneous *Nocardia* can present a diagnostic challenge because lesions may resemble pyogenic bacterial infections. Empiric treatment without culture and failure of the organism to grow in culture before it is thrown away are factors which contribute to treatment failure. *Nocardia* are Gram-positive and variably acid-fast. They are not seen on routine hematoxylin and eosin-stained sections. Gomori methenamine silver (GMS) and Brown-Brenn stains are needed to diagnose the infection histologically. The microbiology laboratory should be alerted if the clinician suspects *Nocardia* so that cultures can be saved for 4 weeks or longer.

A history of inoculation injury, occupational exposure to decaying plant matter, worsening or recurrence of infection despite standard antibiotics, and chronic suppurative infection with negative cultures suggest the possibility of *Nocardia* infection [32]. The coexistence of lung nodules and skin lesions raises the possibility of that diagnosis in an immunocompromised host, as do pleural or pericardial infections [28].

Trimethoprim-sulfamethoxazole is an effective treatment for most *Nocardia*, but *N. farcinica* may be highly resistant to antibiotics.

Gram-Negative Bacteria

Escherichia Coli

Escherichia coli is a Gram-negative aerobic rod which is part of the normal gastrointestinal flora. Cutaneous infection may produce abscesses at sites of inoculation or contaminated surgical wounds. Perirectal phlegmon is seen in neutropenic patients. *E. coli* cellulitis is rare but is more commonly seen in those with neutropenia, corticosteroid treatment, renal or hepatic insufficiency, chronic alcohol use, and diabetes mellitus. Gram-negative cellulitis can be indistinguishable from streptococcal cellulitis, with pain, redness, and fever, though in immunocompromised patients it is frequently described as rapidly progressive. Among transplant patients, hepatic transplant may be a particular risk factor. Spontaneous Gram-negative cellulitis has been well-described in cirrhotic patients due to hypoalbuminemia, edema, and immunosuppression. One reported patient developed spontaneous *E. coli* cellulitis with numerous bullae 8 days after liver transplant for hepatitis C cirrhosis [33].

Ecthyma gangrenosum, classically associated with *Pseudomonas aeruginosa* bacteremia, has been described with many other Gram-negative organisms including *E. coli* [34, 35]. Ecthyma gangrenosum most commonly appears in the gluteal or perineal region (57%) and less frequently on the extremities (30%). For this reason, a thorough skin exam is an indispensable part of the workup of the febrile neutropenic or otherwise immunocompromised patient. Timely diagnosis and treatment are essential; the mortality rate of ecthyma gangrenosum is 10–38% [36].

E. coli septicemia may present with tense serous or hemorrhagic bullae, either on otherwise normal-appearing skin or overlying a cellulitis (Fig. 22.3). These bullae have a predilection for acral sites. Cultures of the bullae, and often of the blood or urine, grow *E. coli* [37, 38].

Malakoplakia is a rare granulomatous skin disease which results from defective killing of bacteria by macrophages. It is most common in immunocompromised patients, particularly those status post renal transplantation. Cutaneous lesions are typically perianal abscesses, nodules, ulcers, or draining sinuses which may be due to *E. coli, Klebsiella, Enterobacter, S. aureus, Streptococcus,* and *Enterococcus* species [39, 40]. Biopsy reveals large macrophages with intracytoplasmic granules known as Michaelis-Gutmann bodies.

Klebsiella, Enterobacter, and *Serratia*

Klebsiella pneumoniae, Enterobacter cloacae, and *Serratia marcescens* are closely related aerobic Gram-negative bacilli that may colonize the gastrointestinal, respiratory, or urinary tracts and are common causes of opportunistic nosocomial infection in debilitated or immunocompromised patients. Like *E. coli,* cutaneous infection with these organisms can cause cellulitis which may progress rapidly to systemic toxicity, hemorrhagic bullae, and necrosis [41]. Cutaneous ulceration, ecthyma gangrenosum, nonclostridial crepitant cellulitis, and necrotizing fasciitis can also occur [42–46]. Like other Gram-negative rods, septicemia with these organisms can cause acral hemorrhagic bullae (Fig. 22.4) [47].

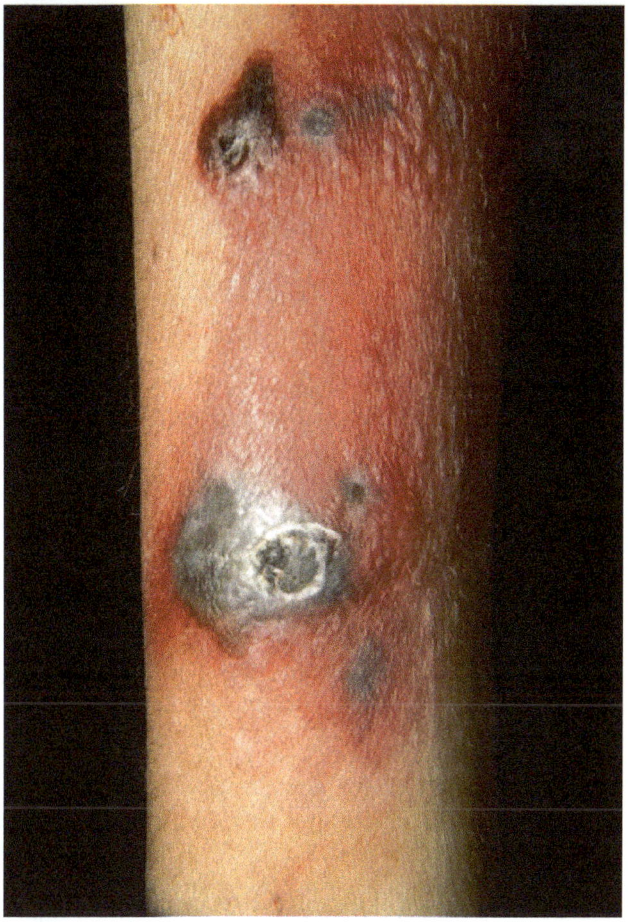

Fig. 22.4 Hemorrhagic necrotic bullae on the forearm. Blood and wound cultures grew *K. pneumoniae.* (Image reprinted from Grossman et al. [284], Fig. 13.21, p. 261, with kind permission from Springer Nature)

Salmonella

Nontyphoidal *Salmonella* species may rarely cause subcutaneous abscesses, hemorrhagic cellulitis, or necrotizing fasciitis in immunocompromised hosts. One woman developed necrotizing fasciitis due to *Salmonella* while on high-dose immunosuppression status post peripheral blood stem cell transplantation for multiple myeloma [48]. *Salmonella* bacteremia in the absence of gastrointestinal infection is a marker of immunosuppression and portends a poor prognosis [49].

Legionella

Legionella is best known as a pulmonary pathogen in immunocompromised patients but may also rarely be a cause of cellulitis and soft tissue infection in those with dysfunctional immune systems. *Legionella* could be considered in the differential diagnosis for cellulitis, which is refractory to conventional antibiotics for skin and soft tissue infections or relapses after therapy. Gram stain and culture of any purulent material may demonstrate neutrophils but no organisms. *Legionella* skin infection, when present, typically occurs without concurrent *Legionella* pneumonia.

Cellulitis caused by *Legionella* is rapidly spreading and necrotizing. Debridement or amputation may be necessary [50]. Relapse of infection in immunocompromised patients can occur even after prolonged therapy with antimicrobials which should ordinarily be curative.

Morganella

Morganella morganii is a Gram-negative rod found in soil, water, and human fecal flora. *Morganella* infection is unusual, but hematologic malignancy, neutropenia, chemotherapy, and systemic steroids, among other things, increase the risk [51]. In reported cases, cellulitis with hemorrhagic bullae is described most often. Gas gangrene with tissue crepitus may occur secondary to fermentation of glucose with production of gas by *Morganella.* As with other Gram-negative organisms, *Morganella* may also present as ecthyma gangrenosum [52].

Helicobacter

Helicobacter cinaedi is a fastidious Gram-negative bacillus which is an unusual pathogen usually affecting only severely immunocompromised patients. Clinical symptoms include fever, rash, arthritis, and leg pain [53]. Common cutaneous manifestations of *H. cinaedi* bacteremia are large, multifocal cellulitic plaques on the extremities with large joint arthritis adjacent to areas of cellulitis [54]. Lesions resembling superficial thrombophlebitis may also occur [55]. By nature, *H. cinaedi* bacteremia is a relapsing condition with recurrent bouts of multifocal cellulitis, which requires prolonged or repeated courses of antibiotics. Growth of the organism in culture can be difficult.

Citrobacter

Citrobacter freundii and *C. koseri* comprise the majority of *Citrobacter* infections, with increased incidence in immunosuppressed patients. Typical cellulitis and "bilateral inflammatory erysipelas" on the legs have been described in patients following organ transplantation or receiving treatment for hematologic malignancy. *Citrobacter* is another bacterium which may cause ecthyma gangrenosum-like ulcers or hemorrhagic bullae [34, 56, 57].

Pseudomonas

P. aeruginosa is a common nosocomial pathogen encountered in patients' immunosuppressed due to organ transplantation or other causes. Dermatologic manifestations of *Pseudomonas* bacteremia include hemorrhagic bullae, gangrenous or bullous cellulitis, and ecthyma gangrenosum, which presents with erythematous or purpuric macules that progress rapidly to become violaceous or "gun metal" gray necrotic plaques or bullae with a red halo [58]. These lesions have a predilection for the anogenital area so may not be readily visible. Pathologically, the violaceous color and necrosis that occur in this condition signal compromise of the underlying cutaneous blood vessels due to invading bacteria.

Though ecthyma gangrenosum is classically due to pseudomonal bacteremia, it has been described in association with many other Gram-negative bacterial, fungal, and viral infections in immunocompromised patients. Furthermore, ecthyma gangrenosum can occur in the absence of bacteremia as a primary and localized infection due to inoculation injury, in which case the prognosis is better [59].

Pseudomonas also causes a necrotizing cellulitis in neutropenic patients which progresses from tense, tender erythema to purpuric, cyanotic, bullous, and ultimately black, necrotic tissue associated with systemic toxicity. The course of this entity is often fulminant and fatal; surgical debridement can be lifesaving but is often performed too late [60, 61].

Subcutaneous nodules and hemorrhagic bullae are other manifestations of *Pseudomonas* bacteremia, which may be solitary or distributed widely over the skin. Some nodules resolve with appropriate antibiotic therapy, but surgical drainage is indicated when nodules or signs of systemic toxicity persist despite antibiotics [62, 63].

Stenotrophomonas

A denizen of moist environs like *Pseudomonas*, and formally a member of that genus, *Stenotrophomonas maltophilia* is an exceedingly resistant nosocomial Gram-negative rod with high mortality rates in immunocompromised patients. Malignancy, neutropenia, chemotherapy, radiation, graft-versus-host disease, antibiotic exposure, central venous catheter, and prolonged hospitalization are risk factors for *Stenotrophomonas* infection [64].

Typical cellulitis, necrotizing cellulitis, ecthyma gangrenosum, metastatic nodules, and multifocal cellulitic plaques are all cutaneous manifestations [65]. These lesions typically manifest with red or violaceous erythema and tenderness and often eventuate in necrosis and ulceration [66–68].

Aeromonas

Aeromonas is another water-loving Gram-negative rod which can cause nosocomial infection in immunosuppressed patients. A rapidly progressive cellulitis can follow trauma with freshwater exposure. Suppuration and necrosis can occur, necessitating debridement of necrotic tissue. Severe infections such as fasciitis, myonecrosis, and ecthyma gangrenosum can result. Septicemia in immunocompromised patients can result in multiple hemorrhagic bullae, followed by extensive necrotizing fasciitis and septic shock [69, 70].

Vibrio

Vibrio vulnificus is the most common member of this genus causing opportunistic wound infection or septicemia in immunocompromised patients. Though classically associated with cirrhosis and chronic iron overload, hematologic malignancy, organ transplantation, and the use of immunosuppressive medications are also risk factors for infection [71, 72]. Infection can occur via primary inoculation injury in a marine environment or through dissemination from the gastrointestinal tract following consumption of raw or inadequately cooked seafood.

Local infection can progress rapidly from edema and cellulitis to hemorrhagic bullae with fever, chills, hypotension, and necrotizing fasciitis. *Vibrio* bacteremia is characterized by fever, chills, hypotension, and shock with rapidly progressive erythematous or ecchymotic plaques and large hemorrhagic bullae on the extremities or trunk. Necrotic ulcers may result in fasciitis and gangrene. Such infections can be rapidly fatal with a mortality >50%. Early diagnosis and aggressive treatment, including surgical debridement, if warranted, are paramount [73–76].

Bartonella

Bartonella species are responsible for cat scratch disease, Oroya fever/verruga peruana, and trench fever as well as bacillary angiomatosis. Though most commonly seen in AIDS patients with CD4 count <100 cells/mm^3, bacillary angiomatosis due to *B. henselae* and *B. quintana* also occurs in patients immunocompromised for other reasons, including solid organ and bone marrow transplant recipients [77], as well as those undergoing chemotherapy for hematologic malignancy. Bacillary angiomatosis typically manifests with nonspecific constitutional symptoms. It can affect multiple organs including the liver, lymphoreticular system, brain, bone marrow, conjunctiva, gastrointestinal, respiratory, oral mucosae, and the skin. Of these, skin lesions are the most common clinical manifestation [78, 79]. Characteristically, single or multiple asymptomatic, firm, red-purple papules are found on the skin. These lesions may be innumerable and disseminated over the entire body surface. They may appear smooth, pedunculated, or verrucous. They resemble pyogenic granuloma and Kaposi sarcoma but do not ulcerate or bleed. Less commonly, bacillary angiomatosis may also present with flesh-colored, subcutaneous nodules. Erythromycin is the therapy of choice.

Mycobacteria

Mycobacterium tuberculosis

M. tuberculosis infection of the skin can occur via inoculation injury, contiguous spread from other infected sites, or hematogenous dissemination. Cutaneous manifestations are on a spectrum from primary cutaneous tuberculosis (tuberculous chancre) to tuberculosis verrucosa cutis, tuberculosis cutis orificialis, scrofuloderma, lupus vulgaris, and miliary cutaneous tuberculosis. Further immunologically driven manifestations include the tuberculids erythema induratum, papulonecrotic tuberculid, lichen scrofulosorum, and nodular tuberculid [80].

Tuberculosis is a serious cause of opportunistic infection among solid organ transplant recipients. It may occur through primary infection or reactivation of latent disease, or it may be acquired through the transplanted organ. Acute miliary tuberculosis can present with a widespread eruption of erythematous or brown macules and papules which evolve into vesiculopustules and can become crusted or necrotic [81]. Signs of systemic infection, including fever, cough, and generalized wasting, may be present. Other reported manifestations of disseminated tuberculosis in immunosuppressed transplant patients include subcutaneous nodules, erythema and edema mimicking cellulitis, and multiple ulcerating nodules [82–84]. Biopsy of such lesions is generally floridly positive with caseating granulomas and numerous acid-fast bacilli.

Nontuberculous Mycobacteria

Nontuberculous or atypical mycobacteria are ubiquitous in the environment [85]. Presentations of cutaneous disease vary markedly between immunocompetent and immunoincompetent patients. In those with normal immune systems, inoculation injury may lead in several weeks to a verrucous nodule or abscess, usually on an extremity, followed in some cases by "sporotrichoid" spread up the regional lymphatics as is seen in the "fish tank" granuloma of *Mycobacterium marinum*. In immunosuppressed patients, a history of trauma may or may not be elicited. Infection may more often lead to multiple localized violaceous subcutaneous nodules with sporotrichoid spread [86, 87] or to widespread disease in the form of nodules, sinus tracts, ulcers, abscesses, or cellulitis (Fig. 22.5) [86, 88–90].

The most common presentations of atypical mycobacterial infection in solid organ transplant patients are cutaneous lesions on the extremities, tenosynovitis, and arthritis, often with skin lesions overlying affected joints [91, 92]. Chronic indwelling central venous catheters are a common cause of atypical mycobacterial infection in solid organ or bone marrow transplant patients [93]. Diagnosis can be difficult since many of these organisms are difficult to grow in culture and hard to demonstrate on histologic sections. Notifying the microbiology lab of suspected pathogens will alert them to use proper plating media and incubate at the correct temperatures. Polymerase chain reaction (PCR) can be performed to aid in diagnosis when suspicion is high. Speciation is essential to guide therapy, as susceptibility profiles differ among the organisms in question.

Viruses

Herpes Simplex

Herpes simplex virus (HSV) infection is exceedingly common among both immunocompetent and immunocompromised hosts. In normal hosts, primary and secondary, or recurrent, infections are self-limited. Typically, 1–2 mm pruritic or painful vesicles arise in the orolabial or anogenital areas, progress to crusted erosions, and resolve over the course of several days. In immunocompromised hosts, HSV

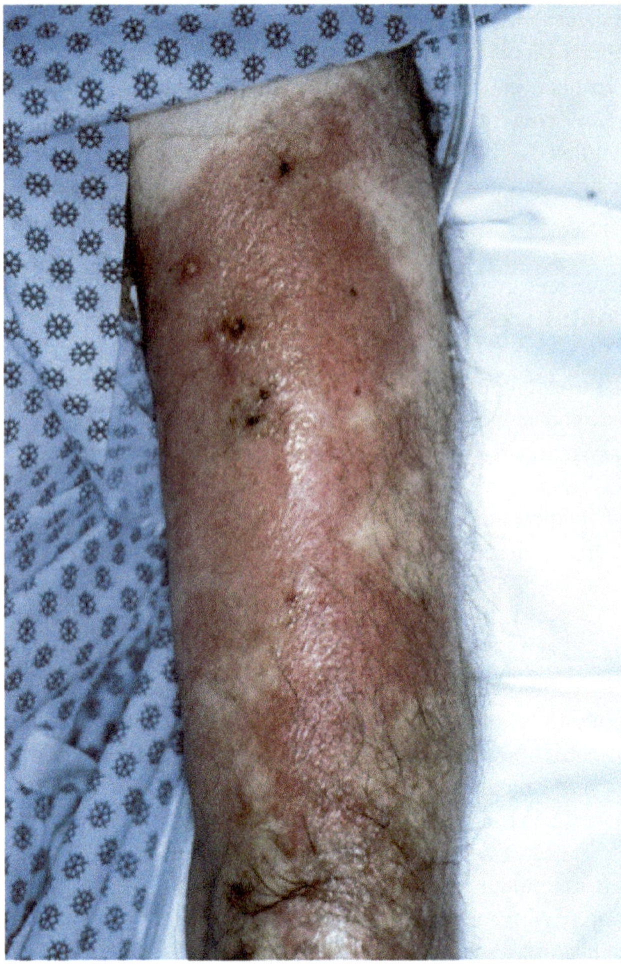

Fig. 22.5 A heart transplant patient presented with a 3-month history of left arm cellulitis. A tender erythematous plaque involved the left arm. Skin biopsy demonstrated sarcoidal granulomas with numerous acid-fast bacilli. Tissue cultures grew *M. haemophilum* after 12 weeks. (Image reprinted from Grossman et al. [285], Fig. 5.23, p. 126, with kind permission from Springer Nature)

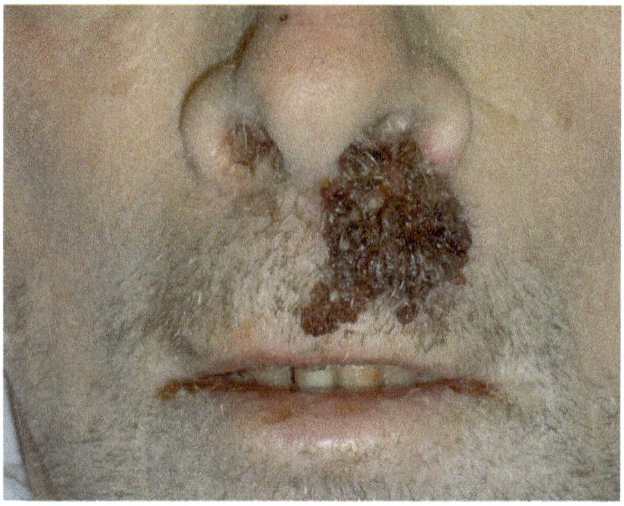

Fig. 22.6 Herpes simplex virus infection manifesting in a heart transplant patient as a chronic, nontender, crusted plaque with scalloped borders extending from the left naris onto the upper lip

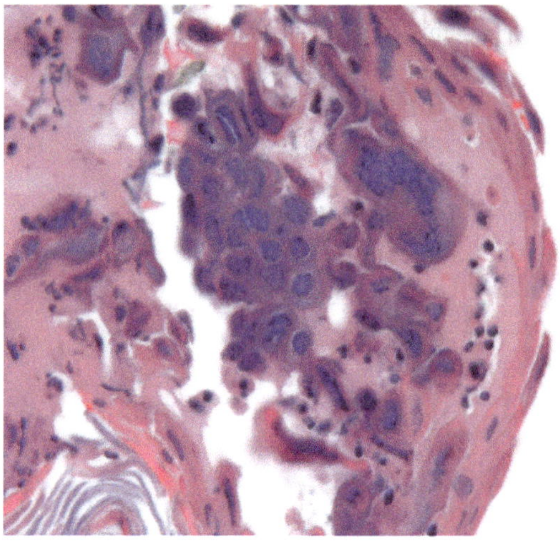

Fig. 22.7 Biopsy of the plaque demonstrated viral cytopathic changes including multinucleation, nuclear molding, and nuclear margination of keratinocytes consistent with herpes simplex virus infection; viral culture confirmed the diagnosis

infections may be chronic and atypical in appearance, belying the diagnosis and leading to therapeutic delay.

In unusual cases of HSV, it is useful to think about the appearance and normal progression of the individual herpetic lesion. The initial 1–2 mm vesicle may become pustular or hemorrhagic; when unroofed, it becomes a wet or weeping 1–2 mm round erosion; then, ultimately, a crust or scab forms. When multiple lesions are present, vesicles or erosions may coalesce to form large areas of open, weeping skin. A scalloped border created by the joining of multiple individual round erosions is a morphologic clue to the origin of such lesions as typical herpetic vesicles. When chronic HSV infection occurs in an area which is moist or macerated, such as the intergluteal cleft, weeping erosions or deeper ulcerations persist. In areas which are drier, such as the cutaneous lips or nose, serous or sanguineous exudate from the erosions dries out and becomes a crusted and heaped-up plaque which may appear exophytic and verrucous (Fig. 22.6). Upon close examination, helpful clues such as a scalloped, friable, eroded, or minute vesicular border may be visible.

Given these myriad presentations, any periorificial ulcer or crust in an immunocompromised host should be considered herpes simplex until proven otherwise. Prompt diagnosis using Tzanck smear, direct immunofluorescence, PCR, culture, or skin biopsy should be used to guide management (Fig. 22.7). Correct technique for performing such tests is important to avoid false-negative results. Vesicles and crusts must be unroofed, and the raw area beneath scraped or swabbed.

Other atypical manifestations of cutaneous HSV infection in immunocompromised patients include intra-oral involvement, an unusual finding among those with intact immune systems. Intra-oral HSV appears as single or multiple erosions or ulcers on the gingiva, palate, tongue, or buccal mucosa with the characteristic scalloped or polycyclic border. Such lesions may occur without herpes labialis, making diagnosis more difficult. In transplant patients, lesions generally develop in the first 4 weeks after transplantation, often following a serious infection or rejection episode [94].

Involvement of the tongue with HSV may result in tender ulcers or linear fissures on the dorsum known as herpetic geometric glossitis [95, 96]. These ulcers may be confused with radiation or chemotherapy-induced mucositis, aphthous stomatitis, erythema multiforme, and other infectious causes. Extension of the infection into the esophagus or respiratory tract may also occur.

Chronic perianal or buttock HSV may be confused with pressure ulcers but tend to be more superficial, have scalloped borders, and involve body fold areas which are not subject to decubitus pressure. Heaped-up granulation tissue may in some cases result in exophytic papules or plaques which mimic condyloma or squamous cell carcinoma. This hypertrophic HSV, also called herpes vegetans, can occur rarely in organ transplant recipients as well as patients with AIDS [97, 98]. Superinfection with bacteria and/or yeast may further complicate the presentation of anogenital HSV and should be considered when ulcers fail to heal with antiviral therapy. Chronic herpetic ulcers in the inguinal or gluteal creases may develop so-called "kissing" lesions on the opposing side of the skin fold, another clue to the diagnosis. Deep linear fissures due to chronic HSV infection can occur in intertriginous areas like the inguinal crease or inframammary or infra-abdominal folds. Termed the "knife-cut sign," this atypical presentation of HSV in immunosuppressed patients should not be confused with other more common types of intertrigo [99].

Digital HSV infection (herpetic whitlow) occurs in immunocompetent patients, often as an occupational hazard of dentists or dental hygienists. In immunosuppressed patients, including transplant patients, digital herpes can produce paronychial inflammation and chronic fingertip ulceration [100]. Such lesions are quite painful and destructive and are frequently incorrectly diagnosed as bacterial infection or paronychia.

Disseminated HSV infection is rare following solid organ transplantation compared with bone marrow transplantation [101]. Dissemination may occur from primary HSV infection, including from the donor organ, as well as through reactivation of donor or recipient virus. Hematogenous dissemination of HSV can result in pneumonitis, hepatitis, pancreatitis, esophagitis, retinitis, encephalitis, and adrenal necrosis [102]. HSV hepatitis should be suspected in an immunocompromised patient presenting with abdominal pain, anicteric transaminitis, fever, and compatible skin lesions [103, 104].

Disseminated cutaneous HSV, also known as Kaposi's varicelliform eruption or eczema herpeticum, presents with widespread 1–2 mm vesicles or punched-out erosions. This eruption can affect immunosuppressed patients and is most likely to occur in those with preexisting skin diseases which result in dysfunctional skin barriers, such as atopic dermatitis or cutaneous T-cell lymphoma [105]. The eruption is associated with fever and malaise and increases the risk of bacterial superinfection with impetigo, cellulitis, or even sepsis. Ocular involvement may be a consequence of widespread facial HSV in this condition.

Acyclovir-resistant HSV is increasingly common among immunocompromised patients with chronic HSV [106]. The degree of immunosuppression and prolonged use of acyclovir are two important factors in the development of drug resistance, as well as erratic or suboptimal dosing or lack of compliance. In patients with profound immunodeficiency, however, lack of response to an antiviral agent does not necessarily correlate with in vitro drug resistance [107]. Acyclovir resistance should be considered when lesions do not decrease in size or when new satellite lesions develop after several days of therapy (Fig. 22.8) [108].

Varicella Zoster

Varicella zoster virus (VZV) is a common cause of vesicular rash in immunocompromised patients. VZV may be dermatomal, disseminated, or chronic. Its incidence increases with advancing age and immunodeficiency, as immunity to the virus wanes and reactivated infection occurs. The condition is increased in both solid organ and particularly bone marrow transplant recipients.

Dermatomal VZV is the most common presentation. Typical presentations are easily recognized by the unilateral distribution of vesicles over patchy erythema in a dermatomal distribution with sharp midline cutoff. One or two contiguous dermatomes may be involved, and few scattered vesicles may occur outside the affected dermatomes. As with HSV, vesicles progress over time and may become pustular, hemorrhagic, or crusted (Fig. 22.9). Pain may be severe but need not be present. Periocular lesions in the distribution of cranial nerve V1, particularly when there are vesicles at the tip of the nose (Hutchinson's sign), are worrisome for ocular involvement. Interestingly, herpes zoster may occur in areas of local immunosuppression such as sites of radiation or surgery or overlying tumors or nodal metastasis. Finally, pain may occur even if skin lesions do not develop (zoster sine herpete).

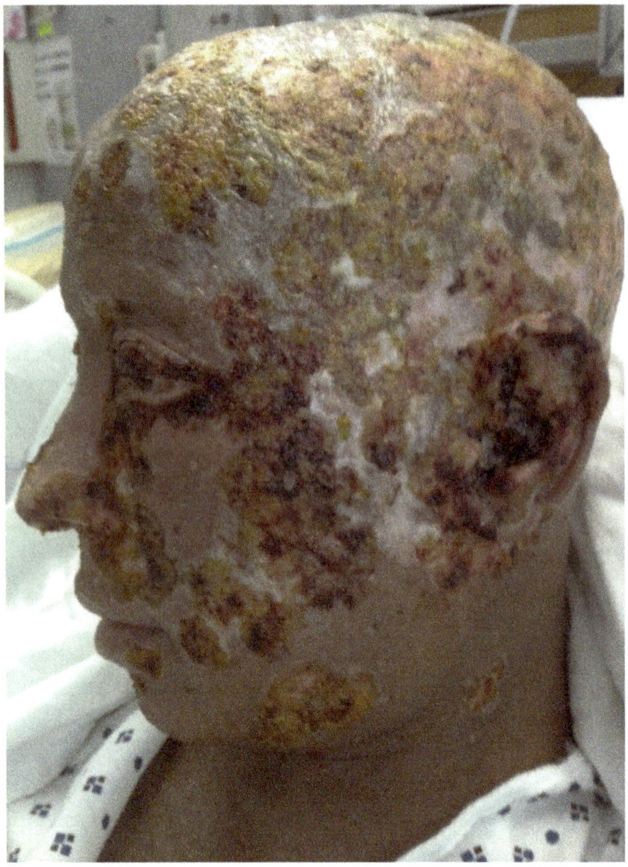

Fig. 22.8 A patient with cutaneous T-cell lymphoma status post stem cell transplant developed chronic herpes simplex virus infection on the face and hands characterized by scalloped borders, scattered intact vesicles, and hemorrhagic and yellow crusts consistent with secondary impetiginization. Refractory to several weeks of intravenous acyclovir therapy, cultures ultimately demonstrated both acyclovir-resistant herpes simplex virus and methicillin-resistant *Staphylococcus aureus*

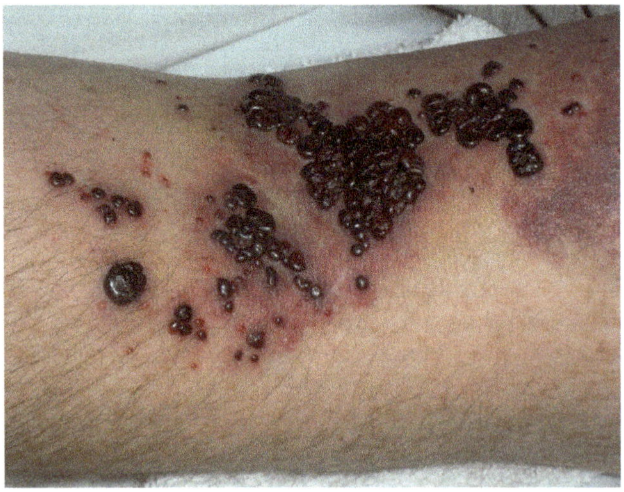

Fig. 22.9 Varicella zoster virus manifesting as coalescing hemorrhagic vesicles in a dermatomal distribution in a patient with severe thrombocytopenia as a complication of chemotherapy

Disseminated zoster is defined as cutaneous VZV in more than three contiguous dermatomes, more than 20 lesions outside the involved dermatome (s), or evidence of systemic involvement. Dissemination to visceral organs usually occurs after the onset of the rash; pneumonitis, meningoencephalitis, and hepatitis due to VZV can be fatal. Rarely, disseminated VZV can present with severe abdominal pain and hyponatremia from the syndrome of inappropriate antidiuretic hormone secretion (SIADH) [109, 110]. Visceral zoster in bone marrow transplant patients can cause abdominal pain and progressive pancreatitis, hepatitis, and paralytic ileus which precede the onset of skin lesions and carry a mortality of 50% despite antiviral therapy [111]. Testing for VZV in the blood by PCR in the appropriate clinical setting may facilitate earlier treatment for disseminated VZV with acyclovir even if vesicles are not seen.

Another form of disseminated VZV seen in immunocompromised patients is referred to as recurrent primary varicella. This presentation is similar to primary varicella (chicken pox) with widespread vesicles on an erythematous base; however, the total number of lesions is far fewer and the course more attenuated than in primary varicella. In the setting of waning, though partial, VZV immunity, endogenous reactivation or exogenous reinfection may explain this presentation [112, 113].

Chronic herpes zoster, characterized by hyperkeratotic thickly crusted plaques, ecthymatous punched-out ulcerations or eschars, or prolonged widespread disseminated vesicles, is defined as active VZV infection that persists longer than 1 month. This presentation is most common in patients with AIDS but may rarely occur in transplant patients or those otherwise immunosuppressed [114, 115]. Many of the reported cases have demonstrated acyclovir resistance.

Cytomegalovirus

Cytomegalovirus (CMV) disease in an immunocompromised host can result from primary infection of a seronegative patient, reactivation of latent virus, or reinfection with a new virus subtype. Most is due to reactivation of latent virus. In cases of iatrogenic immunosuppression, as is seen in organ transplantation, the onset of CMV disease may be rapid. The pattern of organ involvement varies from group to group; in solid organ transplant patients, gastrointestinal ulceration and hepatitis are more common, whereas interstitial pneumonitis and myelosuppression are more common in bone marrow transplant recipients [116]. Cutaneous manifestations of CMV infection are rare in any circumstance.

Lesions of cutaneous CMV are not sufficiently distinctive to allow the diagnosis to be made on clinical grounds alone.

The most common manifestation of CMV skin infection is chronic ulceration of the anogenital area. These ulcers may be single or multiple, small or large, with sharply marginated borders. Because such ulcers can be clinically indistinguishable from those caused by chronic HSV infection, correct diagnosis relies upon culture, PCR, or histopathology. HSV and CMV co-infection in such ulcers may further complicate diagnosis and management.

Chronic ulcers due to CMV may occur elsewhere on the skin and mucous membranes. They may become quite large with purulent exudate or thick black eschar [117, 118]. Oral manifestations include painful erosions or ulcers of the lip, tongue, or buccal mucosa (Fig. 22.10).

Widespread exanthematous morbilliform eruptions due to CMV have also been described in transplant patients [119]. These eruptions, unlike other nonspecific morbilliform eruptions, demonstrate characteristic large intranuclear inclusions with a surrounding halo, the "owl's eye" nuclei of CMV, in dermal vessel endothelial cells, which may be confirmed with an immunoperoxidase stain [120]. This endothelial cell infection may evolve into capillaritis or vasculitis with consequent purpuric appearance or infarction [121–123].

Human Herpes Virus 6

Human herpes virus 6 (HHV-6), along with HSV, VZV, CMV, and EBV, is a member of the *Herpesviridae* family which is the causative agent of exanthema subitum (roseola infantum) in infancy. As with other herpes viruses, HHV-6 can establish latency after primary infection and reactivate in the setting of immunocompromise. Most such reactivations occur 2–4 weeks after transplantation [124]. The use of muromonab-CD3, alemtuzumab, and antithymocyte globulin for prevention of rejection increases the risk of HHV-6 reactivation in solid organ transplant recipients [125]. Symptoms of HHV-6 reactivation include fever, rash, pneumonitis, bone marrow suppression, and encephalitis. Typically, the rash is an erythematous morbilliform eruption not unlike acute GVHD. Because HHV-6 reactivation has been associated with the development of severe acute GVHD, and because the clinical and histologic findings are nonspecific, it is difficult to distinguish between the two entities [126].

Human Papillomavirus

Human papillomavirus (HPV) infection is common in both immunocompetent and immunoincompetent patients. In those with dysfunctional immune systems, lesions of HPV can be extensive, numerous, exuberant, and recalcitrant in addition to exceedingly common. Eighty percent of organ transplant recipients may develop warts [127].

Lesions of HPV classically are exophytic, verrucous papules or plaques which may be flat, sessile or pedunculated, brown, gray, or flesh colored (Fig. 22.11). They are commonly found in the genital region, where they may become large and confluent, locally destructive cauliflower like masses in immunosuppressed patients. Facial, oral, and digital warts, as well as more widespread papules on the extremities and trunk, may be seen.

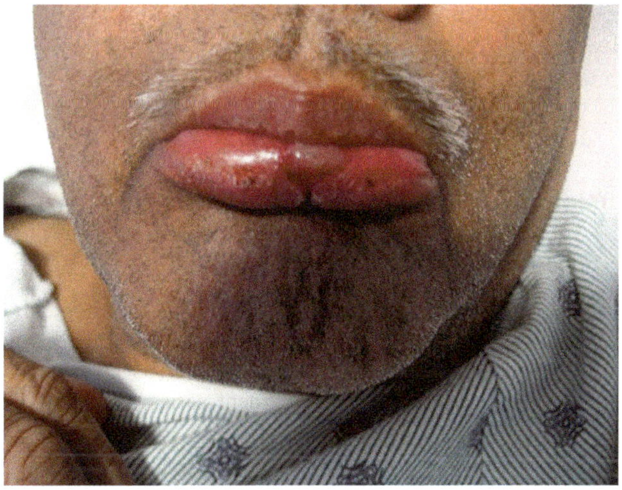

Fig. 22.10 A heart transplant patient presented with an ulcer on the lower lip. Biopsyzrevealed multinucleate giant cells with inclusion bodies and immunoperoxidase staining for cytomegalovirus. (Image reprinted from Grossman et al. [286], Fig. 6.65, p. 168, with kind permission from Springer Nature)

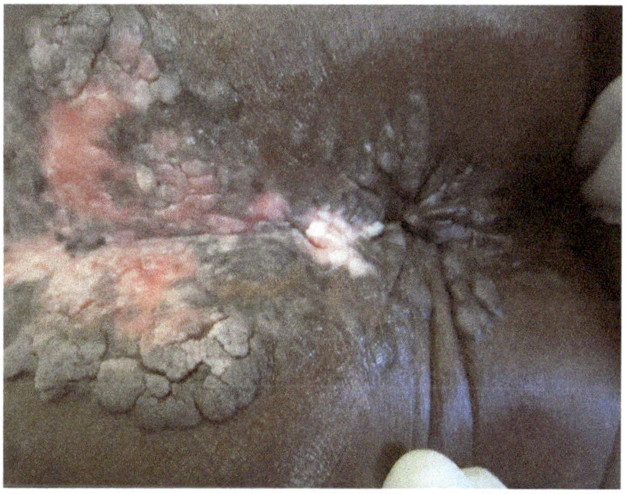

Fig. 22.11 Verrucous perianal papules and plaques of human papilloma virus infection

Molluscum Contagiosum

Typical lesions of molluscum contagiosum are 3–5 mm white or flesh-colored dome-shaped papules with central umbilication (Fig. 22.12). The presence of molluscum, especially widespread or giant molluscum, in an adult patient is a marker of immunosuppression. Such presentations are most common with advanced HIV disease but are also seen in transplant patients and those immunosuppressed for other reasons [128].

Giant molluscum may present as large verrucous or lobulated nodules. Molluscum may also cause a viral folliculitis with multiple reddish papules on the chin and cheeks mimicking tinea barbae [129]. Disseminated cryptococcosis and histoplasmosis can appear molluscoid and should be suspected in the proper clinical setting, particularly when the lesions are atypical and there are signs of systemic illness. In contrast with normal hosts, in whom molluscum is self-limited, molluscum in immunosuppressed patients can be highly recalcitrant, chronic, and resistant to therapy.

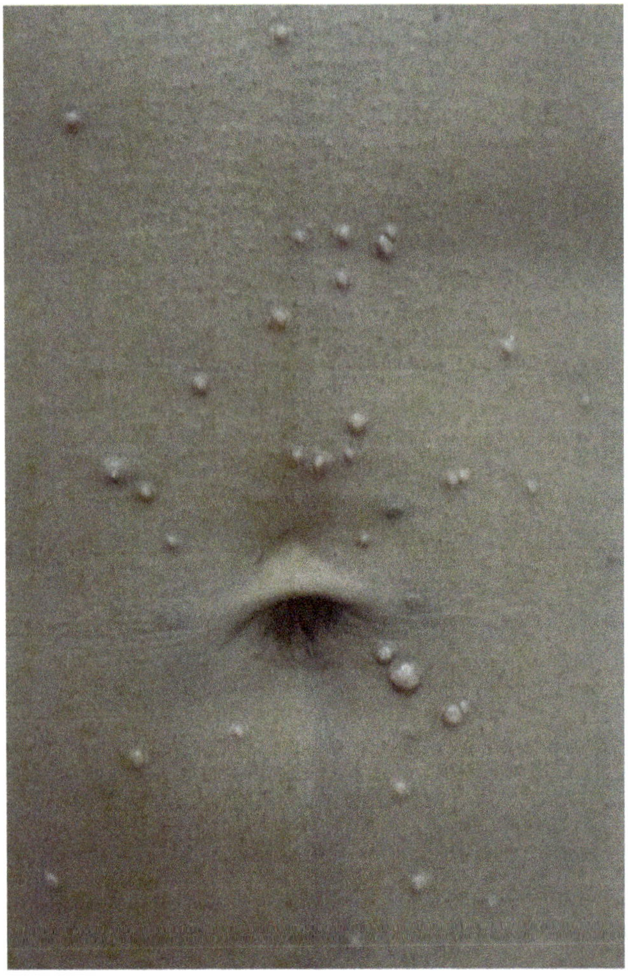

Fig. 22.12 Umbilicated, dome-shaped, flesh-colored and white papules of molluscum contagiosum on the abdomen

Subcutaneous and Deep Mycoses

Aspergillus

Invasive aspergillosis is the most common opportunistic fungal infection following hematopoietic stem cell transplantation [130]. Infection with this ubiquitous mold occurs in the setting of severe or prolonged neutropenia, high-dose corticosteroid therapy for graft-versus-host disease (GVHD), and other states of profound immunosuppression. Following stem cell transplant, invasive aspergillosis is now more commonly seen in the post-engraftment phase due to iatrogenic immunosuppression for GVHD than in the neutropenic period [131]. It is less common, but not infrequently seen, in solid organ transplant recipients.

Cutaneous *Aspergillus* infection can result from primary inoculation injury, in which case *A. flavus* and *A. niger* are the most common causes, or secondary dissemination, most often due to *A. fumigatus* [132]. Primary cutaneous infection generally occurs at sites of iatrogenic trauma or contamination, under arm boards or tape or where intravenous cannulas puncture the skin. Such sites are frequently hidden from view under dressings and are difficult to examine but should be visualized as part of a thorough assessment.

Lesions of cutaneous aspergillosis begin as tender erythematous or purpuric macules or papules that progress to violaceous, edematous plaques with necrotic black or purple centers and a bright purpuric rim. Lesions may become hemorrhagic bullae as the necrotic skin sloughs or ultimately black eschars (Fig. 22.13). Less common presentations include

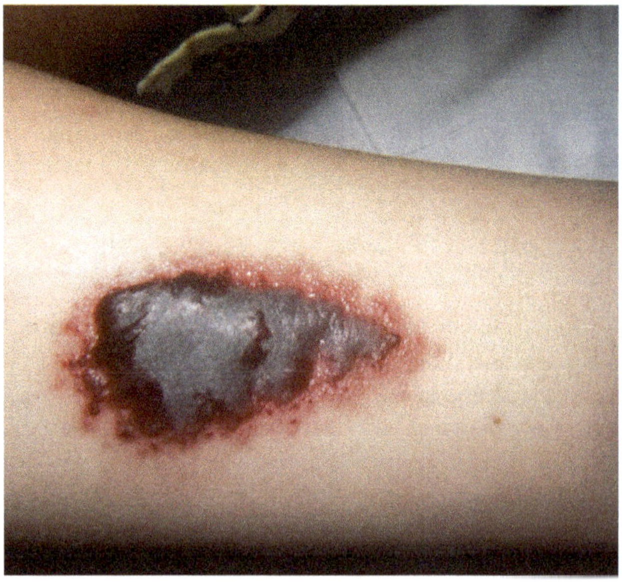

Fig. 22.13 A hemorrhagic bulla on the forearm of a child with ALL. Potassium hydroxide (KOH) preparation, biopsy, and culture all demonstrated *Aspergillus fumigatus*. (Image reprinted from Grossman et al. [287], Fig. 1.5, p. 4, with kind permission from Springer Nature)

erythematous to violaceous plaques studded with pustules, subcutaneous purplish nodules, and cellulitic plaques, among others [133–138].

When such a lesion is noted, it should prompt a thorough examination of the remainder of the skin and mucous membranes to determine whether other lesions are present. Potassium hydroxide (KOH) prep of the blister roof can reveal characteristic broad, regularly septate hyphae dichotomously branching at acute angles, providing an immediate presumptive diagnosis [139]. Otherwise, prompt diagnosis of invasive disease through frozen section biopsy or "rushed" preparation of a fixed specimen, as well as tissue culture, is essential for proper management. Histologic findings may include intravascular thrombosis with masses of angioinvasive hyphae, hemorrhage, necrosis, and inflammatory infiltrate.

While only 10% of cases of disseminated aspergillosis have skin manifestations, cutaneous lesions may be the presenting sign of systemic disease [140]. Thus, in addition to a thorough skin exam, patients with suggestive lesions should undergo further workup, such as CT scans of the chest, abdomen, pelvis, and brain, to determine whether there is evidence of dissemination. Determination of whether a single lesion—or multiple lesions—is present is critical for guiding treatment and predicting outcome.

Single primary lesions have a more favorable prognosis than secondary or disseminated disease. In addition to systemic antifungal therapy with voriconazole, amphotericin B, itraconazole, posaconazole, or caspofungin, surgical excision and debridement may play a critical role. Because *Aspergillus* may secondarily disseminate from primary skin lesions, local control of the infection may be critical to cure. Conversely, if there is more than one cutaneous lesion or radiographic evidence of disseminated disease, there is no role for debridement, and antifungal therapy alone is used. In such cases, mortality is high, particularly without resolution of underlying immunosuppression.

Fusarium

Fusarium is a ubiquitous soil mold which can cause infection in immunocompromised patients which is clinically and histologically similar to that of *Aspergillus*. Major risk factors for *Fusarium* infection include prolonged neutropenia and corticosteroid use as commonly occurring in those with hematologic malignancies who receive stem cell transplantation and require treatment for graft-versus-host disease [141–144].

Primary, locally invasive disease presents at sites of trauma such as that which occurs with intravenous cannula placement or accidental injury to a digit or extremity. Skin lesions evolve rapidly from a painful red macule or papule into a violaceous, necrotic pustule, bulla, ulcer, or eschar with a rim of erythema [145–148].

Disseminated infection occurs almost exclusively in those who are neutropenic or status post bone marrow transplantation. Skin lesions evolve as they do in primary infection. Compared with disseminated *Aspergillus*, cutaneous lesions of *Fusarium* are more common (75–90% versus only 10%) and more numerous and widespread [3]. They appear clinically similar to lesions of other angioinvasive fungi, including *Aspergillus* and *Mucor* species, but they tend to be smaller. Associated sinopulmonary disease is common, as is fungemia.

Disseminated fusariosis is almost uniformly fatal, especially without white blood cell recovery [149]. Compared to neutropenic patients, infection which occurs in the setting of solid organ transplantation is more likely to be localized and has a better prognosis.

Scedosporium and *Pseudallescheria*

Infection with this soil saprophyte (*Scedosporium* is the asexual and *Pseudallescheria* the sexual state of the organism) is typically acquired through inhalation or inoculation. Infection is most commonly associated with hematopoietic stem cell transplants, organ transplants, hematologic malignancies, and HIV. A significant cause of disease, it is responsible for approximately 25% of non-*Aspergillus* mold infections in organ transplant recipients [150]. When infection occurs in this group, it most often does so within 6 months of transplant and with devastating consequences; more than half of patients present with disseminated disease, and around 60% die [150].

One-third of patients with *Scedosporium* infection have cutaneous lesions [151]. Localized lesions may follow trauma, whereas disseminated lesions are secondary to hematogenous spread [151, 152]. *Scedosporium* and *Pseudallescheria* may present with ulcerated dusky nodules, tender pustules, necrotic bullae, or subcutaneous suppurative nodules with spread along cutaneous lymphatics that resembles that of sporotrichosis [153–159].

Scedosporium, *Aspergillus*, and *Fusarium* can be indistinguishable in histologic section; tissue culture is required to differentiate these organisms. Blood cultures may also be positive in 75–80%, in contrast with many other disseminated fungal infections [160, 161]. Itraconazole and voriconazole, as well as surgical debridement, may be effective in some cases of *S. apiospermum* infection, but *S. prolificans* is resistant to almost all antifungals and has a mortality approaching 100% [161].

Mucormycosis/Zygomycosis

Mucormycosis, or zygomycosis, is a term used to describe invasive infection with molds of the genera *Rhizopus*,

Absidia, *Rhizomucor*, and *Mucor*. The organisms in these genera are morphologically identical and cause the same clinical disease.

These fungi are ubiquitous in the environment. In susceptible patients, they can cause rhinocerebral, pulmonary, cutaneous, gastrointestinal, central nervous system, and disseminated infections [162]. Infections most commonly present in the nose and paranasal sinuses or on the palate, from which they spread rapidly to the central nervous system through the orbit and cribriform plate.

Cutaneous mucormycosis most commonly affects patients with significant immunocompromise, including those receiving immunosuppressants following solid organ or stem cell transplantation, as well as those with prolonged neutropenia, and those receiving systemic corticosteroids and other agents for severe graft-versus-host disease [162–165]. An additional risk factor is voriconazole use for fungal prophylaxis after transplantation. Since this agent does not cover zygomycetes, its use may select for zygomycotic infection [166, 167].

Primary inoculation of mucormycosis into the skin most commonly develops at the sites of intravenous catheters, injections, burn injuries, or surgical wounds or in the setting of contaminated tape, dressings, or arm boards. An erythematous papule or plaque initially develops and then becomes purpuric, pustular, hemorrhagic, or ulcerated, ultimately developing into a necrotic eschar [168]. Infection may spread rapidly along tissue planes such that the involved area may far exceed that which is visible clinically. As with *Aspergillus* and other angioinvasive fungi, identification of a single primary cutaneous lesion is critical, as surgical debridement may be curative and systemic dissemination from a primary lesion can occur [169–171].

Secondary cutaneous mucormycosis occurs as a consequence of disseminated infection, most often originating in the lungs or sinuses in the setting of hematologic malignancy, bone marrow transplantation, and prolonged neutropenia. Lesions are most often violaceous and necrotic-appearing plaques with concentric shades of black, yellow, and purple with a thin purpuric red rim, the so-called "bull's-eye infarct" of cutaneous zygomycosis (Fig. 22.14) [172]. Histologically, this clinical appearance corresponds to hyphal invasion and thrombosis of dermal blood vessels with consequent necrosis of surrounding tissue (Fig. 22.15).

Rhinocerebral mucormycosis is the most common presentation of systemic infection. One of the earliest signs is nasal discharge. The nasal mucosa may appear black and necrotic. Invasion into the mouth may cause infarction of the palate, producing a black eschar or ulcer. Necrotic facial lesions suggest aggressive and advanced angioinvasive infection. Extension of infection through the nasal turbinates into the sinuses may result in orbital cellulitis, extraocular muscle paresis, proptosis, chemosis, and eyelid edema.

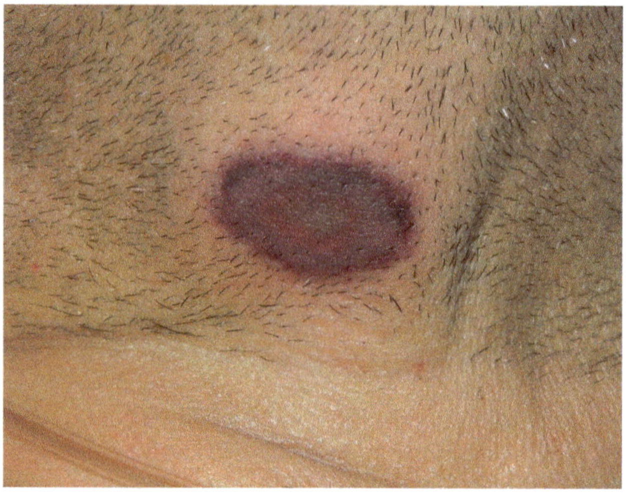

Fig. 22.14 Disseminated mucormycosis manifesting as a rapidly expanding violaceous and necrotic-appearing plaque on the neck with concentric shades of black, yellow, and purple and a peripheral rim of erythema

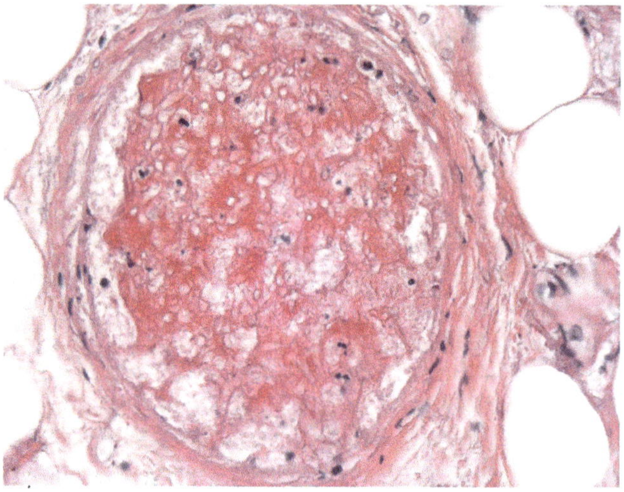

Fig. 22.15 Frozen section and permanent section biopsy demonstrated thick, translucent, ribbon-like, nonseptate hyphae with right-angle branching filling a vessel in the subcutis; findings consistent with mucormycosis. The patient had two other cutaneous lesions and multiple infarcts in the lungs, kidneys, brain, and other organs discovered on computed tomography scan and at autopsy

Diagnosis of cutaneous mucormycosis relies on histologic demonstration of tissue invasion. A touch preparation of a skin biopsy specimen to a glass slide may allow rapid confirmation of infection. Otherwise, frozen section biopsy or "rushed" permanent section processing is vitally important to dictate management [173]. Zygomycetes in tissue appear as wide, ribbon-like, nonseptate hyphae with right-angle branching. Such an appearance is suggestive, if present, but zygomycetes cannot reliably be differentiated from *Aspergillus* on the basis of histologic features alone [174]. Culture is required to identify the particular fungal organism.

The mortality rate of invasive mucormycosis is exceedingly high, on the order of 80–100% [166], particularly in the absence of hematologic recovery or resolution of the underlying immunodeficiency. Prompt initiation of amphotericin B is the therapy of choice, particularly in those already on prophylactic voriconazole. Surgical debridement can play an important role if infection is localized and not widely disseminated. Long-term or even lifelong therapy with posaconazole may be required in those who survive the acute phase of infection.

Hyalohyphomycoses

Together with *Fusarium*, this group of hyaline (nonpigmented) septate molds includes *Paecilomyces*, *Acremonium*, *Trichoderma*, *Scopulariopsis*, and *Trichosporon*. Though less common, these organisms are nonetheless medically important pathogens in the transplant population.

The majority of reported *Paecilomyces* infections involve those with solid organ or bone marrow transplant, chronic steroid use, or lymphoma. *Paecilomyces* enters where there has been a breakdown of the skin barrier, such as occurs with tinea pedis or onychomycosis. Lower extremity involvement is therefore common [175]. Indwelling catheters may provide another portal of entry [176]. Lesions appear as erythematous macules, vesicles, pustules, painful red nodules or furuncles, or cellulitis [177–181]. Culture and histology are necessary for diagnosis, and species identification is important to guide management. Most cases of *Paecilomyces* in immunocompromised patients are localized to the skin and achieve cure with antifungal therapy +/− surgical debridement, but *P. lilacinus* is intrinsically resistant to conventional antifungals such as amphotericin, flucytosine, and fluconazole.

Like *Paecilomyces*, *Acremonium* and *Trichoderma* are increasingly recognized opportunistic pathogens which cause a variety of presentations in immunocompromised patients with hematologic malignancies, prolonged neutropenia, chronic steroid use, or organ transplantation [182]. *Acremonium* may present with widespread painful and necrotic cutaneous papules or nodules in the setting of refractory febrile neutropenia and myalgias [183–185], frequently associated with positive blood cultures [186]. Mycetoma of the extremities with tumefaction and draining sinuses has also been reported as a manifestation of *Acremonium* in transplant patients [187, 188]. *Trichoderma* may present with necrotic, ulcerated plaques at intravenous cannula sites in immunosuppressed transplant or neutropenic patients; from there, the fungus may lead to fatal dissemination to the lungs, liver, and brain [189–192].

Cutaneous manifestations of *Scopulariopsis* infection reported in immunosuppressed transplant patients include a solitary necrotic black eschar at an intravenous cannula site, red-purple, ulcerative, subcutaneous nodules on the extremities, and onychomycosis with necrotic periungual cellulitis [193–196]. Most *Scopulariopsis* species are resistant to amphotericin B, itraconazole, and many other conventional antifungals. Surgical debridement may play an important role in eliminating localized infection.

Trichosporon is a rare but emerging opportunistic pathogen. Invasive infection most commonly affects neutropenic leukemic patients. It presents similarly to candidiasis, with fever, myalgia, endophthalmitis, and multiple necrotizing purpuric papules and nodules in one third of patients [197–201]. However, fungemia, visceral involvement, and death are more common in *Trichosporon* infection. Skin biopsy and tissue culture have high diagnostic yield. Cryptococcal antigen and *Aspergillus* galactomannan may be cross-reactive and falsely positive [202]. Case fatality approaches 80% in disseminated disease despite antifungal treatment unless hematologic recovery occurs [203].

Phaeohyphomycosis

Infection by one of these pigmented fungi, which include such organisms as *Phialophora, Fonseca, Cladosporium, Exophiala, Alternaria, and Scedosporium*, usually results from accidental inoculation of the skin with plant matter, soil, or wood. Lesions may appear up to several years after the event during immunosuppression for transplantation or other causes. A subcutaneous phaeomycotic nodule or abscess may develop, often without pain or other signs of local or systemic inflammation. Suppuration, sinus tract formation, and ulceration may occur less often, or the lesion may become scaly and verrucous [160, 204–208] (Fig. 22.16).

Disseminated phaeohyphomycosis usually occurs in immunosuppressed patients [160]. It is more common for infection to disseminate from the lungs or other viscera to the blood and skin, but secondary dissemination from the skin has also been reported [209]. Disseminated cutaneous lesions may be tender subcutaneous nodules, ulcerated papules, pustules, or nonhealing ulcers (Fig. 22.17) [210].

Surgical debridement is the treatment of choice, if possible, for primary cutaneous phaeohyphomycosis. Amphotericin B, itraconazole, ketoconazole, voriconazole, and terbinafine are antifungal agents which may be useful.

Candidiasis

Behind *Aspergillus*, *Candida* is the second most common invasive fungal infection in patients following hematopoietic stem cell transplantation. Among solid organ transplant recipients, it is the most common cause of invasive fungal

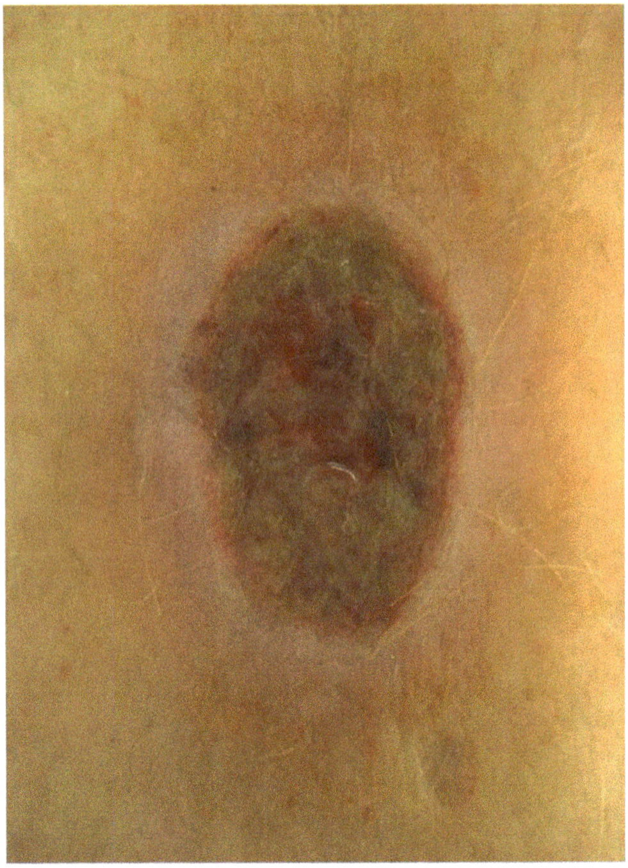

Fig. 22.16 A patient with a history of bilateral lung transplant for α-1 antitrypsin deficiency developed an indurated ulcer and two erythematous nodules on the right lower leg 11 years after transplantation. Pathology and DNA sequencing confirmed the diagnosis of phaeohyphomycosis due to *Exophiala spinifera*

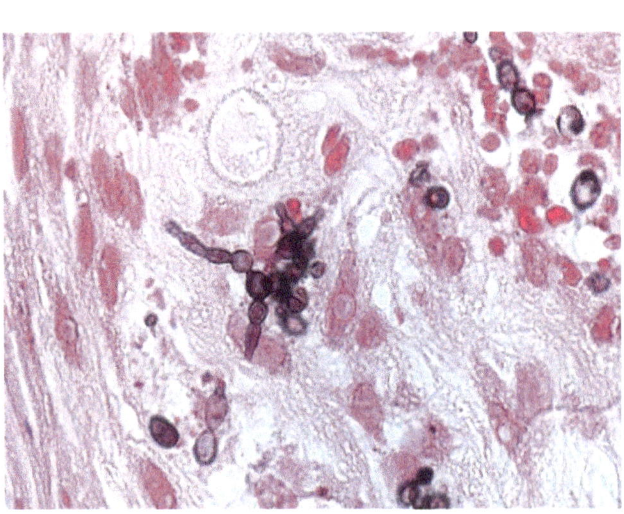

Fig. 22.17 Biopsy of the phaeohyphomycotic ulcer edge demonstrated pigmented yeast-like and pseudohyphal elements highlighted by Fontana Masson stain

infection [211]. The spectrum of infection ranges from thrush to widespread dissemination. Iatrogenic immunosuppression, chemotherapy, hematologic malignancies, neutropenia, and prolonged broad-spectrum antibiotics predispose to disseminated candidiasis. The gastrointestinal tract, indwelling lines, and even a transplanted organ may be the source of dissemination [212].

Candida albicans causes approximately half of disseminated candidiasis—*C. glabrata*, *C. tropicalis*, *C. krusei*, and *C. parapsilosis* account for most of the rest of infections. About 10–13% of the time, disseminated candidiasis is associated with skin lesions [213]. Of these cases, *C. albicans* causes only about 10%, whereas *C. tropicalis* and *C. krusei* make up the majority [131, 214, 215].

Diagnostic delay is a significant contributing factor for the high mortality associated with disseminated candidiasis. Nonspecific symptoms and a frequent lack of positive blood cultures make diagnosis difficult. The presence of cutaneous lesions, however, provides an opportunity for earlier diagnosis and treatment.

Skin lesions may be single or multiple, localized or diffuse, most often involving the trunk and proximal extremities. Morphologically, they are typically erythematous 0.5–1.0 cm papules may be purpuric and can have pale, necrotic, or pustular centers. (Fig. 22.18). Subcutaneous nodules, folliculitis, and cellulitis-like plaques may also occur. Patients are often ill-appearing with fever and clinical deterioration despite therapy with broad-spectrum antibiotics.

Disseminated candidiasis can also cause endophthalmitis with blurred vision and eye pain, as well as muscle abscesses with fever and severe myalgias. Hepatosplenic infection is also characteristic.

Skin biopsy may demonstrate *Candida* in and around dermal blood vessels, but the organism can be difficult to see. Tissue culture is positive in 50% of patients, and potassium hydroxide examination of a touch prep of a tissue specimen may be useful [212, 216]. The mortality associated with *Candida* fungemia is quite high [214, 215]. Fluconazole is the empiric treatment of choice in stable patients, while amphotericin B or echinocandins are preferred in neutropenic or otherwise unstable patients [217].

Cryptococcosis

Cryptococcus neoformans infection is usually acquired via inhalation of spores found in soil or decaying wood contaminated with bird guano. Primary pulmonary infection is the most common form of cryptococcosis. Secondary dissemination most frequently results in central nervous system infection,

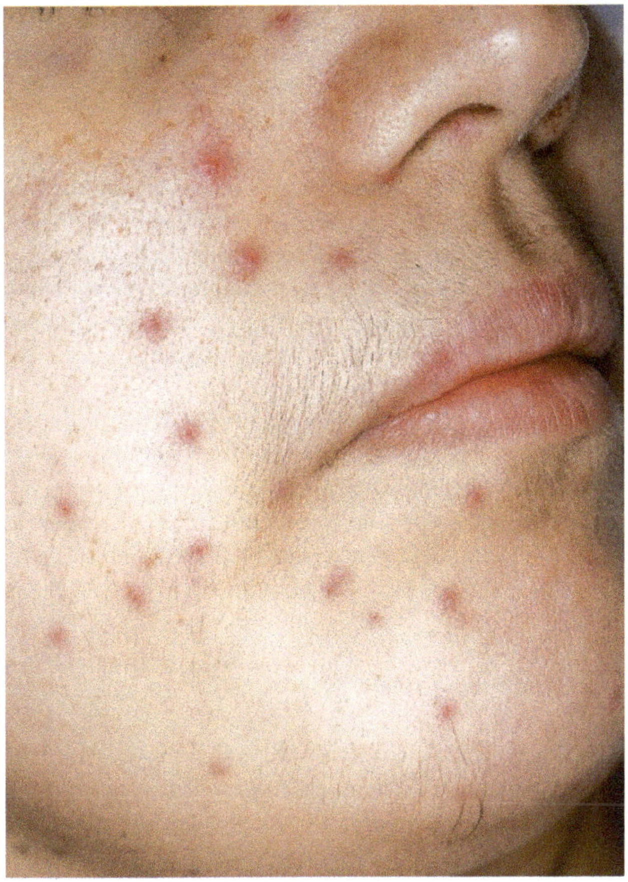

Fig. 22.18 Disseminated erythematous papules with central erosions and crusts due to *Candida parapsilosis*. (Image reprinted from Grossman et al. [287], Fig. 1.21, p. 14, with kind permission from Springer Nature)

followed by the skin in roughly 10–15% of immunocompromised hosts [218]. The combination of meningeal or craniobulbar signs with skin lesions in an immunocompromised patient should raise the possibility of cryptococcal infection. In most cases, this represents reactivation and dissemination of latent infection in the setting of immunosuppression [219].

Primary cutaneous cryptococcosis only rarely occurs. In cases of dissemination, skin lesions can present months before signs of systemic infection. Isolated cutaneous cryptococcosis, therefore, is considered a diagnosis of exclusion, and skin lesions should prompt a thorough workup for extracutaneous disease in all immunosuppressed patients.

Cryptococcal lesions in HIV patients are most often molluscum contagiosum-like umbilicated or crusted papules with a predilection for the head and neck. In non-HIV-related immunosuppression, cutaneous cryptococcosis, whether primary or secondary, most often presents with cellulitis, subcutaneous nodules, or ulcers [220–223]. In solid organ transplant recipients, cellulitis is most common [224] (Fig. 22.19). As with bacterial cellulitis, signs and symptoms include erythema, warmth, and tenderness. Patients with cutaneous cryptococcosis, however, do not respond to typical empiric antibiotics. Necrotizing cellulitis and fasciitis have also been reported in renal and cardiac transplant patients [225, 226].

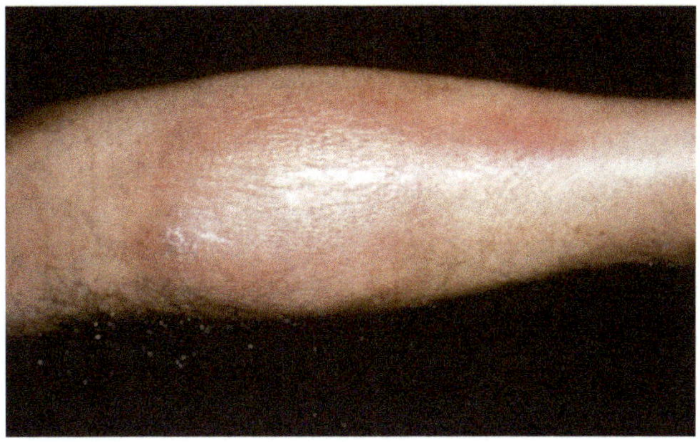

Fig. 22.19 Cryptococcal cellulitis involving the calf of a renal transplant patient. (Image reprinted from Grossman et al. [287], Fig. 1.36, p. 24, with kind permission from Springer Nature)

Patients taking one of the calcineurin inhibitors, which inhibit *C. neoformans* growth in vitro at 37 °C, are more likely to develop cutaneous, soft tissue, bone, joint, or lung involvement than central nervous system or disseminated disease [219, 224, 227–229].

Diagnosis of cutaneous cryptococcosis can be confirmed via biopsy or culture or by visualizing the budding yeast in a Tzanck smear or India ink preparation made from vesicle fluid, ulcer exudate, or skin biopsy touch prep. Serum cryptococcal antigen is always positive in disseminated disease.

Disseminated cryptococcosis is lethal if untreated. Amphotericin B, usually in combination with flucytosine, is the treatment of choice. Lifelong maintenance therapy with fluconazole is often recommended. Reduction of immunosuppression in transplant patients, if feasible, can be lifesaving.

Coccidioidomycosis

Coccidioides immitis is a dimorphic fungus endemic to the soil of the Southwestern United States, as well as Central and South America. Primarily a respiratory pathogen, cutaneous disease can be reactive to the organism (such as erythema nodosum, erythema multiforme, and Sweet syndrome) or due to direct infection (primary inoculation or secondary dissemination) [230].

Disseminated coccidioidomycosis presents with fever, cough, and sweats; involvement of the skin, meninges, bones, and joints is common [230]. Disseminated cutaneous disease is rare even in immunosuppressed patients but may present with verrucous or crusted papules or plaques, subcutaneous abscesses, cellulitic plaques, and ulcers [231–233].

The diagnosis is confirmed through culture, histologic demonstration of the organism, or serologic testing. Treatment with amphotericin B, fluconazole, or itraconazole is recommended for immunocompromised patients in the acute phase of infection. Continuous treatment with an azole antifungal is recommended thereafter for the duration of immunosuppression.

Blastomycosis

Blastomyces dermatitidis is a dimorphic fungus endemic to the Mississippi and Ohio River valleys, the Great Lakes region, and part of Africa and India [234]. Infection usually results from inhalation and is typically asymptomatic. Skin lesions may result from dissemination, which accounts for 60% of cases involving the skin, or primary inoculation.

Primary blastomycosis presents with a solitary plaque with an atrophic, scarred, or ulcerated center and verrucous edges studded with pustules. Associated streaky lymphangitis, lymphadenitis, and red, tender nodules along the cutaneous lymphatics may also be present [218]. In immunosuppressed patients, ulceration and pustulosis may be more prominent features. Disseminated papulopustules and subcutaneous nodules may also occur [235–238].

Though most blastomycosis occurs in immunocompetent patients, severe immunosuppression, including that associated with organ transplantation, may predispose to more severe or disseminated disease and carries a mortality of 29–40% [235, 239]. The skin, bone, genitourinary system, and central nervous system are most commonly involved in cases of disseminated disease [240]. Therapy, which may be lifelong, consists of amphotericin B followed by itraconazole.

Histoplasmosis

Histoplasmosis is most commonly a self-limited primary pulmonary condition which is either asymptomatic or accompanied by flu-like symptoms. Progressive disseminated histoplasmosis can also occur, usually as a consequence of depressed cellular immunity. Symptoms include fever, respiratory symptoms, weight loss, hepatosplenomegaly, and bone marrow suppression. This presentation is most common in patients with AIDS living in endemic areas [241]. Other susceptible patients include those receiving corticosteroids or chemotherapy and those with various hematologic malignancies.

Cutaneous histoplasmosis manifests in three general ways—via primary inoculation, as a reactive erythema, or as a manifestation of disseminated disease. Primary inoculation is rare and results in a nodule or ulcer. Reactive erythema presents as erythema nodosum or erythema multiforme-type lesions. Disseminated cutaneous histoplasmosis may present with macules, papules, necrotic papules, a morbilliform eruption, pustules, nodules, ulcers, panniculitis, cellulitis, and verrucous or vegetative plaques [242].

Skin biopsy of a suspicious lesion reveals the organism within the cytoplasm of histiocytes in the dermis. Urine *Histoplasma* antigen is detected by radioimmunoassay in up to 90% of patients with disseminated disease [243]. Treatment is with amphotericin B or itraconazole. If untreated, the mortality rate of disseminated disease is 95% [241].

Sporotrichosis

Sporothrix schenckii is another dimorphic fungus which is found commonly in plant material and soil. Cutaneous inoculation is classically associated with rose thorns and sphagnum moss [244] and can occur in both immunocompetent and immunoincompetent hosts. Clinical presentations include fixed cutaneous (20%), lymphocutaneous (70%), disseminated, and extracutaneous disease [245, 246]. Disseminated and extracutaneous sporotrichosis are rare, but immunosuppression such as that due to organ transplantation, hematologic malignancy, steroid use, and HIV/AIDS increase the risk. Hematogenous spread can occur from either a primary cutaneous or pulmonary source [247].

Cutaneous sporotrichosis classically presents with a painless papule or ulcerated, draining nodule at the site of inoculation, followed by the appearance of asymptomatic erythematous nodules extending along the cutaneous lymphatics. Lesions may also become fixed verrucous or ulcerated nodules without lymphatic spread [245]. In disseminated disease, cutaneous lesions may be widely distributed ulcerated papules or plaques, crusted nodules, or necrotic ulcers [248]. Dissemination to multiple visceral organs may occur, but involvement of the bones and joints is most characteristic, occurring in 80% of cases [247, 249]. Skin lesions usually precede diagnosis of such widespread involvement.

Yeast cells may be demonstrated as cigar-shaped bodies in histologic sections but should be cultured for definitive diagnosis. Itraconazole is an accepted treatment for localized disease, whereas amphotericin B may be more appropriate in cases of dissemination or immunosuppression.

Superficial Mycoses

Dermatophytosis of the skin, hair, and nails is common in immunocompetent and immunoincompetent patients. Organisms of this group, including *Trichophyton*, *Microsporum*, and *Epidermophyton*, only rarely cause invasive infection but may do so in the severely immunosuppressed. Invasive infection usually occurs at the site of chronic superficial dermatophytosis, presenting with erythematous or violaceous papules or nodules [250–252]. Deep dermal abscesses, draining nodules, or chronic ulcers may also occur [253, 254]. Lesions are typically few but may be many [253].

Because they are rarely suspected and may mimic other cutaneous diseases, widespread, invasive, or otherwise atypical dermatophyte infections are often misdiagnosed. Annular, erythematous, scaling plaques with serpiginous borders are typical of tinea corporis (Fig. 22.20). In the immunocompromised host, a florid presentation may mimic cutaneous lupus or rosacea [255]. Pustular or bullous eruptions may mimic bacterial folliculitis or HSV/VZV, respectively [256]. Application of a topical steroid to a misdiagnosed dermatophyte infection can also produce widespread and atypical-appearing tinea with decreased erythema and scale and follicular papules or pustules [257]. Appropriate history taking and awareness should prompt a scraping for potassium hydroxide (KOH) preparation, skin biopsy, or dermatophyte culture which should, in most cases, readily demonstrate the organism in tissue.

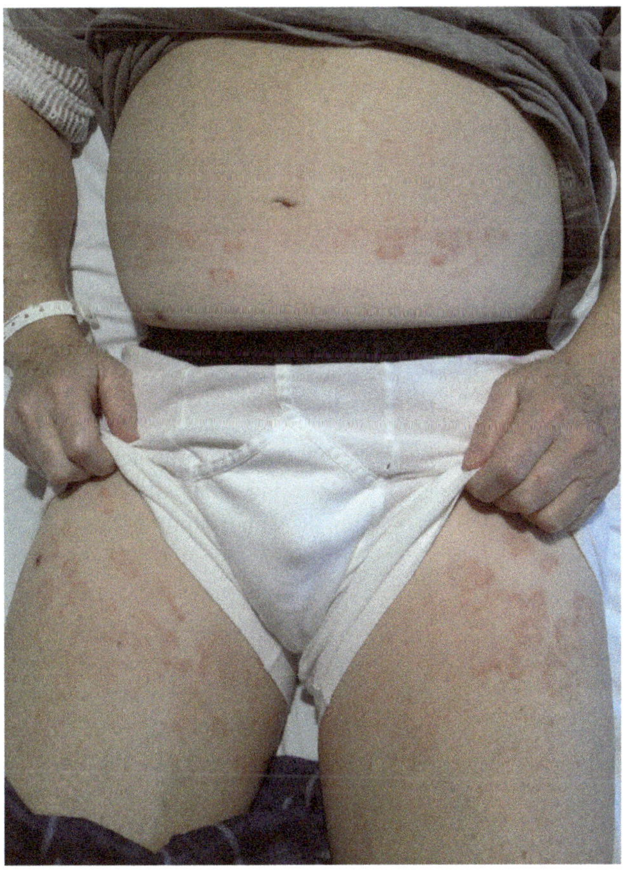

Fig. 22.20 Coalescing annular and arciform scaly pink papules and plaques of tinea corporis on the upper legs and abdomen of a stem cell transplant patient

Superficial dermatophytosis of the skin can be treated with a topical azole antifungal or terbinafine, which may be preferred due to its greater fungicidal activity [258]. Hair and nail infections require systemic antifungals; the same is true of cutaneous dermatophytosis with follicular papules or pustules, indurated papules or plaques, nodules, abscesses, or other signs of deep, invasive, or widespread infection. Oral terbinafine is the most potent systemic drug for dermatophytosis based on in vitro testing, followed by voriconazole, itraconazole, ketoconazole, and griseofulvin. Micafungin and caspofungin also have good activity [259]. Fluconazole has a mean MIC >6 [260]. Though it has excellent in vitro activity against dermatophytes, amphotericin B is ineffective in vivo because it is not secreted in sweat or sebum, and low tissue levels are achieved in the outer layers of the skin through passive diffusion [261].

Protozoa

Trypanosoma cruzi (Chagas disease) reactivation can occur with bone marrow transplantation, solid organ transplantation, and other immunosuppressed states [262]. If the indication for transplantation was Chagas cardiomyopathy, the risk of reactivation is roughly 30% within 3 months of cardiac transplantation [263, 264]. Chagas reactivation can result from transplant-related immunosuppression in a previously infected host. The organism can also be transmitted through an infected organ. Only the donor need have a history of travel to an endemic area. Fever, myocarditis, heart failure, and painful skin lesions are typical, including tender subcutaneous nodules or painful, erythematous, indurated plaques mimicking cellulitis [264–266].

Leishmaniasis in the transplant patient occurs at a median of 18 months after transplantation. It may represent primary infection, reactivation with immunosuppression, or acquisition from an infected organ [267]. Visceral leishmaniasis is the most common form of the disease associated with organ transplantation. Primary skin lesions acquired through the bite of the *Phlebotomus* or *Lutzomyia* sandfly are classically beefy ulcers which develop at the site of inoculation (Fig. 22.21). Skin lesions due to secondary dissemination are rare; they present as erythematous or brown macules and papules and may be the presenting sign of visceral disease.

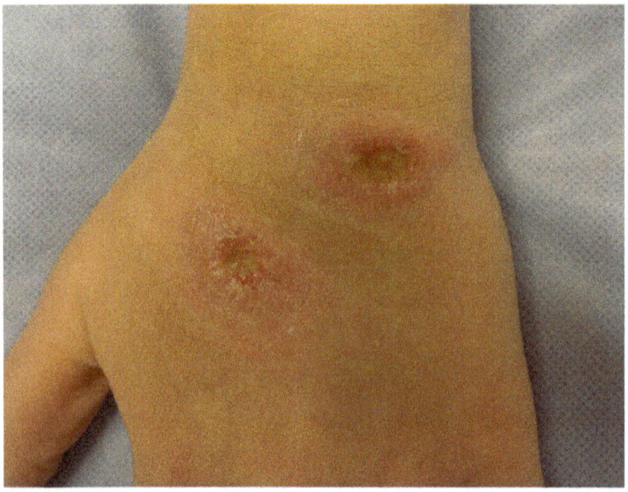

Fig. 22.21 Primary cutaneous leishmaniasis manifesting as beefy ulcerations on the dorsal hand

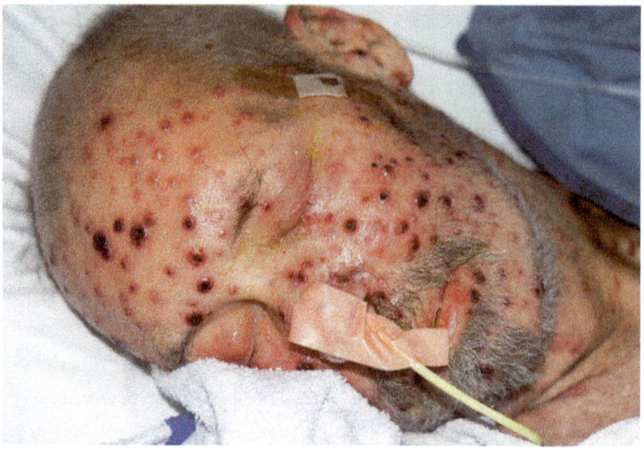

Fig. 22.22 A liver transplant patient with graft versus host disease developed innumerable erythematous papules and pustules with necrotic black crusts on the face, head, and neck. Skin biopsy demonstrated numerous *Acanthamoeba* trophozoites, and polymerase chain reaction testing was positive for *Acanthamoeba* species. (Image reprinted from Grossman et al. [288], Fig. 9.9, p. 198, with kind permission from Springer Nature)

Toxoplasmosis may also occur due to reactivation of past infection or de novo transition via a transplanted organ. Fever, central nervous system, and pulmonary symptoms are common, while cutaneous disease is not. When skin lesions develop, they may be disseminated erythematous papules resembling acute graft-versus-host disease [268–270].

Acanthamoeba may infect the sinuses or lungs and spread hematogenously to the skin, visceral organs, and brain, causing an almost universally fatal meningoencephalitis. Cutaneous lesions are often the presenting sign of disseminated disease. Numerous firm, purulent papulonodules develop into nonhealing, crusted ulcers (Fig. 22.22) [271, 272]. Amoebic trophozoites and cysts are readily seen on biopsy of these lesions, which is often necessary for diagnosis.

Helminths

Strongyloides stercoralis is native to parts of Asia, South America, and Africa, as well as the Southeastern United States [273]. Uniquely, the organism can complete its life cycle in one human host, persisting for years with minimal or no symptoms, sometimes far from the geographic region where it was required. During times of immunosuppression, a fulminant type of strongyloidiasis called hyperinfection syndrome may develop, wherein numerous larvae disseminate throughout the organs of the previously asymptomatic host. Defective cell-mediated immunity, as may occur in hematologic malignancy, organ transplantation, or during treatment for graft rejection or graft-versus-host disease, increases the risk [274, 275]. Organ transplantation confers an additional risk in that *Strongyloides* may be acquired from the organ itself; the concomitant immunosuppression can precipitate hyperinfection syndrome [276].

Complications of hyperinfection syndrome include persistent or recurrent Gram-negative or polymicrobial sepsis, pneumonia, or meningitis. As the larvae migrate across the intestinal wall, they bring enteric bacteria with them to sterile sites. Eosinophilia, abdominal pain, diarrhea or constipation, nausea, gastrointestinal bleeding, cough wheeze, hemoptysis, interstitial pulmonary infiltrates, and acute respiratory distress syndrome may develop. In patients requiring intubation, a dramatic cutaneous manifestation of *Strongyloides* hyperinfection may develop. Due to positive-pressure ventilation, portal venous pressure increases, shunting blood (and numerous larvae) through the periumbilical portal-systemic shunt and into the skin. Extravasation of larvae and red blood cells creates pathognomonic "thumbprint" purpura and innumerable fine petechiae on the abdomen, flanks, and thighs [277, 278]. Examination of bronchoalveolar lavage, stool, and skin biopsy specimens readily reveals the organism. Ivermectin, in addition to supportive care, is the treatment of choice.

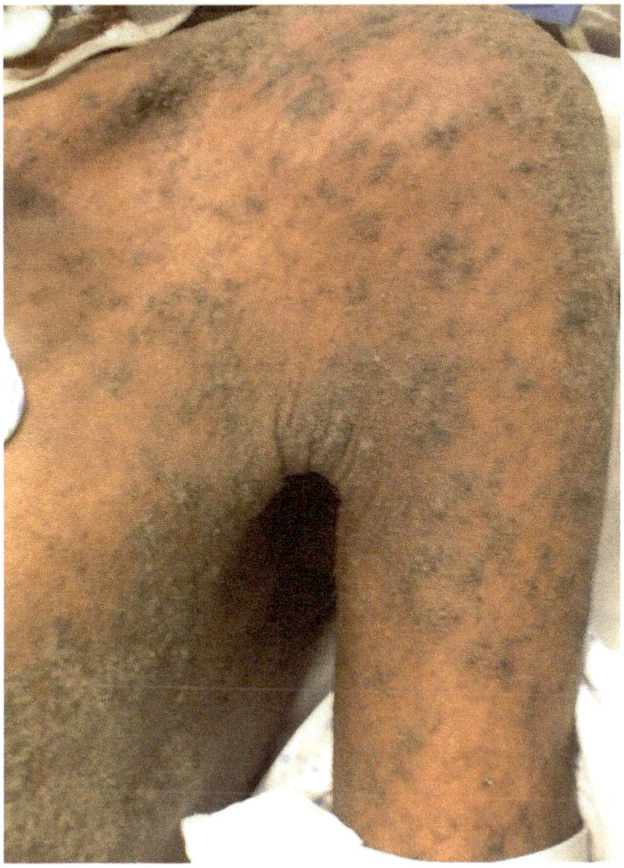

Fig. 22.23 Crusted scabies manifesting as widespread dry scale on most of the body, accentuated in body fold areas such as the finger webs and axillae

Scabies

Crusted scabies, a severe infestation with the scabies mite *Sarcoptes scabiei*, can occur in immunosuppressed patients, including those status post organ transplantation. Crusted scabies, previously called Norwegian scabies, is characterized by widespread thick, crusted, yellow-brown plaques with a predilection for the hands and feet, scalp, ears, groin, and axillae but the potential for involvement of the whole body surface (Fig. 22.23). The condition may be mistaken for severe seborrheic dermatitis or psoriasis [279]. Unlike scabies in a normal host, crusted scabies is paradoxically nonpruritic due to the absence of a normal inflammatory response. Exfoliated scale litters the environment of such patients with thousands of infectious fomites. Failure to diagnosis the condition in a hospitalized patient can therefore become a significant infection control problem.

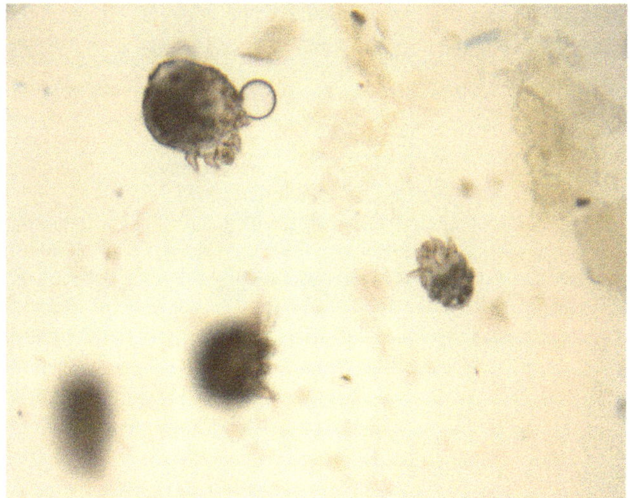

Fig. 22.24 A mineral oil preparation demonstrated numerous mites, ova, and feces

The diagnosis can be confirmed fairly easily due to the high mite burden with either a skin scraping or biopsy demonstrating mites, eggs, or feces (Fig. 22.24). Dual therapy with oral ivermectin and topical permethrin, precipitated sulfur, or other scabicide is required [280]. Repeated treatments and scrapings to demonstrate clearance are often necessary. Bacterial superinfection of the involved skin is a frequent complication that may lead to bacteremia and mortality in some patients [281–283].

Conclusion

In transplant patients, cutaneous infections run the full gamut—they may be common or rare, present typically or atypically, be localized or widespread on the skin, and affect the skin alone or portend widespread visceral dissemination. With this myriad of presentations, the clinician must at all times be alert and aware, maintain appropriate diagnostic suspicion, and note clues suggestive of systemic disease. There should be a low threshold for biopsy and culture of unusual lesions. An understanding of these principles and disease entities hastens diagnosis and the delivery of needed therapy to this vulnerable group (Table 22.1).

Table 22.1 Clinical presentations and complications of skin and soft tissue infections in transplant recipients

Organism	Common cutaneous presentations	Atypical presentations	Complications and prognosis
Gram-positive bacteria			
Staphylococcus	Impetigo, ecthyma, folliculitis/furunculosis, cellulitis	Staph-scalded skin syndrome, botryomycosis (verrucous plaque)	Sepsis, toxic shock
Streptococcus	Similar to staph; most common cause of cellulitis/erysipelas	Necrotizing fasciitis	Sepsis, toxic shock
Clostridium	Myonecrosis (mottled, dusky, crepitus)	Hemorrhagic bullae with numerous Gram-positive rods	Sepsis; 32–79% mortality
Bacillus	Mild food poisoning	Vesicle or pustule with ulceration and rapidly spreading cellulitis	Necrotizing fasciitis, endocarditis, brain abscess; beta-lactam resistance
Corynebacterium	Skin flora; rare cutaneous infection	Cellulitis; nontender subcutaneous nodules, red papules	Skin lesions in nearly half of those with *C. jeikeium* sepsis; 34% mortality
Nocardia	Nodule, abscess, or ulcer with lymphocutaneous spread	Subcutaneous nodules, pustules, pyomyositis	Primary and disseminated skin disease are indistinguishable; must rule out sepsis and CNS/lung infection
Gram-negative bacteria			
Escherichia coli	Abscess, perirectal phlegmon, rapidly progressive cellulitis, ecthyma gangrenosum	Acral hemorrhagic bullae +/− underlying cellulitis a sign of sepsis, malakoplakia perianal or urethral draining nodules	Ecthyma gangrenosum most common in intergluteal cleft; related sepsis with 10–38% mortality
Klebsiella, Enterobacter, Serratia	Similar to *E. coli*; rapidly progressive cellulitis	Acral hemorrhagic bullae, ecthyma gangrenosum, crepitant cellulitis, necrotizing fasciitis	Acral hemorrhagic bullae are a sign of sepsis
Salmonella	Rare cutaneous infection	Subcutaneous abscess, hemorrhagic cellulitis, necrotizing fasciitis	Bacteremia in the absence of GI infection portends a poor prognosis
Legionella	Rare cutaneous infection	Refractory or relapsing necrotizing cellulitis	*Legionella* skin infection typically occurs without concurrent pneumonia
Morganella	Rare cutaneous infection	Cellulitis with hemorrhagic bullae, crepitant gangrene, ecthyma gangrenosum	Increased in hematologic malignancy, neutropenia, chemotherapy
Helicobacter	Rare cutaneous infection	Large, multifocal cellulitic plaques with adjacent large joint arthritis; superficial thrombophlebitis described	Relapsing bacteremia with recurrent multifocal cellulitis; prolonged antibiotics required
Citrobacter	Rare cutaneous infection	Cellulitis and bilateral inflammatory erysipelas of the legs, ecthyma gangrenosum and hemorrhagic bullae	Increased in organ transplantation and hematologic malignancy
Pseudomonas	Hemorrhagic bullous cellulitis, ecthyma gangrenosum (gun metal gray, necrotic plaques)	Necrotizing cellulitis with systemic toxicity and fulminant course; subcutaneous nodules	Better prognosis for isolated ecthyma gangrenosum due to inoculation and not sepsis
Stenotrophomonas	Similar to *Pseudomonas*; necrotizing cellulitis, ecthyma gangrenosum	Metastatic nodules, multifocal cellulitic plaques with eventual necrosis/ulceration	Highly resistant with high mortality rate in immunocompromised patients
Aeromonas	Rapidly progressive necrotic cellulitis	Fasciitis, myonecrosis, ecthyma gangrenosum, multiple hemorrhagic bullae	Sepsis with extensive necrotizing fasciitis and septic shock
Vibrio	Rapidly progressive edema and cellulitis with hemorrhagic bullae	Necrotic ulcers, fasciitis, gangrene	Inoculation injury in seawater or dissemination from GI tract; sepsis with hypotension, shock, >50% mortality
Bartonella	Bacillary angiomatosis with single or multiple asymptomatic red-purple papules	Flesh-colored, subcutaneous nodules	Nonspecific constitutional symptoms, dissemination to multiple organs (skin, most common clinical manifestation)
Mycobacteria			
M. tuberculosis	Acute military TB: erythematous or brown macules and papules evolving to vesiculopustules	Subcutaneous nodules, ulcerating nodules, cellulitis mimic	Generalized wasting, fever, cough with disseminated disease
Nontuberculous mycobacteria	Violaceous subcutaneous nodules with sporotrichoid spread; tenosynovitis and arthritis with lesions overlying affected joints	Widespread nodules, sinus tracts, ulcers, abscesses, cellulitis	Speciation is essential to guide management

Table 22.1 (continued)

Organism	Common cutaneous presentations	Atypical presentations	Complications and prognosis
Viruses			
Herpes simplex	Vesicles or punched-out erosions; periorificial ulcer or crust with a scalloped/polycyclic border	Ulcers of the oral mucosa, herpetic geometric glossitis, linear fissures in body folds, exophytic granulation tissue (herpes vegetans), Kaposi varicelliform eruption	Dissemination with pneumonitis, hepatitis, pancreatitis, esophagitis, retinitis, encephalitis, adrenal necrosis
Varicella zoster	Dermatomal, disseminated	Zoster sine herpete, recurrent primary varicella, chronic hyperkeratotic crusted plaques and punched-out ulcers	Pneumonitis, meningoencephalitis, hepatitis; abdominal pain with hyponatremia and SIADH
Cytomegalovirus	Rare cutaneous infection	Chronic anogenital ulcers with sharp borders; can occur elsewhere on skin, oral mucosa; rare morbilliform exanthem	Gastrointestinal ulceration, hepatitis, pneumonitis, myelosuppression
Human herpes virus 6	Exanthem subitum in infants	Erythematous morbilliform exanthem similar to acute graft-versus-host disease	Fever, pneumonitis, bone marrow suppression, encephalitis
Human papillomavirus	Verrucous papules or plaques	Extensive, numerous, exuberant, recalcitrant; may become large, confluent	Warts develop in 80% of transplant patients; can be locally destructive
Molluscum contagiosum	Small white dome-shaped umbilicated papules	Giant molluscum: verrucous, lobulated nodules; viral folliculitis mimicking tinea barbae; recalcitrant and resistant, chronic	Differentiate from disseminated cryptococcosis and histoplasmosis, which can appear molluscoid
Subcutaneous and deep mycoses			
Aspergillus	Purpuric plaques with black or purple necrotic centers; sites of inoculation or dissemination, of which it may be a presenting sign	Erythematous to violaceous plaques with pustules, subcutaneous nodules, cellulitic plaques	Most common opportunistic fungal infection s/p SCT; consider aggressive surgical management of solitary lesions; high mortality in dissemination
Fusarium	Painful red macules or papules evolving into violaceous, necrotic pustules, ulcers, or eschars; inoculation or dissemination	Acral bullae, flaccid umbilicated pustules, sporotrichoid nodules, localized abscess	Widespread cutaneous lesions more common than in aspergillosis (75–90% vs 10%); sinopulmonary, fungemia; dissemination almost uniformly fatal
Scedosporium/Pseudallescheria	Ulcerated dusky nodules, tender pustules, necrotic bullae; inoculation or dissemination	Suppurative nodules with spread along cutaneous lymphatics	More than half present with disseminated disease; around 60% die; blood cultures frequently positive; *S. prolificans* almost uniformly resistant
Mucormycosis/ zygomycosis	Rhinocerebral disease most common; nasal discharge, black nasal mucosa, palatal infarction, necrotic facial lesions	Erythematous papule or plaque develops into purpuric, hemorrhagic ulcer or necrotic eschar; "bull's-eye infarct"	Rhinocerebral, pulmonary, GI, CNS, and disseminated disease; involved area may far exceed what is visible clinically; 80–100% mortality
Hyalohyphomycosis	Erythematous macules, necrotic, painful papules and nodules, vesiculopustules, cellulitis at portal of entry	Mycetoma with tumefaction and draining sinuses (*Acremonium*), onychomycosis with necrotic periungual cellulitis (*Scopulariopsis*)	*Fusarium, Paecilomyces, Acremonium, Trichoderma, Scopulariopsis, Trichosporon*; fungemia common and mortality high; high-level resistance
Phaeohyphomycosis	Inoculation injury with prolonged incubation period; nodule or abscess	Suppuration, sinus tract formation, ulceration; scaly/verrucous plaques; dissemination from the skin is rare	*Phialophora, Fonseca, Cladosporium, Exophiala, Alternaria, Scedosporium*; surgical debridement if possible
Candida	Local infection versus erythematous, purpuric papules with pale, necrotic, or pustular centers in disseminated disease	Subcutaneous nodules, folliculitis, and cellulitic plaques	Second most common fungal infection in SCT; skin lesions in 10% of dissemination; endophthalmitis, liver/ spleen infection; high mortality
Cryptococcus	Molluscum-like umbilicated or crusted papules, cellulitis, subcutaneous nodules, ulcers	Skin lesions can present months before signs of dissemination; isolated skin lesions rare; can get necrotizing cellulitis, fasciitis	Skin lesions in 10–15% with dissemination; meningeal/ craniobulbar signs plus skin lesions
Coccidioides	Reactive erythema nodosum	Verrucous or crusted papules, plaques, abscesses, cellulitis, ulcers	Fever, cough, sweats; skin, meningeal, bone, and joint disease

(continued)

Table 22.1 (continued)

Organism	Common cutaneous presentations	Atypical presentations	Complications and prognosis
Blastomyces	Annular plaque with atrophic center and verrucous edges, pustules, and lymphatic spread	Ulceration and pustulosis, disseminated papulopustules and subcutaneous nodules	Most blasto in immunocompetent; more severe (29–40% mortality) in immunosuppressed; bone, GU, CNS
Histoplasma	Reactive erythema nodosum; macules, papules, necrotic papules, pustules in dissemination	Morbilliform eruption, ulcers, panniculitis, cellulitis, verrucous or vegetative plaques	Fever, respiratory symptoms, weight loss, hepatosplenomegaly, bone marrow suppression
Sporothrix	Fixed cutaneous (20%) or lymphocutaneous (70%); painless ulcerated papule/nodule at inoculation site	Rare extracutaneous and disseminated disease; widely distributed ulcerated papules or plaques, crusted nodules, necrotic ulcers	Bone and joints most often involved in dissemination (80%); skin lesions usually a presenting sign
Superficial mycoses			
Trichophyton *Microsporum* *Epidermophyton*	Annular pruritic scaling plaques with serpiginous borders typical of tinea corporis	Erythematous or violaceous papules, pustules, nodules, deep abscesses, draining nodules, or ulcers; can mimic folliculitis, lupus, rosacea	Rare invasive infection occurs at sites of chronic superficial dermatophytosis
Protozoa			
Trypanosoma	Tender subcutaneous nodules	Painful erythematous, indurated plaques mimicking cellulitis	Reactivation with immunosuppression or transmission via infected organ
Leishmania	Beefy ulcers at inoculation site	Rare erythematous or brown macules and papules due to dissemination; may be a presenting sign of visceral disease	Reactivation or transmission via infected organ; visceral disease most common form in transplant patients
Toxoplasma	Rare cutaneous infection	Disseminated erythematous papules resembling acute graft versus host disease	Reactivation or transmission via infected organ; fever, CNS, lungs
Acanthamoeba	Rare cutaneous infection	Numerous firm, purulent papulonodules develop into nonhealing crusted ulcers	Sinuses, lungs; spread to skin, viscera, brain; fatal meningoencephalitis
Strongyloides	Larva currens (migratory pruritic serpiginous plaques)	Hyperinfection syndrome with pathognomonic thumbprint purpura on abdomen, flanks, thighs	Reactivation or transmission via infected organ; pulmonary infiltrates, diarrhea, polymicrobial sepsis
Infestations			
Crusted scabies	Widespread thick, crusted, yellow-brown plaques with predilection for body folds	May mimic severe seborrheic dermatitis or psoriasis; can result in erythroderma, involvement of whole body surface	Bacterial superinfection can occur; highly contagious, significant infection control issue

References

1. Nguyen V, Huggins RH, Lertsburapa T, et al. Cutaneous T-cell lymphoma and Staphylococcus aureus colonization. J Am Acad Dermatol. 2008;59(6):949–52.
2. Castano-Molina C, Cockerell CJ. Diagnosis and treatment of infectious diseases in HIV-infected hosts. Dermatol Clin. 1997;15:267–83.
3. Grossman ME, Fox LP, Kovarik C, Rosenbach M. Cutaneous manifestations of infection in the immunocompromised host. 2nd ed. New York: Springer; 2012. 309 pages.
4. Eilers RE Jr, Gandhi M, Patel JD, et al. Dermatologic infections in cancer patients treated with epidermal growth factor receptor inhibitor therapy. J Natl Cancer Inst. 2010;102(1):47–53.
5. Strauss G, Mogensen AM, Rasmussen A, Kirkegaard P. Staphlococcal scalded skin syndrome in a liver transplant patient. Liver Transpl Surg. 1997;3(4):435–6.
6. Ito Y, Funabashi YM, Toda K, et al. Staphlococcal scalded-skin syndrome in an adult due to methicillin-resistant Staphylococcal aureus. J Infect Chemother. 2002;8(3):256–61.
7. Norcross MC Jr, Mitchell DF. Blistering distal dactylitis caused by Staphylococcus aureus. Cutis. 1993;51:353–4.
8. Hewitt WD, Farrar WE. Bacteremia and ecthyma caused by Streptococcus pyogenes in a patient with acquired immunodeficiency syndrome. Am J Med Sci. 1998;295(1):52–4.
9. Cupps TR, Cotton DJ, Schooley RT, Faugi AS. Facial erysipelas in the immunocompormised host. Report of two cases. Arch Dermatol. 1981;117(1):47–9.
10. Sendi P, Johansson L, Norrby-Teglund A. Invasive group B Streptococcal disease in non-pregnant adults: a review with emphasis on skin and soft-tissue infections. Inf Dent. 2008;36(2):100–11.
11. Jansen F, Zelinsky-Gurung A, Caumes E, Decazes JM. Group A streptococcal cellulitis-adenitis in a patient with acquired immunodeficiency syndrome. J Am Acad Dermatol. 1991;24:363–5.
12. Parada JP, Maslow JN. Clinical syndromes associated with adult pneumococcal cellulitis. Scand J Infect Dis. 2000;32(2):133–6.
13. Lawlor MT, Crowe HM, Quintiliani R. Cellulitis due to Streptococcus pneumonia: case report and review. Clin Infect Dis. 1992;14(1):247–50.
14. Burke MP, Opeskin K. Nontraumatic clostridial myonecrosis. Am J Forensic Med Pathol. 1999;20(2):158–62.
15. Smith-Slatas CL, Bourque M, Salazar JC. Clostridium septicum infections in children: a case report and review of the literature. Pediatrics. 2006;117(4):e796–805.

16. Henrickson KJ, Shenep JL, Flynn PM, Pui CH. Primary cutaneous Bacillus cereus infection in neutropenic children. Lancet. 1989;1(8638):601–3.
17. Mori T, Tokuhira M, Takae Y, et al. Successful non-surgical treatment of brain abscess and necrotizing fasciitis caused by Bacillus cereus. Intern Med. 2002;41(8):671–3.
18. Cone LA, Dreisbach L, Potts BE, et al. Fatal Bacillus cereus endocarditis masquerading as an anthrax-like infection in a patient with acute lymphoblastic leukemia: case report. J Heart Valve Dis. 2005;14(1):37–9.
19. Jerdan MS, Shapiro RS, Smith NB, et al. Cutaneous manifestations of Corynebacterium group JK sepsis. J Am Acad Dermatol. 1987;162:444–7.
20. Wan der Lelie H, Leverstein-Van Hall M, Mertens M, et al. Corynebacterium CDC group JK sepsis in hematological patients: a report of three cases and a systematic literature review. Scand J Infect Dis. 1995;27(6):581–4.
21. Guarino MJ, Qazi R, Woll JE, Rubins J. Septicemia, rash, and pulmonary infiltrates secondary to Corynebacterium group JK infection. Am J Med. 1987;82(1):132–4.
22. van der Lelie H, Leverstein-Van Hall M, Mertens M, et al. Corynebacterium CDC Group JK (Corynebacterium jeikeium) sepsis in haematological patients: a report of three cases and a systematic literature review. Scand J Infect Dis. 1995;27(6):581–4.
23. Ambrosioni J, Lew D, Garbino J. Nocardiosis: updated clinical review and experience at a tertiary center. Infection. 2010;38(2):89–97.
24. Peleg AY, Husain S, Qureshi ZA, et al. Risk factors, clinical characteristics, and outcome of Nocardia infection in organ transplant recipients: a matched case-control study. Clin Infect Dis. 2007;44(10):1307–14.
25. Moeller CA, Burton CS III. Primary lymphocutaneous Nocardia brasiliensis infection. Arch Dermatol. 1986;122(10):1180–2.
26. Nishimoto K, Ohno M. Subcutaneous abscesses caused by Nocardia brasiliensis complicated by malignant lymphoma. A survey of cutaneous nocardiosis reported in Japan. Int J Dermatol. 1985;24(7):437–40.
27. Boixeda P, Espana A, Suarez J, et al. Cutaneous nocardiosis and human immunodeficiency virus infection. Int J Dermatol. 1991;30(11):804–5.
28. Case records of the Massachusetts General Hospital. Weekly clinicopathological exercises. Case 29-2000. A 69-year-old renal transplant recipient with low grade fever and multiple pulmonary nodules. N Engl J Med. 2000;343(12):870–7.
29. Freites V, Sumoza A, Bisotti R, et al. Subcutaneous Nocardia asteroides abscess in a bone marrow transplant recipient. Bone Marrow Transplant. 1995;15(1):135–6.
30. Parra IH, Galimberti R, Galimberti G, et al. Lymphocutaneous nocardiosis and cutaneous pheohyphomycosis in a liver transplant recipient. Int J Dermatol. 2008;47(6):571–4.
31. Stamenkovic SA, Madden BP. Nocardia asteroids abscess after heart transplantation. J Heart Lung Transplant. 2001;20(7):789–91.
32. Kalb RE, Kaplan MH, Grossman ME. Cutaneous nocardiosis. Case reports and review. J Am Acad Dermatol. 1985;13(1):125–33.
33. Paterson DL, Gruttadauria S, Lauro A, et al. Spontaneous gram-negative cellulitis in a liver transplant recipient. Infection. 2001;29(6):345–7.
34. Reich HL, Fadeyi DW, Naik NS, et al. Nonpseudomonal ecthyma gangrenosum. J Am Acad Dermatol. 2004;50(5):114–7.
35. Patel JK, Perez OA, Viera MH, et al. Ecthyma gangrenosum caused by Escherichia coli bacteremia: a case report and review of the literature. Cutis. 2009;84:261–7.
36. Elmariah SB, Ubriani R, James WD, et al. Ecthyma gangrenosum. Available at http://www.emedicine.com/derm/topic539.htm. Accessed on 24 May 2007.
37. Hansen EA, Cunha BA. Escherichia coli chest-wall hemorrhagic cellulitis associated with central-line placement. Heart Lung. 2000;29(6):450–2.
38. Fisher K, Berger BW, Keusch GT. Subepidermal bullae secondary to Escherichia coli septicemia. Arch Dermatol. 1974;110(1):105–6.
39. Wittenberg PG, Douglass MC, Azm M, et al. Cutaneous malacoplakia in a patient with the acquired immunodeficiency syndrome. Arch Dermatol. 1998;134(2):244–5.
40. Palou J, Torras H, Baradad M, et al. Cutaneous malakoplakia. Report of a case. Dermatologica. 1988;176(6):288–92.
41. Bonner MJ, Meharg JG Jr. Primary cellulitis due to Serratia marcescens. JAMA. 1983;250(17):2348–9.
42. Rodot S, Lacour JP, van Elslande L, et al. Ecthyma gangrenosum caused by Klebsiella pneumoniae. Int J Dermatol. 1995;34(3):216–7.
43. Gunnarsson GL, Brandt PB, Gad D, et al. Monomicrobial necrotizing fasciitis in a white male caused by hypermucoviscous Klebsiella pneumoniae. J Med Microbiol. 2009;58(Pt 11):1519–21.
44. DiGioia RA, Kane JG, Parker RH. Crepitant cellulitis and myonecrosis caused by Klebsiella. JAMA. 1977;237(19):2097–8.
45. Napgezek MR, Hall WH. Nonclostridial crepitant cellulitis due to Klebsiella. Minn Med. 1975;58(5):377–8.
46. Bachmeyer C, Sanguina M, Turc Y, et al. Necrotizing fasciitis due to Serratia marcescens. Clin Exp Dermatol. 2004;29(6):673–4.
47. Livingston W, Grossman ME, Garvey G. Hemorrhagic bullae in association with Enterobacter cloacae septicemia. J Am Acad Dermatol. 1992;27:637–8.
48. Andriessen MJ, Kotsopoulos AM, Bloemers FW, et al. Necrotizing fasciitis caused by Salmonella enteritidis. Scand J Infect Dis. 2006;38(11–12):1106–7.
49. Gordon MA. Salmonella infections in immunocompromised adults. J Infect. 2008;56(6):413–22.
50. Kilborn JA, Manz LA, O'Brien M, et al. Necrotizing cellulitis caused by Legionella micdadei. Am J Med. 1992;92(1):104–6.
51. Bagel J, Grossman ME. Hemorrhagic bullae associated with Morganella morganii septicemia. J Am Acad Dermatol. 1985;12(3):575–6.
52. Lobo I, Pinto A, Ferreira M, et al. Non-pseudomonal ecthyma gangrenosum present in diclofenac-induced agranulocytosis. Eur J Dermatol. 2008;18(3):350–1.
53. Minauchi K, Takahashi S, Sakai T, et al. The nosocomial transmission of Helicobacter cinaedi infections in immunocompromised patients. Intern Med. 2010;49(16):1733–9. Epub 2010 Aug 13.
54. Sullican AK, Nelson MR, Walsh J, Gazzard BG. Recurrent Helicobacter cinaedi cellulitis and bacteremia in a patient with HIV infection. Int J STD AIDS. 1997;8(1):59–60.
55. Van der Ven AJ, Kullberg BJ, Vandamme P, Meis JF. Helicobacter cinaedi bacteremia associated with localized pain but no with cellulitis. Clin Infect Dis. 1996;22(4):710–1.
56. Schlossberg D, Ricci JA, Fugate JS. Dermatologic manifestations of citrobacter septicemia. J Am Acad Dermatol. 1982;5(5):613–5.
57. Grant MD, Horowitz HI, Lorian V. Gangrenous ulcer and septicemia due to citrobacter. N Engl J Med. 1969;280(23):1286–7.
58. Collini FJ, Spees EK, Munster A, et al. Ecthyma gangrenosum in a kidney transplant recipient with Pseudomonas septicemia. Am J Med. 1986;80(4):729–34.
59. Huminer D, Siegman-Igra Y, Morduchowicz G, Pitlik SD. Ecthyma gangrenosum without bacteremia. Report of six cases and review of the literature. Arch Intern Med. 1987;147(2):299–301.
60. Kusne S, Eibling DE, Yu VL, et al. Gangrenous cellulitis associated with gram-negative bacilli in pancytopenic patients: dilemma with respect to effective therapy. Am J Med. 1988;85(4):490–4.
61. Falagas ME, Pappas VD, Michalopoulos A. Gangrenous, hemorrhagic, bullous cellulitis associated with Pseudomonas aeruginosa in a patient with Waldenstrom's macroglobulinemia. Infection. 2007;35(5):370–3.

62. Bourelly PE. Grossman. Subcutaneous nodule as a manifestation of Pseudomonas sepsis in an immunocompromised host. Clin Infect Dis. 1998;26(1):188–9.
63. Bagel J, Grossman ME. Subcutaneous nodules in Pseudomonas sepsis. Am J Med. 1986;80(3):528–9.
64. Safdar A, Rolston KV. Stenotrophomonas maltophilia: changing spectrum of a serious bacterial pathogen in patients with cancer. Clin Infect Dis. 2007;45(12):1602–9.
65. Teo WY, Chan MY, Lam CM, Chong CY. Skin manifestations of Stenotrophomonas maltophilia infection—a case report and review article. Ann Acad Med Singap. 2006;35(12):897–900.
66. Moser C, Jonsson V, Thomsen K, et al. Subcutaneous lesions and bacteremia due to Stenotrophomonas maltophila in three leukaemic patients with neutropenia. Br J Dermatol. 1997;136(6):949–52.
67. Smeets JG, Lowe SH, Veraart JC. Cutaneous infections with Stenotrophomonas maltophila in patients using immunosuppressive medication. J Eur Acad Dermatol Venereol. 2007;21(9):1298–300.
68. Vartivarian SE, Papadakis KA, Palacious JA, et al. Mucocutaneous and soft tissue infections caused by Xanthomas maltophila. A new spectrum. Ann Intern Med. 1994;121(12):969–73.
69. WC KO, Chuang YC. Aeromonas bacteremia: review of 59 episodes. Clin Infect Dis. 1995;20(5):1298–3034.
70. Cui H, Hao S, Arous E. A distinct cause of necrotizing fasciitis: Aeromonas veronii biovar sobria. Surg Infect. 2007;8(5):523–8.
71. Thodis E, Kriki P, Kakagia D, et al. Rigorous Vibrio vulnificus soft tissue infections of the lower leg in a renal transplant patient managed by vacuum therapy and autologous growth factors. J Cutan Med Surg. 2009;13(4):209–14.
72. Kuhnt-Lenz K, Krengel S, Fetcher S, et al. Sepsis with bullous necrotizing skin lesions due to vibrio vulnificus acquired through recreational activities in the Baltic Sea. Eur J Clin Microbiol Infect Dis. 2004;23(1):49–52.
73. Payinda G. Necrotizing fasciitis due to Vibrio parahaemolyticus. N Z Med J. 2008;121(1283):99–101.
74. Lee CC, Tong KL, Howe HS, Lam MS. Vibrio vulnificus infections: case reports and literature review. Ann Acad Med Singap. 1997;26(5):705–12.
75. Iwata Y, Sato S, Murase Y, et al. Five cases of necrotizing fasciitis: lack of skin inflammatory signs as a clinical clue for the fulminant type. J Dermatol. 2008;35(11):719–25.
76. Kuo Chou TN, Chao WN, Yang C, et al. Predictors of mortality in skin and soft-tissue infections caused by Vibrio vulnificus. World J Surg. 2010;34(7):1669–75.
77. Bonatti H, Mendez J, Guerrero I, et al. Disseminated Bartonella infection following liver transplantation. Transpl Int. 2006;19(8):683–7.
78. Chian CA, Arrese JE, Pierard GE. Skin manifestations of Bartonella infections. Int J Dermatol. 2002;41(8):461–6.
79. Spach DH. Bacillary angiomatosis. Int J Dermatol. 1992;31(1):19–24.
80. Friedman PC, Husain S, Grossman ME. Nodular tuberculid in a patient with HIV. J Am Acad Dermatol. 2005;53:S154–6.
81. Park KW, Kim US, Shin JW, et al. Disseminated erythematous papules in a renal transplant recipient: a case of disseminated tuberculosis. Scand J Infect Dis. 2002;34:775–7.
82. Seyahi N, Apaydin S, Kahveci A, et al. Cellulitis as a manifestation of miliary tuberculosis in a renal transplant recipient. Transpl Infect Dis. 2005;7:80–5.
83. Caroti L, Zanazzi M, Rogasi P, et al. Subbcutaneous nodules and infectious complications in renal allograft recipients. Transplant Proc. 2010;42(4):1146–7.
84. Ram R, Uppin S, Swarnalatha G, et al. Isolated skin ulcers due to Mycobacterium tuberculosis in a renal allograft recipient. Nephrology. 2007;3:688–92.
85. Falkinham JO. Nontuberculous mycobacteria in the environment. Clin Chest Med. 2002;23:529–51.
86. Pandian TK, Deziel PJ, Otley CC, et al. Mycobacterium marinum infections in transplant recipients: case report and review of the literature. Transpl Infect Dis. 2008;10:358–63.
87. Farooqui MA, Berenson C, Lohr JW. Mycobacterium marinum infection in a renal transplant recipient. Transplantation. 1999;67:1495–6.
88. Gombert ME, Goldstein EJ, Corrado ML, et al. Disseminated Mycobacterium marinum infection after renal transplantation. Ann Intern Med. 1981;94:486–7.
89. Wolfson JS, Sober AJ, Rubin RH. Dermatologic manifestations of infections in immunocompromised patients. Medicine (Baltimore). 1985;64:115.
90. Lovric S, Becker JU, Kayser D, et al. Fish, flesh and a good red herring: a case of ascending upper limb infection in a renal transplant patient. Clin Nephrol. 2009;72:402–4.
91. Patel R, Roberts GD, Keating MR, Paya CV. Infections due to nontuberculous mycobacteria in kidney, heart, and liver transplant recipients. Clin Infect Dis. 1993;19:263–73.
92. Lederman C, Spitz JL, Scully B, et al. M. haemophilum cellulitis in a heart transplant recipient. J Am Acad Dermatol. 1994;30:804–6.
93. Doucette K, Fishman JA. Nontuberculous mycobacterial infection in hematopoietic stem cell and solid organ transplant patients. Clin Infect Dis. 2004;38:1428–39.
94. Toback AL, Grossman ME. Chronic intraoral herpes simplex infection in renal transplant recipients. Transplant Proc. 1986;18:966–9.
95. Grossman ME, Stevens AW, Cohen PR. Herpetic geometric glossitis. N Engl J Med. 1993;329:1859–60.
96. Cohen PR, Kazi S, Grossman ME. Herpetic geometric glossitis: a distinctive pattern of lingual herpes simplex virus infection. South Med J. 1995;88:1231–5.
97. Tong P, Mutasim DF. Herpes simplex virus infection masquerading as condyloma acuminate in a patient with HIV disease. Br J Dermatol. 1996;134:797–800.
98. SR N, Calore EE, Manzione CR, et al. Hypertrophic herpes simplex simulating anal neoplasia in AIDS patients: report of five cases. Dis Colon Rectum. 2005;48(12):2289–93.
99. Lieb JA, Brisman S, Herman S, et al. Linear erosive herpes simplex virus infection in immunocompromised patients: the "knifecut sign". Clin Infect Dis. 2008;47:1440–1.
100. Mahmood K, Afzal S. Ulcerating lesions on forearm, fingertips, and tongue in a liver-transplant recipient. Clin Exp Dermatol. 2007;33:91–3.
101. Basse G, Mengelle C, Kamar N, et al. Disseminated herpes simplex type-2 (HSV-2) infection after solid-organ transplantation. Infection. 2008;36:62–4.
102. Dinotta F, De Pasquale R, Nasca MR, et al. Disseminated herpes simplex infection in a HIV+ patient. G Ital Dermatol Venereol. 2009;144:205–9.
103. Arkin LM, Castelo-Soccio L, Kovarik C. Disseminated herpes simplex virus (HSV) hepatitis diagnosed by dermatology evaluation. Int J Dermatol. 2009;48:1017–29.
104. Sevilla J, Fernandez-Plaza S, Gonzalez-Vincent M, et al. Fatal hepatic failure secondary to acute herpes simplex virus infection. J Pediatr Hematol Oncol. 2004;26:686–8.
105. Masessa JM, Grossman ME, Knobler EH, Bank DE. Kaposi's varicelliform eruption in cutaneous t-cell lymphoma. J Am Acad Dermatol. 1989;21(1):133–5.
106. Castelo-Soccio L, Bernardin R, Stern J, et al. Successful treatment of acyclovir-resistant herpes simplex virus with intralesional cidofovir. Arch Dermatol. 2010;146(2):124–6.
107. Sims CR, Thompson K, Chemaly RF, et al. Oral topical cidofovir: novel route of drug delivery in a severely immunosuppressed patient with refractory multidrug-resistant herpes simplex virus infection. Transpl Infect Dis. 2007;9(3):256–9.

108. Bacon TH, Levin MJ, Leary JJ, et al. Herpes simplex virus resistance to acyclovir and penciclovir after two decade of antiviral therapy. Clin Microbiol Rev. 2003;16:114–28.
109. Rau R, Fitzhugh CD, Baird K, et al. Triad of severe abdominal pain, inappropriate antidiuretic hormone secretion, and disseminated varicella-zoster infection preceding cutaneous manifestations after hematopoietic stem cell transplantation: utility of PCR for early recognition and therapy. Pediatr Infect Dis J. 2008;27(3):265–8.
110. Au WY, Ma SY, Cheng VC, et al. Disseminated zoster, hyponatremia, severe abdominal pain and leukemia relapse: recognition of a new clinical quartet after bone marrow transplantation. Br J Dermatol. 2003;149:862–5.
111. David DS, Tegtmeier BR, O'Donnell MR, et al. Visceral varicella-zoster after bone marrow transplantation: report of a case series and review of the literature. Am J Gastroenterol. 1998;93:810–3.
112. Nikkels AF, Simonart T, Kentos A, et al. Atypical recurrent varicella in 4 patients with hemopathies. J Am Acad Dermatol. 2003;188(7):948–53.
113. Baxter JD, DiNubile MJ. Relapsing chickenpox in a young man with non-Hodgkin's lymphoma. Clin Infect Dis. 1994;18:785–8.
114. Jeyaratnam D, Robson AM, Hextall JM, et al. Concurrent verrucous and varicelliform rashes following renal transplantation. Am J Transplant. 2005;5:1777–80.
115. Gallagher JG, Merigan TC. Prolonged herpes-zoster infection associated with immunosuppressive therapy. Ann Intern Med. 1979;91(6):842–6.
116. Kaisar MO, Kirwan RM, Strutton GM, et al. Cutaneous manifestations of cytomegalovirus disease in renal transplant recipients: a case series. Transpl Infect Dis. 2008;10:209–13.
117. Lee JY. Cytomegalovirus infection involving the skin in immunocompromised hosts. Am J Clin Pathol. 1989;92:96–100.
118. Colsky AS, Jegasothy SM, Leonardi C, et al. Diagnosis and treatment of a case of cutaneous cytomegalovirus infection with a dramatic clinical presentation. J Am Acad Dermatol. 1998;38:349–51.
119. Trimarchi H, Casas G, Jordan R, et al. Cytomegalovirus maculopapular eruption in a kidney transplant patient. Transpl Infect Dis. 2001;3(1):47–50.
120. Rees AP, Meadors M, Ventura HO, Pankey GA. Diagnosis of disseminated cytomegalovirus infection and pneumonitis in a heart transplant recipient by skin biopsy: case report. J Heart Lung Transplant. 1991;10:329–32.
121. Konstadt JW, Gatusso P, Eng A, et al. Disseminated cytomegalovirus infection with cutaneous involvement in a heart transplant patient. Clin Cases Dermatol. 1990;2:3.
122. Curtis JL, Egbert BM. Cutaneous cytomegalovirus vasculitis: an unusual presentation of a common opportunistic pathogen. Hum Pathol. 1982;13:1138–41.
123. Golden MP, Hammer SM, Wanke CA, Albrecht MA. Cytomegalovirus vasculitis. Medicine (Baltimore). 1994;73:246–55.
124. Ljungman P, Singh N. Human herpesvirus-g infection in solid organ and stem cell transplant recipients. J Clin Virol. 2006;37:S87–91.
125. Razonable RR, Zerr DM, AST Infectious Diseases Community of Practice. HHV-6, HHV-7 and HHV-8 in solid organ transplant recipients. Am J Transplant. 2009;9:S97–100.
126. Yoshikawa T, Goshima F, Akimoto S, et al. Human herpesvirus 6 infection of human epidermal cell line: pathogenesis of skin manifestation. J Med Virol. 2003;71:62–8.
127. Dharancy S, Catteau B, Mortier L, et al. Conversion to sirolimus: a useful strategy for recalcitrant cutaneous viral warts in liver transplant recipient. Liver Transpl. 2006;12(12):1883–7.
128. Mansur AT, Goktay F, Gunduz S, Serdar ZA. Multiple giant molluscum contagiosum in a renal transplant recipient. Transpl Infect Dis. 2004;6:120–3.
129. Feldmeyer L, Kamarashev J, Boehler A, et al. Molluscum contagiosum folliculitis mimicking tinea barbae in a lung transplant recipient. J Am Acad Dermatol. 2010;63(1):169–71.
130. Groll AH, Shah PM, Mentzel C, et al. Trends in postmortem epidemiology of invasive fungal infections at a university hospital. J Infect. 1996;33:23–32.
131. Nucci M, Marr KA. Emerging fungal diseases. Clin Infect Dis. 2005;41:521–6.
132. Nenoff P, Kliem C, Mittag M, et al. Secondary cutaneous aspergillosis due to Aspergillus flavus in an acute myeloid leukaemia patient following stem cell transplantation. Eur J Dermatol. 2002;12:93–8.
133. Munn S, Keane F, Child F, et al. Primary cutaneous aspergillosis. Br J Dermatol. 1999;141:378–80.
134. Ricci RM, Evans JS, Meffert JJ, et al. Primary cutaneous Aspergillus ustus infection: second reported case. J Am Acad Dermatol. 1998;38:797–8.
135. Chakrabarti A, Gupta V, Biswas G, et al. Primary cutaneous aspergillosis: our experience in 10 years. J infect. 1998;37:24–7.
136. Park SB, Kang MJ, Whang EA, et al. A case of primary cutaneous aspergillosis in a renal transplant recipient. Transplant Proc. 2004;36:2156–7.
137. Mori T, Takae Y, Izaki S, et al. Cutaneous aspergillosis in a patient with follicular lymphoma. Eur J Dermatol. 2003;13:102–3.
138. Szyfelbein K, Lin JY, Bellucci KS, Williams JM. Tender erythema of the left lower extremity. Disseminated Aspergillus fumigatus infection with concurrent active cytomegalovirus infection (CMV). Arch Dermatol. 2007;143:535–40.
139. Grossman ME, Fithian EC, Behrens C, et al. Primary cutaneous aspergillosis in six leukemic children. J Am Acad Dermatol. 1985;12:313–8.
140. Schimmelpfennig C, Naumann R, Zuberbier T, et al. Skin involvement as the first manifestation of systemic aspergillosis in patients after allogeneic hematopoietic cell transplantation. Bone Marrow Transplant. 2001;27:753–5.
141. Polk C, Forrest G, Cross A. Cellulitis in a patient with leukemia. Clin Infect Dis. 2007;44:1240–50.
142. Child FJ, Fuller LC, Higgins EM, et al. Cutaneous presentation of Fusarium solani infection in a bone marrow transplant recipient. J R Soc Med. 1996;89:647–8.
143. Bigley VH, Duarte RF, Gosling RD, et al. Fusarium dimerum infection in a stem cell transplant recipient treated successfully with voriconazole. Bone Marrow Transplant. 2004;34:815–7.
144. Nucci M, Anaissie E. Cutaneous infection by Fusarium species in healthy and immunocompromised hosts: implications for diagnosis and management. Clin Infect Dis. 2002;35:909–19.
145. Bordeaux JS, O'Brien M, Mahalingam M, Wiss K. Clinicopathologic challenge. Int J Dermatol. 2008;47:13–4.
146. Bodey GP, Boktour M, Mays S, et al. Skin lesions associated with Fusarium infection. J Am Acad Dermatol. 2002;437:659–66.
147. Cocuroccia B, Gaido J, Gubinelli E, et al. Localized cutaneous hyalohyphomycosis caused by Fusarium species infection in a renal transplant patient. J Clin Microbiol. 2003;41:905–7.
148. Garder JM, Nelson MM, Hefferman MP. Chronic cutaneous fusariosis. Arch Dermatol. 2005;141:794–5.
149. Nucci M, Anaissie EJ, Queiroz-Telles F, et al. Outcome predictors of 84 patients with hematologic malignancies and Fusarium infection. Cancer. 2003;98:315–9.
150. Husain S, Munoz P, Forrest G, et al. Infections due to Scedosporium apiospermum and Scedosporium prolificans in transplant recipients: clinical characteristics and impact of antifungal agent therapy on outcome. Clin Infect Dis. 2005;40(1):89–99.
151. Cortez KJ, Roilides E, Quiroz-Telles F, et al. Infections caused by Scedosporium spp. Clin Microbiol Rev. 2008;21(1):157–97.

152. Bernstein EF, Schuster MG, Stieritz DD, et al. Disseminated cutaneous Pseudallescheria boydii. Br J Dermatol. 1995;132(3):456–60.
153. Bower CP, Oxley JD, Campbell CK, Archer CB. Cutaneous Scedosporium apiospermum infection in an immunocompromised patient. J Clin Pathol. 1999;52(11):846–8.
154. Castiglioni B, Sutton DA, Rinaldi MG, et al. Pseudallescheria boydii (Anamorph Scedosporium apiospermum). Infection in solid organ transplant recipients in a tertiary medical center and review of the literature. Medicine (Baltimore). 2002;91(5):333–48.
155. Shinohara MM, George E. Scedosporium apiospermum an emerging opportunistic pathogen that must be distinguished from Aspergillus and other hyalohyphomycetes. J Cutan Pathol. 2009;36(S1):39–41.
156. Kusuhara M, Hachisuka H. Lymphocutaneous infection due to Scedosporium apiospermum. Int J Dermatol. 1997;36(9):684–8.
157. Ruxin TA, Steck WD, Helm TN, et al. Pseudallescheria boydii in an immunocompromised host. Successful treatment with debridement and itraconazole. Arch Dermatol. 1996;132(4):382–4.
158. Hagari Y, Ishioka S, Ohyama F, Mihara M. Cutaneous infection showing sporotrichoid spread caused by Pseudallescheria boydii (Scedosporium apiospermum): successful detection of fungal DNA in formalin-fixed, paraffin-embedded sections by seminested PCR. Arch Dermatol. 2002;138(2):271–2.
159. Torok L, Simon G, Csornai A, et al. Scedosporium apiospermum infection imitating lymphocutaneous sporotrichosis in a patient with myeloblastic-monocytic leukaemia. Br J Dermatol. 1995;133(5):805–9.
160. Revanker SG, Patterson JE, Sutton DA, et al. Disseminated phaeohyphomycosis: review of an emerging mycosis. Clin Infect Dis. 2002;34:467–76.
161. Berenguer J, Rodriquez-Tudela JL, Richard C, et al. Deep infections caused by Scedosporium prolificans. A report of 16 cases in Spain and a review of the literature. Scedosporium prolificans Spanish Study Group. Medicine (Baltimore). 1997;76(4):256–65.
162. Moraru RA, Grossman ME. Palatal necrosis in an AIDS patient: a case of mucormycosis. Cutis. 2000;66(1):15–8.
163. Sanchez MR, Pnge-Wilson I, Moy JA, Rosenthal S. Zygomycosis and HIV infection. J Am Acad Dermatol. 1994;30:904–8.
164. Samant JS, Namgoong SH, Parveen T, Katner HP. Cytomegalovirus vasculitis and mucormycosis coinfection in late-stage HIV/AIDS. Am J Med Sci. 2007;333(2):122–4.
165. Micheletti R, Rosenbach M. A violaceous plaque in an immunosuppressed patient. JAMA. 2012;307(24):2635–6.
166. Barnes PD, Marr KA. Risks, diagnosis and outcomes of invasive fungal infections in haematopoietic stem cell transplant recipients. Br J Haematol. 2007;139(4):519–31.
167. Trifilio SM, Bennett CL, Yarnold PR, et al. Breakthrough zygomycosis after voriconazole administration among patients with hematologic malignancies who receive hematopoietic stem-cell transplants or intensive chemotherapy. Bone Marrow Transplant. 2007;39(7):425–9.
168. Mantadakis E, Samonis G. Clinical presentation of zygomycosis. Clin Microbiol Infect. 2009;15(S5):15–20.
169. Takabayashi M, Sakai R, Sakamoto H, et al. Cutaneous mucormycosis during induction chemotherapy for acute lymphocytic leukemia. Leuk Lymphoma. 2004;45(1):199–200.
170. Wirth F, Perry R, Eskenazi A, et al. Cutaneous mucormycosis with subsequent visceral dissemination in a child with neutropenia: a case report and review of the pediatric literature. J Am Acad Dermatol. 1997;36:336–41.
171. Roden MM, Zaoutis TE, Buchanan WL, et al. Epidemiology and outcome of zygomycosis: a review of 929 reported cases. Clin Infect Dis. 2005;41(5):634–53.
172. Rubin AI, Grossman ME. Bull's-eye cutaneous infarct of zygomycosis: a bedside diagnosis confirmed by touch preparation. J Am Acad Dermatol. 2004;51:996–1001.
173. Chamilos G, Lewis RE, Kontoyiannis DP. Delaying amphotericin B-based frontline therapy significantly increases mortality among patients with hematologic malignancy who have zygomycosis. Clin Infect Dis. 2008;47(4):503–9.
174. Sangoi AR, Rogers WM, Longacre TA, et al. Challenges and pitfalls of morphologic identification of fungal infections in histologic and cytologic specimens: a ten-year retrospective review at a single institution. Am J Clin Pathol. 2009;131(3):364–75.
175. Hilmarsdottir I, Thorsteinsson SB, Admundsson P, et al. Cutaneous infection caused by Paecilomyces lilacinus in a renal transplant patient: treatment with voriconazole. Scand J Infect Dis. 2000;32:331–2.
176. Lin WL, Lin WC, Chiu CS. Paecilomyces lilacinus cutaneous infection associated with peripherally inserted central catheter insertion. J Eur Acad Dermatol Venereol. 2008;22:1267–78.
177. Safdar A. Progressive cutaneous hyalohyphomycosis due to Paecilomyces lilacinus: rapid response to treatment with caspofungin and itraconazole. Clin Infect Dis. 2002;43:1415–7.
178. Harris LF, Dan BM, Lefkowitz LB Jr, Alford RH. Paecilomyces cellulitis in a renal transplant patient: successful treatment with intravenous miconazole. South Med J. 1979;72:987.
179. Castro LGM, Salebian A, Sotto MN. Hyalohyphomycosis by Paecilomyces lilacinus in a renal transplant patient and a review of human Paecilomyces species infection. J Med Vet Mycol. 1990;28:15.
180. Lott ME, Sheehan DJ, Davis LS. Paecilomyces lilacinus with a sporotrichoid pattern in a renal transplant patient. J Drugs Dermatol. 2007;6:436–9.
181. Lee J, Yew WW, Chiu CS, et al. Delayed sternotomy wound infection due to Paecilomyces variotii in a lung transplant recipient. J Heart Lung Transplant. 2002;21:1131–4.
182. De Miguel D, Gomez P, Gonzalez R, et al. Nonfatal pulmonary Trichoderma viride infection in an adult patient with acute myeloid leukemia: report of one case and review of the literature. Diagn Microbiol Infect Dis. 2005;53:33–7.
183. Yamazaki R, Mori T, Aisa Y, et al. Systemic infection due to Acremonium after allogeneic peripheral blood stem cell transplantation. Intern Med. 2006;45:989–90.
184. Foell JL, Fischer M, Seibold M, et al. Lethal double infection with Acremonium strictum and Aspergillus fumigatus during induction chemotherapy in a child with ALL. Pediatr Blood Cancer. 2007;49(6):858–61.
185. Mattei D, Mordini N, Lo Nigro C, et al. Successful treatment of Acremonium fungemia with voriconazole. Mycoses. 2003;46:511–4.
186. Schell WA, Perfect JR. Fatal, disseminated Acremonium strictum infection in a neutropenic host. J Clin Microbiol. 1996;34:133–6.
187. Van Etta LL, Peterson LR, Gerding DN. Acremonium falciforme (Cephalosporium falciforme) mycetoma in a renal transplant patient. Arch Dermatol. 1983;119:707–8.
188. Geyer AS, Fox LP, Husain S, et al. Acremonium mycetoma in a heart transplant recipient. J Am Acad Dermatol. 2006;55:1095–100.
189. Gautheret A, Dromer F, Bourhis JH, Andremont A. Trichoderma pseudokoningii as a cause of fatal infection in bone marrow transplant recipient. Clin Infect Dis. 1995;20:1060–3.
190. Munoz FM, Demmler GJ, Travis WR, et al. Trichoderma longibrachiatum infection in a pediatric patient with aplastic anemia. J Clin Microbiol. 1997;35:499–503.
191. Kantarcioglu AS, Celkan T, Yucel A, et al. Fatal Trichoderma harzianum infection in a leukemic pediatric patient. Med Mycol. 2009;47:207–15.
192. Richter S, Cormican MG, Pfaller MA, et al. Fatal disseminated Trichoderma longibrachiatum infection in an adult bone marrow transplant patient: species identification and review of the literature. J Clin Microbiol. 1999;37:1154–60.
193. Sellier P, Monsuez JJ, Lacroix C, et al. Recurrent subcutaneous infection due to Scopulariopsis brevicaulis in a liver transplant recipient. Clin Infect Dis. 2000;30:820–3.

194. Steinbach WJ, Schell WA, Miller JL, et al. Fatal Scopulariopsis brevicaulis infection in a paediatric stem-cell transplant patient treated with voriconazole and caspofungin and a review of Scopulariopsis infections in immunocompromised patients. J Infect. 2004;48:112–6.
195. Patel R, Gustaferro CA, Krom RA, et al. Phaeohyphomycosis due to Scopulariopsis brumptii in a liver transplant recipient. Clin Infect Dis. 1994;19:198–200.
196. Phillips P, Wood WS, Phillips G, Reinaldi MG. invasive hyalohyphomycosis caused by Scopulariopsis brevicaulis in a patient undergoing allogeneic bone marrow transplant. Diagn Microbiol Infect Dis. 1989;12:429–32.
197. Hoy J, Hsu KC, Rolston K, et al. Trichosporon beigelii infection: a review. Rev Infect Dis. 1986;8:959–67.
198. Fournier S, Pavageau W, Feuillhade M, et al. Use of voriconazole to successfully treat disseminated Trichosopron asahii infection in a patient with acute myeloid leukaemia. Eur J Clin Microbiol Infect Dis. 2002;21:892–6.
199. Nahass GT, Rosenberg SP, Leonardi CL, Penneys NS. Disseminated infection with Trichosporon beigelii. Arch Dermatol. 1993;129:1020–3.
200. Hughes CE, Serstock D, Wilson BCD, Payne W. Infection with Trichosporon pullulans. Ann Intern Med. 1988;108:772–3.
201. Winston DJ, Blasley GE, Rhodes J, Linne SR. Disseminated Trichosporon capitatum infection in an immunosuppressed host. Arch Intern Med. 1977;137:1192–5.
202. Fekkar A, Brun S, D'Ussel M, et al. Serum cross-reactivity with Aspergillus galactomannan and cryptococcal antigen during fatal disseminated Trichosporon dermatis infection. Clin Infect Dis. 2009;49:1457–8.
203. Girmenia C, Pagano L, Martino B, et al. Invasive infections caused by Trichosporon species and Geotrichum capitatum in patients with hematological malignancies: a retrospective multicenter study from Italy and review of the literature. J Clin Microbiol. 2005;43:1818–28.
204. Foulet F, Duvoux C, de Bievre C, Hezode C, Bretagne S. Cutaneous phaeohyphomycosis caused by Veronaea bothryosa in a liver transplant recipient successfully treated with itraconazole. Clin Infect Dis. 1999;29(3):689–90.
205. Calabro G, Nino M, Gallo L, Scalvenzi M. Cutaneous alternariosis in a kidney transplantation recipient: report of a case. J Dermatolog Treat. 2008;19:246–8.
206. Segner S, Jouret F, Durant JF, Marot L, Kanaan N. Cutaneous infection by Alternaria infectoria in a renal transplant patient. Transpl Infect Dis. 2009;11:330–2.
207. Martinez-Gonzalez MC, Verea MM, Velasco D, et al. Three cases of cutaneous phaeohyphomycosis by Exophiala jeanselmei. Eur J Dermatol. 2008;18(3):313–6.
208. Brasch J, Busch JO, de Hoog GS. Cutaneous phaeohyphomycosis caused by Alternaria infectoria. Acta Derm Venereol. 2008;88:160–1.
209. O'Quinn RP, Hoffmann JL, Boyd AS. Colletotrichum species as emerging opportunistic fungal pathogens: a report of 3 cases of phaeohyphomycosis and review. J Am Acad Dermatol. 2001;45(1):56–61.
210. Keyser A, Schmid FX, Linde HJ, Merk J, Birnbaum DE. Disseminated Cladophialophora bantiana infection in a heart transplant recipient. J Heart Lung Transplant. 2002;21:503–5.
211. Kriengkauykiat J, Ito JI, Dadwal SS. Epidemiology and treatment approaches in management of invasive fungal infections. Clin Epidemiol. 2011;3:175–91.
212. Virgili A, Zampino MR, Mantovani L. Fungal skin infections in organ transplant recipients. Am J Clin Dermatol. 2002;3:19–35.
213. Bodey GP. Dermatologic manifestations of infections in neutropenic patients. Infect Dis Clin N Am. 1994;8:655–75.
214. Leung AY, Chim CS, Ho PL, et al. Candida tropicalis fungaemia in adult patients with haematological malignancies: clinical features and risk factors. J Hosp Infect. 2002;50:316–9.
215. Munoz P, Sanchez-Somolinos M, Alcala L, et al. Candida krusei fungaemia: antifungal susceptibility and clinical presentation of an uncommon entity during 15 years in a single general hospital. J Antimicrob Chemother. 2005;55:188–93.
216. Held JL, Berkowitz RK, Grossman ME. Use of touch preparation for rapid diagnosis of disseminated candidiasis. J Am Acad Dermatol. 1988;19:1063–6.
217. Spellberg BJ, Filler SG, Edwards JE Jr. Current treatment strategies for disseminated candidiasis. Clin Infect Dis. 2006;42(2):244–51. Epub 2005 Dec 2.
218. Cohen P, Grossman ME, Silvers DN. Mucocutaneous manifestations of systemic fungal infections in the HIV-seropositive patients. AIDS Read. 1993;3:47–60.
219. Sing Y, Ramdial PK. Cryptococcal inflammatory pseudotumors. Am J Surg Pathol. 2007;31:1521–7.
220. Neuville S, Dromer F, Morin O, et al. Primary cutaneous cryptococcosis: a distinct clinical entity. Clin Infect Dis. 2003;36:337–47.
221. Zorman JV, Zupanc TL, Parac Z, Cucek I. Primary cutaneous cryptococcosis in a renal transplant recipient: case report. Mycoses. 2010;53(6):535–7.
222. Hunger RE, Paredes BE, Quattroppani C, Krahenbuhl S, Vraathen LR. Primary cutaneous cryptococcosis in a patient with systemic immunosuppression after liver transplantation. Dermatology. 2000;200:352–5.
223. Baumgarten KL, Valentine VG, Garcia-Diaz JB. Primary cutaneous cryptococcosis in a lung transplant recipient. South Med J. 2004;97:692–5.
224. Husain S, Wagener MM, Singh N. Cryptococcus neoformans infection in organ transplant recipients: variables influencing clinical characteristics and outcome. Emerg Infect Dis. 2001;7(3):375–81.
225. Basaran O, Emiroglu R, Arikan U, Karakayali H, Haberal M. Cryptococcal necrotizing fasciitis with multiple sites of involvement in the lower extremities. Dermatol Surg. 2003;29(11):1158–60.
226. Baer S, Baddley JW, Gnann JW, Pappas PG. Cryptococcal disease presenting as necrotizing cellulitis in transplant recipients. Transpl Infect Dis. 2009;11(4):353–8.
227. Franca AV, Carneiro M, dal Sasso K, Souza Cda S, Martinelli A. Cryptococcosis in cirrhotic patients. Mycoses. 2005;48:68–72.
228. Orsini J, Nowakowski J, Delaney V, Sakoulas G, Wormser GP. Cryptococcal infection presenting as cellulitis in a renal transplant recipient. Transpl Infect Dis. 2009;11:68–71.
229. Moe K, Lotsikas-Baggali AJ, Kupiec-Banasikowska A, Kauffman CL. The cutaneous predilection of disseminated cryptococcal infection in organ transplant recipients. Arch Dermatol. 2005;141(7):913–4.
230. DiCaudo DJ. Coccidioidomycosis: a review and update. J Am Acad Dermatol. 2006;55(6):929–42.
231. Prichard JG, Sorotzkin RA, James RE III. Cutaneous manifestations of disseminated coccidioidomycosis in the acquired immunodeficiency syndrome. Cutis. 1987;39(3):203–5.
232. Braddy CM, Heilman RL, Blair JE. Coccidioidomycosis after renal transplantation in an endemic area. Am J Transplant. 2006;6(2):340–5.
233. Vartivarian SE, Coudron PE, Markowitz SM. Disseminated coccidioidomycosis. Unusual manifestations in a cardiac transplantation patient. Am J Med. 1987;83(5):949–52.
234. Hay RJ. Blastomycosis: what's new? J Eur Acad Dermatol Venereol. 2000;14(4):249–50.
235. Pappas PG. Blastomycosis in the immunocompromised patient. Semin Respir Infect. 1997;12(3):243–51.

236. Fisher KR, Baselski V, Beard G, et al. Pustular blastomycosis. J Am Acad Dermatol. 2009;61:355–8.
237. Smith JA, Kauffman CA. Endemic fungal infections in patients receiving tumor necrosis factor-alpha inhibitor therapy. Drugs. 2009;69:1403–15.
238. Serody JS, Mill MR, Detterbeck FC, Harris DT, Cohen MS. Blastomycosis in transplant recipients: report of a case and review. Clin Infect Dis. 1993;16(1):54–8.
239. Gauthier GM, Safdar H, Klein BS, Andres DR. Blastomycosis in solid organ transplant recipients. Transpl Infect Dis. 2007;9:310–7.
240. Bradsher RW. Clinical features blastomycosis. Semin Respir Infect. 1997;12(3):229–34.
241. Bonifaz A, Chang P, Moreno K, Fernandez-Fernandez V, et al. Disseminated cutaneous histoplasmosis in acquired immunodeficiency syndrome: report of 23 cases. Clin Exp Dermatol. 2009;34(4):481–6.
242. Cohen PR, Bank DE, Silvers DN, Grossman ME. Cutaneous lesions of disseminated histoplasmosis in human immunodeficiency virus-infected patients. J Am Acad Dermatol. 1990;23:422–8.
243. Paul AY, Aldrich S, Scott RS, Ellis MW. Disseminated histoplasmosis in a patient with AIDS: case report and review of the literature. Cutis. 2007;80(4):309–12.
244. Dong JA, Chren MM, Elewski BE. Bonsai tree: risk factor for disseminated sporotrichosis. J Am Acad Dermatol. 1995;33:839–40.
245. Cohen PR, Grossman ME, Silvers DN. Mucocutaneous manifestations of systemic fungal infections in the HIV-seropositive patient. AIDS Read. 1993;3:47–60.
246. Yang DJ, Krishnan RS, Guillen DR, et al. Disseminated sporotrichosis mimicking sarcoidosis. Int J Dermatol. 2006;45:450–3.
247. Ramos-e-Silva M, Vasconcelos C, Carneiro S, Cestari T. Sporotrichosis. Clin Dermatol. 2007;25(2):181–7.
248. Yelverton CB, Stetson CL, Bang RH, Clark JW, Butler DF. Fatal sporotrichosis. Cutis. 2006;78(4):253–6.
249. Severo LC, Festugato M, Bernardi C, Londero AT. Widespread cutaneous lesions due to Sporothrix schenckii in a patient under a long-term steroids therapy. Rev Inst Med Trop Sao Paulo. 1999;41(1):59–62.
250. Squeo RF, Beer R, Silvers D, Weitzman I, Grossman M. Invasive Trichophyton rubrum resembling blastomycosis infection in the immunocompromised host. J Am Acad Dermatol. 1998;39(2 Pt 2):379–80.
251. Baker RL, Para MF. Successful use of ketoconazole for invasive cutaneous Trichophyton rubrum infection. Arch Intern Med. 1984;144(3):615–7.
252. Novick NL, Tapia L, Bottone EJ. Invasive Trichophyton rubrum infection in an immunocompromised host. Am J Med. 1987;82(2):321–5.
253. Demidovich CW, Kornfeld BW, Gentry RH, Fitzpatrick JE. Deep dermatophyte infection with chronic draining nodules in an immunocompromised patient. Cutis. 1995;55(4):237–40.
254. Franco RC. Deep dermatophytosis in a post transplant recipient. Int J Dermatol. 2001;40(5):363–4.
255. Almeida L, Grossman ME. Widespread dermatophyte infections that mimick collagen vascular disease. J Am Acad Dermatol. 1990;23:855–7.
256. Ziemer M, Seyfarth F, Elsner P, Hipler UC. Atypical manifestations of tinea coropois. Mycoses. 2007;50(Suppl 2):31–5.
257. Rallis E, Koumantaki-Mathioudaki E. Pimecrolimus induced tinea incognito masquerading as intertriginous psoriasis. Mycoses. 2008;51(1):71–3.
258. Hazen KC. Fungicidal versus fungistatic activity of terbinafine and itraconazole: an in vitro comparison. J Am Acad Dermatol. 1998;38:S37–41.
259. Bao YQ, Wan Z, RY L. In vitro antifungal activity of micafungin and caspofungin against dermatophytes isolated from China. Mycopathologia. 2013;175(1–2):141–5.
260. Favre B, Hofbauer B, Hildering KS, Ryder NS. Comparison of in vitro activities of 17 antifungal drugs against a panel of 20 dermatophytes by using a microdilution assay. J Clin Microbiol. 2003;41(10):4817–9.
261. Elewski BE, Sullivan J. Dermatophytes as opportunistic pathogens. J Am Acad Dermatol. 1994;30(6):1021–2.
262. Sartori AM, Ibrahim KY, Nunes Westphalen EV, et al. Manifestations of Chagas disease (American trypanosomiasis) in patients with HIV/AIDS. Ann Trop Med Parasitol. 2007;101(1):31–50.
263. Stolf NA, Higushi L, Bocchi E, et al. Heart transplantation in patients with Chagas' disease cardiomyopathy. J Heart Transplant. 1987;6(5):307–12.
264. Godoy HL, Guerra CM, Viegas RF, et al. Infections in heart transplant recipients in Brazil: the challenge of Chagas' disease. J Heart Lung Transplant. 2010;29(3):286–90.
265. Hall CS, Fields K. Cutaneous presentation of Chagas' disease reaction in a heart-transplant patients in Utah. J Am Acad Dermatol. 2008;58(3):529–30.
266. La Forgia MP, Pellerano G, de las Mercedes Portaluppi M, Kien MC, Chouela EN. Cutaneous manifestation of reactivation of Chagas disease in a renal transplant patient: long-term follow-up. Arch Dermatol. 2003;139(1):104–5.
267. Antinori S, Cascio A, Parravicini C, Bianchi R, Corbellino M. Leishmaniasis among organ transplant recipients. Lancet Infect Dis. 2008;8(3):191–9.
268. Lee SA, Diwan AH, Cohn M, Champlin R, Safdar A. Cutaneous toxoplasmosis: a case of confounding diagnosis. Bone Marrow Transplant. 2005;36(5):465–6.
269. Vidal CI, Pollack M, Uliasz A, del Toro G, Emanuel PO. Cutaneous toxoplasmosis histologically mimicking graft-versus-host disease. Am J Dermatopathol. 2008;30(5):492–3.
270. Amir G, Salant H, Resnick IB, Karplus R. Cutaneous toxoplasmosis after bone marrow transplantation with molecular confirmation. J Am Acad Dermatol. 2008;59(5):781–4.
271. May LP, Sidhu GS, Buchness MR. Diagnosis of Acanthamoeba infection by cutaneous manifestations in a man seropositive to HIV. J Am Acad Dermatol. 1992;26(2 Pt 2):352–5.
272. Young AL, Leboeuf NR, Tsiouris SJ, Husain S, Grossman ME. Fatal disseminated Acanthamoeba infection in a liver transplant recipient immunocompromised by combination therapies for graft-versus-host disease. Transpl Infect Dis. 2010;12(6):529–37.
273. Gordon SM, Gal AA, Solomon AR, Bryan JA. Disseminated strongyloidiasis with cutaneous manifestations in an immunocompromised host. J Am Acad Dermatol. 1994;31:255–9.
274. Keiser PB, Nutman TB. Strongyloides stercoralis in the immunocompromised population. Clin Microbiol Rev. 2004;17(1): 208–17.
275. Krishnamurthy R, Dincer HE, Whittemore D. Strongyloides stercoralis hyperinfection in a patient with rheumatoid arthritis after anti-TNF-alpha therapy. J Clin Rheumatol. 2007;13(3):150–2.
276. Weiser JA, Scully BE, Bulman WA, Husain S, Grossman ME. Periumbilical parasitic thumbprint purpura: strongyloides hyperinfection syndrome acquired from a cadaveric renal transplant. Transpl Infect Dis. 2011;13(1):58–62.
277. Bank DE, Grossman ME, Kohn SR, Rabinowitz AD. The thumbprint sign: rapid diagnosis of disseminated strongyloidiasis. J Am Acad Dermatol. 1990;23(2 Pt 1):324–6.
278. Salluh JI, Bozza FA, Pinto TS, et al. Cutaneous periumbilical purpura in disseminated strongyloidiasis in cancer patients: a pathognomonic feature of potentially lethal disease? Braz J Infect Dis. 2005;9(5):419–24.
279. Inserra DW, Bickley LK. Crusted scabies in acquired immunodeficiency syndrome. Int J Dermatol. 1990;29:287–9.
280. Del Giudice P. Ivermectin in scabies. Curr Opin Infect Dis. 2002;15:123–6.

281. Glover R, Young L, Goltz RW. Norwegian scabies in acquired immunodeficiency syndrome: report of a case resulting in death from associated sepsis. J Am Acad Dermatol. 1987;16:396–9.
282. Hulbert TV, Larsen RA. Hyperkeratotic (Norwegian) scabies with gram-negative bacterium as the initial presentation of AIDS. Clin Infect Dis. 1992;14:1164–5.
283. Bonomo RA, Jacobs M, Jacobs G, et al. Norwegian scabies and a toxic shock syndrome toxin 1-producing strain of Staphylococcus aureus endocarditis in a patient with trisomy 21. Clin Infect Dis. 1998;27:645–6.
284. Grossman ME, Fox LP, Kovarik C, Rosenbach M. Gram-negative bacteria. In: Grossman ME, Fox LP, Kovarik C, Rosenbach M, editors. Cutaneous manifestations of infection in the immunocompromised host. 2nd ed. New York: Springer; 2012.
285. Grossman ME, Fox LP, Kovarik C, Rosenbach M. Mycobacteria. In: Grossman ME, Fox LP, Kovarik C, Rosenbach M, editors. Cutaneous manifestations of infection in the immunocompromised host. 2nd ed. New York: Springer; 2012.
286. Grossman ME, Fox LP, Kovarik C, Rosenbach M. Viruses. In: Grossman ME, Fox LP, Kovarik C, Rosenbach M, editors. Cutaneous manifestations of infection in the immunocompromised host. 2nd ed. New York: Springer; 2012.
287. Grossman ME, Fox LP, Kovarik C, Rosenbach M. Subcutaneous and deep mycoses. In: Grossman ME, Fox LP, Kovarik C, Rosenbach M, editors. Cutaneous manifestations of infection in the immunocompromised host. 2nd ed. New York: Springer; 2012.
288. Grossman ME, Fox LP, Kovarik C, Rosenbach M. Protozoa. In: Grossman ME, Fox LP, Kovarik C, Rosenbach M, editors. Cutaneous manifestations of infection in the immunocompromised host. 2nd ed. New York: Springer; 2012.

Cutaneous Lesions that Mimic Infection in Transplant Patients

23

Ana Ciurea and Sharon Hymes

Introduction

Many cutaneous conditions may mimic infectious processes. The ability to diagnose non-infectious skin eruptions, especially in cancer patients, is oftentimes challenging. Using the morphology of the primary skin lesion as a starting point, this section will review the clinical presentation, physical examination, and diagnostic work-up of many of these conditions. This should help the clinician generate a differential diagnosis when evaluating cutaneous lesions in immunosuppressed patients.

Section 1: Pustular Lesions

Pustules are purulent collections which can be solitary or widespread. Not all the pustular processes in the skin are due to infection; pustular psoriasis is one of the non-infectious examples. They may be mistaken for bacterial, fungal, or superinfected herpetic infections.

Reactive Neutrophilic Dermatoses

Reactive neutrophilic dermatoses are a spectrum of diseases mediated by neutrophils manifested by systemic complaints in association with an underlying disease such as inflammatory bowel disorders or internal malignancies.

Differential Diagnosis: Bacterial, Fungal, and Viral Infections

Pyoderma gangrenosum is an uncommon idiopathic ulcerative skin disorder that often is associated with systemic diseases. The ulcerations are distinctive: an irregular, boggy, undermined border surrounding a purulent necrotic base (Fig. 23.1). Culture-negative pulmonary infiltrates are the most common extracutaneous site of disease [1]. PG is associated with a dysregulation of the immune system, in particular altered neutrophil chemotaxis in reaction to various precipitating causes such as inflammatory bowel diseases [2, 3]. Many conditions can be confused with the early pustular stage: folliculitis, furunculosis, carbuncles, and streptococcal gangrene. The ulcerative stage must be differentiated from cutaneous amebiasis, cryptococcosis, blastomycosis, sporotrichosis, and atypical mycobacterial infections [4–6]. PG has a tendency to recur and it usually heals with scarring.

Behcet's syndrome is a chronic relapsing, idiopathic, multisystem disease of recurrent aphthous ulcers, genital ulcers, and uveitis (Fig. 23.2). The cause is unknown; however, current research points toward an autoimmune etiology following exposure to an infectious agent which includes herpes simplex virus, *Streptococcus* and *Staphylococcus* species, and *Escherichia coli*. It has been suggested that the heat shock proteins (HSPs) found in higher concentrations in

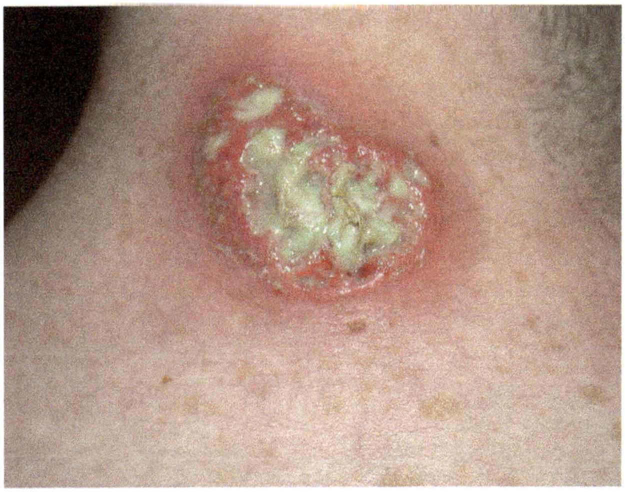

Fig. 23.1 Pyoderma gangrenosum. Painful neck ulceration with an elevated dusky undermined border and fibrinous base

A. Ciurea (✉) · S. Hymes
Department of Dermatology, The University of Texas MD Anderson Cancer Center, Houston, TX, USA
e-mail: amciurea@mdanderson.org; srhymes@mdanderson.org

A. Safdar (ed.), *Principles and Practice of Transplant Infectious Diseases*, https://doi.org/10.1007/978-1-4939-9034-4_23

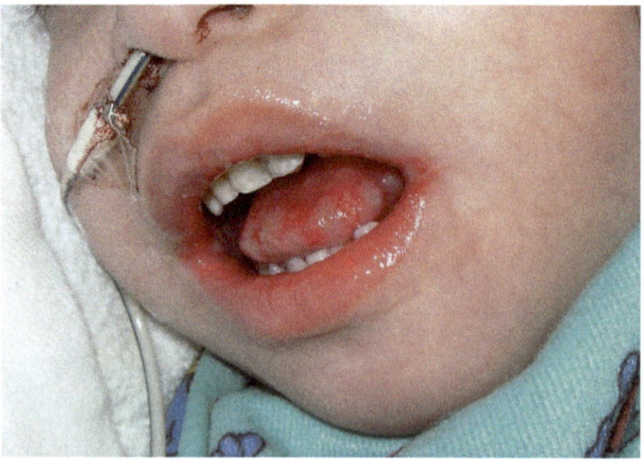

Fig. 23.2 Behcet's disease. Oral ulcerations

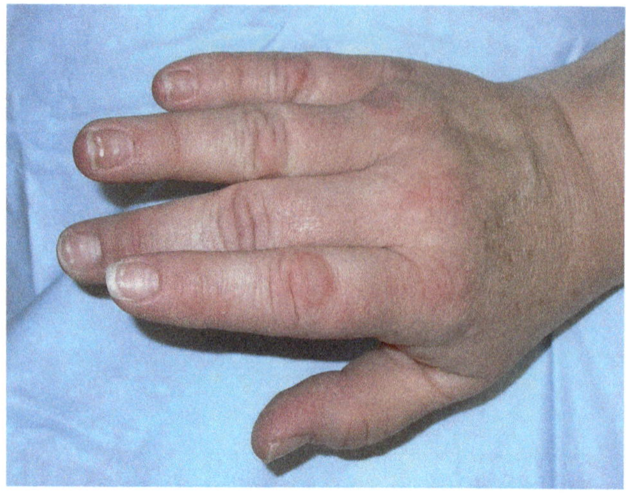

Fig. 23.3 Sweet's syndrome. Erythematous, edematous plaques on the dorsal hand and fingers in a patient with acute myelogenous leukemia

skin lesions and oral aphthae can induce antibody production that cross-react with streptococcal species that are usually found in the mouth [7].

An acneiform papulopustular eruption may be seen on the face, neck, and trunk. The aphthous lesions begin as vesicles and/or pustules and tend to heal with scar formation. Tender, erythematous, recurrent nodules that resemble erythema nodosum are common on the extremities in women. Extragenital ulcerations, if present, are very specific for Behcet's disease [8]. Various treatment regimens have demonstrated benefit including systemic corticosteroids, colchicine, azathioprine, dapsone, interferon-alfa, and infliximab. The disease can be confused with herpetic gingivostomatitis and syphilis.

Acute neutrophilic febrile dermatosis (Sweet's syndrome) is a distinct entity characterized by one or more edematous red, tender, spontaneously painful plaques predominantly on the upper body, accompanied by fever, peripheral leukocytosis, and a variety of constitutional symptoms (Fig. 23.3). It is thought to be a hypersensitivity reaction of unknown cause characterized by infiltration of neutrophils in the skin. It has been associated with various carcinomas and hematopoietic malignancies especially acute myelogenous leukemia (AML) [9]. It responds dramatically to systemic corticosteroids and may resolve with treatment of the underlying disease [9, 10]. Ulcers and bullae are more common in malignancy-associated disease than in other forms. These lesions may be extensive and are generally hard to treat [11]. Sweet's syndrome must be differentiated from erysipelas, cellulitis, arthropod bites, herpetic infections, and drug eruptions.

Bowel bypass syndrome is a constellation of medical complications secondary to intestinal bypass surgery for the treatment of morbid obesity, consisting of fever, asymmetrical polyarthritis, tenosynovitis, sterile skin pustules, mucous membrane ulcerations, retinal vasculitis, and thrombophlebitis [12]. The syndrome is presumed to result from the deposition of circulating immune complexes containing bacterial antigens derived from overgrowth in the bypassed loop of the bowel [13]. Surgical excision of the blind loop or revision of the bowel bypass cures bowel bypass syndrome. The disease may resemble gonococcal sepsis, infectious panniculitis, pyoderma gangrenosum, Behcet's syndrome, and Sweet's syndrome.

Acute Generalized Exanthematous Pustulosis (AGEP)

Differential Diagnosis: Bacterial, Viral, or Fungal Infections

AGEP is a neutrophilic dermatosis characterized by acute-onset monoform, sterile, nonfollicular 1–2-mm pustules on a background of erythema secondary to drug administration, most commonly antibiotics. The lesions have a predilection for the face and intertriginous areas (Fig. 23.4). The eruption is accompanied by fever which can occur several days prior or the same day as the eruption. Widespread desquamation occurs after a few days. Neutrophilia and eosinophilia are commonly seen [14]. The precise mechanism of the disease is unknown. It is suggested that neutrophil-activating cytokines released by drug-specific T lymphocytes (IL-3, IL-8, and G-CSF) are potent triggers for blood neutrophilia and accumulation of neutrophils within the lesions [14]. It is characterized by fever which can occur several days prior to the eruption followed by the onset of classic lesions on the face or intertriginous areas. The withdrawal of the responsible drug is the mainstay of treatment in conjunction with topical corticosteroids [15].

Acneiform Hypersensitivity Drug Eruptions

Differential Diagnosis: Bacterial and Fungal Folliculitis

Acneiform eruptions are characterized by pruritic inflammatory papules or pustules localized primarily on areas with a

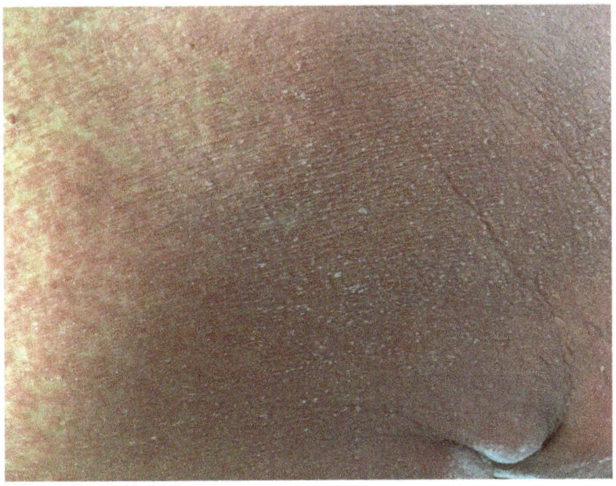

Fig. 23.4 Acute generalized exanthematous pustulosis. Affected individuals show large areas of erythroderma topped with small nonfollicular sterile pustules

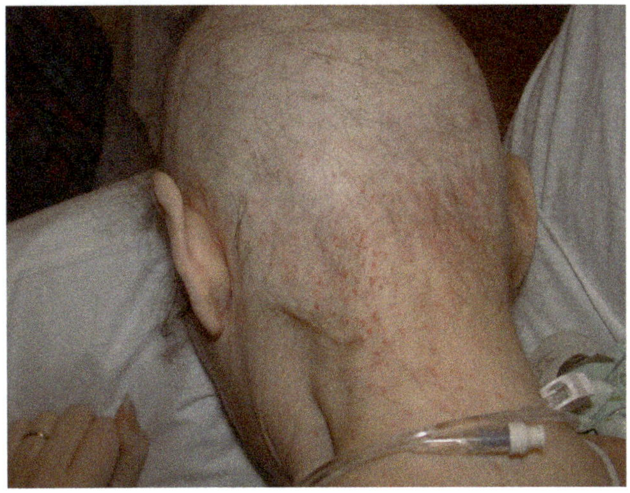

Fig. 23.6 EGFR inhibitor-associated alopecia. Scalp inflammatory papules and scarring alopecia

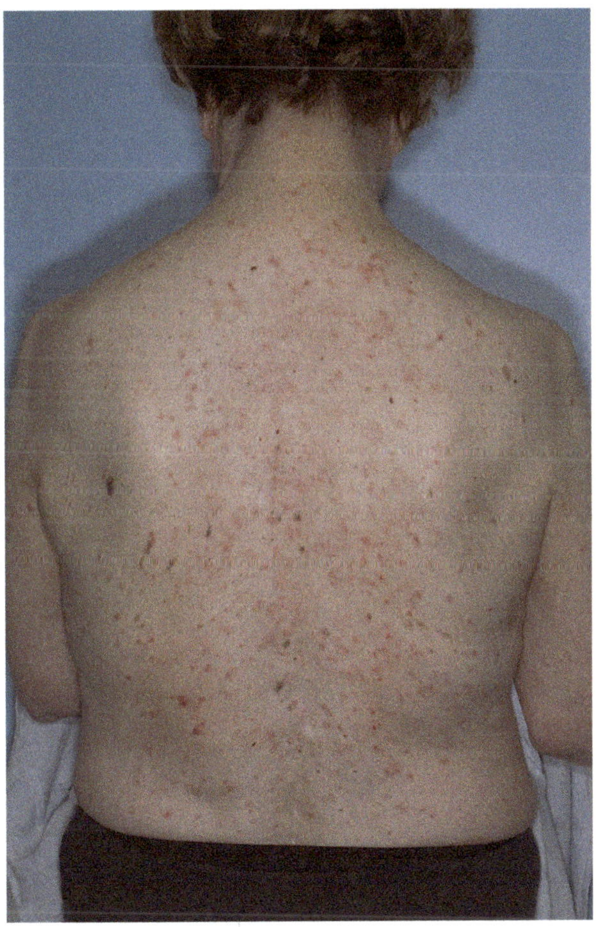

Fig. 23.5 Acneiform drug eruption due to EGFR inhibitor erlotinib. Follicular pustules, located on the skin of the face and trunk in patient with metastatic lung cancer

large number of pilosebaceous units: face, neck, chest, and upper back, sparing the palmar or plantar surfaces (Fig. 23.5). In contrast to acne vulgaris, comedones are absent in acneiform eruptions. The eruption is common in cancer patients treated with systemic corticosteroids. Isoniazid, as well as chemotherapeutic agents including cyclosporine, azathioprine, and sirolimus, may induce acneiform drug eruptions [16, 17]. Cutaneous adverse events associated with epidermal growth factor inhibitors (EGFR) include pustular skin eruptions usually on the scalp, neck, chest, and back along with paronychia, xerosis, and alopecia (Fig. 23.6). Although the exact mechanism of the development of the rash is not completely understood, the inhibitor therapy disrupts the EGFR function by inducing terminal differentiation and apoptosis in the stratum corneum and hair follicles. Patients are often managed symptomatically or by adjusting the dose of the targeted therapy [18]. It is important to promptly identify and treat the adverse events during therapy with EGFR inhibitors to avoid drug suspension. The infectious diseases that enter the differential diagnosis of acneiform drug eruptions are folliculitis, measles, rubeola, rubella, and syphilis.

Eosinophilic Folliculitis

Differential Diagnosis: Bacterial and Fungal Folliculitis

Eosinophilic folliculitis is an uncommon recurrent eosinophilic infiltration of hair follicles manifested by pruritic papules and pustules associated with soft tissue edema seen most commonly on the head, neck, and trunk mostly in immunosuppressed patients [19, 20] (Fig. 23.7). Eosinophilic folliculitis has been classified as an AIDS-defining illness [19]. Although the exact etiology is unknown, an autoimmune reaction against sebocytes or sebum component and an abnormal T-cell immune response to a follicular antigen, such as caused by Demodex species, may be responsible for the eruption [19]. Topical corticosteroids are the mainstay of treatment for eosinophilic folliculitis. Highly active antiretroviral therapy along with isotretinoin therapy is

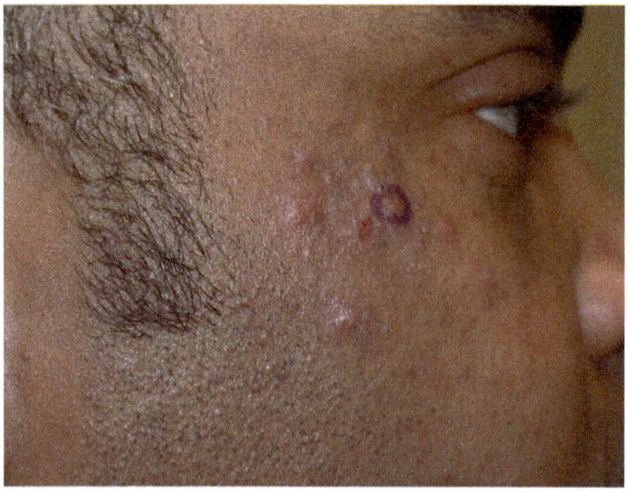

Fig. 23.7 Eosinophilic folliculitis. Crops of sterile papules and pustules on the face

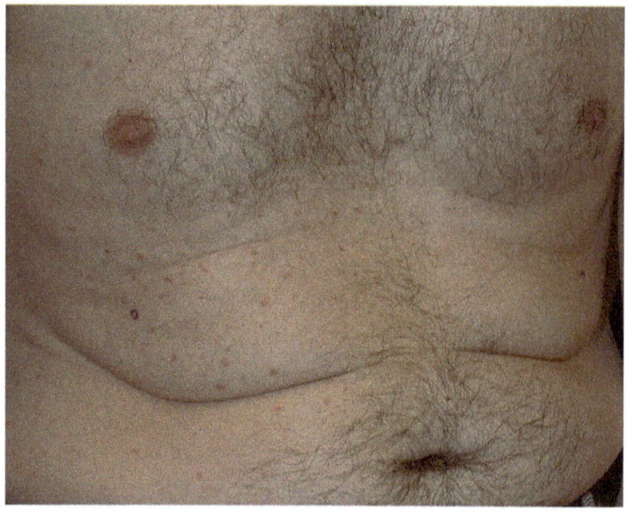

Fig. 23.8 Transient acantholytic dermatosis or Grover's disease. This is an acquired condition that presents with pruritic vesicles and erosions on the upper trunk, most often in men

beneficial for eosinophilic folliculitis in the setting of HIV disease [21]. Clinically, it resembles bacterial folliculitis and candidiasis.

Grover's Disease

Differential Diagnosis: Bacterial and Fungal Folliculitis and Allergic Drug Eruptions

Also known as transient acantholytic dermatosis, this condition is benign, self-limited, exacerbated by heat and sweating, characterized by a sparse eruption of inflammatory papules, and fragile vesicles that erode. It is limited to the chest and upper abdomen, and it can be confused with bacterial folliculitis, herpes simplex and zoster infections, scabies, and syphilis (Fig. 23.8). Viral and bacterial pathogens have been proposed, but no causative role has been established. Potent topical corticosteroids are effective in diminishing inflammation and in controlling pruritus associated with transient acantholytic dermatosis.

Miliaria Rubra

Differential Diagnosis: Bacterial and Fungal Folliculitis

Miliaria rubra is a common anhidrotic disorder in which an obstruction of the sweat duct occurs in the deeper level of the epidermis characterized by minute erythematous macules with a punctate vesicle usually centrally located. The lesions can be seen to be extrafollicular, in contrast to the pustules of folliculitis (Fig. 23.9). It is the only type of miliaria in which the symptom of pruritus is experienced [22]. It occurs primarily at sites of occlusion such as the back of febrile, ill patients. Resident bacteria, such as *Staphylococcus epidermidis and Staphylococcus aureus*, may play a role in the pathogenesis of miliaria [23].

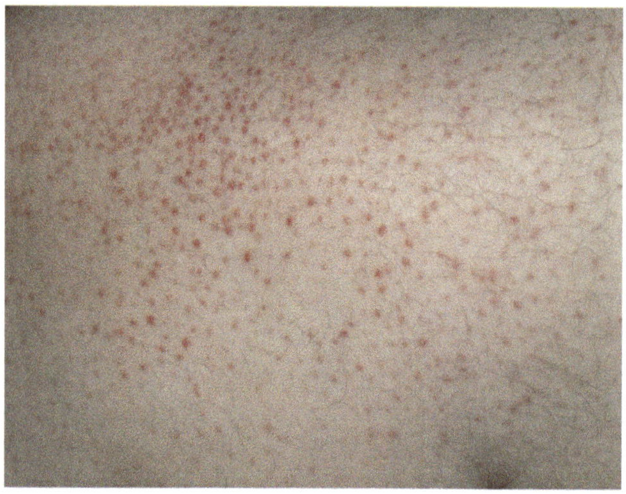

Fig. 23.9 Miliaria rubra. Multiple erythematous pinpoint macules and papules, especially prominent on the occluded surface of the back

Neutrophilic Eccrine Hidradenitis

Differential Diagnosis: Cellulitis

Also known as toxic erythema of chemotherapy, neutrophilic eccrine hidradenitis is a skin condition observed in the setting of AML treated with cytarabine and has been reported in persons with various neoplastic and non-neoplastic conditions and otherwise healthy individuals [24]. It is characterized by solitary or multiple, red and purpuric, macules,

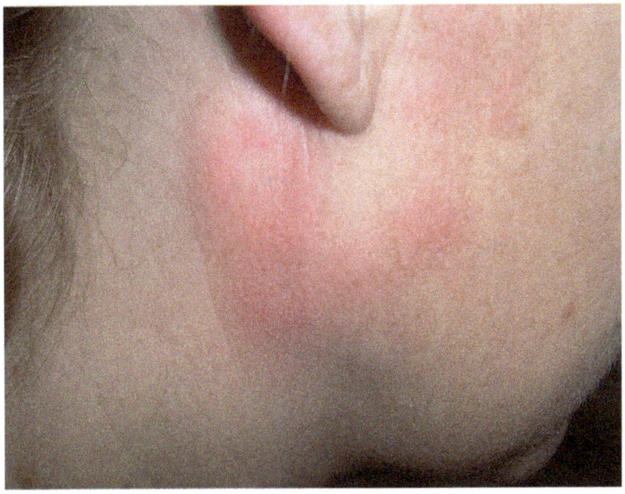

Fig. 23.10 Neutrophilic eccrine hidradenitis. Facial erythematous, indurated plaques

papules, nodules, or plaques most frequently located on the trunk or extremities (Fig. 23.10). The plaques are often tender. Neutrophilic eccrine hidradenitis can simulate orbital and facial cellulitis [24, 25]. Anthracyclines, antimetabolites, taxanes, vinca alkaloids, mitotic inhibitors, and granulocyte colony-stimulating factors may induce this disorder [26].

Section 2: Papulosquamous Lesions

Dermatitis

Dermatitis also known as eczema reflects an inflammatory skin reaction due to exposure to irritants, drugs, and other unknown triggers. It often presents as scaly erythematous plaques and patches, not uncommonly secondarily infected. 90% will be culture positive for *Staphylococcus aureus* [27].

Differential Diagnosis: Superficial Fungal Infection and Cellulitis

Stasis dermatitis presents as erythema and light-brown pigmentation on the lower extremities, especially above malleolus, associated with eczematous dermatitis (Fig. 23.11). It is a cutaneous marker for venous insufficiency and often mistaken for cellulitis. When chronic venous insufficiency is present, patients may present with marked woody induration in a stocking distribution associated with dyspigmentation, termed "lipodermatosclerosis."

Pityriasis alba is a form of dermatitis frequently atopic in origin, characterized by slightly scaly hypopigmented patches on the cheeks, upper arms, and trunk in children (Fig. 23.12). Potassium hydroxide examination of the fine white scale can rule out superficial cutaneous dermatophyte infection.

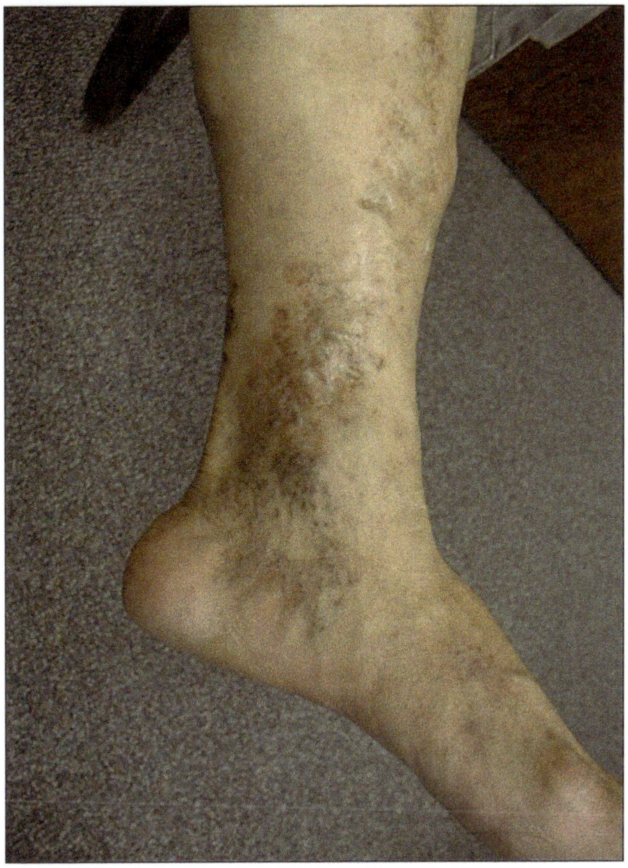

Fig. 23.11 Stasis dermatitis. Post-inflammatory hyperpigmentation over the medial malleolus on the background of varicose veins

Drug eruptions mimic various dermatoses and the morphology includes exanthem (morbilliform), papulosquamous, urticaria, vasculitis, and erythema nodosum. It should be suspected in any patient taking medication who developed a symmetric cutaneous eruption (Fig. 23.13). Chemotherapeutic agents such as busulfan and gentifinib are common causes for intertriginous drug eruption which can be confused with dermatophyte or yeast infection [28, 29].

Acute radiation dermatitis commonly occurs following local radiation therapy for various malignancies, with more than 90% of the patients experiencing erythema and more than 30% experiencing moist desquamation [30] (Fig. 23.14). Intense inflammatory reaction may result in a breakdown of the skin's barrier function and accompanying bacterial colonization, with organisms like *Staphylococcus aureus* [31, 32].

Psoriasis

Differential Diagnosis: Superficial Fungal Infection

Psoriasis is a complex multisystem inflammatory disorder of unknown etiology showing wide variation in severity and

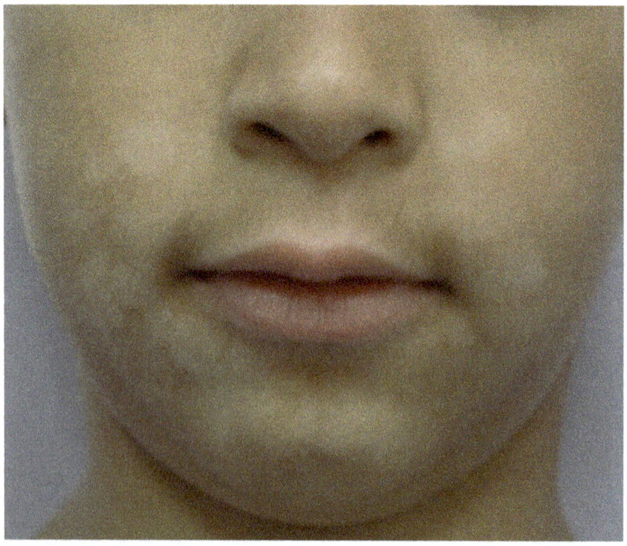

Fig. 23.12 Pityriasis alba. Circumscribed scaly hypopigmented lesions on the face

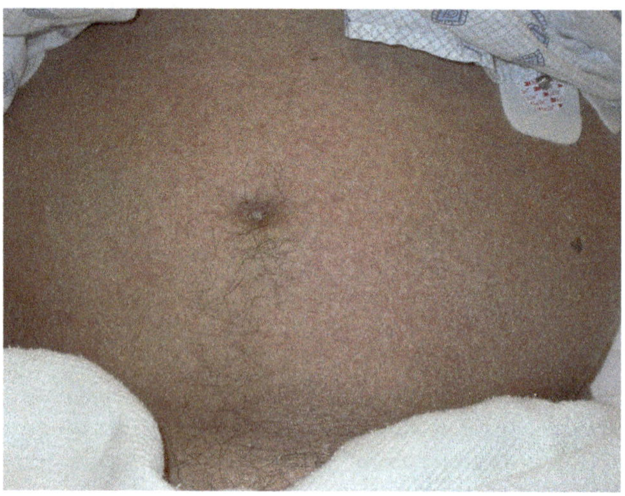

Fig. 23.13 Drug eruption. Morbilliform macules and papules on the abdomen resulting from cefepime

distribution of skin lesions. The most common skin manifestations are erythematous macules, papules, and plaques with thick silvery scale that follow an irregular chronic course marked by remissions and exacerbations of unpredictable onset and duration (Fig. 23.15). Although no region is exempt from involvement, psoriasis has a predilection for the scalp, elbows, and knees [33]. Psoriasis plaques can be mistaken for cutaneous tinea corporis or secondary syphilis.

Pityriasis Rubra Pilaris

Differential Diagnosis: Superficial Fungal Infection

Pityriasis rubra pilaris, a rare scaly, erythematous skin condition of unknown etiology with a preference for the follicular apparatus, is considered a disturbance of keratinization with predilection for the ears, trunk, neck, and extremities. Clinical features include discrete follicular-based reddish papules on the hands dorsum and diffuse palmar exfoliation (Fig. 23.16). Confluent scaly, salmon-colored plaques may appear on the trunk within islands of normal skin. A skin biopsy is mandatory to distinguish this from psoriasis and fungal infection and a search for occult malignancy should be considered if the presentation is atypical or in older patients.

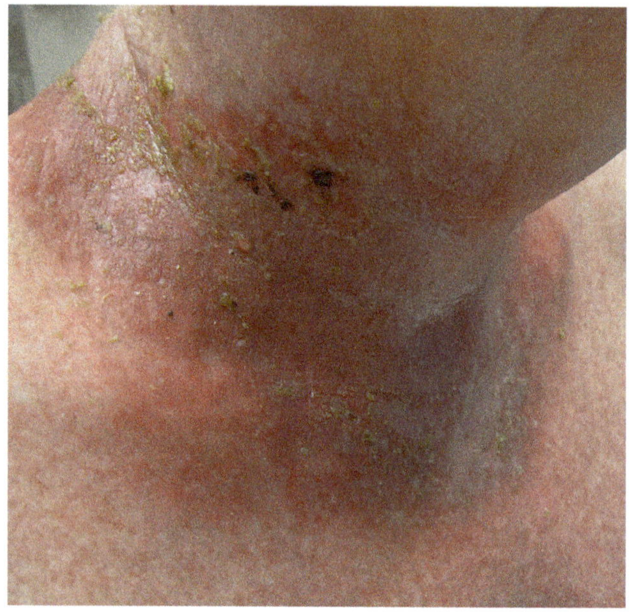

Fig. 23.14 Acute radiation dermatitis. Extensive erythema and crusting with geographic borders defined by the radiation field

Pityriasis Rosea

Differential Diagnosis: Superficial Fungal Infection and Syphilis

This is an acute self-limited, clinically distinctive exanthematous eruption of unknown etiology more commonly seen in adolescents and young adults. A mild prodrome manifested by malaise, fatigue, headache, and sore throat precedes the skin eruption with a few days. The earliest change is the "herald patch," a solitary, oval, or annular plaque on the trunk, arms, and thighs, followed by eruptive erythematous, flat plaques measuring 0.5–1.5 cm in diameter (Fig. 23.17). The clinical features and course of pityriasis rosea strongly suggest a viral etiology; however, no single virus has been proven to cause the disease. The widespread lesions of secondary syphilis and tinea versicolor may resemble pityriasis rosea [34]. Tinea corporis can be confused with the herald patch seen earlier during the course of the disease.

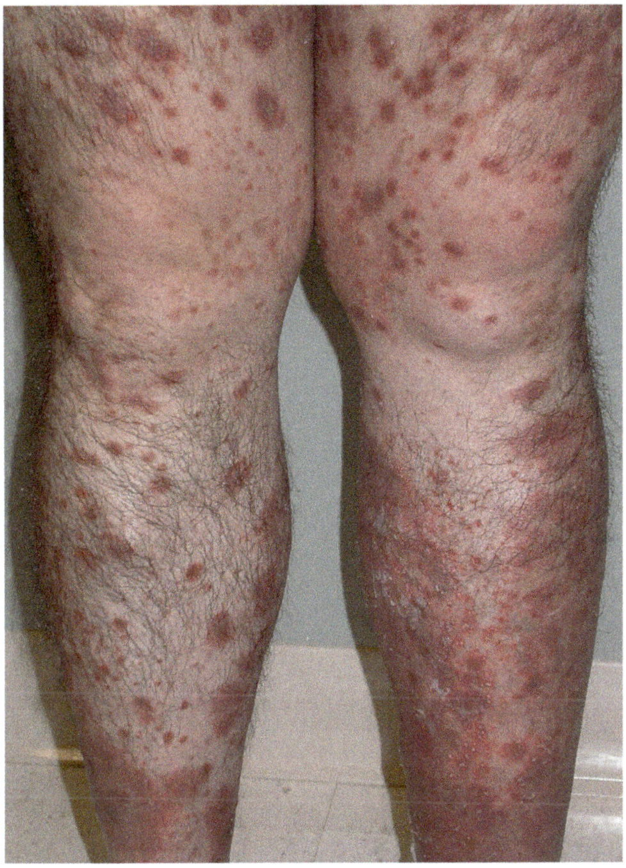

Fig. 23.15 Psoriasis vulgaris. Typical plaques of psoriasis with thick, white scaly overlying erythema

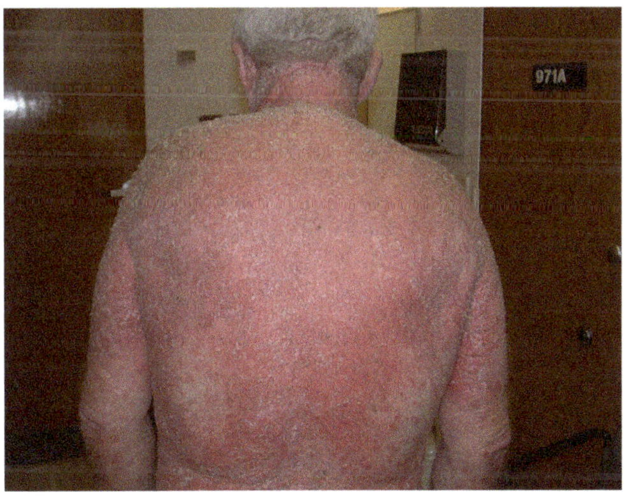

Fig. 23.16 Pityriasis rubra pilaris. Symmetric, diffuse, scaly erythema

Cutaneous T-Cell Lymphoma

Differential Diagnosis: Superficial Fungal Infection

Cutaneous T-cell lymphoma, a class of non-Hodgkin lymphoma, is characterized by infiltration of the skin by clonal malignant T-cells and has many clinical variants, but the classic subtype is characterized by sharply demarcated plaques, uniform in color, ranging from an erythematous to a violaceous hue (Fig. 23.18). The clinical features, histomorphology, and cytomorphology of the lesions are diagnostic clues, and demonstration of a dominant T-cell clone in skin biopsy specimens constitutes an additional diagnostic test to distinguish CTCL from inflammatory dermatoses.

The early stage is typically nonspecific and is often misdiagnosed as eczema, psoriasis and superficial fungal infection.

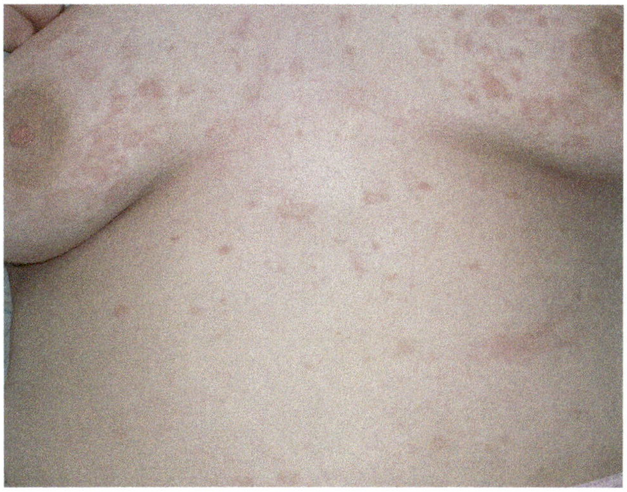

Fig. 23.17 Pityriasis rosea. Truncal involvement with larger plaques and predominantly round patches with peripheral scale

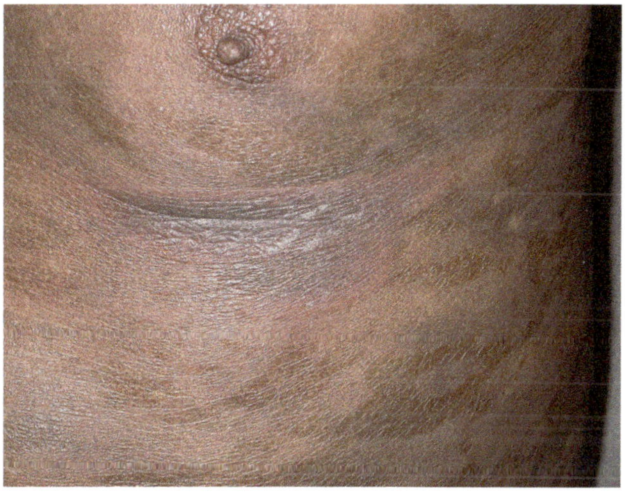

Fig. 23.18 Cutaneous T cell lymphoma. Hyperpigmented scaly patches with minimal scaling

Section 3: Purpuric and Petechial Lesions

Purpura is the multifocal extravasation of blood into the skin or mucous membranes manifested by distinctive red macules a few millimeters in size. Petechiae are superficial, pin-

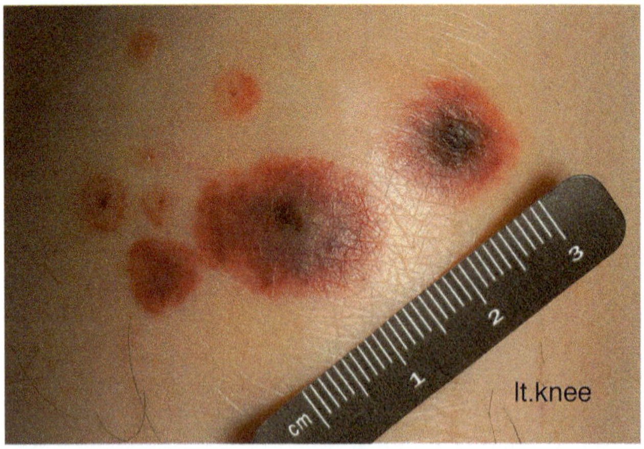

Fig. 23.19 Leukocytoclastic vasculitis. Multiple purpuric papules in a patient with drug-induced hypersensitivity vasculitis

head-sized hemorrhagic macules, bright red at first, seen in the dependent areas. Petechiae most often imply a disorder of platelets.

Leukocytoclastic Vasculitis

Differential Diagnosis: Bacterial and Fungal Infection

Leukocytoclastic vasculitis (LCV) represents a hypersensitivity reaction secondary to immune complex deposition, other autoantibodies, inflammatory mediators, and local factors that involve the endothelial cells. Palpable purpura is the clinical prototype of LCV in which the vascular insult is at the level of arterioles and postcapillary venules. Lesions appear in crops, ranging from 1 to 2 mm in size, and have a predilection for dependent parts. Palpable purpura is generally asymptomatic, but in severe cases (with erosions, bullae, and hemorrhagic vesicles) patients may experience pruritus, edema, and burning [35] (Fig. 23.19). It can be mistaken for systemic bacterial infections including candidiasis and meningococcemia. Skin biopsy reveals the presence of vascular and perivascular infiltration of polymorphonuclear leukocytes with formation of nuclear dust (leukocytoclasis), extravasation of erythrocytes, and fibrinoid necrosis of the vessel walls.

Superficial Thrombophlebitis

Differential Diagnosis: Cellulitis

An inflammatory reaction in which clotting appears on the wall of an inflamed vein in patients with idiopathic venous stasis, prolonged bed rest, local injury to endothelium by trauma, and superficial thrombophlebitis presents with erythema, edema,

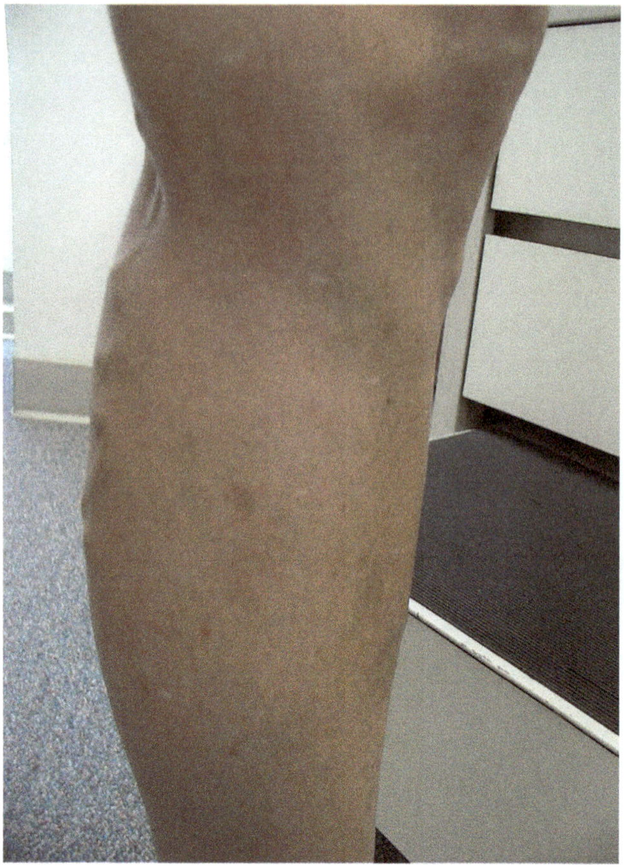

Fig. 23.20 Superficial thrombophlebitis. Erythema and edema along the leg vein

and tenderness in the affected limb (Fig. 23.20). This needs to be distinguished from cellulitis which is a nonnecrotizing inflammation of the skin and subcutaneous tissues.

Calciphylaxis

Differential Diagnosis: Cellulitis, Ecthyma Gangrenosum, and Bacterial and Deep Fungal Infections

This is a highly morbid syndrome characterized by painful ischemic tissue necrosis primarily on fingers, legs, and thighs surrounded by livedo reticularis in patients with chronic renal insufficiency and hyperparathyroidism [36]. Lesions of calciphylaxis typically develop suddenly and progress rapidly. The clinical manifestations of calciphylaxis are similar to those of a significant number of other disorders, including among others cellulitis, necrotizing fasciitis, ecthyma gangrenosum, vibrio vulnificus infection, cholesterol embolization, warfarin necrosis, cryoglobulinemia, and vasculitis [37, 38] (Fig. 23.21).

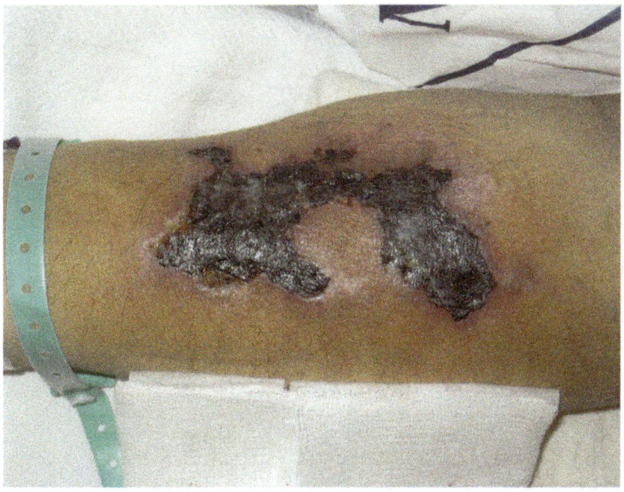

Fig. 23.21 Calciphylaxis. Deep skin necrosis and non-healing ulcer

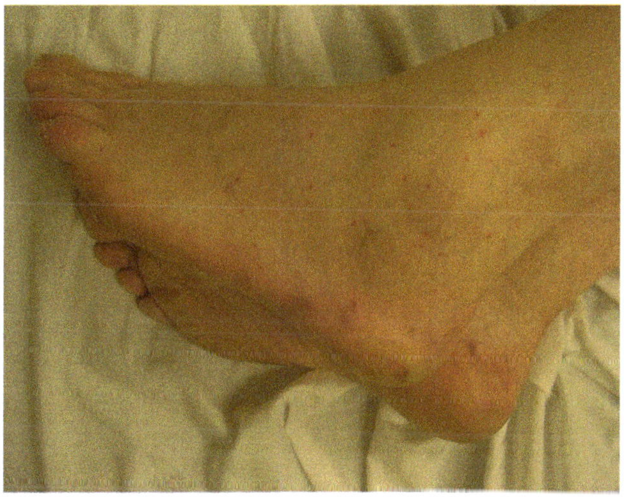

Fig. 23.22 Petechiae. Pinpoint, monoform red macules on the lower legs

Petechiae

Differential Diagnosis: Rickettsial, Bacterial, and Fungal Infection

Petechiae are small purpuric lesions up to 2 mm in size often occurring in crops due to extravasation of red blood cells into the skin. The purpura is not palpable, in contrast to palpable and sometimes tender purpura observed in patients with vasculitis. It tends to form in areas of increased venous pressure, such as the legs (Fig. 23.22). The etiology is multifactorial and includes among others thrombocytopenia, defective platelet function, increased intravascular venous pressure, vitamin C deficiency, and localized trauma or pressure. Purpura is often seen at intravenous injection sites in cancer patients. It must be distinguished from the eruption of Rocky Mountain spotted fever (RMSF), a tick-borne disease caused by the organism *Rickettsia rickettsii.* The hallmark of RMSF is a petechial eruption beginning on the palms of the hands and soles of the feet [39].

Disseminated Intravascular Coagulation

Differential Diagnosis: Bacterial and Fungal Sepsis

Disseminated intravascular coagulation may produce a clinical picture varying from a severe and rapidly fatal disorder (purpura fulminans) to a relatively minor disorder. Varying combinations of bleeding, thromboembolism, and hemolytic anemia are superimposed on the clinical picture caused by primary disorders which include, among others, extensive tissue damage, severe infections, and malignant diseases. The normal inhibitory mechanisms of clotting are overcome so that there is intravenous coagulation, followed by consumption and depletion of platelets and plasma clotting factors. In the most severe cases onset is sudden with fever and a very extensive, symmetrical purpura of the extremities but also on the ears, nose, and lips (Fig. 23.23). Lesser changes include petechiae, purpuric papules, hemorrhagic bullae, and acral cyanosis. Treatment includes that appropriate for the underlying condition, treatment of shock, and replacement therapy as indicated.

Section 4: Lesions of the Adipose Tissue

Differential Diagnosis: Bacterial, Deep Fungal, and Mycobacterial Infections and Cellulitis

Panniculitis is an inflammation occurring within the adipose tissue. It can occur in the septae, lobules, or both. It is often associated with a variety of systemic diseases and clinical syndromes and it often presents as red-to-violaceous nodules and plaques that have a predilection for lower extremities.

Nodular Vasculitis

Nodular vasculitis also called erythema induratum is a vasculitis of the muscular arteries of the deep dermis and fat that result in secondary lobular panniculitis. It occurs in middle-aged women who develop painful, reddish-blue, variably tender nodules and plaques over the lower extremities, especially the calves (Fig. 23.24). A severe small-vessel vasculitis is seen on histologic examination. Nodular panniculitis may be idiopathic but is most commonly due to infections such as tuberculosis and occasionally histoplasmosis,

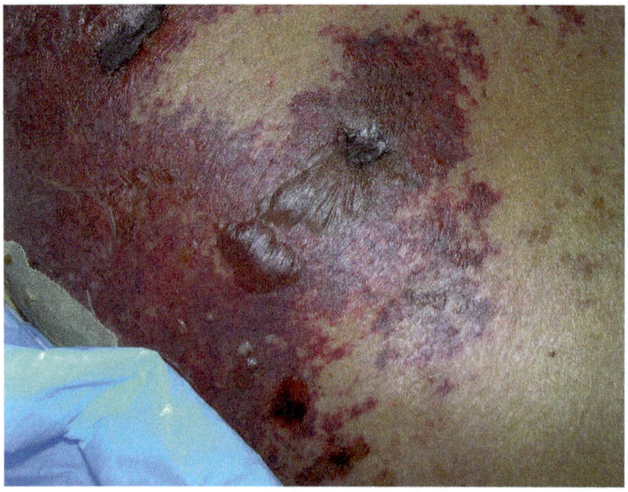

Fig. 23.23 Disseminated intravascular coagulation. Extensive skin necrosis with hemorrhagic bullae

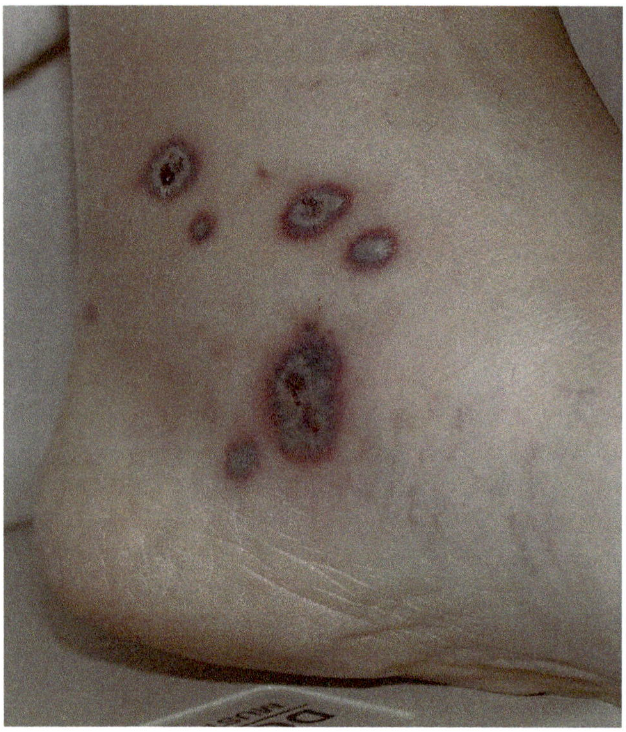

Fig. 23.24 Nodular vasculitis. Tender blue-reddish nodules on the lower legs

HIV, and hepatitis C [40–42]. Painful, indurated red plaques located on the extremities resembling erythema induratum have been reported in patients with chronic myelogenic leukemia undergoing treatment with imatinib [43] and dasatinib [44]. The differential diagnosis of nodular vasculitis includes erythema nodosum, granulomatous vasculitis, and miscellaneous forms of panniculitis.

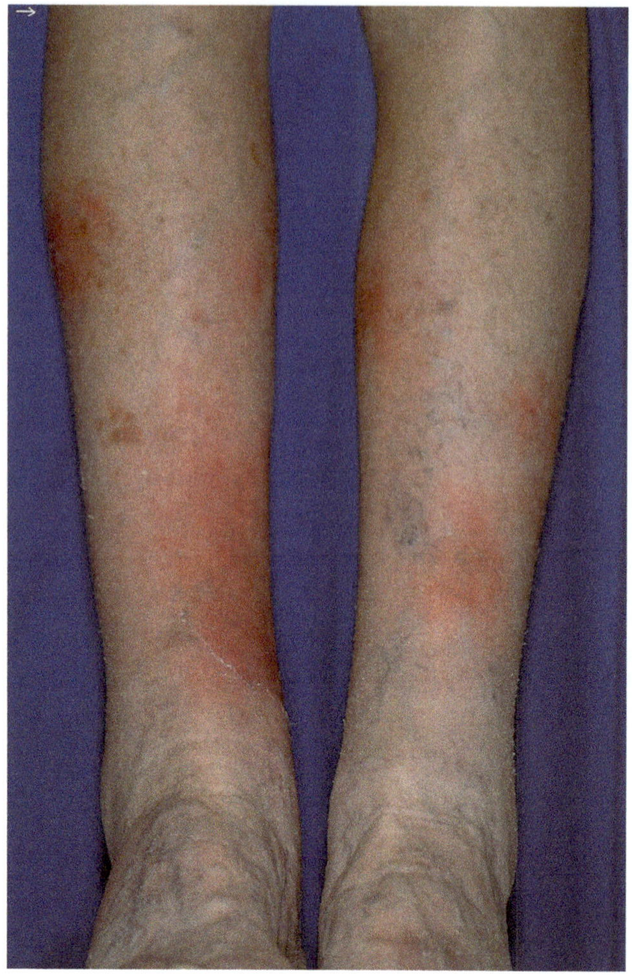

Fig. 23.25 Pancreatic panniculitis. Faint erythematous tender plaques on the lower extremities

Cold Panniculitis

Cold panniculitis is an acute, nodular eruption usually limited to areas exposed to the cold. Cold panniculitis results from a cold injury to the adipose tissue. It is more common in women. The eruptive phase usually begins 48 h (range, 6–72 h) after a cold injury to exposed or poorly protected areas. The lesions should be distinguished from cellulitis and deep fungal or mycobacterial infections.

Pancreatic Panniculitis

Pancreatic panniculitis, acute pancreatitis, and pancreatic tumors may cause fat necrosis of the pancreas and of the subcutaneous tissue. The clinical picture consists of raised, erythematous nodules, 1–3 cm in size, located on the upper and lower extremities (Fig. 23.25). The pathogenic mechanisms underlying the various features of pancreatic panniculitis are unclear.

The histopathology of pancreatic panniculitis is pathognomonic, characterized by ghost adipocytes that are necrotic,

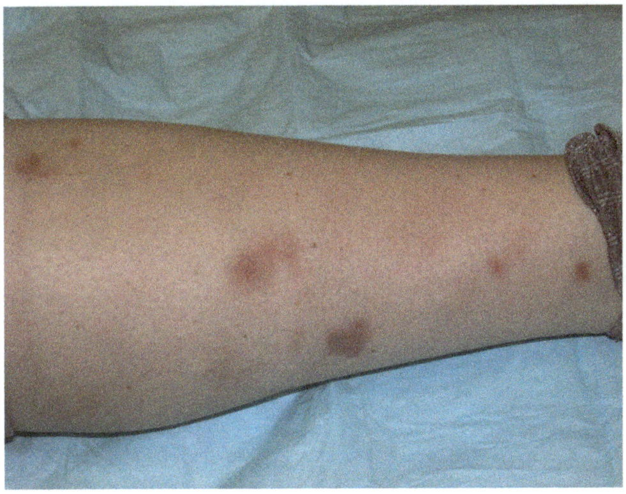

Fig. 23.26 Erythema nodosum. Tender red oval nodules on the extensor aspect of the legs

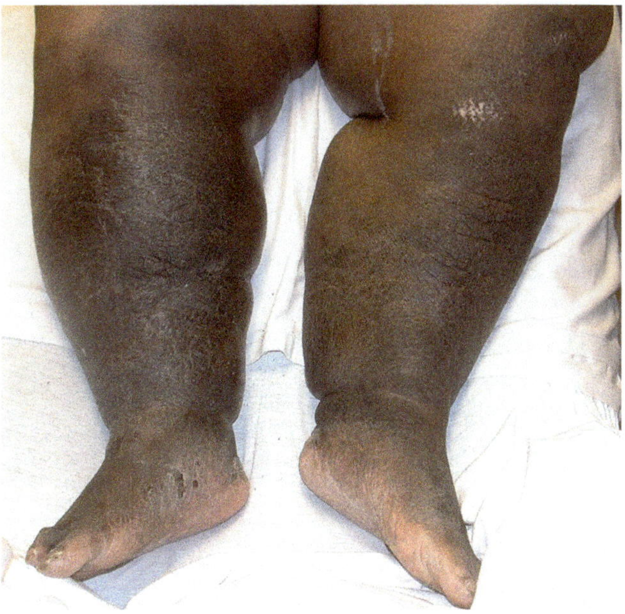

Fig. 23.27 Lipodermatosclerosis. Chronic inflammation and fibrosis of the skin surrounding the entire lower legs

anucleate and contain basophilic material within the cytoplasm indicating dystrophic calcification from the saponification of fat [45]. The exact mechanism is unknown, but it is believed that lipase plays a strong pathogenic role for subcutaneous fat necrosis. The Schmid's triad of panniculitis, polyarthritis, and eosinophilia portends very poor prognosis in a patient with pancreatic carcinoma.

Septal Panniculitis (Erythema Nodosum)

Septal panniculitis (erythema nodosum) is the most common form of inflammatory panniculitis manifested by erythematous, tender nodules on anterior shins, thighs, and lateral aspects of the lower legs and occasionally on the face, accompanied by fever, chills, arthralgias, and leukocytosis (Fig. 23.26). It results from an immunologic reaction triggered by drugs; benign and malignant systemic illness; bacterial, fungal, and viral infections; pregnancy, and medications including oral contraceptives. Circulating immune complexes have not been found in idiopathic and uncomplicated cases but demonstrated in patients with inflammatory bowel disease [46]. It resolves without scarring in 4–6 weeks.

Sclerosing Panniculitis (Lipodermatosclerosis)

Sclerosing panniculitis (lipodermatosclerosis) is a disease process that clinically appears as painful indurated erythematous hyperpigmented plaques and nodules on the lower extremities in middle-aged women. The underlying fibrosis and lobular atrophy give the impression of an inverted champagne bottle with a hard, wood-like appearance which becomes circumferential in well-developed lesions (Fig. 23.27). Occasionally there is overlying ulceration or crusting. Lipodermatosclerosis (LDS) is believed to be associated with chronic venous insufficiency. Abnormal fibrinolysis, an excessive proteolytic activity by matrix metalloproteinase, and the upregulation of an inflammatory response by interleukin-8 are thought to be the causes for this condition [47, 48].

Traumatic Panniculitis

Traumatic panniculitis represents a localized reaction of the subcutaneous tissue following minor trauma. It is most frequently seen in obese women. The lesions consist of indurated, inflamed nodules that undergo necrosis. When localized to the breast, they may clinically simulate a carcinoma or infectious mastitis. Traumatic panniculitis is usually a self-limiting disorder and requires only symptomatic treatment.

Section 5: Vesiculobullous Lesions

A vesicle is a fluid-filled blister less than 0.5 cm in its greatest dimension, while bullae is greater than 0.5 cm. Vesiculobullous lesions may be solitary, grouped, or annular and either localized or widespread in distribution. The etiology of these lesions varies, and valuable clues may be found in the patient's history, clinical presentation, and skin biopsy. From an infectious disease specialist's viewpoint, blistering lesions are often caused by herpetic eruptions or infectious pathogens which produce skin necrosis. However, a variety of non-infectious vesiculobullous lesions may occur in the transplant setting and are reviewed in this section.

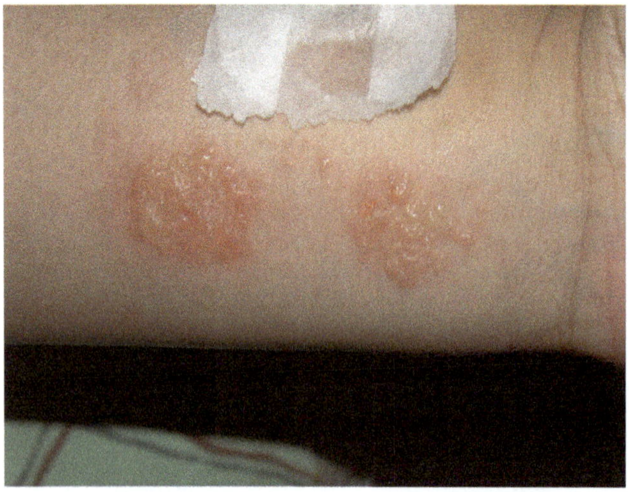

Fig. 23.28 Allergic contact dermatitis. Characterized by well-defined plaques of vesiculopapules overlying erythema and edema. Oozing and secondary infection are common

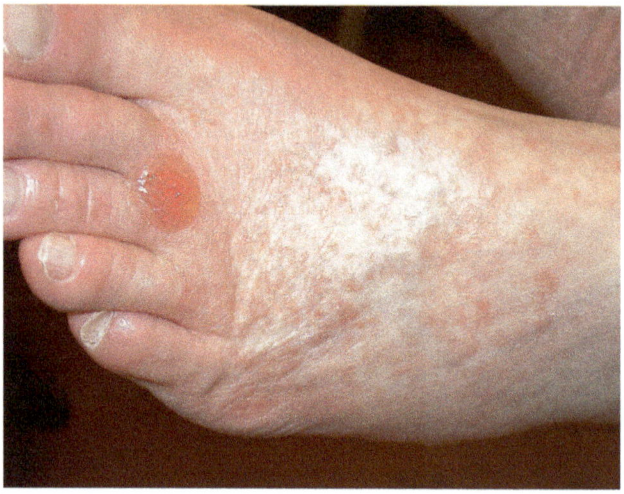

Fig. 23.29 Mechanical blister. Flat bullae on the toe dorsum secondary to trauma

Acute Dermatitis

Differential Diagnosis: Viral Infections and Impetigo

The vesiculobullous eruption associated with acute dermatitis is caused by inter- and intracellular edema in the epidermis, also called spongiosis. The patient may be aware of a preceding irritant or allergen applied to the skin, including surgical preparations, topical antibiotics, or tape. Allergic contact dermatitis may be linear or geometric, corresponding to the application of the precipitating agent (Fig. 23.28). As the blisters rupture, a superficial crust forms, which may be mistaken for impetigo. It is not unusual for the dermatitis to become secondarily infected, especially in the immunosuppressed transplant patient. On occasion, non-infectious vesicular lesions may appear distant to the site of the original dermatitis, a phenomenon known as autosensitization dermatitis. This should be distinguished from a disseminated herpetic process.

Diabetic Blisters

Differential Diagnosis: Viral Infection and Cellulitis

Also known as bullosis diabeticorum [49], this condition is characterized by the spontaneous appearance of intraepidermal or subepidermal, clear, tense bullae on the non-erythematous skin of diabetic patients. These blisters are most often found on the lower extremities and are minimally symptomatic. The pathogenesis may be related to diabetic angiopathy or trauma, and this condition should be distinguished from infectious cellulitis.

Mechanical Blisters

Differential Diagnosis: Cellulitis and Ecthyma

These painful blisters occur in areas of high friction or pressure, which causes epidermal necrosis. The surrounding erythematous rim may mimic cellulitis. Mechanical blisters are also precipitated by burns, extravasations of toxic substances, or vesicants. Hemorrhagic bullae may occur at sites of injections in patients with thrombocytopenia or capillary fragility (Fig. 23.29).

Coma Blister

Differential Diagnosis: Cellulitis and Ecthyma

Skin blisters at sites of pressure and associated with underlying sweat gland necrosis were reported in comatose patients with carbon monoxide intoxication as early as 1812 [50]. Also called barbiturate or neurologic blisters, these lesions are at times associated with surrounding erythema that may look like cellulitis. While barbiturates are the most frequently reported causative agent [51, 52], similar findings have been reported with other medications including tricyclic antidepressants [53] and benzodiazepines [54]. Coma blisters have been associated with central nervous system disorders [55], hypoglycemia [56], and diabetic ketoacidosis [57]. The etiology is multifactorial, but in some cases, a direct toxic drug effect has been implicated, perhaps via drug excretion through the eccrine glands. The bullae may appear as early as 1 h after acute intoxication and usually resolve in 2–4 weeks. They may be clear or hemorrhagic and should be distinguished from ecthyma or cellulitis.

Miliaria Crystallina

Differential Diagnosis: Herpes Infection

Miliaria crystallina, also known as sudamina, occurs in the setting of profuse sweating and epidermal occlusion. It is characterized by 1–2-mm asymptomatic vesicles on a non-inflammatory base, which are easily "wiped away" with pressure. As opposed to grouped herpetic vesicles on a more erythematous base, miliaria crystallina appears on occluded skin, with no underlying erythema (Fig. 23.30).

Edema and Lymphedema Blisters

Differential Diagnosis: Cellulitis

Large dependent bullae may develop in the setting of peripheral edema, anasarca, and lymphedema, especially if the onset of swelling is acute. Although these bullae are usually found on normal-appearing skin, underlying stasis changes may make it difficult to distinguish from bullous cellulitis. Initially, the blisters are tense and clear but may become hemorrhagic or superinfected. Treatment is directed at minimizing the underlying edema.

Bullous Drug Eruptions

Differential Diagnosis: Viral Infections, Ecthyma, and Cellulitis

Bullous drug reactions may be localized or widespread. When localized and recurrent at the same site after drug re-challenge, they are referred to as fixed drug eruptions. Fixed drug eruptions initially appear within 2 weeks of the inciting drug exposure but within 30 min–24 h after re-challenge. The eruption is characterized by erythema, sometimes the formation of bullae, and often characteristic residual "slate-grey" pigmentation as the lesion resolves. Findings suggest that fixed drug eruptions are a form of classic delayed-type hypersensitivity mediated by CD8+ cells [58], although mast cells may play a role [59]. When located on the genitalia the blisters may look like acute herpes simplex infection and, on other sites, cellulitis. Widespread bullous drug reactions have varying etiologies and pathologic features. Certain medications may produce immune-mediated blistering, characterized by the deposition of IgA at the dermal-epidermal junction. This is of special interest to infectious disease specialists as it has been reported with antibiotics like trimethoprim-sulfamethoxazole, penicillin, metronidazole, and rifampicin [60].

Bullous Graft Versus Host Disease

Differential Diagnosis: Viral Infection and Cellulitis

Allogeneic hematopoietic stem cell transplantation is widely used for the treatment of hematologic malignancies, bone marrow failure syndromes, and immunodeficiency. The skin is commonly affected in patients who develop graft-versus-host disease (GVHD). Grade 4 acute GVHD of the skin is characterized by a generalized exfoliative dermatitis, ulcerative dermatitis, and bullae [61] that may be mistaken for disseminated viral infection (Fig. 23.31). In these cases, the damage at the epidermal-dermal junction is severe enough to allow the dermis to separate from the epidermis. Bullae may also appear in the setting of scleroderma like GVHD changes [62, 63].

Fig. 23.30 Miliaria crystallina. Clear, thin-walled vesicles occurring in crops on otherwise normal-appearing skin

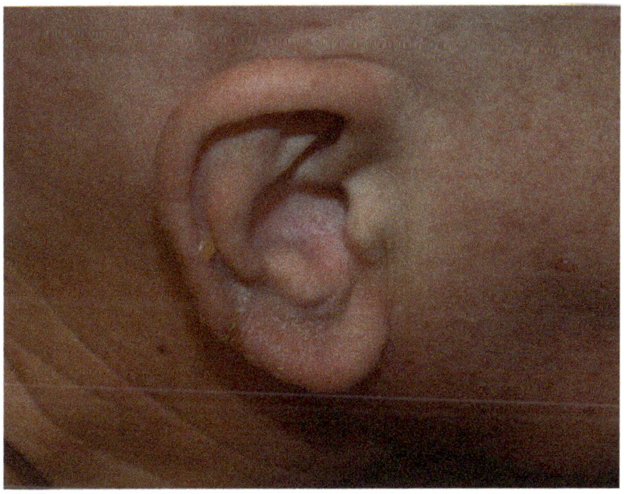

Fig. 23.31 Bullous graft-versus-host disease. Tense bulla and vesicles on the ear in patient with diffuse erythema of the head and neck

Although the pathogenesis is unknown, these cases show significant fibrosis and dermal edema [64, 65].

Porphyria Cutanea Tarda (PCT) and Pseudoporphyria Cutanea Tarda

Differential Diagnosis: Viral and Bacterial Infections

Porphyria cutanea tarda (PCT) is a group of familial and acquired disorders characterized by deficiency in the activity of uroporphyrinogen decarboxylase, an enzyme key in heme synthesis. In the transplant setting, this may be precipitated by exposure to environmental agent such as excess iron [66], coexisting conditions that affect the liver, and infection agents including hepatitis C [67] and HIV [68]. Patients exhibit skin fragility and blistering, especially in sun-exposed areas, as well as hypertrichosis, scleroderma-like changes, milia (small white cysts), and dystrophic calcification (Fig. 23.32). Pseudoporphyria mimics the findings of PCT without demonstrable porphyrin abnormalities. It has been reported in the setting of chronic renal failure and dialysis [69], as well with medications like beta-lactam antibiotics [70], ciprofloxacin [71], voriconazole [72], and tetracycline [73].

Autoimmune Bullous Diseases

Differential Diagnosis: Viral Infection, Cellulitis, and Scabies

This broad category of diseases is characterized as immune-mediated blistering of the skin. Bullous pemphigoid presents with tense skin blisters, urticarial (hive-like) lesions, and variable mucosal involvement. It is characterized by autoantibodies located in the hemidesmosomal complex of the basement membrane zone. It may occur de novo, with other autoimmune diseases, or occasionally with malignancies. Some antibiotics implicated in pathogenesis include amoxicillin [74], cephalexin [75], and ciprofloxacin [76]. The clinical presentation of tense blisters associated with urticaria may be mistaken for cellulitis.

Pemphigus presents on the skin and mucous membranes with intraepidermal flaccid bullae. It is divided into three forms: vulgaris; foliaceus; and paraneoplastic. Patients with pemphigus vulgaris develop painful mucosal erosions and skin lesions, which may resemble a herpetic process. Patients with pemphigus foliaceus develop extensive crusted erosions, easily confused with cutaneous infection (Fig. 23.33). Paraneoplastic pemphigus is associated with underlying neoplasms, and characterized by severe stomatitis, often mistaken for herpetic stomatitis. The lesions on the skin are polymorphous and may resemble lichen planus or erythema multiforme. (These patients may also develop lung involvement characterized by bronchiolitis obliterans [77]). Antibiotics are implicated in the pathogenesis of pemphigus vulgaris, including ampicillin, penicillin, cefadroxil, and rifampicin [60, 78]. In these cases, the eruption usually starts a few weeks after starting the medication. The diagnosis of pemphigus is made by performing a skin biopsy, which demonstrates an intraepidermal vesicle with acantholysis (separation between epidermal cells). Direct immunofluorescence of peri-lesional skin demonstrates IgG and/or C3 binding to the intercellular cement or keratinocyte cell surface [79]. Dermatitis herpetiformis, a cutaneous manifestation of

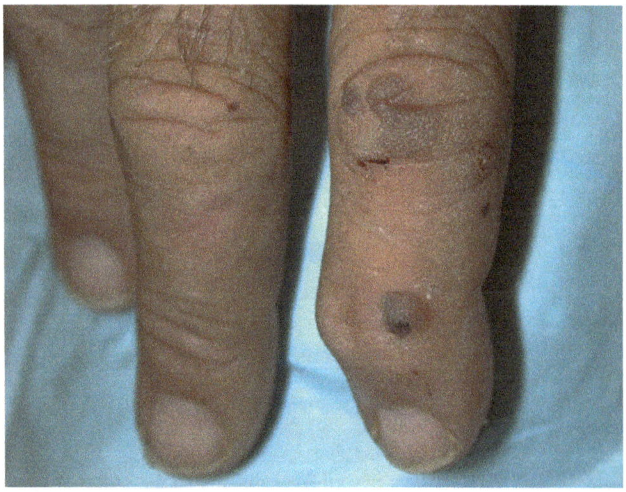

Fig. 23.32 Porphyria cutanea tarda. Vesicles and bullae on light-exposed cutaneous surfaces, especially the dorsal aspects of the hands

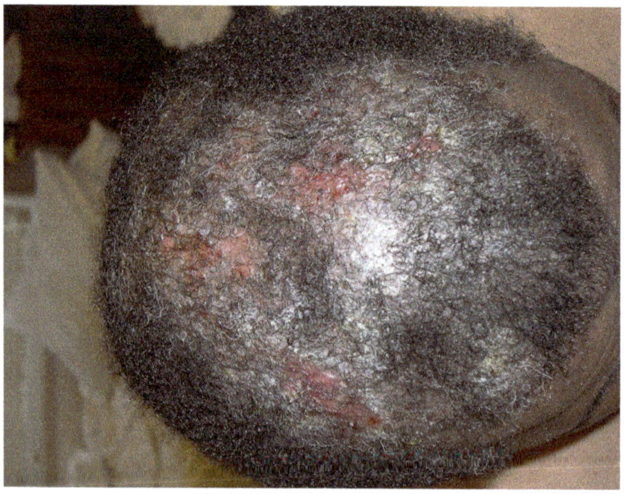

Fig. 23.33 Pemphigus vulgaris. Painful scalp erosions with underlying erythema

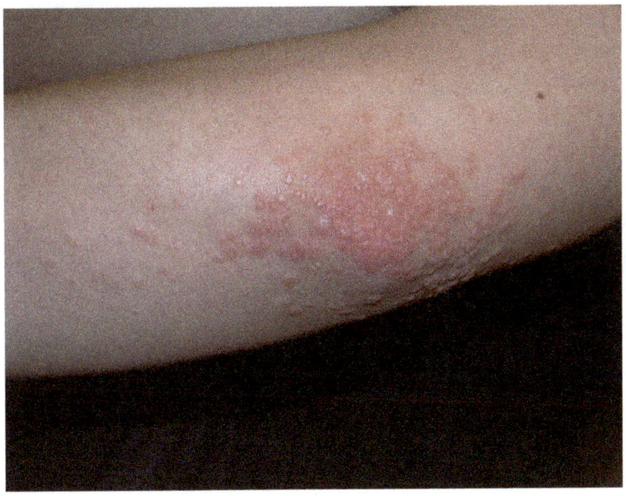

Fig. 23.34 Dermatitis herpetiformis. Grouped, symmetric, and pruritic papules on the elbow

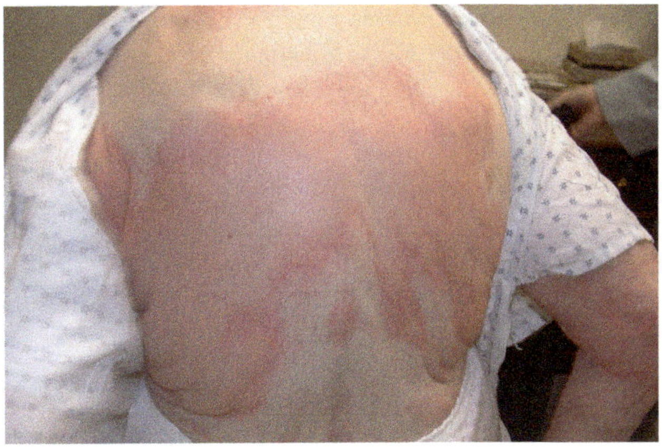

Fig. 23.35 Urticaria. Transient, well-circumscribed erythematous dermal plaques on the trunk

gluten-sensitive enteropathy, is characterized by pruritic, tiny vesicles easily reminiscent of scabies or herpes infections. These are most commonly found on the elbows, back buttocks, and knees (Fig. 23.34). The biopsy shows neutrophils in the dermal papillae and granular deposits of IgA. The eruption may be worsened by ingestion or application of iodide [80].

Bullous Insect Bite Reaction

Differential Diagnosis: Ecthyma, Viral Infection, and Cellulitis

Insect bite reactions may produce varying degrees of erythema and are less commonly vesicles, bullae, and necrosis. Exaggerated bite reactions have been reported in the setting of chronic lymphocytic leukemia as well as other hemato proliferative disorders and human immunodeficiency virus infections [81, 82]. Many patients have no recollection of the bite.

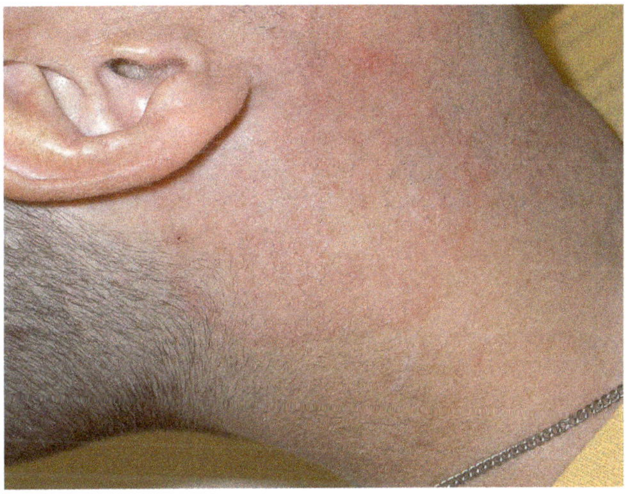

Fig. 23.36 Tinea corporis. An expanding, erythematous annular plaque

Section 6: Erythematous Lesions

Injury, infection, vascular reactivity, and inflammation may cause erythema of the skin. Most of the conditions discussed in this section produce blanchable erythema, that is, resolution of the erythema with pressure. So-called reactive erythema is a cutaneous response to an underlying systemic process, which may be infectious, malignant, or drug related. The primary lesions are red plaques that may be annular, transient, or fixed.

Urticaria

Differential Diagnosis: Cellulitis and Superficial Fungal Infections

Urticaria, commonly referred to as hives or wheals, are well-demarcated, smooth, dermal plaques that may become confluent and demonstrate a variable degree of pruritus. When associated with significant edema and warmth, they are mistaken for cellulitis (Fig. 23.35) and when annular in configuration, for tinea corporis (Fig. 23.36). Because they result from transient dermal edema, they tend to change in size and shape and are rarely present in the same spot for more than 48 h. When persistent, a biopsy may demonstrate urticarial vasculitis, characterized by small vessel destruction.

Angioedema presents with deep and painful swelling, without urticaria. Transplant patients may be at increased risk of angiotensin-converting enzyme (ACE)-associated angioedema because of the effects of immunosuppressants on the activity of circulating dipeptidyl peptidase IV (DPPIV) [83].

Erythema Multiforme (EM)/Stevens-Johnson Syndrome (SJS), and Toxic Epidermal Necrolysis (TEN)

Differential Diagnosis: Disseminated Viral, Bacterial, or Fungal Infections

At the onset, erythema multiforme presents as erythematous macules and plaques on the extensor surfaces of the limbs and on the palms and soles. Other infectious etiologies for palm and sole lesions including rickettsia, spirochetes, or viruses should be considered. The classic target or iris lesion is characterized by a dusky center, red border, and surrounding pallor (Fig. 23.37). If enough epidermal apoptosis is present, the center may appear bullous, hemorrhagic, or necrotic, suggestive of ecthyma or embolic infection. SJS may be complicated by significant mucous membrane involvement of the lips, buccal mucosa palate, conjunctivae, urethra, and vagina. TEN is a life-threatening condition characterized by detachment of the epidermis from the dermis (Fig. 23.38). The differential diagnosis includes staphylococcal scalded skin syndrome (SSSS). However, SSSS causes a more superficial subcorneal skin split that can readily be distinguished by skin biopsy.

EM, SJS, and TEN are associated with many different etiologies. Infectious agents are important precipitating factors in children and young adults [84], whereas drug reactions and malignancy are more important in adults [85, 86]. Herpes simplex, mycoplasma pneumonia, Coxasackie B-5, influenza type A, and echo viruses have all been implicated in pathogenesis [87].

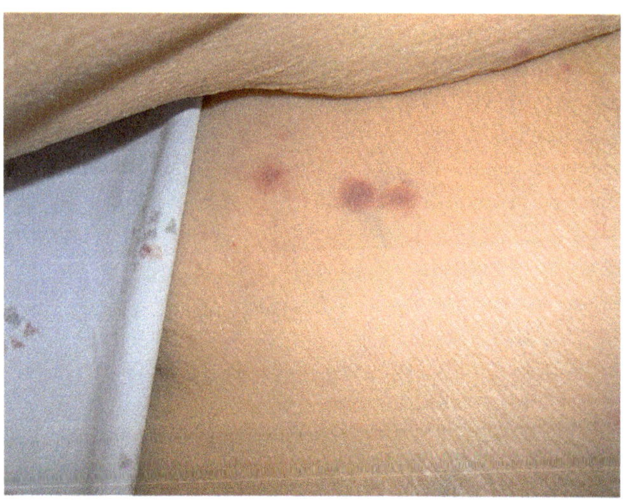

Fig. 23.37 Erythema multiforme. Round lesions in which concentric rings with color variation are present

Gyrate Erythema

Differential Diagnosis: Superficial Fungal, Bacterial, or Rickettsial Infections

A gyrate erythema is characterized by polycyclic erythematous plaques. In the case of erythema annulare centrifugum, the lesions slowly expand, disappear over weeks, and are replaced by new annular lesions (Fig. 23.39). Some cases are associated with dermatophyte infections, but the lesions themselves do not contain fungus. This condition is rarely associated with internal malignancy, and the clinical presentation may mimic secondary syphilis, dermatophytosis, Hansen's disease or erythema migrans, and the gyrate erythema associated with Lyme disease.

Necrolytic migratory erythema, associated with glucagon-secreting tumors of the pancreas, is a gyrate erythema that

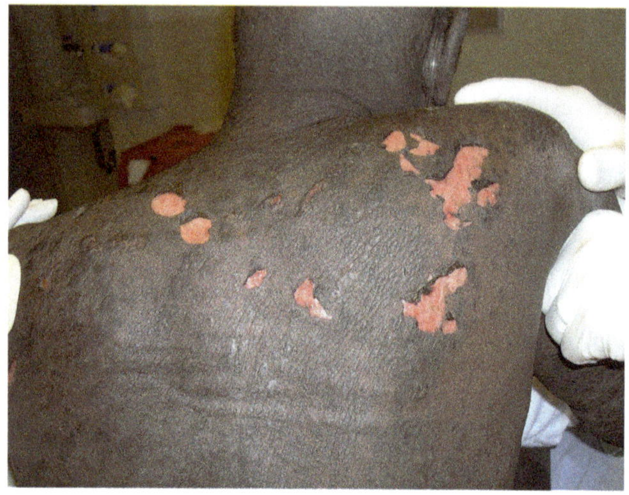

Fig. 23.38 Toxic epidermal necrolysis. Extensive erosions and sloughing of skin resembling wrinkled, wet tissue paper

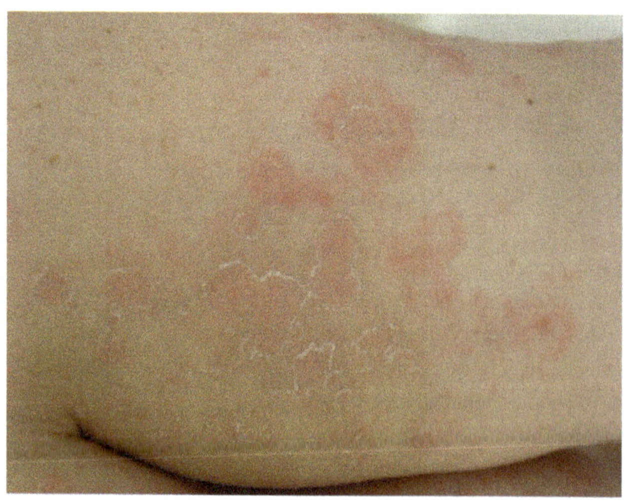

Fig. 23.39 Gyrate erythema. Slowly expanding annular lesions and palpable scaly erythematous borders

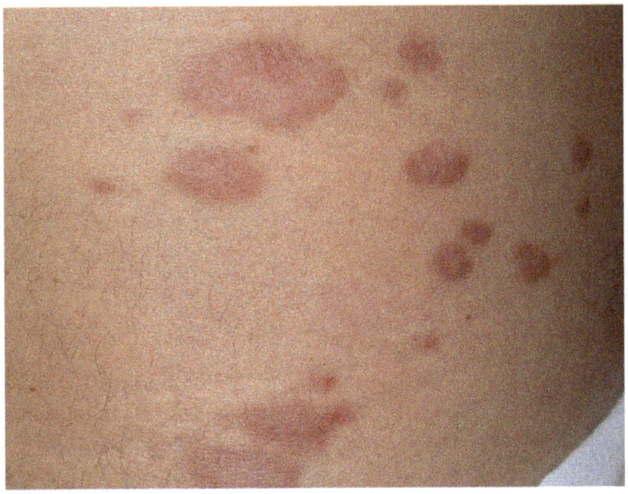

Fig. 23.40 Granuloma annulare. Annular, dusky-red, nonscaly plaques on the trunk

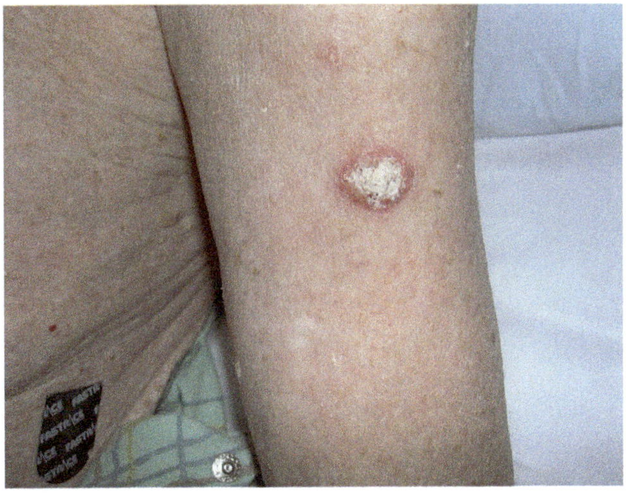

Fig. 23.41 Squamous cell carcinoma. Large, sun-induced, keratotic, non-ulcerated nodule on the arm

occurs in periorificial, flexural, and acral areas. The eruption may resemble chronic mucocutaneous candidiasis, severe seborrheic dermatitis, or acrodermatitis enteropathica associated with zinc deficiency. It has also been associated with hepatitis C [88].

Granuloma Annulare

Differential Diagnosis: Superficial Fungal Infection

This granulomatous process presents with annular and serpiginous plaques with no significant scale (Fig. 23.40). In some studies, GA has been associated with diabetes mellitus [89], but many cases are idiopathic. The lesions may be confused with a superficial fungal infection.

Section 7: Ulcerative Lesions and Skin Tumors

Differential Diagnosis: Bacterial, Fungal, Mycobacterial, or Parasitic Infections

Organ transplantation markedly increases the risk of developing non-melanoma skin cancers, the most common of which are squamous cell carcinoma followed by basal cell carcinoma [90] (Fig. 23.41). Compared to the biologic behavior in non-immunosuppressed individuals, the squamous cell carcinomas tend to be more aggressive, with a higher risk of invasion of surrounding structures as well as metastasis [91, 92]. Kaposi's sarcoma and Merkel cell carcinomas occur with increased frequency [90]. In organ transplant patients with chronic ulcerations, it may be prudent to biopsy for bacterial, fungal, and acid-fast culture as well as for histopathology.

Section 8: Hair and Scalp Lesions

Transplant patients may present with inflammatory lesions of the scalp and alopecia as a result of bacterial and fungal infections. This section will review some of the noninfectious etiologies of hair and scalp lesions.

Tumors

Differential Diagnosis: Bacterial and Deep Fungal Infections

The incidence of squamous cell and basal cell carcinomas of the skin increase with the duration of immunosuppressive therapy in transplant recipients and affect at least 50% of Caucasian transplant patients [93]. Approximately 80% of tumors develop on the head [94] with associated ulceration, crusting, and erosions. Early on, these crusted lesions may be mistaken for bacterial or fungal infections, delaying the diagnosis. Some of these tumors resemble warts and, in fact, human papillomaviruses may be cocarcinogenic [95]. Patients post-organ transplantation may also be at a higher risk for melanoma [96], Kaposi's sarcoma [97], and Merkel cell carcinoma [98].

Plaques and Pustules

Differential Diagnosis: Bacterial and Fungal Infections

While erythematous plaques and pustules on the scalp may be caused by dermatophyte and bacterial infections, this is also a common presentation of scalp psoriasis. The characteristic well-demarcated, scaly plaques may be studded with

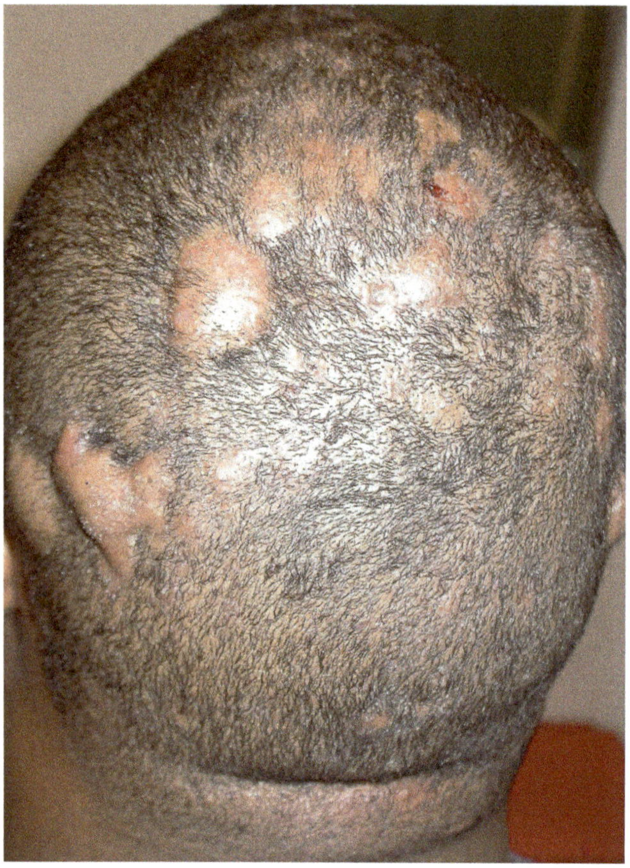

Fig. 23.42 Dissecting cellulitis of the scalp. Painful cutaneous nodules and patchy alopecia

sterile pustules; the latter may be precipitated by systemic corticosteroid withdrawal or taper. Dissecting cellulitis of the scalp, also called perifolliculitis capitis abscedens et suffodiens, produces boggy and fluctuant scalp nodules with interconnecting sinus tracts and sterile, purulent discharge (Fig. 23.42). This disorder often responds better to retinoids than antibiotics [99]. Other common causes of sterile pustules and inflammation on the scalp include acne keloidalis or inflamed cysts.

References

1. Urano S, Kodama H, Kato K, Nogura K. Pyoderma gangrenosum with systemic involvement. J Dermatol. 1995;22(7):515–9.
2. Hurwitz RM, Haseman JH. The evolution of pyoderma gangrenosum. A clinicopathologic correlation. Am J Dermatopathol. 1993;15(1):28–33.
3. Su WP, Davis MD, Weenig RH, Powell FC, Perry HO. Pyoderma gangrenosum: clinicopathologic correlation and proposed diagnostic criteria. Int J Dermatol. 2004;43(11):790–800.
4. Callen JP. Pyoderma gangrenosum. Lancet. 1998;351(9102):581–5.
5. Callen JP, Jackson JM. Pyoderma gangrenosum: an update. Rheum Dis Clin North Am. 2007;33(4):787–802, vi.
6. Powell FC, Su WP, Perry HO. Pyoderma gangrenosum: classification and management. J Am Acad Dermatol. 1996;34(3):395–409; quiz 410–2.
7. Emmi L, Brugnolo F, Salvati G, et al. Immunopathological aspects of Behcet's disease. Clin Exp Rheumatol. 1995;13(6):687–91.
8. Alpsoy E, Zouboulis CC, Ehrlich GE. Mucocutaneous lesions of Behcet's disease. Yonsei Med J. 2007;48(4):573–85.
9. Cohen PR, Kurzrock R. Sweet's syndrome revisited: a review of disease concepts. Int J Dermatol. 2003;42(10):761–78.
10. von den Driesch P. Sweet's syndrome (acute febrile neutrophilic dermatosis). J Am Acad Dermatol. 1994;31(4):535–56.
11. Cohen PR, Kurzrock R. Sweet's syndrome: a neutrophilic dermatosis classically associated with acute onset and fever. Clin Dermatol. 2000;18(3):265–82.
12. Kennedy C. The spectrum of inflammatory skin disease following jejuno-ileal bypass for morbid obesity. Br J Dernatol. 1981;105(4):425–35.
13. Ely P. The bowel bypass syndrome: a response to bacterial peptidoglycans. J Am Acad Dermatol. 1980;2(6):473–87.
14. Revuz J, Valeyrie-Allanore L. Drug reactions. In: Bolognia J, Lorizzo JL, Rapini RP, Callen JP, Horn TD, Mancini AJ, et al., editors. Dermatology. Mosby: Elsevier; 2008. p. 301–20.
15. Roujeau JC, Bioulac-Sage P, Bourseau C, et al. Acute generalized exanthematous pustulosis. Analysis of 63 cases. Arch Dermatol. 1991;127(9):1333–8.
16. Ramdial PK, Naidoo DK. Drug-induced cutaneous pathology. J Clin Pathol. 2009;62(60):493–504.
17. James WD. Clinical practice. Acne. N Engl J Med. 2005;352(14):1463–72.
18. Wnorowski AM, de Souza A, Chachoua A, Cohen DE. The management of EGFR inhibitor adverse events: a case series and treatment paradigm. Int J Dermatol. 2012;51(2):223–32.
19. Nervi SJ, Schwartz RA, Dmochowski M. Eosinophilic pustular folliculitis: a 40 year retrospect. J Am Acad Dermatol. 2006;55(2):285–9.
20. Fraser SJ, Benton EC, Roddie PH, Krajewski AS, Goodlad JR. Eosinophilic folliculitis: an important differential diagnosis after allogeneic bone-marrow transplant. Clin Exp Dermatol. 2009;34(3):369–71.
21. Fukamachi S, Kabashima K, Sugita K, Kobayashi M, Tokura Y. Therapeutic effectiveness of various treatments for eosinophilic pustular folliculitis. Acta Derm Venereol. 2009;89(2):155–9.
22. Wenzel FG, Horn TD. Nonneoplastic disorders of the eccrine glands. J Am Acad Dermatol. 1998;38(1):1–17.
23. Mowad CM, McGinley KJ, Foglia A, Leyden JJ. The role of extracellular polysaccharide substance produced by Staphylococcus epidermidis in miliaria. J Am Acad Dermatol. 1995;33(5. Pt 1):729–33.
24. Bolognia JL, Cooper DL, Glusac EJ. Toxic erythema of chemotherapy: a useful clinical term. J Am Acad Dermatol. 2008;59(3):524–9.
25. Cohen PR. Neutrophilic dermatoses occurring in oncology patients. Int J Dermatol. 2007;46(1):106–11.
26. Alley E, Green R, Schuchter L. Cutaneous toxicities of cancer therapy. Curr Opin Oncol. 2002;14(2):212–6.
27. Kim BS, Kim WJ, Ko HC, Kim MB, Kim DW, Kim JM. Features of Staphylococcus aureus colonization in patients with nummular eczema. Br J Dermatol. 2013;168(3):658–60.
28. Lin SS, Tsai TH, Yang HH. Rare cutaneous side-effect of gefitinib masquerading as superficial dermatophytosis. Clin Exp Dermatol. 2009;34(4):528–30.
29. Wolf R, Oumeish OY, Parish LC. Intertriginous eruption. Clin Dermatol. 2011;29(2):173–9.
30. Pignol JP, Olivotto I, Rakovitch E, et al. A multicenter randomized trial of breast intensity-modulated radiation therapy to reduce acute radiation dermatitis. J Clin Oncol. 2008;26(13):2085–92.

31. Hymes SR, Strom EA, Fife C. Radiation dermatitis: clinical presentation, pathophysiology, and treatment 2006. J Am Acad Dermatol. 2006;54(1):28–46.
32. Hill A, Hanson M, Bogle MA, Duvic M. Severe radiation dermatitis is related to Staphylococcus aureus. Am J Clin Oncol. 2004;27(4):361–3.
33. Johnson MA, Armstrong AW. Clinical and histologic diagnostic guidelines for psoriasis: a critical review. Clin Rev Allergy Immunol. 2013;44(2):166–72.
34. Drago F, Broccolo F, Rebora A. Pityriasis rosea: an update with a critical appraisal of its possible herpesviral etiology. J Am Acad Dermatol. 2009;61(2):303–18.
35. Blanco R, Martínez-Taboada VM, Rodríguez-Valverde V, García-Fuentes M. Cutaneous vasculitis in children and adults. Associated diseases and etiologic factors in 303 patients. Medicine (Baltimore). 1998;77(6):403–18. (review).
36. Wilmer WA, Magro CM. Calciphylaxis: emerging concepts in prevention, diagnosis, and treatment. Semin Dial. 2002;15(3):172–86.
37. Fischer AH, Morris DJ. Pathogenesis of calciphylaxis: study of three cases with literature review. Hum Pathol. 1995;26:1055.
38. Hussein MR, Ali HO, Abdulwahed SR, Argoby Y, Tobeigei FH. Calciphylaxis cutis: a case report and review of literature. Exp Mol Pathol. 2009;86(2):134–5.
39. Buckingham SC, Marshall GS, Schutze GE, et al. Clinical and laboratory features, hospital course, and outcome of Rocky Mountain spotted fever in children. J Pediatr. 2007;150(2):180–4, 184.e1.
40. Winkelmann RK. Panniculitis in connective tissue disease. Arch Dermatol. 1983;119:336.
41. Friedman PC, Husain S, Grossman ME. Nodular tuberculid in a patient with HIV. J Am Acad Dermatol. 2005;53(2. Suppl 1):S154–6.
42. Fernandes SS, Carvalho J, Leite S, Afonso M, Pinto J, Veloso R, et al. Erythema induratum and chronic hepatitis C infection. J Clin Virol. 2009;44(4):333–6.
43. Ugurel S, Lahaye T, Hildenbrand R, Glorer E, Reiter A, Hochhaus A, et al. Panniculitis in a patient with chronic myelogenous leukaemia treated with imatinib. Br J Dermatol. 2003;149(3):678–9.
44. Assouline S, Laneuville P, Gambacorti-Passerini C. Panniculitis during dasatinib therapy for imatinib-resistant chronic myelogenous leukemia. N Engl J Med. 2006;354(24):2623.
45. Ball NJ, Adams SP, Marx LH, et al. Possible origin ofpancreatic fat necrosis as a septal panniculitis. J Am Acad Dermatol. 1996;34:362–4.
46. Nguyen GC, Torres EA, Regueiro M, et al. Inflammatory bowel disease characteristics among African Americans, Hispanics, and non-Hispanic Whites: characterization of a large North American cohort. Am J Gastroenterol. 2006;101(5):1012–23.
47. Miteva M, Romanelli P, Kirsner RS. Lipodermatosclerosis. Dermatol Ther. 2010;23:375–88.
48. Herouy Y, May AE, Pornschlegel G, Stetter C, Grenz H, Preissner KT, et al. Lipodermatosclerosis is characterized by elevated expression and activation on matrix metalloproteinases: implications for venous ulcer formation. J Invest Dermatol. 1998;111:822–7.
49. Cantwell AR Jr, Martz W. Idiopathic bullae in diabetics. Bullosis diabeticorum. Arch Dermatol. 1967;96:42–4.
50. Larrey D. Memoires de Chirurgie Militaire et Campagnes. Paris: Smith and Buisson; 1812.
51. Groschel D, Gerstein AR, Rosenbaum JM. Skin lesions as a diagnostic aid in barbiturate poisoning. N Engl J Med. 1970;283:409–10.
52. Wenzel FG, Horn TD. Nonneoplastic disorders of the eccrine glands. J Am Acad Dermatol. 1998;38:1–17. quiz 8–20.
53. Herschthal D, Robinson MJ. Blisters of the skin in coma induced by amitriptyline and clorazepate dipotassium. Report of a case with underlying sweat gland necrosis. Arch Dermatol. 1979;115:499.
54. Varma AJ, Fisher BK, Sarin MK. Diazepam-induced coma with bullae and eccrine sweat gland necrosis. Arch Intern Med. 1977;137:1207–10.
55. Judge TG, Nisbet NH. Trophoneurotic blisters in elderly hemiplegics. Lancet. 1967;1:811–2.
56. Raymond LW. "Barbiturate blisters" in a case of severe hypoglycaemic coma. Lancet. 1972;2:764.
57. Mehregan DR, Daoud M, Rogers RS 3rd. Coma blisters in a patient with diabetic ketoacidosis. J Am Acad Dermatol. 1992;27:269–70.
58. Shiohara T. Fixed drug eruption: pathogenesis and diagnostic tests. Curr Opin Allergy Clin Immunol. 2009;9:316–21.
59. Teraki Y, Moriya N, Shiohara T. Drug-induced expression of intercellular adhesion molecule-1 on lesional keratinocytes in fixed drug eruption. Am J Pathol. 1994;145:550–60.
60. Ramdial PK, Naidoo DK. Drug-induced cutaneous pathology. J Clin Pathol. 2009;62:493–504.
61. Przepiorka D, Weisdorf D, Martin P, Klingemann HG, Beatty P, Hows J, et al. 1994 Consensus conference on acute GVHD grading. Bone Marrow Transplant. 1995;15:825–8.
62. Hymes SR, Alousi AM, Cowen EW. Graft-versus-host disease: part I. Pathogenesis and clinical manifestations of graft-versus-host disease. J Am Acad Dermatol. 2012;66:515 e1–e18.
63. Schauder CS, Hymes SR, Rapini RP, Zipf TF. Vesicular graft-versus-host disease. Int J Dermatol. 1992;31:509–10.
64. Moreno JC, Valverde F, Martinez F, Velez A, Torres A, Fanego J, et al. Bullous scleroderma-like changes in chronic graft-versus-host disease. J Eur Acad Dermatol Venereol. 2003;17:200–3.
65. Hymes SR, Farmer ER, Burns WH, Morison WL, Tutschka PJ, Walters LL, et al. Bullous sclerodermalike changes in chronic graft-vs-host disease. Arch Dermatol. 1985;121:1189–92.
66. McLaren GD, Muir WA, Kellermeyer RW. Iron overload disorders: natural history, pathogenesis, diagnosis, and therapy. Crit Rev Clin Lab Sci. 1983;19:205–66.
67. Daoud MS, Gibson LE, Daoud S, el-Azhary RA. Chronic hepatitis C and skin diseases: a review. Mayo Clin Proc. 1995;70:559–64.
68. Hogan D, Card RT, Ghadially R, McSheffrey JB, Lane P. Human immunodeficiency virus infection and porphyria cutanea tarda. J Am Acad Dermatol. 1989;20:17–20.
69. Green JJ, Manders SM. Pseudoporphyria. J Am Acad Dermatol. 2001;44:100–8.
70. Phung TL, Pipkin CA, Tahan SR, Chiu DS. Beta-lactam antibiotic-induced pseudoporphyria. J Am Acad Dermatol. 2004;51:S80–2.
71. Degiovanni CV, Darley CR. Pseudoporphyria occurring during a course of ciprofloxacin. Clin Exp Dermatol. 2008;33:109–10.
72. Kwong WT, Hsu S. Pseudoporphyria associated with voriconazole. J Drugs Dermatol. 2007;6:1042–4.
73. Epstein JH, Seibert JS. Porphyria-like cutaneous changes induced by tetracycline hydrochloride photosensitization. Arch Dermatol. 1976;112:661–6.
74. Alcalay J, David M, Ingber A, Hazaz B, Sandbank M. Bullous pemphigoid mimicking bullous erythema multiforme: an untoward side effect of penicillins. J Am Acad Dermatol. 1988;18:345–9.
75. Czechowicz RT, Reid CM, Warren LJ, Weightman W, Whitehead FJ. Bullous pemphigoid induced by cephalexin. Australas J Dermatol. 2001;42:132–5.
76. Kimyai-Asadi A, Usman A, Nousari HC. Ciprofloxacin-induced bullous pemphigoid. J Am Acad Dermatol. 2000;42:847.
77. Nousari HC, Deterding R, Wojtczack H, Aho S, Uitto J, Hashimoto T, et al. The mechanism of respiratory failure in paraneoplastic pemphigus. N Engl J Med. 1999;340:1406–10.
78. Brenner S, Bialy-Golan A, Ruocco V. Drug-induced pemphigus. Clin Dermatol. 1998;16:393–7.
79. Yeh SW, Ahmed B, Sami N. Razzaque Ahmed A. Blistering disorders: diagnosis and treatment. Dermatol Ther. 2003;16:214–23.

80. Blenkinsopp WK, Haffenden GP, Fry L, Leonard JN. Histology of linear IgA disease, dermatitis herpetiformis, and bullous pemphigoid. Am J Dermatopathol. 1983;5:547–54.
81. Rosen LB, Frank BL, Rywlin AM. A characteristic vesiculobullous eruption in patients with chronic lymphocytic leukemia. J Am Acad Dermatol. 1986;15:943–50.
82. Ajithkumar K, George S, Babu PG. Abnormal insect bite reactions: a manifestation of immunosuppression of HIV infection? Indian J Dermatol Venereol Leprol. 2001;67:72–4.
83. Byrd JB, Woodard-Grice A, Stone E, Lucisano A, Schaefer H, Yu C, et al. Association of angiotensin-converting enzyme inhibitor-associated angioedema with transplant and immunosuppressant use. Allergy. 2010;65:1381–7.
84. Choy AC, Yarnold PR, Brown JE, Kayaloglou GT, Greenberger PA, Patterson R. Virus induced erythema multiforme and Stevens-Johnson syndrome. Allergy Proc. 1995;16:157–61.
85. Auquier-Dunant A, Mockenhaupt M, Naldi L, Correia O, Schroder W, Roujeau JC. Correlations between clinical patterns and causes of erythema multiforme majus, Stevens-Johnson syndrome, and toxic epidermal necrolysis: results of an international prospective study. Arch Dermatol. 2002;138:1019–24.
86. Hazin R, Ibrahimi OA, Hazin MI, Kimyai-Asadi A. Stevens-Johnson syndrome: pathogenesis, diagnosis, and management. Ann Med. 2008;40:129–38.
87. French LE, Prins C. Erythema multiforme, Stevens-Johnson syndrome and toxic epidermal necrolysis. In: Bolognia J, Rapini R, editors. Dermatology. St. Louis, MO: Mosby Elsevier; 2008. p. 288.
88. Geria AN, Holcomb KZ, Scheinfeld NS. Necrolytic acral erythema: a review of the literature. Cutis. 2009;83:309–14.
89. Dabski K, Winkelmann RK. Generalized granuloma annulare: clinical and laboratory findings in 100 patients. J Am Acad Dermatol. 1989;20:39–47.
90. Zwald FO, Brown M. Skin cancer in solid organ transplant recipients: advances in therapy and management: part II. Management of skin cancer in solid organ transplant recipients. J Am Acad Dermatol. 2011;65:263–79. quiz 80
91. Lott DG, Manz R, Koch C, Lorenz RR. Aggressive behavior of nonmelanotic skin cancers in solid organ transplant recipients. Transplantation. 2010;90:683–7.
92. Bangash HK, Colegio OR. Management of non-melanoma skin cancer in immunocompromised solid organ transplant recipients. Curr Treat Options Oncol. 2012;13(3):354–76.
93. Euvrard S, Kanitakis J, Claudy A. Skin cancers after organ transplantation. N Engl J Med. 2003;348:1681–91.
94. Euvrard S, Kanitakis J, Pouteil-Noble C, Dureau G, Touraine JL, Faure M, et al. Comparative epidemiologic study of premalignant and malignant epithelial cutaneous lesions developing after kidney and heart transplantation. J Am Acad Dermatol. 1995;33:222–9.
95. Euvrard S, Chardonnet Y, Pouteil-Noble C, Kanitakis J, Chignol MC, Thivolet J, et al. Association of skin malignancies with various and multiple carcinogenic and noncarcinogenic human papillomaviruses in renal transplant recipients. Cancer. 1993;72:2198–206.
96. Hollenbeak CS, Todd MM, Billingsley EM, Harper G, Dyer AM, Lengerich EJ. Increased incidence of melanoma in renal transplantation recipients. Cancer. 2005;104:1962–7.
97. Vajdic CM, van Leeuwen MT. Cancer incidence and risk factors after solid organ transplantation. Int J Cancer. 2009;125:1747–54.
98. Miller DD, Cowen EW, Nguyen JC, McCalmont TH, Fox LP. Melanoma associated with long-term voriconazole therapy: a new manifestation of chronic photosensitivity. Arch Dermatol. 2010;146(3):300–4.
99. Scerri L, Williams HC, Allen BR. Dissecting cellulitis of the scalp: response to isotretinoin. Br J Dermatol. 1996;134:1105–8.

Part III

Etiologic Agents in Infectious Diseases

Staphylococcus, Streptococcus, and *Enterococcus*

24

Amar Safdar and Donald Armstrong

Introduction

Gram-positive bacterial (GPB) infections are an important cause of serious illness in patients undergoing transplantation [1]. In recipients of hematopoietic stem cell transplantation (HSCT), GPB are by far the most common bacterial pathogens isolated. A relative decline in infections due to Gram-negative bacteria (GNB) has been attributed to a variety of factors: (1) frequently used antimicrobial prophylaxis with an emphasis on prevention of systemic infections resulting from these microorgansisms; (2) a rise in drug-resistance among disease-casuing GPB due to extensive exposure to healthcare environment and frequent use of broad-spectrum antibiotics that are often given as preventive or empiric therapy; (3) the necessity for maintenance of vascular access results in retention of intravascular devices for extended duration; (4) orointestinal mucositis associated with conventional preparatory regimens in patients undergoing allogeneic stem cell transplantation; (5) the presence of severe pre-engraftment neutropenia that may result in protracted courses of recovery in certain high-risk transplant groups, such as adults following conventional cord blood stem cell transplantation; (6) the emergence and widespread distribution of community-acquired methicillin-resistant *Staphylococcus aureus* (CA-MRSA) colonization and subsequent risk for invasive disease; (7) acute and chronic graft-versus-host disease (GVHD) involving the skin and orointestinal tract; and (8) hyposplenism noted in patients with chronic GVHD, which promotes the likelihood for serious, invasive pneumococcal disease and infections due to other encapsulated microorganisms [2–4].

Infection prevalance varies among patients undergoing solid organ transplantation (SOT), in most part the risk is a reflection upon the transplanted organ allograft and surgical procedure(s) involved. Deceased donor allograft-derived and organ perfusion fluid (PF)-associated GPB infections are a potential source for such infections. The risk of invasive bacterial infections reflects a proclivity for GPB in this group, and mostly related to surgical procedures that are often long and difficult. Prolonged tissue hypoperfusion, posttransplant allograft ischemia, and retransplantation procedures further increases the risk for bacterial infections. Furthermore, surgical drain(s) that are left in place for a long duration; external biliary tract drains like percutaneous transhepatic biliary catheter; percutaneous nephrostomy catheter, chest tube, and thoracic drains to name a few, promote risk for hospital-acquired bacterial infections; among such infections, GPB are common pathogens encountered. Postsurgical wound infections including wound dehiscence or other early complications following transplant surgery such as the development of primary or secondary hematoma or persistent seroma in the deep surgical bed may provide a nidus for bacterial infection; GPB are also prominent in such post -surgical complications. It is important to note that colonization with MRSA and vancomycin-resistant enterococci (VRE) poses a substantial burden due to a more noticeable risk for subsequent invasive bacterial disease and the risk for potential allograft compromise [5, 6].

Presence of extended-use intravascular access devices that are crucial in patients undergoing transplantation for supportive care that includes and not limited to fluid, electrolyte and mineral supplimentation, hyperalimentation, renal replacement therapy, plasma exchanges, blood and blood product transfusions, and administration of antibiotics among other medications needed to be given parenterally. These intravascular acess devices serve as a direct conduit between skin and blood vessels thereby promoting the risk

A. Safdar (✉)
Clinical Associate Professor of Medicine, Texas Tech University Health Sciences Center El Paso, Paul L. Foster School of Medicine, El Paso, TX, USA
e-mail: amar.safdar@cidimmunology.com

D. Armstrong
Infectious Disease Service, Memorial Sloan-Kettering Cancer Center, New York, NY, USA

Cornell University Medical College (ret), New York, NY, USA

Infectious Disease Society of America, Albuquerque, NM, USA

A. Safdar (ed.), *Principles and Practice of Transplant Infectious Diseases*, https://doi.org/10.1007/978-1-4939-9034-4_24

for bloodstream infections (BSIs). Skin commensals such as coagulase-negative staphylococci (CoNS) and *Corynebacterium jeikeium* are a well-recognized cause of catheter-related bloodstream infection (CR-BSI). Similar to HSCT recipients, patients undergoing SOT are also susceptible to serious invasive disease due to CA-MRSA. Allograft rejection and need for intensified drug-induced immune suppression further promote the risk for invasive disease due to conventional and opportunistic bacterial pathogens. In this regard, *Staphylococcus aureus*, viridans streptococci, and *Enterococcus* spp. are important pathogens [7–10].

Genetic susceptibility for GPB infections may be further accentuated in patients undergoing allograft transplantation. Minor genetic alternations such as single-nucleotide polymorphisms (SNPs) in the essential components of innate immune signaling pathways may become unmasked following trnspantation procedure and are thought to increase hosts' susceptibility for infections. Toll-like receptor 2 (TLR2) is an immune sensor for the components of GPB cell wall. Genetic alterations in the TLR2 gene may render this important pattern recognition receptor with impaired function, thereby enhanced susceptibility for GPB infections in such individuals. In a cohort of 694 liver transplant recipients, it was interesting to note that patients with TLR2 R753Q SNP (an amino acid substitution of arginine for glutamine at position 753) had similar frequency of GPB infections compared with those individuals without this TLR2 SNP. However, the presence of TLR2 R753Q SNP was identified in patients with higher rates of infection recurrence (28% vs. 12%, $P = 0.07$) and initial infection presentation with septic shock was significatly higher in subjects with this TLR2 mutation (11% vs. 1%, $P = 0.04$) versus those without. Important to note that presence of TLR2 R753Q SNP did not result in higher infection-related deaths among liver transplant recipients in this report [11].

Further studies are underway to assess clinical relevance for this and other genetic minor aberrations that may unmask minor immune dysfunction against commonly encountered pathogens, especially in individuals following allograft transplantation.

Staphylococcus Species

Staphylococci are the predominant GPB with the ability to cause serious illness in patients undergoing transplantation [12, 13]. Staphylococci can be divided into two main classes based on their ability to coagulate rabbit plasma. *Staphylococcus aureus* being coagulase positive and all other *Staphylococcus* species are referred to as coagulase negative staphylococci (CoNS). Infections due to *S. aureus* may present as simple cellulitis or bacteremia versus a disseminated disease that features involvement of various organ systems. Patients with disseminated *S. aureus* infection usually present as life-threatening illness with sepsis or severe sepsis and even in non-transplant immunocompetent patients such infections may progress, in short order, to cause multiorgan dysfunction, disseminated intravascular coagulation, hemodynamic collapse and death. Probablity of severe illness is emphasized in transplant recipients with compromised immune defenses and compounded by dysregulation of hosts' immune-inflammatory response. The potential to cause pneumonia, endovascular and prosthetic device infections is an important ability of *S. aureus* and to a lesser extent by species belonging to the CoNS group. In general, infections due to CoNS are less severe, which is a reflection of low inherent virulence of these bacteria to cause disease in humans [14, 15].

Staphylococcus aureus

Epidemiology and Pathogenesis

S. aureus is a common commensal that can be isolated from 10% to 40% of individuals residing in various communities [16]. *S. aureus* has been well-established as a leading cause of both community-onset and nosocomial infections. Prior to the year 2000, a vast majority of MRSA infections were related directly, or indirectly, to the exposure to healthcare environment. *S. aureus* infections acquired in the community, almost exclusively were methicillin-susceptible strains of *S. aureus* (MSSA) [17]. The emergence and global spread of CA-MRSA have resulted in an increased prevalence of these pathogens among the general population and those undergoing transplantation procedures. MRSA colonization has been regarded as an important risk factor among HSCT recipients, and a precursor for subsequent invasive staphylococcal disease [18]. The risk for such infections now extends beyond healthcare exposure and must be entertained when assessing the possibility of illness due to staphylococci in the transplant population [19].

Most invasive *S. aureus* diseases in transplant recipients occur when mechanical defenses are breached, for example, due to break in the skin barrier resulting from catheter placement or bypassing upper airway defenses following insertion of an endotracheal tube [20]. The main risk factors include severe neutropenia, GVHD, allograft rejection, solid allograft retransplantation, treatment with systemic corticosteroids, and complicated allograft transplant surgery. *Staphylococcus aureus* infections are also encountered in a high frequency among patients requiring prolonged intensive care unit stay, mechanical assisted ventilatory support, renal replacement therapy, and those with severe pre-engraftment neutropenia. Diabetic patients with persistent hyperglycemia-induced neutrophil and macrophage dysfunction are also at risk for potentially severe staphylococcal disease [21, 22].

HSCT Recipients

A recent study from Europe in 15,181 neutropenic HSCT patients assessed 2,388 episodes of BSI. The annual incidence of BSI in this population was 16%; 62% had undergone allogeneic and 38% autologous stem cell graft transplants [23]. The authors noted an increase in enterococcal BSI from 2% in 2002 to 3% in 2014 ($P < 0.001$). Whereas the incidence of bacteremia due to CoNS declined from 8% to 5% ($P < 0.001$), in autologous stem cell recipients, this decline was even more pronounced, from 8% to 2% between 2002 and 2011, respectively ($P = 0.02$). No significant change in the trend for MRSA or vancomycin-resistant *Enterococcus* (VRE) bacteremia was evident during the study years. The case fatality rate among 2,388 bacteremia episodes was 3% and remained unchanged over the course of the study [23].

Myeloablative preparative conditioning regimen promotes the risk for bacterial infections. In a recent study of 460 patients, the risk of BSI was assessed during the first year after transplantation between 2008 and 2013. Thirty-four percent of patients who received myeloablative conditioning developed BSI, whereas, in patents, in whom nonmyeloablative stem cell transplantations were performed, BSIs were 17%. Sixty-eight percent of bacteremia episodes were due to GPB [24].

At a comprehensive cancer center in New York, the frequency of late HSCT *S. aureus* bacteremia was reported as 6 episodes per 100,000 patient-days. The median time of onset after transplantation was 137 days, and ranged between 55 and 581 days. Majority of these infections (84%), as expected, were acquired in the community [25]. Risk factors included ongoing acute GVHD, acute or chronic GVHD involving the skin ($P = 0.002$), use of systemic corticosteroids, liver dysfunction, and prolonged transplantation-related hospitalization ($P = 0.02$). *S. aureus* bacteremia in HSCT recipients at this large stem cell transplant center for the most part, occurred in patients with GVHD and/or those receiving systemic corticosteroids [25].

Solid Organ Transplant Recipients

Solid organ transplantation is a high-risk setting for MRSA and VRE colonization, and the carrier state is associated with a heightened risk for subsequent invasive bacterial disease. In a recent meta-analysis of 23 studies, including 17 with reference to liver transplants, the prevalence estimates for MRSA and VRE colonization prior to transplantation surgery were 8.5% and 12%, respectively. After transplantation, the prevalence estimates for MRSA were 9% and 16% for VRE. MRSA colonization significantly increased the risk for invasive bacterial disease both before and after transplantation (risk ratio [RR] 5.5 and RR 10.5, respectively). Similarly, VRE colonization was also associated with a significantly higher risk for subsequent invasive disease (RR 6.6 during pre-transplant and RR 7.9 after transplantation) [6]. In a small study of patients undergoing small bowel and multivisceral transplantation at the University of Nebraska, nearly one-third (36%) of *S. aureus* isolates associated with systemic infection were strains exhibiting resistance to several classes of antimicrobials [26].

Bacterial contamination of solid allograft perfusion fluid has been regarded as a potential source for organ graft contamination, which may result in early postsurgical allograft infection that carries a greater risk for systemic dissemination and sepsis during this period of high immune vulnerability. Microbiological data of 290 PF infections from a single center showed 35% PF had positive cultures for microorgansims, and of these, half (50%) were *Staphylococcus* species. However, it was important to note that invasive bacterial disease seldom resulted following PF contamination graft transplantation compared with patients in whom allografts were transported in PF with no evidence of contamination [27].

Donor-derived infection is an important concern in harvesting organs from donors with a recent history of, or ongoing high-grade *S. aureus* bacteremia, with or without evidence of endovascular infection. Transmission of such infections are well-established by sophisticated epidemiologic analysis and provides a pause for concern in assessing risk of exposure to potentially life-threatening *S. aureus* disease [28]. It is important to note that despite appropriate systemic antibiotics given after such allograft transplantation, patients remain at risk for these infections during or after the antibiotic prophylaxis has ended [29].

In living donor liver transplantation, the prominent risk factors for early bacterial infections were a high serum creatinine level (odds ratio [OR] 1.5), a long anhepatic arterial perfusion phase (OR 1), a reoperation (OR 6.4), young age (OR 1), and recipient who had no history of hepatocellular carcinoma (OR 2) [30].

In patients with cystic fibrosis (CF) undergoing lung transplantation, higher risk of infection is seen in a disease caused by mutations involving endosomal cystic fibrosis transmembrane conductance regulator (*Cftr*), pulmonary *S. aureus* colonization that occurs early in the course of illness and often, prior to colonization with pathogens such as *Pseudomonas aeruginosa*. These patients continue to remain susceptible to *S. aureus* infections as a result of intracellular survival of *S. aureus* in macrophages. In animal experiments, *S. aureus* after being internalized by *Cftr*-deficient macrophages are not killed due to a defect in the fusion of endosomal phagosomes with lysosomes [31]. This defect may persist in CF patients following pulmonary allograft transplant surgery.

A 5-year retrospective study from the University of Pittsburgh evaluated *S. aureus* infections within the first 90 days after lung transplantation [32]. In 596 patients following lung transplantation, 18% developed *S. aureus* infection, of these 38% were MRSA. The study observed an incremental increase in MRSA prevalence over the duration of the study.

Isolation of MRSA from the nares ($P < 0.0001$) or from respiratory tract samples ($P = 0.02$) at the time of transplantation was noted to significantly increase the risk for invasive MRSA disease within 3 months after transplantation [32].

Clinical experience at the University of Pittsburgh endorsed that *S. aureus* screening and decolonization for patients undergoing heart and heart-lung transplantation was fiscally beneficial, and averted 6.7 *S. aureus* infections (4.3 MRSA and 2.4 MSSA) leading to a cost saving of $240,602. The authors found that 89 patients were needed to be screened to prevent one *S. aureus* infection in this at risk organ transplant group [33].

The cross talk between bacterial communities and innate immune cells potentially determines the functional integrity of the transplanted lung allograft. In lung transplant recipients, long-term graft survival depends upon the balance between inflammation and tissue remodeling. Host-microbe interactions after lung transplant determines the immunologic tone of the airways and, consequently, may possibly, impact survival of the pulmonary allograft. In a French and Swiss study, the characteristics of the pulmonary microbiota aligned with distinct innate cell gene expression profiles provided evidence that bacterial dysbiosis could lead to proinflammatory or remodeling profiles in macrophages, whereas a congruous microbial community maintained homeostasis. Such an impact was associated with equitable distribution of bacterial communities with proinflammatory properties such as *Staphylococcus* spp. and *Pseudomonas* spp. versus bacteria like *Prevotella* and *Streptococcus* spp. with low immune-inflammation potential [34]. Further research is underway to assess the impact of host lung and respiratory tract microbiota and its impact on allograft survival.

Clinical Manifestations

S. aureus infections commonly involve the skin and skin structures, and clinical presentations include cellulitis and abscesses; systemic infections and end-organ disease are seen in both immunocompetent and immunocompromised patients [35, 36]. *S. aureus* is a leading cause of catheter-related bacteremia, prosthetic joint infections, and infections following a surgical procedure [15]. Suppurative complications such as infective endocarditis, pneumonia with concurrent bacteremia, osteomyelitis, spinal diskitis, native and prosthetic joint infections, and septic pulmonary emboli from subcutaneous abscesses may occur due to secondary bacterial seeding in patients with high-grade, persistent *S. aureus* bacteremia [37].

Bacteremia is a serious complication in patients undergoing HSCT. A recent 6-year single-center experience in patients with bacteremia following stem cell allograft transplantation, the 2-year overall survival was 46% compared with 60% survival noted among patients without BSI (HR 1.5; $P = 0.07$). *P. aeruginosa* and *E. coli* bacteremia were associated with highest mortality rates of 50% and 33%, respectively [38].

Late *S. aureus* BSIs occurred in HSCT recipients, and 40% involved a focal site of infection. Persistent bacteremia for more than 3 days despite removal of endovascular access was noted in more than 50% of cases. The median survival rate after *S. aureus* bacteremia was 135 days and ranged between 1 and 1,765 days [25].

In a kidney transplant unit in London, England, between 2012 and 2013, graft pyelonephritis was noted as a prominent cause of bacteremia (69%). Methicillin-sensitive *Staphylococcus aureus* was the most common pathogen isolated (26%), followed by, and expectedly, *Escherichia coli* (25%) [39].

Necrotizing pneumonia due to *S. aureus* in transplant patients usually occurs in critically ill patients with respiratory failure requiring prolonged assisted mechanical ventilation; as in general population, superimposed bacterial pneumonia may complicate the course during or after a viral upper respiratory tract infections due to influenza and other respiratory tract viruses [40].

The rise of CA-MRSA has been especially concerning given that CA-MRSA isolates can cause devastating disease including necrotizing fasciitis and necrotizing pneumonia even in otherwise healthy individuals; the potential for such complictions become more pronounced in the immunosuppressed patients undergoing transplantation [41, 42]. It is not uncommon to find *S. aureus* in patients with pyomyositis, septic arthritis, and septic bursitis, which may have occurred due to contiguous infection or from hematogenous bacterial seeding [43, 44].

Nosocomial pneumonia after lung and heart-lung transplantation was assessed between 2008 and 2010 at a surgical unit in France [45]. The authors reported their prospective evaluation of 79 lung or heart-lung transplant recipients, 35 (44%) of whom developed 64 episodes of nosocomial pneumonia. Pneumonia recurrence was seen in 40% of the cases; severities of illness and lung injury were the two main contributors for infection recurrence. *Staphylococcus aureus* accounted for 20% of these episodes, whereas *Enterobacteriaceae* (30%) and *Pseudomonas aeruginosa* (25%) were also common. It was interesting to note that ICU mortality did not greatly differ in patients with nosocomial pneumonia (14%), those with pneumonia recurrence (10%), and patients without pneumonia (11%; $P = 0.9$). It was however, unexpected that diagnosis of pneumonia had no impact on ICU mortality, especially in this high risk transplant group [45].

In 596 patients following lung transplantation at the University of Pittsburgh, *S. aureus* pneumonia (48%) was the most common presentation in 109 lung transplant recipients with *S. aureus* infection. Tracheobronchitis (26%), bacteremia (12%), intrathoracic infections (7%), and skin/soft tissue infections (7%) were also noted. Risk factors included mechanical ventilation for >5 days and isolation of *S. aureus* from recipients' sterility surveillance cultures. Patients with these infections had prolonged hospitalization and intensive care unit stays ($P < 0.0001$). Further, in patients with *S. aureus* infections that occurred after undergoing lung transplantation; acute and chronic allograft rejection at 1 and 3 years ($P = 0.04$ and $P = 0.002$, respectively) and mortality at 1 and 3 years ($P = 0.05$ and $P = 0.009$, respectively) were significantly higher than in other patients in this series without *S. aureus* infection. Mortality rates of 7% on day 30 and 12% by day 90 after *S. aureus* infection was a sobering reminder regarding the severity of this infection in the vulnerable population [32].

In a large study from the Cleveland Clinic in Ohio 2,959 patients with *S. aureus* bacteremia were evaluated; 70 had undergone solid organ transplantation including 26 lung, 19 liver, 18 kidney, and 7 patients following heart allograft transplantation. The overall rate of *S. aureus* BSI was 22.9 per 1000 transplant patients. Early-onset bacteremia within 90 days after the transplant procedure was common in liver allograft recipients (79%) vs. 17% in patients having undergone renal allograft transplants. As expected, the duration of bacteremia was longer in SOT patients vs. non-solid organ transplant population (mean 3.8 days vs. 1.6 days; $P < 0.01$), and SOT recipients had significantly higher frequency of MRSA infection (86% vs. 52% in non-SOT population; $P < 0.0001$). The all-cause 30-day and 1-year mortality rates were 6% and 28% in patients following SOT, respectively. Pneumonia as a source of bacteremia was associated with a higher 30-day mortality (18% vs. 2% nonpulmonary source; $P = 0.04$). It was interesting to note that SOT status was independently associated with a lower risk of 30-day mortality (risk ratio [RR]: 0.37; $P = 0.02$) and may represent high vigilance and prompt institution of empiric antimicrobial therapy in this group [46].

At the University of Nebraska, the first *S. aureus* infection in a liver allograft recipient developed at a median of 29 days after undergoing transplantation. Just over half of these infections occurred during the first month after the liver transplant surgery [47]. As expected, 88% were hospital-acquired infections, 41% were polymicrobial, and nearly half (47%) were due to MRSA. Liver transplant patients with *S. aureus* infection were intubated more frequently (odds ratio [OR] 26.9; $P = 0.0006$), had an indwelling intravascular catheter (OR 11.6; $P = 0.02$), and underwent recent surgery (OR 26.9; $P = 0.0006$). Multivariate analysis revealed a 26.9 times higher risk of developing *S. aureus* infection in patients in whom surgery was performed within 2 weeks prior to infection diagnosis ($P = 0.0006$). Recent surgical procedure was the only significant independent risk factor for *S. aureus* infections after liver transplantation in this analysis [47].

Staphylococcus aureus infections in small bowel and multivisceral transplantation were assessed retrospectively in 22 cases at the University of Nebraska. The median age was 2 years; 43% of the first infection episodes were bacteremia, followed by pneumonia (30%), and surgical site infections (26%). As expected, the time to surgical site infections (41.0; range, 0–89 days) was significantly shorter than that to lung infections (266; range, 130–378 days; $P = 0.01$). When compared with other small bowel and visceral transplant recipients without *S. aureus* infection, the 22 cases studied had higher likelihood of CMV seromismatch (OR 3.0; $P = 0.08$); it was interesting to note that patients with CMV seromismatch had higher probability for developing *S. aureus* infection (OR, 2.9; $P = 0.085$). Patients in this transplant population with *S. aureus* infection were 2.2 times more likely to die ($P = 0.04$) and had a significantly shorter survival (28.5 months) compared with patients without *S. aureus* infection (45.8 months; $P = 0.04$) [26].

Diagnosis

These bacteria are hardy, grow well in enriched laboratory media, and are relatively easy to identify. The presence of *S. aureus* in specimens from sterile body sites in most instances represents microbiologic evidence of an infection. *S. aureus* contamination of blood cultures has been suggested [48]; in authors' view, this phenomenon occurs rarely and must not be entertained, especially in transplant population.

S. aureus has propensity to colonize various body sites, such as the oral and nasal cavities, upper respiratory tract, skin, and lower intestinal and genitourinary tracts. Therefore, isolation of *S. aureus* from endotracheal aspirate or urine sample obtained from an indwelling urinary catheter and even bronchial wash samples must be assessed in context of clinical presentation, pathogen-disease compatibility, and importantly, hosts' susceptibility along with pretest probability for such infections. However, these factors assist mainly in decision-making for individuals with intact immune function and may not necessarily enable determination regarding bacterial colonization versus locally invasive disease in severely immunosuppressed patients undergoing allograft transplantation.

Serologic or antigen assays have not proven to be clinically helpful in the diagnosis of *S. aureus* infection. The new diagnostic assessment including PCR for prompt determination of MRSA represents encouraging development [49]. A detailed review of the advancements in infection diagnosis is presented in the "Diagnoses and Prevention" section.

Treatment

Therapy for systemic *S. aureus* disease constitutes a comprehensive approach toward the patient, which involves (1) lowering the level of immune suppression; (2) identifying and addressing the source and/or primary focus of infection such as (2a) removal of the infected or potentially infected foreign device, when feasible; (2b) surgical drainage of infected collections and debridement of necrotic tissue; and (3) selection of appropriate empiric antibiotic while awaiting culture and drug susceptibility results [50]. The importance of drainage of deep tissue infected collections and surgical removal of devitalized tissue cannot be overemphasized, as in many patients with localized infection, removal of the nidus and primary focus of infection alone may be curative and often supplemented with an abbreviated course of systemic antibiotic therapy [51]. In concert, if an infected foreign material, such as an indwelling intravascular catheter or an infected prosthetic joint, remains in place, then therapeutic success of antibiotic therapy alone tends to be suboptimal [52, 53].

Antibiotic treatment of *S. aureus* infection is complicated by emergence and speard of bacterial starins with extensive antimicrobial drug resistance. When the organism is sensitive, β-lactam antibiotics are the drugs of choice for *S. aureus* infections including nafcillin and oxacillin [54, 55]. Vancomycin is considered by most as optimal treatment for invasive MRSA infections, although increasing frequency of vancomycin treatment failures, especially in oncology and transplant population, have questioned this approach [56]. Treatment of MRSA bacteremia with vancomycin given as a single agent has been associated with a high rate of treatment failure evident as lack of clinical response and complete recovery, or early infection relapse, which may be observed in 15%–20% of the episodes; although overt vancomycin resistance by in vitro drug testing still remains an elusive phenomenon [57]. Failure to vancomycin therapy has motivated a search for alternative treatment options including newer drugs such as linezolid, tedizolid, tigecycline, ceftaroline, and daptomycin, to name a few.

Each of these agents, similar to vancomycin, has significant limitations. Proven treatment efficacy and superiority to vancomycin as a first-line agent for the treatment of systemic MRSA infections such as bacteremia, pneumonia, complicated intra-abdominal infections, and bone and joint infections need further clinical validation. It is imperative to take into account the potential for adverse events and systemic toxicity associated with vancomycin and these newer antibiotics including the following consideration: a) hosts' variables which may at times, influence drug clearance in patients undergoing transplantation; b) drug-drug interactions, with particular emphasis on pharmacokinetics and pharmacodynamics of drugs commonly use to treat allograft rejection GVHD; c) inherent or postexposure development of drug resistance, or selection of less drug susceptible bacterial strains, especially in at risk transplant population, in whom extensive prior exposure to the healthcare environment and the need for periodically given systemic broadspectrum antibiotics for recurrent or suspected infections are routinely priscribed both prior to, and following the transplantation procedure [58–69].

Selection of effective empiric antibiotic therapy for the treatment of glycopeptide-nonsusceptible staphylococci is difficult, as true resistance is rare and isolates exhibiting heterogeneous resistance or vancomycin tolerance may not become evident even after the drug susceptibility profiles are known. In patients undergoing SOT, use of vancomycin has been associated with low therapeutic efficacy and high rates of drug-induced renal impairment, which in part is a reflection of the cumulative nephrotoxicity resulting from standard practice antirejection drug regimens including calcineurin inhibitors given for prolong duration after the allograft transplant surgery.

A study from Spain during 2008 and 2010 enrolled 43 patients mostly after liver and kidney transplantation who received daptomycin for the treatment of GPB infections including CoNS catheter-related bacteremia (23.2%), *S. aureus* skin and skin structure infections (11.5%), and intra-abdominal abscess due to *Enterococcus faecium* (20.9%). The daily daptomycin dose was 6 mg/kg in 74% of the patients. On day 7 of daptomycin treatment, median estimated area under the curve was 1251 μg/mL/h. No changes were observed in tacrolimus serum levels. Daptomycin was not discontinued in any of these patients due to adverse events. Eighty-six percent clinical success with daptomycin therapy was noted in this small group of transplant recipients [63].

The potential role of antibiotics in modulating virulence among *S. aureus* is an intriguing phenomenon and needs further exploration, especially for the treatment of difficult-to-treat infections. The effects of antibacterial agents on pathogens' expression of virulence and on hosts' immune response are currently being explored. A recent review of the literature evaluated relevant articles that explored the effects of antibiotics on staphylococcal toxin production and the impact of these ancillary mechanisms on hosts' immune function. Most in vitro data pointed to a reduced level of expression of bacterial virulence following treatment with ribosomally active antibiotics such as linezolid and clindamycin, whereas cell wall-active antibiotics like beta-lactams were associated with amplified bacterial exotoxin production/release. In vivo studies confirmed the suppressive effect mediated by clindamycin and linezolid on the expression of bacterial virulence, supporting their utilization as a valuable management strategy to improve patient outcomes in cases of toxin-mediated staphylococcal disease [70].

The duration of therapy for *S. aureus* infection is highly individualized. A minimum of 2 weeks is recommended for patients with uncomplicated catheter-related bacteremia [71]. A longer course of antibiotic treatment is generally given ranging from 4 to 8 weeks in patients with complicated infections such as infective endocarditis, necrotizing pneumonia, empyema, septic arthritis, allograft pyelonephritis, intra-abdominal deep tissue abscesses such as liver and splenic abscesses, and osteomyelitis. The antibiotics are usually given intravenous for more serious infections, whereas in select low-risk cases a transition to oral drugs that exhibit dependable enteral bioavailability may be considered as an option. Regardless of treatment duration, *S. aureus* systemic infection-related complications may arise during the course of therapy or long after the antibiotic therapy has ended. New suppurative foci may arise months after a successful resolution of acute *S. aureus* illness. Patients with serious *S. aureus* disease require a close and continued follow-up for the possibility of infection recurrence that may present as a suppurative focus, and may occur remote from the original site of infection; days to months after completing an appropriate course of concordant antibiotic therapy.

Coagulase-Negative Staphylococci

Epidemiology

Coagulase-negative staphylococci (CoNS) are part of the normal hosts' microflora; up to 90% of humans are colonized with these low-virulence environmental organisms [57]. Skin, orointestinal, and genitourinary mucosa are prominent sites of bacterial colonization. Unlike general population, patients undergoing transplantation are vulnerable to invasive disease due to CoNS. This is in most part attributed to breach in protective barriers resulting from (1) indwelling intravascular catheters; (2) surgical wounds; (3) various surgical drainage catheters including percutaneous nephrostomy tubes, external biliary tract catheters, and thoracic cavity drains, among others; (4) implantable left ventricular assist device in patients with advanced heart failure awaiting transplantation; (5) the presence of severe mucositis involving the orointestinal tract resulting from allogeneic HSCT preparatory conditioning regimens or in patients with post-HSCT GVHD; and (6) recently recognized periodontal disease as a risk factor for CoNS bacteremia in patients with pre-engraftment neutropenia following hematopoietic stem cell graft transplantation [23, 72, 73].

When species studies are performed, *S. epidermidis* is generally the leading cause of invasive CoNS infections in the immunosuppressed population [74]. *Staphylococcus lugdunensis* is an emerging member of the CoNS group, which has increasingly been recognized as a cause of severe endovascular infection. Such infections are clinically indistinguishable from that caused by *Staphylococcus aureus*. The potential for endocarditis due to this novel bacterial pathogen in transplant population needs further investigation. *Staphylococcus lugdunensis* has been associated with a variety of infections, especially osteoarticular infections, foreign body-associated infections, and bacteremia. Several putative virulence factors have been identified including adhesion factors, biofilm production, and proteolytic factors appears to proffer opportunistic potential of these newly recognized pathogens, which is in contrast to more insidious, less virulent species of bacteria grouped among CoNS [75]. In a recent retrospective analysis between 2011 and 2014, in only 45 of 2263 CoNS clinical isolates, *S. lugdunensis* was confirmed; skin and skin structure infections being the most common clinical presentation. It was interesting to note that patients with neutropenia did not appear to have a higher frequency of *S. lugdunensis* infections compared with patients with normal peripheral blood neutrophil count [76].

HSCT Recipients

Microbial contamination of hematopoietic stem cell graft derived from peripheral blood or bone marrow is uncommon, albeit, when this does occur, it may potentially lead to devastating systemic graft-acquired infection, especially in patients during pre-engraftment neutropenia. A microbiological evaluation of 291 peripheral blood and 39 bone marrow stem cell samples was conducted at a center in Poland between January 2012 and June 2013; bacterial contamination was demonstrated in nearly 3% of stem cell products. CoNS and *Micrococcus* species were the most frequent organisms detected in their air microbial contamination control environment. The risk for bacterial contamination increased with each step of cell processing, suggesting that least possible manipulation of the stem cells would improve microbial sterility of the transplant material. The authors also endorsed air contamination control environment as essential in the preparation of hematopoietic stem cells in order to reduce the risk for potential bacterial contamination [77].

SOT Recipients

Bacterial contamination of solid organ allograft preservation solution is not uncommon; in some studies, up to 44% of graft preservation fluid may exhibit bacterial and fungal contamination, or both; and as expected, CoNS is the most prevalent (64%) bacteria isolated in this setting [78]. It is important to recognize that only a small number of (~5%) infections after liver transplantation procedure were related to the organisms isolated in the preservation solution [78].

Disease Pathogenesis

The major CoNS diseases in transplant patients include bacteremia associated with an indwelling intravascular device and surgical site infections. The pathogenesis of device-related CoNS infection is thought to stem from bacterial capability to form biofilm on the foreign implanted material [79]. A recent study from Brazil showed that all CoNS strains isolated from patients with bacteremia were biofilm forming phenotypes and exhibited a high prevalence of atlE, indicting an enhanced potential for autolysin/adhesin [80]. The investigators also showed that these blood-borne CoNS had an increased frequency of staphylococcal enterotoxin (SE) A gene and potential for exotoxin production. These heat-stable enterotoxins are a leading cause of gastroenteritis. In addition, SEs are powerful superantigens that stimulate nonspecific T-cell proliferation and indiscriminate lymphocyte activation bypassing the normal, highly regulated antigen presentation process; the resultant unrestraint systemic inflammatory response and hosts' organ damage is often lethal [81]. However, most reports of severe septicemia in transplant patients associated with SE-producing staphylococcus are attributed to *S. aureus* [82].

Clinical Manifestations/Diagnosis

Fever without an apparent focus of infection is the most common clinical presentation in transplant patients with catheter-related CoNS infection including those with a positive blood culture [83]. In the transplant patients, clinical evidence of catheter infection including insertion site inflammation, which is expected to present as pain, erythema, induration, and purulent drainage or an abscess formation along the catheter insertion site, subcutaneous reservoir pocket, or catheter tunnel is frequently absent. Diagnosis requires a high level of suspicion as patients may appear relatively asymptomatic withor without a nonspecific low-grade, persisent febrile illness [84]. Native valve infective endocarditis and hematogenous osteoarticular seeding has been noted in patients with CoNS catheter-related bacteremia, although these complications are far less frequent than those observed with *S. aureus* or GNB indwelling intravascular device infections with or without concurrent bacteremia.

In patients with prosthetic valves, especially those with persistent, recurrent, or relapsing CoNS bacteremia, secondary seeding of the prosthetic heart valves should be taken into consideration [85]. In patients with prosthetic valves, CoNS endocarditis similar to such infections caused by *S. aureus* may present with valve dysfunction and intracardiac abscesses, or both. In such cases, CoNS species evaluation becomes important, with an emphasis for *S. lugdunesis* as a potential pathogen.

Clinical presentation for infections involving nonvascular or non-articular prosthetic devices may also be clinically subtle and often vary based on the type of device used, organ system involved, and the degree of hosts' inflammatory immune response. Patients with CoNS cerebrospinal fluid shunt infection are sicker and have clinical features of bacterial meningitis; subtle clinical presentation such as low-grade fever, alteration in mental status, and shunt malfunction should also alert the treating physician for possible shunt infection; and CoNS are not uncommon pathogens for such device-related infections [86, 87]. The presence of pleocytosis in CSF has limited diagnostic value, as white cell counts in CSF may be either marginally increased or within the normal limits among patients with CoNS shunt infections. Patients with CoNS infection of prosthetic joints may not have significant clinical symptoms and rang from nominal joint discomfort rather than overt joint dysfunction, which is frequently seen in patients with *S. aureus* prosthetic joint septic arthritis. Such infections are less often accompanied with prominent, localized inflammatory response including joint effusion and adjacent tissue inflammation and swelling [88].

Diagnosis

The diagnosis of CoNS infection relies on isolation of the organism from appropriately obtained clinical sample. As expected, false-positive cultures due to bacterial colonization and contamination of the sterile-site samples such as blood cultures are not uncommon and leads to difficulty in interpretation and ascertaining true versus pseudobacteremia [89]. Reliability of blood cultures in reports of CoNS catheter-related bloodstream infections provides an outline for how to approach and determine clinical relevance of CoNS isolated in blood culture specimens [90]. In quantitative cultures, catheter-drawn blood samples exhibit (fourfold) higher number of bacterial colony-forming units compared with blood drawn from a peripheral site and hence regarded as an important diagnostic predictor for infected intrevascular catheter as the source of bacteremia [83]. Similarly, blood drawn through an infected catheter tend to become positive early (~2 h), a reflection on high bacterial inoculum size compared with blood culture samples drawn from a peripheral blood vessel [83, 91]. Isolation of these bacteria from a single blood culture sample or low-grade CoNS growth in quantitative blood cultures often reflects a poor preparation of the blood culture site resulting in inadvertent sample contamination. The diagnosis of CoNS infection from sources other than the blood needs to be considered based on the clinical setting with an understanding that these bacteria are the most common cause of culture contamination, while inversely, also a well-recognized cause of prosthetic joints and other implantable device infections.

Treatment

Removal of the infected device is regarded as the definite therapeutic intervention that is imperative for successful resolution of such infections and importantly, for reduce risk of early and late infection recurrence. The presence of bacteria-induced biofilm on the foreign surfaces and necrotic tissues such as chronically infected bones provides a niche for the bacteria to evade hosts' immune clearance, and commonly used antibiotic classes such as beta-lactams and glycopeptide have limited penetration and significantly reduced antimicrobial activity against non-planktonic bacterial isolates frequently found in the biofilms [92].

Most CoNS isolates from healthcare-associated infections are resistant to β-lactam antibiotics [93]. Almost all clinical CoNS isolates are susceptible to vancomycin, although in vitro drug MICs have been increasing in the recent decades, and now a substantial number of clinical isolates exhibit vancomycin MICs between 1 and 2 μg/ml [94]. As true Vancomycin resistance still remains highly unlikely; most vancomycin clinical failures may result due to heteroresistance, vancomycin tolerance, or yet unknown other potential mechanism(s) at play [95].

Rifampin is active against the non-planktonic CoNS in the biofilms; for serious CoNS infections involving prosthetic heart valves and prosthetic joints that cannot be removed, salvage therapy with the addition of rifampin has been used, although prospective data for assessing efficacy for such intervention is not clear [96, 97]. CoNS are usually susceptible to new antimicrobials such as daptomycin, linezolid, and tedizolid, including recent addition of long-acting lipoglycopeptides like oritavancin and dalbavancin. Daptomycin has the lowest MICs against clinically important bacterial species grouped under CoNS [98].

With the exceptions of prosthetic valve endocarditis, CNS shunt and reservoir, ventricular assist device, and prosthetic joint infections, most CoNS infections respond readily to appropriate antimicrobial therapy. It is prudent and imperative that an infected device, when feasiable, must be removed; this recommendation is for mitigation of patient morbidity and cost of care incurred due to infection recurrence and relapse [99, 100]. Guidelines suggest that 7 days of appropriate concordant antibiotic therapy should be adequate for most uncomplicated CoNS catheter-related bacteremia in nonimmunocompromised patients. Longer treatment duration is suggested for patients with severe immune suppression and those with profound neutropenia; relapse rates of invasive CoNS infections are generally lower than those noted with systemic *S. aureus* disease [90].

Streptococci

The streptococci are a heterogeneous group of Gram-positive disease-causing bacteria with a wide-ranging nomenclature that continues to change [101]. Here we use the clinical microbiology laboratory approach toward these pathogens and consider them as follows: viridans group streptococcus (VGS), β-hemolytic streptococcus, and *Streptococcus pneumoniae*. Streptococci not outlined in these groups rarely cause invasive disease in the immunosuppressed patients undergoing transplantation procedure.

Viridans Group Streptococci

Epidemiology

Viridans group streptococci (VGS) are a diverse group of bacteria. They are often isolated from human orointestinal, upper respiratory, and female genital tracts [102]. Viridans, derived from *viridis*, refers to green color appearance in laboratory blood-enriched culture media due to the breakdown of hemoglobin also known as α-hemolysis. Among α-hemolytic streptococci, the most important pathogen is *Streptococcus pneumoniae*; for most non-*S. pneumoniae* α-hemolytic streptococci, further species determination is performed on request at most microbiology laboratories. The major VGS responsible for invasive disease in patients undergoing transplantation and patients with severe neutropenia belong to the *mitis* group and include *Streptococcus mitis*, *Streptococcus gordonii*, *Streptococcus oralis*, *Streptococcus sanguis*, and *Streptococcus parasanguis* [103–105]. Infections due to *Streptococcus anginosus* group are also seen, albeit less frequently and include *Streptococcus anginosus*, *Streptococcus constellatus*, and *Streptococcus intermedius*.

VGS are considered to have low intrinsic virulence, and in patients with intact immune function, they are mainly associated with endocarditis [106]. Similar to CoNS, VGS are far more likely to cause disease in neutropenic patients with cancer undergoing HSCT. In a recent study among children with cancer undergoing HSCT, diagnosis of leukemia and bacteremia due to *S. mitis* was common. It is important to note that 15% of these infection episodes were associated with Viridans Group Streptococcal Shock Syndrome, resulting in most patients (75%) requiring treatment in ICU, and half of the patients needing ICU care died with multiorgan failure [107].

VGS bacteremia occurs almost exclusively in patients receiving aggressive cytoreduction therapy for conditions such as acute leukemia and patients undergoing allogeneic HSCT preparatory conditioning regimen [108].

Treatment-induced mucosal dysruption of the orointestinal tract has been regarded as a major risk factor for systemic translocation of these low-virulence commensal bacteria, allowing them to gain access into the blood circulation [109]. It is also important to recognize that VGS breakthrough bacteremia are attributed to the widely priscribed antimicrobials for infection prophylaxis with drugs that are known to have limited activity against these organisms such as trimethoprim-sulfamethoxazole and fluorinated quinolones [110].

Clinical Presentation/Diagnosis

Most patients with invasive VGS disease present with fever in the setting of mucositis and profound neutropenia [111]. Approximately 25% of patients may present with a fulminant septic shock syndrome characterized by hypotension, skin rash, and adult respiratory distress syndrome; *S. mitis* is the VGS species most commonly isolated from such patients [103, 111, 112]. This dramatic clinical presentation may represent a combination of hosts' susceptibility due to the underlying severe neutropenia additionally, bacterial exotoxin, which act as superantigen resulting in unrestraint activation of immune-inflammatory pathways resulting is rapidly progressive illness with a substantial risk for multiorgan failure and death [113].

Unlike general population, VGS bacteremia seldom leads to endocarditis in patients with neutropenia and those undergoing a stem cell transplantation procedure. The *risk* of endocarditis in patients following solid organ allograft transplantation who develop high-grade VGS bacteremia is not dissimilar to that observed in general population [114].

Group milleri streptococci (GMS) may cause chronic intra-abdominal and intrathoracic abscesses. Infections due to GMS were reported in 45 SOT recipients between 2001 and 2004. Patients following liver transplantation were prominently respresented (n = 34) in this cohort, followed by four kidney and pancreas; two small bowel; three combined liver and kidney; and combined kidney plus small bowel and a kidney allograft transplants, in one patient each. Most GMS infection episodes (42 cases) were intra-abdominal infections, pleural empyema in two, and one patient with soft tissue infection. It was interesting that unlike neutropenic cancer patients and those undergoing HSCT, only one patient had evidence of bacteremia. It was also of note that 61% of these infections were polymicrobial; recurrent cholangitis (38%) associated with anastomotic and nonanastomotic biliary strictures was the most common intra-abdominal infection, which required a need for repeated stenting or surgical intervention and prolonged antibiotic therapy. In one patient pancreatic allograft failed because of hemorrhagic erosion from bacterial abscess. There were no deaths attributed to MGS infections in the SOT recipients in this report [115].

Intrathoracic GMS infections after thoracic surgery, are an uncommon complication (4%). Most intrathoracic GMS infections present as empyema, infected pleural effusion, whereas bacterial mediastinitis is a rare complication. As seen in patients undergoing intra-abdominal allograft transplantation, GMS intrathoracic infections are frequently polymicrobial (64%), and infection recurrence (27%) may occur in nearly one-thrid of the cases [116].

Diagnosis

The diagnosis of VGS disease relies on isolating the organism from a sterile body site. The presence of VGS in blood cultures obtained adhering to the standard aseptic blood culture techniques may be regarded as a true pathogen. Isolation of VGS from the skin or mucosal sites, as expected, has limited clinical significance, as these organisms are part of the normal cutaneous and mucosal microbiota in humans. It is also important to take note of the possibility of blood cultures contaminated with VGS; however, their presence in blood samples must be considered clinically relevant, especially in high-risk patients such as those with antineoplastic chemotherapy-induced neutropenia and chemotherapy- or radiation-associated mucositis and patients with severe neutropenia and mucositis following condition preparatory regimens for allogenic stem cell transplantation [117]. Serologic or antigen tests have no diagnostic value for invasive VGS disease, even in the high-risk patients undergoing allograft transplantation.

Treatment

Therapy of VGS disease is limited by the high level of β-lactam antimicrobial resistance [118, 119]. The clinical samples isolated from patients with neutropenia, less than half (~40%) of the VGS isolates, exhibit in vitro susceptibility to penicillin [120]. However, for β-lactam-susceptible organisms, these drugs are considered first line of therapy. Vancomycin susceptibility among clinical VGS isolates is close to 100%. In cancer patients with mostly acute leukemia and those undergoing HSCT, nearly 30% of isolates were reported as penicillin resistant, whereas all isolates exhibited in vitro susceptibility to vancomycin [107].

An increasing level of resistance is observed for fluoroquinolone, especially in patients routinely given this class of antibiotics for prophylaxis; empiric therapy with fluoroquinolone to treat systemic or invasive VGS infections is therefore, not recommended [121, 122]. VGS bacteremia is generally treated for 10–14 days; patients with endovascular site of infection including endocarditis should receive treatment for 4 weeks. Patients with septic arthritis and osteomyelitis may be given intravenous antibiotics for 3–4 weeks followed by an oral agent for suppressive therapy for another 4–8 weeks or even longer duration, which depends on the hosts' risk factors, including cumulative immune suppression, severity of infection; and in cases where deferment of excision of necrotic or ischemic debridable tissue leaves the focus of infection unattended. The role of intravenous immunoglobulin and plasmapheresis has been explored for patients with exotoxin-mediated toxic shock syndrome and currently not considered as standard of care for severe VGS infections [113].

GMS were susceptible to penicillin G, carbapenems, and clindamycin, whereas cephalosporins and quinolones showed intermediate activity or resistance in some cases, and it is important to note that GMS bacteria in general tend to be resistant to aminoglycosides [115].

β-Hemolytic Streptococci

The β-hemolytic streptococci reflect upon their ability to cause full red blood cell lysis in the blood-enriched culture media. Group A β-hemolytic streptococci (GAS) or *Streptococcus pyogenes* is a common pathogen followed by group B β-hemolytic streptococci (GBS) or *Streptococcus agalactiae* and groups C and G β-hemolytic streptococci (GCS and GGS, respectively) also known as *Streptococcus dysgalactiae* subspecies *equisimilis* [123–125].

Epidemiology

β-Hemolytic streptococci are ubiquitous in the human and animal population; colonization of the skin and mucous membrane is a common event. They are also an important cause for locally invasive disease such as pharyngitis, lower urinary tract infection, and superficial skin and skin structure infections. Severe systemic disease may occur in the general population and those with immune dysregulation after undergoing allograft transplantation [126]. The oropharynx and skin are the main sites of GAS, GCS, and GGS colonization [127, 128], whereas GBS commonly colonize the perineal area [128–130]. In the general population, majority of β-hemolytic streptococcal infections are acquired and presented from the community [83]. Immunosuppressed patients, especially those undergoing antineoplastic chemotherapy and recipients of HSCT, have a much higher risk for invasive β-hemolytic streptococcal disease compared to the general population [131, 132]. Cancer patients with lymphedema due to cancer infiltration or surgical lymph node dissection or those with radiation-induced tissue scarring impeding lymphatic circulation are especially at risk for such infections [133]. GBS are the most common of the invasive β-hemolytic streptococci isolated from patients with cancer and those undergoing stem cell transplantation [134, 135]. The development of invasive GAS, although less common than GBS, may result in a devastating disease that carries high fatality rates in excess of 50% [125].

Clinical Manifestations

Most β-hemolytic streptococcal infections in immunosuppressed cancer and stem cell transplant patients present with cellulitis and subcutaneous abscesses. In patients undergoing solid organ transplantation procedure, surgical wound infection, deep surgical bed infection, secondary infections of postoperative seromas, and deep tissue hematomas may also be prominent clinical manifestations of β-hemolytic streptococci. It is important to note that number of these infections may accompany other pathogens; appreciation for polymicrobial aspect of such infections is the central tenet in planning and executing a comprehensive treatment approach for deep tissue, and body cavity infections following transplant surgery [136].

Disease may range from relatively uncomplicated cellulitis and superficial wound infection to necrotizing fasciitis with or without exotoxin-induced toxic shock syndrome. The latter two complications are almost exclusively associated with GAS infection. Cellulitis due to β-hemolytic streptococci tends to develop rapidly, spread quickly, and may be accompanied by systemic manifestations such as fatigue, severe prostration, chills, rigors, with high-grade fever [137]. Erysipelas is a form of superficial cellulitis, in which the disease is restricted to the dermis. These lesions are elevated and well-demarcated from the healthy surrounding tissues [138]. Recurrence of erysipelas is a concern and often seen in patients with impaired lymphatic circulation. Infections due to GAS, GCS, and GGS are the leading bacterial causes of pharyngitis in children; most infections are readily treatable, although peritonsillar abscess and cervical lymphadenitis may rarely occur [128].

Invasive, systemic β-hemolytic streptococcal disease causes serious morbidity in patients with a suppressed immune response. Adults with β-hemolytic streptococcal bacteremia, especially patients with advancing age, the risk of death from such infections is high [125]. β-hemolytic streptococcal skin lesions that are greater than 5 cm in diameter, presence of pain that is out of proportion to findings on physical examination, disproporte severity in pain to gentle touch, and signs of systemic toxicity, skin discoloration, and/or presence of bullae on the overlying skin should raise concern for deep tissue involvement; possibility of necrotizing fasciitis, pyomyositis, and compartment syndrome should be entertained in such patients [139]. β-hemolytic streptococci disease via exotoxin production, especially by GAS, leads to extensive destruction of hosts' tissue and usually spreads at an exceedingly fast pace. Streptococcal toxic shock syndrome has also been described in cancer patients with mortality rates exceeding 50% [135]. Patients with diabetes are susceptible to hematogenous bacterial seeding to the bones resulting in remote site acute osteomyelitis [140].

A higher incidence of GAS necrotizing fasciitis was recently observed in Montréal, Canada. The authors reported that varicella and the presence of *speC* gene in GAS strains were associated with necrotizing fasciitis. In patients undergoing transplantation, bacterial genetic factors and potential synergistic or additive effect of concurrent viral infections like varicella on risk of GAS-related necrotizing fasciitis is not known [141].

Diagnosis

β-Hemolytic streptococci are readily isolated from cultures that are appropriately obtained. Rapid antigen tests are reliable for the diagnoses of GAS pharyngitis in patients when such infections are suspected [142]. Recovery of β-hemolytic streptococci from sterile-site samples such as blood, joints, deep tissue, and body cavity abscesses indicates a true infection. In contrast, isolation of β-hemolytic streptococcus species from mucous membranes and skin frequently reflects bacterial colonization.

An exception to the preceding stipulation is the isolation of GAS in mucosal site culture samples to assist in the diagnosis of toxic shock syndrome [143]. Serologic tests are not useful in patients with acute β-hemolytic streptococcal infections. Acute and convalescent serum for antibodies to streptolysin O or DNase can determine a recent infection due to GAS, although such serological tests are now seldom used in clinical practice [144].

Treatment

Penicillin and other β-lactam antibiotics are considered drugs of choice for the treatment of infections due to β-hemolytic streptococci [145]. For patients who cannot receive β-lactams, treatment with vancomycin is recommended. Carbapenems may also be an option in patients with non-life-threatening penicillin allergy [146]. Macrolide and lincosamide should not be used for serious infections as drug resistance is unpredictable and highly variable; these agents should only be used when susceptibility results are available, especially for outpatient transition of therapy [147]. Similarly, resistance to tetracyclines and trimethoprim-sulfamethoxazole warrants the use of these agents empirically to treat β-hemolytic streptococcal disease [148, 149]. Clinical experience with newer gram-positive drugs like daptomycin; the oxazolidinones, such as linezolid and tedizolid; tigecycline; and long-acting lipoglycopeptides such as dalbavancin and oritavancin is encouraging with good in vitro susceptibility data for β-hemolytic streptococcal clinical isolates [150, 151]. In cases of serious soft tissue infection, especially toxic shock syndrome, addition of clindamycin is strongly recommended to attenuate bacterial exotoxin production by slowly dying bacteria after exposure to beta-lactam antibiotics [152]. Uncomplicated bacteremia can be treated with a 10-day course of antibiotics, whereas fiat for complicated β-hemolytic streptococcal disease has traditionally been longer duration of antibiotic therapy. Surgical debridement of devitalized tissue and drainage of large purulent deep tissue collections is, as with any other bacterial or fungal infection, remains important for containment and resolution of infection [139].

Streptococcus pneumoniae

Epidemiology

S. pneumoniae is genetically similar to other bacteria in this category, although it is a prominent pathogen associated with a wide spectrum of invasive disease in immunocompromised patients and those in the general population.

Nasopharynx colonization due to pneumococci occurs more frequently in children (20–40%) compared with healthy adults (10–20%) [153]. *S. pneumoniae* is the leading cause of bacterial pneumonia that commences while patients are in the community [154]. Bacterial meningitis is also an important complication of *S. pneumoniae* in patients with community-onset meningitis [155]. Patients with chronic obstructive pulmonary disease, chronic kidney disease, and deficiencies in humoral immunity such as those following anti-CD20 and other B-cell targeted therapies and patients with chronic lymphocytic leukemia, B cell lymphoma, and plasma cell neoplasms like multiple myeloma; and those with hereditory hypogammaglobulinemia are especially susceptible to pneumococcal invasive disease. Similarly, patients with hyposplenism including those with sickle cell diseases and patients after splenectomy are at risk for, often severe disseminated infection due to *S. pneumoniae* [156]. Patients with chronic graft-versus-host disease following allogenic stem cell transplantation are vulnerable to infections due to encapsulated bacteria; *S. pneumoniae* is prominent in this regard [157].

It has also been suggested that prolonged exposure to systemic corticosteroids increases the risk for pneumococcal infection as is the extremes of age [158–160]. A high prevalence of *S. pneumoniae* in children less than 5 years of age is well recognized; young children with B-cell cancer or those undergoing anti-B-cell-targeted therapy for allogenic hematopoietic or solid organ transplantation are particularly susceptible to serious infection [156].

Clinical Presentation

S. pneumoniae is a major respiratory tract pathogen. Infections in adults involve lower respiratory tracts, and bacterial pneumonia is a common disease presentation; bronchitis and paranasal sinus infections may also occur [161], whereas in children, otitis media is not an uncommon presentation.

Community-onset pneumonia in the immunocompromised transplant recipients is a serious infection. Patients commonly present with chills, fever, and fatigue; cough is generally accompanied by purulent sputum and shortness of breath [162]. Patients with inflammation of the parietal plural with or without bacterial empyema may present with pleuritic chest pain. Bacterial lung abscess due to *S. pneumoniae* is not an uncommon complication of invasive pulmonary pneumococcal disease and often associated with cavitary lung lesions [163].

In recent animal experiments, pneumococcal infection was shown to cause nonspecific ischemic cardiac alterations, myocardial necroptosis, and apoptosis in both acutely ill and convalescent nonhuman primates [164]. *S. pneumoniae* was detected in the myocardium of all animals with acute severe pneumonia. Furthermore, evidence of cardiac scar formation was observed only in convalescent animals [164]. This study suggested a potential role of invasive pulmonary pneumococcal disease in the humans, with the possibility of subclinical bacterial invasion of the myocardium, resulting in cardiac injury from necroptosis and apoptosis, followed by cardiac scarring and remodeling after antibiotic therapy [164]. Clinical importance and cardiac impact in humans with invasive pneumococcal disease need further evaluation.

Patients with bacterial meningitis may often have concurrent bacteremia, whereas pneumonia may not be present. Fever and neck stiffness along with persistent and often severe headache are common clinical features of bacterial meningitis. In patients with advanced pneumococcal meningeal disease, altered sensorium, obtundation, and coma may be the initial presentation.

Other disease manifestations include septic arthritis, usually involving the native large joints. Pneumococcal septic arthritis involving the symphysis pubis is often misdiagnosed as osteitis pubis, a sterile inflammatory condition seen in women following urinary incontinence surgery and sports such as soccer and also in patients with pelvic malignancies. *Staphylococcus aureus* was the major cause among athletes and *Pseudomonas aeruginosa* among intravenous drug users. Septic arthritis in patients with pelvic malignancies are usually polymicrobial infections involving the fecal flora. Antibiotics are recommended for 6 weeks, and surgical debridement is required in nearly half of the patients [165].

Osteomyelitis of spinal and paraspinal tissues caused by *Streptococcus pneumoniae* is an uncommon complication as reported by the group in Houston, Texas. These infections mostly occurred in the absence of recent surgical procedure or presence of a foreign device. The lumbar spine was the frequent site of infection. Such infections complicated by spinal epidural abscess or the presence of a phlegmon were accompanied by neurologic deficits and carried a higher risk for death. Antimicrobial therapy for 6 weeks was effective [166, 167].

In a report from Japan, 6% of patients with invasive pneumococcal disease had evidence of pneumococcal vertebral osteomyelitis. Most infections were acquired in the community and had no recent history of a surgical procedure or trauma. In their experience, the lumbar spine was involved in nearly two-thirds of patients, and the remaining patients had cervical spine involvement. Bacteremia in this group was nearly universal; none of the patients had a primary site of pneumococcal disease. Good response to intravenous beta-lactam therapy in this group was encouraging [168].

HSCT

In HSCT recipients, pneumococcal infections present as late-onset bacteremia. These late-onset BSIs were associated with worse outcomes including septic shock, ICU stays, and high risk for deaths [157, 169]. Early-onset bloodstream infections in patients undergoing HSCT are frequently associated with severe neutropenia, mucositis, and indwelling intravascular catheter infections. Whereas, late-onset BSIs are commonly seen in severely immunosuppressed allogeneic HSCT recipients with GVHD and those undergoing systemic corticosteroid therapy. Since majority of *S. pneumoniae* bacteremia occur during late transplantation period, effective preventive strategies such as immunization with newer, immunogenic conjugated pneumococcal vaccines and drug prophylaxis with agents that have activity against majority of *S. pneumoniae* isolates in the community are considered standard of care. Infection prevention is highly desirable as pneumococcal bacteremia in this population carries unacceptably high case fatality rates.

In patients after undergoing allogeneic HSCT, diagnosis of pneumonia and chronic GVHD was associated with high mortality and a significantly lower probability of survival; this was evident in patients even after a single episode of pneumonia [170]. Pneumococcus is an important bacterial pathogen in allogeneic stem cell transplant recipients and mostly noted as late bacterial pneumonia with or without bloodstream infection. Pneumonia during the first 100 days after allograft stem cell transplantation are significantly more invasive fungal lung disease among individuals with acute GVHD; in such patients acute respiratory failure, and presence of septic shock predicted high risk of death [170].

Memory B-cell defects in allogeneic HSCT recipients increases susceptibility for encapsulated bacterial infections, as effective containment and remedy for these organisms require intact opsonization to promote phagocytosis. In a recent study, circulating IgM memory B cells (CD19+, CD27+, IgM+); and switched memory B cells (CD19+, CD27+, IgM( ), which are indicators of normal B cell activation and development were evaluated in 37 allogeneic HSCT recipients and compared with 35 healthy controls [171]. Among other parameters assessed were T-lymphocyte subpopulations, serum immunoglobulin levels including IgG subclasses, and antibodies to pneumococcal polysaccharides. A significant deficiency in both switched memory and IgM memory B cells was evident in the stem cell transplant cohort compared with the individuals in the healthy control group [171]. This observation was noted throughout the period following transplantation procedure and possibly reflect a switch to impaired B-cell isotype(s) in germinal centers within lymph nodes and other secondary lymphoid tissue. As expected, presence of GVHD was associated with lower IgM memory B-cell counts and lower serum levels of IgG2, IgG4, IgA, and antipneumococcal antibodies. Allogeneic HSCT recipients are susceptible to pneumococcal disease, which in most part is a reflection on the underlying defects in memory B-cell function aggravated in the presence of chronic GVHD [171]. Furthermore, hyposplenism is a frequent feature in HSCT recipients with chronic

GVHD, which further enhances the risk for systemic infections due to encapsulated bacteria.

In a transplant unit in Canada, the probability for pneumococcal disease among HSCT recipients was 30-fold higher than the general population (regression ratio = 30.2; $P < 0.00001$). Serotypes 23F and 6B were most prevalent [172]. All infection-associated serotypes were included in pneumococcal polysaccharide vaccine, whereas only 69% were represented in the conjugate vaccines. It was also important to note that the level of resistance to trimethoprim-sulfamethoxazole was high among the *S. pneumoniae* isolated from the transplant population during this study [172].

At M.D. Anderson Cancer Center between 1989 and 2005, 47 of 7,888 HSCT recipients developed 54 episodes of *S. pneumoniae* infections, accounting for 7 infection episodes per 1000 stem cell transplants [157]. The incidence was significantly higher in the allogeneic vs. autologous stem cell graft recipients, nine vs. five infection episodes per 1000 HSCTs, respectively. Thirty-six percent had graft-versus-host disease, and as expected, 16 of 17 patients had chronic GVHD. The total of 54 episodes of *S. pneumoniae* infection occurred median 433 days after transplntation; 11% of these patients had infection recurrence [157]. All 50 late posttransplant episodes were community-acquired infections and seen 473 ± 671 days after transplantation. Bacteremic pneumonia was the most common presentation (61%), followed by pneumonia without bacteremia (19%) and uncomplicated bacteremia alone (15%) [157]. Regression analysis showed that treatment with corticosteroids significantly increased the risk for bacteremic pneumonia (OR, 11.7; $P \leq 0.025$). In bacterial isolates from 29 episodes, 93% of patients received concordant antimicrobial therapy. It was unexpected that only one of the six patients (13%) who died of *S. pneumoniae* infection had chronic GVHD. The probability of death was higher in patients receiving care in the ICU at the time of infection diagnosis (OR, 15.5; $P \leq 0.007$) and those with each unit increase in APACHE II score (OR, 1.9; $P \leq 0.008$). Vaccine-breakthrough *S. pneumoniae* infection occurred in 5 patients after a median of 546 days following immunization; most such patients (80%) had pneumonia and concurrent bacteremia [157]. It is noteworthy that there were no cases of extrapulmonary focus of pneumococcal disease in HSCT recipients presented in this report.

Nontropical pyomyositis is an uncommon infection, such severe bacterial infections occur mostly in patients with suppressed immune response. *S. aureus* is the prominent pathogen associated with this disease. Pyomyositis due to *S. pneumoniae* is rare [173]. A recent report of hematogenous pneumococcal pyomyositis in an allogeneic stem cell graft recipient involved erector spinae muscles that presented 34 months after the transplantation procedure. Patient had a favorable response to 4 weeks of intravenous benzyl penicillin therapy [173].

SOT

As in HSCT, patients undergoing solid organ transplantation are at a greater risk for IPD compared with general population. Invasive pneumococcal disease is mostly seen in the late posttransplant period, and infections commonly start in the community. A prospective, population-based surveillance from Toronto, Canada, assessed systemic pneumococcal infections in SOT recipients between 1995 and 2004 [174]. The incidence was 146 infections from sterile body sites per 100,000 persons per year compared with 11.5 per 100,000 persons per year in the general population (RR, 12.8; $P < 0.00001$). When they also included the isolates from the respiratory tract, the incidence rate in transplant patients rose to 419 per 100,000 persons per year. Serotypes 23F and 22F were most common; 85% of these infection-associated serotypes were included in the 23-valent pneumococcal vaccine [174]. The antimicrobial resistance in SOT population was similar to that observed in the pneumococcal isolates for the general population and was especially high for penicillin and TMP/SMX.

A large database of 4,458 pediatric heart transplant recipients between 1993 and 2014 showed that the risk of bacterial infection was highest in the first month after transplantation; 25% of patients developed bacteremia. It was not unexpected to notice that community-acquired *S. pneumoniae* (6%) and *Haemophilus influenzae* (3%) were prominent during the late transplant period, whereas within a month following transplant procedure, CoNS (16.97%), *Enterobacter* spp. (12%), and *Pseudomonas* spp. (12%) were the prominent bacterial pathogens [175]. A large proportion of the infections were caused by multidrug-resistant organisms. Patients at risk for bacterial infection following heart transplantation included young age and ventilator or extracorporeal membrane oxygenation during transplantation. Thirty-four percent died due to bacterial infections, and prior cardiac surgery and multiple sites of infection were independent predictors of death [175].

In the Netherlands, a prospective nationwide study between 2006 and the end of 2014 assessed the risk and frequency of community-acquired bacterial meningitis among 16-year-old or older solid organ transplant recipients [176]. Six SOT recipients had bacterial meningitis; interestingly all six had undergone renal allograft transplantation. The annual incidence of bacterial meningitis was sevenfold higher for renal transplant recipients as compared with the general population: 9.5 vs. 1.3 per 100,000 patients per year [176]. It is important to note that in majority of the patients (83%), classic presentation of bacterial meningitis such as fever, neck stiffness, and changes in mental status were not present. Further complicating early diagnosis and prompt institution of appropriate antibiotic therapy for this life-threatening disease in this susceptible population. Seizures were present in 33% of patients. *Streptococcus pneumoniae* and *Listeria monocytogenes* were identified in two patients each, whereas, *Escherichia coli* and *Pseudomonas aeruginosa* were seen in one patient each. Another valuable observation in this report was the high incidence (67%) of unfavorable functional outcomes that probably were a reflection on the hosts' immunocompromised status and, importantly, atypical clinical presentation of bacterial meningitis in patients undergoing solid allograft transplantation [176].

A retrospective review from London, England, assessed long-term outcome in patients who underwent orthotopic cadaveric donor heart and lung transplantation between July 1986 and July 2006 [177]. The mean posttransplant follow-up was 5.4 ± 5.5 years. Bacterial meningitis was diagnosed in 39 adults after receiving 15 heart transplants, 12 lung including 4 bilateral lung transplants, and 12 heart-lung transplants. *Neisseria meningitidis* (54%) and *Streptococcus pneumoniae* (41%) were prominent pathogens followed by *Haemophilus influenzae* (5%). Hospital mortality rate was 10%, and none of these patients developed long-term complications after bacterial meningitis [177].

In a study from South Korea, 14 of 42 episodes of respiratory infections were noted after 1 month following lung transplantation [178]. Six were bacterial, four were viral, and two episodes were fungal infections. Among bacterial infections, two were due to MDR *Acinetobacter baumannii* and one each due to MDR *P. aeruginosa*, ESBL (+) *K. pneumoniae*, MRSA, and *Streptococcus pneumoniae*. Infection-related death occurred in 6 of the 14 episodes (43%) [178].

In a report from Barcelona, Spain, 138 episodes of spontaneous bacterial peritonitis (SBP) in 19 liver transplant recipients and 119 in nontransplant patients showed *Escherichia coli* (35.7%) and *Streptococcus pneumoniae* (21.4%) as the prominent pathogens [179]. It was interesting to note that pathogens associated with SBP were significantly more frequently identified in patients following transplantation (74%), whereas only 39% of nontransplant population with SBP had a positive culture ($P = 0.004$). As expected, renal failure (58% vs. 25%; $P = 0.004$) and hepatic encephalopathy (42% vs. 22%; $P = 0.08$) were more often seen in liver transplant recipients vs. the nontransplant group, respectively [179]. Similarly, deaths during the SBP episodes (53% vs. 13%; $P < 0.001$) and 6 months after the infection diagnosis (71% vs. 35%; $P = 0.005$) were significantly higher in the transplant population. The risk of death associated with the SBP was sixfold higher in patients with a high (>18) Model for End-Stage Liver Disease (MELD) score and fourfold higher in patients who had undergone liver transplantation. Mortality 6 months after SBP was fourfold higher in patients with hepatocellular carcinoma [179].

Orthotopic liver transplantation from a potential donors with active bacterial meningitis has been regarded as a contraindication for allograft procurement from such a donor. Due to a global shortage of liver allografts, in Birmingham, England, orthotopic liver transplants were performed from 33 donors with acute bacterial meningitis, 14 *Neisseria meningitidis*, 4 *Streptococcus pneumoniae*, 2 *Streptococcus* spp., and a single patient with *Haemophilus influenzae*. In 12 donors, a pathogen was not identified [180]. Of 34 recipients, 27 underwent elective and 7 had emergency transplantat surgery including 21 whole liver, 10 reduced-liver, and 3 split-liver allograft transplants. Adequate antimicrobial therapy before organ procurement and after transplant was administrated. The mean duration of follow-up after transplantation was 37 months (ranged from 1 day to 106 months). Overall patient (79% and 77%) and graft survival was; 72% and 65% at 1 and 60 months, respectively [180]. Patients who underwent elective liver transplant had significantly better survival compared with those who underwent emergency transplantation ($P < 0.05$). There was no difference in recipient and graft survival between the 34 patients who had received allograft from a donor with acute bacterial meningitis compared with recipient-matched groups. The authors observed no infectious complications in the recipient due to bacteria associated with meningitis after transplantation. Further data is needed before routine acceptance of liver allografts from donors with active bacterial meningitis becomes an acceptable practice, although study such as this, underscores that lifesaving procedure such as liver transplantation may be safly performed provided both donors and recipients are given adequate antimicrobial therapy. Furthermore, the optimum duration of antibiotic therapy in such recipients is not certain.

Diagnosis

Isolation of *S. pneumoniae* in blood, joint fluid, bronchial wash or lavage samples, and cerebrospinal fluid is regarded as diagnostic. Isolation of *S. pneumoniae* in sputum samples is a challenge, as diagnostic yield is significantly reduced in patients exposed to antibiotic(s) [181]. It has been estimated that only one-fourth of the patients with pneumococcal pneumonia will have a positive blood culture [182]. As with staphylococcal and other streptococcal infections, serologic studies have limited clinical use in assisting with the diagnosis of an acute infection episode. Detection of C-polysaccharide (BINAX-NOW) in the urine of adults with pneumococcal pneumonia is isolated in 75–85% of the patients; this test has high specificity and reliable negative predictive value [183]. Polymorphonuclear-predominant pleocytosis, low glucose, and high protein in the cerebrospinal fluid are the hallmarks of bacterial meningitis that are as expected to be present in most patients with pneumococcal meningitis. Gram-stain, bacterial antigen assays and culture of cerebrospinal fluid obtained promptly prior to extensive antibiotic exposure are essential for establishing the correct diagnosis [182].

Treatment

S. pneumoniae penicillin susceptibility and laboratory breakpoints have been reevaluated as to include the site of infection and the route by which the antibiotics may be administered [184]. For all pneumococcal infections other than the central nervous system, organisms demonstrating in vitro penicillin susceptibility of ≤2 µg/ml, reflecting approximately 95% of clinical pneumococcal cases in the United States, have good probability for attaining a clinical response to high-dose penicillin given intravenously [184]. For treatment of pneumococcal meningitis, penicillin MIC of <0.06 µg/ml is considered susceptible, and others with MIC ≥ 0.12 µg /ml are regarded as resistant bacterial strains; nearly 75% of pneumococci isolated in patients with meningitis in the United States fall in the susceptible category [184]. Pneumococcal isolates are universally susceptible to vancomycin. Respiratory fluorinated quinolones such as levofloxacin and moxifloxacin retain susceptibility for most pneumococcal isolates, although due to limited clinical experience and unpredictable response, authors recommend not to use these agents alone to treat patients with *S. pneumoniae* CNS infections [185, 186]. In *S. pneumoniae* isolated from respiratory specimens in the United States, resistance to macrolides, clindamycin, trimethoprim-sulfamethoxazole, and tetracyclines ranged from 20% to 40% [187]. In the authors' opinion, these drugs should not be used for the treatment of invasive pneumococcal disease in the transplant population.

Linezolid is an effective and safe treatment option for patients with *S. pneumoniae* infections [188]. Linezolid was shown to be effective and well tolerated in severely immunocompromised children with an underlying malignancy including those at young age [189]. The increased susceptibility to bacterial respiratory tract infection following a viral infection was associated with a substantial increase in local and systemic IFN-γ concentrations. Linezolid was shown to reduce IFN-γ and TNF-α production in stimulated peripheral blood mononuclear cells. In mice, linezolid recently showed protection from post influenza pneumococcal infection, and this reversal of immune hyporesponsiveness was attributed to the drug's ability to mitigate exaggerated postviral IFN-γ and TNF-α immune responses [190]. This ancillary immune modulatory effect of linezolid, especially in patients that are susceptibile for postviral superimposed bacterial pneumonia, is intriguing and needs further evaluation.

Daptomycin should not be used to treat lung infections, especially bronchogenic pneumonia because of limited drug diffusion in the alveolar space and inactivation of daptomycin by pulmonary surfactant [191].

Mortality for invasive pneumococcal disease remains around 15% within the first week of hospitalization, and most infections respond to a relatively short course of antibiotic therapy; extended therapy for over 2 weeks is recommended for patients with meningitis, empyema, bone and joint infections, and deep tissue abscesses that are not evacuated and patients with complicated bacteremia with an endovascular focus of infection [182].

S. pneumoniae is the only Gram-positive bacteria for which there are licensed vaccines available globally. The role of pneumococcal vaccine in transplant population is discussed in Chap. 63.

Enterococcus

Epidemiology

Enterococci, not dissimilar to CoNS and VGS, cause a disproportionately higher number of infections in the immunosuppressed cancer and transplant patients compared with the general population [192]. Most enterococcal infections are associated with prolonged exposure to healthcare environment. Enterococci are prominent bacteria in human intestinal microbiome. *E. faecalis* and *E. faecium* are two most frequently isolated species from infections in humans [193]. Patients with cancer and those undergoing transplantation have especially high rates of intestinal colonization and subsequent risk for invasive disease due to vancomycin-resistant enterococci (VRE). The factors promoting selection and persistence for VRE colonization in certain high-risk individuals with cancer and those undergoing transplantation procedure remain unclear, although prior exposure to m antibiotics has been proposed. It was interesting that a recent report indicated transplant unit reconstruction had interrupted endemic transmission of VRE, which resumed with novel enterococcal strains upon reopening of the unit. It was hypothesized that endemic VRE transmission in this transplant unit probably reflected VRE contamination of shared equipment and environmental surfaces [194]. This provides further insight into the possible reason that VRE has been an unabating challenge at certain transplant units, whereas less of a problem in patients undergoing a similar transplantation procedures at other institutions. This hypothesis was further emphasized in a recent study from Buffalo, New York, that active surveillance and contact precautions for VRE colonization were not effective in preventing VRE bacteremia in patients undergoing stem cell transplantation at their institution [195], whereas, a group from Salt Lake City, Utah reported in 2016 that VRE transmission from room surfaces appeared to be an infrequent event, thereby concluding that adherence to VRE surveillance, disinfection strategies, and contact isolation protocols are needed to be adhered to and may reduce VRE colonization rates in patients with hematologic malignancies and those undergoing HSCT [196].

HSCT

A single-center experience among patients admitted for induction chemotherapy or those undergoing HSCT from 2006 to 2014 showed that the incidence of VRE bacteremia was 6.5% of admissions or 2.7 VRE bacteremia per 1000 bloodstream infection at-risk days [192]. Mortality and length of stay were significantly higher in patients in whom VRE bacteremia were to occur. Patients with prior VRE colonization had eightfold higher probability for VRE bacteremia; similarly, patients with renal insufficiency (twofold), aminoglycoside use (~fivefold), and antibiotics with anaerobic activity (~threefold) had significantly higher risk for VRE bacteremia. The authors also reported using a predictive model, which identified severe neutropenia and prior beta-lactam antibiotic use were among prominent risk factors for VRE bloodstream invasion and infection [192].

A recent report from Salt Lake City, Utah, showed that VRE bacteremia after stem cell engraftment and resolution of neutropenia in HSCT recipients was associated with a much higher mortality compared with VRE bacteremia during the neutropenic pre-engraftment period [197]. Pre-engraftment bacteremia from any organism resulted in an increase length of hospitalization and higher cost of care. Mortality was similar for pre-engraftment VRE bacteremia and bacteremia due to other organisms in this neutropenic phase following stem cell transplantation. The authors pointed out that a high VRE bacteremia mortality rate observed during the post-engraftment period was largely associated with severe graft-versus-host disease and relapsed leukemia [197]. It was also interesting to note that frequently VRE strains switched phenotypes when isolated from patients before and after the transplantation procedure [197].

A contrasting review of patients undergoing HSCT at the Mayo Clinic in Rochester, Minnesota concluded that VRE colonization was a surrogate marker and not an independent predictor of mortality in HSCT recipients [198]. They observed high morbidity in their transplant patients with VRE bacteremia, although this had no significant impact on posttransplant survival. The data was generated between 2004 and 2014 by conducting twice-weekly perirectal swab PCR screening for vanA and vanB. In 73 of 203 patients, VRE colonization was noted prior to HSCT and in 11% VRE colonization occurred within the first 100 days after transplantation [198]. There was no significant difference in overall survival based on pretransplant VRE colonization status. However, patients that developed VRE colonization within the first 100 days after HSCT had a significantly worse survival. During the first 30 days following transplant, 91% had screened positive for VRE colonization prior to developing bacteremia. On multivariable analysis, advanced age (≥60 years), high HSCT comorbidity score, and prior VRE colonization were independent risk factors for VRE bacteremia. It was notable that only one patient had died with VRE bacteremia during the first 100 days after HSCT [198].

The findings from a center in Cleveland, Ohio, were in concert with the report from the Mayo Clinic; they found that between 1997 and 2011, the incidence of VRE-B had increased in 800 adult allogeneic HSCT recipients. Seventy-six patients developed VRE-vanB bacteremia after a median of 46 days following transplantation. Multivariable analysis showed that the risk for VRE-vanB bacteremia was higher in patients with high HSCT comorbidity score, with diagnosis of acute lymphoblastic leukemia, and recipients of unrelated donor and umbilical cord blood stem cell allograft transplantation. A fourfold higher probability of death in patients with VRE-vanB bacteremia was a significant finding on multivariate analysis; however, only 6% of 67 deaths within 5 weeks after transplantation were attributed to VRE infection [199], drawing attention to the clinical relevance of VRE bacteremia in high-risk transplant patients as a potential surrogate marker for poor prognosis during the early posttransplant period.

The preceding observation was also noted in a review of 247 adult patients in whom 28% had VRE colonization after allogeneic HSCT between 2008 and 2009 [200]. This report from Memorial Sloan Kettering Cancer Center in New York reported VRE bacteremia (54%) as the leading cause of bloodstream infection within 30 days after HSCT at their institution. Only 57% of patients with VRE bacteremia had VRE colonization during pretransplant screening [200]. Attributable mortality to VRE infection was low (9%), reflecting VRE bacteremia as a surrogate marker for altered host intestinal tract microbiota and perhapse an indicator for a subgroup of high-risk individuals undergoing allogeneic stem cell graft transplantation.

In patients undergoing autologous stem cell transplantation, despite having a high rate of VRE colonization, the risk for invasive bacterial disease is low. High rates of VRE colonization in this group may potentially serve as a reservoir for transmission to other higher-risk patients in a transplant unit or center [201].

In patients following allogeneic stem cell graft transplantation, donor-derived T cells recognize host tissues as foreign and orchestrating an assault on the recipient tissues, clinically known as GVHD. The intestinal tract is the most common site of GVHD, and in recent years, an interest in the composition of gut microbiota and its relationship with the development of GVHD was explored. The loss of intestinal bacterial diversity is common in patients undergoing HSCT due to prophylactic, preemptive, and empiric use of broad-spectrum antibiotics. This loss in intestinal biodiversity and overgrowth of opportunistic pathogens belonging to the phylum *Proteobacteria* and genus *Enterococcus* in patients following HSCT have been linked to enhance the risk for treatment-related mortality including GVHD, systemic infections, and organ failure [202]. In animal experiments, interventions to mitigate alternations in selective intestinal bacterial overgrowth with the use of prebiotic and probiotic strategies have shown favorable results on the risk and severity of GVHD [202]. Further clinical studies are needed to explore these and other interventions that may restore healthy intestinal microbiota, especially in patients undergoing allogeneic stem cell to promote.

In patients undergoing HSCT, 2% chlorhexidine bathing was effective in regards to VRE colonization and infection [203], whereas no similar benefits were noted in protection against MDR-GNB, especially for infections due to *P. aeruginosa*.

A review of 822 autologous and allogeneic HCST recipients at Northwestern Memorial Hospital between 2004 and 2008 noted a 10% incidence in *Clostridium difficile*-associated diarrhea (CDAD) [204]. A significant association became apparent between CDAD and VRE colonization among other prominent risk factors for CDAD such as febrile neutropenia; exposure to ciprofloxacin, vancomycin, and aztreonam; prolonged duration of antibiotic therapy, and allogeneic stem cell transplantation [204].

Experiments have shown the protective significance of the normal microbiota; VRE colonization serves as a surrogate, representing alteration in the intestinal microbiome, especially following the influential perturbation during and after prolonged, broad-spectrum antibiotic therapy. Exogenously administered VRE was shown to efficiently and nearly completely displace the normal microbiota of the small and large intestines in mice after antibiotic therapy [205]. Furthermore, investigators from a comprehensive cancer center in New York showed that VRE colonization preceded bacteremia and sepsis in patients undergoing allogeneic HSCT [205].

SOT

Enterococcus species are recognized for nearly three decades as a potential pathogen in patients undergoing liver and other abdominal visceral transplants. Early on at the Mayo Clinic in Rochester, Minnesota, 405 consecutive liver transplantations were conducted between 1985 and 1993, a selective bowel decontamination prophylaxis regimen was routinely given [206]. In 52 patients (13%), 70 episodes of bacteremia were seen; most infections were due to *Enterococcus faecalis* (n = 50), and 18 isolates of *Enterococcus faecium*; vancomycin resistance in clinical enterococcal isolates was not an issue during the study years. It was important to note that nearly half (49%) of these infections were polymicrobial and one-third (34%) of the patients had complications involving the biliary tract. Not dissimilar to the observation in allogeneic HSCT recipients, most deaths (73%; 11 of 15) were not associated with enterococcal bacteremia. Significant risk factors in this group for enterococcal bacteremia included Roux-en-Y choledochojejunostomy (P = 0.005), a cytomegalovirus-seropositive donor (P = 0.013), prolonged transplantation time (P = 0.02), and strictures in the biliary tract (P = 0.016). On univariate analysis, diagnosis of primary sclerosing cholangitis (P = 0.009) and symptomatic cytomegalovirus infection (P = 0.008) was significantly present in patients in whom bacteremia due to *Enterococcus* spp. was observed [206]. Further underpinning the significance of isolation of these low-virulence pathogens in blood culture samples among patients undergoing liver transplantation, as a potential surrogate for identifying a highly susceptible subgroup of patients who have undergone abdominal visceral allograft transplantation surgery.

Selective bowel decontamination prophylactic regimens were suggested for mitigation of intestinal colonization due to MDR microorganisms. The Mayo Clinic reported isolation of VRE in early 1995 from surveillance cultures obtained from patients undergoing liver and kidney transplantation. By the end of 1997, 52 patients had VRE colonization, importantly with a single vanB clone [207]. VRE infection was observed in six patients (11%) [207].

In a longitudinal study from Pittsburgh, Pennsylvania, between 1990 and 1999, 165 patients underwent liver transplantation. Fifty-one (31%) patients developed posttransplant infection due to one or more MDR bacteria. A substantial number of bacteria (69%) were MDR pathogens. A high level of drug resistance was noted in *S. aureus* (91%) and enterococcal isolates (50%) [208]. During the decade-long study, a significant trend emerged for infections due to MDR bacteria mainly due to GPB infections like MRSA (P = 0.0001) and VRE (P = 0.04). In contrast, no significant increase was reported among MDR-GNB infections during the course of this study [208].

Patients undergoing solid organ transplantation are at an increased risk for colonization due to MRSA and VRE, an observation similar to patients undergoing allogeneic stem cell transplantation. As pointed out in a number of studies, bacterial colonization is an important precursor for invasive disease, especially those undergoing abdominal visceral allograft transplantation. A meta-analysis involving 23 published studies assessed the burden of MRSA and VRE colonization in patients undergoing solid organ transplantation; 17 of these studies were in liver transplant population [6]. The pooled prevalence estimates before transplantation were 8.5% for MRSA and 11.9% for VRE. However, MRSA colonization estimate was lower (4.0%) in studies involving 200 or more patients. The prevalence estimates for bacterial colonization after the transplantation procedure were 9.4% and 16.2% for MRSA and VRE, respectively. The risk for MRSA infection was significantly higher in patients with MRSA colonization before transplantation (RR 5.5) and also for patients in whom colonization occurred after the transplantation procedure (RR 10.56). In concert with the risk for subsequent MRSA infection, VRE colonization before (RR 6.6) and after transplantation (RR 7.9) were associated with significantly higher risk of invasive VRE disease [6].

Most early posttransplant VRE infections are a result of complications arising from transplant surgery, a need for extended stay in transplant or surgical critical unit and prolonged exposure to broad-spectrum antibiotics. Bacteremia, intra-abdominal infections, urinary tract infections, and surgical site infections are common clinical presentation. VRE endovascular infections including endocarditis in the SOT population is rarely seen [114, 209]. Complications involving the biliary tract, such as strictures and biliary leaks, and importantly the interventions to ameliorate these compilations are important risk factors for VRE infection in patients undergoing liver transplantation [209, 210].

In kidney transplant recipients, VRE infections are prominent in patients with HCV infection, those undergoing multivisceral transplantation such as kidney and pancreas allograft surgery, patients requiring renal replacement therapy after transplantation surgery; nephrostomy tube placement, and patients taken back to the operation room for re-exploration surgery [211].

Left ventricular assist devices (LVAD) are used as a bridge to cardiac transplantation in patients with severe life-threatening heart failure awaiting transplant surgery. Pretransplant infection of LVAD increases the risk for post-transplant infections including infections due to VRE. Patients with LVAD infections commonly present as primary bacteremia, pocket and tunnel infection, endovascular infections including LVAD endocarditis, and infections involving the mediastinum. In a report from Rush University Medical Center in Chicago, IL 46 LVAD-related infections were diagnosed in half of patients who underwent LVAD implantation as a bridge to transplantation. Twenty-nine episodes of LVAD-related bacteremia included five patients with LVAD endocarditis; presence of diabetes appeared to increase the risk for bacteremia. VRE infection was diagnosed in six patients with LVAD-related infection who had undergone transplantation surgery; four of these six patients died. It was interesting to note that VRE infections were not seen in patients without pretransplant LVAD-related infection [212].

Diagnosis

Culture is the mainstay of diagnosis, with serologic or antigen tests having no value. The isolation of enterococci from non-sterile specimens such as urine, sputum, or external wound drainage usually represents colonization or subclinical infection rather than infection that requires treatment. Prescribing antibiotics in this situation generally fails to eradicate the organism while promoting the risk for development of antimicrobial resistance and exposing the patient to adverse events and toxicicty plus potentil for drug-drug interactions [213]. Even when isolated from sterile sites such as the abdominal cavity, enterococci are usually present along with one or more other organisms [136], and treatment of more virulent pathogens has been shown to cure such infections even in the absence of targeted anti-enterococcal therapy [214]. This concept is illustrated by the highly effective nature of cephalosporins in treating intra-abdominal infections despite having limited activity against enterococci [215].

Treatment

Treatment of enterococcal infection is complicated; bacterial species and drug resistance profile are the main influence in selection of drug(s) for a specific type of infection. Most clinical *E. faecalis* isolates show in vitro susceptibility to common beta-lactam drugs such as penicillin, ampicillin, amoxicillin, and piperacillin and to carbapenems like imipenem. Nafcillin is not effective against *E. faecalis*. It is important to remember that *E. faecalis* isolates are intrinsically resistant to cephalosporins [216]. In contrast, *E. faecium* isolates exhibit a high level of penicillin resistance, which in most cases exceeds 50% [216]. Macrolides, TMP-SMX, and fluoroquinolones are generally not effective against enterococci [217]. Vancomycin is regarded as the drug of choice for treating enterococci infections in patients with serious hypersensitivity to beta-lactams and those with beta-lactam-resistant isolates. However, with the emergence and spread of vancomycin nonsusceptible strains, the choice(s) of optimum effective therapy remains uncertain [213]. Enterococci may exhibit tolerance to β-lactam antibiotics, meaning that bacterial growth is inhibited in vitro following exposure at low drug concentrations, however bacterial killing induced by autolytic cellular pathways is not achievable following exposure to, even high antibiotic levels that could be given at physiologic doses [218]. Beta-lactam tolerance is an important mechanism underlying treatment failure and/or infection recurrence in severely immunosuppressed patients with neutropenia and those with endovascular infections [213]. A bactericidal effect may be achieved against some isolates by the addition of an aminoglycoside [218]. The bacterial killing after the addition of aminoglycosides only occurs in isolates that show in vitro susceptibility to these drugs, and as expected, no synergistic benefit should be expected among bacterial strains that are tolerant to beta-lactam drugs and also resistant to aminoglycosides [218].

Linezolid, tedizolid, daptomycin, and seldom-used quinupristin/dalfopristin are the drugs active against VRE. Quinupristin/dalfopristin lacks efficacy against *E. faecalis*. Enterococcal bloodstream infection and with rare hematogenous seeding of the meninges resulting in bacterial meningitis that may occasionally occur in severely immunocompromised patients including those undergoing HSCT;

linezolid monotherapy was reported to be effective, although clinical experience is limited [219]. Furthermore, linezolid resistance has emerged as a daunting concern, especially in patients undergoing HSCT. In a study in Essen, Germany, conducted between 2014 and 2015, 20 patients had linezolid-resistant VRE, and 18 of these patients underwent HSCT [220]. Twenty-five percent of patients developed bloodstream infection. Ten patients had bacterial colonization at the time of hospitalization. Eighty percent of patients with hospital-onset linezolid-resistant VRE had prior therapy with linezolid [220]. The authors report no clear evidence of patient-to-patient or environment-to-patient transmission within the transplant unit. It was interesting to note that a single genotype in six patients was noted, and all such patients were referred for the same hospital.

A report from the University of Illinois in Chicago conducted between 2000 and 2008 assessed 48 hospitalized patients being treated with linezolid and reported reduced susceptibility to VRE in these clinical isolates [221]. A significantly high risk for such infections was seen in patients undergoing allogeneic stem cell or solid organ allograft transplantation (OR: 2.6), treatment with immunosuppressive agents (OR: 2.4), both systemic corticosteroids (OR: 2.4) and noncorticosteroid immunosuppressive drugs (OR: 2.3), and exposed to linezolid with 1 year prior to infection diagnosis (OR: 34.5). Multivariable analysis showed that the risk of reduced susceptibility to linezolid among clinical VRE isolates was 32-fold greater in individuals who had received linezolid within 1 year of infection diagnosis. It is important to note that in this report most patients with VRE infections due to reduced linezolid susceptibility had not been treated with linezolid in the year prior and reduced linezolid susceptibility did not impact patient outcomes, which included clinical or microbiological cure, length of hospitalization, and all-cause mortality [221]. Further studies are needed to understand the clinical relevance and potential for treatment failure in patients with the emerging reduced linezolid susceptibility VRE infections and how best to manage such infections.

The in vitro susceptibility data for daptomycin and tigecycline are encouraging. Emergence of daptomycin resistance among clinical VRE isolates, especially in patients undergoing HSCT is of grave concern [222]. Reports of clinical failures with these agents in the setting of high in vitro drug MICs have underscored the potential threat [223]. However, in a recent report among adults with VRE bacteremia following HSCT and those with hematologic malignancies, the duration of bacteremia and microbiological failure rates did not differ by daptomycin MICs [224]. Multivariable analysis indicated an interesting trend that all-cause 30-day mortality was low in patients with VRE bacteremia due to bacterial strains that had high daptomycin MICs (3–4 micrograms/L) [224]. This trend, however, did not reach a level of statistical significance [224]. If this were to be a valid and significant finding, such an observation would put "disease-causing fitness" of such bacterial strains into question and, as mentioned earlier in various reports, and place emphsis on the surrogate nature of enterococcal infections, especially in high-risk patients following allogenic stem cell or solid organ allograft transplantation.

Summary

Gram-positive bacteria (GPB) are an important cause of serious systemic disease in the immunocompromised patients, especially patients after undergoing allograft transplantation. A rise in infections due to GPB in the last two decades has been attributed to a variety of reasons that prominently include antimicrobial prophylaxis with a focus on the prevention of Gram-negative bacterial infections and common use of indwelling intravascular access devices. In solid organ transplant recipients, postsurgical wound and deep tissue infections resulting from tissue ischemia, prolonged and complicated surgical procedures, allograft rejection, and severity of iatrogenic drug-induced immune suppression are important contributing factors. Severe orointestinal mucositis, prolonged pre-engraftment neutropenia, and graft-versus-host disease involving the skin and orointestinal tract are important consideration to promote risk among patients undergoing hematopoietic stem graft transplants. Community-acquired methicillin-resistant *Staphylococcus aureus* is now frequently encountered. Similarly, drug resistance among various pathogenic *Staphylococcus*, *Streptococcus*, and *Enterococcus* species has a substantial impact on selection of empiric antibiotic therapy in this population with suspected bacterial infection. Early diagnosis, prompt institution of appropriate therapy, assessment for outcome prognosticators, and recognizing the potential for early and late infection- and treatment-related complications forms the bases for providing optimum management of GPB infections in the transplant population.

References

1. Berenger BM, Doucette K, Smith SW. Epidemiology and risk factors for nosocomial bloodstream infections in solid organ transplants over a 10-year period. Transpl Infect Dis. 2016;18(2):183–90.
2. Safdar A, Armstrong D. Infections in patients with hematologic neoplasms and hematopoietic stem cell transplantation: neutropenia, humoral, and splenic defects. Clin Infect Dis. 2011;53(8):798–806.
3. Safdar A, Armstrong D. Infectious morbidity in critically ill patients with cancer. Crit Care Clin. 2001;17(3):531–70.

4. Oliveira-Cunha M, Bowman V, di Benedetto G, Mitu-Pretorian MO, Armstrong S, Forgacs B, et al. Outcomes of methicillin-resistant Staphylococcus aureus infection after kidney and/or pancreas transplantation. Transplant Proc. 2013;45(6):2207–10.
5. Moore C, Davis NF, Burke JP, Power R, Mohan P, Hickey D, et al. Colonisation with methicillin-resistant Staphylococcus aureus prior to renal transplantation is associated with long-term renal allograft failure. Transpl Int. 2014;27(9):926–30.
6. Ziakas PD, Pliakos EE, Zervou FN, Knoll BM, Rice LB, Mylonakis E. MRSA and VRE colonization in solid organ transplantation: a meta-analysis of published studies. Am J Transplant. 2014;14(8):1887–94.
7. Nesher L, Chemaly RF, Shah DP, Mulanovich VE, Hosing C, Rolston KV. Utility of routine surveillance blood cultures in asymptomatic allogeneic hematopoietic stem cell transplant recipients with indwelling central venous catheters at a comprehensive cancer center. Am J Infect Control. 2014;42(10):1084–8.
8. Lukenbill J, Rybicki L, Sekeres MA, Zaman MO, Copelan A, Haddad H, et al. Defining incidence, risk factors, and impact on survival of central line-associated blood stream infections following hematopoietic cell transplantation in acute myeloid leukemia and myelodysplastic syndrome. Biol Blood Marrow Transplant. 2013;19(5):720–4.
9. Toro JJ, Morales M, Loberiza F, Ochoa-Bayona JL, Freytes CO. Patterns of use of vascular access devices in patients undergoing hematopoietic stem cell transplantation: results of an international survey. Support Care Cancer. 2007; 15(12):1375–83.
10. Laura R, Degl'Innocenti M, Mocali M, Alberani F, Boschi S, Giraudi A, et al. Comparison of two different time interval protocols for central venous catheter dressing in bone marrow transplant patients: results of a randomized, multicenter study. The Italian Nurse Bone Marrow Transplant Group(GITMO). Haematologica. 2000;85(3):275–9.
11. Lee SO, Brown RA, Kang SH, Abdel-Massih RC, Razonable RR. Toll-like receptor 2 polymorphism and Gram-positive bacterial infections after liver transplantation. Liver Transpl. 2011;17(9):1081–8.
12. Kanamaru A, Tatsumi Y. Microbiological data for patients with febrile neutropenia. Clin Infect Dis. 2004;39(Suppl 1):S7–S10.
13. Wisplinghoff H, Seifert H, Wenzel RP, Edmond MB. Current trends in the epidemiology of nosocomial bloodstream infections in patients with hematological malignancies and solid neoplasms in hospitals in the United States. Clin Infect Dis. 2003;36(9):1103–10.
14. Archer GL, Climo MW. Staphylococcus epidermidis and other coagulase-negative staphylococci. In: Mandell GL, Bennett JE, Dolin R, editors. Principles and practice of infectious diseases. Philadelphia: Elsevier; 2005. p. 2352–9.
15. Moreillon P, YQue YA, Glauser MP. Staphylococcus aureus (including staphylococcal toxic shock). In: Mandell GL, Bennett JE, Dolin R, editors. Principles and practice of infectious diseases. Philadelphia: Elsevier; 2005. p. 2321–51.
16. Kuehnert MJ, Kruszon-Moran D, Hill HA, McQuillan G, McAllister SK, Fosheim G, et al. Prevalence of Staphylococcus aureus nasal colonization in the United States, 2001–2002. J Infect Dis. 2006;193(2):172–9.
17. Boucher HW, Corey GR. Epidemiology of methicillin-resistant Staphylococcus aureus. Clin Infect Dis. 2008;46(Suppl 5):S344–9.
18. Kato N, Tanaka J, Mori A, Tutumi Y, Yonezumi M, Chiba K, et al. The risk of persistent carriage of methicillin-resistant Staphylococcus aureus in hematopoietic stem cell transplantation. Ann Hematol. 2003;82(5):310–2.
19. Navarro MB, Huttner B, Harbarth S. Methicillin-resistant Staphylococcus aureus control in the 21st century: beyond the acute care hospital. Curr Opin Infect Dis. 2008;21(4):372–9.
20. Laupland KB, Ross T, Gregson DB. Staphylococcus aureus bloodstream infections: risk factors, outcomes, and the influence of methicillin resistance in Calgary, Canada, 2000–2006. J Infect Dis. 2008;198(3):336–43.
21. Hodgson K, Morris J, Bridson T, Govan B, Rush C, Ketheesan N. Immunological mechanisms contributing to the double burden of diabetes and intracellular bacterial infections. Immunology. 2015;144(2):171–85.
22. Djaldetti M, Salman H, Bergman M, Djaldetti R, Bessler H. Phagocytosis—the mighty weapon of the silent warriors. Microsc Res Tech. 2002;57(6):421–31.
23. Weisser M, Theilacker C, Tschudin Sutter S, Babikir R, Bertz H, Götting T, et al. Secular trends of bloodstream infections during neutropenia in 15,181 haematopoietic stem cell transplants: 13-year results from a European multicenter surveillance study (ONKO-KISS). Clin Microbiol Infect. 2017;23(11):854–9.
24. Gjaerde LI, Moser C, Sengeløv H. Epidemiology of bloodstream infections after myeloablative and non-myeloablative allogeneic hematopoietic stem cell transplantation: a single-center cohort study. Transpl Infect Dis. 2017;19(5).
25. Mihu CN, Schaub J, Kesh S, Jakubowski A, Sepkowitz K, Pamer EG, et al. Risk factors for late Staphylococcus aureus bacteremia after allogeneic hematopoietic stem cell transplantation: a single-institution, nested case-controlled study. Biol Blood Marrow Transplant. 2008;14(12):1429–33.
26. Florescu DF, Qiu F, Vivekanandan R, Mercer DF, Langnas AN, Kalil AC. Risk factors and outcomes of Staphylococcus aureus infections after small bowel and multivisceral transplantation. Pediatr Infect Dis J. 2012;31(1):25–9.
27. Ranghino A, Diena D, Simonato F, Messina M, Burdese M, Piraina V, et al. Clinical impact of bacterial contamination of perfusion fluid in kidney transplantation. Springerplus. 2016;5:7.
28. Altman DR, Sebra R, Hand J, Attie O, Deikus G, Carpini KW, et al. Transmission of methicillin-resistant Staphylococcus aureus via deceased donor liver transplantation confirmed by whole genome sequencing. Am J Transplant. 2014;14(11):2640–4.
29. Doucette KE, Al-Saif M, Kneteman N, Chui L, Tyrrell GJ, Kumar D, et al. Donor-derived bacteremia in liver transplant recipients despite antibiotic prophylaxis. Am J Transplant. 2013;13(4):1080–3.
30. Soong RS, Chan KM, Chou HS, Wu TJ, Lee CF, Wu TH, et al. The risk factors for early infection in adult living donor liver transplantation recipients. Transplant Proc. 2012;44(3):784–6.
31. Li C, Wu Y, Riehle A, Ma J, Kamler M, Gulbins E, et al. Staphylococcus aureus survives in cystic fibrosis macrophages, forming a reservoir for chronic pneumonia. Infect Immun. 2017;85(5):e00883–16.
32. Shields RK, Clancy CJ, Minces LR, Kwak EJ, Silveira FP, Abdel Massih RC, et al. Staphylococcus aureus infections in the early period after lung transplantation: epidemiology, risk factors, and outcomes. J Heart Lung Transplant. 2012;31(11):1199–206.
33. Clancy CJ, Bartsch SM, Nguyen MH, Stuckey DR, Shields RK, Lee BY. A computer simulation model of the cost-effectiveness of routine Staphylococcus aureus screening and decolonization among lung and heart-lung transplant recipients. Eur J Clin Microbiol Infect Dis. 2014;33(6):1053–61.
34. Bernasconi E, Pattaroni C, Koutsokera A, Pison C, Kessler R, Benden C, et al. Airway microbiota determines innate cell inflammatory or tissue remodeling profiles in lung transplantation. Am J Respir Crit Care Med. 2016;194(10):1252–63.
35. Cordonnier C, Buzny A, Leverger G, Herbrecht R, Hunault M, Leclercq R, et al. Epidemiology and risk factors for gram-positive coccal infections in neutropenia: toward a more targeted antibiotic strategy. Clin Infect Dis. 2003;36(2):149–58.

36. Klevens RM, Morrison MA, Nadle J, Petit S, Gershman K, Ray S, et al. Invasive methicillin-resistant Staphylococcus aureus infections in the United States. JAMA. 2007;298(15):1763–71.
37. Takeda K, Tanaka K, Kumamoto T, Nojiri K, Mori R, Taniguchi K, et al. Septic pulmonary embolism originated from subcutaneous abscess after living donor liver transplantation: a pitfall of postoperative management. Clin J Gastroenterol. 2013;6(5):378–82.
38. Malagola M, Rambaldi B, Ravizzola G, Cattaneo C, Borlenghi E, Polverelli N, et al. Bacterial blood stream infections negatively impact on outcome of patients treated with allogeneic stem cell transplantation: 6 years single-centre experience. Mediterr J Hematol Infect Dis. 2017;9(1):e2017036.
39. Melzer M, Santhakumaran T, Welch C. The characteristics and outcome of bacteraemia in renal transplant recipients and non-transplant renal patients. Infection. 2016;44(5):617–22.
40. Mulcahy ME, McLoughlin RM. Staphylococcus aureus and influenza A virus: partners in coinfection. MBio. 2016;7(6):e02068–16.
41. Obed A, Schnitzbauer AA, Bein T, Lehn N, Linde HJ, Schlitt HJ. Fatal pneumonia caused by Panton-Valentine Leucocidine-positive methicillin-resistant Staphylococcus aureus (PVL-MRSA) transmitted from a healthy donor in living-donor liver transplantation. Transplantation. 2006;81(1):121–4.
42. Audard V, Pardon A, Claude O, Jablonski M, Remy P, Desvaux D, et al. Necrotizing fasciitis during de novo minimal change nephrotic syndrome in a kidney transplant recipient. Transpl Infect Dis. 2005;7(2):89–92.
43. Hachisuka H, Kimori K, Tsuge K. Methicillin-resistant Staphylococcus aureus arthritis of the wrist treated with arthrodesis using vascularized fibular transfer: a case report. J Reconstr Microsurg. 2007;23(5):289–94.
44. Ross JJ. Septic arthritis of native joints. Infect Dis Clin North Am. 2017;31(2):203–18.
45. Dudau D, Camous J, Marchand S, Pilorge C, Rézaiguia-Delclaux S, Libert JM, et al. Incidence of nosocomial pneumonia and risk of recurrence after antimicrobial therapy in critically ill lung and heart-lung transplant patients. Clin Transplant. 2014;28(1):27–36.
46. Malinis MF, Mawhorter SD, Jain A, Shrestha NK, Avery RK, van Duin D. Staphylococcus aureus bacteremia in solid organ transplant recipients: evidence for improved survival when compared with nontransplant patients. Transplantation. 2012;93(10):1045–50.
47. Florescu DF, McCartney AM, Qiu F, Langnas AN, Botha J, Mercer DF, et al. Staphylococcus aureus infections after liver transplantation. Infection. 2012;40(3):263–9.
48. Denniston S, Riordan FA. Staphylococcus aureus bacteraemia in children and neonates: a 10 year retrospective review. J Infect. 2006;53(6):387–93.
49. Malhotra-Kumar S, Haccuria K, Michiels M, Ieven M, Poyart C, Hryniewicz W, et al. Current trends in rapid diagnostics for methicillin-resistant Staphylococcus aureus and glycopeptide-resistant enterococcus species. J Clin Microbiol. 2008;46(5):1577–87.
50. Moellering RC Jr. Current treatment options for community-acquired methicillin-resistant Staphylococcus aureus infection. Clin Infect Dis. 2008;46(7):1032–7.
51. Lowy FD. Staphylococcus aureus infections. N Engl J Med. 1998;339(8):520–32.
52. Zimmerli W, Trampuz A, Ochsner PE. Prosthetic-joint infections. N Engl J Med. 2004;351(16):1645–54.
53. Mermel LA, Farr BM, Sherertz RJ, Raad II, O'Grady N, Harris JS, et al. Guidelines for the management of intravascular catheter-related infections. Clin Infect Dis. 2001;32(9):1249–72.
54. Ruotsalainen E, Kardén-Lilja M, Kuusela P, Vuopio-Varkila J, Virolainen-Julkunen A, Sarna S, et al. Methicillin-sensitive Staphylococcus aureus bacteraemia and endocarditis among injection drug users and nonaddicts: host factors, microbiological and serological characteristics. J Infect. 2008;56(4):249–56.
55. Chang FY, Peacock JE Jr, Musher DM, Triplett P, MacDonald BB, Mylotte JM, et al. Staphylococcus aureus bacteremia: recurrence and the impact of antibiotic treatment in a prospective multicenter study. Medicine (Baltimore). 2003;82(5):333–9.
56. Safdar A, Rolston KV. Vancomycin tolerance, a potential mechanism for refractory gram-positive bacteremia observational study in patients with cancer. Cancer. 2006;106(8):1815–20.
57. Daum RS. Clinical practice. Skin and soft-tissue infections caused by methicillin-resistant Staphylococcus aureus. N Engl J Med. 2007;357(4):380–90.
58. Metzger R, Bonatti H, Sawyer R. Future trends in the treatment of serious Gram-positive infections. Drugs Today (Barc). 2009;45(1):33–45.
59. Liebenstein T, Schulz LT, Viesselmann C, Bingen E, Musuuza J, Safdar N, et al. Effectiveness and safety of tigecycline compared with other broad-spectrum antimicrobials in abdominal solid organ transplant recipients with polymicrobial intraabdominal infections. Pharmacotherapy. 2017;37(2):151–8.
60. Durante-Mangoni E, Andini R, Parrella A, Mattucci I, Cavezza G, Senese A, et al. Safety of treatment with high-dose daptomycin in 102 patients with infective endocarditis. Int J Antimicrob Agents. 2016;48(1):61–8.
61. Matono T, Nagashima M, Mezaki K, Motohashi A, Kutsuna S, Hayakawa K, et al. Molecular epidemiology of β-lactamase production in penicillin-susceptible Staphylococcus aureus under high-susceptibility conditions. J Infect Chemother. 2018; 24(2):153–5.
62. Pea F. Daptomycin in solid organ transplantation: consideration of dosage adjustments in renal impairment. Transpl Infect Dis. 2014;16(5):868–9.
63. Len O, Montejo M, Cervera C, Fariñas MC, Sabé N, Ramos A, Cordero E, et al. Daptomycin is safe and effective for the treatment of gram-positive cocci infections in solid organ transplantation. Transpl Infect Dis. 2014;16(4):532–8.
64. Torre-Cisneros J, Martín-Dávila P, Azanza JR, Pahissa A, Gavaldà J, DAPTOSOT(Daptomycin in Solid Organ Transplantation) Study Group. Daptomycin is safe and effective for the treatment of gram-positive cocci infections in solid organ transplantation. Transpl Infect Dis. 2014;16(4):532–8.
65. Wood ME, Sherrard LJ, Ramsay KA, Yerkovich ST, Reid DW, Kidd TJ, et al. Methicillin-resistant Staphylococcus aureus acquisition in healthcare workers with cystic fibrosis: a retrospective cross-sectional study. BMC Pulm Med. 2016;16(1):78.
66. Samanipour A, Dashti-Khavidaki S, Abbasi MR, Abdollahi A. Antibiotic resistance patterns of microorganisms isolated from nephrology and kidney transplant wards of a referral academic hospital. J Res Pharm Pract. 2016;5(1):43–51.
67. Tessier JM, Puzio T, Young A, Wolfe L, Han J, Duane TM. Thrombocytopenia associated with linezolid therapy in solid organ transplant recipients: a retrospective cohort study. Surg Infect (Larchmt). 2015;16(4):361–7.
68. Radunz S, Juntermanns B, Kaiser GM, Treckmann J, Mathe Z, Paul A, et al. Efficacy and safety of linezolid in liver transplant patients. Transpl Infect Dis. 2011;13(4):353–8.
69. Vernadakis S, Saner FH, Rath PM, Kaiser GM, Mathe Z, Treckmann J, et al. Successful salvage therapy with daptomycin after linezolid and vancomycin failure in a liver transplant recipient with methicillin-resistant Staphylococcus aureus endocarditis. Transpl Infect Dis. 2009;11(4):346–8.
70. Hodille E, Rose W, Diep BA, Goutelle S, Lina G, Dumitrescu O. The role of antibiotics in modulating virulence in Staphylococcus aureus. Clin Microbiol Rev. 2017;30(4):887–917.
71. Kim AI, Adal KA, Schmitt SK. Staphylococcus aureus bacteremia: using echocardiography to guide length of therapy. Cleve Clin J Med. 2003;70(6):517, 520-1, 525-6.

72. Raber-Durlacher JE, Laheij AM, Epstein JB, Epstein M, Geerligs GM, Wolffe GN, et al. Periodontal status and bacteremia with oral viridans streptococci and coagulase negative staphylococci in allogeneic hematopoietic stem cell transplantation recipients: a prospective observational study. Support Care Cancer. 2013;21(6):1621–7.
73. Zakhour R, Chaftari AM, Raad II. Catheter-related infections in patients with haematological malignancies: novel preventive and therapeutic strategies. Lancet Infect Dis. 2016;16(11):e241–50.
74. Persson L, Strid H, Tidefelt U, Söderquist B. Phenotypic and genotypic characterization of coagulase-negative staphylococci isolated in blood cultures from patients with haematological malignancies. Eur J Clin Microbiol Infect Dis. 2006;25(5):299–309.
75. Argemi X, Hansmann Y, Riegel P, Prévost G. Is Staphylococcus lugdunensis significant in clinical samples? J Clin Microbiol. 2017;55(11):3167–74.
76. Nesher L, Tarrand J, Chemaly RF, Rolston KV. Staphylococcus lugdunensis infections, filling in the gaps: a 3-year retrospective review from a comprehensive cancer center. Support Care Cancer. 2017;25(4):1063–9.
77. Kozlowska-Skrzypczak M, Bembnista E, Kubiak A, Matuszak P, Schneider A, Komarnicki M. Microbial contamination of peripheral blood and bone marrow hematopoietic cell products and environmental contamination in a stem cell bank: a single-center report. Transplant Proc. 2014;46(8):2873–6.
78. Garcia-Zamora C, Segura J, Lopez-Lopez V, Salvador C, Cascales Campos PA, Pons Miñano JA, et al. Clinical significance of contamination of the preservation solution in liver transplantation. Transplant Proc. 2015;47(8):2322–3.
79. von Eiff C, Peters G, Heilmann C. Pathogenesis of infections due to coagulase-negative staphylococci. Lancet Infect Dis. 2002;2(11):677–85.
80. Pedroso SHSP, Sandes SHC, Luiz KCM, Dias RS, Filho RAT, Serufo JC, et al. Biofilm and toxin profile: a phenotypic and genotypic characterization of coagulase-negative staphylococci isolated from human bloodstream infections. Microb Pathog. 2016;100:312–8.
81. Paniagua-Contreras GL, Monroy-Pérez E, Vaca-Paniagua F, Rodríguez-Moctezuma JR, Vaca S. Expression of enterotoxin-coding genes in methicillin-resistant Staphylococcus aureus strains isolated from Mexican haemodialysis patients. Ann Clin Microbiol Antimicrob. 2014;13:55.
82. Paterson DL, Singh N, Gayowski T, Marino IR. Rapidly fatal bacteremia due to Staphylococcus aureus producing both enterotoxins A and B in a liver transplant recipient. Clin Infect Dis. 1997;25(6):1481–2.
83. Raad I, Hanna H, Maki D. Intravascular catheter-related infections: advances in diagnosis, prevention, and management. Lancet Infect Dis. 2007;7(10):645–57.
84. Yusuf SW, Ali SS, Swafford J, Durand JB, Bodey GP, Chemaly RF, et al. Culture-positive and culture-negative endocarditis in patients with cancer: a retrospective observational study, 1994–2004. Medicine (Baltimore). 2006;85(2):86–94.
85. Cecchi E, Chirillo F, Castiglione A, Faggiano P, Cecconi M, Moreo A, et al. Clinical epidemiology in Italian Registry of Infective Endocarditis(RIEI): focus on age, intravascular devices and enterococci. Int J Cardiol. 2015;190:151–6.
86. Arnell K, Cesarini K, Lagerqvist-Widh A, Wester T, Sjölin J. Cerebrospinal fluid shunt infections in children over a 13-year period: anaerobic cultures and comparison of clinical signs of infection with Propionibacterium acnes and with other bacteria. J Neurosurg Pediatr. 2008;1(5):366–72.
87. Adams DJ, Rajnik M. Microbiology and treatment of cerebrospinal fluid shunt infections in children. Curr Infect Dis Rep. 2014;16(10):427.
88. Barrett L, Atkins B. The clinical presentation of prosthetic joint infection. J Antimicrob Chemother. 2014;69(Suppl 1):i25–7.
89. Beekmann SE, Diekema DJ, Doern GV. Determining the clinical significance of coagulase-negative staphylococci isolated from blood cultures. Infect Control Hosp Epidemiol. 2005;26(6):559–66.
90. Mermel LA, Farr BM, Sherertz RJ, Raad II, O'Grady N, et al. Guidelines for the management of intravascular catheter-related infections. Clin Infect Dis. 2001;32(9):1249–72.
91. Bouza E, Alvarado N, Alcalá L, Pérez MJ, Rincón C, Muñoz P. A randomized and prospective study of 3 procedures for the diagnosis of catheter-related bloodstream infection without catheter withdrawal. Clin Infect Dis. 2007;44(6):820–6.
92. de Oliveira A, Cataneli Pereira V, Pinheiro L, Moraes Riboli DF, Benini Martins K, Ribeiro de Souza da Cunha Mde L. Antimicrobial resistance profile of planktonic and biofilm cells of Staphylococcus aureus and coagulase-negative staphylococci. Int J Mol Sci. 2016;17(9):pii:E1423.
93. Mutnick AH, Kirby JT, Jones RN. CANCER resistance surveillance program: initial results from hematology-oncology centers in North America. Chemotherapy Alliance for Neutropenics and the Control of Emerging Resistance. Ann Pharmacother. 2003;37(1):47–56.
94. García de la Mària C, Cervera C, Pericàs JM, Castañeda X, Armero Y, Soy D, et al. Epidemiology and prognosis of coagulase-negative staphylococcal endocarditis: impact of vancomycin minimum inhibitory concentration. PLoS One. 2015;10(5):e0125818.
95. Decousser JW, Desroches M, Bourgeois-Nicolaos N, Potier J, Jehl F, Lina G, et al. Susceptibility trends including emergence of linezolid resistance among coagulase-negative staphylococci and meticillin-resistant Staphylococcus aureus from invasive infections. Int J Antimicrob Agents. 2015;46(6):622–30.
96. Chu V, Miro JM, Hoen B, Cabell CH, Pappas PA, Jones P, et al. Coagulase-negative staphylococcal prosthetic valve endocarditis: a contemporary update based on the International Collaboration on Endocarditis: prospective cohort study. Heart. 2009;95(7):570–6.
97. Karchmer AW, Archer GL, Dismukes WE. Rifampin treatment of prosthetic valve endocarditis due to Staphylococcus epidermidis. Rev Infect Dis. 1983;5(Suppl 3):S543–8.
98. Stuart JI, John MA, Milburn S, Diagre D, Wilson B, Hussain Z. Susceptibility patterns of coagulase-negative staphylococci to several newer antimicrobial agents in comparison with vancomycin and oxacillin. Int J Antimicrob Agents. 2011;37(3):248–52.
99. Ortega M, Ortega M, Rovira M, Almela M, Marco F, de la Bellacasa JP, Martínez JA, et al. Bacterial and fungal bloodstream isolates from 796 hematopoietic stem cell transplant recipients between 1991 and 2000. Ann Hematol. 2005;84(1):40–6.
100. Elting LS, Rubenstein EB, Rolston KV, Bodey GP. Outcomes of bacteremia in patients with cancer and neutropenia: observations from two decades of epidemiological and clinical trials. Clin Infect Dis. 1997;25(2):247–59.
101. Facklam R. What happened to the streptococci: overview of taxonomic and nomenclature changes. Clin Microbiol Rev. 2002;15(4):613–30.
102. Johnson CC, Tunkel AR. Viridans group streptococci, groups C and G streptococci, and Gemella morbilliform. In: Mandell GL, Bennett JE, Dolin R, editors. Principles and practice of infectious diseases. Philadelphia: Elsevier; 2005. p. 2434–50.
103. Han XY, Kamana M, Rolston KV. Viridans streptococci isolated by culture from blood of cancer patients: clinical and microbiologic analysis of 50 cases. J Clin Microbiol. 2006;44(1):160–5.
104. Husain E, Whitehead S, Castell A, Thomas EE, Speert DP. Viridans streptococci bacteremia in children with malignancy: relevance of species identification and penicillin susceptibility. Pediatr Infect Dis J. 2005;24(6):563–6.

105. Lyytikainen O, Rautio M, Carlson P, Anttila VJ, Vuento R, Sarkkinen H, et al. Nosocomial bloodstream infections due to viridans streptococci in haematological and non-haematological patients: species distribution and antimicrobial resistance. J Antimicrob Chemother. 2004;53(4):631–4.
106. Fowler VG Jr, Miro JM, Hoen B, Cabell CH, Abrutyn E, Rubinstein E, et al. Staphylococcus aureus endocarditis: a consequence of medical progress. JAMA. 2005;293(24):3012–21.
107. Nielsen MJ, Claxton S, Pizer B, Lane S, Cooke RP, Paulus S, et al. Viridans group streptococcal infections in children after chemotherapy or stem cell transplantation: a 10-year review from a Tertiary Pediatric Hospital. Medicine (Baltimore). 2016;95(9):e2952.
108. Almyroudis NG, Fuller A, Jakubowski A, Sepkowitz K, Jaffe D, Small TN, et al. Pre- and post-engraftment bloodstream infection rates and associated mortality in allogeneic hematopoietic stem cell transplant recipients. Transpl Infect Dis. 2005;7(1):11–7.
109. Richard P, Amador Del Valle G, Moreau P, Milpied N, Felice MP, Daeschler T, et al. Viridans streptococcal bacteraemia in patients with neutropenia. Lancet. 1995;345(8965):1607–9.
110. Prabhu RM, Piper KE, Litzow MR, Steckelberg JM, Patel R. Emergence of quinolone resistance among viridans group streptococci isolated from the oropharynx of neutropenic peripheral blood stem cell transplant patients receiving quinolone antimicrobial prophylaxis. Eur J Clin Microbiol Infect Dis. 2005;24(12):832–8.
111. Marron A, Carratala J, Gonzalez-Barca E, Fernandez-Sevilla A, Alcaide F, Gudiol F. Serious complications of bacteremia caused by viridans streptococci in neutropenic patients with cancer. Clin Infect Dis. 2000;31(5):1126–30.
112. Elting LS, Bodey GP, Keefe BH. Septicemia and shock syndrome due to viridans streptococci: a case-control study of predisposing factors. Clin Infect Dis. 1992;14(6):1201–7.
113. Ohuoba EF, Kansal RG, Hayden RT, Kotb M, Adderson EE. Failure of viridans group streptococci causing bacteremia in pediatric oncology patients to express superantigens. J Pediatr Hematol Oncol. 2006;28(9):627–9.
114. Paterson DL, Dominguez EA, Chang FY, Snydman DR, Singh N. Infective endocarditis in solid organ transplant recipients. Clin Infect Dis. 1998;26(3):689–94.
115. Stelzmueller I, Berger N, Wiesmayr S, Eller M, Tabarelli W, Fille M, et al. Group milleri streptococci: significant pathogens in solid organ recipients. Transpl Int. 2007;20(1):51–6.
116. Stelzmueller I, Biebl M, Berger N, Eller M, Mendez J, Fille M, et al. Relevance of group Milleri streptococci in thoracic surgery: a clinical update. Am Surg. 2007;73(5):492–7.
117. Richter SS, Beekmann SE, Croco JL, Diekema DJ, Koontz FP, Pfaller MA, et al. Minimizing the workup of blood culture contaminants: implementation and evaluation of a laboratory-based algorithm. J Clin Microbiol. 2002;40(7):2437–44.
118. Huang WT, Chang LY, Hsueh PR, Lu CY, Shao PL, Huang FY, et al. Clinical features and complications of viridans streptococci bloodstream infection in pediatric hemato-oncology patients. J Microbiol Immunol Infect. 2007;40(4):349–54.
119. Collin BA, Leather HL, Wingard JR, Ramphal R. Evolution, incidence, and susceptibility of bacterial bloodstream isolates from 519 bone marrow transplant patients. Clin Infect Dis. 2001;33(7):947–53.
120. Tunkel AR, Sepkowitz KA. Infections caused by viridans streptococci in patients with neutropenia. Clin Infect Dis. 2002;34(11):1524–9.
121. Hughes WT, Armstrong D, Bodey GP, Bow EJ, Brown AE, Calandra T, et al. 2002 guidelines for the use of antimicrobial agents in neutropenic patients with cancer. Clin Infect Dis. 2002;34(6):730–51.
122. Razonable RR, Litzow MR, Khaliq Y, Piper KE, Rouse MS, Patel R. Bacteremia due to viridans group streptococci with diminished susceptibility to levofloxacin among neutropenic patients receiving levofloxacin prophylaxis. Clin Infect Dis. 2002;34(11):1469–74.
123. Sylvetsky N, Raveh D, Schlesinger Y, Rudensky B, Yinnon AM. Bacteremia due to beta-hemolytic Streptococcus group G: increasing incidence and clinical characteristics of patients. Am J Med. 2002;112(8):622–6.
124. Nielsen HU, Kolmos HJ, Frimodt-Moller N. Beta-hemolytic streptococcal bacteremia: a review of 241 cases. Scand J Infect Dis. 2002;34(7):483–6.
125. Colford JM Jr, Mohle-Boetani J, Vosti KL. Group B streptococcal bacteremia in adults. Five years' experience and a review of the literature. Medicine (Baltimore). 1995;74(4):176–90.
126. Bisno AL, Ruoff KL. Streptococcus pyogenes. In: Mandell GL, Bennett JE, Dolin R, editors. Principles and practice of infectious diseases. Philadelphia: Elsevier; 2005. p. 2362–79.
127. Peter G, Smith AL. Group A streptococcal infections of the skin and pharynx (second of two parts). N Engl J Med. 1977;297(7):365–70.
128. Peter G, Smith AL. Group A streptococcal infections of the skin and pharynx (first of two parts). N Engl J Med. 1977;297(6):311–7.
129. Edwards MS, Rench MA, Palazzi DL, Baker CJ. Group B streptococcal colonization and serotype-specific immunity in healthy elderly persons. Clin Infect Dis. 2005;40(3):352–7.
130. McDonald MI, Towers RJ, Andrews RM, Benger N, Currie BJ, Carapetis JR. Low rates of streptococcal pharyngitis and high rates of pyoderma in Australian aboriginal communities where acute rheumatic fever is hyperendemic. Clin Infect Dis. 2006;43(6):683–9.
131. Lamagni TL, Darenberg J, Luca-Harari B, Siljander T, Efstratiou A, Henriques-Normark B, et al. Epidemiology of severe Streptococcus pyogenes disease in Europe. J Clin Microbiol. 2008;46(7):2359–67.
132. Phares CR, Lynfield R, Farley MM, Mohle-Boetani J, Harrison LH, Petit S, et al. Epidemiology of invasive group B streptococcal disease in the United States, 1999–2005. JAMA. 2008;299(17):2056–65.
133. Simon MS, Cody RL. Cellulitis after axillary lymph node dissection for carcinoma of the breast. Am J Med. 1992;93(5):543–8.
134. Awada A, van der Auwera P, Meunier F, Daneau D, Klastersky J. Streptococcal and enterococcal bacteremia in patients with cancer. Clin Infect Dis. 1992;15(1):33–48.
135. Ekelund K, Skinhoj P, Madsen J, Konradsen HB. Invasive group A, B, C and G streptococcal infections in Denmark 1999–2002: epidemiological and clinical aspects. Clin Microbiol Infect. 2005;11(7):569–76.
136. Rolston KV, Bodey GP, Safdar A. Polymicrobial infection in patients with cancer: an underappreciated and underreported entity. Clin Infect Dis. 2007;45(2):228–33.
137. Gabillot-Carre M, Roujeau JC. Acute bacterial skin infections and cellulitis. Curr Opin Infect Dis. 2007;20(2):118–23.
138. Bonnetblanc JM, Bedane C. Erysipelas: recognition and management. Am J Clin Dermatol. 2003;4(3):157–63.
139. Wong CH, Wang YS. The diagnosis of necrotizing fasciitis. Curr Opin Infect Dis. 2005;18(2):101–6.
140. Solis-Garcia del Pozo J, Martinez-Alfaro E, Abad L, Solera J. Vertebral osteomyelitis caused by Streptococcus agalactiae. J Infect. 2000;41(1):84–90.
141. Minodier P, Bidet P, Rallu F, Tapiero B, Bingen E, Ovetchkine P. Clinical and microbiologic characteristics of group A streptococcal necrotizing fasciitis in children. Pediatr Infect Dis J. 2009;28(6):541–3.
142. Bisno AL, Gerber MA, Gwaltney JM, Kaplan EL, Schwartz RH. Practice guidelines for the diagnosis and management of

group A streptococcal pharyngitis. Infectious Diseases Society of America. Clin Infect Dis. 2002;35(2):113–25.
143. Defining the group A streptococcal toxic shock syndrome. Rationale and consensus definition. The Working Group on Severe Streptococcal Infections. JAMA. 1993;269(3):390–1.
144. Shet A, Kaplan EL. Clinical use and interpretation of group A streptococcal antibody tests: a practical approach for the pediatrician c. Pediatr Infect Dis J. 2002;21(5):420–6; quiz 427–30.
145. Kaplan EL. Recent evaluation of antimicrobial resistance in beta-hemolytic streptococci. Clin Infect Dis. 1997;24(Suppl 1):89–92.
146. Sodhi M, Axtell SS, Callahan J, Shekar R. Is it safe to use carbapenems in patients with a history of allergy to penicillin? J Antimicrob Chemother. 2004;54(6):1155–7.
147. Martin JM, Green M, Barbadora KA, Wald ER. Erythromycin-resistant group A streptococci in schoolchildren in Pittsburgh. N Engl J Med. 2002;346(16):1200–6.
148. Ayer V, Tewodros W, Manoharan A, Skariah S, Luo F, Bessen DE. Tetracycline resistance in group A streptococci: emergence on a global scale and influence on multiple-drug resistance. Antimicrob Agents Chemother. 2007;51(5):1865–8.
149. Traub WH, Leonhard B. Comparative susceptibility of clinical group A, B, C, F, and G beta-hemolytic streptococcal isolates to 24 antimicrobial drugs. Chemotherapy. 1997;43(1):10–20.
150. King A, Phillips I. The in vitro activity of daptomycin against 514 Gram-positive aerobic clinical isolates. J Antimicrob Chemother. 2001;48(2):219–23.
151. Jones RN, Ross JE, Castanheira M, Mendes RE. United States resistance surveillance results for linezolid (LEADER Program for 2007). Diagn Microbiol Infect Dis. 2008;62(4):416–26.
152. Russell NE, Pachorek RE. Clindamycin in the treatment of streptococcal and staphylococcal toxic shock syndromes. Ann Pharmacother. 2000;34(7–8):936–9.
153. Garcia-Rodriguez JA, Fresnadillo Martinez MJ. Dynamics of nasopharyngeal colonization by potential respiratory pathogens. J Antimicrob Chemother. 2002;50(Suppl S2):59–73.
154. Mandell LA, Wunderink RG, Anzueto A, Bartlett JG, Campbell GD, Dean NC, et al. Infectious Diseases Society of America/American Thoracic Society consensus guidelines on the management of community-acquired pneumonia in adults. Clin Infect Dis. 2007;44(Suppl 2):S27–72.
155. Scarborough M, Gordon SB, Whitty CJ, French N, Njalale Y, Chitani A, et al. Corticosteroids for bacterial meningitis in adults in sub-Saharan Africa. N Engl J Med. 2007;357(24):2441–50.
156. Torda A, Chong Q, Lee A, Chen S, Dodds A, Greenwood M, et al. Invasive pneumococcal disease following adult allogeneic hematopoietic stem cell transplantation. Transpl Infect Dis. 2014;16(5):751–9.
157. Youssef S, Rodriguez G, Rolston KV, Champlin RE, Raad II, Safdar A. Streptococcus pneumoniae infections in 47 hematopoietic stem cell transplantation recipients: clinical characteristics of infections and vaccine-breakthrough infections, 1989–2005. Medicine (Baltimore). 2007;86(2):69–77.
158. Kyaw MH, Rose CE Jr, Fry AM, Singleton JA, Moore Z, Zell ER, et al. The influence of chronic illnesses on the incidence of invasive pneumococcal disease in adults. J Infect Dis. 2005;192(3):377–86.
159. Kulkarni S, Powles R, Treleaven J, Riley U, Singhal S, Horton C, et al. Chronic graft versus host disease is associated with long-term risk for pneumococcal infections in recipients of bone marrow transplants. Blood. 2000;95(12):3683–6.
160. Engelhard D, Cordonnier C, Shaw PJ, Parkalli T, Guenther C, Martino R, et al. Early and late invasive pneumococcal infection following stem cell transplantation: a European Bone Marrow Transplantation survey. Br J Haematol. 2002;117(2):444–50.
161. Said MA, Johnson HL, Nonyane BA, Deloria-Knoll M, O'Brien KL, AGEDD Adult Pneumococcal Burden Study Team, et al. Estimating the burden of pneumococcal pneumonia among adults: a systematic review and meta-analysis of diagnostic techniques. PLoS One. 2013;8(4):e60273.
162. Principi N, Marchisio P, Rosazza C, Sciarrabba CS, Esposito S. Acute otitis media with spontaneous tympanic membrane perforation. Eur J Clin Microbiol Infect Dis. 2017;36(1):11–8.
163. Nicolini A, Cilloniz C, Senarega R, Ferraioli G, Barlascini C. Lung abscess due to Streptococcus pneumoniae: a case series and brief review of the literature. Pneumonol Alergol Pol. 2014;82(3):276–85.
164. Reyes LF, Restrepo MI, Hinojosa CA, Soni NJ, Anzueto A, Babu BL, et al. Severe pneumococcal pneumonia causes acute cardiac toxicity and subsequent cardiac remodeling. Am J Respir Crit Care Med. 2017;196(5):609–20.
165. Ross JJ, Hu LT. Septic arthritis of the pubic symphysis: review of 100 cases. Medicine (Baltimore). 2003;82(5):340–5.
166. Siddiq DM, Musher DM, Darouiche RO. Spinal and paraspinal pneumococcal infections-a review. Eur J Clin Microbiol Infect Dis. 2014;33(4):517–27.
167. Kutas LM, Duggan JM, Kauffman CA. Pneumococcal vertebral osteomyelitis. Clin Infect Dis. 1995;20(2):286–90.
168. Suzuki H, Shichi D, Tokuda Y, Ishikawa H, Maeno T, Nakamura H. Pneumococcal vertebral osteomyelitis at three teaching hospitals in Japan, 2003–2011: analysis of 14 cases and a review of the literature. BMC Infect Dis. 2013;13:525.
169. Gudiol C, Garcia-Vidal C, Arnan M, Sánchez-Ortega I, Patiño B, Duarte R, et al. Etiology, clinical features and outcomes of pre-engraftment and post-engraftment bloodstream infection in hematopoietic SCT recipients. Bone Marrow Transplant. 2014;49(6):824–30.
170. Aguilar-Guisado M, Jiménez-Jambrina M, Espigado I, Rovira M, Martino R, Oriol A, et al. Pneumonia in allogeneic stem cell transplantation recipients: a multicenter prospective study. Clin Transplant. 2011;25(6):E629–38.
171. D'Orsogna LJ, Wright MP, Krueger RG, McKinnon EJ, Buffery SI, Witt CS, et al. Allogeneic hematopoietic stem cell transplantation recipients have defects of both switched and igm memory B cells. Biol Blood Marrow Transplant. 2009;15(7):795–803.
172. Kumar D, Humar A, Plevneshi A, Siegal D, Franke N, Green K, et al. Invasive pneumococcal disease in adult hematopoietic stem cell transplant recipients: a decade of prospective population-based surveillance. Bone Marrow Transplant. 2008;41(8):743–7.
173. Kurosawa S, Doki N, Sekiya N, Senoo Y, Ikuta S, Takaki Y, et al. Pyomyositis caused by Streptococcus pneumoniae after allogeneic hematopoietic stem cell transplantation. J Infect Chemother. 2017;23(4):250–2.
174. Kumar D, Humar A, Plevneshi A, Green K, Prasad GV, Siegal D, et al. Invasive pneumococcal disease in solid organ transplant recipients–10-year prospective population surveillance. Am J Transplant. 2007;7(5):1209–14.
175. Rostad CA, Wehrheim K, Kirklin JK, Naftel D, Pruitt E, Hoffman TM, et al. Bacterial infections after pediatric heart transplantation: Epidemiology, risk factors and outcomes. J Heart Lung Transplant. 2017;36(9):996–1003.
176. van Veen KE, Brouwer MC, van der Ende A, van de Beek D. Bacterial meningitis in solid organ transplant recipients: a population-based prospective study. Transpl Infect Dis. 2016;18(5):674–80.
177. Bahrami T, Vohra HA, Shaikhrezai K, Tadjkarimi S, Banner N, Amrani M, et al. Intrathoracic organ transplantation from donors with meningitis: a single-center 20-year experience. Ann Thorac Surg. 2008;86(5):1554–6.
178. Kim SY, Shin JA, Cho EN, Byun MK, Kim HJ, Ahn CM, et al. Late respiratory infection after lung transplantation. Tuberc Respir Dis (Seoul). 2013;74(2):63–9.

179. Pérez-Cameo C, Vargas V, Castells L, Bilbao I, Campos-Varela I, Gavaldà J, et al. Etiology and mortality of spontaneous bacterial peritonitis in liver transplant recipients: a cohort study. Liver Transpl. 2014;20(7):856–63.
180. Satoi S, Bramhall SR, Solomon M, Hastings M, Mayer AD, de Goyet JV, et al. The use of liver grafts from donors with bacterial meningitis. Transplantation. 2001;72(6):1108–13.
181. Le Monnier A, Carbonnelle E, Zahar JR, Le Bourgeois M, Abachin E, Quesne G, et al. Microbiological diagnosis of empyema in children: comparative evaluations by culture, polymerase chain reaction, and pneumococcal antigen detection in pleural fluids. Clin Infect Dis. 2006;42(8):1135–40.
182. Musher DM. Streptococcus pneumoniae. In: Mandell GL, Bennett JE, Dolin R, editors. Principles and practice of infectious diseases. Philadelphia: Elsevier; 2005. p. 2392–410.
183. Klugman KP, Madhi SA, Albrich WC. Novel approaches to the identification of Streptococcus pneumoniae as the cause of community-acquired pneumonia. Clin Infect Dis. 2008;47(Suppl 3):S202–6.
184. Centers for Disease Control and Prevention (CDC). Effects of new penicillin susceptibility breakpoints for Streptococcus pneumoniae–United States, 2006–2007. MMWR Morb Mortal Wkly Rep. 2008;57(50):1353–5.
185. Fernandez J, Hilliard JJ, Morrow BJ, Melton JL, Flamm RK, Barron AM, et al. Efficacy of a new fluoroquinolone, JNJ-Q2, in murine models of Staphylococcus aureus and Streptococcus pneumoniae skin, respiratory, and systemic infections. Antimicrob Agents Chemother. 2011;55(12):5522–8.
186. Hameed N, Tunkel AR. Treatment of drug-resistant Pneumococcal Meningitis. Curr Infect Dis Rep. 2010;12(4):274–81.
187. Sahm DF, Brown NP, Draghi DC, Evangelista AT, Yee YC, Thornsberry C. Tracking resistance among bacterial respiratory tract pathogens: summary of findings of the TRUST Surveillance Initiative, 2001–2005. Postgrad Med. 2008;120(3 Suppl 1):8–15.
188. San Pedro GS, Cammarata SK, Oliphant TH, Todisco T, Linezolid Community-Acquired Pneumonia Study Group. Linezolid versus ceftriaxone/cefpodoxime in patients hospitalized for the treatment of Streptococcus pneumoniae pneumonia. Scand J Infect Dis. 2002;34(10):720–8.
189. Moschovi M, Trimis G, Tsotra M, Chatzi F, Karamolegou K, Santou A, et al. Efficacy and safety of linezolid in immunocompromised children with cancer. Pediatr Int. 2010;52(5):694–8.
190. Breslow-Deckman JM, Mattingly CM, Birket SE, Hoskins SN, Ho TN, Garvy BA, et al. Linezolid decreases susceptibility to secondary bacterial pneumonia postinfluenza infection in mice through its effects on IFN-γ. J Immunol. 2013;191(4):1792–9.
191. Baltz RH. Daptomycin: mechanisms of action and resistance, and biosynthetic engineering. Curr Opin Chem Biol. 2009;13(2):144–51.
192. Webb BJ, Healy R, Majers J, Burr Z, Gazdik M, Lopansri B, et al. Prediction of bloodstream infection due to vancomycin-resistant Enterococcus in patients undergoing leukemia induction or hematopoietic stem-cell transplantation. Clin Infect Dis. 2017;64(12):1753–9.
193. Ghanem G, Hachem R, Jiang Y, Chemaly RF, Raad I. Outcomes for and risk factors associated with vancomycin-resistant Enterococcus faecalis and vancomycin-resistant Enterococcus faecium bacteremia in cancer patients. Infect Control Hosp Epidemiol. 2007;28(9):1054–9.
194. Ford CD, Gazdik Stofer MA, Coombs J, Lopansri BK, Webb BJ, Motyckova G, et al. Decrease in vancomycin-resistant Enterococcus colonization after extensive renovation of a unit dedicated to the treatment of hematologic malignancies and hematopoietic stem-cell transplantation. Infect Control Hosp Epidemiol. 2017;38(9):1055–61.
195. Almyroudis NG, Osawa R, Samonis G, Wetzler M, Wang ES, McCarthy PL, et al. Discontinuation of systematic surveillance and contact precautions for Vancomycin-Resistant Enterococcus (VRE) and its impact on the incidence of VRE faecium bacteremia in patients with hematologic malignancies. Infect Control Hosp Epidemiol. 2016;37(4):398–403.
196. Ford CD, Lopansri BK, Gazdik MA, Webb B, Snow GL, Hoda D, et al. Room contamination, patient colonization pressure, and the risk of vancomycin-resistant Enterococcus colonization on a unit dedicated to the treatment of hematologic malignancies and hematopoietic stem cell transplantation. Am J Infect Control. 2016;44(10):1110–5.
197. Ford CD, Gazdik MA, Lopansri BK, Webb B, Mitchell B, Coombs J, et al. Vancomycin-resistant Enterococcus colonization and bacteremia and hematopoietic stem cell transplantation outcomes. Biol Blood Marrow Transplant. 2017;23(2):340–6.
198. Hefazi M, Damlaj M, Alkhateeb HB, Partain DK, Patel R, Razonable RR, et al. Vancomycin-resistant Enterococcus colonization and bloodstream infection: prevalence, risk factors, and the impact on early outcomes after allogeneic hematopoietic cell transplantation in patients with acute myeloid leukemia. Transpl Infect Dis. 2016;18(6):913–20.
199. Tavadze M, Rybicki L, Mossad S, Avery R, Yurch M, Pohlman B, et al. Risk factors for vancomycin-resistant enterococcus bacteremia and its influence on survival after allogeneic hematopoietic cell transplantation. Bone Marrow Transplant. 2014;49(10):1310–6.
200. Kamboj M, Chung D, Seo SK, Pamer EG, Sepkowitz KA, Jakubowski AA, et al. The changing epidemiology of vancomycin-resistant Enterococcus (VRE) bacteremia in allogeneic hematopoietic stem cell transplant (HSCT) recipients. Biol Blood Marrow Transplant. 2010;16(11):1576–81.
201. Ford CD, Lopansri BK, Gazdik MA, Snow GL, Webb BJ, Konopa KL, Petersen FB. The clinical impact of vancomycin-resistant Enterococcus colonization and bloodstream infection in patients undergoing autologous transplantation. Transpl Infect Dis. 2015;17(5):688–94.
202. Staffas A, Burgos da Silva M, van den Brink MR. The intestinal microbiota in allogeneic hematopoietic cell transplant and graft-versus-host disease. Blood. 2017;129(8):927–33.
203. Mendes ET, Ranzani OT, Marchi AP, Silva MT, Filho JU, Alves T, et al. Chlorhexidine bathing for the prevention of colonization and infection with multidrug-resistant microorganisms in a hematopoietic stem cell transplantation unit over a 9-year period: Impact on chlorhexidine susceptibility. Medicine (Baltimore). 2016;95(46):e5271.
204. Trifilio SM, Pi J, Mehta J. Changing epidemiology of Clostridium difficile-associated disease during stem cell transplantation. Biol Blood Marrow Transplant. 2013;19(3):405–9.
205. Ubeda C, Taur Y, Jenq RR, Equinda MJ, Son T, Samstein M, et al. Vancomycin-resistant Enterococcus domination of intestinal microbiota is enabled by antibiotic treatment in mice and precedes bloodstream invasion in humans. J Clin Invest. 2010;120(12):4332–41.
206. Patel R, Badley AD, Larson-Keller J, Harmsen WS, Ilstrup DM, Wiesner RH, et al. Relevance and risk factors of enterococcal bacteremia following liver transplantation. Transplantation. 1996;61(8):1192–7.
207. Patel R, Allen SL, Manahan JM, Wright AJ, Krom RA, Wiesner RH, et al. Natural history of vancomycin-resistant enterococcal colonization in liver and kidney transplant recipients. Liver Transpl. 2001;7(1):27–31.
208. Singh N, Gayowski T, Rihs JD, Wagener MM, Marino IR. Evolving trends in multiple-antibiotic-resistant bacteria in liver transplant recipients: a longitudinal study of antimicrobial susceptibility patterns. Liver Transpl. 2001;7(1):22–6.

209. Papanicolaou GA, Meyers BR, Meyers J, Mendelson MH, Lou W, Emre S, et al. Nosocomial infections with vancomycin-resistant Enterococcus faecium in liver transplant recipients: risk factors for acquisition and mortality. Clin Infect Dis. 1996;23(4):760–6.
210. McNeil SA, Malani PN, Chenoweth CE, Fontana RJ, Magee JC, Punch JD, et al. Vancomycin-resistant enterococcal colonization and infection in liver transplant candidates and recipients: a prospective surveillance study. Clin Infect Dis. 2006;42(2):195–203.
211. Linares L, Cervera C, Cofán F, Ricart MJ, Esforzado N, Torregrosa V, et al. Epidemiology and outcomes of multiple antibiotic-resistant bacterial infection in renal transplantation. Transplant Proc. 2007;39(7):2222–4.
212. Simon D, Fischer S, Grossman A, Downer C, Hota B, Heroux A, et al. Left ventricular assist device-related infection: treatment and outcome. Clin Infect Dis. 2005;40(8):1108–15.
213. Murray BE. Vancomycin-resistant enterococcal infections. N Engl J Med. 2000;342(10):710–21.
214. Maki DG, Agger WA. Enterococcal bacteremia: clinical features, the risk of endocarditis, and management. Medicine (Baltimore). 1988;67(4):248–69.
215. Fry DE. Third generation cephalosporin antibiotics in surgical practice. Am J Surg. 1986;151(2):306–13.
216. Weinstein MP. Comparative evaluation of penicillin, ampicillin, and imipenem MICs and susceptibility breakpoints for vancomycin-susceptible and vancomycin-resistant Enterococcus faecalis and Enterococcus faecium. J Clin Microbiol. 2001;39(7):2729–31.
217. Deshpande LM, Fritsche TR, Moet GJ, Biedenbach DJ, Jones RN. Antimicrobial resistance and molecular epidemiology of vancomycin-resistant enterococci from North America and Europe: a report from the SENTRY antimicrobial surveillance program. Diagn Microbiol Infect Dis. 2007;58(2):163–70.
218. Kristich CJ, Rice LB, Arias CA. Enterococcal infection—treatment and antibiotic resistance. In: Gilmore MS, Clewell DB, Ike Y, Shankar N, editors. Enterococci: from commensals to leading causes of drug resistant infection [Internet]. Boston: Massachusetts Eye and Ear Infirmary; 2014. Available from http://www.ncbi.nlm.nih.gov/books/NBK190420/PubMed.
219. Frasca KL, Schuster MG. Vancomycin-resistant enterococcal meningitis in an autologous stem cell transplant recipient cured with linezolid. Transpl Infect Dis. 2013;15(1):E1–4.
220. Krull M, Klare I, Ross B, Trenschel R, Beelen DW, Todt D, et al. Emergence of linezolid- and vancomycin-resistant Enterococcus faecium in a department for hematologic stem cell transplantation. Antimicrob Resist Infect Control. 2016;5:31.
221. Santayana EM, Grim SA, Janda WM, Layden JE, Lee TA, Clark NM. Risk factors and outcomes associated with vancomycin-resistant Enterococcus infections with reduced susceptibilities to linezolid. Diagn Microbiol Infect Dis. 2012;74(1):39–42.
222. Wudhikarn K, Gingrich RD, de Magalhaes Silverman M. Daptomycin nonsusceptible enterococci in hematologic malignancy and hematopoietic stem cell transplant patients: an emerging threat. Ann Hematol. 2013;92(1):129–31.
223. Grim SA, Hong I, Freeman J, Edwards C, Clark NM. Daptomycin for the treatment of vancomycin-resistant enterococcal infections. J Antimicrob Chemother. 2009;63(2):414–6.
224. Chong PP, van Duin D, Bangdiwala A, Ivanova A, Miller WC, Weber DJ, et al. Vancomycin-resistant Enterococcal bloodstream infections in hematopoietic stem cell transplant recipients and patients with hematologic malignancies: impact of daptomycin MICs of 3 to 4 mg/L. Clin Ther. 2016;38(11):2468–76.

Enterobacteriaceae in Transplantation

25

Kathryn Whitaker, Valerie Cluzet, and Emily A. Blumberg

Introduction

Enterobacteriaceae, Gram-negative, facultative anaerobes that ferment sugars, are common causes of infection and colonization in solid organ transplant (SOT) recipients and have become increasingly important pathogens in hematopoietic stem cell recipients (HSCT). The group comprises diverse organisms including *Escherichia coli*, *Klebsiella* spp., *Enterobacter* spp., *Serratia* spp., *Citrobacter* spp., *Proteus* spp., *Salmonella* spp., *Shigella* spp., and *Yersinia* spp., among others (Table 25.1). Of particular concern is the rise of multidrug-resistant organisms within the *Enterobacteriaceae* family, resulting in difficult-to-treat infections in an already immunosuppressed population of patients. Additionally, due to their immunosuppressed state, solid organ transplant recipients and hematopoietic stem cell recipients can have true infections with typically nonpathogenic bacteria in the *Enterobacteriaceae* family. This chapter will review the epidemiology and risk factors for these infections as well as specific syndromes commonly found in transplant recipients.

Table 25.1 Organisms in the *Enterobacteriaceae* family

Organism
Escherichia coli
Klebsiella spp.
Enterobacter spp.
Serratia marcescens
Citrobacter spp.
Morganella morganii
Proteus spp.
Providencia spp.
Edwardsiella spp.
Salmonella spp.
Shigella spp.
Yersinia spp.

Epidemiology and Risk Factors

Solid organ transplant recipients are at particular risk for infection with *Enterobacteriaceae* and other bacteria, given end-organ failure, surgical intervention, and immunosuppression. In fact, solid organ transplantation is an independent risk factor for acquiring infection with *Klebsiella pneumoniae* [1]. These infections are most commonly seen in the first 30 days following transplantation but can also occur later in the post-transplant period. They can be donor derived, nosocomial, or community acquired. The development of antimicrobial resistance in *Enterobacteriaceae* is a growing problem worldwide [2, 3]. This increase has been noted in the transplant population as well. Moreover, it appears that SOT recipients may be at greater risk than the general population for the development of infections with resistant organisms.

Infections with *Enterobacteriaceae* can occur at multiple sites, including the urinary tract, bloodstream, respiratory tract, intra-abdominal region, and wounds. The most common sites of infection differ depending on the type of transplant. Kidney and kidney-pancreas transplant recipients are at highest risk for urinary tract infections (UTIs) [4–8]. The most common infection after lung or heart transplant is pneumonia [9–11]. Intra-abdominal and wound infections are the predominant bacterial infections seen in liver and small bowel transplant recipients [12, 13]. Liver and kidney transplant recipients are also at high risk of developing bloodstream infections [7, 12–14].

K. Whitaker · E. A. Blumberg (✉)
Division of Infectious Diseases, Hospital of the University of Pennsylvania, Perelman School of Medicine at the University of Pennsylvania, Philadelphia, PA, USA
e-mail: kathryn.whitaker@uphs.upenn.edu; blumbere@pennmedicine.upenn.edu

V. Cluzet
Health Quest Medical Practice, Department of Infectious Diseases, Poughkeepsie, NY, USA
e-mail: vcluzet@health-quest.org

A. Safdar (ed.), *Principles and Practice of Transplant Infectious Diseases*, https://doi.org/10.1007/978-1-4939-9034-4_25

Hematopoietic stem cell transplant recipients (HSCT) are also at increased risk for infections with *Enterobacteriaceae*, with different patterns of infection related to the timing of the infection [15]. Early infections during the pre-engraftment phase are secondary to loss of host defenses, including neutropenia and mucosal surface breakdown, thus increasing the risk of Gram-negative rod (GNR) bacteremia. Prior to the 1980s and 1990s, GNRs were the most common organisms associated with BSI in patients undergoing HSCT; however, with antibacterial prophylaxis and the increased use of central venous catheters, Gram-negative infections including those due to *Enterobacteriaceae* have become less frequent. This decline has been counteracted by the increase in antimicrobial resistance. Early post-engraftment bacterial infections with GNR are most commonly related to enteric GVHD allowing for translocation, as well as the immunosuppression associated with the treatment of GVHD.

Enterobacteriaceae can cause a variety of infections in the HSCT population. Bloodstream infections are the most commonly documented bacterial infection in the adult HSCT population, and pneumonia is the second most frequent, followed by gastrointestinal infections [16, 17]. *Enterobacteriaceae* contribute between 25% and 30% of BSIs in this population [17]. In a study of pediatric HSCT patients, *Enterobacteriaceae* were the most common cause of bacterial infections in matched related and unrelated donors, most frequently in association with enteritis and UTI [18].

Urinary Tract Infections

The urinary tract is the most common site of infection in kidney and kidney-pancreas transplant patients with a reported frequency of 4–86% but is also a source of infection in other SOT recipients [4–8, 19]. The highest risk is in the 30 days following the transplantation procedure, likely related to urinary tract instrumentation, with the exception of kidney transplant recipients whose major at-risk period extends at least to the first 6 months following transplant [7]. Patients with kidney and liver transplants are more likely to develop upper tract infections than other SOT recipients [7]. Additionally, kidney transplant recipients are also more likely to develop bacteremia related to UTI [6]. Risk factors for the development of UTI include female gender, age, diabetes, length of hospitalization, and presence of urinary catheters; additional factors specific to kidney transplant patients include deceased donor organ and posttransplant dialysis [7, 8, 19]. Studies have not shown increased mortality due to bacterial UTI [7].

Similar to normal hosts, *Enterobacteriaceae* are the most common organisms causing UTIs in transplant recipients. *Escherichia coli* is the most commonly identified organism, followed by *Klebsiella* species; *Enterobacter* species are also commonly seen [7, 19]. Resistance to trimethoprim-sulfamethoxazole is seen in most of these organisms, probably related to the use of this agent for *Pneumocystis jirovecii* infection prophylaxis [20]. Fluoroquinolone resistance is seen in over one-third of infections, and greater than one-quarter are extended-spectrum beta-lactamase (ESBL)-producing organisms [21–23]. Recent reports also noted the increasing presence of carbapenemase-producing *Enterobacteriaceae* UTIs [24, 25].

Special Consideration: Kidney Transplant

Although bacterial UTI is not associated with increased mortality [14], it is potentially important in kidney transplant patients as infections may lead to graft dysfunction and potentially rejection [26, 27]. Studies evaluating this association have noted contradictory results. A few studies found that episodes of pyelonephritis are associated with an increased risk of graft failure or death at 5 years [28, 29]. Additionally, investigators using data from the United States Renal Data System (USRDS) demonstrated that late infections (occurring after 6 months following transplantation) are associated with similarly poor outcomes [30]. However, other investigators found no association between graft pyelonephritis and graft dysfunction [31, 32]. Because measures of renal function vary with methodology, some of the differences may be explained by the assessment measures [33]; preexisting medical comorbidities likely play a role as well. Risk factors for UTI following kidney transplant include factors unrelated to transplant such as female sex and diabetes mellitus and those related to immunosuppression, especially the use of antimetabolites and cell-depleting agents, and instrumentation including prolonged use of urinary stents and other foreign devices [19].

Intra-abdominal Infections

Intra-abdominal infections are usually related to technical problems with surgery, resulting in lacerations, perforations, or anastomotic leaks. These are most commonly seen after liver, pancreas, and small bowel transplants. *Enterobacteriaceae* are a major component of gut flora and, therefore, are predominant pathogens in these infections.

Special Consideration: Liver Transplant

Intra-abdominal infections due to *Enterobacteriaceae* are especially common following liver transplant, with incidence rates ranging from 53% to 79%, with most occurring in the first 2 months after transplantation [12, 13, 34]. Infections with *Enterobacteriaceae* can involve the liver, biliary tract, or peritoneal cavity. Most of these infections are related to surgical complications or biliary tract complications [35]. Patients who develop graft ischemia secondary to hepatic artery thrombosis and those experiencing biliary tract complications are at increased risk of developing hepatic abscesses, which are most frequently caused by *Enterobacteriaceae* [36]. Risk factors for intra-abdominal infections after liver transplantation include prolonged surgical time, high intraoperative transfusion requirement, reoperation or re-transplantation, prolonged hospitalization, acute rejection, CMV infection, and elevated preoperative creatinine and bilirubin levels [12, 34, 35].

The choice of biliary anastomosis can also predispose the liver transplant patient to intra-abdominal infections. Choledochocholedochostomy is the preferred method of anastomosis, as compared to the Roux-en-Y choledochojejunostomy, which is used in patients who have anatomic abnormalities of the extrahepatic biliary system such as primary sclerosing cholangitis, patients undergoing re-transplantation, and those with a history of prior bile duct surgeries [37–40]. The choledochocholedochostomy preserves the sphincter of Oddi, whereas the Roux-en-Y anatomy facilitates reflux of enteric organisms into the biliary system, thereby increasing the risk of infections with these organisms. In live donor liver transplantation, lower graft-to-recipient weight ratio has also been noted to be a risk factor for surgical site infection in liver transplantation [41].

Respiratory Tract Infections

Lower respiratory tract infections (LRTI) are the leading cause of morbidity and mortality after transplant and the most common infection following lung and heart transplants [42–45]. They also occur frequently following liver transplant, perhaps related to the presence of right-sided pleural effusions and atelectasis, and are frequently seen in stem cell recipients with graft versus host disease [34, 46–48]. As many as 55–75% of the LRTIs identified in SOT recipients are hospital acquired or health-care associated, usually related to aspiration [44, 47, 49]. Bacterial pneumonia occurs most commonly in the first 3 months after transplantation [47], with GNRs among the more common organisms identified. One study found that infections with *Enterobacteriaceae* such as *E. coli*, *Klebsiella* spp., *Enterobacter* spp., and *Serratia* spp. were equally common as those with non-fermentative organisms, such as *Pseudomonas aeruginosa* [47]. Transplant recipients are at higher risk of acquiring infections with resistant organisms [49]. Mortality from bacterial LRTI is high, especially when the infection occurs in the immediate posttransplant period and in patients with nosocomial infection and recurrent pneumonia, those requiring prolonged mechanical ventilation, and those admitted with sepsis related to pneumonia [42, 46, 48, 50–52]. *Enterobacteriaceae* are common causes of nosocomial pneumonia and contribute significantly to this mortality risk.

Special Consideration: Lung Transplant

Historically, the incidence of pneumonia following lung transplantation ranged from 22% to 39% [44, 52, 53]. A more recent prospective multicenter cohort demonstrated 72 episodes per 100 lung transplant years; 82.7% were due to bacteria and the median onset of bacterial pneumonia occurred at 31 days after transplantation [54]. Studies specifying the microbiologic causes of pneumonia in lung transplant recipients identify *Enterobacteriaceae* as common etiologic agents [54, 55]. Deusch et al. reported that *Klebsiella pneumoniae* was the most commonly identified pathogen, with *Escherichia coli* and *Enterobacter cloacae* also making up a significant proportion of very early post-lung transplant LRTIs [53]. In a lung transplant subset of the RESITRA cohort, a large Spanish registry focused on transplant-related infections, and *Enterobacteriaceae* were also commonly seen as causes of pneumonia, although they were less frequently noted than the non-fermentative GNRs [54].

Wound/Surgical Site Infections

In SOT recipients, wound infections after transplant occur with the same frequency as with other surgeries, with incidences of 5–51% [56–67]. Gram-negative wound infections, including members of the *Enterobacteriaceae* family, are more commonly seen in wound infections after transplants involving organs below the diaphragm, specifically small bowel [59, 60], kidney, pancreas or simultaneous kidney-pancreas [5, 61, 63, 64], and liver [13, 34, 35, 66] transplants. Recently, surgical site infections are increasingly due to multidrug-resistant organisms, including ESBL- and *K. pneumoniae* carbapenemase (KPC)-producing organisms [35]. Of additional concern are reports of necrotizing skin infections due to *Klebsiella* spp. in liver transplant patients [67]. Risk factors for surgical site infections in transplant recipients mirror those seen in non-transplant patients and include increased BMI, reoperation, diabetes mellitus, and increased operative time [62, 65, 68–73]. Transplant-specific factors include prior transplantation, surgical approach such as choledocho- or hepaticojejunostomy, choice of immunosuppression, especially the use of mTOR inhibitors, graft rejection, prolonged ischemic time, increased packed red blood cell transfusion requirement, dialysis, and delayed graft function [64, 65, 68–74].

Bloodstream Infections

Bloodstream infections in SOT recipients are common. Mortality is higher with Gram-negative infections compared with Gram-positive BSI [75–79]. Over 75% of these infections are nosocomial. *Enterobacteriaceae* are among the most common etiologic agents. Al-Hasan and colleagues conducted a retrospective study of GNR BSI in 3367 diverse SOT recipients (kidney, liver, kidney-pancreas, pancreas, heart, and lung transplant recipients) followed for 12 years and found a declining incidence; nevertheless, GNR BSI occurred at a 20-fold higher rate than that in the general population [78]. The highest incidence is in the early posttransplant period during the first 30 days, with a sharp decline thereafter. Importantly, however, the incidence of GNR BSI 12 months after transplant is still notably higher than the general population, especially in kidney transplant recipients. In contrast to earlier studies [76, 77, 79], Al-Hasan et al. found a lower 28-day mortality in their cohort of patients (4.9% vs. 25–59%), which may be related to advances in medical care [78]. However, SOT recipients who developed GNR BSI in the first year after the transplantation procedure continue to have higher 1-year mortality than those who do not [78].

Similar to the general population, the most common GNR organism seen in BSI in SOT patients is *Escherichia coli*, followed by *Klebsiella pneumoniae*; other important *Enterobacteriaceae* seen commonly in BSI are *Enterobacter cloacae* and *Citrobacter freundii*. *Escherichia coli*, along with *Pseudomonas aeruginosa*, account for most of the infections in the early posttransplant period, while *Escherichia coli* and *Klebsiella pneumoniae* are seen more commonly 12 months or later after transplantation [78]. The rates of resistance to antimicrobials, including ampicillin for *Escherichia coli*, fluoroquinolones, and trimethoprim-sulfamethoxazole, and ESBL-producing strains are increasing in GNR BSI; this is an important consideration for empiric selection of antimicrobial therapy [78, 80].

The urinary tract is the most common source of GNR BSI, followed by the gastrointestinal (GI) tract, respiratory tract, intravenous catheters, and skin and soft tissue [78]. Females are more likely than males to have a urinary source of GNR BSI [78]. A urinary source is more common in kidney transplant patients, whereas liver transplant patients are more likely to have a GI source and lung transplant recipients a respiratory tract source [76, 78].

Bacteremia is also common in HSCT recipients, with an incidence between 21% and 43% and an attributable mortality of 3.3–22.6%; overall mortality is substantially higher in HSCT recipients than in the general population [81–83]. Most BSIs are noted during the pre-engraftment period represented by severe neutropenia, compared to the post-engraftment period [81, 83]. However, the occurrence of grade 2 or greater GVHD in the post-engraftment period has been associated with an increased risk of bacteremia, as well [81, 82]. Additional risk factors for bloodstream infection include reduced intensity allogeneic stem cell transplantation [83, 84]. Bloodstream infections have been reported frequently in both allogeneic and autologous stem cell recipients. The timing of infection may vary however, and in at least one study, later infections such as those occurring at least 180 days after transplant were more common in allogeneic stem cell graft recipients [85].

Depending on the study, *Enterobacteriaceae* make up a majority of the GNRs isolated in HSCT recipients, with a median incidence of 30%. Within the *Enterobacteriaceae* group, *E. coli* is the most common isolated organism, approximately 25%, although with great variability in studies [16, 81, 82]. As described with other sites and solid organ transplant recipients, antimicrobial resistance has been increasingly described and may reflect the near-universal use of fluoroquinolone prophylaxis during periods of neutropenia [16, 82, 85].

Multidrug-Resistant *Enterobacteriaceae*

Multidrug-resistant *Enterobacteriaceae* (MDRE) are a growing problem worldwide. Solid organ and hematopoietic stem cell transplantation are independent risk factors for acquiring infection with MDRE [86–89]. Other risk factors include antibiotic exposure, surgery, hospitalization, mechanical ventilation, renal replacement therapy, and the presence of indwelling devices, all of which are common in SOT recipients [89, 90]. MDRE, specifically those that have plasmid-encoded genes that produce extended-spectrum beta-lactamases, AmpC beta-lactamases, and carbapenemases, are a particularly important problem given their rapidly rising rates and limited treatment options. Extended-spectrum beta-lactamase- and AmpC beta-lactamase-producing organisms confer resistance to penicillins and cephalosporins and are often only susceptible to carbapenems. Carbapenemase-producing organisms produce an even larger problem, as they are more globally resistant with even fewer treatment options. Not unexpectedly, infection with drug-resistant

Enterobacteriaceae is associated with increased cost of care, treatment failure, and risk for death [90–93].

Solid organ transplantation is an independent risk factor specifically for infection with ESBL-producing *Enterobacteriaceae* and carbapenem-resistant *Klebsiella pneumoniae* [87, 90]. Infections with ESBL-producing strains of *Enterobacteriaceae* are extremely common in SOT recipients, with rates of up to 53% identified in some studies [4, 66, 89]. Outbreaks within institutions, particularly on transplant wards and in intensive care units, are often reported [94–99], the majority of which involve liver and kidney transplant recipients. Patel and Bergamasco found that 35–41% of the cases in carbapenem-resistant *Klebsiella pneumoniae* outbreaks occurred in SOT patients and all transplant patients who were colonized with KPC later developed infection [90, 94]. Even more worrisome is a report of pelvic abscess in a renal transplant recipient which grew New Delhi metallo-b-lactamase-1-producing *Klebsiella oxytoca* [100]. Infection with carbapenemase-producing organisms confers a high mortality rate in the transplant population as well as the general population, and 30-day and 1-year mortality rates in posttransplant cohorts have been reported between 30% and 79% [90, 94, 101–104].

Similar to that seen in SOT recipients, there has been a rise in resistant GNR infections in HSCT recipients [81, 82], from 3% to 11% in one study [105]. Mechanisms of resistance vary; there have been report of ESBL producers and Amp C beta lactamases in addition to diverse mechanisms of carbapenem resistance and fluoroquinolone resistance. ESBL-producing *Enterobacteriaceae* are frequent, with prevalence ranging from 13% to 48% [16]. Some studies have shown that MDR Gram-negative bacterial bloodstream infections are more common in allogeneic HSCT compared to those who underwent autologous stem cell transplantation. This is likely due to underlying malignancies that require allogeneic HSCT compared to autologous HSCT. Patients undergoing allogeneic stem cell transplants frequently have more prolonged periods of neutropenia and have had more courses of treatment with broad-spectrum antibiotics [85]. In one study comparing allogeneic HSCT to autologous HSCT, GN bacterial infections caused by MDR pathogens represented 78% of infections in allogeneic graft recipients compared to 20% in autologous HSCT. Of those in the allogeneic HSCT group, 72.5% were ESBL-positive, and 5.5% were AmpC-positive [106]. Another potential risk factor for resistance may be the use of prophylactic antimicrobials, and the use of fluoroquinolones, per guidelines, in high-risk neutropenic populations has been associated with increased resistance to fluoroquinolones [82, 107]. In one study, in an institution using fluoroquinolone prophylaxis for neutropenic patients, all isolated GNR bacteria were resistant to fluoroquinolones, and 92.8% were multidrug-resistant organisms [82]. The rate of fluoroquinolone resistance in *E. coli* has increased, irrespective of the use of fluoroquinolones for prophylaxis [16]. As with SOT recipients, infection with resistant *Enterobacteriaceae* has been associated with increased mortality; in some cases, mortality in HSCT has exceeded that seen in SOT [108]. Of special concern has been pneumonia due to carbapenemase-producing *Klebsiella pneumonia* in HSCT recipients, which has a reported attributable mortality rate between 38% and 67% [16].

Mechanisms of Resistance

Mechanisms of resistance are diverse and can be encoded on plasmids or chromosomes. Resistance may be intrinsic or inducible. All types of resistance have been encountered in transplant recipients [80, 93–100, 109]. Almost all species of *Enterobacteriaceae* can produce ESBL. They are plasmid-encoded genes and are therefore easily transmissible among organisms. The types of ESBL include TEM, SHV, and CTX-M, which is currently the most commonly seen [110]. Plasmid-encoded AmpC beta-lactamases have been identified in *Escherichia coli*, *Klebsiella pneumoniae*, and *Proteus mirabilis*. Certain *Enterobacteriaceae*, including *Enterobacter*, *Citrobacter*, and *Serratia* species, have chromosomally encoded AmpC beta-lactamases, which confer resistance to third-generation cephalosporins and may be inducible, an important consideration when choosing antimicrobials. Several distinct carbapenemases have been described, including chromosomal- and plasmid-encoded types. The most common carbapenemases seen in the United States are various types of KPC. Worldwide, other types are geographically distributed, such as metallo-beta-lactamases including VIM in Southern Europe and Asia and NDM-1 in the United Kingdom, India, and Pakistan and oxacillinase-48-type carbapenemases in Mediterranean countries, Europe, and India [111]. However, these types are not geographically isolated and global spread is increasing. Fluoroquinolone resistance generally results from chromosomal mutations leading to target enzyme modifications or efflux pumps. However, there is also a plasmid-encoded qnr gene that is associated with fluoroquinolone resistance in *Escherichia coli* and *Klebsiella pneumoniae*. Table 25.2 outlines diagnostic and treatment considerations for MDRE.

Donor-Derived Infections

Donor-derived *Enterobacteriaceae* infections have been reported most frequently involving abdominal organs and donors with abdominal trauma [112, 113]. With the rising rates of colonization and infection with multidrug-resistant *Enterobacteriaceae* in hospitalized patients as well as increasing rates of community-acquired MDRE,

Table 25.2 Multidrug-resistant *Enterobacteriaceae*

Organism	Diagnosis	Treatment
Extended-spectrum beta-lactamase producers	Double-disk diffusion assay Microbroth dilution Refer to new CLSI breakpoints	Carbapenems
Carbapenemase producers	Disk diffusion assay: screen using ertapenem or meropenem Microbroth dilution: screen using imipenem, meropenem, or ertapenem Automated susceptibility testing: screen using ertapenem	Ceftazidime avibactam Colistin or polymyxin B (IV)[a] Aminoglycoside[a] Tigecycline[b] Fosfomycin (only available in oral formulation in the United States, for uncomplicated UTI)

[a]May be given in combination with either carbapenem or tigecycline
[b]Second-line therapy. Avoid for urinary tract infections and bloodstream infections

donor-derived infections with MDRE are also being more frequently reported.

Donor-derived infection with MDRE is particularly concerning because of the high mortality rate associated with these infections as well as the risks related to treatment. There have been several case reports detailing donor-derived infections with MDRE [114–117]. These include transmission of MDR *E. coli* to two kidney transplant recipients from one donor, with resultant graft loss due to infection in one recipient [114]. There have also been case reports of donor-derived carbapenem-resistant *K. pneumoniae* infections [115–117]. Transmission of resistant pathogens has been variable and may not be related to the presence of infection versus colonization in the donor [115]. In one report, the recipient of one of the lungs became infected and died, whereas the two kidney recipients, the liver recipient and the other lung recipient, did not develop infection [118]. In a second case report, the recipient of simultaneous kidney-liver transplant developed infection with KPC, whereas the other kidney, heart, and vein graft recipients did not develop signs of infection [119]. Cases in which single recipients are involved primarily involve donors in whom the infection is localized to a single organ without evidence of bloodstream infection at the time of procurement [119].

It is unclear whether organs from donors infected with MDRE should be used; currently, there is no standard approach to the use of these organs. In some cases, prompt initiation of effective antimicrobials may improve outcomes, although the impact of antimicrobial prophylaxis may be variable, even among recipients of the same donor [115]. Because of variable outcomes in recipients of these organs, recipients of organs from donors known to have Gram-negative bacterial infections, especially those with resistant *Enterobacteriaceae*, should be warned about the potential risk of transmission [120]. Additionally, it is important to tailor antimicrobial prophylaxis to include the resistant pathogen to minimize the risk of poor recipient outcome.

Notably, delays in communication between the reference laboratories that receive bacterial cultures at the time of organ procurement and the clinicians caring for the recipient have resulted in delayed initiation of appropriate therapy and increased risk of transmission [121]. This delay in communication of culture information is highlighted in the report of transmission of MDR *E. coli* described above. The Organ Procurement and Transplantation Network mandates reporting of potential donor-transmissible infections when initially suspected, in part to mitigate risks of donor-derived infection to other recipients of organs from the same donor [122].

Infection Diagnosis

Diagnosis of infection with *Enterobacteriaceae* first involves assessment of the source of the culture and the method of collection. Cultures from sterile sites indicate true infection, whereas cultures from wounds, the respiratory tract, or intravenous lines need to be interpreted in the context of the clinical scenario in order to distinguish infection from colonization. In patients who are mechanically ventilated, distal sputum samples obtained through bronchoscopy and bronchoalveolar lavage are more specific than standard tracheal aspirates and have been shown to have high diagnostic yield in solid organ and stem cell transplant patients [123–126]. In one randomized study, patients who underwent invasive procedures to gather sputum samples had improved outcomes over those whose samples were procured via tracheal aspirate [127]. It is also important to distinguish asymptomatic bacteriuria from true urinary tract infection, even in the setting of kidney transplantation (see below) [128].

Both broth dilution and disk diffusion methods are recommended by the Clinical and Laboratory Standards Institute (CLSI) for susceptibility testing in *Enterobacteriaceae* [129]. CLSI updated MIC and diffusion cephalosporin and aztreonam breakpoints for *Enterobacteriaceae* in 2014 to reflect the increasing problem of resistance via multiple

Table 25.3a Laboratory breakpoints for *Enterobacteriaceae*[a]. MIC breakpoints (μg/ml)

Agent	Susceptible	Intermediate	Resistant
Cefazolin	≤2	4	≥8
Cefuroxime (IV)	≤8	16	≥32
Cefotetan	≤16	32	≥64
Cefoxitin	≤8	16	≥32
Cefotaxime	≤1	2	≥4
Ceftizoxime	≤1	2	≥4
Ceftriaxone	≤1	2	≥4
Ceftazidime	≤4	8	≥16
Cefepime	≤2	4–8	≥16
Aztreonam	≤4	8	≥16

[a]Clinical and Laboratory Standards Institute criteria

Table 25.3b Laboratory breakpoints for *Enterobacteriaceae*[a] zones of inhibition (mm)

Agent	Susceptible	Intermediate	Resistant
Cefazolin (non-UTI)	≥23	20–22	≤19
Cefotaxime	≥26	23–25	≤22
Ceftizoxime	≥25	22–24	≤21
Ceftriaxone	≥23	20–22	≤19
Ceftazidime	≥21	18–20	≤17
Aztreonam	≥21	18–20	≤17

Disk diffusion breakpoints (mm)
[a]Clinical and Laboratory Standards Institute criteria

mechanisms and treatment failure with traditional antibiotics, despite "susceptible" MICs. The revised breakpoints eliminated the need to perform ESBL screening and confirmatory tests. Screening for carbapenemase-producing organisms can be done using ertapenem or meropenem for disk diffusion susceptibility testing; using imipenem, meropenem, or ertapenem for microbroth dilution; or using ertapenem in automated susceptibility testing. All require special interpretive criteria. Production of KPC can be detected using the modified Hodge test. Laboratories should be familiar with these new guidelines and breakpoints in order to correctly identify multidrug-resistant *Enterobacteriaceae*. If the laboratory is not experienced with the evaluation of unusual susceptibility patterns, referral to a reference laboratory may be warranted (Tables 25.3a and 25.3b).

Treatment

Prompt recognition of infection with *Enterobacteriaceae*, particularly multidrug-resistant organisms, and initiation of appropriate antimicrobials are essential. Removal of known foci of infection such as indwelling catheters or drainage of abscesses is strongly recommended, when possible. Initial empiric therapy should be guided by the hospital or region's known *Enterobacteriaceae* resistance patterns, and definitive antimicrobial therapy should be chosen based on susceptibility testing.

Carbapenems are the mainstay of treatment for infections with ESBL-producing *Enterobacteriaceae* [110, 130]. Cephalosporins and penicillins should be avoided in AmpC-producing organisms as they can induce hyper-production of beta-lactamase; in these cases, a non-beta-lactam antibiotic should be chosen [110, 130]. Agents that are active against carbapenemase-producing *Enterobacteriaceae* include ceftazidime avibactam, polymyxins like colistin and polymyxin B, the aminoglycosides, fosfomycin for urinary tract infections, and tigecycline [108, 110, 130]. Use of tigecycline is no longer routinely recommended as there is a trend toward increased mortality when this antibiotic is used due to low drug concentrations in the blood and urinary tract [131]. There are no good data on optimum therapy or combination therapy for these infections. In vitro studies show synergy when using colistin with carbapenems [132–134], but, thus far, there have been no definitive studies showing significant difference in clinical outcomes when "synergistic" combinations are used [135–137].

Special Consideration: Asymptomatic Bacteriuria

Due to the severity of the potential outcomes of graft pyelonephritis, as well as the higher level of immunosuppression in the first few months following transplant, some experts recommend treatment of asymptomatic bacteriuria during the early posttransplant period [138]. In the general population, treatment of asymptomatic bacteriuria is not recommended, and at least one prospective trial has failed to confirm any benefit from treating asymptomatic bacteriuria in renal transplant recipients [128, 139]. Consequently, there is no consensus on whether to treat asymptomatic bacteriuria, at least in the early posttransplant period, and the benefits from routine screening are unknown.

Special Consideration: Febrile Neutropenia

Neutropenic patients represent a specific group at risk for infection, most commonly seen in the pre-engraftment period following HSCT. Because *Enterobacteriaceae* are common pathogens in neutropenic patients, high-risk groups should be admitted and started on empiric IV antibiotics with cefepime, a carbapenem, or piperacillin-tazobactam, depending on local resistance patterns [140]. Low-risk populations, as defined by the Multinational Association for Supportive Care in Cancer (MASCC) score, may be managed with empiric enteral antibiotics. Modification of the empiric regimen should be made if organisms are isolated and susceptibilities are available; otherwise empiric treatment is recommended until engraftment and recovery of peripheral blood granulocyte count [140].

Prevention

Prophylaxis

Given the diversity of timing and sources of infections with *Enterobacteriaceae* in SOT recipients, there is limited data regarding prevention of infections with these organisms during the extended posttransplant period. Most reports have focused on early infections. Historically, several studies have shown that prophylaxis with co-trimoxazole given mainly for prophylaxis against *Pneumocystis jirovecii* infection has reduced the incidence of UTI and bacteremia after solid organ transplantation [141, 142]; however, in a study by Vidal et al. [7], co-trimoxazole prophylaxis did not demonstrate a protective effect. Interestingly, the use of co-trimoxazole has not contributed to increased colonization with MDRE organisms, although the rates of co-trimoxazole resistance are expectedly high [7, 20, 141, 142]. Selective bowel decontamination prior to liver transplant has been evaluated in several randomized controlled trials, which have produced conflicting results, although the regimens and time courses varied from study to study [143–146]. A systematic analysis by Safdar et al. [146] showed that selective bowel decontamination reduces infections with Gram-negative organisms. None of the studies were adequately powered to detect a difference in mortality, however, and Gram-positive infections have been noted with this approach [143]. The emergence of antimicrobial resistance was not explored. Based on the limited impact on survival and the risk for resistance, this strategy is not routinely recommended [146].

In HSCT recipients, antibiotic prophylaxis with fluoroquinolones has demonstrated reduction in the incidence of Gram-negative sepsis during neutropenia, albeit no mortality benefit has been consistently demonstrated [147]. Moreover, fluoroquinolone resistance has been noted in patients receiving this prophylaxis [82, 107]. Current recommendations still include antibacterial prophylaxis for high-risk neutropenic patients with anticipated prolonged neutropenia (ANC <100 cells/mm^3) for a minimum of 7 days [140, 147]. Antimicrobial prophylaxis is not currently recommended for low-risk neutropenia patients with a short duration of anticipated neutropenia, especially those undergoing uncomplicated autologous stem cell transplantation.

In SOT and HSCT recipients, colonization with CRE has been associated with subsequent infections with CRE [108, 148, 149]. There are no data available to recommend either alteration of antimicrobial prophylaxis or exclusion from transplantation. As noted previously, the use of CRE-infected or CRE-colonized donors is not specifically contraindicated; adjustment in prophylactic regimens to cover resistant pathogens should be considered [108, 115]. Regardless, greater emphasis on infection control measures is recommended for patients known to have prior infection or colonization with CRE, especially to prevent spread of resistant organisms on transplant units [108, 130].

Infection Control

Cross-transmission of ESBL-producing and carbapenem-resistant *Enterobacteriaceae* is common, as evidenced by the previously mentioned outbreaks. Therefore, it is crucial that institutions introduce strict infection control policies in order to prevent the nosocomial spread of highly resistant organisms. In HSCT recipients, current recommendations include screening for MDR bacteria, especially in institutions with known high prevalence, and instituting contact precautions to prevent cross-patient transfer of such organisms [150]. There are no specific recommendations with respect to screening SOT recipients, although many centers with increased prevalence of CRE are screening candidates and recipients in transplant units. The Centers for Disease Control and Prevention has developed a tool kit for facilities and clinicians outlining procedures to prevent spread of resistant *Enterobacteriaceae*, and current guidelines designed for solid organ transplant recipients recommend adherence to this tool kit [130, 151]. Procedures include cohorting patients and staff with known MDRE colonization or infection, use of contact precautions including gown and gloves, strict enforcement of hand hygiene, minimization of invasive device use, promotion of antimicrobial stewardship in order to curb the development of resistance, and implementation of surveillance and screening protocols [151].

Infectious Diarrhea with *Enterobacteriaceae*

Epidemiology

Diarrhea is common among SOT recipients and most frequently attributed to the direct effects of immunosuppression. However, these recipients are also at increased risk for infections with pathogens that cause gastroenteritis. Transplant patients tend to be symptomatic for longer and have less abdominal pain, which may make it difficult to assess for secondary complications [152]. Transplant recipients are at risk for acquisition of community-acquired infectious diarrhea with viral and bacterial organisms, including those in the *Enterobacteriaceae* family such as *Escherichia coli*, *Salmonella* spp., *Shigella* spp., and *Yersinia* spp. as well as extraintestinal manifestations of these infections [153, 154]. Arslan et al. reported that the rate of infectious diarrhea in SOT recipients caused by *Enterobacteriaceae* was similar to the general population [154]. *Salmonella* was the most common bacterial etiologic agent, causing 42% of infectious diarrhea cases that were attributed to bacteria other than *Clostridium difficile*. Additional causes included *Campylobacter* (not in the *Enterobacteriaceae* family) (27%), *Shigella* (15%), pathogenic *E. coli* (35), and *Yersinia* (<1%). Although the incidence of *Salmonella* as a cause of infectious diarrhea did not seem to differ from the general population, the incidence of extraintestinal infections with non-typhoidal *Salmonella* species was much greater in renal transplant recipients, approximately 20 times higher than in the non-transplant population [155].

Diagnosis

Determination of the etiology of diarrhea in a solid organ transplant patient is complicated due to the diversity of pathogens in this population as well as the immunosuppressive medications that often have diarrhea as a side effect. A thorough history, including timing, volume, and presence of bloody diarrhea and/or fever, exposure history, and full physical exam should be completed. Stool samples should be sent for routine culture and, based on clinical presentations such as the presence of bloody diarrhea, fever, and exposure history, may include special culture for Shiga toxin-producing *E. coli*, *Campylobacter* spp., and *Yersinia* spp., as well as multiplex PCR for enteric pathogens and Shiga toxin (Table 25.4a) [153]. In addition, stool should be tested for non-*Enterobacteriaceae* bacterial pathogens including *Clostridium difficile*; parasitic infections such as *Giardia*, *Cryptosporidium*, *Isospora*, and *Cyclospora*; microsporidiosis; and both community-acquired and opportunistic viruses.

Treatment

Given the multiple potential causes of diarrhea in SOT recipients, empiric treatment recommendations vary with individual circumstances. Empiric treatment is generally withheld until an etiologic agent is identified. However, if shigellosis or *Campylobacter* spp. infection is suspected in a patient with bloody diarrhea, fever, and appropriate exposure history, it is advisable to provide empiric treatment. In the immunocompetent host, most gastrointestinal infections caused by *Enterobacteriaceae* are self-limited illnesses and do not require treatment with antibacterials; however, transplant recipients with more severe infection should receive treatment [153, 156]. Anti-motility agents should be avoided in patients with bloody diarrhea due to the risk of prolonging infection. Table 25.4b outlines diagnostic and treatment considerations in patients with diarrhea due to *Enterobacteriaceae*.

Emerging Pathogens

Due to their immunosuppressed state, SOT recipients are at risk for infections with organisms that do not usually cause infection in immunocompetent individuals. There

Table 25.4a *Enterobacteriaceae* causing infectious diarrhea: organisms and clinical presentation

Organism	Common subtypes	Symptoms/signs	Seasonality	Exposures	Complications
Salmonella	Non-typhoidal: *S. enteritidis*, *S. typhimurium* Typhoidal: *S. typhi*, *S. paratyphi*	Nausea, vomiting, nonbloody diarrhea, abdominal cramping Typhoid fever: Fever, rose spots, hepatosplenomegaly	None	Raw eggs, poultry, pork, beef; reptiles	Extra-intestinal disease (bone and joint, bacteremia, meningitis, myocarditis Reactive arthritis
Shigella	*S. sonnei* (most common), *S. dysenteriae*, *S. flexneri*, *S. boydii*	Diarrhea with blood or mucous, crampy abdominal pain, fever	Summer/ fall	Sick contacts, contaminated food (salads, dairy products, raw vegetables, seafood, raw meat)	HUS Reactive arthritis, seizures, perforation
E. coli	Enterotoxigenic (ETEC) Enteroadherent (EAEC), Enteropathogenic (EPEC), Enterohemorrhagic (EHEC), Enteroinvasive (EIEC)	Varies Nonbloody diarrhea: ETC, EAEC Bloody diarrhea: EIEC, EHEC, and EPEC Fever: EIEC, EHEC	None	ETEC, traveler's diarrhea, waterborne, soft cheeses, raw vegetables; EAEC, children with chronic diarrhea in developing countries; EPEC, infants and nurseries; EIEC, person-to-person, fecal-oral; EHEC, undercooked meat, raw milk, unpasteurized juices, raw vegetables, waterborne	Hemorrhagic colitis (EHEC), HUS (*E. coli* 0157:H7)
Yersinia	*Y. Enterocolitica*	Watery or bloody diarrhea, fever	Winter	Pork (chitterlings), beef, poultry, lamb, seafood, waterborne	Pseudoappendicitis, perforation, intussusception, peritonitis, toxic megacolon, cholangitis, bacteremia, reactive arthritis

Table 25.4b Diagnosis and treatment of infectious diarrhea caused by *Enterobacteriaceae*

Organism	Diagnostic considerations	Treatment	Treatment considerations
Salmonella	Routine stool culture	Empiric: Fluoroquinolone or third-generation cephalosporin for 5–7 days	Duration of treatment for extraintestinal, dependent on site of infection Typhoid vaccine should be administered to travelers
Shigella	Routine stool culture	Fluoroquinolone or TMP-SMX for 3–7 days	Avoid anti-motility agents
E. coli	Request special medium to isolate E O157:H7	Fluoroquinolone for moderate to severe traveler's diarrhea (ETEC), EPEC, or EIEC	NO antibiotics if E O157:H7 confirmed, unless septic
Yersinia	Request special medium	Doxycycline, TMP-SMX, aminoglycosides, fluoroquinolones	

are several members of the *Enterobacteriaceae* family that are commensal or environmental organisms that have been shown to cause infection in patients undergoing transplantation. Notably, infections with *Hafnia alvei*, a commensal organism in soil, water, and the GI tract of mammals, reptiles, birds, and fish, have been reported in kidney, liver, and lung transplant patients [157–161]. *Pantoea agglomerans* formerly *Enterobacter agglomerans*, an organism found in the environment, usually on plants, fruits, and vegetables, has been described as a cause of pneumonia in a heart-lung transplant patient [162]. Finally, *Kluyvera*, another member of the *Enterobacteriaceae* family that inhabits the human gastrointestinal and respiratory tracts, has been found to be one of the etiologic agents of a polymicrobial liver abscess in a transplanted liver as well as of pyelonephritis in a transplanted kidney [163].

Summary

Enterobacteriaceae are important etiologic agents of bacterial infections in transplant recipients. They are prominent pathogens in both the early and late posttransplant periods and can cause infection at any site. Antimicrobial resistance among *Enterobacteriaceae* is increasing, and this is reflected in the transplant population as well. Given that transplantation is an independent risk factor for infection with resistant *Enterobacteriaceae*, providers should have a high level of suspicion and choose empiric therapy accordingly in order to improve outcomes.

References

1. Meatherall BL, Gregson D, Ross T, et al. Incidence, risk factors, and outcomes of Klebsiella pneumoniae bacteremia. Am J Med. 2009;122:866.
2. Centers for Disease Control and Prevention. Surveillance for Emerging Antimicrobial Resistance Connected to Healthcare (S.E.A.R.C.H.) http://www.cdc.gov/hai/. Accessed 4/12/2017.
3. Antimicrobial resistance surveillance in Europe 2015. http://ecdc.europa.eu/en/publications/_layouts/forms/Publication_DispForm.aspx?List=4f55ad51-4aed-4d32-b960-af70113dbb90&ID=1637. Accessed 4/12/2017.
4. Kawecki D, Kwiatkowski A, Sawicka-Grzelak A, et al. Urinary tract infections in the early posttransplant period after kidney transplantation: etiologic agents and their susceptibility. Transplant Proc. 2011;43:2991–3.
5. Dantas SR, Kuboyama RH, Mazzali M, et al. Nosocomial infections in renal transplant patients: risk factors and treatment implications associated with urinary tract and surgical site infections. J Hosp Infect. 2006;63(2):117–23.
6. Giral M, Pascuariello G, Karam G, et al. Acute graft pyelonephritis and long-term kidney allograft outcome. Kidney Int. 2002;61:1880–6.
7. Vidal E, Torre-Cisneros J, Blanes M, et al. Bacterial urinary tract infection after solid organ transplantation in the RESITRA cohort. Transpl Infect Dis. 2012;14:595–603.
8. Herrero-Martínez JM, Lumbreras C, Manrique A, et al. Epidemiology, risk factors and impact on long-term pancreatic function of infection following pancreas-kidney transplantation. Clin Microbiol Infect. 2013;19:1132–9.
9. Brooks RG, Hofflin JM, Jamieson SW, et al. Infectious complications in heart-lung transplant recipients. Am J Med. 1985;79:412–22.
10. Gullestad L, Eisjkauer H, Gustafsson F, et al. Long-term outcomes of thoracic transplant recipients following conversion to everolimus with reduced calcineurin inhibitor in a multicenter, open-label, randomized trial. Transpl Int. 2016;29:819–29.
11. Yun JH, Kee S-O, Jo K-W, et al. Infections after lung transplantation: time of occurrence, sites, and microbiologic etiologies. Korean J Intern Med. 2015;30:506–14.bl.
12. Paya CV, Wiesner RH, Herman PE, et al. Risk factors for cytomegalovirus and severe bacterial infections following liver transplantation: a prospective multivariate time-dependent analysis. J Hepatol. 1993;18:185–95.
13. Lumbreras C, Lizasoin M, Moreno E, et al. Major bacterial infections following liver transplantation: a prospective study. Hepatogastroenterol. 1992;39:362–5.
14. Linares L, García GJ, Cervera C, et al. Early bacteremia after solid organ transplantation. Transplant Proc. 2009;41:2262–4.
15. Wingard JR, Hsu J, Hiemenz JW. Hematopoietic stem cell transplantation: an overview of infection risks and epidemiology. Infect Dis Clin North Am. 2010;24:257–72.
16. Mikulska M, Del Bono V, Viscoli C. Bacterial infections in hematopoietic stem cell transplantation recipients. Curr Opin Hematol. 2014;21:451–8.
17. Balletto E, Mikulska M. Bacterial infections in hematopoietic stem cell transplant recipients. Mediterr J Hematol Infect Dis. 2015;7:e2015045.
18. Zając-Spychała O, Wachowiak J, Pieczonka A, Siewiera K, Frączkiewicz J, Kałwak K, et al. Bacterial infections in pediatric hematopoietic stem cell transplantation recipients: incidence, epidemiology, and spectrum of pathogens: report of the Polish Pediatric Group for hematopoietic stem cell transplantation. Transpl Infect Dis. 2016;18:690–8.

19. Parasuraman R, Julian K. Urinary tract infections in solid organ transplantation. Am J Transplant. 2013;13:327–36.
20. Green H, Rahamimov R, Gafter U, Leibovitci L, Paul M. Antibiotic prophylaxis for urinary tract infections in renal transplant recipients: systematic review and meta-analysis. Transpl Infect Dis. 2011;13:441–7.
21. Espinar EJ, Miranda IM, Costa-de-Oliveira S, Rocha R, Rodrigues AG, Pina-Vaz C. Urinary tract infections in kidney transplant patients due to Escherichia coli and Klebsiella pneumoniae-producing extended-spectrum β-lactamases: risk factors and molecular epidemiology. PLoS One. 2015;10(8):e0134737.
22. Azap Ö, Togan T, Yesilkaya A, Arslan H, Haberal M. Antimicrobial susceptibilities of uropathogen Escherichia coli in renal transplant recipients: dramatic increase in ciprofloxacin resistance. Transplant Proc. 2013;45:956–7.
23. Gołębiewska J, Tarasewicz A, Dębska-Ślizień A, Rutkowski B. Klebsiella spp urinary tract infections during first year after renal transplantation. Transplant Proc. 2014;46:2748–51.
24. Freire MP, Abdala E, Moura ML, et al. Risk factors and outcome of infections with Klebsiella pneumoniae carbapenemase-producing K. pneumoniae in kidney transplant recipients. Infection. 2015;43:315–23.
25. Brizendine KD, Richter SS, Cober ED, van Duin D. Carbapenem-resistant Klebsiella pneumoniae urinary tract infection following solid organ transplantation. Antimicrob Agents Chemother. 2015;59:553–7.
26. Pelle G, Vimont S, Levy PP, et al. Acute pyelonephritis represents a risk factor impairing long-term kidney graft function. Am J Transplant. 2007;7:899–907.
27. Audard V, Amor M, Desvaux D, et al. Acute graft pyelonephritis: a potential cause of acute rejection in renal transplant. Transplantation. 2005;80:1128–30.
28. Kamath NS, John GT, Neelakantan N, et al. Acute graft pyelonephritis following renal transplantation. Transpl Infect Dis. 2006;8:140–7.
29. Naik AS, Dharnidharka VR, Schnitzler MA, et al. Clinical and economic consequences of first-year urinary tract infections, sepsis, and pneumonia in contemporary kidney transplantation practice. Transpl Int. 2016;29:241–52.
30. Abbott KC, Swanson SJ, Richter ER, et al. Late urinary tract infection after renal transplantation in the United States. Am J Kidney Dis. 2004;44:353–62.
31. Fiorante S, Fernández-Ruiz M, López-Medrano F, et al. Acute graft pyelonephritis in renal transplant recipients: incidence, risk factors and long-term outcome. Nephrol Dial Transplant. 2011;26:1065–73.
32. Camargo LF, Esteves ABA, Ulisses LRS, Rivelli GG, Mazzali M. Urinary tract infection in renal transplant recipients: incidence, risk factors, and impact on graft function. Transplant Proc. 2014;46:1757–9.
33. Ariza-Heredia EJ, Beam EN, Lesnick TG, Cosio FG, Kremers WK, Razonable RR. Impact of urinary tract infection on allograft function after kidney transplantation. Clin Transpl. 2014;28:683–90.
34. George DL, Arnow PM, Fox AS, et al. Bacterial infection as a complication of liver transplantation: epidemiology and risk factors. Rev Infect Dis. 1991;3:287–96.
35. Viehman JA, Clancy CJ, Clarke L, et al. Surgical site infections after liver transplantation: emergence of multidrug-resistant bacteria and implications for prophylaxis and treatment strategies. Transplantation. 2016;100:2107–14.
36. Kornasiewicz O, Hołówko W, Grąt M, et al. Hepatic abscess: a rare complication after liver transplant. Clin Transpl. 2016;30:1230–5.
37. Wade JJ, Rolando N, Hayllar K, et al. Bacterial and fungal infections after liver transplantation: an analysis of 284 patients. Hepatology. 1995;21:1328–36.
38. Bubak ME, Porayko MK, Krom RAF, et al. Complications of liver biopsy in liver transplant patients: increased sepsis associated with choledochojejunostomy. Hepatology. 1991;14:1063–5.
39. Krom RAF, Kingma LM, Haagsma EB, et al. Choledochocholedochostomy, a relatively safe procedure in orthotopic liver transplantation. Surgery. 1985;97:552–6.
40. Arnow PM, Zachary KC, Thistlethwaite JR, Thompson KD, Bova JL, Newell KA. Pathogenesis of early operative site infections after orthotopic liver transplantation. Transplantation. 1998;65:1500–3.
41. Yamamoto M, Takakura S, Iinuma Y, et al. Changes in surgical site infections after living donor liver transplantation. PLoS One. 2015;10(8):e0136559.
42. Kotloff RM, Ahya VN, Crawford SW. Pulmonary complications of solid organ and hematopoietic stem cell transplantation. Am J Respir Crit Care Med. 2004;170(1):22–48.
43. Kramer MR, Marshall SE, Starnes VA, et al. Infectious complications in heart-lung transplantation. Analysis of 200 episodes. Arch Intern Med. 1993;153(17):2010–6.
44. Maurer JR, Tullis DE, Grossman RF, et al. Infectious complications following isolated lung transplantation. Chest. 1992;101(4):1056–9.
45. Cisneros JM, Munoz P, Torre-Cisneros J, et al. Pneumonia after heart transplantation: a multi-institutional study. Spanish Transplantation Infection Study Group. Clin Infect Dis. 1998;27(2):324–31.
46. Cervera C, Augusti C, Marcos MA, et al. Microbiologic features and outcome of pneumonia in transplanted patients. Diagn Microbiol Infect Dis. 2006;55:47–54.
47. Bonatti H, Pruett TL, Brandacher G, et al. Pneumonia in solid organ recipients: Spectrum of pathogens in 217 episodes. Transplant Proc. 2009;41:371–4.
48. Aguilar-Guisado M, Jiménez-Jambrina M, Espigado I, et al. Pneumonia in allogeneic stem cell transplantation recipients: a multicenter prospective study. Clin Transpl. 2011;25:E629–38.
49. Giannella M, Muñoz P, Alarcón JM, et al. Pneumonia in solid organ transplant recipients: a prospective multicenter study. Transpl Infect Dis. 2014;16:232–41.
50. Bige N, Zafrani L, Lambert J, et al. Severe infections requiring intensive care unit admission in kidney transplant recipients: impact on graft outcome. Transpl Infect Dis. 2014;16:588–96.
51. Mermel LA, Maki DG. Bacterial pneumonia in solid organ transplantation. Semin Respir Infect. 1990;5(1):10–29.
52. Patel SR, Kirby TJ, McCarthy PM, et al. Lung transplantation: the Cleveland Clinic experience. Cleve Clin J Med. 1993;60:303–19.
53. Deusch E, End A, Grimm M, et al. Early bacterial infections in lung transplant recipients. Chest. 1993;104:1412–6.52.
54. Aguilar-Guisado M, Givalda J, Ussetti P. Pneumonia after lung transplantation in the Resitra Cohort: a multicenter prospective study. Am J Transplant. 2007,7.1989–96.
55. Dudau D, Camous J, Marchand S, et al. Incidence of nosocomial pneumonia and risk of recurrence after antimicrobial therapy in critically ill lung and heart–lung transplant patients. Clin Transpl. 2014;28:27–36.
56. Lumbreras C, Fernandez I, Velosa J, et al. Infectious complications following pancreatic transplantation: incidence, microbiological and clinical characteristics, and outcome. Clin Infect Dis. 1995;20:514–20.
57. Paya CV, Hermans PE. Bacterial infections after liver transplantation. Eur J Clin Microbiol Infect Dis. 1989;8:499–504.
58. Ramos A, Asensio A, Muñez E, et al. Incisional surgical infection in heart transplantation. Transpl Infect Dis. 2008;10:298–302.
59. Zanfi C, Cescon M, Lauro A, et al. Incidence and management of abdominal closure-related complications in adult intestinal transplantation. Transplantation. 2008;85:1607–9.
60. Loinaz C, Kato T, Nishida S, et al. Bacterial infections after intestine and multivisceral transplantation. The experience of the University of Miami (1994-2001). Hepatogastroenterology. 2006;53:234–42.
61. Linhares MM, Gonzalez AM, Triviño T. Simultaneous pancreas-kidney transplantation: infectious complications and microbiological aspects. Transplant Proc. 2004;36:980–1.

62. Hellinger WC, Crook JE, Heckman MG, et al. Surgical site infection after liver transplantation: risk factors and association with graft loss or death. Transplantation. 2009;87:1387–93.
63. Michalak G, Kwiatkowski A, Bieniasz M, et al. Infectious complications after simultaneous pancreas-kidney transplantation. Transplant Proc. 2005;37:3560–3.
64. Perdiz LB, Furtado GH, Linhares MM, et al. Incidence and risk factors for surgical site infection after simultaneous pancreas-kidney transplantation. J Hosp Infect. 2009;72:326–31.
65. Shields RK, Clancy CJ, Minces L, et al. Epidemiology and outcomes of deep surgical site infections following lung transplantation. Am J Transplant. 2013;13:2137–45.
66. Kawecki D, Chmura A, Pacholczyk M, et al. Surgical site infections in liver recipients in the early posttransplantation period: etiological agents and susceptibility profiles. Transplant Proc. 2007;39:2800–6.
67. Rana MM, Sturdevant M, Patel G, Huprikar S. Klebsiella necrotizing soft tissue infections in liver transplant recipients: a case series. Transpl Infect Dis. 2013;15:157–63.
68. Menezes FG, Wey SB, Peres CA, et al. Risk factors for surgical site infection in kidney transplant recipients. Infect Control Hosp Epidemiol. 2008;29(8):771–3.
69. Asensio A, Ramos A, Cuervas-Mons V, et al. Effect of antibiotic prophylaxis on the risk of surgical site infection in orthotopic liver transplant. Liver Transpl. 2008;14(6):799–805.
70. Peraira JR, Segovia J, Arroyo R, et al. High incidence of severe infections in heart transplant recipients receiving tacrolimus. Transplant Proc. 2003;35:1999–2000.
71. Freire MP, Antonopoulos IM, Piovesan AC, et al. Amikacin prophylaxis and risk factors for surgical site infection after kidney transplantation. Transplantation. 2015;99:521–7.
72. Freire MP, Soares Oshiro IC, Bonazzi PR, et al. Surgical site infections in liver transplant recipients in the model for end-stage liver disease era: an analysis of the epidemiology, risk factors, and outcomes. Liver Transpl. 2013;19:1011–9.
73. Zuckermann A, Barten MJ. Surgical wound complications after heart transplantation. Transpl Int. 2011;24:627–36.
74. Kuppahally S, Al-Khaldi A, Weisshaar D, et al. Wound healing complications with de novo sirolimus versus mycophenolate mofetil-based regimen in cardiac transplant recipients. Am J Transplant. 2006;6:986–92.
75. Husain S, Chan KM, Palmer SM, et al. Bacteremia in lung transplant recipients in the current era. Am J Transplant. 2006;6:3000–7.
76. Wagener MM, Yu VL. Bacteremia in transplant recipients: a prospective study of demographics, etiologic agents, risk factors, and outcomes. Am J Infect Control. 1992;20:239–47.
77. Rodriguez C, Munoz P, Rodriguez-Creixems M, et al. Bloodstream infections among heart transplant recipients. Transplantation. 2006;81:384–91.
78. Al-Hasan MN, Razonable RR, Eckel-Passowd JE, et al. Incidence rate and outcome of gram-negative bloodstream infection in solid organ transplant recipients. Am J Transplant. 2009;9:835–43.
79. Singh N, Gayowski T, Wagener MM, et al. Bloodstream infections in liver transplant recipients receiving tacrolimus. Clin Transpl. 1997;11:275–81.
80. Ye QF, Zhao J, Wan QQ, et al. Frequency and clinical outcomes of ESKAPE bacteremia in solid organ transplantation and the risk factors for mortality. Transpl Infect Dis. 2014;16:767–74.
81. Blennow O, Ljungman P, Sparrelid E, Mattsson J, Remberger M. Incidence, risk factors, and outcome of bloodstream infections during the pre-engraftment phase in 521 allogeneic hematopoietic stem cell transplantations. Transpl Infect Dis. 2014;16:106–14.
82. Wang CH, Chang FY, Chao TY, Kao WY, Ho CL, Chen YC, et al. Characteristics comparisons of bacteremia in allogeneic and autologous hematopoietic stem cell-transplant recipients with levofloxacin prophylaxis and influence on resistant bacteria emergence. J Microbiol Immunol Infect. 2016;pii: S1684–1182(16)30003–30002.
83. Poutsiaka DD, Price LL, Ucuzian A, Chan GW, Miller KB, Snydman DR. Blood stream infection after hematopoietic stem cell transplantation is associated with increased mortality. Bone Marrow Transplant. 2007;40:63–70.
84. Shigematsu A, Yamamoto S, Sugita J, et al. Increased risk of bacterial infection after engraftment in patients treated with allogeneic bone marrow transplantation following reduced-intensity conditioning regimen. Transpl Infect Dis. 2010;12:412–20.
85. Hong J, Moon SM, Ahn HK, et al. Comparison of characteristics of bacterial bloodstream infection between adult patients with allogeneic and autologous hematopoietic stem cell transplantation. Biol Blood Marrow Transplant. 2013;19:988–99.
86. Qureshi ZA, Paterson DL, Pakstis DL, et al. Risk factors and outcome of extended-spectrum beta-lactamase producing bloodstream infections. Int J Antimicrob Agents. 2011;37(1):26–32.
87. Qureshi ZA, Paterson DL, Peleg AY, et al. Clinical characteristics of bacteremia caused by extended-spectrum beta-lactamase-producing Enterobacteriaceae in the era of CTX-M-type and KPC-type beta-lactamases. Clin Microbiol Infect. 2012;18(9):887–93.
88. Mills JP, Talati NJ, Alby K, Han JH. The epidemiology of Carbapenem-Resistant Klebsiella pneumoniae colonization and infection among long-term acute care hospital residents. Infect Control Hosp Epidemiol. 2016;37:55–60.
89. Linares L, Cervera C, Hoyo I, et al. Klebsiella pneumoniae infection in solid organ transplant recipients: epidemiology and antibiotic resistance. Transplant Proc. 2010;42:2941–3.
90. Patel G, Huprikar S, Factor SH, et al. Outcomes of carbapenem-resistant Klebsiella pneumoniae infection and the impact of antimicrobial and adjunctive therapies. Infect Control Hosp Epidemiol. 2008;29:1099–106.
91. Schwaber MJ, Navon-Venezia S, Kaye KS, et al. Clinical and economic impact of bacteremia with extended-spectrumβ –lactamase-producing Enterobacteriaceae. Antimicrob Agents Chemother. 2006;50:1257–62.
92. Lee SY, Kotapati S, Kuti JL, et al. Impact of extended-spectrum β-lactamase–producing Escherichia coli and Klebsiella species on clinical outcomes and hospital costs: a matched cohort study. Infect Control Hosp Epidemiol. 2006;27:1226–32.
93. Bodro M, Sabé N, Tubau F, et al. Risk factors and outcomes of bacteremia caused by drug-resistant ESKAPE pathogens in solid-organ transplant recipients. Transplantation. 2013;96:843–9.
94. Bergamasco MD, Barroso Barbosa M, de Oliveira GD, et al. Infection with Klebsiella pneumoniae carbapenemase (KPC)-producing K. pneumoniae in solid organ transplantation. Transpl Infect Dis. 2012;14(2):198–205.
95. Paterson DL, Singh N, Rihs JD, et al. Control of an outbreak of infection due to extended-spectrum beta-lactamase-producing Escherichia coli in a liver transplantation unit. Clin Infect Dis. 2001;33:126–8.
96. Rebuck JA, Olsen KM, Fey PD, et al. Characterization of an outbreak due to extended-spectrum beta-lactamase-producing Klebsiella pneumoniae in a pediatric intensive care unit transplant population. Clin Infect Dis. 2000;31:1368–72.
97. Martins IS, Moreira BM, Riley LW, et al. Outbreak of extended-spectrum beta-lactamase-producing Klebsiella pneumoniae infection among renal transplant recipients. J Hosp Infect. 2006;64:305–8.
98. Zárate MS, Gales AC, Picão RC, et al. Outbreak of OXY-2 producing Klebsiella oxytoca in a renal transplant unit. J Clin Microbiol. 2008;46:2099–101.
99. Mathers AJ, Cox HL, Bonatti H, et al. Fatal cross infection by carbapenem-resistant Klebsiella in two liver transplant recipients. Transpl Infect Dis. 2009;11(3):257–65.

100. Lai CC, Lin TL, Tseng SP, et al. Pelvic abscess caused by New Delhi metallo-beta-lactamase-1-producing Klebsiella oxytoca in Taiwan in a patient who underwent renal transplantation in China. Diagn Microbiol Infect Dis. 2011;71(4):474–5.
101. Mouloudi E, Protonotariou E, Zagorianou A, et al. Bloodstream infections caused by metallo-beta-lactamase/Klebsiella pneumoniae carbapenemase-producing K. pneumoniae among intensive care unit patients in Greece: risk factors for infection and impact of type of resistance on outcomes. Infect Control Hosp Epidemiol. 2010;31(12):1250–6.
102. Pouch SM, Kubin CJ, Satlin MJ, et al. Epidemiology and outcomes of carbapenem-resistant Klebsiella pneumonia bacteriuria in kidney transplant recipients. Transpl Infect Dis. 2015;17:800–9.
103. Pereira MR, Scully BF, Pouch SM, et al. Risk factors and outcomes of carbapenem-resistant Klebsiella pneumonia infections in liver transplant recipients. Liver Transpl. 2015;21:1511–9.
104. Simkins J, Muggia V, Cohen HW, Minamoto GY. Carbapenem-resistant Klebsiella pneumoniae infections in kidney transplant recipients: a case-control study. Transpl Infect Dis. 2014;16:775–82.
105. Balletto E, Mikulska M. Bacterial infections in hematopoietic stem cell transplant recipients. Mediterr J Hematol Infect Dis. 2015;7(1):e2015045.
106. Zając-Spychała O, Wachowiak J, Pieczonka A, Siewiera K, Frączkiewicz J, Kałwak K, et al. Bacterial infections in pediatric hematopoietic stem cell transplantation recipients: incidence, epidemiology, and spectrum of pathogens: report of the Polish Pediatric Group for hematopoietic stem cell transplantation. Transpl Infect Dis. 2016;18(5):690–8.
107. Bonadio M, Morelli G, Mori S, Riccioni R, Papineschi F, Petrini M. Fluoroquinolone resistance in hematopoietic stem cell transplant recipients with infectious complications. Biomed Pharmacother. 2005;59(9):511–6.
108. Satlin MJ, Jenkins SG, Walsh TJ. The global challenge of carbapenem-resistant Enterobacteriaceae in transplant recipients and patients with hematologic malignancies. Clin Infect Dis. 2014;58:1274–83.
109. Baker TM, Satlin MJ. The growing threat of multidrug-resistant gram-negative infections in patients with hematologic malignancies. Leuk Lymphoma. 2016;57:2245–58.
110. Iredell J, Brown J, Tagg K. Antibiotic resistance in Enterobacteriaceae: mechanisms and clinical implications. BMJ. 2016;352:h6420.
111. Nordmann P, Naas T, Poirel L. Global spread of Carbapenemase-producing Enterobacteriaceae. Emerg Infect Dis. 2011;17:1791–8.
112. Blumberg E, Green M, Covington SG, et al. Donor derived bacterial infections: report from the Disease Transmission Advisory Committee (DTAC). In: 48th Annual meeting of the Infectious Diseases Society of America. Vancouver. 2010. Available at https://idsa.confex.com/idsa/2010/webprogram/Paper3060.html.
113. Watkins AC, Vedula GV, Horan J, et al. The deceased organ donor with an "open abdomen": proceed with caution. Transpl Infect Dis. 2012;14:311–5.
114. Chung W, Pascoe N, Heseltine G, Qazi Y, Bower WA, Kuehnert M, Wise M, Zheteyeva Y. Transmission of multidrug-resistant Escherichia coli through kidney transplantation – California and Texas, 2009. MMWR. 2010;59(50):1642–6.
115. Mularoni A, Bertani A, Vizzini G, et al. Outcome of transplantation using organs from donors infected or colonized with carbapenem-resistant gram-negative bacteria. Am J Transplant. 2015;15:2674–82.
116. Mills JP, Wilck MB, Weikert BC, et al. Successful treatment of a disseminated infection with extensively drug-resistant Klebsiella pneumoniae in a liver transplant recipient with a fosfomycin-based multidrug regimen. Transpl Infect Dis. 2016;18:777–81.
117. Giani T, Conte V, Mandalà S, et al. Cross-infection of solid organ transplant recipients by a multidrug-resistant Klebsiella pneumoniae isolate producing the OXA-48 carbapenemase, likely derived from a multiorgan donor. J Clin Microbiol. 2014;52:2702–5.
118. Goldberg E, Bishara J, Lev S, et al. Transplantation from a donor colonized with a multidrug-resistant organism: a case report. Transpl Infect Dis. 2012;14(3):296–9.
119. Ariza-Heredia EJ, Patel R, Blumberg EA, et al. Outcomes of transplantation using organs from a donor infected with Klebsiella pneumoniae carbapenemase (KPC)-producing K. pneumoniae. Transpl Infect Dis. 2012;14(3):229–36.
120. Ison MG, Grossi P. AST Infectious Diseases Community of Practice. Donor-derived infections in solid organ transplantation. Am J Transplant. 2013;13(Suppl 4):22–30.
121. Miller R, Covington S, Taranto S, et al. Communication gaps associated with donor-derived infections. Am J Transplant. 2015;15:259–64.
122. https://optn.transplant.hrsa.gov/media/1200/optn_policies.pdf.
123. Craven DE. 2005 IDSA/ATS Hospital-acquired pneumonia guidelines: new principles for improving management. Johns Hopkins Adv Stud Med Proc. 2006;6(6C):S541–8.
124. Chan CC, Abi-Saleh WJ, Arroliga AC, et al. Diagnostic yield and therapeutic impact of flexible bronchoscopy in lung transplant recipients. J Heart Lung Transplant. 1996;15(2):196–205.
125. Harris B, Geyer AI. Diagnostic evaluation of pulmonary abnormalities in patients with hematologic malignancies and hematopoietic cell transplantation. Clin Chest Med. 2017;38:317–31.
126. Kupeli E, Akcay S, Ulubay G, Ozyurek BA, Ozdemirel TS, Haberal M. Diagnostic utility of flexible bronchoscopy in recipients of solid organ transplants. Transplant Proc. 2011;43:543–6.
127. Fagon JY, Chastre J, Wolff M, et al. Invasive and noninvasive strategies for management of suspected ventilator-associated pneumonia. A randomized trial. Ann Intern Med. 2000;132:621–30.
128. Origüen J, López-Medrano F, Fernández-Ruiz M, et al. Should asymptomatic bacteriuria be systematically treated in kidney transplant recipients? Results from a randomized controlled trial. Am J Transplant. 2016;16:2943–53.
129. http://clsi.org/standards/micro/microbiology-files/.
130. van Duin D, van Delden C. AST Infectious Diseases Community of Practice. Multidrug-resistant gram-negative bacteria infections in solid organ transplantation. Am J Transplant. 2013;13(Suppl 4):31–41.
131. van Duin D, Cober E, Richter SS, et al. Impact of therapy and strain type on outcomes in urinary tract infections caused by carbapenem-resistant Klebsiella pneumoniae. J Antimicrob Chemother. 2015;70:1203–11.
132. Souli M, Rekatsina PD, Chryssouli Z, et al. Does the activity of the combination of imipenem and colistin in vitro exceed the problem of resistance in metallo-beta-lactamase-producing Klebsiella pneumoniae isolates? Antimicrob Agents Chemother. 2009;53:2133–35.1.
133. Urban C, Mariano N, Rahal JJ. In vitro double and triple bactericidal activities of doripenem, polymyxin B, and rifampin against multidrugresistant Acinetobacter baumannii, Pseudomonas aeruginosa, Klebsiella pneumoniae, and Escherichia coli. Antimicrob Agents Chemother. 2010;54:2732–4.
134. Lin KH, Chuang YC, Lee SH, Yu WL. In vitro synergistic antimicrobial effect of imipenem and colistin against an isolate of multidrugresistant Enterobacter cloacae. J Microbiol Immunol Infect. 2010;43:317–22.
135. Falagas ME, Rafailidis PI, Ioannidou E, et al. Colistin therapy for microbiologically documented multidrug-resistant gram-negative bacterial infections: a retrospective cohort study of 258 patients. Int J Antimicrob Agents. 2010;35:194–9.

136. Kasiakou SK, Michalopoulos A, Soteriades ES, et al. Combination therapy with intravenous colistin for management of infections due to multidrug-resistant gram-negative bacteria in patients without cystic fibrosis. Antimicrob Agents Chemother. 2005;49: 3136–46.
137. Michalopoulos AS, Tsiodras S, Rellos K, et al. Colistin treatment in patients with ICU-acquired infections caused by multiresistant gram-negative bacteria: the renaissance of an old antibiotic. Clin Microbiol Infect. 2005;11:115–21.
138. Yacoub R, Akl NK. Urinary tract infections and asymptomatic bacteriuria in renal transplantrecipients. J Glob Infect Dis. 2011;3(4):383–9.
139. Nicolle LE, Bradley S, Colgan R, Rice JC, Schaeffer A, Hooton TM. Infectious Diseases Society of America; American Society of Nephrology; American Geriatric Society. Infectious Diseases Society of America guidelines for the diagnosis and treatment of asymptomatic bacteriuria in adults. Clin Infect Dis. 2005;40:643–54.
140. Freifeld AG, Freifeld AG, Bow EJ, et al. Clinical practice guideline for the use of antimicrobial agents in neutropenic patients with cancer: 2010 update by the Infectious Diseases Society of America. Clin Infect Dis. 2011;52:e56–93.
141. Tolkoff-Rubin NE, Cosimi AB, Russell PS, et al. A controlled study of trimethoprim-sulfamethoxazole prophylaxis of urinary tract infection in renal transplant recipients. Rev Infect Dis. 1982;4:614–8.
142. Fox BC, Sollinger HW, Belzer FO, Maki DG. A prospective, randomized, double-blind study of trimethoprimsulfamethoxazole for prophylaxis of infection in renal transplantation: clinical efficacy, absorption of trimethoprimsulfamethoxazole, effects on the microflora, and the cost-benefit of prophylaxis. Am J Med. 1990;89:255–74.
143. Resino E, San-Juan R, Aguado JM. Selective intestinal decontamination for the prevention of early bacterial infections after liver transplantation. World J Gastroenterol. 2016;22:5950–7.
144. Badger IL, Crosby HA, Kong KL, et al. Is selective bowel decontamination of the digestive tract beneficial in liver transplant patients? Interim results of a prospective, randomized trial. Transplant Proc. 1991;23:1460–1.
145. Smith SD, Jackson RJ, Hannakan CJ, et al. Selective decontamination in pediatric liver transplants. A randomized prospective study. Transplantation. 1993;55:1306–9.
146. Safdar N, Said A, Lucey MR. The role of selective digestive decontamination for reducing infection in patients undergoing liver transplantation: a systematic review and meta-analysis. Liver Transpl. 2004;10:817–27.
147. Wingard JR, Hsu J, Hiemenz JW. Hematopoietic stem cell transplantation: an overview of infection risks and epidemiology. Infect Dis Clin North Am. 2010;24(2):257–72.
148. Bert F, Larroque B, Paugam-Burtz C, et al. Pretransplant fecal carriage of extended-spectrum β-lactamase-producing Enterobacteriaceae and infection after liver transplant, France. Emerg Infect Dis. 2012;18:908–16.
149. Lübbert C, Becker-Rux D, Rodloff AC, et al. Colonization of liver transplant recipients with KPC-producing Klebsiella pneumoniae is associated with high infection rates and excess mortality: a case-control analysis. Infection. 2014;42:309–16.
150. Ullmann AJ, Schmidt-Hieber M, Bertz H, et al. Infectious diseases in allogeneic haematopoietic stem cell transplantation: prevention and prophylaxis strategy guidelines 2016. Ann Hematol. 2016;95(9):1435–55.
151. Facility Guidance for Control of Carbapenem-resistant Enterobacteriaceae (CRE) – November 2015 Update CRE Toolkit. https://www.cdc.gov/hai/pdfs/cre/CRE-guidance-508.pdf.
152. Sellin JH. The pathophysiology of diarrhea. Clin Transplant. 2001;15(Supple 4):29–35.
153. Angarone M, Ison MG. Diarrhea in solid organ transplant recipients. Curr Opin Infect Dis. 2015;28:308–16.
154. Arslan H, Inci EK, Azap OK, et al. Etiologic agents of diarrhea in solid organ recipients. Transpl Infect Dis. 2007;9:270–5.
155. Dhar JM, Al-Khader AA, Al-Sulaiman M, et al. Non-typhoid Salmonella in renal transplant recipients: a report of twenty cases and review of the literature. Q J Med. 1991;78:235–50.
156. Lübbert C. Antimicrobial therapy of acute diarrhoea: a clinical review. Expert Rev Anti Infect Ther. 2016;14(2):193–206.
157. Washington JA 2nd, Birk RJ, Ritts RE Jr. Bacteriologic and epidemiologic characteristics of Enterobacter hafniae and Enterobacter liquefaciens. J Infect Dis. 1971;124:379–86.
158. Günthard H, Pennekamp A. Clinical significance of extraintestinal Hafnia alvei isolates from 61 patients and review of the literature. Clin Infect Dis. 1996;22:1040–5.
159. Barry JW, Dominguez EA, Boken DJ, Preheim LC. Hafnia alvei infection after liver transplantation. Clin Infect Dis. 1997;24:1263–4.
160. Benito MH, Hernández RS, Fernàndez-Reyes MJ, Hernando S. Sepsis induced by Hafnia alvei in a kidney transplant patient. Nefrologia. 2008;28:470–1.
161. Cardile AP, Forbes D, Cirigliano V, et al. Hafnia alvei pyelonephritis in a renal transplant recipient: case report and review of an under-recognized nosocomial pathogen. Transpl Infect Dis. 2011;13:407–10.
162. Shubov A, Jagannathan P, Chin-Hong PV. Pantoea agglomerans pneumonia in a heart-lung transplant recipient: case report and a review of an emerging pathogen in immunocompromised hosts. Transpl Infect Dis. 2011;13(5):536–9.
163. Cheruvattath R, Balan V, Stewart R, et al. Kluyvera co-infection in two solid organ transplant recipients: an emerging pathogen or a colonizer bystander? Transpl Infect Dis. 2007;9(1):83–6.

Pseudomonas, *Stenotrophomonas*, *Acinetobacter*, and Other Nonfermentative Gram-Negative Bacteria and Medically Important Anaerobic Bacteria in Transplant Recipients

26

Kenneth V. I. Rolston and Amar Safdar

Introduction

Aerobic gram-negative bacilli currently account for 15–20% of monomicrobial bacterial infections in neutropenic patients, including patients with hematologic malignancies and those undergoing stem cell allograft transplantation [1, 2]. Furthermore, 80% of polymicrobial infections have a gram-negative component [3]. Since polymicrobial infections now account for 25–30% of documented bacterial infections, a trend that has been increasing in recent years, gram-negative bacilli are isolated from nearly 50% of bacterial infections in this patient population. This occurs despite the use of antimicrobial prophylaxis directed primarily against gram-negative bacilli in high-risk patient groups. The majority of gram-negative pathogens are residents of the human gastrointestinal or skin microflora, although some are acquired from environmental or other sources. In general, monomicrobial gram-negative and polymicrobial infections are associated with greater morbidity and mortality than infections due to gram-positive bacteria. Consequently, the prompt administration of empiric broad-spectrum, parenteral, antimicrobial therapy is considered the standard of care for febrile neutropenic patients, who are at increased risk for developing such infections [4]. Unfortunately, neutropenic episodes occur often, and the frequent use of antimicrobial agents for prophylaxis and therapy often leads to the emergence and/or selection of resistant microorganisms [5–7]. Some organisms acquire several mechanisms of drug resistance that render them nonsusceptible to a number of antimicrobials belonging to different classes of antibiotic. Multidrug resistant (MDR) bacteria are defined as exhibiting resistance to three or more classes of antimicrobial agents that are expected to be active against a particular pathogen. MDR gram-negative pathogens such as *Pseudomonas aeruginosa*, *Stenotrophomonas maltophilia*, and *Acinetobacter* species pose a significant problem, especially since the research and clinical development of novel antimicrobial agents remains relatively scarce as outlined by several recent monographs and publications from Infectious Diseases Society of America (IDSA) [8, 9].

Current Spectrum of Gram-Negative Infections

Most cancer and transplant centers have documented a decline in the proportion of bacterial infections caused by aerobic gram-negative bacilli over the past three decades, with a corresponding increase in gram-positive and polymicrobial infections [1, 2, 10]. Of late, some centers are reporting a shift back toward a predominance of gram-negative infections with an alarming increase in the frequency of MDR organisms [11, 12]. Unfortunately, most epidemiologic studies have focused primarily on monomicrobial bacteremia and have failed to provide data on polymicrobial infections and on sites of infections other than the bloodstream such as the respiratory tract, urinary tract, skin/skin structure, hepatobiliary, and intestinal tract infections [1, 13]. Since bacteremia account for only 15–25% of infections in such patients, these data underscore an incomplete picture regarding the epidemiology of gram-negative infections including those caused by NFGNB, and perhaps substantially underestimating their true frequency [2], whereas bacteremic infections including catheter-related bacteremia are caused predominantly by skin-dwelling gram-positive organisms in up to 75–80% in some

K. V. I. Rolston
Department of Infectious Diseases, Infection Control & Employee Health, The University of Texas MD Anderson Cancer Center, Houston, TX, USA
e-mail: krolston@mdanderson.org

A. Safdar (✉)
Clinical Associate Professor of Medicine, Texas Tech University Health Sciences Center El Paso, Paul L. Foster School of Medicine, El Paso, TX, USA
e-mail: amar.safdar@cidimmunology.com

A. Safdar (ed.), *Principles and Practice of Transplant Infectious Diseases*, https://doi.org/10.1007/978-1-4939-9034-4_26

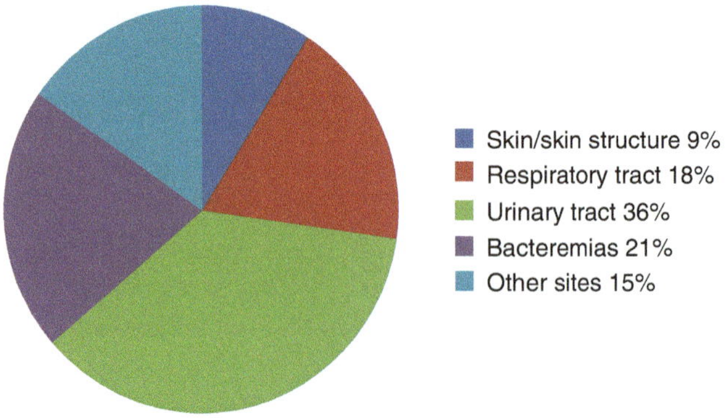

Fig. 26.1 The most common sites of gram-negative infections in patients with hematologic malignancies and in HSCT recipients. (Data are from the M.D. Anderson Cancer Center (2011–2012))

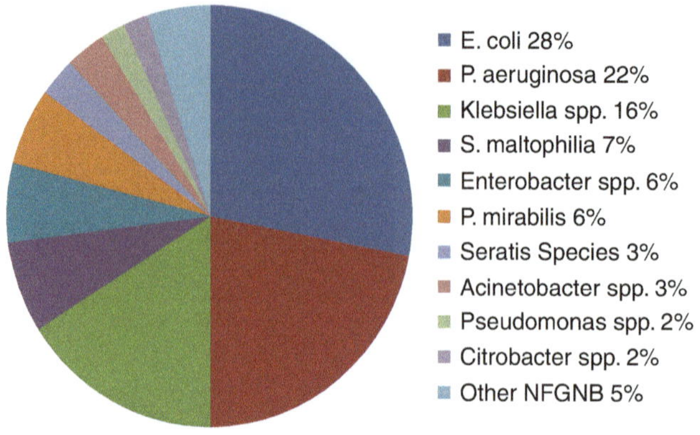

Fig. 26.2 Proportion of various gram-negative bacilli causing infection in patients with hematologic malignancies and in HSCT recipients. (Data are from the M.D. Anderson Cancer Center (2011–2012) and include adult and pediatric patients)

reports. Gram-negative bacteria predominate at most other sites of infection. Additionally, 80% of polymicrobial infections have a gram-negative component, and 30–35% are caused by multiple gram-negative bacterial species [3, 14].

Consequently, when all sites of infections and polymicrobial infections are taken into account, a substantially different epidemiologic picture emerges, with a greater proportion of infections being caused by gram-negative organisms. The most common sites of bacterial infection in HSCT recipients are depicted in Fig. 26.1. These include urinary tract infections, bacteremia, and respiratory tract infections. Other less common but important sites include the hepatobiliary and intestinal tracts such as cholangitis; neutropenic enterocolitis; perirectal infections; and infections involving pleura, peritoneum, synovium, and meninges.

A number of studies from various parts of the globe have consistently shown that *Escherichia coli*, *P. aeruginosa*, and *Klebsiella* species are the most common gram-negative pathogens isolated from patients undergoing stem cell graft transplantation and solid organ allograft, especially kidney, intestinal, liver, and lung transplantation both in adults and in children [1, 13, 15, 16]. Local and institutional differences do occur. It is therefore important to conduct periodic epidemiologic surveillance studies in order to determine the most current spectrum of infections and antimicrobial drug susceptibility profile of clinically prominent bacteria, particularly at institutions that care for a large number of immunosuppressed transplant population (Fig. 26.2). The rest of this chapter will focus on specific infections caused by NFGNB.

Nonfermentative Gram-Negative Bacilli

Despite the overall decline in the frequency of gram-negative infections in cancer patients, there has been an increase in the proportion of such infections caused by NFGNB [17, 18]. Collectively, NFGNB caused 36–38% of documented gram-negative infections in this setting, a proportion that has steadily increased over the past three decades—Table 26.1 [19–22].

P. aeruginosa is the most frequently isolated and the most important pathogen in this group. Non-*aeruginosa Pseudomonas* species such as *Pseudomonas putida and Pseudomonas fluorescens* are much less common and considered less serious compared with infections due to *P. aeruginosa* [17, 18, 23]. The frequency of infections caused by *S. maltophilia* has risen dramatically over the past two decades and may be related to the widespread use of the carbapenems and broad-spectrum beta-lactams as monotherapy in febrile neutropenic patients [24]. *S. maltophilia* is now the second most common NFGNB isolated from patients being treated in our intensive care unit (unpublished data from the MDACC antimicrobial stewardship program and infection control service). These isolates are often multidrug resistant and appear to be causing infections in patients without classic predisposing factors [25]. *Acinetobacter* species are still relatively uncommon, particularly if only bacteremic infections are considered and poses a serious challenge, as most hospital-onset infections are resistant to a number of broad-spectrum antibacterial drugs. Other NFGNB including *Achromobacter* spp. and *Alcaligenes* spp. are distinctly uncommon but do cause serious infections. These pathogens will be discussed in greater detail below.

Pseudomonas aeruginosa

P. aeruginosa has emerged as a common cause of bacterial infections in neutropenic patients in the 1900s, and before the availability of antipseudomonal agents such as carbenicillin, infections due to *P. aeruginosa* were associated with mortality rates in excess of 90%. Since then, the development of potent antipseudomonal agents such as aminoglycosides,

Table 26.1 Increasing frequency of infections caused by NFGNB in patients with cancer [19–22 + MDACC[a]]

References	Year	Total no. of gram-negative isolates	NFGNB, no. (%)
Bodey et al. [19]	1985	941	245 (26)
Bodey et al. [19]	1986	851	220 (26)
Rolston et al. [20]	1993	679	159 (23)
Jacobson et al. [21]	1996	758	225 (30)
Rolston et al. [22]	2002	903	329 (36)
Unpublished data[a]	2011	831	319 (38)

Approximately 90% of episodes occurred in patients with hematologic malignancies and/or HSCT recipients

[a]Unpublished data from epidemiologic/surveillance study conducted in 2011 at the M.D. Anderson Cancer Center

Table 26.2 The spectrum of infections caused by *Pseudomonas aeruginosa* and other NFGNB

Bacteremia—primary and catheter related
Pneumonia, empyema, lung abscess[a]
Urinary tract infection—primary and catheter related
Neutropenic enterocolitis (typhlitis)
Perirectal infection/abscess[a]
Skin and skin structure infection (ecthyma)
Cholangitis/biliary tract infection
Abdominal/pelvic/hepatic abscess[a]
Otitis externa/mastoiditis
Keratitis/endophthalmitis
Osteomyelitis/septic arthritis
Prostatitis

Data from Infectious Diseases consultation records at M.D. Anderson Cancer Center

[a]Abscess formation is uncommon in patients with severe and prolonged neutropenia

penicillins, cephalosporins, and carbapenems along with advances in critical and supportive care have resulted in markedly reduced mortality to less than 20%. Substantial regional and institutional variation in the frequency of pseudomonal infections has been documented [15]. Some institutions have reported a decline in the frequency of infections caused by *P. aeruginosa* possibly related to the use of fluoroquinolone prophylaxis in the high-risk patient population. However, at most major cancer and stem cell transplant treatment centers, *P. aeruginosa* remains among the three most common gram-negative pathogens and causes between 15% and 20% of all gram-negative invasive bacterial disease [1, 2, 10, 11]. Additionally it is the most common gram-negative organism isolated among immunosuppressed patients with polymicrobial bacterial infections [3, 14]. Drug susceptibility and resistance patterns also differ from institution to institution. Consequently, knowledge of local epidemiology and susceptibility and resistance patterns is critical, particularly since the administration of empiric therapy in high-risk patients with fever or suspected sepsis is the standard of care. A recent review of *P. aeruginosa* infection episodes in cancer patients identified several risk factors [26]. Most patients (54%) had an underlying hematologic malignancy; usually a variant of acute leukemia. *P. aeruginosa* bacteremia was 27 times more common in patients with acute leukemia than in patients with solid tumors. During the 2 weeks prior to documentation of *P. aeruginosa* bacteremia, 89% of patients received some form of antineoplastic therapy, prominently myelosuppressive chemotherapy, and 43% underwent an invasive procedure or placement of a medical device such as urinary or intravascular catheter or an ommaya reservoir. Additionally, during the 7 days preceding the onset of *P. aeruginosa* bacteremia, 36% of patients had received antibiotics for presumed or documented infections. The practice of administering intensive chemotherapy in the outpatient setting, and of outpatient-early discharge following hospitalization for the transplantation procedure, has had an impact on *P. aeruginosa* infections. In the study cited above, 50% of patients with *P. aeruginosa* bacteremia were not hospitalized. However, 9% had been discharged during the preceding 3 days, and 25% had been discharged during the preceding week.

The spectrum of clinical disease caused by *P. aeruginosa* is wide (Table 26.2). Pneumonia, primary and catheter-related bacteremia, and urinary tract infections are common. Other serious, often life-threatening infections include neutropenic enterocolitis, perirectal infections, and meningitis. When central venous catheters, or other foreign medical devices are infected, removal of the device, in addition to antipseudomonal therapy, is almost always necessary [27]. Colonization of the respiratory tract often precedes infection. Some experts recommend the use of aerosolized antimicrobial agents, especially the aminoglycosides in addition to systemic agents, in patients with pseudomonal pneumonia, although definitive evidence of the usefulness of this approach is lacking [28]. True abscess formation is uncommon in patients with neutropenia, and surgical incision and drainage are often beneficial in patients with perirectal infections [29]. Complicated urinary tract infections are difficult to cure, especially if foreign bodies such as stents or anatomical diversions are present. Recurrent episodes of infection are common, and long-term suppressive therapy may occasionally be necessary.

P. aeruginosa has the potential for developing resistance to antimicrobial agents by multiple cellular mechanisms of resistance [30, 31]. A recent study demonstrated that the risk factors associated with multidrug-resistant *P. aeruginosa* infections were the use of a carbapenem as monotherapy for >7 days, a history of *P. aeruginosa* during the preceding year, and a history of chronic obstructive pulmonary disease [32]. Data from M.D. Anderson Cancer Center Infection Control and Antimicrobial Stewardship Programs demonstrated that the frequency of multidrug-resistant pseudomonal infections at this institution was 0.16 per 1000 patient days from 2009 to mid-2011. Consequently, the Antimicrobial Stewardship team started monitoring carbapenem usage since July 2011. Patients receiving carbapenems, except ertapenem, were identified and the primary team caring for the patient were asked to (a) justify further usage of the agent usually based on microbiologic criteria, (b) discontinue the agent, or (c) seek the advice of the consulting Infectious Diseases team for possible alternative treatment options. Compliance with these options was about 70% and resulted in a substantial reduction in carbapenem usage; furthermore, a decline in the frequency of MDR infections to 0.10 per 1000 patient days was encouraging [33].

Table 26.3 Frequency of moderate- to high-grade bacteremia[a] caused by NFGNB in cancer patients at M.D. Anderson Cancer Center

	Moderate- to high-grade bacteremia No. (%) of isolates		
Organisms	1998	2004	2011
NFGNB isolates	111 (39)[b]	75 (42)[c]	117 (52)[d]
Stenotrophomonas maltophilia	4 (4)	13 (17)	26 (22)
Pseudomonas aeruginosa	14 (13)	8 (10)	37 (31)
Acinetobacter spp.	7 (6)	8 (10)	11 (9)

[a]Moderate grade: 101–500 CFU/ml. High grade: >500 CFU/ml, using quantitative cultures
[b]From a total of 284 gram-negative bacilli
[c]From a total of 186 gram-negative bacilli
[d]From a total of 224 gram-negative bacilli

Stenotrophomonas maltophilia

S. maltophilia colonization and infection rates in patients with cancer and HSCT have progressively increased over the past two to three decades. Surveillance studies conducted at the University of Texas M.D. Anderson Cancer Center have documented an increase in the proportion of *S. maltophilia* from 2% of all gram-negative bacilli isolated in 1986 to 7% in 2012. During this period, *S. maltophilia* increased from being the ninth most common gram-negative bacteria isolated to the fifth most common. Patients with prolonged neutropenia, those exposed to broad-spectrum antibiotics, especially the carbapenems, and those requiring mechanical ventilation have a higher risk for such infections [34–36]. The shift from TMP/SMX, which has potent activity against *S. maltophilia* to the fluoroquinolones and are far less active against *S. maltophilia,* as the standard agent for antibacterial prophylaxis in high-risk patients may also have contributed to the rise in infections caused by *S. maltophilia* (K. Rolston – unpublished data). *S. maltophilia* infections are also being documented more often in patients without traditional risk factors [25]. Some of these infections appear to be community onset, as they are being encountered in patients not previously exposed to the healthcare environment. The most common clinical manifestations of *S. maltophilia* infections in HSCT recipients include bacteremia, which is often related to an indwelling intravascular device, pneumonia, tracheitis, or airway anastomosis site infection in lung transplant recipients, skin and skin structure infections, and complicated urinary tract infections that is often noted in patients with obstructive uropathy or presence of indwelling foreign medical devices such as percutaneous nephrostomy tubes, among others [34, 37, 38]. Rapidly progressive hemorrhagic pneumonia is not an uncommon clinical presentation, particularly in patients who have failed to engraft allogenic stem cell infusion and remain severely neutropenic [39, 40]. This condition is often fatal despite prompt therapy and appropriate supportive care. Furthermore, at the author's (K. Rolston) institution, *S. maltophilia* bacteremia has been associated with a significant increase in moderate- to high-grade bacteremia, defined as greater than 100 CFU/ml in quantitative blood culture measurements, and may reflect a heightened severity for these infections (Table 26.3).

Recovery of *S. maltophilia* on microbiological cultures does not always indicate the presence of infection. Skin and intestinal colonization are not uncommon, especially in patients with extensive exposure to healthcare environment. Intestinal colonization may occur after fluroquinolone prophylaxis. In a recent study, *S. maltophilia* intestinal colonization was demonstrated in 10% of hospitalized neutropenic patients [41]. *S. maltophilia* colonization of the respiratory tract occurs frequently in patients with (a) prolonged stay in an intensive care unit, (b) presence of a tracheostomy, (c) prolonged exposure to broad-spectrum antibiotics, and (d) those with cystic fibrosis being considered for lung transplantation. Colonization often precedes infection.

For decades, trimethoprim/sulfamethoxazole (TMP-SMX) has been the agent with the most potent and reliable activity against *S. maltophilia*, but resistance appears to be increasing [42]. Several beta-lactams including ceftazidime, cefepime, ticarcillin-clavulanate, and piperacillin-tazobactam, have been reported to have variable activity, ranging from 35% to 70% against clinical *S. maltophilia* isolates [43]. The organisms are uniformly resistant to the carbapenems and the aminoglycosides also have poor activity against them. The fluoroquinolones have variable activity, with newer agents such as moxifloxacin being more active than ciprofloxacin and levofloxacin [17, 44]. Minocycline and the novel glycycline, like tigecycline, are also active against many *S. maltophilia* isolates [45]. TMP/SMX still represents the agent of choice for the treatment of infections caused by *S. maltophilia*. Some experts recommend high doses of TMP/SMX similar to doses used for pneumonia caused by *Pnemonocysits jiroveci*. Combination regimens based on the susceptibility of individual isolates are often employed.

Acinetobacter baumannii Complex

Acinetobacter baumannii is being increasingly recognized worldwide as a significant cause of morbidity and mortality in hospitalized patients, especially those with hematologic malignancies and neutropenia [46–48]. Many centers are reporting high rates of *Acinetobacter* spp. isolation. In one Brazilian cancer center, *A. baumannii* represented 9.3% of bloodstream infections over a 2-year period [49]. This rate slightly surpassed that of *P. aeruginosa* isolated in clinical specimens. Similarly, at the National Taiwan University hospital, the *A. baumannii* isolation rate was 6%, being higher than those of *P. aeruginosa* and *Enterobacter* spp. [47]. At the National Cancer Institute in Cairo, Egypt, *Acinetobacter* spp. comprised 6.9% of over 770 isolates from patients with hematologic malignancies and/or solid tumors [50]. *Acinetobacter* is also seen in the pediatric population. In one report, 92 bloodstream infections were caused by *Acinetobacter* spp. over a 5-year period, including nearly 50% of cases in children [51].

The clinical manifestations of *Acinetobacter* spp. infection are similar to those seen with other gram-negative bacillary infections, with pneumonia, bacteremia, urinary tract infections, and wound infections being predominant [52–54]. Although having an underlying malignancy is an important risk factor for the development of *Acinetobacter* spp. infection, it is not clear whether patients with cancer have a higher attributable mortality due to these infections compared with non-immunosuppressed oncology population despite the fact that a number of such infections may be due to multidrug-resistant isolates [46, 55].

The rising levels of antimicrobial resistance that have been documented among other gram-negative bacilli are also being seen in clinical *Acinetobacter* isolates [56]. In a large European study of antimicrobial susceptibility of bacterial isolates collected between 2004 and 2007, approximately 16% of the *A. baumannii* isolates were noted to be MDR organisms [57]. Due to the development of MDR gram-negative isolates, older drugs such as colistin and other polymyxin compounds, which have been long disfavored mainly due to systemic drug toxicity, are making a comeback [58]. In an attempt to reduce toxicity and maintain, or even enhance efficacy, strategies such as aerosolized/inhaled colistin administration are being evaluated and, to some extent, have been shown to be successful [59, 60]. Unfortunately, resistance to colistin among *A. baumannii* isolates has also been reported. In a recent study looking at colistin resistance among *A. baumannii* isolates collected from across the globe, 23% were found to be colistin heteroresistant [61]. In another recent study, the in vitro activity of tigecycline, minocycline, and a colistin/tigecycline combination against *A. baumannii* including colistin-resistant strains was evaluated [62]. Tigecycline showed better activity than minocycline even against pandrug-resistant bacterial strains. As with other antimicrobial agents, resistance to tigecycline is emerging [63].

Other NFGNB

Approximately 4–7% of all gram-negative infections in HSCT recipients are caused by other less common, albeit clinically important NFBNB such as *Achromobacter* species, *Alcaligenes* species, *Burkholderia* species, *Chryseobacterium* species, and non*aeruginosa Pseudomonas* species like *P. fluorescens* and *P. putida*. *Achromobacter* sp. and *Alcaligenes* species are ubiquitous organisms and most infections can be traced to sources such as contaminated dialysis fluid, chlorhexidine solution, deionized water, mechanical ventilators, and incubators [64]. Patients with cancer, those undergoing HSCT or solid organ transplantation, and those with HIV/AIDs or other immune compromised states are at increased risk. These infections are often life threatening. The most common clinical manifestation is primary uncomplicated bacteremia, although infected indwelling catheters and other foreign medical devices, pneumonia, and meningitis have also been reported. Although uncommon, the clinical importance of these organisms has increased in recent years, as they may occur in outbreak clusters and due to infecting organisms may not be susceptible to commonly used antibiotics.

These organisms are uniformly resistant to the fluoroquinolones, and the impact of near-universal use of fluorinated quinolone prophylaxis in HSCT and high-risk solid organ allograft recipients, the frequency of such infections, needs to be formally studied. Most isolates are susceptible to TMP-SMX, and the frequency of these infections appears to have increased, albeit slowly, since TMP-SMX was abandoned in favor of the quinolones for routine antibacterial prophylaxis [65]. Most isolates are also susceptible to the carbapenems. Of concern is the detection of IMP-type metallo-B-lactamases from these organisms in the past decade, conferring carbapenem resistance [66]. Some combination regimens have been shown to be synergistic in vitro and may be preferred for therapy in neutropenic patients with severe sepsis and multiorgan dysfunction [67].

Burkholderia cepacia complex (BCC) are opportunistic pathogens that occasionally cause outbreaks in patients with cancer including HSCT recipients [68, 69]. These outbreaks can generally be traced to contaminated intravenous solutions, disinfectants such as chlorhexidine and povidone–iodine solutions, ultrasound gel, mouthwashes, and aerosols [70]. Infection of central venous catheters is common. The organisms are often susceptible to TMP-SMX, the carbapenems, fluroquinolones, and extended-spectrum cephalosporins including cefepime, ceftazidime and semisynthetic penicillin such as piperacillin, piperacillin-tazobactam. These infections are especially of concern among patients with advanced cystic fibrosis and those undergoing lung transplantation with severe long-standing structural lung disease. Presence of biofilm plays an important role in prolonged BCC colonization of the respiratory tract in such induvuduls and poses a serious risk of potentially life-threatening infection of the pulmonary allograft following transplantation. Aerosolized aminoglycoside have played an important role in ameliorating this complication and recurrent infections due to *B. cepacia* complex. Early recognition of outbreaks and strict implementation of infection control measures, once an outbreak has been identified, is an essential component of management.

Chrysobacterium species such as *Chrysobacterium meningosepticum* and *Chrysobacterium indologenes* are rare pathogens; however, life-threatening infections such as bacteremia, pneumonia, and meningitis, especially in immunocompromised individuals, may occasionally be seen [71–74]. Previously considered *Flavobacterium* species, some *Chrysobacterium* species, have now been regrouped as *Elizabethkingia* gen. nov., which was based on 16s r RNA gene sequencing analysis with the names as *Elizabethkingia meningoseptica* and *Elizabethkingia minuscola* [75]. They are waterborne, saprophytic microorganisms, ubiquitous in nature including plants, water, soil, and the hospital environment. Primary and catheter-related bacteremia, pneumonia, meningitis, and skin and skin structure infections have been reported [76]. *E. meningoseptica* displays a strong biofilm-forming phenotype, which may play a role in its pathogenicity [77]. Carbapenem resistance has been described and appears to be mediated by metallo-B-lactamase Bla B [78]. The organisms are susceptible to TMP-SMX, fluoroquinolones, rifampin, minocycline, tigecycline, vancomycin, and piperacillin-tazobactam [79–81]. The overall mortality is approximately 25%, and combination drug therapy may be the prudent option in most cases [82].

P. fluorescens and *P. putida* are members of the fluorescent-pseudomonad group. Unlike *P. aeruginosa*, these organisms have low levels of inherent virulence. They do colonize the skin in some individuals and can cause pseudo-bacteremia and procedure-related infections [83]. The association between *P. fluorescens* and contaminated blood products has been well established [84–86]. They are also present in commercial bottled water, which can be a source of infection in neutropenic HSCT recipients [87–89]. Catheter-related bacteremia and pneumonia are the most common clinical manifestations [23]. Carbapenems have the most reliable activity against these organisms. The activity of other beta-lactams and fluoroquinolones is variable [17]. The overall mortality associated with these organisms is low. Many patients respond to the removal of the offending catheter alone, and most respond to appropriate antimicrobial therapy.

Anaerobic Gram-Negative Bacterial Infections

Stem cell and solid organ transplantation is a lifesaving medical intervention in patients with aggressive hematologic malignancies and end-stage solid organ dysfunction and organ failure [90–94]. Iatrogenic drug-induced immune suppression is needed for the maintenance of a functioning solid organ allograft; to harness and sustain the delicate balance between potentially devastating graft-versus-host disease and the much desired, allogenic stem cell-assisted graft-versus -leukemia/lymphoma or antitumor effect; the resultant immune suppression contributes significantly toward hosts' susceptibility for opportunistic infections [94–99]. In patients undergoing solid organ transplantation, surgical site and deep tissue infections are mostly seen during the early (≤1 month) post-transplantation period [90]. Most bacterial infections in such patients, despite having severe immune defects, are due to conventional aerobic bacteria. Anaerobic gram-positive or gram-negative bacteria, on the other hand, are a seldom cause for systemic disease. In this section, a brief review of anaerobic infections is provided.

In prior reports, the four prominent anaerobic bacterial genera isolated from HSCT recipients included *Propionibacterium* spp. [100], *Bacteroides* spp. [101], *Clostridium* spp. [102], and *Prevotella* spp. [96]. Whereas, in patients undergoing solid organ transplantation, *Bacteroides* spp. [97], *Clostridium* spp. [92], and *Prevotella* spp. [92] are dominant anaerobic bacterial genera isolated.

Stem Cell Transplantation

In a retrospective 4-year review of BSIs following HSCT, 17% of infections were due to anaerobic bacteria [103]. In this report, *Fusobacterium nucleatum* (n = 17) followed by *Leptotrichia buccalis* (n = 4) were prominent, whereas *Clostridium septicum* (n = 1) and *Clostridium tertium* (n = 1) were rarely isolated [103]. Presence of severe mucositis was associated with a greater than fourfold higher probability of infection due to anaerobes [102–104]. Interventions that reduce severity and duration of early post-transplant mucositis are important factors for risk mitigation for such infections [103]. This was supported by higher frequency of invasive bacterial infections due to commensal anaerobic bacteria noted during mid and late 1990s, a period during which high-dose methotrexate was routinely used for pre-HSCT conditioning and its well-established risk for debilitating mucositis. Furthermore, others have observed an association between the risk of post-transplant bacteremia and high-dose preparatory conditioning regimens given prior to transplantation [105].

A novel anaerobe, *Leptotrichia hongkongensis,* was isolated in five of eight patients with multiple myeloma undergoing autologous stem cell infusion after high-dose chemotherapy. This commensal bacterium that primarily resides in the orointestinal and female genital tracts is difficult to isolate in routine laboratory anaerobic cultures. Molecular diagnostic assays are needed for identification and confirmation of this fastidious pathogen [105, 106]. *Leptotrichia* infections are rare in the general population;

risk for these uncommon pathogens increases in patients with suppressed immune response and along with other risk factors stated earlier for invasive anaerobic bacterial disease [107, 108]. It is important to emphasize that on Gram staining, *Leptotrichia* may be misidentified as a gram-positive rod and disregarded as probable *Bacillus* spp. contamination [109]. Along with other difficult-to-culture pathogens, 16S rRNA analysis has become the gold standard in the diagnosis of *Leptotrichia* spp. infection [110, 111].

Patients with impaired cell-mediated immune response are at an increased risk for *Legionella* spp. infection. In recipients of allogeneic stem cell or solid organ transplantation, legionella infection frequently presents as serious systemic illness involving lungs as well as life-threatening extra-pulmonary disease. In transplant patients with *Legionella pneumophila* infection, secondary infection(s) may involve an anaerobic bacteria such as *Prevotella* spp. [112]. As with other immunosuppressed patients, those undergoing transplantation, who develop lung abscess or empyema, a heightened awareness for polymicrobial infection with mixed aerobic and/or anaerobic bacteria will assist in appropriate empiric selection of antibiotics. The authors are of the opinion that early surgical therapeutic drainage of lung abscesses and empyema will also provide a desirable specimen for microbiological diagnosis. When anaerobes are suspected, use of advanced molecular diagnostic assays such as 16SrRNA analysis will improve the diagnostic yield compared with conventional anaerobic laboratory culture methods.

Acute GVHD is a serious complication after allogeneic stem cell transplantation. The composition of the intestinal microflora of patients, especially prevalence of anaerobic microbiota, was investigated as a potential predictor for the risk of acute GVHD [113]. A favorable impact for GVHD risk in nonprimates and nonhuman primates was demonstrated by creating a germ-free or decontaminated intestinal microenvironment [114–116]. Results of these experiments encouraged clinical evaluation for such interventions in patients undergoing allogeneic HSCT. In 194 patients undergoing identical sibling bone marrow stem cell transplantation, influence of intestinal bacterial decontamination and strict isolation protocol on the risk of moderate to severe acute GVHD was assessed [113]. Acute GVHD was noted in 23% of patients after a median of 33 days following transplantation; sustained suppression of intestinal anaerobic bacteria microflora favorably influenced the cumulative incidence of acute GVHD in this study ($P < 0.006$) [113]. Further large scale clinical assesssment is needed for validation of this hypothesis.

Intestinal anaerobic microflora from the domain Archaea are methanogens or methane producers that have evolved to adapt to extremes of environment conditions. The predominant methanogen in the human intestinal tract is a gram-negative anaerobe, *Methanobrevibacter smithii* [117]. These bacteria are nonsusceptible to most antibiotics, although they retain susceptibility to metronidazole [118]. Metronidazole prophylaxis has been associated with reduced frequency of moderate to severe acute GVHD [119, 120]. The underlying hypothesis is based on reduced immunostimulation caused by bacterial products, especially by methanogens. Eleven of 13 patients undergoing HSCT treated with metronidazole showed reduced methane gas in feces [121]. In all 11 patients with post-metronidazole treatment-negative fecal methane detection observed at 2 and 5 weeks after transplantation, risk for acute GVHD was significantly modified [121]. The authors caution regarding drug-induced suppression of anaerobic microbiota in the lower intestinal tract, especially in the immunosuppressed patients undergoing allogeneic stem cell transplantation. The extended alteration in homeostasis of patients' intestinal microflora may compromise the physiologic protection proffered by the gram-negative anaerobes in the large intestine, thereby creating a niche for colonization and subsequent disease due to microoragnisms such as MDR GNB, vancomycin-resistant enterococci and exotoxin-producing *Clostridium difficile*, to name a few.

Solid Organ Transplantation

In the past three decades, overall survival and quality of life after solid organ allograft transplantation have greatly improved. Advances in surgical techniques, sophistication in prevention and treatment of allograft rejection, progress in infection prophylaxis and management, and additionally improved comprehensive supportive care have all contributed favorably toward this trend. Infections are either due to microorganisms that are endogenous to the host microbiota or acquired from the environment of patients [122]. The overall frequency of infection varies among various solid allograft recipients: 33–68% after liver transplantation; 21–30% after heart; 35% following pancreas; 47% in kidney; and 54% in patients undergoing lung transplantation [90]. Enteric pathogens such as *Enterococcus* spp. and gram-negative aerobic and anaerobic bacteria are prominent bacterial pathogens in patients after liver transplantation. In many transplant centers, selective bowel decontamination sparing the gut anaerobic flora has been used to reduce the risk for early post-transplant infections due to aerobic gram-negative bacteria; this is an important consideration in patients who are considered at increased risk for such infections [123, 124]. However, the data supporting selective bowel decontamination as a routine practice remain controversial. Furthermore, concern for selection and colonization with drug-resistant pathogens like MDR *Pseudomonas*, extended-spectrum beta-lactamase-producing *Enterobacteriaceae*, vancomycin-resistant enterococci, yeast overgrowth, and expansion of microaerophilic gram-positive bacteria like *Lactobacillus* spp. are a hypothetical, albeit, serious concern [125, 126]. It is appealing that selective bowel decontamination has shown reduced risk for GNB infections during the early post-transplant period in patients undergoing solid organ allograft transplant surgery [100, 101, 127–130].

In 103 patients following orthotopic liver transplantation, half of 115 bacterial infections observed in 68% of patients were noted within 2 weeks following transplant surgery [131]. Among 190 organisms recovered from 115 infection sites, gram-negative bacteria as expected were common (65%), with *E. coli* being the most prominent aerobic gram-negative pathogen. *Enterococcus* spp. were prevalent in 38% of gram-positive organisms. Eight percent anaerobes other than *C. difficile* included 4% *Bacteroides fragilis*. It is important to recognize that polymicrobial infections were observed in 37% of the episodes [131]. Intra-abdominal infections were common (69%), followed by surgical wounds (42%) and lung infections (36%) [131].

Pulmonary infections are considerably prominent in patients undergoing heart and heart–lung transplantation [132, 133]. In 12 heart–lung allograft recipients, 29 infection episodes accounted for 2.4% of infections per patient [133]. Among 18 of 29 bacterial infections, only one episode was due to *Bacteroides melaninogenicus* and presented as polymicrobial infection with aerobic bacteria. In the recipients of heart–lung allografts, anaerobic bacterial infections are often related to transtracheal and transthoracic aspiration; however, these infections are rarely observed [133].

The incidence of urinary tract infections after allograft renal transplantation ranges from 28% to as high as 90% in high-risk subgroups. Bacterial contamination of cadaveric renal grafts may be as high as 25%, although its association with post-transplant graft pyelonephritis is not convincing. In an earlier study, UTIs in renal transplant population due to anaerobic bacteria were 8%, which included *B. fragilis* and *B. melaninogenicus*; aerobic bacteria accounted for 24% of infections [134]. It appeared that most of these anaerobic infections were seen in patients following cadaveric renal grafts and associated with infections in the early post-transplant period; in contrast, post-transplant UTIs due to anaerobic bacteria were not noted following living donor renal graft transplantation. Since the introduction of routine prophylaxis with trimethoprim–sulfamethoxazole (TMP-SMX) in patients receiving comprehensive antirejection regimens after kidney transplantation, the overall frequency of bacterial UTIs with or without concurrent bacteremia have declined significantly [135–137].

Newer Agents

The emergence of resistant gram-negative bacilli including NFGNB as well as the *Enterobacteriaceae* created substantial therapeutic problems as outlined in several monographs and publications [8, 9]. These problems were made worse by the fact that new drug developments had come to a virtual standstill. In response to this, a global initiative termed "the 10 by 20 initiative" was launched with the goal of developing 10 agents with activity against resistant microorganisms by the year 2020 [138]. This initiative has encouraged the development of several novel agents, some of which have been approved by the FDA while others are in advanced stages of development (Table 26.4). Many of these agents have provided newer options for the treatment of resistant gram-negative infections and, to some extent, have replaced or supplanted older and more toxic agents such as the polymyxins [139]. Unfortunately, there already are reports of resistance to some of these newer agents, which have raised caution and as with all other antimicrobial agents, in vitro susceptibility should be performed when an infection-causing GNB is isolated in cultures [140–142]. It is important to recognize the advantage the new combination drugs offer against bacteria; they have acquired capability to produce serine carbapenemase including KCP, extended-spectrum beta-lactamase, and MDR *Pseudomonas*; these drugs, however, lack activity against metallo-beta-lactamase-producing organisms, including bacteria that are mostly seen as sporadic, nonoutbreak infections in the US hospitals [142]. Additional agents that are in early stages of development are in the pipeline and continue to provide hope for the future.

Table 26.4 Newer agents for the treatment of gram-negative bacterial infections[a]

Beta-lactam/beta-lactamase inhibitor combinations
Ceftazidime/avibactam[b]
Ceftolozane/tazobactam[c]
Meropenem/vaborbactam[c]
Imipenem-cilastatin/relebactam
Aztreonam/avibactam
Other agents
Cefiderocol (a novel siderophore cephalosporin)
Plazomicin (aminoglycoside derivative)
Eravacycline (a synthetic tetracycline derivative)

[a]Several other agents are in earlier phases of development (Phases 1 and 2)
[b]Ceftazidime/avibactam has been approved by the US Food and Drug Administration (FDA) and the European Medicines Agency
[c]Ceftolozane/tazobactam and meropenem/vaborbactam have been approved by the US FDA

Summary

An increasing proportion of bacterial infections in patients following stem cell and high-risk organ allograft recipients are due to NFGNB, which is despite the overall decline in the frequency of microbiologically proven invasive gram-negative bacterial disease in the immunosuppressed population. The spectrum and clinical manifestations of these infections are similar to those caused by *Enterobacteriaceae*. A common theme among many NFGNB is the development of resistance to multiple antimicrobial agents. Strategies to combat these infections include (a) judicious use of currently available antimicrobial agents with assistance and adherence to the antimicrobial stewardship protocols; (b) encourage and promote development of novel antimicrobial drug classes with nonredundant target of antibacterial activity, (c) revival of older antimicrobial agents with combination of novel classes of antibacterial hydrolyzing enzyme inhibitors, (d) development of novel antimicrobial agents, and (e) strict adherence to infection prevention guidelines and infection control policies designed to limit the spread of such infections, when they do occur. Nevertheless, infections caused by NFGNB, especially in the highly diverse and complicated transplant population, will continue to challenge clinicians in the foreseeable future.

References

1. Wisplinghoff H, Seifert H, Wenzel RP, et al. Current trends in the epidemiology of nosocomial bloodstream infections in patients with hematological malignancies and solid neoplasms in hospitals in the United States. Clin Infect Dis. 2003;36:1103–10.
2. Yadegarynia D, Tarrand J, Raad I, Rolston K. Current spectrum of bacterial infections in patients with cancer. Clin Infect Dis. 2003;37:1144–5.
3. Rolston KV, Bodey GP, Safdar A. Polymicrobial infection in patients with cancer: an underappreciated and underreported entity. Clin Infect Dis. 2007;45:228–33.
4. Freifeld AG, Bow EJ, Sepkowitz KA, et al. Clinical practice guideline for the use of antimicrobial agents in neutropenic patients with cancer: 2010 update by the Infectious Diseases Society of America. Clin Infect Dis. 2011;52:427–31.
5. Rangaraj G, Granwehr BP, Jiang Y, et al. Perils of quinolone exposure in cancer patients: breakthrough bacteremia with multidrug-resistant organisms. Cancer. 2010;116:967–73.
6. Cattaneo C, Quaresmini G, Casari S, et al. Recent changes in bacterial epidemiology and the emergence of fluoroquinolone-resistant Escherichia coli among patients with haematological malignancies: results of a prospective study on 823 patients at a single institution. J Antimicrob Chemother. 2008;61:721–8.
7. Mihu CN, Rhomberg PR, Jones RN, et al. Escherichia coli resistance to quinolones at a comprehensive cancer center. Diagn Microbiol Infect Dis. 2010;67:266–9.
8. Boucher HW, Talbot GH, Bradley JS, et al. Bad bugs, no drugs: no ESKAPE! An update from Infectious Diseases Society of America. Clin Infect Dis. 2009;48:1–12.
9. Talbot GH, Bradley J, Edwards JE Jr, et al. Bad bugs need drugs: an update on the development pipeline from the Antimicrobial Availability Task Force of the Infectious Diseases Society of America. Clin Infect Dis. 2006;42:657–68.
10. Klastersky J, Ameye L, Maertens J, et al. Bacteraemia in febrile neutropenic cancer patients. Int J Antimicrob Agents. 2007;30(Suppl 1):S51–9.
11. Mikulska M, Del Bono V, Bruzzi P, et al. Mortality after bloodstream infections in allogeneic haematopoietic stem cell transplant (HSCT) recipients. Infection. 2012;40:271–8.
12. Oliveira AL, de Souza M, Carvalho-Dias VM, et al. Epidemiology of bacteremia and factors associated with multi-drug-resistant gram-negative bacteremia in hematopoietic stem cell transplant recipients. Bone Marrow Transplant. 2007;39:775–81.
13. Zinner SH. Changing epidemiology of infections in patients with neutropenia and cancer: emphasis on gram-positive and resistant bacteria. Clin Infect Dis. 1999;29:490–4.
14. Elting LS, Bodey GP, Fainstein V. Polymicrobial septicemia in the cancer patient. Medicine (Baltimore). 1986;65:218–25.
15. Rolston KV, Tarrand JJ. Pseudomonas aeruginosa --still a frequent pathogen in patients with cancer: 11-year experience at a comprehensive cancer center. Clin Infect Dis. 1999;29:463–4.
16. Safdar A, Rodriguez GH, De Lima MJ, et al. Infections in 100 cord blood transplantations: spectrum of early and late posttransplant infections in adult and pediatric patients 1996-2005. Medicine (Baltimore). 2007;86:324–33.
17. Rolston KV, Kontoyiannis DP, Yadegarynia D, et al. Nonfermentative gram-negative bacilli in cancer patients: increasing frequency of infection and antimicrobial susceptibility of clinical isolates to fluoroquinolones. Diagn Microbiol Infect Dis. 2005;51:215–8.
18. Martino R, Martinez C, Pericas R, et al. Bacteremia due to glucose non-fermenting gram-negative bacilli in patients with hematological neoplasias and solid tumors. Eur J Clin Microbiol Infect Dis. 1996;15:610–5.
19. Bodey GP, Ho DH, Elting L. Survey of antibiotic susceptibility among gram-negative bacilli at a cancer hospital. Am J Med. 1988;85:49–51.
20. Rolston KV, Elting L, Waguespack S, et al. Survey of antibiotic susceptibility among gram-negative bacilli at a cancer center. Chemotherapy. 1996;42:348–53.
21. Jacobson K, Rolston K, Elting L, et al. Susceptibility surveillance among gram-negative bacilli at a cancer center. Chemotherapy. 1999;45:325–34.
22. Rolston KKD, Raad I, LeBlanc BJ, et al. Susceptibility surveillance among gram-negative bacilli at a comprehensive cancer center [A-004]. In: Program and abstracts of the 103rd general meeting of American Society of Microbiology. Washington, DC: American Society of Microbiology; 2003.
23. Anaissie E, Fainstein V, Miller P, et al. Pseudomonas putida. Newly recognized pathogen in patients with cancer. Am J Med. 1987;82:1191–4.
24. Sanyal SC, Mokaddas EM. The increase in carbapenem use and emergence of Stenotrophomonas maltophilia as an important nosocomial pathogen. J Chemother. 1999;11:28–33.
25. Aisenberg G, Rolston KV, Dickey BF, et al. Stenotrophomonas maltophilia pneumonia in cancer patients without traditional risk factors for infection, 1997-2004. Eur J Clin Microbiol Infect Dis. 2007;26:13–20.
26. Chatzinikolaou I, Abi-Said D, Bodey GP, et al. Recent experience with Pseudomonas aeruginosa bacteremia in patients with cancer: retrospective analysis of 245 episodes. Arch Intern Med. 2000;160:501–9.
27. Mermel LA, Allon M, Bouza E, et al. Clinical practice guidelines for the diagnosis and management of intravascular catheter-related infection: 2009 update by the Infectious Diseases Society of America. Clin Infect Dis. 2009;49:1–45.
28. Safdar A. Feasibility of aerosolized colistin in the era of escalating drug-resistant Pseudomonas pneumonia: pressing need for validation clinical trials. Intensive Care Med. 2010;36:1110–1.
29. Barnes SG, Sattler FR, Ballard JO. Perirectal infections in acute leukemia. Improved survival after incision and debridement. Ann Intern Med. 1984;100:515–8.
30. Aboufaycal H, Sader HS, Rolston K, et al. blaVIM-2 and blaVIM-7 carbapenemase-producing Pseudomonas aeruginosa isolates detected in a tertiary care medical center in the United States: report from the MYSTIC program. J Clin Microbiol. 2007;45:614–5.
31. Toleman MA, Rolston K, Jones RN, et al. blaVIM-7, an evolutionarily distinct metallo-beta-lactamase gene in a Pseudomonas aeruginosa isolate from the United States. Antimicrob Agents Chemother. 2004;48:329–32.
32. Ohmagari N, Hanna H, Graviss L, et al. Risk factors for infections with multidrug-resistant Pseudomonas aeruginosa in patients with cancer. Cancer. 2005;104:205–12.
33. Tverdek FP, Rolston KV, Chemaly RF. Antimicrobial stewardship in patients with cancer. Pharmacotherapy. 2012;32:722–34.
34. Safdar A, Rolston KV. Stenotrophomonas maltophilia: changing spectrum of a serious bacterial pathogen in patients with cancer. Clin Infect Dis. 2007;45:1602–9.

35. Safdar A, Rodriguez GH, Balakrishnan M, et al. Changing trends in etiology of bacteremia in patients with cancer. Eur J Clin Microbiol Infect Dis. 2006;25:522–6.
36. Micozzi A, Venditti M, Monaco M, et al. Bacteremia due to Stenotrophomonas maltophilia in patients with hematologic malignancies. Clin Infect Dis. 2000;31:705–11.
37. Vartivarian SE, Papadakis KA, Anaissie EJ. Stenotrophomonas (Xanthomonas) maltophilia urinary tract infection. A disease that is usually severe and complicated. Arch Intern Med. 1996;156:433–5.
38. Papadakis KA, Vartivarian SE, Vassilaki ME, et al. Stenotrophomonas maltophilia meningitis. Report of two cases and review of the literature. J Neurosurg. 1997;87:106–8.
39. Araoka H, Fujii T, Izutsu K, et al. Rapidly progressive fatal hemorrhagic pneumonia caused by Stenotrophomonas maltophilia in hematologic malignancy. Transpl Infect Dis. 2012;14:355–63.
40. Tada K, Kurosawa S, Hiramoto N, et al. Stenotrophomonas maltophilia infection in hematopoietic SCT recipients: high mortality due to pulmonary hemorrhage. Bone Marrow Transplant. 2013;48:74–9.
41. Apisarnthanarak A, Fraser VJ, Dunne WM, et al. Stenotrophomonas maltophilia intestinal colonization in hospitalized oncology patients with diarrhea. Clin Infect Dis. 2003;37:1131–5.
42. Vartivarian S, Anaissie E, Bodey G, et al. A changing pattern of susceptibility of Xanthomonas maltophilia to antimicrobial agents: implications for therapy. Antimicrob Agents Chemother. 1994;38:624–7.
43. Krueger TS, Clark EA, Nix DE. In vitro susceptibility of Stenotrophomonas maltophilia to various antimicrobial combinations. Diagn Microbiol Infect Dis. 2001;41:71–8.
44. Lecso-Bornet M, Pierre J, Sarkis-Karam D, et al. Susceptibility of Xanthomonas maltophilia to six quinolones and study of outer membrane proteins in resistant mutants selected in vitro. Antimicrob Agents Chemother. 1992;36:669–71.
45. Noskin GA. Tigecycline: a new glycylcycline for treatment of serious infections. Clin Infect Dis. 2005.;41Suppl 5;41:S303–14.
46. Rolston K, Guan Z, Bodey GP, et al. Acinetobacter calcoaceticus septicemia in patients with cancer. South Med J. 1985;78(6):647–51.
47. Chen CY, Tsay W, Tang JL, et al. Epidemiology of bloodstream infections in patients with haematological malignancies with and without neutropenia. Epidemiol Infect. 2010;138:1044–51.
48. Wisplinghoff H, Paulus T, Lugenheim M, et al. Nosocomial bloodstream infections due to Acinetobacter baumannii, Acinetobacter pittii and Acinetobacter nosocomialis in the United States. J Infect. 2012;64:282–90.
49. Velasco E, Byington R, Martins CA, et al. Comparative study of clinical characteristics of neutropenic and non-neutropenic adult cancer patients with bloodstream infections. Eur J Clin Microbiol Infect Dis. 2006;25:1–7.
50. Ashour HM, El-Sharif A. Species distribution and antimicrobial susceptibility of gram-negative aerobic bacteria in hospitalized cancer patients. J Transl Med. 2009;7:14.
51. Segal SC, Zaoutis TE, Kagen J, et al. Epidemiology of and risk factors for Acinetobacter species bloodstream infection in children. Pediatr Infect Dis J. 2007;26:920–6.
52. Gales AC, Jones RN, Forward KR, et al. Emerging importance of multidrug-resistant Acinetobacter species and Stenotrophomonas maltophilia as pathogens in seriously ill patients: geographic patterns, epidemiological features, and trends in the SENTRY Antimicrobial Surveillance Program (1997-1999). Clin Infect Dis. 2001;32(Suppl 2):S104–13.
53. Cayô R, Yañez San Segundo L, Pérez del Molino Bernal IC, et al. Bloodstream infection caused by Acinetobacter junii in a patient with acute lymphoblastic leukaemia after allogenic haematopoietic cell transplantation. J Med Microbiol. 2011;60:375–7.
54. Turkoglu M, Mirza E, Tunçcan OG, et al. Acinetobacter baumannii infection in patients with hematologic malignancies in intensive care unit: risk factors and impact on mortality. J Crit Care. 2011;26:460–7.
55. Turkoglu M, Dizbay M. Multidrug-resistant Acinetobacter baumannii infection is not an independent risk factor for mortality in critically ill patients with hematologic malignancy. J Crit Care. 2011;26:526–7.
56. Queenan AM, Pillar CM, Deane J, et al. Multidrug resistance among Acinetobacter spp. in the USA and activity profile of key agents: results from CAPITAL Surveillance 2010. Diagn Microbiol Infect Dis. 2012;73:267–70.
57. Nørskov-Lauritsen N, Marchandin H, Dowzicky MJ. Antimicrobial susceptibility of tigecycline and comparators against bacterial isolates collected as part of the TEST study in Europe (2004-2007). Int J Antimicrob Agents. 2009;34:121–30.
58. Vila J, Pachón J. Therapeutic options for Acinetobacter baumannii infections: an update. Expert Opin Pharmacother. 2012;13:2319–36.
59. Kuo SC, Lee YT, Yang SP, et al. Eradication of multidrug-resistant Acinetobacter baumannii from the respiratory tract with inhaled colistin methanesulfonate: a matched case-control study. Clin Microbiol Infect. 2012;18:870–6.
60. Dalfino L, Puntillo F, Mosca A, et al. High-dose, extended-interval colistin administration in critically ill patients: is this the right dosing strategy? A preliminary study. Clin Infect Dis. 2012;54:1720–6.
61. Yau W, Owen RJ, Poudyal A, et al. Colistin hetero-resistance in multidrug-resistant Acinetobacter baumannii clinical isolates from the Western Pacific region in the SENTRY antimicrobial surveillance programme. J Infect. 2009;58:138–44.
62. Arroyo LA, Mateos I, González V, et al. In vitro activities of tigecycline, minocycline, and colistin-tigecycline combination against multi- and pandrug-resistant clinical isolates of Acinetobacter baumannii group. Antimicrob Agents Chemother. 2009;53:1295–6.
63. Sun Y, Cai Y, Liu X, et al. The emergence of clinical resistance to tigecycline. Int J Antimicrob Agents. 2013;41:110–6.
64. Aisenberg G, Rolston KV, Safdar A. Bacteremia caused by Achromobacter and Alcaligenes species in 46 patients with cancer (1989-2003). Cancer. 2004;101:2134–40.
65. Rolston KV, Messer M. The in-vitro susceptibility of Alcaligenes denitrificans subsp. xylosoxidans to 40 antimicrobial agents. J Antimicrob Chemother. 1990;26:857–60.
66. Yamamoto M, Nagao M, Hotta G, et al. Molecular characterization of IMP-type metallo-β-lactamases among multidrug-resistant Achromobacter xylosoxidans. J Antimicrob Chemother. 2012;67:2110–3.
67. Saiman L, Chen Y, Gabriel PS, et al. Synergistic activities of macrolide antibiotics against Pseudomonas aeruginosa, Burkholderia cepacia, Stenotrophomonas maltophilia, and Alcaligenes xylosoxidans isolated from patients with cystic fibrosis. Antimicrob Agents Chemother. 2002;46:1105–7.
68. Mann T, Ben-David D, Zlotkin A, et al. An outbreak of Burkholderia cenocepacia bacteremia in immunocompromised oncology patients. Infection. 2010;38:187–94.
69. Yamagishi Y, Fujita J, Takigawa K, et al. Clinical features of Pseudomonas cepacia pneumonia in an epidemic among immunocompromised patients. Chest. 1993;103:1706–9.
70. Heo ST, Kim SJ, Jeong YG. Hospital outbreak of Burkholderia stabilis bacteraemia related to contaminated chlorhexidine in haematological malignancy patients with indwelling catheters. J Hosp Infect. 2008;70:241–5.
71. Bloch KC, Nadarajah R, Jacobs R. Chryseobacterium meningosepticum: an emerging pathogen among immunocompromised adults. Report of 6 cases and literature review. Medicine. 1997;76:30–41.
72. Chen FL, Wang GC, Teng SO, et al. Clinical and epidemiological features of Chryseobacterium indologenes infections: analysis of 215 cases. J Microbiol Immunol Infect. 2013;46:425–32.

73. Lin JT, Wang WS, Yen CC, et al. Chryseobacterium indologenes bacteremia in a bone marrow transplant recipient with chronic graft-versus-host disease. Scand J Infect Dis. 2003;35:882–3.
74. Adachi A, Mori T, Shimizu T, et al. Chryseobacterium meningosepticum septicemia in a recipient of allogeneic cord blood transplantation. Scand J Infect Dis. 2004;36:539–40.
75. Kim KK, Kim MK, Lim JH, et al. Transfer of Chryseobacterium meningosepticum and Chryseobacterium miricola to Elizabethkingia gen. nov. as Elizabethkingia meningoseptica comb. nov. and Elizabethkingia miricola comb. nov. Int J Syst Evol Microbiol. 2005;55:1287–93.
76. Hsu MS, Liao CH, Huang YT, et al. Clinical features, antimicrobial susceptibilities, and outcomes of Elizabethkingia meningoseptica (Chryseobacterium meningosepticum) bacteremia at a medical center in Taiwan, 1999-2006. Eur J Clin Microbiol Infect Dis. 2011;30:1271–8.
77. Jacobs A, Chenia HY. Biofilm formation and adherence characteristics of an Elizabethkingia meningoseptica isolate from Oreochromis mossambicus. Eur J Clin Microbiol Infect Dis. 2011;30:1271–8.
78. González LJ, Vila AJ. Carbapenem resistance in Elizabethkingia meningoseptica is mediated by metallo-β-lactamase BlaB. Antimicrob Agents Chemother. 2012;56:1686–92.
79. Hsueh PR, Hsiue TR, Wu JJ, et al. Flavobacterium indologenes bacteremia: clinical and microbiological characteristics. Clin Infect Dis. 1996;23:550–5.
80. Chang JC, Hsueh PR, Wu JJ, et al. Antimicrobial susceptibility of flavobacteria as determined by agar dilution and disk diffusion methods. Antimicrob Agents Chemother. 1997;41:1301–6.
81. Jiang X, Wang D, Wang Y, et al. Occurrence of antimicrobial resistance genes sul and dfrA12 in hospital environmental isolates of Elizabethkingia meningoseptica. World J Microbiol Biotechnol. 2012;28:3097–102.
82. Green O, Murray P, Gea-Banacloche JC. Sepsis caused by Elizabethkingia miricola successfully treated with tigecycline and levofloxacin. Diagn Microbiol Infect Dis. 2008;62:430–2.
83. Simor AE, Ricci J, Lau A, et al. Pseudobacteremia due to Pseudomonas fluorescens. Pediatr Infect Dis. 1985;4:508–12.
84. Scott J, Boulton FE, Govan JR, et al. A fatal transfusion reaction associated with blood contaminated with Pseudomonas fluorescens. Vox Sang. 1988;54:201–4.
85. Puckett A, Davison G, Entwistle CC, et al. Post transfusion septicaemia 1980-1989: importance of donor arm cleansing. J Clin Pathol. 1992;45:155–7.
86. Gershman MD, Kennedy DJ, Noble-Wang J, et al. Multistate outbreak of Pseudomonas fluorescens bloodstream infection after exposure to contaminated heparinized saline flush prepared by a compounding pharmacy. Clin Infect Dis. 2008;47:1372–9.
87. Wilkinson FH, Kerr KG. Bottled water as a source of multiresistant Stenotrophomonas and Pseudomonas species for neutropenic patients. Eur J Cancer Car (Engl). 1998;7:12–4.
88. Wong V, Levi K, Baddal B, et al. Spread of Pseudomonas fluorescens due to contaminated drinking water in a bone marrow transplant unit. J Clin Microbiol. 2011;49:2093–6.
89. Patel R, Paya C. Infections in solid organ transplant recipients. Clin Microbiol Rev. 1997;10:86–124.
90. CDC. Guidelines for preventing opportunistic infections among hematopoietic cell transplant recipients. MMWR Recomm Rep. 2000;49(RR-10):1–125, CE1-7.
91. Boulad F, Sands S, Sklar C. Late complications after bone marrow transplantation in children and adolescents. Curr Probl Pediatr. 1998;28:273–97.
92. Chawla R. Infections after bone marrow transplantation. 2009. emedicine.medscope.com/article/1013470.
93. Appelbaum FR. The use of bone marrow and peripheral blood stem cell transplantation in the treatment of cancer. CA Cancer J Clin. 1996;46:142–64.
94. Thomas ED, Clift RA, Fefer A, et al. Marrow transplantation for the treatment of chronic myelogenous leukemia. Ann Intern Med. 1986;104:155–63.
95. Van Burik J, Weisdorf D. Infections in recipients of blood and marrow transplantation. In: Mandell GL, Bennet JE, Dolin R, editors. Principals and practice of infectious diseases 5th ed. Philadelphia: Churchill Livingstone; 2000. p. 3136–47.
96. Sable CA, Donowitz GR. Infections in bone marrow transplant recipients. Clin Infect Dis. 1994;18:273–81.
97. Engels EA, Ellis CA, Supran SE, et al. Early infection in bone marrow transplantation: quantitative study of clinical factors that affect risk. Clin Infect Dis. 1999;28:256–66.
98. Busca A, Saroglia EM, Giacchino M, et al. Analysis of early infectious complications in pediatric patients undergoing bone marrow transplantation. Support Care Cancer. 1999;7:253–9.
99. Lark R, Mcneel S, VanderHyde K, et al. Risk factors for anaerobic bloodstream infections on bone marrow transplant recipients. Clin Infect Dis. 2001;35:338–43.
100. Wyner LM. The evaluation and management of urinary tract infections in recipients of solid organ transplants. Semin Urol. 1994;12:134–9.
101. Prokurut S, Drabik E, Genda R, et al. Ganciclovir in cytomegalovirus prophylaxis in high risk pediatric renal transplant recipients. Transplant Proc. 1993;25:2577.
102. Couturier M, Slechta E, Goulston C, et al. Leptotrichia bacteremia in patients recovering high dose chemotherapy. J Clin Microbiol. 2012;50:1228–32.
103. Vidal A, Sarria J, Kimbrough RR, et al. Anaerobic bacteremia in a neutropenic patient with oral mucositis. Am J Med Sci. 2000;319:189–90.
104. DePauw B, Bowden R, Paya C. Management of the febrile patient in hematopoietic stem cell and solid organ transplant recipients. In: Bowden R, Ljungman P, Paya C, editors. Transplant infection. Philadelphia: Lippincott-Raven; 1998. p. 153–65.
105. Winn WC, Koneman EW. Konemans's color atlas and textbook of diagnostic microbiology. 6th ed. Philadelphia: Lippincott/The Williams & Wilkins Co.; 2006.
106. Cooreman S, Schuermans C, Van Schaeren J, et al. Bacteremia caused by Leptotrichia trevisanii in a neutropenic patient. Anaerobe. 2011;17:1–3.
107. Tee W, Midolo P, Janssen PH, et al. Bacteremia due to Leptotrichia Trevisanii sp. Nov. Eur J Clin Microbiol Infect Dis. 2001;20:765–9.
108. Patel JB, Clarridge J, Schuster MS, et al. Bacteremia caused by novel isolate resembling Leptotrichia species in a neutropenic patient. J Clin Microbiol. 1999;37:2064–7.
109. Justesen US, Skov MN, Knudsen E, et al. 16S rRNA gene sequencing in routine identification of anaerobic bacteria isolated from bloodstream infections. J Clin Microbiol. 2008;46:1596–601.
110. Simmon KE, Mirrett S, Relle LB, et al. Genotypic diversity of anaerobic isolates from bloodstream infections. J Clin Microbiol. 2008;46:1596–601.
111. Schindel C, Siepman U, Han SR, et al. Persistant legionella infection in a patient after bone marrow transplantation, vol. 38; 2000. p. 4294–5.
112. Beelen DW, Haralambie E, et al. Evidence that sustained growth suppression of intestinal anaerobic bacteria reduces the risk of acute graft-versus-host disease after sibling marrow transplantation. Blood. 1992;80:2668–76.
113. Jones JM, Wilson R, Bealmear PM. Mortality and gross pathology of secondary disease in germfree mouse radiation chimeras. Radiat Res. 1971;45:577.
114. Truit RL, Winter M, Winter S. Application of germfree techniques to the treatment of leukemia in AKR mice by allogeneic bone marrow transplantation. In: Waters H, editor. The handbook of can-

cer immunology. Volume 5: immunotherapy. New York: Garland STPM; 1978. p. 431.

115. Van Bekkum DW, Roodenburg J, Heidt PJ, et al. Mitigation of secondary disease of allogeneic mouse radiation chimeras by modification of the intestinal microflora. J Natl Cancer Inst. 1974;52:401.
116. Miller TL, Wolin MJ. Methanogens in human and animal intestinal tracts. Syst Appl Microbiol. 1986;7:223–9.
117. Dermoumi HL, Ansong RAM. Isolation and antimicrobial susceptibility testing of fecal strains of the archaeon Methanobrevibacter smithii. Chemotherapy. 2001;47:177–83.
118. Beelen DW, Haralambie E, Brandt H, et al. Evidence that sustained growth suppression of intestinal anaerobic bacteria reduces the risk of acute graft-versus-host-disease after sibling bone marrow transplantation. Blood. 1192;80:2668.
119. Beelen DW, Elmaagacli A, Muller KD, et al. Influence of intestinal bacterial decontamination using metronidazole and ciprofloxacin or ciprofloxacin alone on the development of acute graft-versus-host-disease after bone marrow transplantation in patients with hematologic malignancies: final results and long-term follow-up of an open-label prospective randomized trail. Blood. 1999;93:3267–75.
120. Ansorg R, Rath PM, Runde V, et al. Influence of intestinal decontamination using metronidazole on the detection of methanogenic archaea in bone marrow transplant recipients. Bone Marrow Transplant. 2003;31:117–9.
121. Paya CV, Hermans PE, Smith TF, et al. Efficacy of ganciclovir in liver and kidney transplant recipients with severe cytomegalovirus infection. Transplantation. 1988;46:229–34.
122. Stouteanbeek C, Van Saens H, Mirande D, et al. A new technique of infection prevention in the intensive care unit by selective decontamination of the digestive tract. Acta Anaesthesiol Belg. 1983;34:209–21.
123. Van Der Waaij D. Colonization resistance of the digestive tract: clinical consequences and implications. J Antimicrob Chemother. 1982;10:263–70.
124. Patel R, Cockerill F, Porayko M, et al. Lactobacillemia in liver transplantation patients. Clin Infect Dis. 1994;18:207–12.
125. Paya CV, Hermans PE, Washington JA, et al. Incidence, distribution, and outcome of episodes of infection in 100 orthotopic liver transplantation. Mayo Clin Proc. 1989;64:555–64.
126. Gorensek M, Carey WD, Vogt D, et al. A multivariate analysis of risk factors for cytomegalovirus infection in liver transplantation recipients. Gastroenterology. 1990;98:1326–32.
127. Gorensek MJ, Carey WD, Washington JA, et al. Selective bowel decontamination with quinolones and nystatin reduces gram negative and fungal infections in orthotropic liver transplant recipients. Cleve Clin J Med. 1993;60:139–44.
128. Wolinsky E. Mycobacterial disease other than tuberculosis. Clin Infect Dis. 1990;5:80–9.
129. Zeluff BJ. Fungal Pneumonia in Transplant Recipients. Semin Respir Infect. 1990;5:50–89.
130. George D, Arnow P, Fox A, et al. Bacterial infections a complication of the liver transplantation. Rev Infect Dis. 1991;13:387–96.
131. Kusne S, Dummer JS, Singh N, et al. Infections after liver transplantation. An analysis of 101 consecutive cases. Medicine. 1988;67:132–43.
132. Waser M, Maggiorini M, Luthy A, et al. Infectious complications in 100 consecutive heart transplant recipients. Eur J Clin Microbiol Infect Dis. 1994;13:12–8.
133. Brooks R, Hofflin J, Jamieson S, et al. Infectious complications in heart-lung transplant recipients. Am J Med. 1985;79:412–22.
134. Krieger J, Senterfit L, Muecke E, et al. Anaerobic bacterium in renal transplantation. Urology. 1978;12:635–40.
135. Fox BC, Sollinger HW, Belzer FO, et al. A prospective, randomized, double-blind study of trimethoprim-sulfamethoxazole for prophylaxis of infection in renal transplantation: clinical efficacy, absorption of trimethoprim-sulfamethoxazole, effects on the microflora, and the cost-benefit of prophylaxis. Am J Med. 1990;89:255–74.
136. Maki DG, Fox BC, Kuntz J, et al. A prospective, randomized, double-blind study of trimethoprim-sulfamethoxazole for prophylaxis of infection in renal transplantation: side effects of trimethoprim-sulfamethoxazole, interaction with cyclosporine. J Lab Clin Med. 1992;119:11–24.
137. Tolkoff-Rubin NE, Cosimi AB, Russell PS, et al. A controlled study of trimethoprim-sulfamethoxazole prophylaxis of urinary tract infection in renal transplant recipients. Rev Infect Dis. 1982;4:614–8.
138. Infectious Diseases Society of America. The 10 x '20 initiative: pursuing a global commitment to develop 10 new antibacterial drugs by 2020. Clin Infect Dis. 2010;50(8):1081–3.
139. Wright H, Bonomo RA, Paterson DL. New agents for the treatment of infections with Gram-negative bacteria: restoring the miracle or false dawn? Clin Microbiol Infect. 2017;23:704–12.
140. Munita JM, Aitken SL, Miller WR, et al. Multicenter evaluation of ceftolozane/tazobactam for serious infections caused by carbapenem-resistant Pseudomonas aeruginosa. Clin Infect Dis. 2017;65:158–61.
141. Fraile-Ribot PA, Cabot G, Mulet X, et al. Mechanisms leading to in vivo ceftolozane/tazobactam resistance development during the treatment of infections caused by MDR Pseudomonas aeruginosa. J Antimicrob Chemother. 2017;73(3):658–63.
142. Aitken SL, Tarrand JJ, Deshpande LM, et al. High rates of non-susceptibility to ceftazidime-avibactam and identification of New Delhi metallo-β-lactamase production in Enterobacteriaceae bloodstream infections at a major cancer center. Clin Infect Dis. 2016;63(7):954–8.

Nocardiosis and Actinomycosis

27

Heather E. Clauss and Bennett Lorber

Nocardiosis

Microbiology

Nocardia are informally known as "aerobic nocardioform actinomycetes," along with *Corynebacterium*, *Gordonia*, *Rhodococcus*, *Tsukamurella*, *Actinomadura*, and *Mycobacterium* [1]. There are more than 50 known species of *Nocardia*, less than half of which are human pathogens. Newer molecular methods of identification have expanded the spectrum of *Nocardia* species known. The most important causes of *Nocardia* infection in transplantation are *Nocardia asteroides* sensu stricto, *N. nova*, *N. farcinica*, and *N. brasiliensis* [2]. *Nocardia asteroides* sensu stricto are distinct from "*N. asteroides* complex," which is an older designation.

Typical findings on Gram stain include gram-positive, beaded, branching rods with acute pyogenic inflammatory reaction. Sulfur granules may be found in nocardial lesions, similar to those seen in actinomycosis.

There are several known virulence factors that play a role in the pathogenesis of nocardiosis. One of the most important factors is *Nocardia*'s cell wall and its components, including peptidoglycan and mycolic acid polymers. Another factor in virulent *Nocardia* strains is the innate resistance to neutrophil-mediated killing. *Nocardia* have resistance to the oxidative burst within the phagosomes of neutrophils and macrophages. There is a well-documented association between nocardiosis and chronic granulomatous disease (CGD) for this reason [3]. Also, pathogenic *Nocardia* species secrete superoxide dismutase (SOD) into growth media, while nonpathogenic species do not [4]. This contributes to the protection of *Nocardia* species within the host. Finally, the ability of some *Nocardia* species to exhibit tropism for the cerebral tissue is evident and may vary between strains.

The response of the host to *Nocardia* species is determined by the portal of entry of the organism, the tissue tropism, growth rates in vivo, and the ability to survive the phagocytic attack. The key host defenses against developing nocardiosis are T cell mediated. There is little effective humoral response.

Epidemiology

Nocardia are ubiquitous in the environment, living in soil, water, and vegetable matter. Infection occurs most commonly via inhalation, with hematogenous dissemination to other tissues including the brain. Also, direct inoculation of the skin can occur via penetrating injuries. *Nocardia* infections have increased in the last 20 years, due to both increased detection and identification by molecular methods and the expanding use of immunosuppressive agents [1]. The use of immunosuppressive medications is the hallmark of organ transplantation, and these procedures have increased in recent years. *Nocardia* are considered opportunistic pathogens, causing infection in patients with impaired cell-mediated immune response, including patients with organ transplantation, lymphoreticular neoplasia, HIV/AIDS (CD4 counts <100 cells/mm^3), diabetes mellitus, alcoholism, and patients treated with chronic corticosteroid therapy. More than 60% of *Nocardia* cases occur in these settings [5]. *Nocardia* cases in transplant recipients typically occur within the first year following transplantation, although cases in the first month, prior to the period of heaviest immunosuppression, following transplant are rare. However, if aggressive immunosuppression is used, this diagnosis should be considered even in the first month posttransplant. However, in a published 30-year experience of 19 cases of *Nocardia* in 4600 adult solid organ transplants, 2 occurred after 1 month, 4 after more than 3 months, and 13 after over 1 year [6].

H. E. Clauss (✉) · B. Lorber
Section of Infectious Diseases, Lewis Katz School of Medicine at Temple University, Philadelphia, PA, USA

Temple University, Philadelphia, PA, USA

Temple University Hospital, Department of Infectious Diseases, Philadelphia, PA, USA
e-mail: heather.clauss@tuhs.temple.edu; bennett.lorber@tuhs.temple.edu

A. Safdar (ed.), *Principles and Practice of Transplant Infectious Diseases*, https://doi.org/10.1007/978-1-4939-9034-4_27

The incidence of *Nocardia* infection varies somewhat by the organ transplanted. In a review of over 5000 transplant recipients, lung transplant recipients had the greatest incidence of *Nocardia* (3.5%), followed by heart (2.5%), intestine (1.3%), kidney (0.2%), and liver (0.1%) recipients [7]. The overall rate of *Nocardia* in this group, from 1995 to 2005, was 0.6%. These numbers were similar to a 30-year experience in Spain of 4600 adult solid organ transplants where lung transplant recipients had a slightly higher incidence (1.78%) than heart recipients, renal recipients, and liver recipients (0.65%, 0.26%, and 0.18%, respectively) [6]. Lung transplant recipients may have a higher rate of this infection due to the fact that the respiratory tract is the natural access route and also the higher immunosuppression given to lung transplant recipients. In the first paper mentioned, the species of *Nocardia* causing infections in transplant recipients were as follows: *N. nova* in 49%, *N. farcinica* in 28%, *N. asteroides* in 23%, and *N. brasiliensis* in 3% [7].

Risk Factors

Several risk factors for *Nocardia* infection in organ transplant recipients were determined via a matched case control study. These include receipt of high-dose steroids, a high median calcineurin inhibitor level in the preceding 30 days (15 mcg/mL for tacrolimus and >300 ng/mL for cyclosporine), and cytomegalovirus (CMV) disease in the preceding 6 months [7]. In another paper, CMV coinfection was present in 53% of *Nocardia* cases, 47% of cases were dialysis patients, and 26% of cases had diabetes mellitus [6]. Newer immunosuppressive therapies may also be risk factors for *Nocardia* infections. First, alemtuzumab, a humanized monoclonal antibody against CD52 found on B and T lymphocytes, monocytes, and natural killer cells, is being used commonly as induction immunosuppression prior to solid organ transplantation as well as treatment for rejection. It causes lymphopenia and is most commonly associated with CMV infection but also is associated with *Nocardia* infections [8]. Rituximab is a monoclonal antibody directed against the CD20 antigen found on B cells and has been used to treat or prevent antibody-mediated rejection. This agent has been described as a risk factor for cerebral nocardiosis in a non-transplant recipient [9]. Additionally, hypogammaglobulinemia in the setting of transplant immunosuppression has been implicated as a risk factor for the development of *Nocardia* infections [10]. These are intriguing findings, given that there is thought to be little humoral response to *Nocardia* infection. Perhaps, antibody-dependent cellular cytotoxicity plays more of a role in the defense against nocardiosis. Finally, there have been reports of *Nocardia* infections in patients with rheumatologic diseases treated with tumor necrosis factor (TNF) blockers [11].

Clinical Syndromes

Clinical syndromes caused by *Nocardia* species include pulmonary masses, nodules, infiltrates and cavities, brain abscesses, systemic disease, and nodular lymphangitis. Primary infection occurs via inhalation or direct inoculation of skin and soft tissues. Then, bloodstream dissemination can cause metastatic infection throughout the body, most commonly to the central nervous system (CNS). Sites of metastasis can include virtually any other anatomic site.

The most important site of primary infection is the lung. Pulmonary nocardiosis is the predominant clinical manifestation, seen in over 40% of nocardiosis cases in organ transplant recipients [7]. The *N. asteroides* complex are the main species causing pulmonary nocardiosis. Common clinical symptoms include a subacute course (from days to weeks) of fever, cough, purulent sputum production, malaise, anorexia, dyspnea on exertion, and sometimes pleuritic chest pain. Oxygenation is usually preserved at rest until disease has advanced. This is commonly a suppurative infection but may be granulomatous. Chest radiograph findings can include focal or multifocal disease, nodules, or consolidations that can progress to cavities [12]. Additionally, there can be necrotizing lung abscess and cavitary disease with contiguous extension to the surface and deep structures, including effusion and empyema. The "halo sign," typically associated with pulmonary aspergillosis, has been described [1]. On bronchoscopy, endobronchial masses can be visualized in some cases. In one Spanish study, predisposing conditions for 31 pulmonary nocardiosis patients were transplantation (29%), HIV infection (19%), and treatment with steroids (64.5%) [13]. In this study, the median time to diagnosis was 42 days, and the mortality rate for pulmonary nocardiosis was 41% and 64% for disseminated nocardiosis. Progressive fibrosis may develop if pulmonary nocardiosis is incorrectly or inadequately treated. This infection should be considered in the differential diagnosis of indolent pulmonary disease in organ transplant recipients. Evidence pointing to a diagnosis of pulmonary nocardiosis may be spread of infection to contiguous structures within the chest.

Disseminated infection involving two or more body sites can occur in nocardiosis. There is local and hematogenous spread, but *Nocardia* species are isolated from blood cultures only rarely. When *Nocardia* species are isolated from patients, it is typically in association with central venous catheters, not disseminated disease. *Nocardia* species can erode into blood vessels and disseminate to the retina, skin, subcutaneous tissues, kidneys, joints, bones, and heart. Most commonly, *Nocardia* species spread to the CNS.

Nocardia species have a particular tropism for the brain and spinal cord. In all cases of pulmonary and disseminated nocardiosis, an MRI of the brain should be performed to evaluate for CNS infection. The differential diagnosis of pulmonary-CNS syndromes in organ transplant recipients includes *Nocardia*, *Cryptococcus*, *Aspergillus*, *Rhodococcus*, and posttransplant lymphoproliferative disease (PTLD).

CNS involvement is seen in 44% of cases of disseminated nocardiosis. A third of *Nocardia* cases in the literature involved the CNS without evidence of other infections [5]. CNS lesions can be seen throughout the brain, and there may be meningitis with or without involvement of other portions of the brain and spinal cord. Clinical presentation is usually subacute to chronic (months to years), as with the pulmonary infection. Location of the abscess or granulomas determines the clinical manifestations seen in patients with CNS nocardiosis. Chronic behavioral and psychiatric disturbances can be seen. Tissue diagnosis of a brain mass may not be necessary in the setting of pulmonary nocardiosis [12]. However, one should consider brain biopsy for definitive diagnosis in an organ transplant recipient with an isolated CNS lesion, as the differential diagnosis is broad and includes many bacterial, mycobacterial, fungal pathogens, PTLD, and other malignancies and rarely *Acanthamoeba* or toxoplasmosis.

Nocardia species can also cause cutaneous, subcutaneous, and lymphocutaneous (sporotrichoid) disease following direct, traumatic inoculation of the organism into the skin. *N. brasiliensis* is the most common case of these conditions. These can occur after animal or insect bites, puncture wounds, and contaminated abrasions [1]. These may appear to be *staphylococcal* abscesses, which are much more common. The diagnosis of *Nocardia* may be confused or missed. In transplant patients, self-limited infections may be treated initially as *staphylococcal* abscesses, but if these do not improve, less common infections such as cutaneous nocardiosis should be considered. Mycetomas can form, which can be suppurative or necrotic and may form sinus tracts. *Nocardia* can spread through the lymphatics causing sporotrichoid nocardiosis in immunocompromised hosts. Inoculation injuries can also occasionally affect the cornea [1].

Nocardiosis in Cancer Patients and Hematopoietic Stem Cell Recipients

In a study at MD Anderson Cancer Center conducted between 1988 and 2001, 42 cancer patients were diagnosed with nocardiosis, in the first large series of patients of this type [14]. Twenty-seven (64%) patients had hematologic malignancies, and in 13 patients, nocardiosis complicated bone marrow transplantation (BMT). Patients had received steroids in 25 (58%) episodes of nocardiosis and had received chemotherapy within 30 days before the onset of nocardiosis in 10 (23%) episodes. Pulmonary nocardiosis was diagnosed in 30 of 43 cases (70%), while only 1 (2%) patient developed CNS nocardial infection. The mortality rate in this study was 60%.

In bone marrow transplant patients at one institution, the rate of nocardiosis was 1/554 (0.2%) among autologous BMT recipients and 5/302 (1.7%) in allogeneic BMT recipients from 1980 to 1994 [15]. All but one of the six cases had graft-versus-host disease. Four of the cases had extensive exposure to soil or dust prior to their nocardial infection. Also, nocardial infection in this BMT population was associated with a high rate of invasive fungal infection. In a retrospective study of 27 patients with nocardiosis at 3 centers, the median time to the diagnosis of nocardiosis after bone marrow transplantation was 210 days, and all of the infections occurred in allogeneic marrow recipients [16]. In this paper, 96% of the isolates were *N. asteroides* complex. The survival rate from *Nocardia* infection was 84%. Forty percent of these patients had taken trimethoprim-sulfamethoxazole (TMP-SMX) regularly prior to developing nocardiosis. Interestingly, 3/6 patients in the first paper mentioned developed nocardiosis despite taking TMP-SMX for *Pneumocystis jiroveci* prophylaxis. TMP-SMX may not be protective against nocardial infections in immunosuppressed patients the same way it is protective against *Listeria monocytogenes* and other gastrointestinal and genitourinary infections.

Diagnosis

The mainstay of diagnosing nocardiosis is to inform the laboratory this diagnosis is being considered. The diagnosis can be missed by routine laboratory methods. The organism must be isolated from a clinical specimen, noting that *Nocardia* species are not common lab contaminants or oral flora. However, some patients with chronic lung disease can have transient nocardial carriage which must be interpreted with caution. Often this diagnosis requires an invasive procedure such as a lung biopsy, skin biopsy, or brain biopsy. All biopsies should be evaluated by Gram stain, modified acid-fast staining, culture, and pathology. Gram staining can reveal fine gram-positive, beaded, branching rods surrounded by white blood cells. Acid-fast staining by modified Kinyoun stain can be weakly positive. Blood cultures for *Nocardia* species require prolonged incubation (up to 14 days), and selective media such as Thayer-Martin agar or Buffered Charcoal Yeast Extract (BCYE) agar should be used. The organism will grow in 3–5 days. Molecular methods may be needed to accurately identify species of *Nocardia*. It is important to accurately identify the species causing infection in order to predict antimicrobial susceptibility. Techniques that have been developed include ribotyping, polymerase chain reaction (PCR), restriction fragment length polymorphism (RFLP) analyses, and DNA sequencing [2]. There is genetic variation within the *Nocardia* heat shock protein 65 (hsp65) gene and the 16S rRNA gene region that can be used in these analyses [1].

Treatment

The mainstay of treatment of nocardiosis is antibiotic therapy. The Transplant Infectious Disease Guidelines published in 2009 recommend antimicrobial susceptibility testing for all nocardial isolates against amikacin, amoxicillin-clavulanate, ceftriaxone, ciprofloxacin, clarithromycin, imipenem, linezolid, minocycline, TMP-SMX, and tobramycin [17]. TMP-SMX is the preferred treatment for most forms of nocardiosis, given its high tissue concentrations in the lungs, brain, skin, and bone [18]. The recommended dosage is 15 mg/kg of TMP divided into 3–4 doses/day. Higher doses are used for patients with high disease burden in the central nervous system. Side effects include nausea and vomiting (especially with oral therapy) and rash but can include more serious issues such as myelosuppression, hyperkalemia, and erythema multiforme. Of note, some species of *Nocardia* are sulfonamide resistant, such as *N. farcinica* and *N. nova*.

In immunosuppressed patients and patients with CNS involvement or disseminated disease, the combination of imipenem/cilastatin and amikacin is recommended empirically until sensitivities are known [17]. There may be synergism between these agents. The toxicities of imipenem include rash and seizures, while the toxicities of amikacin include renal failure and ototoxicity. Of note, there may be enhanced nephrotoxicity in patients taking aminoglycosides in conjunction with calcineurin inhibitors. Meropenem may be a better choice for those patients with CNS disease, as there is good blood-brain barrier penetration and fewer seizures with this agent. Also, meropenem may have better activity against *N. brasiliensis*, but it may be less active against *N. asteroides* complex organisms than imipenem [17]. Ertapenem has significantly less activity in vitro than imipenem and meropenem [19].

Another option for treating CNS nocardiosis includes third-generation cephalosporins such as ceftriaxone and cefotaxime [17]. There are case reports of their success, usually in combination with other agents [20]. There are minimal side effects to these medications. Minocycline has been used as an alternative to TMP-SMX for *Nocardia* treatment, at doses of 200 mg twice daily orally or intravenously [21]. However, several strains of *Nocardia* are resistant, so susceptibility testing should be used to determine if this antibiotic would be successful. Toxicities include photosensitivity, dizziness, nausea, and ulceration of the esophagus. A 2003 report describes six cases of nocardiosis, including CNS infection, successfully treated with linezolid [22]. The dosage is 600 mg twice daily, either intravenously or orally. Side effects include nausea and rash, as well as more severe adverse effects such as thrombocytopenia, aplastic anemia, peripheral neuropathy, and lactic acidosis.

Surgical drainage should be considered in patients with cerebral disease and maybe other large soft tissue abscesses. In patients with CNS abscess, drainage should be considered when the patient's condition deteriorates, if the abscesses are accessible and relatively large, if the lesions progress despite 2 weeks of therapy, or if there is no reduction in abscess size within a month of therapy [23]. Surgical therapy should be performed in conjunction with pharmacologic treatment.

Common recommendations for treatment of nocardiosis include 3–4 weeks of intravenous therapy, followed by several months of oral therapy, especially in particularly ill patients [1]. In patients with CNS infection, a minimum of 9–12 months would be appropriate [17]. Pulmonary and soft tissue infection can be treated within 6–12 months depending on the response to therapy [17]. If graft rejection and increased immunosuppression are required, therapy may need to be extended to 12 months or longer. Patients with cerebral *Nocardia* infection should have repeat CT or MRI of the brain to follow the response to therapy.

Prevention/Prophylaxis

Primary prophylaxis against *Nocardia* infections is not indicated due to the low overall incidence of nocardiosis; however, some centers initiate secondary prophylaxis for this infection. One study suggests that when solid organ transplant recipients take TMP-SMX daily to prevent *Pneumocystis jiroveci* pneumonia, it reduces the rate of nocardiosis [24]. This observation has also been made in the HIV-infected population. However, as discussed above, in two studies of nocardiosis in bone marrow transplant recipients, 40–50% of patients who developed nocardiosis were taking TMP-SMX prophylaxis [15, 16]. Also, in a study of *Nocardia* infection in solid organ transplant recipients, 69% (24/35) of the patients developed their infection while on TMP-SMX [7]. On univariate analysis in this paper, TMP-SMX was not shown to be protective against the development of nocardiosis. This may be because organ transplant recipients tend to take a regimen of TMP-SMX two to three times per week or because of the strength of posttransplant immunosuppression combined with the coexistence of opportunistic infections in this population. Many breakthrough infections in patients taking TMP-SMX cast doubt on its prevention of nocardiosis in the transplant population.

Cure Rates/Prognosis

Clinical improvement of nocardiosis should be expected within 3 5 days from the initiation of appropriate therapy, at least within 10 days [25]. Reasons for failure of initial antimicrobial therapy include inadequate penetration of drug to the site of infection, primary drug resistance, or a focus of infection requiring surgical drainage. In organ transplant recipients, reasons could also include a coexisting opportunistic infection or overwhelming nocardial sepsis. Nearly 100% of cutaneous nocardiosis is treated successfully while pulmonary nocardiosis slightly less so (90%). In one study, 31/35 cases (89%) of both pulmonary and disseminated nocardiosis, including CNS infection, were cured [7]. Of note, most transplant patients are cured despite immunosuppression being continued.

Infection Control

Inhalation of *Nocardia* species from environmental sources is the main route of transmission, followed by direct inoculation via penetrating cutaneous injury. There have been reports of outbreaks of nocardiosis around construction sites; however, most infections are sporadic in nature [5]. Also, reports of nosocomial outbreaks of *Nocardia* infection have been published, but did not include strain testing with molecular methods to document the relationship between infections [3]. Person-to-person transmission and common source environmental transmission have been shown by pulsed-field gel electrophoresis in healthcare facilities [26]. However, there is no data to support respiratory isolation of patients with nocardiosis while they are in a hospital, and there is no effective measure to prevent inhalation. It is controversial if TMP-SMX reduces the incidence of *Nocardia* infections in high-risk transplant recipients.

Actinomycosis

Microbiology

Actinomycetes are gram-positive branching rods which are anaerobic or microaerophilic. On Gram stain, these are indistinguishable from *Nocardia*; however, *Nocardia* will weakly stain with an acid-fast Kinyoun stain, while actinomycetes will not. The most common species causing human disease is *Actinomyces israelii*. Less common species that cause actinomycosis include *A. naeslundii*, *A. odontolyticus*, *A. viscosus*, and *A. meyeri*. Most evidence supports that most actinomycotic infections are polymicrobial in nature [27]. Commonly isolated in combination with actinomycetes are *Eikenella corrodens*, *Fusobacterium*, *Bacteroides*, *Capnocytophaga*, *Staphylococci*, *Streptococci*, and *Enterobacteriaceae*. These organisms may inhibit host defenses or reduce oxygen tension allowing actinomycetes to thrive.

The virulence factors for actinomycetes and their ability to grow contiguously, ignoring tissue planes, have not been well defined in vitro or in animal models. Also it is unclear which arm of host defenses is necessary to prevent and control these infections.

Epidemiology/Risk Factors

Actinomycetes are part of the endogenous flora of the mucous membranes of humans [28]. These organisms can be cultured from the gastrointestinal tract as well as the female genital tract. Oral cavity colonization is nearly 100% by 2 years of age [29]. There has never been documented person-to-person transmission of actinomycetes, and this organism has never been cultured from the environment [30]. The incidence of actinomycosis was 1 in 100,000 persons in Europe in the 1960s [28]. The highest incidence is from ages 10–60. Cases outside of that age range are less frequent. Males are more frequently infected than females at a 3:1 ratio [27]. Possible reasons for this imbalance have been hypothesized, including poorer dental hygiene among men as well as increased oral trauma in this population. These hypotheses remain unproven. Risk factors for actinomycosis in the general population may be lack of access to dental care and bisphosphonate use (cervicofacial actinomycosis), as well as long-term use of intrauterine devices (IUDs) (abdominal actinomycosis) [27].

Disruption of the mucosal barrier is an important step in the pathogenesis of actinomycosis. Dental procedures, trauma, oral surgery, and radiation of the head and neck are associated with the development of oral and cervicofacial actinomycosis [31]. Pulmonary actinomycosis occurs due to aspiration. Abdominal actinomycosis is associated with foreign bodies in the gastrointestinal/genital tracts as well as gastrointestinal surgery for diverticulitis or appendicitis.

It is unclear whether immunosuppression is a risk factor for actinomycosis. There are cases reported to be associated with HIV [32] and infliximab [33] use for Crohn's disease. Also there have been reported cases with steroid use [34] and cancer chemotherapy [35]. Case reports of actinomycosis in solid organ transplant recipients are slightly more frequent, but far from common. There have been documented cases in renal transplant recipients including a patient with an abdominal mass 4 years posttransplantation who was found to have abdominal actinomycosis [36] and a patient with actinomycosis of the posterior glottis involving both vocal processes [37]. Additionally, a patient was found to have pulmonary actinomycosis 6 months following a cadaveric liver transplant [38]. Finally, one lung and one heart-lung recipient each developed thoracopulmonary actinomycosis following transplant [39]. However, it is uncertain the role of organ transplantation and its associated immunosuppression played in these cases.

Clinical Syndromes

Actinomycetes cause several types of infections including oral-cervicofacial disease, thoracopulmonary disease, abdominal disease, pelvic disease, CNS disease, musculoskeletal disease, and, rarely, disseminated disease. Oral-cervicofacial actinomycosis is the most common variety, accounting for 55% of cases [40]. The typical presentation is a soft-tissue swelling, mass, or abscess that is mistaken for malignancy. The angle of the jaw is the most common location for cervicofacial actinomycosis, but these masses can present anywhere in the head and neck and are often painless. Often these masses will temporarily respond to short courses of antibiotics, then relapse. Associated lymphadenopathy is rare. Extension to any contiguous structure may occur, without regard for tissue planes. Dental infections can also occur and are typically periapical. Spread to the skin from a dental focus with sinus tract formation is the hallmark of this infection. Infected osteoradionecrosis, a complication of radiation therapy, and bisphosphonate-associated osteonecrosis have both been associated with cervicofacial actinomycosis. These conditions may alter host defenses, which, if followed by dental procedures disrupting the mucosa, can lead to infection with actinomycetes. Actinomycosis is also an uncommon cause of otitis media, which, if untreated, can spread to the CNS.

Thoracopulmonary actinomycosis is less common, in about 15% of cases, and can present with chest pain, fever, and weight loss. Cough and hemoptysis may be present as well. This infection can involve the chest wall, the pleural space, or the lung parenchyma itself. On radiography, there can be a consolidation or a mass lesion, and cavitary disease and/or hilar lymphadenopathy can develop as well. Lung disease that crosses lobes or fissures or invades the mediastinum or the bones and muscles of the chest well or a sinus tract should make one consider the diagnosis of pulmonary actinomycosis. The usual source of this infection is aspiration of oral organisms. Again this infection can be mistaken for malignancy. Mediastinal actinomycosis is very uncommon.

Approximately 20% of cases of actinomycosis involve the abdomen [40]. The inciting conditions are not always obvious, but they involve a breach in the gastrointestinal mucosa. Months to years usually pass from the inciting event to the diagnosis of abdominal actinomycosis [41]. These events include, but are not limited to, appendicitis (most commonly), peptic ulcer disease, diverticulitis, bowel surgery, foreign body perforation, or ascension from IUD-associated pelvic disease. Any organ, region, or space can be involved due to the flow of peritoneal fluid and direct extension of primary disease [41]. These infections can be mistaken for malignancy and present often as a mass or abscess fixed to the underlying tissue. As in oral-cervicofacial disease and pulmonary disease, sinus tracts to the body wall can form. Liver infection can present as single or multiple abscesses. Renal disease can present as perinephric abscess or pyelonephritis. The diagnosis of abdominal actinomycosis is rarely considered until pathologic specimens are obtained and evaluated.

Pelvic actinomycosis is most commonly associated with ascending infection from a uterus containing an IUD. It may also occur after perforated appendicitis. The likelihood of infection from an IUD increases with time. Pelvic actinomycosis rarely occurs when an IUD has been in place for less than a year. Often, this infection is seen in the setting of the "forgotten" IUD. This infection can also occur as a consequence of other pelvic foreign bodies such as pessaries and contraceptive devices. Pelvic actinomycosis can present in an indolent fashion, with fever, weight loss, abdominal pain, and vaginal bleeding or discharge. The first stage is an endometritis, which can be followed by a tuboovarian abscess. The diagnosis is often delayed, sometimes until there is a "frozen pelvis" which can mimic malignancy or endometriosis. Seven percent of women who use an IUD can have actinomycetes on their Papanicolaou-stained cervical specimens [42]. This finding alone, in the absence of symptoms, has a low predictive value for pelvic disease and does not warrant the removal of the IUD. However, if pain, abnormal bleeding, or discharge are present and cannot be attributed to another condition, the removal of the IUD may be necessary, along with a 14-day course of a penicillin or a tetracycline for treatment of possible early pelvic actinomycosis [28].

CNS actinomycosis is rare and may be from a hematogenous source or from the direct extension of oral-cervicofacial disease. Brain abscess is the most common presentation [28]. Clinical features include headache and focal neurologic findings. Fever can also be present. On radiography, there can be single or multiple lesions, which are most often ring enhancing and irregular. Diagnosis can be made by biopsy or examination of the cerebrospinal fluid, having low to normal glucose, elevated protein, pleocytosis (lymphocyte predominant), and a negative culture.

Musculoskeletal actinomycosis is also rare and may result from the spread of soft tissue infection, trauma, or hematogenous spread of infection. It also may be associated with osteoradionecrosis and bisphosphonate use. The most frequent bones involved in this infection are the mandible and maxilla [43]. However, contiguous spread from oral-cervicofacial, thoracopulmonary, or abdominal actinomycosis can cause osteomyelitis of many bones. Cutaneous sinus tracts may develop. As discussed above, the presentation is often indolent and can be confused with other infections as well as malignancy.

Actinomycetes are capable of hematogenous dissemination resulting in multisystem involvement of infection [28]. Disease in any of the areas described can result in widespread infection. The liver and the lungs are the most common organs involved, again mimicking malignancy.

Diagnosis

The diagnosis of actinomycosis is not often considered until pathologic specimens have been obtained and evaluated. This is particularly true when actinomycosis causes mass lesions or nodules that mimic malignancy. Since medical therapy is typically sufficient for cure, the key is to maintain an index of suspicion for this infection, prior to invasive debulking procedures. Fine needle aspiration or biopsy may give enough sample to make the diagnosis. The diagnosis is most commonly made by microscopic identification of sulfur granules, which are in vivo matrices of bacteria and host material [41]. These can be missed, however, when only small samples are available, making a surgical diagnosis necessary at times. Microbiological identification is less common, but when actinomycetes are isolated in culture of a sterile site, the diagnosis is confirmed. These organisms are normal flora of the oral cavity and the female genital tract, so isolation of the bacteria alone, without sulfur granules or clinical symptoms, is of little significance.

In order to grow actinomycetes in culture, strict anaerobic processing must be used. The microbiology lab should be notified that this diagnosis is being considered. These organisms will grow in 5–7 days, but it may take longer to confirm the diagnosis. Specialized media are not required. Gram staining may be more sensitive than culture, especially if the patient received antibiotics prior to the specimen being obtained [28]. Amplification and sequencing of 16S rRNA genes is beginning to be used in the diagnosis of actinomycosis.

Treatment

The mainstay of treatment of actinomycosis is penicillin; it is necessary to use high doses of this antibiotic for a prolonged period of time. Commonly recommended therapy is 18–24 million units of intravenous penicillin for 2–6 weeks followed by oral penicillin or amoxicillin for 6–12 months, depending on the severity of disease. Treatment should continue until radiologic resolution of disease to minimize relapse of infection. For penicillin-allergic patients, tetracycline is the antibiotic of choice. Possible alternative therapies include erythromycin, doxycycline, minocycline, or clindamycin [28]. Agents that should be avoided are metronidazole, aminoglycosides, oxacillin, dicloxacillin, and cephalexin.

Other bacteria isolated along with actinomycetes may require therapy as well. If these do not grow in culture, it is important for the clinician to consider the site of actinomycosis when selecting an empiric regimen. In many cases, medical therapy alone is sufficient for cure. Surgical therapy often can be avoided or a less extensive procedure can be performed. The same principles apply when treating organ transplant recipients with actinomycosis of any area.

Prevention/Prophylaxis

Actinomycosis is rarely reported in organ transplant recipients. Therefore, no specific prophylaxis is recommended or required for these, or any, patients. However, this diagnosis must be considered when evaluating organ transplant recipients with cutaneous draining sinus tracts, nodules, or mass lesions of uncertain etiology.

Cure Rates/Prognosis

Nearly all infections with actinomycetes can be cured with medical therapy. Refractory disease has been described in patients with HIV as well as normal hosts. If medical therapy does fail, surgical resection of the infection, especially in critical areas of the body, will often be curative in combination with antibiotic therapy. However, surgery can often be avoided, at least initially. Prognosis is good, but if extensive surgery is necessary, there can be sequelae, depending on the location of the infection and the extent of the procedure.

Infection Control

There have been no reported cases of person-to-person transmission of actinomycosis. Therefore, no particular infection control measures need to be taken in hospitalized patients or outpatients. There is minimal to no risk to organ transplant recipients who have a household contact with a person with actinomycosis.

References

1. Sorrell TC, Mitchell DH, Iredell JR, Chen SCA. *Nocardia* Species. In: Mandell GL, Bennett JE, Dolin R, editors. Principles and practice of infectious diseases. 7th ed. Philadelphia: Churchill Livingstone; 2010. p. 3199–207.
2. Brown-Elliott BA, Brown JM, Conville PS, Wallace PJ Jr. Clinical and laboratory features of the *Nocardia* species based on current molecular taxonomy. Clin Microbiol Rev. 2006;19(2):259–82.
3. Dorman SE, Guide SV, Conville PS, DeCarlo ES, Malech HL, Gallin JI, Witebsky FG, Holland SM. *Nocardia* infection in chronic granulomatous disease. Clin Infect Dis. 2002;35(4):390–4.
4. Beaman L, Beaman BL. Monoclonal antibodies demonstrate that superoxide dismutase contributes to protection of *Nocardia asteroides* within the intact host. Infect Immun. 1990;58(9):3122–8.
5. Beaman BL, Beaman L. *Nocardia* species: host-parasite relationships. Clin Microbiol Rev. 1994;7(2):213–64.
6. Santos M, Gil-Brusola A, Morales P. Infection by *Nocardia* in solid organ transplantation: thirty years of experience. Transplant Proc. 2011;43(6):2141–4.
7. Peleg AY, Husain S, Qureshi ZA, Silveira FP, Sarumi M, Shutt KA, Kwak EJ, Paterson DL. Risk factors, clinical characteristics, and outcome of *Nocardia* infection in organ transplant recipients: a matched case-control study. Clin Infect Dis. 2007;44(10):1307–14.
8. Peleg AY, Husain S, Kwak EJ, Silveira FP, Ndirangu M, Tran J, et al. Opportunistic infections in 547 organ transplant recipients receiving alemtuzumab, a humanized monoclonal CD-52 antibody. Clin Infect Dis. 2007;44(2):204–12.

9. Kundranda MN, Spiro TP, Muslimani A, Gopalakrishna KV, Melaragno MJ, Daw HA. Cerebral nocardiosis in a patient with NHL treated with rituximab. Am J Hematol. 2001;82(11):1033–4.
10. Corales R, Chua J, Mawhorter S, Young JB, Starling R, Tomford JW, et al. Significant post-transplant hypogammaglobulinemia in six heart transplant recipients: an emerging clinical phenomenon? Transpl Infect Dis. 2000;2(3):133–9.
11. Doraiswamy VA. *Nocardia* infection with adalimumab in rheumatoid arthritis. J Rheumatol. 2008;35(3):542–3.
12. Lerner PI. Nocardiosis. Clin Infect Dis. 1996;22(6):891–903.
13. Martínez TR, Menéndez VR, Reyes CS, Santos DM, Vallés Tarazona JM, Modesto AM, Gobernado SM. Pulmonary nocardiosis: risk factors and outcomes. Respirology. 2007;12(3):394–400.
14. Torres HA, Reddy BT, Raad II, Tarrand J, Bodey GP, Hanna HA, Rolston KV, Kontoyiannis DP. Nocardiosis in cancer patients. Medicine. 2002;81(5):388–97.
15. Chouciño C, Goodman SA, Greer JP, Stein RS, Wolff SN, Dummer JS. Nocardial infections in bone marrow transplant recipients. Clin Infect Dis. 2002;23(5):1012–9.
16. Van Burik J, Hackman RC, Nadeem SQ, Hiemenz JW, White MH, Flowers ME, Bowden RA. Nocardiosis after bone marrow transplantation: a retrospective study. Clin Infect Dis. 1997;24(6):1154–60.
17. Clark NM. *Nocardia* in solid organ transplant recipients. Am J Transplant. 2009;9(Suppl 4):S70–7.
18. Smego RA Jr, Moeller MB, Gallis HA. Trimethoprim-sulfamethoxazole for treatment of Nocardia infections. Arch Intern Med. 1983;143(4):711–8.
19. Cercenado E, Marin M, Sanchez-Martinez M, Cuevas O, Martinez-Alarcon J, Bouza E. *In vitro* activities of tigecycline and eight other antimicrobials against different *Nocardia* species identified by molecular methods. Antimicrob Agents Chemother. 2007;51(3):1102–4.
20. Garlando F, Bodmer T, Lee C, Zimmerli W, Pirovino M. Successful treatment of disseminated nocardiosis complicated by cerebral abscess with ceftriaxone and amikacin: case report. Clin Infect Dis. 1992;15(6):1039–40.
21. Wren MV, Savage AM, Alford RH. Apparent cure of intracranial *Nocardia asteroides* infection by minocycline. Arch Intern Med. 1979;139(2):249–50.
22. Moylett EH, Pacheco SE, Brown-Elliott BA, Perry TR, Buescher ES, Birhimngham MC, et al. Clinical experience with linezolid for the treatment of Nocardia infection. Clin Infect Dis. 2003;36(3):313–8.
23. Mamelak AN, Obana WG, Flaherty JF, Rosenblum ML. Nocardial brain abscess: treatment and factors influencing outcome. Neurosurgery. 1994;35(4):622–31.
24. Arduino RC, Johnson PC, Mirando AG. Nocardiosis in renal transplant recipients undergoing immunosuppression with cyclosporine. Clin Infect Dis. 1993;16(4):505–12.
25. McNeil MM, Brown JM, Hutwagner LC, Schiff TA. Evaluation of therapy for Nocardia asteroides complex infections. Infect Dis Clin Pract. 1995;4:287–92.
26. Blumel J, Blumel E, Yassin AF, Schmidt-Rotte H, Schaal KP. Typing of *Nocardia farcinica* by pulsed-field gel electrophoresis reveals an endemic strain as source of hospital infections. J Clin Microbiol. 1998;36(1):118–22.
27. Pulverer G, Schutt-Gerowitt H, Schaal KP. Human cervicofacial actinomycoses: microbiological data for 1997 cases. Clin Infect Dis. 2003;37(4):490–7.
28. Russo TA. Agents of Actinomycosis. In: Mandell GL, Bennett JE, Dolin R, editors. Principles and practice of infectious diseases. 7th ed. Philadelphia: Churchill Livingstone; 2010. p. 3209–19.
29. Sarkonen N, Kononen E, Summanen P, Kinervo A, Takala A, Jousimies-Somer H. Oral colonization with Actinomyces species in infants by two years of age. J Dent Res. 2000;79(3):864–7.
30. Smego RA Jr, Foglia G. Actinomycosis. Clin Infect Dis. 1998;26(6):1255–61.
31. Zitch RP 3rd, Bothwell M. Actinomycosis: a potential complication of head and neck surgery. Am J Otolaryngol. 1999;20(4):260–2.
32. Chaudhry SI, Greenspan JS. Actinomycosis in HIV infection: a review of a rare complication. Int J STD AIDS. 2000;11(6):349–55.
33. Cohen RD, Bowie WR, Enns R, Flint J, Fitzgerald JM. Pulmonary actinomycosis complicating infliximab therapy for Crohn's disease. Thorax. 2007;62(11):1013–4.
34. Gaffney R, Walsh M. Cervicofacial actinomycosis: an unusual cause of submandibular swelling. J Laryngol Otol. 1993;107(12):1169–70.
35. Chen CY, Chen YC, Tang JL, Lin WC, Su IJ, Tien HF. Splenic actinomycotic abscess in a patient with acute myeloid leukemia. Ann Hematol. 2002;81(9):532–4.
36. Leach TD, Sadek SA, Mason HC. An unusual abdominal mass in a renal transplant recipient. Transpl Infect Dis. 2002;4(4):218–22.
37. Sims HS, Heywood BB. Post-transplant actinomycosis of the posterior glottis involving both vocal processes. Otolaryngology. 2007;137(6):967.
38. Galaria II, Marcos A, Orloff M, Mieles L, Bozorgadeh KS, Tan HP. Pulmonary Actinomycosis in solid organ transplantation. Transplantation. 2003;75(11):1914.
39. Bassiri AG, Girgis RE, Theodore J. *Actinomyces odontolyticus* thoracopulmonary infections: two cases in lung and heart-lung transplant recipients and a review of the literature. Chest. 1996;109(4):1109–11.
40. Bennhoff D. Actinomycosis: diagnostic and therapeutic considerations and a review of 32 cases. Laryngocope. 1984;94(9):1198–217.
41. Russo TA. Actinomycosis. In: Schlossberg D, editor. Clinical infectious disease. Hong Kong: Cambridge University Press; 2008. p. 881–5.
42. Westhoff C. IUDs and colonization or infection with Actinomyces. Contraception. 2007;75(6 Suppl):S48–50.
43. Hansen T, Kunkel M, Springer E, Walter C, Weber A, Siegel E, Kirkpatrick CJ. Actinomycosis of the jaws—histopathological study of 45 patients shows significant involvement in bisphosphonate-associated osteonecrosis and infected osteoradionecrosis. Virchows Arch. 2007;451(6):1009–17.

Listeriosis

28

Heather E. Clauss and Bennett Lorber

Introduction

The bacterium *Listeria monocytogenes* infrequently causes illness in the general population. In some groups, however, including pregnant women, newborns, elderly persons, and those with impaired cell-mediated immunity, including many transplant recipients, it is an important cause of invasive disease, particularly bacteremia, meningoencephalitis, and brain abscess [1–3]. Additionally, listeriae may cause other clinical syndromes, including in utero infection typically resulting in miscarriage or stillbirth, as well as focal infections of heart valves, joints, liver, and peritoneum. Growing interest in this organism has resulted from foodborne outbreaks, concerns about food safety, and the recognition that foodborne infection can result in self-limited febrile gastroenteritis in healthy persons [4].

Listeria monocytogenes is a short, non-branching, gram-positive rod that is facultatively anaerobic and nonsporulating and grows readily on blood agar where it produces incomplete beta-hemolysis [5]. The bacterium exhibits characteristic tumbling motility at room temperature and, unlike most bacteria, grows well at refrigerator temperatures (4 °C–10 °C). In clinical specimens, the organisms may be gram-variable and may look like diphtheroids, cocci, or diplococci leading to misdiagnosis. The isolation of a "diphtheroid" from blood or CSF always should alert one to the possibility that the organism is really *L. monocytogenes*.

H. E. Clauss (✉) · B. Lorber
Section of Infectious Diseases, Lewis Katz School of Medicine at Temple University, Philadelphia, PA, USA

Temple University, Philadelphia, PA, USA

Temple University Hospital, Department of Infectious Diseases, Philadelphia, PA, USA
e-mail: heather.clauss@tuhs.temple.edu; bennett.lorber@tuhs.temple.edu

Pathogenesis

Human-to-human transmission of *L. monocytogenes* has not been reported aside from vertical transmission between mother and child and sporadic cross contamination in neonatal nurseries [6]. Most commonly, listeriae are transmitted via the ingestion of contaminated food with subsequent mucosal invasion and systemic infection. In mammals, $\geq 10^9$ organisms are required for infection [7]. Alkalinization of the stomach with antacids, H_2 blockers, proton pump inhibitors, or achlorhydria associated with advanced age may promote infection [8]. The incubation period for invasive disease (bacteremia, meningitis) is not well established, but evidence from cases related to specific ingestions points to a range from 11 to 70 days (mean 31 days) [9].

Once inside an enterocyte or macrophage, *L. monocytogenes*, a facultative intracellular parasite, uses its major virulence factor, listeriolysin O, to escape from the phagosome [10]. Through other novel mechanisms, it then can move from cell to cell without entering the extracellular space, thus avoiding contact with complement, antibodies, and neutrophils [11]. There is no increased frequency of listeriosis in those with deficiencies in neutrophil numbers or function, splenectomy, complement deficiency, or immunoglobulin disorders, the latter not surprising given that *L. monocytogenes* can be passed from cell to cell without being exposed to antibody.

Listeriae have a particular predilection for the central nervous system (CNS). Experimental data indicate that *L. monocytogenes* can use several different mechanisms to invade the CNS: (1) transportation of bacteria to the CNS within circulating leukocytes in a phagocyte-facilitated (Trojan horse) mechanism, (2) via direct invasion of endothelial cells of the blood-brain barrier by blood-borne bacteria, or (3) via a neural route whereby bacteria are inoculated into oral tissues when abrasive food is chewed, followed by tissue macrophage phagocytosis of the bacteria making possible the invasion of cranial nerves [12]. In the latter case, bacteria move in a retrograde direction through the nerve

A. Safdar (ed.), *Principles and Practice of Transplant Infectious Diseases*, https://doi.org/10.1007/978-1-4939-9034-4_28

axons, eventually reaching the CNS where they continue to spread intercellularly to the parenchyma.

Another important virulence factor for *L. monocytogenes* is the ability to scavenge iron. In vitro, iron enhances organism growth [13]. In animal models of listeria infection, iron overload is associated with enhanced susceptibility to infection and iron supplementation with enhanced lethality, whereas prolonged survival results from iron depletion [14]. Iron overload states are risk factors for listerial infection, and clinical correlates include outbreaks of listerial infection in patients receiving hemodialysis who have transfusion-induced iron overload and patients with hemochromatosis [9].

Epidemiology

Listeria monocytogenes is readily isolated from soil and vegetation and has been found to be present in the feces of many mammals [15]. The organism has been isolated from the stool of ~5% of healthy adults [16]. In three healthy, asymptomatic adults followed up for 1 year, *L. monocytogenes* was present transiently in 3.5% of stool specimens [17]. Many foods are contaminated with *L. monocytogenes*; recovery rates of 15–70% have been found from raw vegetables, unpasteurized milk, fish, poultry, and meats [18]. Ingestion of listeriae must be a common occurrence. Nonperinatal listeriosis is almost always the result of foodborne infection. Listeriosis is a relatively rare foodborne illness (~1% of US cases) but is associated with a case fatality rate of 16–20% (second only to *Vibrio vulnificus* at 35–39%) and causes 19–28% of all foodborne disease-related deaths [19, 20]. Mortality risk factors in nonperinatal cases include nonhematological cancers, steroid medication, and renal disease.

Numerous foodborne outbreaks have occurred with vehicles including unpasteurized soft cheeses, hot dogs, and deli-style ready-to-eat sliced poultry products. In October 2002, *L. monocytogenes* was found in sliced deli-style turkey meat, the ingestion of which produced illness in 54 patients in 9 states, resulting in the largest recall of meat ever in the United States (more than 30 million pounds of food products) [21]. In 2011, cantaloupes contaminated by *L. monocytogenes* were responsible for the deadliest foodborne outbreak in US history with 28 states reporting cases [22]. The epidemic affected 146 persons, 30 of whom died (21% mortality).

The highest infection rates of invasive listeriosis are seen in adults >60 years of age and in infants <1 month old [23]. The rate of infection declines sharply between the ages of 1 and 11 months. Pregnant women account for approximately 30% of all cases of listerial bacteremia and 60% of cases in the 10- to 40-year age group. It is noteworthy that although pregnancy is a clear risk factor for bacteremia, for unknown reasons, listerial meningitis is exceedingly rare during pregnancy unless a second risk factor, such as corticosteroid therapy, is present. Seventy percent of nonperinatal infections occur in patients with impairments in cell-mediated immunity. Seemingly normal persons may develop invasive disease, particularly those older than age 60.

The major risk factor for listeriosis is impaired cell-mediated immunity whether due to a specific disease or due to immunosuppressive therapy. Specific risk factors for developing listeriosis include corticosteroid treatment, organ transplantation, malignancy, AIDS, pregnancy, liver failure, diabetes, and age >60 [24]. In a review of almost 2000 cases of listeriosis reported in France from 2001 to 2008, when compared with healthy persons under the age of 65, those with chronic lymphocytic leukemia had a >1000-fold increased risk of acquiring listeriosis, and those with hepatic cancer; myeloproliferative disorder; myeloma; acute leukemia; giant cell arteritis; dialysis; esophageal, stomach, pancreas, lung, and brain cancer; cirrhosis; organ transplantation; and pregnancy had a 100- to 1000-fold increased risk of listeriosis [25]. Reports continue to be published of *L. monocytogenes* meningitis presenting as an opportunistic infection in AIDS [26] and as a complication of solid organ transplantation [27]. One new risk factor for listerial infection is the use of antitumor necrosis factor alpha (TNF-α) agents. Case reports describe listerial meningitis complicating infliximab treatment for Crohn's disease [28] as well as etanercept treatment for Still's disease [29]. An interesting basic science correlate of these clinical events is the observation that, in a murine model, TNF was found to play a crucial role in the intracerebral control of *L. monocytogenes* infection [30].

Major Clinical Syndromes

The species name derives from the fact that an extract of the *L. monocytogenes* cell membrane has potent monocytosis-producing activity in rabbits [31], but monocytosis is a very rare feature of human infection.

Infection in Pregnancy and the Neonatal Period

Pregnant women are prone to develop listerial bacteremia with an estimated 17-fold increase in risk [32]; clinical illness most often occurs in the third trimester. Listeriae proliferate in the placenta in areas that appear to be unreachable by usual defense mechanisms [33], and cell-to-cell spread facilitates maternal-fetal transmission [34]. For unexplained reasons, CNS infection, a commonly recognized form of listeriosis in other groups, is extremely rare during pregnancy in the absence of other risk factors [9, 16, 35]. Bacteremia is manifested clinically as an acute febrile illness, often accompanied by myalgias, arthralgias, headache, and backache. Twenty-two percent of human perinatal infections result in stillbirth or neonatal death; spontaneous abortion is common. Untreated bacteremia is generally self-limited, although if there is a complicating amnionitis, fever in the mother may persist until the fetus is spontaneously or therapeutically aborted. Among women who have listeriosis during pregnancy, two thirds of surviving infants develop clinical neonatal listeriosis. Early diagnosis and antimicrobial treatment of the infected woman can result in the birth of a healthy infant [9, 32].

Similar to disease due to Group B streptococcus, neonatal infections manifest as early-onset sepsis with disseminated infection, typically in premature infants, or late-onset meningitis, typically in term infants who were healthy at birth.

Bacteremia

Bacteremia without an evident focus is the most common manifestation of listeriosis after the neonatal period [2, 24]. Clinical manifestations are similar to those seen in bacteremia with other causes and typically include fever and myalgias; a prodromal illness with diarrhea and nausea may occur [9].

Central Nervous System Infection

The organisms that cause bacterial meningitis most frequently (*Streptococcus pneumoniae*, *Neisseria meningitidis*, *Haemophilus influenzae*) rarely cause parenchymal brain infections such as cerebritis and brain abscess. In contrast, *L. monocytogenes* has tropism for the brain itself, particularly the brain stem, as well as for the meninges [2, 3, 36]. Many patients with meningitis have altered consciousness, seizures, or movement disorders, or all of these, and truly have a meningoencephalitis.

Meningitis

In an active meningitis surveillance study [37], *L. monocytogenes* accounted for 20% of cases in neonates and 20% in those older than 60 years. Worldwide, *L. monocytogenes* is one of the three major causes of neonatal meningitis, is second only to pneumococcus as a cause of bacterial meningitis in adults older than 50 years, and is the most common cause of bacterial meningitis in patients with lymphomas [38], organ transplant recipients, or those receiving corticosteroid immunosuppression for any reason [9].

Clinically, meningitis caused by *L. monocytogenes* is usually similar to that due to more common causes [39, 40]; features particular to listerial meningitis are summarized in Table 28.1. Despite the name "monocytogenes," the CSF pleocytosis is more often neutrophilic than monocytic.

Table 28.1 Features particular to listerial meningitis as compared to more common bacterial etiologies[a]

Feature	Frequency (%)
Presentation can be subacute >24[b]	~60
Absence of stiff neck is more common	25
Movement disorders (ataxia, tremors, myoclonus) are more common	15–20
Seizures are more common	10–25
Fluctuating mental status is more common	~75
Focal neurologic findings are more common	35–40
Positive blood culture is more common	50–75
Cerebrospinal fluid (CSF):	
Positive Gram stain is less common	30–40
Normal CSF glucose is more common	>60
Mononuclear cell predominance is more common	~30

[a]Adapted from [9, 39, 41]

[b]May be several days or more and mimic tuberculous meningitis in ~10–30%

The first prospective study of meningitis due to *L. monocytogenes* recently was reported from the Netherlands [41]. In this nationwide cohort study of 30 adults, notable clinical features of listerial meningitis included headache in 88%, nausea in 83%, and fever in 90%; but only 75% of patients had a stiff neck at the time of presentation. A focal neurologic deficit was present in 37% (many patients with meningitis have simultaneous infection of the brain parenchyma and truly have a meningoencephalitis). Only 43% had the classic meningitis triad of fever, neck stiffness, and change in mental status. At the time of presentation, 19 out of 30 patients had symptoms persisting for greater than 24 h, and 8 had symptoms for ≥4 days. Remarkable CSF findings included a median white blood cell count of 620 (range 24–16,003) and protein of 2.52 g/L. Spinal fluid Gram stain revealed a gram-positive rod in only 28% of patients, while blood cultures were positive for *L. monocytogenes* in 46% of patients. These data illustrate how difficult it can be to make a definitive diagnosis of listerial meningitis at initial presentation.

Mortality from listerial meningitis has variously been reported at 15% in a CDC active surveillance study [37], 27% in the Massachusetts General Hospital review [39], and 17% in the prospective study from the Netherlands [41]. In the last report, all deaths occurred within 3 days of being admitted to the hospital. Mortality is low (zero to 13%) for adults without serious underlying disease or immunosuppressive treatment [36].

Brain Stem Encephalitis (Rhombencephalitis)

An unusual form of listerial encephalitis involves the brain stem [42]. In contrast to other listerial CNS infections, this illness usually occurs in healthy adults. The typical clinical picture is one of a biphasic illness with a prodrome of fever, headache, nausea, and vomiting lasting about 4 days followed by the abrupt onset of asymmetric cranial nerve deficits, cerebellar signs, and hemiparesis or hemisensory deficits, or both. About 40% of patients develop respiratory failure. Nuchal rigidity is present in about one half, and CSF findings are only mildly abnormal with a positive CSF culture in about one-third. Almost two-thirds of patients are bacteremic. Magnetic resonance imaging is superior to computed tomography for demonstrating brain stem encephalitis [43]. Mortality is high, and serious sequelae are common in survivors.

Brain Abscess

Macroscopic brain abscesses account for about 10% of CNS listerial infections. Bacteremia is almost always present, and concomitant meningitis with isolation of *L. monocytogenes* from the CSF is found in 25–40%; both these features are rare in other forms of bacterial brain abscess [44]. Most cases occur in known risk groups for listerial infection [45]. Subcortical abscesses located in the thalamus, pons, and medulla are common; these sites are exceedingly rare when abscesses are caused by other bacteria. Mortality is high, and survivors usually have serious sequelae.

Febrile Gastroenteritis

Many patients with invasive listeriosis have a history of antecedent gastrointestinal illness, often accompanied by fever. Isolated cases of gastrointestinal illness due to *L. monocytogenes* are rare, but at least seven outbreaks of foodborne gastroenteritis due to *L. monocytogenes* have been documented [4]. Illness typically occurs 24 h (range 6 h to 10 days) after ingestion of a large inoculum of bacteria and usually lasts 1–3 days (range 1–7 days); attack rates have been quite high (52–100%). Common symptoms include fever, watery diarrhea, nausea, headache, and pains in joints and muscles. Vehicles of infection have included chocolate milk, cold corn and tuna salad, cold smoked trout, and delicatessen meat. *Listeria monocytogenes* should be considered to be a possible etiology in outbreaks of febrile gastroenteritis when routine cultures fail to yield a pathogen.

Listeriosis in Cancer Patients

Louria, in 1967 [46], was the first to point out the strong association between opportunistic listerial infection and malignancies, particularly Hodgkin's disease being treated with corticosteroids. He described 18 cases of invasive listerial infection, 16 of which had underlying hematologic malignancies. Twelve of the 18 cases were receiving corticosteroids at the time of diagnosis.

Listeria monocytogenes infection occurred in 94 patients during 1955–1997 at the Memorial Sloan Kettering Cancer Center; the incidence was 0.5 (1955–1966), 0.96 (1970–1979), and 0.14 (1985–1997) cases per 1000 new admissions [38]. Eighty-five of 94 (90%) patients had listerial bacteremia, and 34/94 (36%) had evidence of intracranial infection. Listeriosis in these patients with cancer occurred most often in individuals receiving antineoplastic therapy for advanced or relapsed malignancy (77%) and systemic corticosteroids (68%). In another study, combined treatment with fludarabine and prednisone in patients with chronic lymphocytic leukemia decreased their CD4+ T lymphocyte counts and increased their incidence of listeriosis; fludarabine alone was not associated with listeriosis [47].

In a comprehensive review [39] of 33 years of experience at the Massachusetts General Hospital with CNS listeriosis outside of the neonatal period and pregnancy, including a case series of 41 patients and 776 episodes from the literature, the most common predisposing factor for developing listerial meningitis was malignancy (both solid tumor and hematologic), occurring in 24% of patients.

At another institution, from 1990 to 2001, 34 cancer patients with listeriosis were reviewed, and 20 (59%) had an underlying hematologic malignancy [48]. In 11 patients, listeriosis complicated bone marrow transplantation. Twenty-six patients received prior corticosteroids. Here again, bacteremia was the most common presentation of listeriosis (74%), followed by meningoencephalitis (21%). The rate of response to antimicrobial therapy was 79%, and no relapses were identified. Listeriosis contributed to death in 9 (75%) of the 12 patients who died. In the Memorial Sloan-Kettering study [38], 37 (39%) of the 94 patients died of listeriosis; more than one-third of deaths occurred within the first 48 h after *L. monocytogenes* cultures were obtained.

In a recent study of all listeriosis cases in France over an 8-year period, having chronic lymphocytic leukemia, myeloproliferative disorders, liver cancer, myeloma, acute leukemia, or cancers of the esophagus, pancreas, and lung was associated with a 100- to 1000-fold risk of listeriosis, when compared with persons less than 65 years of age with no underlying conditions [25]. Mortality from listeriosis in those with hematological malignancies was increased by more than fivefold compared with those without underlying disease.

In the elderly, listerial meningitis may serve as a marker for cancer. In a recent Danish study [49], adult survivors of meningitis had an increase in cancer-related deaths during the 5-year period after the diagnosis of meningitis. Another interesting relationship exists between listeriosis and cancer. Listerial endocarditis, not bacteremia per se, in an otherwise healthy person, may be an indicator of underlying gastrointestinal tract pathology, including colon cancer [50].

Listeriosis in Transplant Recipients

A little more than 30 years ago, Nieman and Lorber, in a case series and review of listeriosis in the preceding decade [36], pointed out an emerging association between transplantation and the risk of listeriosis. The last three decades have strengthened this association with numerous reports and reviews of invasive *L. monocytogenes* infection in both solid organ and bone marrow transplants. A recent nationwide review of listeriosis in France during an 8-year period showed that, when compared with healthy persons under age 65, the risk of acquiring infection in patients with solid organ transplants was increased 164-fold; all were receiving immunosuppressive therapy [25].

Two other observations illustrate well the strong link between transplantation and listeriosis risk. Firstly, of the six species of *Listeria*, *L. monocytogenes* is almost exclusively responsible for human disease. But, as shown in well-documented instances of bacteremia due to *L. grayi* in a heart transplant recipient [51] and a stem cell recipient [52], along with bacteremia due to *L. ivanovii* in a renal transplant recipient [53], transplanted individuals are at particular risk for listeriosis, even when due to species other than *L. monocytogenes*. Secondly, recurrent listerial infection is exceedingly rare, but again, reports of recurrent *L. monocytogenes* meningitis in heart transplant recipients [54] and of recurrent bacteremia in a liver transplant recipient [55] show the high risk of listeriosis in transplanted persons.

Both solid organ and bone marrow transplant recipients are considered to be at increased risk for listeriosis due to immunosuppressive therapy-related defects in cellular immune function. In a matched case-control study of risk factors for listeriosis in solid organ transplant recipients [56], independent risk factors for infection included diabetes, cytomegalovirus infection or disease in the preceding 6 months, and high-dose corticosteroid therapy in the preceding 6 months; trimethoprim-sulfamethoxazole prophylaxis was protective. In this study, CMV disease or infection carried the highest risk; the immunomodulatory effects of CMV infection and associated infection risk due to a variety of agents are increasingly recognized. The median time to diagnosis for listeriosis after transplantation was 202 days (range, 16–5189 days); 50% of cases occurred more than 6 months following transplantation. The 30-day mortality rate was 27%.

The impact of antecedent or concurrent CMV infection on listeriosis risk has also been noted in the setting of allogeneic blood and marrow transplantation. Six systemic *L. monocytogenes* infections were seen on the bone marrow transplantation service at one cancer center during a 13-year period; four of the six were being treated for acute CMV viremia [57]. Bacteremia is more common than CNS infection, and most listerial infections are seen more than 60 days after bone marrow transplantation. Hemophagocytosis syndrome has been reported as an unusual complication of listerial infection in a bone marrow transplant recipient [58].

An early series of listeriosis complicating renal transplantation was reported by Stamm and colleagues in 1982 [59]. They described an outbreak involving six cases in a 10-week period and reviewed 102 cases. Meningitis was the presenting illness in 50% of patients, parenchymal brain infection in 10%, combined meningeal and parenchymal CNS infection in 9%, and primary bacteremia in 30%. Mortality rate was 26%. In a large review of 820 cases of CNS listeriosis at a single institution, hematologic cancers and renal transplantation were the two most common predisposing factors [32].

A 2007 review of *L. monocytogenes* infection following orthotopic liver transplantation described a case of meningitis and reviewed 14 cases from the English language literature [27]. Time from transplantation to infection ranged from 7 days to 32 months; ten patients presented with bacteremia and five with CNS infection. Diagnosis in the index patient in this report was delayed because the severe headache that developed on day 5 posttransplant was initially thought to represent tacrolimus encephalopathy.

Listerial infection following lung transplantation has been reported rarely. In one case [60], a 59-year-old man developed a pleural effusion 8 days after bilateral lung transplantation. Pleural fluid contained 3900 white blood cells/mm^3 (85% neutrophils) and had a pH of 7.29; cultures of blood and pleural fluid grew *L. monocytogenes*. Pleuropulmonary listeriosis is rare. Most cases have been associated with hematological malignancies and presented with isolated pleural effusion or empyema.

Another unusual manifestation of listerial infection is myocarditis which has been reported in two heart transplant recipients who presented with heart failure that was initially attributed to graft rejection [61].

Although transplant recipients are at markedly increased risk for listeriosis when compared with the general population, the overall risk remains small and has been reported to be 0.12% [56] in solid organ recipients and 0.47% in allogeneic marrow recipients [57].

All transplant recipients should be given information on foodborne illnesses including listeriosis and should be instructed in the importance of handwashing along with food safety and handling (see Prevention section).

Diagnosis

The key to making a diagnosis of listerial infection and initiating early, appropriate treatment is to know when it should be considered. CNS listeriosis should be a major consideration as part of the differential diagnosis in the following clinical settings:

1. Meningitis or parenchymal brain infection in:
   - Patients with organ or bone marrow transplantation, corticosteroid immunosuppression, hematologic malignancy, or AIDS or those receiving anti-TNF agents.
   - Patients with a subacute presentation of meningitis.
   - Neonates and adults >50 years of age.
   - Those in whom CSF shows gram-positive rods or is reported to have "diphtheroids" on Gram stain or culture.
2. Simultaneous infection of the meninges and brain parenchyma.
3. Subcortical brain abscess.
4. Spinal symptoms in the setting of acute bacterial meningitis of uncertain etiology.
5. Fever during pregnancy, particularly in the third trimester.
6. Blood, CSF, or other normally sterile specimen reported to have "diphtheroids" on Gram stain or culture.
7. Foodborne outbreak of febrile gastroenteritis when routine cultures fail to identify a pathogen.

Diagnosis requires isolation of *L. monocytogenes* from a normally sterile site such as blood or CSF and identification through standard microbiologic techniques. Antibodies to listeriolysin O have proved useful during investigation of outbreaks of febrile gastroenteritis [62] but have not proved useful in invasive disease [63]. *Listeria monocytogenes* DNA in CSF and tissue can be detected specifically by polymerase chain reaction (PCR) assays [64]. Real-time PCR of CSF for the *hly* gene, which encodes listeriolysin O, has been useful in diagnosing CNS listeriosis, including cases in which the routine bacterial cultures were negative [65], but this test is not yet commercially available. MRI is superior to CT for demonstrating parenchymal brain involvement, especially in the brainstem [42, 43].

Treatment

Many antimicrobials show in vitro activity against listerial isolates, but only a few agents have been proved clinically efficacious. Ampicillin has been the most widely used agent in the treatment of *L. monocytogenes* infections and generally is considered the preferred agent [2, 40]. Synergy has been demonstrated both in vitro and in animal models when an aminoglycoside is added to ampicillin or penicillin, and many authorities recommend the addition of an aminoglycoside to ampicillin for at least the first week in treatment of CNS infection [9].

In the absence of a positive CSF Gram stain, initial therapy for bacterial meningitis in adults older than age 50 should include an anti-listerial agent (either ampicillin or trimethoprim-sulfamethoxazole) [2]. Due to the high affinity of *L. monocytogenes* for the CNS, meningitis doses of the chosen antibiotic should be used for all bacteremic patients, even in the absence of CNS findings, until the CSF is examined. An exception is bacteremia in pregnancy without another risk factor, since, in this group, CNS infection is almost never present. Relapses are reported in those with meningitis treated for less than 2 weeks; therefore, treatment for 3 weeks is recommended for all cases of listerial meningitis. Bacteremic patients with normal CSF may be treated for 2 weeks. Patients with brain abscess, cerebritis, or rhombencephalitis should be treated for at least 6 weeks and followed up with repeated brain imaging studies. In cases of listerial brain abscess, surgical intervention may not be necessary; numerous case reports describe successful treatment with antimicrobial therapy alone.

In those with penicillin hypersensitivity, trimethoprim-sulfamethoxazole is the treatment of choice and appears to be bactericidal and as effective as the combination of ampicillin and gentamicin. Cephalosporins have limited activity against listeriae. Many reports document treatment failures with cephalosporins, and patients have developed listerial meningitis while receiving cephalosporins for other reasons. Chloramphenicol has also been shown to have an unacceptable failure rate and should not be used. Erythromycin and tetracycline have been reported to be effective but are unreliable therapeutic options and should be avoided. Vancomycin has been used successfully in penicillin-allergic patients, but listerial meningitis has developed in patients being treated with vancomycin. Both imipenem and meropenem have also been used with success to treat cases of listeriosis, but caution is advised because both drugs lower the seizure threshold, imipenem was less effective than ampicillin in a mouse model [66], and meropenem clinical failure has been documented [67].

In an animal model of listerial meningitis, the addition of rifampin to ampicillin was no better than ampicillin alone. While some newer quinolones and linezolid show good in vitro activity, clinical experience is mixed [68–70] and, to date, too limited to support recommending these antimicrobials.

Although adjunctive corticosteroids have become the standard of care in the initial management of bacterial meningitis, their value in listerial infection remains unknown. Listeriae use iron as a virulence factor; therefore, in patients with iron deficiency, it seems prudent to withhold iron replacement until treatment of infection is completed.

Prevention

Food industry regulations were instituted in the United States over 20 years ago to minimize the risk of foodborne listeriosis and cut foodborne infection rates by more than one-half; rates have been relatively stable for several years [71, 72]. In contrast, rates of listerial infection appear to be rising in Europe [73].

Transplant recipients, cancer patients with hematological malignancies, and/or those on corticosteroids should be advised to avoid certain foods. Detailed recommendations from the CDC concerning food handling and avoidance for those at risk for listeriosis can be found on the CDC website at (http://www.cdc.gov/listeria/prevention.html#melonsafety). Major recommendations are summarized in Table 28.2.

Except from infected mother to fetus, human-to-human transmission of listeriosis does not occur; therefore, patients do not need to be isolated.

Listerial infections are effectively prevented by trimethoprim-sulfamethoxazole given as *Pneumocystis* prophylaxis to those on long-term corticosteroids [74].

Table 28.2 Recommendations for preventing foodborne listeriosis

General recommendations:
Washing and handling food
Rinse raw produce thoroughly under running tap water before eating, cutting, or cooking. Even if the produce will be peeled, it should still be washed first
Scrub firm produce, such as melons and cucumbers, with a clean produce brush
Dry the produce with a clean cloth or paper towel
Keep your kitchen and environment cleaner and safer
Wash hands, knives, countertops, and cutting boards after handling and preparing uncooked foods
Be aware that *Listeria monocytogenes* can grow in foods in the refrigerator. The refrigerator should be 40 °F or lower and the freezer 0 °F or lower.
Clean up all spills in your refrigerator right away—especially juices from hot dogs and lunchmeat packages, raw meat, and raw poultry
Cook meat and poultry thoroughly
Thoroughly cook raw food from animal sources, such as beef, pork, or poultry, to a safe internal temperature
Use precooked or ready-to-eat food as soon as you can. Do not store the product in the refrigerator beyond the use-by date
Use leftovers within 3–4 days
Choose safer foods
Do not drink raw (unpasteurized) milk, and do not eat foods that have unpasteurized milk in them
Recommendations for persons at higher risk, such as pregnant women, persons with weakened immune systems, and older adults in addition to the recommendations listed above, include:
Meats
Do not eat hot dogs, luncheon meats, cold cuts, other deli meats (e.g., bologna), or fermented or dry sausages unless they are heated to an internal temperature of 165 °F or until steaming hot just before serving
Avoid getting fluid from hot dog and lunchmeat packages on other foods, utensils, and food preparation surfaces, and wash hands after handling hot dogs, luncheon meats, and deli meats
Do not eat refrigerated pâté or meat spreads from a deli or meat counter or from the refrigerated section of a store. Foods that do not need refrigeration, like canned or shelf-stable pâté and meat spreads, are safe to eat. Refrigerate after opening
Cheeses
Do not eat soft cheese such as feta, queso blanco, queso fresco, brie, Camembert, blue-veined, or panela (queso panela) unless it is labeled as made with pasteurized milk. Make sure the label says, "*made with pasteurized milk.*"
Seafood
Do not eat refrigerated smoked seafood, unless it is contained in a cooked dish, such as a casserole, or unless it is a canned or shelf-stable product
Canned and shelf-stable tuna, salmon, and other fish products are safe to eat
Melons
Wash hands with warm water and soap for at least 20 s *before* and *after* handling any whole melon
Scrub the surface of melons with a clean produce brush under running water, and dry them with a clean cloth or paper towel before cutting. Be sure that your scrub brush is sanitized after each use
Promptly consume cut melon or refrigerate promptly. Keep your cut melon refrigerated for no more than 7 days
Discard cut melons left at room temperature for more than 4 h

References

1. Bucholz U, Mascola L. Transmission, pathogenesis, and epidemiology of Listeria monocytogenes. Infect Dis Clin Pract. 2001;10:34–41.
2. Lorber B. Listeria monocytogenes. In: Mandell GL, Bennett JE, Dolin R, editors. Principles and practice of infectious diseases. 7th ed. Philadelphia: Churchill Livingstone Inc; 2009. p. 2707–14.
3. Painter J, Slutsker L. Listeriosis in humans. In: Ryser ET, Marth EH, editors. Listeria, listeriosis and food safety. 3rd ed. Boca Raton: CRC Press; 2007. p. 85–109.
4. Ooi ST, Lorber B. Gastroenteritis due to Listeria monocytogenes. Clin Infect Dis. 2005;40:1327–32.
5. Bille J. Listeria and Erysipelothrix. In: Murray PR, Baron EJ, Jorgensen JH, et al., editors. Manual of clinical microbiology. 9th ed. Washington, DC: American Society for Microbiology Press; 2007. p. 474–84.
6. Colodner R, Sakran W, Miron D, Teitler N, Khavalevsky E, Kopelowitz J. Listeria monocytogenes cross-contamination in a nursery. Am J Infect Control. 2003;31:322–4.
7. Farber JM, Daley E, Coates F, Beausoleil N, Fournier J. Feeding trials of Listeria monocytogenes with a nonhuman primate model. J Clin Microbiol. 1991;29:2606–8.
8. Schlech WF 3rd, Chase DP, Badley A. A model of food-borne Listeria monocytogenes infection in the Sprague-Dawley rat using

gastric inoculation: development and effect of gastric acidity on infective dose. Int J Food Microbiol. 1993;18:15–24.
9. Lorber B. Listeriosis. Clin Infect Dis. 1997;24:1–11.
10. Schnupf P, Portnoy DA. Listeriolysin O: a phagosome-specific lysin. Microbes Infect. 2007;9:1176–87.
11. Hamon M, Bierne H, Cossart P. Listeria monocytogenes: a multi-faceted model. Nature Rev. 2006;4:423–34.
12. Drevets DA, Bronze MS. Listeria monocytogenes: epidemiology, human disease, and mechanisms of brain invasion. FEMS Immunol Med Microbiol. 2008;53:151–65.
13. Dramsi S, Lévi S, Triller A, Cossart P. Entry of Listeria monocytogenes into neurons occurs by cell-to-cell spread: an in vitro study. Infect Immun. 1998;66:4461–8.
14. Ampel NM, Bejarano GC, Saavedra M Jr. Deferoxamine increases the susceptibility of beta-thalassemic, iron-overloaded mice to infection with Listeria monocytogenes. Life Sci. 1992;50:1327–3132.
15. Schuchat A, Swaminathan B, Broome CV. Epidemiology of human listeriosis. Clin Microbiol Rev. 1991;4:169–83.
16. Schlech WF 3rd, Lavigne PM, Bortolussi RA, Allen AC, Haldane EV, Wort AJ, et al. Epidemic listeriosis—evidence for transmission by food. N Engl J Med. 1983;308:203–6.
17. Grif K, Patscheider G, Dierich MP, Allerberger F. Incidence of fecal carriage of Listeria monocytogenes in three healthy volunteers: a one-year prospective stool survey. Eur J Clin Microbiol Infect Dis. 2003;22:16–20.
18. Farber JM, Peterkin PI. Listeria monocytogenes, a food-borne pathogen. Microbiol Rev. 1991;55:476–511.
19. Guevara RE, Mascola L, Sorvillo F. Risk factors for mortality among patients with nonperinatal listeriosis in Los Angeles County, 1992-2004. Clin Infect Dis. 2009;48:1507–15.
20. Scallan E, Griffin PM, Angulo FJ, Tauxe RV, Hoekstra RM. Foodborne illness acquired in the United States--unspecified agents. Emerg Infect Dis. 2011;17:16–22.
21. Gottlieb SL, Newbern EC, Griffin PM, Graves LM, Hoekstra RM, Baker NL, et al, Listeriosis Outbreak Working Group. Multistate outbreak of listeriosis linked to turkey deli meat and subsequent changes in US regulatory policy. Clin Infect Dis 2006;42:29–36.
22. United States Centers for Disease Control and Prevention. Multistate outbreak of listeriosis linked to whole cantaloupes from Jensen Farms, Colorado. December 8, 2011 (final update). http://www.cdc.gov/listeria/outbreaks/cantaloupes-jensen-farms/120811/index.html. Accessed 18 May 2012.
23. Tappero JW, Schuchat A, Deaver KA, Mascola L, Wenger JD. Reduction in the incidence of human listeriosis in the United States. Effectiveness of prevention efforts? JAMA. 1995;273:1118–22.
24. Swaminathan B, Gerner-Smidt P. The epidemiology of human listeriosis. Microbes Infect. 2007;9:1236–43.
25. Goulet V, Hebert M, Hedberg C, Laurent E, Vaillant V, De Valk H, Desenclos J-C. Incidence of listeriosis and related mortality among groups at risk of acquiring listeriosis. Clin Infect Dis. 2012;54:652–60.
26. Patil AB, Nadiger S, Chandrasekhar MR, Halesh LH, Kumar M. Listeria monocytogenes meningitis: an uncommon opportunistic infection in HIV/AIDS. Ind J Pathol Microbiol. 2007;50:671–3.
27. Mizuno S, Zendejas IR, Reed AI, Kim RD, Howard RJ, Hemming AW, et al. Listeria monocytogenes following orthotopic liver transplantation: central nervous system involvement and review of the literature. World J Gastroenterol. 2007;13:4391–3.
28. Williams G, Khan AA, Schweiger F. Listeria meningitis complicating infliximab treatment for Crohn's disease. Can J Infect Dis Microbiol. 2005;16:289–92.
29. La Montagna G, Valentini G. Listeria monocytogenes meningitis in a patient receiving etanercept for Still's disease. Clin Exp Rheumatol. 2005;23:121.
30. Virna S, Deckert M, Lütjen S, Soltek S, Foulds KE, Shen H, et al. TNF is important for pathogen control and limits brain damage in murine cerebral listeriosis. J Immunol. 2006;177:3972–82.
31. Stanley NF. Studies of Listeria monocytogenes: I. Isolation of a monocytosis-producing agent (MPA). Aust J Exp Biol Med Sci. 1949;27:123–31.
32. Mylonakis E, Paliou M, Hohmann EL, Calderwood SB, Wing EJ. Listeriosis during pregnancy: a case series and review of 222 cases. Medicine. 2002;81:260–9.
33. Bakardjiev AI, Theriot JA, Portnoy D. Listeria monocytogenes traffics from maternal organs to the placenta and back. PLoS Pathog. 2006;2:e66.
34. Bakardjiev AI, Stacy BA, Portnoy DA. Growth of Listeria monocytogenes in the guinea pig placenta and role of cell-to-cell spread in fetal infection. J Infect Dis. 2005;191:1889–97.
35. Ciesielski CA, Hightower AW, Parsons SK, Broome CV. Listeriosis in the United States: 1980–1982. Arch Intern Med. 1988;148:1416–9.
36. Nieman RE, Lorber B. Listeriosis in adults: a changing pattern. Report of eight cases and review of the literature, 1968–1978. Rev Infect Dis. 1980;2:207–27.
37. Schuchat A, Robinson K, Wenger JD, Harrison LH, Farley M, Reingold AL, et al. Bacterial meningitis in the United States in 1995. Active surveillance team. N Engl J Med. 1997;337:970–6.
38. Safdar A, Armstrong D. Listeriosis in patients at a comprehensive cancer center, 1955–1997. Clin Infect Dis. 2003;37:359–64.
39. Mylonakis E, Hohmann EL, Calderwood SB. Central nervous system infection with Listeria monocytogenes. 33 years' experience at a general hospital and review of 776 episodes from the literature. Medicine. 1998;77:313–36.
40. Clauss HE, Lorber B. CNS infection with Listeria monocytogenes. Curr Infect Dis Rep. 2008;10:300–6.
41. Brouwer MC, van de Beek D, Heckenberg SG, Spanjaard L, de Gans J. Community-acquired Listeria monocytogenes meningitis in adults. Clin Infect Dis. 2006;43:1233–8.
42. Armstrong RW, Fung PC. Brainstem encephalitis (rhombencephalitis) due to Listeria monocytogenes: case report and review. Clin Infect Dis. 1993;16:689–702.
43. Alper G, Knepper L, Kanal E. MR findings in listerial rhombencephalitis. AJNR. 1996;17:593–6.
44. Eckburg PB, Montoya JG, Vosti KL. Brain abscess due to Listeria monocytogenes. Five cases and a review of the literature. Medicine. 2001;80:223–35.
45. Cone LA, Leung MM, Byrd RG, Annunziata GM, Lam RY, Herman BK. Multiple cerebral abscesses because of Listeria monocytogenes: three case reports and a literature review of supratentorial listerial brain abscess(es). Surg Neurol. 2003;59:320–8.
46. Louria DB, Hensle T, Armstrong D, Collins HS, Blevins A, Krugman D, Buse M. Listeriosis complicating malignant disease. A new association. Ann Intern Med. 1967;67:261–81.
47. Anaissie E, Kontoyiannis DP, O'Brien S, Kantarjian H, Robertson L, Lerner S, Keating MJ. Listeriosis in patients with chronic lymphocytic leukemia who were treated with fludarabine and prednisone. Ann Intern Med. 1992;117:466–9.
48. Rivero GA, Torres HA, Rolston KV, Kontoyiannis DP. Listeria monocytogenes infection in patients with cancer. Diagn Microbiol Infect Dis. 2003;47:393–8.
49. Roed C, Engsig FN, Omland LH, Skinhoj P, Obel N. Long-term mortality in patients diagnosed with Listeria monocytogenes meningitis: a Danish nationwide cohort study. J Infect. 2012;64:34–40.
50. Lorber B. Clinical listeriosis-implications for pathogenesis. In: Miller AJ, Smith JL, Somkuti GA, editors. Foodborne Listeriosis. New York: Elsevier; 1990. p. 41–9.
51. Rapose A, Lick SD, Ismail N. Listeria grayi bacteremia in a heart transplant recipient. Transplant Infect Dis. 2008;10:434–6.

52. Salimnia H, Patel D, Lephart PR, Fairfax MR, Chandrasekar PH. Listeria grayi: vancomycin-resistant, gram-positive rod causing bacteremia in a stem cell transplant recipient. Transplant Infect Dis. 2010;12:526–8.
53. Guillet C, Join-Lambert O, Le Monnier A, Leclercq A, Mechaï F, Mamzer-Bruneel M-F, et al. Human listeriosis caused by Listeria ivanovii. Emerg Infect Dis. 2010;16:136–8.
54. Larner AJ, Conway MA, Mitchell RG, Forfar JC. Recurrent Listeria monocytogenes meningitis in a heart transplant recipient. J Infect. 1989;19:263–6.
55. Peetermans WE, Endtz HP, Janssens AR, vand den Broek PJ. Recurrent Listeria monocytogenes bacteraemia in a liver transplant patient. Infection. 1990;18:107–8.
56. Fernandez-Sabé N, Cervera C, López-Medrano F, Llano M, Sáez E, Len Ó, et al. Risk factors, clinical features, and outcomes of listeriosis in solid-organ transplant recipients: a matched case-control study. Clin Infect Dis. 2009;49:1153–9.
57. Safdar A, Papadopoulous EB, Armstrong D. Listeriosis in recipients of allogeneic blood and marrow transplantation: thirteen year review of disease characteristics, treatment outcomes and a new association with human cytomegalovirus infection. Bone Marrow Transplant. 2002;29:913–6.
58. Lambotte O, Fihman V, Poyart C, Buzyn A, Berche P, Soumelis V. Listeria monocytogenes skin infection with cerebritis and haemophagocytosis syndrome in a bone marrow transplant recipient. J Infect. 2004;50:356–8.
59. Stamm AM, Dismukes WE, Simmons BP, Cobbs CG, Elliott A, Budrich P, Harmon J. Listeriosis in renal transplant recipients: report of an outbreak and review of 102 cases. Rev Infect Dis. 1982;4:665–82.
60. Janssens W, Van Raemdonck D, Dupont L, Verleden GM. Listeria pleuritis 1 week after lung transplantation. J Heart Lung Transplant. 2006;25:734–7.
61. Stamm AM, Smith SH, Kirklin JK, McGiffin DC. Listerial myocarditis in cardiac transplantation. Rev Infect Dis. 1990;12:820–3.
62. Dalton CB, Austin CC, Sobel J, Hayes PS, Bibb WF, Graves LM, et al. An outbreak of gastroenteritis and fever due to Listeria monocytogenes in milk. N Engl J Med. 1997;336:100–5.
63. Chatzipanagiotou S, Hof H. Sera from patients with high titers of antibody to streptolysin 0 react with listeriolysin. J Clin Microbiol. 1988;26:1066–7.
64. Greisen K, Loeffelholz PA, Leong D. PCR primers and probes for the 16S rRNA gene of most species of pathogenic bacteria, including bacteria found in cerebrospinal fluid. J Clin Microbiol. 1994;32:335–51.
65. Le Monnier A, Abachin E, Beretti J-L, Berche P, Kayal S. Diagnosis of Listeria monocytogenes meningoencephalitis by real-time PCR for the hly gene. J Clin Microbiol. 2011;49:3917–23.
66. Kim KS. In vitro and in vivo studies of imipenem—cilastatin alone and in combination with gentamicin against Listeria monocytogenes. Antimicrob Agents Chemother. 1986;29:289–93.
67. Stepanović S, Lazarević G, Ješić M, Kos R. Meropenem therapy failure in Listeria monocytogenes infection. Eur J Clin Microbiol Infect Dis. 2004;23:484–6.
68. Grumbach NM, Mylonakis E, Wing EJ. Development of listerial meningitis during ciprofloxacin treatment. Clin Infect Dis. 1999;29:1340–1.
69. Viale P, Furlanut M, Cristini F, Cadeo B, Pavan F, Pea F. Major role of levofloxacin in the treatment of a case of Listeria monocytogenes meningitis. Diagn Microbiol Infect Dis. 2007;58:137–9.
70. Leiti O, Gross JW, Tuazon CU. Treatment of brain abscess caused by Listeria monocytogenes in a patient with allergy to penicillin and trimethoprim-sulfamethoxazole. Clin Infect Dis. 2005;40:907–8.
71. Voetsch AC, Angulo FJ, Jones TF, Moore MR, Nadon C, McCarthy P, et al. Centers for Disease Control and Prevention Emerging Infections Program Foodborne Diseases Active Surveillance Network Working Group. Reduction in the incidence of invasive listeriosis in foodborne diseases active surveillance network sites, 1996–2003. Clin Infect Dis. 2007;44:513–20.
72. Goulet V. What can we do to prevent listeriosis in 2006? Clin Infect Dis. 2007;44:529–30.
73. Allerberger F, Wagner M. Listeriosis: a resurgent foodborne infection. Clin Microbiol Infect. 2010;16:16–23.
74. Dworkin MS, Williamson J, Jones JL, Kaplan JE. Prophylaxis with trimethoprim-sulfamethoxasole for human immunodeficiency virus-infected patients: impact on risk for infectious diseases. Clin Infect Dis. 2001;33:393–8.

Tuberculosis

29

Cynthia Portal-Celhay and Jennifer A. Philips

Mycobacterium Tuberculosis Pathogenesis and Host Response

Basic Biology of Mycobacterium Tuberculosis

Robert Koch identified *Mycobacterium tuberculosis* (Mtb) as the causative agent of tuberculosis (TB) nearly 130 years ago, and it is estimated to infect one third of the world's population. It is a rod-shaped bacterium with a very high lipid and mycolic acid content in its cell wall. This makes it stain poorly with Gram stain, but it retains certain dyes such as Ziehl-Neelsen after acid treatment, resulting in characteristic "acid-fast" staining. Other unique features are its exceptionally slow growth, dividing approximately every 20 h, and its ability to establish latent infection. While few people infected with Mtb develop acute disease upon infection, most individuals, even those with a seemingly normal immune system, are unable to eradicate infection.

People are initially infected via an aerosol route. In contrast to infections with non-tuberculous mycobacteria (NTM), there is no known environmental reservoir, so infection only occurs after contact with a person with active disease. It is thought that the infectious dose is quite low, perhaps on the order of several bacilli, and the initial infection generally is not clinically recognized. The initial site of infection in the lungs, referred to as a Ghon complex, is most often in the upper part of the lower lobe or the lower part of the upper lobe. Inhaled bacteria are deposited in the distal alveoli where they encounter and are taken up by alveolar macrophages. Additional phagocytic cells recruited to the infected lung, including neutrophils, monocyte-derived macrophages, and dendritic cells (DCs), ingest bacteria and play an important role in the outcome of the infection [1].

The initial interaction between bacteria and cells of the innate immune system occurs through pattern recognition receptors such as Toll-like receptors, complement receptors, mannose receptors, and C-type lectin receptors, such as Dectin-1 and the macrophage-inducible C-type lectin, Mincle [2–4]. Unlike pathogens that avoid uptake into host cells, Mtb appears to take advantage of multiple possible receptors to enter phagocytic cells. Bacteria are taken up into the macrophage phagosome, a compartment that ordinarily becomes acidified and fuses with lysosomes forming a phagolysosome. However, the phagosome containing mycobacteria does not fully acidify or acquire features of mature phagolysosomes [5, 6]. Mycobacteria have long been thought to persist and grow within this specialized cellular compartment that resembles an early endosome, which allows the bacteria to acquire nutrients, such as iron via recycling endosomes, while avoiding the acidic, degradative environment of the lysosome [7]. More recent work has shown that the bacteria also gain access to the host cell cytoplasm [8, 9], which activates host cytosolic sensors and alternative pathways for phagosome maturation [10–12].

In contrast to their usual role in protecting the host, macrophages appear to be an important determinant of bacterial spread and dissemination. For example, studies performed using a zebrafish model and *Mycobacterium marinum*, a close genetic relative of Mtb, revealed that uninfected macrophages are actively recruited to the area surrounding an infected cell [13]. Following replication of mycobacteria in the initial macrophage, bacteria released into the extracellular space are rapidly ingested by the recruited, surrounding macrophages, allowing further expansion and dissemination of the pathogen population [14].

Based upon work in mice, DCs, myeloid cells that are specialized for antigen presentation, transport Mtb from the lungs to the local draining lymph nodes to present antigen to naive T cells. T helper (Th)1 cells that are activated in the

C. Portal-Celhay
Division of Infectious Diseases, Department of Medicine, NYU Langone Medical Center, NYU School of Medicine, New York, NY, USA
e-mail: cynthia.portal@nyumc.org

J. A. Philips (✉)
Division of Infectious Diseases, Department of Medicine, Washington University School of Medicine, St. Louis, MO, USA
e-mail: philips.j.a@wustl.edu

A. Safdar (ed.), *Principles and Practice of Transplant Infectious Diseases*, https://doi.org/10.1007/978-1-4939-9034-4_29

draining lymph node then travel back to the lung, where they can subsequently activate infected macrophages. T cell activation is delayed compared to other infections, which may be important in allowing the bacteria to establish their initial niche [15]. T-cells activate infected macrophages by secreting cytokines such as interferon-gamma (IFN-γ) and tumor necrosis factor-alpha (TNF-α), which promote the ability of macrophages to restrict mycobacterial growth. IFN-γ promotes production of reactive nitrogen intermediates [16], enhances phagosome maturation in a manner dependent upon the immunity related GTPases [17, 18], and promotes autophagy, a host cellular mechanism recently appreciated to clear certain intracellular pathogens including Mtb [10, 12, 19, 20]. Nonetheless, the host is ultimately ineffective at eradicating infection. One reason for this may be is that although there is a robust immune response to Mtb antigens, there may be limited availability or recognition of antigen within the infected tissue [21–23]. In addition, although cytokines can improve the antimycobacterial capacity of macrophages, Mtb impairs the responsiveness of the infected macrophage [24, 25].

In addition to activating a Th1 response, Th17 cells, which are characterized by the secretion of IL-17, IL-21, and IL-22, are also induced in the draining lymph node and return to the lung where they exert effector function. The balance of Th1 and Th17 responses appears to be important in the outcome of Mtb infection [26]. One way in which Th17 cells and IL-17 influence immunity and immunopathology in TB is the recruitment of neutrophils, a cell type whose role in TB infection is increasingly appreciated. Neutrophils are recruited early during initial infection, are a dominant infected cell population, and promote granuloma formation [27]. In addition, infected apoptotic bodies are transferred from neutrophils to DCs, which promotes T cell priming in the draining lymph node, although Mtb appears to impair this process by inhibiting apoptosis and promoting cellular necrosis [28–31]. Although neutrophils appear to have a role in host protection early during infection, mouse models and recent human data suggest they are also associated with immunopathology and poor outcome in Mtb infection. Neutrophilia may indicate a failed Th1 immune response, as IFN-γ inhibits pathogenic neutrophil accumulation and impairs neutrophil survival in a mouse model [32]. In humans, an analysis of gene transcriptional responses in Mtb-infected patients found that patients with active tuberculosis exhibit a signature reflecting a neutrophil-driven type I IFN-α,β and IFN-γ signaling that was reversed with drug treatment [33].

The histological response to Mtb infection is characterized by granuloma formation. Granulomas contain an organized aggregate of macrophages [34], which exhibit a variety of phenotypes, including epithelioid macrophages, foamy macrophages, and multinucleated giant cells formed by the fusion of multiple macrophages, along with other cell types such as lymphocytes, neutrophils, and dendritic cells. Classically, granulomas have been thought to "wall off" infection, implying they are primarily of benefit to the host. However, more recent data suggest that granulomas may also benefit the pathogen, and several mycobacterial components promote granuloma formation. Granulomas may benefit the bacilli by serving as a site for macrophage recruitment and concomitant bacterial expansion [14]. In addition, during the early stages of granuloma formation, a fraction of infected macrophages may depart from the nascent granuloma and initiate infection at distant sites. Granulomas are also probably important for immune control of TB, since they are a site for interactions between antigen-presenting cells and effector T cells. Therefore, granulomas may more accurately be thought of as a site of the stalemate between bacteria and host, providing benefit to both.

Latent TB infection (LTBI) is characterized by absent or very limited bacterial replication and no clinical symptoms. The only evidence of infection is an immune response to Mtb antigens. A striking feature of tuberculosis is that this situation can persist for decades. However, while the host immune response is inadequate to eradicate bacteria, it is important in preventing active disease. Approximately 5% of people will become sick in the first 2 years after initial infection, and an additional 5% will reactivate infection sometime during their lifetime. In apparently normal hosts, reactivation most commonly occurs in the lungs, resulting in characteristic cavitary disease. However, since the bacteria are able to disseminate during infection, they can also reactivate in distant tissues. Unlike the détente of latent infection where the bacterial burden is low and tissue injury is minimal, during active disease, the granuloma becomes necrotic, resulting in the tissue damage that is necessary to promote transmission. Thus, while Mtb appears to be minimally inflammatory during latent infection, it must generate a robust immune response to successfully transmit. Thus, it must be exquisitely adept at manipulating the host immune response in two seemingly distinct manners [35].

Host Determinants of Disease

The host immune response is critical in susceptibility to tuberculosis infection. Animal models have shown that both CD4+ and CD8+ T-cells are required for protection against disease [36, 37], an observation borne out clinically in patients who lack adequate T cell function. Individuals with reduced CD4+ T cells, such as those infected with HIV, have markedly increased susceptibility to tuberculosis [38, 39]. Similarly, chemotherapy that impairs T cell function, such as fludarabine, results in enhanced susceptibility to Mtb [40]. T cells are essential for the maintenance of organized granulomas and the control of infection. Thus, the highest frequency of disseminated disease is found in those HIV-infected patients with the lowest CD4+ T cell counts. At least part of the importance of T cells is to activate infected macrophages, making them more potently bactericidal. Hence, cytokines that mediate the interaction between T cells and macrophages have also been shown to be critically important in host immunity. For example, mice lacking IFN-γ die rapidly of Mtb infection [41]. Likewise, children with mutations in genes involved in IFN-γ-mediated immunity, including interferon gamma receptor 1 (IFNGR1), interferon gamma receptor 2 (IFNGR2), signal transducer and activator of transcription 1 (STAT1), interleukin 12B (IL12B), interleukin 12 receptor, beta 1 (IL12RB1), NF-κB essential modulator (NEMO), cytochrome b-245, beta polypeptide (CYBB), interferon regulatory factor 8 (IRF8), and ubiquitin-like protein ISG15, suffer from susceptibility to weakly virulent mycobacteria such as *Mycobacterium bovis*-bacillus Calmette-Guerin (BCG), a vaccine strain, as well as to *Salmonella* and Mtb [42–45]. In addition, neutralizing anti-IFN-γ-autoantibodies have been found in Asian patients with an adult onset immunodeficiency syndrome that makes them highly susceptible to mycobacterial infection [46]. Vitamin D is important in the ability of macrophages to respond to IFN-γ [47], and clinical studies have linked serum 25-hydroxyvitamin D levels with susceptibility to tuberculosis [48–51]. Detailed studies of human macrophages have illuminated the mechanism by which vitamin D improves clearance of intracellular bacteria, a pathway that appears to operate both in response to Toll-like receptor signaling [52] and IFN-γ signaling, suggesting vitamin D is important in both the innate and acquired response to Mtb.

In addition to IFN-γ, tumor necrosis factor-alpha (TNF-α) is essential for control of Mtb. Mice lacking TNF-α are highly susceptible to Mtb [53]. TNF-α activates macrophages and modulates apoptosis of infected cells [54, 55]. At the same time, excess TNF-α contributes to the immunopathology of TB [56, 57], and Mtb has developed specific mechanisms to modulate macrophage production of TNF-α [58]. Patients who receive TNF-α inhibitors for rheumatoid arthritis or Crohn's disease are at increased risk of reactivation of latent tuberculosis, often presenting with disseminated disease [59]. Use of infliximab, an anti-TNF-α antibody, has illustrated the importance of TNF-α in humans, as well as pointing to the importance of a particular set of CD8+ T-cells. Patients treated with infliximab have a significantly higher risk of reactivating Mtb than those treated with etanercept, a soluble TNF receptor that functions as a decoy receptor to block TNF signaling [60, 61]. This may be explained by the fact that infliximab binds much better than etanercept does to transmembrane TNF, which is found on a specific population of CD8+ T-cells that exhibit antimicrobial activity against Mtb. Infliximab binding to these cells makes them susceptible to complement-mediated lysis [62], and they are depleted in patients treated with infliximab. This is consistent with additional literature pointing to the role of CD8+ T cells in host defense against Mtb. To conclude, animal models and human studies all support the fact that T cells, IFN-γ, and TNF-α play central roles in host defense against Mtb. When these are impaired—by disease states, genetic mutations, or therapeutic intervention—the risk of developing active tuberculosis rises substantially. There are certain to be other critical determinants, for example, the inflammasome and IL-1β, which are actively under investigation, but their contribution in human infection has yet to be fully elucidated [63].

Bacterial Determinants of Disease

Determinants of Mtb virulence include secreted proteins and biologically active lipids. These components interact with the host to modulate intracellular bacterial trafficking, host cellular signaling, host cell death pathways, and granuloma formation. Mycobacteria have an unusual lipid-rich cell envelope containing distinctive long-chain fatty acids such as mycolic acids. These lipids play an important role in bacterial pathogenesis and have been an active focus for research on interactions with the host. For example, a complex lipid (phthiocerol dimycoserate) is required for bacterial growth in the lungs of mice [64, 65]. An abundant cell wall lipoglycan, mannose-capped lipoarabinomannan (ManLAM), is implicated in affecting intracellular bacterial trafficking. ManLAM has been extensively investigated as a potential virulence factor because LAM is mannosylated in pathogenic mycobacteria, whereas in the cell wall of environmental mycobacteria, LAM is capped by arabinose or inositol phosphate [66]. Trehalose dimycolate (TDM), a glycolipid historically known as cord factor, has profound immunomodulatory roles. It induces inflammatory cell recruitment and granuloma formation, and its receptor, Mincle, was recently identified [3, 4, 67]. TDM and other mycobacterial glycolipids can promote the formation of multinucleated giant cells found in granulomas, and ManLAM can mediate the aggregation of mononuclear cells [68]. Thus, the unique and complex cell envelope of Mtb is central to the biology of the organism.

In addition to being a source of bioactive molecules, the cell envelope also represents a hurdle for bacteria to secrete virulence factors, and recent work has shed light on a specialized protein secretion system that enables mycobacteria to transport virulence factors across their complex and impermeable cell envelope [69]. This secretion apparatus came to light based upon a direct genomic comparison between the avirulent vaccine strain, BCG, and Mtb [70, 71]. Although there is considerable sequence identity between these strains, several genomic regions are deleted in BCG. Among these is a region that encodes a type VII secretion apparatus (TSSS), called ESAT-6 system 1 (Esx-1), and several associated secreted proteins, including EsxA and EsxB. EsxA and EsxB also known as early secreted antigen target-6 (ESAT-6) and 10-kDa culture filtrate protein (CFP-10), respectively, are highly secreted, prominent antigens recognized by CD4+ and CD8+ T cells [72]. The absence of this region in BCG largely accounts for why the vaccine strain is attenuated [73–75], so it has been the focus of intense study. Esx-1 plays a central although incompletely understood role in Mtb pathogenesis that includes effects on intracellular trafficking and innate and adaptive immune responses. The Mtb genome encodes five separate TSSSs, but less is known about the others. The Esx-5 locus is required for transport of many proteins from two gene families found uniquely in mycobacteria termed PE and PPE proteins named for their conserved proline and glutamic acid (PE) and proline-proline-glutamic acid (PPE) motifs [76]. Remarkably, approximately 10% of the coding capacity of Mtb is dedicated to these gene families, which remain poorly understood. Thus, the secreted effectors of the TSSSs are likely to be critical in the pathogenesis of Mtb infection, but currently there is limited insight into their mechanism of action.

In addition, a growing number of proteins have been implicated in modulating the cell biology of macrophages. For example, the secreted bacterial proteins phosphotyrosine protein phosphatase (PtpA), dihydrolipoamide dehydrogenase (LpdC), secreted acid phosphatase (SapM), zinc-dependent metalloprotease (Zmp1), and nucleoside diphosphate kinase (NdkA) are implicated in arresting phagosome maturation, creating the early endosome-like niche of Mtb [77–79]. Mtb appears to impair apoptosis of infected cells, and bacterial mutants defective in this activity are attenuated [29]. Molecules such as the abundantly secreted 19-kDa lipoprotein antigen blunts IFN-γ signaling in macrophages [80], and a secreted bacterial adenylate cyclase modulates macrophage production of TNF-α [58]. It is not surprising that a bacterium that has evolved to make its home in human macrophages has a complex set of tools to remodel its residence. Currently, we are developing a better understanding of the tool set and how the individual components work together to orchestrate the complex life cycle of the bacteria under active investigation.

Tuberculosis in the Transplant Population

Epidemiology

Transplant patients are highly susceptible to Mtb infection. Most posttransplant TB cases occur due to reactivation of latent infection, but acquisition from donor tissue and primary infection are also seen, although they are relatively rare. Donor transmission was the proposed source in 4% of cases based upon a review of the literature from 1967 to 1997 [81] and has been described even in countries with a low overall TB incidence because of global immigration [82]. The overall incidence of posttransplant tuberculosis varies by geographic region based upon the local prevalence of Mtb (http://www.who.int/tb/publications/global_report/2010/en/index.html) and has been reported to be 20–74-fold higher in solid organ transplant (SOT) patients than the general population. Across different studies from developed countries, the frequency of TB in SOT patients ranged from 0.25% to 6.4% [81, 83–85], while in countries where tuberculosis is highly endemic, such as India and Pakistan, it has been reported to be as high as 15% [86, 87]. In bone marrow transplant (BMT) patients, the prevalence of active tuberculosis has been reported to be in the range of 0.23–0.79%. As for SOTs, regions of high TB endemicity, such as Taiwan and Hong Kong, report much higher rates (1.4–5.5%) [88–92]. A review of the literature between 1967 and 1997 indicated that active tuberculosis infection was diagnosed in 0.35–1.2% of kidney, 1–1.4% of heart, 0.9–2.3% of liver, and 2–6.5% of lung transplant recipients [81]. The type of graft influences risk, but which type is at highest risk may depend upon the local population; a large cohort of patients from 16 centers in Spain were followed prospectively, and the highest frequency was found in lung transplant recipients [84]. In contrast, the largest series of SOTs from a single US center comes from Columbia University College of Physicians and Surgeons in New York City, where renal transplant patients had the highest risk of tuberculosis [93]. In that study, Hispanic patients were overrepresented among kidney transplants as compared with those receiving other SOTs, suggesting the higher rate among renal transplant patients may, at least in part, reflect a higher rate of prior TB exposure in that population. In endemic areas such as Taiwan, it was recently reported that kidney transplant recipients were also found to have a higher risk of TB infection compared to other SOTs such as liver and heart [94].

Risk Factors

Since most posttransplant tuberculosis is due to reactivation of latent infection, the risk depends upon the likelihood of pre-transplant infection. Risk factors for Mtb infection and for progression to active tuberculosis infection in the general population are provided below.

Individuals at higher risk for latent tuberculosis infection are as follow:

(a) Close contacts of persons with known or suspected active tuberculosis, infections including residents and employees of congregate settings where residents are at increased risk for active tuberculosis such as correctional and long-term care facilities, homeless shelters, and healthcare workers who serve patients at higher risk for active tuberculosis infection.

(b) Foreign-born persons from regions with high rates of active tuberculosis infection including Africa, Asia, Eastern Europe, Latin America, and Russia; individuals from low tuberculosis-endemic regions become at increased risk for tuberculosis infection if they visit high tuberculosis-endemic regions frequently and for an extended duration.

(c) Local populations considered at risk for latent tuberculosis infection possibly include medically underserved, low-income population or those with a history of chronic alcohol abuse and/or illicit recreation drug use.

Risk factors for progression of latent tuberculosis infection to active tuberculosis are outlined below:

(a) Persons with primary tuberculosis exposure and latent infection of less than 24-month duration.

(b) Patients with active tuberculosis that was not treated or received inadequate antituberculosis therapy, especially in individuals with evidence of pulmonary fibrosis.

(c) Patients with underlying medical conditions such as silicosis, chronic renal disease, diabetes mellitus, leukemia, lymphoma, head and neck or lung cancer. Patients who have undergone gastrectomy or jejunoileal bypass surgery are also at an increased risk for developing active tuberculosis infection.

(d) Individuals with history of cigarette smoking and alcohol and drug abuse and those with severe emaciation (<90% of ideal body weight) are considered at risk.

A subgroup of patients not only have higher risk for active tuberculosis infection, but such an infection, when it occurs, carries poor prognosis including tuberculous meningitis, disseminated multiorgan involvement, and death. In this group, infants and children aged <5 years, persons with HIV/AIDS, those receiving TNF inhibitors, high-dose systemic corticosteroids, and solid organ transplant recipients on antirejection regimens are prominent.

In transplant patients, the risk has been shown to be related to similar factors, such as history of exposure to Mtb based upon positive TST results or radiographic evidence of previously untreated Mtb, as well as clinical conditions present in this population, including chronic renal insufficiency or hemodialysis, diabetes mellitus, chronic liver disease, and other co-existing opportunistic infections. In a study in Spain, the recipient's age was a risk factor, likely reflecting the decrease in TB in the general population in recent years, such that older people are more likely to be latently infected [84]. Although positive TST results are a significant risk factor, it is important to note that only 20–25% of cases of posttransplant tuberculosis occur in patients with positive TSTs before transplant, reflecting the poor sensitivity of this test in patients with underlying end-organ failure [95].

A consistent finding has been that immunosuppressive regimens that contain (muromonab-CD3) OKT3 or antithymocyte globulin (ATG) enhance the risk of tuberculosis. OKT3 is an antibody that blocks T cell function by binding the surface molecule, CD3, on T cells. ATG is either pooled rabbit or horse antibodies against human T cells and results in T cell depletion. It is not surprising that these agents enhance the risk of tuberculosis given the importance of T cells in preventing reactivation of latent infection. In addition, intensification of immunosuppression to treat graft rejection is also a predisposing factor. In BMT patients, risk factors include graft-versus-host disease and total body irradiation [88].

Timing of Diagnosis

More than two-thirds of posttransplant tuberculosis in SOT patients are diagnosed in the first year posttransplant, with a median time to diagnosis of ~ 6–9 months (range 0.5–144 months) [81, 83, 84, 96]. The fact that the majority of patients develop tuberculosis in the first year posttransplant is consistent with the idea that most disease is due to reactivation of latent infection. Late cases presumably reflect a mix of both late reactivation and new infection and therefore may be more common in settings with a high local prevalence of tuberculosis where reinfection is more likely to occur [97]. Although rare, nosocomial transmission posttransplant has also been reported. In one instance, active tuberculosis occurred in ten renal transplant patients over an 11-month period. The median incubation period was only 7.5 weeks and 5 of the patients died a median of 8 weeks after diagnosis [98], pointing to the high susceptibility of transplant patients to primary infection.

Risk factors for diagnosis in the first year of transplant include non-renal transplant, history of early allograft rejection, immunosuppressive therapy with OKT3 or anti-T cell antibodies, and clinical and/or radiographic evidence of prior tuberculosis [81, 83]. Other immunosuppressive reagents also influence the time to diagnosis. In an Egyptian study, the introduction of cyclosporine A (CsA) in 1987 resulted in a shorter time to TB diagnosis than in previous patients who had received azathioprine and steroids (64 months versus 130 months) [99]. In a series of renal transplant patients in Turkey, the use of tacrolimus and/or mycophenolate mofetil was associated with earlier development of TB posttransplant than regimens with azathioprine, CsA, and prednisolone [100].

In bone marrow transplant patients, tuberculosis occurs with a mean time to presentation of ~9 months [88–90]. Few patients are diagnosed during the period of neutropenia, and most cases (75%) occur after day 100. This pattern may reflect that fact that bacteria reactivate during the early phase of the BMT due to immunosuppressive therapy and total body irradiation, but given the slow growth of Mtb and the lack of a robust immune response, disease rarely manifests until later during periods of immune reconstitution [88].

Clinical Manifestations

Regardless of transplant type, the organ most frequently with tuberculosis is the lung, but approximately one third to one half of patients present with extrapulmonary or disseminated disease, compared with ~15% in immunocompetent individuals [101, 102]. Extrapulmonary and disseminated disease can involve nearly any organ with atypical and varied clinical presentations. Thus, tuberculosis should be considered in all patients with fever of unknown origin. The frequency of disseminated disease does not differ significantly based upon the type of SOT, but is more likely to occur if patients receive OKT3.

Fever is nearly a universal finding in patients with disseminated disease (>90%), and also occurs with localized infection in ~60% of patients [81]. Night sweats and weight loss are often present. Hepatic involvement has been reported in ~50% of liver transplant patients, and it has been reported at a similar rate in renal, heart, and lung transplant patients in whom liver tissue samples were studied by biopsy or at autopsy [81]. Gastrointestinal disease outside of the liver can have a wide variety of forms including gastrointestinal bleeding, peritonitis, and abscess formation. It often presents with abdominal pain and gastrointestinal bleeding that can be exsanguinating. It is often unsuspected until laparotomy or colonoscopy and most often involves the ileocecal area. Colonic disease can present as a perforated abscess or mimic a tumor. Isolated pancreatic tuberculosis has also been reported. Septic arthritis, cutaneous abscesses, and pyomyositis can occur, most commonly in the context of disseminated disease. Vertebral osteomyelitis is relatively rare, and more often occurs as localized infection and early symptoms may be atypical [103]. Central nervous system disease can present as either meningitis, which is most often associated with disseminated disease, or as focal abscesses, which can be the only site of infection or as part of disseminated illness. The most common symptoms of TB meningitis include fever, headache, vomiting, and altered consciousness. Involvement of the basilar meninges and cistern can cause cranial nerve dysfunction [104]. Renal and genitourinary disease occurs both in renal transplant patients as well as other SOT recipients. Lymphadenitis most often occurs as part of disseminated infection but can be localized. In summary, tuberculosis can involve almost any tissue, and other less commonly reported sites of infection include the pericardium, spleen, larynx, tonsil, and ocular choroid. Co-infections occur in up to 20% of patients; cytomegalovirus infection, *Nocardia* infection, community-acquired pneumonia, urinary tract infection, and invasive mold infections may modify the nonspecific symptomatology and further delay tuberculosis diagnosis [95].

Although acquisition from donors is relatively rare, it does occur and can present with various manifestations [81]. In one example, an American-born woman underwent a double lung transplant. Routine BAL on postoperative day 1 grew Mtb in culture, as did bronchial washing from postoperative day 10. The donor had no known Mtb risk factors except recent immigration from Guatemala. Retrospectively, a faint opacity was seen in the donor's chest radiograph prior to transplant, which corresponded with a left upper lobe micronodular infiltrate on the recipients CT scan. Genotypic analysis of the isolate suggested it was related to strains in Guatemala, not to those in California where the transplant was performed [105]. In another case, the donor had active pulmonary tuberculosis, and the sole site of Mtb in the recipient was an abscess in the hepatic allograft [106]. Graft-related infections need not involve the transplanted graft as in the cases above. For example, in one case, separate grafts from a single donor resulted in genitourinary infection in the renal transplant recipient, but osteomyelitis in a liver transplant patient. Interestingly, a third patient who received a renal graft from the same donor was asymptomatic and was treated for LTBI [107].

Radiographic Findings

Although posttransplant tuberculosis often involves the lungs, there is no characteristic radiographic pattern seen, which makes diagnosis difficult. In fact, as few as 4% of patients present with cavitary disease. Instead, focal infiltrates, a miliary pattern, nodules, and pleural effusions are more common. Diffuse interstitial infiltrates can also be seen [81]. The findings can be subtle, such as bronchial narrowing caused by an endobronchial granulomatous mass [108].

Diagnosis

It is important to diagnose LTBI in donor and recipient pretransplant in order to consider pre- or posttransplant chemoprophylaxis. The decision to treat LTBI requires weighing the risk of reactivation with the possible drug toxicities and drug-drug interactions [109]. Careful screening of donors has become increasingly important as the donor pool has become more ethnically diverse, and a recent international working group formulated consensus recommendations for screening of donors [110–112].

Unfortunately, there is no gold standard to detect LTBI. Clinical history is useful in assessing the risk of latent TB infection, and questions about country of origin, travel, exposure to patients with active tuberculosis, and social and medical risk factors should be evaluated. In addition, CXR may reveal old granulomatous disease or apical scaring as evidence of prior TB. Evidence of latent TB infection can be obtained by tuberculin skin testing (TST) or IFN-γ release assays (IGRAs) [113]. When conventional TST is used, ≥5 mm of induration at 48–72 h should be considered positive in transplant patients [114]. Repeating the test 7–10 days after an initial negative TST may reveal that the first test was falsely negative, as the first administration of PPD can boost the response in individuals with remote TB exposure. There are two FDA-approved IGRAs available in the United States: QuantiFERON-TB Gold In-tube test (QFT-GIT, Cellestis Ltd) and T-SPOT.TB test (T-Spot, Oxford Immunotec Ltd). Guidelines on their use is available from the CDC [115], and the American Academy of Pediatrics has published guidance for their use in children [116]. Like TST, IGRAs detect an immunological response to Mtb antigens. TSTs detect a delayed type hypersensitivity response to purified protein derivative (PPD) in vivo. PPD is a crude mix of Mtb antigens that can also elicit responses due to prior vaccination with BCG or exposure to non-tuberculous mycobacteria. In contrast, IGRAs detect IFN-γ release in vitro from T cells in response to TB antigens, EsxA and EsxB, which are absent from BCG and most environmental mycobacteria. *M. kansasii*, *M. szulgai*, and *M. marinum* are exceptions as they encode homologs of Mtb EsxA and EsxB, so sensitization to these organisms might cause false-positive results in IGRAs. Importantly, unlike TST, positive test results using IGRAs are not confounded by prior BCG vaccination. Thus, IGRAs offer higher specificity than TSTs, particularly in BCG vaccinated populations, although they do not provide a major increase in sensitivity.

Unfortunately, TST performs poorly in transplant populations, both prior to transplant, due to anergy related to end organ disease or long-term corticosteroid treatment, and after transplant due to immunosuppressive agents. The data on IGRAs in immunocompromised patients is more limited than TSTs, but IGRAs appear to perform similarly to or slightly better than TST in SOT patients prior to transplant [117–122]. Only two studies have looked at hematopoietic stem cell transplant patients prior to transplant, and there was a poor correlation between the TST and GTF-GIT, regardless of BCG vaccination history [123, 124]. Thus, although testing for LTBI should be performed prior to transplant, a negative TST or IGRA prior to or after transplant does not rule out prior infection with Mtb [125]. In fact, only 20–25% of cases of active tuberculosis after transplantation occur in patients with positive TST reactions before transplant [95].

Data on the ability of IGRAs to predict subsequent active tuberculosis are limited, particularly in immunocompromised individuals. However, they appear to perform similarly to TST in studied populations, and IGRA can detect some TST-negative subjects who go on to active disease [126]. Routine testing with both TST and IGRAs is not generally recommended, but it might be useful in high-risk transplant patients, when indeterminate results are obtained with one test or when active tuberculosis is suspected [115]. If both TST and IGRA are performed, a positive result in either should be taken as evidence of infection. Since TST and IGRAs detect an immune response to Mtb, they cannot distinguish latent from active infection. Thus, in the case of a positive result, active infection must be ruled out. If clinical or radiographic data suggest TB, sputum smears and cultures or, if necessary, bronchoalveolar aspirate or lavage should be performed. Additional imaging and biopsy may be necessary depending upon the clinical history. TST and IGRAs cannot rule out active infection, as only 75–90% of patients with active tuberculosis are TST positive and the sensitivity drops in patients with underlying immunosuppression [127]. In the case of disseminated disease, approximately 50% of patients have negative TSTs. Therefore, these tests can neither "rule in" nor "rule out" active infection.

Diagnosis of tuberculosis in the posttransplant setting requires a high index of suspicion as the cases are often extrapulmonary and may present with minimal or atypical symptomatology. In addition, diagnostic tests perform poorly, and tuberculosis is also frequently associated with other infections, which may complicate the picture. It should be considered in any patient with fevers of unknown origin, constitutional symptoms, or pulmonary infiltrates. Sputum and biopsy specimens should be sent for acid-fast bacilli staining and culture. Since most cases do not involve cavitary lung disease, invasive procedures are often required to obtain a diagnostic specimen, such as bronchoscopy, mediastinoscopy, laparoscopy, and tissue biopsy. Cerebral spinal fluid (CSF) culture is the gold standard for diagnosing TB meningitis. Direct examination of specimens by means of an acid-fast stain provides supportive evidence of tuberculosis weeks before the culture and species identification may be available. Although microscopic examination is rapid, it is relatively insensitive. Culture is the gold standard, although results take weeks and approximately 20% of clinically suspected pulmonary Mtb infections remain culture negative. The false negative rate is likely to be even higher in extrapulmonary disease. Growth on solid media (such as Lowenstein-Jensen or Middlebrook agar) takes 3–6 weeks. Broth detection systems that detect early changes in the media due to growth of bacteria provide a more rapid turnaround time, often becoming positive after 2 weeks.

Since acid-fast staining and growth on solid or liquid media cannot distinguish Mtb from NTM, once an isolate is recovered, further testing is required for species identification. Growth of a mycobacterial isolate after several days in culture excludes the diagnosis of Mtb, as it is invariably a rapid grower, most commonly *M. fortuitum*, *M. abscesses*, or *M. chelonae*. For slow-growing mycobacteria, molecular approaches can speed the process of species identification. These tests detect mycobacterial nucleic acids directly from clinical specimens. Thus, nucleic acid amplification tests are useful to quickly determine whether the acid-fast bacilli seen on smear or biopsy are a member of the Mtb complex weeks before cultures are available. In addition, nucleic acid amplification tests can detect Mtb in 50–80% of smear-negative, culture-positive specimens. Guidance on the use of such tests has been recently updated [128], which recommend that nucleic acid amplification tests be performed on at least one respiratory specimen from each patient in whom a diagnosis of TB is being considered but has not been established.

A new diagnostic test, Xpert MTF/RIF (Cepheid), uses PCR and molecular beacon technology to identify Mtb in sputum samples within several hours, while simultaneously detecting rifampin resistance [129]. Rifampin resistance is a marker of other drug resistance, so this allows a rapid way to identify suspected MDR cases, which would otherwise take months with conventional drug susceptibility testing. It is highly sensitive in smear-negative sputum samples, and the World Health Organization has endorsed its use as first line in HIV-infected patients in TB-endemic countries. It also appears promising for diagnosing extra-pulmonary disease [130]. One study showed a sensitivity of >85% from CSF, biopsy, urine, pus, and fine needle aspirates, although it may be lower (40–50%) in pleural and cavitary fluids. Further evaluation is necessary in extra-pulmonary disease and in the transplant setting, but it is likely to enter clinical practice given its high sensitivity, rapid turn-around time, and ability to quickly identify rifampin resistance. More novel diagnostic tests, such as TB ID/R [131], pyrosequencing assays [132], whole genome sequencing (WGS) [133], and next-generation sequencing [134, 135] are being configured in a low-cost platform to provide rapid diagnosis and drug susceptibility information.

Outcomes

The mortality rate associated with tuberculosis in transplant patients is 25–40% [81]. The high incidence of extrapulmonary disease and atypical presentations, coupled with the poor performance of diagnostic tests and the slow growth of the bacilli in culture result in diagnostic delays. At the same time, profound immunosuppression can lead to rapid disease progression. Predictors of mortality include disseminated disease, prior rejection, receipt of OKT3 or ATG, and presence of other opportunistic infections [83]. Treatment is complicated by drug interactions with immunosuppressive agents, particularly calcineurin inhibitors. Subtherapeutic immunosuppressive drug levels can result in organ rejection, and allograft loss has been reported in up to 33% of transplant patients on antituberculous therapy. In addition, side effects such as hepatotoxicity can be difficult to manage particularly in liver transplant patients [83]. Given the complexity of treatment and drug interactions, they are covered in detail in the therapeutic section.

Conclusion

Tuberculosis is an important cause of morbidity and mortality in the transplant patient. Our understanding of the basic biology of tuberculosis has made significant advances. It is clear that T cells, IFN-γ, and TNF-α play central roles in host defense against Mtb. On the bacterial side, work has pointed to the importance of the complex cell envelope and the type VII secretion system. Newer molecular techniques have made incremental improvements in diagnosis, although they have not been well studied in the transplant population. Despite these gains, the understanding of TB pathogenesis and host immunity has yet to translate into an efficacious vaccine, robust diagnostics for latent and active tuberculosis, or shorter and less toxic therapies. Therefore, tuberculosis is likely to remain a significant cause of disease in transplant patients for the foreseeable future.

References

1. Wolf AJ, Linas B, Trevejo-Nuñez GJ, Kincaid E, Tamura T, Takatsu K, et al. Mycobacterium tuberculosis infects dendritic cells with high frequency and impairs their function in vivo. J Immunol. 2007;179(4):2509–19.
2. Schäfer G, Jacobs M, Wilkinson RJ, Brown GD. Non-opsonic recognition of Mycobacterium tuberculosis by phagocytes. J Innate Immun. 2009;1(3):231–43.
3. Ishikawa E, Ishikawa T, Morita YS, Toyonaga K, Yamada H, Takeuchi O, et al. Direct recognition of the mycobacterial glycolipid, trehalose dimycolate, by C-type lectin Mincle. J Exp Med. 2009;206(13):2879–88.
4. Schoenen H, Bodendorfer B, Hitchens K, Manzanero S, Werninghaus K, Nimmerjahn F, et al. Cutting edge: mincle is essential for recognition and adjuvanticity of the mycobacterial cord factor and its synthetic analog trehalose-dibehenate. J Immunol. 2010;184(6):2756–60.
5. Armstrong JA, Hart PD. Response of cultured macrophages to Mycobacterium tuberculosis, with observations on fusion of lysosomes with phagosomes. J Exp Med. 1971;134(3 Pt 1): 713–40.
6. Sturgill-Koszycki S, Schlesinger PH, Chakraborty P, Haddix PL, Collins HL, Fok AK, et al. Lack of acidification in Mycobacterium phagosomes produced by exclusion of the vesicular proton-ATPase. Science. 1994;263(5147):678–81.
7. Russell DG. Mycobacterium tuberculosis: here today, and here tomorrow. Nat Rev Mol Cell Biol. 2001;2(8):569–77.

8. van der Wel N, Hava D, Houben D, Fluitsma D, van Zon M, Pierson J, et al. M. tuberculosis and M. leprae translocate from the phagolysosome to the cytosol in myeloid cells. Cell. 2007;129(7):1287–98.
9. McDonough KA, Kress Y, Bloom BR. Pathogenesis of tuberculosis: interaction of Mycobacterium tuberculosis with macrophages. Infect Immun. 1993;61(7):2763–73.
10. Watson RO, Manzanillo PS, Cox JS. Extracellular M. tuberculosis DNA targets bacteria for autophagy by activating the host DNA-sensing pathway. Cell. 2012;150(4):803–15.
11. Manzanillo PS, Shiloh MU, Portnoy DA, Cox JS. Mycobacterium tuberculosis activates the DNA-dependent cytosolic surveillance pathway within macrophages. Cell Host Microbe. 2012;11(5):469–80.
12. Sakowski ET, Koster S, Portal Celhay C, Park HS, Shrestha E, Hetzenecker SE, et al. Ubiquilin 1 promotes IFN-gamma-induced xenophagy of Mycobacterium tuberculosis. PLoS Pathog. 2015;11(7):e1005076.
13. Davis JM, Clay H, Lewis JL, Ghori N, Herbomel P, Ramakrishnan L. Real-time visualization of mycobacterium-macrophage interactions leading to initiation of granuloma formation in zebrafish embryos. Immunity. 2002;17(6):693–702.
14. Davis JM, Ramakrishnan L. The role of the granuloma in expansion and dissemination of early tuberculous infection. Cell. 2009;136(1):37–49.
15. Wolf AJ, Desvignes L, Linas B, Banaiee N, Tamura T, Takatsu K, et al. Initiation of the adaptive immune response to Mycobacterium tuberculosis depends on antigen production in the local lymph node, not the lungs. J Exp Med. 2008;205(1):105–15.
16. Chan J, Xing Y, Magliozzo RS, Bloom BR. Killing of virulent Mycobacterium tuberculosis by reactive nitrogen intermediates produced by activated murine macrophages. J Exp Med. 1992;175(4):1111–22.
17. MacMicking JD, Taylor GA, McKinney JD. Immune control of tuberculosis by IFN-gamma-inducible LRG-47. Science. 2003;302(5645):654–9.
18. Kim BH, Shenoy AR, Kumar P, Das R, Tiwari S, MacMicking JD. A family of IFN-γ-inducible 65-kD GTPases protects against bacterial infection. Science. 2011;332(6030):717–21.
19. Gutierrez MG, Master SS, Singh SB, Taylor GA, Colombo MI, Deretic V. Autophagy is a defense mechanism inhibiting BCG and Mycobacterium tuberculosis survival in infected macrophages. Cell. 2004;119(6):753–66.
20. Levine B, Mizushima N, Virgin HW. Autophagy in immunity and inflammation. Nature. 2011;469(7330):323–35.
21. Egen JG, Rothfuchs AG, Feng CG, Horwitz MA, Sher A, Germain RN. Intravital imaging reveals limited antigen presentation and T cell effector function in mycobacterial granulomas. Immunity. 2011;34(5):807–19.
22. Bold TD, Banaei N, Wolf AJ, Ernst JD. Suboptimal activation of antigen-specific CD4+ effector cells enables persistence of M. tuberculosis in vivo. PLoS Pathog. 2011;7(5):e1002063.
23. Srivastava S, Grace PS, Ernst JD. Antigen export reduces antigen presentation and limits T cell control of M. tuberculosis. Cell Host Microbe. 2016;19(1):44–54.
24. Banaiee N, Kincaid EZ, Buchwald U, Jacobs WR, Ernst JD. Potent inhibition of macrophage responses to IFN-gamma by live virulent Mycobacterium tuberculosis is independent of mature mycobacterial lipoproteins but dependent on TLR2. J Immunol. 2006;176(5):3019–27.
25. Harding CV, Boom WH. Regulation of antigen presentation by Mycobacterium tuberculosis: a role for Toll-like receptors. Nat Rev Microbiol. 2010;8(4):296–307.
26. Torrado E, Cooper AM. IL-17 and Th17 cells in tuberculosis. Cytokine Growth Factor Rev. 2010;21(6):455–62.
27. Seiler P, Aichele P, Bandermann S, Hauser AE, Lu B, Gerard NP, et al. Early granuloma formation after aerosol Mycobacterium tuberculosis infection is regulated by neutrophils via CXCR3-signaling chemokines. Eur J Immunol. 2003;33(10):2676–86.
28. Blomgran R, Desvignes L, Briken V, Ernst JD. Mycobacterium tuberculosis inhibits neutrophil apoptosis, leading to delayed activation of naive CD4 T cells. Cell Host Microbe. 2012;11(1):81–90.
29. Velmurugan K, Chen B, Miller JL, Azogue S, Gurses S, Hsu T, et al. Mycobacterium tuberculosis nuoG is a virulence gene that inhibits apoptosis of infected host cells. PLoS Pathog. 2007;3(7):e110.
30. Hinchey J, Lee S, Jeon BY, Basaraba RJ, Venkataswamy MM, Chen B, et al. Enhanced priming of adaptive immunity by a proapoptotic mutant of Mycobacterium tuberculosis. J Clin Invest. 2007;117(8):2279–88.
31. Keane J, Remold HG, Kornfeld H. Virulent Mycobacterium tuberculosis strains evade apoptosis of infected alveolar macrophages. J Immunol. 2000;164(4):2016–20.
32. Nandi B, Behar SM. Regulation of neutrophils by interferon-γ limits lung inflammation during tuberculosis infection. J Exp Med. 2011;208(11):2251–62.
33. Berry MP, Graham CM, McNab FW, Xu Z, Bloch SA, Oni T, et al. An interferon-inducible neutrophil-driven blood transcriptional signature in human tuberculosis. Nature. 2010;466(7309):973–7.
34. Adams DO. The granulomatous inflammatory response. A review. Am J Pathol. 1976;84(1):164–92.
35. Ernst JD. The immunological life cycle of tuberculosis. Nat Rev Immunol. 2012;12(8):581–91.
36. Mogues T, Goodrich ME, Ryan L, LaCourse R, North RJ. The relative importance of T cell subsets in immunity and immunopathology of airborne Mycobacterium tuberculosis infection in mice. J Exp Med. 2001;193(3):271–80.
37. Caruso AM, Serbina N, Klein E, Triebold K, Bloom BR, Flynn JL. Mice deficient in CD4 T cells have only transiently diminished levels of IFN-gamma, yet succumb to tuberculosis. J Immunol. 1999;162(9):5407–16.
38. Havlir DV, Barnes PF. Tuberculosis in patients with human immunodeficiency virus infection. N Engl J Med. 1999;340(5):367–73.
39. Kwan CK, Ernst JD. HIV and tuberculosis: a deadly human syndemic. Clin Microbiol Rev. 2011;24(2):351–76.
40. Silva FA, Matos JO, de Q Mello FC, Nucci M. Risk factors for and attributable mortality from tuberculosis in patients with hematologic malignances. Haematologica. 2005;90(8):1110–5.
41. Flynn JL, Chan J, Triebold KJ, Dalton DK, Stewart TA, Bloom BR. An essential role for interferon gamma in resistance to Mycobacterium tuberculosis infection. J Exp Med. 1993;178(6):2249–54.
42. Alcaïs A, Abel L, Casanova JL. Human genetics of infectious diseases: between proof of principle and paradigm. J Clin Invest. 2009;119(9):2506–14.
43. Bustamante J, Arias AA, Vogt G, Picard C, Galicia LB, Prando C, et al. Germline CYBB mutations that selectively affect macrophages in kindreds with X-linked predisposition to tuberculous mycobacterial disease. Nat Immunol. 2011;12(3):213–21.
44. Hambleton S, Salem S, Bustamante J, Bigley V, Boisson-Dupuis S, Azevedo J, et al. IRF8 mutations and human dendritic-cell immunodeficiency. N Engl J Med. 2011;365(2):127–38.
45. Bogunovic D, Byun M, Durfee LA, Abhyankar A, Sanal O, Mansouri D, et al. Mycobacterial disease and impaired IFN-γ immunity in humans with inherited ISG15 deficiency. Science. 2012;337(6102):1684–8.
46. Browne SK, Burbelo PD, Chetchotisakd P, Suputtamongkol Y, Kiertiburanakul S, Shaw PA, et al. Adult-onset immunodeficiency in Thailand and Taiwan. N Engl J Med. 2012;367(8):725–34.
47. Fabri M, Stenger S, Shin DM, Yuk JM, Liu PT, Realegeno S, et al. Vitamin D is required for IFN-gamma-mediated antimicrobial activity of human macrophages. Sci Transl Med. 2011;3(104):104ra2.
48. Wilkinson RJ, Llewelyn M, Toossi Z, Patel P, Pasvol G, Lalvani A, et al. Influence of vitamin D deficiency and vitamin D receptor polymorphisms on tuberculosis among Gujarati Asians in west London: a case-control study. Lancet. 2000;355(9204):618–21.

49. Grange JM, Davies PD, Brown RC, Woodhead JS, Kardjito T. A study of vitamin D levels in Indonesian patients with untreated pulmonary tuberculosis. Tubercle. 1985;66(3):187–91.
50. Talat N, Perry S, Parsonnet J, Dawood G, Hussain R. Vitamin d deficiency and tuberculosis progression. Emerg Infect Dis. 2010;16(5):853–5.
51. Martineau AR, Leandro AC, Anderson ST, Newton SM, Wilkinson KA, Nicol MP, et al. Association between Gc genotype and susceptibility to TB is dependent on vitamin D status. Eur Respir J. 2010;35(5):1106–12.
52. Liu PT, Stenger S, Li H, Wenzel L, Tan BH, Krutzik SR, et al. Toll-like receptor triggering of a vitamin D-mediated human antimicrobial response. Science. 2006;311(5768):1770–3.
53. Flynn JL, Goldstein MM, Chan J, Triebold KJ, Pfeffer K, Lowenstein CJ, et al. Tumor necrosis factor-alpha is required in the protective immune response against Mycobacterium tuberculosis in mice. Immunity. 1995;2(6):561–72.
54. Balcewicz-Sablinska MK, Keane J, Kornfeld H, Remold HG. Pathogenic Mycobacterium tuberculosis evades apoptosis of host macrophages by release of TNF-R2, resulting in inactivation of TNF-alpha. J Immunol. 1998;161(5):2636–41.
55. Clay H, Volkman HE, Ramakrishnan L. Tumor necrosis factor signaling mediates resistance to mycobacteria by inhibiting bacterial growth and macrophage death. Immunity. 2008;29(2):283–94.
56. Bekker LG, Moreira AL, Bergtold A, Freeman S, Ryffel B, Kaplan G. Immunopathologic effects of tumor necrosis factor alpha in murine mycobacterial infection are dose dependent. Infect Immun. 2000;68(12):6954–61.
57. Tobin DM, Vary JC Jr, Ray JP, Walsh GS, Dunstan SJ, Bang ND, et al. The lta4h locus modulates susceptibility to mycobacterial infection in zebrafish and humans. Cell. 2010;140(5):717–30.
58. Agarwal N, Lamichhane G, Gupta R, Nolan S, Bishai WR. Cyclic AMP intoxication of macrophages by a Mycobacterium tuberculosis adenylate cyclase. Nature. 2009;460(7251):98–102.
59. Keane J, Gershon S, Wise RP, Mirabile-Levens E, Kasznica J, Schwieterman WD, et al. Tuberculosis associated with infliximab, a tumor necrosis factor alpha-neutralizing agent. N Engl J Med. 2001;345(15):1098–104.
60. Solovic I, Sester M, Gomez-Reino JJ, Rieder HL, Ehlers S, Milburn HJ, et al. The risk of tuberculosis related to tumour necrosis factor antagonist therapies: a TBNET consensus statement. Eur Respir J. 2010;36(5):1185–206.
61. Wallis RS, Broder MS, Wong JY, Hanson ME, Beenhouwer DO. Granulomatous infectious diseases associated with tumor necrosis factor antagonists. Clin Infect Dis. 2004;38(9):1261–5.
62. Bruns H, Meinken C, Schauenberg P, Harter G, Kern P, Modlin RL, et al. Anti-TNF immunotherapy reduces CD8+ T cell-mediated antimicrobial activity against Mycobacterium tuberculosis in humans. J Clin Invest. 2009;119(5):1167–77.
63. Mayer-Barber KD, Barber DL, Shenderov K, White SD, Wilson MS, Cheever A, et al. Caspase-1 independent IL-1beta production is critical for host resistance to mycobacterium tuberculosis and does not require TLR signaling in vivo. J Immunol. 2010;184(7):3326–30.
64. Cox JS, Chen B, McNeil M, Jacobs WR Jr. Complex lipid determines tissue-specific replication of Mycobacterium tuberculosis in mice. Nature. 1999;402(6757):79–83.
65. Camacho LR, Ensergueix D, Perez E, Gicquel B, Guilhot C. Identification of a virulence gene cluster of Mycobacterium tuberculosis by signature-tagged transposon mutagenesis. Mol Microbiol. 1999;34(2):257–67.
66. Briken V, Porcelli SA, Besra GS, Kremer L. Mycobacterial lipoarabinomannan and related lipoglycans: from biogenesis to modulation of the immune response. Mol Microbiol. 2004;53(2):391–403.
67. Matsunaga I, Moody DB. Mincle is a long sought receptor for mycobacterial cord factor. J Exp Med. 2009;206(13):2865–8.
68. Puissegur MP, Botanch C, Duteyrat JL, Delsol G, Caratero C, Altare F. An in vitro dual model of mycobacterial granulomas to investigate the molecular interactions between mycobacteria and human host cells. Cell Microbiol. 2004;6(5):423–33.
69. Abdallah AM, Gey van Pittius NC, Champion PA, Cox J, Luirink J, Vandenbroucke-Grauls CM, et al. Type VII secretion--mycobacteria show the way. Nat Rev Microbiol. 2007;5(11):883–91.
70. Mahairas GG, Sabo PJ, Hickey MJ, Singh DC, Stover CK. Molecular analysis of genetic differences between Mycobacterium bovis BCG and virulent M. bovis. J Bacteriol. 1996;178(5):1274–82.
71. Gordon SV, Brosch R, Billault A, Garnier T, Eiglmeier K, ST C. Identification of variable regions in the genomes of tubercle bacilli using bacterial artificial chromosome arrays. Mol Microbiol. 1999;32(3):643–55.
72. Brodin P, Rosenkrands I, Andersen P, Cole ST, Brosch R. ESAT-6 proteins: protective antigens and virulence factors? Trends Microbiol. 2004;12(11):500–8.
73. Guinn KM, Hickey MJ, Mathur SK, Zakel KL, Grotzke JE, Lewinsohn DM, et al. Individual RD1-region genes are required for export of ESAT-6/CFP-10 and for virulence of Mycobacterium tuberculosis. Mol Microbiol. 2004;51(2):359–70.
74. Hsu T, Hingley-Wilson SM, Chen B, Chen M, Dai AZ, Morin PM, et al. The primary mechanism of attenuation of bacillus Calmette-Guerin is a loss of secreted lytic function required for invasion of lung interstitial tissue. Proc Natl Acad Sci U S A. 2003;100(21):12420–5.
75. Pym AS, Brodin P, Brosch R, Huerre M, Cole ST. Loss of RD1 contributed to the attenuation of the live tuberculosis vaccines Mycobacterium bovis BCG and Mycobacterium microti. Mol Microbiol. 2002;46(3):709–17.
76. Abdallah AM, Verboom T, Weerdenburg EM, Gey van Pittius NC, Mahasha PW, Jimenez C, et al. PPE and PE_PGRS proteins of Mycobacterium marinum are transported via the type VII secretion system ESX-5. Mol Microbiol. 2009;73(3):329–40.
77. Philips JA. Mycobacterial manipulation of vacuolar sorting. Cell Microbiol. 2008;10(12):2408–15.
78. Wong D, Bach H, Sun J, Hmama Z, Av-Gay Y. Mycobacterium tuberculosis protein tyrosine phosphatase (PtpA) excludes host vacuolar-H+-ATPase to inhibit phagosome acidification. Proc Natl Acad Sci U S A. 2011;108(48):19371–6.
79. Sun J, Wang X, Lau A, Liao TY, Bucci C, Hmama Z. Mycobacterial nucleoside diphosphate kinase blocks phagosome maturation in murine RAW 264.7 macrophages. PLoS One. 2010;5(1):e8769.
80. Fortune SM, Solache A, Jaeger A, Hill PJ, Belisle JT, Bloom BR, et al. Mycobacterium tuberculosis inhibits macrophage responses to IFN-gamma through myeloid differentiation factor 88-dependent and -independent mechanisms. J Immunol. 2004;172(10):6272–80.
81. Singh N, Paterson DL. Mycobacterium tuberculosis infection in solid-organ transplant recipients: impact and implications for management. Clin Infect Dis. 1998;27(5):1266–77.
82. Bucher JN, Schoenberg MB. Donor-derived tuberculosis after solid organ transplantation in two patients and a staff member. Infection. 2016;44(3):365–70.
83. Aguado JM, Herrero JA, Gavaldá J, Torre-Cisneros J, Blanes M, Rufí G, et al. Clinical presentation and outcome of tuberculosis in kidney, liver, and heart transplant recipients in Spain. Spanish Transplantation Infection Study Group, GESITRA. Transplantation. 1997;63(9):1278–86.
84. Torre-Cisneros J, Doblas A, Aguado JM, San Juan R, Blanes M, Montejo M, et al. Tuberculosis after solid-organ transplant: incidence, risk factors, and clinical characteristics in the RESITRA (Spanish Network of Infection in Transplantation) cohort. Clin Infect Dis. 2009;48(12):1657–65.
85. Yoo JW, Jo KW, Kim SH, Lee SO, Kim JJ, Park SK, et al. Incidence, characteristics, and treatment outcomes of mycobacterial diseases in transplant recipients. Transpl Int. 2016;29(5):549–58.

86. Naqvi A, Rizvi A, Hussain Z, Hafeez S, Hashmi A, Akhtar F, et al. Developing world perspective of posttransplant tuberculosis: morbidity, mortality, and cost implications. Transplant Proc. 2001;33(1-2):1787–8.
87. Sakhuja V, Jha V, Varma PP, Joshi K, Chugh KS. The high incidence of tuberculosis among renal transplant recipients in India. Transplantation. 1996;61(2):211–5.
88. Yuen KY, Woo PC. Tuberculosis in blood and marrow transplant recipients. Hematol Oncol. 2002;20(2):51–62.
89. Cordonnier C, Martino R, Trabasso P, Held TK, Akan H, Ward MS, et al. Mycobacterial infection: a difficult and late diagnosis in stem cell transplant recipients. Clin Infect Dis. 2004;38(9):1229–36.
90. Russo RL, Dulley FL, Suganuma L, França IL, Yasuda MA, Costa SF. Tuberculosis in hematopoietic stem cell transplant patients: case report and review of the literature. Int J Infect Dis. 2010;14(Suppl 3):e187–91.
91. Ip MS, Yuen KY, Woo PC, Luk WK, Tsang KW, Lam WK, et al. Risk factors for pulmonary tuberculosis in bone marrow transplant recipients. Am J Respir Crit Care Med. 1998;158(4):1173–7.
92. Ku SC, Tang JL, Hsueh PR, Luh KT, Yu CJ, Yang PC. Pulmonary tuberculosis in allogeneic hematopoietic stem cell transplantation. Bone Marrow Transplant. 2001;27(12):1293–7.
93. Lopez de Castilla D, Schluger NW. Tuberculosis following solid organ transplantation. Transpl Infect Dis. 2010;12(2):106–12.
94. Chen CH, Shu KH, Ho HC, Cheng SB, Lin CC, Wei HJ, et al. A nationwide population-based study of the risk of tuberculosis in different solid organ transplantations in Taiwan. Transplant Proc. 2014;46(4):1032–5.
95. Muñoz P, Rodríguez C, Bouza E. Mycobacterium tuberculosis infection in recipients of solid organ transplants. Clin Infect Dis. 2005;40(4):581–7.
96. Ulubay G, Kupeli E, Duvenci Birben O, Seyfettin EP, Dogrul MI, Ozsancak Ugurlu A, et al. A 10-year experience of tuberculosis in solid-organ transplant recipients. Exp Clin Transplant. 2015;13(Suppl 1):214 8.
97. Hsu MS, Wang JL, Ko WJ, Lee PH, Chou NK, Wang SS, et al. Clinical features and outcome of tuberculosis in solid organ transplant recipients. Am J Med Sci. 2007;334(2):106–10.
98. Jereb JA, Burwen DR, Dooley SW, Haas WH, Crawford JT, Geiter LJ, et al. Nosocomial outbreak of tuberculosis in a renal transplant unit: application of a new technique for restriction fragment length polymorphism analysis of Mycobacterium tuberculosis isolates. J Infect Dis. 1993;168(5):1219–24.
99. el-Agroudy AF, Refaie AF, Moussa OM, Ghoneim MA. Tuberculosis in Egyptian kidney transplant recipients: study of clinical course and outcome. J Nephrol. 2003;16(3):404–11.
100. Atasever A, Bacakoglu F, Toz H, Basoglu OK, Duman S, Basak K, et al. Tuberculosis in renal transplant recipients on various immunosuppressive regimens. Nephrol Dial Transplant. 2005;20(4):797–802.
101. Bodro M, Sabe N, Santin M, Cruzado JM, Llado L, Gonzalez-Costello J, et al. Clinical features and outcomes of tuberculosis in solid organ transplant recipients. Transplant Proc. 2012;44(9):2686–9.
102. Olithselvan A, Rajagopala S, Vij M, Shanmugam V, Shanmugam N, Rela M. Tuberculosis in liver transplant recipients: experience of a South Indian liver transplant center. Liver Transpl. 2014;20(8):960–6.
103. Lou XF, Wu RH, Xu SZ, Lin XJ. Spinal tuberculosis in post-liver transplantation patients: case reports. Transpl Infect Dis. 2010;12(2):132–7.
104. Nelson CA, Zunt JR. Tuberculosis of the central nervous system in immunocompromised patients: HIV infection and solid organ transplant recipients. Clin Infect Dis. 2011;53(9):915–26.
105. Winthrop KL, Kubak BM, Pegues DA, Hufana C, Costamagna P, Desmond E, et al. Transmission of mycobacterium tuberculosis via lung transplantation. Am J Transplant. 2004;4(9):1529–33.
106. Kiuchi T, Inomata Y, Uemoto S, Satomura K, Egawa H, Okajima H, et al. A hepatic graft tuberculosis transmitted from a living-related donor. Transplantation. 1997;63(6):905–7.
107. Graham JC, Kearns AM, Magee JG, El-Sheikh MF, Hudson M, Manas D, et al. Tuberculosis transmitted through transplantation. J Infect. 2001;43(4):251–4.
108. Schulman LL, Scully B, McGregor CC, Austin JH. Pulmonary tuberculosis after lung transplantation. Chest. 1997;111(5):1459–62.
109. Aguado JM, Torre-Cisneros J, Fortún J, Benito N, Meije Y, Doblas A, et al. Tuberculosis in solid-organ transplant recipients: consensus statement of the group for the study of infection in transplant recipients (GESITRA) of the Spanish Society of Infectious Diseases and Clinical Microbiology. Clin Infect Dis. 2009;48(9):1276–84.
110. Morris MI, Daly JS, Blumberg E, Kumar D, Sester M, Schluger N, et al. Diagnosis and management of tuberculosis in transplant donors: a donor-derived infections consensus conference report(†). Am J Transplant. 2012;12:2288–300.
111. Bumbacea D, Arend SM, Eyuboglu F, Fishman JA, Goletti D, Ison MG, et al. The risk of tuberculosis in transplant candidates and recipients: a TBNET consensus statement. Eur Respir J. 2012;40(4):990–1013.
112. Tomblyn M, Chiller T, Einsele H, Gress R, Sepkowitz K, Storek J, et al. Guidelines for preventing infectious complications among hematopoietic cell transplant recipients: a global perspective. Preface. Bone Marrow Transplant. 2009;44(8):453–5.
113. Pai M, Denkinger CM, Kik SV, Rangaka MX, Zwerling A, Oxlade O, et al. Gamma interferon release assays for detection of Mycobacterium tuberculosis infection. Clin Microbiol Rev. 2014;27(1):3–20.
114. Targeted tuberculin testing and treatment of latent tuberculosis infection. American Thoracic Society. MMWR Recomm Rep. 2000;49(RR-6):1–51.
115. Mazurek GH, Jereb J, Vernon A, LoBue P, Goldberg S, Castro K, et al. Updated guidelines for using Interferon Gamma Release Assays to detect Mycobacterium tuberculosis infection - United States, 2010. MMWR Recomm Rep. 2010;59(RR-5):1–25.
116. Red book: 2009 report of the Committee on Infectious Disease. 28th ed ed. Pickering LK BC, Kimberlin DW, Long SS, eds, editor. Elk Grove Villiage, IL: American Academy of Pediatrics; 2009.
117. Lindemann M, Dioury Y, Beckebaum S, Cicinnati VR, Gerken G, Broelsch CE, et al. Diagnosis of tuberculosis infection in patients awaiting liver transplantation. Hum Immunol. 2009;70(1):24–8.
118. Manuel O, Humar A, Preiksaitis J, Doucette K, Shokoples S, Peleg AY, et al. Comparison of quantiferon-TB gold with tuberculin skin test for detecting latent tuberculosis infection prior to liver transplantation. Am J Transplant. 2007;7(12):2797–801.
119. Kim SY, Jung GS, Kim SK, Chang J, Kim MS, Kim YS, et al. Comparison of the tuberculin skin test and interferon-γ release assay for the diagnosis of latent tuberculosis infection before kidney transplantation. Infection. 2013;41(1):103–10.
120. Theodoropoulos N, Lanternier F, Rassiwala J, McNatt G, Preczewski L, DeMayo E, et al. Use of the QuantiFERON-TB Gold interferon-gamma release assay for screening transplant candidates: a single-center retrospective study. Transpl Infect Dis. 2012;14(1):1–8.
121. Sester M, van Leth F, Bruchfeld J, Bumbacea D, Cirillo DM, Dilektasli AG, et al. Risk assessment of tuberculosis in immunocompromised patients. A TBNET study. Am J Respir Crit Care Med. 2014;190(10):1168–76.
122. Hadaya K, Bridevaux PO, Roux-Lombard P, Delort A, Saudan P, Martin PY, et al. Contribution of interferon-gamma release assays (IGRAs) to the diagnosis of latent tuberculosis infection after renal transplantation. Transplantation. 2013;95(12):1485–90.

123. Moon SM, Lee SO, Choi SH, Kim YS, Woo JH, Yoon DH, et al. Comparison of the QuantiFERON-TB Gold In-Tube test with the tuberculin skin test for detecting latent tuberculosis infection prior to hematopoietic stem cell transplantation. Transpl Infect Dis. 2013;15(1):104–9.
124. Qin LL, Wang QR, Wang Q, Yao H, Wen LJ, Wu LL, et al. T-SPOT. TB for detection of tuberculosis infection among hematological malignancy patients and hematopoietic stem cell transplant recipients. Asian Pac J Cancer Prev. 2013;14(12):7415–9.
125. Horne DJ, Narita M, Spitters CL, Parimi S, Dodson S, Limaye AP. Challenging issues in tuberculosis in solid organ transplantation. Clin Infect Dis. 2013;57(10):1473–82.
126. Kim SH, Lee SO, Park JB, Park IA, Park SJ, Yun SC, et al. A prospective longitudinal study evaluating the usefulness of a T-cell-based assay for latent tuberculosis infection in kidney transplant recipients. Am J Transplant. 2011;11(9):1927–35.
127. Huebner RE, Schein MF, Bass JB. The tuberculin skin test. Clin Infect Dis. 1993;17(6):968–75.
128. (CDC) CfDCaP. Updated guidelines for the use of nucleic acid amplification tests in the diagnosis of tuberculosis. MMWR Morb Mortal Wkly Rep. 2009;58(1):7–10.
129. Boehme CC, Nabeta P, Hillemann D, Nicol MP, Shenai S, Krapp F, et al. Rapid molecular detection of tuberculosis and rifampin resistance. N Engl J Med. 2010;363(11):1005–15.
130. Tortoli E, Russo C, Piersimoni C, Mazzola E, Dal Monte P, Pascarella M, et al. Clinical validation of Xpert MTB/RIF for the diagnosis of extrapulmonary tuberculosis. Eur Respir J. 2012;40(2):442–7.
131. Ao W, Aldous S, Woodruff E, Hicke B, Rea L, Kreiswirth B, et al. Rapid detection of rpoB gene mutations conferring rifampin resistance in Mycobacterium tuberculosis. J Clin Microbiol. 2012;50(7):2433–40.
132. Lin SY, Rodwell TC, Victor TC, Rider EC, Pham L, Catanzaro A, et al. Pyrosequencing for rapid detection of extensively drug-resistant Mycobacterium tuberculosis in clinical isolates and clinical specimens. J Clin Microbiol. 2014;52(2):475–82.
133. Ocheretina O, Shen L, Escuyer VE, Mabou MM, Royal-Mardi G, Collins SE, et al. Whole genome sequencing investigation of a tuberculosis outbreak in Port-au-Prince, Haiti caused by a strain with a "low-level" rpoB mutation L511P - insights into a mechanism of resistance escalation. PLoS One. 2015;10(6):e0129207.
134. Daum LT, Rodriguez JD, Worthy SA, Ismail NA, Omar SV, Dreyer AW, et al. Next-generation ion torrent sequencing of drug resistance mutations in Mycobacterium tuberculosis strains. J Clin Microbiol. 2012;50(12):3831–7.
135. Koser CU, Bryant JM, Becq J, Torok ME, Ellington MJ, Marti-Renom MA, et al. Whole-genome sequencing for rapid susceptibility testing of M. tuberculosis. N Engl J Med. 2013;369(3):290–2.

30 Nontuberculous Mycobacterial Disease in Transplant Recipients

Julie V. Philley, Amar Safdar, and Charles L. Daley

Introduction

Nontuberculous mycobacteria (NTM) include over 170 species and subspecies many of which have been reported to cause disease in transplant recipients. The frequency of NTM disease among transplant recipients varies from center to center ranging from 1.4% to 22.4% [1–4] among lung transplant recipients; however, actual NTM disease occurs in less than 5% of patients [1, 2, 4]. Posttransplant infection can occur through several ways including reactivation of prior infection, donor-derived infection, contamination at the time of transplant, or posttransplant environmental contamination. The most common site of infection is the lung although these nearly ubiquitous mycobacteria can produce disease at any site in immunocompromised individuals, so a high index of suspicious is necessary in order to make an early diagnosis and initiate appropriate therapy promptly [5]. Treatment of NTM is complicated because of the multiple drugs required for treatment, drug-related toxicity, potential for drug-drug interactions, and long duration of therapy. Untreated NTM can produce significant morbidity and mortality with outcomes varying by mycobacterial species, drug resistance patterns, and type of transplant. This chapter will review the diagnosis and treatment of NTM disease among transplant candidates and recipients.

J. V. Philley (✉)
University of Texas Health Science Center at Tyler, Department of Pulmonary and Critical Care Medicine, Tyler, TX, USA
e-mail: julie.philley@uthct.edu

A. Safdar
Clinical Associate Professor of Medicine, Texas Tech University Health Sciences Center El Paso, Paul L. Foster School of Medicine, El Paso, TX, USA
e-mail: amar.safdar@cidimmunology.com

C. L. Daley
Division of Mycobacterial and Respiratory Infections, National Jewish Health and University of Colorado, Denver, CO, USA
e-mail: daleyc@njhealth.org

Epidemiology

The prevalence of NTM disease in the general population is increasing in many areas [6–10]. However, lack of mandated reporting and difficulty in distinguishing clinically significant disease from colonization or indolent infection make the prevalence of NTM disease hard to determine. The prevalence of NTM disease in transplant recipients is equally difficult to establish although case series and retrospective cohort studies have provided estimates of the prevalence of disease in this high-risk population.

The proportion of mycobacterial infections due to NTM varies depending on the prevalence of tuberculosis (TB). Among 7342 solid organ transplant (SOT) and 1266 hematopoietic stem cell transplant (HSCT) recipients at a center in South Korea where TB is prevalent, there were 152 patients identified with a mycobacterial infection of whom 22 (15%) had NTM isolated [11]. The overall incidence of TB was 257.4 per 100,000 patient-years compared to 42.7 per 100,000 patient-years for NTM. In areas with lower rates of TB, the proportion of mycobacterial infections due to NTM is typically 80–90% [3, 12, 13].

The type of transplant is an important factor determining the risk of NTM disease with higher rates of NTM disease reported among HSCT than SOT recipients in some studies [14]. For example, in a study from South Korea, the incidence of NTM in HSCT recipients was 258.7 per 100,000 patient-years, significantly higher than that seen in SOT recipients (27.1 per 100,000 patient-years) [11].

Solid Organ Transplants

The overall incidence of NTM disease among SOT recipients varies by the type of transplant with the highest rate among lung (0.46–8.0%) [2–4, 13, 15] and heart (0.24–2.8%) [16, 17] transplant recipients followed by kidney (0.16–0.38%) [18–24] and liver transplants (0.04–0.1%) [15, 25].

A. Safdar (ed.), *Principles and Practice of Transplant Infectious Diseases*, https://doi.org/10.1007/978-1-4939-9034-4_30

Lung Transplants

Lung transplant recipients have the highest rate of developing NTM infection after undergoing transplantation [26]. Much of the data concerning the epidemiology of NTM disease in lung transplants comes from large retrospective series, primarily from low TB prevalence areas. In general, between 3.8% and 22% of lung transplant recipients undergoing surveillance bronchoscopies have NTM isolated from bronchoalveolar lavage samples [2–4, 13]. However, most of these patients were not thought to have invasive NTM disease; only 10–14% of such patients were considered to have NTM disease [4, 27].

One of the first studies to describe the frequency of NTM in lung transplant recipients was published in 1999 and described a 12-year experience at a single center in Australia [13]. Of 261 transplants, there were 23 mycobacterial infections detected (8%) and all but two of whom had NTM isolated. The most common site of NTM disease was the lung (83%) and the most common causative organism was *M. avium* complex (MAC). Median time from transplant to diagnosis of NTM infection was 450 days and ranged between 50 and 3272 days [13]. A case series from the United States reported 34 patients with NTM disease over 7.5 years from all solid organ transplants. Nineteen occurred in lung transplants, 6 single and 13 bilateral allograft transplants [15]. The median time of occurrence was 8 months following transplantation procedure. In another series from the United States, 15 (22.4%) of 237 lung transplant recipients over a 15-year period developed NTM disease corresponding to an incidence of NTM isolation of 9 per 100 person-years and incidence rate of NTM disease of 1.1 per 100 person-years [4]. The most common NTM isolated was MAC (70%) followed by *Mycobacterium abscessus* (9%).

M. abscessus has become an increasingly common and challenging NTM infection in transplant recipients. An international survey of 31 of 62 transplant centers that responded reported that 17 of 5200 (0.33%) transplant recipients were identified to have *M. abscessus* after transplantation with two patients known to have pretransplant "colonization" [28]. Disease developed in the allograph in 12 patients, in the skin/soft tissue in 3 patients, and in both in 2 patients. Median time to diagnosis was 18.5 months, ranged between 1 and 111 months.

NTM can be isolated from 6% to 13% of patients with CF, and up to 20% of CF patients awaiting transplantation become infected [1, 29]. In several studies invasive NTM infections have been reported to occur in 0.5–3.4% of CF patients after undergoing lung transplantation [1, 28, 30]. In a review of both CF ($n = 60$) and non-CF ($n = 60$) lung transplants, mycobacteria were isolated from 7.2% and 9.1% of recipients, respectively [31]. *M. abscessus* is a particularly challenging pathogen to treat in patients with CF. Among 13 patients with pretransplant cultures positive for *M. abscessus*, all of whom met ATS criteria for disease, 3 developed posttransplant complications, and all 3 responded to treatment [32]. Survival posttransplant was 77% 1 year after transplantation, 64% at 3 years, and 50% at 5 years with no deaths related to *M. abscessus*. Additionally, there was no significant difference in survival when compared with other transplanted patients.

Other SOT

The frequency of NTM disease in other types of SOT is less common than with lung transplants. Among renal transplants, the incidence of NTM has been reported between 0.16% and 0.38% [12, 14, 15, 18–24, 33]. Of 3921 renal transplants between 1984 and 2002, 18 were identified as having mycobacterial infections after undergoing allograft transplantation, only 3 of which were due to TB. Thirteen of the patients were alive and well at a mean follow-up of 9.2 years since the infection diagnosis [12]. In Spain, between 1980 and 2000, there were 27 renal transplant patients (2.1%) with mycobacterial infections, 20 had TB, 5 had *M. kansasii*, and 2 patients had *M. fortuitum* infection [34].

The incidence of NTM infection among heart transplant recipients ranges between 0.24% and 2.8% [16, 35]. Novick and colleagues reported a 17-year experience at Stanford and noted that only 14 of 502 heart transplant recipients developed NTM infections over a mean of 3.5 years of follow-up [16]. The rate was higher among those receiving azathioprine and prednisone than cyclosporine alone. Additional heart transplant patients with pulmonary and extrapulmonary disease have been reported with various NTM species including *M. abscessus*, *M. xenopi*, and *M. scrofulaceum*. The estimates for NTM disease in liver transplants have been reported to be quite low at 0.1% [15, 25] although a recent study from Korea reported an incidence of 14.7 per 100,000 patient-years [11].

HSCT

The incidence of NTM infection among HSCT recipients has ranged from 0.4% to 4.9%; however, the reported incidence in allogenic stem cell graft recipients has been as high as 3–9.7% [36–41]. Among 6259 HSCT recipients at the University of Washington over a 20-year period, 40 were identified as having NTM infection (0.64%) of which 28 were considered to have invasive mycobacterial disease (0.44%) [37]. The median time to diagnosis was 251 days following transplantation. All three patients with definitive pulmonary disease were treated successfully.

A retrospective study from the University of Toronto reported that 4% of their 1097 allogenic HSCT patients had NTM isolated with 2.7% having NTM disease [42]. The median time to diagnosis was 343 days. All had pulmonary

NTM disease with 93% experiencing pulmonary-only involvement. In general, the rate of NTM disease in HSCT recipients has been higher than that in SOT recipients but not in all studies. A recent study from Korea reported an incidence of NTM in HSCT recipients at 258.7 per 100,000 patient-years, higher than that seen in SOT recipients (27.1 per 100,000 patient-years) [11].

Risk Factors for NTM Disease

Risk factors for development of NTM disease vary from study to study but recipients of lung transplant are at highest risk for NTM disease compared with other SOT recipients [15]. In a case-control study of 34 post-lung transplant recipients matched to 102 control patients, lung transplant was strongly associated with NTM disease (56% vs. 10%; OR 11.49) [15]. Among HSCT recipients a number of risk factors for NTM disease have been reported including a higher risk with allografts versus autografts, myeloablative versus nonmyeloablative transplants, matched unrelated donor over sibling allografts, underlying GVHD, use of steroids to treat GVHD, leukemia relapse, and the existence of bronchiolitis obliterans [36]. A recent study from Toronto reported that severe chronic graft-versus-host disease and CMV viremia were factors associated with an increased risk of NTM [42].

Immunologic Susceptibility to NTM Disease

Immunity to mycobacterial infection requires an effective interplay between the myeloid and lymphoid cells through the interleukin 12-interferon-gamma pathway [43]. A complicated cascade of events is set into effect following exposure to mycobacterial antigens, and organism-specific antigen primed T cells at the infection site orchestrate events leading to cell death of these intracellular pathogens. The critical effector cell for controlling NTM is the macrophage, which ingests mycobacteria, and once engulfed by the macrophage, the bacteria's fate is determined by the cell's state of immune activation, which is determined by interactions between cells in the TH1 pathway and their associated cytokines, particularly the IL-12/IFN-gamma axis [44]. Mononuclear phagocytes produce interleukin-12 which stimulates T cells and natural killer cells through the interleukin-12 receptor [43]. Signal transducer and activator of transcription (STAT)4 is activated leading to induction of interferon-gamma production which binds to its receptor causing activation and differentiation of macrophages [45, 46]. IFN gamma via cytokine receptor activates Janus kinase (JAK1 and JAK2) tyrosine-phosphorylation and stimulation of STAT1, which mediates activation of interferon-stimulated genes. In vitro experiments have shown that addition of IFN-γ promotes killing of microbes by upregulating T_H1 responses through neutrophils, monocytes, and macrophages [47]. IFN-γ activation of macrophages via T_H1 lymphocyte activation induces macrophages to overcome inhibition of mycobacteria containing phagolysosome maturation [48]. IFN-γ has also been noted to prime macrophages for enhanced microbial killing and activation of inflammatory response via Toll-like receptor (TRL) pathway [49, 50]. Furthermore, as a response to TLR signaling, IFN-γ alters epigenetic governance of macrophages, inducing and priming enhancers to increase transcriptional output [51].

The activated macrophages are then able to kill relatively avirulent intracellular organisms like NTM. Numerous other cytokines such as IL-18, IL-23, and IL-29, receptors like vitamin D receptor, and unidentified cofactors may also be important in garnering hosts' effective containment and elimination of immune-inflammatory response against NTM. Novel influences on macrophage lysosomal activity due to IL-12, IL-27, and STAT-3 were demonstrated by Jung et al. [52]. These adjunct cytokine and transcription signals promote enhanced trafficking of mycobacteria to lysosomes in human macrophages. This may have important implications in future approaches for effective containment of mycobacterial infection.

HIV-associated acquired immunodeficiency has demonstrated the critical role of CD4-positive T-helper lymphocytes (CD4+ cells) in maintaining host resistance to MAC and other NTM. CD4 cell decline is also associated with a cascade of dysfunction within the cell-mediated immune, or TH1 pathway, including alterations in cytokine levels and hosts' immune responsiveness [53, 54].

Interleukin-12 (IL-12) [55], IFN-γ, and tumor necrosis factor alpha are important for sustained macrophage activation and regulation of effective intracellular microbicidal activity. Reactive nitrogen and oxygen species are a family of toxic antimicrobial molecules derived from nitric oxide and superoxide, respectively. They assist in intracellular mycobacterial killing; IFN-γ is the principal cytokine in promoting nitrosative stress and bacterial cell death [56]. Recently, the important influence of restricted IFN-γ-mediated activation of pulmonary macrophages by the local suppressor of cytokine signaling (SOCS)1 was reported [57]. Additionally, this group showed that factors secreted by alveolar epithelial cells enhanced the microbicidal capacities of macrophages by mechanisms independent of reactive nitrogen species transcribed under the influence of IFN-γ; the clinical significance for such processes in physiologic clearance of environmental NTM that are routinely exposed to the human respiratory tract needs further investigation [57].

Transplant recipients are treated with immunosuppressive drugs in order to prevent and treat solid organ allograft rejection. In recipients of stem cell allograft, intragenic immune suppression is the mainstay of therapy for graft sustenance and treatment of acute or chronic graft-versus-host disease.

Immunosuppression is achieved through depleting lymphocytes, diverting lymphocyte traffic, or blocking their response pathways described above [58]. Besides the therapeutic effect of these drugs, there is also the undesirable effect of increasing the risk of infection from numerous pathogens including NTM.

Microbiology

NTM consists of over 170 species and subspecies that are found throughout the environment including from soil and water, both natural and treated. NTM are traditionally divided into two groups based on their rate of growth on subculture; rapid growers show visible growth by 7 days and slow growers after 7 days (Table 30.1). Many of these organisms have been reported to cause disease in transplant recipients. Most infections are caused by more virulent organisms such as *M. avium* complex, *M. kansasii*, and *M. abscessus*. Isolation of low-virulence mycobacteria is not uncommon, and in immunologically intact, nonsusceptible individuals, they frequently represent either laboratory/environmental contaminant or nondisease-associated colonization. However, in the setting of allogeneic transplantation, all organisms must be considered as potential pathogens until proven otherwise.

The most clinically important slowly growing NTM include *Mycobacterium avium* complex (MAC) and *Mycobacterium kansasii* although numerous other slow growers have been reported to cause disease in transplant recipients (Table 30.1). MAC currently consists of at least ten species; the most common to cause infection in humans are *M. avium*, *M. intracellulare*, and *M. chimaera* [59]. MAC isolates are usually susceptible to the macrolides like azithromycin and clarithromycin and clofazimine with variable susceptibility to rifamycins, ethambutol, amikacin, and streptomycin. *Mycobacterium kansasii* is a slowly growing organism that is considered one of the most virulent NTM. *M. kansasii* is usually susceptible in vitro to the first-line anti-tuberculosis agents except pyrazinamide as well as to the macrolides and fluoroquinolones [60–62].

Rapidly growing mycobacteria are particularly common among HSCT recipients and include *Mycobacterium fortuitum*, *Mycobacterium chelonae*, and members of the *Mycobacterium abscessus* complex. Rapid growers are more resistant to current antimicrobials than most slow growers and some species contain an erythromycin ribosomal methylase gene (*erm*) that can lead to inducible macrolide resistance [63]. *M. abscessus* is further subdivided into three subspecies (ssp) including ssp. *abscessus*, ssp. *massiliense*, and the least common ssp. *bolletii* [64, 65]. Approximately 80% of isolates of *M. abscessus* ssp. *abscessus* carry a functional *erm*(41) gene that results in inducible macrolide resistance in the presence of a macrolide; this resistance is not reflected by the initial 3-day in vitro MIC reported by some laboratories [63]. *M. abscessus* ssp. *massiliense* does not undergo inducible macrolide resistance as the *erm*(41) gene is nonfunctional and, hence, the disease is easier to treat [66–68]. Depending on the organism, the following antimicrobials show variable in vitro susceptibility: macrolides, aminoglycosides, clofazimine, fluoroquinolones, tigecycline, cefoxitin, and imipenem/meropenem [69].

Table 30.1 Nontuberculous mycobacteria reported to have caused disease in transplant recipients

Slowly Growing mycobacteria	Rapidly growing mycobacteria
Mycobacterium asciaticum	*Mycobacterium abscessus*
M. avium	*M. bolletii*
M. celatum	*M. chelonae*
M. genevense	*M. fortuitum*
M. haemophilum	*M. margeritense*
M. intracellulare	*M. massiliense*
M. gastri	*M. mucogenicum*
M. gordonae	*M. neoaurum*
M. kansasii	*M. smegmatis*
M. malmoense	
M. marinum	
M. scrofulaceum	
M. szulgai	
M. terrae	
M. thermoresistable	
M. triplex	
M. xenopi	

Clinical Presentation

The clinical presentation of NTM disease in transplant patients varies depending on the type of transplant, degree of immunosuppression, patient comorbidities, and species of NTM involved [70]. Patients may present with pleuropulmonary, skin and soft tissue, bone and joint, catheter-related, as well as disseminated disease [5]. Among HSCT recipients, catheter-related infections are one of the most common infections followed by skin and soft tissue infections [36–41, 71, 72]. In lung transplant recipients, pleuropulmonary infections are most common ranging from 54% to 82% followed by skin and soft tissue infections [14, 73]. Cough and sputum production are common and more common in transplant recipients with NTM than TB. Skin, soft tissue, and disseminated infections are the most common types of NTM infections in heart and kidney transplants.

Time to presentation varies between types of transplants and tends to be longer for NTM than TB. A recent study from South Korea reported a median time to diagnosis of 24.2 months for NTM and 8.5 months for TB. For HSCT recipients the median time to presentation is 5 months and over 10 months for SOT [70]. Among SOT patients, the median time to diagnosis has ranged from 15 to 30 months for heart, 20 to 24 months for kidney, 15 months for lung, and 10 months for liver transplants [5, 33, 70].

Pulmonary Disease

Pleuropulmonary disease is the most common presentation in lung transplant recipients but occurs in other transplants as well [74]. In fact, pleuropulmonary infections account for about one-third of NTM infections in recipients of HSCT with MAC being the most common causative organism. Cough, with or without sputum production, is the most prominent symptom although weight loss, fatigue, hemoptysis, night sweats, dyspnea, and chills also occur [75]. Chronic lung disease is a well-recognized predisposing factor in immunosuppressed patients, including transplant recipients. The radiographic features suggestive of pulmonary NTM include small nodules, tree-in-bud opacities, and/or small cavitary lesions with bronchiectasis [2]. Infections due to *M. kansasii* frequently involve the upper-lung lobes, and thin-wall cavities are seen commonly. Other pleuropulmonary manifestations include empyema as well as chest wall and surgical wound infections [76].

Skin, Soft Tissue, and Musculoskeletal Infections

While most NTM disease affects the lung in lung transplant recipients, skin and soft tissue infections are also a major concern post surgically [4, 13, 25, 33, 77, 78]. In one series, 4 of the 53 lung transplant patients had soft tissue infections (3 with *M. abscessus* and 1 with *M. chelonae*) and 1 died from progressive disseminated disease [4]. Typical findings include painful to minimally painful erythematous to violaceous subcutaneous nodules usually on the extremities or near the site of surgical wounds [4, 77]. Lesions will often ulcerate and may follow lymphatic distribution resembling sporotrichosis. The most common species to cause skin and soft tissue involvement are the rapidly growing mycobacteria and *Mycobacterium marinum* [33, 79].

M. fortuitum produces skin and soft tissue infection in immunologically competent patients; most infections occur due to accidental inoculation. In transplant recipients, surgical sites and scars may become sites of infection. Most infections due to *M. chelonae* are seen in patients with underlying predisposing conditions such as chronic corticosteroid use, rheumatoid arthritis, lupus, and cancer [80, 81], while *M. abscessus* has notably caused surgical infections surrounding transplant sites [25, 77, 82]. Health-related infections occur sporadically and have been seen in patients after deep intramuscular injection, sternal wound infection following cardiac surgery, and after a variety of reconstructive and plastic surgical procedures including augmentation mammoplasty and chest wall reconstruction after tumor resection [83].

Musculoskeletal infections may present as septic arthritis, tenosynovitis, or osteomyelitis. These infections may involve noncontiguous sites due to disseminated disease. In one review of NTM in SOT recipients, 67% presented with soft tissue and musculoskeletal involvement with over 50% involving noncontiguous sites [25].

Catheter-Related Infections

Catheter-related infections have become the most common healthcare-related infections due to RGM with most infections occurring in patients with long-term indwelling intravascular catheters. In immunosuppressed patients, *M. chelonae* and *M. abscessus* are among the most common NTM isolates [84]. RGM species are increasingly reported in immunosuppressed patients with catheter-related infection and include uncommon NTM like *M. smegmatis* [85], *Mycobacterium neoaurum* [86], *Mycobacterium aurum* [87], *Mycobacterium lacticola* [88], and *Mycobacterium brumae* [89]. Catheter-related infections are the most commonly encountered infectious complication in HSCT recipients accounting for approximately one-third of all NTM infections in this setting and most are due to rapidly growing NTM. Median time to presentation is approximately 2 months [37]. It is important to emphasize that RGM are frequently isolated in hospital and laboratory water supplies, and numerous pseudo-outbreaks involving contaminated blood culture materials and fiberoptic bronchoscope sterilizing machine contamination have been described [90, 91].

Disseminated Disease

Disseminated disease has been reported with all types of SOT but is most common in kidney and heart transplant recipients [14, 25, 77, 92]. In some series, approximately half of patients with pulmonary disease have evidence of dissemination [14, 33]. Disseminated disease can involve almost any body site including skin, soft tissues, musculoskeletal sites, lymph nodes, blood, bone marrow, and lung. Patients may present with fever of unknown origin often with subcutaneous nodules. The rapidly growing mycobacteria are the most common species to disseminate followed by *M. kansasii* and *M. haemophilum*.

Diagnosis

Clinical Diagnosis

The diagnosis of pulmonary disease is based on the American Thoracic Society (ATS) and Infectious Diseases Society of America (IDSA) criteria (Table 30.2), which involve the assessment of clinical, radiographic, and microbiological factors [69]. Given the variable clinical presentation noted in transplant recipients with NTM disease, the clinician should have a high index of suspicion and send appropriate clinical specimens for culture and histopathologic examination.

Table 30.2 Clinical and microbiologic criteria for diagnosing nontuberculous mycobacterial lung disease [69]

Clinical (both required)
1. Pulmonary symptoms, nodular or cavitary opacities on chest radiograph, or a high-resolution computed tomography scan that shows multifocal bronchiectasis with multiple small nodules
and
2. Appropriate exclusion for other diagnoses.
Microbiologic
1. Positive culture results from at least two separate expectorated sputum samples. If results are nondiagnostic, consider repeat sputum AFB smears and cultures.
or
2. Positive culture result from at least one bronchial wash or lavage.
or
3. Transbronchial or other lung biopsy with mycobacterial histopathologic features (granulomatous inflammation or AFB) and positive culture for NTM or biopsy showing mycobacterial histopathologic features (granulomatous inflammation or AFB) and one or more sputum or bronchial washings that are culture positive for NTM.

Typical chest computed tomography findings of NTM pulmonary disease include the presence of bronchiectasis and centrilobular nodules with a tree-in-bud appearance [5, 70]. In the transplant setting, bronchiolitis obliterans and rejection may produce similar findings although the presence of nodules is more suggestive of NTM disease [93].

Laboratory Diagnosis

Laboratory diagnosis of NTM disease is based on isolation of these organisms from culture of clinical specimens. Both solid and broth media are recommended for growth of mycobacteria [69]. Slow-growing mycobacteria (SGM) take between 3 and 8 weeks to grow, whereas in the case of rapidly growing mycobacteria (RGM) growth often becomes evident within 7 days on subculture. Some organisms such as *M. genavense* can take up to 12 weeks of incubation to detect growth. For most NTM species, the optimal temperature for growth is 28 to 37 °C, although some species require either higher or lower temperatures for optimal growth. Specimens obtained from cutaneous sites should be incubated at 35 and 28–32 °C. In addition, some fastidious species such as *M. haemophilum* require addition of hemin or ferric ammonium citrate for growth.

The clinical usefulness of antimicrobial drug susceptibility testing remains unclear because of the lack of correlation between the in vitro activity of some antimycobacterial drugs and clinical outcomes. A broth-based culture method with both microdilution and macrodilution methods is considered acceptable for testing against MAC[69]. Initial isolates and treatment failures should be tested against clarithromycin because of the good correlation between identification of macrolide resistance and poor treatment outcomes. Recent studies also suggest correlation between amikacin and treatment outcomes with an MIC >64 ug/ml associated with lack of microbiologic response [94]. Isolates of *M. kansasii* should be tested for susceptibility to rifampin and if resistant, additional drugs should be tested such as macrolides and fluoroquinolones [69]. For rapidly growing mycobacteria, broth microdilution minimal inhibitory concentration determination is recommended [69].

Molecular methods such as gene sequencing and line probe assays are becoming increasingly available for rapid speciation and even identification of genetic mutations that confer drug resistance. A line probe assay is commercially available (Hain, Germany) that can detect several common NTM species and identify mutations which cause macrolide and aminoglycoside resistance [95]. While whole genome sequencing is the gold standard, the test remains expensive and not widely available.

Treatment

Treatment of NTM disease requires a multidrug regimen in order to achieve cure and prevent the emergence of resistance. In addition, surgical excision/debridement may be required in extrapulmonary disease and in some cases lessening of the immunosuppressive regimen is required [74]. The optimal combination of drugs (Table 30.3) and duration of therapy are not known for any NTM species. Given the high recurrence rate seen in non-immunosuppressed patients, the current ATS/IDSA recommendation to treat pulmonary NTM disease for 12 months of negative cultures should be considered the minimal duration [69]. Cutaneous and disseminated disease should be treated for a minimum of 6 months although longer durations may be required depending on the infecting species, site of disease, resistance pattern, and response to therapy [70]. Treatment of catheter-related infections includes prompt removal of infected devices and combination antimicrobial therapy for a minimum of 6–12 weeks [70]. Prolonged therapy greater than 12 weeks may be necessary depending on the infecting organism and clinical response to treatment. Lessening of immunosuppression increases the risk of solid organ graft rejection, stem cell graft compromise or graft loss, and potential worsening of graft-versus-host disease. Unlike patients with HIV/AIDS, immune reconstitution syndrome has not been a concern in transplant population.

As in non-immunosuppressed patients, isolation of an NTM from a clinical specimen does not necessarily indicate

Table 30.3 Commonly used drugs for nontuberculous mycobacterial infections

Drug	Route of administration	Dosage	Adverse reactions
Amikacin	Intravenous	10–15 mg/kg once daily or 15–25 mg/kg three times weekly	Nephrotoxicity, auditory-vestibular toxicity
Azithromycin	Oral	250–500 mg daily	Nausea, vomiting, diarrhea, auditory-vestibular toxicity Prolonged QT
Cefoxitin	Intravenous	50 mg/kg/dose 2–3 times daily	Fever, rash, cytopenias
Clarithromycin	Oral	500 mg twice daily	Hepatitis, taste disturbance, inhibits metabolism of rifabutin
Clofazimine	Oral	100 mg once daily	Discoloration of skin, enteropathy, nausea, vomiting, prolonged QT
Ethambutol	Oral	15 mg/kg/dose once daily	Optic neuritis, peripheral neuropathy
Imipenem	Intravenous	500–1000 mg 2–3 times daily	Nausea, vomiting, diarrhea, hepatitis, fever, rash
Isoniazid	Oral	5 mg/kg/dose once daily	Hepatitis, peripheral neuropathy
Linezolid	Oral, intravenous	600 mg once or twice daily	Cytopenias, peripheral neuropathy, optic neuritis
Minocycline	Oral	100 mg twice daily	Photosensitivity, nausea, vomiting, diarrhea, vertigo, tooth discoloration
Moxifloxacin	Oral	400 mg daily	Nausea, vomiting, diarrhea, insomnia, agitation, tendonitis, photosensitivity, prolonged QT
Rifabutin	Oral	300 mg daily	Cytopenias, orange discoloration of fluids, hepatitis, nausea, vomiting, diarrhea, hypersensitivity/flu-like syndrome, increased metabolism of many drugs, uveitis for rifabutin
Rifampin	Oral	600 mg daily	Cytopenias, orange discoloration of fluids, hepatitis, nausea, vomiting, diarrhea, hypersensitivity/flu-like syndrome, increased metabolism of many drugs
Tigecycline	Intravenous	50 mg once or twice daily	Nausea, vomiting, diarrhea, pancreatitis, hypoproteinemia, hepatitis
Trimethoprim-sulfamethoxazole	Oral	10–20 mg/kg/dose twice daily	Nausea, vomiting, diarrhea, cytopenia, fever, rash

that treatment is required. Studies in lung transplant recipients have reported that 75% or more of patients who have NTM isolated from the respiratory tract are "colonized" [2, 4, 26]. Repeated isolation of a more virulent species is more suggestive of NTM-related disease although in extrapulmonary disease it may not be possible to obtain additional samples for culture.

Despite the difficulties faced when treating NTM disease, most patients who have developed NTM disease after undergoing transplantation have survived and been cured with less than 5% of deaths related to the NTM disease. However, in many cases, treatment is prolonged and requires surgical debridement, and adverse reactions including hearing loss in those receiving aminoglycosides are common [33]. Consultation with an expert in the treatment of NTM disease is advised.

Slowly Growing NTM

Mycobacterium avium Complex

The ATS/IDSA recommend treatment with three to four drugs depending on the radiographic extent of disease (Table 30.4) [69]. For immunocompetent patients with nodular lung disease and bronchiectasis, three times weekly dosing of clarithromycin (1000 mg) or azithromycin (500 mg), ethambutol (25 mg/kg), and rifampin (600 mg) are recommended. However, for fibrocavitary or severe nodular/bronchiectatic disease, or in the transplant setting, medications should be administered daily instead of three times weekly with adjustment in doses where necessary (clarithromycin 500–1000 mg/day or azithromycin 250–500 mg/day, ethambutol 15 mg/kg per day, and rifampin 10 mg/kg per day (maximum 600 mg) or rifabutin 150–300 mg/day). For patients with cavitary changes or other severe forms of infection, amikacin or streptomycin given intravenously or intramuscularly at a dose of approximately 15–25 mg/kg three times weekly is recommended for the first 2–3 months [69]. Because of drug interactions (described below), rifabutin and azithromycin are preferred over rifampin and clarithromycin, respectively.

In the transplant setting, there are no specific recommendations for the duration of therapy. For pulmonary disease, the patient should be treated for at least 12 months of negative cultures although longer durations may be needed in transplant recipients. Patients are considered treatment failures if

Table 30.4 Treatment regimens for nontuberculous mycobacterial infections in transplant recipients

Organism	Example regimens	Dose	Alternative
M. avium complex *(noncavitary)*	Azithromycin Rifabutin Ethambutol	250–500 mg daily 300 mg daily 15 mg/kg daily	Moxifloxacin 400 mg daily Clofazimine 100 mg daily
M. avium complex *(cavitary)*	Azithromycin Rifabutin Ethambutol Amikacin	250–500 mg daily 300 mg daily 15 mg/kg/day per day 10–15 mg/kg once daily or 15–25 mg/kg three times weekly	Moxifloxacin 400 mg daily Clofazimine 100 mg daily
M. haemophilum	Azithromycin Rifabutin Moxifloxacin	250–500 mg daily 300 mg daily 400 mg daily	Ethambutol 15 mg/kg daily Clofazimine 100 mg daily
M. kansasii	Isoniazid Rifabutin Ethambutol	300 mg daily 300 mg daily 15 mg/kg per day	Azithromycin 250–500 mg daily Moxifloxacin 400 mg once daily Clofazimine 100 mg daily
M. marinum	Azithromycin Ethambutol	250–500 mg daily 15 mg/kg per day	Rifabutin 300 mg daily Moxifloxacin 400 mg daily Trimethoprim-sulfamethoxazole DS twice daily Doxycycline 100 mg twice daily Minocycline 100 mg daily
M. abscessus spp. *abscessus or bolletii*	Azithromycin Imipenem Amikacin Clofazimine	250–500 mg daily 500–1000 mg 2–3 times daily 10–15 mg/kg once daily or 15–25 mg/kg three times weekly 100 mg daily	Cefoxitin 12 gm in divided doses 3–4 times daily Tigecycline 50 mg 1–2 times daily Linezolid 600 mg 1–2 times daily
M. abscessus spp. massiliense	Azithromycin Imipenem Amikacin	250–500 mg daily 500–1000 mg 2–3 times daily 10–15 mg/kg once daily or 15–25 mg/kg three times weekly	Cefoxitin 12 gm in divided doses 3–4 times daily Clofazimine 100 mg daily Tigecycline 50 mg 1–2 times daily Linezolid 600 mg 1–2 times daily
M. chelonae	Azithromycin Imipenem Amikacin	250–500 mg daily 500–1000 mg 2–3 times daily 10–15 mg/kg once daily or 15–25 mg/kg three times weekly	Clofazimine 100 mg daily Tigecycline 50 mg 1–2 times daily Linezolid 600 mg 1–2 times daily
M. fortuitum	Imipenem Moxifloxacin Trimethoprim-sulfamethoxazole DS	500–1000 mg 2–3 times daily 400 mg daily 1 table twice daily	Cefoxitin 12 gm in divided doses 3–4 times daily Tigecycline 50 mg 1–2 times daily Doxycycline 100 mg twice daily Minocycline 100 mg twice daily Linezolid 600 mg 1–2 times daily

they have not responded after 6 months of appropriate therapy or achieved culture negativity of sputum after 12 months of therapy. Common factors in such patients include medication nonadherence, the use of inadequate regimens (e.g., clarithromycin with a fluoroquinolone only), and emergence of macrolide-resistant MAC isolates. Use of a macrolide alone or in combination with a fluoroquinolone is not recommended due to poor response and the frequent emergence of resistance [96, 97].

Mycobacterium kansasii

The ATS/IDSA guidelines recommend a daily three-drug regimen of isoniazid, rifampin, and ethambutol (Table 30.4) [69]. Although the role of isoniazid in this regimen is not clear (the MICs are 100x higher than with MTB), excellent results have been obtained in clinical studies using this regimen [60, 61]. Clarithromycin is highly active against *M. kansasii*, and clarithromycin-containing regimens have been associated with good treatment outcomes [98–100]. Rifabutin and azithromycin are preferred over rifampin and clarithromycin, respectively, because of drug interactions with some immunosuppressive medications.

The recommended duration of treatment is 12 months of negative cultures, although good results with 12 months of therapy have been reported [61]. As with MAC, a longer duration may be appropriate in the transplant setting but this has not been studied. Other drugs usually given in three-drug combinations are effective for the retreatment of disease that has become resistant to rifampin; they include macrolides, fluoroquinolones, trimethoprim/sulfamethoxazole, streptomycin, and amikacin [69]. At least in non-transplant populations, relapse after treatment with rifampin-containing regimens is uncommon.

Other Slow-Growing Mycobacteria

A number of other slowly growing mycobacteria have been reported to cause NTM disease in transplant recipients (Table 30.1). A detailed discussion of the treatment of these less common NTM is beyond the scope of this chapter. However, a few comments regarding treatment of *M. haemophilum* and *M. marinum* follow. *M. haemophilum* has been almost exclusively seen in patients with severe immune dysfunction either due to HIV-associated AIDS or in recipients of hematopoietic stem cell transplantation [101]. Disseminated infections are reported and predilection for tendon sheaths, bone, and joints is similar to infections seen with RGM. Drug susceptibility testing is not standardized and the correlation between susceptibility test results and clinical outcomes is uncertain. Current recommendations are to treat with a fluoroquinolone, macrolide, and rifamycin which has led to successful treatment (Table 30.4) [69, 102].

M. marinum is a slowly growing mycobacteria found in aquatic environments. Infection usually occurs when traumatized skin is exposed to water containing the organism. At least seven cases of *M. marinum* have been reported in transplant recipients including both SOT and HSCT patients [79, 103, 104]. Most have presented with erythematous tender cutaneous nodules on the extremities after exposure to fish tanks. Treatment regimens have included combinations of macrolides, rifamycins, fluoroquinolones, and cycline derivatives with cure in most patients including a patient with disseminated disease. The ATS currently recommends treatment of cutaneous disease with two active agents for approximately 1–2 months after resolution of the nodules (Table 30.4) [69]. However, most transplant recipients have been treated successfully for 3–9 months with one relapse after 6 months of ciprofloxacin and ethambutol.

Rapidly Growing NTM

M. abscessus Complex

Combination therapy including intravenous agents is necessary for clinically significant disease. Drug combinations including oral azithromycin, clofazimine, or linezolid/tedizolid plus intravenous cefoxitin, imipenem, tigecycline, or amikacin can be successful; however, refractory *M. abscessus* infections are common and remain difficult to treat (Table 30.4) [69]. Patients are begun on three or four of the above antibiotics during an initial multidrug intensive phase including intravenous antibiotics that are usually transitioned to a multidrug regimen of oral and possibly inhaled antibiotics. Long-term sputum conversion is difficult to achieve in patients with *M. abscessus ssp abscessus* lung disease with a functional *erm*(41) gene [68, 105, 106]. Sputum conversion rates among nonimmunocompromised patients with pulmonary disease due to *M. abscessus* ssp *abscessus* have been approximately 25% [66–68]. However, in patients infected with subspecies *M. massiliense* that lacks a functional *erm*(41) gene, culture conversion rates have reached over 80%. Among 16 patients with *M. abscessus* following lung transplantation that were treated, 11 (73%) had a radiographic or microbiologic response to treatment and 10 were considered cured [28]. Death was attributed to *M. abscessus* in two patients. Of note, the strains were not subspeciated so some patients may have been infected with the easier-to-treat *M. massiliense*.

M. chelonae

Mycobacterium chelonae causes skin and soft tissue disease similar to that of *M. abscessus* [69]. Unlike *M. abscessus* and *M. fortuitum*, *M chelonae* does not carry an *erm* gene and therefore effective therapy with a macrolide-based regimen may be more obtainable in these individuals [63]. *M. chelonae* is typically susceptible to macrolides, clofazimine, and tobramycin and resistant to cefoxitin with variable activity to fluoroquinolones, doxycycline, linezolid, and imipenem [81, 107]. Treatment usually involves a combination of three of the antibiotics above (Table 30.4).

M. fortuitum

Mycobacterium fortuitum is a rapid grower similar to *M. abscessus* and *M. chelonae*. It is a rare cause of lung disease, sometimes identified in patients with achalasia and other gastroesophageal reflux disorders [69, 108]. *M. fortuitum* isolates are usually susceptible to fluoroquinolones, doxycycline and minocycline, sulfonamides and trimethoprim/sulfamethoxazole, amikacin, imipenem, and tigecycline, and approximately one-half of the isolates are susceptible to cefoxitin [81, 107, 109]. Like *M. abscessus*, most *M. fortuitum* isolates have a functional *erm* gene so macrolides should not be counted on to treat this infection. Multidrug therapy with agents shown to be susceptible in vitro should be given for 12 months or until clinical resolution of the disease (Table 30.4).

Drug Interactions

Significant drug-drug interactions may occur between antimycobacterial drugs and immunosuppressive drugs used to prevent rejection (Table 30.5). Rifampin is a potent inducer of the CYPA3A4 pathway and thus can decrease the serum concentrations of calcineurin inhibitors and mTOR inhibitors such as sirolimus [70, 77]. Use of rifampin has been associated with acute rejection rates as high as 35% [110, 111]. Rifabutin, which is a less potent inhibitor of cytochrome p450, is the preferred rifamycin in these settings. Clarithromycin is an inhibitor of the CYP3A4 pathway and p-glycoprotein and thus raises the concentration of calcineurin and m-TOR inhibitors. In order to avoid this drug interaction, azithromycin is recommended over clarithromycin.

Table 30.5 Drug interactions between antimycobacterial and antirejection drugs[a]

Antibiotic class/ antibiotics	Cyclosporine	Sirolimus/everolimus	Tacrolimus
Azalide/macrolide			
Azithromycin	Possible mild increase in cyclosporine levels	No significant interaction	Possible mild increase in tacrolimus levels
Clarithromycin	Increase in cyclosporine levels	Increase in sirolimus/everolimus levels	Increase in tacrolimus levels
Fluoroquinolones			
Ciprofloxacin	No significant interaction	No significant interaction	No significant interaction
Levofloxacin	Possible mild increase in serum concentration	No significant interaction	No significant interaction
Moxifloxacin	No significant interaction	No significant interaction	No significant interaction
Rifamycins			
Rifampin	Decrease in cyclosporine levels	Decrease in sirolimus/everolimus levels	Decrease in tacrolimus levels
Rifabutin	Mild decrease in cyclosporine levels	Mild decrease in sirolimus/ everolimus levels	Mild decrease in tacrolimus levels

[a]Serum drug concentrations should be measured and doses adjusted as needed to effectively treat the NTM infection and avoid rejection or drug-related toxicity

Because of the many potential drug interactions, therapeutic drug monitoring should be strongly considered in order to maintain adequate serum drug concentrations and avoid unwanted toxicity [33].

When rifamycin is not used, an alternative drug should be selected. Studies in nontransplant populations have reported similar microbiologic outcomes in patients receiving a three-drug regimen including clofazimine instead of rifampin [112], and there is some evidence of activity in patients with refractory disease [113, 114]. A small study in five SOT patients reported good tolerance to clofazimine [115] although one pediatric bone marrow transplant patient has been reported to have developed an enteropathy [116].

Monitoring for Adverse Reactions and Treatment Response

Multidrug treatment regimens used for NTM infections are frequently associated with drug-related adverse events so monitoring of patients for toxicity is essential. The most common adverse reactions associated with antimycobacterial agents are included in Table 30.3. Transplant patients are often on other drugs that could have overlapping toxicities with antimycobacterial drugs; thus, close monitoring for adverse reactions is even more critical in this population. All patients who are being treated for NTM disease should have periodic assessment of complete blood counts, liver function tests, and creatinine. For patients receiving ethambutol or linezolid, a baseline assessment of visual acuity and color discrimination testing are recommended with periodic reassessments during the course of therapy. In addition, a baseline audiogram is needed for patients on an aminoglycoside and should be repeated during the course of treatment.

Response to treatment should be documented through periodic clinical, radiographic, and microbiologic evaluations. For pulmonary disease, treatment duration is based on the time of culture conversion so monthly cultures should be obtained to document the time of conversion. For patients with extrapulmonary disease, clinical and radiographic evaluation are most critical as resampling of extrapulmonary sites may not be possible or practical.

Survival

The impact of NTM infections on survival has varied between studies although in most the direct impact has been minimal. In a cohort of 237 lung transplant recipients from a center in the United States, NTM infection was not associated with an increased mortality [4]. In a retrospective cohort study to evaluate the impact of NTM on survival, 33 patients with NTM infection post-SOT were evaluated [92]. Surprisingly, there was not an increased mortality in patients with *M. abscessus* disease compared with other NTM disease. However, development of NTM infection during the first year after transplantation was strongly associated with decreased survival, independent of organ type. NTM infection was considered a contributing cause of death in only three of the nine patients whose death certificates were available for review. A recent study from a large Midwestern center reported that among 3338 SOT recipients, 50 (1.5%) had NTM infection, 43 of whom were lung transplant recipients. However, NTM infection was not associated with mortality in infected lung transplant recipients versus those not infected although NTM disease was associated with increased mortality compared with colonization in lung transplant recipients [26]. There was no difference in survival between NTM-infected and NTM-uninfected lung transplant recipients: the former were more likely to develop bronchiolitis obliterans (80 vs. 52%, $p = 0.02$) although this finding was not noted in multivariate analysis. One study reported that NTM colonization and NTM pulmonary disease increased the risk of death after lung transplantation although NTM pulmonary disease was not considered the direct cause of disease [2]. The increased risk of death persisted even after adjusting for single-lung transplantation and presence of bronchiolitis obliterans.

Isolation of NTM Before Transplantation

Isolation of NTM during pretransplant period is not uncommon in patients undergoing lung transplant given their underlying lung disease, and pretransplant isolation of NTM has been associated with a greater risk of NTM disease after undergoing transplantation [1]. The International Society for Heart and Lung Transplantation (ISHLT) states that "chronic infection with highly virulent and/or resistant microbes that are poorly controlled pretransplant" is an absolute contraindication for transplantation [117]. However, "colonization or infection with highly resistant or highly virulent bacteria, fungi, and certain strains of mycobacteria…" is considered a relative contraindication. Furthermore, infection with multidrug resistant *M. abscessus* is considered a relative contraindication if the infection is "sufficiently treated" preoperatively and there is a reasonable expectation for adequate control postoperatively. Unfortunately, none of these recommendations provide clear guidance to providers or patients as it is difficult to distinguish "colonization" from indolent infection and active disease and sufficiently treated are not defined.

NTM are commonly isolated in patients with CF but the risk of NTM infections posttransplantation is not well defined. The Cystic Fibrosis Foundation (CFF), European Cystic Fibrosis Society (ECFS), and the ISHLT recommend that individuals with CF who are being considered for lung transplantation be evaluated for NTM pulmonary disease and the presence of current or previous history of respiratory tract samples with NTM should not preclude consideration for transplantation [117, 118]. Those who are found to have NTM lung disease should be started on treatment prior to transplant listing, and once they have achieved sequential negative cultures, they should be considered eligible for transplantation. This includes patients who have completed therapy. ISHLT states that progressive pulmonary or extrapulmonary disease secondary to NTM despite optimal therapy or an inability to tolerate optimal therapy is a contraindication for transplant listing; however, the CFF and ECFS state that even if the NTM cannot be cleared from the respiratory tract, this is not an absolute contraindication for transplant in patients with CF [118, 119]. Isolation of NTM prior to HSCT is also not a contraindication to transplant as patients have been successfully transplanted [14].

Prevention

Recent outbreaks of NTM infections in transplant patients and patients who have undergone cardiac surgery have highlighted the potential for nosocomial acquisition of NTM [120, 121]. Most nosocomial infections can be traced back to contamination with tap water containing NTM, so avoidance of tap water during and after transplantation surgery is critical. Person-to-person transmission of *Mycobacterium abscessus* ssp. *massiliense* may have occurred among patients with CF as described in two CF clinics in the United States and United Kingdom [122, 123], and a recent study suggested global transmission of two clones of *M. abscessus* and one of *M. massiliense* among CF patients [124]. To date, person-to-person transmission of NTM has not been described in other settings. Because of the possibility of transmission among CF patients, current CF foundation infection control and prevention guidelines should be adhered to [125].

Effective chemoprophylactic treatment including azithromycin, clarithromycin, and rifabutin has been demonstrated through randomized clinical trials to prevent disseminated MAC in advanced AIDS patients [126, 127]. Not surprisingly, some physicians have called for posttransplant prophylaxis with azithromycin for CF patients "colonized" with rapidly growing mycobacteria [77]. However, there is no evidence to support this practice and it is unlikely to be effective given the presence of an *erm*(41) gene in most *M. abscessus* complex strains. Multidrug treatment regimens to decrease the bacterial load as much as possible are likely to be more effective at preventing development of NTM disease in the posttransplant setting.

Summary

Nontuberculous mycobacteria (NTM) are common in the environment, being most often associated with soil and water sources. NTM isolation does not always portray clinically significant disease, albeit, in patients with severe immune dysfunction following allogeneic transplantation, these near-ubiquitous environmental bacteria may lead to serious and potentially life-threatening systemic disease. The true prevalence of NTM among transplant recipients is largely unknown. Correct laboratory identification of NTM species, adequate genetic analysis, and susceptibility testing are essential for identification of mycobacteria and are necessary in assembling effective antimicrobial treatment regimens. Reference laboratory evaluation may be required depending on local laboratory capabilities. Antibiotic regimens are chosen according to NTM species, site of infection, and drug susceptibility profile, which can vary greatly according to the NTM species isolated. The treatment of NTM involves multiple antibiotics given for a prolonged period of time and is often accompanied by side effects and drug-drug interactions, especially in transplant patients on antirejection drugs and other agents given for suppressing hosts' immune response for prevention or treatment of graft-versus-host disease. Treatment by experienced NTM physicians is often necessary. It is essential for transplant providers to maintain a low index of suspicion in order to promptly and correctly diagnose NTM infections in the susceptible transplant population and provide host- and pathogen-specific treatment options.

References

1. Chalermskulrat W, Sood N, Neuringer IP, et al. Non-tuberculous mycobacteria in end stage cystic fibrosis: implications for lung transplantation. Thorax. 2006;61:507–13.
2. Huang HC, Weigt SS, Derhovanessian A, et al. Non-tuberculous mycobacterium infection after lung transplantation is associated with increased mortality. J Heart Lung Transplant. 2011;30:790–8.
3. Kesten S, Chaparro C. Mycobacterial infections in lung transplant recipients. Chest. 1999;115:741–5.
4. Knoll BM, Kappagoda S, Gill RR, et al. Non-tuberculous mycobacterial infection among lung transplant recipients: a 15-year cohort study. Transpl Infect Dis. 2012;14:452–60.
5. Daley CL. Nontuberculous mycobacterial disease in transplant recipients: early diagnosis and treatment. Curr Opin Organ Transplant. 2009;14:619–24.
6. Adjemian J, Olivier KN, Seitz AE, Holland SM, Prevots DR. Prevalence of nontuberculous mycobacterial lung disease in U.S. Medicare beneficiaries. Am J Respir Crit Care Med. 2012;185:881–6.
7. Prevots DR, Marras TK. Epidemiology of human pulmonary infection with nontuberculous mycobacteria: a review. Clin Chest Med. 2015;36:13–34.
8. Prevots DR, Shaw PA, Strickland D, et al. Nontuberculous mycobacterial lung disease prevalence at four integrated health care delivery systems. Am J Respir Crit Care Med. 2010;182:970–6.
9. Marras TK, Chedore P, Ying AM, Jamieson F. Isolation prevalence of pulmonary non-tuberculous mycobacteria in Ontario, 1997 2003. Thorax. 2007;62:661–6.
10. Marras TK, Mendelson D, Marchand-Austin A, May K, Jamieson FB. Pulmonary nontuberculous mycobacterial disease, Ontario, Canada, 1998-2010. Emerg Infect Dis. 2013;19:1889–91.
11. Yoo JW, Jo KW, Kim SH, et al. Incidence, characteristics, and treatment outcomes of mycobacterial diseases in transplant recipients. Transpl Int. 2016;29:549–58.
12. Jie T, Matas AJ, Gillingham KJ, Sutherland DE, Dunn DL, Humar A. Mycobacterial infections after kidney transplant. Transplant Proc. 2005;37:937–9.
13. Malouf MA, Glanville AR. The spectrum of mycobacterial infection after lung transplantation. Am J Respir Crit Care Med. 1999;160:1611–6.
14. Doucette K, Fishman JA. Nontuberculous mycobacterial infection in hematopoietic stem cell and solid organ transplant recipients. Clin Infect Dis. 2004;38:1428–39.
15. Longworth SA, Vinnard C, Lee I, Sims KD, Barton TD, Blumberg EA. Risk factors for nontuberculous mycobacterial infections in solid organ transplant recipients: a case-control study. Transpl Infect Dis. 2014;16:76–83.
16. Novick RJ, Moreno-Cabral CE, Stinson EB, et al. Nontuberculous mycobacterial infections in heart transplant recipients: a seventeen-year experience. J Heart Transplant. 1990;9:357–63.
17. Munoz RM, Pulpon LA, Yebra M, Segovia J, San Martin M, Salas C. Three cases of tuberculosis after heart transplantation in Spain. Eur J Clin Microbiol Infect Dis. 1998;17:801–6.
18. Hall CM, Willcox PA, Swanepoel CR, Kahn D, Van Zyl Smit R. Mycobacterial infection in renal transplant recipients. Chest. 1994;106:435–9.
19. Lloveras J, Peterson PK, Simmons RL, Najarian JS. Mycobacterial infections in renal transplant recipients. Seven cases and a review of the literature. Arch Intern Med. 1982;142:888–92.
20. Delaney V, Sumrani N, Hong JH, Sommer B. Mycobacterial infections in renal allograft recipients. Transplant Proc. 1993;25:2288–9.
21. Costa JM, Meyers AM, Botha JR, Conlan AA, Myburgh A. Mycobacterial infections in recipients of kidney allografts. A seventeen-year experience. Acta Medica Port. 1988;1:51–7.
22. Higgins RM, Cahn AP, Porter D, et al. Mycobacterial infections after renal transplantation. Q J Med. 1991;78:145–53.
23. Vandermarliere A, Van Audenhove A, Peetermans WE, Vanrenterghem Y, Maes B. Mycobacterial infection after renal transplantation in a Western population. Transpl Infect Dis. 2003;5:9–15.
24. Spence RK, Dafoe DC, Rabin G, et al. Mycobacterial infections in renal allograft recipients. Arch Surg. 1983;118:356–9.
25. Patel R, Roberts GD, Keating MR, Paya CV. Infections due to nontuberculous mycobacteria in kidney, heart, and liver transplant recipients. Clin Infect Dis. 1994;19:263–73.
26. George IA, Santos CA, Olsen MA, Bailey TC. Epidemiology and outcomes of nontuberculous mycobacterial infections in solid organ transplant recipients at a Midwestern Center. Transplantation. 2016;100:1073–8.
27. Shah SK, McAnally KJ, Seoane L, et al. Analysis of pulmonary non-tuberculous mycobacterial infections after lung transplantation. Transpl Infect Dis. 2016;18:585–91.
28. Chernenko SM, Humar A, Hutcheon M, et al. Mycobacterium abscessus infections in lung transplant recipients: the international experience. J Heart Lung Transplant. 2006;25:1447–55.
29. Qvist T, Gilljam M, Jonsson B, et al. Epidemiology of nontuberculous mycobacteria among patients with cystic fibrosis in Scandinavia. J Cyst Fibros. 2015;14:46–52.
30. Aguilar-Guisado M, Givalda J, Ussetti P, et al. Pneumonia after lung transplantation in the RESITRA Cohort: a multicenter prospective study. Am J Transplant. 2007;7:1989–96.
31. Bonvillain RW, Valentine VG, Lombard G, LaPlace S, Dhillon G, Wang G. Post-operative infections in cystic fibrosis and non-cystic fibrosis patients after lung transplantation. J Heart Lung Transplant. 2007;26:890–7.
32. Lobo LJ, Chang LC, Esther CR Jr, Gilligan PH, Tulu Z, Noone PG. Lung transplant outcomes in cystic fibrosis patients with pre-operative Mycobacterium abscessus respiratory infections. Clin Transpl. 2013;27:523–9.
33. Piersimoni C. Nontuberculous mycobacteria infection in solid organ transplant recipients. Eur J Clin Microbiol Infect Dis. 2012;31:397–403.
34. Queipo JA, Broseta E, Santos M, Sanchez-Plumed J, Budia A, Jimenez-Cruz F. Mycobacterial infection in a series of 1261 renal transplant recipients. Clin Microbiol Infect. 2003;9:518–25.
35. Munoz RM, Alonso-Pulpon L, Yebra M, Segovia J, Gallego JC, Daza RM. Intestinal involvement by nontuberculous mycobacteria after heart transplantation. Clin Infect Dis. 2000;30:603–5.

36. Au WY, Cheng VC, Ho PL, et al. Nontuberculous mycobacterial infections in Chinese hematopoietic stem cell transplantation recipients. Bone Marrow Transplant. 2003;32:709–14.
37. Gaviria JM, Garcia PJ, Garrido SM, Corey L, Boeckh M. Nontuberculous mycobacterial infections in hematopoietic stem cell transplant recipients: characteristics of respiratory and catheter-related infections. Biol Blood Marrow Transplant. 2000;6:361–9.
38. Roy V, Weisdorf D. Mycobacterial infections following bone marrow transplantation: a 20 year retrospective review. Bone Marrow Transplant. 1997;19:467–70.
39. Navari RM, Sullivan KM, Springmeyer SC, et al. Mycobacterial infections in marrow transplant patients. Transplantation. 1983;36:509–13.
40. Weinstock DM, Feinstein MB, Sepkowitz KA, Jakubowski A. High rates of infection and colonization by nontuberculous mycobacteria after allogeneic hematopoietic stem cell transplantation. Bone Marrow Transplant. 2003;31:1015–21.
41. Kurzrock R, Zander A, Vellekoop L, Kanojia M, Luna M, Dicke K. Mycobacterial pulmonary infections after allogeneic bone marrow transplantation. Am J Med. 1984;77:35–40.
42. Beswick J, Shin E, Michelis F, et al. Incidence and risk factors for nontuberculous mycobacterial infection after allogeneic hematopoietic cell transplantation. Biol Blood Marrow Transplant. 2018;24(2):366–72. pii: S1083–8791(17)30748–6.
43. Wu UI, Holland SM. Host susceptibility to non-tuberculous mycobacterial infections. Lancet Infect Dis. 2015;15:968–80.
44. Rook GA. Macrophages and Mycobacterium tuberculosis: the key to pathogenesis. Immunol Ser. 1994;60:249–61.
45. Casanova JL, Holland SM, Notarangelo LD. Inborn errors of human JAKs and STATs. Immunity. 2012;36:515–28.
46. Rosenzweig SD, Holland SM. Defects in the interferon-gamma and interleukin-12 pathways. Immunol Rev. 2005;203:38–47.
47. Liles WC. Immunomodulatory approaches to augment phagocyte-mediated host defense for treatment of infectious diseases. Semin Respir Infect. 2001;16:11–7.
48. Deretic V, Singh S, Master S, et al. Mycobacterium tuberculosis inhibition of phagolysosome biogenesis and autophagy as a host defence mechanism. Cell Microbiol. 2006;8:719–27.
49. Karim AF, Reba SM, Li Q, Boom WH, Rojas RE. Toll like Receptor 2 engagement on CD4+ T cells promotes TH9 differentiation and function. Eur J Immunol. 2017;47:1513–24.
50. Su X, Yu Y, Zhong Y, et al. Interferon-gamma regulates cellular metabolism and mRNA translation to potentiate macrophage activation. Nat Immunol. 2015;16:838–49.
51. Ostuni R, Piccolo V, Barozzi I, et al. Latent enhancers activated by stimulation in differentiated cells. Cell. 2013;152:157–71.
52. Jung JY, Robinson CM. IL-12 and IL-27 regulate the phagolysosomal pathway in mycobacteria-infected human macrophages. Cell Commun Signal. 2014;12:16.
53. Safdar A, Armstrong D, Murray HW. A novel defect in interferon-gamma secretion in patients with refractory nontuberculous pulmonary mycobacteriosis. Ann Intern Med. 2003;138:521.
54. Safdar A, White DA, Stover D, Armstrong D, Murray HW. Profound interferon gamma deficiency in patients with chronic pulmonary nontuberculous mycobacteriosis. Am J Med. 2002;113:756–9.
55. Silva RA, Florido M, Appelberg R. Interleukin-12 primes CD4+ T cells for interferon-gamma production and protective immunity during Mycobacterium avium infection. Immunology. 2001;103:368–74.
56. Bhattacharyya A, Pathak S, Kundu M, Basu J. Mitogen-activated protein kinases regulate Mycobacterium avium-induced tumor necrosis factor-alpha release from macrophages. FEMS Immunol Med Microbiol. 2002;34:73–80.
57. Petursdottir DH, Chuquimia OD, Freidl R, Fernandez C. Macrophage control of phagocytosed mycobacteria is increased by factors secreted by alveolar epithelial cells through nitric oxide independent mechanisms. PLoS One. 2014;9:e103411.
58. Halloran PF. Immunosuppressive drugs for kidney transplantation. N Engl J Med. 2004;351:2715–29.
59. Tortoli E. Microbiological features and clinical relevance of new species of the genus Mycobacterium. Clin Microbiol Rev. 2014;27:727–52.
60. Ahn CH, Lowell JR, Ahn SS, Ahn S, Hurst GA. Chemotherapy for pulmonary disease due to Mycobacterium kansasii: efficacies of some individual drugs. Rev Infect Dis. 1981;3:1028–34.
61. Ahn CH, Lowell JR, Ahn SS, Ahn SI, Hurst GA. Short-course chemotherapy for pulmonary disease caused by Mycobacterium kansasii. Am Rev Respir Dis. 1983;128:1048–50.
62. Pezzia W, Raleigh JW, Bailey MC, Toth EA, Silverblatt J. Treatment of pulmonary disease due to Mycobacterium kansasii: recent experience with rifampin. Rev Infect Dis. 1981;3:1035–9.
63. Nash KA, Brown-Elliott BA, Wallace RJ Jr. A novel gene, erm(41), confers inducible macrolide resistance to clinical isolates of Mycobacterium abscessus but is absent from Mycobacterium chelonae. Antimicrob Agents Chemother. 2009;53:1367–76.
64. Cho YJ, Yi H, Chun J, et al. The genome sequence of 'Mycobacterium massiliense' strain CIP 108297 suggests the independent taxonomic status of the Mycobacterium abscessus complex at the subspecies level. PLoS One. 2013;8:e81560.
65. Tortoli E, Kohl TA, Brown-Elliott BA, et al. Emended description of Mycobacterium abscessus, Mycobacterium abscessus subsp. abscessus and Mycobacterium abscessus subsp. bolletii and designation of Mycobacterium abscessus subsp. massiliense comb. nov. Int J Syst Evol Microbiol. 2016;66:4471–9.
66. Harada T, Akiyama Y, Kurashima A, et al. Clinical and microbiological differences between Mycobacterium abscessus and Mycobacterium massiliense lung diseases. J Clin Microbiol. 2012;50:3556–61.
67. Koh WJ, Jeon K, Lee NY, et al. Clinical significance of differentiation of Mycobacterium massiliense from Mycobacterium abscessus. Am J Respir Crit Care Med. 2011;183:405–10.
68. Lyu J, Jang HJ, Song JW, et al. Outcomes in patients with Mycobacterium abscessus pulmonary disease treated with long-term injectable drugs. Respir Med. 2011;105:781–7.
69. Griffith DE, Aksamit T, Brown-Elliott BA, et al. An official ATS/IDSA statement: diagnosis, treatment, and prevention of nontuberculous mycobacterial diseases. Am J Respir Crit Care Med. 2007;175:367–416.
70. Knoll BM. Update on nontuberculous mycobacterial infections in solid organ and hematopoietic stem cell transplant recipients. Curr Infect Dis Rep. 2014;16:421.
71. Wallace RJ Jr, Tanner D, Brennan PJ, Brown BA. Clinical trial of clarithromycin for cutaneous (disseminated) infection due to Mycobacterium chelonae. Ann Intern Med. 1993;119:482–6.
72. Heironimus JD, Winn RE, Collins CB. Cutaneous nonpulmonary Mycobacterium chelonei infection. Successful treatment with sulfonamides in an immunosuppressed patient. Arch Dermatol. 1984;120:1061–3.
73. Fan MH, Hadjiliadis D. Incidence and management of mycobacterial infection in solid organ transplant recipients. Curr Infect Dis Rep. 2009;11:216–22.
74. Meije Y, Piersimoni C, Torre-Cisneros J, Dilektasli AG, Aguado JM, Hosts ESGoIiC. Mycobacterial infections in solid organ transplant recipients. Clin Microbiol Infect. 2014;20(Suppl 7):89–101.
75. Abad CLRR. Non-tuberculous mycobacterial infections in solid organ transplant recipients: an update. J Clin Tuberc Other Mycobact Dis. 2016;4:1–8.
76. Fairhurst RM, Kubak BM, Shpiner RB, Levine MS, Pegues DA, Ardehali A. Mycobacterium abscessus empyema in a lung transplant recipient. J Heart Lung Transplant. 2002;21:391–4.

77. Keating MR, Daly JS, Practice ASTIDCo. Nontuberculous mycobacterial infections in solid organ transplantation. Am J Transplant. 2013;13(Suppl 4):77–82.
78. Dorman S, Subramanian A, Practice ASTIDCo. Nontuberculous mycobacteria in solid organ transplant recipients. Am J Transplant. 2009;9(Suppl 4):S63–9.
79. Pandian TK, Deziel PJ, Otley CC, Eid AJ, Razonable RR. Mycobacterium marinum infections in transplant recipients: case report and review of the literature. Transpl Infect Dis. 2008;10:358–63.
80. Jacobson K, Garcia R, Libshitz H, et al. Clinical and radiological features of pulmonary disease caused by rapidly growing mycobacteria in cancer patients. Eur J Clin Microbiol Infect Dis. 1998;17:615–21.
81. Wallace RJ Jr, Brown BA, Onyi GO. Skin, soft tissue, and bone infections due to Mycobacterium chelonae chelonae: importance of prior corticosteroid therapy, frequency of disseminated infections, and resistance to oral antimicrobials other than clarithromycin. J Infect Dis. 1992;166:405–12.
82. Shields RK, Clancy CJ, Minces LR, et al. Epidemiology and outcomes of deep surgical site infections following lung transplantation. Am J Transplant. 2013;13:2137–45.
83. Safdar A, Bains M, Polsky B. Clinical microbiological case: refractory chest wall infection following reconstructive surgery in a patient with relapsed lung cancer. Clin Microbiol Infect. 2001;7:563–4. 77–9.
84. Engler HD, Hass A, Hodes DS, Bottone EJ. Mycobacterium chelonei infection of a Broviac catheter insertion site. Eur J Clin Microbiol Infect Dis. 1989;8:521–3.
85. Skiest DJ, Levi ME. Catheter-related bacteremia due to Mycobacterium smegmatis. South Med J. 1998;91:36–7.
86. Woo PC, Tsoi HW, Leung KW, et al. Identification of Mycobacterium neoaurum isolated from a neutropenic patient with catheter-related bacteremia by 16S rRNA sequencing. J Clin Microbiol. 2000;38:3515–7.
87. Koranyi KI, Ranalli MA. Mycobacterium aurum bacteremia in an immunocompromised child. Pediatr Infect Dis J. 2003;22:1108–9.
88. Kiska DL, Turenne CY, Dubansky AS, Domachowske JB. First case report of catheter-related bacteremia due to "Mycobacterium lacticola". J Clin Microbiol. 2004;42:2855–7.
89. Lee SA, Raad II, Adachi JA, Han XY. Catheter-related bloodstream infection caused by Mycobacterium brumae. J Clin Microbiol. 2004;42:5429–31.
90. Ashford DA, Kellerman S, Yakrus M, et al. Pseudo-outbreak of septicemia due to rapidly growing mycobacteria associated with extrinsic contamination of culture supplement. J Clin Microbiol. 1997;35:2040–2.
91. Fraser VJ, Jones M, Murray PR, Medoff G, Zhang Y, Wallace RJ Jr. Contamination of flexible fiberoptic bronchoscopes with Mycobacterium chelonae linked to an automated bronchoscope disinfection machine. Am Rev Respir Dis. 1992;145:853–5.
92. Longworth SA, Blumberg EA, Barton TD, Vinnard C. Nontuberculous mycobacterial infections after solid organ transplantation: a survival analysis. Clin Microbiol Infect. 2015;21:43–7.
93. Al-Anazi KA, Al-Jasser AM, Al-Anazi WK. Infections caused by non-tuberculous mycobacteria in recipients of hematopoietic stem cell transplantation. Front Oncol. 2014;4:311.
94. Olivier KN, Griffith DE, Eagle G, et al. Randomized trial of liposomal amikacin for inhalation in nontuberculous mycobacterial lung disease. Am J Respir Crit Care Med. 2017;195:814–23.
95. van Ingen J. Microbiological diagnosis of nontuberculous mycobacterial pulmonary disease. Clin Chest Med. 2015;36:43–54.
96. Meier A, Heifets L, Wallace RJ Jr, et al. Molecular mechanisms of clarithromycin resistance in Mycobacterium avium: observation of multiple 23S rDNA mutations in a clonal population. J Infect Dis. 1996;174:354–60.
97. Griffith DE, Brown-Elliott BA, Langsjoen B, et al. Clinical and molecular analysis of macrolide resistance in Mycobacterium avium complex lung disease. Am J Respir Crit Care Med. 2006;174:928–34.
98. Griffith DE. Management of disease due to Mycobacterium kansasii. Clin Chest Med. 2002;23:613–21. vi
99. Griffith DE, Brown-Elliott BA, Wallace RJ Jr. Thrice-weekly clarithromycin-containing regimen for treatment of Mycobacterium kansasii lung disease: results of a preliminary study. Clin Infect Dis. 2003;37:1178–82.
100. Shitrit D, Baum GL, Priess R, et al. Pulmonary Mycobacterium kansasii infection in Israel, 1999-2004: clinical features, drug susceptibility, and outcome. Chest. 2006;129:771–6.
101. White MH, Papadopoulos EB, Small TN, Kiehn TE, Armstrong D. Mycobacterium haemophilum infections in bone marrow transplant recipients. Transplantation. 1995;60:957–60.
102. Baluch A, Pasikhova Y, Snyder M. Successful management of Mycobacterium haemophilum lower extremity cutaneous infection in a matched-unrelated donor stem cell transplant recipient. Transpl Infect Dis. 2017;19(1):e12627. https://doi.org/10.1111/tid.12627.
103. Gombert ME, Goldstein EJ, Corrado ML, Stein AJ, Butt KM. Disseminated Mycobacterium marinum infection after renal transplantation. Ann Intern Med. 1981;94:486–7.
104. Jacobs S, George A, Papanicolaou GA, et al. Disseminated Mycobacterium marinum infection in a hematopoietic stem cell transplant recipient. Transpl Infect Dis. 2012;14:410–4.
105. Jeon K, Kwon OJ, Lee NY, et al. Antibiotic treatment of Mycobacterium abscessus lung disease: a retrospective analysis of 65 patients. Am J Respir Crit Care Med. 2009;180:896–902.
106. Jarand J, Levin A, Zhang L, Huitt G, Mitchell JD, Daley CL. Clinical and microbiologic outcomes in patients receiving treatment for Mycobacterium abscessus pulmonary disease. Clin Infect Dis. 2011;52:565–71.
107. Brown BA, Wallace RJ Jr, Onyi GO, De Rosas V, Wallace RJ 3rd. Activities of four macrolides, including clarithromycin, against Mycobacterium fortuitum, Mycobacterium chelonae, and M. chelonae-like organisms. Antimicrob Agents Chemother. 1992;36:180–4.
108. Hadjiliadis D, Adlakha A, Prakash UB. Rapidly growing mycobacterial lung infection in association with esophageal disorders. Mayo Clin Proc. 1999;74:45–51.
109. Wallace RJ Jr, Brown BA, Onyi GO. Susceptibilities of Mycobacterium fortuitum biovar. Fortuitum and the two subgroups of Mycobacterium chelonae to imipenem, cefmetazole, cefoxitin, and amoxicillin-clavulanic acid. Antimicrob Agents Chemother. 1991;35:773–5.
110. Aguado JM, Herrero JA, Gavalda J, et al. Clinical presentation and outcome of tuberculosis in kidney, liver, and heart transplant recipients in Spain. Spanish Transplantation Infection Study Group, GESITRA. Transplantation. 1997;63:1278–86.
111. Finch CK, Chrisman CR, Baciewicz AM, Self TH. Rifampin and rifabutin drug interactions: an update. Arch Intern Med. 2002;162:985–92.
112. Jarand J, Davis JP, Cowie RL, Field SK, Fisher DA. Long-term follow-up of Mycobacterium avium complex lung disease in patients treated with regimens including Clofazimine and/or Rifampin. Chest. 2016;149:1285–93.
113. Martiniano SL, Wagner BD, Levin A, Nick JA, Sagel SD, Daley CL. Safety and effectiveness of Clofazimine for primary and refractory nontuberculous mycobacterial infection. Chest. 2017;152(4):800–9.
114. Yang B, Jhun BW, Moon SM, et al. Clofazimine-containing regimen for the treatment of Mycobacterium abscessus lung disease. Antimicrob Agents Chemother. 2017;61(6):e02052–16.
115. Cariello PF, Kwak EJ, Abdel-Massih RC, Silveira FP. Safety and tolerability of clofazimine as salvage therapy for atypical

mycobacterial infection in solid organ transplant recipients. Transpl Infect Dis. 2015;17:111–8.

116. Parizhskaya M, Youssef NN, Di Lorenzo C, Goyal RK. Clofazimine enteropathy in a pediatric bone marrow transplant recipient. J Pediatr. 2001;138:574–6.

117. Weill D, Benden C, Corris PA, et al. A consensus document for the selection of lung transplant candidates: 2014--an update from the pulmonary transplantation Council of the International Society for heart and lung transplantation. J Heart Lung Transplant. 2015;34:1–15.

118. Floto RA, Olivier KN, Saiman L, et al. US Cystic Fibrosis Foundation and European Cystic Fibrosis Society consensus recommendations for the management of non-tuberculous mycobacteria in individuals with cystic fibrosis: executive summary. Thorax. 2016;71:88–90.

119. Qvist T, Pressler T, Thomsen VO, Skov M, Iversen M, Katzenstein TL. Nontuberculous mycobacterial disease is not a contraindication to lung transplantation in patients with cystic fibrosis: a retrospective analysis in a Danish patient population. Transplant Proc. 2013;45:342–5.

120. Sax H, Bloemberg G, Hasse B, et al. Prolonged outbreak of Mycobacterium chimaera infection after open-chest heart surgery. Clin Infect Dis. 2015;61:67–75.

121. Baker AW, Lewis SS, Alexander BD, et al. Two-phase hospital-associated outbreak of Mycobacterium abscessus: investigation and mitigation. Clin Infect Dis. 2017;64:902–11.

122. Aitken ML, Limaye A, Pottinger P, et al. Respiratory outbreak of Mycobacterium abscessus subspecies massiliense in a lung transplant and cystic fibrosis center. Am J Respir Crit Care Med. 2012;185:231–2.

123. Bryant JM, Grogono DM, Greaves D, et al. Whole-genome sequencing to identify transmission of Mycobacterium abscessus between patients with cystic fibrosis: a retrospective cohort study. Lancet. 2013;381:1551–60.

124. Bryant JM, Grogono DM, Rodriguez-Rincon D, et al. Emergence and spread of a human-transmissible multidrug-resistant nontuberculous mycobacterium. Science. 2016;354:751–7.

125. Saiman L, Siegel J. Cystic Fibrosis Foundation Consensus Conference on Infection Control P. Infection control recommendations for patients with cystic fibrosis: microbiology, important pathogens, and infection control practices to prevent patient-to-patient transmission. Am J Infect Control. 2003;31:S1–62.

126. Havlir DV, Dube MP, Sattler FR, et al. Prophylaxis against disseminated Mycobacterium avium complex with weekly azithromycin, daily rifabutin, or both. California Collaborative Treatment Group. N Engl J Med. 1996;335:392–8.

127. Pierce M, Crampton S, Henry D, et al. A randomized trial of clarithromycin as prophylaxis against disseminated Mycobacterium avium complex infection in patients with advanced acquired immunodeficiency syndrome. N Engl J Med. 1996;335:384–91.

Invasive Fungal Disease in the Transplant Population: An Overview

31

Jennifer L. Saullo, John R. Perfect, and Barbara D. Alexander

Abbreviations

5-FC	5-Flucytosine
5-FU	5-Fluorouracil
ABD	Amphotericin B deoxycholate
ABLC	Amphotericin B lipid complex
AML	Acute myelogenous leukemia
AST	American Society of Transplantation
CI	Cumulative incidence
CMV	Cytomegalovirus
CNI	Calcineurin inhibitor
CNS	Central nervous system
GVHD	Graft-versus-host disease
HCT	Hematopoietic cell transplant
IA	Invasive aspergillosis
IC	Invasive candidiasis
IDSA	Infectious Diseases Society of America
IFI	Invasive fungal infection
IRS	Immune reconstitution syndrome
LAMB	Liposomal amphotericin B
MDS	Myelodysplastic syndrome
MMRD	Mismatched-related donor
MRD	Matched-related donor
mTOR	Mammalian target of rapamycin
MVT	Multivisceral transplant
OHT	Orthotopic heart transplant
OLT	Orthotopic liver transplant
PATH	Prospective antifungal therapy
SBT	Small bowel transplant
SOT	Solid organ transplant
TLR	Toll-like receptor
TRANSNET	Transplant-Associated Infection Surveillance Network
URD	Unrelated donor
UTI	Urinary tract infection

J. L. Saullo (✉) · J. R. Perfect
Duke University Medical Center, Department of Medicine, Division of Infectious Diseases and International Health, Durham, NC, USA
e-mail: jennifer.horan@duke.edu; john.perfect@duke.edu

B. D. Alexander
Duke University Medical Center, Departments of Medicine and Pathology, Division of Infectious Diseases and International Health, Durham, NC, USA
e-mail: alexa011@duke.edu

Introduction

In the latter half of the twentieth century, considerable progress occurred in transplantation including improvements in donor selection and screening, surgical techniques, immunosuppression, and antimicrobial therapy. Despite these advances, infection persists as a common complication post-transplant and fungal infections in particular are associated with significant morbidity and mortality. The number of individuals receiving either a hematopoietic cell transplant (HCT) or solid organ transplant (SOT) continues to rise, resulting in an ever-expanding at-risk population for invasive fungal infections (IFIs). This chapter will provide a broad overview of the fungal pathogens affecting both the HCT and SOT populations inclusive of the changing epidemiology and unique considerations in the transplant recipient.

Fungal Pathogens in HCT and SOT

The list of fungi capable of affecting this population seems infinite with new pathogens continuing to emerge. For simplification, fungal pathogens can be classified into three categories: yeasts, filamentous molds, and endemic fungi. Yeasts are fungi that grow as single, rounded, or elongated cells and reproduce by budding or sometimes fission; chains of these elongated cells are called pseudohyphae. In contrast, molds are multicellular fungi with spores that germinate to produce branching hyphae. The third category, endemic fungi, are dimorphic fungi capable of existing as molds at room temperature and yeast or yeast-like forms at body temperature in the human host [1].

A. Safdar (ed.), *Principles and Practice of Transplant Infectious Diseases*, https://doi.org/10.1007/978-1-4939-9034-4_31

Table 31.1 Currently documented agents of hyalohyphomycosis[a] [13]

Acremonium spp.	*Emmonsia parva*	*Paecilomyces* spp.	*Trichoderma* spp.
A. alabamense	*Engyodontium album*	*P. lilacinus*	*T. harzianum*
A. atrogriseum	*Fusarium* spp.	*P. variotii*	*T. longibrachiatum*
A. curvulum	*F. chlamydosporum*	*Penicillium* spp	*Tritirachium oryzae*
A. falciforme	*F. dimerum*	*P. chrysogenum*	*Verticillium serrae*
A. kiliense	*F. incarnatum*	*P. citrinum*	*Volutella cinerescens*
A. potronii	*F. moniliforme*	*P. commune*	
A. roseogriseum	*F. napiforme*	*P. decumbens*	
A. strictum	*F. nivale*	*P. expansum*	
Aphanoascus fulvescens	*F. nygamai*	*P. marneffei*[b]	
Arthrographis kalrae	*F. oxysporum*	*Phaeoacremonium parasiticum*	
Aspergillus spp.	*F. pallidoroseum*	*P. inflatipes*	
Beauveria spp.			
B. alba	*F. proliferatum*	*P. rubrigenum*	
B. bassiana	*F. solani*	*Phialemonium obovatum*	
Cephaliophora irregularis	*F. veriticillioides*	*Phialemonium curvatum*	
Chrysonilia sitophila	*Gymnascella dankaliensis*	*Polycytella hominis*	
Chrysosporium spp.	*Lecythophora hoffmannii*	*Schizophyllum commune*	
C. pannicola	*Lecythophora mutabilis*	*Scedosporium* spp	
C. zonatum	*Metarhizium anisopliae*	*S. apiospermum*[c]	
Coprinus cinereus	*Myceliophthora thermophila*	*S. prolificans*[d]	
Cylindrocarpon spp.	*Onychocola canadensis*	*Scopulariopsis* spp.	
C. destructans	*Ovadendron sulphureoochraceum*	*S. brevicaulis*	
C. lichenicola	*Neocosmospora vasinfecta*	*Scytalidium dimidiatum*	
C. vaginae			

Adapted with permission from: Alexander and Schell [13]
[a]List not inclusive
[b]Most authorities refer to disease as penicilliosis
[c]Sexual anamorph of *Pseudallescheria boydii*
[d]Some experts consider this a dematiaceous mold, recently reclassified as *Lomentospora prolificans*

The most common yeasts associated with infection in SOT and HCT are *Candida* species, although numerous other pathogens are seen including, but not limited to, *Cryptococcus*, *Hansenula*, *Malassezia*, *Rhodotorula*, *Saccharomyces*, and *Trichosporon* [2–5]. Non-*albicans Candida* species such as *C. glabrata*, *C. parapsilosis*, and *C. krusei* account for an increasing proportion of infections with evolving trends in antifungal resistance and are associated with worse outcomes in specific populations [6–9]. Infections with the encapsulated yeast *Cryptococcus* occur more frequently in SOT as compared to HCT. While *C. neoformans* var *grubii* (serotype A) is the predominant pathogen in both SOT and HCT populations, infections with *C. neoformans* var *neoformans* (serotype D) can be seen in Northern Europe, and *C. gattii* has emerged in both immunocompetent and immunocompromised hosts in Canada and the northwest United States and continues to cause disease in subtropical climates [10–12].

Molds include the hyaline and dematiaceous hyphomycetes as well as those from the subphylum *Mucormycotina*. Hyalohyphomycosis describes infections caused by the hyaline molds, a large group of septate molds that present as colorless or lightly pigmented hyphae in tissue. There are numerous molds in this group but the most common in the transplant population are *Aspergillus*, *Fusarium*, and *Scedosporium* species [13] (see Table 31.1). These molds are widely distributed and associated with an array of infections. Fungemia is a relatively rare occurrence with *Aspergillus* but is frequently seen in invasive fusariosis as it is capable of adventitious sporulation which probably aids its entry into the bloodstream. Other molds including *Acremonium*, *Scedosporium*, and *Paecilomyces* also demonstrate this phenomenon [14]. The dematiaceous fungi represent an assorted group of molds containing prominent amounts of melanin in their cell walls which contributes directly to their pathogenicity and is responsible for the light or dark brown color frequently seen in culture and/or histopathology [15]. Furthermore, these fungi are responsible for phaeohyphomycoses which often present as skin and soft tissue, ocular, and/or disseminated infections. *Alternaria*, *Bipolaris*, *Cladophialophora*, *Curvularia*, *Dactylaria*, *Exophiala*, and *Phialophora* are some of the more common black molds associated with infection in the transplant recipient [16, 17] (see Table 31.2). Many of these molds are also neurotropic and associated with severe and often fatal central nervous system (CNS) infections [2, 3]. Therefore, it is essential that there is proper and accurate identification of all molds from both sterile and non-sterile sites so prediction of disease and choice of therapy can be predicated on experience.

Table 31.2 Currently documented agents of phaeohyphomycosis[a] [16]

Alternaria spp.	*Exophiala* spp.	*Phaeoacremonium parasiticum*
A. alternate *A. chartarum*	*E. dermatitidis* *E. jeanselmei*	*Phaeoannellomyces werneckii* *Phialemonium curvatum*
Aureobasidium pullulans	*Exserohilum* spp.	*Phialophora* spp.
Bipolaris spp.	*E. rostratum*	*P. richardsiae*
B. spicifera	*E. longirostratum*	*P. verrucosa*
B. hawaiiensis	*E. mcginnisii*	*Phoma* spp.
Chaetomium spp.	*Fonsecaea* spp.	*Piedraia hortae*
Cladophialophora spp.	*F. compacta*	*Ramichloridium mackenzei*
C. bantiana	*F. pedrosoi*	*Scedosporium prolificans*[b]
C. carrionii	*Hormonema dematioides*	*Stenella araguata*
Curvularia spp.	*Madurella* spp.	*Tetraploa aristata*
C. clavata	*M. grisea*	*Thermomyces lanuginosa*
C. lunata	*M. mycetomatis*	*Trichomaris invadens*
Dactylaria gallopava (formerly *Ochroconis gallopavum*)		*Ulocladium chartarum* *Veronaea botryosa*

Adapted with permission from: Revankar [16]

[a]List not inclusive

[b]Some experts consider this a hyaline mold, recently reclassified as *Lomentospora prolificans*

Mucormycosis refers to infection caused by molds in the order *Mucorales* in the subphylum *Mucormycotina* [18]. They are characterized by broad, irregularly branching hyphae with few septations in contrast to the more commonly seen narrow, regularly branching septate hyphae with *Aspergillus* and the other hyphomycetes [1]. Expert pathologists can generally tell the difference between these two groups of molds by histopathology. The genera most frequently associated with infections include *Rhizopus* and *Mucor*; however, infections with *Apophysomyces*, *Cunninghamella*, *Rhizomucor*, *Saksenaea*, and *Syncephalastrum* are reported [2, 19–21]. These molds are abundant in soil as well as decaying plant material and often gain entrance into the host via inhalation or direct skin penetration. They are associated with localized skin and soft tissue infections from trauma as well as rhinocerebral, gastrointestinal, and pulmonary infections from aerosolized or ingested spores and in the immunocompromised host have the ability to disseminate to other organs [21, 22].

The primary endemic mycoses include histoplasmosis, blastomycosis, and coccidioidomycosis and are an infrequent but important cause of transplant fungal infections particularly in the SOT population [23]. Inhalation serves as the primary mode of acquisition with clinical presentations ranging from isolated pneumonia to disseminated disease. Given their geographic predilection, obtaining a comprehensive exposure history in the transplant recipient remains critical to diagnosis as both primary infection and reactivation from prior infection can occur. Moreover, donor-derived infections have been reported with both histoplasmosis and coccidioidomycosis making links to exposure further complex in transplant patients [24–26].

A brief discussion of the immune reconstitution syndrome (IRS) is warranted in the introduction of fungal pathogens in transplantation. In an acute, life-threatening IFI in an immunocompromised host, it seems logical to attempt to restore the immune system to combat the infection. However, this must be approached in a careful and step-wise fashion as abrupt withdrawal of immunosuppression alongside institution of antifungal therapy has been associated with IRS in the transplant recipient with a number of fungal pathogens. It is most commonly reported in *Cryptococcus* and *Aspergillus* infections but has been associated with other IFIs including *Candida*, *Dipodascus capitatus*, and *Histoplasma capsulatum* [27]. The interactions are complex given the immunomodulatory effects of antifungals as well as the antifungal properties of certain immunosuppressives. However, in general the underlying pathogenesis involves a conversion of T-cell regulatory pathways to a proinflammatory state when antifungal therapy is initiated and immunosuppression is reduced. The net effect of this proinflammatory state is paradoxical worsening clinical signs and symptoms often misinterpreted as progressive infection in the transplant recipient as well as potential for allograft loss [28–30]. Presently guidelines detailing how to most appropriately manage these patients are lacking, but the challenging interplay of immunosuppressants and antifungals creates marked potential for future innovative strategies.

Epidemiology of IFIs in Transplantation

Inherent to understanding the epidemiology of IFIs is first an acknowledgement of the limitations of the available literature. For instance, studies in transplantation are often single-center, retrospective, and transplant organ-specific and lack uniform definitions of disease, thereby hampering epidemiologic assessments. However, attempts to optimize standardized definitions and incorporate study designs with detailed prospective data collection have advanced more recent estimations. The originally proposed definitions of IFIs applied only to patients with cancer and/or undergoing HCT but were revised to extend application to individuals with primary immunodeficiencies as well as SOT recipients [31, 32]. Current definitions include three categories, proven, probable, and possible IFIs, and attempt to incorporate the less common fungi and yet maintain the focus on patients with the highest likelihood of an IFI. While imperfect, these definitions serve as starting point with ongoing efforts in place to further refine. There is at least one major prospectively maintained database to assist in defining the burden of IFIs in HCT and SOT. The Transplant-Associated Infection Surveillance Network (TRANSNET) [4, 5, 17, 23, 33] contains information regarding IFIs from 23 transplant centers in the United States. Published data from TRANSNET encompasses a 5-year period from 2001 to 2006 and provides the most recent and comprehensive prospective evaluation in the transplant groups regarding the characteristics and appearance of IFIs in this risk group. The Prospective Antifungal Therapy (PATH) [20, 21] Alliance is an additional large multicenter observational registry of IFIs inclusive of HCT/SOT recipients in North America.

Epidemiology in HCT

Incidence and Types of IFIs

Changes in the incidence of IFIs in HCT have occurred over the last few decades for a multitude of reasons including modifications in stem cell sources and conditioning regimens, utilization of hematopoietic growth factors, as well as advances in diagnosis, prevention, and treatment of infections [19, 34–40]. Previous studies report IFI incidence rates upwards of 15% [41, 42]. However, more recent data from TRANSNET found a 12-month cumulative incidence (CI) for any IFI of 3.4% (range 0.9–13.2%) in 15,820 patients undergoing HCT from March 2001 through September 2005 [5]. Among transplant types, the incidence was lowest in autologous HCT recipients (1.2%) when compared to rates of 5.8%, 7.7%, and 8.1% in allogeneic HCT recipients with matched-related donors (MRDs), unrelated donors (URD), and mismatched-related donors (MMRD), respectively.

Modifications in the practice of HCT have also resulted in shifts in the primary fungal pathogens associated with IFIs (see Table 31.3). While *Candida* maintains an imposing presence, it has been superseded by *Aspergillus* as the primary fungal pathogen in this risk group. Institution of antifungal prophylaxis directed against *Candida* species, increased utilization of alternate donor sources, and changes in HCT conditioning regimens are a few of the contributing factors for *Aspergillus* supplanting *Candida* as the most common IFI [43]. We can expect that as practices continue to change, the future will likely bring another group of leading fungal pathogens. For instance, alongside declining *Candida* infections since the early 1990s following institution of fluconazole prophylaxis in HCT patients, the concerning trend toward infections with more resistant non-*albicans Candida* species emerged [7, 44–50]. Invasive candidiasis (IC) typically manifests as bloodstream infections related to neutropenia and mucosal injury with the potential for dissemination. Hepatosplenic candidiasis, a distinct form of disseminated *Candida* infection seen in this population, is often referred to as chronic disseminated candidiasis as it can affect other organs in addition to the liver and spleen. Among *Aspergillus* species, *A. fumigatus* remains the most common pathogen in part due to specific virulence factors and its ubiquitous ecology [51]. However, non-*fumigatus* types are increasingly recognized to produce disease in the mammalian host including *A. terreus* which typically exhibits *in vitro* resistance to amphotericin B and *A. lentulus* which harbors *in vitro* and clinical resistance to most present antifungal therapies [52–54]. *Aspergillus* infections present as invasive pulmonary infections, rhinosinusitis, and disseminated disease involving the skin and/or CNS [55]. *Aspergillus* tracheobronchitis, an early presentation in the lung transplant recipient, is also reported, albeit rare, in HCT recipients [56, 57]. In the HCT recipient, neutrophil recovery can also be associated with worsening clinical and radiologic findings alongside declining serum *Aspergillus* galactomannan levels signaling the possibility of IRS associated with invasive aspergillosis (IA) treatment [58].

Non-*Aspergillus* molds, although less common, are emerging pathogens in HCT and unfortunately are often relatively resistant to most conventional antifungal agents. Marr et al. [59] retrospectively evaluated 5589 patients undergoing HCT at single center from 1985 to 1992 and of 144 proven

Table 31.3 Primary fungal pathogens in hematopoietic cell transplantation [5, 17, 23, 33]

Fungal pathogen	12-month CI[a,b] (%)	Total IFIs[b] (%)	Predominant pathogens[b]	12-month survival[b] (%)
Aspergillus	1.6	43.2	*A. fumigatus, A. niger, A. flavus*	25.4
Candida	1.1	28.1	*C. glabrata, C. albicans, C. parapsilosis*	33.6
Mucormycosis	0.3	7.8	*Rhizopus, Mucor, Rhiozomucor, Cunninghamella*	28.0
Fusarium and *Scedosporium*	~0.2	4.8	*F. solani, F. proliferatum, S. apiospermum* complex, *S. prolificans*[d]	6.3[c]
Endemic mycoses	NA	0.6	*Histoplasma capsulatum, Coccidioides immitis, Blastomyces dermatitidis*	NA
Cryptococcus	NA	0.6	NA[e]	NA

NA: Data not available

[a]12-month cumulative incidence (CI) for first invasive fungal infection (IFI)

[b]Based on Transplant-Associated Infection Surveillance Network (TRANSNET)-derived data [5, 17, 23, 33]

[c]For *Fusarium* only (*Scedosporium* outcomes not available)

[d]Recently reclassified as *Lomentospora prolificans*

[e]Clinically *C. neoformans* var. *grubii* most common

or probable infections with non-*Aspergillus* molds, *Fusarium* and *Scedosporium* were the most common. Surveillance data from TRANSNET confirm stable 12-month CI for both *Scedosporium* and *Fusarium* infections but increases in mucormycosis [5, 33]. Kontoyiannis et al. [60] also reported increasing rates of mucormycosis at a major cancer center in the late 1980s to 1990s. This same center later reported continued increases after the institution of voriconazole prophylaxis in their HCT population [61], and this report coincided with multiple reports of "breakthrough" mucormycosis at other institutions utilizing voriconazole [62–66]. As the increase was seen before and after the introduction of voriconazole, many propose this association is multifactorial, including changes in immunosuppression and patient survival, rather than a simple direct stimulatory effect on the fungus [5, 53]. Furthermore, similar breakthrough infections have been reported with other azole antifungals including posaconazole which has extended coverage against some but not all of the *Mucorales* species [67–69]. *F. solani* is the most commonly identified *Fusarium* species. Retrospective characterization of *Fusarium* infections in HCT recipients by Nucci et al. [70] at 2 US and 7 Brazilian transplant centers found an overall incidence of 5.97 cases per 1000 transplants with an approximate fourfold to tenfold increase in incidence when comparing autologous to allogeneic MRD and MMRD HCT recipients, respectively. The overall incidence of fusariosis did not differ between the two countries; however, Brazilian patients tended to be younger with underlying diagnosis of chronic myelogenous leukemia or aplastic anemia and received primarily MRDs as opposed to patients in the United States wherein AML (acute myelogenous leukemia) and non-MRD transplants predominated. Of the 61 cases identified, invasive fusariosis most often presented as disseminated disease including skin and pulmonary involvement with fungemia occurring in 28% of patients. *Scedosporium,* another prominent pathogen in HCT recipients, was first identified as a human pathogen in the early 1900s. Husain et al. [71] found that *S. apiospermum* complex (the sexual anamorph of *Pseudallescheria boydii*) infections occurred most commonly in all transplant groups, but infections with *S. prolificans* (recently reclassified as *Lomentospora prolificans*) and its presence in fungemias were clearly more common in the HCT as compared to the SOT population [72]. Moreover, severe presentations including sepsis-like syndromes with scedosporiosis were reported primarily in patients with hematologic malignancy or undergoing HCT.

The primary endemic mycoses, namely, histoplasmosis, coccidioidomycosis, and blastomycosis, are uncommon in HCT patients as evidenced by only six cases reported in TRANSNET [5, 23]. Data regarding histoplasmosis, the most common of this group, predominate in the form of case reports and series of pneumonia and disseminated infections [73–79]. However, Vail et al. [78] found no cases of histoplasmosis among 137 allogeneic HCT recipients at a single center in a "hyperendemic" region, 5% of which were identified with positive complement-fixation titers to *Histoplasma* antigens pre-transplant, suggesting it is not an overwhelming problem even in areas with substantial exposure. Coccidioidomycoses is the second most common endemic mycosis in the transplant population overall [76, 80–82]. Blair et al. [82] reported incidence rates of 0.9% and 2.1% in autologous and allogeneic HCT, respectively, in an endemic region where routine pre- and post-transplant recipient screening and prophylaxis is employed. In a separate report by this same group, 55 cases of coccidioidomycoses were described in patients with underlying hematologic malignancies. Pulmonary involvement was most common (95%) and 22% of the infections were disseminated [83]. Infections with blastomycoses are even more rare in HCT recipients [76, 84]. In sum, endemic mycoses must be considered in recipients, but they do not represent an overwhelming problem in the HCT population.

Risk Factors for IFIs

Multiple factors unique to HCT modify the IFI risk and typically depend upon the host, transplant, as well as post-transplant complications [40]. The impact of these variables is often time dependent, thereby preferentially increasing risks in the early or late post-transplant period. Early risk of infection is often mediated by abnormal mucosal barriers and neutropenia, whereas late infections following engraftment involve complications such as graft-versus-host disease (GVHD), cytomegalovirus (CMV), and delayed immune reconstitution. Identified risk factors for IFIs are most often directly applicable to *Candida* and *Aspergillus* infections and then extrapolated to other fungal pathogens with less precision. In addition, while we typically associate antineoplastic and other immunosuppressive therapy as additive in the risk of IFIs, it is important to recall that some of these agents may have antifungal properties. As an example, 5-flucytosine (5-FC), the precursor of 5-fluorouracil (5-FU), is used clinically for its synergistic effects with amphotericin B against *Cryptococcus* and less commonly against *Candida* species. Prior studies have also shown synergistic effects of agents such as 5-FU, methotrexate, mitomycin C, and doxorubicin when combined with polyenes against *Candida* species [85]. The antifungal properties of the calcineurin inhibitors (CNIs, e.g., tacrolimus and cyclosporine) and mammalian targets of rapamycin (mTOR) inhibitors (e.g., sirolimus) will be discussed further in the section on risks for IFIs in SOT.

Multiple host-related factors increasing IFI risk include (1) the recipient age, (2) underlying disease, (3) polymorphisms in host genes, (4) "biological factors," and (5) history of prior IFI(s). Older age at transplant is a well-established risk factor impacting both the early and late transplant periods [34, 35, 59, 86, 87]. Autologous HCT recipients have less IFIs overall than allogeneic recipients. With respect to underlying disease, chronic myelogenous leukemia in chronic phase has been associated with fewer IFIs post-transplant [35, 59, 87]. Increased risks for IFIs including IA, mucormycosis, and fusariosis have been reported in patients with underlying multiple myeloma, aplastic anemia, AML, or myelodysplastic syndrome (MDS) [35, 59, 88]. Specific genetic polymorphisms in constituents of the immune system such as toll-like receptors (TLRs) 1–6, interleukin-10 promoter, tumor necrosis factor-alpha receptor, and plasminogen may play a role in susceptibility to IFIs [89–99]. Clearly the future will be to validate and quantitate these risks within the individual patient. "Biologic" host factors associated with increased IFI risk include iron overload and diabetes [100, 101]. Finally, patients undergoing evaluation for HCT are often heavily pre-treated with chemotherapy and other immunosuppressive modalities resulting in the development of IFIs prior to HCT. A previous IFI has already marked the patient for the potential of either reactivation or susceptibility to new IFIs. In a retrospective analysis of 48 HCT recipients with IA prior to transplant, Offner et al. [102] found evidence of relapse in 33% of patients with an associated 88% mortality. Given this and other reports of high rates of relapse or progression and potential increased mortality, in the past some centers considered pre-transplant IFIs a contraindication to HCT [102–104]. However, other centers have demonstrated that successful transplantation is feasible in patients with prior and even active IFIs and thus management of pre-transplant IFIs continues to evolve [105–114]. Remaining IFI risk factors associated with the transplant and post-transplant complications are summarized in Table 31.4 [115–127].

Table 31.4 Risk factors for invasive fungal infections in hematopoietic stem cell transplantation[a] [5, 7, 34, 35, 87, 88, 115–127]

Risk factor	Details	References
Transplant related		
Donor HLA similarity	Autologous < Allogeneic (MRD < MMRD/URD)	[5, 88, 115]
Stem cell source	Peripheral blood < bone marrow < cord blood; increased risk with T cell-depleted/CD34 selected cells	[35, 116–120]
Conditioning regimen	NMA < MA in early infections, NMA ≥ MA in late infections	[121–124]
Post-transplant related		
Neutropenia	Especially during early risk period	[7, 34, 35]
Viral illness	CMV (most commonly associated), RSV, parainfluenza, +/− influenza	[34, 35]
GVHD	Both acute (particularly grade III–IV) and chronic GVHD and associated treatment (e.g., corticosteroids, TNF-alpha blockers)	[87, 88, 125–127]

CMV cytomegalovirus, *GVHD* graft-versus-host disease, *HLA* human-leukocyte antigen, *MA* myeloablative, *MRD* matched-related donor, *MMRD* mismatched-related donor, *NMA* non-myeloablative, *RSV* respiratory syncytial virus, *TNF* tumor necrosis factor, *URD* unrelated donor

[a]List of risk factors not fully inclusive

Timeline and Outcomes for IFIs

For simplification, the timeline for infections post-HCT can be broken into three periods corresponding with an early (0–30 days), late (31–180 days), and very late (greater than 180 days) onset of infection (see Fig. 31.1) [4, 5, 128]. *Candida* infections tend to occur earliest, when neutropenia and mucositis predominate, but of course these IFIs can be seen throughout the transplant course with widespread use of antibiotics and foreign bodies such as catheters. Invasive candidiasis typically occurs earlier in autologous as compared to allogeneic HCT recipients as illustrated by PATH Alliance generated data with a median onset of IC at day 28 versus day 108, respectively [19]. Furthermore, in allogeneic HCT recipients, a myeloablative conditioning regimen tends to be associated with an earlier onset of IC (median 65 days) compared to a non-myeloablative regimen (median 590 days) with no differences seen among the donor types (e.g., MRD, URD, MMRD) [19].

Aspergillus infections are bimodal occurring in both the early and more commonly in the late post-transplant period with important implications for certain fungal diagnostics whose sensitivity vary pre- and post-engraftment. For example, invasion and thrombosis of the vasculature seen with angioinvasive fungi such as *Aspergillus* often result in a classic "halo" of surrounding ground-glass attenuation secondary to hemorrhage on computed tomographic imaging of the chest and are more commonly found in the neutropenic host [129]. In addition, screening diagnostics such as *Aspergillus* galactomannan, an enzyme-linked immunosorbent assay that detects galactomannan, a component of the fungal cell wall released during hyphal growth, has been found to be a more sensitive screening tool in the neutropenic versus non-neutropenic HCT recipient [130]. In general, IA occurs later than IC with a median onset of 99 days post-transplant in the TRANSNET cohort [5]. Similar to IC, an earlier onset was found in autologous versus allogeneic HCT recipients. Within the first month, 50% of the total IA cases in autologous HCT recipients had occurred compared to only 22% in allogeneic HCT recipients. Furthermore, the conditioning regimen and donor type have not consistently been shown to impact the timing of IA in the allogeneic HCT recipient [19].

Non-*Aspergillus* molds, including mucormycosis, *Fusarium*, and *Scedosporium*, also tend to occur later in the transplant period as compared to IC, although timing is variable dependent upon the pathogen and clinical scenario. For HCT recipients in the TRANSNET cohort, 67 (54.4%) of

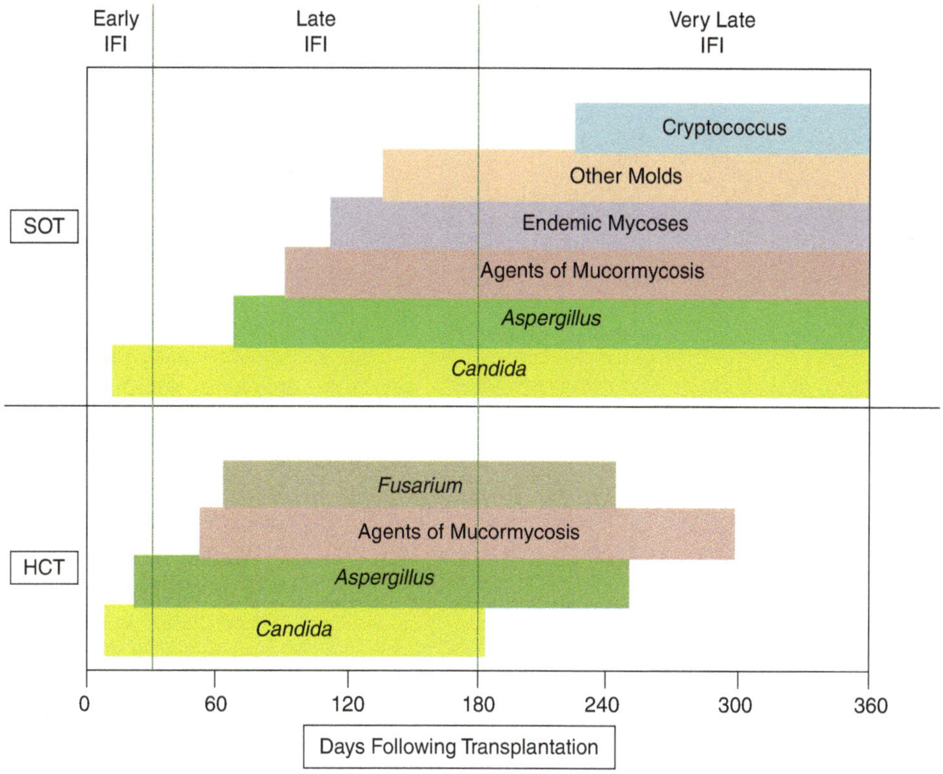

Fig. 31.1 Timeline of infections following hematopoietic and solid organ transplantation [4, 5, 128]. Based on Transplant-Associated Infection Surveillance Network (TRANSNET)-derived data for invasive fungal infections (IFIs) in solid organ transplantation (SOT) from Pappas et al. [4]) and hematopoietic stem cell transplantation (Kontoyiannis et al. [5]). (Adapted with permission from: Low and Rotstein [128]

invasive non-*Aspergillus* mold infections occurred within 6 months of transplant, though onset was quite delayed in some cases, with an appreciable number (13.8%) of infections with mucormycosis, *Fusarium*, and *Scedosporium* developing 2 or more years post-transplant [33]. In a smaller retrospective evaluation of *Fusarium* infections in HCT recipients involving nine transplant centers, Nucci et al. [70] described a trimodal timeline in allogeneic recipients wherein peak infections occurred a median of 16 days (pre-engraftment) and 62 days post-transplant with another peak after day 360. *Scedosporium* infections have been described earlier in the post-transplant course as well. For instance, in the study by Marr et al. [59] characterizing invasive mold infections in HCT recipients, the majority of *Scedosporium* infections occurred on or before post-transplant day 40 and Husain et al. [71] reported a median onset of 1.3 months after transplant with 75% of infections occurring within 6 months.

Outcomes in HCT continue to improve with the advances in transplantation and management of IFIs but remain sub-optimal (see Table 31.3). In general, IC has been associated with the best survival outcomes followed by IA and the non-*Aspergillus* molds, but it is often difficult to differentiate the impact of the IFI versus the underlying disease on outcomes. However, clearly the IFIs contribute to morbidity and mortality. Pagano et al. [41] evaluated proven/probable IFIs in 3228 patients undergoing HCT from 1999 to 2003 and found an attributable mortality of 50% (IC), 72.1% (IA), and 65.3% (overall). Of note, among the cases of IC, non-*albicans* *Candida* infections were associated with the worst outcomes. Attributable mortality for IA was significantly higher in allogeneic (77.2%) compared with autologous HCT recipients (14.3%) whereas IC outcomes were similar among the two groups. Low survival associated with infections due to non-*Aspergillus* molds alongside possible increased frequency imparts significant concern for future trends. Neofytos et al. [19] evaluated 250 IFIs in adult HCT recipients and found the highest 12-week mortality rates with mucormycosis and other molds (inclusive of *Fusarium* species) at 64.3% and 80%, respectively. Husain et al. [71] similarly reported high overall mortality rates with *Scedosporium* infections, particularly *S. prolificans* (77.8%). In contrast to other studies, Neofytos et al. [19] found overall higher mortality rates with IC compared to IA, similar to findings in a more contemporary retrospective single-center review of IFIs by Corzo-León et al. [131], possibly related to the inherent difficulties in delineating true attributable mortality with specific pathogens in this complex patient population.

Epidemiology in SOT

Incidence and Types of IFIs

The spectrum of IFIs in SOT depends upon a multitude of variables including the transplanted organ(s). The section that follows will discuss selective epidemiologic characteris-

Table 31.5 Primary fungal pathogens in solid organ transplantation (SOT) [4, 33]

SOT group	12-month CI (%)[a,b]	Primary fungal pathogens (total % of IFIs)[b]
Lung	8.6[c]	*Candida* (23) *Aspergillus* (44) Cryptococcus (2) Endemic mycoses (1) Agents of mucormycosis (3) Other molds (20)
Liver	4.7	*Candida* (68) *Aspergillus* (11) Cryptococcus (6) Endemic mycoses (5) Agents of mucormycosis (2) Other molds (2)
Heart	3.4	*Candida* (49) *Aspergillus* (23) Cryptococcus (10) Endemic mycoses (3) Agents of mucormycosis (3) Other molds (7)
Kidney	1.3	*Candida* (49) *Aspergillus* (14) Cryptococcus (15) Endemic mycoses (10) Agents of mucormycosis (2) Other molds (3)
Pancreas	4.0[d]	*Candida* (76) *Aspergillus* (5) Cryptococcus (5) Endemic mycoses (6) Agents of mucormycosis (0) Other molds (3)
Small bowel	11.6	*Candida* (85) *Aspergillus* (0) Cryptococcus (5) Endemic mycoses (0) Agents of mucormycosis (0) Other molds (0)

[a]12-month cumulative incidence (CI) for first invasive fungal infection (IFI)

[b]Based on Transplant-Associated Infection Surveillance Network (TRANSNET)-derived data [4, 33]

[c]12-month CI reflects lung and heart-lung transplant recipients

[d]12-month CI reflects pancreas and kidney-pancreas transplant recipients

tics of the individual SOT groups, namely lung, liver, heart, renal, pancreas, and small bowel/multivisceral transplant. TRANSNET-generated data provide a broad overview of IFIs in this population [4] (see Table 31.5). A 12-month CI for the first IFI in the cohort of 16,459 SOT recipients was 3.1% overall and among SOT groups was highest in small bowel (11.6%) and lowest in kidney (1.3%) transplant recipients. Overall trends suggested an increase in IFIs in the SOT population driven primarily by the occurrence of IC.

With the exception of the lung transplant population, *Candida* remains the most common fungal pathogen in SOT recipients. In contrast to HCT in which non-*albicans Candida* predominated, *C. albicans* remained the most common yeast, accounting for 46% of the cases of IC in TRANSNET. However, increasing infections with non-*albicans Candida* species have been reported. The types of IC vary across SOT groups. In orthotopic liver transplantation (OLT), *Candida* often presents as intra-abdominal infections inclusive of peritonitis, recurrent cholangitis, and intra-abdominal abscesses with or without associated candidemia. Surgical site infections are also common [8, 132–134]. The spectrum of infections in lung transplantation includes isolated mucocutaneous involvement, candidemia, bronchial and aortic anastomotic infections, mediastinitis, empyema, and dissemination [135–138]. Schaenman et al. [139] reviewed 921 orthotopic heart transplant (OHT) recipients from a single center from 1980 to 2004 and found a decreasing overall incidence of IC (from 6.1% to 2.1%) with bloodstream (41%), disseminated (21%), gastrointestinal (14%), and urinary tract infections (UTIs) (11%) occurring most commonly. Although a sizeable number of infections were attributed to non-*albicans Candida*, the proportion did not change significantly over time. In renal transplantation, candiduria occurs commonly. Safdar et al. [140] reviewed 1738 renal recipients from a single center and found an 11% incidence of candiduria with *C. glabrata* predominating (53%). *Candida* infections of the renal allograft can also manifest as *Candida* arteritis of the renal and/or iliac arteries [141]. In pancreas transplant recipients, the site of IC varies based on multiple factors inclusive of transplant type and exocrine drainage site; however, intra-abdominal, surgical site, and UTIs predominate with or without accompanying bloodstream infections [142–146]. Finally, among all SOT groups, IC occurs most often in small bowel (SBT) and multivisceral transplant (MVT) owing to the heightened immunosuppression and altered gastrointestinal tract mucosa. One of the largest series in SBT and liver-SBT found that *Candida* bloodstream infections occurred most commonly followed by intra-abdominal infections [147].

Aspergillus is the second most common fungal pathogen overall and the lung transplant recipient remains most susceptible to this airborne pathogen. In lung transplantation, early infections can manifest as tracheobronchitis and often involve the bronchial anastomotic sites with the potential for devastating complications including bronchopleural fistulas. Later in the post-transplant period invasive pulmonary and disseminated *Aspergillus* infections predominate [138, 148–150]. IA in OLT consists primarily of pulmonary, cutaneous, and CNS disease with historically higher rates of dissemination, occurring in upwards of 50–60% of OLT recipients [55]. Singh et al. [151] compared OLT cohorts from 1990–1995 to 1998–2001 and despite improvements in transplantation techniques over time, the overall incidence of IA remained unchanged; however, significant reductions in CNS and disseminated IA were noted. IA occurs in up to 14% of heart transplant patients and pulmonary infections predominate although extrapulmonary infection inclusive of mediastinitis and endocarditis as well as dissemination can occur [55, 152–157]. A descriptive analysis of IA in OHT at a single center over a 24-year period showed a decrease in overall incidence across time from 8.7% (1988–1999) to 3.5% (2000–2011) wherein pulmonary infections again predominated but later onset of infection (>3 months) in both cohorts was associated with a higher number of disseminated and/or atypical sites of infection [158].

Cryptococcal infections are more common in SOT as compared to HCT, but they remain overall infrequent constituting approximately 8% of IFIs in the TRANSNET dataset [4]. In SOT recipients, cryptococcal disease can manifest at multiple sites including pulmonary, skin, or soft tissue infections; however, over 50% of SOT recipients will have CNS involvement or disseminated disease, and cryptococcemia has been seen in roughly one-third of patients [28, 159]. Interestingly, lung transplant recipients may have an overall decreased burden of disease. They have been found to have lower rates of positive serum cryptococcal antigen testing in isolated pulmonary infections and have the lowest rates of dissemination of the SOT groups [159, 160]. It is possible that this is related to the removal of latent cryptococcal infections in the native lungs or earlier detection secondary to frequent pulmonary radiographic imaging and sampling, but this remains unanswered. Conversely, liver transplant recipients often have severe disease with dissemination and septic shock [160–162].

The non-*Aspergillus* molds, namely, mucormycosis, *Fusarium*, and *Scedosporium*, are increasingly recognized, together accounting for approximately 4% of IFIs in the TRANSNET surveillance cohort [33]. Mucormycosis is the most common of these pathogens and presentations in SOT range from isolated cutaneous infections due to direct trauma to invasive pulmonary and rhino-orbital-cerebral disease. Endobronchial anastomotic infections with potential for dissemination occur more commonly in the lung transplant recipient [163, 164]. Direct involvement of a non-pulmonary transplanted organ, such as a renal allograft, can occur with devastating consequences [165–167]. *Fusarium* infections in SOT range from isolated cutaneous and ocular involvement to severe pulmonary and disseminated infections with fungemia occurring in over 40% of reported cases [168]. Hussain et al. [71] evaluated 57 cases of *Scedosporium* infections in SOT and found pulmonary and disseminated infections occurring frequently. Moreover, SOT recipients with *S. prolificans* were more likely to have associated fungemia than those infected with the more commonly isolated *S. apiospermum* complex (40% vs. 4.7%, respectively).

Histoplasmosis is the most common endemic mycosis occurring in SOT, accounting for 75% of infections of this type in the TRANSNET-generated data, but overall IFIs with the endemic fungi are rare. Among SOT groups, renal transplant recipients are affected most often, with endemic fungal infections constituting 10% of IFIs in this SOT group [4, 23]. Disseminated disease in SOT is often seen with all of the endemic fungi. Cuellar-Rodriguez et al. [24] reviewed 3436 patients undergoing SOT in an endemic region for histoplasmosis and identified 14 patients with proven active infection and all had disseminated infection with pulmonary involvement. Gauthier et al. [169] reported 11 cases of blastomycosis in SOT recipients from a single center. Pulmonary infections occurred most commonly (82% of cases), and infections were often severe, with respiratory distress syndrome in 67% and dissemination in over one-third of patients. Blair et al. [170] reviewed the literature for cases of coccidioidomycosis in SOT and found incidence rates ranging from 3.8% to 8.7% in renal and heart transplant recipients from endemic regions. Pulmonary infection predominated and dissemination was seen in upwards of 75% in one case series, often to multiple sites, including the transplanted allograft, skin, meninges, genitourinary tract, and spleen.

Donor-derived fungal infections in SOT are rare but important considerations when caring for a transplant recipient. A donor source should at least be considered in early infections, particularly those involving the transplanted allograft. Multiple fungal pathogens have been associated with donor-derived infection and guidelines have been published by the American Society of Transplantation (AST) to guide both recognition and management [171]. Issues of transplant tourism may further impact the incidence of donor-derived IFIs [172, 173]. Donor-derived *Candida* infections are often a result of contaminated preservation fluid and are seen most commonly in the renal transplant population. Digestive tract disruption at the time of procurement is often identified. Resultant complications in the renal transplant recipient include *Candida* arteritis of the graft vasculature as previously mentioned [141]. Unrecognized candidemia in the donor may have significant impact on the graft including mycotic aneurysms with potential for rupture. In lung transplant recipients, heavy donor airway colonization with *Candida* has been associated with complicated early infections such as mediastinitis, empyema, and *Candida* arteritis involving the aortic anastomosis [174, 175]. Cases with *Aspergillus* have involved contamination of preservation fluid and unrecognized infection in the donor with complications including multiple renal abscesses and *Aspergillus* arteritis in the renal allograft as well as *Aspergillus* endocarditis with ultimate dissemination in a heart transplant recipient [171, 176, 177]. Rare reports of donor-derived infections in near-drowning accidents have also been reported with *S. apiospermum* complex and *Apophysomyces elegans* [178, 179]. Case reports of cryptococcal infection include transmission in a donor with unrecognized cryptococcal meningitis with resultant cryptococcemia and pneumonia and/or meningitis in the SOT recipients [180]. In addition, Sun et al. [181] described five cases of early-onset (defined as less than 30 days post-transplant) donor-derived cryptococcal infections involving the allograft or surgical site. Finally, as previously mentioned, the endemic mycoses, namely histoplasmosis and coccidioidomycosis, have been transmitted from donors either from or with extensive travel to endemic areas inclusive of a rare case of *Coccidioides immitis* endocarditis [182].

Risk Factors for IFIs

Many IFI risks are relevant across transplant groups; however, some remain specific to the organ transplanted. In all SOT groups, the importance of rejection and resultant augmentation of immunosuppression and specific agents utilized therein cannot be underemphasized, increasing the risk across the spectrum of pathogens. However, as in HCT, it is important to keep in mind that some immunosuppressive agents used in SOT, such as CNIs and mTOR inhibitors, may impart a protective effect against IFIs. Calcineurin is a calcium- and calmodulin-dependent phosphatase involved in T-cell signaling and is the primary target of the CNIs (tacrolimus and cyclosporine). Based on their effects on the highly conserved mammalian and fungal calcineurin, these agents paradoxically possess both immunosuppressive and antifungal properties with the potential to both increase susceptibility to IFIs and reduce the severity and extent of fungal infections in the transplant recipient. The CNIs have been shown to impair fungal cell stress response, growth, and virulence and have demonstrated *in vitro* and *in vivo* synergistic activity with other antifungal agents against *Candida* and *Aspergillus* species [85]. In addition, the CNIs have been shown to impair the growth of *C. neoformans* at higher temperatures (e.g., body temperature) as well as inhibit hyphal elongation necessary for mating with resultant decreased infectivity. Moreover, tacrolimus has exhibited synergistic activity against *Cryptococcus* in combination with azoles and echinocandins [85, 183]. Clinically, the protective effects of CNIs were demonstrated by Singh et al. [160] in a multicenter, prospective study of *Cryptococcus* infections in SOT. In the 111 identified SOT recipients with cryptococcal infections, receipt of a CNI was independently associated with a lower mortality. Infections in those receiving a CNI also less frequently involved the CNS and were more often isolated to the lungs. These effects were more pronounced in the group receiving tacrolimus, perhaps at least partially explained by better penetration of the tacrolimus into the CNS as compared to cyclosporine. Rapamycin targets the kinase mTOR with a single homolog in humans, *Candida*, and *Cryptococcus* species. *In vitro* studies show fungicidal activity against both *C. albicans* and *C. neoformans* [184]; however, activity against *Aspergillus* is less clear with conflicting *in vitro* susceptibility results. Positive interactions were seen *in vitro* with disc-diffusion testing when used in combination with caspofungin against isolates of *A. fumigatus*, *A. flavus*, and *A. terreus* [185]. In addition, reports from *in vitro* testing against agents of mucormycosis (including both *Mucor* and *Rhizopus* species) with CNI and mTOR inhibitors in combination with antifungal agents suggest variable synergy against this fungal pathogen [186, 187]. These data support future studies examining potential therapeutic combinations for both prevention and treatment of IFIs in the transplant recipient.

In OLT, risks for IFIs in the pre-transplant period include prolonged intensive care unit stays, receipt of broad-spectrum antimicrobial therapy including spontaneous bacterial peritonitis antimicrobial prophylaxis, indwelling catheters, fungal colonization, and fulminant hepatic failure. Perioperative risks include prolonged operation times, significant intraoperative transfusion requirements, and choledochojejunostomy biliary anastomoses. Key post-transplant risks include renal failure (particularly the requirement of renal replacement therapy), early graft failure, retransplantation, and surgical re-exploration [8, 132, 151, 188–194]. As surgical techniques and procedures continue to advance, the perioperative risks have decreased in importance; however, post-transplant complications, particularly the need for retransplantation and renal failure requiring hemodialysis, remain prominent IFI risks [8, 195].

In lung transplantation, receipt of a single-lung transplant carries the unique risk of the remaining native lung serving as a nidus for fungal pathogens [150, 174, 196, 197]. However, double-lung transplant results in greater impairment in respiratory protective mechanisms and increased at-risk anastomotic area [138, 150]. The significance of airway colonization both pre- and post-transplant remains unclear as invasive disease can evolve with or without preceding colonization [198]. However, patients with cystic fibrosis developing IA post-transplant have been shown to be significantly more likely to have been colonized pre-transplant [199]. Furthermore, Cahill et al. [200] found that recipients with *Aspergillus* isolated from the airways in the 6-month period post-transplant were 11 times more likely to develop IA. Additional risk factors in lung transplantation for IFIs include advanced age, hypogammaglobulinemia, anastomotic airway stenosis and ischemia, and receipt of extracorporeal membrane oxygenation post-operatively [55, 150, 198–207].

Detailed evaluation of risk factors unique to heart transplant recipients is less robust than the previously discussed transplant populations. Munoz et al. [157] looked at risks for IA in 287 patients undergoing OHT between 1988 and 2002 confirming previously recognized factors such as re-operation and renal dysfunction and also demonstrating elevated risk with identification of an episode of IA in the heart transplant program within 2 months of the transplant. The latter finding signaled the importance of center-specific environmental exposures, another shared risk in SOT groups [208]. A single-center cohort study of IFIs in heart transplant recipients from 1995 to 2012 identified further risks including delayed chest closure and the addition of OKT3, anti-thymocyte globulin, or daclizumab to standard corticosteroid induction [209]. Risks specific to the renal transplant recipient include prolonged pre-transplant hemodialysis, underlying diabetes, advanced donor age, delayed graft function, CMV infection, previous antibiotic exposure, and disruption of the intestinal and bladder mucosa [210–212]. In pancreas transplantation, enteric anastomotic drainage is particularly important in the context of intra-abdominal infections [142]. Finally, in SBT/MVT, the receipt of total parenteral nutrition and long-term antibiotic therapy both play a significant role [213]. These risk factors and epidemiologic characteristics are critical for each transplant program to review for both their diagnostic awareness and potential need for prophylactic or pre-emptive interventions.

Geographical differences in risk of IFIs are perhaps most notable among the endemic mycoses including blastomycosis, coccidioidomycosis, and histoplasmosis as infections typically occur in those residing in, or with extensive travel to, an endemic area. Knowledge of the geographic exposure in both patients and their donors is important in SOT given the potential for reactivation and donor-derived infections with these pathogens. *Blastomyces* species are found primarily in North America in midwestern, southern, and southeastern states, especially those bordering the Ohio and Mississippi river valleys, and in provinces bordering the Great Lakes and Saint Lawrence Riverway in Canada [214]. *Coccidioides* species are found in arid desert regions in the Western Hemisphere including California's south-central valley, southern Arizona and New Mexico, West Texas, and parts of Mexico and Central and South America [215]. *Histoplasma capsulatum* is endemic in North America, most notably the Ohio and the Mississippi River valleys within the United States, as well as Central and South America and areas in Africa and Europe [216].

Timeline and Outcomes of IFIs

As discussed in HCT, general periods of infection corresponding with early, late, and very late fungal infections ascribed to differing fungal pathogens are proposed in SOT (see Fig. 31.1). However, more recent epidemiologic data in SOT suggests a need to modify this timeline as the majority of IFIs tend to occur greater than 90 days post-transplant. Reasons for this shift to later in the post-transplant course are multifactorial and include utilization of antifungal prophylaxis, a topic discussed later in this chapter. The predominant IFIs early in the transplant course are IC and IA. Overall *Candida* infections occur earliest with a median onset of 130 days as compared to 184 days with IA based on the TRANSNET cohort [4]. Neofytos et al. found the median onset of IC post-transplant was earliest in lung (day 52) and heart transplant (day 67) and much later in renal transplant recipients (day 896) [20]. In contrast, IA occurred earliest in OLT with approximately 75% of OLT recipients developing infection within 6 months post-transplant. In lung transplant recipients, most cases of IA presented greater than 1 year post-transplant although infections at the tracheobronchial anastomoses are typically reported in the early transplant period.

Non-*Aspergillus* molds occurred later post-transplant with a collective median onset post-transplant of 467 days based on TRANSNET data. Combining IFIs with mucormycosis, *Scedosporium,* and *Fusarium*, only 37.8% occurred within 6 months of transplant with an additional approximate one-third occurring at 2 years and beyond. Similar to IA, OLT recipients had an earlier onset with these infections, with a median time to onset of 81 days as compared to 533 days for the non-liver SOT groups [33]. As in HCT, infections with *Scedosporium* may occur earlier than other non-*Aspergillus* molds. Husain et al. [71] reported a median post-transplant onset of 4 months in 57 SOT recipients with *Scedosporium* infections with over 60% occurring within 6 months. In general, IFIs associated with the endemic fungi and *Cryptococcus* tend to occur much later in the transplant course; the median onset of *Cryptococcus* is well beyond the first post-transplant year [4].

Survival outcomes with IFIs in SOT vary based on the pathogen, the host, and the site of infection. TRANSNET-generated data showed that 12-month survival rates, inclusive of all SOT recipients with IFIs, were lowest with IA (59%) followed by non-*Aspergillus* molds (61%), IC (66%), and cryptococcosis (73%) [4]. Among the SOT groups, Neofytos et al. [20] found the poorest overall survival outcomes in OLT recipients. Similar to IFI risks, the preponderance of outcomes-related data is with *Candida* and *Aspergillus* infections. When comparing outcomes specifically with IC among the groups, PATH Alliance data showed the highest 12-week survival rates in the lung transplant population; in contrast, OHT recipients fared the worst although not reaching statistical significance [20]. The increasingly common non-*albicans Candida* has been associated with decreased survival in OLT [8, 217]. In a multicenter, case-controlled study in 103 OLT recipients consisting of 34 cases with IC and 69 non-infected controls, Husain et al. [8] reported that infections with non-*albicans Candida* ($n = 12$) including *C. glabrata* (7), *C. tropicalis* (3), *C. parapsilosis* (1), and *C. guilliermondii* (1) were associated with higher mortality rates (58.3%) than those with *C. albicans* (22.7%). Similarly, in a more recent retrospective single-center evaluation of IFIs in OLT recipients, Raghuram et al. [217] reported 1-year survival rates of 27.8% and 50% in OLT recipients with *C. parapsilosis* ($n = 16$) and other non-*albicans Candida* [$n = 16$, *C. dubliniensis* (3), *C. glabrata* (10), *C. krusei* (2), and *C. tropicalis* (1)] infections, respectively, in contrast to 75% with *C. albicans* infections (n = 15). The lower survival reported with *C. parapsilosis* in this study is surprising as *C. parapsilosis* has been shown to be less virulent in comparison to other *Candida* species in animal models and correspondingly has been associated with less severe outcomes in the clinical setting [7, 218]. However, all six isolates of *C. parapsilosis* in this study were fluconazole resistant, and the collective data beget the question of whether higher mortality associated with infections with non-*albicans Candida* reflects increasingly resistant and virulent organisms or is simply a surrogate marker for a more debilitated and complex transplant patient. Worse outcomes with IA are particularly seen in OLT recipients undergoing late retransplantation e.g., more than 30 days from the initial transplant, with a reported mortality of 100% [219]. In lung transplant, *Aspergillus* infections have been associated with mortality rates from 23% with isolated tracheobronchitis up to 82% in invasive pulmonary infections, and single-lung transplant recipients often have inferior survival outcomes [55]. Potential reasons for worse outcomes in the single-lung transplant recipient include older age at transplant as well as increased proportions of infections with invasive pulmonary aspergillosis as compared to tracheobronchitis with the native lung often serving as the source [55, 150]. *Scedosporium* and *Fusarium* infections have been associated with overall mortality rates of 54% and 33%, respectively, the latter much lower than reported rates in HCT [71, 220].

The impact of IFIs on overall graft function and survival is also a crucial consideration in SOT. In the lung transplant recipient, fungal pneumonias and even fungal colonization have been associated with the development of bronchiolitis obliterans syndrome and chronic allograft dysfunction [221, 222]. Albano et al. [141] conducted a multicenter, retrospective evaluation of graft site *Candida* infections in renal transplant recipients wherein 14 of the 18 infections were identified as *Candida* arteritis of either renal and/or iliac arteries. Local aneurysm developed in all but one patient, with three deaths due to rupture, and 82% of the remaining patients required nephrectomy. Based on their findings, the authors argue for empiric nephrectomy in this setting; however, varying reports with improved outcomes including retained graft function make management unclear [223]. Intra-abdominal fungal infections in pancreas transplant recipients were also associated with significantly lower 1-year graft survival rates compared to those without infection (17% vs. 65%, respectively) [142].

Antifungal Prophylaxis

Addressing fungal infections early, at the time of lowest fungal burden, is essential to the management of these infections and this is especially true with immunocompromised hosts. Given the present difficulties in early diagnosis of IFIs, prophylaxis has been a frequently utilized strategy in the transplant population. Antifungal prophylaxis in the HCT and SOT recipient is predicated on multiple variables including transplant and disease-related risk factors, prior history of fungal infections, screening strategies employed for early IFI diagnosis, and the local environment and epidemiology. In the future, additional risks that may be incorporated into the decision for antifungal prophylaxis include previously mentioned genetic polymorphisms in the transplant donor and recipient. For example, TLRs are proteins that reside on immune cells' surfaces and are important in fungal recognition and immune activation in response to infection. Bochud et al. [90] evaluated specific single-nucleotide polymorphisms in four TLR genes in HCT donors and recipients to assess whether they were associated with increased IA risk. In their initial discovery and subsequent validation cohorts they identified that the TLR4 haplotype S4 in the donor was associated with increased risk of IA in unrelated donor-recipient pairs. While research in this area remains ongoing, identification of genetic polymorphisms modifying risks for IFIs may significantly impact our future designation of the high-risk recipient meriting prophylaxis. Table 31.6 provides a summary of some of the genes wherein specific polymorphisms

Table 31.6 Genetic determinants of fungal risk[a] [97–99, 224, 225]

Gene	*Candida*	*Aspergillus*
CXCL10		Invasive aspergillosis
Dectin-1	Candida colonization	Invasive aspergillosis
DEFB1	Candida colonization	
IL-4	Chronic disseminated candidiasis Recurrent vulvo-vaginal candidiasis	ABPA (IL-4Rα)
IL-10	Candidemia/invasive candidiasis	Invasive aspergillosis
IL-12B	Candidemia/invasive candidiasis	
MBL2	Recurrent vulvo-vaginal candidiasis	Invasive aspergillosis Chronic pulmonary aspergillosis, ABPA
PLG		Invasive aspergillosis
PTPN22	Chronic mucocutaneous candidiasis	
TLR1/ TLR4	Candidemia/invasive candidiasis	Invasive aspergillosis
TLR2	Candidemia/invasive candidiasis	
TLR3	Chronic mucocutaneous candidiasis	Invasive aspergillosis
TLR6		Invasive aspergillosis

ABPA allergic bronchopulmonary aspergillosis, *CXCL10* C-X-C motif chemokine 10, *DEFB* beta defensin gene cluster, *IL* interleukin, *MBL* mannose-binding lectin, *PLG* plasminogen, *PTPN* protein tyrosine phosphatase nonreceptor, *TLR* toll-like receptor

[a]List is not fully inclusive

impact the risk associated with two common fungal pathogens, *Candida* and *Aspergillus* [97–99, 224, 225].

In general, prophylaxis consists of two types: primary prophylaxis occurs in patients at high risk but without prior history of an IFI, whereas secondary prophylaxis is given to patients with a prior IFI and impending heightened immunosuppression (e.g., transplantation) at increased risk for relapsed or new IFI. Strategies utilized by transplant centers include administration of prophylaxis to all patients (universal) versus those at increased risk (targeted). Limiting prophylaxis to a select high-risk population is important for a variety of reasons including reduced costs, drug interactions, drug toxicities, and the emergence of resistance. Data regarding prophylaxis in HCT and SOT continue to evolve and regimens are highly variable across centers but principles need to be explored and validated.

In HCT there are essentially two time points when prophylaxis is considered: early post-transplant when neutropenia predominates and following engraftment in high-risk patients with GVHD. Early prophylactic studies focused primarily on fluconazole. Goodman et al. [45] performed the first randomized controlled trial in HCT showing a reduction in superficial and systemic fungal infections with prophylactic fluconazole. Further evaluation by Slavin et al. [226] and Marr et al. [227] confirmed these findings along with both acute and long-term beneficial effects on survival, respectively. Epidemiologic changes in HCT, including the emergence of *Aspergillus* as the primary fungal pathogen and increasing non-*Aspergillus* molds and non-*albicans Candida* species, have expanded prophylactic considerations to echinocandins, polyenes, and the extended spectrum azoles (primarily posaconazole and voriconazole although data are likely to emerge with newly introduced agents such as isavuconazole) [228].

Robenshtok et al. [229] conducted the largest meta-analysis of antifungal prophylaxis in patients receiving chemotherapy or undergoing HCT. Sixty-four trials of prophylactic regimens inclusive of amphotericin B, fluconazole, itraconazole, posaconazole, voriconazole, and non-systemic antifungals were evaluated. Prophylactic therapy was associated with a reduction in all-cause and fungal-related mortality and total IFIs in allogeneic HCT patients but there was insufficient power to show significant benefit in the autologous HCT population. Ethier et al. [230] compared fluconazole with systemic mold-active prophylactic regimens (e.g., amphotericin B, caspofungin, micafungin, anidulafungin, posaconazole, itraconazole, voriconazole, and ketoconazole) in a meta-analysis which included 20 randomized controlled trials of antifungal prophylaxis in patients receiving chemotherapy or undergoing HCT. These authors found that mold-active regimens reduced proven or probable IFIs, IA, and IFI-related mortality when compared to fluconazole but did not significantly impact overall mortality and were associated with increased adverse effects. Data summarizing secondary prophylactic regimens are less common with no randomized controlled trials or meta-analyses to guide recommendations. However, a prospective, open-label, multicenter trial evaluated voriconazole for secondary prophylaxis in allogeneic HCT recipients with prior proven or probable IFI with a resultant 1-year cumulative incidence of IFI of 6.7 +/− 3.6% compared to prior clinical experience wherein relapsed infection occurred in 30–50% of patients suggesting overall benefit in this patient population [231, 232]. Certainly considerations for secondary prophylaxis are dependent on the previous offending pathogens, sites of infection, and available susceptibility data.

Guidelines available for antifungal prophylaxis in HCT include the Infectious Diseases Society of America (IDSA) [233], the European Conference on Infection in Leukemia [234], and the National Comprehensive Cancer Network [235]. For *Candida* infections, fluconazole remains a drug of choice before engraftment in allogeneic and high-risk autologous HCT recipients. Echinocandins are an alternative option and are often chosen due to their favorable side effect profile, lack of significant drug interactions, as well as their expanded antifungal coverage, particularly for patients known to be colonized or previously infected with non-*albicans Candida* species. In a randomized, double-blind, multicenter trial, micafungin was compared to fluconazole during the neutropenic phase following HCT and was superior to fluconazole in the primary endpoint of the absence of suspected, proven, and probable IFIs with overall fewer cases of IA in the micafungin arm [236]. In allogeneic HCT recipients at high risk for mold infections (e.g., those with GVHD), the guidelines support utilization of posaconazole. This recommendation is primarily based on the study by Ullmann et al. [237] comparing posaconazole to fluconazole which showed posaconazole was equivalent to fluconazole in IFI prevention and superior in prevention of proven and probable IA. Of note, the study did not show an overall survival advantage in the posaconazole arm. Posaconazole and isavuconazole have not yet been studied as primary prophylaxis in the early pre-engraftment period in the HCT population. However, posaconazole prophylaxis in patients with AML or MDS with prolonged neutropenia secondary to remission-induction chemotherapy was associated with a reduction in IFIs and improved survival [238]. Since these studies were published, posaconazole became available in an extended release tablet and intravenous formulation, thereby bypassing some of the previous concerns regarding overall posaconazole exposure with the suspension formulation. In addition, two studies evaluating voriconazole both pre-engraftment and during GVHD in allogeneic HCT recipients resulted in some advocating provisional use in this setting [239, 240].

In SOT, data for antifungal prophylaxis resides predominantly in liver and lung transplantation but continues to emerge in other populations. In OLT, the primary pathogens targeted are *Candida* and *Aspergillus* and a variety of prophylactic agents have been utilized. Amphotericin B is among the first drugs studied for prophylaxis, and available data suggest that low-dose amphotericin B [e.g., 0.1 to 0.5 mg/kg/day amphotericin B or 1 mg/kg/day liposomal amphotericin B (LAMB) preparations] may not be effective, perhaps due to lack of adequate *Aspergillus* coverage [241–243]. However, treatment doses of LAMB (e.g., 3–5 mg/kg) have been shown to be effective in high-risk OLT recipients including a study in those requiring renal replacement therapy [244]. The frequently cited prophylactic study with fluconazole by Winston et al. [245] was a prospective, randomized, double-blind controlled trial comparing 10 weeks of fluconazole 400 mg daily to placebo and showed reductions in fungal colonization (from 70% to 28%) as well as significant reductions in proven IFIs in the prophylaxis arm without perceptible increases in colonization with non-*albicans Candida* species. Although prophylaxis did not impact overall mortality, there were fewer deaths due to IFIs. Utilization of echinocandin prophylaxis is appealing due to the lack of significant drug interactions or hepatotoxicity and potential activity against both fluconazole-resistant *Candida* and *Aspergillus* [246–249]. Saliba et al. [249] performed an international, multicenter, randomized, open-label trial of antifungal prophylaxis in high-risk OLT recipients comparing micafungin to institutional standard of care (fluconazole, LAMB, or caspofungin) and demonstrated non-inferiority with respect to the primary composite efficacy endpoint defined as the absence of a proven or probable IFI and no initiation of antifungal treatment at the end of prophylaxis. Furthermore, the side effect profile was comparable to standard of care with less renal toxicity during the course of prophylaxis.

With the trend of increasing non-*albicans Candida* infections in the setting of fluconazole prophylaxis alongside isolated reports of increased mortality associated with these infections in OLT recipients, the importance of targeted prophylactic therapy must be underscored [8]. Available IDSA and AST guidelines support the use of targeted prophylaxis in this population for patients with defined risk factors for *Candida* and *Aspergillus* infections [195, 250, 251]. As previously discussed, risk factors for *Candida* infections include choledochojejunostomy anastomoses, complicated surgical procedures (e.g., high intraoperative transfusion requirements, prolonged intraoperative times), and demonstrated colonization with *Candida* spp. Risks for both *Candida* and *Aspergillus* infections include the need for retransplantation, renal failure (particularly the need for renal replacement therapy), and reoperation. The duration of therapy and the most appropriate agents in this setting (e.g., fluconazole and extended spectrum azoles, amphotericin B products, and echinocandins) continue to be defined [250–253].

Most lung transplant centers utilize some form of prophylaxis in the early post-transplant period given the overall high level of immunosuppression applied and exposure of the transplanted organ to the outside environment [254–256]. Risks such as ischemia at the anastomotic site and pre- and post-transplant fungal colonization are among other considerations. However, consensus regarding the most appropriate strategy (targeted vs. universal), specific agents, and duration has not been reached. In the past the most common agents utilized were polyenes and azoles, namely, itraconazole and voriconazole, with increasing utilization now at some centers of posaconazole and the echinocandins [256]. Amphotericin B prophylaxis in the lung transplant population primarily consists of inhaled formulations owing to the potential to protect the transplanted organ without systemic drug exposure, thereby avoiding nephrotoxicity [257–261]. However, the localized nature of this therapy limits prevention of systemic complications such as pleural space infections. Lipid preparations of amphotericin B for nebulization were introduced to reduce the side effects associated with nebulized amphotericin B deoxycholate (ABD), namely wheezing and bronchospasm, as well as to optimize pharmacokinetic parameters including intrapulmonary concentration and half-life [262]. After the safety of nebulized amphotericin B lipid complex (ABLC) was demonstrated [259], Drew et al. [260] conducted the only available prospective, randomized controlled trial with nebulized ABLC comparing it to ABD. This study showed similar efficacy between the groups and significantly less adverse effects with nebulized ABLC. Both itraconazole and voriconazole alone and in combination with nebulized amphotericin have shown efficacy as IFI prophylaxis [263, 264]; however, concerns of increased voriconazole-associated hepatotoxicity are reported and issues around drug interactions as well as associated skin malignancies (e.g., squamous cell carcinoma) with long-term use are concerning [264, 265]. Robust studies evaluating agents such as posaconazole and echinocandins as primary prophylaxis within the lung transplant population are lacking. On the basis of available data, IDSA guidelines recommend antifungal prophylaxis in this group [250].

A final comment on prophylaxis for the endemic mycoses is to some extent applicable in both the HCT and SOT groups. The primary endemic mycosis for which routine screening and/or prophylaxis is performed in endemic areas is coccidioidomycosis; however, individual transplant centers vary in their screening practice as well as application and duration of prophylaxis. With coccidioidomycosis, risks are greatest among recipients with a prior history of infection or positive serologies, and donor exposure is also critical in decisions for initiating prophylaxis. Blair et al. [82] evaluated the impact of fluconazole prophylaxis at a single transplant center in an endemic region and found that prophylaxis contributed to a decrease in incidence of coccidioidomycosis from historical rates of up to 9% down to 1% to 2% in the HCT and SOT transplant groups. The need for screening for histoplasmosis in recipients from endemic regions is less straightforward and is not routinely employed given the low rates of infection post-transplant and unclear benefit [266]. However, practice areas that remain controversial include appropriate prophylactic management in recipients with evidence of disease in the explanted organ and/or donor tissue and in recipients with recent active infection (e.g., within 2 years of transplantation). Cuellar-Rodriguez [24] reported their center's findings over a 10-year period during which they found 14 recipients with histopathologic evidence of histoplasmosis in either the explanted organ (ten cases) or donor tissue (four cases) and in whom long-term prophylaxis with either itraconazole (in lung transplant recipients) or fluconazole (in one liver transplant recipient) was administered. The authors found no evidence of active histoplasmosis in these patients after a mean of 13.5 months of follow-up and argue that long-term prophylaxis is necessary in this scenario. However, others cite experience in transplant patients with both serologic and radiographic evidence suggestive of prior histoplasmosis who did not develop infection despite lack of routine antifungal prophylaxis post-transplant suggesting therapy is not warranted [78]. In patients with recent active infection (e.g., within 2 years of transplant), present IDSA guidelines do not lend specific recommendations but suggest consideration of prophylaxis. In those with a history of completed treatment for histoplasmosis, recommendations are to check a urinary *Histoplasma* antigen prior to transplantation and to monitor frequently during the time of heightened immunosuppression with thorough investigation and potential therapy if increases in urinary antigen testing are appreciated [267]. The current recommendations regarding management for potential donor-derived infection with endemic mycoses including histoplasmosis and coccidioidomycosis in both living and deceased donors is beyond the scope of this chapter but is provided in the guidelines put forth by the AST on donor-derived fungal infections [171].

There are also important non-pharmacologic strategies utilized for preventing IFIs [233, 268]. Transplant recipients must incorporate healthy habits into their post-transplant routine and be counseled to identify and avoid high-risk activities and environments. The importance of maintaining good hand hygiene via frequent washing and/or alcohol-based rubs (for non-soiled hands) and the use of gloves and masks when in contact with substances such as soil and plants must be emphasized. Avoidance of smoking is also important, including tobacco and marijuana, particularly as the latter has been associated with pulmonary IFIs due to inhalation of fungal spores such as *Aspergillus*. Transplant recipients should attempt to avoid environments that may be associated with a high inoculum of fungal spores such construction sites, caves, horse barns, bird aviaries, and chicken coups. Limiting direct involvement in activities such as home remodeling, mulching, or spelunking is also important [268]. Certain beverages, spices, and foods associated with high quantities of fungal contamination should be avoided, particularly in neutropenic hosts. This list includes (but is not limited to) cold-brewed teas, pepper, unwashed raw fruits (particularly those with downy skins such as apricots and peaches), unroasted raw nuts, and many soft cheeses [233, 269]. The United States Department of Agriculture and the Food Safety and Inspection Service also have comprehensive food safety recommendations specifically for transplant recipients available online [270].

Conclusions

In summary, IFIs remain a vexing issue in HCT and SOT populations despite many advances in the field of transplantation. Multicenter collaboration with prospective monitoring and randomized controlled trials of diagnostics, prevention, and treatment are vital, particularly as we face new and increasingly resistant pathogens with less traditional presentations.

References

1. Kwon-Chung KJ, Bennett JE. The fungi. In: Medical mycology. Philadelphia: Lea & Febiger; 1992.
2. Huprikar S, Shoham S. Emerging fungal infections in solid organ transplantation. Am J Transplant. 2013;13(Suppl 4):262–71.
3. Walsh TJ, Groll AH. Emerging fungal pathogens: evolving challenges to immunocompromised patients for the twenty-first century. Transpl Infect Dis. 1999;1(4):247–61.
4. Pappas PG, Alexander BD, Andes DR, Hadley S, Kauffman CA, Freifeld A, et al. Invasive fungal infections among organ transplant recipients: results of the Transplant-Associated Infection Surveillance Network (TRANSNET). Clin Infect Dis. 2010;50(8):1101–11.
5. Kontoyiannis DP, Marr KA, Park BJ, Alexander BD, Anaissie EJ, Walsh TJ, et al. Prospective surveillance for invasive fungal infections in hematopoietic stem cell transplant recipients, 2001-2006: overview of the Transplant-Associated Infection Surveillance Network (TRANSNET) Database. Clin Infect Dis. 2010;50(8):1091–100.
6. Pappas PG, Kauffman CA, Andes DR, Clancy CJ, Marr KA, Ostrosky-Zeichner L, et al. Clinical practice guideline for the management of candidiasis: 2016 update by the Infectious Diseases Society of America. Clin Infect Dis. 2016;62(4):e1–50.
7. Pfaller M, Neofytos D, Diekema D, Azie N, Meier-Kriesche HU, Quan SP, et al. Epidemiology and outcomes of candidemia in 3648 patients: data from the prospective antifungal therapy (PATH Alliance®) registry, 2004-2008. Diagn Microbiol Infect Dis. 2012;74(4):323–31.
8. Husain S, Tollemar J, Dominguez EA, Baumgarten K, Humar A, Paterson DL, et al. Changes in the spectrum and risk factors for invasive candidiasis in liver transplant recipients: prospective, multicenter, case-controlled study. Transplantation. 2003;75(12): 2023–9.

9. Pfaller MA, Moet GJ, Messer SA, Jones RN, Castanheira M. Candida bloodstream infections: comparison of species distributions and antifungal resistance patterns in community-onset and nosocomial isolates in the SENTRY Antimicrobial Surveillance Program, 2008-2009. Antimicrob Agents Chemother. 2011;55(2):561–6.
10. Byrnes EJ 3rd, Bartlett KH, Perfect JR, Heitman J. Cryptococcus gattii: an emerging fungal pathogen infecting humans and animals. Microbes Infect. 2011;13(11):895–907.
11. Mitchell DH, Sorrell TC, Allworth AM, Heath CH, McGregor AR, Papanaoum K, et al. Cryptococcal disease of the CNS in immunocompetent hosts: influence of cryptococcal variety on clinical manifestations and outcome. Clin Infect Dis. 1995;20(3):611–6.
12. Perfect JR, Dismukes WE, Dromer F, Goldman DL, Graybill JR, Hamill RJ, et al. Clinical practice guidelines for the management of cryptococcal disease: 2010 update by the infectious diseases society of america. Clin Infect Dis. 2010;50(3):291–322.
13. Alexander BD, Schell WA. Hyalohyphomycosis. In: Kaufmann CA, Mandell GL, editors. Atlas of fungal infections. 2nd ed. Philadelphia: Springer Publishing; 2006.
14. Liu K, Howell DN, Perfect JR, Schell WA. Morphologic criteria for the preliminary identification of Fusarium, Paecilomyces, and Acremonium species by histopathology. Am J Clin Pathol. 1998;109(1):45–54.
15. Jacobson ES. Pathogenic roles for fungal melanins. Clin Microbiol Rev. 2000;13(4):708–17.
16. Revankar SG. Phaeohyphomycosis. In: Kaufmann CA, Mandell GL, editors. Atlas of fungal infections. 2nd ed. Philadelphia: Springer Publishing; 2006.
17. McCarty TP, Baddley JW, Walsh TJ, Alexander BD, Kontoyiannis DP, Perl TM, et al. Phaeohyphomycosis in transplant recipients: Results from the Transplant Associated Infection Surveillance Network (TRANSNET). Med Mycol. 2015;53(5):440–6.
18. Kwon-Chung KJ. Taxonomy of fungi causing mucormycosis and entomophthoramycosis (zygomycosis) and nomenclature of the disease: molecular mycologic perspectives. Clin Infect Dis. 2012;54(Suppl 1):S8–S15.
19. Neofytos D, Horn D, Anaissie E, Steinbach W, Olyaei A, Fishman J, et al. Epidemiology and outcome of invasive fungal infection in adult hematopoietic stem cell transplant recipients: analysis of Multicenter Prospective Antifungal Therapy (PATH) Alliance registry. Clin Infect Dis. 2009;48(3):265–73.
20. Neofytos D, Fishman JA, Horn D, Anaissie E, Chang CH, Olyaei A, et al. Epidemiology and outcome of invasive fungal infections in solid organ transplant recipients. Transpl Infect Dis. 2010;12(3):220–9.
21. Petrikkos G, Skiada A, Lortholary O, Roilides E, Walsh TJ, Kontoyiannis DP. Epidemiology and clinical manifestations of mucormycosis. Clin Infect Dis. 2012;54(Suppl 1):S23–34.
22. Roden MM, Zaoutis TE, Buchanan WL, Knudsen TA, Sarkisova TA, Schaufele RL, et al. Epidemiology and outcome of zygomycosis: a review of 929 reported cases. Clin Infect Dis. 2005;41(5):634–53.
23. Kauffman CA, Freifeld AG, Andes DR, Baddley JW, Herwaldt L, Walker RC, et al. Endemic fungal infections in solid organ and hematopoietic cell transplant recipients enrolled in the Transplant-Associated Infection Surveillance Network (TRANSNET). Transpl Infect Dis. 2014;16(2):213–24.
24. Cuellar-Rodriguez J, Avery RK, Lard M, Budev M, Gordon SM, Shrestha NK, et al. Histoplasmosis in solid organ transplant recipients: 10 years of experience at a large transplant center in an endemic area. Clin Infect Dis. 2009;49(5):710–6.
25. Tripathy U, Yung GL, Kriett JM, Thistlethwaite PA, Kapelanski DP, Jamieson SW. Donor transfer of pulmonary coccidioidomycosis in lung transplantation. Ann Thorac Surg. 2002;73(1):306–8.
26. Wright PW, Pappagianis D, Wilson M, Louro A, Moser SA, Komatsu K, et al. Donor-related coccidioidomycosis in organ transplant recipients. Clin Infect Dis. 2003;37(9):1265–9.
27. Sun HY, Singh N. Opportunistic infection-associated immune reconstitution syndrome in transplant recipients. Clin Infect Dis. 2011;53(2):168–76.
28. Baddley JW, Forrest GN. Cryptococcosis in solid organ transplantation. Am J Transplant. 2013;13(Suppl 4):242–9.
29. Singh N, Lortholary O, Alexander BD, Gupta KL, John GT, Pursell K, et al. Allograft loss in renal transplant recipients with cryptococcus neoformans associated immune reconstitution syndrome. Transplantation. 2005;80(8):1131–3.
30. Sun HY, Alexander BD, Huprikar S, Forrest GN, Bruno D, Lyon GM, et al. Predictors of immune reconstitution syndrome in organ transplant recipients with cryptococcosis: implications for the management of immunosuppression. Clin Infect Dis. 2015;60(1): 36–44.
31. Ascioglu S, Rex JH, de Pauw B, Bennett JE, Bille J, Crokaert F, et al. Defining opportunistic invasive fungal infections in immunocompromised patients with cancer and hematopoietic stem cell transplants: an international consensus. Clin Infect Dis. 2002;34(1):7–14.
32. De Pauw B, Walsh TJ, Donnelly JP, Stevens DA, Edwards JE, Calandra T, et al. Revised definitions of invasive fungal disease from the European Organization for Research and Treatment of Cancer/Invasive Fungal Infections Cooperative Group and the National Institute of Allergy and Infectious Diseases Mycoses Study Group (EORTC/MSG) Consensus Group. Clin Infect Dis. 2008;46(12):1813–21.
33. Park BJ, Pappas PG, Wannemuehler KA, Alexander BD, Anaissie EJ, Andes DR, et al. Invasive non-Aspergillus mold infections in transplant recipients, United States, 2001-2006. Emerg Infect Dis. 2011;17(10):1855–64.
34. Garcia-Vidal C, Upton A, Kirby KA, Marr KA. Epidemiology of invasive mold infections in allogeneic stem cell transplant recipients: biological risk factors for infection according to time after transplantation. Clin Infect Dis. 2008;47(8):1041–50.
35. Marr KA, Carter RA, Boeckh M, Martin P, Corey L. Invasive aspergillosis in allogeneic stem cell transplant recipients: changes in epidemiology and risk factors. Blood. 2002;100(13):4358–66.
36. van Burik JA, Carter SL, Freifeld AG, High KP, Godder KT, Papanicolaou GA, et al. Higher risk of cytomegalovirus and aspergillus infections in recipients of T cell-depleted unrelated bone marrow: analysis of infectious complications in patients treated with T cell depletion versus immunosuppressive therapy to prevent graft-versus-host disease. Biol Blood Marrow Transplant. 2007;13(12):1487–98.
37. Labbe AC, Su SH, Laverdiere M, Pepin J, Patino C, Cohen S, et al. High incidence of invasive aspergillosis associated with intestinal graft-versus-host disease following nonmyeloablative transplantation. Biol Blood Marrow Transplant. 2007;13(10):1192–200.
38. Ben-Ami R, Lewis RE, Kontoyiannis DP. Invasive mould infections in the setting of hematopoietic cell transplantation: current trends and new challenges. Curr Opin Infect Dis. 2009;22(4):376–84.
39. Mihu CN, King E, Yossepovitch O, Taur Y, Jakubowski A, Pamer E, et al. Risk factors and attributable mortality of late aspergillosis after T-cell depleted hematopoietic stem cell transplantation. Transpl Infect Dis. 2008;10(3):162–7.
40. Bow EJ. Invasive fungal infection in haematopoietic stem cell transplant recipients: epidemiology from the transplant physician's viewpoint. Mycopathologia. 2009;168(6):283–97.
41. Pagano L, Caira M, Nosari A, Van Lint MT, Candoni A, Offidani M, et al. Fungal infections in recipients of hematopoietic stem cell transplants: results of the SEIFEM B-2004 study--Sorveglianza Epidemiologica Infezioni Fungine Nelle Emopatie Maligne. Clin Infect Dis. 2007;45(9):1161–70.
42. Baddley JW, Stroud TP, Salzman D, Pappas PG. Invasive mold infections in allogeneic bone marrow transplant recipients. Clin Infect Dis. 2001;32(9):1319–24.

43. Marr KA. Fungal infections in hematopoietic stem cell transplant recipients. Med Mycol. 2008;46(4):293–302.
44. Sipsas NV, Lewis RE, Tarrand J, Hachem R, Rolston KV, Raad II, et al. Candidemia in patients with hematologic malignancies in the era of new antifungal agents (2001-2007): stable incidence but changing epidemiology of a still frequently lethal infection. Cancer. 2009;115(20):4745–52.
45. Goodman JL, Winston DJ, Greenfield RA, Chandrasekar PH, Fox B, Kaizer H, et al. A controlled trial of fluconazole to prevent fungal infections in patients undergoing bone marrow transplantation. N Engl J Med. 1992;326(13):845–51.
46. Marr KA, Seidel K, White TC, Bowden RA. Candidemia in allogeneic blood and marrow transplant recipients: evolution of risk factors after the adoption of prophylactic fluconazole. J Infect Dis. 2000;181(1):309–16.
47. Marr KA. The changing spectrum of candidemia in oncology patients: therapeutic implications. Curr Opin Infect Dis. 2000;13(6):615–20.
48. van Burik JH, Leisenring W, Myerson D, Hackman RC, Shulman HM, Sale GE, et al. The effect of prophylactic fluconazole on the clinical spectrum of fungal diseases in bone marrow transplant recipients with special attention to hepatic candidiasis. An autopsy study of 355 patients. Medicine (Baltimore). 1998;77(4):246–54.
49. Wingard JR. Importance of Candida species other than C. albicans as pathogens in oncology patients. Clin Infect Dis. 1995;20(1):115–25.
50. Pfaller MA, Castanheira M, Lockhart SR, Ahlquist AM, Messer SA, Jones RN. Frequency of decreased susceptibility and resistance to echinocandins among fluconazole-resistant bloodstream isolates of Candida glabrata. J Clin Microbiol. 2012;50(4):1199–203.
51. Latge JP. Aspergillus fumigatus and aspergillosis. Clin Microbiol Rev. 1999;12(2):310–50.
52. Hachem RY, Kontoyiannis DP, Boktour MR, Afif C, Cooksley C, Bodey GP, et al. Aspergillus terreus: an emerging amphotericin B-resistant opportunistic mold in patients with hematologic malignancies. Cancer. 2004;101(7):1594–600.
53. Nucci M, Marr KA. Emerging fungal diseases. Clin Infect Dis. 2005;41(4):521–6.
54. Steinbach WJ, Benjamin DK Jr, Kontoyiannis DP, Perfect JR, Lutsar I, Marr KA, et al. Infections due to Aspergillus terreus: a multicenter retrospective analysis of 83 cases. Clin Infect Dis. 2004;39(2):192–8.
55. Singh N, Paterson DL. Aspergillus infections in transplant recipients. Clin Microbiol Rev. 2005;18(1):44–69.
56. Tang TC, Chuang WY. Aspergillus tracheobronchitis in allogeneic stem cell transplanted recipient. Eur J Haematol. 2012;88(2):183.
57. Tasci S, Glasmacher A, Lentini S, Tschubel K, Ewig S, Molitor E, et al. Pseudomembranous and obstructive Aspergillus tracheobronchitis - optimal diagnostic strategy and outcome. Mycoses. 2006;49(1):37–42.
58. Miceli MH, Maertens J, Buve K, Grazziutti M, Woods G, Rahman M, et al. Immune reconstitution inflammatory syndrome in cancer patients with pulmonary aspergillosis recovering from neutropenia: proof of principle, description, and clinical and research implications. Cancer. 2007;110(1):112–20.
59. Marr KA, Carter RA, Crippa F, Wald A, Corey L. Epidemiology and outcome of mould infections in hematopoietic stem cell transplant recipients. Clin Infect Dis. 2002;34(7):909–17.
60. Kontoyiannis DP, Wessel VC, Bodey GP, Rolston KV. Zygomycosis in the 1990s in a tertiary-care cancer center. Clin Infect Dis. 2000;30(6):851–6.
61. Kontoyiannis DP, Lionakis MS, Lewis RE, Chamilos G, Healy M, Perego C, et al. Zygomycosis in a tertiary-care cancer center in the era of Aspergillus-active antifungal therapy: a case-control observational study of 27 recent cases. J Infect Dis. 2005;191(8): 1350–60.
62. Trifilio SM, Bennett CL, Yarnold PR, McKoy JM, Parada J, Mehta J, et al. Breakthrough zygomycosis after voriconazole administration among patients with hematologic malignancies who receive hematopoietic stem-cell transplants or intensive chemotherapy. Bone Marrow Transplant. 2007;39(7):425–9.
63. Trifilio S, Singhal S, Williams S, Frankfurt O, Gordon L, Evens A, et al. Breakthrough fungal infections after allogeneic hematopoietic stem cell transplantation in patients on prophylactic voriconazole. Bone Marrow Transplant. 2007;40(5):451–6.
64. Imhof A, Balajee SA, Fredricks DN, Englund JA, Marr KA. Breakthrough fungal infections in stem cell transplant recipients receiving voriconazole. Clin Infect Dis. 2004;39(5):743–6.
65. Marty FM, Cosimi LA, Baden LR. Breakthrough zygomycosis after voriconazole treatment in recipients of hematopoietic stem-cell transplants. N Engl J Med. 2004;350(9):950–2.
66. Siwek GT, Dodgson KJ, de Magalhaes-Silverman M, Bartelt LA, Kilborn SB, Hoth PL, et al. Invasive zygomycosis in hematopoietic stem cell transplant recipients receiving voriconazole prophylaxis. Clin Infect Dis. 2004;39(4):584–7.
67. Lerolle N, Raffoux E, Socie G, Touratier S, Sauvageon H, Porcher R, et al. Breakthrough invasive fungal disease in patients receiving posaconazole primary prophylaxis: a 4-year study. Clin Microbiol Infect. 2014;20(11):952–9.
68. Kang SH, Kim HS, Bae MN, Kim J, Yoo JY, Lee KY, et al. Fatal breakthrough Mucormycosis in an Acute Myelogenous Leukemia patient while on Posaconazole Prophylaxis. Infect Chemother. 2015;47(1):49–54.
69. Lekakis LJ, Lawson A, Prante J, Ribes J, Davis GJ, Monohan G, et al. Fatal rhizopus pneumonia in allogeneic stem cell transplant patients despite posaconazole prophylaxis: two cases and review of the literature. Biol Blood Marrow Transplant. 2009;15(8):991–5.
70. Nucci M, Marr KA, Queiroz-Telles F, Martins CA, Trabasso P, Costa S, et al. Fusarium infection in hematopoietic stem cell transplant recipients. Clin Infect Dis. 2004;38(9):1237–42.
71. Husain S, Munoz P, Forrest G, Alexander BD, Somani J, Brennan K, et al. Infections due to Scedosporium apiospermum and Scedosporium prolificans in transplant recipients: clinical characteristics and impact of antifungal agent therapy on outcome. Clin Infect Dis. 2005;40(1):89–99.
72. Lackner M, Sybren de Hoog G, Yang L, Moreno L, Ahmed S, Lopes L, et al. Proposed nomenclature for Pseudallescheria, Scedosporium and related genera. Fungal Divers. 2014;67:1–10.
73. Peterson MW, Pratt AD, Nugent KM. Pneumonia due to Histoplasma capsulatum in a bone marrow transplant recipient. Thorax. 1987;42(9):698–9.
74. Walsh TJ, Catchatourian R, Cohen H. Disseminated histoplasmosis complicating bone marrow transplantation. Am J Clin Pathol. 1983;79(4):509–11.
75. Morrison VA, Haake RJ, Weisdorf DJ. The spectrum of non-Candida fungal infections following bone marrow transplantation. Medicine (Baltimore). 1993;72(2):78–89.
76. Torres HA, Rivero GA, Kontoyiannis DP. Endemic mycoses in a cancer hospital. Medicine (Baltimore). 2002;81(3):201–12.
77. Jones O, Cleveland KO, Gelfand MS. A case of disseminated histoplasmosis following autologous stem cell transplantation for Hodgkin's lymphoma: an initial misdiagnosis with a false-positive serum galactomannan assay. Transpl Infect Dis. 2009;11(3): 281–3.
78. Vail GM, Young RS, Wheat LJ, Filo RS, Cornetta K, Goldman M. Incidence of histoplasmosis following allogeneic bone marrow transplant or solid organ transplant in a hyperendemic area. Transpl Infect Dis. 2002;4(3):148–51.
79. Haydoura S, Wallentine J, Lopansri B, Ford CD, Saad D, Burke JP. Disseminated histoplasmosis in allogeneic bone marrow transplant: a diagnosis not to be missed. Transpl Infect Dis. 2014;16(5):822–6.

80. Glenn TJ, Blair JE, Adams RH. Coccidioidomycosis in hematopoietic stem cell transplant recipients. Med Mycol. 2005;43(8):705–10.
81. Riley DK, Galgiani JN, O'Donnell MR, Ito JI, Beatty PG, Evans TG. Coccidioidomycosis in bone marrow transplant recipients. Transplantation. 1993;56(6):1531–3.
82. Blair JE. Coccidioidomycosis in patients who have undergone transplantation. Ann N Y Acad Sci. 2007;1111:365–76.
83. Blair JE, Smilack JD, Caples SM. Coccidioidomycosis in patients with hematologic malignancies. Arch Intern Med. 2005;165(1):113–7.
84. Serody JS, Mill MR, Detterbeck FC, Harris DT, Cohen MS. Blastomycosis in transplant recipients: report of a case and review. Clin Infect Dis. 1993;16(1):54–8.
85. Chen SC, Lewis RE, Kontoyiannis DP. Direct effects of non-antifungal agents used in cancer chemotherapy and organ transplantation on the development and virulence of Candida and Aspergillus species. Virulence. 2011;2(4):280–95.
86. Meyers JD. Fungal infections in bone marrow transplant patients. Semin Oncol. 1990;17(3 Suppl 6):10–3.
87. Wald A, Leisenring W, van Burik JA, Bowden RA. Epidemiology of Aspergillus infections in a large cohort of patients undergoing bone marrow transplantation. J Infect Dis. 1997;175(6):1459–66.
88. Jantunen E, Ruutu P, Niskanen L, Volin L, Parkkali T, Koukila-Kahkola P, et al. Incidence and risk factors for invasive fungal infections in allogeneic BMT recipients. Bone Marrow Transplant. 1997;19(8):801–8.
89. Kesh S, Mensah NY, Peterlongo P, Jaffe D, Hsu K, M VDB, et al. TLR1 and TLR6 polymorphisms are associated with susceptibility to invasive aspergillosis after allogeneic stem cell transplantation. Ann N Y Acad Sci. 2005;1062:95–103.
90. Bochud PY, Chien JW, Marr KA, Leisenring WM, Upton A, Janer M, et al. Toll-like receptor 4 polymorphisms and aspergillosis in stem-cell transplantation. N Engl J Med. 2008;359(17):1766–77.
91. Seo KW, Kim DH, Sohn SK, Lee NY, Chang HH, Kim SW, et al. Protective role of interleukin-10 promoter gene polymorphism in the pathogenesis of invasive pulmonary aspergillosis after allogeneic stem cell transplantation. Bone Marrow Transplant. 2005;36(12):1089–95.
92. Sainz J, Hassan L, Perez E, Romero A, Moratalla A, Lopez-Fernandez E, et al. Interleukin-10 promoter polymorphism as risk factor to develop invasive pulmonary aspergillosis. Immunol Lett. 2007;109(1):76–82.
93. Sainz J, Perez E, Hassan L, Moratalla A, Romero A, Collado MD, et al. Variable number of tandem repeats of TNF receptor type 2 promoter as genetic biomarker of susceptibility to develop invasive pulmonary aspergillosis. Hum Immunol. 2007;68(1):41–50.
94. Mezger M, Steffens M, Beyer M, Manger C, Eberle J, Toliat MR, et al. Polymorphisms in the chemokine (C-X-C motif) ligand 10 are associated with invasive aspergillosis after allogeneic stem-cell transplantation and influence CXCL10 expression in monocyte-derived dendritic cells. Blood. 2008;111(2):534–6.
95. Zaas AK, Liao G, Chien JW, Weinberg C, Shore D, Giles SS, et al. Plasminogen alleles influence susceptibility to invasive aspergillosis. PLoS Genet. 2008;4(6):e1000101.
96. Mezger M, Einsele H, Loeffler J. Genetic susceptibility to infections with Aspergillus fumigatus. Crit Rev Microbiol. 2010;36(2):168–77.
97. Pana ZD, Farmaki E, Roilides E. Host genetics and opportunistic fungal infections. Clin Microbiol Infect. 2014;20(12):1254–64.
98. Wójtowicz A, Bochud PY. Host genetics of invasive Aspergillus and Candida infections. Semin Immunopathol. 2015;37(2):173–86.
99. Maskarinec SA, Johnson MD, Perfect JR. Genetic susceptibility to fungal infections: what is in the genes? Curr Clin Microbiol Rep. 2016;3(2):81–91.
100. Maertens J, Demuynck H, Verbeken EK, Zachee P, Verhoef GE, Vandenberghe P, et al. Mucormycosis in allogeneic bone marrow transplant recipients: report of five cases and review of the role of iron overload in the pathogenesis. Bone Marrow Transplant. 1999;24(3):307–12.
101. Miceli MH, Dong L, Grazziutti ML, Fassas A, Thertulien R, Van Rhee F, et al. Iron overload is a major risk factor for severe infection after autologous stem cell transplantation: a study of 367 myeloma patients. Bone Marrow Transplant. 2006;37(9):857–64.
102. Offner F, Cordonnier C, Ljungman P, Prentice HG, Engelhard D, De Bacquer D, et al. Impact of previous aspergillosis on the outcome of bone marrow transplantation. Clin Infect Dis. 1998;26(5):1098–103.
103. Robertson MJ, Larson RA. Recurrent fungal pneumonias in patients with acute nonlymphocytic leukemia undergoing multiple courses of intensive chemotherapy. Am J Med. 1988;84(2):233–9.
104. Cordonnier C, Beaune J, Offner F, Marinus A, Ljungman P, Meunier F. Aspergillosis prior to bone marrow transplantation. Infectious Diseases Working Party of the EBMT and the EORTC Invasive Fungal Infections Cooperative Group. Bone Marrow Transplant. 1995;16(2):323–4.
105. Hill BT, Kondapalli L, Artz A, Smith S, Rich E, Godley L, et al. Successful allogeneic transplantation of patients with suspected prior invasive mold infection. Leuk Lymphoma. 2007;48(9):1799–805.
106. Aki ZS, Sucak GT, Yegin ZA, Guzel O, Erbas G, Senol E. Hematopoietic stem cell transplantation in patients with active fungal infection: not a contraindication for transplantation. Transplant Proc. 2008;40(5):1579–85.
107. Richard C, Romon I, Baro J, Insunza A, Loyola I, Zurbano F, et al. Invasive pulmonary aspergillosis prior to BMT in acute leukemia patients does not predict a poor outcome. Bone Marrow Transplant. 1993;12(3):237–41.
108. Michailov G, Laporte JP, Lesage S, Fouillard L, Isnard F, Noel-Walter MP, et al. Autologous bone marrow transplantation is feasible in patients with a prior history of invasive pulmonary aspergillosis. Bone Marrow Transplant. 1996;17(4):569–72.
109. Singhal S, Safdar A, Chiang KY, Godder K, van Rhee F, Garner F, et al. Non-myeloablative allogeneic transplantation ('microallograft') for refractory myeloma after two preceding autografts: feasibility and efficacy in a patient with active aspergillosis. Bone Marrow Transplant. 2000;26(11):1231–3.
110. Hermann S, Klein SA, Jacobi V, Thalhammer A, Bialleck H, Duchscherer M, et al. Older patients with high-risk fungal infections can be successfully allografted using non-myeloablative conditioning in combination with intensified supportive care regimens. Br J Haematol. 2001;113(2):446–54.
111. Eibl M, Auner HW, Zinke-Cerwenka W, Sill H, Dornbusch HJ, Linkesch W. High-risk AML complicated by pulmonary aspergillosis: successful treatment with nonmyeloablative stem cell transplantation and long-term administration of voriconazole. Ann Hematol. 2004;83(2):133–6.
112. Martino R, Nomdedeu J, Altes A, Sureda A, Brunet S, Martinez C, et al. Successful bone marrow transplantation in patients with previous invasive fungal infections: report of four cases. Bone Marrow Transplant. 1994;13(3):265–9.
113. Liu M, Li Y, Zhang Y, Zhao X, Zhai B, Zhang Q, et al. Secondary antifungal prophylaxis in hematological malignancy patients with previous invasive fungal disease: a retrospective analysis. PLoS One. 2014;9(12):e115461.
114. Georgiadou SP, Lewis RE, Best L, Torres HA, Champlin RE, Kontoyiannis DP. The impact of prior invasive mold infections in leukemia patients who undergo allo-SCT in the era of triazole-based secondary prophylaxis. Bone Marrow Transplant. 2013 Jan;48(1):141–3.
115. Ochs L, Shu XO, Miller J, Enright H, Wagner J, Filipovich A, et al. Late infections after allogeneic bone marrow transplantations: comparison of incidence in related and unrelated donor transplant recipients. Blood. 1995;86(10):3979–86.

116. Storek J, Dawson MA, Storer B, Stevens-Ayers T, Maloney DG, Marr KA, et al. Immune reconstitution after allogeneic marrow transplantation compared with blood stem cell transplantation. Blood. 2001;97(11):3380–9.
117. Powles R, Mehta J, Kulkarni S, Treleaven J, Millar B, Marsden J, et al. Allogeneic blood and bone-marrow stem-cell transplantation in haematological malignant diseases: a randomised trial. Lancet. 2000;355(9211):1231–7.
118. Parody R, Martino R, Rovira M, Vazquez L, Vazquez MJ, de la Camara R, et al. Severe infections after unrelated donor allogeneic hematopoietic stem cell transplantation in adults: comparison of cord blood transplantation with peripheral blood and bone marrow transplantation. Biol Blood Marrow Transplant. 2006;12(7):734–48.
119. Saavedra S, Sanz GF, Jarque I, Moscardo F, Jimenez C, Lorenzo I, et al. Early infections in adult patients undergoing unrelated donor cord blood transplantation. Bone Marrow Transplant. 2002;30(12):937–43.
120. Crippa F, Holmberg L, Carter RA, Hooper H, Marr KA, Bensinger W, et al. Infectious complications after autologous CD34-selected peripheral blood stem cell transplantation. Biol Blood Marrow Transplant. 2002;8(5):281–9.
121. Martino R, Subira M, Rovira M, Solano C, Vazquez L, Sanz GF, et al. Invasive fungal infections after allogeneic peripheral blood stem cell transplantation: incidence and risk factors in 395 patients. Br J Haematol. 2002;116(2):475–82.
122. Junghanss C, Marr KA, Carter RA, Sandmaier BM, Maris MB, Maloney DG, et al. Incidence and outcome of bacterial and fungal infections following nonmyeloablative compared with myeloablative allogeneic hematopoietic stem cell transplantation: a matched control study. Biol Blood Marrow Transplant. 2002;8(9):512–20.
123. Hagen EA, Stern H, Porter D, Duffy K, Foley K, Luger S, et al. High rate of invasive fungal infections following nonmyeloablative allogeneic transplantation. Clin Infect Dis. 2003;36(1):9–15.
124. Fukuda T, Boeckh M, Carter RA, Sandmaier BM, Maris MB, Maloney DG, et al. Risks and outcomes of invasive fungal infections in recipients of allogeneic hematopoietic stem cell transplants after nonmyeloablative conditioning. Blood. 2003;102(3):827–33.
125. Sayer HG, Longton G, Bowden R, Pepe M, Storb R. Increased risk of infection in marrow transplant patients receiving methylprednisolone for graft-versus-host disease prevention. Blood. 1994;84(4):1328–32.
126. Marty FM, Lee SJ, Fahey MM, Alyea EP, Soiffer RJ, Antin JH, et al. Infliximab use in patients with severe graft-versus-host disease and other emerging risk factors of non-Candida invasive fungal infections in allogeneic hematopoietic stem cell transplant recipients: a cohort study. Blood. 2003;102(8):2768–76.
127. Mackall C, Fry T, Gress R, Peggs K, Storek J, Toubert A. Background to hematopoietic cell transplantation, including post transplant immune recovery. Bone Marrow Transplant. 2009;44(8):457–62.
128. Low CY, Rotstein C. Emerging fungal infections in immunocompromised patients. F1000 Med Rep. 2011;3:14.
129. Pinto PS. The CT Halo Sign. Radiology. 2004;230(1):109–10.
130. Marr KA, Balajee SA, McLaughlin L, Tabouret M, Bentsen C, Walsh TJ. Detection of galactomannan antigenemia by enzyme immunoassay for the diagnosis of invasive aspergillosis: variables that affect performance. J Infect Dis. 2004;190(3):641–9.
131. Corzo-León DE, Satlin MJ, Soave R, Shore TB, Schuetz AN, Jacobs SE, et al. Epidemiology and outcomes of invasive fungal infections in allogeneic haematopoietic stem cell transplant recipients in the era of antifungal prophylaxis: a single-centre study with focus on emerging pathogens. Mycoses. 2015;58(6):325–36.
132. Karchmer AW, Samore MH, Hadley S, Collins LA, Jenkins RL, Lewis WD. Fungal infections complicating orthotopic liver transplantation. Trans Am Clin Climatol Assoc. 1995;106:38–47.
133. Kusne S, Blair JE. Viral and fungal infections after liver transplantation--part II. Liver Transpl. 2006;12(1):2–11.
134. Zicker M, Colombo AL, Ferraz-Neto BH, Camargo LF. Epidemiology of fungal infections in liver transplant recipients: a six-year study of a large Brazilian liver transplantation centre. Mem Inst Oswaldo Cruz. 2011;106(3):339–45.
135. Dowling RD, Baladi N, Zenati M, Dummer JS, Kormos RL, Armitage JM, et al. Disruption of the aortic anastomosis after heart-lung transplantation. Ann Thorac Surg. 1990;49(1):118–22.
136. Palmer SM, Alexander BD, Sanders LL, Edwards LJ, Reller LB, Davis RD, et al. Significance of blood stream infection after lung transplantation: analysis in 176 consecutive patients. Transplantation. 2000;69(11):2360–6.
137. Palmer SM, Perfect JR, Howell DN, Lawrence CM, Miralles AP, Davis RD, et al. Candidal anastomotic infection in lung transplant recipients: successful treatment with a combination of systemic and inhaled antifungal agents. J Heart Lung Transplant. 1998;17(10):1029–33.
138. Hadjiliadis D, Howell DN, Davis RD, Lawrence CM, Rea JB, Tapson VF, et al. Anastomotic infections in lung transplant recipients. Ann Transplant. 2000;5(3):13–9.
139. Schaenman JM, Rosso F, Austin JM, Baron EJ, Gamberg P, Miller J, et al. Trends in invasive disease due to Candida species following heart and lung transplantation. Transpl Infect Dis. 2009;11(2):112–21.
140. Safdar N, Slattery WR, Knasinski V, Gangnon RE, Li Z, Pirsch JD, et al. Predictors and outcomes of candiduria in renal transplant recipients. Clin Infect Dis. 2005;40(10):1413–21.
141. Albano L, Bretagne S, Mamzer-Bruneel MF, Kacso I, Desnos-Ollivier M, Guerrini P, et al. Evidence that graft-site candidiasis after kidney transplantation is acquired during organ recovery: a multicenter study in France. Clin Infect Dis. 2009;48(2):194–202.
142. Benedetti E, Gruessner AC, Troppmann C, Papalois BE, Sutherland DE, Dunn DL, et al. Intra-abdominal fungal infections after pancreatic transplantation: incidence, treatment, and outcome. J Am Coll Surg. 1996;183(4):307–16.
143. Fontana I, Bertocchi M, Diviacco P, De Negri A, Magoni Rossi A, Santori G, et al. Infections after simultaneous pancreas and kidney transplantation: a single-center experience. Transplant Proc. 2009;41(4):1333–5.
144. Berger N, Wirmsberger R, Kafka R, Margreiter C, Ebenbichler C, Stelzmueller I, et al. Infectious complications following 72 consecutive enteric-drained pancreas transplants. Transpl Int. 2006;19(7):549–57.
145. Lumbreras C, Fernandez I, Velosa J, Munn S, Sterioff S, Paya CV. Infectious complications following pancreatic transplantation: incidence, microbiological and clinical characteristics, and outcome. Clin Infect Dis. 1995;20(3):514–20.
146. Berger N, Guggenbichler S, Steurer W, Margreiter C, Mayer G, Kafka R, et al. Bloodstream infection following 217 consecutive systemic-enteric drained pancreas transplants. BMC Infect Dis. 2006;6:127.
147. Florescu DF, Islam KM, Grant W, Mercer DF, Langnas A, Botha J, et al. Incidence and outcome of fungal infections in pediatric small bowel transplant recipients. Transpl Infect Dis. 2010;12(6):497–504.
148. Nathan SD, Shorr AF, Schmidt ME, Burton NA. Aspergillus and endobronchial abnormalities in lung transplant recipients. Chest. 2000;118(2):403–7.
149. Kramer MR, Denning DW, Marshall SE, Ross DJ, Berry G, Lewiston NJ, et al. Ulcerative tracheobronchitis after lung transplantation. A new form of invasive aspergillosis. Am Rev Respir Dis. 1991;144(3. Pt 1):552–6.
150. Singh N, Husain S. Aspergillus infections after lung transplantation: clinical differences in type of transplant and implications for management. J Heart Lung Transplant. 2003;22(3):258–66.

151. Singh N, Avery RK, Munoz P, Pruett TL, Alexander B, Jacobs R, et al. Trends in risk profiles for and mortality associated with invasive aspergillosis among liver transplant recipients. Clin Infect Dis. 2003;36(1):46–52.
152. Montoya JG, Giraldo LF, Efron B, Stinson EB, Gamberg P, Hunt S, et al. Infectious complications among 620 consecutive heart transplant patients at Stanford University Medical Center. Clin Infect Dis. 2001;33(5):629–40.
153. Montoya JG, Chaparro SV, Celis D, Cortes JA, Leung AN, Robbins RC, et al. Invasive aspergillosis in the setting of cardiac transplantation. Clin Infect Dis. 2003;37(Suppl 3):S281–92.
154. Morio F, Treilhaud M, Lepelletier D, Le Pape P, Rigal JC, Delile L, et al. Aspergillus fumigatus endocarditis of the mitral valve in a heart transplant recipient: a case report. Diagn Microbiol Infect Dis. 2008;62(4):453–6.
155. Levin T, Suh B, Beltramo D, Samuel R. Aspergillus mediastinitis following orthotopic heart transplantation: case report and review of the literature. Transpl Infect Dis. 2004;6(3):129–31.
156. Florescu DF, Iwen PC, Hill LA, Dumitru I, Quader MA, Kalil AC, et al. Cerebral aspergillosis caused by Aspergillus ustus following orthotopic heart transplantation: case report and review of the literature. Clin Transpl. 2009;23(1):116–20.
157. Muñoz P, Rodriguez C, Bouza E, Palomo J, Yanez JF, Dominguez MJ, et al. Risk factors of invasive aspergillosis after heart transplantation: protective role of oral itraconazole prophylaxis. Am J Transplant. 2004;4(4):636–43.
158. Muñoz P, Cerón I, Valerio M, Palomo J, Villa A, Eworo A, et al. Invasive aspergillosis among heart transplant recipients: a 24-year perspective. J Heart Lung Transplant. 2014;33(3):278–88.
159. Singh N, Alexander BD, Lortholary O, Dromer F, Gupta KL, John GT, et al. Pulmonary cryptococcosis in solid organ transplant recipients: clinical relevance of serum cryptococcal antigen. Clin Infect Dis. 2008;46(2):e12–8.
160. Singh N, Alexander BD, Lortholary O, Dromer F, Gupta KL, John GT, et al. Cryptococcus neoformans in organ transplant recipients: impact of calcineurin-inhibitor agents on mortality. J Infect Dis. 2007;195(5):756–64.
161. Jean SS, Fang CT, Shau WY, Chen YC, Chang SC, Hsueh PR, et al. Cryptococcaemia: clinical features and prognostic factors. QJM. 2002;95(8):511–8.
162. Alexander J, Limaye AP, Ko CW, Bronner MP, Kowdley KV. Association of hepatic iron overload with invasive fungal infection in liver transplant recipients. Liver Transpl. 2006;12(12):1799–804.
163. McGuire FR, Grinnan DC, Robbins M. Mucormycosis of the bronchial anastomosis: a case of successful medical treatment and historic review. J Heart Lung Transplant. 2007;26(8):857–61.
164. Lanternier F, Sun HY, Ribaud P, Singh N, Kontoyiannis DP, Lortholary O. Mucormycosis in organ and stem cell transplant recipients. Clin Infect Dis. 2012;54(11):1–8.
165. Godara SM, Kute VB, Goplani KR, Gumber MR, Gera DN, Shah PR, et al. Mucormycosis in renal transplant recipients: predictors and outcome. Saudi J Kidney Dis Transpl. 2011;22(4):751–6.
166. Almyroudis NG, Sutton DA, Linden P, Rinaldi MG, Fung J, Kusne S. Zygomycosis in solid organ transplant recipients in a tertiary transplant center and review of the literature. Am J Transplant. 2006;6(10):2365–74.
167. Einollahi B, Lessan-Pezeshki M, Aslani J, Nemati E, Rostami Z, Hosseini MJ, et al. Two decades of experience in mucormycosis after kidney transplantation. Ann Transplant. 2011;16(3):44–8.
168. Nucci M, Anaissie E. Fusarium infections in immunocompromised patients. Clin Microbiol Rev. 2007;20(4):695–704.
169. Gauthier GM, Safdar N, Klein BS, Andes DR. Blastomycosis in solid organ transplant recipients. Transpl Infect Dis. 2007;9(4):310–7.
170. Blair JE, Logan JL. Coccidioidomycosis in solid organ transplantation. Clin Infect Dis. 2001;33(9):1536–44.
171. Singh N, Huprikar S, Burdette SD, Morris MI, Blair JE, Wheat LJ. Donor-derived fungal infections in organ transplant recipients: guidelines of the American Society of transplantation, infectious diseases community of practice. Am J Transplant. 2012;12(9):2414–28.
172. Shoham S, Hinestrosa F, Moore JJ, O'Donnell S, Ruiz M, Light J. Invasive filamentous fungal infections associated with renal transplant tourism. Transpl Infect Dis. 2010;12(4):371–4.
173. Babik JM, Chin-Hong P. Transplant tourism: understanding the risks. Curr Infect Dis Rep. 2015;17(4):473.
174. Avery RK. Antifungal prophylaxis in lung transplantation. Semin Respir Crit Care Med. 2011;32(6):717–26.
175. Zenati M, Dowling RD, Dummer JS, Paradis IL, Arena VC, Armitage JM, et al. Influence of the donor lung on development of early infections in lung transplant recipients. J Heart Transplant. 1990;9(5):502–8.
176. Mueller NJ, Weisser M, Fehr T, Wuthrich RP, Mullhaupt B, Lehmann R, et al. Donor-derived aspergillosis from use of a solid organ recipient as a multiorgan donor. Transpl Infect Dis. 2010;12(1):54–9.
177. Keating MR, Guerrero MA, Daly RC, Walker RC, Davies SF. Transmission of invasive aspergillosis from a subclinically infected donor to three different organ transplant recipients. Chest. 1996;109(4):1119–24.
178. van der Vliet JA, Tidow G, Kootstra G, van Saene HF, Krom RA, Sloof MJ, et al. Transplantation of contaminated organs. Br J Surg. 1980;67(8):596–8.
179. Alexander BD, Schell WA, Siston AM, Rao CY, Bower WA, Balajee SA, et al. Fatal Apophysomyces elegans infection transmitted by deceased donor renal allografts. Am J Transplant. 2010;10(9):2161–7.
180. Baddley JW, Schain DC, Gupte AA, Lodhi SA, Kayler LK, Frade JP, et al. Transmission of Cryptococcus neoformans by organ transplantation. Clin Infect Dis. 2011;52(4):e94–8.
181. Sun HY, Alexander BD, Lortholary O, Dromer F, Forrest GN, Lyon GM, et al. Unrecognized pretransplant and donor-derived cryptococcal disease in organ transplant recipients. Clin Infect Dis. 2010;51(9):1062–9.
182. Nelson JK, Giraldeau G, Montoya JG, Deresinski S, Ho DY, Pham M. Donor-derived Coccidioides immitis endocarditis and disseminated infection in the setting of solid organ transplantation. Open Forum Infect Dis. 2016;3(3):ofw086.
183. Steinbach WJ, Reedy JL, Cramer RA Jr, Perfect JR, Heitman J. Harnessing calcineurin as a novel anti-infective agent against invasive fungal infections. Nat Rev Microbiol. 2007;5(6):418–30.
184. Singh N, Heitman J. Antifungal attributes of immunosuppressive agents: new paradigms in management and elucidating the pathophysiologic basis of opportunistic mycoses in organ transplant recipients. Transplantation. 2004;77(6):795–800.
185. Kontoyiannis DP, Lewis RE, Osherov N, Albert ND, May GS. Combination of caspofungin with inhibitors of the calcineurin pathway attenuates growth in vitro in Aspergillus species. J Antimicrob Chemother. 2003;51(2):313–6.
186. Narreddy S, Manavathu E, Chandrasekar PH, Alangaden GJ, Revankar SG. In vitro interaction of posaconazole with calcineurin inhibitors and sirolimus against zygomycetes. J Antimicrob Chemother. 2010;65(4):701–3.
187. Dannaoui E, Schwarz P, Lortholary O. In vitro interactions between antifungals and immunosuppressive drugs against zygomycetes. Antimicrob Agents Chemother. 2009;53(8):3549–51.
188. Patel R, Portela D, Badley AD, Harmsen WS, Larson-Keller JJ, Ilstrup DM, et al. Risk factors of invasive Candida and non-Candida fungal infections after liver transplantation. Transplantation. 1996;62(7):926–34.

189. Singh N. Fungal infections in the recipients of solid organ transplantation. Infect Dis Clin N Am. 2003;17(1):113–34.
190. George MJ, Snydman DR, Werner BG, Griffith J, Falagas ME, Dougherty NN, et al. The independent role of cytomegalovirus as a risk factor for invasive fungal disease in orthotopic liver transplant recipients. Boston Center for Liver Transplantation CMVIG-Study Group Cytogam, MedImmune, Inc Gaithersburg, Maryland. Am J Med. 1997;103(2):106–13.
191. Hadley S, Karchmer AW. Fungal infections in solid organ transplant recipients. Infect Dis Clin N Am. 1995;9(4):1045–74.
192. Collins LA, Samore MH, Roberts MS, Luzzati R, Jenkins RL, Lewis WD, et al. Risk factors for invasive fungal infections complicating orthotopic liver transplantation. J Infect Dis. 1994;170(3):644–52.
193. Wade JJ, Rolando N, Hayllar K, Philpott-Howard J, Casewell MW, Williams R. Bacterial and fungal infections after liver transplantation: an analysis of 284 patients. Hepatology. 1995;21(5):1328–36.
194. Singh N, Wagener MM, Marino IR, Gayowski T. Trends in invasive fungal infections in liver transplant recipients: correlation with evolution in transplantation practices. Transplantation. 2002;73(1):63–7.
195. Singh N, Husain S. AST Infectious Diseases Community of Practice. Aspergillosis in solid organ transplantation. Am J Transplant. 2013;13(Suppl 4):228–41.
196. Westney GE, Kesten S, De Hoyos A, Chapparro C, Winton T, Maurer JR. Aspergillus infection in single and double lung transplant recipients. Transplantation. 1996;61(6):915–9.
197. Speziali G, McDougall JC, Midthun DE, Peters SG, Scott JP, Daly RC, et al. Native lung complications after single lung transplantation for emphysema. Transpl Int. 1997;10(2):113–5.
198. Gavalda J, Len O, San Juan R, Aguado JM, Fortun J, Lumbreras C, et al. Risk factors for invasive aspergillosis in solid-organ transplant recipients: a case-control study. Clin Infect Dis. 2005;41(1):52–9.
199. Nunley DR, Ohori P, Grgurich WF, Iacono AT, Williams PA, Keenan RJ, et al. Pulmonary aspergillosis in cystic fibrosis lung transplant recipients. Chest. 1998;114(5):1321–9.
200. Cahill BC, Hibbs JR, Savik K, Juni BA, Dosland BM, Edin-Stibbe C, et al. Aspergillus airway colonization and invasive disease after lung transplantation. Chest. 1997;112(5):1160–4.
201. Husni RN, Gordon SM, Longworth DL, Arroliga A, Stillwell PC, Avery RK, et al. Cytomegalovirus infection is a risk factor for invasive aspergillosis in lung transplant recipients. Clin Infect Dis. 1998;26(3):753–5.
202. Paterson DL, Singh N. Invasive aspergillosis in transplant recipients. Medicine (Baltimore). 1999;78(2):123–38.
203. Alexander BD, Tapson VF. Infectious complications of lung transplantation. Transpl Infect Dis. 2001;3(3):128–37.
204. Goldfarb NS, Avery RK, Goormastic M, Mehta AC, Schilz R, Smedira N, et al. Hypogammaglobulinemia in lung transplant recipients. Transplantation. 2001;71(2):242–6.
205. Higgins R, McNeil K, Dennis C, Parry A, Large S, Nashef SA, et al. Airway stenoses after lung transplantation: management with expanding metal stents. J Heart Lung Transplant. 1994;13(5):774–8.
206. Helmi M, Love RB, Welter D, Cornwell RD, Meyer KC. Aspergillus infection in lung transplant recipients with cystic fibrosis: risk factors and outcomes comparison to other types of transplant recipients. Chest. 2003;123(3):800–8.
207. Gordon SM, Avery RK. Aspergillosis in lung transplantation: incidence, risk factors, and prophylactic strategies. Transpl Infect Dis. 2001;3(3):161–7.
208. Bouza E, Pelaez T, Perez-Molina J, Marin M, Alcala L, Padilla B, et al. Demolition of a hospital building by controlled explosion: the impact on filamentous fungal load in internal and external air. J Hosp Infect. 2002;52(4):234–42.
209. Rabin AS, Givertz MM, Couper GS, Shea MM, Peixoto D, Yokoe DS, et al. Risk factors for invasive fungal disease in heart transplant recipients. J Heart Lung Transplant. 2015;34(2):227–32.
210. Abbott KC, Hypolite I, Poropatich RK, Hshieh P, Cruess D, Hawkes CA, et al. Hospitalizations for fungal infections after renal transplantation in the United States. Transpl Infect Dis. 2001;3(4):203–11.
211. Badiee P, Alborzi A. Invasive fungal infections in renal transplant recipients. Exp Clin Transplant. 2011;9(6):355–62.
212. Altiparmak MR, Apaydin S, Trablus S, Serdengecti K, Ataman R, Ozturk R, et al. Systemic fungal infections after renal transplantation. Scand J Infect Dis. 2002;34(4):284–8.
213. Florescu DF, Qiu F, Mercer DF, Langnas AN, Shafer LR, Kalil AC. Risk factors for systemic Candida infections in pediatric small bowel transplant recipients. Pediatr Infect Dis J. 2012;31(2):120–3.
214. Saccente M, Woods GL. Clinical and laboratory update on blastomycosis. Clin Microbiol Rev. 2010;23(2):367–81.
215. Brown J, Benedict K, Park BJ, Thompson GR 3rd. Coccidioidomycosis: epidemiology. Clin Epidemiol. 2013;5:185–97.
216. Knox KS, Histoplasmosis HCA. Proc Am Thorac Soc. 2010;7(3):169–72.
217. Raghuram A, Restrepo A, Safadjou S, Cooley J, Orloff M, Hardy D, et al. Invasive fungal infections following liver transplantation 2003-2007: incidence, risk factors, survival and the impact of fluconazole-resistant Candida parapsilosis. Liver Transpl. 2012;18(9):1100–9.
218. van Asbeck EC, Clemons KV, Stevens DA. Candida parapsilosis: a review of its epidemiology, pathogenesis, clinical aspects, typing and antimicrobial susceptibility. Crit Rev Microbiol. 2009;35(4):283–309.
219. Singh N, Pruett TL, Houston S, Munoz P, Cacciarelli TV, Wagener MM, et al. Invasive aspergillosis in the recipients of liver retransplantation. Liver Transpl. 2006;12(8):1205–9.
220. Sampathkumar P, Paya CV. Fusarium infection after solid-organ transplantation. Clin Infect Dis. 2001;32(8):1237–40.
221. Valentine VG, Gupta MR, Walker JE Jr, Seoane L, Bonvillain RW, Lombard GA, et al. Effect of etiology and timing of respiratory tract infections on development of bronchiolitis obliterans syndrome. J Heart Lung Transplant. 2009;28(2):163–9.
222. Weigt SS, Elashoff RM, Huang C, Ardehali A, Gregson AL, Kubak B, et al. Aspergillus colonization of the lung allograft is a risk factor for bronchiolitis obliterans syndrome. Am J Transplant. 2009;9(8):1903–11.
223. Matignon M, Botterel F, Audard V, Dunogue B, Dahan K, Lang P, et al. Outcome of renal transplantation in eight patients with Candida sp. contamination of preservation fluid. Am J Transplant. 2008;8(3):697–700.
224. Smeekens SP, van de Veerdonk FL, Kullberg BJ, Netea MG. Genetic susceptibility to Candida infections. EMBO Mol Med. 2013;5(6):805–13.
225. Cunha C, Rodrigues F, Zelante T, Aversa F, Romani L, Carvalho A. Genetic susceptibility to aspergillosis in allogeneic stem-cell transplantation. Med Mycol. 2011;49(Suppl 1):S137–43.
226. Slavin MA, Osborne B, Adams R, Levenstein MJ, Schoch HG, Feldman AR, et al. Efficacy and safety of fluconazole prophylaxis for fungal infections after marrow transplantation--a prospective, randomized, double-blind study. J Infect Dis. 1995;171(6):1545–52.
227. Marr KA, Seidel K, Slavin MA, Bowden RA, Schoch HG, Flowers ME, et al. Prolonged fluconazole prophylaxis is associated with persistent protection against candidiasis-related death in allogeneic marrow transplant recipients: long-term follow-up of a randomized, placebo-controlled trial. Blood. 2000;96(6):2055–61.
228. Miceli MH, Kauffman CA. Isavuconazole: A New Broad-Spectrum Triazole Antifungal Agent. Clin Infect Dis. 2015;61(10):1558–65.

229. Robenshtok E, Gafter-Gvili A, Goldberg E, Weinberger M, Yeshurun M, Leibovici L, et al. Antifungal prophylaxis in cancer patients after chemotherapy or hematopoietic stem-cell transplantation: systematic review and meta-analysis. J Clin Oncol. 2007;25(34):5471–89.
230. Ethier MC, Science M, Beyene J, Briel M, Lehrnbecher T, Sung L. Mould-active compared with fluconazole prophylaxis to prevent invasive fungal diseases in cancer patients receiving chemotherapy or haematopoietic stem-cell transplantation: a systematic review and meta-analysis of randomised controlled trials. Br J Cancer. 2012;106(10):1626–37.
231. Cordonnier C, Rovira M, Maertens J, Olavarria E, Faucher C, Bilger K, et al. Voriconazole for secondary prophylaxis of invasive fungal infections in allogeneic stem cell transplant recipients: results of the VOSIFI study. Haematologica. 2010;95(10):1762–8.
232. Cordonnier C, Maury S, Pautas C, Bastie JN, Chehata S, Castaigne S, et al. Secondary antifungal prophylaxis with voriconazole to adhere to scheduled treatment in leukemic patients and stem cell transplant recipients. Bone Marrow Transplant. 2004;33(9):943–8.
233. Freifeld AG, Bow EJ, Sepkowitz KA, Boeckh MJ, Ito JI, Mullen CA, et al. Clinical practice guideline for the use of antimicrobial agents in neutropenic patients with cancer: 2010 update by the infectious diseases society of america. Clin Infect Dis. 2011;52(4):e56–93.
234. Maertens J, Marchetti O, Herbrecht R, Cornely OA, Fluckiger U, Frere P, et al. European guidelines for antifungal management in leukemia and hematopoietic stem cell transplant recipients: summary of the ECIL 3--2009 update. Bone Marrow Transplant. 2011;46(5):709–18.
235. National Comprehensive Cancer Network (NCCN) clinical practice guidelines in oncology. Prevention and treatment of cancer-related infections. Version 2.2016.[internet] Available from: http://www.nccn.org/professionals/physicians_gls/pdf/infections.pdf [cited 2016 Aug 1].
236. van Burik JA, Ratanatharathorn V, Stepan DE, Miller CB, Lipton JH, Vesole DH, et al. Micafungin versus fluconazole for prophylaxis against invasive fungal infections during neutropenia in patients undergoing hematopoietic stem cell transplantation. Clin Infect Dis. 2004;39(10):1407–16.
237. Ullmann AJ, Lipton JH, Vesole DH, Chandrasekar P, Langston A, Tarantolo SR, et al. Posaconazole or fluconazole for prophylaxis in severe graft-versus-host disease. N Engl J Med. 2007;356(4):335–47.
238. Cornely OA, Maertens J, Winston DJ, Perfect J, Ullmann AJ, Walsh TJ, et al. Posaconazole vs. fluconazole or itraconazole prophylaxis in patients with neutropenia. N Engl J Med. 2007;356(4):348–59.
239. Marks DI, Pagliuca A, Kibbler CC, Glasmacher A, Heussel CP, Kantecki M, et al. Voriconazole versus itraconazole for antifungal prophylaxis following allogeneic haematopoietic stem-cell transplantation. Br J Haematol. 2011;155(3):318–27.
240. Wingard JR, Carter SL, Walsh TJ, Kurtzberg J, Small TN, Baden LR, et al. Randomized, double-blind trial of fluconazole versus voriconazole for prevention of invasive fungal infection after allogeneic hematopoietic cell transplantation. Blood. 2010;116(24):5111–8.
241. Lorf T, Braun F, Ruchel R, Muller A, Sattler B, Ringe B. Systemic mycoses during prophylactical use of liposomal amphotericin B (Ambisome) after liver transplantation. Mycoses. 1999;42(1–2):47–53.
242. Singh N, Mieles L, Yu VL, Gayowski T. Invasive aspergillosis in liver transplant recipients: association with candidemia and consumption coagulopathy and failure of prophylaxis with low-dose amphotericin B. Clin Infect Dis. 1993;17(5):906–8.
243. Eschenauer GA, Lam SW, Carver PL. Antifungal prophylaxis in liver transplant recipients. Liver Transpl. 2009;15(8):842–58.
244. Singh N, Paterson DL, Gayowski T, Wagener MM, Marino IR. Preemptive prophylaxis with a lipid preparation of amphotericin B for invasive fungal infections in liver transplant recipients requiring renal replacement therapy. Transplantation. 2001;71(7):910–3.
245. Winston DJ, Pakrasi A, Busuttil RW. Prophylactic fluconazole in liver transplant recipients. A randomized, double-blind, placebo-controlled trial. Ann Intern Med. 1999;131(10):729–37.
246. Kishino S, Ohno K, Shimamura T, Furukawatodo H. Optimal prophylactic dosage and disposition of micafungin in living donor liver recipients. Clin Transpl. 2004;18(6):676–80.
247. Fortun J, Martin-Davila P, Montejo M, Munoz P, Cisneros JM, Ramos A, et al. Prophylaxis with caspofungin for invasive fungal infections in high-risk liver transplant recipients. Transplantation. 2009;87(3):424–35.
248. Winston DJ, Limaye AP, Pelletier S, Safdar N, Morris MI, Meneses K, et al. Randomized, double-blind trial of anidulafungin versus fluconazolefor prophylaxis of invasive fungal infections in high-risk liver transplant recipients. Am J Transplant. 2014;14(12):2758–64.
249. Saliba F, Pascher A, Cointault O, Laterre PF, Cervera C, De Waele JJ, et al. TENPIN Liver Transplant European Study Into the Prevention of Fungal Infection Investigators. Randomized trial of micafungin for the prevention of invasive fungal infection in high-risk liver transplant recipients. Clin Infect Dis. 2015;60(7):997–1006.
250. Patterson TF, Thompson GR 3rd, Denning DW, Fishman JA, Hadley S, Herbrecht R, et al. Practice guidelines for the diagnosis and management of aspergillosis: 2016 update by the Infectious Diseases Society of America. Clin Infect Dis. 2016;63(4):e1–e60.
251. Silveira FP, Kusne S, AST Infectious Diseases Community of Practice. Candida infections in solid organ transplantation. Am J Transplant. 2013;13(Suppl 4):220–7.
252. Eschenauer GA, Kwak EJ, Humar A, Potoski BA, Clarke LG, Shields RK, et al. Targeted versus universal antifungal prophylaxis among liver transplant recipients. Am J Transplant. 2015;15(1):180–9.
253. Giannella M, Bartoletti M, Morelli M, Cristini F, Tedeschi S, Campoli C, et al. Antifungal prophylaxis in liver transplant recipients: one size does not fit all. Transpl Infect Dis. 2016;18(4):538–44.
254. Dummer JS, Lazariashvilli N, Barnes J, Ninan M, Milstone AP. A survey of anti-fungal management in lung transplantation. J Heart Lung Transplant. 2004;23(12):1376–81.
255. Husain S, Zaldonis D, Kusne S, Kwak EJ, Paterson DL, McCurry KR. Variation in antifungal prophylaxis strategies in lung transplantation. Transpl Infect Dis. 2006;8(4):213–8.
256. Neoh CF, Snell GI, Kotsimbos T, Levvey B, Morrissey CO, Slavin MA, et al. Antifungal prophylaxis in lung transplantation--a world-wide survey. Am J Transplant. 2011;11(2):361–6.
257. Reichenspurner H, Gamberg P, Nitschke M, Valantine H, Hunt S, Oyer PE, et al. Significant reduction in the number of fungal infections after lung-, heart-lung, and heart transplantation using aerosolized amphotericin B prophylaxis. Transplant Proc. 1997;29(1–2):627–8.
258. Monforte V, Roman A, Gavalda J, Bravo C, Tenorio L, Ferrer A, et al. Nebulized amphotericin B prophylaxis for Aspergillus infection in lung transplantation: study of risk factors. J Heart Lung Transplant. 2001;20(12):1274–81.
259. Palmer SM, Drew RH, Whitehouse JD, Tapson VF, Davis RD, McConnell RR, et al. Safety of aerosolized amphotericin B lipid complex in lung transplant recipients. Transplantation. 2001;72(3):545–8.
260. Drew RH, Dodds Ashley E, Benjamin DK Jr, Duane Davis R, Palmer SM, Perfect JR. Comparative safety of amphotericin B lipid complex and amphotericin B deoxycholate as aerosolized antifungal prophylaxis in lung-transplant recipients. Transplantation. 2004;77(2):232–7.

261. Monforte V, Ussetti P, Gavalda J, Bravo C, Laporta R, Len O, et al. Feasibility, tolerability, and outcomes of nebulized liposomal amphotericin B for Aspergillus infection prevention in lung transplantation. J Heart Lung Transplant. 2010;29(5):523–30.
262. Husain S, Capitano B, Corcoran T, Studer SM, Crespo M, Johnson B, et al. Intrapulmonary disposition of amphotericin B after aerosolized delivery of amphotericin B lipid complex (Abelcet; ABLC) in lung transplant recipients. Transplantation. 2010;90(11):1215–9.
263. Minari A, Husni R, Avery RK, Longworth DL, DeCamp M, Bertin M, et al. The incidence of invasive aspergillosis among solid organ transplant recipients and implications for prophylaxis in lung transplants. Transpl Infect Dis. 2002;4(4):195–200.
264. Husain S, Paterson DL, Studer S, Pilewski J, Crespo M, Zaldonis D, et al. Voriconazole prophylaxis in lung transplant recipients. Am J Transplant. 2006;6(12):3008–16.
265. Cadena J, Levine DJ, Angel LF, Maxwell PR, Brady R, Sanchez JF, et al. Antifungal prophylaxis with voriconazole or itraconazole in lung transplant recipients: hepatotoxicity and effectiveness. Am J Transplant. 2009;9(9):2085–91.
266. Miller R, Assi M, AST Infectious Diseases Community of Practice. Endemic fungal infections in solid organ transplantation. Am J Transplant. 2013;13(Suppl 4):250–61.
267. Wheat LJ, Freifeld AG, Kleiman MB, Baddley JW, McKinsey DS, Loyd JE, et al. Clinical practice guidelines for the management of patients with histoplasmosis: 2007 update by the Infectious Diseases Society of America. Clin Infect Dis. 2007;45(7):807–25.
268. Avery RK, Michaels MG, AST Infectious Diseases Community of Practice. Strategies for safe living after solid organ transplantation. Am J Transplant. 2013;13(Suppl 4):304–10.
269. Lund BM, O'Brien SJ. The occurrence and prevention of foodborne disease in vulnerable people. Foodborne Pathog Dis. 2011;8(9):961–73.
270. FSIS/USDA. Food safety for transplant recipients. 2006 [updated 2011 Sept, cited 2016 Aug 23]. Available from: http://www.fda.gov/Food/FoodborneIllnessContaminants/PeopleAtRisk/ucm312570.htm.

Candida Infections in Hematopoietic and Solid Organ Transplant Recipients

32

Alison G. Freifeld and Carol A. Kauffman

Introduction

Candida spp. are a major cause of morbidity and mortality among immunocompromised patients, especially recipients of hematopoietic stem cell transplant (HCT) or solid organ transplants (SOT). *Candida* spp. are the most common etiology of fungal infections in SOT recipients and the second most common among HCT recipients, after aspergillosis [1, 2]. Clinical signs of candidiasis range from mucosal colonization to invasive and/or systemic fungal disease. Candidemia is the most common manifestation of invasive candidiasis. Deep tissue *Candida* infections, including intra-abdominal abscesses, hepatosplenic, and urinary tract infections, are less common than candidemia, but they cause important syndromes in SOT and HCT patients. The immunosuppressive agents required to prevent organ rejection or graft-versus-host disease in transplant recipients can blunt immune responses to *Candida* spp. and predispose transplant recipients to developing invasive candidiasis. Other general risk factors include neutropenia, systemic antibiotic exposure, central venous catheters, parenteral nutrition, renal or hepatic insufficiency, a prolonged intensive care unit (ICU) stay, treatment with systemic corticosteroids, GVHD, immunosuppressive antirejection therapy, etc.

The diagnosis of invasive candidiasis is often hampered by the low sensitivity of traditional blood culture techniques for *Candida* spp. and by the lack of specific clinical findings associated with candidemia or deep tissue infection. Presenting clinical signs include fever, leukocytosis, and, less commonly, hypotension, none of which differentiate between *Candida* and bacterial infections. Furthermore, distinguishing *Candida* colonization, which is very common, from invasive disease complicates accurate diagnosis. Due to these confounding factors, reliable longitudinal incidence data about fungal infections have been difficult to obtain. The Mycoses Study Group (MSG) and the European Organisation for Research in Treatment of Cancer (EORTC) have provided consensus definitions for the diagnosis of invasive mycoses including candidiasis (Table 32.1) [3]. These definitions are now widely used and have greatly clarified epidemiologic, clinical, and drug susceptibility data, as they provide a common basis for diagnosing mycoses.

With the expanding repertoire of medical and surgical transplantation approaches that require adjunctive immunosuppression, it is not surprising that a recent study found that the incidence of systemic *Candida* infections has been rising in recent years [4]. Disturbingly, it was also found that despite the availability of potent antifungal agents, outcomes have not improved concomitantly. Candidemia remains one of the deadliest causes of bloodstream infection, with an attributable mortality rate ranging from 20 to 40% [5–7].The clinical manifestations, diagnostic methods, and antifungal prophylaxis and treatment approaches to *Candida* infections in transplant patients are reviewed herein to help clinicians in the management and prevention of these infections.

Pathogenesis and Risk Factors

Candida colonization of skin, gut, and mucosal surfaces is a frequent prerequisite for the development of invasive disease. *Candida* species colonize the oropharynx, axillary, groin, perineal skin folds, and genital and intestinal mucosa of 30–70% of healthy individuals, notably without causing any illness [8]. Effective and intact host immunological mechanisms prevent invasion and permit microorganisms to exist innocuously on mucosal and skin surfaces. Perturbations of this host-pathogen interaction at the mucosal surfaces can lead to oral thrush, colonic overgrowth, and

A. G. Freifeld (✉)
Infectious Diseases Division, University of Nebraska Medical Center, Omaha, NE, USA
e-mail: afreifeld@unmc.edu

C. A. Kauffman
University of Michigan Medical School, Infectious Diseases Section, Veterans Affairs Ann Arbor Healthcare System, Ann Arbor, MI, USA
e-mail: ckauff@umich.edu

A. Safdar (ed.), *Principles and Practice of Transplant Infectious Diseases*, https://doi.org/10.1007/978-1-4939-9034-4_32

Table 32.1 MSG/EORTC definitions for the diagnosis of proven or probable invasive candidiasis [3]

Proven	Histopathologic, cytopathologic, or direct microscopic examination of a specimen obtained by needle aspiration or biopsy from a normally sterile site (other than mucous membranes) showing yeast cells, pseudohyphae, or true hyphae compatible with *Candida* spp. Recovery of a *Candida* spp. by culture of a sample obtained by a sterile procedure (including a freshly placed [<24 h ago] drain) from a normally sterile site showing a clinical or radiological abnormality consistent with an infectious disease process. Blood culture that yields *Candida* spp.
Probable	Disseminated candidiasis: at least one of the following two entities is identified after an episode of candidemia within the previous 2 weeks: Small, target-like abscesses (bull's-eye lesions) in the liver or spleen on CT and/or ultrasound Progressive retinal exudates on ophthalmologic examination

Modified from De Pauw et al. [3]

candiduria. These conditions are usually benign and readily treated, but further immunologic and physical impairments of skin or mucosal barriers may allow entry of colonizing yeast into the bloodstream or tissues.

Mucosal damage due to radiation or chemotherapy in HCT recipients and surgical wounds or incompetent anastomotic sites in SOT recipients are examples of barrier breaches that predispose to tissue infiltration by colonizing *Candida* spp. Indwelling intravenous catheters are ubiquitous in recently transplanted patients, and they create an important portal of entry for *Candida* into the bloodstream. The foreign materials comprising venous catheters appear to inhibit immune cell function, allowing uninhibited fungal growth on internal and external surfaces. Furthermore, *Candida* is able to produce a complex polysaccharide biofilm on these foreign surfaces, creating a protective matrix around the yeast and hyphal forms that grow inside [9, 10]. Parenteral nutrition via an indwelling venous catheter is linked to development of candidemia, perhaps due to enhanced yeast growth by component nutrients [11, 12]. *Candida* derived from contaminated organ preservative fluids postharvest is a rare source of infection in SOT recipients [13, 14].

Immunosuppressive drugs, particularly corticosteroids, are key risk factors for serious *Candida* infections [15–17]. They can significantly impair lymphocyte and neutrophil recognition and attack functions needed to eradicate *Candida* yeast and hyphal forms. Furthermore, co-colonizing bacteria at skin and mucosal sites appear to help control yeast numbers through competition for nutrients. Bacterial production of toxic substances such as hydrogen peroxide, lactic acid, and bacteriocins may also serve to keep local concentrations of colonizing *Candida* low [18]. However, when these resident bacterial populations are reduced by systemic broad-spectrum antibiotic treatment, as so often happens in transplant patients, yeast colonization increases, creating an increased opportunity for systemic invasion [9]. Other risk factors include renal insufficiency, dialysis, cytomegalovirus reactivation, overall severity of illness, mechanical ventilation, prolonged ICU stay, and malnutrition (Table 32.2).

Initial host responses to yeast invasion are mediated by the innate immune system. This rapidly active, evolutionarily ancient and conserved pathway is based on the broad recognition of fungal-specific small molecular targets (pathogen-associated molecular patterns, PAMPs) by host cell surface pattern recognition receptors (PRRs) that are located on phagocytes (granulocytes, monocytes/macrophages) and dendritic cells [19, 20]. Subsequent activation of intracellular signaling pathways and stimulation of inflammatory mediators then lead to an accumulation of inflammatory effector cells at the site of *Candida* invasion. Neutrophils and macrophages are the critical effector cells responsible for phagocytosis and killing of *Candida* through both oxidative and non-oxidative mechanisms. Accordingly, a lack of these key cells (i.e., neutropenia) occurring as a consequence of cytotoxic chemotherapy, underlying hematologic malignancy, or any other etiology is a strong risk factor for the development of invasive *Candida* infections [9].

Table 32.2 Risk factors for invasive candidiasis

Host factors	Medical interventions
Neutropenia	Cytotoxic cancer chemotherapy
Extremes of age	Dialysis
Renal failure	Central venous catheter or nasogastric tube
Trauma or burns	Prior antibiotic use
Bowel perforation	Prior surgery (especially abdominal)
High APACHE II score	Parenteral nutrition
Candida colonization	ICU stay >7 days

Epidemiology

Candida species are the fourth leading cause of hospital-acquired bloodstream infection (BSI) in the United States, accounting for nearly 10% of all healthcare-associated BSIs [21]. Data from the Transplant-Associated Infection Surveillance Network (TRANSNET), a consortium of 23 transplant centers in the United States that prospectively studied the epidemiology of invasive fungal infections in SOT and HCT recipients from 2001 to 2006, revealed that, in the SOT cohort, invasive candidiasis had the highest 12-month cumulative incidence (1.9%) followed by invasive aspergillosis (0.7%) [2]. Similarly, in the HCT TRANSNET cohort, the cumulative incidence was 1.1% at 12 months for invasive candidiasis [1]. Crude mortality rates for *Candida* bloodstream infections, the most common form of invasive candidiasis, have often been reported to be more than 30% [6, 22–24]. Longitudinal studies indicate that despite advances in diagnosis and antifungal therapy, there has been no overall decline in either incidence or mortality associated with invasive candidiasis in the last decade [2, 4, 25, 26].

The timing and incidence of *Candida* infections vary by type of organ or hematopoietic cell transplant procedure, as well as by prior antifungal therapy, transplant center, time post-transplant, and aforementioned patient risk factors [1, 2, 15]. Most episodes of candidiasis occur early after SOT or HCT, generally within the first 2–3 months. Later episodes post-transplant are largely related to the use of corticosteroids and other immunosuppressive drugs for graft rejection in SOT or for graft-versus-host disease in HCT recipients [17, 27, 28].

Abdominal organ transplant recipients have the highest rates of invasive candidiasis among patients undergoing organ transplantation; rates of infection are highest in those receiving small bowel, liver, pancreas, or multi-organ transplants [29–33]. Candidemia predominates in this group and is often related to a vascular access device source [17]. Intra-abdominal candidiasis (e.g., peritoneal and biliary infection) is also common, however, and likely due to bile or intestinal fluid leakage during biliary anastomosis or translocation of intestinal flora into peritoneal fluid. Technical difficulty and prolonged time of abdominal surgery, primary graft failure, and early surgical re-exploration contribute to the risk of invasive candidiasis after abdominal organ transplantation [15, 31, 32]. Liver recipients appear to be especially susceptible to candidiasis, and higher risk is conferred by a number of pre- and postoperative factors, including choledochojejunostomy anastomosis, preoperative renal failure/dialysis, low serum albumin, CMV viremia, substantial infusions of intraoperative cellular blood products, as well as re-transplantation and surgical re-exploration after transplantation [29, 31, 32]. Enteric drainage in pancreas transplant recipients predisposes to a greater risk of invasive candidiasis than does bladder drainage [34]. Candidiasis is relatively infrequent among kidney transplant recipients, and it typically occurs later in the first year post-transplant [17]. A syndrome of early, within 1 month, graft-transmitted candidiasis resulting in fungal arteritis, with high morbidity and mortality after renal transplantation, is related to organ contamination during recovery of the donor kidney [13]. A recent study showed the overall incidence of candidiasis was 4.8% in heart and 8.3% in lung plus heart-lung transplant recipients and that the incidence has declined dramatically over the last 20 years. Candidemia was most often seen following heart transplant while tracheobronchitis due to *Candida* species was a more common manifestation in lung transplant recipients [35, 36].

The overall incidence of *Candida* infection, which is primarily candidemia, in HCT recipients is low, about 1% overall. Notably, the incidence is similar between autologous (1.2%) and allogeneic (0.8%) HCT [28]. The widespread use of antifungal prophylaxis may be credited with this reduction in invasive candidiasis in HCT populations over the last 20 years. In allogeneic HCT patients, two periods of risk for invasive candidiasis and other invasive fungal infections are identified: pre-engraftment and, subsequently, in the first 100 days post-engraftment. During the pre-engraftment period, mucositis, broad-spectrum antibiotics, and neutropenia are significant risk factors, but fluconazole prophylaxis effectively prevents most *C. albicans* infections. However, fluconazole prophylaxis clearly plays a significant role in the increase in breakthrough infections with non-*albicans* species that have lower azole susceptibility [26–28]. The second risk period is post-engraftment after allogeneic HCT, in the setting of GVHD. Corticosteroid use and CMV reactivation during GVHD treatment are both linked to increases in bacterial and fungal infections. In autologous transplantation, virtually all candidemias occur during pre-engraftment and are related to indwelling central venous catheters.

Candida albicans has traditionally been the most frequently isolated yeast pathogen. An important epidemiologic phenomenon over the last two decades has been the well-documented shift from *C. albicans* to non-*albicans Candida* as the most common infecting *Candida* species in some tertiary care centers [6, 37, 38]. This shift is especially prominent in immunosuppressed populations and is of great concern because *Candida glabrata* and *Candida krusei* are relatively or totally resistant to many azole agents, respectively. Increasing resistance to these agents limits their utility for both prophylaxis and treatment in immunosuppressed patients. Between 2001 and 2007 at MD Anderson Cancer Center, 75% of invasive candidiasis cases that occurred in patients with hematologic malignancy or undergoing HCT were due to non-*albicans Candida* species [26]. In the TRANSNET cohort, only 20% of isolates from HCT recipients were *C. albicans*. In this population, the majority of isolates were non-*albicans* species: *C. glabrata* (34%), *C. parapsilosis* (21%), or *C. krusei* (15%) [39]. *C. krusei* is intrinsically resistant to fluconazole but remains susceptible to voriconazole and to echinocandins. The routine use of azole prophylaxis in high-risk cancer populations, particularly in allogeneic HCT recipients, has been responsible for a decrease in invasive candidiasis, but it is also undoubtedly responsible for the rise in non-*albicans Candida* infections [26, 27, 40].

In the SOT population, *C. albicans* remains the most frequently isolated *Candida* species, although a shift toward more non-*albicans Candida* infections has been identified in two nationwide surveys [6, 39]. In the TRANSNET SOT cohort, *C. glabrata* accounted for 30%

of all isolates and *C. parapsilosis* for 9% [39]. Overall, 16% of the 915 *Candida* isolates from this SOT cohort, including several *C. tropicalis* and *C. albicans* isolates, were fluconazole resistant. Prior fluconazole use was a significant risk factor for nonsusceptibility to the drug. Clinicians should be especially aware of the relative or intrinsic fluconazole resistance patterns of *C. glabrata and C. krusei* in transplant populations. Since these and most other non-*albicans* isolates are typically susceptible to echinocandins, it is recommended that an echinocandin be initiated when yeast is isolated in blood cultures, pending species identification.

Clinical Manifestations

Candidemia

Candidemia simply means *Candida* species in the blood. Candidemia can be a transient event associated with colonization of an indwelling central venous catheter, but it is also the most common manifestation of disseminated infection involving multiple organs. The initial clinical presentation of these two different events may be similar; thus, one can never assume that an episode of candidemia is a transient event not requiring antifungal therapy. The clinical manifestations vary from mild fever to symptoms and signs of overwhelming sepsis that include hypotension, tachypnea, tachycardia, and confusion. The initial presentation is non-localizing, but focal signs later point to specific organ involvement. The appearance of multiple pustular skin lesions is a manifestation of widespread disseminated infection. Symptoms and signs associated with candidemia are the same, irrespective of the causative *Candida* species, and they mimic those seen with bacteremia. At autopsy, in severely immunosuppressed patients, widespread infection is characterized by microabscesses noted in many organs.

In SOT recipients, indwelling venous catheters and intra-abdominal processes related to surgery are likely sources for candidemia. In HCT patients, the greatest risk for candidemia is when neutropenia is present or during periods of maximum immune suppression during treatment of GVHD. Often, the source of the organisms is the gut because of damage to the mucosa from chemotherapy, but it can also be from indwelling central venous catheters that are present in almost all HCT patients.

A recent retrospective review of bloodstream infections in hospitalized patients found that mixed infections including bacteria plus *Candida* spp. are very rare, accounting for about 0.7% of all bloodstream infections. Outcomes from these mixed infections were similar to those with candidemia alone [41].

Hepatosplenic (Chronic Disseminated) Candidiasis

This form of invasive candidiasis is seen almost entirely in patients who have hematological cancers and who have been previously neutropenic. HCT recipients can manifest this form of candidiasis after engraftment when they have a return of their neutrophils, but more often, this syndrome occurs in the course of chemotherapy for acute leukemia before transplantation occurs [42]. *C. albicans* is the most likely pathogen, but all species have been found to cause this syndrome. The return of neutrophils triggers the symptoms of high fever, right upper quadrant discomfort, nausea, and fatigue. The symptoms can persist for weeks, but blood cultures usually remain negative. There may be documentation of a previous episode of candidemia, but in many patients, candidemia had not been documented. Imaging studies reveal the characteristic punched out lesions representing multiple small abscesses throughout the liver and the spleen. It has been postulated that hepatosplenic candidiasis could represent a form of immune reconstitution inflammatory syndrome (IRIS) because cultures from lesions often are negative, the illness begins when neutrophils return to normal levels, and symptoms respond to corticosteroids when they are added to antifungal agents [42].

Intra-abdominal Infections

Intra-abdominal infections with *Candida* species are usually seen in the immediate postoperative period in SOT recipients, especially those who received a liver, pancreas, or small bowel transplant [34, 43]. Infections are generally polymicrobial, involving facultative aerobic and anaerobic bacteria from the bowel, along with yeasts. *C. albicans* and *C. glabrata* are the yeasts most commonly isolated. The usual source is perforation of the bowel or mechanical problems with the anastomosis of the biliary tract in liver transplant recipients. The symptoms of intra-abdominal infection include fever, chills, abdominal pain, and distention; if the biliary tract is obstructed, nausea, vomiting, and jaundice occur. Signs of peritonitis may be present, especially with bowel perforation, and focal pain and fevers occur when a localized abscess is present. Imaging is essential to define the site of infection.

Biliary stents are often required after liver transplantation. When these devices remain in place for long periods, they are often colonized persistently with *Candida* species. A complication of this colonization is development of fungus balls, which can cause further obstruction and require revision of the stent [44].

Neutropenic enterocolitis is a life-threatening abdominal complication that occurs rarely after intensive chemotherapy for acute leukemias and solid tumors. Gram-negative bacteria are the most common cause, but a recent review of published cases showed that the pooled frequency of fungal involvement in neutropenic enterocolitis from all reported patients was calculated to be 6.2% [45]. The vast majority was due to *Candida* spp. Antifungal coverage should be considered in the setting of neutropenic enterocolitis although bacteria are the predominant pathogens.

Urinary Tract Infections

Candiduria is common, but symptomatic urinary tract infections are uncommon in transplant recipients [46]. Many transplant recipients have candiduria in the postoperative period because of the use of indwelling urinary catheters and broad-spectrum antibiotics. The most common species found in the urine are *C. albicans* and *C. glabrata* [46]. Previously, it was thought that candiduria contributed to poor outcomes among kidney transplant recipients, and it was standard practice to treat with fluconazole when candiduria was documented. However, it has been shown in a large, nested, case-control study that those who had candiduria had a higher mortality rate, but the candiduria did not contribute to death, and treatment of candiduria had no effect on outcomes [47]. In this study, as in others, it was thought that candiduria merely was a marker for the severity of underlying illness [48].

Although most patients with candiduria have colonization of the bladder and do not require treatment, ascending infection leading to pyelonephritis can occur, especially in a kidney transplant recipient. In this case, symptoms of dysuria, frequency, and pain over the transplanted kidney will be present and may be accompanied by systemic signs of infection, such as chills, fever, and malaise. These patients require prompt treatment with an antifungal agent, almost always fluconazole. Patients who have candiduria and require ureteral stent placement are at increased risk for persistent *Candida* colonization of the stent and kidney infection.

An uncommon manifestation of *Candida* infection seen specifically in kidney transplant recipients is infection of the graft. This is manifested most often by fungal arteritis with aneurysm formation at the anastomosis site and less often as a graft site abscess [13]. In this circumstance, it has been shown that the kidney was infected at the time it was harvested from the donor, and this infection was directly transmitted with the organ to the recipient. The outcomes are poor with loss of the graft in the majority of patients.

The situation is different in HCT recipients who are neutropenic and who have candiduria. In these patients, candiduria may well be a marker for invasive candidiasis [49]. Symptoms are minimal if the patient is neutropenic and cannot be relied upon to define infection. In this circumstance, treatment is appropriate.

Pulmonary Candidiasis

Candida species rarely cause pneumonia. HCT patients who are markedly immunosuppressed can develop diffuse nodular infiltrates as part of widely disseminated candidiasis, but this is uncommon [50, 51]. In this type of patient, it is more common for pneumonia to be due to molds. Most patients have pulmonary involvement with *Candida* species discovered at autopsy. Sputum and bronchoalveolar lavage samples that yield *Candida* species have low specificity and should not be interpreted as evidence of invasive disease. Lung biopsy is needed to establish the diagnosis of *Candida* pneumonia [52].

Tracheobronchitis due to *Candida* species is the most common form of invasive candidiasis in lung and heart-lung transplant recipients [36]. Patients present with fever, productive cough, and shortness of breath; exam may reveal labored breathing and scattered rhonchi can be heard. Visualization of the airway by bronchoscopy and histologic confirmation are the usual methods of diagnosis.

Endophthalmitis

Endogenous *Candida* endophthalmitis occurs when the organism is hematogenously seeded into the highly vascular choroid layer of the eye [53]. It is not more common in the transplant population than in others who have been candidemic. The most common organism causing this infection is *C. albicans*, but all species have been reported to cause ocular infection [54]. Treatment is most effective if given early in the course of infection. Because the length of therapy and choice of antifungal agent for candidemia will vary if endophthalmitis is present, the Infectious Diseases Society of America (IDSA) guidelines for the management of invasive candidiasis recommend that a dilated ophthalmoscopic examination be performed on all patients who have candidemia to establish whether ocular involvement is present [7]. In patients who have neutropenia, it is recommended that a retinal examination be repeated after neutropenia resolves when lesions are more likely to be manifested [7]. Patients may have no complaints early in the course when typical white lesions are seen in the retina. If not found at this stage, patients seek attention later for changes in visual acuity; at this point, extension to the vitreous is common, and active vitritis is seen on examination. Treatment is more difficult, and the outcomes are less good at this stage of the infection.

Less Common Invasive *Candida* Infections

Endocarditis, osteomyelitis, and meningitis are uncommon complications of candidemia. None of these occur with greater frequency in transplant recipients than in other patients who have had candidemia. The clue to the presence of endocarditis is persistently positive blood cultures with or without manifestations of cardiac dysfunction or peripheral stigmata of endocarditis [55]. The vegetations tend to be large, and the disease may present with an embolus to a major vessel. All species have been implicated, but most commonly, endocarditis is due to *C. albicans* or *C. parapsilosis*. Echocardiographic studies are essential for establishing the diagnosis and defining valvular dysfunction and complications, such as paravalvular abscesses.

Osteomyelitis as a result of hematogenous spread usually involves the vertebral column [56]. The disc space is seeded during the course of candidemia, and then extension to the adjacent vertebral bodies occurs. Patients often do not develop symptoms until weeks after the candidemic episode, and then back pain is the main complaint. CT and MRI imaging studies are essential to identify infection, and needle aspiration or open biopsy, when feasible, are essential to define this process as due to *Candida*.

Candida meningitis, a common finding in neonates who have invasive candidiasis, is very uncommon in adults [57]. The manifestations vary from an acute presentation to a subacute process similar to that seen with cryptococcosis. This complication of invasive candidiasis can occur at the time of candidemia or several weeks later with the subacute form. Symptoms are headache, visual symptoms, and confusion; examination shows mild nuchal rigidity, occasionally papilledema, and lethargy, confusion, or stupor. Diagnosis is made by lumbar puncture after a CT or MRI scan to rule out an associated brain abscess.

Mucosal Candidiasis

Oropharyngeal candidiasis (thrush) is a superficial infection that used to be extremely common in transplant recipients, but is seen infrequently now because of the routine use of fluconazole for prophylaxis against fungal infections in these patients. Patients are often asymptomatic, but may complain of a cottony feeling in their mouth or pharyngeal pain when they swallow. Older patients who wear upper dentures are at increased risk for denture stomatitis due to *Candida*. Examination reveals white, plaque-like lesions on the buccal mucosa, tongue, and palate. Ulcerations are unusual and are usually due to mucositis or atypical herpes infections, and not *Candida*. Patients with denture stomatitis have erythema of the hard palate but no plaques.

Candida vaginitis is a very common infection in the general population and can be problematic in patients who are immunosuppressed. Vaginal discharge, vulvar pruritus, and dysuria are common manifestations. The discharge may be curd-like, but also can be thin. Examination shows vulvar erythema and plaque-like lesions on the vaginal mucosa.

Esophagitis is usually manifested by odynophagia; patients can generally point to a specific substernal area where they experience pain with swallowing. The patient may or may not have concomitant thrush. Endoscopy is diagnostic, but most physicians initiate treatment with an oral azole based on the clinical symptoms and make the diagnosis by noting a therapeutic response within several days.

Outcomes

Invasive candidiasis is associated with high crude mortality rates [6, 15, 22–24]. For many patients, *Candida* infection is a marker for serious underlying illness, but is not the cause of death. Attributable mortality has been difficult to evaluate, and estimates have varied from 30 to 62% in the general hospital population [58, 59]. Multicenter surveillance studies have provided crude, but not attributable mortality rates for candidiasis in transplant recipients [1, 2, 15]. A prospective observational study in French ICUs found that independent factors associated with mortality from invasive candidiasis included diabetes mellitus, immunosuppression, and mechanical ventilation [60], whereas a study that included all hospitalized patients in four medical centers in Sao Paulo, Brazil, found the highest risk factors were advanced age and high APACHE II score [24]. The association of a high APACHE II score and increased mortality in patients with candidemia has been noted by others, as has increased mortality with increasing age [22, 38].

Several studies have shown that prompt treatment of candidemia significantly decreases the mortality rate, and delay for as long as 48 h after the blood culture is performed is associated with increased mortality [61, 62]. A recent study noted a crude mortality rate of 63.5% among patients who had septic shock associated with candidemia [63]. In those in whom antifungal therapy was given within 24 h and who had adequate source control (removal of catheters, drainage of abscesses), the mortality rate was 52.8%; for those in whom these parameters were not met, the mortality was 97.6%.

Mortality appears to be higher in patients with candidemia due to *C. krusei*, but this likely reflects the fact that this species is seen most often in patients who have hematological malignancies or have received an HCT [6, 64]. *C. tropicalis* is known to be more virulent in animal models and has also been associated with worse outcomes in immunosuppressed patients, especially those who have a hematological malignancy [65]. Mortality associated with candidemia due to *C. parapsilosis* appears to be consistently lower than that found with other species [22, 66, 67]. In some studies, mortality rates for patients who have *C. glabrata* fungemia have been noted to be higher than that seen with *C. albicans* [6], but in other studies, there was no difference or the rates were lower [22, 68, 69]. In general, the most important factors for outcome in transplant recipients are the extent of immunosuppression and the susceptibility of the organism to antifungal agents, rather than the virulence factors of the specific species causing infection.

Diagnosis

The diagnosis of invasive candidiasis requires clinical suspicion that *Candida* infection could be the cause of a patient's symptoms. The manifestations are similar to those seen with many bacterial infections, but several clinical clues should raise suspicion for candidemia and invasive candidiasis. The sudden appearance of non-tender, non-pruritic skin lesions is a strong clue to the presence of fungemia with *Candida* species. The lesions vary from a few millimeters to a centimeter in diameter and are usually manifested as a pustule on an erythematous base (Fig. 32.1). Similarly, a new complaint of focal muscle pain with tenderness noted on palpation should raise suspicion for the possibility of invasive candidiasis in an immunosuppressed host. Eye pain or visual loss should prompt an immediate workup for endogenous *Candida* endophthalmitis resulting from candidemia.

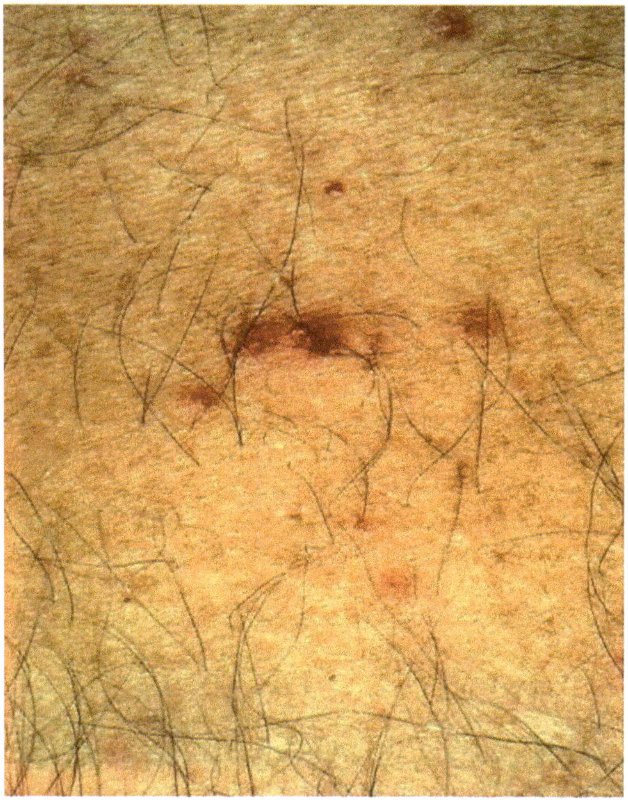

Fig. 32.1 Skin lesions that developed on the back of a 65 year-old man who was neutropenic after receiving an allogeneic stem cell transplant. Blood cultures yielded *C. albicans*

Cultures

By definition, candidemia is the presence of *Candida* species in the bloodstream, and this is usually established by growth of the organism in cultures obtained from blood. At least two sets of blood cultures from a peripheral vein should be obtained, and if the patient has a central venous catheter in place, blood also should be taken from the catheter for culture. The automated blood culture systems routinely used in most hospital laboratories are able to isolate *Candida* species, but it takes a minimum of 1–3 days for growth to occur. Overall, blood cultures are relatively insensitive, and invasive disease can be present without blood cultures yielding the organism.

After growth occurs in blood culture bottles, it generally takes another 1–2 days for the organism to be identified to the species level. This delay can be shortened with the use of several new techniques. One technique uses peptide nucleic acid fluorescence in situ hybridization (PNA-FISH), which can identify *C. albicans* and *C. glabrata* within several hours of a blood culture turning positive [70, 71]. Another technique uses mass spectrometry to quickly identify species of yeast once growth has occurred in blood culture bottles [72]. It is essential to identify *Candida* to the species level in all cases of candidemia and invasive disease because of differences in susceptibility to antifungal agents among the various species. It is especially important to identify *C. glabrata* and *C. krusei* because of resistance to fluconazole and other azoles [25, 73].

Candida species are part of the human microbiota, so that growth of yeasts from samples obtained from non-sterile sites documents only colonization. For example, sputum and bronchoalveolar lavage fluid cultures yielding *Candida* species cannot be used to establish a diagnosis of *Candida* pneumonia. However, finding organisms in lung tissue obtained by biopsy establishes the diagnosis. Growth of yeast from material aspirated through an indwelling drainage tube almost always reflects colonization of the tube and not what is in an abscess. In contrast, growth of *Candida* species from normally sterile body fluids, such as cerebrospinal fluid or synovial fluid, establishes a diagnosis of invasive candidiasis. Material obtained by biopsy of a newly developed skin lesion or a muscle abscess should be submitted for culture and also for histopathological examination with special stains to detect fungi-invading tissues.

Non-Culture-Based Techniques

Substantial work has gone into the development of non-culture-based techniques to enhance the rapid diagnosis of candidemia and invasive candidiasis. These include antigen detection and DNA-based techniques.

Several different assays are commercially available to detect the presence of beta-D-glucan, a cell wall component of many fungi, not just *Candida* species. Many studies have been performed, and results show wide variations in sensitivity and specificity of this assay. A recent meta-analysis that included 16 studies with a total of 2979 patients who had probable or proven invasive fungal infections, not just *Candida* infections, calculated that the pooled sensitivity of the assay was 77% and specificity was 85% [74]. There was large heterogeneity among studies, including the use of different commercial products for the assay, different cutoff points for positivity, and different patient populations. When these investigators analyzed the 295 patients who were identified as having invasive candidiasis in 11 different studies, the sensitivity appeared to be 75%; it is not clear how many of these patients were transplant recipients. A study among 20 lung transplant recipients found modest sensitivity (71%) and poor specificity (59%) [75], and another in liver transplant recipients found poor sensitivity (58%) and moderately good specificity (83%) [74]. All studies have noted that this assay has poor positive predictive value and good negative predictive value.

Real-time PCR techniques continue to hold promise for rapid diagnosis, but to date, there is no standardized PCR test commercially available for the diagnosis of candidiasis [76]. Newer studies suggest that this technique may be more sensitive than both blood cultures and the beta-D-glucan assay for the diagnosis of invasive candidiasis [77]. A new more rapid system uses magnetic biosensor technology to identify different *Candida* species from whole blood [78].

Histopathology

Histopathology is used less often in the diagnosis of candidiasis than in the diagnosis of mold infections, most likely because *Candida* species are easily grown in the laboratory. Tissue biopsy with histopathological examination of skin lesions is useful for documenting disseminated infection

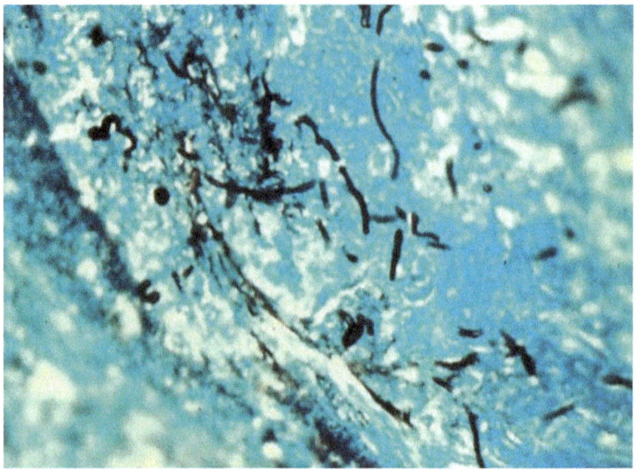

Fig. 32.2 Silver stain performed on the biopsy of a skin lesion shown in Fig. 32.1. Both yeast forms and hyphae, the typical picture noted with *C. albicans*, are present in the biopsy

(Fig. 32.2). Lung biopsy is essential for diagnosis of *Candida* pneumonia, and liver biopsy can document hepatosplenic *Candida* infection as cultures often fail to grow. Silver stains are used most often to visualize the yeast and hyphal elements that are usually both seen with tissue invasion. One cannot differentiate species of *Candida* by tissue biopsy, but it should be noted that *C. glabrata* remains a yeast in tissues and cannot produce hyphae.

Imaging Studies

In contrast to mold infections, imaging techniques are not useful in the diagnosis of infections due to *Candida*. The one exception is hepatosplenic candidiasis (chronic disseminated candidiasis), which occurs almost entirely in patients who are recovering from an episode of neutropenia. In this form of invasive candidiasis, ultrasound, computerized tomography (CT) scans, and magnetic resonance imaging (MRI) all are useful to establish the diagnosis [79]. The picture is characteristic, especially on CT scan, the modality used most often for this type of candidiasis. Multiple, discrete low-attenuation lesions representing small abscesses are typically seen in the liver, spleen, and, sometimes, kidneys and other organs (Fig. 32.3). Similarly, CT scans are useful for visualizing small abscesses that can occur in muscles during an episode of candidemia (Fig. 32.4).

Imaging studies are extremely useful for patients who have focal *Candida* infections. Examples include the use of trans-esophageal echocardiography to help establish the diagnosis and define the extent of disease in a patient with *Candida* endocarditis. CT or MRI scans are essential for evaluation

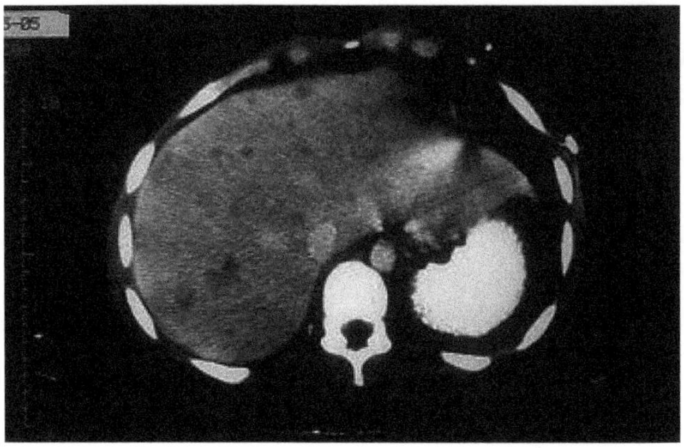

Fig. 32.3 Abdominal CT scan of a 25-year-old patient who had been neutropenic during induction therapy for acute leukemia and developed nausea, fever, and pain in the right upper quadrant. Discrete punched out lesions are evident throughout the liver, which is typical for hepatosplenic candidiasis

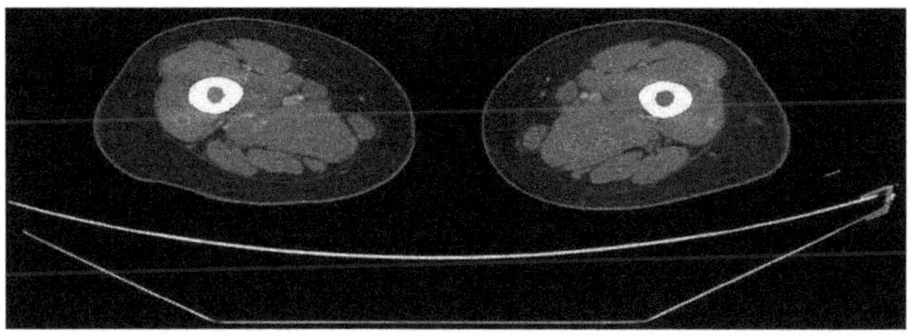

Fig. 32.4 CT scan of the thigh muscles of a 31-year-old woman who had undergone an allogeneic stem cell transplant and who developed muscle tenderness and persistent fever following *C. tropicalis* fungemia that was identified several days before. Multiple ring-enhancing lesions are noted

of abscesses and hydrocephalus in patients with central nervous system candidiasis and to define the presence of vertebral osteomyelitis due to *Candida* species. Additionally, ultrasound and CT scans are used routinely to define the location and response to therapy of polymicrobial bacterial/fungal intra-abdominal abscesses that occur in the postoperative period in recipients of small bowel, liver, or pancreas transplants.

Treatment

The treatment of *Candida* infections has changed markedly in the last 10–15 years. Amphotericin B is now rarely used, and most patients are treated with an echinocandin or an azole. As a result, toxicity is much less frequently seen. Guidelines for the treatment of candidemia and invasive candidiasis have been established by the IDSA, and these guidelines are applicable to transplant recipients, as well as other patient populations [7]. The American Society of Transplantation (AST) also has issued guidelines for treatment of *Candida* infections in SOT recipients [80].

Candidemia

All patients whose blood cultures yield *Candida* species should be treated with an antifungal agent for a minimum of 2 weeks after the blood cultures become negative. Removal of a central venous catheter is, by itself, not adequate therapy. Outcomes have been noted to be improved when antifungal therapy is begun as early as possible [61, 62]. Thus, in some patients, especially those who are severely ill, pre-emptive or empirical therapy with an antifungal agent is appropriate [81, 82].

Choice of Antifungal Agents

The choice of antifungal agents is usually either fluconazole or an echinocandin. Numerous randomized controlled trials have shown the efficacy of azoles and echinocandins, when compared with one another and when compared with amphotericin B [83–91]. When the infecting species is *C. glabrata* or *C. krusei*, the agent of choice is an echinocandin because of increasing resistance to fluconazole among *C. glabrata* isolates and the inherent resistance of *C. krusei* to fluconazole [64, 68, 69, 92, 93]. Cross-resistance to voriconazole is common among strains of *C. glabrata* that are fluconazole resistant, and for many strains, there is cross-resistance noted among all of the azoles when the isolate is shown to be resistant to fluconazole [25]. The cross-resistance to voriconazole does not occur in strains of *C. krusei*; they remain susceptible to this azole.

When empiric therapy in a high-risk transplant patient is deemed prudent before culture results are known, an echinocandin is the drug of choice [7]. After the organism has been identified and susceptibilities determined, therapy can be changed if needed. Switching to fluconazole from an echinocandin allows oral dosing and is less costly. In the transplant population, it is necessary to consider whether prophylactic antifungal agents had been given to the patient prior to the episode of candidemia. Prophylaxis has the potential to select out for species that are resistant to that class of drug.

Duration

The total length of therapy for candidemia without the development of other focal infections is 2 weeks from the time of the first negative blood culture. However, in patients who are neutropenic, therapy should be continued until the neutropenia has resolved [7]. Follow-up daily blood cultures should be obtained to document when candidemia has cleared.

Other Measures

All patients who have candidemia should have a dilated eye examination by an ophthalmologist. The presence of endophthalmitis will require longer therapy with drugs that achieve adequate levels within the posterior compartment of the eye. For neutropenic patients, it is important to repeat the retinal examination after their neutrophils return to normal levels when eye manifestations are more likely to be noted.

Management of Central Venous Catheters

The IDSA guidelines for both the management of invasive candidiasis and the management of intravascular catheter-associated infections recommend removing central venous catheters in patients with candidemia [7, 94]. Several small series and post-hoc reviews of clinical treatment trials for candidemia show faster clearance rates of candidemia and better outcomes when catheters are removed [67, 95, 96]. However, there are clinicians who believe that for certain patient groups, especially those who have received chemotherapy and are neutropenic, the source of the candidemia is likely to be the bowel and the catheter need not be removed [97]. A retrospective review of two randomized treatment trials showed that early removal of central venous catheters was not associated with improved treatment success and survival [98]. In contrast, a larger retrospective review of individual patient-level data from seven randomized treatment trials found that removal of a central venous catheter was associated with decreased mortality [67]. This subject remains controversial, but the strength of opinion and the recommendations of the guidelines are on the side of removing the catheter whenever feasible in a patient who has candidemia.

Hepatosplenic Candidiasis

For patients who have moderate to severe disease manifestations, it is recommended that therapy begin with a lipid formulation of amphotericin B, 3–5 mg/kg/day, or an echinocandin for several weeks and then go to step-down therapy with oral fluconazole, 400 mg daily [7]. Therapy should continue until there is resolution of the lesions on follow-up CT scans performed every 2–3 months. Importantly, if hepatosplenic candidiasis occurred prior to HCT, antifungal therapy must be continued throughout the period of engraftment and maximal immunosuppression in order to prevent relapse of the fungal infection.

The hypothesis that this syndrome is related to an IRIS phenomenon led to the use of oral glucocorticoids in addition to antifungal therapy [42, 99–101]. Patients given prednisone had prompt resolution of their fever and abdominal pain, and their inflammatory response markers more quickly returned to normal. However, lesions seen on CT scan did not resolve any faster. The dose of prednisone usually given has been 0.5–1.0 mg/kg daily for several weeks. However, the role of corticosteroids is still not established [7].

Intra-abdominal Candidiasis

An important factor in improving outcomes of patients who have an intra-abdominal abscess is either percutaneous or open surgical drainage. Antifungal therapy should be directed at the *Candida* species isolated from the abscess. When the patient has peritonitis or a diffuse phlegmon and a surgical procedure is not contemplated, antimicrobial therapy should be directed toward the most likely pathogens including *Candida* species. In the most common scenario in which *C. albicans* is isolated, either an echinocandin or fluconazole, 400 mg daily, can be used. If *C. glabrata* is isolated, the most appropriate therapy is with an echinocandin. Echinocandin doses used are micafungin, 100 mg daily; caspofungin 70 mg loading dose and then 50 mg daily; and anidulafungin, 200 mg loading dose and then 100 mg daily. Voriconazole should not be used until the isolate has been shown to be susceptible by in vitro testing. Treatment duration will be dependent on improvement of signs and symptoms and resolution of any abscesses noted on CT scan.

Treatment of candidiasis in liver transplant recipients who have biliary tract obstruction and indwelling stents is difficult. Colonization of the stent is common, and the major decision is to determine whether these organisms are causing infection. Just isolating yeast from a percutaneous drain is not adequate evidence that an antifungal agent is needed. If infection is deemed likely, then stent replacement, in addition to antifungal therapy, is usually required.

Urinary Tract Infections

Only patients in whom there is a high likelihood that symptomatic urinary tract infection is due to *Candida* species should receive antifungal therapy. Patients who are in hospital post-transplant and with an indwelling catheter rarely need to be treated for candiduria, which almost always reflects asymptomatic colonization of the catheter and bladder. When infection is present, fluconazole is the agent of choice as no other azoles and no echinocandins achieve adequate concentrations in the urine [102]. Most infections are due to *C. albicans* and respond nicely to oral fluconazole, 200 mg daily. In contrast, *C. glabrata* and *C. krusei* urinary tract infections are very difficult to treat. The agent of choice is amphotericin B deoxycholate, not a lipid formulation of amphotericin B. Therapy with as low as 0.3 mg/kg daily for just a few days may be adequate [7]. Regardless of the species and the agent used, if obstruction is present, therapy will likely fail. Ureteral stents that are colonized generally will have to be removed to eradicate candiduria.

Endophthalmitis

For *Candida* endophthalmitis, use of systemic antifungal agents that achieve adequate concentrations in the vitreous is recommended. The agents that achieve the best concentrations are fluconazole, voriconazole, and flucytosine [103]. Amphotericin B does not penetrate into the vitreous well, but there is a long experience using this agent in combination with flucytosine for *Candida* endophthalmitis [7]. However, for susceptible organisms, most clinicians use fluconazole, 400–800 mg daily, or voriconazole, loading dose 6 mg/kg bid for 1 day and then 4 mg/kg bid thereafter, rather than amphotericin B. The echinocandins and posaconazole do not achieve good intra-vitreal concentrations and are not recommended.

For patients who have *Candida* chorioretinitis with no vitreal involvement, systemic antifungal agents are appropriate as long as repeated examinations show no extension into the vitreous or the macula. Initial intravenous administration seems prudent to establish high concentrations in the vitreous [103]. When using voriconazole, serum concentrations should be monitored carefully to ensure that adequate levels have been achieved and to minimize toxicity.

For sight-threatening macular involvement and mild vitritis, in addition to systemic therapy, intravitreal injection of either voriconazole or amphotericin B deoxycholate should be performed to ensure immediate achievement of appropriate levels in the posterior compartment. For more extensive vitritis, in addition to systemic and intra-vitreal antifungal therapy, pars plana vitrectomy is recommended.

Mucosal Candidiasis

Oropharyngeal candidiasis can be treated with clotrimazole troches, nystatin swish and swallow suspension, or oral antifungal agents, such as fluconazole. Fluconazole is generally used as it is effective, simple to take once daily, more effective than local suspensions and troches in profoundly immunosuppressed patients, and inexpensive. The dose is 100 mg daily for 7 days. Other oral azole agents are also effective, but more costly and either absorbed less well or with more drug-drug interactions.

Vaginal candidiasis is almost always treated with oral fluconazole. Many local creams and vaginal suppositories are available, but patients prefer oral therapy, and it generally is more effective. Infection with *C. glabrata* is uncommon, but problematic to treat and requires consultation with an expert in the treatment of complicated vaginal candidiasis.

Esophagitis cannot be treated with local agents and requires systemic therapy. Fluconazole is the agent of choice at a dosage of 200 mg daily for at least 14 days. Echinocandins, voriconazole, and amphotericin B formulations are also effective, but generally only used if fluconazole fails to clear the infection.

Prophylaxis in Immunocompromised Hosts

Prevention of invasive candidiasis using antifungal agents during the pre-engraftment period is standard practice in patients undergoing allogeneic HCT [104]. Fluconazole is the most commonly used agent as it has a long track record of efficacy (Table 32.3). In a randomized double-blinded study, voriconazole proved to be no more effective than fluconazole in preventing invasive candidiasis among allogeneic HCT recipients [105]. Micafungin and presumably the other echinocandins are alternative prophylactic agents, comparable to fluconazole. However, their use is limited by the need for intravenous infusion and high costs [106]. Solid tumor patients undergoing autologous HCT generally do not require anti-yeast prophylaxis. However, many experts recommend that prophylaxis be given to the considerably larger population of patients who have underlying hematologic malignancies (e.g., lymphoma, leukemia, or myeloma). Other autologous HCT recipients for whom antifungal prophylaxis might be warranted are those who have or will have prolonged neutropenia and mucosal damage from intense conditioning regimens or graft manipulation, and those who have received purine analog therapy within the 6 months prior to HCT [104]. The choice of prophylactic agent ultimately depends on tolerability and cost. Fluconazole is the mostly widely used drug.

Guidelines for antifungal prophylaxis in SOT have been delineated by the American Society of Transplantation [80]. Antifungal prophylaxis against *Candida* should be provided to high-risk liver transplant recipients, specifically those with two or more of the following risk factors: prolonged surgical time, repeated abdominal surgery or re-transplantation, renal failure, high transfusion needs (≥40 units of cellular blood products), choledochojejunostomy, and *Candida* colonization in the perioperative period. Fluconazole is the standard agent used (Table 32.3). A recent meta-analysis demonstrated that antifungal prophylaxis in these patients significantly reduced invasive candidiasis as well as fungal-related mortality, but not overall mortality [107]. Lower-risk liver transplant recipients do not require routine antifungal prophylaxis as their risk of invasive candidiasis is very low.

In contrast, patients receiving intestinal transplants have very high rates of *Candida* infection. Despite a lack of randomized clinical trial evidence, antifungal prophylaxis is recommended, especially for those who have graft rejection, increased immunosuppression or anastomotic incompetence. Pancreas transplant recipients whose transplants are drained via the enteric route or who have vascular thrombosis or

Table 32.3 Prophylaxis against *Candida* infections in solid organ transplant and hematopoietic cell transplant recipients

Transplant type	Risk factors	Antifungal prophylaxis	Notes/duration
Liver	Prolonged operation time Repeat operation Retransplantation	Fluconazole 400 mg/day *or* Lipid formulation of amphotericin B 3–5 mg/kg/day	Selected high-risk patients (see Risk Factors) should receive prophylaxis Up to 4 weeks of duration
Small bowel	Renal failure Choledochojejunostomy *Candida* colonization High transfusion requirement Graft rejection/dysfunction Enhanced immunosuppression	Fluconazole 400 mg/day *or* Lipid formulation of amphotericin B 3–5 mg/kg/day[a]	All recipients should receive prophylaxis At least 4 weeks of duration and/or healing of anastomosis and absence of rejection
Pancreas	Anastomotic disruption Abdominal reoperation Multivisceral transplantation Enteric drainage Vascular thrombosis	Fluconazole 400 mg/day *or* Lipid formulation of amphotericin B 3–5 mg/kg/day[a]	All patients should receive prophylaxis At least 4 weeks of duration
Allogeneic HCT	Neutropenia Mucositis Broad-spectrum antibiotics Hematologic malignancy	Fluconazole 400 mg/day *or* Micafungin 50 mg IV/day *or* Posaconazole 300 mg qd *or* Voriconazole 200 mg bid	All patients should receive prophylaxis up to day +75 Fluconazole is the drug of choice during pre-engraftment and post-engraftment Posaconazole is the drug of choice during therapy for severe GVHD; voriconazole is an acceptable alternative
Autologous HCT	Neutropenia Mucositis Broad-spectrum antibiotics Hematologic malignancy	Fluconazole 400 mg/day *or* Micafungin 50 mg IV/day	Prophylaxis is NOT routinely recommended Consider for patients who will have prolonged neutropenia (> 10 days) and/or extensive mucositis

[a]If high rates of non-*albicans Candida* sp. or risk factors for *Aspergillus*

postoperative pancreatitis are at higher risk for invasive candidiasis and should be considered candidates for antifungal prophylaxis [34].

Although the airways of lung and heart-lung transplant recipients are frequently colonized with *Candida* species, invasive infection is rare. Prophylaxis practices vary considerably among different centers, and there is no consensus. Candidiasis is relatively uncommon in heart and kidney recipients, and antifungal prophylaxis is not recommended as a routine practice in these patients [80].

References

1. Kontoyiannis DP, Marr KA, Park BJ, Alexander BD, Anaissie EJ, Walsh TJ, et al. Prospective surveillance for invasive fungal infections in hematopoietic stem cell transplant recipients, 2001-2006: overview of the Transplant-Associated Infection Surveillance Network (TRANSNET) Database. Clin Infect Dis. 2010;50(8):1091–100.
2. Pappas PG, Alexander BD, Andes DR, Hadley S, Kauffman CA, Freifeld A, et al. Invasive fungal infections among organ transplant recipients: results of the Transplant-Associated Infection Surveillance Network (TRANSNET). Clin Infect Dis. 2010;50(8):1101–11.
3. De Pauw B, Walsh TJ, Donnelly JP, Stevens DA, Edwards JE, Calandra T, et al. Revised definitions of invasive fungal disease from the European Organization for Research and Treatment of Cancer/Invasive Fungal Infections Cooperative Group and the National Institute of Allergy and Infectious Diseases Mycoses Study Group (EORTC/MSG) Consensus Group. Clin Infect Dis. 2008;46(12):1813–21.
4. Fortun J, Martin-Davila P, Gomez-Garcia de la Pedrosa E, Pintado V, Cobo J, Fresco G, et al. Emerging trends in candidemia: a higher incidence but a similar outcome. J Infect. 2012;65(1):64–70.
5. Gonzalez de Molina FJ, Leon C, Ruiz-Santana S, Saavedra P, the CAVA I Study Group. Assessment of candidemia-attributable mortality in critically ill patients using propensity score matching analysis. Crit Care. 2012;16(3):R105.
6. Horn DL, Neofytos D, Anaissie EJ, Fishman JA, Steinbach WJ, Olyaei AJ, et al. Epidemiology and outcomes of candidemia in 2019 patients: data from the prospective antifungal therapy alliance registry. Clin Infect Dis. 2009;48(12):1695–703.
7. Pappas PG, Kauffman CA, Andes DR, Clancy CJ, Marr KA, Ostrosky-Zeichner L, et al. Clinical practice guideline for the management of candidiasis: 2016 update by the Infectious Diseases Society of America. Clin Infect Dis. 2016;62:409–17.
8. Perlroth J, Choi B, Spellberg B. Nosocomial fungal infections: epidemiology, diagnosis, and treatment. Med Mycol. 2007;45(4):321–46.
9. van der Meer JW, van de Veerdonk FL, Joosten LA, Kullberg BJ, Netea MG. Severe *Candida* spp. infections: new insights into natural immunity. Int J Antimicrob Agents. 2010;36 Suppl 2:S58–62.

10. Blankenship JR, Mitchell AP. How to build a biofilm: a fungal perspective. Curr Opin Microbiol. 2006;9(6):588–94.
11. Chow JK, Golan Y, Ruthazer R, Karchmer AW, Carmeli Y, Lichtenberg D, et al. Factors associated with candidemia caused by non-albicans *Candida* species versus *Candida albicans* in the intensive care unit. Clin Infect Dis. 2008;46(8):1206–13.
12. Muskett H, Shahin J, Eyres G, Harvey S, Rowan K, Harrison D. Risk factors for invasive fungal disease in critically ill adult patients: a systematic review. Crit Care. 2011;15(6):R287.
13. Albano L, Bretagne S, Mamzer-Bruneel MF, Kacso I, Desnos-Ollivier M, Guerrini P, et al. Evidence that graft-site candidiasis after kidney transplantation is acquired during organ recovery: a multicenter study in France. Clin Infect Dis. 2009;48(2):194–202.
14. Botterel F, Foulet F, Legrand P, Soria AM, Farrugia C, Grimbert P, et al. Yeast contamination of kidney, liver and cardiac preservation solutions before graft: need for standardisation of microbial evaluation. J Hosp Infect. 2010;76(1):52–5.
15. Neofytos D, Fishman JA, Horn D, Anaissie E, Chang CH, Olyaei A, et al. Epidemiology and outcome of invasive fungal infections in solid organ transplant recipients. Transpl Infect Dis. 2010;12(3):220–9.
16. Cheng MF, Yang YL, Yao TJ, Lin CY, Liu JS, Tang RB, et al. Risk factors for fatal candidemia caused by *Candida albicans* and non-albicans *Candida* species. BMC Infect Dis. 2005;5:22.
17. van Hal SJ, Marriott DJ, Chen SC, Nguyen Q, Sorrell TC, Ellis DH, et al. Candidemia following solid organ transplantation in the era of antifungal prophylaxis: the Australian experience. Transpl Infect Dis. 2009;11(2):122–7.
18. Shekh RM, Roy U. Biochemical characterization of an anti-Candida factor produced by *Enterococcus faecalis*. BMC Microbiol. 2012;12(1):132.
19. Netea MG, Marodi L. Innate immune mechanisms for recognition and uptake of *Candida* species. Trends Immunol. 2010;31(9):346–53.
20. Moyes DL, Naglik JR. Mucosal immunity and *Candida albicans* infection. Clin Dev Immunol. 2011;2011:346307.
21. Wisplinghoff H, Bischoff T, Tallent SM, Seifert H, Wenzel RP, Edmond MB. Nosocomial bloodstream infections in US hospitals: analysis of 24,179 cases from a prospective nationwide surveillance study. Clin Infect Dis. 2004;39(3):309–17.
22. Pappas PG, Rex JH, Lee J, Hamill RJ, Larsen RA, Powderly W, et al. A prospective observational study of candidemia: epidemiology, therapy, and influences on mortality in hospitalized adult and pediatric patients. Clin Infect Dis. 2003;37(5):634–43.
23. Morgan J, Meltzer MI, Plikaytis BD, Sofair AN, Huie-White S, Wilcox S, et al. Excess mortality, hospital stay, and cost due to candidemia: a case-control study using data from population-based candidemia surveillance. Infect Control Hosp Epidemiol. 2005;26(6):540–7.
24. Colombo AL, Guimaraes T, Silva LR, de Almeida Monfardini LP, Cunha AK, Rady P, et al. Prospective observational study of candidemia in Sao Paulo, Brazil: incidence rate, epidemiology, and predictors of mortality. Infect Control Hosp Epidemiol. 2007;28(5):570–6.
25. Pfaller MA, Diekema DJ, Gibbs DL, Newell VA, Ellis D, Tullio V, et al. Results from the ARTEMIS DISK Global Antifungal Surveillance Study, 1997 to 2007: a 10.5-year analysis of susceptibilities of Candida Species to fluconazole and voriconazole as determined by CLSI standardized disk diffusion. J Clin Microbiol. 2010;48(4):1366–77.
26. Sipsas NV, Lewis RE, Tarrand J, Hachem R, Rolston KV, Raad II, et al. Candidemia in patients with hematologic malignancies in the era of new antifungal agents (2001-2007): stable incidence but changing epidemiology of a still frequently lethal infection. Cancer. 2009;115(20):4745–52.
27. Marr KA, Seidel K, Slavin MA, Bowden RA, Schoch HG, Flowers ME, et al. Prolonged fluconazole prophylaxis is associated with persistent protection against candidiasis-related death in allogeneic marrow transplant recipients: long-term follow-up of a randomized, placebo-controlled trial. Blood. 2000;96(6):2055–61.
28. Pagano L, Caira M, Nosari A, Van Lint MT, Candoni A, Offidani M, et al. Fungal infections in recipients of hematopoietic stem cell transplants: results of the SEIFEM B-2004 study – Sorveglianza Epidemiologica Infezioni Fungine Nelle Emopatie Maligne. Clin Infect Dis. 2007;45(9):1161–70.
29. Collins LA, Samore MH, Roberts MS, Luzzati R, Jenkins RL, Lewis WD, et al. Risk factors for invasive fungal infections complicating orthotopic liver transplantation. J Infect Dis. 1994;170(3):644–52.
30. Patel R, Portela D, Badley AD, Harmsen WS, Larson-Keller JJ, Ilstrup DM, et al. Risk factors of invasive Candida and non-Candida fungal infections after liver transplantation. Transplantation. 1996;62(7):926–34.
31. Husain S, Tollemar J, Dominguez EA, Baumgarten K, Humar A, Paterson DL, et al. Changes in the spectrum and risk factors for invasive candidiasis in liver transplant recipients: prospective, multicenter, case-controlled study. Transplantation. 2003;75(12):2023–9.
32. Hadley S, Huckabee C, Pappas PG, Daly J, Rabkin J, Kauffman CA, et al. Outcomes of antifungal prophylaxis in high-risk liver transplant recipients. Transpl Infect Dis. 2009;11(1):40–8.
33. Florescu DF, Qiu F, Mercer DF, Langnas AN, Shafer LR, Kalil AC. Risk factors for systemic Candida infections in pediatric small bowel transplant recipients. Pediatr Infect Dis J. 2012;31(2):120–3.
34. Benedetti E, Gruessner AC, Troppmann C, Papalois BE, Sutherland DE, Dunn DL, et al. Intra-abdominal fungal infections after pancreatic transplantation: incidence, treatment, and outcome. J Am Coll Surg. 1996;183(4):307–16.
35. Hsu RB, Chang CI, Fang CT, Chang SC, Wang SS, Chu SH. Bloodstream infection in heart transplant recipients: 12-year experience at a university hospital in Taiwan. Eur J Cardiothorac Surg. 2011;40(6):1362–7.
36. Schaenman JM, Rosso F, Austin JM, Baron EJ, Gamberg P, Miller J, et al. Trends in invasive disease due to Candida species following heart and lung transplantation. Transpl Infect Dis. 2009;11(2).112–21.
37. Nucci M, Marr KA. Emerging fungal diseases. Clin Infect Dis. 2005;41(4):521–6.
38. Playford EG, Marriott D, Nguyen Q, Chen S, Ellis D, Slavin M, et al. Candidemia in nonneutropenic critically ill patients: risk factors for non-albicans *Candida* spp. Crit Care Med. 2008;36(7):2034–9.
39. Lockhart SR, Wagner D, Iqbal N, Pappas PG, Andes DR, Kauffman CA, et al. Comparison of in vitro susceptibility characteristics of Candida species from cases of invasive candidiasis in solid organ and stem cell transplant recipients: Transplant-Associated Infections Surveillance Network (TRANSNET), 2001 to 2006. J Clin Microbiol. 2011;49(7):2404–10.
40. Riddell J 4th, Kauffman CA. The evolution of resistant Candida species in cancer centers: implications for treatment and prophylaxis. Cancer. 2008;112(11):2334–7.
41. Bouza E, Burillo A, Munoz P, Guinea J, Marin M, Rodriguez-Creixems M. Mixed bloodstream infections involving bacteria and Candida spp. J Antimicrob Chemother. 2013;68(8):1881–8.
42. Legrand F, Lecuit M, Dupont B, Bellaton E, Huerre M, Rohrlich PS, et al. Adjuvant corticosteroid therapy for chronic disseminated candidiasis. Clin Infect Dis. 2008;46(5):696–702.
43. Guaraldi G, Cocchi S, Codeluppi M, Di Benedetto F, De Ruvo N, Masetti M, et al. Outcome, incidence, and timing of infectious complications in small bowel and multivisceral organ transplantation patients. Transplantation. 2005;80(12):1742–8.

44. Story B, Gluck M. Obstructing fungal cholangitis complicating metal biliary stent placement in pancreatic cancer. World J Gastroenterol. 2010;16(24):3083–6.
45. Gorschluter M, Mey U, Strehl J, Schmitz V, Rabe C, Pauls K, et al. Invasive fungal infections in neutropenic enterocolitis: a systematic analysis of pathogens, incidence, treatment and mortality in adult patients. BMC Infect Dis. 2006;6:35.
46. Kauffman CA, Vazquez JA, Sobel JD, Gallis HA, McKinsey DS, Karchmer AW, et al. Prospective multicenter surveillance study of funguria in hospitalized patients. The National Institute for Allergy and Infectious Diseases (NIAID) Mycoses Study Group. Clin Infect Dis. 2000;30(1):14–8.
47. Safdar N, Slattery WR, Knasinski V, Gangnon RE, Li Z, Pirsch JD, et al. Predictors and outcomes of candiduria in renal transplant recipients. Clin Infect Dis. 2005;40(10):1413–21.
48. Simpson C, Blitz S, Shafran SD. The effect of current management on morbidity and mortality in hospitalised adults with funguria. J Infect. 2004;49(3):248–52.
49. Sobel JD, Fisher JF, Kauffman CA, Newman CA. Candida urinary tract infections – epidemiology. Clin Infect Dis. 2011;52(Suppl 6):S433–6.
50. Barkauskas C, Perfect J. *Candida* pneumonia: what we know and what we don't. Curr Fungal Infect Rep. 2009;3(1):21–31.
51. Franquet T, Muller NL, Lee KS, Oikonomou A, Flint JD. Pulmonary candidiasis after hematopoietic stem cell transplantation: thin-section CT findings. Radiology. 2005;236(1):332–7.
52. Kontoyiannis DP, Reddy BT, Torres HA, Luna M, Lewis RE, Tarrand J, et al. Pulmonary candidiasis in patients with cancer: an autopsy study. Clin Infect Dis. 2002;34(3):400–3.
53. Lingappan A, Wykoff CC, Albini TA, Miller D, Pathengay A, Davis JL, et al. Endogenous fungal endophthalmitis: causative organisms, management strategies, and visual acuity outcomes. Am J Ophthalmol. 2012;153(1):162–6.e1.
54. Oude Lashof AM, Rothova A, Sobel JD, Ruhnke M, Pappas PG, Viscoli C, et al. Ocular manifestations of candidemia. Clin Infect Dis. 2011;53(3):262–8.
55. Baddley JW, Benjamin DK Jr, Patel M, Miro J, Athan E, Barsic B, et al. Candida infective endocarditis. Eur J Clin Microbiol Infect Dis. 2008;27(7):519–29.
56. Gamaletsou MN, et al. Candida osteomyelitis: analysis of 207 pediatric and adult cases (1970-2011). Clin Infect Dis. 2012;55:1338–51.
57. Voice RA, Bradley SF, Sangeorzan JA, Kauffman CA. Chronic candidal meningitis: an uncommon manifestation of candidiasis. Clin Infect Dis. 1994;19(1):60–6.
58. Gudlaugsson O, Gillespie S, Lee K, Vande Berg J, Hu J, Messer S, et al. Attributable mortality of nosocomial candidemia, revisited. Clin Infect Dis. 2003;37(9):1172–7.
59. Zaoutis TE, Argon J, Chu J, Berlin JA, Walsh TJ, Feudtner C. The epidemiology and attributable outcomes of candidemia in adults and children hospitalized in the United States: a propensity analysis. Clin Infect Dis. 2005;41(9):1232–9.
60. Leroy O, Gangneux JP, Montravers P, Mira JP, Gouin F, Sollet JP, et al. Epidemiology, management, and risk factors for death of invasive Candida infections in critical care: a multicenter, prospective, observational study in France (2005-2006). Crit Care Med. 2009;37(5):1612–8.
61. Morrell M, Fraser VJ, Kollef MH. Delaying the empiric treatment of candida bloodstream infection until positive blood culture results are obtained: a potential risk factor for hospital mortality. Antimicrob Agents Chemother. 2005;49(9):3640–5.
62. Garey KW, Rege M, Pai MP, Mingo DE, Suda KJ, Turpin RS, et al. Time to initiation of fluconazole therapy impacts mortality in patients with candidemia: a multi-institutional study. Clin Infect Dis. 2006;43(1):25–31.
63. Kollef M, Micek S, Hampton N, Doherty JA, Kumar A. Septic shock attributed to Candida infection: importance of empiric therapy and source control. Clin Infect Dis. 2012;54(12):1739–46.
64. Hachem R, Hanna H, Kontoyiannis D, Jiang Y, Raad I. The changing epidemiology of invasive candidiasis: *Candida glabrata* and *Candida krusei* as the leading causes of candidemia in hematologic malignancy. Cancer. 2008;112(11):2493–9.
65. Kontoyiannis DP, Vaziri I, Hanna HA, Boktour M, Thornby J, Hachem R, et al. Risk factors for *Candida tropicalis* fungemia in patients with cancer. Clin Infect Dis. 2001;33(10):1676–81.
66. Trofa D, Gacser A, Nosanchuk JD. *Candida parapsilosis*, an emerging fungal pathogen. Clin Microbiol Rev. 2008;21(4):606–25.
67. Andes DR, Safdar N, Baddley JW, Playford G, Reboli AC, Rex JH, et al. Impact of treatment strategy on outcomes in patients with candidemia and other forms of invasive candidiasis: a patient-level quantitative review of randomized trials. Clin Infect Dis. 2012;54(8):1110–22.
68. Klevay MJ, Ernst EJ, Hollanbaugh JL, Miller JG, Pfaller MA, Diekema DJ. Therapy and outcome of *Candida glabrata* versus *Candida albicans* bloodstream infection. Diagn Microbiol Infect Dis. 2008;60(3):273–7.
69. Malani A, Hmoud J, Chiu L, Carver PL, Bielaczyc A, Kauffman CA. *Candida glabrata* fungemia: experience in a tertiary care center. Clin Infect Dis. 2005;41(7):975–81.
70. Gherna M, Merz WG. Identification of *Candida albicans* and *Candida glabrata* within 1.5 hours directly from positive blood culture bottles with a shortened peptide nucleic acid fluorescence in situ hybridization protocol. J Clin Microbiol. 2009;47(1):247–8.
71. Shepard JR, Addison RM, Alexander BD, Della-Latta P, Gherna M, Haase G, et al. Multicenter evaluation of the *Candida albicans/ Candida glabrata* peptide nucleic acid fluorescent in situ hybridization method for simultaneous dual-color identification of C. albicans and C. glabrata directly from blood culture bottles. J Clin Microbiol. 2008;46(1):50–5.
72. Iriart X, Lavergne RA, Fillaux J, Valentin A, Magnaval JF, Berry A, et al. Routine identification of medical fungi by the new vitek MS matrix-assisted laser desorption ionization-time of flight system with a new time-effective strategy. J Clin Microbiol. 2012;50(6):2107–10.
73. Pfaller MA, Castanheira M, Lockhart SR, Ahlquist AM, Messer SA, Jones RN. Frequency of decreased susceptibility and resistance to echinocandins among fluconazole-resistant bloodstream isolates of *Candida glabrata*. J Clin Microbiol. 2012;50(4):1199–203.
74. Karageorgopoulos DE, Vouloumanou EK, Ntziora F, Michalopoulos A, Rafailidis PI, Falagas ME. beta-D-glucan assay for the diagnosis of invasive fungal infections: a meta-analysis. Clin Infect Dis. 2011;52(6):750–70.
75. Alexander BD, Smith PB, Davis RD, Perfect JR, Reller LB. The (1,3){beta}-D-glucan test as an aid to early diagnosis of invasive fungal infections following lung transplantation. J Clin Microbiol. 2010;48(11):4083–8.
76. Kourkoumpetis TK, Fuchs BB, Coleman JJ, Desalermos A, Mylonakis E. Polymerase chain reaction-based assays for the diagnosis of invasive fungal infections. Clin Infect Dis. 2012;54(9):1322–31.
77. Nguyen MH, Wissel MC, Shields RK, Salomoni MA, Hao B, Press EG, et al. Performance of candida real-time polymerase chain reaction, beta-D-glucan assay, and blood cultures in the diagnosis of invasive candidiasis. Clin Infect Dis. 2012;54(9):1240–8.
78. Mylonakis E, Clancy CJ, Ostrosky-Zeichner L, et al. T2 magnetic resonance assay for the rapid diagnosis of candidemia in whole blood: a clinical trial. Clin Infect Dis. 2015;60:892–9.
79. Vazquez JA, Sobel JD. Candidiasis. In: Kauffman CA, Pappas PG, Sobel JD, Dismukes WE, editors. Essentials of clinical mycology. 2nd ed. New York: Springer; 2011. p. 167–206.

80. Pappas PG, Silveira FP, AST Infectious Diseases Community of Practice. Candida in solid organ transplant recipients. Am J Transplant. 2009;9 Suppl 4:S173–9.
81. Schuster MG, Edwards JE Jr, Sobel JD, Darouiche RO, Karchmer AW, Hadley S, et al. Empirical fluconazole versus placebo for intensive care unit patients: a randomized trial. Ann Intern Med. 2008;149(2):83–90.
82. Piarroux R, Grenouillet F, Balvay P, Tran V, Blasco G, Millon L, et al. Assessment of preemptive treatment to prevent severe candidiasis in critically ill surgical patients. Crit Care Med. 2004;32(12):2443–9.
83. Rex JH, Bennett JE, Sugar AM, Pappas PG, van der Horst CM, Edwards JE, et al. A randomized trial comparing fluconazole with amphotericin B for the treatment of candidemia in patients without neutropenia. Candidemia Study Group and the National Institute. N Engl J Med. 1994;331(20):1325–30.
84. Phillips P, Shafran S, Garber G, Rotstein C, Smaill F, Fong I, et al. Multicenter randomized trial of fluconazole versus amphotericin B for treatment of candidemia in non-neutropenic patients. Canadian Candidemia Study Group. Eur J Clin Microbiol Infect Dis. 1997;16(5):337–45.
85. Rex JH, Pappas PG, Karchmer AW, Sobel J, Edwards JE, Hadley S, et al. A randomized and blinded multicenter trial of high-dose fluconazole plus placebo versus fluconazole plus amphotericin B as therapy for candidemia and its consequences in nonneutropenic subjects. Clin Infect Dis. 2003;36(10):1221–8.
86. Mora-Duarte J, Betts R, Rotstein C, Colombo AL, Thompson-Moya L, Smietana J, et al. Comparison of caspofungin and amphotericin B for invasive candidiasis. N Engl J Med. 2002;347(25):2020–9.
87. Kuse ER, Chetchotisakd P, da Cunha CA, Ruhnke M, Barrios C, Raghunadharao D, et al. Micafungin versus liposomal amphotericin B for candidaemia and invasive candidosis: a phase III randomised double-blind trial. Lancet. 2007;369(9572): 1519–27.
88. Reboli AC, Rotstein C, Pappas PG, Chapman SW, Kett DH, Kumar D, et al. Anidulafungin versus fluconazole for invasive candidiasis. N Engl J Med. 2007;356(24):2472–82.
89. Pappas PG, Rotstein CM, Betts RF, Nucci M, Talwar D, De Waele JJ, et al. Micafungin versus caspofungin for treatment of candidemia and other forms of invasive candidiasis. Clin Infect Dis. 2007;45(7):883–93.
90. Betts RF, Nucci M, Talwar D, Gareca M, Queiroz-Telles F, Bedimo RJ, et al. A multicenter, double-blind trial of a high-dose caspofungin treatment regimen versus a standard caspofungin treatment regimen for adult patients with invasive candidiasis. Clin Infect Dis. 2009;48(12):1676–84.
91. Kullberg BJ, Sobel JD, Ruhnke M, Pappas PG, Viscoli C, Rex JH, et al. Voriconazole versus a regimen of amphotericin B followed by fluconazole for candidaemia in non-neutropenic patients: a randomised non-inferiority trial. Lancet. 2005;366(9495):1435–42.
92. Ruan SY, Lee LN, Jerng JS, Yu CJ, Hsueh PR. *Candida glabrata* fungaemia in intensive care units. Clin Microbiol Infect. 2008;14(2):136–40.
93. Alexander BD, Schell WA, Miller JL, Long GD, Perfect JR. Candida *glabrata fungemia* in transplant patients receiving voriconazole after fluconazole. Transplantation. 2005;80(6):868–71.
94. Mermel LA, Allon M, Bouza E, Craven DE, Flynn P, O'Grady NP, et al. Clinical practice guidelines for the diagnosis and management of intravascular catheter-related infection: 2009 update by the Infectious Diseases Society of America. Clin Infect Dis. 2009;49(1):1–45.
95. Karlowicz MG, Hashimoto LN, Kelly RE Jr, Buescher ES. Should central venous catheters be removed as soon as candidemia is detected in neonates? Pediatrics. 2000;106(5):E63.
96. Rex JH, Bennett JE, Sugar AM, Pappas PG, Serody J, Edwards JE, et al. Intravascular catheter exchange and duration of candidemia. NIAID Mycoses Study Group and the Candidemia Study Group. Clin Infect Dis. 1995;21(4):994–6.
97. Nucci M, Anaissie E. Should vascular catheters be removed from all patients with candidemia? An evidence-based review. Clin Infect Dis. 2002;34(5):591–9.
98. Nucci M, Anaissie E, Betts RF, Dupont BF, Wu C, Buell DN, et al. Early removal of central venous catheter in patients with candidemia does not improve outcome: analysis of 842 patients from 2 randomized clinical trials. Clin Infect Dis. 2010;51(3):295–303.
99. Rammaert B, Desjardins A, Lortholary O. Mycoses. 2012;55(3):e74–84.
100. De Castro N, Mazoyer E, Porcher R, Raffoux E, Suarez F, Ribaud P, et al. Hepatosplenic candidiasis in the era of new antifungal drugs: a study in Paris 2000-2007. Clin Microbiol Infect. 2012;18(6):E185–7.
101. Chaussade H, Bastides F, Lissandre S, Blouin P, Bailly E, Chandenier J, et al. J Antimicrobi Chemoter. 2012;67:1493–5.
102. Fisher JF, Sobel JD, Kauffman CA, Newman CA. *Candida* urinary tract infections – treatment. Clin Infect Dis. 2011;52(Suppl 6):S457–66.
103. Riddell J 4th, Comer GM, Kauffman CA. Treatment of endogenous fungal endophthalmitis: focus on new antifungal agents. Clin Infect Dis. 2011,52(5):648–53.
104. Tomblyn M, Chiller T, Einsele H, Gress R, Sepkowitz K, Storek J, et al. Guidelines for preventing infectious complications among hematopoietic cell transplantation recipients: a global perspective. Biol Blood Marrow Transplant. 2009;15(10):1143–238.
105. Wingard JR, Carter SL, Walsh TJ, Kurtzberg J, Small TN, Baden LR, et al. Randomized, double-blind trial of fluconazole versus voriconazole for prevention of invasive fungal infection after allogeneic hematopoietic cell transplantation. Blood. 2010;116(24):5111–8.
106. van Burik JA, Ratanatharathorn V, Stepan DE, Miller CB, Lipton JH, Vesole DH, et al. Micafungin versus fluconazole for prophylaxis against invasive fungal infections during neutropenia in patients undergoing hematopoietic stem cell transplantation. Clin Infect Dis. 2004;39(10):1407–16.
107. Cruciani M, Mengoli C, Malena M, Bosco O, Serpelloni G, Grossi P. Antifungal prophylaxis in liver transplant patients: a systematic review and meta-analysis. Liver Transpl. 2006;12(5):850–8.

Aspergillosis

33

Michael J. Satlin, Samantha E. Jacobs, and Thomas J. Walsh

Introduction

Aspergillus species are ubiquitous, saprophytic fungi that are important causes of morbidity and mortality in transplant recipients [1]. Although their primary ecologic location is in soil and decaying environmental matter, *Aspergillus* produce small asexual spores called conidia or microconidia that disperse easily into the air and survive in a broad range of environmental conditions. Humans become infected with *Aspergillus* after conidia are inhaled and deposited in bronchioles, in alveolar spaces, and less commonly in paranasal sinuses [1].

Although there are approximately 250 species of *Aspergillus*, fewer than 20 cause human disease [2]. *Aspergillus fumigatus* is the most common cause of invasive aspergillosis in transplant recipients [3, 4] and other immunocompromised hosts [5]. However, the proportion of infections caused by other species is increasing [6]. In transplant recipients, *Aspergillus flavus* and *Aspergillus niger* are the next most common pathogens, followed by *Aspergillus terreus* [3, 4].

M. J. Satlin (✉)
Transplantation-Oncology Infectious Diseases Program, Division of Infectious Diseases, Weill Cornell Medicine, New York, NY, USA
e-mail: mjs9012@med.cornell.edu

S. E. Jacobs
Transplantation-Oncology Infectious Diseases Program, Division of Infectious Diseases, Weill Cornell Medicine, New York, NY, USA

Transplant Infectious Diseases Program, Division of Infectious Diseases, Icahn School of Medicine at Mount Sinai, Department of Medicine, New York, NY, USA
e-mail: samantha.jacobs1@mssm.edu

T. J. Walsh
Transplantation-Oncology Infectious Diseases Program, New York-Presbyterian/Weill Cornell Medical Center, New York, NY, USA

Department of Pediatrics, New York-Presbyterian/Weill Cornell Medical Center, New York, NY, USA

Department of Microbiology and Immunology, New York-Presbyterian/Weill Cornell Medical Center, New York, NY, USA

Transplant Infectious Diseases Program, Division of Infectious Diseases, Icahn School of Medicine at Mount Sinai, New York, NY, USA
e-mail: thw2003@med.cornell.edu

Pathogenesis and Host Defenses

Innate immunity plays an important role in preventing infection from inhaled *Aspergillus* conidia. Respiratory epithelial cells are the first lines of defense. These cells provide an anatomic barrier to invasion by *Aspergillus*, promote mucociliary clearance, and ingest inhaled conidia [7]. Conidia that are not removed by epithelial cells encounter alveolar macrophages [1]. These cells are responsible for phagocytosis and killing of mainly the metabolically active *Aspergillus* conidia with the potential for germination into filamentous tissue-invasive mold. These cells are also critical in initiating a proinflammatory response. Neutrophils are the primary inflammatory cells recruited by alveolar macrophages and serve as the dominant host defense against conidia that have evaded macrophage killing and have germinated to become hyphae, the tissue-invasive form of *Aspergillus* [7]. Histopathologically, invasive disease is characterized by progression of infection across tissue planes and vascular invasion with subsequent infarction and tissue necrosis [1].

The primary host deficiencies that are responsible for the increased risk of invasive aspergillosis in transplant recipients are neutropenia, corticosteroid-induced immunosuppression, and immune dysregulation resulting from graft-versus-host disease (GVHD). The absence of neutrophils allows unchecked proliferation of hyphae through tissue planes, including the walls of blood vessels. This leads to thrombosis and hemorrhage from rapid and extensive hyphal growth with scant inflammatory response [8]. Without neutrophil recovery, angioinvasion and dissemination to other organs via the bloodstream occur.

A. Safdar (ed.), *Principles and Practice of Transplant Infectious Diseases*, https://doi.org/10.1007/978-1-4939-9034-4_33

The pathology of invasive aspergillosis in non-neutropenic patients who are receiving corticosteroids is different from that of neutropenic patients. Invasive disease in these patients is typically not angioinvasive, but is instead characterized by only limited hyphal proliferation with neutrophilic and monocytic infiltrates, tissue necrosis, and excessive inflammation [8]. Corticosteroids impair the ability of phagocytes to kill *Aspergillus* conidia by interfering with phagocytosis, intracellular oxidative burst, production of cytokines and chemokines, and cellular migration [9]. Despite the deleterious effects of corticosteroids on innate immune cell function, phagocytes are typically successful in being recruited and preventing hyphal angioinvasion, but create an inflammatory environment that results in tissue injury and necrosis [8]. This exacerbated inflammatory response is generally regarded as the direct cause of pathology, in contrast to uncontrolled fungal growth observed in neutropenic hosts [1, 8]. Of note, the histopathologic patterns of non-neutropenic hematopoietic stem cell transplant (HSCT) recipients with invasive aspergillosis resemble that of neutropenic patients, with no influx of neutrophils into the lung tissue [8]. This lack of neutrophil migration may be related to delayed function of innate and adaptive immunity after HSCT, despite recovery of white blood cells [10].

Epidemiology

Aspergillosis is the most common invasive fungal infection in HSCT recipients [4]. The incidence of invasive aspergillosis after allogeneic HSCT ranges from 4% to 24%, with most centers reporting rates between 11% and 15% [6, 11]. In contrast, reported rates in autologous HSCT recipients are 1–2% [6, 11, 12]. Recent data suggest that although aspergillosis remains the most common invasive fungal infection after HSCT, its incidence may be lower than previously reported. In a study of 3288 adult HSCT recipients at 11 Italian sites from 1999 to 2003, the overall incidence of invasive aspergillosis was 6.3% after allogeneic transplant and 0.4% after autologous transplant [13]. In the Transplant-Associated Infection Surveillance Network (TRANSNET), a prospective study of 16,200 allogeneic and autologous HSCT recipients at 23 US sites from 2001 through 2005, invasive aspergillosis occurred within 6 months and within 12 months of transplant in 1.3% and 1.6% of patients, respectively [4]. These lower rates of invasive aspergillosis may be related to increasing use of broad-spectrum mold-active triazoles for prophylaxis and empirical therapy.

There are three distinct periods of risk for invasive aspergillosis after HSCT. The first period is during neutropenia before engraftment and is present after both allogeneic and autologous transplants. The next two periods, early post-engraftment in the setting of acute GVHD and late post-engraftment in the setting of chronic GVHD, pertain primarily to allogeneic transplants. Overall, the median time from transplantation to onset of invasive aspergillosis in TRANSNET was 99 days. However, this median time was shorter in autologous transplants and longer in allogeneic transplants. In autologous HSCT recipients, 50% of *Aspergillus* infections occurred within 1 month after transplant. In contrast, only 22% occurred during this time period after allogeneic transplant and nearly half occurred more than 4 months after transplant [4].

Baseline risk factors for invasive aspergillosis in allogeneic HSCT recipients include older age, mismatched or unrelated donor grafts, and use of cord blood or T cell-depleted grafts. Transplant complications that are independently associated with invasive aspergillosis include neutropenia, acute or chronic GVHD, use of high doses of glucocorticoids, cytomegalovirus (CMV) disease, and respiratory viral infections [6, 14].

Aspergillosis is less common after solid organ transplantation than after HSCT. While glucocorticoids predispose to invasive aspergillosis [9], calcineurin and mammalian target of rapamycin inhibitors are mechanistically less immunosuppressive in regard to the risk of aspergillosis [15, 16]. Calcineurin inhibitors may even exert an inhibitory effect against *Aspergillus* spp. [17]. However, aspergillosis is still the second most common cause of invasive fungal infection in solid organ transplant recipients, after candidiasis. The cumulative incidence of invasive aspergillosis in 11,014 solid organ transplant recipients in the Spanish Network for Research on Infection in Transplantation (RESISTRA) who had at least 18 months of follow-up was 1.4% [18]. Among 16,459 solid organ transplant recipients who were followed up in TRANSNET, the 12-month cumulative incidence of invasive aspergillosis was 0.7% [3]. The median time to development of invasive aspergillosis in TRANSNET was longer after solid organ transplantation than after HSCT (184 days vs. 99 days) and 20% occurred more than 3 years after transplant [3]. The exception to this timing is in liver transplant recipients, who are more likely to develop invasive aspergillosis early in the post-transplant period [18–20]. The major risk factors for aspergillosis after liver transplantation are re-transplantation and the need for renal replacement therapy, which each confer a 20- to 30-fold increased risk [21].

Risk factors for invasive aspergillosis after solid organ transplantation depend on the timing of infection. Independent risk factors for early invasive aspergillosis (during the first 3 months after transplant) are postoperative complications including re-operations, repeated bacterial infections, CMV disease, and renal failure. Risk factors for late invasive aspergillosis which is observed more than 3 months after transplantation procedure include older age, an immunosuppressed state because of chronic transplant rejection or allograft dysfunction, and renal failure [18].

Lung transplant recipients have a higher risk of aspergillosis than recipients of other organs, and aspergillosis is the most common invasive fungal infection in this population [3, 18]. Between 3% and 12% of lung transplant recipients develop invasive aspergillosis, compared to 1% and 8% of liver transplant recipients and less than 1% of kidney transplant recipients [3, 18, 22–24]. This relatively high incidence is likely related to continuous exposure of the transplanted organ to the environment and impaired mechanical defenses from decreased mucociliary clearance and blunted cough reflex [25]. Risk factors for invasive aspergillosis in lung transplant recipients include transplant of a single lung, CMV infection, rejection with augmented immunosuppression, and bronchiolitis obliterans [22, 26, 27].

Clinical Manifestations

Although *Aspergillus* infection has been reported at virtually all organs and sites, invasive aspergillosis most commonly occurs in the lungs. Clinical manifestations are nonspecific and include fever and nonproductive cough. The classic triad of fever, pleuritic chest pain, and hemoptysis is occasionally seen in neutropenic patients, but is rarely seen in non-neutropenic patients. In addition to invasive pulmonary disease, *Aspergillus* can also cause tracheobronchitis. This disease is most common in lung transplant recipients, but has also been described in other transplant recipients.

Common clinical manifestations of tracheobronchitis are productive cough and dyspnea, followed by fever, wheezing, and acute respiratory distress. Three different patterns of *Aspergillus* tracheobronchitis have been described: (1) obstructive bronchial aspergillosis, in which thick mucus plugs filled with fungal hyphae are found in the airways within minimal or no tissue invasion; (2) ulcerative tracheobronchitis, in which there is focal invasion of tracheobronchial mucosa by fungal hyphae; and (3) pseudomembranous tracheobronchitis, in which a pseudomembrane of necrotic debris and fungal hyphae overlie extensive inflammation and invasion of the tracheobronchial tree [28]. Chronic forms of pulmonary aspergillosis, such as aspergilloma, chronic necrotizing aspergillosis, and chronic cavitary pulmonary aspergillosis, are relatively uncommon in transplant recipients.

Inhalation of *Aspergillus* conidia can also lead to invasive rhinosinusitis. Common presenting symptoms include fever, facial pain, and nasal congestion. If disease progresses to the orbit, patients may develop blurred vision, proptosis, and chemosis. Facial numbness and diplopia can occur in the setting of cranial nerve involvement. It is essential to note, however, that findings may be subtle in neutropenic patients because of a blunted inflammatory response [29, 30]. Therefore, a high suspicion must be maintained in neutropenic transplant recipients with any of these symptoms or signs. Early endoscopic evaluation of the nares and oral cavity to look for areas of necrosis is essential to establish the diagnosis early and initiate timely therapy [31].

In the setting of angioinvasive disease, *Aspergillus* can disseminate from the respiratory tract to multiple organs, including the brain, eyes, skin, liver, and kidneys. Central nervous system (CNS) aspergillosis can occur in the setting of hematogenous dissemination or local extension from paranasal sinuses and should be considered in patients with acute onset of focal neurologic deficits or seizures. CNS aspergillosis can present as meningitis, encephalitis, brain abscess, subarachnoid hemorrhage, or mycotic aneurysm [32, 33]. *Aspergillus* endophthalmitis can be a presenting feature of disseminated disease and is typically associated with eye pain, visual changes, and destruction of multiple components of the eye [34]. Cutaneous aspergillosis can occur as primary disease in an area of skin breakdown or as multiple cutaneous lesions in the setting of disseminated disease [35, 36].

Diagnosis

General Considerations

Aspergillus conidia are ubiquitous and frequently inhaled into the airways. Many patients effectively clear these organisms without developing disease, and thus, culturing *Aspergillus* species from respiratory specimens does not necessarily indicate disease. Therefore, the diagnosis of invasive aspergillosis is not solely based on isolating the organism (or markers of the organism) but also on the probability that it is causing disease, which is a reflection on host's functional status and clinical presentation. Based on this uncertainty, the European Organisation for Research and Treatment of Cancer (EORTC) and the Mycoses Study Group (MSG) of the National Institute of Allergy and Infectious Diseases established definitions of "proven," "probable," and "possible" invasive aspergillosis. Disease is "proven" when hyphal invasion is identified in tissue. "Probable" disease requires presence of a host factor such as neutropenia, use of glucocorticoids or T-cell immunosuppressant, compatible clinical disease, and either detection of *Aspergillus* directly (e.g., culture, direct microscopy) or indirectly via detection of aspergillus galactomannan and/or [1 → 3]-β-D-glucan tests or both. Cases that meet criteria for a host factor and a clinical criterion, but for which mycological criteria are absent, are considered "possible" disease.

Importantly, these definitions were designed to maintain consistency in research studies and were not designed to drive clinical decision-making [37]. Notably, all recent allogeneic HSCT recipients, neutropenic autologous HSCT recipients, and most solid organ transplant recipients satisfy EORTC/MSG host criteria. Unfortunately, transplant recipients often cannot undergo invasive procedures to obtain tissue and establish "proven" disease because of thrombocytopenia, advanced coagulation deficits, hemodynamic instability, or severe hypoxia.

Direct Examination and Culture

Respiratory specimens of patients being evaluated for aspergillosis should be stained where possible with calcofluor white, a fluorescent stain that binds to chitin, and 10% potassium hydroxide to detect the presence of fungal elements. Gomori methenamine silver (GMS) and periodic acid-Schiff (PAS) stains should be used on cytology preparations [38]. Organisms are typically seen as narrow as 3–6-micron-wide, septated hyphae with dichotomous acute angle branching [39]. Importantly, these characteristics are not diagnostic of *Aspergillus*, as they can be seen with other filamentous fungi, such as *Scedosporium* and *Fusarium* species.

Aspergillus grows rapidly in the laboratory and is often visible in culture within 1–3 days of incubation. Culture confirmation, where possible, is important to differentiate aspergillosis from other filamentous fungi, such as scedosporiosis and fusariosis. Identification to the species levels requires sporulation in order to examine the morphology of spore-bearing structures on lactophenol cotton blue wet mount preparations (Fig. 33.1a) [39].

Unfortunately, cultures of respiratory tract secretions lack sensitivity and specificity for invasive aspergillosis. *Aspergillus* is grown from sputum specimens in only 8–34% and from bronchoalveolar lavage (BAL) specimens in 45–62% of patients with invasive aspergillosis [40]. Thus, confirmation of invasive aspergillosis often requires histopathology. However, obtaining a biopsy is often not feasible in

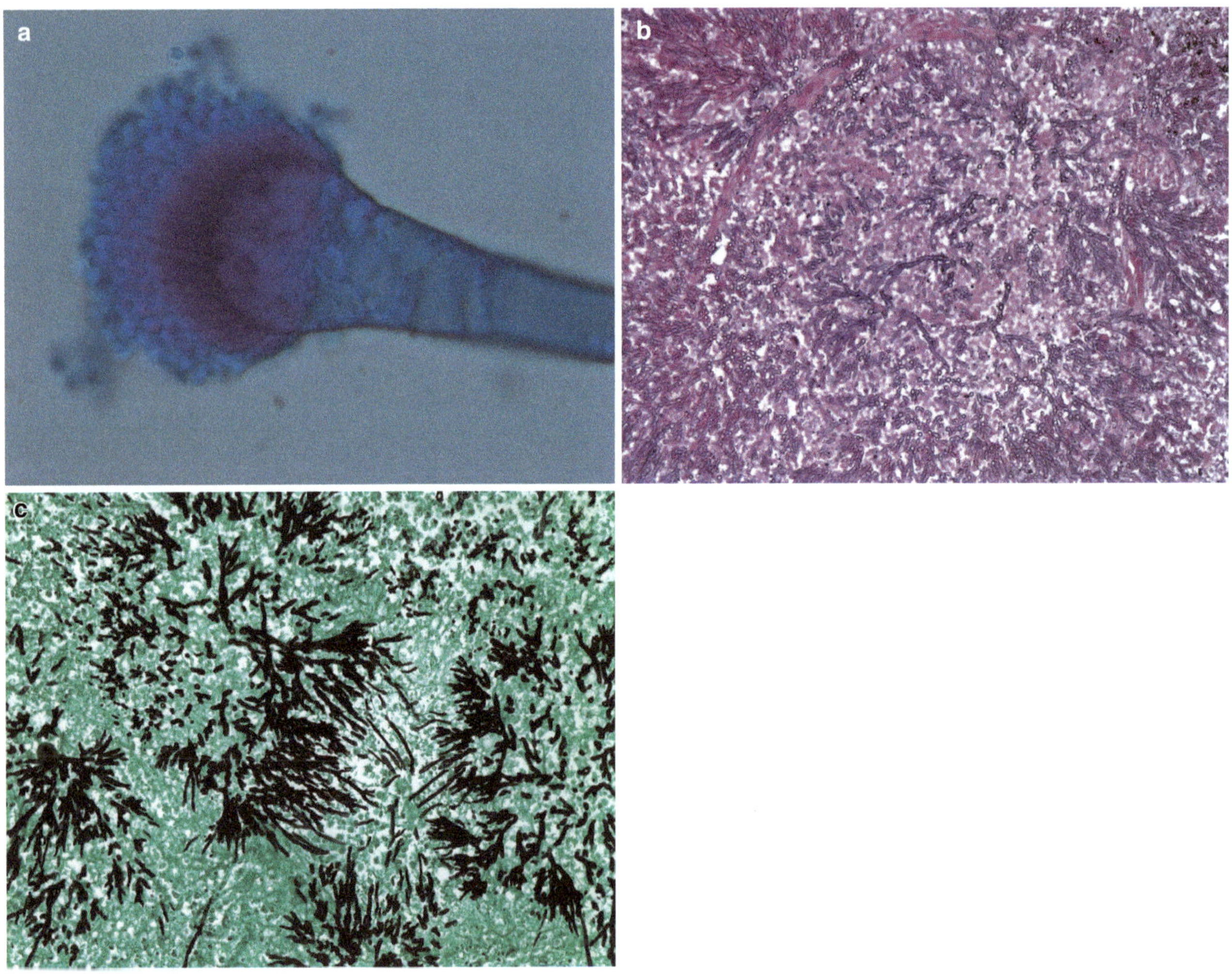

Fig. 33.1 *Aspergillus fumigatus*. (**a**) uniseriate vesicle with columnar phialides that encompass two-thirds of the vesicle on lactophenol cotton blue wet mount preparation (magnification ×100). (**b**) lung tissue demonstrating narrow, acutely branching septated hyphae and vascular invasion on hematoxylin-eosin stain; (**c**) lung tissue section showing narrow, acutely branching hyphae on Gomori methenamine silver stain. (All photomicrographs are courtesy of Audrey N. Schuetz, MD, MPH)

transplant recipients, particularly in HSCT recipients, because of thrombocytopenia. As such, negative fungal cultures should not preclude treatment in a clinical setting concerning for invasive aspergillosis. Although growth of *Aspergillus* from lower respiratory tract cultures does not necessarily indicate invasive infection, the positive predictive value of a positive lower respiratory tract culture is very high in HSCT recipients [41, 42]. Conversely, the positive predictive value in solid organ transplant recipients may be as low as 58% [41]. Of note, blood cultures have no role in the diagnosis of invasive aspergillosis and are negative even in the setting of disseminated infection.

Histopathology

The visualization of organisms on GMS or PAS stains of histopathology that resemble *Aspergillus* provides the strongest evidence of infection. As with direct microscopy, organisms are septated, hyaline hyphae with dichotomous, acute angle branching (Fig. 33.1b, c), features that can also be seen with other filamentous fungi. An important distinction is to differentiate *Aspergillus* from molds of the *Mucorales* order, because voriconazole is the treatment of choice against aspergillosis, but has no activity against the agents of mucormycosis. This distinction is usually possible from histopathology because, in contrast to *Aspergillus*, *Mucorales* typically appear as broad, nonseptate hyphae with right angle branching.

Serologic Markers

Given the limited sensitivities of microscopy and culture-based techniques and the difficulties of obtaining tissue histopathology in transplant recipients, the use of alternate modalities to diagnose invasive aspergillosis, such as serum biomarkers, is warranted. Galactomannan is a heteropolysaccharide found in the cell wall of *Aspergillus* species that is released into the serum and BAL fluid during hyphal growth and cell wall turnover. An enzyme-linked immunosorbent assay (ELISA) to detect galactomannan has been approved by the US Food and Drug Administration (FDA) for serum and BAL fluid. The assay is performed with an optical readout that is interpreted as a ratio relative to the optical density (OD) of a control, called the OD index. The FDA has recommended that an OD index of more than 0.5 should be considered a positive result. A meta-analysis demonstrates that the galactomannan serum ELISA has a sensitivity of 82% and specificity of 86% for invasive aspergillosis in HSCT recipients [43]. The performance of this test in solid organ transplant recipients has not been thoroughly evaluated. Among lung transplant recipients, the sensitivity appears to be lower, possibly because of a smaller fungal burden associated with infection in these hosts [44]. Conversely, in a study of 199 liver transplant recipients at high risk for invasive fungal infection who were randomized to fluconazole or anidulafungin for antifungal prophylaxis, the baseline serum galactomannan was positive in 47% of patients, suggesting poor test specificity in this population [45].

There are a number of limitations to the serum galactomannan assay. First, the sensitivity of the test is decreased by concurrent administration of mold-active antifungal therapy [46]. Second, there are a number of settings where false-positive tests may occur. False-positive results have traditionally been seen in patients receiving piperacillin-tazobactam and may persist for up to 5 days after discontinuation of the drug [47]. However, a recent study demonstrates that current preparations of piperacillin-tazobactam do not lead to false-positive galactomannan results [48]. False-positive results are common during the first 100 days after HSCT and in patients with chronic GVHD [49]. The likely explanation of these findings is that galactomannan in food or bacteria have cross-reactive epitopes and may translocate across intestinal mucosa in the setting of mucosal damage [50]. Third, fungi other than *Aspergillus*, such as *Penicillium* species, also have galactomannan on their cell walls [51]. A recent report demonstrated that nine of 11 hematology patients with *Fusarium* infection had positive serum galactomannan tests [52]. These limitations should be considered when using this assay to diagnose invasive aspergillosis in transplant recipients.

The galactomannan assay can also be performed on BAL fluid and provides additional sensitivity for the detection of pulmonary aspergillosis compared to culture and serum galactomannan. A study of high-risk hematology patients demonstrated that the sensitivity of BAL galactomannan to diagnose proven and probable invasive aspergillosis was 91%, compared to 50% and 53% for culture and microscopy, respectively [53]. Additional studies have confirmed the high sensitivity of BAL galactomannan in this population [54]. Data supporting the use of BAL galactomannan in solid organ transplant recipients are limited, but studies in lung transplant recipients have demonstrated sensitivities of 60–82% and specificities of 95–96% [55, 56].

(1 → 3)-β-D-glucan (BDG) is an integral component of the cell wall of many fungi, including *Aspergillus* and *Candida*, and can be detected in serum. The Fungitell assay is approved by the US FDA for the diagnosis of invasive fungal infections. This assay reports BDG concentrations as measured by optical density. Results are interpreted as positive (>80 pg/mL), intermediate (60–79 pg/mL), or negative (<60 pg/mL) [57]. In addition to aspergillosis and candidiasis, this test also detects infections caused by *Pneumocystis*, *Fusarium*, and *Trichosporon*. It does not detect mucormycosis, cryptococcosis, or mucosal candidiasis. A meta-analysis evaluating the use of serum BDG for the diagnosis of invasive

fungal infections demonstrated a sensitivity of 77% and specificity of 86% [58]. However, a more recent meta-analysis demonstrated a lower sensitivity (50%) and higher specificity (99%) in patients with hematologic malignancies, including HSCT recipients [59]. Its use in solid organ transplant recipients has not been well studied. A major limitation of the BDG assay is that false-positive results are seen in a number of settings. These include the use of hemodialysis with cellulose membranes [60], intravenous (IV) immunoglobulin [61], albumin [62] and amoxicillin-clavulanate [63], gauze packing of serosal surfaces [64], and bloodstream infections with certain bacteria, such as *Pseudomonas aeruginosa* [65].

Polymerase chain reaction (PCR) may be a powerful tool for early diagnosis of invasive aspergillosis, particularly in high-risk patients not receiving mold-active antifungal prophylaxis [66]. However, the lack of standardized and validated procedures for PCR detection of invasive aspergillosis remains a limitation of its wider usage [37].

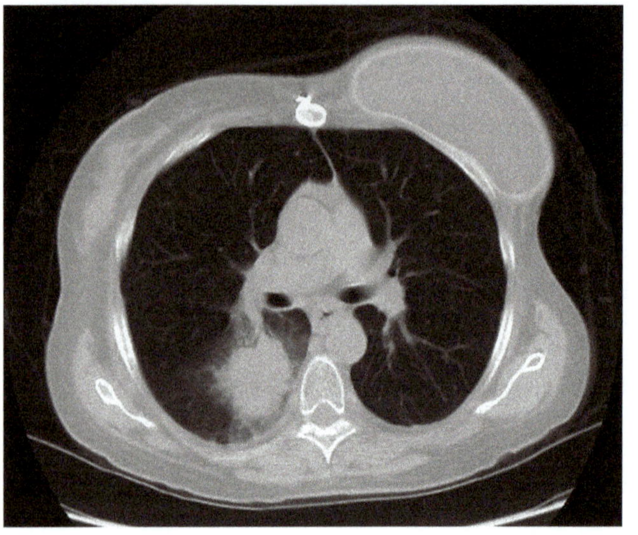

Fig. 33.2 Chest CT scan that demonstrates a halo sign (well-circumcised dense lesion with a surrounding area of ground-glass attenuation), a characteristic radiographic appearance of invasive pulmonary aspergillosis in a neutropenic patient

Imaging

Chest radiographs are insensitive for detecting the earliest stages of invasive pulmonary aspergillosis. On the other hand, computed tomography (CT) scanning of the lungs is an important and sensitive diagnostic screening method. Although radiographic abnormalities of invasive pulmonary aspergillosis are variable, focal lesions are typically seen on CT. In a review of baseline chest CT findings of 235 patients with invasive pulmonary aspergillosis, 94% had a nodule ≥1 cm in diameter, 61% had a halo sign, 30% had a consolidation including infarct (wedge)-shaped consolidations, and 20% had a cavitary lesion [67].

The CT halo sign is an area of ground-glass attenuation surrounding the circumference of a nodule or mass (Fig. 33.2) and was initially described in neutropenic patients with acute leukemia and invasive pulmonary aspergillosis [68]. Histopathologically, it represents a focus of pulmonary infarction as a nodule surrounded by hemorrhage represented as ground-glass attenuation. Although the halo sign may be seen in a variety of pulmonary infections, it is highly suggestive of aspergillosis in neutropenic patients with hematologic malignancies, including HSCT recipients [69–71]. The halo sign is commonly seen in early stages of invasive pulmonary aspergillosis but tends to disappear over time. In a study of 25 patients with hematologic malignancies, neutropenia, and invasive pulmonary aspergillosis who underwent serial CT scans, the prevalence of the halo sign on days 0, 3, 7, and 14 after initial diagnosis was 96%, 68%, 22%, and 19%, respectively [72]. The natural history of nodules caused by *Aspergillus* in neutropenic patients is to enlarge, even during appropriate therapy, and often cavitate. An air-crescent sign within a cavity is a finding that is highly suggestive of invasive aspergillosis. This finding results from air accumulation that separates necrotic tissue from normal lung parenchyma during cavitation [72].

Chest CT findings in solid organ transplant recipients with invasive pulmonary aspergillosis may differ from those of neutropenic patients. Among 92 solid organ transplant recipients who developed pulmonary aspergillosis in RESISTRA, nearly two-thirds presented with segmental areas of consolidation, rather than classic nodule progression to cavitation [18].

The role of CT pulmonary angiography for diagnosing invasive mold infections is unclear. One study found that this technique could distinguish between mold infections and other causes of pulmonary infiltrates, by virtue of detection of angioinvasion [73]. However, the study was small, conducted at a single center, and only included patients with hematologic malignancies. Given the risks associated with IV contrast and limited data to support its benefit compared to a noncontrast CT, the routine use of CT pulmonary angiography to diagnose invasive aspergillosis is not currently recommended.

Treatment

Primary Antifungal Therapy

Due to difficulties in obtaining an exact microbiologic diagnosis and the threat of clinical deterioration and death without treatment in immunocompromised transplant recipients, treatment of invasive aspergillosis should not be withheld while conducting a diagnostic evaluation [74]. Typically, therapy is initiated based on risk profile, clinical presentation, imaging studies, and serological markers. This section will focus on therapy as it relates to the treatment of invasive aspergillosis. A treatment algorithm for suspected or documented invasive aspergillosis is shown in Fig. 33.3, and Table 33.1 reviews dosing, pharmacokinetic parameters, adverse effects, and notable drug interactions for antifungal agents used in the treatment of aspergillosis.

Triazoles, polyenes, and echinocandins all have in vitro and in vivo activity against *Aspergillus*. Voriconazole is recommended as the drug of choice for the initial treatment of invasive pulmonary aspergillosis by the Infectious Diseases Society of America (IDSA) [74]. This recommendation is based on a randomized, open-label trial of primary therapy of proven or probable invasive aspergillosis in 277 adult patients. The trial compared voriconazole 6 mg/kg IV every 12 h for two doses, followed by 4 mg/kg IV every 12 h for the first 7 days, followed by 200 mg twice daily thereafter to 1.0–1.5 mg/kg/day of IV amphotericin B deoxycholate [75]. Approximately 90% of patients had pneumonia, 30% were HSCT recipients, and 5% were solid organ transplant recipients. The treating clinician

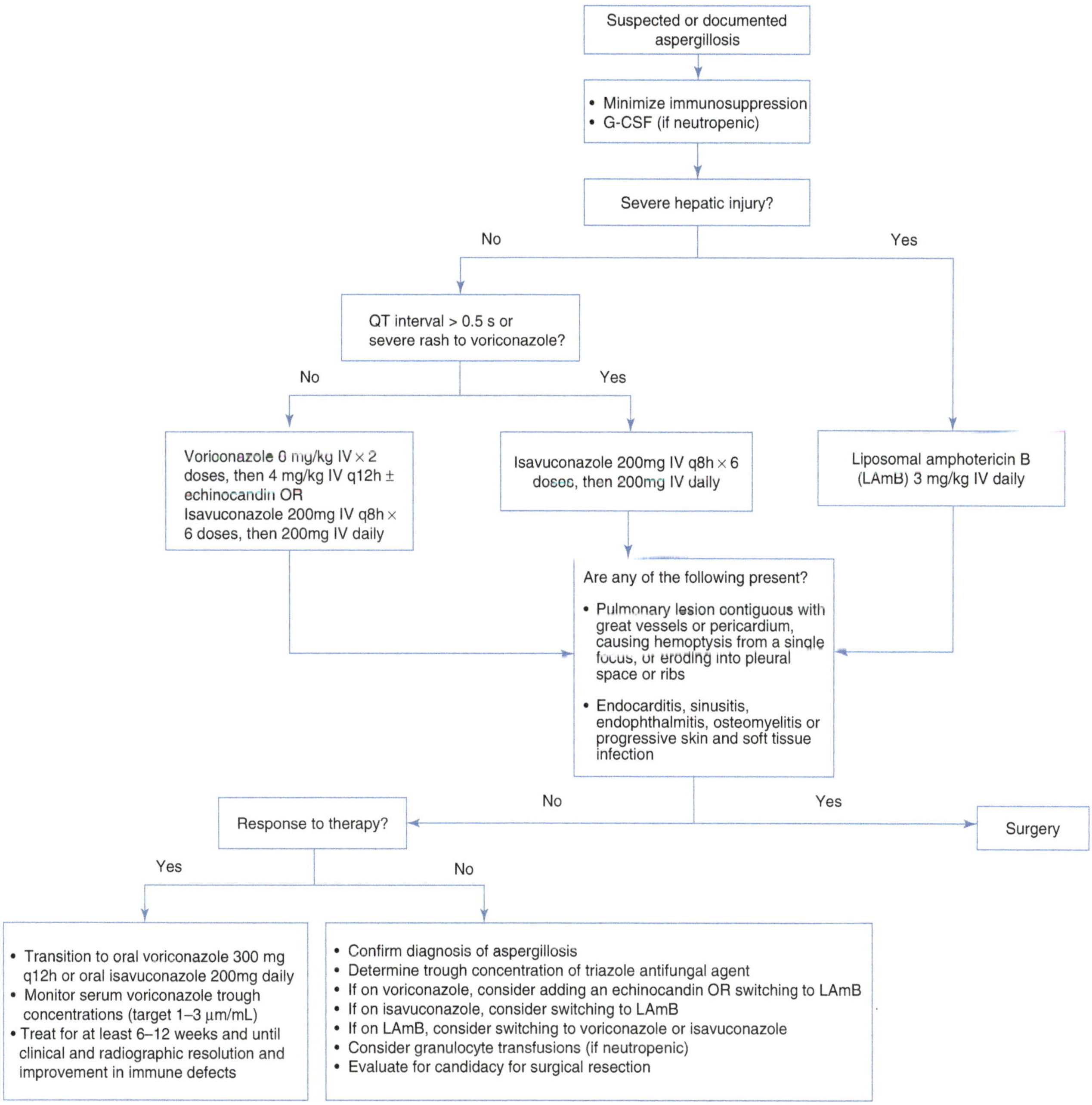

Fig. 33.3 Treatment algorithm for suspected or documented invasive aspergillosis

Table 33.1 Antifungal agents for aspergillosis

Antifungal agent	Adult dosing	Administration	Adverse effects	Notable drug interactions
First-line agents				
Voriconazole	IV: 6 mg/kg every 12 h ×2 doses and then 4 mg/kg every 12 h Oral: 300 mg every 12 h	IV: contains cyclodextrin, which may accumulate in patients with impaired renal function[a] Oral: absorption maximized if taken on an empty stomach (bioavailability up to 90%)	Hepatotoxicity Vision changes: photopsia, photophobia, or color changes Hallucinations Rash, photosensitivity QT prolongation Gastrointestinal Periostitis (prolonged use) Possible increased risk of squamous cell carcinoma and melanoma (prolonged use)	Rifampin and anticonvulsants (phenytoin, carbamazepine, phenobarbital): severely decrease voriconazole concentrations Warfarin, HIV protease inhibitors, simvastatin, atorvastatin, calcineurin inhibitors: voriconazole increases concentrations of these drugs Sirolimus: contraindicated with voriconazole
Isavuconazole	IV and oral: 200 mg every 8 h ×6 doses and then 200 mg daily		Gastrointestinal Hepatotoxicity Rash QT shortening	Similar to voriconazole Mycophenolate mofetil: isavuconazole may increase concentration
Liposomal amphotericin B (LAMB)	3 mg/kg IV daily	Acetaminophen, diphenhydramine, and low-dose hydrocortisone may limit infusion-related reactions 0.5–1 L of isotonic saline prior to drug administration may limit nephrotoxicity	Infusion-related reactions: Chest pain, dyspnea, hypoxia OR Severe abdominal, flank, or leg pain OR Rigors, chills, nausea, flushing, urticaria (less common) Nephrotoxicity: Azotemia (glomerular) Hypokalemia and hypomagnesemia (tubular) Metabolic acidosis (tubular)	Nephrotoxicity risk increases with concurrent use of other nephrotoxic agents Digoxin: Hypokalemia from amphotericin B may lead to digoxin toxicity
Second-line agents				
Echinocandins				
Caspofungin	70 mg IV ×1 dose and then 50 mg IV daily		Hepatotoxicity (rare: less common than with azole antifungal agents) Infusion and hypersensitivity reactions (very rare) Gastrointestinal (mild)	Cyclosporine: modestly increases caspofungin concentrations Rifampin and anticonvulsants: modestly decrease caspofungin concentrations (use 70 mg IV daily dose) Tacrolimus: caspofungin decreases tacrolimus concentrations by ~20%
Micafungin	150 mg IV daily		Similar to caspofungin	Cyclosporine and sirolimus: Caspofungin modestly increases concentrations of these drugs but does not affect tacrolimus concentrations
Anidulafungin	200 mg IV ×1 dose and then 100 mg IV daily		Similar to caspofungin	None
Amphotericin derivatives				
Amphotericin B lipid complex (ABLC)	5 mg/kg IV daily	Similar to LAMB	Infusion-related reactions: fever, rigors, nausea, and vomiting – higher rate than with LAMB Nephrotoxicity: rate likely higher than with LAMB	Similar to LAMB
Amphotericin B colloidal dispersion (ABCD)	3–4 mg/kg IV daily	Similar to ABLC	Similar to LAMB and ABLC, except higher rate of infusion-related reactions	Similar to LAMB

Table 33.1 (continued)

Antifungal agent	Adult dosing	Administration	Adverse effects	Notable drug interactions
Amphotericin B deoxycholate	1–1.5 mg/kg IV daily	Similar to ABLC	Higher rates of infusion-related reactions and nephrotoxicity than with LAMB or ABLC	Similar to LAMB
Posaconazole	IV: 300 mg every 12 h ×2 doses and then 300 mg daily Delayed-release tablet: 300 mg every 12 h ×2 doses and then 300 mg daily Oral suspension: 200 mg 4 times daily. Switch to 400 mg twice daily once disease has stabilized	IV: contains cyclodextrin, which may accumulate in patients with impaired renal function[b]; must be administered via a central venous catheter Tablet formulation preferred due to higher bioavailability, less food effect, fewer adverse effects Oral suspension must be taken with food, optimally with a high-fat meal, to ensure effective absorption	Hepatotoxicity Gastrointestinal	Drugs that increase gastric pH (proton pump inhibitors, histamine-2 receptor antagonists, and antacids) decrease absorption and serum concentrations (oral suspension only) Rifampin and phenytoin: severely decrease posaconazole concentrations Warfarin, HIV protease inhibitors, simvastatin, atorvastatin, calcineurin, and mTOR inhibitors: posaconazole increases concentrations of these drugs
Itraconazole	Capsule: 200 mg twice daily Oral solution: 2.5 mg/kg twice daily	Capsule: take with food and acidic beverages (cola or cranberry juice) to optimize absorption (55% bioavailability) Oral solution: take on an empty stomach to optimize absorption	Nausea, bloating, diarrhea, and weight loss (especially with the oral solution) Hepatotoxicity Hypertension, hypokalemia, and peripheral edema (use cautiously in patients with heart failure)	Drugs that increase gastric pH decrease absorption and serum levels of the capsule form, but not the oral solution Rifampin and phenytoin: severely decrease posaconazole concentrations Warfarin, HIV protease inhibitors, simvastatin, atorvastatin, calcineurin, and mTOR inhibitors: itraconazole increases concentrations of these drugs

mTOR mammalian target of rapamycin, *HIV* human immunodeficiency virus

[a]The clinical significance of the accumulation of cyclodextrin in patients with renal insufficiency is unclear

had the opportunity to switch to an alternate antifungal agent for drug intolerance or clinical failure. Patients who received voriconazole vs. amphotericin B deoxycholate had significantly improved survival (71% vs. 58%) and higher likelihood of complete or partial response (53% vs. 32%) at 12 weeks, respectively. They were also less likely to be switched to another antifungal agent because of intolerance or poor response (36% vs. 80%) and had significantly fewer drug-related adverse events. The results of this landmark trial demonstrated the superiority of voriconazole compared to amphotericin B deoxycholate for the treatment of invasive pulmonary aspergillosis.

The role and optimal dosing of oral voriconazole for invasive aspergillosis in transplant recipients are unclear. In the aforementioned trial, patients were eligible to receive 200 mg of oral voriconazole twice daily after 1 week of IV therapy. However, there is substantial variability in serum drug concentrations in patients receiving oral voriconazole. Serum trough concentrations at this dose are often <0.5–1 μg/mL (the minimum inhibitory concentrations at which, for most *Aspergillus* species, 90% of isolates are susceptible) [76, 77]. Trough concentrations ≤1 μg/mL have been associated with a lack of response to therapy, and concentrations >5.5 μg/mL have been associated with neurological toxicity. A randomized trial provides further support for monitoring voriconazole levels in patients receiving treatment for invasive aspergillosis [78]. One hundred ten patients receiving voriconazole for invasive fungal infection or empirical treatment were randomly assigned to therapeutic drug monitoring of voriconazole levels or no monitoring. In the monitored group, the dosage was adjusted to target a trough level between 1.0 and 5.5 μg/mL. Patients randomized to the therapeutic drug monitoring arm had a significantly higher rate of complete or partial response (81% vs. 57%) and a significantly lower rate of voriconazole discontinuation due to adverse events (4% vs. 17%) compared with patients randomized to no serum drug level monitoring.

The development of voriconazole represented a major advance in the therapy of aspergillosis. However, nonlinear pharmacokinetics, drug-drug interactions, adverse effects, and need for therapeutic drug monitoring may pose management challenges in immunocompromised patients with multiple comorbid conditions. Isavuconazole is a new-generation azole with potent activity against *Aspergillus* species. Similar to other azoles, isavuconazole prevents fungal cell wall synthesis via inhibition of lanosterol 14α-demethylase. The thiazolyl cyanophenyl moiety of the active isavuconazole molecule allows greater avidity of isavuconazole for the binding pocket in the fungal cytochrome P450 51 protein, conferring broader antifungal spectrum. In animal studies and human trials, isavuconazole has comparable efficacy to voriconazole for the treatment of aspergillosis; yet, it has a more favorable safety, tolerability, and pharmacokinetic profile.

IDSA recommends isavuconazole as an alternative primary therapy for invasive aspergillosis based on the SECURE trial, a randomized, double-blind, noninferiority trial of isavuconazole versus voriconazole for the treatment of invasive fungal infections due to *Aspergillus* species and other filamentous fungi [79]. Adult patients with proven, probable, or possible invasive fungal infection according to EORTC/MSG criteria were randomized in a 1:1 ratio to treatment with isavuconazole given as 200 mg IV three times per day for six doses followed by 200 mg IV or orally daily thereafter or voriconazole administered as 6 mg/kg IV twice daily for two doses followed by 4 mg/kg IV twice daily or 200 mg orally twice daily thereafter. The primary outcome measure of the trial was day 42 all-cause mortality in the intention-to-treat (ITT) arm. The median durations of treatment were 45 and 47 days for patients receiving isavuconazole and voriconazole, respectively. All-cause mortality through day 42 in the ITT population of 516 subjects was 18.6% and 20.2% in the isavuconazole and voriconazole treatment groups, respectively, meeting the prespecified 10% noninferiority margin.

Treatment with isavuconazole is generally well-tolerated. The relatively greater safety and tolerability of isavuconazole as compared to voriconazole are key distinguishing features of this drug. The most common adverse events observed in clinical trials include nausea, diarrhea, vomiting, pyrexia, constipation, and hypokalemia [79, 80]. In the SECURE trial, significantly fewer drug-related treatment-emergent adverse events (TEAEs) occurred in patients treated with isavuconazole (42%) versus voriconazole (60%; $P < 0.001$). In particular, fewer adverse events occurred in the following system organ classes in patients receiving isavuconazole versus voriconazole: hepatobiliary disorders (9% versus 16%), eye disorders (15% versus 27%), and skin and subcutaneous tissue disorders (33% versus 42%). Permanent drug discontinuation due to drug-related TEAEs was 8% and 14% in patients taking isavuconazole and voriconazole, respectively. Also, of note, isavuconazole causes QTc shortening, as opposed to most triazoles that are associated with QT prolongation. The clinical significance of this observed QT shortening is unknown; in clinical trials, no ventricular arrhythmias were observed, and no medical interventions were required.

In patients who are intolerant of triazoles or have contraindications to their use, liposomal amphotericin B is a valid alternate option for initial treatment of invasive aspergillosis [74]. This recommendation is based on a randomized, double-blind trial of 201 adult patients with proven or probable invasive mold infection who received liposomal amphotericin B at either 3 mg/kg or 10 mg/kg per day for 14 days, followed by 3 mg/kg per day [81]. Invasive aspergillosis accounted for 97% of cases and 90% were pulmonary infections. Approximately 20% of patients were HSCT recipients and only one had received a solid organ transplant. A favorable response was achieved in 50% and 46% of patients in the 3- and 10-mg/kg groups, a difference that was not statistically significant. However, in the 3 mg/kg arm, there was a trend toward overall improved survival (72% vs. 59%; $P = 0.09$) and significantly lower rates of hypokalemia and renal failure. The results of this trial demonstrate the efficacy of 3 mg/kg of daily liposomal amphotericin B as first-line therapy for invasive aspergillosis, yielding similar outcomes to those of the pivotal trial that established the efficacy of voriconazole [75]. This study also establishes that increasing the dose of liposomal amphotericin B beyond 3 mg/kg daily for invasive pulmonary aspergillosis yields no additional clinical benefit, but higher rates of nephrotoxicity.

Unfortunately, there are no randomized comparisons of liposomal amphotericin B and voriconazole or isavuconazole for invasive aspergillosis and few between lipid formulations of amphotericin B and conventional amphotericin B deoxycholate. A randomized trial of 66 patients with neutropenia-associated invasive fungal infections, of which 40 had pulmonary aspergillosis, demonstrated that liposomal amphotericin B had a strong trend toward improved response rates and significantly lower mortality and renal failure compared to amphotericin B deoxycholate [82]. Another study randomized 174 patients with invasive aspergillosis to receive amphotericin B colloidal dispersion (ABCD) versus amphotericin B deoxycholate [83]. Patients randomized to either arm had poor, but similar, complete or partial response rates of 18% and 23%, respectively. Patients who received ABCD had lower rates of nephrotoxicity (25% vs. 49%) but higher rates of infusion-related chills and fevers. Lipid formulations of amphotericin B are less nephrotoxic than conventional amphotericin B deoxycholate, and amphotericin B lipid complex and liposomal amphotericin B have fewer infusion-related side effects [82–84]. This improved side effect profile, combined with data that suggest superior efficacy [81, 82], provides a strong rationale for using lipid formulations of amphotericin B instead of amphotericin B deoxycholate for invasive aspergillosis.

Second-Line Antifungal Therapy

Alternate antifungal agents for patients who are intolerant of or not responding to voriconazole, isavuconazole, or liposomal amphotericin B include amphotericin B lipid complex, posaconazole, itraconazole and echinocandins. Amphotericin B lipid complex has not been compared in a randomized trial to liposomal amphotericin B for the treatment of aspergillosis. However, a randomized comparison for empirical therapy of prolonged fever and neutropenia and an observational study suggest that amphotericin B lipid complex may be associated with greater rates of infusion-related reactions and nephrotoxicity [85, 86]. Posaconazole demonstrates activity comparable to amphotericin B in animal models, and clinical data are consistent with these laboratory findings [87, 88]. In an open-label study of 107 patients with invasive aspergillosis refractory to or intolerant of amphotericin B or itraconazole, treatment with posaconazole given as 800 mg/day oral suspension in divided doses was successful in 42% of patients [89]. This response rate was greater than that of 86 historical controls with similar demographic and disease features and is similar to those observed with other agents in the salvage setting. Posaconazole was approved in Europe for salvage treatment of patients with invasive aspergillosis who are refractory to amphotericin B or itraconazole, but not for patients refractory to voriconazole.

Itraconazole is a second-line agent for the treatment of aspergillosis and has less intrinsic activity against *Aspergillus* than voriconazole [90]. IDSA guidelines do not recommend using itraconazole for salvage therapy in patients with invasive aspergillosis that is refractory to primary therapy with voriconazole because of its inferior in vitro activity, bioavailability, and toxicity profile, compared to voriconazole [74].

Caspofungin is the only echinocandin approved by the US FDA for the treatment of invasive aspergillosis in patients intolerant of or refractory to standard therapy [91]. A study of 83 patients with invasive aspergillosis who were mostly refractory to amphotericin B or a triazole demonstrated a favorable response rate of 45% [92]. Although not FDA-approved for salvage therapy, micafungin and anidulafungin are at least as potent as caspofungin in vitro against *Aspergillus* [93]. Studies using micafungin alone for salvage therapy are small but show similar response rates to that of caspofungin [94, 95].

Although not formally investigated in a clinical trial, when a change in antifungal therapy is considered necessary because of refractory disease, switching to a different class is prudent. Given suboptimal response rates to salvage therapy using single-agent therapy, combination therapy is often employed. Combination therapy using an echinocandin and a triazole is an attractive option because this combination inhibits both cell wall and cell membrane biosynthesis and both drug classes have favorable toxicity profiles. Furthermore, this combination demonstrates a synergistic interaction in neutropenic animal models of pulmonary aspergillosis [96, 97]. A study of 47 patients with invasive aspergillosis who failed therapy with amphotericin B compared outcomes of those who switched to voriconazole alone to that of those who switched to the combination of voriconazole and caspofungin [98]. Salvage therapy with this combination was associated with improved 3-month survival in multivariate analysis.

An antifungal combination that is not recommended is the use of amphotericin B and triazoles. Antagonism between these agents has been demonstrated both in vitro and in animal models [99]. A proposed mechanism for this antagonism is that amphotericin B binding to fungal cell membranes is reduced in the setting of triazole inhibition of the ergosterol biosynthetic pathway. Confirmatory clinical data of the significance of this antagonism are limited, but one observational study demonstrated no benefit to adding itraconazole to a lipid formulation of amphotericin B [100].

Combination Antifungal Therapy for Primary Treatment

The aforementioned in vitro, animal, and clinical observational data that suggest the potential benefit of combining a triazole and an echinocandin provided rationale for testing this hypothesis in a clinical trial [96–98]. A multicenter, randomized, double-blind trial compared outcomes among patients with invasive aspergillosis who received primary therapy with combination voriconazole and anidulafungin versus voriconazole alone [101]. The study population consisted of allogeneic HSCT recipients (32%) and patients with hematologic malignancies with proven or probable invasive aspergillosis. Voriconazole was given for a minimum of 1 week intravenously, after which the investigator could switch to 300 mg of twice daily oral voriconazole. After 2 weeks, patients in the combination therapy arm could have been switched to voriconazole monotherapy, to complete 6 weeks of antifungal treatment. Mortality at 6 weeks was 19.3% in the combination arm and 27.5% in the monotherapy arm and at 12 weeks was 29.3% in the combination arm and 39.4% in the monotherapy arm. The *P* value for these differences was 0.09 and 0.08, respectively. The rate of adverse events was not higher in the combination arm.

Although these findings did not reach statistical significance, the strong and consistent trend toward a mortality benefit with combination therapy, combined with the apparent lack of significant added toxicity and supportive in vitro and laboratory animal data, provides a compelling rationale for adding an echinocandin to voriconazole as initial therapy for invasive aspergillosis. Assuming that the survival differences are not due to chance, then this trial suggests that for every 12 patients who have an echinocandin added to voriconazole in their initial regimen, one life will be saved. It is unclear how long the echinocandin should be continued in the trial; it was given for 2–4 weeks, and it is reasonable to discontinue it upon discharge from an inpatient setting.

Extrapulmonary Aspergillosis

The optimal treatment of aspergillosis at sites other than the lungs has not been well studied because most patients in randomized trials had pulmonary aspergillosis. The trial comparing voriconazole to amphotericin B deoxycholate included 37 patients with extrapulmonary infection [75]. Of these 37 patients, successful outcome occurred in 43% of those randomized to voriconazole, compared to 13% of those randomized to amphotericin B ($P < 0.05$). Based on these data, the IDSA recommends voriconazole for the primary treatment of extrapulmonary manifestations of invasive aspergillosis [74].

Aspergillus dissemination to the CNS is a devastating complication of invasive aspergillosis. Unlike amphotericin B, echinocandins, and itraconazole, voriconazole achieves therapeutic levels in the cerebrospinal fluid (CSF) and brain tissue [102–104]. The CSF penetration of isavuconazole is not well studied. Mortality rates for CNS disease prior to the availability of voriconazole were >90% [105, 106]. In contrast, 35% of patients with CNS aspergillosis who received voriconazole combined with surgical intervention had a complete or partial response, with long-term survival observed in 31% of patients [107]. These findings provide strong rationale for using voriconazole as the cornerstone of therapy for CNS aspergillosis.

The sinuses are also common sites of extrapulmonary aspergillosis. Therapy for invasive sinus aspergillosis often consists of systemic antifungal therapy and surgical debridement. Although voriconazole is recommended for invasive sinus aspergillosis, amphotericin B formulations should be used until sinus mucormycosis has been excluded by culture or histopathologic examination [74]. Because of its high degree of water solubility, voriconazole is also a reasonable option for endophthalmitis, peritonitis, and joint infections. A detailed discussion of site-directed treatments can be found in the IDSA guidelines [74].

Antifungal Resistance

The vast majority of *Aspergillus* isolates are susceptible to amphotericin B, voriconazole, isavuconazole, posaconazole, itraconazole, and echinocandins. However, there are exceptions that make identifying the species from growth of a clinical specimen helpful in deciding on treatment. Most isolates of *Aspergillus terreus* are resistant to amphotericin B, but susceptible to voriconazole [108]. Furthermore, observational data and data from animal models demonstrate poor efficacy of amphotericin B against infections caused by *Aspergillus terreus* compared to voriconazole [109, 110]. Therefore, amphotericin B derivatives should not be used for antifungal resistance to treat infections due to *A. terreus*.

Certain uncommon *Aspergillus* species such as *A. lentulus* and *Neosartorya udagawae* have decreased in vitro susceptibility to antifungal resistance in antifungal agents commonly used for aspergillosis [111, 112]. Recently, *Aspergillus fumigatus* isolates with elevated minimum inhibitory concentrations of voriconazole have been reported [113]. However, these isolates are extremely rare and the vast majority of clinically significant *Aspergillus* antifungal resistance isolates remain highly susceptible to voriconazole [114].

Duration of Antifungal Therapy

Antifungal therapy for invasive aspergillosis should be continued for at least 6–12 weeks, until all signs and symptoms of infection have resolved and until all radiographic abnormalities have stabilized [7, 74]. Transplant recipients with invasive aspergillosis may need to remain on therapy for longer periods of time because of persistent immune defects. Long-term therapy is facilitated by the excellent bioavailability of oral voriconazole and isavuconazole.

Adjunctive Therapies

Reversal of immunosuppression is an important component of the treatment of invasive aspergillosis. In a review of 405 HSCT recipients with invasive aspergillosis, neutropenia and receipt of high doses of corticosteroids were independently associated with mortality [115]. Dose reduction or discontinuation of corticosteroids is recommended, when feasible. In neutropenic patients, recovery of bone marrow function is essential for control of the infection [116]. Granulocyte colony-stimulating factors (G-CSF) shorten the duration of chemotherapy-induced neutropenia and lead to fewer episodes of fever and neutropenia and infection [117, 118]. Although it is not clear that G-CSF improves response rates or decreases mortality in patients with invasive fungal infections, IDSA guidelines support their use in neutropenic patients with aspergillosis [74].

The role of granulocyte transfusions in the management of neutropenic patients with aspergillosis is not well defined, but favorable responses have been reported [119]. The Resolving Infection in Neutropenia with Granulocytes (RING) trial was an open-label, multicenter, randomized trial to investigate the efficacy and safety of granulocyte transfusions for bacterial and fungal infections in patients who were neutropenic (absolute neutrophil count <500 cells/μL) due to chemotherapy, HSCT, or underlying disease [120]. The primary outcome was clinical success, defined as survival at day 42 and clinical response of the study-qualifying infection. This endpoint was met in 20/48 (42%)

and 21/49 (43%) of patients in the granulocyte and control arms, respectively. Twenty percent of patients had transfusion reactions of grade 3 and 4 severity including hypoxia (n = 7), tachycardia (n = 1), hypotension (n = 1), and an allergic reaction (n = 1). No deaths were attributable to transfusion reactions. Unfortunately, this study had low subject accrual, enrolling less than half of its intended sample size of 118 patients per study arm; therefore, statistical power was limited to detect a difference in the primary outcome if one truly existed. In persistently neutropenic patients with invasive aspergillosis who are not responding to medical and (when appropriate) surgical therapy, administration of granulocyte transfusions from G-CSF-stimulated healthy donors may be considered.

Surgical resection of a pulmonary lesion of aspergillosis can provide a definitive diagnosis and eradicate a localized infection. Surgery may be indicated in the setting of recurrent hemoptysis from a single cavitary lesion, lesions contiguous with the great vessels or pericardium, or lesions that invade the chest wall (Fig. 33.3) [74]. Surgical resection may also be considered in appropriate HSCT candidates prior to transplant. Multiple case series suggest that surgery can be safely and effectively performed in patients with localized infections, even during neutropenia [121, 122].

Surgery is essential for the treatment of *Aspergillus* endocarditis and should be strongly considered in endophthalmitis, osteomyelitis, and necrotic, progressive skin and soft tissue infections [74]. Neurosurgical interventions have been independently associated with survival in CNS aspergillosis and should be pursued when feasible [107]. Similarly, surgical debridement of infected tissues is an important component of the management of invasive sinusitis [123].

Prevention

Antifungal Prophylaxis

Primary prophylaxis against *Aspergillus* and other mold infections is not indicated in autologous HSCT recipients because of the low rate of these infections in this population [13]. Current data are inconclusive as to whether antimold prophylaxis should be routinely administered to allogeneic HSCT recipients. A randomized, double-blind trial of 600 allogeneic HSCT recipients compared the efficacy of voriconazole to that of fluconazole in preventing invasive fungal infections after myeloablative transplant [124]. These agents were administered for either 100 or 180 days after transplant, depending on the risk of invasive fungal infection, and serum galactomannan was routinely monitored until day 100. There were no significant differences between groups in rates of invasive fungal infection, survival, or toxicities, although there was a trend toward a lower rate of invasive aspergillosis in the voriconazole arm (3% vs. 6%; P = 0.09). Another blinded study randomized 882 HSCT recipients of autologous and allogeneic stem cell grafts to intravenous micafungin or fluconazole during the neutropenic phase after transplant [125]. Patients randomized to micafungin had less use of empirical antifungal therapy and a trend toward fewer cases of aspergillosis (1 vs. 7; P = 0.07), but there were no differences in the rate of breakthrough fungal infection. These studies suggest that mold-active primary prophylaxis may not be necessary for allogeneic HSCT recipients in the setting of empirical antifungal therapy for prolonged fever and neutropenia and structured galactomannan screening. However, many experts favor the use of a mold-active agent for prophylaxis in high-risk HSCT recipients with anticipated prolonged neutropenic periods, such as cord blood transplant recipients or those with lengthy duration of neutropenia immediately prior to HSCT [74].

HSCT recipients with GVHD are at high risk of invasive mold infections and merit consideration for prophylaxis with mold-active agents [6, 14]. In a double-blind trial, 600 patients with GVHD who were receiving immunosuppressive therapies were randomized to 112 days of posaconazole (200 mg three times daily) or 400 mg of daily fluconazole for antifungal prophylaxis [126]. Patients randomized to posaconazole had a lower rate of invasive aspergillosis (2.3% vs. 7.0%; P = 0.006) and death from an invasive fungal infection (1% vs. 4%, P = 0.046) and a strong trend toward a lower rate of invasive fungal infection overall (5.3% vs. 9.0%; P = 0.07). The incidence of treatment-related adverse events and overall mortality were similar in both arms. Voriconazole has also been shown to be effective in preventing invasive aspergillosis in HSCT recipients with GVHD who are receiving glucocorticoids [127]. These data support the use of prophylactic posaconazole or voriconazole, instead of fluconazole, in patients with GVHD who are receiving corticosteroids.

Patients with prior invasive aspergillosis are at high risk for relapse of fungal disease after HSCT [128]. Secondary prophylaxis with voriconazole is effective in preventing relapse after transplantation and is recommended for this indication by the American Society for Blood and Marrow Transplantation (ASBMT) [129, 130].

Aspergillosis is generally less common after solid organ transplantation than after HSCT, and prophylaxis against aspergillosis is not routinely recommended in this population [3, 25]. However, mold-active prophylaxis may be warranted in high-risk patients, such as lung, heart, and heart-lung transplant recipients. Prophylaxis options in these patients include nebulized amphotericin B and oral mold-active triazoles. The administration of nebulized amphotericin B delivers drug to the site of *Aspergillus* exposure, with minimal systemic drug exposure, and its use has been associated with lower rates of invasive aspergillosis in observational studies [131, 132].

Common adverse effects of nebulized amphotericin B include nausea, vomiting, taste alterations, and bronchospasm. Nebulized lipid formulations of amphotericin B may also be effective in preventing aspergillosis and have better lung penetration and longer half-lives than conventional nebulized amphotericin B deoxycholate [133]. In a randomized trial, nebulized amphotericin B lipid complex was as effective as nebulized amphotericin B deoxycholate and associated with fewer adverse events [132]. The primary disadvantage of using nebulized amphotericin for prophylaxis against aspergillosis is that it does not prevent systemic fungal infections, such as candidemia, and pleural space infections [134]. A retrospective study showed that voriconazole is also effective in preventing pulmonary aspergillosis in lung transplant recipients [135]. However, liver enzyme abnormalities developed in over 40% of patients who received voriconazole. Regular monitoring of liver enzymes and serum concentrations of calcineurin inhibitors is required when using voriconazole as primary prophylaxis in solid organ transplant recipients.

Mold-active prophylaxis may also be warranted in high-risk liver transplant recipients. The American Society of Transplantation recommends consideration of targeted prophylaxis in patients who are receiving a second or third liver transplant, receive renal replacement therapy, require reoperation involving the thoracic or intraabdominal cavity, or are transplanted for fulminant hepatic failure [25]. Both lipid formulations of amphotericin B and echinocandins appear to be effective for this indication [136, 137], whereas voriconazole has not typically been used because of concerns of hepatotoxicity.

Limiting Exposures

Invasive aspergillosis among transplant recipients results from respiratory exposure to and direct contact with fungal spores. Transplant recipients should avoid construction, excavation, and other dust-laden environments during at-risk periods [130, 138]. Physical barriers should be used in the hospital to prevent airborne transmission of *Aspergillus* from construction sites to transplant wards [23]. The use of high-efficiency particulate air (HEPA) filters has been shown to reduce the incidence of aspergillosis in neutropenic patients [139]. The ASBMT recommends the use of HEPA filters and at least 12 air exchanges per hour in all rooms housing HSCT recipients [130]. The need for HEPA filters in rooms of solid organ transplant recipients is not well established [23].

Prognosis

In a study of 642 patients in TRANSNET who developed invasive aspergillosis from 2001 through 2006, the 12-week all-cause mortality rate was 58% in HSCT recipients and 34% in solid organ transplant recipients [140]. Factors independently associated with mortality in HSCT recipients included persistent neutropenia, renal or hepatic insufficiency, onset of disease within 30 days of transplant, and corticosteroid use. Factors independently associated with mortality in solid organ transplant recipients included hepatic insufficiency, malnutrition, and CNS disease. Use of an amphotericin B formulation for treatment was associated with increased mortality in both groups. Other studies of HSCT recipients with invasive aspergillosis have found that poor pulmonary function prior to transplant, use of human leukocyte antigen-mismatched stem cells, and disseminated disease are associated with increased mortality and that survival has improved in recent years [115, 141, 142].

The serum galactomannan assay may also have prognostic value. A meta-analysis of 27 studies showed a strong correlation between the galactomannan index level at the time of diagnosis and mortality [143]. Other studies have confirmed the prognostic value of the initial serum galactomannan and demonstrated that the rate of galactomannan decline after starting antifungal therapy is also correlated with survival [144, 145].

References

1. Dagenais TR, Keller NP. Pathogenesis of *Aspergillus fumigatus* in invasive aspergillosis. Clin Microbiol Rev. 2009;22(3):447–65.
2. Bennett JW. *Aspergillus*: a primer for the novice. Med Mycol. 2009;47(Suppl 1):S5–12.
3. Pappas PG, Alexander BD, Andes DR, et al. Invasive fungal infections among organ transplant recipients: results of the Transplant-Associated Infection Surveillance Network (TRANSNET). Clin Infect Dis. 2010;50(8):1101–11.
4. Kontoyiannis DP, Marr KA, Park BJ, et al. Prospective surveillance for invasive fungal infections in hematopoietic stem cell transplants, 2001-2006: overview of the Transplant-Associated Infection Surveillance Network (TRANSNET) Database. Clin Infect Dis. 2010;50(8):1091–100.
5. Perkhofer S, Lass-Florl C, Hell M, et al. The Nationwide Austrian Aspergillus Registry: a prospective data collection on epidemiology, therapy and outcome of invasive mould infections in immunocompromised and/or immunosuppressed patients. Int J Antimicrob Agents. 2010;36(6):531–6.
6. Marr KA, Carter RA, Boeckh M, Martin P, Corey L. Invasive aspergillosis in allogeneic stem cell transplant recipients: changes in epidemiology and risk factors. Blood. 2002;100(13):4358–66.
7. Segal BH. Aspergillosis. N Engl J Med. 2009;360(18):1870–84.
8. Stergiopoulou T, Meletiadis J, Roilides E, et al. Host-dependent patterns of tissue injury in invasive pulmonary aspergillosis. Am J Clin Pathol. 2007;127(3):349–55.
9. Lionakis MS, Kontoyiannis DP. Glucocorticoids and invasive fungal infections. Lancet. 2003;362(9398):1828–38.
10. Auletta JJ, Lazarus HM. Immune restoration following hematopoietic stem cell transplantation: an evolving target. Bone Marrow Transplant. 2005;35(9):835–57.
11. Wirk B, Wingard JR. Current approaches in antifungal prophylaxis in high risk hematologic malignancy and hematopoietic stem cell transplant patients. Mycopathologia. 2009;168(6):299–311.

12. Gil L, Styczynski J, Komarnicki M. Infectious complication in 314 patients after high-dose therapy and autologous hematopoietic stem cell transplantation: risk factors analysis and outcome. Infection. 2007;35(6):421–7.
13. Pagano L, Caira M, Nosari A, et al. Fungal infections in recipients of hematopoietic stem cell transplants: results of the SEIFEM B-2004 study—Sorveglianza Epidemiologica Infezioni Fungine Nelle Emopatie Maligne. Clin Infect Dis. 2007;45(9):1161–70.
14. Garcia-Vidal C, Upton A, Kirby KA, Marr KA. Epidemiology of invasive mold infections in allogeneic stem cell transplants: biological risk factors for infection according to time after transplantation. Clin Infect Dis. 2008;47(8):1041–50.
15. Roilides E, Robinson T, Sein T, Pizzo PA, Walsh TJ. *In vitro* and *ex vivo* effects of cyclosporin a on phagocytic host defenses against *Aspergillus fumigatus*. Antimicrob Agents Chemother. 1994;38(12):2883–8.
16. Berenguer J, Allende MC, Lee JW, et al. Pathogenesis of pulmonary aspergillosis. Granulocytopenia versus cyclosporine and methylprednisolone-induced immunosuppression. Am J Respir Crit Care Med. 1995;152(3):1079–86.
17. Steinbach WJ, Reedy JL, Cramer RA Jr, Perfect JR, Heitman J. Harnessing calcineurin as a novel anti-infective agent against invasive fungal infections. Nat Rev Microbiol. 2007;5(6):418–30.
18. Gavalda J, Len O, San Juan R, et al. Risk factors for invasive aspergillosis in solid-organ transplant recipients: a case-control study. Clin Infect Dis. 2005;41(1):52–9.
19. Singh N, Arnow PM, Bonham A, et al. Invasive aspergillosis in liver transplant recipients in the 1990s. Transplantation. 1997;64(5):716–20.
20. Singh N, Avery RK, Munoz P, et al. Trends in risk profiles for and mortality associated with invasive aspergillosis among liver transplant recipients. Clin Infect Dis. 2003;36(1):46–52.
21. Fortun J, Martin-Davila P, Moreno S, et al. Risk factors for invasive aspergillosis in liver transplant recipients. Liver Transpl. 2002;8(11):1065–70.
22. Singh N, Husain S. *Aspergillus* infections after lung transplantation: clinical differences in type of transplant and implications for management. J Heart Lung Transplant. 2003;22(3):258–66.
23. Singh N, Paterson DL. *Aspergillus* infections in transplant recipients. Clin Microbiol Rev. 2005;18(1):44–69.
24. Minari A, Husni R, Avery RK, et al. The incidence of invasive aspergillosis among solid organ transplant recipients and implications for prophylaxis in lung transplants. Transpl Infect Dis. 2002;4(4):195–200.
25. Singh N, Husain S. Invasive aspergillosis in solid organ transplant recipients. Am J Transplant. 2009;9(Suppl 4):S180–91.
26. Husni RN, Gordon SM, Longworth DL, et al. Cytomegalovirus infection is a risk factor for invasive aspergillosis in lung transplant recipients. Clin Infect Dis. 1998;26(3):753–5.
27. Paradowski LJ. Saprophytic fungal infections and lung transplantation – revisited. J Heart Lung Transplant. 1997;16(5):524–31.
28. Fernandez-Ruiz M, Silva JT, San-Juan R, et al. *Aspergillus* tracheobronchitis: report of 8 cases and review of the literature. Medicine (Baltimore). 2012;91(5):261–73.
29. Drakos PE, Nagler A, Or R, et al. Invasive fungal sinusitis in patients undergoing bone marrow transplantation. Bone Marrow Transplant. 1993;12(3):203–8.
30. Savage DG, Taylor P, Blackwell J, et al. Paranasal sinusitis following allogeneic bone marrow transplant. Bone Marrow Transplant. 1997;19(1):55–9.
31. DelGaudio JM, Clemson LA. An early detection protocol for invasive fungal sinusitis in neutropenic patients successfully reduces extent of disease at presentation and long term morbidity. Laryngoscope. 2009;119(1):180–3.
32. Walsh TJ, Hier DB, Caplan LR. Aspergillosis of the central nervous system: clinicopathological analysis of 17 patients. Ann Neurol. 1985;18(5):574–82.
33. Pagano L, Ricci P, Montillo M, et al. Localization of aspergillosis to the central nervous system among patients with acute leukemia: report of 14 cases. Gruppo Italiano Ematologiche dell'Adulto Infection Program. Clin Infect Dis. 1996;23(3):628–30.
34. Hunt KE, Glasgow BJ. *Aspergillus* endophthalmitis. An unrecognized endemic disease in orthotopic liver transplantation. Ophthalmology. 1996;103(5):757–67.
35. Walsh TJ. Primary cutaneous aspergillosis – an emerging infection among immunocompromised patients. Clin Infect Dis. 1998;27(3):453–7.
36. van Burik JA, Colven R, Spach DH. Cutaneous aspergillosis. J Clin Microbiol. 1998;36(11):3115–21.
37. De Pauw B, Walsh TJ, Donnelly JP, et al. Revised definitions of invasive fungal disease from the European Organization for Research and Treatment of Cancer/Invasive Fungal Infections Cooperative Group and the National Institute of Allergy and Infectious Diseases Mycoses Study Group (EORTC/MSG) Consensus Group. Clin Infect Dis. 2008;46(12):1813–21.
38. Gray LD, Roberts GD. Laboratory diagnosis of systemic fungal diseases. Infect Dis Clin N Am. 1988;2(4):779–803.
39. Larone D. Medically important fungi: a guide to identification. 5th ed. Washington (D.C.): ASM Press; 2011.
40. Paterson DL, Singh N. Invasive aspergillosis in transplant recipients. Medicine (Baltimore). 1999;78(2):123–38.
41. Horvath JA, Dummer S. The use of respiratory-tract cultures in the diagnosis of invasive pulmonary aspergillosis. Am J Med. 1996;100(2):171–8.
42. Wald A, Leisenring W, van Burik JA, Bowden RA. Epidemiology of *Aspergillus* infections in a large cohort of patients undergoing bone marrow transplantation. J Infect Dis. 1997;175(6):1459–66.
43. Pfeiffer CD, Fine JP, Safdar N. Diagnosis of invasive aspergillosis using a galactomannan assay: a meta-analysis. Clin Infect Dis. 2006;42(10):1417–27.
44. Husain S, Kwak EJ, Obman A, et al. Prospective assessment of Platelia *Aspergillus* galactomannan antigen for the diagnosis of invasive aspergillosis in lung transplant recipients. Am J Transplant. 2004;4(5):796–802.
45. Singh N, Winston DJ, Limaye AP, et al. Performance characteristics of galactomannan and β-d-glucan in high-risk liver transplant recipients. Transplantation. 2015;99(12):2543–50.
46. Marr KA, Laverdiere M, Gugel A, Leisenring W. Antifungal therapy decreases sensitivity of the *Aspergillus* galactomannan enzyme immunoassay. Clin Infect Dis. 2005;40(12):1762–9.
47. Walsh TJ, Shoham S, Petraitiene R, et al. Detection of galactomannan antigenemia in patients receiving piperacillin-tazobactam and correlations between *in vitro*, *in vivo*, and clinical properties of the drug-antigen interaction. J Clin Microbiol. 2004;42(10):4744–8.
48. Mikulska M, Furfaro E, Del Bono V, et al. Piperacillin/tazobactam (Tazocin) seems to be no longer responsible for false-positive results of the galactomannan assay. J Antimicrob Chemother. 2012;67(7):1746–8.
49. Asano-Mori Y, Kanda Y, Oshima K, et al. False-positive *Aspergillus* galactomannan antigenaemia after haematopoietic stem transplantation. J Antimicrob Chemother. 2008;61(2):411–6.
50. Mennink-Kersten MA, Donnelly JP, Verweij PE. Detection of circulating galactomannan for the diagnosis and management of invasive aspergillosis. Lancet Infect Dis. 2004;4(6):349–57.
51. Swanink CM, Meis JF, Rijs AJ, Donnelly JP, Verweij PE. Specificity of a sandwich enzyme-linked immunosorbent assay for detecting *Aspergillus* galactomannan. J Clin Microbiol. 1997;35(1):257–60.

52. Tortorano AM, Esposto MC, Prigitano A, et al. Cross-reactivity of *Fusarium* spp. in the *Aspergillus* galactomannan enzyme-linked immunosorbent assay. J Clin Microbiol. 2012;50(3):1051–3.
53. Maertens J, Maertens V, Theunissen K, et al. Bronchoalveolar lavage fluid galactomannan for the diagnosis of invasive pulmonary aspergillosis in patients with hematologic diseases. Clin Infect Dis. 2009;49(11):1688–93.
54. D'Haese J, Theunissen K, Vermeulen E, et al. Detection of galactomannan in bronchoalveolar lavage fluid samples of patients at risk for invasive pulmonary aspergillosis: analytical and clinical validity. J Clin Microbiol. 2012;50(4):1258–63.
55. Husain S, Clancy CJ, Nguyen MH, et al. Performance characteristics of the platelia *Aspergillus* enzyme immunoassay for detection of *Aspergillus* galactomannan antigen in bronchoalveolar lavage fluid. Clin Vaccine Immunol. 2008;15(12):1760–3.
56. Husain S, Paterson DL, Studer SM, et al. *Aspergillus* galactomannan antigen in the bronchoalveolar lavage fluid for the diagnosis of invasive aspergillosis in lung transplant recipients. Transplantation. 2007;83(10):1330–6.
57. Pickering JW, Sant HW, Bowles CA, Roberts WL, Woods GL. Evaluation of a (1->3)-beta-D-glucan assay for diagnosis of invasive fungal infections. J Clin Microbiol. 2005;43(12):5957–62.
58. Karageorgopoulos DE, Vouloumanou EK, Ntziora F, Michalopoulos A, Rafailidis PI, Falagas ME. Beta-D-glucan assay for the diagnosis of invasive fungal infections: a meta-analysis. Clin Infect Dis. 2011;52(6):750–70.
59. Lamoth F, Cruciani M, Mengoli C, et al. Beta-glucan antigenemia assay for the diagnosis of invasive fungal infections in patients with hematologic malignancies: a systematic review and meta-analysis of cohort studies from the Thrid European Conference on Infections in Leukemia (ECIL-3). Clin Infect Dis. 2012;54(5):633–43.
60. Kato A, Takita T, Furuhashi M, Takahashi T, Maruyama Y, Hishida A. Elevation of blood (1-->3)-beta-D-glucan concentrations in hemodialysis patients. Nephron. 2001;89(1):15–9.
61. Ogawa M, Hori H, Niiguchi S, Azuma E, Komada Y. False-positive plasma (1-->3)-beta-D-glucan test following immunoglobulin product replacement in an adult bone marrow recipient. Int J Hematol. 2004;80(1):97–8.
62. Usami M, Ohata A, Horiuchi T, Nagasawa K, Wakabayashi T, Tanaka S. Positive (1-->3)-beta-D-glucan in blood components and release of (1-->3)-beta-D-glucan from depth-type membrane filters for blood processing. Transfusion. 2002;42(9):1189–95.
63. Mennink-Kersten MA, Warris A, Verweij PE. 1,3-beta-D-glucan in patients receiving intravenous amoxicillin-clavulanic acid. N Engl J Med. 2006;354(26):2834–5.
64. Nakao A, Yasui M, Kawagoe T, Tamura H, Tanaka S, Takagi H. False-positive endotoxemia derives from gauze glucan after hepatectomy for hepatocellular carcinoma with cirrhosis. Hepato-Gastroenterology. 1997;44(17):1413–8.
65. Mennink-Kersten MA, Ruegebrink D, Verweij PE. *Pseudomonas aeruginosa* as a cause of 1,3-beta-D-glucan assay reactivity. Clin Infect Dis. 2008;46(12):1930–1.
66. Springer J, Lackner M, Nachbaur D, et al. Prospective multicentre PCR-based aspergillus DNA screening in high-risk patients with and without primary antifungal prophylaxis. Clin Microbiol Infect. 2016;22(1):80–6.
67. Greene RE, Schlamm HT, Oestmann JW, et al. Imaging findings in acute invasive pulmonary aspergillosis: clinical significance of the halo sign. Clin Infect Dis. 2007;44(3):373–9.
68. Kuhlman JE, Fishman EK, Siegelman SS. Invasive pulmonary aspergillosis in acute leukemia: characteristic findings on CT, the CT halo sign, and the role of CT in early diagnosis. Radiology. 1985;157(3):611–4.
69. Kami M, Kishi Y, Hamaki T, et al. The value of the chest computed tomography halo sign in the diagnosis of invasive pulmonary aspergillosis. An autopsy-based retrospective study of 48 patients. Mycoses. 2002;45(8):287–94.
70. Bruno C, Minniti S, Vassanelli A, Pozzi-Mucelli R. Comparison of CT features of *Aspergillus* and bacterial pneumonia in severely neutropenic patients. J Thorac Imaging. 2007;22(2):160–5.
71. Georgiadou SP, Sipsas NV, Marom EM, Kontoyiannis DP. The diagnostic value of halo and reversed halo signs for invasive mold infections in compromised hosts. Clin Infect Dis. 2011;52(9):1144–55.
72. Caillot D, Couaillier JF, Bernard A, et al. Increasing volume and changing characteristics of invasive pulmonary aspergillosis on sequential thoracic computed tomography scans in patients with neutropenia. J Clin Oncol. 2001;19(1):253–9.
73. Stanzani M, Battista G, Sassi C, et al. Computed tomographic pulmonary angiography for diagnosis of invasive mold diseases in patients with hematological malignancies. Clin Infect Dis. 2012;54(5):610–6.
74. Patterson TF, Thompson GR 3rd, Denning DW, et al. Practice guidelines for the diagnosis and management of aspergillosis: 2016 update by the Infectious Diseases Society of America. Clin Infect Dis. 2016;63(4):e1–e60.
75. Herbrecht R, Denning DW, Patterson TF, et al. Voriconazole versus amphotericin B for primary therapy of invasive aspergillosis. N Engl J Med. 2002;347(6):408–15.
76. Pascual A, Calandra T, Bolay S, Buclin T, Bille J, Marchetti O. Voriconazole therapeutic drug monitoring in patients with invasive mycoses improves efficacy and safety outcomes. Clin Infect Dis. 2008;46(2):201–11.
77. Johnson LB, Kauffman CA. Voriconazole: a new triazole antifungal agent. Clin Infect Dis. 2003;36(5):630–7.
78. Park WB, Kim NH, Kim KH, et al. The effect of therapeutic drug monitoring on safety and efficacy of voriconazole in invasive fungal infections: a randomized controlled trial. Clin Infect Dis. 2012;55(8):1080–7.
79. Maertens JA, Raad II, Marr KA, et al. Isavuconazole versus voriconazole for primary treatment of invasive mould disease caused by *Aspergillus* and other filamentous fungi (SECURE): a phase 3, randomised-controlled, non-inferiority trial. Lancet. 2016;387(10020):760–9.
80. Marty FM, Ostrosky-Zeichner L, Cornely OA, et al. Isavuconazole treatment for mucormycosis: a single-arm open-label trial and case-control analysis. Lancet Infect Dis. 2016;16(7):828–37.
81. Cornely OA, Maertens J, Bresnik M, et al. Liposomal amphotericin B as initial therapy for invasive mold infection: a randomized trial comparing a high-loading dose regimen with standard dosing (AmBiLoad trial). Clin Infect Dis. 2007;44(10):1289–97.
82. Leenders AC, Daenen S, Jansen RL, et al. Liposomal amphotericin B compared with amphotericin B deoxycholate in the treatment of documented and suspected neutropenia-associated invasive fungal infections. Br J Haematol. 1998;103(1):205–12.
83. Bowden R, Chandrasekar P, White MH, et al. A double-blind, randomized, controlled trial of amphotericin B colloidal dispersion versus amphotericin B for treatment of invasive aspergillosis in immunocompromised patients. Clin Infect Dis. 2002;35(4):359–66.
84. Walsh TJ, Finberg RW, Arndt C, et al. Liposomal amphotericin B for empirical therapy in patients with persistent fever and neutropenia. National Institute of Allergy and Infectious Diseases Mycoses Study Group. N Engl J Med. 1999;340(10):764–71.
85. Wingard JR, White MH, Anaissie E, Raffalli J, Goodman J, Arrieta A. A randomized, double-blind comparative trial evaluating the safety of liposomal amphotericin B versus amphotericin B lipid complex in the empirical treatment ofrile neutropenia. L Amph/ABLC Collaborative Study Group. Clin Infect Dis. 2000;31(5):1155–63.
86. Hachem RY, Boktour MR, Hanna HA, et al. Amphotericin B lipid complex versus liposomal amphotericin B monotherapy for

invasive aspergillosis in patients with hematologic malignancy. Cancer. 2008;112(6):1282–7.
87. Kirkpatrick WR, McAtee RK, Fothergill AW, Loebenberg D, Rinaldi MG, Patterson TF. Efficacy of SCH56592 in a rabbit model of invasive aspergillosis. Antimicrob Agents Chemother. 2000;44(3):780–2.
88. Petraitiene R, Petraitis V, Groll AH, et al. Antifungal activity and pharmacokinetics of posaconazole (SCH 56592) in treatment and prevention of experimental invasive pulmonary aspergillosis: correlation with galactomannan antigenemia. Antimicrob Agents Chemother. 2001;45(3):857–69.
89. Walsh TJ, Raad I, Patterson TF, et al. Treatment of invasive aspergillosis with posaconazole in patients who are refractory to or intolerant of conventional therapy: an externally controlled trial. Clin Infect Dis. 2007;44(1):2–12.
90. Pfaller MA, Messer SA, Hollis RJ, Jones RN. Antifungal activities of posaconazole, ravuconazole, and voriconazole compared to those of itraconazole and amphotericin B against 239 clinical isolates of *Aspergillus* spp. and other filamentous fungi: report from SENTRY Antimicrobial Surveillance Program, 2000. Antimicrob Agents Chemother. 2002;46(4):1032–7.
91. Cappelletty D, Eiselstein-McKitrick K. The echinocandins. Pharmacotherapy. 2007;27(3):369–88.
92. Maertens J, Raad I, Petrikkos G, et al. Efficacy and safety of caspofungin for treatment of invasive aspergillosis in patients refractory to or intolerant of conventional antifungal therapy. Clin Infect Dis. 2004;39(11):1563–71.
93. Wiederhold NP, Cota JM, Frei CR. Micafungin in the treatment of invasive candidiasis and invasive aspergillosis. Infect Drug Resist. 2008;1:63–77.
94. Denning DW, Marr KA, Lau WM, et al. Micafungin (FK463), alone or in combination with other systemic antifungal agents, for the treatment of acute invasive aspergillosis. J Infect. 2006;53(5):337–49.
95. Kontoyiannis DP, Ratanatharathorn V, Young JA, et al. Micafungin alone or in combination with other systemic antifungal therapies in hematopoietic stem cell transplant recipients with invasive aspergillosis. Transpl Infect Dis. 2009;11(1):89–93.
96. Petraitis V, Petraitiene R, Sarafandi AA, et al. Combination therapy in treatment of experimental pulmonary aspergillosis. J Infect Dis. 2003;187(12):1834–43.
97. Kirkpatrick WR, Perea S, Coco BJ, Patterson TF. Efficacy of caspofungin alone and in combination with voriconazole in a Guinea pig model of invasive aspergillosis. Antimicrob Agents Chemother. 2002;46(8):2564–8.
98. Marr KA, Boeckh M, Carter RA, Kim HW, Corey L. Combination antifungal therapy for invasive aspergillosis. Clin Infect Dis. 2004;39(6):797–802.
99. Meletiadis J, Petraitis V, Petraitiene R, et al. Triazole-polyene antagonism in experimental invasive pulmonary aspergillosis: *in vitro* and *in vivo* correlation. J Infect Dis. 2006;194(7):1008–18.
100. Kontoyiannis DP, Boktour M, Hanna H, Torres HA, Hachem R, Raad II. Itraconazole added to a lipid formulation of amphotericin B does not improve outcome of primary treatment of invasive aspergillosis. Cancer. 2005;103(11):2334–7.
101. Marr KA, Sclamm HT, Hebrecht R, et al. Combination antifungal therapy for invasive aspergillosis: a randomized trial. Ann Intern Med. 2015;162(2):81–9.
102. Collette N, Van der Auwera P, Meunier F, Lambert C, Sculier JP, Coune A. Tissue distribution and bioactivity of amphotericin B administered in liposomes to cancer patients. J Antimicrob Chemother. 1991;27(4):535–48.
103. Hajdu R, Thompson R, Sundelof JG, et al. Preliminary animal pharmacokinetics of the parenteral antifungal agent MK-0991 (L-743,872). Antimicrob Agents Chemother. 1997;41(11):2339–44.
104. Lutsar I, Roffey S, Troke P. Voriconazole concentrations in the cerebrospinal fluid and brain tissue of Guinea pigs and immunocompromised patients. Clin Infect Dis. 2003;37(5):728–32.
105. Denning DW. Therapeutic outcome in invasive aspergillosis. Clin Infect Dis. 1996;23(3):608–15.
106. Lin SJ, Schranz J, Teutsch SM. Aspergillosis case-fatality rate: systematic review of the literature. Clin Infect Dis. 2001;32(3):358–66.
107. Schwartz S, Ruhnke M, Ribaud P, et al. Improved outcome in central nervous system aspergillosis, using voriconazole treatment. Blood. 2005;106(8):2641–5.
108. Sutton DA, Sanche SE, Revankar SG, Fothergill AW, Rinaldi MG. *In vitro* amphotericin B resistance in clinical isolates of *Aspergillus terreus*, with a head-to-head comparison to voriconazole. J Clin Microbiol. 1999;37(7):2343–5.
109. Walsh TJ, Petraitis V, Petraitiene R, et al. Experimental pulmonary aspergillosis due to *Aspergillus terreus*: pathogenesis and treatment of an emerging fungal pathogen resistant to amphotericin B. J Infect Dis. 2003;188(2):305–19.
110. Steinbach WJ, Benjamin DK Jr, Kontoyiannis DP, et al. Infections due to *Aspergillus terreus*: a multicenter retrospective analysis of 83 cases. Clin Infect Dis. 2004;39(2):192–8.
111. Balajee SA, Nickle D, Varga J, Marr KA. Molecular studies reveal frequent misidentification of *Aspergillus fumigatus* by morphotyping. Eukaryot Cell. 2006;5(10):1705–12.
112. Vinh DC, Shea YR, Sugui JA, et al. Invasive aspergillosis due to *Neosartorya udagawae*. Clin Infect Dis. 2009;49(1):102–11.
113. Verweij PE, Mellado E, Melchers WJ. Multiple-triazole-resistant aspergillosis. N Engl J Med. 2007;356(14):1481–3.
114. Alanio A, Sitterle E, Liance M, et al. Low prevalence of resistance to azoles in *Aspergillus fumigatus* in a French cohort of patients treated for hematological malignancies. J Antimicrob Chemother. 2011;66(2):371–4.
115. Upton A, Kirby KA, Carpenter P, Boeckh M, Marr KA. Invasive aspergillosis following hematopoietic cell transplantation: outcomes and prognostic factors associated with mortality. Clin Infect Dis. 2007;44(4):531–40.
116. Sipsas NV, Kontoyiannis DP. Clinical issues regarding relapsing aspergillosis and the efficacy of secondary antifungal prophylaxis in patients with hematological malignancies. Clin Infect Dis. 2006;42(11):1584–91.
117. Lowenberg B, Suciu S, Archimbaud E, et al. Use of recombinant GM-CSF during and after remission induction chemotherapy in patients aged 61 years or older with acute myeloid leukemia: final report of AML-11, a phase III randomized study of the Leukemia Cooperative Group of European Organisation for the Research and Treatment of Cancer in Dutch Belgian Hemato-Oncology Cooperative Group. Blood. 1997;90(8):2952–61.
118. Sung L, Nathan PC, Alibhai SM, Tomlinson GA, Beyene J. Meta-analysis: effect of prophylactic hematopoietic colony-stimulating factors on mortality and outcomes of infection. Ann Intern Med. 2007;147(6):400–11.
119. Dignani MC, Anaissie EJ, Hester JP, et al. Treatment of neutropenia-related fungal infections with granulocyte colony-stimulating factor-elicited white blood cell transfusions: a pilot study. Leukemia. 1997;11(10):1621–30.
120. Price TH, Boeckh M, Harrison RW, et al. Efficacy of transfusion with granulocytes from G-CSF/dexamethasone-treated donors in neutropenic patients with infection. Blood. 2015;126(18):2153–61.
121. Caillot D, Mannone L, Cuisenier B, Couaillier JF. Role of early diagnosis and aggressive surgery in the management of invasive pulmonary aspergillosis in neutropenic patients. Clin Microbiol Infect. 2001;7(Suppl 2):54–61.
122. Matt P, Bernet F, Habicht J, et al. Predicting outcome after lung resection for invasive pulmonary aspergillosis in patients with neutropenia. Chest. 2004;126(6):1783–8.

123. Suslu AE, Ogretmenoglu O, Suslu N, Yucel OT, Onerci TM. Acute invasive fungal rhinosinusitis: our experience with 19 patients. Eur Arch Otorhinolaryngol. 2009;266(1):77–82.
124. Wingard JR, Carter SL, Walsh TJ, et al. Randomized, double-blind trial of fluconazole versus voriconazole for prevention of invasive fungal infection after allogeneic hematopoietic cell transplantation. Blood. 2010;116(24):5111–8.
125. van Burik JA, Ratanatharathorn V, Stepan DE, et al. Micafungin versus fluconazole for prophylaxis against invasive fungal infections during neutropenia in patients undergoing hematopoietic stem cell transplantation. Clin Infect Dis. 2004;39(10): 1407–16.
126. Ullmann AJ, Lipton JH, Vesole DH, et al. Posaconazole or fluconazole for prophylaxis in severe graft-versus-host disease. N Engl J Med. 2007;356(4):335–47.
127. Gergis U, Markey K, Greene J, et al. Voriconazole provides effective prophylaxis for invasive fungal infection in patients receiving glucocorticoid therapy for GVHD. Bone Marrow Transplant. 2010;45(4):662–7.
128. Offner F, Cordonnier C, Ljungman P, et al. Impact of previous aspergillosis on the outcome of bone marrow transplantation. Clin Infect Dis. 1998;5:1098–103.
129. Cordonnier C, Rovira M, Maertens J, et al. Voriconazole for secondary prophylaxis of invasive fungal infections in allogeneic stem cell transplant recipients: results of the VOSIFI study. Haematologica. 2010;95(10):1762–8.
130. Tomblyn M, Chiller T, Einsele H, et al. Guidelines for preventing infectious complications among hematopoietic cell transplantation recipients: a global perspective. Biol Blood Marrow Transplant. 2009;15(10):1143–238.
131. Reichenspurner H, Gamberg P, Nitschke M, et al. Significant reduction in the number of fungal infections after lung-, heart-lung, and heart transplantation using aerosolized amphotericin B prophylaxis. Transplant Proc. 1997;29(1–2):627–8.
132. Drew RH, Dodds Ashley E, Benjamin DK Jr, Duane Davis R, Palmer SM, Perfect JR. Comparative safety of amphotericin B lipid complex and amphotericin B deoxycholate as aerosolized antifungal prophylaxis in lung-transplant recipients. Transplantation. 2004;77(2):232–7.
133. Sole A. Invasive fungal infections in lung transplantation: role of aerosolised amphotericin B. Int J Antimicrob Agents. 2008;32(Suppl 2):S161–5.
134. Wahidi MM, Willner DA, Snyder LD, Hardison JL, Chia JY, Palmer SM. Diagnosis and outcome of early pleural space infection following lung transplantation. Chest. 2009;135(2):484–91.
135. Husain S, Paterson DL, Studer S, et al. Voriconazole prophylaxis in lung transplant recipients. Am J Transplant. 2006;6(12):3008–16.
136. Fortun J, Martin-Davila P, Moreno S, et al. Prevention of invasive fungal infections in liver transplant recipients: the role of prophylaxis with lipid formulations of amphotericin B in high-risk patients. J Antimicrob Chemother. 2003;52(5):813–9.
137. Fortun J, Martin-Davila P, Montejo M, et al. Prophylaxis with caspofungin for invasive fungal infections in high-risk liver transplant recipients. Transplantation. 2009;87(3):424–35.
138. Praz-Christinaz SM, Lazor-Blanchet C, Binet I, Boillat MA, Danuser B. Occupational risk assessment of aspergillosis after renal transplantation. Transpl Infect Dis. 2007;9(3):175–81.
139. Oren I, Haddad N, Finkelstein R, Rowe JM. Invasive pulmonary aspergillosis in neutropenic patients during hospital construction: before and after chemoprophylaxis and institution of HEPA filters. Am J Hematol. 2001;66(4):257–62.
140. Baddley JW, Andes DR, Marr KA, et al. Factors associated with mortality in transplant patients with invasive aspergillosis. Clin Infect Dis. 2010;50(12):1559–67.
141. Nivoix Y, Velten M, Letscher-Bru V, et al. Factors associated with overall and attributable mortality in invasive aspergillosis. Clin Infect Dis. 2008;47(9):1176–84.
142. Parody R, Martino R, Sanchez F, Subira M, Hidalgo A, Sierra J. Predicting survival in adults with invasive aspergillosis during therapy for hematological malignancies or after hematopoietic stem cell transplantation: single-center analysis and validation of the Seattle, French, and Strasbourg prognostic indexes. Am J Hematol. 2009;84(9):571–8.
143. Miceli MH, Grazziutti ML, Woods G, et al. Strong correlation between serum *Aspergillus* galactomannan index and outcome of aspergillosis in patients with hematological cancer: clinical and research implications. Clin Infect Dis. 2008;46(9):1412–22.
144. Woods G, Miceli MH, Grazziutti ML, Zhao W, Barlogie B, Anaissie E. Serum *Aspergillus* galactomannan antigen values strongly correlate with outcome of invasive aspergillosis: a study of 56 patients with hematologic cancer. Cancer. 2007;110(4):830–4.
145. Koo S, Bryar JM, Baden LR, Marty FM. Prognostic features of galactomannan antigenemia in galactomannan-positive invasive aspergillosis. J Clin Microbiol. 2010;48(4):1255–60.

Mucormycosis

34

Brad Spellberg and Johan Maertens

Taxonomy

Previously, the class *Zygomycetes* encompassed both fungi of the order *Mucorales* and *Entomophthorales*. However, recent reclassification has abolished the class *Zygomycetes* and placed the order *Mucorales* in the subphylum *Mucoromycotina* and the order *Entomophthorales* in the subphylum *Entomophthoromycotina*, both in the phylum *Glomeromycota* [1] (Table 34.1). Therefore, infection caused by the *Mucorales* is most accurately referred to as mucormycosis, although the term zygomycosis may be still used by some sources. Infections caused by the *Entomophthoromycotina* are referred to as entomophthoromycosis, but may be clinically indistinguishable from cases of mucormycosis.

Fungi belonging to the order *Mucorales* are distributed into six families, all of which can cause clinical infections [2]. These families include (1) the *Mucoraceae* (genera *Rhizopus, Mucor, Cokeromyces*), (2) the *Lichtheimaceae* (genera *Lichtheimia* [formerly *Absidia*]), *Rhizomucor*), (3) the *Cunninghamellaceae* (genus *Cunninghamella*), (4) the *Mortierellaceae* (genus *Mortierella*), (5) the *Saksenaeaceae* (genera *Saksenaea, Apophysomyces*), and (6) the *Syncephalastraceae* (genus *Syncephalastrum*). The latter three families are rare causes of infection and are more frequently encountered in highly immunocompromised patients, such as in the transplant setting [3].

Table 34.1 Taxonomy of Mucormycosis Etiologic Fungi; Subphylum *Mucormycotina*, Order *Mucorales*

Family	Genus (species listed for some)
Mucoraceae	*Rhizopus oryzae* *Rhizopus microsporus* *Rhizomucor* *Mucor* *Actinomucor*
Lichtheimaceae	*Lichtheimia* (formerly *Mycocladus,* formerly *Absidia*)
Cunninghamellaceae	*Cunninghamella*
Thamnidiaceae	*Cokeromyces*
Mortierellaceae	*Mortierella*
Saksenaeaceae	*Saksenaea* *Apophysomyces*
Syncephalastraceae	*Syncephalastrum*

Species belonging to the family *Mucoraceae* are isolated more frequently from patients with mucormycosis than those of any other family. Among the *Mucoraceae*, *Rhizopus oryzae* (*Rhizopus arrhizus*) is by far the most common cause of infection [2, 4]. Other less frequently isolated species of the *Mucoraceae* family that cause a similar spectrum of infections include *Rhizopus microsporus* var. *rhizopodiformis, Lichtheimia* spp., *Apophysomyces elegans, Mucor* species, and *Rhizomucor pusillus* [2–4]. It is important to emphasize that the syndrome name, mucormycosis, derives from the order *Mucorales* and family *Mucoraceae*, not from the genus *Mucor*, which itself is a rare cause of infection. Increasing cases of mucormycosis have been also reported due to infection with *Cunninghamella* spp. [4–8]. As mentioned, to date, rare case reports have demonstrated the ability of species belonging to other families to cause mucormycosis [2, 3, 9–12].

Incidence

Mucormycosis is far less common than other opportunistic fungal infections, such as those caused by *Candida* and *Aspergillus spp*. An older population-based study estimated

B. Spellberg (✉)
Los Angeles County+University of Southern California (LAC+USC) Medical Center, Los Angeles, CA, USA

Division of Infectious Diseases, Keck School of Medicine at USC, Los Angeles, CA, USA
e-mail: bspellberg@dhs.lacounty.gov

J. Maertens
Department of Hematology, Acute Leukemia and Stem Cell Transplantation Unit, University Hospital Gasthuisberg, K. U. Leuven, Leuven, Belgium
e-mail: johan.maertens@uzleuven.be

A. Safdar (ed.), *Principles and Practice of Transplant Infectious Diseases*, https://doi.org/10.1007/978-1-4939-9034-4_34

the incidence of mucormycosis to be 1.7 cases per million people per year, which translates to approximately 500 cases per year in the United States [13]. In autopsy series, the prevalence of mucormycosis has ranged from 1 to 5 cases per 10,000 autopsies, making the infection 10–50 fold less common than invasive *Candida* or *Aspergillus* infections [14–16]. Most recently, a 10-year study of mucormycosis in France based on the International Classification of Diseases, 10th Revision (ICD-10) codes, found a doubling of incidence, from 2001 to 2010, to 2.1 cases per million population [17].

In recent years, the epidemiology of mucormycosis has shown an alarming trend. Mucormycosis, formerly virtually always community-acquired and often in the setting of diabetic ketoacidosis (DKA), has rapidly become a nosocomial infection in patients with malignancy or undergoing organ transplantation or HSCT [18]. Indeed, in patients undergoing allogeneic bone marrow transplantation, the prevalence of mucormycosis has been described to be as high as 2–3% [19, 20]. However, rates as low as 0.4% have also been reported [21].

Epidemiology and Risk Factors

While in previous years poorly controlled diabetes mellitus was the most common risk factor, more recent series have found that in developed countries, immunocompromise caused by transplantation, prolonged corticosteroid courses, and neutropenia are collectively more common risk factors than diabetes mellitus [22–25]. However, in underdeveloped countries, diabetes mellitus remains the most common risk factor [26, 27].

At transplant centers, the incidence of mucormycosis has been rising since the late 1990s, although rates still remain low relative to other fungal infections [28, 29]. For example, at the Fred Hutchinson Cancer Research Center, Marr et al. described a doubling in the number of cases from 1985–1989 to 1995–1999 [30]. Kontoyiannis et al. described a greater than doubling in the incidence of mucormycosis in transplant patients over a similar time span [31]. Similarly, a single-center study from Belgium found a marked increase in probable or proven mucormycosis (from 0.019 to 0.148 cases per 10,000 patient-days) between 2000 and 2009, driven mostly by changes between the years 2005 and 2009 [25]. The increase in cases in the latter study was most likely explained by an increase in the at-risk population, rather than other factors (e.g., changes in antifungal prophylaxis, etc.).

In patients undergoing hematological stem cell transplantation, mucormycosis develops at least as commonly in nonneutropenic periods as in neutropenic periods. For example, more than half the cases of mucormycosis occur more than 90 days after transplantation [19, 21, 30]. Nevertheless, mucormycosis remains relatively uncommon in the setting of solid organ transplantation (SOT). For example, in the recent, multicenter, TRANSNET study, the incidence of mucormycosis in recipients of solid organ transplants in the United States was less than 1 per 1000 (0.07%) at 1 year of follow-up [32], and mucormycosis accounted for only 2% of invasive fungal infections in this setting (versus >50% for invasive candidiasis and nearly 20% for invasive aspergillosis) [33].

The major risk factors for mucormycosis in the transplant setting include underlying myelodysplastic syndrome (possibly due to iron overload from repeated blood transfusions) and graft-versus-host disease (GVHD) treated with steroids [19, 28, 30, 34, 35]. Administration of antithymocyte globulin may also be a risk for mucormycosis [28]. Although less than half of these patients are neutropenic at the time of disease onset, prolonged neutropenia is a risk factor for mucormycosis in this setting [36], as are diabetes mellitus and steroid use [36].

The possible role of antifungal prophylaxis in predisposing patients to developing mucormycosis is increasingly being described, but remains uncertain. Prophylaxis with either itraconazole [36] or voriconazole [20, 29, 37–39] has been implicated in predisposing to mucormycosis, and these cases have typically presented with disseminated mucormycosis, the most lethal form of disease. However, other studies have indicated that the primary factor driving increased cases is the increased population at risk, rather than exposure to specific prophylactic regimens [25].

Mucormycosis of the lung occurs most commonly in leukemic patients who are receiving chemotherapy or in patients undergoing HSCT. Indeed, the pulmonary form of the disease is the most common form found in neutropenic or stem cell transplant patients [30, 40]. In contrast, soft tissue infections occur in patients with disrupted cutaneous barriers, either as a result of traumatic implantation of soil, maceration of skin by a moist surface [41, 42], or in nosocomial settings via direct access through intravenous catheters or subcutaneous injections [43–45]. Contaminated surgical dressings and linens have also been implicated as a source of outbreaks of cutaneous mucormycosis [46–49]. Cutaneous mucormycosis has also occurred in the context of contaminated tape used to secure an endotracheal tube in a ventilated patient [41]. Recently, an iatrogenic outbreak of gastric mucormycosis occurred due to contamination of the wooden applicators used to mix drugs that were poured down the patients' nasogastric feeding tubes [50]. These patients presented with acute severe gastric bleeding. The diagnosis was established by demonstration of the pathogen in cultures of samples taken from gastric aspirates and the box of wooden tongue depressors.

Clinical Manifestations

In large studies, the median time to onset of mucormycosis after SOT has been reported to be 5–7 months [21, 32, 51], underscoring that the disease most commonly occurs after the immediate post-transplant period, often in association with corticosteroid therapy for GVHD. Based on clinical presentation and the involvement of a particular anatomic site, mucormycosis can be divided into at least six clinical categories: (1) rhinocerebral, (2) pulmonary, (3) cutaneous, (4) gastrointestinal, (5) disseminated, and (6) miscellaneous [4, 22, 24, 27, 31, 51–53]. These categories of invasive mucormycosis tend to occur in patients with specific defects in host defense (Table 34.2). For example, patients with DKA typically develop the rhinocerebral form of the disease and much more rarely develop pulmonary or disseminated disease. In contrast, pulmonary mucormycosis occurs most commonly in leukemic patients who are receiving chemotherapy or in patients undergoing HSCT.

Table 34.2 Risk factors and clinical manifestations of mucormycosis

Clinical risk factor[a]	Immune defect	Typical disease manifestation
Diabetes mellitus[b]	Increased available iron Increased expression of host receptor for *Mucorales* invasion [58] Possible phagocytic defects	Rhino-orbital-cerebral
Neutropenia	Disruption of predominant innate immune host defense mechanism against the fungus (phagocytic killing)	Pulmonary disease, occasionally disseminated
Corticosteroids	Suppression of phagocytic defense mechanisms Unmasking or inducing diabetes mellitus	Rhino-orbital-cerebral, pulmonary, or disseminated
Iron overload states and deferoxamine therapy during renal failure	Elaboration of free iron to enhance fungal growth	Disseminated or local
Injection drug use	Bypassing anatomical barriers to directly access the bloodstream	Cerebral or disseminated
Trauma or cutaneous breakdown	Bypassing anatomical barrier	Subcutaneous or deeper to fascia and muscle
Severe malnutrition	Unclear	Gastrointestinal

[a]Multiple risk factors are often coexistent. For example, patients with malignancy or undergoing transplantation are often treated with corticosteroids which cause diabetes mellitus. Such patients are also often neutropenic and undergo multiple blood transfusions which can create iron overload and also have multiple areas of skin disruption (via catheters, tape, etc.)

[b]Contrary to historical teaching, the predominant mechanism by which diabetes mellitus predisposes to mucormycosis is not acidosis, since the majority of diabetic patients with mucormycosis do not present with acidosis. Diabetes disrupts normal iron sequestering mechanisms, and hyperglycemia upregulates expression of a host receptor used by *Mucorales* to penetrate into epithelia. Acidosis exacerbates the likelihood of infection by further disrupting iron sequestration

Rhinocerebral mucormycosis is the most common form of the disease generally, but is less common than lung disease in the transplant setting [33, 35]. Most rhinocerebral mucormycosis cases occur in patients with diabetes, although such cases are increasingly being described in the transplant setting, likely due to corticosteroid use. The initial symptoms of rhinocerebral mucormycosis are nonspecific and include eye or facial pain and facial numbness, followed by the onset of conjunctival suffusion, blurry vision, and soft tissue swelling. Fever may be absent in up to half of cases, while white blood cell counts are typically elevated, as long as the patient has functioning bone marrow. If untreated, infection usually spreads from the ethmoid sinus to the orbit, resulting in loss of extraocular muscle function and proptosis, typically with chemosis. Onset of signs and symptoms in the contralateral eye, with resulting bilateral proptosis, chemosis, vision loss, and ophthalmoplegia, is an ominous sign that suggests the development of cavernous sinus thrombosis.

Upon visual inspection, the infected tissue may appear normal during the earliest stages of spread of the fungus. The infected tissue then progresses through an erythematous phase, with or without edema, before onset of a violaceous appearance, and finally the development of a black, necrotic eschar. Infection can sometimes extend from the sinuses into the mouth and produce painful, necrotic ulcerations of the hard palate, but this is a late finding and suggests extensive, well-established infection.

Pulmonary mucormycosis is the most common manifestation in the setting of SOT [35], accounting for more than half of mucormycosis cases in some series [25, 33, 54]. Symptoms of pulmonary mucormycosis include dyspnea, cough, and chest pain; fever is often, but not invariably, present. Fungal invasion of blood vessels results in thrombosis and subsequent tissue necrosis, cavitation, resulting in potentially life-threatening hemoptysis. Lobar consolidation, isolated masses, nodular disease, cavities, or wedge-shaped infarcts may be seen on chest radiography. High-resolution chest CT scan is the best method for determining the extent of pulmonary mucormycosis and may demonstrate evidence of infection before it is seen on the chest x-ray. In the setting of cancer, where mucormycosis may be difficult to differentiate from aspergillosis, multiple pulmonary nodules (i.e., ≥10), pleural effusion, or concomitant sinusitis makes mucormycosis more likely [55]. It is critical to distinguish mucormycosis from aspergillosis as rapidly as possible, as treatments for these infections differ. Indeed voriconazole, the first-line treatment for aspergillosis, exacerbates the severity of mucormycosis in mouse and fly models [56, 57].

Cutaneous mucormycosis may occur as a result of external implantation of the fungus or, conversely, as a result of hematogenous dissemination. External implantation infection has been described from soil exposure resulting from trauma (e.g., motor vehicle accident), penetrating injury with plant material (e.g., thorn), injections of medications (e.g., insulin), catheter insertion, contaminated surgical dressings, and use of tape to secure endotracheal tubes. Cutaneous disease can be very invasive, penetrating into the muscle, fascia, and even bone. Mucormycosis necrotizing fasciitis has a mortality rate approaching 80%. However, isolated cutaneous mucormycosis (i.e., not disseminated disease) has a favorable prognosis and a low mortality rate with prompt, aggressive surgical debridement. In contrast, necrotic cutaneous lesions in the setting of hematogenous dissemination are associated with an extremely high mortality rate.

Gastrointestinal mucormycosis has been seen in premature neonates in association with disseminated disease and necrotizing enterocolitis; more rarely, it has been described in adults with neutropenia or other immune-compromised states. It has also been described as a nosocomial process after administration to patients of medications mixed with contaminated wooden applicator sticks. Nonspecific abdominal pain and distention associated with nausea and vomiting are the most common symptoms. Gastrointestinal bleeding is common, and fungating masses may be seen in the stomach at endoscopy. The disease may progress to visceral perforation, with extremely high mortality rates.

Hematogenous dissemination of mucormycosis may originate from any primary site of infection. For unclear reasons, patients receiving liver transplants are at higher risk for dissemination [51]. The most common site of dissemination is the brain, but metastatic lesions may also be found in any other organ. The mortality associated with dissemination to the brain approaches 100%. Even without central nervous system involvement, disseminated mucormycosis has a mortality rate of >90%. Miscellaneous mucormycosis may affect any body site including the bones, mediastinum, trachea, kidneys, and peritoneum associated with dialysis.

Diagnosis

A high index of suspicion is required to make the diagnosis of mucormycosis. The median time to diagnosis after onset of symptoms in the setting of SOT was 6 weeks in the retrospective study from France [24]. A concept that is frequently poorly grasped by clinicians inexperienced with mucormycosis is that the initial imaging study is frequently negative or has subtle findings [52]. Radiographic findings are often not in pace with clinical progression of mucormycosis, and a negative imaging study result does not provide a rationale to delay a more aggressive diagnostic approach including tissue biopsy via sinus endoscopy or bronchoscopy in appropriate at-risk transplant recipients.

Disease manifestations of invasive aspergillosis and mucormycosis may be similar, and both diseases affect similar populations of high-risk cancer or transplant patients. However, it is critical to determine if antifungal coverage for mucormycosis must be included, since therapy for mucormycosis tends to be active against aspergillosis, but therapy for aspergillosis is not necessarily active against mucormycosis (discussed below). In this regard, Chamilos et al. performed a retrospective comparison of cancer patients who developed pulmonary mucormycosis or pulmonary invasive aspergillosis to determine if clinical or radiographic findings could distinguish the two diseases [55]. By logistic regression analysis, cancer patients with concomitant invasive sinusitis were 25-fold more likely to have pulmonary mucormycosis than aspergillosis, and patients receiving voriconazole prophylaxis were almost eightfold more likely to have mucormycosis. On the initial pulmonary CT scan, the presence of multiple nodules or pleural effusion imparted a 20-fold or fivefold increased risk of mucormycosis compared to aspergillosis, respectively. No other clinical or radiographic findings could distinguish the two diseases, not even the so-called reverse halo-sign on chest CT scan. Galactomannan, particularly from bronchoalveolar lavage (BAL) in a patient with lung infection, appears to be able to distinguish invasive aspergillosis (positive galactomannan) from mucormycosis (negative galactomannan) [59]. However, a recent case report of positive galactomannan in a patient with infection caused by *Lichtheimia* underscores that false-positive results may occur or the patient may have concurrent polymicrobial fungal disease [25, 60]. The true specificity of galactomannan in cases of potential mucormycosis is not well defined.

Because the *Mucorales* are environmental isolates, establishing a definitive diagnosis requires a positive culture from a sterile site (e.g., needle aspirate, tissue biopsy specimen, or pleural fluid) or histopathological evidence of invasive mucormycosis. A probable diagnosis of mucormycosis can be established by culture from a non-sterile site (e.g., sputum or bronchoalveolar lavage) in a patient with appropriate risk factors and clinical and radiographic evidence of disease. However, given the urgency to administer therapy early, therapy should be given while awaiting confirmation of the diagnosis from pending studies.

Biopsy with histopathology remains the most sensitive and specific modality to definitively establish the diagnosis (Fig. 34.1). The biopsy should demonstrate the characteristic-wide (e.g., ≥6–30 μm in diameter), thick-walled, ribbonlike, aseptate, hyphal elements that branch at right angles. Other fungi including *Aspergillus, Fusarium,* or *Scedosporium* spp. have septae, are thinner, and branch at acute angles. The width and ribbonlike form of the fungus is most reliable to

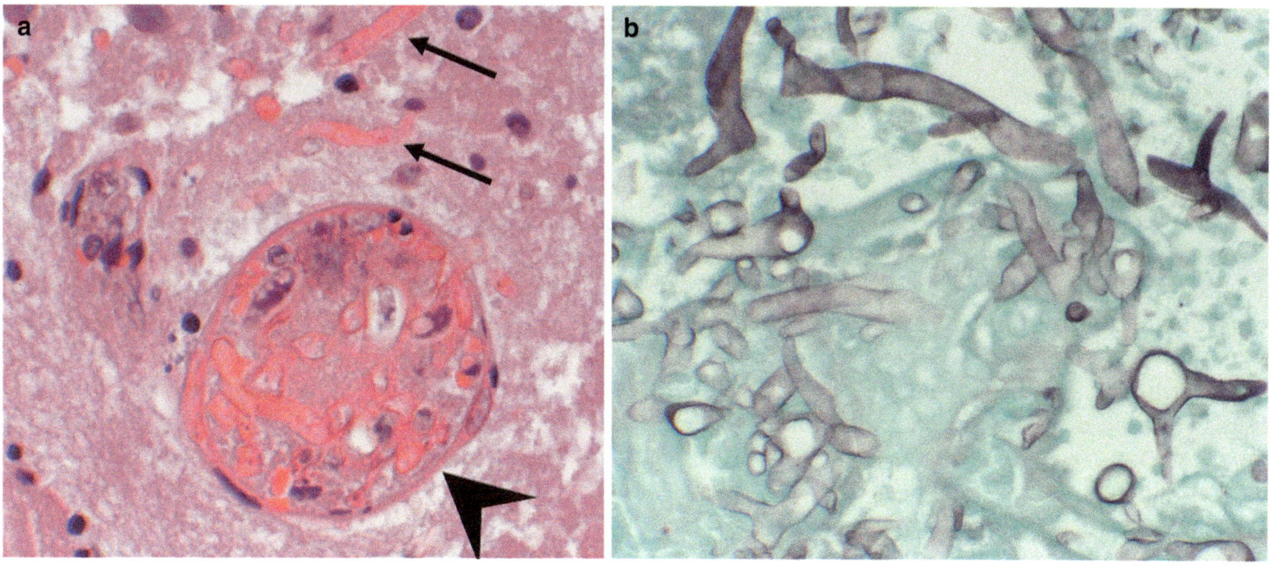

Fig. 34.1 Histopathology sections of *R. oryzae* in infected brain. (**a**) H&E stain of the brain showing broad, ribbonlike, non-septate hyphae in parenchyma (arrows) and a thrombosed blood vessel with extensive intravascular hyphae (arrowhead). (**b**) Gomori methenamine silver (GMS) stain of the brain showing extensive broad, ribbonlike hyphae invading the parenchyma

distinguish mucormycosis, since artificial septae may be apparent due to folding of the tissue during processing, which may also alter the appearance of the angle of branching. The *Mucorales* are visualized most effectively with periodic acid-Schiff (PAS) or methenamine silver stain and, if the organism burden is high, with hematoxylin and eosin (H&E) stain (Fig. 34.1). While histopathology can identify *Mucorales*, species identification can only be made from positive cultures. PCR is under investigation as a diagnostic tool and may be available at certain sites, but it is not yet approved by the US Food and Drug Administration as a diagnostic test for mucormycosis and is not generally available. A recent intriguing study suggested that immune-based assays may be available to detect mucormycosis in the future [61].

Unfortunately, cultures are positive in less than half of cases of mucormycosis. Nevertheless, the *Mucorales* are not fastidious organisms and tend to grow quickly (i.e., <48 h) on culture media. The likely explanation for the low sensitivity of culture is that the *Mucorales* form long filamentous structures that are killed by tissue homogenization, the standard method for preparing tissue cultures in the clinical microbiology laboratory. When processing tissues for culture, the microbiology laboratory should be advised that a diagnosis of mucormycosis is suspected and the tissue should be cut into sections which are placed in the center of culture dishes, rather than being homogenized.

Imaging techniques often have subtle findings which underestimate the extent of disease. For example, the most common finding on CT or MRI scanning of the head or sinuses in a patient with rhino-orbital mucormycosis is sinusitis which is indistinguishable from bacterial sinusitis [62]. It is also common to detect no abnormalities in sinus bones despite clinical evidence of progressive disease. MRIs are more sensitive than CT scans for detecting orbital and CNS involvement [62]. CT scans are useful for early detection of pulmonary mucormycosis, particularly in patients with cancer. By logistic regression, pulmonary mucormycosis in patients with cancer could be distinguished from aspergillosis on the basis of sinusitis, presence of multiple (≥10) nodules by CT scan, and pleural effusion [55]. Endoscopy and/or surgical exploration with biopsy of the areas of suspected infection should always be performed in high-risk patients. If mucormycosis is suspected, initial empiric therapy with a polyene antifungal agent should begin while the diagnosis is being confirmed.

Treatment of Mucormycosis

The successful treatment of mucormycosis requires four steps [52]: (1) early diagnosis; (2) reversal of underlying predisposing risk factors, if possible; (3) surgical debridement where applicable; and (4) prompt antifungal therapy.

Early Diagnosis

A recent study from Chamilos et al. quantified the benefit of early initiation of polyene antifungal therapy in the setting of hematologic malignancies [63]. They reported that if treatment was initiated within 5 days of diagnosis of mucormycosis, survival was markedly improved compared to initiation of polyene therapy at ≥6 days after diagnosis (83% vs. 49% survival). Hence establishing an early diagnosis of mucormycosis is critical to enable early initiation of active antifungal therapy. Given the overlap of clinical syndromes caused by mucormycosis and other pathogens or noninfectious syndromes in the lung and other body sites, a high index of suspicion is required to enable an early diagnosis.

Reversal of Underlying Disease

It is critical to reverse/prevent underlying defects in host defense when treating patients with mucormycosis. Immunosuppressive medications, particularly corticosteroids, should be dose reduced or stopped if at all possible. Aggressive management to rapidly restore euglycemia and normal acid-base status is critical in diabetics in ketoacidosis. Administration of iron should be avoided, as it exacerbates the severity of infection in animal models of mucormycosis [64–66]. For the same reason, it may be advisable to minimize blood transfusions [67], if feasible. Deferoxamine use should also be avoided due to its ability to exacerbate mucormycosis [64, 65, 68–70].

Surgical Management

Blood vessel thrombosis and resulting tissue necrosis during mucormycosis can result in poor penetration of antifungal agents to the site of infection. Therefore, debridement of necrotic tissues may be critical for complete eradication of mucormycosis. In a recent study, surgery was found to be an independent variable by logistic regression for favorable outcome in patients with mucormycosis [4]. Furthermore, in multiple case series, patients who did not undergo surgical debridement of mucormycosis had a far higher mortality rate than patients who underwent surgery [31, 34, 42, 71–76]. While there is potential selection bias in these case series, as patients who did not undergo surgery likely differed in disease severity or comorbidities from those who did, these data support the concept that surgical debridement is necessary to optimize cure rates.

The extent and timing of surgical debridement necessary to maximize outcomes of mucormycosis has never been defined. Data from a recent retrospective review of patients with rhino-orbital-cerebral mucormycosis [62] support the use of intraoperative frozen sections to delineate the margins of infected tissues so that uninvolved tissues can be spared from debridement. The use of calcofluor fluorescence microscopy has also been reported to increase the sensitivity of frozen sections for guiding the extent of surgical revision [77].

Antifungal Therapy

First-Line Monotherapy Options

In general, primary antifungal therapy for mucormycosis should be based on a polyene, if possible (Table 34.3). While amphotericin B deoxycholate (AmB) was the cornerstone of mucormycosis therapy for decades, lipid formulations of AmB are significantly less nephrotoxic and can be safely administered at higher doses for a longer period of time than AmB [62, 78]. Furthermore, treatment of mucormycosis with liposomal amphotericin B (LAmB) was associated with a 67% survival rate, compared to 39% survival rate when patients were treated with AmB ($p = 0.02$) [79]. Multiple other, more recent case series also found initial therapy with LAmB to be substantially more effective than other options, particularly in transplant settings [51, 80, 81]. Therefore, most experts now prefer to use lipid polyenes rather than AmB for the treatment of mucormycosis. Indeed, lipid polyenes are recommended as first-line therapy in the recently released European treatment guidelines for this disease [82].

Available data indicate advantages of LAmB over ABLC for the treatment of central nervous system (CNS) mucormycosis. For example, LAmB levels achieved in rabbit brain were fivefold above ABLC levels [83]. Furthermore, while similarly effective in neutropenic mice, LAmB was markedly superior to ABLC in mice with induced diabetic ketoacidosis (DKA) who were infected with *R. oryzae*, primarily due to superior clearance of fungus from the brain [84]. These animal studies are complemented by a recent, relatively small retrospective case series, in which the outcomes of patients with rhino-orbital-cerebral mucormycosis were found to be worse when ABLC was used as initial therapy versus AmB or LAmB [62]. In contrast, a recent murine study found that ABLC achieved superior lung levels compared to LAmB, resulting in superior clearance of fungus from the lungs [85]. When a higher dose of LAmB was used than that of ABLC, the efficacy was similar. No clinical studies are available yet to validate these intriguing murine data.

In the absence of definitive data on dose selection, 5–7.5 mg/kg/day of lipid polyenes are reasonable for most cases of mucormycosis. A recent randomized study of 339 patients with various mold infections found no clinical benefit of LAmB dosed at 10 mg/kg/day versus 3 mg/kg/day [86]. However, there were only five total cases of mucormycosis in the study, none of which involved the CNS. Given the low CNS penetration of polyenes, some experts prefer dose escalation to 10 mg/kg/day of LAmB for CNS mucormycosis. Doses of LAmB higher than 10 mg/kg/day do not result in pharmacokinetic advantage [87].

Recently, a new triazole, isavuconazonium sulfate, was approved for the treatment of mucormycosis in the United

Table 34.3 First-line antifungal options for mucormycosis

Drug	Recommended dosage	Advantages and supporting studies	Disadvantages
Primary antifungal therapy			
Liposomal amphotericin B (LAmB)	5–10 mg/kg/day	Less nephrotoxic than AmB Better CNS penetration than AmB and ABLC Improved outcomes vs. AmB in murine models and a retrospective clinical review	Expensive
Amphotericin B lipid complex (ABLC)	5–7.5 mg/kg/day	Less nephrotoxic than AmB Murine and retrospective clinical data suggest benefit of combination therapy with echinocandins	Expensive Possibly less efficacious than LAmB for CNS infection
Primary combination therapy[a]			
Caspofungin plus lipid polyene	70 mg IV load, then 50 mg/day for ≥2 weeks 50 mg/m^2 IV in children	Favorable toxicity profile Synergistic in murine disseminated mucormycosis Retrospective clinical data suggested superior outcomes with combination caspofungin-lipid polyene therapy for rhino-orbital-cerebral mucormycosis	Clinical data of combination therapy are very limited
Micafungin or anidulafungin plus lipid polyene	100 mg/day for ≥2 weeks Micafungin 4 mg/kg/day in children Micafungin 10 mg/kg/day in low-birth-weight infants Anidulafungin 1.5 mg/kg/day in children	Favorable toxicity profile Synergistic with LAmB in murine model of disseminated mucormycosis	No clinical data

Primary therapy should generally include a lipid formulation polyene. Non-polyene-based regimens may be appropriate for patients who refuse polyene therapy or for patients with mild disease in relatively immune-competent hosts that can be surgically eradicated (e.g., isolated suprafascial cutaneous infection)

[a]Prospective, randomized trials are necessary to confirm the suggestion of benefit of combination therapy from animal and small, retrospective human studies of mucormycosis. Also, dose escalation of any of the echinocandins is not recommended based on paradoxical loss of benefit of combination therapy at echinocandin doses ≥3 mg/kg/day

States (US) and for salvage treatment in Europe. Isavuconazole does have in vitro activity against the *Mucorales,* but with MICs that are about fourfold higher than those of posaconazole (discussed below); however, blood levels achieved are more than fourfold above those of posaconazole [88–92]. The FDA approval as therapy of mucormycosis was based on the positive results of a 37-patient, open-label, single armed study in which isavuconazole was used to treat patients with mucormycosis [93]. Outcomes were compared to a historical cohort treated with polyenes and were similar in the open-label isavuconazole cohort and the historical cohort. While these results provide reassurance that isavuconazole has merit as a therapeutic agent for mucormycosis, the study design cannot establish isavuconazole as a first-line option [94, 95]. The trial was small, underpowered, and inherently subject to bias in the absence of an active control group [94]. Furthermore, most patients in the open-label study had been pretreated with lipid polyenes. Thus, isavuconazole may be best considered as a second-line option in patients intolerant of lipid polyenes, for salvage therapy or possibly for combination therapy (as discussed below).

Fluconazole, voriconazole, and itraconazole do not have reliable activity against mucormycosis [20, 29, 36–39, 96–100]. The reported in vitro MIC_{90} of posaconazole against the *Mucoromycotina* has ranged from 1 to ≥4 μg/ml [96, 101–104]. However, in patients with febrile neutropenia or invasive fungal infections, posaconazole oral solution dosed at 400 mg twice daily resulted in serum levels <1 μg/ml, with considerable variability [105–107]. These data raise concerns about the reliability of achieving adequate in vivo levels of posaconazole to treat mucormycosis. Furthermore, posaconazole is relatively ineffective for the treatment of mucormycosis in preclinical animal models [98, 108–110]. The efficacy of posaconazole as a treatment option is further called into question by reports of mucormycosis developing as a breakthrough infection while on posaconazole prophylaxis [111–113]. Thus, posaconazole cannot be recommended as a first-line treatment for mucormycosis.

In contrast, Van Burik et al. reported 60% response rates (45% partial response, 15% complete response) for salvage therapy in patients with mucormycosis who were refractory to or intolerant of polyenes [114]. Greenberg et al. reported similar results [115]. Hence, posaconazole is an option for salvage therapy for these infections. Given its variable absorption, therapeutic drug monitoring for posaconazole should be considered, although precise therapeutic or toxicity targets have not been defined [116, 117]. Some experts have recommended serum levels of 0.7 μg/ml [117].

Combination Antifungal Therapy for Mucormycosis

Among patients with mucormycosis in the setting of hematologic malignancies, a recent retrospective study used propensity matching to assess if patients who received combination therapy had improved survival compared to those who received monotherapy [118]. Among 106 patients, 44% received monotherapy and 56% received combination therapy. By propensity matching, patients who received combination therapy did not have superior survival compared to patients who received monotherapy. These data cast some doubt on the role of combination therapy in patients with hematologic malignancy. However, the study was retrospective, and various combination therapy regimens were evaluated, and so it is not possible to say if one combination regimen might be more favorable than others. Definitive answers regarding the role of combination therapy await prospective randomized trials.

Among combination regimens, the one with the most promising preclinical and retrospective data is lipid polyenes with echinocandins. It is now known that *R. oryzae* expresses the target enzyme for echinocandins [119]. In DKA mice infected with *R. oryzae*, combination caspofungin plus ABLC therapy markedly improved survival compared to either monotherapy or placebo [120]. Combination therapy with LAmB plus either micafungin or anidulafungin was also synergistic in either neutropenic or DKA mice with disseminated mucormycosis [121].

In a recent retrospective review from two institutions, combination polyene-caspofungin therapy was associated with significantly improved outcomes in patients with rhino-orbital and rhino-orbital-cerebral mucormycosis compared to polyene monotherapy [62]. Most of the patients were diabetic, although there were patients with neutropenia or status post solid organ transplant in the series. In multivariate analysis, only combination therapy was significantly associated with superior outcomes (OR = 10.9 for success vs. monotherapy, $p = 0.02$).

Echinocandins have extremely favorable toxicity profiles. Furthermore, at an average hospitalization cost of ~$100,000 per case of mucormycosis [122], addition of an echinocandin at ~$100 per day for 2–4 weeks would increase hospital costs by a small amount (i.e., < 3%). Thus, neither toxicity nor cost is a compelling reason to avoid combination polyene-echinocandin therapy for patients with mucormycosis. If used as combination therapy, echinocandins should be administered at standard doses—dose escalation is not recommended, due to paradoxical loss of efficacy during murine mucormycosis at doses ≥3 mg/kg/day [119, 121, 123]. A large-scale, definitive, phase III clinical trial is necessary to determine if combination lipid polyene-echinocandin therapy is superior to monotherapy.

The central role of iron in pathogenesis of mucormycosis has been confirmed based on in vitro, in vivo animal models and retrospective human studies [64, 66, 70, 124, 125]. The requirement for iron acquisition for *R. oryzae* growth and pathogenesis suggested that abrogation of iron uptake could be an important therapeutic adjunct for mucormycosis infections. Unfortunately, despite promising preclinical [66, 70, 125] and observational clinical data in the setting of diabetes mellitus [126, 127], a recent randomized, double-blinded, placebo-controlled trial found that patients treated with iron chelation therapy plus LAmB had higher mortality rates than patients treated with LAmB plus placebo [128]. These data do not preclude an advantage of iron chelation therapy in the setting of diabetes mellitus since no patient enrolled had isolated diabetes mellitus as a risk factor [128], but they preclude routine use of adjunctive iron chelation therapy in the setting of active malignancy.

There are few clinical data to address the role of combination azole-polyene therapy for mucormycosis. However, two recent preclinical studies evaluated the efficacy of posaconazole combination therapy during murine mucormycosis. In the first study, Rodriguez et al... found that combining posaconazole with AmB enhanced the survival of neutropenic mice infected with *R. oryzae* only when compared to a subtherapeutic dose of AmB monotherapy (0.3 mg/kg/day) [109]. In contrast, combination therapy was of no advantage compared to AmB monotherapy at a standard dose (0.8 mg/kg/day). Similarly, we recently reported that combination posaconazole plus LAmB was of no benefit compared to monotherapy with LAmB alone in either neutropenic or DKA mice with mucormycosis [110]. Based on available data, posaconazole does not have a clear role as adjunctive therapy in combination with lipid polyenes. Whether isavuconazole combinations with lipid polyenes are of advantage is not known.

Ben-Ami et al. recently reported that the antibacterial agent, colistin, has activity against the *Mucorales* [129]. Colistin was cidal in vitro, although regrowth of the fungus occurred unless subinhibitory AmB was added for synergy. Colistin mechanism of action appeared to involve disruption of the cytoplasmic and intracellular vacuolar membrane integrity. The drug had limited activity as a prophylactic agent during inhalational challenge, but did not have systemic therapeutic activity. Its potential role as a second agent in a combination regimen merits further study.

Proinflammatory cytokines, such as IFN-γ and GM-CSF, enhance the ability of granulocytes to damage the agents of mucormycosis [130]. Adjunctive immune therapy with recombinant G-CSF and GM-CSF, or with recombinant IFN-γ, has been used successfully in conjunction with lipid formulations of amphotericin B in the treatment of mucormycosis [131–133]. Whether recombinant cytokines have a role in the primary treatment of mucormycosis in immunocompromised patients is not well defined.

G-CSF-mobilized granulocyte transfusions have been increasingly used for refractory mycoses, including mucormycosis [134]. While the reported experience in the management of mucormycosis with granulocyte transfusions is limited, such transfusion use may contain the infection and be lifesaving in persistently neutropenic hosts with this infection. Finally, based on limited experimental and clinical data, hyperbaric oxygen therapy may be also useful in centers with the appropriate technical expertise and facilities, although the precise mechanism by which hyperbaric oxygen would be effective is not well described [135].

Salvage Therapy

Posaconazole and deferasirox are reasonable salvage options for patients with mucormycosis refractory to or intolerant of polyene or isavuconazole therapy. Substantially, more clinical data are available for posaconazole in this setting [114, 115]. Posaconazole appears to be quite safe despite dosing for months to years of administration [114, 115].

Deferasirox is cidal against *Mucorales*, killing the fungi by inducing iron starvation [66]. Deferasirox cannot be used by *Mucorales* as an iron siderophore as is deferoxamine, to which the fungi bind and from which they strip iron. This explains why deferasirox kills *Mucorales* while deferoxamine actually enhances growth [70]. There is limited experience with deferasirox as salvage therapy. However, in case series and case reports, its addition to patients progressing on previous therapy has resulted in favorable outcomes without substantive toxicity [126, 127, 136]. Nevertheless, the majority of patients treated with deferasirox in these studies did not have active malignancy and had not undergone hematopoietic stem cell transplantation. If deferasirox is used as salvage, it should be limited to patients with diabetes mellitus or possibly steroid therapy in the setting of solid organ transplantation, and it should be used cautiously and with regular monitoring of renal and hepatic function. Administration at a dose of 20 mg/kg/day for 2–4 weeks is reasonable for salvage therapy, since in preclinical studies of non-iron-overloaded primates, deferasirox toxicity increased beyond 4 weeks of therapy [137].

G-CSF-mobilized granulocyte transfusions may provide additional support for persistently neutropenic patients until recovery from neutropenia. Administration of GM-CSF or IFN-γ may further augment host response and antifungal effect in non-neutropenic patients with refractory infection. In a recent murine study, addition of GM-CSF to LAmB therapy, but not IFN-γ, improved the survival of mice with mucormycosis [138].

References

1. Hibbett DS, Binder M, Bischoff JF, Blackwell M, Cannon PF, Eriksson OE, et al. A higher-level phylogenetic classification of the Fungi. Mycolog Res. 2007;111(Pt 5):509–47.
2. Ribes JA, Vanover-Sams CL, Baker DJ. Zygomycetes in human disease. Clin Microbiol Rev. 2000;13(2):236–301.
3. Gomes MZ, Lewis RE, Kontoyiannis DP. Mucormycosis caused by unusual mucormycetes, non-Rhizopus, –Mucor, and -Lichtheimia species. Clin Microbiol Rev. 2011;24(2):411–45.
4. Roden MM, Zaoutis TE, Buchanan WL, Knudsen TA, Sarkisova TA, Schaufele RL, Sein M, Sein T, Chiou CC, Chu JH, et al. Epidemiology and outcome of zygomycosis: a review of 929 reported cases. Clin Infect Dis. 2005;41(5):634–53.
5. Cohen-Abbo A, Bozeman PM, Patrick CC. Cunninghamella infections: review and report of two cases of Cunninghamella pneumonia in immunocompromised children. Clin Infect Dis. 1993;17(2):173–7.
6. Kwon-Chung KJ, Young RC, Orlando M. Pulmonary mucormycosis caused by Cunninghamella elegans in a patient with chronic myelogenous leukemia. Am J Clin Pathol. 1975;64(4):544–8.
7. Kontoyianis DP, Vartivarian S, Anaissie EJ, Samonis G, Bodey GP, Rinaldi M. Infections due to Cunninghamella bertholletiae in patients with cancer: report of three cases and review. Clin Infect Dis. 1994;18(6):925–8.
8. Ventura GJ, Kantarjian HM, Anaissie E, Hopfer RL, Fainstein V. Pneumonia with Cunninghamella species in patients with hematologic malignancies. A case report and review of the literature. Cancer. 1986;58(7):1534–6.
9. Bearer EA, Nelson PR, Chowers MY, Davis CE. Cutaneous zygomycosis caused by Saksenaea vasiformis in a diabetic patient. J Clin Microbiol. 1994;32(7):1823–4.
10. Lye GR, Wood G, Nimmo G. Subcutaneous zygomycosis due to Saksenaea vasiformis: rapid isolate identification using a modified sporulation technique. Pathology. 1996;28(4):364–5.
11. Kemna ME, Neri RC, Ali R, Salkin IF. Cokeromyces recurvatus, a mucoraceous zygomycete rarely isolated in clinical laboratories. J Clin Microbiol. 1994;32(3):843–5.
12. Kamalam A, Thambiah AS. Cutaneous infection by Syncephalastrum. Sabouraudia. 1980;18(1):19–20.
13. Rees JR, Pinner RW, Hajjeh RA, Brandt ME, Reingold AL. The epidemiological features of invasive mycotic infections in the San Francisco Bay area, 1992-1993: results of population-based laboratory active surveillance. Clin Infect Dis. 1998;27(5):1138–47.
14. Hotchi M, Okada M, Nasu T. Present state of fungal infections in autopsy cases in Japan. Am J Clin Pathol. 1980;74(4):410–6.
15. Tietz HJ, Brehmer D, Janisch W, Martin H. Incidence of endomycoses in the autopsy material of the Berlin Charite Hospital. Mycoses. 1998;41(Suppl 2):81–5.
16. Yamazaki T, Kume H, Murase S, Yamashita E, Arisawa M. Epidemiology of visceral mycoses: analysis of data in annual of the pathological autopsy cases in Japan. J Clin Microbiol. 1999;37(6):1732–8.
17. Bitar D, Lortholary O, Le Strat Y, Nicolau J, Coignard B, Tattevin P, et al. Population-based analysis of invasive fungal infections, France, 2001-2010. Emerg Infect Dis. 2014;20(7):1163–9.
18. Nussbaum ES, Hall WA. Rhinocerebral mucormycosis: changing patterns of disease. Surg Neurol. 1994;41(2):152–6.
19. Maertens J, Demuynck H, Verbeken EK, Zachee P, Verhoef GE, Vandenberghe P, Boogaerts MA. Mucormycosis in allogeneic bone marrow transplant recipients: report of five cases and review of the role of iron overload in the pathogenesis. Dermatology, Bone Marrow Transplant. 1999;24(3):307–12.
20. Marty FM, Cosimi LA, Baden LR. Breakthrough zygomycosis after voriconazole treatment in recipients of hematopoietic stem-cell transplants. N Engl J Med. 2004;350(9):950–2.
21. Xhaard A, Lanternier F, Porcher R, Dannaoui E, Bergeron A, Clement L, et al. Mucormycosis after allogeneic haematopoietic stem cell transplantation: a French Multicentre Cohort Study (2003-2008). Clin Microbiol Infect. 2012;18(10): E396–400.
22. Rammaert B, Lanternier F, Zahar JR, Dannaoui E, Bougnoux ME, Lecuit M, Lortholary O. Healthcare-associated mucormycosis. Clin Infect Dis. 2012;54(Suppl 1):S44–54.
23. Lanternier F, Sun HY, Ribaud P, Singh N, Kontoyiannis DP, Lortholary O. Mucormycosis in organ and stem cell transplant recipients. Clin Infect Dis. 2012;54(11):1629–36.

24. Lanternier F, Dannaoui E, Morizot G, Elie C, Garcia-Hermoso D, Huerre M, et al. A global analysis of mucormycosis in France: the RetroZygo study (2005-2007). Clin Infect Dis. 2012;54(Suppl 1):S35–43.
25. Saegeman V, Maertens J, Meersseman W, Spriet I, Verbeken E, Lagrou K. Increasing incidence of mucormycosis in University Hospital, Belgium. Emerg Infect Dis. 2010;16(9):1456–8.
26. Chakrabarti A, Das A, Sharma A, Panda N, Das S, Gupta KL, Sakhuja V. Ten years' experience in zygomycosis at a tertiary care centre in India. J Infect. 2001;42(4):261–6.
27. Chakrabarti A, Das A, Mandal J, Shivaprakash MR, George VK, Tarai B, et al. The rising trend of invasive zygomycosis in patients with uncontrolled diabetes mellitus. Med Mycol. 2006;44(4):335–42.
28. Siwek GT, Dodgson KJ, de Magalhaes-Silverman M, Bartelt LA, Kilborn SB, Hoth PL, et al. Invasive zygomycosis in hematopoietic stem cell transplant recipients receiving voriconazole prophylaxis. Clin Infect Dis. 2004;39(4):584–7.
29. Kauffman CA. Zygomycosis: reemergence of an old pathogen. Clin Infect Dis. 2004;39(4):588–90.
30. Marr KA, Carter RA, Crippa F, Wald A, Corey L. Epidemiology and outcome of mould infections in hematopoietic stem cell transplant recipients. Clin Infect Dis. 2002;34(7):909–17.
31. Kontoyiannis DP, Wessel VC, Bodey GP, Rolston KV. Zygomycosis in the 1990s in a tertiary-care cancer center. Clin Infect Dis. 2000;30(6):851–6.
32. Park BJ, Pappas PG, Wannemuehler KA, Alexander BD, Anaissie EJ, Andes DR, et al. Invasive non-aspergillus mold infections in transplant recipients, United States, 2001-2006. Emerg Infect Dis. 2011;17(10):1855–64.
33. Pappas PG, Alexander BD, Andes DR, Hadley S, Kauffman CA, Freifeld A, et al. Invasive fungal infections among organ transplant recipients: results of the Transplant-Associated Infection Surveillance Network (TRANSNET). Clin Infect Dis. 2010;50(8):1101–11.
34. Pavie J, Lafaurie M, Lacroix C, Marie Zagdanski A, Debrosse D, Socie G, et al. Successful treatment of pulmonary mucormycosis in an allogenic bone-marrow transplant recipient with combined medical and surgical therapy. Scand J Infect Dis. 2004;36(10):767–9.
35. Almyroudis NG, Sutton DA, Linden P, Rinaldi MG, Fung J, Kusne S. Zygomycosis in solid organ transplant recipients in a tertiary transplant center and review of the literature. Am J Transplant. 2006;6(10):2365–74.
36. Rickerts V, Bohme A, Just-Nubling G. Risk factor for invasive zygomycosis in patients with hematologic malignancies. Mycoses. 2002;45(Suppl 1):27–30.
37. Imhof A, Balajee SA, Fredricks DN, Englund JA, Marr KA. Breakthrough fungal infections in stem cell transplant recipients receiving voriconazole. Clin Infect Dis. 2004;39(5):743–6.
38. Ide L, Buysschaert I, Demuynck H, De Man R, Verlinde A, De Laere E, Surmont I. Zygomycosis in neutropenic patients with past aspergillus infection: a role for posaconazole? Clin Microbiol Infect. 2004;10(9):862–3.
39. Vigouroux S, Morin O, Moreau P, Mechinaud F, Morineau N, Mahe B, et al. Zygomycosis after prolonged use of voriconazole in immunocompromised patients with hematologic disease: attention required. Clin Infect Dis. 2005;40(4):e35–7.
40. Morrison VA, McGlave PB. Mucormycosis in the BMT population. Bone Marrow Transplant. 1993;11(5):383–8.
41. Alsuwaida K. Primary cutaneous mucormycosis complicating the use of adhesive tape to secure the endotracheal tube. Can J Anaesth. 2002;49(8):880–2.
42. Petrikkos G, Skiada A, Sambatakou H, Toskas A, Vaiopoulos G, Giannopoulou M, Katsilambros N. Mucormycosis: ten-year experience at a tertiary-care center in Greece. Eur J Clin Microbiol Infect Dis. 2003;22(12):753–6.
43. Adam RD, Hunter G, DiTomasso J, Comerci G Jr. Mucormycosis: emerging prominence of cutaneous infections. Clin Infect Dis. 1994;19(1):67–76.
44. Kerr OA, Bong C, Wallis C, Tidman MJ. Primary cutaneous mucormycosis masquerading as pyoderma gangrenosum. Br J Dermatol. 2004;150(6):1212–3.
45. Quinio D, Karam A, Leroy JP, Moal MC, Bourbigot B, Masure O, et al. Zygomycosis caused by Cunninghamella bertholletiae in a kidney transplant recipient. Med Mycol. 2004;42(2):177–80.
46. Gartenberg G, Bottone EJ, Keusch GT, Weitzman I. Hospital-acquired mucormycosis (Rhizopus rhizopodiformis) of skin and subcutaneous tissue: epidemiology, mycology and treatment. N Engl J Med. 1978;299(20):1115–8.
47. Mead JH, Lupton GP, Dillavou CL, Odom RB. Cutaneous Rhizopus infection. Occurrence as a postoperative complication associated with an elasticized adhesive dressing. JAMA. 1979;242(3):272–4.
48. Teal LJ, Schultz KM, Weber DJ, Gergen MF, Miller MB, DiBiase LM, et al. Invasive cutaneous Rhizopus infections in an immunocompromised patient population associated with hospital laundry carts. Infect Control Hosp Epidemiol. 2016;37(10):1251–3.
49. Duffy J, Harris J, Gade L, Sehulster L, Newhouse E, O'Connell H, et al. Mucormycosis outbreak associated with hospital linens. Pediatr Infect Dis J. 2014;33(5):472–6.
50. Maravi-Poma E, Rodriguez-Tudela JL, de Jalon JG, Manrique-Larralde A, Torroba L, Urtasun J, et al. Outbreak of gastric mucormycosis associated with the use of wooden tongue depressors in critically ill patients. Intensive Care Med. 2004;30(4):724–8.
51. Singh N, Aguado JM, Bonatti H, Forrest G, Gupta KL, Safdar N, et al. Zygomycosis in solid organ transplant recipients: a prospective, matched case-control study to assess risks for disease and outcome. J Infect Dis. 2009;200(6):1002–11.
52. Spellberg B, Edwards J Jr, Ibrahim A. Novel perspectives on mucormycosis: pathophysiology, presentation, and management. Clin Microbiol Rev. 2005;18(3):556–69.
53. Petrikkos G, Skiada A, Lortholary O, Roilides E, Walsh TJ, Kontoyiannis DP. Epidemiology and clinical manifestations of mucormycosis. Clin Infect Dis. 2012;54(Suppl 1):S23–34.
54. Sun HY, Aguado JM, Bonatti H, Forrest G, Gupta KL, Safdar N, et al. Pulmonary zygomycosis in solid organ transplant recipients in the current era. Am J Transplant. 2009;9(9):2166–71.
55. Chamilos G, Marom EM, Lewis RE, Lionakis MS, Kontoyiannis DP. Predictors of pulmonary zygomycosis versus invasive pulmonary aspergillosis in patients with cancer. Clin Infect Dis. 2005;41(1):60–6.
56. Lewis RE, Liao G, Wang W, Prince RA, Kontoyiannis DP. Voriconazole pre-exposure selects for breakthrough mucormycosis in a mixed model of aspergillus fumigatus-Rhizopus oryzae pulmonary infection. Virulence. 2011;2(4):348–55.
57. Lamaris GA, Ben-Ami R, Lewis RE, Chamilos G, Samonis G, Kontoyiannis DP. Increased virulence of Zygomycetes organisms following exposure to voriconazole: a study involving fly and murine models of zygomycosis. J Infect Dis. 2009;199(9):1399–406.
58. Liu M, Spellberg B, Phan QT, Fu Y, Fu Y, Lee AS, et al. The endothelial cell receptor GRP78 is required for mucormycosis pathogenesis in diabetic mice. J Clin Invest. 2010;120(6):1914–24.
59. Lutterloh EC, Opal SM, Pittman DD, Keith JC Jr, Tan XY, Clancy BM, et al. Inhibition of the RAGE products increases survival in experimental models of severe sepsis and systemic infection. Crit Care. 2007;11(6):R122.
60. Liliensiek B, Weigand MA, Bierhaus A, Nicklas W, Kasper M, Hofer S, et al. Receptor for advanced glycation end products

(RAGE) regulates sepsis but not the adaptive immune response. J Clin Invest. 2004;113(11):1641–50.
61. Ramsgaard L, Englert JM, Manni ML, Milutinovic PS, Gefter J, Tobolewski J, et al. Lack of the receptor for advanced glycation end-products attenuates E. coli pneumonia in mice. PLoS One. 2011;6(5):e20132.
62. C R, Bryant R, Ibrahim AS, Edwards J Jr, Filler SG, Goldberg R, Spellberg B. Combination polyene-caspofungin treatment of rhino-orbital-cerebral mucormycosis. Clin Infect Dis. 2008;47:364–71.
63. Chamilos G, Lewis RE, Kontoyiannis DP. Delaying amphotericin B-based frontline therapy significantly increases mortality among patients with hematologic malignancy who have zygomycosis. Clin Infect Dis. 2008;47(4):503–9.
64. Boelaert JR, de Locht M, Van Cutsem J, Kerrels V, Cantinieaux B, Verdonck A, et al. Mucormycosis during deferoxamine therapy is a siderophore-mediated infection. In vitro and in vivo animal studies. J Clin Investig. 1993;91(5):1979–86.
65. Van Cutsem J, Boelaert JR. Effects of deferoxamine, feroxamine and iron on experimental mucormycosis (zygomycosis). Kidney Int. 1989;36(6):1061–8.
66. Ibrahim AS, Gebermariam T, Fu Y, Lin L, Husseiny MI, French SW, et al. The iron chelator deferasirox protects mice from mucormycosis through iron starvation. J Clin Invest. 2007;117(9):2649–57.
67. Spellberg B, Kontoyiannis DP, Fredricks D, Morris MI, Perfect JR, Chin-Hong PV, et al. Risk factors for mortality in patients with mucormycosis. Med Mycol. 2012;50(6):611–8.
68. Daly AL, Velazquez LA, Bradley SF, Kauffman CA. Mucormycosis: association with deferoxamine therapy. Am J Med. 1989;87(4):468–71.
69. Boelaert JR, de Locht M, Schneider YJ. The effect of deferoxamine on different zygomycetes. J Infect Dis. 1994;169(1):231–2.
70. Boelaert JR, Van Cutsem J, de Locht M, Schneider YJ, Crichton RR. Deferoxamine augments growth and pathogenicity of Rhizopus, while hydroxypyridinone chelators have no effect. Kidney Int. 1994;45(3):667–71.
71. Nithyanandam S, Jacob MS, Battu RR, Thomas RK, Correa MA, D'Souza O. Rhino-orbito-cerebral mucormycosis. A retrospective analysis of clinical features and treatment outcomes. Indian J Ophthalmol. 2003;51(3):231–6.
72. Peterson KL, Wang M, Canalis RF, Abemayor E. Rhinocerebral mucormycosis: evolution of the disease and treatment options. Laryngoscope. 1997;107(7):855–62.
73. Khor BS, Lee MH, Leu HS, Liu JW. Rhinocerebral mucormycosis in Taiwan. J Microbiol Immunol Infect. 2003;36(4):266–9.
74. Tedder M, Spratt JA, Anstadt MP, Hegde SS, Tedder SD, Lowe JE. Pulmonary mucormycosis: results of medical and surgical therapy. Ann Thorac Surg. 1994;57(4):1044–50.
75. Reid VJ, Solnik DL, Daskalakis T, Sheka KP. Management of bronchovascular mucormycosis in a diabetic: a surgical success. Ann Thorac Surg. 2004;78(4):1449–51.
76. Asai K, Suzuki K, Takahashi T, Ito Y, Kazui T, Kita Y. Pulmonary resection with chest wall removal and reconstruction for invasive pulmonary mucormycosis during antileukemia chemotherapy. Jpn J Thorac Cardiovasc Surg. 2003;51(4):163–6.
77. McDermott NE, Barrett J, Hipp J, Merino MJ, Richard Lee CC, Waterman P, et al. Successful treatment of periodontal mucormycosis: report of a case and literature review. Oral Surg Oral Med Oral Pathol Oral Radiol Endod. 2010;109(3):e64–9.
78. Walsh TJ, Hiemenz JW, Seibel NL, Perfect JR, Horwith G, Lee L, et al. Amphotericin B lipid complex for invasive fungal infections: analysis of safety and efficacy in 556 cases. Clin Infect Dis. 1998;26(6):1383–96.
79. Gleissner B, Schilling A, Anagnostopolous I, Siehl I, Thiel E. Improved outcome of zygomycosis in patients with hematological diseases? Leuk Lymphoma. 2004;45(7):1351–60.
80. Ruping MJ, Heinz WJ, Kindo AJ, Rickerts V, Lass-Florl C, Beisel C, et al. Forty-one recent cases of invasive zygomycosis from a global clinical registry. J Antimicrob Chemother. 2010;65(2):296–302.
81. Pagano L, Valentini CG, Posteraro B, Girmenia C, Ossi C, Pan A, et al. Zygomycosis in Italy: a survey of FIMUA-ECMM (Federazione Italiana di Micopatologia Umana ed Animale and European Confederation of Medical Mycology). J Chemother. 2009;21(3):322–9.
82. Cornely OA, Arikan-Akdagli S, Dannaoui E, Groll AH, Lagrou K, Chakrabarti A, et al. ESCMID and ECMM joint clinical guidelines for the diagnosis and management of mucormycosis 2013. Clin Microbiol Infect. 2014;20(Suppl 3):5–26.
83. Groll AH, Giri N, Petraitis V, Petraitiene R, Candelario M, Bacher JS, et al. Comparative efficacy and distribution of lipid formulations of amphotericin B in experimental Candida albicans infection of the central nervous system. J Infect Dis. 2000;182(1):274–82.
84. Ibrahim AS, Gebremariam T, Husseiny MI, Stevens DA, Fu Y, Edwards JE Jr, Spellberg B. Comparison of lipid amphotericin B preparations in treating murine zygomycosis. Antimicrob Agents Chemother. 2008;52(4):1573–6.
85. Lewis RE, Liao G, Hou J, Chamilos G, Prince RA, Kontoyiannis DP. Comparative analysis of amphotericin B lipid complex and liposomal amphotericin B kinetics of lung accumulation and fungal clearance in a murine model of acute invasive pulmonary aspergillosis. Antimicrob Agents Chemother. 2007;51(4):1253–8.
86. Cornely OA, Maertens J, Bresnik M, Ebrahimi R, Ullmann AJ, Bouza E, et al. Liposomal amphotericin B as initial therapy for invasive mold infection: a randomized trial comparing a high-loading dose regimen with standard dosing (AmBiLoad trial). Clin Infect Dis. 2007;44(10):1289–97.
87. Walsh TJ, Goodman JL, Pappas P, Bekersky I, Buell DN, Roden M, et al. Safety, tolerance, and pharmacokinetics of high-dose liposomal amphotericin B (AmBisome) in patients infected with aspergillus species and other filamentous fungi: maximum tolerated dose study. Antimicrob Agents Chemother. 2001;45(12):3487–96.
88. Perkhofer S, Lechner V, Lass-Florl C. European committee on antimicrobial susceptibility T. in vitro activity of Isavuconazole against aspergillus species and zygomycetes according to the methodology of the European committee on antimicrobial susceptibility testing. Antimicrob Agents Chemother. 2009;53(4):1645–7.
89. Verweij PE, Gonzalez GM, Wiedrhold NP, Lass Florl C, Warn P, Heep M, et al. In vitro antifungal activity of isavuconazole against 345 mucorales isolates collected at study centers in eight countries. J Chemother. 2009;21(3):272–81.
90. Castanheira M, Messer SA, Rhomberg PR, Dietrich RR, Jones RN, Pfaller MA. Isavuconazole and nine comparator antifungal susceptibility profiles for common and uncommon Candida species collected in 2012: application of new CLSI clinical breakpoints and epidemiological cutoff values. Mycopathologia. 2014;178(1–2):1–9.
91. Arendrup MC, Jensen RH, Meletiadis J. In vitro activity of isavuconazole and comparators against clinical isolates of the mucorales order. Antimicrob Agents Chemother. 2015;59(12):7735–42.
92. Kovanda LL, Desai AV, Lu Q, Townsend RW, Akhtar S, Bonate P, Hope WW. Isavuconazole population pharmacokinetic analysis using nonparametric estimation in patients with invasive fungal disease (results from the VITAL study). Antimicrob Agents Chemother. 2016;60(8):4568–76.
93. Marty FM, Ostrosky-Zeichner L, Cornely OA, Mullane KM, Perfect JR, Thompson GR 3rd, et al. Isavuconazole treatment for mucormycosis: a single-arm open-label trial and case-control analysis. Lancet Infect Dis. 2016;16(7):828–37.
94. Spellberg B, Brass EP. The VITAL study: case control studies are hypothesis-generating. Lancet Infect Dis. 2016;16(8):886.

95. Miceli MH, Kauffman CA. Isavuconazole: a new broad-spectrum triazole antifungal agent. Clin Infect Dis. 2015;61(10):1558–65.
96. Sun QN, Fothergill AW, McCarthy DI, Rinaldi MG, Graybill JR. In vitro activities of posaconazole, itraconazole, voriconazole, amphotericin B, and fluconazole against 37 clinical isolates of zygomycetes. Antimicrob Agents Chemother. 2002;46(5):1581–2.
97. Trifilio SM, Bennett CL, Yarnold PR, McKoy JM, Parada J, Mehta J, et al. Breakthrough zygomycosis after voriconazole administration among patients with hematologic malignancies who receive hematopoietic stem-cell transplants or intensive chemotherapy. Bone Marrow Transplant. 2007;39(7):425–9.
98. Dannaoui E, Meis JF, Loebenberg D, Verweij PE. Activity of posaconazole in treatment of experimental disseminated zygomycosis. Antimicrob Agents Chemother. 2003;47(11):3647–50.
99. Dannaoui E, Meletiadis J, Mouton JW, Meis JF, Verweij PE. In vitro susceptibilities of zygomycetes to conventional and new antifungals. J Antimicrob Chemother. 2003;51(1):45–52.
100. Van Cutsem J, Van Gerven F, Fransen J, Janssen PA. Treatment of experimental zygomycosis in Guinea pigs with azoles and with amphotericin B. Chemotherapy. 1989;35(4):267–72.
101. Pfaller MA, Messer SA, Hollis RJ, Jones RN. Antifungal activities of posaconazole, ravuconazole, and voriconazole compared to those of itraconazole and amphotericin B against 239 clinical isolates of Aspergillus spp. and other filamentous fungi: report from SENTRY Antimicrobial Surveillance Program, 2000. Antimicrob Agents Chemother. 2002;46(4):1032–7.
102. Almyroudis NG, Sutton DA, Fothergill AW, Rinaldi MG, Kusne S. In vitro susceptibilities of 217 clinical isolates of zygomycetes to conventional and new antifungal agents. Antimicrob Agents Chemother. 2007;51(7):2587–90.
103. Lass-Florl C, Mayr A, Perkhofer S, Hinterberger G, Hausdorfer J, Speth C, Fille M. The activities of antifungal agents against yeasts and filamentous fungi: assessment according to EUCAST methodology. Antimicrob Agents Chemother. 2008;52:3637–41.
104. Arikan S, Sancak B, Alp S, Hascelik G, McNicholas P. Comparative in vitro activities of posaconazole, voriconazole, itraconazole, and amphotericin B against Aspergillus and Rhizopus, and synergy testing for Rhizopus. Med Mycol. 2008;12:1–7.
105. Ullmann AJ, Cornely OA, Burchardt A, Hachem R, Kontoyiannis DP, Topelt K, et al. Pharmacokinetics, safety, and efficacy of posaconazole in patients with persistent febrile neutropenia or refractory invasive fungal infection. Antimicrob Agents Chemother. 2006;50(2):658–66.
106. Krishna G, Sansone-Parsons A, Martinho M, Kantesaria B, Pedicone L. Posaconazole plasma concentrations in juvenile patients with invasive fungal infection. Antimicrob Agents Chemother. 2007;51(3):812–8.
107. Krishna G, Martinho M, Chandrasekar P, Ullmann AJ, Patino H. Pharmacokinetics of oral posaconazole in allogeneic hematopoietic stem cell transplant recipients with graft-versus-host disease. Pharmacotherapy. 2007;27(12):1627–36.
108. Sun QN, Najvar LK, Bocanegra R, Loebenberg D, Graybill JR. In vivo activity of posaconazole against Mucor spp. in an immunosuppressed-mouse model. Antimicrob Agents Chemother. 2002;46(7):2310–2.
109. Rodriguez MM, Serena C, Marine M, Pastor FJ, Guarro J. Posaconazole combined with amphotericin B, an effective therapy for a murine-disseminated infection caused by Rhizopus oryzae. Antimicrob Agents Chemother. 2008;52:3786–8.
110. Ibrahim AS, Gebremariam T, Schwartz JA, Edwards JE Jr, Spellberg B. Posaconazole mono- or combination therapy for treatment of murine zygomycosis. Antimicrob Agents Chemother. 2009;53:772–5.
111. Lekakis LJ, Lawson A, Prante J, Ribes J, Davis GJ, Monohan G, et al. Fatal rhizopus pneumonia in allogeneic stem cell transplant patients despite posaconazole prophylaxis: two cases and review of the literature. Biol Blood Marrow Transplant. 2009;15(8):991–5.
112. Mousset S, Bug G, Heinz WJ, Tintelnot K, Rickerts V. Breakthrough zygomycosis on posaconazole prophylaxis after allogeneic stem cell transplantation. Transpl Infect Dis. 2010;12(3):261–4.
113. Schlemmer F, Lagrange-Xelot M, Lacroix C, de La Tour R, Socie G, Molina JM. Breakthrough Rhizopus infection on posaconazole prophylaxis following allogeneic stem cell transplantation. Bone Marrow Transplant. 2008;42(8):551–2.
114. van Burik JA, Hare RS, Solomon HF, Corrado ML, Kontoyiannis DP. Posaconazole is effective as salvage therapy in zygomycosis: a retrospective summary of 91 cases. Clin Infect Dis. 2006;42(7):e61–5.
115. Greenberg RN, Mullane K, van Burik JA, Raad I, Abzug MJ, Anstead G, et al. Posaconazole as salvage therapy for zygomycosis. Antimicrob Agents Chemother. 2006;50(1):126–33.
116. National Diabetes Fact Sheet, 2011. Atlanta: US Centers for Disease Control and Prevention; 2012.
117. Joshi N, Caputo GM, Weitekamp MR, Karchmer AW. Infections in patients with diabetes mellitus. N Engl J Med. 1999;341(25):1906–12.
118. Kyvernitakis A, Torres HA, Jiang Y, Chamilos G, Lewis RE, Kontoyiannis DP. Initial use of combination treatment does not impact survival of 106 patients with haematologic malignancies and mucormycosis: a propensity score analysis. Clin Microbiol Infect. 2016;22(9):811.e1–8.
119. Ibrahim AS, Bowman JC, Avanessian V, Brown K, Spellberg B, Edwards JE Jr, Douglas CM. Caspofungin inhibits Rhizopus oryzae 1,3-beta-D-glucan synthase, lowers burden in brain measured by quantitative PCR, and improves survival at a low but not a high dose during murine disseminated zygomycosis. Antimicrob Agents Chemother. 2005;49(2):721–7.
120. Spellberg B, Fu Y, Edwards JE Jr, Ibrahim AS. Combination therapy with amphotericin B lipid complex and caspofungin acetate of disseminated zygomycosis in diabetic ketoacidotic mice. Antimicrob Agents Chemother. 2005;49(2):830–2.
121. Ibrahim AS, Gebremariam T, Fu Y, Edwards JE Jr, Spellberg B. Combination echinocandin-polyene treatment of murine mucormycosis. Antimicrob Agents Chemother. 2008;52(4):1556–8.
122. Ibrahim AS, Bryant R, Edwards JE, Spellberg B. Economic burden of mucormycosis in the United States: can a vaccine be cost-effective? Med Mycol. 2009;47(6):592–600.
123. Ibrahim AS, Gebremariam T, Lin L, Luo G, Husseiny MI, Skory CD, et al. The high affinity iron permease is a key virulence factor required for Rhizopus oryzae pathogenesis. Mol Microbiol. 2010;77(3):587–604.
124. de Locht M, Boelaert JR, Schneider YJ. Iron uptake from ferrioxamine and from ferrirhizoferrin by germinating spores of Rhizopus microsporus. Biochem Pharmacol. 1994;47(10):1843–50.
125. Ibrahim AS, Edwards JE Jr, Fu Y, Spellberg B. Deferiprone iron chelation as a novel therapy for experimental mucormycosis. J Antimicrob Chemother. 2006;58:1070–3.
126. Reed C, Ibrahim A, Edwards JE Jr, Walot I, Spellberg B. Deferasirox, an iron-chelating agent, as salvage therapy for rhinocerebral mucormycosis. Antimicrob Agents Chemother. 2006;50(11):3968–9.
127. Spellberg B, Andes D, Perez M, Anglim A, Bonilla H, Mathisen GE, et al. Safety and outcomes of open-label deferasirox iron chelation therapy for mucormycosis. Antimicrob Agents Chemother. 2009;53(7):3122–5.
128. Spellberg B, Ibrahim AS, Chin-Hong PV, Kontoyiannis DP, Morris M, Perfect JR, Fredricks D, Brass EP. The Deferasirox-AmBisome Therapy for Mucormycosis (DEFEAT Mucor) Study: A Randomized, Double-Blinded Placebo Controlled Trial. J Antimicrob Chemother. 2012;67:715–22.

129. Ben-Ami R, Lewis RE, Tarrand J, Leventakos K, Kontoyiannis DP. Antifungal activity of colistin against mucorales species in vitro and in a murine model of Rhizopus oryzae pulmonary infection. Antimicrob Agents Chemother. 2010;54(1):484–90.
130. Gil-Lamaignere C, Simitsopoulou M, Roilides E, Maloukou A, Winn RM, Walsh TJ. Interferon- gamma and granulocyte-macrophage colony-stimulating factor augment the activity of polymorphonuclear leukocytes against medically important zygomycetes. J Infect Dis. 2005;191(7):1180–7.
131. Abzug MJ, Walsh TJ. Interferon-gamma and colony-stimulating factors as adjuvant therapy for refractory fungal infections in children. Pediatr Infect Dis J. 2004;23(8):769–73.
132. Gonzalez CE, Couriel DR, Walsh TJ. Disseminated zygomycosis in a neutropenic patient: successful treatment with amphotericin B lipid complex and granulocyte colony-stimulating factor. Clin Infect Dis. 1997;24(2):192–6.
133. Kullberg BJ, Anaissie EJ. Cytokines as therapy for opportunistic fungal infections. Res Immunol. 1998;149(4–5):478–88; discussion 515.
134. Grigull L, Beilken A, Schmid H, Kirschner P, Sykora KW, Linderkamp C, et al. Secondary prophylaxis of invasive fungal infections with combination antifungal therapy and G-CSF-mobilized granulocyte transfusions in three children with hematological malignancies. Support Care Cancer. 2006;14(7):783–6.
135. John BV, Chamilos G, Kontoyiannis DP. Hyperbaric oxygen as an adjunctive treatment for zygomycosis. Clin Microbiol Infect. 2005;11(7):515–7.
136. Busca A, Marmont F, Locatelli F, Limerutti G, Sorrentino MT, Barbui A, et al. Combined antifungal therapy, iron chelation and surgical resection as treatment of hepatic zygomycosis in a patient with haematological malignancy. Mycoses. 2010;53(3):275–8.
137. Nick H, Wong A, Acklin P, Faller B, Jin Y, Lattmann R, et al. ICL670A: preclinical profile. Adv Exp Med Biol. 2002;509:185–203.
138. Rodriguez MM, Calvo E, Marine M, Pastor FJ, Fernandez-Ballart J, Guarro J. Efficacy of liposomal amphotericin B combined with gamma interferon or granulocyte-macrophage colony-stimulating factor for treatment of systemic zygomycosis in mice. Antimicrob Agents Chemother. 2009;53(8):3569–71.

Cryptococcus Infections in Transplant Recipients

35

Raymund R. Razonable and Pearlie P. Chong

Introduction

Cryptococcus species are group of closely related basidiomycetous encapsulated yeasts. Distributed worldwide, there are over 50 species belonging to the genus *Cryptococcus*. However, only *Cryptococcus neoformans* (which includes *C. neoformans* var *grubii* and var *neoformans*) and *Cryptococcus gattii* (formerly known as *C. neoformans* var *gattii*) are well known pathogens causing human illness [1, 2]. There have been only few reports of human disease due to other members, such as *Cryptococcus albidus* and *Cryptococcus laurentii*, especially in immunocompromised hosts [3–5].

C. neoformans var. *grubii* and var. *neoformans* are present in soil, especially enriched with droppings of birds, including pigeons and chickens [6]. These fungi have been cultured from roosting sites of pigeons and from rotting vegetation [7]. *C. neoformans* var *grubii* and var *neoformans* account for the large majority of human cryptococcosis in the United States and other temperate climates of the world [1]. On the other hand, *C. gattii* is endemic in tropical and subtropical regions of Africa and Australia, Southeast Asia, and Brazil. *C. gattii* has been cultured from eucalyptus (red gum) trees in Australia [8]. Recently, *C. gattii* has been reported in the Pacific Northwest of the United States and Canada, as a cause of an outbreak of human cryptococcosis [2, 9]. *C. gattii* has been cultured from trees native in California and British Columbia [2, 9].

Cryptococcus species cause infections in immunocompetent and immunocompromised individuals. Most serious infections, however, occur in individuals with defective cell-mediated immunity, such as patients with acquired immunodeficiency syndrome (AIDS) and transplant recipients [10, 11]. *C. neoformans* causes most infections occurring in immunocompromised hosts, while most infections due to *C. gattii* has been reported in immunocompetent hosts [9].

Epidemiology of Cryptococcosis After Transplantation

Cryptococcosis is the third most common fungal infection after solid organ transplantation (SOT), following *Candida* and *Aspergillus* species. In a recent multicenter epidemiologic study, cryptococcosis accounts for 8% of all invasive fungal infections after SOT [12, 13]. However, the overall incidence of cryptococcal disease after SOT ranges from as low as 0.2% to as high as 5%, depending on the type of organ transplant and the duration of follow-up [12, 13]. In contrast to the SOT population, cryptococcal disease is rarely seen among hematopoietic stem cell transplant (HSCT) recipients. The TRANSNET database reported that cryptococcal disease occurred in 0% of the HSCT recipients, while it accounted for 8% of all invasive fungal infections in SOT recipients [13, 14]. This difference is probably due to the widespread use of *Cryptococcus*-active azole prophylaxis routinely given to the recipients of hematopoietic stem cell transplantation such as fluconazole for the prevention of invasive candidiasis or voriconazole and posaconazole for the prevention of invasive mold disease among high-risk transplant recipients [15].

R. R. Razonable (✉)
Division of Infectious Diseases, Department of Medicine, and the William J. von Liebig Center for Transplantation and Clinical Regeneration, College of Medicine, Mayo Clinic, Rochester, MN, USA
e-mail: razonable.raymund@mayo.edu

P. P. Chong
Division of Infectious Diseases, University of Texas Southwestern Medical Center, Dallas, TX, USA
e-mail: pearlie.chong@UTSouthwestern.edu

A. Safdar (ed.), *Principles and Practice of Transplant Infectious Diseases*, https://doi.org/10.1007/978-1-4939-9034-4_35

Transmission and Patterns of Disease After Transplantation

Transmission of *Cryptococcus* sp. occurs through inhalation of the fungus, either in yeast form or as basidiophores, from an environmental source such as bird droppings or soil. Following inhalation, the fungus may remain localized in the lungs or it may disseminate hematogenously, with particular predilection to infect the central nervous system (CNS).

Three patterns of cryptococcal infection occur in transplant recipients. First, it may result from the reactivation of subclinical (and latent) cryptococcus infection [16]. This pattern of infection was suggested in a study where pre- and post-transplant cryptococcal serology was evaluated with the risk of fungal disease [17]. Transplant recipients with detectable pretransplant serum cryptococcal antibodies had an earlier onset of cryptococcal disease indication for the potential of reactivation of previously acquired infection [17]. The factors associated with reactivation of latent cryptococcal infection are not yet defined, although it may reflect an overall net state of immunosuppression and fungal burden. Second, de novo acquisition of cryptococcal infection may occur after transplantation, as a result of natural transmission via inhalation of the fungus [18, 19]. The majority of de novo cryptococcal disease occurs after the first year following transplantation, and the median time to the onset of cryptococcal disease ranges from 16 to 21 months [13, 20, 21]. Third, cryptococcus may rarely be acquired from the donor (i.e., donor-derived cryptococcus) [22–24]. Donor-derived cryptococcus infection manifests early, and the symptoms generally occur between 14 and 24 days after transplantation [22]. Hence, donor-derived cryptococcal disease should be considered in any transplant recipient with diagnosis within 30 days after transplantation. Occurrence of donor-transmitted cryptococcal disease in one transplant recipient should alert surveillance and management of possible disease in the other organ recipients from the same donor. Occurrence of cryptococcal disease in multiple recipients from a single donor raises the suspicion for donor-derived infection. Donor-derived cryptococcal disease is however so infrequent that routine screening of donors for latent cryptococcal infection is not recommended [10].

Risk Factors and Pathogenesis

Transplant candidates with liver cirrhosis and end-stage liver disease have impaired host defenses, including compromised cell mediated immunity, phagocytic dysfunction, decreased antibody and immunoglobulins, and complement deficiency that may increase their risk of cryptococcosis [25]. Indeed, liver cirrhosis is a recognized risk factor for the development of cryptococcal disease [25]. Mortality in liver cirrhotic patients with cryptococcosis is high, and previous studies have reported this to range from 81% to 100% [26, 27]. Patients with pretransplant cryptococcal disease should be treated aggressively. Improvement of clinical signs and symptoms of cryptococcal disease, stable and improving cryptococcal antigen titers, and sterility of fungal cultures should be demonstrated before these patients are considered for organ transplantation.

The primary host defense against cryptococcal infections is cell-mediated immunity, of which T helper CD4+ cells play a central role [10, 11]. Impairment in cell-mediated immunity may therefore predispose to cryptococcal disease. An over-immunosuppressed state is generally considered as a risk factor for cryptococcal disease. Use of lymphocyte-depleting drugs such as alemtuzumab and antithymocyte globulin has been associated with cryptococcosis [28, 29]. Use of high doses of corticosteroids has also been suggested as a risk factor for cryptococcal infection [30, 31]. In contrast, use of calcineurin inhibitors appears to influence the clinical manifestation of cryptococcosis. For example, patients on tacrolimus or other calcineurin inhibitors were less likely to have disseminated cryptococcal disease and more likely to present with disease localized to the lungs or skin. Tacrolimus has anticryptococcal activity at temperatures of 37–39 °C but not at environmental temperatures. This property could account for the higher ratio of skin and soft tissue infections compared to CNS infections in patients receiving tacrolimus-based immunosuppressive regimens [32].

Cryptococcal disease is rarely encountered in HSCT recipients. In one review, there have only been nine HSCT patients identified in the literature [12]. In this small cohort, there were more autologous that allogeneic HSCT recipients with cryptococcal disease. The precise reasons for this observation are largely unknown. Prophylaxis with cryptococcus-active azoles may account for this difference, since it is given for longer periods of time in allogeneic HSCT recipients. In the same context, the routine use of antifungal prophylaxis in HSCT recipients may also account for the lower incidence of cryptococcosis in HSCT compared to SOT recipients. In our review of invasive fungal infections after lung transplantation, where prolonged universal azole prophylaxis is provided, no cases of cryptococcal disease was observed [15].

Clinical Disease and Its Manifestations

Cryptococcus neoformans may affect any organ system, but it most commonly involves the lungs and CNS as shown in Table 35.1. Disseminated invasive disease is a very common presentation and was documented in up to 61% of SOT recipients with cryptococcal infection, especially liver recipients [21]. Pulmonary disease is the most common organ

Table 35.1 Clinical manifestations of cryptococcosis

Respiratory	Nodules Infiltrates (lobar, interstitial) Cavitation Effusions/empyema Adenopathy (mediastinal, hilar) Acute respiratory distress syndrome Pneumothorax Endobronchial lesions
Neurologic	Meningitis Encephalitis Cryptococcoma (more common with *C. gattii* infection) Hydrocephalus Spinal cord granuloma
Cutaneous	Nodules (classically with central umbilication) Vesicles Plaques Purpura Ulcers Cellulitis
Other organs	Musculoskeletal (arthritis, myositis, osteomyelitis) Ocular (keratitis, chorioretinitis, endophthalmitis) Genitourinary (prostatitis, renal abscess) Gastrointestinal (hepatitis, peritonitis, mucosal ulcers) Cardiovascular (endocarditis, cryptococcemia) Lymph (lymphadenopathy)

involved with cryptococcus infection in transplant recipients [33–35]. It may present as an asymptomatic infection that is detected incidentally on chest radiograph [33, 34] or as a severe pneumonia and respiratory failure [35]. Depending on the pulmonary syndrome, patients may present with fever, cough, sputum production, pleurisy, and weight loss. Radiographic findings vary depending on the syndrome and may include an isolated pulmonary nodule, nodular infiltrates, consolidation, or pleural effusions [33–35].

Extra pulmonary involvement is common in transplant patients with cryptococcosis, and the CNS is the most common extra-pulmonary site [20, 21, 36]. Accordingly, transplant recipients with cryptococcal infection should undergo spinal fluid examination. Cryptococcal meningitis or meningoencephalitis is the most frequent CNS disease, and it may have an acute or subacute clinical presentation with headache, fever, neck pain, nuchal rigidity, altered mental status, lethargy, coma, cranial nerve palsies, and memory loss. An isolated CNS parenchymal lesion is observed less frequently. However, focal parenchymal mass lesions may be observed in neuroimaging studies of 10–25% of patients with cryptococcal meningitis. Findings consistent with meningeal enhancement, hydrocephalus, and cerebral edema may occur in 15%, 10%, and 3%, respectively [37]. CNS parenchymal lesion is reported to be a more common presentation of *C. gattii* compared to *C. neoformans* infection.

Skin and soft tissues is the third most common organ involved in cryptococcal disease. Eight percent of patients with cryptococcosis have skin, soft tissue, or osteoarticular involvement [21]. Cutaneous involvement is generally indicative of a widely disseminated disease, and the skin was involved through hematogenous dissemination from a primary pulmonary focus. Rarely, primary cutaneous cryptococcosis may occur as a result of direct inoculation or exposure from the environment, and these skin lesions may serve as foci for hematogenous dissemination. The typical cryptococcal skin lesion is characterized as a papule or maculopapule with central umbilication (that is easily mistaken for molluscum contagiosum). However, cryptococcus may produce almost any type of skin lesion, including nodules, cellulitis, and ulcerations [38]. The diagnosis is confirmed by demonstrating the fungus on skin biopsy, either using histopathology or fungal culture.

Other sites of the body may be involved in cryptococcosis, usually as part of a disseminated disease. Cryptococcal disease affecting the prostate gland, kidney, liver, tendons, bones, and joints has been observed [39]. Kidney and prostatic involvement may be indicated by detection of cryptococcus in urine [40]. Systemic spread from the prostate may occur during urologic manipulation and with a longer duration of antifungal treatment in patients with prostatic involvement since the organ may serve as a sanctuary site. Ocular cryptococcosis may also occur, although it is rare [41]. The two distinct clinical patterns of ocular cryptococcosis are rapid and slow visual loss. Rapid visual loss is due to optic neuritis resulting from the direct invasion of the optic nerve by *C. neoformans*. This illness is rapidly progressive, with a clinical course of as short as 12 h [42]. Slow visual loss occurs later, often during antifungal therapy, secondary to raised intracranial pressure. Endophthalmitis has also been reported in patients with disseminated cryptococcosis [43]. Cryptococcal peritonitis has been reported in patients undergoing peritoneal dialysis and those with underlying liver disease and cirrhosis [27, 44].

Diagnosis of Cryptococcal Infection

Transplant recipients and candidates suspected to have cryptococcal disease should undergo thorough clinical evaluation to confirm the diagnosis and to ascertain the extent of the disease. The evaluation may include blood and urine culture and antigen detection in clinical samples such as blood, respiratory secretions, tissues, and cerebrospinal fluid (CSF). Lumbar puncture to detect cryptococcal meningitis should be performed in all patients with documented cryptococcosis. The opening pressure should be obtained (to evaluate for hydrocephalus) and the CSF should be evaluated for pleocytosis (white cell count), protein, glucose, and microbiology including cryptococcal antigen [10]. Imaging studies such as brain CT or MRI may be performed to determine the presence of mass lesions or hydrocephalus [10]. MRI is more sensitive that CT scan in detecting cerebral cryptococcomas, which may be present in up to 33% of patients with CNS disease [10]. Biopsy of affected tissues such as the prostate or kidney should be performed if feasible when cryptococcus infection is suspected in these sites [10].

Several methods are available for the diagnosis of cryptococcal infection. Isolation of the fungi for culture of clinical specimens is considered the gold standard for diagnosis of cryptococcal infection. *Cryptococcus* species grows easily, usually within 3–7 days on most bacterial and fungal culture media. Colonies of *C. neoformans* usually appear within 48–72 h after plating a specimen on routine laboratory agar media. Macroscopically, they appear as white- to cream-colored opaque colonies which usually become mucoid in appearance with prolonged incubation.

Detection of cryptococcal antigen in the serum and CSF, using either latex agglutination or enzyme immunoassay method, is an accurate and rapidly available method for the detection of cryptococcal infection. The sensitivity and specificity with either method is more than 90% [45]. In a review of SOT recipients, the serum cryptococcal antigen had a sensitivity of 88–98% in patients with cryptococcosis, while the CSF cryptococcal antigen has a sensitivity of 98–100% in patients with cryptococcal meningitis [46]. The mean titers have ranged from 1:2 to 1:512 [46]. The sensitivity of cryptococcal antigen testing over culture (33–39%) has been demonstrated [46], and several studies reporting cases of cryptococcal meningitis in which CSF cryptococcal antigen is detected before CSF culture is positive [20, 21, 47]. Cryptococcal antigen is also more sensitive compared to India Ink preparation (50–80%) in the diagnosis of cryptococcal meningitis [46]. Cryptococcal antigen testing relies on the detection of capsular polysaccharide antigens from *Cryptococcus* species, which allows for its detection in lower fungal burden states and earlier in the course of the infection. Serum cryptococcal antigen may be negative in cases of isolated pulmonary cryptococcosis [47]. However, a positive serum cryptococcal antigen should trigger evaluation for extrapulmonary disease, including the CNS. In patients at high risk for dissemination, such as transplant recipients, a lumbar puncture should be performed even if neurologic symptoms are absent. Early spread to the CNS may be asymptomatic and be manifested only by a positive CSF fungal culture or cryptococcal antigen. Indeed, CSF cryptococcal antigen may be useful in detecting early CNS cryptococcal disease, before there is sufficient fungal burden to result in a positive fungal culture.

Measurement of cryptococcal antigen titers carries prognostic information. A high initial cryptococcal titer indicates high fungal burden, disseminated disease, poor host immunity, and higher likelihood of treatment failure [20, 21, 47]. In one review, the serum cryptococcal antigen titer was higher in patients with symptomatic pulmonary cryptococcosis compared to those with asymptomatic or incidentally detected cases (1:128 versus 1:32) [35]. Notably, the titers are usually lower in patients with *C. gattii* compared to *C. neoformans* infections [2]. Cryptococcal antigen titers are also generally useful in following antifungal treatment responses. However, this may not be as reliable as fungal culture in differentiating clinical disease progression due to treatment failure versus immune reconstitution inflammatory syndrome (IRIS) [10, 48]. A rising cryptococcal antigen titer is generally indicative of clinical progression, while it is stable or decreasing antigen levels in patients with IRIS, although this is not generally the case (see below). Other fungal antigen tests such as serum galactomannan or the (1- > 3) ß-D-glucan tests are not reliable for the detection of cryptococcus and should not be used for diagnosis of and monitoring cryptococcosis.

Several stains are used to identify cryptococcus in biopsy samples and other clinical specimens. Traditionally, India ink preparation was used as a readily available tool for the rapid diagnosis of cryptococcal infection. *Cryptococcus* species are yeasts, measuring 5–10 μm in diameter, that contain a polysaccharide capsule that appears as clear halo or space in specimens treated with India ink stain. The sensitivity of India ink preparation is only in the 50% in patients with cryptococcal meningitis in the non-AIDS population [49]. Alcian blue stains are also used and may provide better specificity for cryptococcus infection. Mucicarmine staining will stain the cryptococcal capsule to rose or burgundy color [49]. Gram stain usually shows poorly stained Gram-positive yeast, while Gomori methenamine silver (GMS) fungal stain may demonstrate the narrow-based budding oval yeast of cryptococcus in tissue specimens [49].

Treatment of Cryptococcal Disease in Transplant Recipients

Treatment of cryptococcal disease in transplant recipients entails the use of antifungal drugs and reduction in pharmacologic immunosuppression. The antifungal drugs that are recommended for the treatment of cryptococcal disease in transplant recipients are amphotericin B products, preferably lipid formulations, flucytosine, and fluconazole (Table 35.2) [10, 50]. Voriconazole, itraconazole, and posaconazole are also active against cryptococcus, but they offer no additional benefit compared to fluconazole and have higher potential for drug-drug interactions, especially drugs used for prevention of graft rejection and prevention and treatment of GVDH [5, 43]. The basis of the treatment recommendations in transplant recipients is extrapolated from retrospective studies in SOT recipients and from clinical trials performed in patients with AIDS [10, 50]. There are no randomized, prospective clinical treatment trials in transplant recipients with cryptococcosis.

Antifungal susceptibility testing is not generally recommended in cryptococcosis, unless there is persistent infection and relapsed infection or the infection is due to *C. gattii*, which may sometimes be associated with high minimum

Table 35.2 Treatment of cryptococcosis in transplant recipients

Therapy	Drug and dose	Duration
Asymptomatic pulmonary disease	Fluconazole, 400 mg per day	6–12 months
Mild to moderate isolated pulmonary disease	Fluconazole, 400 mg per day	6–12 months
All other cases, including CNS disease, severe pulmonary disease, and disseminated disease		
Induction therapy		
(a) Preferred therapy	Liposomal amphotericin B, 3–4 mg/kg per day; or amphotericin B lipid complex, 5 mg/kg per day, plus flucytosine, 100 mg/kg per day	Minimum of 2 weeks
(b) Alternative therapy	Liposomal amphotericin B, 3–4 mg/kg per day, or amphotericin B lipid complex, 5 mg/kg per day	Minimum of 4–6 weeks
Consolidation therapy	Fluconazole, 400–800 mg per day	8 weeks
Maintenance therapy	Fluconazole, 200–400 mg per day	6–12 months

inhibitory concentration to fluconazole [51–53]. In vitro *resistance* to amphotericin B and fluconazole among cryptococcal isolates is very uncommon [53].

With the exception of mild-to-moderate pulmonary cryptococcosis, all other cryptococcal diseases in transplant recipients should be treated using induction therapy with fungicidal liposomal amphotericin B (3–4 mg/kg per day) or amphotericin B lipid complex (5 mg/kg per day) and flucytosine (100 mg/kg per day) for a total of 14 days (Table 35.2) [10, 50]. This combination therapy should be used to treat patients with CNS disease, disseminated disease, or severe respiratory disease. Lipid formulations of amphotericin B are preferred over amphotericin B deoxycholate, as it confers survival benefit and is less nephrotoxic, especially in transplant patients who are already receiving several nephrotoxic medications [54]. Mortality at 90 days is lower in SOT patients with cryptococcosis treated with lipid formulation compared to the deoxycholate formulation of amphotericin B [54]. Flucytosine is an essential component of induction therapy. The lack of flucytosine use and its use for <14 days have been associated with treatment failure at 2 weeks and 90 days, respectively [55, 56].

The 2-week induction phase with amphotericin B plus flucytosine should be followed by a consolidation phase using oral fluconazole (400–800 mg per day) for 8 weeks and finally maintenance therapy phase using oral fluconazole (200–400 mg per day) for at least 6–12 months [10, 50]. The duration of antifungal treatment may be prolonged as guided by serial serum cryptococcal antigen monitoring [50]. Transplant clinicians generally continue treatment for a duration that exceeds the time of positive cryptococcal antigen in the blood.

Patients with isolated (localized) mild-to-moderate pulmonary disease have lower fungal burden and may be treated upfront with fluconazole (400 mg per day) for 6–12 months. The duration of treatment may be prolonged until the serum cryptococcal antigen is negative [10]. Prior to embarking on this treatment regimen, disseminated cryptococcal disease should be excluded with a lumbar puncture and culture of the blood and urine [10].

Monitoring of drug levels during antifungal therapy may be needed to avoid drug-associated toxicities. Flucytosine is a common cause of bone marrow suppression, especially in the setting of renal impairment. Therefore, routine monitoring of flucytosine levels is recommended, with the goal of 2-h postdose level being 30–80 μg/mL. The potential for drug-drug interaction should be considered when fluconazole is used, since azoles are potent inhibitors of CYP 3A4, which decreases hepatic metabolism of calcineurin inhibitors, thereby resulting in supratherapeutic levels of tacrolimus and cyclosporine. Voriconazole, itraconazole, and posaconazole have greater potential for drug-drug interactions compared to fluconazole and do not offer additional benefit compared to fluconazole [5].

Cryptococcal meningitis causes significant inflammation with the development of a film that prevents the absorption of the CSF, and this may result in the elevation of the intracranial pressure. Patients with cryptococcal meningitis should therefore have routine measurement of the intracranial pressure during lumbar puncture. Patients with initial opening pressure >25 mmHg should have therapeutic lumbar punctures to reduce the intracranial pressure to <20 mmHg [10]. If the intracranial pressure remains high, either a lumbo-peritoneal or an external ventricular drain can be placed as a bridge to eventual ventriculoperitoneal shunt placement. Uncontrolled and prolonged raised intracranial pressure from cryptococcal meningitis may lead to hydrocephalus, blindness, and death [57].

Cautious reduction in immunosuppression is another component of therapy that is essential in the successful management of cryptococcal disease. However, there should be gradual reduction of net immunosuppression during antifungal therapy, since drastic reduction has been associated with organ rejection for SOT recipients, worsening of graft-versus-host disease in HSCT recipients, and development of IRIS [10].

Cryptococcal Immune Reconstitution Inflammatory Syndrome

Cryptococcal IRIS may occur in some patients treated for cryptococcal disease, especially if there is an abrupt restoration of host immunity. IRIS is characterized clinically by exacerbation of the signs and symptoms, and it has been mistaken as treatment failure or clinical relapse [37]. The incidence of cryptococcus-associated IRIS in SOT recipients is estimated to be 5–10% [58]. The pathogenesis of cryptococcus-associated IRIS represents an intricate relationship between the fungus, immunosuppressive agent, and the type of host inflammatory immune response. Experimental studies have shown that *C. neoformans* has immunomodulatory characteristics and preferentially inhibits Th1 while inducing Th2 responses. Immunosuppressive agents used to maintain graft function such as tacrolimus, cyclosporine, and corticosteroids suppress the production of cytokines stimulated by Th1 cells to a varying degree. Withdrawal of these agents, especially tacrolimus, may lead to an increase in proinflammatory cytokines and subsequent development of IRIS.

Cryptococcus-associated IRIS often presents clinically between 4 and 6 weeks upon initiation of antifungal therapy [58]. Risk factors include potent baseline immunosuppression and disseminated cryptococcal disease. In one study, the risk of IRIS was higher in patients receiving triple immunosuppressive regimen [59]. Clinical manifestation is highly variable, and this may include exacerbation of hydrocephalus, aseptic meningitis, cerebral mass lesions, pulmonary nodules, cellulitis, and lymphadenitis [37]. The clinical manifestation may be so severe that it may cause significant morbidity. There are currently no laboratory markers or clinical criteria that can reliably distinguish IRIS from worsening cryptococcosis. However, IRIS may be considered if there is (1) new or worsening appearance of clinical manifestations, (2) symptoms occurred during receipt of appropriate antifungal therapy and could not be explained by a newly acquired infection, and (3) negative results of cultures for *C. neoformans* during the diagnostic workup for the inflammatory process [48]. An increase in serum cryptococcal antigen titer and/or visualization of cryptococcus in histopathology specimens are not strictly indicative of treatment failure, as both have been described in SOT recipients with crypto-associated IRIS [58]. Maintaining a high index of clinical suspicion for IRIS is crucial to avoid unnecessary adjustments and changes in antifungal therapy. Ultimately, the key feature that distinguishes cryptococcal IRIS from treatment failure is the persistently negative fungal cultures with IRIS.

The management of cryptococcal-associated IRIS in transplant recipients is similar to that in nontransplant patient population and is symptom centric. If symptoms are minor, they usually resolve spontaneously within a few weeks. Corticosteroids (e.g., prednisone 0.5–1 mg/kg) may be considered for more severe manifestations of pulmonary and other sites, especially if the CNS involved. If used, the corticosteroids are generally tapered over 6–8 weeks [10].

Prognosis of Cryptococcal Disease in Transplant Recipients

The overall mortality rates in SOT recipients with cryptococcosis is about 14% [21], although other studies have reported as high as 33–42% [20]. In HSCT recipients, the assessment of outcomes is limited due to a small number of reported cases. Long-term outcomes were only reported in four of nine HSCT patients; two were alive and two had died at the end of the follow-up, suggesting a mortality rate of 50% [12].

The mortality rate varies according to extent of organ involvement; it may be as high as 49% in patients with CNS involvement, while it can be as low as 2.8% in isolated pulmonary cryptococcal disease [20]. Risk factors for higher mortality are altered mental status, absence of headache, and liver and renal failure [47]. For CNS disease, patients with brain parenchymal lesions had a mortality rate of 50%, while those with leptomeningeal lesions had a mortality rate of 12.5% [37, 60]. Serum and CSF cryptococcal antigen titers have not been found to correlate with outcomes. Patients on calcineurin inhibitors appear to be at lower risk of death [61].

Conclusions

Cryptococcosis is the third most common invasive fungal infection in SOT recipients, whereas seldom seen in HSCT recipients. Most infections in transplant recipients are due to *C. neoformans*. Pulmonary disease is the most common clinical presentation, although extrapulmonary disease such as CNS infection is a well-recognized extrapulmonary complication of cryptococcosis. Diagnosis can be confirmed with the use of culture and antigen testing. Depending on disease severity and extent of infection, treatment consists of lipid formulations of amphotericin B, flucytosine, and fluconazole. Reduction in immunosuppression should also be considered as an important component of infection management. This, however, should be approached with some caution due to the concern for the potential risk of cryptococcus-associated IRIS.

References

1. Kwon-Chung KJ, Bennett JE. Epidemiologic differences between the two varieties of Cryptococcus neoformans. Am J Epidemiol. 1984;120(1):123–30.
2. Harris JR, Lockhart SR, Debess E, et al. Cryptococcus gattii in the United States: clinical aspects of infection with an emerging pathogen. Clin Infect Dis. 2011;53(12):1188–95.
3. Banerjee P, Haider M, Trehan V, et al. Cryptococcus laurentii fungemia. Indian J Med Microbiol. 2013;31(1):75–7.
4. Shankar EM, Kumarasamy N, Bella D, et al. Pneumonia and pleural effusion due to Cryptococcus laurentii in a clinically proven case of AIDS. Can Respir J. 2006;13(5):275–8.

5. Cleveland KO, Gelfand MS, Rao V. Posaconazole as successful treatment for fungemia due to Cryptococcus albidus in a liver transplant recipient. QJM. 2013;106(4):361–2.
6. Emmons CW. Saprophytic sources of Cryptococcus neoformans associated with the pigeon (Columba livia). Am J Hyg. 1955;62(3):227–32.
7. Lazera MS, Pires FD, Camillo-Coura L, et al. Natural habitat of Cryptococcus neoformans var. neoformans in decaying wood forming hollows in living trees. J Med Vet Mycol. 1996;34(2):127–31.
8. Ellis DH, Pfeiffer TJ. Natural habitat of Cryptococcus neoformans var. gattii. J Clin Microbiol. 1990;28(7):1642–4.
9. Kidd SE, Hagen F, Tscharke RL, et al. A rare genotype of Cryptococcus gattii caused the cryptococcosis outbreak on Vancouver Island (British Columbia, Canada). Proc Natl Acad Sci U S A. 2004;101(49):17258–63.
10. Baddley JW, Forrest GN. Cryptococcosis in solid organ transplantation. Am J Transplant. 2013;13(Suppl 4):242–9.
11. Brizendine KD, Baddley JW, Pappas PG. Predictors of mortality and differences in clinical features among patients with Cryptococcosis according to immune status. PLoS One. 2013;8(3):e60431.
12. Sun HY, Wagener MM, Singh N. Cryptococcosis in solid-organ, hematopoietic stem cell, and tissue transplant recipients: evidence-based evolving trends. Clin Infect Dis. 2009;48(11):1566–76.
13. Kontoyiannis DP, Marr KA, Park BJ, et al. Prospective surveillance for invasive fungal infections in hematopoietic stem cell transplant recipients, 2001-2006: overview of the Transplant-Associated Infection Surveillance Network (TRANSNET) Database. Clin Infect Dis. 2010;50(8):1091–100.
14. Pappas PG, Alexander BD, Andes DR, et al. Invasive fungal infections among organ transplant recipients: results of the Transplant-Associated Infection Surveillance Network (TRANSNET). Clin Infect Dis. 2010;50(8):1101–11.
15. Arthurs SK, Eid AJ, Deziel PJ, et al. The impact of invasive fungal diseases on survival after lung transplantation. Clin Transpl. 2010;24(3):341–8.
16. Garcia-Hermoso D, Janbon G, Dromer F. Epidemiological evidence for dormant Cryptococcus neoformans infection. J Clin Microbiol. 1999;37(10):3204–9.
17. Saha DC, Goldman DL, Shao X, et al. Serologic evidence for reactivation of cryptococcosis in solid-organ transplant recipients. Clin Vaccine Immunol. 2007;14(12):1550–4.
18. Kapoor A, Flechner SM, O'Malley K, Paolone D, File TM Jr, Cutrona AF. Cryptococcal meningitis in renal transplant patients associated with environmental exposure. Transpl Infect Dis. 1999;1(3):213–7.
19. Neuville S, Dromer F, Morin O, Dupont B, Ronin O, Lortholary O. Primary cutaneous cryptococcosis: a distinct clinical entity. Clin Infect Dis. 2003;36(3):337–47.
20. Husain S, Wagener MM, Singh N. Cryptococcus neoformans infection in organ transplant recipients: variables influencing clinical characteristics and outcome. Emerg Infect Dis. 2001;7(3):375–81.
21. Singh N, Alexander BD, Lortholary O, et al. Cryptococcus neoformans in organ transplant recipients: impact of calcineurin-inhibitor agents on mortality. J Infect Dis. 2007;195(5):756–64.
22. Baddley JW, Schain DC, Gupte AA, et al. Transmission of Cryptococcus neoformans by Organ Transplantation. Clin Infect Dis. 2011;52(4):e94–8.
23. Ooi BS, Chen BT, Lim CH, Khoo OT, Chan DT. Survival of a patient transplanted with a kidney infected with Cryptococcus neoformans. Transplantation. 1971;11(4):428–9.
24. Kanj SS, Welty-Wolf K, Madden J, et al. Fungal infections in lung and heart-lung transplant recipients. Report of 9 cases and review of the literature. Medicine (Baltimore). 1996;75(3):142–56.
25. Singh N. How I treat cryptococcosis in organ transplant recipients. Transplantation. 2012;93(1):17–21.
26. Chuang YM, Ho YC, Chang HT, Yu CJ, Yang PC, Hsueh PR. Disseminated cryptococcosis in HIV-uninfected patients. Eur J Clin Microbiol Infect Dis. 2008;27(4):307–10.
27. Singh N, Husain S, De Vera M, Gayowski T, Cacciarelli TV. Cryptococcus neoformans infection in patients with cirrhosis, including liver transplant candidates. Medicine (Baltimore). 2004;83(3):188–92.
28. Silveira FP, Husain S, Kwak EJ, et al. Cryptococcosis in liver and kidney transplant recipients receiving anti-thymocyte globulin or alemtuzumab. Transpl Infect Dis. 2007;9(1):22–7.
29. Peleg AY, Husain S, Kwak EJ, et al. Opportunistic infections in 547 organ transplant recipients receiving alemtuzumab, a humanized monoclonal CD-52 antibody. Clin Infect Dis. 2007;44(2):204–12.
30. Baddley JW, Perfect JR, Oster RA, et al. Pulmonary cryptococcosis in patients without HIV infection: factors associated with disseminated disease. Eur J Clin Microbiol Infect Dis. 2008;27(10):937–43.
31. Pappas PG, Perfect JR, Cloud GA, et al. Cryptococcosis in human immunodeficiency virus-negative patients in the era of effective azole therapy. Clin Infect Dis. 2001;33(5):690–9.
32. Singh N, Gayowski T, Wagener MM, Marino IR. Clinical spectrum of invasive cryptococcosis in liver transplant recipients receiving tacrolimus. Clin Transpl. 1997;11(1):66–70.
33. Mueller NJ, Fishman JA. Asymptomatic pulmonary cryptococcosis in solid organ transplantation: report of four cases and review of the literature. Transpl Infect Dis. 2003;5(3):140–3.
34. Paterson DL, Singh N, Gayowski T, Marino IR. Pulmonary nodules in liver transplant recipients. Medicine (Baltimore). 1998;77(1):50–8.
35. Singh N, Alexander BD, Lortholary O, et al. Pulmonary cryptococcosis in solid organ transplant recipients: clinical relevance of serum cryptococcal antigen. Clin Infect Dis. 2008;46(2):e12–8.
36. Jabbour N, Reyes J, Kusne S, Martin M, Fung J. Cryptococcal meningitis after liver transplantation. Transplantation. 1996;61(1):146–9.
37. Singh N, Lortholary O, Dromer F, et al. Central nervous system cryptococcosis in solid organ transplant recipients: clinical relevance of abnormal neuroimaging findings. Transplantation. 2008;86(5):647–51.
38. Baer S, Baddley JW, Gnann JW, Pappas PG. Cryptococcal disease presenting as necrotizing cellulitis in transplant recipients. Transpl Infect Dis. 2009;11(4):353–8.
39. Bruno KM, Farhoomand L, Libman BS, Pappas CN, Landry FJ. Cryptococcal arthritis, tendinitis, tenosynovitis, and carpal tunnel syndrome: report of a case and review of the literature. Arthritis Rheum. 2002;47(1):104–8.
40. Siddiqui TJ, Zamani T, Parada JP. Primary cryptococcal prostatitis and correlation with serum prostate specific antigen in a renal transplant recipient. J Infect. 2005;51(3):e153–7.
41. Okun E, Butler WT. Ophthalmologic complications of cryptococcal meningitis. Arch Ophthalmol. 1964;71:52–7.
42. Rex JH, Larsen RA, Dismukes WE, Cloud GA, Bennett JE. Catastrophic visual loss due to Cryptococcus neoformans meningitis. Medicine (Baltimore). 1993;72(4):207–24.
43. Denning DW, Armstrong RW, Fishman M, Stevens DA. Endophthalmitis in a patient with disseminated cryptococcosis and AIDS who was treated with itraconazole. Rev Infect Dis. 1991;13(6):1126–30.
44. Mocan H, Murphy AV, Beattie TJ, McAllister TA. Fungal peritonitis in children on continuous ambulatory peritoneal dialysis. Scott Med J. 1989;34(4):494–6.
45. Kauffman CA, Bergman AG, Severance PJ, McClatchey KD. Detection of cryptococcal antigen. Comparison of two latex agglutination tests. Am J Clin Pathol. 1981;75(1):106–9.
46. Singh N, Dromer F, Perfect JR, Lortholary O. Cryptococcosis in solid organ transplant recipients: current state of the science. Clin Infect Dis. 2008;47(10):1321–7.

47. Wu G, Vilchez RA, Eidelman B, Fung J, Kormos R, Kusne S. Cryptococcal meningitis: an analysis among 5,521 consecutive organ transplant recipients. Transpl Infect Dis. 2002;4(4):183–8.
48. Singh N, Forrest G. Cryptococcosis in solid organ transplant recipients. Am J Transplant. 2009;9 Suppl 4:S192–8.
49. Gazzoni AF, Severo CB, Salles EF, Severo LC. Histopathology, serology and cultures in the diagnosis of cryptococcosis. Rev Inst Med Trop Sao Paulo. 2009;51(5):255–9.
50. Perfect JR, Dismukes WE, Dromer F, et al. Clinical practice guidelines for the management of cryptococcal disease: 2010 update by the infectious diseases society of america. Clin Infect Dis. 2010;50(3):291–322.
51. Thompson GR 3rd, Wiederhold NP, Fothergill AW, Vallor AC, Wickes BL, Patterson TF. Antifungal susceptibilities among different serotypes of Cryptococcus gattii and Cryptococcus neoformans. Antimicrob Agents Chemother. 2009;53(1):309–11.
52. Thompson GR 3rd, Fothergill AW, Wiederhold NP, Vallor AC, Wickes BL, Patterson TF. Evaluation of Etest method for determining isavuconazole MICs against Cryptococcus gattii and Cryptococcus neoformans. Antimicrob Agents Chemother. 2008;52(8):2959–61.
53. Brandt ME, Pfaller MA, Hajjeh RA, et al. Trends in antifungal drug susceptibility of Cryptococcus neoformans isolates in the United States: 1992 to 1994 and 1996 to 1998. Antimicrob Agents Chemother. 2001;45(11):3065–9.
54. Sun HY, Alexander BD, Lortholary O, et al. Lipid formulations of amphotericin B significantly improve outcome in solid organ transplant recipients with central nervous system cryptococcosis. Clin Infect Dis. 2009;49(11):1721–8.
55. Dromer F, Mathoulin-Pelissier S, Launay O, Lortholary O. Determinants of disease presentation and outcome during cryptococcosis: the CryptoA/D study. PLoS Med. 2007;4(2):e21.
56. Dromer F, Bernede-Bauduin C, Guillemot D, Lortgercllholary O. Major role for amphotericin B-flucytosine combination in severe cryptococcosis. PLoS One. 2008;3(8):e2870.
57. Graybill JR, Sobel J, Saag M, et al. Diagnosis and management of increased intracranial pressure in patients with AIDS and cryptococcal meningitis. The NIAID Mycoses Study Group and AIDS Cooperative Treatment Groups. Clin Infect Dis. 2000;30(1):47–54.
58. Singh N, Lortholary O, Alexander BD, et al. An immune reconstitution syndrome-like illness associated with Cryptococcus neoformans infection in organ transplant recipients. Clin Infect Dis. 2005;40(12):1756–61.
59. Singh N, Lortholary O, Alexander BD, et al. Allograft loss in renal transplant recipients with cryptococcus neoformans associated immune reconstitution syndrome. Transplantation. 2005;80(8):1131–3.
60. Charlier C, Dromer F, Leveque C, et al. Cryptococcal neuroradiological lesions correlate with severity during cryptococcal meningoencephalitis in HIV-positive patients in the HAART era. PLoS One. 2008;3(4):e1950.
61. Kontoyiannis DP, Lewis RE, Alexander BD, et al. Calcineurin inhibitor agents interact synergistically with antifungal agents in vitro against Cryptococcus neoformans isolates: correlation with outcome in solid organ transplant recipients with cryptococcosis. Antimicrob Agents Chemother. 2008;52(2):735–8.

Histoplasmosis, Coccidioidomycosis, and Diseases Due to Other Endemic Fungi in Transplant Recipients

36

Pascalis Vergidis, Chadi A. Hage, and L. Joseph Wheat

Introduction

Endemic mycoses are a diverse group of fungal infections that can cause disease in both healthy and immunocompromised individuals. Histoplasmosis, coccidioidomycosis, and blastomycosis are the three major endemic mycoses encountered in North America. Paracoccidioidomycosis is endemic in South America and penicilliosis in Southeast Asia. Sporotrichosis, typically a lymphocutaneous infection, can disseminate in the immunocompromised host. Endemic fungi occur naturally in the environment in specific geographic areas and are thermally dimorphic; they exist as molds at ambient temperature and as yeasts or spherules in the case of coccidioidomycosis, at body temperature.

Among transplant recipients, endemic mycoses are less commonly encountered compared to infection caused by opportunistic fungi. Based on data from the Transplant-Associated Infection Surveillance Network (TRANSNET), 1208 invasive fungal infections occurred among 1063 solid organ transplant (SOT) recipients in 15 US centers for the period 2001–2006 [1]. Of those, 18.8% were caused by *Aspergillus* spp. and 5.3% by endemic fungi. Among hematopoietic stem cell transplant (HSCT) recipients, endemic mycoses are less common. Based on the TRANSNET database, 983 invasive fungal infections occurred among 875 HSCT recipients in 22 centers [2]. Of those, 43% were caused by *Aspergillus* spp. and only 0.6% by endemic fungi. Because each endemic fungal infection is unusual outside of a specific geographic area, a careful travel and residence history should be obtained, preferably at the time of pretransplant evaluation. Otherwise, the diagnosis may be missed and appropriate treatment may be delayed or not given.

P. Vergidis
University Hospital of South Manchester, University of Manchester, Department of Medicine, Manchester, UK
e-mail: paschalis.vergidis@uhsm.nhs.uk

C. A. Hage
Indiana University School of Medicine, Pulmonary-Critical Care, Thoracic Transplantation Program, Methodist Professional Center-2, Indianapolis, IN, USA
e-mail: chage@iu.edu

L. J. Wheat (✉)
MiraVista Diagnostics, Indianapolis, IN, USA
e-mail: jwheat@miravistalabs.com

Histoplasmosis

Histoplasma capsulatum is the causative agent of histoplasmosis. There are two varieties causing human disease: var. *capsulatum* and var. *duboisii*. These vary in their geographic distribution. In the mold phase, septate hyphae produce microconidia and macroconidia. Tuberculated macroconidia with their thick wall and radial, fingerlike projections are used for identification of the organism in culture. Budding yeast cells of *Histoplasma* are small (2–4 μm), narrow, and ovoid in shape.

Epidemiology

Soil contaminated with bird droppings or excrements of bats is the common natural habitat. The disease is endemic in the Mississippi and Ohio River valleys, Central America, the Caribbean, several countries in South America, and parts of Southeast Asia and Africa. *H. duboisii* is the cause of African histoplasmosis. Histoplasmosis is the most common endemic mycosis among transplant recipients in North America. This may be explained by the large geographic area that harbors the mold. However, even in endemic areas, the incidence is low and has been estimated to be 1 case per 1000 transplant-person-years [3]. In 586 patients undergoing solid organ or allogeneic bone marrow transplantation in Indianapolis, a hyperendemic area, none of them developed histoplasmosis after a mean follow-up period exceeding 16 months [4]. On the other hand, during two large outbreaks that occurred in Indianapolis between 1978 and 1981, rates of 2.1% were reported among allograft recipients [5].

A. Safdar (ed.), *Principles and Practice of Transplant Infectious Diseases*, https://doi.org/10.1007/978-1-4939-9034-4_36

Pathogenesis

Cell-mediated immunity provides the primary host defense against *H. capsulatum*, explaining the severity of disease in transplant recipients who receive potent T-cell immunosuppressants. Following transplantation, histoplasmosis is predominantly acquired from the environment via inhalation of molds. As the organism remains in tissue for prolonged periods following infection, it has been proposed that disease can occur following endogenous reactivation. However, there is no clear evidence supporting this mechanism of disease acquisition. In a study of autopsy specimens, *Histoplasma* could not be grown from calcified pulmonary granulomas in which yeast cells were seen and granulomas failed to cause histoplasmosis when injected into mice [6]. Rather than reactivation, conversion of latent infection-acquired pretransplant into symptomatic disease is a plausible mechanism of posttransplant histoplasmosis. Far less commonly, infection may be derived from the allograft if the disease went unrecognized in the donor [7].

Clinical Manifestations

Respiratory disease presents with fever, chills, cough, and dyspnea, which can progress to severe hypoxemia. Imaging usually reveals miliary or diffuse reticulonodular infiltrates. Mediastinal and hilar adenopathy is rarely seen in immunosuppressed patients. Disseminated disease is more likely to develop in the immunocompromised host. Besides fever and chills, manifestations include malaise, anorexia, and weight loss. Hepatomegaly and splenomegaly are common physical findings. Gastrointestinal manifestations include painful, nonhealing mucosal ulcers, abdominal pain, and diarrhea. Cutaneous manifestations include erythematous macules, necrotic or hyperkeratotic papules, and nodules. Central nervous system (CNS) involvement occurs in 5–10%, presenting as chronic meningitis or focal brain lesions. Patients with severe infection may present with shock, respiratory failure, or disseminated intravascular coagulation. Laboratory abnormalities include pancytopenia due to bone marrow involvement and elevated liver enzymes, particularly alkaline phosphatase. Symptom onset may range from months to years after transplantation [3, 8]. If the donor has unrecognized active histoplasmosis at the time of transplantation, disease in the recipient typically manifests within months after transplantation [7].

Among transplant recipients an immune reconstitution inflammatory syndrome (IRIS) has been described, mainly in association with cryptococcal infection [9]. Patients present with new or worsening clinical or radiographic manifestations or an inflammatory mass while receiving appropriate antifungal therapy [10]. Culture results are negative and biomarker levels are stable or decreasing. For histoplasmosis, the syndrome has been described among patients with AIDS initiating antiretroviral treatment and patients discontinuing tumor necrosis factor-α blocker therapy. Among transplant recipients, IRIS associated with histoplasmosis could occur after reduction in potent immunosuppressive therapy.

Diagnosis

Diagnosis is established by growing the organism from respiratory secretions, blood, other body fluids, or biopsy tissue. Typically culture methods require up to 4 weeks for growth and hence do not provide a rapid diagnosis. The yield from blood cultures is enhanced by using the lysis-centrifugation system (Isolator tube system) [11]. Automated blood culture systems have a lower yield and take a longer time to show growth. Cutaneous, oral, or gastrointestinal lesions may also be sources for isolation of the fungus. Detection of yeast cells on tissue biopsy allows for rapid identification. Periodic acid-Schiff stain or methenamine silver stain should be used in biopsy specimens. Appropriate tissues include lung, mucocutaneous lesions, liver, and bone marrow. For direct detection from respiratory specimens, calcofluor white staining can be used. This binds with chitin and allows for detection of fungi using fluorescent microscopy. Potassium hydroxide is added to hasten clearing of viscous specimens. Yeast cells may also be detected using Wright's stain in peripheral blood smears within polymorphonuclear cells and/or monocytes.

The *Histoplasma* enzyme-linked immunoassay (EIA) can detect the cell wall polysaccharide antigen in serum, urine, bronchoalveolar lavage (BAL) fluid, or cerebrospinal fluid (CSF), and has become a useful diagnostic tool, especially in immunosuppressed patients who may not be able to mount an immunologic response. Results are available within 1–2 days after collection of the specimen allowing for rapid diagnosis. To increase the yield of the assay, both serum and urine should be tested in suspected cases. Repeated testing is recommended in patients with suspected disease progression, if initial results are negative. In a multicenter study, antigenuria was present in 91.8% of 158 patients with disseminated disease and 96.3% of patients who had undergone solid organ transplantation [12]. Urine antigen was detected more often and at higher levels in immunosuppressed patients and those with severe disease.

Cross-reactivity in the *Histoplasma* antigen assay can occur in infections due to other endemic fungi, such as *Paracoccidioides brasiliensis*, *Penicillium marneffei*, *Blastomyces dermatitidis* [13], and *Coccidioides immitis* [14]. Of note, *Histoplasma* and *Blastomyces* antigens are immunologically identical. In patients with disseminated histoplasmosis, false-positive reactions with the *Aspergillus* galactomannan assay have been reported [15]. There have been no reports of false-positive *Histoplasma* antigen in the serum of patients with invasive aspergillosis, but 8.3% of BAL fluid specimens positive for *Aspergillus* galactomannan were positive for low levels of *Histoplasma* antigen (below the limit of quantification) [16]. Patients with histoplasmosis may have a positive beta-D-glucan assay [17]. Hence, *Histoplasma* antigen should be determined in patients with positive results for *Aspergillus* galactomannan or beta-D-glucan assays if they have a relevant epidemiologic history.

Antibody detection by means of immunodiffusion (ID) or complement fixation (CF) is a useful diagnostic tool. In the ID test, results are reported as M or H precipitin bands. Most patients will develop an M band. The H band is seen in less than 20% of patients, mainly in those with disseminated infection, chronic cavitary pulmonary histoplasmosis, or more severe acute pulmonary histoplasmosis. The M band becomes positive sooner than the H band and persists longer [18]. The CF test uses antigen from the yeast and mycelial forms. Titers of 1:32 or higher are highly suggestive of active infection. With the currently used immunosuppressive regimens, antibody is detected in only 18–33% of infected SOT recipients [3, 12]. Antibodies may persist for several years following recovery and may not indicate active disease. Furthermore, cross-reactions are possible in patients with other endemic mycoses.

Molecular detection methods are not standardized and their role remains limited. Using two nested PCR assays, *H. capsulatum* was detected in 20/29 (68.9%) formalin-fixed, paraffin-embedded tissue specimens [19]. Using a real-time PCR assay, the organism was directly detected in 11/15 (73.3%) clinical specimens, but in only 2 of 6 (33.3%) specimens of BAL fluid [20]. Finally, PCR is less sensitive than *Histoplasma* antigen. PCR was positive in urine in 7.8% [21], BAL fluid in two of nine (22.2%), serum in none of ten, and CSF in none of ten patients with positive *Histoplasma* antigen in the respective body fluids [22].

Treatment

The Infectious Disease Society of America (IDSA) has published guidelines for the treatment of histoplasmosis [23]. Antifungal agents are presented in Table 36.1. Treatment should be initiated with a lipid formulation of amphotericin B.

Table 36.1 Antifungal agents used for the treatment of endemic mycoses

Antifungal agent	Dosage and duration of treatment	Comment
Liposomal AmB	3 mg/kg/d for 1–2 weeks For CNS disease: 5 mg/kg/day for 4–6 weeks Dose adjustment not needed for renal dysfunction	Lipid formulations are preferred in transplant recipients due to the lower risk of nephrotoxicity After a favorable clinical response to AmB, treatment can be transitioned to an oral azole
AmB lipid complex	5 mg/kg/day for 1–2 weeks Dose may be adjusted for acute renal dysfunction	
AmB deoxycholate	0.7–1 mg/kg/day If renal dysfunction, one may need to reduce dose or take the dose every other day to reduce risk of further nephrotoxicity	
Itraconazole capsule or oral solution	Loading dose 200 mg po q8h for the first 3 days, followed by 200 mg po q12h thereafter Higher doses may be used based on serum concentrations Dose unchanged for $Cl_{cr} > 10$ mL/min $Cl_{cr} \leq 10$ mL/min: 50% of normal dose Prophylaxis: 200 mg/day	Preferred agent for histoplasmosis and blastomycosis Administer capsule with food or acidic beverage Target serum concentration (random): 1–10 μg/mL (combined itraconazole and hydroxy-itraconazole) by HPLC or 3–10 μg/mL by bioassay
Fluconazole	200–800 mg po daily Consider loading with 2× maintenance dose Cl_{cr} 50–80 mL/min: Dose unchanged Cl_{cr} 10–49 mL/min: Usual load and then 50% of normal dose $Cl_{cr} < 10$ mL/min: Usual load and then 25% of normal dose	Preferred agent for central nervous system coccidioidomycosis Drug-level monitoring is typically not required
Voriconazole	≥40 kg: 200 mg po q12h (increase to 300 mg q12h if inadequate response) <40 kg: 100 mg po q12h (increase to 150 mg q12h if inadequate response) Dose unchanged for renal dysfunction	Drug-level monitoring recommended, target trough concentration: 1–5 μg/mL
Posaconazole	600–800 mg po daily in 2–4 divided doses Dose unchanged for renal dysfunction Prophylaxis: 200 mg three times daily	Obtain with fatty meal Drug-level monitoring recommended, target trough concentration: 0.5–1.5 μg/mL
Echinocandins	Not indicated for endemic mycoses	Their role in combination with other antifungals against endemic mycoses has not been established

AmB amphotericin B, Cl_{cr} creatinine clearance, *HPLC* high-performance liquid chromatography

In a randomized controlled trial, the liposomal formulation was more effective and less nephrotoxic than amphotericin B deoxycholate in patients with AIDS [24]. In a recent case series of posttransplant histoplasmosis, 94% of patients treated with amphotericin B had a favorable response [3, 8]. Nephrotoxicity remains a problem even in patients treated with the lipid formulations.

After intravenous therapy, transition to an azole antifungal can be made if the patient is afebrile, clinically stable, and able to take oral medications. Itraconazole is the treatment of choice and is available in capsule form and as oral solution. Capsules require food and an acidic gastric pH for solubilization. Absorption can be increased by concurrent ingestion of cola or cranberry juice and is impaired by drugs that interfere with gastric acidification (such as proton pump inhibitors). The oral solution has better bioavailability but is more commonly associated with gastrointestinal upset. Serum concentrations should be measured after achieving steady-state levels (typically after the second week of therapy). Because of the long half-life of itraconazole, serum samples may be obtained independent of the drug administration time. Concentrations are determined by high-performance liquid chromatography (HPLC) or bioassay. Combined drug concentrations (parent drug and hydroxy-itraconazole metabolite) as determined by HPLC of at least 1 mcg/mL and lower than 10 mcg/mL are recommended. Concentrations determined by bioassay vary among different laboratories and are higher than the concentrations determined by HPLC. Concentrations of at least 3 mcg/mL determined by bioassay are recommended. Serum concentration should be measured after starting treatment and repeated if initial values are low, if the dose is modified, and if there is concern about compliance, absorption, or relapse. Of note, itraconazole may increase the levels of cyclosporine, tacrolimus, and sirolimus. Monitoring immunosuppressant concentrations is recommended.

Fluconazole is a second-line agent and should be used only in patients who cannot tolerate itraconazole or are unable to achieve therapeutic concentrations. Voriconazole and posaconazole are active in vitro and have been studied in a few patients intolerant of or who have failed other therapies [25, 26]. Their effectiveness in comparison to itraconazole is unknown. Of note, *Histoplasma* may develop resistance to fluconazole and voriconazole during therapy [27]. Echinocandins are not active and should not be used [28, 29].

Most patients respond quickly to appropriate antifungal therapy. High mortality rates may be related to delays in timely disease recognition. Antigenemia declines during the first month of treatment, followed by a decline in antigenuria [8, 30]. Monitoring antigen concentration is useful in assessing response to treatment and diagnosing relapse. Antifungal treatment is recommended for at least 12 months, but may not be required for life. The safety of discontinuation of life-long suppressive therapy has been demonstrated in patients with AIDS. In patients who have responded to antiretroviral treatment with an increase in their CD_4 count above 150 cells/mm^3, and have no clinical or laboratory signs of histoplasmosis, itraconazole therapy can be safely stopped [31]. The safety of treatment discontinuation has not been established in transplant recipients, but feasibility has been reported [8]. Decisions should be based on appraisal of the net state of immunosuppression in individual patients.

Prevention

Transplant recipients should be informed about activities that carry a high risk of acquiring histoplasmosis. These include excavation, demolition, or remodeling of old buildings, cleaning debris from attics or barns, shoveling bird or bat manure, cutting or burning wood, tearing down structures on which birds and bats may have roosted, and spelunking [32].

Candidates for transplantation who reside or have traveled to areas endemic for histoplasmosis should be carefully evaluated for a history of pneumonia or systemic illness characterized by fever and weight loss. Radiographic abnormalities consistent with histoplasmosis form the basis for further testing. If the clinical and laboratory findings indicate active disease during the 2 years preceding transplantation, itraconazole treatment for a few months before transplantation, if feasible, and 6–12 months following transplantation should be considered. Studies in SOT and HSCT recipients have shown that pretransplant recipient serologies or radiographic findings of prior infection (such as pulmonary nodules or calcified mediastinal lymph nodes) are not associated with posttransplant histoplasmosis [4, 33]. As such, routine pretransplant screening in the absence of history of active disease is not recommended.

Potential living donors should be evaluated before organ donation. If there is prior history of histoplasmosis, undiagnosed pneumonia in the last 2 years, clinical or radiographic findings suggestive of disease, further testing should be performed. The presence of an H band, CF titers of 1:32 or higher, antigenuria, or antigenemia suggest active infection. M bands and CF titers of 1:8 to 1:16 may represent active or inactive infection. In the presence of active disease, the donor should be treated for 3–6 months before organ donation. Antifungal therapy and close monitoring for 1 year following transplantation should be considered in the recipient. For deceased or living donors, organs should be inspected for the presence of granulomas at the time of procurement (Fig. 36.1). Suspicious lesions should be examined by histopathology and fungal culture. Additionally, antigen and antibody testing of the donor should be performed. If cultures or

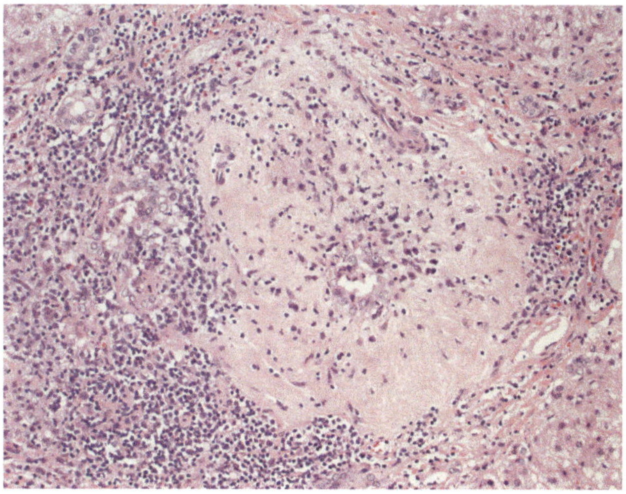

Fig. 36.1 Donor liver biopsy demonstrating scattered non-necrotizing granulomas (hematoxylin and eosin stain, ×200). No yeast cells were detected. The recipient developed disseminated histoplasmosis 1 month posttransplant

antigen tests are positive, the recipient should be treated for 12 months. If cultures and antigen tests are negative but antibodies are detected, a 3–6-month course of itraconazole is recommended.

Coccidioidomycosis

The genus *Coccidioides* contains two species, *C. immitis* and *C. posadasii*. These are morphologically identical but genetically and epidemiologically distinct. Hyphae and arthroconidia are produced at ambient temperature. Hyphae are hyaline, septate, and thin. Arthroconidia are thick-walled and barrel-shaped. At body temperature, large, round, thick-walled spherules (10–80 μm in diameter) filled with endospores (2–5 μm in diameter) are observed.

Epidemiology

Coccidioides is found in soil particularly at warm and dry areas with low rainfall, mild winters, and high summer temperatures. It is endemic in the desert Southwestern United States (mainly southern Arizona and Central California), Northern Mexico, and certain areas in Central and South America. *C. immitis* is the predominant species in California. *C. posadasii* is mainly found in the remainder of the endemic areas. Infection is common as the organism is easily dispersed by desert winds. Skin test positivity rates of 30% were reported in a study conducted between 1977 and 1979 in Tucson [34]. The rate of reported coccidioidomycosis in Arizona has increased from 21 cases per 100,000 population in 1997 to 91 cases per 100,000 in 2006 [35]. Besides mandatory reporting, this increase in incidence may be explained by climatic changes.

From 1970 to 1979, coccidioidomycosis occurred in 6.9% of renal transplant recipients residing in Arizona [36]. After 1999, the overall infection rate among transplant recipients was 1.5% (1.3% in renal, 2.1% in allogeneic bone marrow, and 2.5% in liver transplant recipients), which is similar to the estimated rate among all residents of the endemic area [37]. Among 37 liver transplant recipients who received their allograft at an area of low endemicity and moved to an endemic area, only one (2.7%) developed coccidioidomycosis within at least 1 year of follow-up [38]. Disease has also been reported in transplant recipients who visited endemic areas [39, 40], but the actual risk is unknown.

Pathogenesis

Infection is acquired by inhalation of the spores (arthroconidia) that transform into spherules within the airways. The rupture of mature spherules releases endospores, which can settle in the lung parenchyma or spread via blood circulation. Disease progresses as each endospore forms a new spherule. In the normal host, disease is usually self-limited and results in long-lived immunity, which protects from a second infection. For unclear reasons, individuals of Filipino or African ancestry have a higher risk of developing disseminated disease. Patients with impaired cell-mediated immunity, such as transplant recipients, are also at increased risk for dissemination. Disease may occur after primary infection and reactivation or may be transmitted from the donor.

Clinical Manifestations

In the normal host, disease is usually asymptomatic or manifests as a mild respiratory illness. In the immunocompromised host, pulmonary disease presents with high fever, cough, dyspnea, and hypoxemia. Skin rash may be accompanied by muscle and joint pain. Disease may progress to fulminant respiratory failure. Typical radiographic findings include diffuse reticulonodular infiltrates. Cavitary lesions may be seen. Some patients may present with fatigue, anorexia, and weight loss. The most frequently involved extrapulmonary sites are the skin, osteoarticular structures, and meninges. Skin lesions include papules, pustules, or nodules that commonly ulcerate. Meningeal involvement results in headache, cranial nerve palsies, and signs of increased intracranial pressure. Hydrocephalus may occur, especially in children. The most feared complication is CNS vasculitis leading to cerebral ischemia, infarction, and hemorrhage.

In the transplant recipient, disease can occur at any time but is more common during the first year after transplantation [41]. Donor-derived disease has been reported within the first posttransplant month in patients not receiving antifungals, as the disease was not recognized in the donor [42–44]. Donor-transmitted infection has also been manifested after antifungals were discontinued [45].

Diagnosis

Diagnosis is established by growing the organism from sputum, BAL fluid, blood and other body fluids, or biopsy tissue. *Coccidioides* usually grows on routine laboratory media within 7 days. When coccidioidomycosis is suspected, the clinician should alert the microbiology laboratory since the organism is highly contagious. In respiratory specimens, spherules can be detected using calcofluor white staining. Spherules can be detected in tissue biopsy using hematoxylin and eosin or special stains such as methenamine silver. Notably, spherules do not take up Gram stain.

Anti-coccidioidal antibody titers, although specific, may take several weeks or months to rise after the onset of illness, especially in patients with impaired immunity. Moreover, in immunosuppressed patients with disseminated disease, serologic tests may remain negative. ID methods for both IgM and IgG antibodies are commonly used. Available assays are qualitative and quantitative [46]. A positive qualitative test should be confirmed with CF or quantitative ID. Tube precipitin-type antibodies, considered to be IgM, develop relatively early during infection (within the first 3 weeks of symptoms). Complement-fixing antibodies, considered to be IgG, are typically detected later in the course of the disease. Antibody detection in CSF is useful in diagnosing meningitis. Finally, an EIA for IgM and IgG antibodies is highly sensitive, but less specific than ID [47]. Combining the results of serologic tests can increase the diagnostic yield. Among 62 immunosuppressed patients with coccidioidomycosis, 84% were seropositive using all methods [48].

For moderate to severe disease, detection of urine *Coccidioides* antigen by means of an EIA was found to have a sensitivity of 70.8% [49]. Cross-reactions with other endemic mycoses can occur. The role of molecular methods has not been established. A real-time PCR assay has been validated in clinical specimens [50] and is offered in reference laboratories. The assay demonstrated a sensitivity of 75% and specificity of 99% compared with culture of respiratory specimens [51].

Treatment

The Infectious Diseases Society of America has published treatment guidelines [52]. Clinicians who practice in the Southwestern United States are familiar with this disease. Seeking advice from a specialist with experience in treating coccidioidomycosis may be of benefit. All transplant recipients should receive antifungal treatment (Table 36.1). The choice of intravenous versus oral therapy depends on the degree of respiratory compromise or rate of disease progression. The use of amphotericin B is favored in more severe disease. Lipid formulations are preferred due to the lower risk of nephrotoxicity, even though these agents have not been specifically studied for coccidioidomycosis in clinical trials. After a favorable clinical response, treatment can be transitioned to an oral azole. In a randomized trial of oral itraconazole (200 mg twice daily) versus oral fluconazole (400 mg daily) for the treatment of nonmeningeal progressive coccidioidomycosis, there was a trend toward greater efficacy with itraconazole at 12 months [53]. Regarding fluconazole use, higher doses (800 mg daily) are preferred and are generally well tolerated. Even for widespread disease, there is no evidence that combination treatment with amphotericin B and an azole is superior to treatment with a single agent. There are anecdotal reports of successful use of voriconazole for the treatment of coccidioidomycosis [54–56]. In small series, posaconazole has been used for refractory disease [57–59]. Overall, experience with the newer triazoles is limited in transplant recipients. Echinocandins should not be used. Patients should receive antifungal treatment for at least 1 year. Lifelong azole prophylaxis to prevent disease relapse should be considered.

For meningeal disease, the treatment of choice is fluconazole. Currently, most experts treat with daily doses of 800 mg or higher. In clinical trials, the dose used was 400 mg per day [60]. Some experts combine azole treatment with a lipid formulation of amphotericin B on the basis of the belief that responses are more prompt with this approach. In a small series of patients with refractory disease, itraconazole therapy was also found effective [61]. Patients who respond to azole therapy should continue this treatment indefinitely [62]. Hydrocephalus, a complication which frequently requires shunt decompression, does not per se indicate the need for alternative antifungal treatment.

Clinical and laboratory follow-up at frequent intervals to assess treatment response is advised. Fluconazole has high oral bioavailability and predictable pharmacokinetics; hence, serum drug concentrations are rarely obtained. If itraconazole is used, concentrations of at least 1 μg/mL by HPLC (combined itraconazole and hydroxy-itraconazole) and 3 μg/mL by bioassay are recommended. If serology was positive at diagnosis, response to treatment should be monitored using quantitative ID or CF assays. Coccidioidomycosis can be fatal, especially in transplant recipients who are at risk for dissemination. As the number of infected recipients is small, mortality rates have varied widely. In a single-center retrospective study (1999–2007), mortality was 13% (2/15) among liver transplant recipients [41]. In a literature review (1966–2002), mortality was 55% (18/33) among renal transplant recipients [63].

Prevention

Exposure to dust is an established risk factor for coccidioidomycosis. Activities related to disturbance of the soil, such as agricultural work, appear to be associated with development of disease, and transplant recipients should be informed about the risk. However, exposure to contaminated dust cannot be totally prevented in areas of endemicity.

For the transplant candidate diagnosed with active disease, transplantation should be postponed until clinical manifestations and radiographic abnormalities have resolved with antifungal treatment. Ideally, CF titer should decrease to 1:2 or less before considering transplantation. If there is evidence of active disease at the time of transplantation, antifungals should be continued lifelong. There is no clear consensus about the optimal posttransplant prophylactic strategy for recipients residing in an endemic area who do not have a history of active disease. Some experts recommend universal prophylaxis for all patients in endemic areas while others base it on evidence for active disease including seropositivity. Evidence is not available to determine if prophylaxis prevents posttransplant coccidioidomycosis. At the Mayo Clinic in Arizona, targeted antifungal prophylaxis was administered to those with a history of coccidioidomycosis or positive serologic studies at the time of transplantation. Using this approach, de novo coccidioidomycosis developed in 3% of liver transplant recipients who did not meet the criteria for targeted prophylaxis [41]. More than half of the cases occurred in the first posttransplant year. The authors currently recommend universal antifungal prophylaxis for 6–12 months for those residing in endemic areas.

Potential living donors with a history of travel to or residence in an endemic area should be evaluated for active or past infection. Serologic studies (EIA, CF, and ID), cultures of respiratory secretions, and chest imaging should be obtained. If there is evidence of active infection, the donor is not suitable for organ procurement. Lung transplant recipients from a seropositive donor require long-term antifungal prophylaxis due to the high likelihood of a quiescent granuloma in the lung parenchyma. For deceased or living donors, organs should be inspected for the presence of granulomas at the time of procurement. Suspicious lesions should be examined by histopathology and fungal culture. Serologic studies should also be obtained. If there is evidence of active disease in the donor, fluconazole should be administered indefinitely in the recipient.

Blastomycosis

Blastomycosis is a pyogranulomatous systemic mycosis caused by *Blastomyces dermatitidis*. In the mold phase, narrow branching septate hyphae bear small conidia on a short stalk. The yeast cell (8–15 μm in diameter) has a doubly refractile thick wall and produces a characteristic single, broad-based daughter bud. Two serotypes have been identified based on the presence of the A-antigen.

Epidemiology

The organism exists in warm, moist soil enriched by organic debris including decaying vegetation and wood. Endemic areas include the Southern, Central, and Midwestern United States, especially areas around the Great Lakes and the Ohio and Mississippi River valleys. It also occurs in Canadian provinces that border the Great Lakes and St. Lawrence River. Outside North America, blastomycosis is most common in Africa (typically A-antigen negative strains). Fewer cases have been reported from Central and South America and Western Europe. Blastomycosis is commonly associated with recreational or occupational activities that take place around rivers or lakes. In endemic areas, disease commonly occurs in dogs. Owning an infected pet may provide a useful diagnostic clue, as the dog and its owner may inhale conidia from the same source. Disease transmission to humans following dog bites has been reported [64]. The disease is rarely reported after solid organ transplantation. In two retrospective studies, the cumulative incidence was 0.13% (1996–2008) [65] and 0.14% (1986–2004) [66], respectively. Newly acquired infection typically occurs long after transplantation when patients resume their normal activities.

Pathogenesis

As with other endemic mycoses, the disease occurs after inhalation of conidia from the environment. The lungs are the primary site of involvement. Hematogenous spread can cause focal manifestations at a distant site or disseminated infection. Patients with defective cell-mediated immunity are at highest risk for severe disease. In transplant recipients, blastomycosis may result from conversion of latent infection-acquired pretransplant into symptomatic disease. Donor-derived infections have not been reported but could potentially occur.

Clinical Manifestations

In the normal host, pulmonary disease typically presents with a non-specific flu-like syndrome. In the immunocompromised host, multilobar disease is more common and may progress to adult respiratory distress syndrome (ARDS) which is associated with high mortality. Extrapulmonary manifestations usually involve the skin, osteoarticular structures, or the genitourinary system. The disease presents with pustular, nodular, or ulcerative skin lesions. The typical verrucous cutaneous lesions of blastomycosis are not seen in immunosuppressed patients. Osteomyelitis may occur contiguously to or separately from cutaneous lesions. Prostate infection presents with dysuria, perineal pain, or obstructive symptoms. CNS infection typically presents with lymphocytic meningitis. Other manifestations include epidural abscess and intracranial mass lesions [67].

Diagnosis

Blastomyces grows within 2–5 weeks on most culture media at room temperature. The fungus is isolated from respiratory secretions in most cases of pulmonary infection [68]. Direct specimen examination allows for rapid diagnosis. Respiratory specimens should be treated with potassium hydroxide or calcofluor white or stained with Papanicolaou stain. Similarly, exudate from cutaneous or subcutaneous lesions should be examined by wet prep or special stain. Direct CSF examination typically does not reveal the organism in cases of meningitis. Diagnosis can be established by detection of yeast cells consistent with *Blastomyces* in pulmonary or extrapulmonary tissue specimens. These may be difficult to identify with routine hematoxylin and eosin stains. Special stains, such as methenamine silver or periodic acid-Schiff, should be used. The presence of pyogranulomas on biopsy should raise the suspicion for blastomycosis.

Serologic testing includes techniques for detection of antibody to the A-antigen. CF and ID methods lack both sensitivity and specificity. EIAs have shown improved sensitivity, but there are insufficient clinical data to recommend their use as a routine diagnostic tool [69, 70]. Detection of the cell wall polysaccharide antigen by means of an EIA is available. Antigen can be detected in urine, serum, and other body fluids. The sensitivity of the quantitative urine antigen assay is 90% [71–73]. Antigen concentrations are highest in patients with ARDS. Specificity is 99% in patients with nonfungal infections and healthy subjects. The assay shows cross-reactivity with other fungi, particularly *H. capsulatum*, which is endemic in the same areas as *Blastomyces*. Similar to *Histoplasma* antigen, levels decline with successful treatment and increase with disease relapse.

Molecular methods are not widely available and have not been studied extensively. In a real-time PCR assay, detection directly from clinical specimens (mainly respiratory secretions and pleural fluid) demonstrated a sensitivity of 86% and a specificity of 99% [20]. The assay provides a rapid method for the detection of *B. dermatitidis*. Molecular methods may prove useful in detecting the organism from formalin-fixed paraffin-embedded tissue [74].

Treatment

The Infectious Diseases Society of America has published guidelines for the treatment of blastomycosis [75]. All immunocompromised patients should be treated. For moderately severe to severe pulmonary or disseminated disease, treatment should be started with amphotericin B. In transplant recipients, lipid formulations of the drug are preferred due to the lower risk of nephrotoxicity. Treatment can be transitioned to oral itraconazole after clinical improvement. In immunosuppressed patients, antifungal therapy is recommended for at least 12 months. Indefinite treatment may be needed in patients who remain on immunosuppressive agents or those who experience relapse. For CNS disease, a lipid formulation of amphotericin B should be administered for 4–6 weeks followed by an oral azole. Itraconazole is the preferred azole [76]. Fluconazole (400–800 mg daily) is an alternative agent [77, 78]. The newer triazoles are active in vitro. The successful use of voriconazole [65, 79, 80] and posaconazole [81] has been reported in small series or case reports. As with other endemic mycoses, echinocandins are not active. Large abscesses should be drained and devitalized tissue should be debrided in the setting of extensive osteomyelitis. Surgical resection of residual pulmonary cavities is not indicated. In the two published case series, overall mortality among transplant recipients was approximately 36% [65, 66], reaching 67% (4/6) in SOT recipients with ARDS.

Prevention

Transplant recipients should be educated about the risk associated with recreational or occupational activities along waterways in areas of endemicity. Due to the rarity of disease in transplant recipients, the role of pretransplant screening and posttransplant antifungal prophylaxis to prevent blastomycosis has not been defined. In the absence of robust data, an approach similar to the one followed for histoplasmosis seems reasonable.

Other Endemic Mycoses

Paracoccidioidomycosis is a systemic fungal infection caused by *Paracoccidioides brasiliensis*. The organism is endemic in areas of Central and Latin America.

Most cases have been reported from Brazil, particularly among individuals involved in agricultural activities [82]. The lungs are the primary site of involvement but disease can disseminate. Ulcerated painful mucocutaneous lesions are characteristic. Radiographically, diffuse alveolar and interstitial pulmonary infiltrates are seen in acute disease. Paracoccidioidomycosis has been described in single case reports among kidney transplant recipients [83–85]. The organism may be visualized in direct specimens or biopsy tissue. Antibody and antigen detection are useful tools in diagnosing disease and following treatment response [86, 87]. Sulfonamides, amphotericin B, and itraconazole are active against *Paracoccidioides*. The rarity of the infection among transplant recipients may be explained by the routine prophylactic use of trimethoprim-sulfamethoxazole.

Penicilliosis is caused by *Penicillium marneffei*, a dimorphic fungus endemic in most countries in Southeast Asia, Southern China, Taiwan, and Northeast India. Patients may present with pulmonary involvement, diffuse lymphadenopathy, hepatomegaly, and splenomegaly. Skin lesion characteristics of the disease are found on the face, upper trunk, and extremities. Papules may have a necrotic center which gives an umbilicated appearance. The disease has been well described in HIV-infected individuals. Cases of penicilliosis have been reported in renal transplant recipients [88–90]. As with HIV-infected patients, disease has been reported in a transplant recipient after a brief visit to an endemic area [91]. Diagnosis is established by culture and histopathology. Standard treatment involves a formulation of amphotericin B followed by azole therapy.

Sporothrix schenckii is a dimorphic fungus with worldwide distribution. Most commonly, infection presents with ulcerated, verrucous, or erythematous skin nodules which can spread locally via the lymphatic route. Pulmonary involvement, systemic dissemination, and meningeal involvement may occur in the immunocompromised host. Lymphocutaneous infection results from inoculation of the organism into the skin and subcutaneous tissues. Pulmonary disease is acquired via inhalation of arthroconidia. Activities such as landscaping, gardening, or farming have been associated with sporotrichosis. Recurrent systemic disease [92] and urinary sporotrichosis [93] have been reported in renal transplant recipients. Diagnosis is established by culture and histopathology. Treatment guidelines have been published by IDSA [94]. Itraconazole is the treatment of choice for lymphocutaneous and osteoarticular disease. For meningeal, severe pulmonary, and disseminated disease, a lipid formulation of amphotericin B should be used. After the initial clinical response, treatment with itraconazole is recommended.

References

1. Pappas PG, Alexander BD, Andes DR, et al. Invasive fungal infections among organ transplant recipients: results of the Transplant-Associated Infection Surveillance Network (TRANSNET). Clin Infect Dis. 2010;50(8):1101–11.
2. Kontoyiannis DP, Marr KA, Park BJ, et al. Prospective surveillance for invasive fungal infections in hematopoietic stem cell transplant recipients, 2001-2006: overview of the Transplant-Associated Infection Surveillance Network (TRANSNET) Database. Clin Infect Dis. 2010;50(8):1091–100.
3. Cuellar-Rodriguez J, Avery RK, Lard M, et al. Histoplasmosis in solid organ transplant recipients: 10 years of experience at a large transplant center in an endemic area. Clin Infect Dis. 2009;49(5):710–6.
4. Vail GM, Young RS, Wheat LJ, et al. Incidence of histoplasmosis following allogeneic bone marrow transplant or solid organ transplant in a hyperendemic area. Transpl Infect Dis. 2002;4(3):148–51.
5. Wheat LJ, Smith EJ, Sathapatayavongs B, et al. Histoplasmosis in renal allograft recipients. Two large urban outbreaks. Arch Intern Med. 1983;143(4):703–7.
6. Straub M, Schwarz J. The healed primary complex in histoplasmosis. Am J Clin Pathol. 1955;25(7):727–41.
7. Limaye AP, Connolly PA, Sagar M, et al. Transmission of *Histoplasma capsulatum* by organ transplantation. N Engl J Med. 2000;343(16):1163–6.
8. Freifeld AG, Iwen PC, Lesiak BL, et al. Histoplasmosis in solid organ transplant recipients at a large Midwestern university transplant center. Transpl Infect Dis. 2005;7(3–4):109–15.
9. Singh N, Lortholary O, Alexander BD, et al. An immune reconstitution syndrome-like illness associated with Cryptococcus neoformans infection in organ transplant recipients. Clin Infect Dis. 2005;40(12):1756–61.
10. Singh N, Perfect JR. Immune reconstitution syndrome associated with opportunistic mycoses. Lancet Infect Dis. 2007;7(6):395–401.
11. Vetter E, Torgerson C, Feuker A, et al. Comparison of the BACTEC MYCO/F lytic bottle to the isolator tube, BACTEC plus aerobic F/bottle, and BACTEC anaerobic lytic/10 bottle and comparison of the BACTEC plus aerobic F/bottle to the isolator tube for recovery of bacteria, mycobacteria, and fungi from blood. J Clin Microbiol. 2001,39(12):4380–6.
12. Hage CA, Ribes JA, Wengenack NL, et al. A multicenter evaluation of tests for diagnosis of histoplasmosis. Clin Infect Dis. 2011;53(5):448–54.
13. Wheat J, Wheat H, Connolly P, et al. Cross-reactivity in *Histoplasma capsulatum* variety *capsulatum* antigen assays of urine samples from patients with endemic mycoses. Clin Infect Dis. 1997;24(6):1169–71.
14. Kuberski T, Myers R, Wheat LJ, et al. Diagnosis of coccidioidomycosis by antigen detection using cross-reaction with a *Histoplasma* antigen. Clin Infect Dis. 2007;44(5):e50–4.
15. Vergidis P, Walker RC, Kaul DR, et al. False-positive *Aspergillus* galactomannan assay in solid organ transplant recipients with histoplasmosis. Transpl Infect Dis. 2012;14(2):213–7.
16. Hage CA, Davis TE, Fuller D, et al. Diagnosis of histoplasmosis by antigen detection in BAL fluid. Chest. 2010;137(3):623–8.
17. Egan L, Connolly P, Wheat LJ, et al. Histoplasmosis as a cause for a positive Fungitell (1→3)-beta-D-glucan test. Med Mycol. 2008;46(1):93–5.
18. Wheat LJ. Approach to the diagnosis of the endemic mycoses. Clin Chest Med. 2009;30(2):379–89, viii.
19. Bialek R, Feucht A, Aepinus C, et al. Evaluation of two nested PCR assays for detection of *Histoplasma capsulatum* DNA in human tissue. J Clin Microbiol. 2002;40(5):1644–7.

20. Babady NE, Buckwalter SP, Hall L, et al. Detection of *Blastomyces dermatitidis* and *Histoplasma capsulatum* from culture isolates and clinical specimens by use of real-time PCR. J Clin Microbiol. 2011;49(9):3204–8.
21. Tang YW, Li H, Durkin MM, et al. Urine polymerase chain reaction is not as sensitive as urine antigen for the diagnosis of disseminated histoplasmosis. Diagn Microbiol Infect Dis. 2006;54(4):283–7.
22. Wheat LJ. Improvements in diagnosis of histoplasmosis. Expert Opin Biol Ther. 2006;6(11):1207–21.
23. Wheat LJ, Freifeld AG, Kleiman MB, et al. Clinical practice guidelines for the management of patients with histoplasmosis: 2007 update by the Infectious Diseases Society of America. Clin Infect Dis. 2007;45(7):807–25.
24. Johnson PC, Wheat LJ, Cloud GA, et al. Safety and efficacy of liposomal amphotericin B compared with conventional amphotericin B for induction therapy of histoplasmosis in patients with AIDS. Ann Intern Med. 2002;137(2):105–9.
25. Freifeld A, Proia L, Andes D, et al. Voriconazole use for endemic fungal infections. Antimicrob Agents Chemother. 2009;53(4):1648–51.
26. Restrepo A, Tobon A, Clark B, et al. Salvage treatment of histoplasmosis with posaconazole. J Infect. 2007;54(4):319–27.
27. Wheat LJ, Connolly P, Smedema M, et al. Activity of newer triazoles against *Histoplasma capsulatum* from patients with AIDS who failed fluconazole. J Antimicrob Chemother. 2006;57(6):1235–9.
28. Kohler S, Wheat LJ, Connolly P, et al. Comparison of the echinocandin caspofungin with amphotericin B for treatment of histoplasmosis following pulmonary challenge in a murine model. Antimicrob Agents Chemother. 2000;44(7):1850–4.
29. Hage CA, Connolly P, Horan D, et al. Investigation of the efficacy of micafungin in the treatment of histoplasmosis using two north American strains of *Histoplasma capsulatum*. Antimicrob Agents Chemother. 2011;55(9):4447–50.
30. Hage CA, Kirsch EJ, Stump TE, et al. *Histoplasma* antigen clearance during treatment of histoplasmosis in patients with AIDS determined by a quantitative antigen enzyme immunoassay. Clin Vaccine Immunol. 2011;18(4):661–6.
31. Goldman M, Zackin R, Fichtenbaum CJ, et al. Safety of discontinuation of maintenance therapy for disseminated histoplasmosis after immunologic response to antiretroviral therapy. Clin Infect Dis. 2004;38(10):1485–9.
32. Cano MV, Hajjeh RA. The epidemiology of histoplasmosis: a review. Semin Respir Infect. 2001;16(2):109–18.
33. Kang SH, Deziel PJ, Razonable RR. Pre-transplant serology, lung nodules, calcified mediastinal lymph nodes, and the risk of histoplasmosis after liver transplantation. 49th interscience conference on antimicrobial agents and chemotherapy. San Francisco; 2009.
34. Dodge RR, Lebowitz MD, Barbee R, et al. Estimates of *C. immitis* infection by skin test reactivity in an endemic community. Am J Public Health. 1985;75(8):863–5.
35. Sunenshine RH, Anderson S, Erhart L, et al. Public health surveillance for coccidioidomycosis in Arizona. Ann N Y Acad Sci. 2007;1111:96–102.
36. Cohen IM, Galgiani JN, Potter D, et al. Coccidioidomycosis in renal replacement therapy. Arch Intern Med. 1982;142(3):489–94.
37. Blair JE. Coccidioidomycosis in patients who have undergone transplantation. Ann N Y Acad Sci. 2007;1111:365–76.
38. Blair JE, Douglas DD. Coccidioidomycosis in liver transplant recipients relocating to an endemic area. Dig Dis Sci. 2004;49(11–12):1981–5.
39. Cha JM, Jung S, Bahng HS, et al. Multi-organ failure caused by reactivated coccidioidomycosis without dissemination in a patient with renal transplantation. Respirology. 2000;5(1):87–90.
40. Vartivarian SE, Coudron PE, Markowitz SM. Disseminated coccidioidomycosis. Unusual manifestations in a cardiac transplantation patient. Am J Med. 1987;83(5):949–52.
41. Vucicevic D, Carey EJ, Blair JE. Coccidioidomycosis in liver transplant recipients in an endemic area. Am J Transplant. 2011;11(1):111–9.
42. Miller MB, Hendren R, Gilligan PH. Posttransplantation disseminated coccidioidomycosis acquired from donor lungs. J Clin Microbiol. 2004;42(5):2347–9.
43. Tripathy U, Yung GL, Kriett JM, et al. Donor transfer of pulmonary coccidioidomycosis in lung transplantation. Ann Thorac Surg. 2002;73(1):306–8.
44. Wright PW, Pappagianis D, Wilson M, et al. Donor-related coccidioidomycosis in organ transplant recipients. Clin Infect Dis. 2003;37(9):1265–9.
45. Brugiere O, Forget E, Biondi G, et al. Coccidioidomycosis in a lung transplant recipient acquired from the donor graft in France. Transplantation. 2009;88(11):1319–20.
46. Wieden MA, Galgiani JN, Pappagianis D. Comparison of immunodiffusion techniques with standard complement fixation assay for quantitation of coccidioidal antibodies. J Clin Microbiol. 1983;18(3):529–34.
47. Zartarian M, Peterson EM, de la Maza LM. Detection of antibodies to *Coccidioides immitis* by enzyme immunoassay. Am J Clin Pathol. 1997;107(2):148–53.
48. Blair JE, Coakley B, Santelli AC, et al. Serologic testing for symptomatic coccidioidomycosis in immunocompetent and immunosuppressed hosts. Mycopathologia. 2006;162(5):317–24.
49. Durkin M, Connolly P, Kuberski T, et al. Diagnosis of coccidioidomycosis with use of the *Coccidioides* antigen enzyme immunoassay. Clin Infect Dis. 2008;47(8):e69–73.
50. Binnicker MJ, Buckwalter SP, Eisberner JJ, et al. Detection of *Coccidioides* species in clinical specimens by real-time PCR. J Clin Microbiol. 2007;45(1):173–8.
51. Vucicevic D, Blair JE, Binnicker MJ, et al. The utility of *Coccidioides* polymerase chain reaction testing in the clinical setting. Mycopathologia. 2010;170(5):345–51.
52. Galgiani JN, Ampel NM, Blair JE, et al. Coccidioidomycosis. Clin Infect Dis. 2005;41(9):1217–23.
53. Galgiani JN, Catanzaro A, Cloud GA, et al. Comparison of oral fluconazole and itraconazole for progressive, nonmeningeal coccidioidomycosis. A randomized, double-blind trial. Mycoses *Study Group*. Ann Intern Med. 2000;133(9):676–86.
54. Proia LA, Tenorio AR. Successful use of voriconazole for treatment of *Coccidioides* meningitis. Antimicrob Agents Chemother. 2004;48(6):2341.
55. Prabhu RM, Bonnell M, Currier BL, et al. Successful treatment of disseminated nonmeningeal coccidioidomycosis with voriconazole. Clin Infect Dis. 2004;39(7):e74–7.
56. Cortez KJ, Walsh TJ, Bennett JE. Successful treatment of coccidioidal meningitis with voriconazole. Clin Infect Dis. 2003;36(12):1619–22.
57. Anstead GM, Corcoran G, Lewis J, et al. Refractory coccidioidomycosis treated with posaconazole. Clin Infect Dis. 2005;40(12):1770–6.
58. Catanzaro A, Cloud GA, Stevens DA, et al. Safety, tolerance, and efficacy of posaconazole therapy in patients with nonmeningeal disseminated or chronic pulmonary coccidioidomycosis. Clin Infect Dis. 2007;45(5):562–8.
59. Stevens DA, Rendon A, Gaona-Flores V, et al. Posaconazole therapy for chronic refractory coccidioidomycosis. Chest. 2007;132(3):952–8.
60. Galgiani JN, Catanzaro A, Cloud GA, et al. Fluconazole therapy for coccidioidal meningitis. The NIAID-Mycoses Study Group. Ann Intern Med. 1993;119(1):28–35.
61. Tucker RM, Denning DW, Dupont B, et al. Itraconazole therapy for chronic coccidioidal meningitis. Ann Intern Med. 1990;112(2):108–12.

62. Dewsnup DH, Galgiani JN, Graybill JR, et al. Is it ever safe to stop azole therapy for *Coccidioides immitis* meningitis? Ann Intern Med. 1996;124(3):305–10.
63. Antony SJ, Dummer SJ, McNeil KK, et al. Coccidioidomycosis in Renal Transplant Recipients. Infect Dis Clin Pract. 2005;13(5):250–4.
64. Gnann JW Jr, Bressler GS, Bodet CA 3rd, et al. Human blastomycosis after a dog bite. Ann Intern Med. 1983;98(1):48–9.
65. Gauthier GM, Safdar N, Klein BS, et al. Blastomycosis in solid organ transplant recipients. Transpl Infect Dis. 2007;9(4):310–7.
66. Grim SA, Proia L, Miller R, et al. A multicenter study of histoplasmosis and blastomycosis after solid organ transplantation. Transpl Infect Dis. 2012;14(1):17–23.
67. Bariola JR, Perry P, Pappas PG, et al. Blastomycosis of the central nervous system: a multicenter review of diagnosis and treatment in the modern era. Clin Infect Dis. 2010;50(6):797–804.
68. Martynowicz MA, Prakash UB. Pulmonary blastomycosis: an appraisal of diagnostic techniques. Chest. 2002;121(3):768–73.
69. Klein BS, Kuritsky JN, Chappell WA, et al. Comparison of the enzyme immunoassay, immunodiffusion, and complement fixation tests in detecting antibody in human serum to the A antigen of *Blastomyces dermatitidis*. Am Rev Respir Dis. 1986;133(1):144–8.
70. Bradsher RW, Pappas PG. Detection of specific antibodies in human blastomycosis by enzyme immunoassay. South Med J. 1995;88(12):1256–9.
71. Bariola JR, Hage CA, Durkin M, et al. Detection of *Blastomyces dermatitidis* antigen in patients with newly diagnosed blastomycosis. Diagn Microbiol Infect Dis. 2011;69(2):187–91.
72. Durkin M, Witt J, Lemonte A, et al. Antigen assay with the potential to aid in diagnosis of blastomycosis. J Clin Microbiol. 2004;42(10):4873–5.
73. Connolly P, Hage CA, Bariola JR, et al. *Blastomyces dermatitidis* antigen detection by quantitative enzyme immunoassay. Clin Vaccine Immunol. 2012;19(1):53–6.
74. Bialek R, Cirera AC, Herrmann T, et al. Nested PCR assays for detection of *Blastomyces dermatitidis* DNA in paraffin-embedded canine tissue. J Clin Microbiol. 2003;41(1):205–8.
75. Chapman SW, Dismukes WE, Proia LA, et al. Clinical practice guidelines for the management of blastomycosis: 2008 update by the Infectious Diseases Society of America. Clin Infect Dis. 2008;46(12):1801–12.
76. Dismukes WE, Bradsher RW Jr, Cloud GC, et al. Itraconazole therapy for blastomycosis and histoplasmosis. NIAID Mycoses Study Group. Am J Med. 1992;93(5):489–97.
77. Pappas PG, Bradsher RW, Kauffman CA, et al. Treatment of blastomycosis with higher doses of fluconazole. The National Institute of Allergy and Infectious Diseases *Mycoses Study Group*. Clin Infect Dis. 1997;25(2):200–5.
78. Pappas PG, Bradsher RW, Chapman SW, et al. Treatment of blastomycosis with fluconazole: a pilot study. The National Institute of Allergy and Infectious Diseases Mycoses Study Group. Clin Infect Dis. 1995;20(2):267–71.
79. Bakleh M, Aksamit AJ, Tleyjeh IM, et al. Successful treatment of cerebral blastomycosis with voriconazole. Clin Infect Dis. 2005;40(9):e69–71.
80. Borgia SM, Fuller JD, Sarabia A, et al. Cerebral blastomycosis: a case series incorporating voriconazole in the treatment regimen. Med Mycol. 2006;44(7):659–64.
81. Proia LA, Harnisch DO. Successful use of posaconazole for treatment of blastomycosis. Antimicrob Agents Chemother. 2012;56(7):4029.
82. Blotta MH, Mamoni RL, Oliveira SJ, et al. Endemic regions of paracoccidioidomycosis in Brazil: a clinical and epidemiologic study of 584 cases in the southeast region. Am J Trop Med Hyg. 1999;61(3):390–4.
83. Zavascki AP, Bienardt JC, Severo LC. Paracoccidioidomycosis in organ transplant recipient: case report. Rev Inst Med Trop Sao Paulo. 2004;46(5):279–81.
84. Shikanai-Yasuda MA, Duarte MI, Nunes DF, et al. Paracoccidioidomycosis in a renal transplant recipient. J Med Vet Mycol. 1995;33(6):411–4.
85. Sugar AM, Restrepo A, Stevens DA. Paracoccidioidomycosis in the immunosuppressed host: report of a case and review of the literature. Am Rev Respir Dis. 1984;129(2):340–2.
86. de Camargo ZP. Serology of paracoccidioidomycosis. Mycopathologia. 2008;165(4–5):289–302.
87. da Silva SH, Grosso Dde M, Lopes JD, et al. Detection of *Paracoccidioides brasiliensis* gp70 circulating antigen and follow-up of patients undergoing antimycotic therapy. J Clin Microbiol. 2004;42(10):4480–6.
88. Chan YH, Wong KM, Lee KC, et al. Pneumonia and mesenteric lymphadenopathy caused by disseminated *Penicillium marneffei* infection in a cadaveric renal transplant recipient. Transpl Infect Dis. 2004;6(1):28–32.
89. Lin JN, Lin HH, Lai CH, et al. Renal transplant recipient infected with *Penicillium marneffei*. Lancet Infect Dis. 2010;10(2):138.
90. Wang JL, Hung CC, Chang SC, et al. Disseminated *Penicillium marneffei* infection in a renal-transplant recipient successfully treated with liposomal amphotericin B. Transplantation. 2003;76(7):1136–7.
91. Hart J, Dyer JR, Clark BM, et al. Travel-related disseminated *Penicillium marneffei* infection in a renal transplant patient. Transpl Infect Dis. 2012;14(4):434–9. Epub 2011 Dec 20.
92. Gullberg RM, Quintanilla A, Levin ML, et al. Sporotrichosis: recurrent cutaneous, articular, and central nervous system infection in a renal transplant recipient. Rev Infect Dis. 1987;9(2):369–75.
93. Agarwal SK, Tiwari SC, Dash SC, et al. Urinary sporotrichosis in a renal allograft recipient. Nephron. 1994;66(4):485.
94. Kauffman CA, Bustamante B, Chapman SW, et al. Clinical practice guidelines for the management of sporotrichosis: 2007 update by the Infectious Diseases Society of America. Clin Infect Dis. 2007;45(10):1255–65.

Cytomegalovirus

37

Amar Safdar and Donald Armstrong

Introduction

Cytomegalovirus (CMV) is a herpesvirus, and similar to other viruses in this group, after an acute infection, the virus establishes lifelong asymptomatic residency referred to as "viral latency". Primary or initial infection in the general population with intact immune response is often a brief and mild illness that requires no therapy. Individuals with latent CMV infection may experience subclinical viral reactivation and unwittingly shed the virus in bodily fluids, such as saliva, tears, semen, breast milk, and urine. In the United States, by the age of 40 years, more than half of adults show serologic evidence of prior CMV infection (www.CDC.gov) [1]. CMV is not considered highly contagious, although the common mode of viral transmission within the members of a shared household, close contacts including children in daycare centers, is via exchange of saliva; it is important to recognize that CMV infection may be acquired after sexual intercourse. Cytomegalovirus infection during pregnancy is a leading cause of permanent birth defects (www.CDC.gov) [1].

Only 8 herpesviruses among more than 100 discovered so far cause disease in humans. These include herpes simplex virus types 1 and 2, varicella-zoster virus, cytomegalovirus, Epstein-Barr virus, human herpesvirus 6 variants A and B, human herpesvirus 7, and Kaposi's sarcoma virus or human herpesvirus 8 that also causes primary effusion lymphomas and the rare multicentric Castleman's disease. A simian virus, called B virus, occasionally infects humans.

A. Safdar (✉)
Clinical Associate Professor of Medicine, Texas Tech University Health Sciences Center El Paso, Paul L. Foster School of Medicine, El Paso, TX, USA
e-mail: amar.safdar@cidimmunology.com

D. Armstrong
Infectious Disease Service, Memorial Sloan-Kettering Cancer Center, New York, NY, USA

Cornell University Medical College (ret), New York, NY, USA

Infectious Disease Society of America, Albuquerque, NM, USA

Patients with dysfunctional adaptive immune response are at a higher risk for severe CMV infection and end-organ disease [2, 3]. Since it is a common childhood infection, most viremia in immunocompromised patients represents reactivation of a remotely acquired latent infection [2]. End-organ viral disease poses an existential threat for patients with severe immune dysregulation and/or suppression of adaptive cellular immune response [4]. A newly acquired CMV infection in seronegative transplant recipients from an allograft harvested from CMV-seropositive donor has emerged as the most serious risk for post-transplant CMV infection and disease after blood or marrow hematopoietic stem cell or solid organ allograft transplantation (HSCT and SOT, respectively) [3, 5].

In transplant recipients, viral infection or recurrence of a remotely acquired infection is a well-recognized risk factor for end-organ disease that has the potential to involve any organ system. In patients undergoing HSCT, viral pneumonitis, myelosuppression, encephalitis, enterocolitis, hepatitis, and rarely retinitis or adrenalitis may be encountered [3]. CMV organ disease may occur in patients despite effective anti-CMV prophylaxis. Stem cell graft compromise or loss of allograft is another life-threatening complication resulting from direct virus-induced suppression of hematopoiesis. In addition, CMV infection was noted to elevate the risk for graft-versus-host disease (GVHD) [6]. In solid organ allograft recipients, CMV infection and end-organ disease is a well-recognized and serious post-transplant complication that has far-reaching impact on the allograft function and survival [5].

CMV infection is increasingly recognized to influence and elicit multifaceted modifications in hosts' immune response. This appears to be more pronounced in yet unpredictable select group of individuals that undergo allograft transplantation. The virus-induced immune dysregulation has been implicated in fostering vulnerability for secondary fungal and bacterial infections, which additionally influence poor transplant outcomes [7].

A. Safdar (ed.), *Principles and Practice of Transplant Infectious Diseases*, https://doi.org/10.1007/978-1-4939-9034-4_37

In this chapter, a comprehensive review of cytomegalovirus is presented with pertinent aspects of this opportunistic viral pathogen in patients undergoing transplantation procedures.

CMV Structure

CMV is a double-stranded DNA virus encased in an icosahedral capsid and belongs to the beta (β) subfamily of the *Herpesviridae*. The viral DNA is composed of nearly 230,000 base pairs that encode for approximately 200 proteins [8]. CMV genes are named after their position within each segment of the genome like UL97 is the 97th open reading frame in the unique long segment.

CMV tegument or matrix is composed of a cluster of proteins that lines the space between the envelope and nucleocapsid.

In laboratory cell line cultures, diploid human fibroblasts, endothelial cells, and macrophages support CMV growth ex vivo, whereas, during infection, CMV is found in a variety of cells such as endothelial cells, epithelial cells, smooth muscle cells, and peripheral blood neutrophils [9]. The diverse hosts' tissue tropism for cytomegalovirus plays an important role in viral disease involvement of a wide spectrum of hosts' organ systems.

Like other herpesviruses, CMV persist within the cells in a latent state for the life span of the host and periodically replicated resulting in low-level viremia and viral shedding at various body sites. Latent CMV virus has been shown to exist within neutrophils and monocytes [10, 11]. It is possible that the virus also maintains latent residency in other tissues and abdominothoracic viscera.

CMV Cell Entry

CMV infection of human fibroblasts and epithelial cells requires glycoprotein complexes composed of gB and gH/gL/gO. In addition, for epithelial cell infection, the viral envelope pentamer complex consisting of gH, gL, UL128, UL130, and UL131A is required. Data from vaccine development showed that neutralizing antibodies to gB or gH epitopes can interfere with CMV entry in fibroblasts and epithelial cells [12]. It was interesting that neutralizing antibodies targeting conformational epitopes such as UL128/130/131A that are important components of the viral unit that interacts with hosts' immune receptors did not prevent viral entry into the fibroblasts, although these antibodies were able to cease viral entry into epithelial cells [12]. However, the envelope pentamer complex is highly immunogenic in eliciting neutralizing antibody response against UL128/130/131A subunits and gH, which can effectively block CMV entry into both epithelial cells and fibroblasts [12]. This has been an area of keen interest in designing a novel immunogen construct for effective and durable CMV vaccine.

CMV Immunity

Innate Anti-CMV Immunity

CMV triggers cellular inflammatory cytokine production via TLR pathway. It is known that viral glycoproteins B and gH that are also a part of CMV envelope pentamer complex cause TLR2 activation [13, 14]. Certain genetic polymorphisms in TLR2 were explored to identify potential host vulnerabilities for the risk of CMV infection. In patients undergoing orthotopic liver transplantation, a multivariate Cox hazard model demonstrated a possible link between higher risk of CMV disease after transplantation in patients exhibiting homozygous TLR2 Arg753Gln polymorphism (hazard ratio, 1.9) [15]. This risk for cytomegalovirus remained after adjusting for age, CMV serostatus, and allograft rejection [15].

TLR3 and TLR9 are important in eliciting innate immune defense against CMV replication and infection in mice [16, 17]. In the murine CMV experiments, TLR9 assures rapid antiviral response; this was in concert with other TLR-dependent and TLR-independent innate immune events assisting to garner subsequent adaptive anti-CMV response in the animals studied [17].

Natural killer cells are marrow-derived lymphoid cells that play an integral role in hosts' innate immune response needed to contain an infection after the initial exposure. NK cells are also constituent in orchestrating adaptive immune response. It has been known for some time that patients with various deficiencies in NK cell function are predisposed to serious herpesvirus infections that include CMV and EBV [18, 19]. Activating killer Ig-like receptor (aKIR) plays a central role in NK cell-mediated anti-CMV immunity, and certain stem cell donor aKIR genotypes appear to modify risk for post-transplant CMV infection [20, 21]. One hundred and fifty-two patients with CMV reactivation were compared with 59 with no viral reactivation after HSCT [22]. Presence of specific aKIR haplotypes in the donor, but not in the recipient, were significantly associated with protection from CMV reactivation and the degree of CMV viremia during post-transplant period [22]. A donor aKIR profile exhibiting aKIR2DS2 and aKIR2DS4 predicted low risk of CMV reactivation after transplantation; this was independent of CD4 and cytotoxic T cell-mediated CMV protection [22]. It needs to be further investigated if pre-transplant selection of donor aKIR haplotypes may optimize the risk of post-transplant CMV infection, especially in patients undergoing stem cell transplantation that are known to have high risk for CMV infection and end-organ disease after transplantation.

NK cells have recently been shown to exert regulatory effect on antiviral T cell response. In part, this is achieved by direct NK cell-mediated killing of activated, CMV-targeted T cells for the purpose of modifying risk of tissue injury from an untamed antiviral cellular immune response [23]. NK cells modify antiviral immune response by destroying dendritic cells, which also serves to restrain continuous antigen presentation and T cell activation in patients with persistent viral infection [24]. It is likely that overall or net immunoregulatory NK cell function is contingent up on the location and extent of inflammation elicited by adaptive antiviral immune response [25].

NK cells are the first lymphoid cells to repopulate after allogeneic HSCT. Innate immunity is axiomatically thought to lack recall or memory function. It was therefore interesting and unexpected to see reports that certain NK cell subsets (Ly49H) exhibit memory following re-exposure to pathogens like cytomegalovirus [26].

In addition, the association between post-transplant risk of CMV reactivation and disease and presence of simple genetic aberrations in chemokine receptor 5, IL-10, and monocyte chemoattractant protein 1 is intriguing and needs further clinical verification [27].

Adaptive Immunity

CD8 cytotoxic T lymphocyte (CTL) response is an important feature of adaptive immune response against cytomegalovirus [28]. CTL responses against viral epitopes like UL123 (IE-1), UL122 (IE-2), and UL83 (pp65) are most prominent and robust [28–31]. The clinical significance of CMV cellular immunity in controlling viral replication is demonstrated in studies that show causal relationship between viremia and lack of CMV-specific CTLs, whereas post HSCT reconstitution and recovery of CMV-specific cytotoxic T cell provide protection from CMV infection and end-organ viral disease [32–34].

CMV-specific CD4 helper T cells also play an important role in protection from CMV disease in patients undergoing allogeneic stem cell transplantation [35–37]. In patients with late post-transplant CMV infection, inadequate CMV-specific helper T cell responses were noted as a risk for late CMV disease and death [38]. Since cytotoxic response forms the backbone of adaptive cellular immunity against CMV infection and disease, it was proposed that a virus-specific helper T cell in most part assists in sustaining a forceful cytotoxic antiviral response [34]. The emerging role of gamma delta ($\gamma\delta$) T cells in protection against CMV infection is of interest and needs to be explored further [25].

The role of humoral immunity against CMV disease in patients after allograft transplants remains uncertain. Following naturally acquired CMV infection, antibodies are produced against various viral proteins, and anti-gB and anti-gH antibodies are thought to limit the extent of CMV disease progression after the initial infection [39, 40]. However, anti-CMV antibodies thus far have shown to play a limited or no role in containment or prevention of CMV disease after stem cell allograft transplantation.

CMV Immune Evasion

Cytomegalovirus has developed and refined a number of evolutionary mechanisms to elude and avoid mammalian immune surveillance. In the past three decades, a number of sophisticated viral methods have come to light. Some of the salient functional features of CMV genes to achieve this goal include (a) impede apoptosis of CMV infected [41], (b) MHC-I restricted antigen presentation [42], and (c) blocking interferon-assisted antiviral response [43–45].

CMV also encodes proteins that are homologues to hosts' cellular proteins. Among them, proteins that resemble MHC Class-I molecules, IL-10, TNF receptors, and chemokines including CXC-1 help CMV to dodge hosts' immune surveillance [46–51].

NK cells are effective deterrent against viral infection, although CMV among other herpesviruses have developed means to avoid NK cell attack by pirating MHC-like domains, thereby attenuating an important element of host's innate antiviral immune defense [52]. It is important to note that CMV has the capability to modulate NK cell functions including cell maturity; and possibly recall or memory after the initial viral exposure, the later obervation needs further investigation [53].

CMV and Hematopoiesis

Since early 1990, CMV DNA could be isolated from the marrow cells in healthy CMV-seropositive individuals being considered for stem cell harvest [54]. It was also shown that CMV can render severe and potentially irremediable damage to the bone marrow stroma, crippling the rate of regeneration of pluripotent stem cell necessary for repopulation and engraftment hematopoiesis [55]. Others in the late 1980s showed that CMV can impair hematopoiesis either through infection of bone marrow stromal cells influencing hematopoietic growth factor production or by a direct viral infection of myeloid cells and their precursors [56].

CMV Diagnosis and Viral Surveillance

CMV IgG and IgM are measured to assess acute or latent infection due to cytomegalovirus. These tests probe the potential risk for post-transplant CMV infection and disease;

however, by itself serology provides no meaningful information for the presence of infection (viremia) or end-organ disease. The ex vivo cultures cannot be clinically relied upon due to slow viral growth in cell lines that may take weeks to identify virus-induced cytopathic effects. It is important to note that culture-proven viremia is highly predictive of CMV disease and probably a reflection of high viral load at the time specimens were collected [57]. The limited utility of CMV cultures has yielded to innovative assays such as shell vial test, which is now seldom used due to lack of sensitivity; however, shell vial when positive could provide evidence of viable replicating cytomegalovirus in the clinical sample, and results could be available within 18–24 h [58, 59].

Tissue samples when obtained may exhibit characteristic "owl's eye" CMV nuclear inclusions, although more sensitive immunohistochemical techniques are now routinely used to identify CMV antigens within the infected cells. It is not uncommon to find intracellular CMV antigens by immunohistochemical test in samples that do not exhibit intracellular or intracytoplasmic viral inclusions.

Advances in molecular techniques that are independent of viral growth in tissue cultures have boosted ability to diagnose CMV infection. Identification of CMV tegument phosphoprotein that is 65 kilodalton in weight (pp65; UL83) in peripheral blood leukocytes by fluorescent anti-pp65 antibodies has become a standard clinical practice for rapid diagnosis of CMV infection, especially in high-risk transplant recipients. CMV pp65 antigenemia assay has adequate sensitivity and specificity, with reliable predictive values. The number of positive cells over the total number of leukocytes per slide provides a semi-quantitative estimation of the CMV viral load in the peripheral blood. A positive CMV pp65 antigenemia has reliable predictive value for end-organ CMV disease in patients undergoing allogeneic HSCT [60]. Conditions with low-peripheral blood leukocyte counts including pre-engraftment severe neutropenia or other post-transplant disorders with low blood neutrophils limit this test's utility. CMV antigenemia test is not valid for diagnosis of CMV infection in other bodily fluid such as CSF, BAL, pleural, and peritoneal aspirate samples. Use of pp65 antigenemia to assess treatment response should include the forethought that once neutrophils are infected by cytomegalovirus, the viral antigens will remain present through the lifespan of these cells and may not be construed as an indicator of real-time viral kinetics in the peripheral blood. Therefore, a decline in pp65 antigenemia may lag behind actual resolution of viremia while on anti-CMV therapy.

Quantitative PCR relies on quantitative amplification of viral DNA. This test has now become the standard for assessing level of CMV viremia in whole blood or plasma. CMV DNA PCR is also used in CSF along with other routine viral PCR for HSV and VZV. PCR is the most sensitive method for detecting CMV viremia and may capture cases where pp65 antigenemia either cannot be performed due to severe neutropenia or provides false-negative result [61]. The results are usually available within 24 h, and the test shows high specificity for presence of cytomegalovirus. It is a direct measurement of viral load and illustrates oscillations in CMV viremia that could reliably predict the risk for CMV end-organ disease [62].

In patients with suspected CMV pneumonitis, CMV PCR in BAL fluid appears to be a sensitive test with good negative predictive values. Due to limited specificity for viral lung disease and inability to distinguish CMV lung disease versus asymptomatic respiratory tract viral shedding, use of CMV PCR in BAL samples is discouraged [63].

Nucleic acid sequence-based amplification (NASBA) is a new technology that measures early-immediate CMV mRNA and appears to be comparable to DNA PCR or pp65 antigenemia for the diagnosis of viremia; providing real-time guidance for preemptive antiviral therapy in patients following stem cell allograft transplantation [64]. Most transplant centers, however, still use pp65 antigenemia or CMV DNA PCR assays. A detailed review of diagnosis of CMV infection and disease is provided in Chaps. 47 and 49.

Risk Factors

Hematopoietic Stem Cell Transplantation

Allograft Stem Cell Transplants

Despite universal screening for CMV viremia and the institution of prophylactic or preemptive antiviral therapy in patients undergoing allogeneic HSCT, a small number of patients end up developing CMV end-organ disease during post-transplant period [65]. Donor and recipient CMV serostatus continues to be an essential factor in selection of stem cell grafts, with an appreciation for potential variability in engraftment kinetics, preparatory conditioning regimens, GVHD prophylaxis, and the underlying malignant versus non-malignant disorders.

The lowest risk of CMV infection and disease during post-transplant period is among seronegative donor and recipient (D−/R−) allograft transplantation. The highest risk (~30%) of newly acquired CMV infection is among seronegative patients undergoing HSCT from a CMV (+) donor (D+/R−). Primary CMV infection that is not transmitted via allograft now rarely occurs in patients given blood and blood products from CMV (+) donor(s) or acquired by natural transmission. It is important to recognize that heightened awareness and strict adherence to CMV screening, antiviral prophylaxis and preemptive therapy protocols, and recent addition of effective and safe antiviral drugs all contribute favorably toward improved outcomes in these high-risk (D+/R−) transplant recipients. However, in a study, mortality due to bacterial and fungal infections was noted to be significantly higher in this group (18%; D+/R−) compared with 10% mortality due to such infection observed in patients undergoing allograft stem cell transplantation with a low risk of newly acquired CMV infection (D−/R−) [66].

Patients with D+/R+ CMV serostatus often exhibit a complex dynamic of CMV transmission from the donor; it was interesting to note that in such patients transmission or reactivation of multiple CMV strains can occur [67]. Clinical significance of viremia due to newly acquired donor-specific viral strain(s) and reactivation of recipients' latent viral strains, or both, may influence outcome in a yet uncertain manner. The genetic variety and potential for a wide-ranging phenotypic viral variance may potentially influence viral kinetics, risk for end-organ disease, and importantly risk of drug resistance and response to antiviral drug therapy. Further investigation is needed.

Up to 80% of CMV-seropositive stem cell allograft recipients may have viral infection if no antiviral prophylaxis is given. The overall risk of CMV infection in allogeneic transplant recipients has been between 20% and 35%; however, it is important to underscore that advancement in risk estimation and intervention with preventive strategies has significantly modified such a risk [68]. Despite these highly effective interventions to prevent CMV disease in seropositive HSCT recipients, several investigators have reported that non-cancer relapse mortality remains high compared with CMV-seronegative recipient [69, 70]. The impact of donor CMV serostatus in seropositive HSCT recipients continues to be tendentious. Some studies have reported a beneficial effect of having seropositive donor with regards to a reduction in cancer relapse or non-cancer relapse mortality, whereas other studies have found no such advantage [71–79]. Despite the controversy for non-cancer relapse mortality and overall survival, transplantation in D−/R+ patients has resulted in delayed CMV-specific immune reconstitution, increased risk of CMV reactivation, CMV recurrence during late transplant period, and risk for end-organ CMV disease [80–85].

Patients undergoing mismatched or unrelated donor graft transplants, indication for HSCT (cancer vs. other disorders), T cell depletion, acute GVHD, and high-dose (1 mg/kg per day) corticosteroid use are all recognized as factors that promote risk for CMV infection in this population [86–90]. Similarly, it is uncertain if the source of stem cell graft either from peripheral blood or marrow-derived stem cells makes a significant impact on the risk for CMV infection in the post-transplant period. There are reports of CMV risk divergence based on the source of allograft; however, others have controverted such findings [85, 87, 90–92]. Mechanistic target of rapamycin such as sirolimus appears to modify cellular signaling pathways that are influenced or assimilated by CMV-encoded viral proteins; use of sirolimus for GVHD prophylaxis has been observed to protect against CMV infection and disease [85, 93].

Late CMV Infections

In the era of preemptive ganciclovir therapy during early (<100 days) transplant period, CMV infections are gaining increasing, albeit, dubious recognition during the late (≥100 days) transplant period [94, 95]. CMV infection 100 days after transplantation was strongly associated with the risk for non-cancer relapse mortality [84]. In 15–30% of allogeneic HSCT recipients, late CMV infection may occur if no antiviral measures are put in place, resulting in CMV end-organ disease in approximately 6–18% of such patients [96–98]. Those at risk for late CMV infection are (a) patients who developed CMV infection or disease within first 100 days after transplantation, (b) patients exhibiting a lack of CMV-specific immune reconstitution, (c) patients with presence of persistently low lymphocytes in the peripheral blood, and (d) patients with acute or (e) chronic GVHD [84, 88, 99, 100]. In select group of patients with such risk factors, anti-CMV prophylaxis may be extended beyond 100 days after transplantation. It is also imperative to continue weekly viral surveillance using pp65 antigenemia or CMV blood PCR, and in patients with the evidence of continued viremia, preemptive therapy may reduce the burden of late transplant CMV disease [98, 101].

Nonmyeloablative Transplants

The risk of CMV infection and disease in the early post-transplant period is substantially lower in patients undergoing nonmyeloablative conditioning in preparation for matched, related donor stem cell graft compared with patients given conventional myeloablative preparatory regimens [101, 102]. However, the risk of CMV infection and disease appeared to be similar among nonmyeloablative and myeloablative groups after the first year following transplantation [101, 102]. It is important to recognize that in T cell depletion and transplantation using matched, unrelated donor grafts, the risk reduction for early CMV infection becomes unnoticeable between nonmyeloablative and myeloablative transplantation procedures [101, 103].

Autologous Stem Cell Transplantation

It has long been recognized that cytomegalovirus infection influences engraftment capacity of autografts during the aplastic period. A significant predictive relationship was shown between CMV infection and delay in granulocyte recovery, whereas such a relationship was not evident for the recovery in platelet counts after autologous transplantation. In nearly 40% of CMV-seropositive patients undergoing autologous transplantation, CMV can be detected by pp65 antigenemia or viral DNA in the peripheral blood [104, 105]. However, despite these high rates of CMV viremia, end-organ disease is seldom seen in patients undergoing autologous SCT [106–108]. In this group, when CMV pneumonia does occur, the outcome for such a devastating viral lung disease is similar to that seen in allogeneic HSCT recipients [109]. CD34+ selected grafts, treatment with high-dose corticosteroids, and conditioning regimen with fludarabine or total-body irradiation increases the risk for CMV disease following autologous SCT [91]. CMV does not pose a serious risk for patients undergoing autologous SCT and routine antiviral prophylaxis, and viral surveillance is therefore not recommended. However, a select group of high-risk patients following autologous stem cell transplant may benefit from routine surveillance and preemptive anti-CMV therapy.

Cord Blood Stem Cell Transplants

Umbilical cord blood provides a novel source of stem cell for suitable recipients [110]. Such allografts are virtually always CMV-negative. Among CMV-seropositive recipients of cord blood stem cell transplantation (CBT), lack of antiviral prophylaxis would result in an unacceptable rate of CMV infection, which is reported between 40% and 80% although in one report, all patients undergoing such transplants developed CMV reactivation [111–115]. High-dose valacyclovir prophylaxis was shown to reduce increased CMV risk after cord blood transplantation to what has been known for patients undergoing peripheral blood or marrow stem cell allograft transplantation [116].

In a report of 100 CBT, the overall incidence of infection was 2.4 times higher in adults compared with children undergoing transplants with cord blood stem cell allografts [117]. In adults, overall infection risk was significantly higher in the presence of severe neutropenia (3 × higher) and GVHD (1.9 × higher). Late (>100 days) cytomegalovirus infections occurred only in children with chronic GVHD [117]. Multivariate analysis showed that resolution of lymphocytopenia (≥1000 cells/ml) and successful stem cell engraftment were significantly protective against the risk of serious infection (hazard ratio 0.71 and 0.20, respectively) [117]. Due to the substantial risk and potential burden of CMV infections in patients undergoing CBT, continued viral surveillance, especially in patients with acute or chronic GVHD, necessitates optimized CMV prevention and preemptive treatment strategies.

CMV Disease in HSCT

CMV infection in transplant patients implies presence of CMV in blood by direct qualitative or quantitative measurement of viral DNA or by measurement of viral surrogate like pp65 antigenemia. It is also important to recognize that transplant patients similar to general population, despite having a noteworthy vulnerability for viremia and end-organ disease, may develop asymptomatic viral shedding at various body sites. Therefore, isolation of cytomegalovirus DNA in bodily fluids such as urine, tears, nasal, upper respiratory tract secretions, and orointestinal tract may not necessarily indicate viral organ disease. This is in contrast to viral isolation in CSF and BAL culture samples in patients with a compatible clinical illness [118]. It is important to note presence of CMV DNA by PCR in CSF and especially BAL samples are of value due to its high negative predictive value that may assist in ruling out CMV infection or end-organ viral disease.

CMV can cause disease in almost any organ system, although CMV disease designation should be approached with great caution as other infections and non-infectious complications may be misconstrued as CMV disease. This is further complicated by the fact that protean clinical presentation of cytomegalovirus infection most commonly presents as a nonspecific febrile illness.

The first step is to identify hosts' immunologic susceptibility for end-organ CMV disease. In such patients, isolation of cytomegalovirus in tissue cultures is important; for example, in patients suspected to have CMV-related loss of stem cell graft, culture isolation of the virus in marrow aspirate or biopsy sample is highly suggestive, whereas a positive PCR for CMV DNA is not considered adequate to establish viral causality for the loss of stem cell graft [119].

CMV pneumonitis in symptomatic patients with a suggestive radiographic presentation of viral interstitial pneumonitis or, at times, nodular infiltrates needs to be differentiated from other pulmonary infections such as common respiratory tract viral infections, drug toxicity, and PCP, in addition to the growing recognition of various syndromes associated with pulmonary GVHD. Detection of CMV by viral culture in lower respiratory tract samples such as bronchoalveolar lavage fluid is encouraged. Lung biopsy samples are seldom available in stem cell transplant recipients due to severe thrombocytopenia and dysregulation in coagulation pathways, or limited functional respiratory reserve; although these potential contraindications for lung biopsy do not exist in most SOT patients in whom CMV pneumonitis may be suspected. Presence of CMV by (+) PCR is not adequate; diagnosis of CMV pneumonitis requires isolation of virus in lower respiratory tract fluid or tissue culture samples along with evidence of viral inclusions and/or immunohistochemical viral confirmation in lung biopsy samples [119]. It has been proposed that in HSCT recipients, isolation of other opportunistic pathogens like filamentous fungi in the setting radiologic features consistent with IFD probably indicates fungal pneumonia rather than CMV pneumonia, when such a diagnosis is based on (+) CMV PCR alone [119]. The authors would like to emphasize that various immunologic aberrations and compromised structural respiratory tract barrier as a consequence of cytomegalovirus infection promote the risk for secondary superimposed bacterial and fungal lung disease that may occur concurrently or sequentially after viral lung infection.

Suspected viral eye disease including retinitis requires detailed examination by an ophthalmologist or a specialist in retinal disease. Similarly, in patients with orointestinal CMV disease, the diagnosis is predicated upon isolation of cytomegalovirus in tissue cultures along with histologically compatible disease with immunohistochemical confirmation. Detection of CMV by PCR by itself is considered insufficient for the diagnosis of CMV gastrointestinal disease [119].

CNS disease should be suspected in patients with acute or chronic changes in mentation or cognition, persistent headaches, and other symptoms eluding to intracranial disease process. Isolation of CMV in CSF cultures is highly suggestive although most experts agree that isolation of CMV DNA by PCR in CSF sample in a susceptible patient with clinical and radiographic features consistent with CMV encephalitis or myelitis is adequate for diagnosis. In certain patients, brain biopsy may be approached to confirm diagnosis, especially in individuals with localized or focal brain lesions. This is attempted to exclude other potential causes like neurotropic molds, dimorphic fungi, tuberculous or nontuberculous mycobacteria, *Nocardia*, parasite like *Toxoplasma gondii*, and among noninfectious conditions like primary CNS lymphoma or metastatic cancers.

CMV Pneumonia

Cytomegalovirus lung infection that often presents as multifocal interstitial pneumonitis is an important CMV disease in patients undergoing high-risk blood and marrow stem cell transplantation and is historically associated with an unacceptably high mortality rate ranging between 60% and 90% [120].

The incidence and risk for developing fatal CMV pneumonia were assessed after a review of 999 autopsies [121]. Twenty-five patients who died with CMV pneumonia were compared with 34 similar patients. The incidence of CMV pneumonia was 3.5% during 1990–1997 at a major Comprehensive Cancer Center in the United States; a sizeable decline in the incidence of CMV pneumonitis (0.8%) during 1997 through 2004 was encouraging [121]. Sustained and prolonged lymphopenia was a well-recognized risk factor for CMV infection and disease. Routine anti-CMV prophylaxis in susceptible population and preemptive antiviral treatment approach based on sensitive new-generation quantitative viral assays have greatly improved the overall incidence of end-organ CMV disease including viral lung disease [122].

Most patients present with fever, cough without sputum production, dyspnea and hypoxia on exertion that subsequently progresses to disabling shortness of breath at rest. Onset of symptoms are usually insidious; if the diagnosis and treatment is delayed, the disease in vast majority of cases progresses to severe hypoxemia and respiratory failure requiring assisted ventilatory support within 1–2 weeks after the process commenced. Chest rays are not sensitive for the diagnosis of CMV pneumonitis [123]. A high-resolution CT scan without IV contrast may show early interstitial viral infiltrates (Fig. 37.1a, b) [124]. Rarely, pulmonary nodules

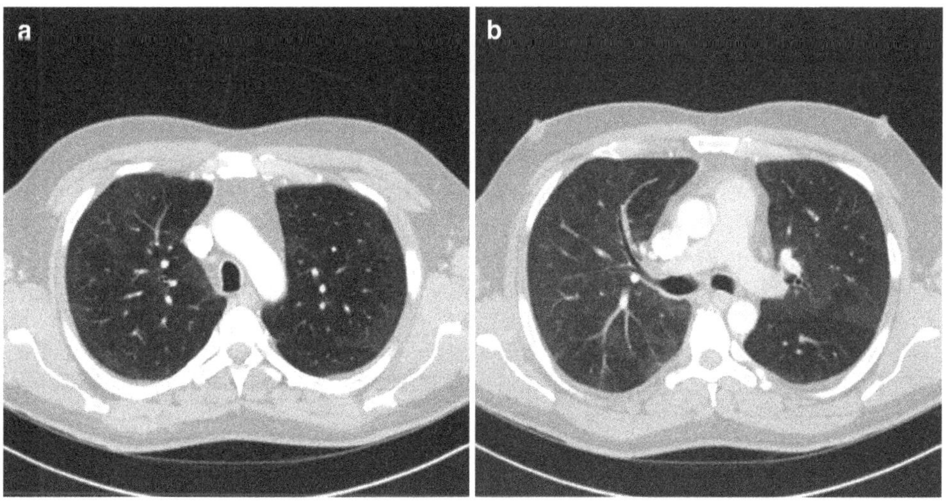

Fig. 37.1 (**a**) Computed tomography scan of the lungs without intravenous contrast showing characteristic early multicentric bilateral acute interstitial lung disease in a patient with cytomegalovirus pneumonitis. (**b**) Computed tomography scan of the lungs without intravenous contrast showing characteristic advanced multicentric bilateral acute interstitial lung disease in the same patient with cytomegalovirus pneumonitis (**a**). (Images courtesy of Dr. Edmundo Calleros, MD, DABR, of Texas Tech University Health Sciences Center El Paso, Paul L. Foster School of Medicine)

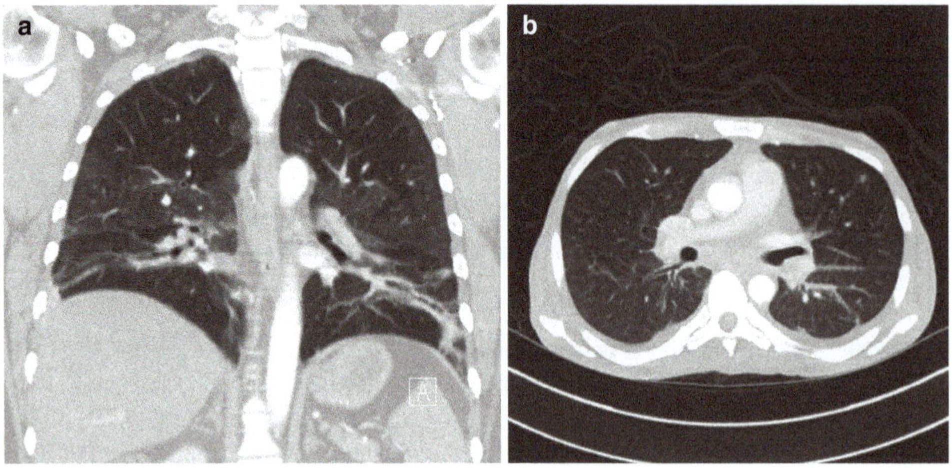

Fig. 37.2 (**a**) Computed tomography scan of the lungs without intravenous contrast showing not so uncommonly seen bilateral acute interstitial lung disease with peribronchial thickening and nodular lung disease with cytomegalovirus pneumonitis. (**b**) Computed tomography scan of the lungs without intravenous contrast showing anterolateral, peripheral left lung nodule in a severely immunosuppressed patient with cytomegalovirus pneumonitis. (Images courtesy of Dr. Edmundo Calleros, MD, DABR, of Texas Tech University Health Sciences Center El Paso, Paul L. Foster School of Medicine)

and cavitary pneumonia are attributed to cytomegalovirus lung disease, especially in severely immunosuppressed individuals (Fig. 37.2a, b).

The diagnosis of CMV pneumonia requires demonstration of viable, replicating virus in BAL or lung biopsy samples by shell vial or cultures. In the event biopsy is a possibility, presence of CMV in the lung tissue by immunohistochemical assays is considered diagnostic. CMV shedding in the lower respiratory tract is not uncommon among transplant population and should not be used for the diagnosis of CMV pneumonia.

In a randomized, controlled trial of ganciclovir prophylaxis for CMV pneumonia in patients undergoing HSCT, strongest predictors of CMV pneumonia was CMV-positive culture in BAL and blood samples [125]. Nearly two-thirds of asymptomatic patients developed CMV pneumonia subsequently [125]. As mentioned earlier, performing CMV DNA PCR in BAL fluid samples for the purpose of diagnosing CMV pneumonia is discouraged. A negative BAL CMV DNA PCR carries high negative predictive value which may assist in ruling out CMV as a cause of pneumonia [63].

CMV Retinitis

Major ocular complications in allogeneic HSCT recipients include chronic GVHD, dry eye syndrome in the absence of GVHD, corneal ulcers, cataract, and glaucoma [126]. CMV retinitis, varicella zoster virus, and fungal endophthalmitis are rare but devastating infections. It is also interesting that in some patients allergic conjunctivitis may be acquired from atopic donors and may be mistaken for acute viral infection, since the recipient had no prior history of allergic conjunctivitis before undergoing transplantation [126].

In CMV retinitis, though uncommon in allogeneic HSCT recipients, clinical presentation is not dissimilar to that observed in patients with advanced HIV/AIDS. CMV eye disease presents with gradual and progressive loss of vision; however, sudden blindness has also been reported. CMV, like varicella zoster virus posterior eye chamber involvement, includes retinitis, retinal hemorrhage, vitritis; whereas, anterior chamber infection presents as uveitis, or iridocyclitis. Patients with initial single eye involvement have greater than 50% risk for contralateral eye to become involved, if not treated preemptively [127]. Most cases of CMV retinitis are seen after 100 days following transplantation and often associated with the evidence of GVHD, delayed lymphocyte engraftment, and early (<100 days) CMV reactivation [127].

In 2014, five cases of CMV retinitis were a significant increase in children undergoing allogeneic HSCT at a transplant center in the United States [128]. These sporadic cluster of cases may occur from time to time, although there have been no reports of systematic increase in the incidence of CMV retinitis in HSCT population. Continued ophthalmic assessment and screening are part of routine comprehensive care provided for transplant recipients.

CMV Hepatitis

CMV hepatitis like other viral infections such as adenovirus, HHV6, and EBV among others is difficult to distinguish clinically from non-infectious causes of liver injury including drug toxicity, and GVHD [129, 130]. Among allogeneic HSCT recipients, high-dose corticosteroids, T cell-depleted graft, acute and chronic GVHD, and mismatched or unrelated donor stem cell grafts are well-recognized risk factors for CMV infection and end-organ disease. Diagnosis requires histologic and CMV identification by immunohistochemical stain performed on liver tissue biopsy samples. As obtaining liver biopsy may not be always feasible, a high degree of suspicion, along with presence of CMV viremia, that have coincided with acute hepatocellular injury may provide an indication for possible CMV etiology in patients with acute hepatitis. Post-transplant reactivation of chronic, latent HBV and HCV infections should always be an essential part of such investigations.

CMV Encephalitis

Viral encephalitis is most notably seen during the late post-transplant period. The median time from HSCT to diagnosis was recently reported as 145 days [131]. In a report from China, RSV was the most prominent pathogen (50%), whereas cytomegalovirus (7%), and HHV6 and HSV (3% each) were less common. Clinical presentation included alterations in mentation and new-onset seizures. Neuroimaging showed abnormality in close to 80% of patients. Elevated protein in cerebral spinal fluid was present in 60%, whereas pleocytosis and elevated or normal glucose levels were noted in less than one-third of patients. Multivariate analyses revealed high-grade acute GVHD, presence of CMV viremia, and engraftment syndrome as significant risk factors for viral encephalitis [131].

The classic histologic feature of CMV brain infection is non-lethal cytotoxic edema due to intracellular viral inclusions (Figs. 37.3 and 37.4). This edema forms the basis of highly suggestive long-lasting diffusion restriction findings noted in brain MRI scans in patients with CMV cerebritis [132].

Punctiform lesions on diffusion-weighted MRI images appear to have a clear ventricle wall tropism, validated on classical autopsy findings in patients with CMV encephalitis [132].

Subependymal and periventricular punctiform-restricted diffusion lesions on IV contrast-enhanced MRI in patients with clinical features of meningoencephalitis are highly suggestive of CMV encephalitis [132].

It is important to note that encephalitis due to other neurotropic viruses like adenovirus, EBV, VZV, HSV, and HHV-6 may elicit a clinical syndrome that is difficult to distinguish from CMV brain disease. HHV6 encephalitis is mostly seen during early post-transplant period and patients appear to have high-grade HHV6 viremia [133].

CMV Myelosuppression

CMV-induced myelosuppression or hematopoietic stem cell graft failure needs to be distinguished from recipients' immunologic rejection of the stem cell allograft, myelotoxicity resulting from a cornucopia of drug cocktails given to patients following transplantation. Furthermore, alternative causes of myelosuppression like (a) recurrence of hematologic malignancy, (b) bone marrow infiltration due to lymphoproliferative disorders among others, and (c) infection

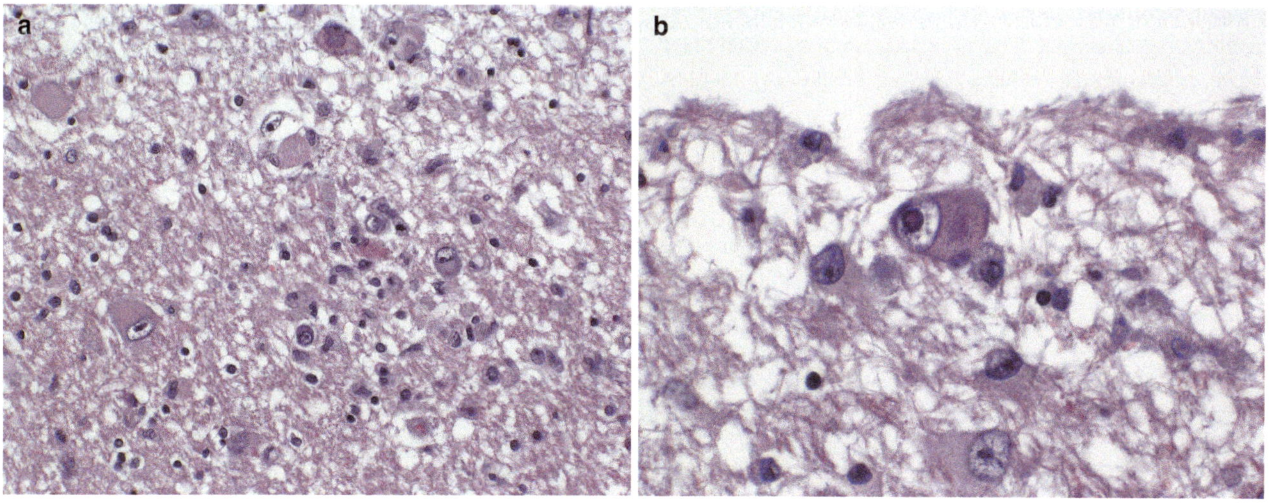

Fig. 37.3 Hematoxylin and eosin stain of subependymal white matter, the lower power (**a**; 40×) showing multiple enlarged astrocytes with prominent inclusion bodies in the nuclei. There is also lymphocytic infiltration in the tissue indicating inflammation. The higher power (**b**; 100×) emphasizes an enlarged astrocyte bearing both a large intranuclear inclusion and basophilic stippling of the cytoplasm representing cytoplasmic inclusions also characteristic of cytomegalovirus encephalitis. (Images courtesy of Dr. Marc K. Rosenblum of Memorial Sloan-Kettering Cancer Center, New York, NY)

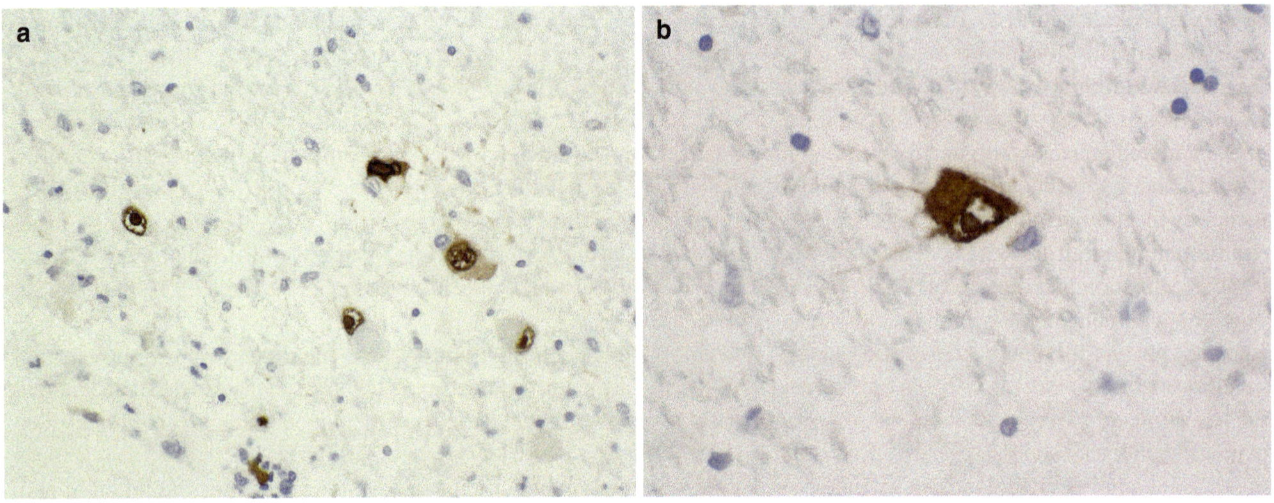

Fig. 37.4 Immunohistochemistry for cytomegalovirus in brain sample at (**a**) 40× and (**b**) 100× magnification. The higher magnification shows antibody labeling of both the intranuclear inclusion and the viral inclusions in the cytoplasm. (Images courtesy of Dr. Marc K. Rosenblum of Memorial Sloan-Kettering Cancer Center, New York, NY)

due to myelotoxic viruses like HHV6, EBV, adenovirus, and parvovirus B19 should be part of such an evaluation. Patients with severe peripheral blood pancytopenia thought to result from CMV-associated graft failure need demonstration of (a) bone marrow hypoplasia, (b) detection of cytomegalovirus in marrow sample culture, (c) exclusion of stem cell graft rejection, and (d) recurrence of cancer [119].

CMV Gastrointestinal Tract Disease

CMV can affect any part of orointestinal tract. Viral esophagitis similar to HSV or *Candida* esophagitis may occur without significant disease in the oral cavity. Difficulty in swallowing, substernal chest pain, and epigastric discomfort are common clinical features. On endoscopic examination, confluent or nonconfluent pseudomembranous lesions, confluent or nonconfluent deep mucosal ulcers that may be more pronounced in the distal esophagus are prominent findings.

Patients with CMV enteritis and colitis may present with abdominal pain, diarrhea, and abdominal distention; these patients are often febrile. Presence of hematochezia heralds underlying severe ulcerative CMV colitis. In such patients, viral ulcers may extend deep into the submucosa. Clinically, and by visual inspection on endoscopic examination, gastrointestinal viral disease is difficult to distinguish from GVHD. Diagnosis require culture isolation of CMV in tissue biopsy samples and immunohistologic evidence of viral disease; albeit both of these diagnostic approaches lack sensitivity. Diagnosis of CMV gastrointestinal disease is further complicated as patients may not have evidence of CMV viremia or antigenemia at the time of clinical presentation [134, 135]. CMV gastritis, gastric and duodenal viral ulcers, when suspected, also require biopsy of the affected site for viral culture and immunohistologic assessment.

Solid Organ Transplantation

Risk Factors

A recent report of CMV infection using the Scientific Registry of Transplant Receipts data published between 2005 and 2014 showed the overall rates of donor and recipient CMV seropositivity have remained constant over the reported period. It was encouraging that among living donor transplantation, there were more CMV-seronegative donors and recipients over the span of this data registry [136]. This probably reflected a donor selection bias and a preference for CMV-seronegative living donors for seronegative patients awaiting transplantation with stable end-stage organ disease.

Patients receiving calcineurin inhibitor, mycophenolate mofetil, and corticosteroid-based regimens intended for solid organ allograft preservation have high susceptibility for CMV infection and disease. The drugs that inhibit mechanistic target of rapamycin (mTOR) such as sirolimus and everolimus exhibit indirect protection against cytomegalovirus. This has propelled the hypothesis for use of such agents in calcineurin inhibitor-sparing antirejection regimen to reduce the risk for CMV infection and disease, especially among at risk population. A recent review of existing literature regarding potential benefit of mTOR inhibitors on the risk for opportunistic viral infection after transplantation showed a favorable impact on the risk of CMV, polyomavirus, and HHV8 infections, whereas there was no advantage noted for post-transplant infections due to EBV and HCV [137].

Presently, calcineurin inhibitor-based regimen is preferred, specifically for patients considered at high risk for allograft rejection. However, calcineurin inhibitor-sparing regimen that includes mTOR inhibitor with various permutations including or excluding mycophenolate mofetil, corticosteroids, and thymocyte globulins are under investigation.

It was recently demonstrated that in patients undergoing solid organ allograft transplantation, risk of post-transplant CMV reactivation and disease can be measured by evaluating subpopulation of active CMV-specific CD8 cells that produce IFN-γ [138]. Patients who exhibited ≥0.25% CMV-specific active CD8 cells prior to transplantation and 0.15% or 0.25% 2 and 4 weeks following transplantation, respectively, had adequate control of CMV infection and were purposed to require less viral monitoring. Others have also reported that monitoring CMV-specific T cell kinetics, especially against CMV major early immediate protein (IE-1) before and after transplantation in patients receiving CMV discordant (D+/R−) renal allograft, may provide a better risk stratification for appraising the risk of post-transplant CMV infection [139]. The authors reported that pre- and post-transplant declining or undetectable CMV IE1-specific T cells identified a subgroup of patients that have high frequency of CMV viremia (81%) after kidney transplantation, in whom graft was harvested from CMV-seropositive donor ($P < 0.001$) [139].

Heart & Lung Transplants

In lung transplant recipients, infections are a significant complication. Within first year after transplantation, infections are the leading cause of death [140]. In lung transplant reipients, allograft rejection also continues to be an important challenge that presents as either acute graft failure or chronic allograft dysfunction due to bronchiolitis obliterans syndrome. Nearly half of long-term transplant survivors develop bronchiolitis obliterans syndrome within 5 years after undergoing lung transplantation [140]. CMV infection remains a serious complication in SOT population; recipients of pulmonary allograft are regarded as a high-risk group. It is daunting to ascertain a delicate balance between iatrogenic antirejection drug-induced, cumulative immunosuppression, which is necessary for the allograft preservation, and, on the other hand, an attempt to preserve hosts' adaptive immune surveillance needed to protect against opportunistic infections among whom, CMV leads the stage as the protagonist. This is certainly the case in patients after high-risk allograft transplantation and those who need aggressive treatment for moderate to severe allograft rejection.

In 378 consecutive heart transplant recipients, CMV infections were significantly more common in older patients [141]. Treatment with rabbit thymoglobulin or with T-cell acute lymphoblastic leukemia cell line Jurkat-derived ATG-Fresenius had twofold higher risk for CMV infection compared with patients in whom such induction regimens were not used [141]. Everolimus compared with azathioprine or mycophenolate significantly lowered the risk of CMV infection (OR 0.19; $p < 0.0001$). It is also pertinent to note that other major opportunistic infections were significantly more common in patients with CMV infection or viral end-organ disease following heart transplantation [141].

In lung transplant recipients, mycophenolate-sparing antirejection regimen with everolimus was noted to reduce the incidence of CMV infection [142]. These patients also had lower rates of lower respiratory tract infection, leukopenia, post-transplant bronchiolitis obliterans syndrome, and biopsy-proven acute pulmonary allograft rejection [142]. The increased dropout rate in everolimus treatment group was in most part due to drug intolerability.

Liver Transplantation

A recent meta-analysis included 21 retrospective observational studies that included over 8000 patients and showed no survival benefit in hepatic graft donor/recipient ABO blood group concordance [143]. However, patients undergoing orthotopic liver transplantation from AOB blood type incompatible donor had significant high risk for CMV infection (OR = 2.6), incidence in antibody-mediated rejection (OR = 74), risk of chronic rejection (OR = 2.3), overall biliary (OR = 1.5), and hepatic artery complications (OR = 4.2) compared with patients given liver graft from ABO compatible donor [143].

HHV6 infections in liver transplant recipients are known to cause hepatitis, encephalitis, and graft dysfunction. The indirect effects of HHV6 infection in this population were reported to increase risk for (a) CMV disease, (b) post-transplant HCV progression, (c) greater fibrosis scores, and (d) death [144].

Kidney and Pancreases Transplant

As with other visceral allograft transplantation, donor and recipient CMV discordance (D+/R−) is the most important determinant for CMV infection and organ disease following transplantation. In early antiviral prophylaxis trials, 48–67% of kidney transplant recipients that were randomized in the placebo group developed CMV disease within first year after transplant procedure [145, 146]. The risk was highest among D+/R− (48%) compared with D+/R+ (6%) renal allograft recipients [145]. Additionally, more than half of the patients without antiviral prophylaxis developed acute graft rejection within 6 months after transplant surgery [145, 146].

In a large prospective study that assessed 609 kidney and kidney-pancreas recipients, 18% developed CMV viremia after a median 5.6 months after transplantation [147]. Patients were given standardized CMV prophylaxis, and close to 90% of patients with CMV infection were asymptomatic [147]. In multivariate analysis, D+/R− serostatus, older donor age more than >50 years, high tacrolimus, and mycophenolic doses were significant risk factors for CMV infection [147]. As expected, D−/R− status yielded lowest risk for CMV infection after transplantation. Patients who did develop symptomatic CMV disease had 3.5 times higher risk for allograft loss [147]. As noted with other transplants, pooled analysis of randomized controlled trials found that risk of CMV viremia and end-organ disease was significantly reduced in patients given mTOR inhibitors versus mycophenolate [148].

A similar CMV disease rate was observed in patients undergoing pancreas transplants. The overall CMV infection rate in this group was 24% among 130 pancreas-kidney or pancreas after kidney allograft recipients, in whom antiviral prophylaxis was continued for a median of 49 days [149]. CMV-seronegative recipient status (D+/R−) was associated with the highest risk (44%) for CMV infection during the post-transplant period, whereas only 8% had CMV infection in pre-transplant CMV-seropositive group [149].

In 407 pancreas allograft recipients, the incidence of CMV infection was highest in D+/R− (20%), followed by 17% in D+/R+ and 5% in D−/R+, and lowest (3%) when transplants were performed in seronegative donor and recipients [150]. Most infections occurred 90 days after transplantation, and despite no reduction in immune suppression in most patients (72%), none of these patients experienced adverse outcomes that included CMV-related deaths or loss of the allograft [150].

Intestinal and Multivisceral Transplant

Intestinal transplant recipients are especially vulnerable to serious CMV-related complications. The incidence of CMV infection is close to 40%, and most infections are seen within 60 days after transplantation [151]. A vast majority (81%) of CMV disease affects intestinal allograft. Risk of CMV disease is greater in (a) D+/R−, (b) isolated intestinal transplant recipients, patients with high net state of immune suppression resulting from (c) high tacrolimus serum levels, and (d) higher cumulative corticosteroid dose [151]. It is important to note that over half of the patients with clinical and histopathologically proven CMV visceral disease did not have detectable CMV viremia by DNA PCR analysis [151].

In children undergoing intestinal transplantation, incidence of CMV is lower (24%) compared with adults following similar allograft transplants [152]. Most infections are also noted within 2 months after transplantation, and 90% CMV disease involves the visceral transplanted allograft [152]. In children, no CMV disease was noted when both donor and recipients were seronegative [152]. As with adults, high cumulative corticosteroid dose was associated with greater risk of CMV disease in children [152]. Recent studies have shown a lower incidence of CMV infection (18%) and disease (7%) in pediatric transplant recipients [153]. As noted, most end-organ CMV disease in patients undergoing intestinal transplantation involve the transplanted allograft, and disease recurrence occurs in 50–86% of patients, in whom an initial response to antiviral therapy was observed [152, 153]. Presence of CMV disease increases the risk of death by 11-fold in patients undergoing intestinal transplantation and, indirectly, enhances their vulnerability for EBV infection and PTLD [153].

Face, Limbs, and Integument Transplant

CMV infection in patients receiving composite tissue allotransplantation has evolved as one the most important infection challenges during the post-transplant period [154, 155]. Seronegative receipts following allograft harvested from seropositive donor are at the greatest risk for CMV infection and disease. Due to elevated iatrogenic immune suppression needed in such patients, response to anti-CMV therapy is often erratic; infection and viral disease relapse are common [154, 155].

Biologics and Risk of CMV

The risk of CMV infection in patients receiving conventional chemotherapy for hematological malignancies is low [156]. Therefore, routine CMV screening in the asymptomatic patients receiving fludarabine, hyperfractionated cyclophosphamide, vincristine, doxorubicin and dexamethasone, or rituximab is not recommended. In non-HSCT patients, rate of CMV infection or viral reactivation ranges between 2% and 67% [157]. Some of the prominent although putative risk factors include treatment with high-dose corticosteroids, advanced malignancy, poor performance status, and treatment with alemtuzumab, fludarabine, Velcade, and rituximab [157]. CMV prophylaxis and preemptive therapy are reserved for only high-risk patients and not given routinely in non-transplant patients undergoing treatment with biologic immune suppressive agents.

Alemtuzumab (Campath)

Alemtuzumab is a recombinant DNA-derived humanized monoclonal antibody directed against CD52, a cell surface glycoprotein. It is used in the treatment of chronic lymphocytic leukemia, T cell prolymphocytic leukemic, cutaneous T cell lymphoma, and T cell lymphoma. CMV reactivation after Campath usually occurs within 3–6 weeks following therapy and the incidence ranges between 10% and 66% [158, 159]. Up to one-third of CMV infections in patients after Campath therapy are symptomatic and may present with a nonspecific febrile illness [160]. Patients at risk for CMV reactivation being treated with Campath may benefit from anti-CMV drug prophylaxis. The data regarding valganciclovir is encouraging. In a randomized trial, 35% of patients given valacyclovir (500 mg daily) prophylaxis developed CMV reactivation, where none had CMV reactivation in valganciclovir (450 mg bid) treatment group [161]. Valganciclovir three times a week was also reported to be effective in preventing CMV reactivation [162].

Preemptive anti-CMV therapy instead of prophylaxis is another approach, which is similar to all preemptive antiviral regimens and requires close monitoring for early and sustained viral reactivation using pp65 antigenemia or viral DNA PCR in blood [163]. CMV monitoring should be continued for 8 weeks after treatment with Campath has been discontinued [164]. In patients with evidence of CMV viremia during Campath therapy, it is suggested to withhold further treatment with the biologic agent until viremia has resolved. A thorough assessment for possible end-organ CMV disease should be undertaken and treated according to the established standards [165].

Pancreas-kidney dual organ transplant recipients in whom alemtuzumab induction therapy was compared with historical controls that received induction with basiliximab at a single transplant center in the US. There was no difference in patients, renal, or pancreas allograft survival, or renal allograft delayed graft function, incidence of PTLD, and sepsis in the two groups [166]. Infections due to EBV or BKV were not significantly dissimilar in the cohorts studied [166]. It is, however, important to note that the incidence of CMV infection was significantly higher in the alemtuzumab-treatment group vs. patients in whom basiliximab induction was given [166]. This observation resulted in modification of induction protocol at this center from two-dose alemtuzumab to a single 30 mg-dose induction therapy [166]. Alemtuzumab was still considered desirable due to low drug cost and few acute drug-related toxicities during induction for abdominal visceral transplantation.

Rituximab

Rituximab is a human-mouse chimeric monoclonal antibody that has been successfully used to treat B-cell non-Hodgkin's lymphoma, certain autoimmune diseases, and dermatologic disorders like Pemphigus vulgaris, post-transplant B-cell-mediated allograft rejection, and PTLD which are among other constantly emerging uses for this effective anti-CD20 biologic immune-modulatory drug.

The risk of cytomegalovirus infection is considerable in allogeneic HSCT and solid organ transplantation recipients receiving high-dose rituximab therapy. However, it was interesting to note that in 49 patients with primary post-transplant CMV infection, 32 patients received low-dose rituximab therapy and exhibited no clinical or immunologic difference compared with 17 such patients in whom rituximab was not given [167].

In a literature review, 64 reported cases of serious viral infection after rituximab therapy in patients with lymphoma, the median time from the start of rituximab treatment and diagnosis of viral infection was 5 months and ranged between 1 and 20 months [168]. Infections due to HBV (39%), CMV (23%), and varicella-zoster virus (9%) were the three prominent viral infections. Among HBV-seropositive patients, just over half of the patients had developed fatal liver failure. In contrast, nearly one-third of the patients with other severe systemic viral illness following rituximab therapy including CMV, had died [168]. The cause of death in the latter group could not be fully attributed to CMV or varicella zoster disease.

In allograft CMV-seropositive transplant patients undergoing rituximab therapy, risk for CMV infection and disease is much higher than in patients undergoing autologous SCT [169]. In a report of nearly 1000 autologous SCT recipients, 239 patients had clinical suspicion for symptomatic CMV reactivation. Among these, only 3% had confirmation of CMV viremia that developed after a median of 32 days following transplantation [169]. CMV viremia was detected in 4% of patients in whom rituximab was given, whereas 2% in patients without rituximab therapy. In this report, rituximab therapy in autologous stem cell graft recipients did not contribute to significant increase in CMV reactivation, end-organ disease, or death [169].

In 182 patient experience following T cell depleted matched unrelated or haploidentical donor stem cell transplant was recently reported [170]. In this high-risk group, half of the patients developed CMV viremia, whereas end-organ viral disease was noted in 6% of the patients. High-grade acute GVHD, D−/R+ CMV serology, and cancer as an indication for transplantation were prominent risk factors for CMV viremia. Treatment with rituximab significantly reduced risk for EBV reactivation in whom high B cell-containing stem cell grafts were given. The authors reported an increase in the rate of CMV viremia following TCR-α/β and CD19-depleted stem cell allografts; however, rituximab therapy did not result in unfavorable survival or risk for end-organ CMV disease. Furthermore, in this group, use of CD19-depleted allografts and rituximab combination in select high-risk patients eliminated the risk of PTLD [170].

CMV antiviral drug prophylaxis is not routinely recommended for transplant patients undergoing treatment with rituximab. It is however recommended that in high-risk allogeneic stem cell graft recipients, a greater degree of vigilance for CMV reactivation and viremia, or both should be maintained during and 3 months after completing anti-CD20 antibody therapy. As with any other at-risk transplant group, clinical suspicion for viral end-organ disease should prompt appropriate investigation and commencement of effective antiviral drug therapy.

Basiliximab

Basiliximab is a chimeric mouse-human monoclonal antibody that has high affinity against CD25, the α chain of the IL-2 receptor expressed on T lymphocytes. It is indicated for the prevention of acute renal allograft rejection. Basiliximab was shown to significantly reduce acute renal allograft rejection compared with cyclosporine and corticosteroids or triple antirejection therapy [171]. The efficacy of basiliximab was similar to that of equine antithymocyte globulin and daclizumab and perhaps superior to muromonab-CD3. The incidence of adverse events had been similar in basiliximab-treated patients versus those given conventional induction. Secondary malignancies and PTLD after transplants were rare and were similar in basiliximab vs. the control group [171]. It is important to note that incidence of CMV infection did not increase after basiliximab preparatory antirejection therapy compared with conventional dual or triple drug combinations [171]. The incidence of CMV infection was also similar with basiliximab, compared with patients given induction therapy using equine or rabbit antithymocyte globulin [171].

In heart transplant recipients, the results of 22 randomized clinical trials were systematically assessed for immunosuppressive T cell antibody induction; these trials had data in 1427 heart-transplant recipients [172]. Chronic allograft vasculopathy, renal dysfunction, PTLD, and risk of other cancers were not significantly dissimilar across these studies. There was also no noteworthy difference in the risk of infections, including CMV infection and risk of death [172]. It was important to note that acute cardiac allograft rejection occurred less frequently when IL-2 receptor antagonist was given (33%) compared with no induction (45%; RR 0.73) [172].

CMV Prevention

CMV Risk Reduction

CMV-seronegative patients should ideally receive an allograft from a CMV-negative donor. This is true for patients awaiting hematopoietic blood or marrow stem cells or solid organ allograft transplantation. In patients undergoing allogeneic stem cell transplantation, major human leukocyte antigen compatibility is regarded as of greater significance than discordance between donor and recipient CMV serostatus (D+/R−). However, taking into account the risks that newly, graft-acquired CMV infection poses in such patients, some experts have questioned the current practice and advocated that CMV-negative donor being more preferential than graft concordance based on minor HLA antigen such as allele-mismatches or mismatches for HLA-C, DQ, or DP. CMV-seronegative donor status has also been considered more important than other risk factors such as advanced donor age or blood group disparity. Clinical validation for these largely anecdotal although plausible recommendations still need validation via prospective randomized trials that should include ethnically diverse cohort of patients.

Newly acquired CMV infection in D−/R− HSCT recipients was less likely due to naturally acquired infection in the adult life, whereas CMV transmission via transfusion of unscreened blood and blood products was reported as an important source of infection in older studies [173]. Use of blood products from CMV-seronegative blood donors is of foremost significance in prevention of newly acquired CMV infection during the post-transplant period. Reports of leukocyte-reduced or filtered blood products were an alternative approach to mitigate risk of CMV infection from blood transfusions in CMV + donor pool [174, 175].

In authors' opinion, all CMV-seronegative transplant recipients should receive adequately screened blood and blood products from CMV-seronegative donors, as newly acquired CMV infection via transfusion poses a devastating complication in this vulnerable population.

CMV Drug Prophylaxis

Ganciclovir prophylaxis was a major breakthrough in prevention of CMV infection and end-organ viral disease in patients undergoing HSCT. Though it was well tolerated in most patients, drug toxicity, selection of drug-resistant viral mutants after prolonged exposure with low drug dose, subsequent risk for breakthrough, and often difficult-to-treat infections and potential for end-organ disease became limiting concerns. Valganciclovir was a welcome addition.

A search for more potent antiviral drugs with a low likelihood for the risk of breakthrough CMV infections, infections due to drug-resistant viral stains, has propelled research in the past decades. After a less than stellar performance by maribavir in phase III trials [176], the recently concluded trial using a new anti-CMV agent was an encouraging gain in the existing antiviral drug armamentarium. Letermovir is a novel antiviral drug that inhibits the CMV-terminase complex. In phase II dose escalation trial, a significant benefit was noted in incidence of CMV infection and end-organ disease plus lower discontinuation of prophylaxis for any reason at 240 mg daily dose vs. 60 mg, 120 mg, or when no drug prophylaxis given [177].

A phase III trial in CMV (+) adult HSCT recipients with no evidence of CMV infection and/or disease, letermovir prophylaxis with 480 mg, or half that daily dose in patients taking cyclosporine was assessed for 14 weeks after patients underwent transplantation [178]. The primary end point was the proportion of patients in whom clinically significant CMV infection became evident within 24 weeks after transplant. Patients were followed through week 48 after HSCT. In 495 patients, 38% randomized to receive high-dose letermovir prophylaxis developed clinically significant CMV infection, whereas a significantly higher proportion of patients (61%) developed such episodes in the group given placebo [178]. Letermovir was well tolerated; no episodes of drug-related myelotoxicity or renal dysfunction were observed. Vomiting, edema, and atrial fibrillation or flutter were low-grade adverse events that were possibly attributed to letermovir prophylaxis. All-cause mortality, 48 weeks after transplantation, was 21% in letermovir group compared with 26% in patients randomized to receive no anti-CMV prophylaxis [178]. This trial has provided a much-needed new approach for preventing CMV infection in patients undergoing allogeneic stem cell transplantation.

Immunoprophylaxis

Use of intravenous immune globulin (IVIG) has shown variable efficacy in prevention of CMV viremia during post-transplant period, especially among at-risk population. In addition, even target-specific, enriched anti-CMV hyperimmunoglobulins or CMV-specific monoclonal immunoglobulins have also been disappointing in this regard [179–181].

The lack of therapeutic efficacy of IVIG in reducing CMV risk after D+/R− and D+/R+ allogeneic HSCT was known in earlier studies and was validated in a recent meta-analysis [182]. Use of enriched or monoclonal CMV antibodies is a high-price alternative for antiviral drug prophylaxis and currently not recommended for routine use in prevention of post-transplant CMV infection [183, 184].

In patients undergoing solid organ transplantation, treatment with hyperimmunoglobulins or target-enriched immunoglobulins, especially for CMV and HBV infections, may have ancillary immune modulatory effect(s) [185]. It was interesting to note in orthotopic liver transplant recipients, HBV hyperimmunoglobulin prophylaxis had an unexpected favorable influence on the risk of graft rejection resulting in improved graft and patient survival compared with patients given antiviral drug therapy alone [185]. Similarly, anti-CMV hyperimmunoglobulin prophylaxis in patients following lung transplantation had resulted in reduced frequency of bronchiolitis obliterans syndrome [185]. These additional host-immune-modifying events attributed to hyperimmunoglobulin prophylaxis given during early post-transplant period may not be a direct treatment-induced modification of allograft recipients' immune-inflammation response. It could be contended that such benefit, if valid, arises from an indirect effect from suppression of opportunistic, possibly immune-modulating viral infections.

Preemptive Therapy in HSCT

Prevention of CMV end-organ disease in patients with early and sustained CMV viremia has spearheaded the evolution of preemptive therapy in the last three decades. Implementation of effective preemptive anti-CMV therapy that reduces the need for universal antiviral drug prophylaxis relies upon predictor(s) that confidently portend CMV disease risk in patients undergoing allogeneic transplantation. Such preemptive strategies in a select group of allogeneic transplant recipients have been a notable intervention that resulted in a considerable decline in early post-transplant CMV disease and reflected upon improved patient survival [61].

However, the premise of anti-CMV drug prophylaxis, as with prevention strategies for other opportunistic infections, is to routinely provide antimicrobial drug, often given in lower doses during high-risk periods. Unlike preemptive therapy, prophylaxis is administered regardless of the evidence of CMV infection (antigenemia or viremia). Empiric therapy is regarded as systemic full-dose anti-CMV therapy given in patients when CMV end-organ disease is suspected and confirmation is either pending or not attainable.

A suitable agent for prophylaxis must (a) have favorable toxicity profile, (b) be easy to administer, (c) not require frequent dose administration, (d) demonstrate efficacy in prevention of infection and tissue invasive disease, and importantly (e) have low potential to influence emergence of drug-resistant mutants or (f) breakthrough infections due to organisms inherently nonsusceptible to the class of drug being used for prophylaxis. Another important consideration is reliable bioavailability of such an agent that would make routine blood/serum drug monitoring dispensable. CMV prophylaxis, unlike preemptive approach, is offered to all at-risk transplant patients and not selected for patients that demonstrate CMV infection, therefore exposing a subgroup of low-risk patients to systemic toxicity of ganciclovir or foscarnet, in whom post-transplant CMV infection or disease would not have occurred. Unlike preemptive approach, in patients given drug prophylaxis, routine viral monitoring is not required. Both strategies have demonstrated comparable efficacy in preventing CMV end organ disease [61]. It was therefore considered desirable to opt for preemptive approach using CMV pp65 antigenemia or viral DNA PCR techniques to avoid more generalized use of an antiviral drug prophylaxis, especially in transplant receipients with suboptimum restitution of post-trasnplant antiviral immune surveillance [186, 187].

Assessing CMV-specific immune reconstitution after allogenic stem cell allograft transplantation is a novel approach to objectively stratifying patients at risk for CMV infection and end-organ disease. The utility of CMV-specific adaptive T cell response as a guide for withholding preemptive anti-CMV therapy was assessed in 58 patients 3–6 months after allogeneic HSCT [188]. In 19 CMV episodes, this strategy was applied, treatment was deferred in 5/19 patients and none of these five patients developed CMV disease [80]. This approach has not become the standard of care at most transplant centers barring cost, feasibility, and limited clinical experience.

The current approach for preemptive therapy after allogeneic HSCT is based on regular, once a week measurement of

CMV pp65 antigenemia, or viremia by new-generation sensitive PCR DNA analysis, or RNA amplification using nucleic acid sequence-based amplification (NASBA). These measurements are performed during first 100 days after transplantation and may be extended beyond 100 days in patients with sustained risk for late CMV disease. It is important that patients assigned to receive preemptive anti-CMV therapy should be periodically assessed for subclinical or modestly symptomatic end-organ viral disease.

A short 2- to 3-week course of ganciclovir is frequently adequate in resolving CMV viremia although close to one-third of patients given short anti-CMV preemptive therapy will have infection recurrence [189]. Currently, preemptive therapy is given for 6–8 weeks or for 100 days after engraftment [190]. In patients with persistent viremia or pp65 antigenemia after 2 weeks of anti-CMV therapy, treatment needs to be extended until viral clearance is achieved. A gradual decline in CMV viremia after institution of preemptive antiviral therapy was noticeable as an important prognosticator of CMV disease during the late transplant period [191].

In authors' opinion, in patients in whom, rise in CMV PCR or antigenemia is observed for 2 consecutive weeks after commencing ganciclovir preemptive therapy, a genetic drug mutation analysis should be performed. This is especially pertinent for patients with prior and extensive exposure to ganciclovir. A change to an alternative antiviral drug should also be considered without delay in patients with the earliest clinical and/or radiographic evidence of CMV end-organ disease, while receiving ganciclovir preemptive therapy. However, it should be emphasized that a number of patients will exhibit protracted or gradual response to anti-CMV preemptive therapy, which is more a reflection on patients' ineffective T cell antiviral immune response and possibily, yet undermined, hosts' minor genetic polymorphism(s) that curtails ability to suppress viral replication during the post-transplant period. It has also been sugested that such immune vulnerablity for CMV infection may only become clinically evident, after an allogenic transplantation procedure has been undertake.

Management of CMV Disease

CMV sporadically activates from viral latency in most non-immunosuppressed individuals with or without periods of physical and/or immunologic stress with no certain clinical consequence. Even in immunosuppressed patients, diagnosis for CMV end-organ disease requires fulfilment of certain criteria, such as (1) isolation of cytomegalovirus in viral cultures, (2) clinical and radiologic features of CMV disease, (3) identifying susceptible transplantation population, and, most importantly, (4) demonstration of cytomegalovirus in tissue biopsy samples.

Gastrointestinal Disease

For gastrointestinal CMV disease, induction parenteral drug therapy with intravenous ganciclovir is given for 2–3 weeks followed by 4–6 weeks of low-dose maintenance therapy, which needs to be continued well after resolution of CMV viremia and clinical and/or radiographic evidence of viral disease. Historically, short course (≤2 weeks) antiviral therapy was associated with the risk of treatment failure and viral disease relapse [192]. In patients with orointestinal CMV disease, tissue damage is a direct result of virus-mediated cell damage; therefore, immunomodulation with adjunct IVIG for harnessing or modifying immune-inflammatory response is not recommended [193].

Nearly one-third of HSCT recipients may experience disease recurrence after demonstrating a clinical response to anti-CMV drug therapy. The authors suggest a reinduction with systemic antiviral drug given for 3–4 weeks and maintained until precipitating risk factors, if present, such as high-grade acute or chronic GVHD, graft rejection, high-dose anti-GVHD or allograft rejection therapy, and treatment for cancer recurrence including donor lymphocyte infusion mediated severe immune suppression has improved. Despite limited data, prolonged suppression with oral valganciclovir was encouraged in patients with end-organ CMV disease, including recurrent CMV enteritis or colitis. It is important to assess for potential malabsorption state even in the setting of well-controlled chronic enteric GVHD or visceral graft rejection. In such circumstances, drugs even with otherwise high oral bioavailability like valganciclovir may fail to achieve adequate therapeutic drug concentration.

CMV Pneumonitis

Response to antiviral drug therapy by itself for treatment of CMV pneumonia, particularly in patients undergoing allogeneic HSCT, has been disappointing. CMV pneumonia has dual components, direct virus-mediated cytopathic effects on pneumocytes, and additional virus-elicited tissue damage via an exaggerated hosts' inflammatory response. Therefore, combination therapy has long since become the standard of care that comprises of an effective anti-CMV drug like ganciclovir or foscarnet along with IVIG [194, 195]. This approach has resulted in a substantial improvement yeilding good clinical response and improved patient survival compared with historic outcomes following antiviral drug therapy alone. It was not unexpected that no additional benefit occurred by substituting CMV-enriched immune globulin compared to pooled IVIG from community blood donors [196]. In patients with pulmonary edema and circulatory volume overload that may be exacerbated by IVIG, a reduced volume CMV-enriched immunoglobulins may exert less intravascular oncotic pressure and can be substituted in select clinical situations.

Immunopathogenesis of CMV pneumonitis is predicated on hosts' exaggerated inflammatory response triggered by cytomegalovirus infection involving the lungs [197]. Systematic review in a number of studies has provided support for IVIGtherapy in recipients of allogeneic HSCT with CMV pneumonitis; ergo addition of IVIG is presently regarded as standard of care, despite limited controversies that may surface periodically.

CMV Retinitis

Treatment of CMV retinitis involves systemic treatment with an antiviral drug like ganciclovir, foscarnet, or cidofovir. Intraocular, posterior chamber instillation of ganciclovir via injections or implantation of slow drug-release devices has evolved as the mainstay of therapy for this devastating CMV disease that threatens to compromise vision and in some patients resulting in permanent blindness, despite best possible, intensive multimodality treatment measures [198, 199]. It is also important to recognize that initially uninvolved contralateral eye is at risk for CMV disease in most patients with CMV retinitis initially involving a single eye.

Cidofovir has permitted biweekly maintenance therapy. Local ophthalmic treatment options such as intraocular devices for sustained ganciclovir delivery or intravitreal instillation of cidofovir, fomivirsen, and ganciclovir have been used to circumvent systemic drug toxicity while maintaining high drug concentration at the site of viral disease [200]. The intraocular cidofovir is desirable due to its long half-life, and patients may be spared from implantation of intraocular devices that are needed for ganciclovir sustained local delivery. Safety and pharmacokinetics of the cidofovir prodrug was evaluated in rabbits [201, 202]. The drug was well tolerated, and gradually dissolved, yielding free drug accumulation in the retina and vitreous; half life of 25 days. The status of future development of cidofovir prodrugs for potential clinical use is presently not known.

It is important to recognize that acute uveitis may complicate systemic cidofovir therapy, similar to ophthalmic toxicity noted with rifabutin. Discontinuation of the offending drug and topical steroids along with mydriatic cycloplegic agents are ameliorative in most patients [203]. Since patients commonly present with painful red eye and signs of anterior segment inflammation accompanied by fibrinous exudate and possibly vitritis, a lack of awareness of this drug-induced toxicity that may rarely complicate cidofovir therapy may misdirect a cumbersome and fruitless exploration for possible infection.

Ocular hypotony is another rare complication of systemic cidofovir therapy [204]. Anterior uveitis or iridocyclitis and ocular hypotony are a result from a direct interaction between cidofovir and the ciliary body [205]. Most reports of this cidofovir ophthalmic toxicity is reported in patients with HIV/AIDS receiving treatment for CMV retinitis. Alternatively, inflammation of anterior eye chamber and vitreous body may be a reflection of immune restoration in patients with AIDS and not a direct consequence of cidofovir on the ciliary apparatus [206].

Fomivirsen is a phosphorothioate oligonucleotide that inhibits CMV replication via an antisense mechanism that targets mRNA encoded by CMV. This drug is approved as second-line intraocular instillation therapy for CMV retinitis in patients with HIV/AIDS [207]. Therapeutic feasibility and efficacy of fomivirsen in treatment of CMV retinitis in non-HIV patients, especially those undergoing allograft transplantation is not certain.

Other Organ Diseases

CMV hepatitis, encephalitis, myelitis/myeloradiculitis, and adrenalitis are not common, and management with an antiviral agent like ganciclovir is often adequate. It has been proposed, barring adequate clinical experience, that intravenous foscarnet may penetrate physiological blood-brain barrier better than that occurs after intravenous ganciclovir therapy. The potential superiority of one drug versus the other has not been systematically studied and at best is regarded as anecdotal opinion. In transplant patients with CMV disease, high degree of clinical suspicion, early and correct diagnosis, and appropriate supportive care is what determines a favorable outcome along with the implementation of effective and well-tolerated anti-CMV drug therapy.

Antiviral Agents

Drugs that are active against cytomegalovirus are given for infection prevention and preemptive therapy prior to development of end-organ cytomegalovirus disease. These agents are also effective for the treatment of CMV disease. In patients undergoing transplantation, all resources are focused on identifying patients at risk for CMV organ disease such as high risk transplant procedures, and post-transplant complication that increase vulnerability for this devastating potentially life-threatening complication.

Acyclovir

Acyclovir is active against herpes simplex viruses and regarded as the cornerstone of antiviral prevention and treatment since its approval by FDA in 1982. The initial critical step in intracellular drug activation is dependent on phosphorylation by viral thymidine kinase that exhibits >3000 times higher avidity for acyclovir than mammalian host enzymes; cellular thymidine kinase then converts acyclovir to triphosphate form, which is a potent inhibitor of viral DNA polymerase. Acyclovir despite showing less than optimal anti-CMV activity in vitro tests, when given to patients undergoing stem cell transplantation was noted to reduce the overall risk for CMV infection and perhaps favorably influenced the risk for CMV organ disease [208].

Valacyclovir

Valacyclovir is a valine-ester prodrug of acyclovir with a greater than 50% oral bioavailability compared with 10–20% oral bioavailability achieved with traditional oral acyclovir therapy. Valacyclovir is converted to acyclovir after first-pass hepatic metabolism by hosts' esterase enzymes yielding a high-serum drug concertation. It was therefore, not unexpected that prophylaxis with valacyclovir was more effective than acyclovir in reducing the risk of CMV infection, as noted by a decline in the need for ganciclovir preemptive therapy in patients undergoing allogeneic HSCT [209]. The impact of valacyclovir prophylaxis on overall survival after allogeneic HSCT remains uncertain. It is recommended that allogeneic transplant recipients at risk for CMV disease, while on valacyclovir prophylaxis should undergo routine surveillance for CMV infection and be treated preemptively with appropriate anti-CMV drug should there be evidence of CMV antigenemia or viremia [210].

Ganciclovir

Ganciclovir is competitive inhibitor of deoxyguanosine triphosphate and interferes with the incorporation of this essential nucleoside into viral DNA. Ganciclovir is a synthetic nucleoside analogue 9-(1,3-dihydroxy-2-propoxymethyl) guanine (DHPG) that is converted to ganciclovir monophosphate by a CMV gene (UL97)-encoded phosphotransferase. Further phosphorylation of ganciclovir monophosphate into the active triphosphate form is undertaken by hosts' cellular enzymes. Presently, ganciclovir is regarded as the first-line drug for prevention and preemptive treatment of CMV infection in patients undergoing transplantation. Intravenous ganciclovir significantly reduces the risk of CMV disease in patients undergoing allogeneic HSCT [211, 212].

One of the major treatment limiting toxicity of ganciclovir is suppression of marrow granulocytopoiesis; the resultant peripheral blood neutropenia is noted in nearly one-third of the stem cell allograft recipients being treated with ganciclovir [213]. As expected, presence of drug-induced severe neutropenia (ANC < 500 cells/ml), if it remains unabated, significantly increases the risk for secondary superimposed bacterial infections and tissue invasive fungal disease [213].

Ganciclovir dose reduction and additional support with recombinant myeloid growth factor may help mitigate this potential life-threatening complication, although in a number of patients the drug may have to be discontinued. Most often, such patients are switched over to foscarnet. Ganciclovir serum drug concentration analysis may help guide drug dosing in select patients, especially those with renal impairment, although this is not a common practice in transplant centers in the United States and elsewhere. Another important observation in clinical trials showed a lack of overall survival benefit from ganciclovir prophylaxis or preemptive therapy; this was noted despite a significant reduction in the risk for end-organ CMV disease.

Valganciclovir

Oral valganciclovir has better bioavailability compared with oral ganciclovir; in HSCT recipients, serum drug levels may be comparable to those seen after intravenous ganciclovir therapy [214]. The efficacy and tolerability of valganciclovir preemptive therapy are now regarded as analogous to intravenous ganciclovir therapy in patients undergoing allogeneic stem cell transplantation [215, 216].

In patients following solid organ transplantation, oral valganciclovir showed a safe, easy to administer, and potentially effective option for CMV therapy nearly comperable to intravenous ganciclovir [217]. It was cautioned that in allograft recipients with specific organ transplants that were not represented in the comparison trials, extrapolating valganciclovir feasibility data in such transplant recipients should be approached with caution [217]. The VICTOR trial showed comparable efficacy of oral valganciclovir vs. intravenous ganciclovir for the treatment of CMV disease in recipients of solid organ transplantation [218]. Oral anti-CMV therapy is now recommended in SOT patients for the treatment of CMV disease. VICTOR biobank was used in a series of post hoc analyses that yielded important information regarding treatment of CMV disease in SOT population. These included the following: (a) modifying antiviral therapy with the initial CMV viral load, (b) the effect of immune suppression on anti-CMV treatment outcomes, and (c) importantly, for prevention of disease recurrence and emergence of drug resistance, antiviral treatment should be continued until CMV viral load has become undetectable [218].

A multicenter randomized study assessed intravenous ganciclovir in patients undergoing alemtuzumab reduced intensity conditioning HSCT vs. oral valganciclovir; 67% of 27 patients cleared CMV viremia after a median 14 days of therapy [219]. By measuring serum ganciclovir levels, bioavailability of oral valganciclovir was 73%. It was interesting to note that average drug exposure was higher in the valganciclovir group compared with patients given ganciclovir intravenously (37 ± 15 and 28 ± 7 μg h/ml, respectively).

Taking into account the existing data, systemic drug exposure and safety of valganciclovir has emerged as comparable to traditional intravenous ganciclovir given preemptively in both solid organ and hematopoietic stem cell allograft recipients. An important exception includes the lack of such data in high-risk HSCT recipients and those with CMV infection while undergoing treatment for severe GVHD or visceral allograft cellular immune rejection.

Foscarnet

Foscarnet, trisodium phosphonoformate, is a pyrophosphate analog that binds reversibly near the pyrophosphate-binding site of viral DNA polymerase or reverse transcriptase. Foscarnet unlike nucleoside analogues does not require modification for antiviral activity. Foscarnet binding with viral DNA polymerase, blocks DNA chain elongation. Foscarnet selectively inhibits viral DNA polymerase; cross-over inhibition of mammalian DNA polymerase would require 100-fold greater drug concentration than that needed for blocking CMV replication. It is active in vitro against herpes viruses, HBV and HIV. Foscarnet is presently used as a second-line agent for the treatment of CMV infection in transplant patients intolerant to ganciclovir or those with ganciclovir nonsusceptible or unresponsive CMV, HSV, and VZV infection. In vitro activity and limited clinical data also foster use of foscarnet in patients with end-organ disease due to human herpesvirus 6A and 6B [220].

Foscarnet is considered as effective as ganciclovir for pre-emptive anti-CMV therapy in patients undergoing allogeneic stem cell transplantation [221, 222]. However, as all currently licensed antiviral drugs, breakthrough infection is not unique to treatment with foscarnet. In most such cases, lack of clinical response reflects a combination of less drug-susceptible viral strains and viral escape due to profound hosts' cellular immune dysfunction.

In 20 high-risk HSCT recipients including unrelated donors, or T cell-depleted stem cell grafts, and/or transplant for advanced malignancy, foscarnet prophylaxis was assessed during first 100 days after transplantation [223]. CMV pp65 antigenemia was seen in 80% of patients with low dose and less than 20% with high-dose foscarnet prophylaxis. CMV disease occurred in 33% receiving lower two-dose schedule, where none of the patients assigned to high two-dose approach developed end-organ viral disease. Increased serum creatinine was noted in 75% of these patients, and in nearly half, the drug needed to be stopped. Authors reported dose-dependent prophylactic effect of foscarnet in prevention of CMV antigenemia, and despite high incidence of nephrotoxicity, it was reversible after the treatment was discontinued [223].

Compared with ganciclovir, foscarnet anti-CMV therapy is given preemptively to individuals undergoing allogeneic blood or marrow stem cell transplantation. In this randomized study involving 213 patients, the primary efficacy endpoint was the occurrence of CMV disease or death from any cause within 180 days after transplantation [190]. The event-free 180-day survival estimates were similar in the two treatment groups. As anticipated, significantly more patients (11%) developed severe neutropenia in ganciclovir group versus 4% in those receiving foscarnet prophylaxis. Renal impairment was not significantly different among the two groups; 5% in foscarnet-treated patients and 2% in the ganciclovir-treated patients. Ganciclovir was discontinued in 6% of patients due to hematopoietic toxicity such as neutropenia or severe thrombocytopenia, whereas no such treatment interruptions were noted in foscarnet-treated group.

A report in 39 patients in whom 22 had undergone SOT and 17 HSCT received foscarnet for treatment of ganciclovir-resistant CMV infection (n = 15) and other exhibiting lack of clinical response to ganciclovir therapy. Patients were given foscarnet for well over a month (median 32 days). Virologic failure occurred in 33%, and viremia relapsed in 31% of the patients. More patients died (31%) in HSCT group compared with SOT, whereas significantly more SOT recipients had ganciclovir-resistant CMV virus [224]. It was not unexpected to see that nearly half of the patients (51%) developed impaired renal function by the end of foscarnet therapy. It is important to take into account that end-organ CMV disease was documented in 28% of the 39 patients [224].

Drug treatment refractory CMV viremia, viral recurrence, and risk of end-organ disease are more of a reflection on hosts' genetic and immunologic viral susceptibility, type of allograft transplantation, and post-transplant complication(s) resulting in hosts' immune dysregulation. This concept has given way to handling CMV infection in transplantation population with novel approaches such as adaptive cellular immunotherapy and search for vaccine candidates and constructs that may yield effective and durable anti-CMV immune response.

Cidofovir

Cidofovir or hydroxyphosphonylmethoxypropylcytosine (HPMPC) is a phosphonate containing cyclic cytosine analogue. Cidofovir phosphonate group mimics deoxycytidine monophosphate. This drug does not require viral kinases for phosphorylation to furnish its antiviral potential [225]. Therefore, cidofovir is active against the viral mutants that are deficient in viral kinase including ganciclovir-resistant CMV strains. Hosts' cellular enzymes phosphorylate cidofovir twice to its active form. The resulting cidofovir diphosphate remains within the cells for an extended duration. The diphosphate cidofovir competitively inhibits incorporation of deoxycytidine triphosphate into viral DNA by viral DNA polymerase. Incorporation of the drug in viral DNA disrupts further chain elongation [225]. Tenofovir and adefovir are two related phosphonate-containing drugs that are acyclic deoxyadenosine analogue and are active against HIV and HBV. The mechanism of antiviral activity of these drugs is similar to that of cidofovir against CMV.

Acute renal tubular necrosis is a major drug toxicity that can be, in part, muted by optimizing intravascular hydration before and after cidofovir infusion to maximize glomerular filtration, and probenecid is given to reduce active cidofovir secretion in proximal renal tubules. Despite these measures, acute renal failure limits first- or second-line use of cidofovir in most transplant recipients with CMV infection and/or disease.

Cidofovir is a broad-spectrum agent that exhibits in vitro activity against a variety of human pathogenic viruses including human herpesviruses, adenovirus, HPV, polyomaviruses, and human poxviruses [226]. Potential clinical application other than the standard indication for CMV retinitis in patients with AIDS is not presently approved. Intravenous cidofovir has been used as salvage therapy for treatment of progressive multifocal leukoencephalopathy and Kaposi's sarcoma. Intraocular injection for treatment of CMV retinitis, intralesional cidofovir injections for treatment of respiratory papillomatosis, topical application for treatment of aggressive molluscum contagiosum, anogenital condyloma acuminata, and recurrent genital herpes have been used with some success. Topical ophthalmic instillation of cidofovir for treatment of viral keratoconjunctivitis has also been well tolerated and with good results [227].

Maribavir

Maribavir is a benzimidazole l-riboside compound with potent activity against CMV including ganciclovir-resistant viral strains. The mechanism of action against ganciclovir-resistant CMV isolates include drug-induced inhibition of UL97 kinase and viral DNA synthesis [228]. Viral UL97 kinase is involved in viral DNA synthesis and viral capsids' exit from cell nuclei. Maribavir shows in vitro activity against ganciclovir- foscarnet-and cidofovir-resistant strains of CMV [228].

In a study, clinical CMV isolates and laboratory viral stains exhibiting mutations in UL97 and UL54 DNA polymerase were tested in vitro by plaque reduction assay. All 17 CMV stains resistant to ganciclovir ($n = 11$), foscarnet ($n = 4$), and cidofovir showing UL97 and UL54 DNA polymerase mutations were susceptible to maribavir [229]. A laboratory mutant CMV virus with UL97 L397R mutation showed high-level maribavir resistance; however, this strain was sensitive to other three antiviral drugs tested. Maribavir demonstrates rapid absorption after oral administration and linear pharmacokinetics and has effective in vivo activity against cytomegalovirus [230]. In phase I trials, based on urinary drug recovery, 25–45% of maribavir was noted to be absorbed when given orally [231].

In a phase II dose-ranging trial conducted in patients following HSCT, CMV infection and disease were reduced with all three drug doses tested, although this antiviral benefit was not evident in phase III trial among patients randomized to receive maribavir 100 mg twice daily [232]. Inadequate low-dose maribavir was thought to be a potential flaw in this phase III trial [232].

In 120 patients following stem cell or solid organ transplantation, safety, antiviral activity, and pharmacokinetics of different oral doses of maribavir for up to 24 weeks for treatment of CMV infections resistant or refractory to treatment with ganciclovir, valganciclovir, or foscarnet were studied. A number of participants with confirmed undetectable plasma CMV within 6 weeks after being randomized to receive 400 mg, 800 mg, and 1200 mg twice daily dose was 70%, 63%, and 71%, respectively. Serious adverse events were not widely different among the three groups (70%, 68%, and 65%, respectively) (clinicaltrials.gov NCT01611974).

Another phase II European randomized dose-ranging trial to assess safety and efficacy of maribavir vs. valganciclovir for the treatment of CMV infection in transplant patients without CMV end-organ disease has ended in 2014 (EudraCT: 2010-024247-32); results from this trial are not known. Overall, Maribavir has been safe and well tolerated; alteration in taste was the most frequently reported adverse event.

Letermovir

Letermovir is a novel antiviral drug that inhibits the CMV-terminase complex that can be given orally or intravenously. In vitro data has shown letermovir remains active against drug-resistant CMV mutant strains. Limited clinical experience for treatment of multidrug-resistant CMV infection or disease in allograft transplant recipients was encouraging [233]. In a phase II dose-escalation study in 131 CMV (+) stem cell HLA-matched allograft recipients, letermovir was given at doses of 60, 120, or 240 mg daily and compared with similar patients that were given placebo. Prophylaxis and placebo were continued for 12 weeks after stem cell engraftment. The primary end point was "all-cause prophylaxis failure" which was defined as stopping study drug due to CMV antigenemia or viremia, viral end-organ disease, or any other cause [177]. The "all-cause prophylaxis failure" was 48% in patients given 60 mg dose versus 64% in the placebo group. It was 32% in patients given 120 mg ($P = 0.01$) and 29% in patients given 240 mg letermovir daily dose ($P = 0.007$). A difference in time-to-onset for prophylaxis failure for letermovir 240 mg daily dose vs. placebo was a significant finding ($P = 0.002$) [177]. There were no episodes of drug-induced hematologic or renal toxicity. The drug was well tolerated, and the safety profile of letermovir was comparable to patients who were randomly assigned to receive placebo.

In a phase III trial in adult CMV (+) HSCT recipients without CMV viremia, letermovir prophylaxis 480 mg daily, or half that dose in patients taking cyclosporine, was assessed during the first 14 weeks after transplantation. In 495 patients, 24 weeks after transplantation, 38% randomized in letermovir treatment group developed clinically significant CMV infection, whereas such events were observed in 61% among the placebo group ($P < 0.001$) [178]. Letermovir was well tolerated, with no drug-related myelotoxicity or renal dysfunction. Vomiting, edema, and atrial fibrillation or flutter were low-grade adverse events possibly associated with letermovir use. The 48-week all-cause mortality in letermovir group was 21% comparted with 26% in patients who did not receive this anti-CMV drug for prophylaxis [178].

Brincidofovir

Brincidofovir (CMX-001) is a lipid acyclic nucleoside phosphonate prodrug of cidofovir that exhibits excellent oral bioavailability and expected long half-life allowing twice-weekly dosing schedule. Brincidofovir crosses cell membrane via facilitated and passive diffusion; once inside the cell, it is converted into cidofovir after cleavage from its lipid moiety and phosphorylated to cidofovir diphosphate by intracellular kinases [234]. In experimental CMV infections, brincidofovir is 400 times more potent than cidofovir [235]. The spectrum of antiviral activity of this cidofovir prodrug includes all five families of DNA viruses that causes human disease including the herpesviruses and adenoviruses [236, 237]. Brincidofovir has shown potent activity against Ebola virus in vitro, and in experimental Ebola virus disease results were cautiously encouraging [238]. Unlike cidofovir, brincidofovir is not a substrate for the human organic anion transporters, which favorably contributes to its low nephrotoxicity potential [239].

A phase II dose-escalation study in HSCT recipients showed reduced CMV infection and/or disease in patients given brincidofovir prophylaxis with 200 mg per week dose started at the time of stem cell engraftment. The most common side effect was diarrhea that became notable in patients given 200 mg or higher weekly doses. Due to the dose-limiting toxicity noted at 200 mg twice weekly, the protocol was amended to 100 mg twice weekly dose for phase III trial. In the phase III trial with amended protocol conducted at 27 centers, 230 evaluable CMV (+) patients undergoing HSCT were randomized to receive oral brincidofovir 100 mg twice weekly versus placebo [240]. It is important to note that randomization was stratified according to the presence or absence of GVHD and CMV viremia. Anti-CMV prophylaxis commenced after stem cell engraftment for a duration of 9–11 weeks and until 13th week post-transplant. CMV DNA PCR was performed weekly, and in patients with presence of CMV breakthrough viremia, drug was discontinued and switched to standard preemptive anti-CMV therapy. The primary end point was presence of CMV disease or viremia (>200 copies per ml) at the time study drug prophylaxis was discontinued. The incidence of CMV events was 27% points lower in patients in whom brincidofovir was given prophylactically (10% vs. 37% in placebo; $P = 0.002$) [240]. Diarrhea was common adverse event in patients receiving brincidofovir at doses of 200 mg or higher weekly doses and was the dose-limiting adverse event associated with brincidofovir prophylaxis [240]. According to the manufacturer website, brincidofovir has not been associated with kidney or bone marrow toxicity in over 1000 patients. Brincidofovir has received Fast Track designation from the FDA for CMV, adenovirus, and smallpox (http://www.chimerix.com) [241].

Leflunomide

Leflunomide is a disease-modifying antirheumatic drug that has shown effectiveness in various autoimmune disorders [242]. Leflunomide has exhibited in vitro anti-CMV activity and dose-dependent anti-CMV response in humans [242]. In HSCT recipients with MDR CMV infection or end-organ viral disease due to such difficult-to-treat drug-resistant strains, options for effective and sustainable therapy remain severely curtailed. Leflunomide has been exploited for possible salvage therapy in such select cases. Leflunomide adjuvant, salvage therapy in three HSCT recipients with MDR CMV infections assessed anti-CMV efficacy of leflunomide based on virologic response and proposed therapeutic drug monitoring [243].

Leflunomide salvage therapy has also resulted in favorable outcome in two SOT recipients with systemic and local antiviral combination therapy refractory CMV retinitis [244]. A kidney allograft recipient with treatment refractory (UL97 mutation) CMV retinitis involving both eyes responded after oral leflunomide was added. This patient had disease worsening despite intravitreal instillation of ganciclovir and foscarnet in addition to IV foscarnet and oral valganciclovir therapy. Following addition of leflunomide, CMV retinitis became inactive for 22 months. CMV retinitis in a lung transplant patient worsened despite intravitreal foscarnet injections and oral valganciclovir. Retinitis was controlled with the addition of oral leflunomide that allowed discontinuation of intravitreal therapy. In this patient, CMV retinitis remained inactive until his death [244].

Experience with leflunomide for CMV infection in nine patients following lung transplantation three such allograft recipients received leflunomide for secondary CMV prophylaxis [245]. In 67% of 12 patients, demonstrable genetic antiviral mutations were noted that are known to confer drug resistance. Leflunomide therapy in 78% of patients resulted in a decline in the level of CMV viremia. Long-term viral suppression was achieved in 58% of these patients. In one-fourth of patients, leflunomide had to be discontinued due to drug toxicity [245]. Leflunomide experimental therapy is currently reserved for patients with ganciclovir-resistant CMV infection that has failed second- and third-line agents.

Artesunate

Artesunate is an antimalarial agent that also exhibits a wide-ranging in vitro activity against a variety of viruses such as herpesviruses, hepatitis, and HIV [246].

Mechanistically, arsenate antiviral activity is linked with interference in essential steps in the host cell kinase cascades. It was shown that DNA-binding activity of the two virus-induced cellular transcription factors Sp1 and NF-kappa B were markedly reduced in the presence of artesunate. The investigators showed noticeable drug-induced inhibition of cellular signaling kinase phosphoinositide 3-kinase, which is required for activation of factors such as Sp1 and NF-kappa B in CMV-infected fibroblasts [247]. Artesunate inhibits CMV replication in human fibroblasts and astrocytes by these mechanisms including strains susceptible or resistant to ganciclovir. Artesunate exhibits anti-CMV activity similar to ganciclovir in astrocytoma and fibroblast cell lines [248].

Limited clinical experience includes a study involving six HSCT patients; preemptive artesunate treatment for CMV infection showed a rapid decline in viral load (0.8–2.1 logs) in two patients a week after therapy commenced. In the other four patients, artesunate therapy resulted in a stunted CMV growth slope. In this preliminary observation, lack of adverse events among six HSCT recipients treated over 7–56 days with artesunate therapy was encouraging and indicated further safety feasibility studies, especially exploring alternative options for drug-resistant CMV infection [249].

Response to salvage artesunate therapy for MDR-CMV infection late after HSCT forms the repertoire of experience with this agent that at best are anecdotal and arbitrary [250]. No systematic evaluation of artesunate feasibility for the treatment of CMV infection or of viral end-organ disease precludes this drug to be recommended for routine use.

Others

The monoclonal antibody MSL-109 when added to traditional anti-CMV therapy did not result in a significant advantage. Further development of cyclic cidofovir and lobucavir has been placed on hold by their respective manufacturers. Adefovir is a nucleotide analogue that possesses anti-CMV activity; however, presently it is only approved for the treatment of HBV infection. Other compounds with anti-CMV activity include BAY 38-4766 and GW1263W94; these are in early stages of development [251].

It is well recognized that infections due to drug-resistant CMV pose a serious management challenge, especially in patients undergoing allogeneic stem cell or visceral allograft transplantation. Response to salvage combination of antiviral drugs including ganciclovir, foscarnet, and cidofovir may only result in a transient response in some patients, and experimental treatment with leflunomide and artesunate appears to provide no clear additional benefit [252]. In order to trounce this daunting obstacle that non-treatment responsive CMV infection presents; one alternative appoach is based on adaptive cellular immunotherapy to achieve sustainable target-specific immune restoration in patients undergoing livesaving transplantation procedures. This is discussed briefly in the later text.

Antiviral Resistance

In recent years, a remarkable progress has been made in deciphering viral genomics. The diversity of CMV virus is much higher among other viruses belonging to *Herpesviridae* group; an individual may be infected with >20,000 single nucleotide polymorphisms, thereby CMV can rapidly evolve after exposure to and under influence of an antiviral drug. It is thought that selection of preexisting viral variant(s) rather than development of a new mutant strain confers drug nonsusceptibility, especially after a prolonged exposure to a drug [253].

Resistance to ganciclovir is linked with the presence of mutations in viral protein kinase, UL97. Such viral mutants prevent intracellular conversion of ganciclovir-monophosphate at a varying degree. Therefore, care must be taken in interpretation of viral genotype analysis, as UL97 mutations do not uniformly disrupt the antiviral effect of ganciclovir on CMV DNA synthesis. In some instances, higher ganciclovir drug concentration may overcome CMV strains exhibiting certain types of UL97 mutations [254].

The active antiviral forms of ganciclovir, foscarnet, and cidofovir share the common molecular viral target, UL54, the viral DNA polymerase. Therefore, CMV-encoding UL54 mutations have the potential to confer phenotypic resistance for all three drugs. It is important to note that cross-resistance between foscarnet and ganciclovir is not common, as mutations in UL54 conferring foscarnet resistance is in a distinct region of DNA polymerase than that for ganciclovir resistance. Some viral stains do exhibit cross-resistance to second- and third-line anti-CMV agents thereby critically limiting options for effective therapy. De novo emergence for CMV resistance to cidofovir while patients are on cidofovir therapy is seldom seen. Similarly, cross-resistance between cidofovir- and foscarnet-resistant CMV strains is not a common occurrence. It is important to note that CMV strains that exhibit certain DNA polymerase mutations that confer resistance to ganciclovir may also make these viral strains less susceptible or resistant to cidofovir [255]. Since clinical experience with cidofovir for treatment of ganciclovir-resistant CMV infection or disease is limited, probably due to risk of nephrotoxicity, cidofovir is not recommended as a second-line drug for the treatment for such infections. A detailed review of molecular bases of antiviral resistance is provided in Chap. 54.

Ganciclovir-resistant CMV has emerged in patients undergoing solid organ allograft transplants. Infections due to such viral strains are difficult to manage. A series of 15 patients at a single transplant center in whom ganciclovir resistance was demonstrated in clinical CMV isolates and a review the literature on treatment for such infection showed UL97 and UL54 viral genome mutations were present in 100% and 40% of clinical viral strains, respectively [256]. Most of these infections (73%) occurred within 1 year after transplant surgery. Lowering of valganciclovir dose prior to isolation of ganciclovir-resistant CMV was noted in all such patients, thereby suggesting a possible viral escape during low ganciclovir serum concentration; it is possible that multiplication of less drug-susceptible viral mutants may have taken place under the influence of subtherapeutic drug concentration. High-risk CMV serostatus, and history of valganciclovir dose reduction were prominent hosts' risk factors. After diagnosis of drug-resistant CMV infection, half of the patients developed organ rejection, resulting in allograft loss in 27% and death in 20% of patients. Readmissions were common; requiring three or more hospitalizations for treatment of drug-resistant CMV infection. All patients exhibited a major complication including graft rejection (60%), loss of allograft (20%), and death (40%). It appears that hospital readmission rate was reduced when such infections were first approached with reduced immunosuppression, treatment with foscarnet, intravenous immunoglobulins, and leflunomide [256].

Prolonged exposure to antiviral drugs, especially intermittent drug exposure either due to antiviral dose reduction, noncompliance, acute or chronic enteric malabsorption states such as chronic diarrheal diseases, or intestinal GVHD or allograft rejection, may play a role in promoting the risk for viral drug resistance. Resulting intermittent low-level viral replication in the presence of profound drug-induced (antirejection) immune suppression or lack of CMV immunity following allogeneic HSCT promotes a milieu that emboldens possibility for emergence and repopluation with drug resistant viral mutant strain(s) [257].

Drug resistance should be suspected in patients with increasing CMV viral loads by quantitative blood PCR after 10–14 days of adequately dosed, appropriate systemic antiviral therapy. A viral rebound during the first week of antiviral therapy may be noted in one-third of treatment-naïve patients and should not be construed as an evidence of drug resistance [60]. However, in patients with prior ganciclovir therapy, a rising CMV viral load upon reintroduction of intravenous ganciclovir should alert for the probability of infection with ganciclovir nonsusceptible viral mutant strain; switch to foscarnet should be considered while awaiting CMV UL97 and UL54 genotype mutation analysis. Some centers add foscarnet to ganciclovir with hopes for a better viral control; however, studies have shown that addition of foscarnet along with ganciclovir for treatment of ganciclovir-resistant CMV infection or disease adds no clear benefit [258]. Ganciclovir-based combination therapy for the treatment of known ganciclovir-resistant CMV viral infection is presently not recommended.

The new anti-CMV drugs with a favorable toxicity profile such as high-dose maribavir, brincidofovir, letermovir need to be explored further as potential first-line agents for the treatment of CMV infection or end-organ disease. The role of other disease-modifying agents such as leflunomide and artesunate is presently unknown and need to be studied to devise future optimum anti-CMV combination regimen.

Lowering the point state of immune suppression by modification in immunosuppressive drug regimens, such measures may include: (a) lowering corticosteroid dose and (b) calcineurin inhibitor dose reduction; (c) discontinuation of mycophenolate mofetil for the duration of severe clinical illness; d) interrupting treatment with immunosuppressive biologics; and (e), if feasible, switch calcineurin inhibitor to mTOR inhibitor such as sirolimus or everolimus that have shown to impair CMV replication by regulating hosts' cellular signaling pathways that are exploited by cytomegalovirus-encoded homologous proteins.

Adoptive Immunotherapy

Adoptive transfer of T cell as individualized treatment for cancer was heralded as a major breakthrough in 2003 and regarded as "T cells on the attack" [259]. Sophistication in developing validation animal models have also evolved for the adaptive T cell therapy against opportunistic viral infections such as CMV, adenovirus, and EBV [260–262]. CMV-specific T cells generated ex vivo by various different techniques and the adoptive anti-CMV immunity garnered by such an intervention was shown in a number of reports to favorably influence the risk of CMV viremia and end-organ viral disease in patients undergoing allograft transplantation [263, 264].

One major limitation of current approach for anti-CMV adaptive cellular therapy is that most cells are terminally differentiated effector, CMV-specific CD8$^+$ T cells that despite furnishing much needed immediate effector anti-CMV cellular response; such responses are relatively short-lived. Due to the absence of self-renewing memory T cells, borrowed immune restoration via terminally differentiated effector cell have limited life span [265]. Adaptive T cell therapy that consists of a subset of CMV-specific memory T cell population would yield a long-lasting anti-CMV CD8$^+$ T cell repertoire with highly desirable, on-demand capacity to expand and differentiate in events of viral recrudescence.

A bank of 32 virus-specific T cell lines was created at the Center for Cell and Gene Therapy in Houston, Texas. These cell lines were established from individuals with common HLA polymorphisms who were immune to EBV, CMV, or adenovirus. The investigators reported clinical experience for 18 T cell lines that were used in 50 HSCT recipients with severe, or treatment-refractory, intractable viral illness [266]. The cumulative rate of complete or partial response 6 weeks after T cell infusion was 74% for the entire group [266]. Adaptive T cell therapy resulted in encouraging response for adenovirus (78%), CMV (74%), and EBV (67%) infections [266]. It was important to note that among patients who exhibited a response, only four patients had evidence of infection recurrence or disease progression. There were no reports of immediate infusion-related toxicity. Two patients developed new-onset GVHD. It was noted that despite immunologic discordance between the T cell lines and transplant recipients in whom such investigational antiviral therapy was given, post-infusion virus-specific T cell frequency increased significantly and coincided with conspicuous decline in viremia and resolution of clinical symptoms [266].

The main limitation of "third-party" derived pathogen-specific T cell lines is that specific patterns of HLA expression within a given population probably have widespread geographic and ethnic variations [25]. Nonetheless, virus-specific T cell adaptive immunotherapy from unrelated donors with common HLA polymorphisms offers an important advantage for rapid delivery of virus-specific CD8 T cells to a patient with incompetent pathogen-specific cellular immune response and an intractable systemic CMV infection after transplantation procedure.

Furthermore, adaptive cellular immunotherapy for viral infections has thus far focused on terminally differentiated cytotoxic T cells. Harnessing other T cell subsets including target-specific memory T cell, γδ T cells, and the keen recognition of the role of NK cells play in pathogen-specific recall against opportunistic viruses like CMV are the directions for future research that may further advance the field in providing a durable, on-demand, targeted immune recovery in the high-risk allograft transplant recipients [25].

Adoptive immunotherapy continues to remain an area of great interest for severely immunosuppressed stem cell transplant patients with difficult to treat CMV infection and for prevention of life-threatening end-organ viral disease. The optimum cell type, and infusion dose, along with limited technical personale expertise, technological proficiency, and the current astronomical cost are among the salient issues that have prevented such interventions to gain popularity in broader clinical scrutiny and research.

CMV Vaccines

Presently there is no licensed CMV vaccine [267]. Despite propitious advancement in development and licensing of new anti-CMV drugs like letermovir, and brincidofovir, the financial burden for prolonged drug therapy for prevention and preemptive antiviral approach should provide encouragement for prioritization and incentive for developing and launching a safe and effective CMV vaccine [268]. A vaccine that effectively reconstitutes a durable anti-CMV immune response following transplantation has the potential to transform the existing practice paradigm in transplant medicine.

Potential vaccine candidates such as CMV glycoprotein B showed modest efficacy in preventing CMV infection in young women and adolescents in early stage clinical trial [269]. In a phase-II randomized trial in adults awaiting kidney or liver transplantation, 70 CMV (−) and 70 CMV (+) patients were randomly assigned to receive either three-dose CMV gB vaccine with MF59 adjuvant or placebo. Sixty-seven patients received vaccine, and 73 were randomized to placebo arms. The CMV gB Ab titers were significantly increased in both CMV (−) and CMV (+) vaccine recipients. In patients in whom CMV viremia was demonstrated after transplantation, gB Ab titers correlated inversely with duration of viremia ($p = 0.002$). In CMV-seronegative patients with CMV-seropositive allografts, duration of viremia and duration of ganciclovir therapy were also significantly less among novel vaccine recipients prior to transplant surgery [270]. Vaccines containing CMV gB appears encouraging when boosted with a potent adjuvant and needs further immunogenicity and safety assessment in patients undergoing visceral allograft transplantation.

So far, only one CMV vaccine has been evaluated in a randomized, placebo-controlled phase II study. ASP0113 is a bivalent product containing two plasmids that encode CMV gB and the most abundant constituent of the viral matrix or tegument, phosphoprotein 65 [271]. In an open-label, phase II trial between 2013 and 2014 undertaken at three centers in Japan [272], the safety and tolerability of this combination -immunogen vaccine were assessed in patients undergoing HSCT for hematologic disorders. Nine of ten patients between ages 22 and 61 years were enrolled. Five (5 mg) doses of recombinant vaccine were given before and after transplantation in six patients. No serious adverse events were attributed to the experimental vaccine. CMV antigenemia was observed in seven patients. None of the patients developed CMV end-organ disease. Adverse events associated with recombinant CMV vaccine were fever and injection site skin reaction; hyperuricemia was noted in one individual. Although there was no significant difference in rate of initiation of anti-CMV therapy, rates of CMV viremia were lower, and time-to-first episode of viremia was longer in patients given this investigational vaccine. These findings facilitated the ongoing placebo-controlled phase III trial that is expected to enroll 500 subjects [271].

In patients undergoing visceral allograft transplants, prevention of graft-transmitted CMV infection is of high priority. Recently, two randomized controlled trials, one with active immunization of recipients prior to undergoing transplant surgery and another using monoclonal anti-CMV antibodies for passive immunization at the time of transplantation, showed reduced incidence of CMV viremia during post-transplant period [273]. Further studies and immunization strategies that completely or significantly interrupt CMV transmission from organ donor graft to seronegative recipient are needed.

Dendritic cell vaccines were shown to enhance tumor-specific cytotoxic T cell polyfunctionality. Dendritic cell vaccine has also been shown to garner potent ex vivo antiviral response against the influenza virus and resulted in significant protection against experimental influenza infection in immunosuppressed animals [274, 275]. An interesting anti-CMV vaccine construct with CMV pp65 RNA-loaded dendritic cells was evaluated on polyfunctional CMV pp65-specific cytotoxic T cells. In a pilot trial, 17 patients with newly diagnosed glioblastoma multiforme were randomized to receive CMV pp65-specific T cells with CMV-DC vaccination or saline. Patients who received dendritic cell vaccination plus specific T cells regimen experienced a significant increase in the overall frequencies of polyfunctional (IFNγ+, TNFα+, and CCL3+) cytotoxic T cell that were specific against cytomegalovirus [276]. Generation of polyfunctional T cell responses after recombinant DC vaccine given with target specific T cells is an emerging field. A lot needs to be done before this potential approach is considered for clinical use.

Some of the predictable issues for exploring the potential for new vaccines including the DC vaccine platform with or without specific T cell construct may include the following: (a) production applications need to be fine-tuned, (b) thorough assessment of clinical safety in the short-term and the long term, (c) durability and specificity of such an adaptive immune response, (d) strength of recall following viral exposure (D+/R−), re-exposure (D+/R+) or in the event of viral recrudescence of a remotely acquired infection (D−/R+), (e) influence on de novo or existing GVHD or solid organ allograft rejection, (f) viral disease modification or potential worsening in scenarios where hosts' inflammatory response perpetuates clinical illness/disease, (g) infection-free survival, and (h) patients' overall well-being all need to be taken into keen consideration.

Summary

CMV is a serious infection, which, if remain unchecked, will result in serious illness in patients undergoing transplantation. Recently, a major stride forward in recognizing at-risk subpopulation among solid organ and stem cell allograft transplant recipients has underscored selective allocation of resources where they are most needed. Highly sensitive PCR-based, viral DNA screening tools are now widely used to identify early CMV viremia and better risk-assessment for end-organ viral disease. Awareness regarding drug resistance in clinical practice appears to have now caught up with the development of new antiviral drugs with novel mechanisms of action and are entering advanced clinical validation stages. Understanding the viral immunopathogenesis involved in various end-organ CMV disease including viral pneumonitis has vastly improved treatment outcomes for what used to be a dreaded illness with high fatality rates. Future refinement in adaptive immunotherapy, research in CMV vaccine development with novel vaccine delivery platforms, and multifacted vaccine constructs have the potential to favorably change the current role cytomegalovirus plays in transplant medicine.

References

1. CDC. www.CDC.gov. Accessed 1 Dec 2017.
2. Safdar A, Armstrong D. Infectious morbidity in critically ill patients with cancer. Crit Care Clin. 2001;17(3):531–70, vii–viii
3. Safdar A, Armstrong D. Infections in patients with hematologic neoplasms and hematopoietic stem cell transplantation: neutropenia, humoral, and splenic defects. Clin Infect Dis. 2011;53(8):798–806.
4. Merigan TC, Resta S. Cytomegalovirus: where have we been and where are we going? Rev Infect Dis. 1990;12(Suppl 7):S693–700.
5. Fishman JA. Infection in solid-organ transplant recipients. N Engl J Med. 2007;357(25):2601–14.
6. Lönnqvist B, Ringdén O, Wahren B, et al. Cytomegalovirus infection associated with and preceding chronic graft-versus-host disease. Transplantation. 1984;38(5):465–8.
7. Boeckh M, Fries B, Nichols WG. Recent advances in the prevention of CMV infection and disease after hematopoietic stem cell transplantation. Pediatr Transplant. 2004;8(Suppl 5):19–27.
8. Murphy E, Yu D, Grimwood J, et al. Coding potential of laboratory and clinical strains of human cytomegalovirus. Proc Natl Acad Sci U S A. 2003;100(25):14976–81.
9. Sinzger C, Digel M, Jahn G. Cytomegalovirus cell tropism. Curr Top Microbiol Immunol. 2008;325:63–83.
10. Bolovan-Fritts CA, Mocarski ES, Wiedeman JA. Peripheral blood CD14(+) cells from healthy subjects carry a circular conformation of latent cytomegalovirus genome. Blood. 1999;93(1):394–8.
11. Taylor-Wiedeman J, Sissons JG, Borysiewicz LK, Sinclair JH. Monocytes are a major site of persistence of human cytomegalovirus in peripheral blood mononuclear cells. J Gen Virol. 1991;72(9):2059–64.
12. Wussow F, Chiuppesi F, Contreras H, et al. Neutralization of human cytomegalovirus entry into fibroblasts and epithelial cells. Vaccines (Basel). 2017;5(4):pii: E39.
13. Boehme KW, Guerrero M, Compton T. Human cytomegalovirus envelope glycoproteins B and H are necessary for TLR2 activation in permissive cells. J Immunol. 2006;177(10):7094–102.
14. Compton T, Kurt-Jones EA, Boehme KW, et al. Human cytomegalovirus activates inflammatory cytokine responses via CD14 and Toll-like receptor 2. J Virol. 2003;77(8):4588–96.
15. Kijpittayarit S, Eid AJ, Brown RA, Paya CV, Razonable RR. Relationship between Toll-like receptor 2 polymorphism and cytomegalovirus disease after liver transplantation. Clin Infect Dis. 2007;44(10):1315–20.
16. Tabeta K, Georgel P, Janssen E, et al. Toll-like receptors 9 and 3 as essential components of innate immune defense against mouse cytomegalovirus infection. Proc Natl Acad Sci U S A. 2004;101(10):3516–21.
17. Delale T, Paquin A, Asselin-Paturel C, et al. MyD88-dependent and -independent murine cytomegalovirus sensing for IFN-alpha release and initiation of immune responses in vivo. J Immunol. 2005;175(10):6723–32.
18. Biron CA, Byron KS, Sullivan JL. Severe herpesvirus infections in an adolescent without natural killer cells. N Engl J Med. 1989;320(26):1731–5.
19. Orange JS. Natural killer cell deficiency. J Allergy Clin Immunol. 2013;132(3):515–25.

20. Chen C, Busson M, Rocha V, et al. Activating KIR genes are associated with CMV reactivation and survival after non-T-cell depleted HLA-identical sibling bone marrow transplantation for malignant disorders. Bone Marrow Transplant. 2006;38(6):437–44.
21. Cook M, Briggs D, Craddock C, et al. Donor KIR genotype has a major influence on the rate of cytomegalovirus reactivation following T-cell replete stem cell transplantation. Blood. 2006;107(3):1230–2.
22. Zaia JA, Sun JY, Gallez-Hawkins GM, et al. The effect of single and combined activating killer immunoglobulin-like receptor genotypes on cytomegalovirus infection and immunity after hematopoietic cell transplantation. Biol Blood Marrow Transplant. 2009;15(3):315–25.
23. Waggoner SN, Cornberg M, Selin LK, Welsh RM. Natural killer cells act as rheostats modulating antiviral T cells. Nature. 2012;481:394–8.
24. Andrews DM, Estcourt MJ, Andoniou CE, et al. Innate immunity defines the capacity of antiviral T cells to limit persistent infection. J Exp Med. 2010;207:1333–43.
25. Boeckh M, Murphy WJ, Peggs KS. Recent advances in cytomegalovirus: an update on pharmacologic and cellular therapies. Biol Blood Marrow Transplant. 2015;21(1):24–9.
26. Sun JC, Beilke JN, Lanier LL. Adaptive immune features of natural killer cells. Nature. 2009;457:557–61.
27. Loeffler J, Steffens M, Arlt EM, et al. Polymorphisms in the genes encoding chemokine receptor 5, interleukin-10, and monocyte chemoattractant protein 1 contribute to cytomegalovirus reactivation and disease after allogeneic stem cell transplantation. J Clin Microbiol. 2006;44(5):1847–50.
28. Khan N, Cobbold M, Keenan R, Moss PA. Comparative analysis of CD8+ T cell responses against human cytomegalovirus proteins pp65 and immediate early 1 shows similarities in precursor frequency, oligoclonality, and phenotype. J Infect Dis. 2002;185(8):1025–34.
29. Kern F, Bunde T, Faulhaber N, et al. Cytomegalovirus (CMV) phosphoprotein 65 makes a large contribution to shaping the T cell repertoire in CMV-exposed individuals. J Infect Dis. 2002;185(12):1709–16.
30. Khan N, Best D, Bruton R, Nayak L, Rickinson AB, Moss PA. T cell recognition patterns of immunodominant cytomegalovirus antigens in primary and persistent infection. J Immunol. 2007;178(7):4455–65.
31. Sylwester AW, Mitchell BL, Edgar JB, et al. Broadly targeted human cytomegalovirus-specific CD4+ and CD8+ T cells dominate the memory compartments of exposed subjects. J Exp Med. 2005;202(5):673–85.
32. Quinnan GV Jr, Kirmani N, Rook AH, et al. Cytotoxic t cells in cytomegalovirus infection: HLA-restricted T-lymphocyte and non-T-lymphocyte cytotoxic responses correlate with recovery from cytomegalovirus infection in bone-marrow-transplant recipients. N Engl J Med. 1982;307(1):7–13.
33. Reusser P, Cathomas G, Attenhofer R, Tamm M, Thiel G. Cytomegalovirus (CMV)-specific T cell immunity after renal transplantation mediates protection from CMV disease by limiting the systemic virus load. J Infect Dis. 1999;180(2):247–53.
34. Reusser P, Riddell SR, Meyers JD, Greenberg PD. Cytotoxic T-lymphocyte response to cytomegalovirus after human allogeneic bone marrow transplantation: pattern of recovery and correlation with cytomegalovirus infection and disease. Blood. 1991;78(5):1373–80.
35. Hebart H, Daginik S, Stevanovic S, et al. Sensitive detection of human cytomegalovirus peptide-specific cytotoxic T-lymphocyte responses by interferon-gamma-enzyme-linked immunospot assay and flow cytometry in healthy individuals and in patients after allogeneic stem cell transplantation. Blood. 2002;99(10):3830–7.
36. Ljungman P, Aschan J, Azinge JN, et al. Cytomegalovirus viraemia and specific T-helper cell responses as predictors of disease after allogeneic marrow transplantation. Br J Haematol. 1993;83(1):118–24.
37. Ciáurriz M, Beloki L, Zabalza A, et al. Functional specific-T-cell expansion after first cytomegalovirus reactivation predicts viremia control in allogeneic hematopoietic stem cell transplant recipients. Transpl Infect Dis. 2017;19(6)
38. Boeckh M, Leisenring W, Riddell SR, et al. Late cytomegalovirus disease and mortality in recipients of allogeneic hematopoietic stem cell transplants: importance of viral load and T-cell immunity. Blood. 2003;101(2):407–14.
39. Marshall GS, Rabalais GP, Stout GG, Waldeyer SL. Antibodies to recombinant-derived glycoprotein B after natural human cytomegalovirus infection correlate with neutralizing activity. J Infect Dis. 1992;165(2):381–4.
40. Rasmussen L, Matkin C, Spaete R, Pachl C, Merigan TC. Antibody response to human cytomegalovirus glycoproteins gB and gH after natural infection in humans. J Infect Dis. 1991;164(5):835–42.
41. Goldmacher VS, Bartle LM, Skaletskaya A, et al. A cytomegalovirus-encoded mitochondria-localized inhibitor of apoptosis structurally unrelated to Bcl-2. Proc Natl Acad Sci U S A. 1999;96(22):12536–41.
42. Basta S, Bennink JR. A survival game of hide and seek: cytomegaloviruses and MHC class I antigen presentation pathways. Viral Immunol. 2003;16(3):231–42.
43. Abate DA, Watanabe S, Mocarski ES. Major human cytomegalovirus structural protein pp65 (ppUL83) prevents interferon response factor 3 activation in the interferon response. J Virol. 2004;78(20):10995–1006.
44. Child SJ, Hakki M, De Niro KL, Geballe AP. Evasion of cellular antiviral responses by human cytomegalovirus TRS1 and IRS1. J Virol. 2004;78(1):197–205.
45. Taylor RT, Bresnahan WA. Human cytomegalovirus immediate-early 2 gene expression blocks virus-induced beta interferon production. J Virol. 2005;79(6):3873–7.
46. Chapman TL, Heikeman AP, Bjorkman PJ. The inhibitory receptor LIR-1 uses a common binding interaction to recognize class I MHC molecules and the viral homolog UL18. Immunity. 1999;11(5):603–13.
47. Kotenko SV, Saccani S, Izotova LS, Mirochnitchenko OV, Pestka S. Human cytomegalovirus harbors its own unique IL-10 homolog (cmvIL-10). Proc Natl Acad Sci U S A. 2000;97(4):1695–700.
48. Benedict CA, Butrovich KD, Lurain NS, et al. Cutting edge: a novel viral TNF receptor superfamily member in virulent strains of human cytomegalovirus. J Immunol. 1999;162(12):6967–70.
49. Penfold ME, Dairaghi DJ, Duke GM, et al. Cytomegalovirus encodes a potent alpha chemokine. Proc Natl Acad Sci U S A. 1999;96(17):9839–44.
50. Taylor RT, Bresnahan WA. Human cytomegalovirus immediate-early 2 protein IE86 blocks virus-induced chemokine expression. J Virol. 2006;80(2):920–8.
51. Gao JL, Murphy PM. Human cytomegalovirus open reading frame US28 encodes a functional beta chemokine receptor. J Biol Chem. 1994;269(46):28539–42.
52. Lisnic VJ, Krmpotic A, Jonjic S. Modulation of natural killer cell activity by viruses. Curr Opin Microbiol. 2010;13:530–9.
53. Marcenaro E, Notarangelo LD, Orange JS, et al. Editorial: NK cell subsets in health and disease: new developments. Front Immunol. 2017;8:1363.
54. Torok-Storb B, Simmons P, Khaira D, et al. Cytomegalovirus and marrow function. Ann Hematol. 1992;64(Suppl):A128–31.
55. Reddehase MJ, Dreher-Stumpp L, Angele P, et al. Hematopoietic stem cell deficiency resulting from cytomegalovirus infection of bone marrow stroma. Ann Hematol. 1992;64(Suppl):A125–7.
56. Simmons P, Kaushansky K, Torok-Storb B. Mechanisms of cytomegalovirus-mediated myelosuppression: perturbation of stromal cell function versus direct infection of myeloid cells. Proc Natl Acad Sci U S A. 1990;87(4):1386–90.

57. Meyers JD, Ljungman P, Fisher LD. Cytomegalovirus excretion as a predictor of cytomegalovirus disease after marrow transplantation: importance of cytomegalovirus viremia. J Infect Dis. 1990;162(2):373–80.
58. Boeckh M, Boivin G. Quantitation of cytomegalovirus: methodologic aspects and clinical applications. Clin Microbiol Rev. 1998;11(3):533–54.
59. Einsele H, Ehninger G, Hebart H, et al. Polymerase chain reaction monitoring reduces the incidence of cytomegalovirus disease and the duration and side effects of antiviral therapy after bone marrow transplantation. Blood. 1995;86(7):2815–20.
60. Nichols WG, Corey L, Gooley T, et al. Rising pp65 antigenemia during preemptive anticytomegalovirus therapy after allogeneic hematopoietic stem cell transplantation: risk factors, correlation with DNA load, and outcomes. Blood. 2001;97(4):867–74.
61. Boeckh M, Gooley TA, Myerson D, et al. Cytomegalovirus pp65 antigenemia-guided early treatment with ganciclovir versus ganciclovir at engraftment after allogeneic marrow transplantation: a randomized double-blind study. Blood. 1996;88(10):4063–71.
62. Gor D, Sabin C, Prentice HG, et al. Longitudinal fluctuations in cytomegalovirus load in bone marrow transplant patients: relationship between peak virus load, donor/recipient serostatus, acute GVHD and CMV disease. Bone Marrow Transplant. 1998;21(6):597–605.
63. Cathomas G, Morris P, Pekle K, et al. Rapid diagnosis of cytomegalovirus pneumonia in marrow transplant recipients by bronchoalveolar lavage using the polymerase chain reaction, virus culture, and the direct immunostaining of alveolar cells. Blood. 1993;81(7):1909–14.
64. Gerna G, Lilleri D, Baldanti F, et al. Human cytomegalovirus immediate-early mRNAemia versus pp65 antigenemia for guiding pre-emptive therapy in children and young adults undergoing hematopoietic stem cell transplantation: a prospective, randomized, open-label trial. Blood. 2003;101(12):5053–60.
65. Chan ST, Logan AC. The clinical impact of cytomegalovirus infection following allogeneic hematopoietic cell transplantation: why the quest for meaningful prophylaxis still matters. Blood Rev. 2017;31(3):173–83.
66. Nichols WG, Corey L, Gooley T, et al. High risk of death due to bacterial and fungal infection among cytomegalovirus (CMV)-seronegative recipients of stem cell transplants from seropositive donors: evidence for indirect effects of primary CMV infection. J Infect Dis. 2002;185(3):273–82.
67. Manuel O, Pang XL, Humar A, et al. An assessment of donor-to-recipient transmission patterns of human cytomegalovirus by analysis of viral genomic variants. J Infect Dis. 2009; 199(11):1621–8.
68. Boeckh M. Current antiviral strategies for controlling cytomegalovirus in hematopoietic stem cell transplant recipients: prevention and therapy. Transpl Infect Dis. 1999;1(3):165–78.
69. Broers AE, van Der Holt R, van Esser JW, et al. Increased transplant-related morbidity and mortality in CMV- seropositive patients despite highly effective prevention of CMV disease after allogeneic T-cell-depleted stem cell transplantation. Blood. 2000;95(7):2240–5.
70. Craddock C, Szydlo RM, Dazzi F, et al. Cytomegalovirus seropositivity adversely influences outcome after T- depleted unrelated donor transplant in patients with chronic myeloid leukaemia: the case for tailored graft-versus-host disease prophylaxis. Br J Haematol. 2001;112(1):228–36.
71. Boeckh M, Nichols WG. The impact of cytomegalovirus serostatus of donor and recipient before hematopoietic stem cell transplantation in the era of antiviral prophylaxis and preemptive therapy. Blood. 2004;103(6):2003–8.
72. Cwynarski K, Roberts IA, Iacobelli S, et al. Stem cell transplantation for chronic myeloid leukemia in children. Blood. 2003;102(4):1224–31.
73. Erard V, Guthrie KA, Riddell S, Boeckh M. Impact of HLA A2 and cytomegalovirus serostatus on outcomes in patients with leukemia following matched-sibling myeloablative allogeneic hematopoietic cell transplantation. Haematologica. 2006;91(10):1377–83.
74. Grob JP, Grundy JE, Prentice HG, et al. Immune donors can protect marrow-transplant recipients from severe cytomegalovirus infections. Lancet. 1987;1(8536):774–6.
75. Jacobsen N, Badsberg JH, Lonnqvist B, et al. Graft-versus-leukaemia activity associated with CMV-seropositive donor, post-transplant CMV infection, young donor age and chronic graft-versus-host disease in bone marrow allograft recipients. The Nordic Bone Marrow Transplantation Group. Bone Marrow Transplant. 1990;5(6):413–8.
76. Kollman C, Howe CW, Anasetti C, et al. Donor characteristics as risk factors in recipients after transplantation of bone marrow from unrelated donors: the effect of donor age. Blood. 2001;98(7):2043–51.
77. Ljungman P, Einsele H, Frassoni F, et al. Donor CMV serological status influences the outcome of CMVseropositive recipients after unrelated donor stem cell transplantation; an EBMT megafile analysis. Blood. 2003;102:4255–60.
78. Nachbaur D, Clausen J, Kircher B. Donor cytomegalovirus seropositivity and the risk of leukemic relapse after reduced-intensity transplants. Eur J Haematol. 2006;76(5):414–9.
79. Ringden O, Schaffer M, Le Blanc K, et al. Which donor should be chosen for hematopoietic stem cell transplantation among unrelated HLA-A, -B, and -DRB1 genomically identical volunteers? Biol Blood Marrow Transplant. 2004;10(2):128–34.
80. Avetisyan G, Aschan J, Hagglund H, et al. Evaluation of intervention strategy based on CMV-specific immune responses after allogeneic SCT. Bone Marrow Transplant. 2007;40(9):865–9.
81. Ganepola S, Gentilini C, Hilbers U, et al. Patients at high risk for CMV infection and disease show delayed CD8+ T-cell immune recovery after allogeneic stem cell transplantation. Bone Marrow Transplant. 2007;39(5):293–9.
82. Moins-Teisserenc H, Busson M, Scieux C, et al. Patterns of cytomegalovirus reactivation are associated with distinct evolutive profiles of immune reconstitution after allogeneic hematopoeitic stem cell transplantation. J Infect Dis. 2008;198(6):818–26.
83. Lin TS, Zahrieh D, Weller E, Alyea EP, Antin JH, Soiffer RJ. Risk factors for cytomegalovirus reactivation after CD6+ T-cell-depleted allogeneic bone marrow transplantation. Transplantation. 2002;74(1):49–54.
84. Ozdemir E, Saliba R, Champlin R, et al. Risk factors associated with late cytomegalovirus reactivation after allogeneic stem cell transplantation for hematological malignancies. Bone Marrow Transplant. 2007;40(2):125–36.
85. Marty FM, Bryar J, Browne SK, et al. Sirolimus-based graft-versus-host disease prophylaxis protects against cytomegalovirus reactivation after allogeneic hematopoietic stem cell transplantation: a cohort analysis. Blood. 2007;110(2):490–500.
86. Miller W, Flynn P, McCullough J, et al. Cytomegalovirus infection after bone marrow transplantation: an association with acute graft-v-host disease. Blood. 1986;67(4):1162–7.
87. Walker CM, van Burik JA, De For TE, Weisdorf DJ. Cytomegalovirus infection after allogeneic transplantation: comparison of cord blood with peripheral blood and marrow graft sources. Biol Blood Marrow Transplant. 2007;13(9):1106–15.
88. Ljungman P, Aschan J, Lewensohn-Fuchs I, et al. Results of different strategies for reducing cytomegalovirus-associated mortality in allogeneic stem cell transplant recipients. Transplantation. 1998;66(10):1330–4.
89. Martino R, Rovira M, Carreras E, et al. Severe infections after allogeneic peripheral blood stem cell transplantation: a matched-pair comparison of unmanipulated and CD34+ cell-selected transplantation. Haematologica. 2001;86(10):1075–86.

90. Nakamae H, Kirby KA, Sandmaier BM, et al. Effect of conditioning regimen intensity on CMV infection in allogeneic hematopoietic cell transplantation. Biol Blood Marrow Transplant. 2009;15(6):694–703.
91. Holmberg LA, Boeckh M, Hooper H, et al. Increased incidence of cytomegalovirus disease after autologous CD34-selected peripheral blood stem cell transplantation. Blood. 1999;94(12):4029–35.
92. Trenschel R, Ross S, Husing J, et al. Reduced risk of persisting cytomegalovirus pp65 antigenemia and cytomegalovirus interstitial pneumonia following allogeneic PBSCT. Bone Marrow Transplant. 2000;25(6):665–72.
93. Kudchodkar SB, Yu Y, Maguire TG, Alwine JC. Human cytomegalovirus infection alters the substrate specificities and rapamycin sensitivities of raptor- and rictor-containing complexes. Proc Natl Acad Sci U S A. 2006;103(38):14182–7.
94. Einsele H, Steidle M, Vallbracht A, et al. Early occurrence of human cytomegalovirus infection after bone marrow transplantation as demonstrated by the polymerase chain reaction technique. Blood. 1991;77(5):1104–10.
95. Nguyen Q, Champlin R, Giralt S, et al. Late cytomegalovirus pneumonia in adult allogeneic blood and marrow transplant recipients. Clin Infect Dis. 1999;28(3):618–23.
96. Machado CM, Menezes RX, Macedo MC, et al. Extended antigenemia surveillance and late cytomegalovirus infection after allogeneic BMT. Bone Marrow Transplant. 2001;28(11):1053–9.
97. Osarogiagbon RU, Defor TE, Weisdorf MA, et al. CMV antigenemia following bone marrow transplantation: risk factors and outcomes. Biol Blood Marrow Transplant. 2000;6(3):280–8.
98. Peggs KS, Preiser W, Kottaridis PD, et al. Extended routine polymerase chain reaction surveillance and pre-emptive antiviral therapy for cytomegalovirus after allogeneic transplantation. Br J Haematol. 2000;111(3):782–90.
99. Li CR, Greenberg PD, Gilbert MJ, et al. Recovery of HLA-restricted cytomegalovirus (CMV)-specific T-cell responses after allogeneic bone marrow transplant: correlation with CMV disease and effect of ganciclovir prophylaxis. Blood. 1994;83(7):1971–9.
100. Krause H, Hebart H, Jahn G, et al. Screening for CMV-specific T cell proliferation to identify patients at risk of developing late onset CMV disease. Bone Marrow Transplant. 1997;19(11):1111–6.
101. Junghanss C, Boeckh M, Carter RA, et al. Incidence and outcome of cytomegalovirus infections following nonmyeloablative compared with myeloablative allogeneic stem cell transplantation, a matched control study. Blood. 2002;99(6):1978–85.
102. Safdar A, Rodriguez GH, Mihu CN, et al. Infections in non-myeloablative hematopoietic stem cell transplantation patients with lymphoid malignancies: spectrum of infections, predictors of outcome and proposed guidelines for fungal infection prevention. Bone Marrow Transplant. 2010;45(2):339–47.
103. Chakrabarti S, Mackinnon S, Chopra R, et al. High incidence of cytomegalovirus infection after nonmyeloablative stem cell transplantation: potential role of Campath-1H in delaying immune reconstitution. Blood. 2002;99(12):4357–63.
104. Boeckh M, Stevens-Ayers T, Bowden RA. Cytomegalovirus pp65 antigenemia after autologous marrow and peripheral blood stem cell transplantation. J Infect Dis. 1996;174(5):907–12.
105. Hebart H, Schroder A, Loffler J, et al. Cytomegalovirus monitoring by polymerase chain reaction of whole blood samples from patients undergoing autologous bone marrow or peripheral blood progenitor cell transplantation. J Infect Dis. 1997;175(6):1490–3.
106. Bilgrami S, Aslanzadeh J, Feingold JM, et al. Cytomegalovirus viremia, viruria and disease after autologous peripheral blood stem cell transplantation: no need for surveillance. Bone Marrow Transplant. 1999;24(1):69–73.
107. Boeckh M, Gooley TA, Reusser P, Buckner CD, Bowden RA. Failure of high-dose acyclovir to prevent cytomegalovirus disease after autologous marrow transplantation. J Infect Dis. 1995;172(4):939–43.
108. Singhal S, Powles R, Treleaven J, et al. Cytomegaloviremia after autografting for leukemia: clinical significance and lack of effect on engraftment. Leukemia. 1997;11(6):835–8.
109. Reusser P, Fisher LD, Buckner CD, et al. Cytomegalovirus infection after autologous bone marrow transplantation: occurrence of cytomegalovirus disease and effect on engraftment. Blood. 1990;75(9):1888–94.
110. Schoemans H, Theunissen K, Maertens J, et al. Adult umbilical cord blood transplantation: a comprehensive review. Bone Marrow Transplant. 2006;38(2):83–93.
111. Albano MS, Taylor P, Pass RF, et al. Umbilical cord blood transplantation and cytomegalovirus: posttransplantation infection and donor screening. Blood. 2006;108(13):4275–82.
112. Matsumura T, Narimatsu H, Kami M, et al. Cytomegalovirus infections following umbilical cord blood transplantation using reduced intensity conditioning regimens for adult patients. Biol Blood Marrow Transplant. 2007;13(5):577–83.
113. Saavedra S, Sanz GF, Jarque I, et al. Early infections in adult patients undergoing unrelated donor cord blood transplantation. Bone Marrow Transplant. 2002;30(12):937–43.
114. Takami A, Mochizuki K, Asakura H, et al. High incidence of cytomegalovirus reactivation in adult recipients of an unrelated cord blood transplant. Haematologica. 2005;90(9):1290–2.
115. Tomonari A, Takahashi S, Ooi J, et al. Preemptive therapy with ganciclovir 5 mg/kg once daily for cytomegalovirus infection after unrelated cord blood transplantation. Bone Marrow Transplant. 2008;41(4):371–6.
116. Beck JC, Wagner JE, DeFor TE, et al. Impact of cytomegalovirus (CMV) reactivation after umbilical cord blood transplantation. Biol Blood Marrow Transplant. 2010;16(2):215–22.
117. Safdar A, Rodriguez GH, De Lima MJ, et al. Infections in 100 cord blood transplantations: spectrum of early and late posttransplant infections in adult and pediatric patients 1996-2005. Medicine (Baltimore). 2007;86(6):324–33.
118. Hebart H, Ljungman P, Klingebiel T, et al. Prospective comparison of PCR-based versus late mRNA-based preemptive antiviral therapy for HCMV infection in patients after allogeneic stem cell transplantation. Blood. 2003;102(11):195a.
119. Ljungman P, Griffiths P, Paya C. Definitions of cytomegalovirus infection and disease in transplant recipients. Clin Infect Dis. 2002;34(8):1094–7.
120. Konoplev S, Champlin RE, Giralt S, et al. Cytomegalovirus pneumonia in adult autologous blood and marrow transplant recipients. Bone Marrow Transplant. 2001;27(8):877–81.
121. Torres HA, Aguilera E, Safdar A, et al. Fatal cytomegalovirus pneumonia in patients with haematological malignancies: an autopsy-based case-control study. Clin Microbiol Infect. 2008;14(12):1160–6.
122. Ison MG, Fishman JA. Cytomegalovirus pneumonia in transplant recipients. Clin Chest Med. 2005;26(4):691–705, viii
123. Ketai L, Jordan K, Busby KH. Imaging infection. Clin Chest Med. 2015;36(2):197–217, viii
124. Green ML. Viral pneumonia in patients with hematopoietic cell transplantation and hematologic malignancies. Clin Chest Med. 2017;38(2):295–305.
125. Schmidt GM, Horak DA, Niland JC, et al. A randomized, controlled trial of prophylactic ganciclovir for cytomegalovirus pulmonary infection in recipients of allogeneic bone marrow transplants; The City of Hope-Stanford-Syntex CMV Study Group. N Engl J Med. 1991;324(15):1005–11.
126. Tabbara KF, Al-Ghamdi A, Al-Mohareb F, et al. Ocular findings after allogeneic hematopoietic stem cell transplantation. Ophthalmology. 2009;116(9):1624–9.
127. Crippa F, Corey L, Chuang EL, et al. Virological, clinical, and ophthalmologic features of cytomegalovirus retinitis after hematopoietic stem cell transplantation. Clin Infect Dis. 2001;32(2):214–9.

128. Larochelle MB, Phan R, Craddock J, et al. Cytomegalovirus retinitis in pediatric stem cell transplants: report of a recent cluster and the development of a screening protocol. Am J Ophthalmol. 2017;175:8–15.
129. Greco R, Crucitti L, Noviello M, et al. Human herpesvirus 6 infection following haploidentical transplantation: immune recovery and outcome. Biol Blood Marrow Transplant. 2016;22(12):2250–5.
130. Clark DA, Emery VC, Griffiths PD. Cytomegalovirus, human herpesvirus-6, and human herpesvirus-7 in hematological patients. Semin Hematol. 2003;40(2):154–62.
131. Zhang XH, Zhang JM, Han W, et al. Viral encephalitis after haplo-identical hematopoietic stem cell transplantation: causative viral spectrum, characteristics, and risk factors. Eur J Haematol. 2017;98(5):450–8.
132. Renard T, Daumas-Duport B, Auffray-Calvier E, et al. Cytomegalovirus encephalitis: undescribed diffusion-weighted imaging characteristics. Original aspects of cases extracted from a retrospective study, and from literature review. J Neuroradiol. 2016;43(6):371–7.
133. Inazawa N, Hori T, Yamamoto M, et al. HHV-6 encephalitis may complicate the early phase after allogeneic hematopoietic stem cell transplantation: detection by qualitative multiplex PCR and subsequent quantitative real-time PCR. J Med Virol. 2016;88(2):319–23.
134. Jang EY, Park SY, Lee EJ, et al. Diagnostic performance of the cytomegalovirus (CMV) antigenemia assay in patients with CMV gastrointestinal disease. Clin Infect Dis. 2009;48(12):e121–4.
135. Mori T, Okamoto S, Matsuoka S, et al. Risk-adapted pre-emptive therapy for cytomegalovirus disease in patients undergoing allogeneic bone marrow transplantation. Bone Marrow Transplant. 2000;25(7):765–9.
136. Kotton CN, Huprikar S, Kumar D. Transplant infectious diseases: a review of the scientific registry of transplant recipients published data. Am J Transplant. 2017;17(6):1439–46.
137. Pascual J, Royuela A, Fernández AM, et al. Role of mTOR inhibitors for the control of viral infection in solid organ transplant recipients. Transpl Infect Dis. 2016;18(6):819–31.
138. Mena-Romo JD, Pérez Romero P, Martín-Gandul C, et al. CMV-specific T-cell immunity in solid organ transplant recipients at low risk of CMV infection. Chronology and applicability in preemptive therapy. J Infect. 2017;75(4):336–45.
139. Schachtner T, Stein M, Reinke P. CMV-specific T cell monitoring offers superior risk stratification of CMV-seronegative kidney transplant recipients of a CMV-seropositive donor. Transplantation. 2017;101(10):e315–25.
140. Costa J, Benvenuto LJ, Sonett JR. Long-term outcomes and management of lung transplant recipients. Best Pract Res Clin Anaesthesiol. 2017;31(2):285–97.
141. Durante-Mangoni E, Andini R, Pinto D, et al. Effect of the immunosuppressive regimen on the incidence of cytomegalovirus infection in 378 heart transplant recipients: a single center, prospective cohort study. J Clin Virol. 2015;68:37–42.
142. Strueber M, Warnecke G, Fuge J, et al. Everolimus versus mycophenolate mofetil de novo after lung transplantation: a prospective, randomized, open-label trial. Am J Transplant. 2016;16(11):3171–80.
143. Lee EC, Kim SH, Park SJ. Outcomes after liver transplantation in accordance with ABO compatibility: a systematic review and meta-analysis. World J Gastroenterol. 2017;23(35):6516–33.
144. Phan TL, Lautenschlager I, Razonable RR, et al. HHV-6 in liver transplantation: a literature review. Liver Int. 2018;38(2):210–23.
145. Lowance D, Neumayer HH, Legendre CM, et al. Valacyclovir for the prevention of cytomegalovirus disease after renal transplantation. International Valacyclovir Cytomegalovirus Prophylaxis Transplantation Study Group. N Engl J Med. 1999;340(19):1462–70.
146. Reischig T, Jindra P, Mares J, et al. Valacyclovir for cytomegalovirus prophylaxis reduces the risk of acute renal allograft rejection. Transplantation. 2005;79(3):317–24.
147. Elfadawy N, Flechner SM, Liu X, et al. CMV viremia is associated with a decreased incidence of BKV reactivation after kidney and kidney-pancreas transplantation. Transplantation. 2013;96(12):1097–103.
148. Malvezzi P, Jouve T, Rostaing L. Use of everolimus-based immunosuppression to decrease cytomegalovirus infection after kidney transplant. Exp Clin Transplant. 2016;14(4):361–6.
149. Fallatah SM, Marquez MA, Bazerbachi F, et al. Cytomegalovirus infection post-pancreas-kidney transplantation--results of antiviral prophylaxis in high-risk patients. Clin Transpl. 2013; 27(4):503–9.
150. Shah AP, Chen JM, Fridell JA. Incidence and outcomes of cytomegalovirus in pancreas transplantation with steroid-free immunosuppression. Clin Transpl. 2015;29(12):1221–9.
151. Manez R, Kusne S, Green M, et al. Incidence and risk factors associated with the development of cytomegalovirus disease after intestinal transplantation. Transplantation. 1995;59(7):1010–4.
152. Bueno J, Green M, Kocoshis S, et al. Cytomegalovirus infection after intestinal transplantation in children. Clin Infect Dis. 1997;25(5):1078–83.
153. Florescu DF, Langnas AN, Grant W, et al. Incidence, risk factors, and outcomes associated with cytomegalovirus disease in small bowel transplant recipients. Pediatr Transplant. 2012;16(3):294–301.
154. Gordon C, Siemionow M, Papay F, et al. The world's experience with facial transplantation: what have we learned thus far? Ann Plast Surg. 2009;63:572–8.
155. Schneeberger S, Lucchina S, Lanzetta M, et al. Cytomegalovirus-related complications in human hand transplantation. Transplantation. 2005;80:441–7.
156. Ng AP, Worth L, Chen L, et al. Cytomegalovirus DNAemia and disease: incidence, natural history and management in settings other than allogeneic stem cell transplantation. Haematologica. 2005;90(12):1672–9.
157. Marchesi F, Pimpinelli F, Ensoli F, et al. Cytomegalovirus infection in hematologic malignancy settings other than the allogeneic transplant. Hematol Oncol. 2018;36(2):381–91.
158. O'Brien SM, Keating MJ, Mocarski ES. Updated guidelines on the management of cytomegalovirus reactivation in patients with chronic lymphocytic leukemia treated with alemtuzumab. Clin Lymphoma Myeloma. 2006;7(2):125–30.
159. Orlandi EM, Baldanti F, Citro A, et al. Monitoring for cytomegalovirus and Epstein-Barr virus infection in chronic lymphocytic leukemia patients receiving i.v. fludarabine-cyclophosphamide combination and alemtuzumab as consolidation therapy. Haematologica. 2008;93(11):1758–60.
160. Laurenti L, Piccioni P, Cattani P, et al. Cytomegalovirus reactivation during alemtuzumab therapy for chronic lymphocytic leukemia: incidence and treatment with oral ganciclovir. Haematologica. 2004;89(10):1248–52.
161. O'Brien S, Ravandi F, Riehl T, et al. Valganciclovir prevents cytomegalovirus reactivation in patients receiving alemtuzumab-based therapy. Blood. 2008;111(4):1816–9.
162. Hwang YY, Cheung WW, Leung AY, et al. Valganciclovir thrice weekly for prophylaxis against cytomegalovirus reactivation during alemtuzumab therapy. Leukemia. 2009;23(4):800–1.
163. Gonzalez H, Vernant JP, Caumes E. Successful oral valganciclovir treatment of cytomegalovirus infection during Campath-1H therapy. Leukemia. 2005;19(3):478.
164. Thursky KA, Worth LJ, Seymour JF, et al. Spectrum of infection, risk and recommendations for prophylaxis and screening among patients with lymphoproliferative disorders treated with alemtuzumab. Br J Haematol. 2006;132(1):3–12.

165. Osterborg A, Foà R, Bezares RF, et al. Management guidelines for the use of alemtuzumab in chronic lymphocytic leukemia. Leukemia. 2009;23(11):1980–8.
166. Magliocca JF, Odorico JS, Pirsch JD, et al. A comparison of alemtuzumab with basiliximab induction in simultaneous pancreas-kidney transplantation. Am J Transplant. 2008;8(8):1702–10.
167. Ishihara H, Ishida H, Toki D, et al. Effects of low-dose rituximab therapy in patients with primary cytomegalovirus infection. Exp Clin Transplant. 2015;13(6):573–80.
168. Aksoy S, Harputluoglu H, Kilickap S, et al. Rituximab-related viral infections in lymphoma patients. Leuk Lymphoma. 2007;48(7):1307–12.
169. Jain T, John J, Kotecha A, et al. Cytomegalovirus infection in autologous stem cell transplant recipients in the era of rituximab. Ann Hematol. 2016;95(8):1323–7.
170. Laberko A, Bogoyavlenskaya A, Shelikhova L, et al. Risk factors for and the clinical impact of cytomegalovirus and Epstein-Barr virus infections in pediatric recipients of TCR--α/β- and CD19-depleted grafts. Biol Blood Marrow Transplant. 2017;23(3):483–90.
171. Chapman TM, Keating GM. Basiliximab: a review of its use as induction therapy in renal transplantation. Drugs. 2003;63(24):2803–35.
172. Penninga L, Møller CH, Gustafsson F, et al. Immunosuppressive T-cell antibody induction for heart transplant recipients. Cochrane Database Syst Rev. 2013;(12):CD008842.
173. Bowden RA, Sayers M, Flournoy N, et al. Cytomegalovirus immune globulin and seronegative blood products to prevent primary cytomegalovirus infection after marrow transplantation. N Engl J Med. 1986;314(16):1006–10.
174. Bowden R, Cays M, Schoch G, et al. Comparison of filtered blood (FB) to seronegative blood products (SB) for prevention of cytomegalovirus (CMV) infection after marrow transplant. Blood. 1995;86:3598–603.
175. Nichols WG, Price TH, Gooley T, et al. Transfusion-transmitted cytomegalovirus infection after receipt of leukoreduced blood products. Blood. 2003;101(10):4195–200.
176. Marty FM, Ljungman P, Papanicolaou GA, et al. Maribavir prophylaxis for prevention of cytomegalovirus disease in recipients of allogeneic stem-cell transplants: a phase 3, double-blind, placebo-controlled, randomized trial. Lancet Infect Dis. 2011;11(4):284–92.
177. Chemaly RF, Ullmann AJ, Stoelben S, et al. Letermovir for cytomegalovirus prophylaxis in hematopoietic-cell transplantation. N Engl J Med. 2014;370(19):1781–9.
178. Marty FM, Ljungman P, Chemaly RF, et al. Letermovir prophylaxis for cytomegalovirus in hematopoietic-cell transplantation. N Engl J Med. 2017;377(25):2433–44.
179. Ruutu T, Ljungman P, Brinch L, et al. No prevention of cytomegalovirus infection by anti-cytomegalovirus hyperimmune globulin in seronegative bone marrow transplant recipients. The Nordic BMT Group. Bone Marrow Transplant. 1997;19(3):233–6.
180. Bowden RA, Fisher LD, Rogers K, et al. Cytomegalovirus (CMV)-specific intravenous immunoglobulin for the prevention of primary CMV infection and disease after marrow transplant. J Infect Dis. 1991;164(3):483–7.
181. Boeckh M, Bowden R, Storer B, et al. Randomized, placebo-controlled, double-blind study of a cytomegalovirus-specific monoclonal antibody (MSL-109) for prevention of cytomegalovirus infection after allogeneic hematopoietic stem cell transplantation. Biol Blood Marrow Transplant. 2001;7(6):343–51.
182. Messori A, Rampazzo R, Scroccaro G, et al. Efficacy of hyperimmune anti-cytomegalovirus immunoglobulins for the prevention of cytomegalovirus infection in recipients of allogeneic bone marrow transplantation: a metaanalysis. Bone Marrow Transplant. 1994;13:163–8.
183. Sullivan KM, Kopecky KJ, Jocom J, et al. Immunomodulatory and antimicrobial efficacy of intravenous immunoglobulin in bone marrow transplantation. N Engl J Med. 1990;323(11):705–12.
184. Tomblyn M, Chiller T, Einsele H, et al. Guidelines for preventing infectious complications among hematopoietic cell transplantation recipients: a global perspective. Biol Blood Marrow Transplant. 2009;15(10):1143–238.
185. van Gent R, Metselaar HJ, Kwekkeboom J. Immunomodulation by hyperimmunoglobulins after solid organ transplantation: beyond prevention of viral infection. Transplant Rev (Orlando). 2017;31(2):78–86.
186. Safdar A, Bruorton M, Henslee-Downey JP, et al. Role of quantitative human cytomegalovirus PCR in predicting antiviral treatment response among high-risk hematopoietic stem-cell transplant recipients. Bone Marrow Transplant. 2004;33(4):463–4.
187. Boeckh M, Ljungman P. How we treat cytomegalovirus in hematopoietic cell transplant recipients. Blood. 2009;113(23):5711–9.
188. Lacey SF, Diamond DJ, Zaia JA. Assessment of cellular immunity to human cytomegalovirus in recipients of allogeneic stem cell transplants. Biol Blood Marrow Transplant. 2004;10(7):433–47.
189. Ljungman P, Lore K, Aschan J, et al. Use of a semi-quantitative PCR for cytomegalovirus DNA as a basis for pre-emptive antiviral therapy in allogeneic bone marrow transplant patients. Bone Marrow Transplant. 1996;17(4):583–7.
190. Reusser P, Einsele H, Lee J, et al. Randomized multicenter trial of foscarnet versus ganciclovir for preemptive therapy of cytomegalovirus infection after allogeneic stem cell transplantation. Blood. 2002;99(4):1159–64.
191. Ljungman P, Perez-Bercoff L, Jonsson J, et al. Risk factors for the development of cytomegalovirus disease after allogeneic stem cell transplantation. Haematologica. 2006;91(1):78–83.
192. Reed EC, Wolford JL, Kopecky KJ, et al. Ganciclovir for the treatment of cytomegalovirus gastroenteritis in bone marrow transplant patients. A randomized, placebo-controlled trial. Ann Intern Med. 1990;112(7):505–10.
193. Ljungman P, Cordonnier C, Einsele H, et al. Use of intravenous immune globulin in addition to antiviral therapy in the treatment of CMV gastrointestinal disease in allogeneic bone marrow transplant patients: a report from the European Group for Blood and Marrow Transplantation (EBMT). Infectious Diseases Working Party of the EBMT. Bone Marrow Transplant. 1998;21(5):473–6.
194. Reed EC, Bowden RA, Dandliker PS, et al. Treatment of cytomegalovirus pneumonia with ganciclovir and intravenous cytomegalovirus immunoglobulin in patients with bone marrow transplants. Ann Intern Med. 1988;109(10):783–8.
195. Emanuel D, Cunningham I, Jules-Elysee K, et al. Cytomegalovirus pneumonia after bone marrow transplantation successfully treated with the combination of ganciclovir and high-dose intravenous immune globulin. Ann Intern Med. 1988;109(10):777–82.
196. Ljungman P, Engelhard D, Link H, et al. Treatment of interstitial pneumonitis due to cytomegalovirus with ganciclovir and intravenous immune globulin: experience of European Bone Marrow Transplant Group. Clin Infect Dis. 1992;14(4):831–5.
197. Machado CM, Dulley FL, Boas LS, et al. CMV pneumonia in allogeneic BMT recipients undergoing early treatment of pre-emptive ganciclovir therapy. Bone Marrow Transplant. 2000;26(4):413–7.
198. Chang M, Dunn JP. Ganciclovir implant in the treatment of cytomegalovirus retinitis. Expert Rev Med Devices. 2005;2(4):421–7.
199. Okamoto T, Okada M, Mori A, et al. Successful treatment of severe cytomegalovirus retinitis with foscarnet and intraocular infection of ganciclovir in a myelosuppressed unrelated bone marrow transplant patient. Bone Marrow Transplant. 1997;20(9):801–3.
200. Rahhal FM. Treatment advances for CMV retinitis. AIDS Read. 1999;9(1):28, 31–4
201. Wang H, Chhablani J, Freeman WR, et al. Intraocular safety and pharmacokinetics of hexadecyloxypropyl-cidofovir (HDP-CDV)

as a long-lasting intravitreal antiviral drug. Invest Ophthalmol Vis Sci. 2011;52(13):9391–6.

202. Cheng L, Beadle JR, Tammewar A, et al. Intraocular pharmacokinetics of a crystalline lipid prodrug, octadecyloxyethyl-cyclic-cidofovir, for cytomegalovirus retinitis. J Ocul Pharmacol Ther. 2011;27(2):157–62.
203. Bazewicz M, Fikri J, Martin CH, et al. Drug-induced uveitis in aids patients: two case reports. Bull Soc Belge Ophtalmol. 2011;318:19–23.
204. Wang L, Damji KF, Chialant D, Hodge WG. Hypotony after intravenous cidofovir therapy for the treatment of cytomegalovirus retinitis. Can J Ophthalmol. 2002;37(7):419–22.
205. Scott RA, Pavesio C. Ocular side-effects from systemic HPMPC (cidofovir) for a non-ocular cytomegalovirus infection. Am J Ophthalmol. 2000;130(1):126–7.
206. Ambati J, Wynne KB, Angerame MC, et al. Anterior uveitis associated with intravenous cidofovir use in patients with cytomegalovirus retinitis. Br J Ophthalmol. 1999;83(10):1153–8.
207. Biron KK. Antiviral drugs for cytomegalovirus diseases. Antivir Res. 2006;71(2–3):154–63.
208. Meyers JD, Reed EC, Shepp DH, et al. Acyclovir for prevention of cytomegalovirus infection and disease after allogeneic marrow transplantation. N Engl J Med. 1988;318(2):70–5.
209. Ljungman P, De La Camara R, Milpied N, et al. A randomised study of valaciclovir as prophylaxis against CMV reactivation in allogeneic bone marrow transplant recipients. Blood. 2002;73:930–6.
210. Sullivan KM, Dykewicz CA, Longworth DL, et al. Preventing opportunistic infections after hematopoietic stem cell transplantation: the Centers for Disease Control and Prevention, Infectious Diseases Society of America, and American Society for Blood and Marrow Transplantation Practice Guidelines and beyond. Hematology Am Soc Hematol Educ Program. 2001:392–421.
211. Goodrich JM, Bowden RA, Fisher L, Keller C, Schoch G, Meyers JD. Ganciclovir prophylaxis to prevent cytomegalovirus disease after allogeneic marrow transplant. Ann Intern Med. 1993;118(3):173–8.
212. Winston DJ, Yeager AM, Chandrasekar PH, Snydman DR, Petersen FB, Territo MC. Randomized comparison of oral valacyclovir and intravenous ganciclovir for prevention of cytomegalovirus disease after allogeneic bone marrow transplantation. Clin Infect Dis. 2003;36(6):749–58.
213. Salzberger B, Bowden RA, Hackman RC, et al. Neutropenia in allogeneic marrow transplant recipients receiving ganciclovir for prevention of cytomegalovirus disease: risk factors and outcome. Blood. 1997;90(6):2502–8.
214. Einsele H, Reusser P, Bornhauser M, et al. Oral valganciclovir leads to higher exposure to ganciclovir than intravenous ganciclovir in patients following allogeneic stem cell transplantation. Blood. 2006;107(7):3002–8.
215. Allice T, Busca A, Locatelli F, et al. Valganciclovir as pre-emptive therapy for cytomegalovirus infection post-allogenic stem cell transplantation: implications for the emergence of drug-resistant cytomegalovirus. J Antimicrob Chemother. 2009;63(3):600–8.
216. Ayala E, Greene J, Sandin R, et al. Valganciclovir is safe and effective as pre-emptive therapy for CMV infection in allogeneic hematopoietic stem cell transplantation. Bone Marrow Transplant. 2006;37(9):851–6.
217. Asberg A, Humar A, Rollag H, et al. Oral valganciclovir is noninferior to intravenous ganciclovir for the treatment of cytomegalovirus disease in solid organ transplant recipients. Am J Transplant. 2007;7(9):2106–13.
218. Åsberg A, Humar A, Rollag H, et al. Lessons learned from a randomized study of oral valganciclovir versus parenteral ganciclovir treatment of cytomegalovirus disease in solid organ transplant recipients: the VICTOR trial. Clin Infect Dis. 2016;62(9):1154–60.
219. Lim ZY, Cook G, Johnson PR, et al. Results of a phase I/II British Society of Bone Marrow Transplantation study on PCR-based pre-emptive therapy with valganciclovir or ganciclovir for active CMV infection following alemtuzumab-based reduced intensity allogeneic stem cell transplantation. Leuk Res. 2009;33(2):244–9.
220. Safdar A, Brown AE, Malkin M. Acute febrile myelodysplasia and pneumonitis due to human herpesvirus 6 after accelerated chemotherapy. Am J Med. 2001;111(4):329–30.
221. Bacigalupo A, Tedone E, Van Lint MT, et al. CMV prophylaxis with foscarnet in allogeneic bone marrow transplant recipients at high risk of developing CMV infections. Bone Marrow Transplant. 1994;13(6):783–8.
222. Reusser P, Gambertoglio JG, Lilleby K, et al. Phase I-II trial of foscarnet for prevention of cytomegalovirus infection in autologous and allogeneic marrow transplant recipients [see comments]. J Infect Dis. 1992;166(3):473–9.
223. Bregante S, Bertilson S, Tedone E, et al. Foscarnet prophylaxis of cytomegalovirus infections in patients undergoing allogeneic bone marrow transplantation (BMT): a dose-finding study. Bone Marrow Transplant. 2000;26(1):23–9.
224. Avery RK, Arav-Boger R, Marr KA, et al. Outcomes in transplant recipients treated with foscarnet for ganciclovir-resistant or refractory cytomegalovirus infection. Transplantation. 2016;100(10):e74–80.
225. Lea AP, Bryson HM. Cidofovir. Drugs. 1996;52:225.
226. Safrin S, Cherrington J, Jaffe HS. Clinical uses of cidofovir. Rev Med Virol. 1997;7(3):145–56.
227. Evers DL, Komazin G, Ptak RG, et al. Inhibition of human cytomegalovirus replication by benzimidazole nucleosides involves three distinct mechanisms. Antimicrob Agents Chemother. 2004;48:3918–27.
228. Drew WL, Miner RC, Marousek GI, et al. Maribavir sensitivity of cytomegalovirus isolates resistant to ganciclovir, cidofovir or foscarnet. J Clin Virol. 2006;37:124–7.
229. Lalezari JP, Aberg JA, Wang LH, et al. Phase I dose escalation trial evaluating the pharmacokinetics, anti-human cytomegalovirus (HCMV) activity, and safety of 1263W96 in human immunodeficiency virus-infected men with asymptomatic HCMV shedding. Antimicrob Agents Chemother. 2002;46:2969–76.
230. Wang LH, Peck RW, Yin Y, et al. Phase I safety and pharmacokinetic trials of 1263W94, a novel oral anti-human cytomegalovirus agent, in healthy and human immunodeficiency virus-infected subjects. Antimicrob Agents Chemother. 2003;47:1334–42.
231. Marty FM, Ljungman P, Papanicolaou GA, et al. Maribavir prophylaxis for prevention of cytomegalovirus disease in recipients of allogeneic stem-cell transplants: a phase 3, double-blind, placebo-controlled, randomised trial. Lancet Infect Dis. 2011;11:284–92.
232. Marty FM, Boeckh M. Maribavir and human cytomegalovirus-what happened in the clinical trials and why might the drug have failed? Curr Opin Virol. 2011;1:555–62.
233. Kaul DR, Stoelben S, Cober E, et al. First report of successful treatment of multidrug-resistant cytomegalovirus disease with the novel anti-CMV compound AIC246. Am J Transplant. 2011;11(5):1079–84.
234. Aldern KA, Ciesla SL, Winegarden KL, et al. Increased antiviral ac- tivity of 1-O-hexadecyloxypropyl-[2-(14)C] cidofovir in MRC-5 human lung fibro- blasts is explained by unique cellular up- take and metabolism. Mol Pharmacol. 2003;63:678–81.
235. Bidanset DJ, Beadle JR, Wan WB, Hostetler KY, Kern ER. Oral activity of ether lipid ester prodrugs of cidofovir against experimental human cytomegalovirus infection. J Infect Dis. 2004;190:499–503.
236. Painter W, Robertson A, Trost LC, et al. First pharmacokinetic and safety study in humans of the novel lipid antiviral conjugate CMX001, a broad-spectrum oral drug active against

double-stranded DNA viruses. Antimicrob Agents Chemother. 2012;56:2726–34.
237. Hiwarkar P, Amrolia P, Sivaprakasam P, et al. Brincidofovir is highly efficacious in controlling adenoviremia in pediatric recipients of hematopoietic cell transplant. Blood. 2017;129(14):2033–7.
238. Dunning J, Kennedy SB, Antierens A, et al. Experimental treatment of Ebola virus disease with brincidofovir. PLoS One. 2016;11(9):e0162199.
239. Ciesla SL, Trahan J, Wan WB, et al. Esterification of cidofovir with alkoxyalkanols increases oral bioavailability and diminishes drug accumulation in kidney. Antivir Res. 2003;59:163–71.
240. Marty FM, Winston DJ, Rowley SD, et al. CMX001 to prevent cytomegalovirus disease in hematopoietic-cell transplantation. N Engl J Med. 2013;369(13):1227–36.
241. Clinical Trials. http://www.chimerix.com/?s=Brincidofovir. Accessed 27 Dec 2017.
242. Lu CH, Tsai JH, Wu MZ, Yu CL, Hsieh SC. Can leflunomide play a role in cytomegalovirus disease prophylaxis besides its antirheumatic effects? Antivir Ther. 2015;20(1):93–6.
243. El Chaer F, Mori N, Shah D, et al. Adjuvant and salvage therapy with leflunomide for recalcitrant cytomegalovirus infections in hematopoietic cell transplantation recipients: a case series. Antivir Res. 2016;135:91–6.
244. Rifkin LM, Minkus CL, Pursell K, et al. Utility of leflunomide in the treatment of drug resistant cytomegalovirus retinitis. Ocul Immunol Inflamm. 2017;25(1):93–6.
245. Silva JT, Pérez-González V, López-Medrano F, et al. Experience with leflunomide as treatment and as secondary prophylaxis for cytomegalovirus infection in lung transplant recipients: a case series and review of the literature. Clin Transpl. 2018;32(2)
246. Sellar RS, Ward KN, Thomson KJ, et al. Evidence for clinical activity of artesunate in multidrug-resistant herpes simplex infection following HSCT. Bone Marrow Transplant. 2012;47:1482–3.
247. Efferth T, Marschall M, Wang X, et al. Antiviral activity of artesunate towards wild-type, recombinant, and ganciclovir-resistant human cytomegaloviruses. J Mol Med (Berl). 2002;80(4):233–42.
248. Schnepf N, Corvo J, Pors MJ, et al. Antiviral activity of ganciclovir and artesunate towards human cytomegalovirus in astrocytoma cells. Antivir Res. 2011;89(2):186–8.
249. Wolf DG, Shimoni A, Resnick IB, et al. Human cytomegalovirus kinetics following institution of artesunate after hematopoietic stem cell transplantation. Antivir Res. 2011;90:183–6.
250. Shapira MY, Resnick IB, Chou S, et al. Artesunate as a potent antiviral agent in a patient with late drug-resistant cytomegalovirus infection after hematopoietic stem cell transplantation. Clin Infect Dis. 2008;46:1455–7.
251. Hoffman VF, Skiest DJ. Therapeutic developments in cytomegalovirus retinitis. Expert Opin Investig Drugs. 2000;9(2):207–20.
252. Stuehler C, Stüssi G, Halter J, et al. Combination therapy for multidrug-resistant cytomegalovirus disease. Transpl Infect Dis. 2015;17(5):751–5.
253. Vere Hodge RA. Meeting report: 29th International Conference on Antiviral Research in La Jolla, CA, USA. Antiviral Res. 2017;137:23–40.
254. Iwasenko JM, Scott GM, Rawlinson WD, Keogh A, Mitchell D, Chou S. Successful valganciclovir treatment of post-transplant cytomegalovirus infection in the presence of UL97 mutation N597D. J Med Virol. 2009;81(3):507–10.
255. Chou S, Lurain NS, Thompson KD, et al. Viral DNA polymerase mutations associated with drug resistance in human cytomegalovirus. J Infect Dis. 2003;188(1):32–9.
256. Rolling KE, Jorgenson MR, Descourouez JL, et al. Ganciclovir-resistant cytomegalovirus infection in abdominal solid organ transplant recipients: case series and review of the literature. Pharmacotherapy. 2017;37(10):1258–71.
257. Chou SW. Cytomegalovirus drug resistance and clinical implications. Transpl Infect Dis. 2001;3(Suppl 2):20–4.
258. Drew WL. Is combination antiviral therapy for CMV superior to monotherapy? J Clin Virol. 2006;35(4):485–8.
259. Couzin-Frankel J. Breakthrough of the year 2013. Cancer immunotherapy. Science. 2013;342(6165):1432–3.
260. Lemmermann NA, Reddehase MJ. Refining human T-cell immunotherapy of cytomegalovirus disease: a mouse model with "humanized" antigen presentation as a new preclinical study tool. Med Microbiol Immunol. 2016;205(6):549–61.
261. Hanley PJ, Cruz CR, Savoldo B, et al. Functionally active virus-specific T cells that target CMV, adenovirus, and EBV can be expanded from naive T-cell populations in cord blood and will target a range of viral epitopes. Blood. 2009;114(9):1958–67.
262. Neuenhahn M, Albrecht J, Odendahl M, et al. Transfer of minimally manipulated CMV-specific T cells from stem cell or third-party donors to treat CMV infection after allo-HSCT. Leukemia. 2017;31(10):2161–71.
263. Einsele H, Kapp M, Grigoleit GU. CMV-specific T cell therapy. Blood Cells Mol Dis. 2008;40(1):71–5.
264. Pei XY, Zhao XY, Chang YJ, et al. Cytomegalovirus-specific T-cell transfer for refractory cytomegalovirus infection after haploidentical stem cell transplantation: the quantitative and qualitative immune recovery for cytomegalovirus. J Infect Dis. 2017;216(8):945–56.
265. Smith CJ, Quinn M, Snyder CM. CMV-specific CD8 T cell differentiation and localization: implications for adoptive therapies. Front Immunol. 2016;7:352.
266. Leen AM, Bollard CM, Mendizabal AM, et al. Multicenter study of banked third-party virus-specific T cells to treat severe viral infections after hematopoietic stem cell transplantation. Blood. 2013;121(26):5113–23.
267. Anderholm KM, Bierle CJ, Schleiss MR. Cytomegalovirus vaccines: current status and future prospects. Drugs. 2016;76(17):1625–45.
268. Arvin AM, Fast P, Myers M, et al. Vaccine development to prevent cytomegalovirus disease: report from the National Vaccine Advisory Committee. Clin Infect Dis. 2004;39(2):233–9.
269. Bernstein DI, Munoz FM, Callahan ST, et al. Safety and efficacy of a cytomegalovirus glycoprotein B (gB) vaccine in adolescent girls: a randomized clinical trial. Vaccine. 2016;34(3):313–9.
270. Griffiths PD, Stanton A, McCarrell E, et al. Cytomegalovirus glycoprotein-B vaccine with MF59 adjuvant in transplant recipients: a phase 2 randomised placebo-controlled trial. Lancet. 2011;377(9773):1256–63.
271. Kharfan-Dabaja MA, Nishihori T. Vaccine therapy for cytomegalovirus in the setting of allogeneic hematopoietic cell transplantation. Expert Rev Vaccines. 2015;14(3):341–50.
272. Mori T, Kanda Y, Takenaka K, et al. Safety of ASP0113, a cytomegalovirus DNA vaccine, in recipients undergoing allogeneic hematopoietic cell transplantation: an open-label phase 2 trial. Int J Hematol. 2017;105(2):206–12.
273. Baraniak IA, Reeves MB, Griffiths PD. Criteria to define interruption of transmission of human cytomegalovirus from organ donor to recipient. Rev Med Virol. 2018;28(1)
274. Safdar A, Decker WK, Li S, et al. De novo T-lymphocyte responses against baculovirus-derived recombinant influenzavirus hemagglutinin generated by a naïve umbilical cord blood model of dendritic cell vaccination. Vaccine. 2009;27(10):1479–84.
275. Konduri V, Decker WK, Halpert MM, et al. Modeling dendritic cell vaccination for influenza prophylaxis: potential applications for niche populations. J Infect Dis. 2013;207(11):1764–72.
276. Reap E, Suryadevara CM, Batich KA, et al. Dendritic cells enhance polyfunctionality of adoptively transferred T cells which target cytomegalovirus in glioblastoma. Cancer Res. 2018;78(1):256–64.

Epstein-Barr Virus Infection and Posttransplant Lymphoproliferative Disease

38

Benjamin E. Gewurz, Elizabeth Moulton, Amy Bessnow, David M. Weinstock, and Sheila Bond

Abbreviation

AIM	Acute infectious mononucleosis
AP-1	Activating protein-1
ATG	Antithymocyte globulin
BCR	B-cell receptor
ChIP-Seq	Chromatin immunoprecipitation-sequencing
CIITA	Class II, major histocompatibility complex, transactivator
CNS	Central nervous system
CR	Complete response
CT	Computed tomography
CTL	Cytotoxic lymphocytes
D	Diffuse
DLBCL	Diffuse large B-cell lymphoma
DLI	Donor lymphocyte infusion
DNA	Deoxyribonucleic acid
EA	Early antigen
EBER	Epstein-Barr virus-encoded ribonucleic acid
EBNA	Epstein-Barr virus nuclear antigen
EBV	Epstein-Barr virus
ELISA	Enzyme-linked immunosorbent assays
GC	Germinal center
gp350	Glycoprotein 350
GVHD	Graft versus host disease
HDACi	Histone deacetylation inhibitors
HIV	Human immunodeficiency virus
HL	Hodgkin lymphoma
HLA	Human leukocyte antigen
HSCT	Hematopoietic stem cell transplantation
IC50	Half maximal inhibitory concentration
IF	Immunofluorescence
IL-10	Interleukin 10
LCL	Lymphoblastoid cell line
LMP	Latent membrane protein
MHC	Major histocompatibility complex
miRNA	MicroRNA
NIH	National Institutes of Health
NK	Natural killer
NPC	Nasopharyngeal carcinoma
ORR	Objective response rate
PCR	Polymerase chain reaction
PET	Positron emission tomography
PR	Partial response
PTLD	Posttransplant lymphoproliferative disease
R	Restricted
RI	Reduction of immunosuppression
RNA	Ribonucleic acid
RR	Response rate
RS	Reed-Sternberg
SOT	Solid-organ transplantation
TAP	Transporter associated with antigen processing
UCBT	Umbilical cord blood transplantation
VCA	Viral capsid antigen
VZV	Varicella zoster virus
WHO	World Health Organization
XLP	X-linked lymphoproliferative disease

B. E. Gewurz · S. Bond
Brigham and Women's Hospital, Division of Infectious Diseases, Boston, MA, USA
e-mail: bgewurz@partners.org; smitsuma@partners.org

E. Moulton
Baylor College of Medicine, Department of Pediatrics, Infectious Diseases, Houston, TX, USA
e-mail: emoulton@bcm.edu

A. Bessnow · D. M. Weinstock (✉)
Dana-Farber Cancer Institute, Division of Medical Oncology, Boston, MA, USA
e-mail: amy_sievers@dfci.harvard.edu; dweinstock@partners.org

Taxonomy, Structure, and Genome

Epstein-Barr virus (EBV), or human herpesvirus-4, is a member of the herpes virus family. EBV is the only human member of the gamma-1 herpes virus subfamily and the prototype of the *Lymphocryptovirus* genus. The latter designation refers to the virus's ability to establish infection

A. Safdar (ed.), *Principles and Practice of Transplant Infectious Diseases*, https://doi.org/10.1007/978-1-4939-9034-4_38

in lymphocytes. Structurally, EBV is similar to other herpesviruses. EBV's double-stranded DNA genome is wrapped around a toroid-shaped protein core and enclosed in a nucleocapsid composed of 162 capsomeres. The nucleocapsid is surrounded by a protein tegument, which is housed in a glycoprotein envelope [2].

The genome is 184 kilobase pairs in length and contains both internal and terminal repeat sequences. The repeat sequences divide the genome into short and long unique sequence domains. Most of the nearly 100 open reading frames are found within the unique sequences, though the exact number and identity of all EBV-encoded genes are not yet known [2, 3]. Most EBV genes encode viral proteins important for lytic replication, including enzymes that function in viral DNA replication and viral structural components and noncoding RNAs.

Viral Life Cycle

EBV and all other herpesviruses have both a lytic and a latent phase. In the lytic cycle, the EBV-encoded DNA polymerase replicates the viral episome, and progeny virions are produced. In the latent cycle, a cellular polymerase replicates the viral genome, which persists as a nuclear episome for the lifetime of the host B cell. While lytic phase genes tend to be conserved among *Herpesviridae*, proteins important for the establishment and maintenance of latent infection vary greatly.

Lytic Infection

EBV lytic replication is necessary for the production of infectious virions and for the establishment of persistent latent infection in the B cell. However, once latency is established, lytic replication is not needed for the maintenance of this persistent infection. Thus, EBV latent infection cannot be eliminated by lytic replication inhibitors, such as acyclovir or ganciclovir [4]. Reactivation of lytic replication does occur from latent EBV-infected cells, and the virus is shed more or less continuously into the saliva, which serves as the major source of transmission from one host to the next [5].

The physiologic signals that reactivate EBV lytic replication are not yet well defined. In vitro, lytic infection can be triggered by phorbol esters and n-butyrate or by cross-linking of surface immunoglobulin [6–8]. In vivo, viral replication may occur in Waldeyer's ring memory B cells undergoing differentiation into antibody-secreting plasma cells, as well as in the associated epithelium [5]. Two immediate early EBV transcription factors, BZLF1 and BRLF1, orchestrate the transition from latent to lytic growth. BZLF1, which is related to the cellular activating protein 1 (AP-1) family of transcription factors, is sufficient to activate the lytic replication cycle [9, 10]. In response to BZLF1 and BRLF1, approximately 80 EBV lytic genes are expressed. RNA sequencing has detected transcription of additional EBV genes [11] and demonstrated that EBV transcripts comprise 7% of all mapped reads from the B cell during reactivation. Early antigens (E) include multiple enzymes important for EBV DNA replication, including the viral thymidine kinase, DNA polymerase, ribonucleotide reductase, and alkaline exonuclease. Most virion structural components are produced during the late phase, including the viral capsid antigens (VCA). During the late phase, linear double-stranded DNA genomes are packaged into icosahedral protein nucleocapsids, which are then encased in a lipid envelope laden with viral glycoproteins. These virions can then be transmitted from one cell to another or to a new human host.

Latent Infection

Following resolution of acute primary EBV infection, between 1 and 50 per million B cells remain EBV-infected [12–14]. EBV spends much of its life cycle thereafter in the B-cell compartment, partially hidden in a state of viral latency. While latently infected B cells do not produce progeny viruses, the EBV genome is not entirely quiescent. A limited subset of gene products that promote viral genome propagation and infected cell survival are expressed. This strategy allows EBV to evade immune detection while maintaining persistent infection for the lifetime of the host.

There are four principal patterns of EBV latency. Upon initial B-cell infection, EBV initiates the Latency III growth program, in which all nine latency viral proteins and several noncoding RNAs are expressed. These include three latent membrane proteins (LMPs), six Epstein-Barr nuclear antigens (EBNA), two small non-polyadenylated EBV-encoded RNAs (EBERs), and the BamA genome fragment region-encoded BART transcripts (Table 38.1). Latency III cells morphologically resemble antigen-stimulated B lymphocytes [15]. Latency III proteins comprise over 4000 amino acids and thus provide numerous epitopes for T-cell detection. Furthermore, EBV latency proteins activate NF-kB and interferon pathways, which in turn upregulate numerous T-cell and natural-killer (NK)-cell ligands. The robust immune response to Latency III cells is likely responsible for many of the symptoms of acute infectious mononucleosis (AIM). CD8+ T cells and NK cells responding to Latency III cells comprise the atypical lymphocytes seen in the peripheral blood during AIM [16–19]. Fortunately, most Latency III cells are eliminated by immune surveillance. However, if left unchecked by the host immune system, Latency III B cells are oncogenic. In vitro, EBV uses the Latency III program to efficiently convert resting B cells into immortalized lymphoblastoid cell lines (LCL). Likewise, in the setting of immune suppression such as following hematopoietic stem cell or solid-organ transplant, Latency III cells can give

Table 38.1 EBV genome expression programs and associated characteristics

EBV program	EBV gene products expressed	Cell type	Immunogenicity	EBV-associated malignancy
Latency 0	RNA: EBERs	Resting peripheral blood memory B cell	None	–
Latency I	EBNAs: 1 RNAs: EBERs, BARTs	Dividing peripheral blood memory cell	Low	Burkitt lymphoma
Latency II	EBNA: 1 LMPs: 1, 2A, 2B RNAs: EBERs, BARTs	Germinal center B cell	Moderate	Hodgkin lymphoma, NK- and T-cell lymphoma, DLBCL of elderly, nasopharyngeal carcinoma
Latency III	EBNAs: 1, 2, 3A, 3B, 3C, LP LMPs: 1, 2A, 2B RNAs: EBERs, BARTs, BHRF1	Naïve B cell	High	PTLD, HIV-associated lymphoma, DLBCL of elderly
Lytic	>80 lytic gene products	Plasma cell, Waldeyer's ring epithelial cell	High	–

rise to posttransplant lymphoproliferative disorders (see below). Latency III expression is nearly always present in EBV-associated central nervous system (CNS) lymphomas of patients with human immunodeficiency virus (HIV) infection. Perhaps due to immune senescence of aging, the Latency III pattern is again found in a subset of EBV-associated diffuse large B-cell lymphoma (DLBCL) of the elderly [20].

To establish persistent host infection, EBV must reach the memory B-cell compartment, the site of long-term EBV residence. EBV uses its Latency II program to accomplish this [21, 22]. In Latency II, the viral genome expresses only EBNA1, LMP1, LMP2A, EBER, and BART RNAs. In a ligand-independent fashion, LMP1 and LMP2A mimic signals from CD40 and B-cell immunoglobulin receptors, respectively. LMP2A promotes germinal center (GC) formation, and transgenic LMP2A expression in mice causes spontaneous germinal center formation in the gut-associated lymphoid tissue [21]. Interestingly, LMP2A expression rescues germinal center formation in B-cell receptor (BCR)-deficient mice, and conditional LMP2A expression in germinal center B cells resulted in preferential selection of low-affinity antibody-producing B cells and a lupus-like illness [23]. Meanwhile, EBNA1 tethers the EBV episome to host chromosomes and ensures that the EBV genome is maintained in dividing B cells [22]. Expression of only these three EBV-encoded proteins limits the immunogenicity of Latency II cells.

Upon transition to the peripheral blood memory B-cell compartment, EBV enters the Latency 0 program, in which EBV gene products are not expressed [22]. This EBV B-cell reservoir appears to be a long-lived IgD-, CD27+ resting memory cell [12, 24, 25]. Cell surface phenotype and expression profile analysis suggest that these cells have transited through the germinal center [22], and 90% of these quiescent B cells are in the G0 cell cycle stage at any given time [26, 27]. However, they do divide approximately once per month, at which point EBV switches to the Latency I program. In Latency I, only EBNA1 and the EBER and BART RNAs are expressed. An EBNA1 glycine-alanine repeat domain limits EBNA1 biosynthesis and proteasomal turnover and, thereby, limits presentation of EBNA1 peptide epitopes by the HLA (human leukocyte antigen) class I antigen presentation pathway [28].

Oncogenesis

EBV efficiently converts B lymphocytes into immortalized LCL in cell culture. Recombinant EBV genetic studies have demonstrated that only six EBV protein-encoding genes and several microRNAs (miRNA) are crucial for B-cell transformation: the oncogene LMP1 and the nuclear antigens EBNA1, EBNA2, EBNA-LP, EBNA3A, and EBNA3C. LMP1 is an integral membrane protein that constitutively signals from two C-terminal cytoplasmic tail domains in a ligand-independent fashion [29–31]. LMP1 mimics the immune receptor CD40, and the LMP1 signaling domains can substitute for the CD40 signaling domains in mouse B cells [32]. Forced LMP1 expression causes loss of contact inhibition and anchorage-independent growth in soft agar [33]. Similarly, multiple transgenic mouse models have highlighted an important role for LMP1 in B-cell growth and survival. LMP1 expression produces an activated B-cell phenotype and drives B-cell growth [34]. LMP1 expression, under the control of an immunoglobulin heavy-chain promoter and enhancer, produces lymphoma at a threefold higher incidence than in LMP1-negative control littermates [35]. When LMP1 is inducibly expressed in mouse B cells, T cells efficiently recognize and eliminate the newly LMP1+ cells [36]. Strikingly, in the absence of CD8+ T-cell surveillance, LMP1 drives rapid and fatal lymphoproliferation and lymphomagenesis [36].

Although not required for EBV-mediated B-cell transformation, LMP2A nonetheless plays an important role in vivo. LMP2A also constitutively signals in the absence of ligand and further promotes B-cell development and survival [21, 37]. LMP2A provides an important B-cell survival signal, in particular for B cells that have not successfully rearranged their BCRs. LMP2A expression rescues such

BCR-negative, "crippled" GC B cells that would otherwise undergo apoptosis [38]. The LMP2A N-terminal cytoplasmic tail contains multiple signaling domains, including an immunoreceptor tyrosine-based activation motif homologous to the ones present in the BCR Igα and Igβ signaling chains. LMP2A thereby acts as a BCR surrogate, albeit signaling at lower levels than an activated BCR. At the same time, LMP2A competes with the BCR for recruitment of tyrosine kinases and thereby maintains B-cell latency by preventing antigen stimulation-mediated lytic cycle activation [39].

LMP2A, together with LMP1, may rescue GC B cells that would ordinarily be slated for apoptosis. Such LMP1- and LMP2-mediated rescue of pre-apoptotic cells may play an important pathogenic role in classical Hodgkin disease malignant transformation. Indeed, LMP1 and LMP2A are highly expressed in EBV+ Reed-Sternberg (RS) cells, the malignant B cell of classical Hodgkin lymphoma (HL). RS cells are dependent on constitutive NF-κB pathway activation. Interestingly, the tumor suppressor and NF-κB negative regulator A20/TNFAIP3 is frequently inactivated by somatic mutations in the 50% of HL cases that lack EBV, but is only rarely mutated in LMP1+ RS cells [40]. This observation suggests that EBV LMP1 and NF-κB pathway activating somatic mutations serve redundant functions in HL pathogenesis. Likewise, LMP1 and LMP2A cooperatively promote epithelial tumor development in murine carcinogenesis models [41], and they are frequently co-expressed in nasopharyngeal carcinoma tumor cells in vivo.

The nuclear antigens EBNA2, EBNA3A, and EBNA3C further promote B-cell growth. EBNA2 is an acidic transcriptional transactivator that upregulates expression of both EBV and cell genes, including *LMP1* and *MYC* [42, 43]. EBNA2 associates with DNA, in part through association with RBP-J kappa, a cellular transcription factor that is a downstream component of the cellular Notch pathway [44–46]. LCL chromatin immunoprecipitation-sequencing (ChIP-Seq) analysis suggests that EBNA2 predominantly binds to non-promoter sequences and may frequently regulate gene transcription through long-range DNA interactions [46]. EBNA3A and EBNA3C are both critical for EBV-mediated B-cell transformation, perhaps by jointly repressing expression of the tumor suppressors p16 (INK4A) and p14 (ARF). When EBNA3A or EBNA3C are functionally inactivated, p16 and p14 expression increases, and LCL growth ceases [47]. Reminiscent of adenovirus E1A and human papillomavirus E6/7, EBNA3C also blocks p53-dependent apoptosis and enhances proteasomal turnover of the pRb and p27KIP1 tumor suppressors [48, 49]. EBNA2, EBNA3A, EBNA3C, and EBNA-LP combine with LMP1-activated NF-kB transcription factors to form EBV super-enhancers that target 187 host genes. EBV super-enhancer targets include c-Myc and the anti-apoptosis proteins BCL2 and cFLIP [50].

EBV encodes two Bcl-2 family proteins, BHRF1 and BALF1 [10]. Both are highly, but transiently, expressed upon B-cell infection and are important for EBV-mediated B-cell transformation. BHRF1/BALF1 may function by inhibiting apoptosis of newly EBV-infected cells undergoing the transition into latency [51]. Interestingly, once latency has been established, both EBV Bcl-2 proteins are dispensable for maintenance of latency and for viral reactivation, perhaps since LMP1 highly upregulates cellular Bcl-2 family pro-survival proteins.

EBV also encodes 44 mature miRNAs, more than any other human virus studied thus far [52]. Recent studies have implicated EBV-encoded miRNAs in B-cell transformation. A cluster of miRNAs located near the BHRF1 open reading frame (and therefore called BHRF1 miRNAs) are highly expressed in Latency III and in a range of B-cell tumors [53]. All three BHRF1 miRNAs are important for EBV-mediated B-cell transformation in vitro, and genetic disruption of all miRNAs impairs transformation by 20-fold [54]. The BHRF1 miRNAs may reduce levels of the tumor suppressors PTEN and p27 through incompletely understood mechanisms [55].

Host Immune Response

EBV has coevolved with the human species and its antecedents over millions of years [56, 57]. Over this time period, the virus developed a complex relationship with the human immune system that permits its persistence in the memory B-cell compartment for the lifetime of the host. The host immune response to EBV is robust and equally complex; infected B cells are under constant surveillance by circulating immune cells.

Innate Immunity

Little is known about the innate immune response to primary infection with EBV, though several lines of evidence suggest that innate immunity limits early lytic infection [58]. In AIM, there is an expansion of NK cells, and NK-cell peripheral blood count is inversely proportional to EBV viral loads [59–61]. In vitro, NK cells inhibit EBV-infected B-cell growth [62]. An EBV miRNA, miR-BART2, reduces micB expression, an NK-cell activating ligand [63]. In vivo, patients with X-linked lymphoproliferative disease (XLP) have a specific immune defect that may lead to a fatal inflammatory illness, characterized by marked expansions of EBV-infected B cells and reactive T cells following primary EBV infection [64]. Though still incompletely characterized, XLP may in part arise from inadequate initial NK-cell control of EBV-infected B cells [65–67]. Individuals with immunodeficiencies preferentially affecting NK-cell function, such as CD16 mutations, are also prone to EBV-driven lymphoproliferative disorders [68, 69].

CD8+ T-cell Immunity

The importance of T-cell surveillance against EBV growth-transforming infection is supported by the high frequency with which T-cell-immunodeficient transplant recipients develop PTLD and by the fact that adoptive transfer of polyclonal EBV-specific T cells has proven successful in the treatment of this disease [70].

A large expansion of oligoclonal EBV-specific CD8+ T cells has been observed in patients with infectious mononucleosis at the time of symptom onset [17]. Similar expansions have not been observed in persons with primary asymptomatic infection [71, 72]. In some persons with infectious mononucleosis, the expanded T-cell population may account for up to 50% of the total peripheral blood CD8+ T-cell population [14, 17, 60]. The dominant CD8 T-cell responses are against the lytic immediate early and early antigens. The response to latent antigens is approximately tenfold less in number, and it accounts for 0.1–5% of the total CD8+ T-cell population [14, 17]. In most persistently infected individuals, the strongest response is directed against the Latency III EBNA3 antigens [19] though there is some variability depending on HLA background [14, 17]. As infection progresses, EBV downregulates both lytic and latent antigen expression. Subsequently, antigen stimulation decreases, and the bulk of CD8+ T cells reactive to these antigens undergoes apoptosis. In long-term asymptomatic carriers, MHC (major histocompatibility complex) class I tetramer analyses have shown that 0.2–2% of CD8+ T cells are specific for lytic antigens, versus 0.05–1% for latent antigens [14, 17]. In the carrier state, the majority of T cells have a resting phenotype, as compared to the activated phenotype seen in early primary infection.

In addition to progressive downregulation of antigen expression, EBV employs several strategies to evade CD8+ T-cell detection. As examples, the EBV lytic protein BNLF2A binds to the transporter associated with antigen processing (TAP) and thereby inhibits MHC class I antigen processing [73, 74]. Lytic proteins BGLF5 and BILF1 also function to reduce cell surface HLA I levels by, respectively, reducing new HLA antigen expression and impairing export of new MHC I complexes [75–77]. EBV miRNAs also inhibit TAP expression and downregulate the expression of cytokines that aid in EBV-specific CD8+ T-cell antigen recognition [78, 79]. Latent antigens LMP1 and EBNA1 have also devised strategies to decrease the efficacy by which they are presented on HLA class I molecules [80–82]. Notably, as EBV infection progresses from the acute to the persistent state, the EBV-specific T-cell repertoire becomes less skewed toward early lytic antigens and also encompasses late lytic antigens [83]. This phenomenon suggests that the aforementioned MHC class I immune evasion strategies may have evolved to allow viral replication in the acute phase and to facilitate the establishment of persistent EBV infection [83].

CD4+ T-cell Immunity

The CD4+ T-cell expansion in acute EBV infection appears to be at least tenfold less than that of CD8+ T cells [14, 17, 60]. The hierarchy of immunodominant epitopes is less well studied in the CD4+ than in the CD8+ T-cell population, though the available data suggests CD4+ T-cell responses are more often directed at latent antigens. Among CD4+ T-cell responses directed at lytic antigens, there is a more uniform distribution across the immediate early, early, and late lytic antigens [17, 84]. In contrast to the CD8+ T-cell response, the EBV-specific CD4+ T-cell response is lower in magnitude, and the role of CD4+ T cells is less well defined. However, CD4+ T-cell responses are likely important, as evidenced by the high frequency of EBV-associated lymphomas that arise with waning CD4+ T-cell count in patients with HIV. In vitro, EBV-specific CD4+ T-cell clones exert cytotoxic function and prevent the proliferation of newly EBV-infected B cells [84, 85]. Virus-specific CD4+ T cells may also be necessary for the persistence of adoptively transferred CD8+ T cells in immunotherapy products used for the treatment of PTLD [86].

Several EBV proteins interfere with MHC II antigen presentation and subsequent CD4+ T-cell activation. As examples, BZLF1, an immediate-early lytic protein, downregulates CD74 expression, a chaperone for MHC II dimers [87], and may also reduce surface class II expression by downregulating the class II transactivator, CIITA [88]. BZLF2 also subverts CD4+ T-cell activation by obstructing MHC II and T-cell receptor interactions [89]. The EBV lytic protein BCRF1 encodes an interleukin-10 (IL-10) homolog, which blocks many interferon-gamma-mediated functions, such as upregulated expression of MHC II and other costimulatory molecules needed for CD4+ T-cell activation. Unlike the human IL-10 homolog, viral IL-10 has a reduced ability to stimulate T cells [90].

Humoral Immunity

The humoral response to acute infection is characterized by polyclonal B-cell activation and marked immunoglobulin response to both lytic and latent viral antigens [91]. Antibodies to glycoprotein 350 (gp350), one of the major outer envelope glycoproteins, have been shown to have neutralizing effects [92–94]; generation of antibodies to gp350 is impaired during acute infectious mononucleosis [95]. These features support gp350's use in vaccine strategies. The pattern of antibody development to viral antigens and heterophile antibodies have long been used to diagnose EBV infection and are further reviewed below.

Epidemiology

EBV is ubiquitous and infects over 90% of the world's population [1]. A large portion of the population will acquire infection during youth. Higher rates of acquisition in early childhood are seen in developing nations, where over three quarters of children acquire EBV infection by age 6 [96]. By contrast, in developed nations, EBV infection is detected in less than half of school-aged children [96, 97]. Prevalence increases with age, and by late adulthood, 89–100% of the population harbors latent EBV infection [97–103]. These numbers suggest that a substantial number of pediatric and young adult transplant recipients will be seronegative for EBV at the time of transplantation and thus susceptible to primary infection as well as PTLD. Humans are the only natural host for EBV infection. The major vehicles for transmission to the non-transplant host are saliva and oropharyngeal secretions. Most infected individuals will shed virus in saliva near continuously over their lifetimes, and this appears to be the major reservoir for transmission from one individual to another [5]. Thus, contact with an acutely infected individual is not necessary for EBV spread. However, the degree of contact does play a role. Casual household contact appears to be largely insufficient for transmission [60, 104]. More intimate contact including kissing, mouth-to-mouth transfer of food, or transmission via saliva-contaminated toys, cups, or other fomites as occurs in daycare settings is likely required [105]. In a single study undertaken in the daycare setting, the rate of EBV seroconversion was 9% per month; the likelihood of acquiring infection was proportional to the duration of time spent in daycare [106]. This may have important implications for the pediatric EBV-seronegative transplant host as the likelihood of acquiring primary EBV infection in certain settings is not small.

Several reports of EBV shedding in genital secretions exist [107–110], and the risk of EBV seropositivity increases proportionally with number of sexual partners [111], suggesting that the virus may also be sexually transmitted. However, definitive evidence is lacking. Rare cases of primary EBV infection being transmitted via blood transfusion have also been reported [112]. Leukoreduction significantly reduces the number of B cells in packed red blood cells [113] but may not completely eliminate B cells from packed red blood cell products [114, 115], making blood transfusion a biologically plausible but unlikely source of transmission. One of the major sources of transmission in the transplant recipient is the transplanted organ. Higher rates of PTLD are reported in organ transplants in which a large reservoir of lymphoid cells are transplanted with the organ, such as with intestinal transplantation [116]. However, it is unclear whether this increased prevalence is due to the transfer of an increased number of allogeneic EBV-infected B cells, the higher degree of immunosuppression that often accompanies such transplantation, or the interplay of these two factors.

There are two major EBV strains, type 1 (or A) and type 2 (or B) [117]. An important difference between the two strains is their differential growth-transforming capacity. Type 1 EBV has greater growth-transforming efficiency than the type 2 strain [118, 119]. Type 1 is the more prevalent strain, although there is some suggestion that type 2 EBV may preferentially infect immunocompromised hosts [120]. To date, studies that have addressed whether PTLD is associated with type 1 or 2 have predominantly detected type 1 EBV in PTLD tumor tissue [121, 122].

EBV Diagnostics

An overview of the serologic and virologic assays used to diagnose EBV infection is presented below. As humoral immunity may be impaired in the transplant population, serologic testing may be less reliable in these hosts. Transfusion of blood or immunoglobulin may also result in false-positive serologic testing in the population [123].

Heterophile Antibody Testing

Heterophile antibodies are a group of antibodies, primarily of the IgM class [124], that are produced in acute EBV infection. The precise nature of the antigen, termed the Paul-Bunnel antigen, is not known, but it is believed to be an infection-induced cell membrane glycoconjugate [124]. Heterophile antibodies have the ability to agglutinate sheep and horse erythrocytes and are adsorbed by cattle erythrocytes. The most common clinical heterophile antibody test is the monospot assay, which tests for the presence of antibodies in sera that agglutinate purified bovine antigen bound to latex particles. The reported sensitivity of the test ranges from 81% to 95% and the specificity from 94% to 100% in the setting of symptoms of AIM [125, 126]. Heterophile antibodies are positive in 75% of patients during the first week of symptoms and in 90–95% of patients during weeks 2–5 and then decline rapidly thereafter; in some, heterophile antibodies may persist for years [126–128]. The sensitivity of the heterophile assay appears to be reduced in young children [129, 130]. Although the specificity of the test is high, false-positive heterophile antibody testing has been reported in patients with leukemia, lymphoma, systemic lupus erythematosus, viral hepatitis, and acute HIV infection [127, 131–134].

Virus-Specific Antibodies

The humoral response to EBV is composed of a vast number of antibodies to both lytic and latent cycle antigens. Three of these antibodies are routinely used for diagnostic purposes and can distinguish acute from prior infection. Antibodies expressed during lytic viral infection develop during acute infection; antibodies expressed during latent infection develop thereafter.

Antibodies to Lytic Cycle Antigens

The VCA consists of several viral proteins that comprise EBV's capsomers. VCA IgM is a marker of recent EBV infection. It is typically present at the time of AIM symptom onset and then disappears within a few weeks. VCA IgG is frequently detected at the time of presentation or shortly thereafter, peaks, and then declines to a steady state. As VCA IgG persists for life and the assay is relatively sensitive, testing for VCA IgG alone is an appropriate pretransplant screening test for the detection of prior EBV infection.

The early antigen (EA) complex is expressed early in EBV's lytic life cycle. There are two patterns of anti-EA antibodies, diffuse (D) and restricted (R). These designations refer to the pattern of immunofluorescence (IF) observed when these antibodies were first detected [135]. The EA-D IgG arises at the onset of symptoms and typically decreases 3–4 weeks after illness. However, in some the antibody may persist for years. EA-D antibodies have also been detected in 10–20% of the healthy population [136]. Thus, although EA-D IgG arises early in acute EBV infection, it is not a clear indicator of primary EBV infection. The EA-R IgG is detected in only a small subset of patient with AIM and may correlate with severe disease [135].

Antibodies to Latent Cycle Antigens

Anti-EBNA antibody arises 1–3 months following acute infection and persists for life. EBNA1 is the primary antigen targeted by anti-EBNA antibody. Approximately 5% of those infected with EBV will not develop the anti-EBNA antibody [137].

Traditionally, the above EBV-specific antibodies have been detected by indirect IF assays. Though IF assays are more specific, they are technically demanding, and most clinical laboratories are now using enzyme-linked immunosorbent assays (ELISA) in their place. Avidity assays had been used to help distinguish acute primary infection versus prior infection in the past, but their accuracy is uncertain [138].

Viral Load Testing

EBV DNA viral loads are routinely monitored by quantitative polymerase chain reaction (PCR) in patients at risk for the development of PTLD. Presently, there is no FDA-approved assay for the quantitation of EBV DNA. Each assay is developed and validated by each individual laboratory and subject to its standards. Use of the World Health Organization (WHO) International Standard for EBV viral loading testing can help mitigate some of the variability among laboratories [139, 140]. However, specimen handling, DNA extraction methods, primers, probes, and gene targets may all vary between laboratories. Consequently, the upper and lower limits of quantitation, linear range, precision, accuracy, and reported units may also differ. These differences preclude comparison of test results and cutoff values between laboratories. Interpreting viral load results, thus, requires knowledge of the performance characteristics of the specific assay used.

The type of specimen assayed will also affect results. Most commercial laboratories perform viral load testing on either whole blood or plasma. Whole blood-based assays detect intracellular DNA as well as cell-free DNA, which may include both DNA released during lytic viral replication and from dying tumor cells. By contrast, plasma-based assays measure only cell-free DNA. Consistent with the fact that whole blood-based assays detect both intracellular and cell-free DNA, viral loads from whole blood tend to be higher than those from plasma [141–145]. While whole blood-based assays may be more sensitive for the detection of EBV DNA, the significance of viremia depends upon the clinical setting.

EBV DNA is typically not detectable in the plasma of healthy individuals but may be detectable in whole blood at low levels as approximately 0.0001% of circulating leukocytes are estimated to harbor latent EBV infection [141, 143, 146]. In asymptomatic primary infection or AIM, viral loads in plasma may be undetectable or quickly decline after the onset of symptoms [141, 143]. By contrast, virus is frequently detected in whole blood in patients with infectious mononucleosis, and viral loads may remain elevated up to 180 days [141, 143]. It should be stressed that serologies are the preferred diagnostic for acute primary EBV infection and that viral load assay is not licensed for the diagnosis of AIM. However in the immunocompromised host, serologies may be unreliable and a whole blood-based PCR assay may be a useful alternative assay.

The optimal specimen type for PTLD screening has not been determined, though several studies have addressed this issue [141–143, 147–150]. While viremia may be more frequently detected from whole blood, it may not be the test of choice. In a prospective trial by Tsai et al., the sensitivity of both whole blood- and plasma-based assays for the detection of PTLD was similar. However, the plasma-based assay had greater specificity and positive predictive value for diagnosing PTLD. Higher false-positive rates were found with the whole blood assay [142]. Of note, false-negative test results have been reported for patients with CNS PTLD with both whole blood- and plasma-based assays [151, 152]. Some researchers advocate that testing both plasma and whole blood viral loads concurrently may have the greatest predictive value [150]. Finally, because of the lack of standardization of EBV viral load testing, following viral load treads in patients over time using a single assay from a single laboratory may have greater value than attempting to interpret a specific result at a single time point.

Posttransplant Lymphoproliferative Disease

EBV-seronegative solid-organ transplantation (SOT) or hematopoietic stem cell transplantation (HSCT) recipients are at high risk from primary EBV infection. As in the immunocompetent host, primary infection may be asymptomatic or may present with features of AIM, such as fever, pharyngitis and lymphadenopathy, or other systemic symptoms. More severe complications of primary EBV infection include hepatitis, aseptic meningitis, encephalitis, and more rarely cerebellar ataxia and transverse myelitis. Review of the literature at this point in time does not suggest that these complications are more frequent in transplant recipients. The most serious and common clinical manifestation of EBV infection following transplantation is PTLD (Fig. 38.1).

PTLD refers to any abnormal proliferation of lymphocytes that occurs following HSCT or SOT. The spectrum of disease ranges from a benign and self-limited expansion of lymphocytes to fulminant, fatal lymphoma. The majority of PTLD is of B-cell origin, though T-cell disease also occurs.

Incidence

Estimated incidences of PTLD vary among institutions, with the type of transplantation and with the degree of immunosuppression. The true incidence of PTLD is difficult to ascertain, as the disorder itself is heterogenous and approaches to diagnosis differ between institutions. A review of 100,000 adult SOT recipients in the United States found PTLD to be the most common posttransplantation malignancy in kidney and liver transplant recipients with rates of 1.6% and 2.4%, respectively [153]. PTLD was the third most common malignancy in heart transplantation recipients with a frequency of 2.2%. The highest rates for PTLD were reported in lung transplantation recipients at 5.7%, though the incidence of lung cancers still exceeded that of PTLD in this population. Equally comprehensive data is not available in the pediatric SOT recipient population; however, reported PTLD rates are often substantially higher in this population, ranging from 1% to 19% depending on the type of organ transplanted [154–160].

The frequency of PTLD in the allogeneic HSCT population at large is approximately 1% [161], though this

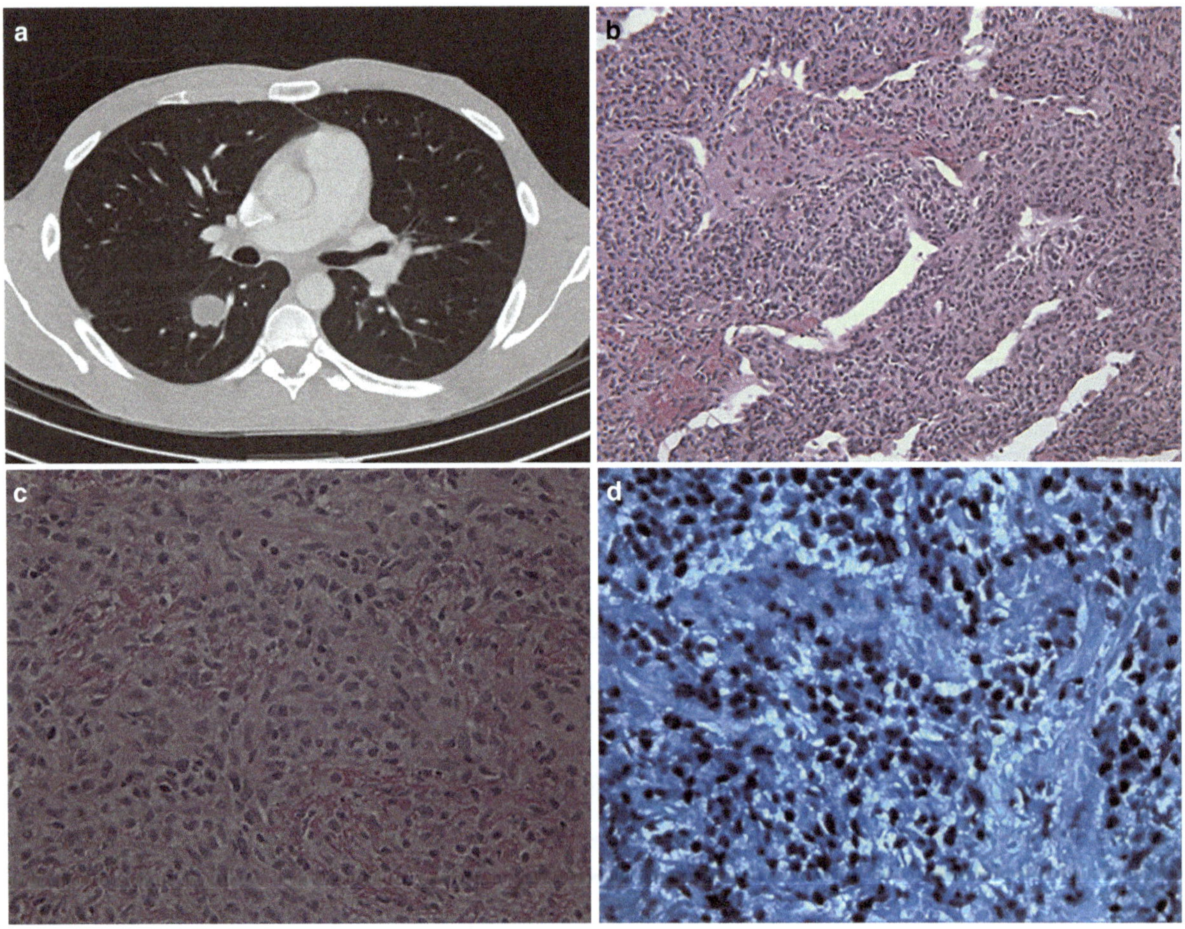

Fig. 38.1 Posttransplant lymphoproliferative disease: (**a**) CT scan of a right lower lobe lung nodule in HSCT recipient. (**b**) The nodule is composed of a sheet-like infiltrate of a relatively monotonous population of lymphocytes. (**c**) Higher-power image of medium to large lymphoid cells with marked nuclear atypia, consistent with DLBCL. (**d**) In situ hybridization for EBER, the dark blue nuclear stain, is positive confirming the presence of EBV in the tumor tissue. (*Photos courtesy of Leona Doyle*)

varies with the type of transplant and conditioning regimen. Higher rates have been reported in the setting of allograft T-cell depletion by in vitro selection or by in vivo treatment with T-cell-depleting antibody preparations [162, 163]. Within the allogeneic stem cell transplantation populations, the umbilical cord blood transplantation (UCBT) population appears to be at particularly high risk, with reported rates as high as 21% [164–166]. This may not be unexpected, as the majority of UCBT recipients are EBV-seropositive and the transplanted immune system is by nature EBV-naïve. At present, there is not sufficient data to suggest that PTLD rates are higher in pediatric allogeneic HSCT recipients compared with adults. The incidence of PTLD among recipients of autologous HSCT is extremely low.

The majority of PTLD is associated with EBV [167]. This association is strengthened in early-onset PTLD (i.e., PTLD occurring within the first year posttransplant) and in pediatric transplant recipients [168, 169]. Early-onset PTLD is associated with EBV and younger age, while late-onset PTLD appears to be associated with both younger (<20 years of age) and older age (>50 years of age) [168]. The diminished EBV association and increased risk in older age groups suggest that the pathogenesis of late-onset PTLD may be distinct from early-onset disease and more akin to lymphomagenesis in the general population. Late-onset PTLD tends to have a worse prognosis than early disease [170].

Pathogenesis

The oncogenic potential of the virus may best be illustrated by its in vitro activity. The growth of EBV-transformed B cells can be inhibited in tissue culture by the addition of autologous T cells from EBV-seropositive hosts [171–173]. In healthy humans with persistent EBV infection, approximately 0.2–3% of circulating CD8+ T cells are devoted to continually controlling EBV infection [14, 17, 174]. Thus, in the setting of T-cell immunodeficiency, control of the virus-infected B cells may be lost. As detailed above, several EBV proteins inhibit apoptosis, which may further contribute to the outgrowth of EBV-infected B cells in PTLD. Early in the process, this outgrowth may be polymorphic, polyclonal, and largely driven by EBV's latent genes. However, as growth persists, the likelihood of acquiring mutations increases, and monomorphic, monoclonal lymphomas may arise.

Most PTLD lesions exhibit a Latency III growth pattern, though more restricted as well as heterogeneous patterns of latency have also been reported [175–178]. As PTLD arises in the setting of T-cell immunodeficiency and can be controlled by the adoptive transfer of EBV-specific T cells, it is clear that inadequate T-cell immunity plays a significant pathogenic role. However, the events that initiate the development of PTLD have not been fully elucidated, and this remains an area of active investigation. In particular, the role of lytic infection in pathogenesis is poorly defined. PTLD has been reported to arise in both cells of donor and recipient origin [175, 179]. In support of an intervening period of lytic replication, PTLD can arise in recipient B cells in hosts who were EBV-seronegative at the time of transplantation and who received organs from EBV-seropositive donors [179]. Further, strain typing demonstrates that EBV-seronegative transplant recipients often acquire EBV from their donor [175].

Risk Factors

Risk factors for the development of PTLD mirror its pathogenesis and may be broadly categorized into three groups: (1) agents that disrupt T-cell immunity, such as antithymocyte globulin (ATG), OKT3, or calcineurin inhibitors; (2) interventions that either donate or leave behind a reservoir of EBV-infected B cells, such as receipt of an organ from an EBV-seropositive donor or receipt of nonmyeloablative transplantation; and (3) lack of underlying EBV-specific immunity, as is frequently seen in the pediatric SOT recipients or with receipt of UCBT.

The most clearly defined risk factor for the development of PTLD in SOT recipients is EBV seronegativity at the time of transplantation [154, 159, 168, 180]; the highest risk is conferred in EBV-seronegative recipients who receive organs from EBV-seropositive donors [159]. Multiple studies also describe young age as a risk factor for the development of PTLD in SOT recipients [168, 181–183], though this association often weakens in multivariate analyses, suggesting that young age may be a reflection of EBV seronegativity [168]. Intense T-cell immunosuppression is also a commonly reported risk factor for PTLD [184–189], and for all organs, risk seems to be greatest during the first 12 months following transplantation when immunosuppression is at its peak [189]. Though there is little evidence to implicate one induction or maintenance immunosuppressive drug or regimen over another, an increased risk of PTLD with a predilection for CNS disease in EBV-seronegative SOT recipients was reported in Phase III trials of belatacept, a T-cell costimulatory blocker, suggesting that this drug carries particular risk in the EBV-seronegative population [190–192].

In a survey of 235 transplant centers, which included over 18,000 HSCT recipients worldwide, risk factors for the development of PTLD in the first year following transplant included (1) unrelated or HLA-mismatched donors, (2) in vitro T-cell depletion, and (3) the use of ATG or CD3 monoclonal antibodies for the treatment of graft rejection and/or graft versus host disease (GVHD) [161]. Subsequent studies found nonmyeloablative conditioning regimens, especially those containing ATG, to confer risk [163, 193]. Each of these risk factors is consistent with the central role T cells play in controlling the proliferation of latent EBV-infected B cells. To further illustrate this point, methods of

T-cell depletion that selectively target T-cell or T- and NK-cell populations impart greater risk than those that deplete both T and B cells, such as anti-CD52 monoclonal antibodies (e.g., alemtuzumab) [161, 193, 194]. The importance of maintaining balanced T- and B-cell populations has also been found in the UCBT population, where rates of PTLD are as low as 2% in those who receive myeloablative conditioning regimens [165, 195] but rise to as high as 21% in those who receive nonmyeloablative conditioning regimens and ATG [165].

Clinical Presentation

The clinical manifestations of PTLD are protean. Thus, maintaining a high index of clinical suspicion and knowledge of predisposing factors are critical to making the diagnosis. Patients may be asymptomatic or may present with systemic signs that range from fever to frank systemic inflammatory response syndrome. Mononucleosis-type syndromes are not infrequently reported. Symptoms associated with the site or sites of disease may also be present.

As with lymphoma, PTLD may present in lymph nodes or in the lymphoid tissue of other organs. In SOTs, PTLD has a propensity to arise in the transplanted organ [179, 196]; therefore, graft dysfunction should raise suspicion for PTLD. The incidence of localization to the allograft diminishes with time and is significantly less likely beyond the first year after transplantation [197]. The gastrointestinal tract is another common site of involvement, though virtually any organ can be involved [197]. Compared to lymphomas within the general populations, PTLD seems to have a greater propensity to involve the CNS [198].

The majority of PTLD arises in the first year posttransplantation [189] and has been reported to occur as early as 15 days following transplantation. PTLD occurring in the first year following transplantation is termed early PTLD. PTLD occurring thereafter is termed late PTLD. Greater than 90% of early PTLD is associated with EBV, whereas only about half of late PTLD is associated with EBV [199], indicating that a subset of late PTLD may be a distinct disorder.

Pretransplant Screening and Posttransplant Surveillance

Prior to transplantation, both donor and recipient should be screened by serologic testing for EBV infection to assess risk status. Following transplantation, peripheral blood viral load monitoring is commonly used to monitor for elevated levels of EBV DNA. The intent of monitoring is to identify patients who are at higher risk for developing PTLD and afford enough time to intervene by adjusting immunosuppressive regimens and/or by preemptively treating to avert progression to PTLD. Approaches to surveillance differ among transplant centers and society guidelines [200–207].

Conflicting data exist on what constitutes a significantly elevated viral load and to what extent the height of elevation correlates with risk for PTLD [208–212]. Patients with PTLD tend to have higher EBV viral loads than those without [144]. However, many patients with detectable viremia will not progress to PTLD [213, 214]. Sustained high-level viremia without progression to PTLD is particularly prominent in the pediatric population [215–217]. Which populations require routine monitoring is also a matter of debate. Some transplantation centers will monitor all transplant recipients, while others will limit routine monitoring to high-risk groups (e.g., UCBT recipients, in vitro T-cell depletion).

The frequency with which viral loads should be monitored is also unclear and may depend on the risk status of the patient and the type of transplant received. As an example, a renal transplant work group recommended that high-risk renal transplant recipients be monitored once during the first week after transplant, monthly for 3–6 months, and then every 3 months for the first year. Monitoring should then be reinstituted if T-cell immunosuppression for acute rejection is needed [218]. By contrast, another renal transplant work group found that there is insufficient data to suggest that patient outcomes differ with routine monitoring and recommended that testing be individualized [205]. Recommendations from a leukemia working group were for weekly monitoring for a minimum of 3 months in high-risk HSCT recipients [200]. The 2013 American Society of Transplantation guidelines and the 2017 National Cancer Care Network guidelines make no definitive recommendation on whom to monitor and with what frequency [206, 207].

Until standardized approaches are developed through prospective trials, many of the above questions may remain unanswered. Importantly, preemptive viral load testing alone is not 100% effective at predicting disease. In order to augment the positive predictive value of viral load testing, various adjunct assays have been investigated, including measuring specific peripheral blood B- and T-cell subsets, interferon-gamma release to EBV antigens, and cytokine expression levels [219–230], though none are routinely employed in the clinical setting. As PTLD is likely a consequence of impaired cellular immunity, most adjunct assays focus on measuring T-cell number, function, or phenotype. Several studies have used MHC I tetramers for the detection of EBV-specific CD8+ cells in conjunction with viral load monitoring in both SOT and HSCT recipients [231–235]. Though most studies are limited by small sample sizes, many have found that expansion of EBV-specific T cells may indicate appropriate immune control and predict a lack of progression to PTLD despite elevated EBV viral load [231, 232]. Conversely, lack of expansion of EBV-specific T cells in response to elevated viral load correlates with the development of PTLD [234, 235]. A major disadvantage with MHC class I tetramer monitoring is that the reagent is HLA-specific. Therefore, it is only applicable to patients with common HLA alleles. At present, this diagnostic is not available outside the research setting.

Prevention of EBV-Associated Disease

Several studies have addressed the use of antiviral medications for the prevention of PTLD. Available antiviral medications target lytic cycle replication. It is plausible that lytic cycle replication contributes to the pathogenesis of PTLD; though as described above, the disorder is largely a result of latent gene effects on B-cell growth and survival. The greatest role for antivirals may, therefore, be in the prevention of primary infection (i.e., transmission from an EBV-infected organ or from another infected person) in EBV-seronegative transplant recipients and possibly the mitigation of severe AIM in immunocompromised individuals.

EBV encodes its own DNA polymerase, which replicates viral DNA as linear concatemers. The EBV DNA polymerase is only expressed during lytic replication. In latently infected cells, the host cell DNA polymerase replicates the EBV episome. Thus, available antiviral agents, such as acyclovir, ganciclovir, and foscarnet, each block EBV lytic but not latent replication. Acyclovir and ganciclovir are guanine nucleoside analogues that are converted into nucleotides by the EBV-encoded protein thymidine kinase [236]. The monophosphorylated form is then incorporated into viral DNA and terminates viral DNA chain synthesis.

Acyclovir is the most well-studied drug for the prevention of PTLD. The results of these studies have been mixed [237–243]. Notably, in most cases, the study populations included both EBV-seronegative and EBV-seropositive patients. The effect of acyclovir on prevention of primary infection in the seronegative population may have been obscured. Further, 800 mg of oral acyclovir was used in most of these studies, and the peak serum concentration of this dosage may not be consistently greater than the half maximal inhibitory concentration (IC50) for EBV replication [236, 244]. Valacyclovir, the esterified form of acyclovir, has greater bioavailability, and its peak serum concentration with the commonly used 1000 mg dose exceeds EBV's IC50 [236]. Valacyclovir's use has nonetheless not yet been as rigorously studied for the prevention of PTLD in the transplant population.

Ganciclovir may be more effective than acyclovir in treating or preventing EBV lytic infection. Both peak serum concentrations of the oral form of ganciclovir and the esterified form, valganciclovir, exceed the IC50 of the virus by 4- to 20-fold [236, 245]. Two studies have evaluated the use of ganciclovir or valganciclovir in high-risk EBV-seronegative pediatric SOT recipients. The first found a significant reduction in the incidence of PTLD in high-risk patients treated with 100 days of IV ganciclovir, when compared to historic controls. However, this finding may have been confounded by concurrent intense viral load monitoring with a reduction of immunosuppression for viremia in the treatment group [240]. A small prospective cohort study found that primary EBV infection was significantly decreased in patients who received ganciclovir or valganciclovir compared to those who received no prophylaxis (45% versus 100%, $p < 0.0001$) [246].

Results from some of these trials were included in a meta-analysis of 31 studies, largely observational in nature; no significant difference in rate of EBV-associated PTLD in SOT recipients was observed among those who received prophylaxis (acyclovir, valacyclovir, ganciclovir, valganciclovir) compared with those who did not receive prophylaxis [247]. Overall, use of antiviral prophylaxis remains a controversial area, and as ganciclovir and its derivatives are not without toxicity, further research is needed.

Preemptive Therapy

EBV viral load monitoring has become routine in many transplant centers. However, how to best manage subclinical EBV viremia detected by routine screening remains a major quandary. Present approaches include reduction in immunosuppression and/or treatment with anti-CD20 monoclonal antibodies, such as rituximab. Numerous studies have evaluated the role of rituximab in preemptive treatment, where rituximab is given for EBV reactivation or primary infection with a goal of destroying infected B cells before clinical PTLD can develop. This strategy may be particularly effective in HSCT recipients [217, 248, 249], although not every patient with EBV viremia will progress to PTLD. Thus, this strategy comes at the cost of additional humoral immune deficits in an already immunocompromised population. Adoptive transfer of EBV-specific T cells has also been shown to be effective prophylaxis [250–253], but its use has historically been limited by the technical difficulty of generating an individualized product for each transplant recipient. Each of these management strategies is further detailed below.

Diagnosis

The accurate diagnosis of PTLD requires tissue biopsy. When safe and clinically feasible, excisional biopsy is preferred over needle core biopsy or fine needle aspiration. Elevated or rising EBV viral load within the peripheral blood or sterile fluid, such as cerebrospinal fluid, raises the likelihood of disease, but it is not diagnostic. Likewise, radiographic evidence of PET (positron emission tomography)-avid lesions increases the likelihood of disease, but again is not diagnostic of PTLD. As with lymphomas in the non-transplant population, CT (computed tomography)/PET imaging should be used to stage disease at diagnosis and may be used to assess for interval change with treatment. Of note, CNS PTLD is less likely to present with an elevated peripheral blood viral load [151, 152]. Tissue biopsy remains the gold standard for diagnosis of CNS PTLD. However, diagnosis may be inferred from the presence of malignant lymphocytes in the cerebrospinal fluid if biopsy cannot be performed [237].

In situ hybridization for EBERs is the gold standard for confirming the presence of EBV in tumor tissue. EBER1 and EBER2 are noncoding RNAs that are expressed at roughly one million transcripts per latently infected cell making them readily amenable hybridization targets [254]. Immunohistochemical detection of EBNA1, EBNA2, LMP1, LMP2, and BZLF1 can also be used to confirm the presence of EBV in tumor tissue, as well as to distinguish EBV latency patterns. However, these assays are typically less sensitive and are also prone to cross reaction with human proteins [240, 254]. Further, it is not typically necessary to distinguish the latency pattern when diagnosing PTLD.

Pathology

The pathologic diagnosis of PTLD is based on the WHO classification [255]. There are four major categories: (1) early lesions, (2) polymorphic PTLD, (3) monomorphic PTLD, and (4) classical Hodgkin lymphoma-like PTLD (see Table 38.2). Early lesions typically arise in the first year following transplantation. A variety of B-cell types can become malignant in early lesions, though the underlying tissue architecture tends to be preserved in this type of PTLD. There are two subtypes of early lesions, plasmacytic hyperplasia and infectious mononucleosis-type PTLD, though some morphological overlap occurs between the two. Both the abnormal B cells and the latent EBV strain tend to be oligoclonal or polyclonal, and chromosomal karyotypes are typically normal in early lesions [204, 255]. By contrast, in polymorphic PTLD, the underlying tissue architecture is effaced by an expansion of B cells in various stages of differentiation. Additionally, there may be a higher degree of nuclear atypia, mitosis, and necrosis [204]. Both B cells and EBV tend to be clonal in polymorphic PTLD, and chromosomal karyotypes are commonly abnormal [146, 204].

Table 38.2 WHO classification of PTLD

WHO classification of PTLD
Early lesions
Plasmacytic hyperplasia
Infectious mononucleosis-like PTLD
Polymorphic PTLD
Monomorphic PTLD
B-cell neoplasms
Diffuse large B-cell lymphoma
Burkitt lymphoma
Plasma cell myeloma
Plasmacytoma-like lesion
Others
T-cell neoplasms
Peripheral T-cell lymphoma, not otherwise specified
Hepatosplenic lymphoma
Other
Classical Hodgkin lymphoma-type PTLD

Monomorphic PTLD is the most commonly detected form of PTLD and refers to a heterogenous group of monoclonal malignancies of B- or T-cell origin. The most common form of monomorphic PTLD is DLBCL [255]. Monomorphic PTLD may also take the form of Burkitt lymphoma. As in the sporadic form of Burkitt lymphoma, proliferation rates are high and *MYC* mutations are common. Rarely, monomorphic PTLD manifests as a plasma cell neoplasm. Like their counterparts in the non-transplant population, monoclonal immunoglobulins may be found in the serum or urine in patients with this form of PTLD [204].

Up to 15% of PTLD may be of T-cell origin. The association with EBV is weaker, with only 30% of T-cell PTLD harboring the EBV genome [256]. NK-cell disease is even less common than T-cell disease, but the majority of these lesions are EBV positive [257]. In the majority of cases of monomorphic T-cell PTLD, both the malignant cell and EBV are clonal. Classical Hodgkin lymphoma-type PTLD is a rare form of PTLD and tends to occur in the late posttransplant course, though is often EBV positive [258]. Notably, while PTLD appears morphologically similar to many lymphomas arising in the non-transplant population, the gene expression profiles of both polymorphic and monoclonal PTLD appear more similar to one another than to B-cell lymphomas arising in the non-transplant population [259].

Management

There are several strategies for treatment of PTLD, ranging from reduction of immune suppression, local therapy with surgery or radiation, EBV-directed antiviral therapy, rituximab with or without cytotoxic chemotherapy, and adoptive T-cell immunotherapy. A general principle of treatment of PTLD is to start with the best tolerated therapies and proceed to more toxic therapies only if initial management attempts prove inadequate. However, with highly aggressive disease, rapid disease progression and clinical decline may limit attempts at conservative treatment strategies.

Reduction of Immune Suppression

The mainstay of initial treatment for PTLD is reduction of immunosuppression (RI). The goal of RI is to restore the host immune response to EBV infection and, thereby, regain control of Latency III B-cell outgrowth. Thus, RI is a more effective strategy in SOT recipients or in HSCT recipients later in their transplant course once some level of immune reconstitution has been achieved. In addition, RI is typically more effective in polymorphic PTLD than in monomorphic PTLD. As RI can potentially increase the risk of graft rejection in SOT recipients or graft-versus-host disease in HSCT recipients, the risks and benefits must be weighed carefully on a patient-by-patient basis. For SOT recipients, graft function must be monitored closely with RI, especially in recipients of critical organs such as the heart, liver, and lung, where rejection can be fatal.

Although response to RI will vary depending on the immunosuppressive regimen, type of transplant, and pathologic subtype of PTLD, data suggest that lowering immunosuppression as in initial management step can lead to a salutary effect on PTLD, and in some cases it is sufficient for resolution of disease [260, 261]. In one of the largest study to date, 162 SOT recipients with PTLD were analyzed for response to RI [262]. Sixty-seven patients were treated with RI alone, and an additional 30 were treated with complete surgical resection of a localized PTLD lesion followed by adjuvant RI. Of the 67 patients receiving RI monotherapy, the vast majority had monomorphic PTLD, predominately DLBCL-like. RI resulted in an overall response rate (RR) of 45% and complete response rate (CR) of 37%. Of the 67 total patients treated with RI, 60% required further systemic therapy. However, the relapse rate among complete responders was only 17%. Additionally, 32% of treated patients experienced acute rejection, some leading to loss of allograft. Risk factors for lack of response to RI alone included advanced age, presence of B symptoms, hepatitis C coinfection, elevated lactate dehydrogenase, and liver and bone marrow involvement. Conversely, the Southwest and Eastern Cooperative Oncology Groups published results of a protocol starting with a 50% RI for 2 weeks followed by an additional 50% RI if no response, which resulted in only a single partial response among 16 patients [263].

In sum, RI alone is a reasonable initial strategy for patients with PTLD who are not early in their transplant course. Risk factors, such as markers of poor performance status or aggressive disease, have been identified for situations where RI alone may not be effective, but these are not universally accepted.

Local Therapies

In rare cases, focal PTLD lesions may be amenable to either surgical resection or radiotherapy with a curative goal. Local treatments are often followed by adjuvant RI.

Antiviral Therapy

Available antiviral drugs target viral lytic cycle replication and are not appropriate monotherapy for PTLD. However, lytic replication can be induced by histone deacetylation inhibitors (HDACi) such as arginine butyrate [8]. Using HDACi to induce lytic replication followed by treatment with high-dose ganciclovir is a novel PTLD treatment strategy. Notably, unlike acyclovir, phosphorylated ganciclovir also inhibits the cellular DNA polymerase and induces cell death which may also contribute to its effect on PTLD [264, 265]. In a Phase I/II trial of 15 patients with EBV-associated lymphoproliferative disorders refractory to at least 1 prior systemic regimen, 10 patients had a response to arginine butyrate and standard doses of ganciclovir, with 4 complete responses (CR) and 6 partial responses (PR) [266]. Of the six transplant recipients (three HSCT, three SOT), two achieved a CR and three achieved a PR. Adverse effects included tumor lysis syndrome and reversible CNS depression. Although encouraging, there are limited follow-up data; arginine butyrate is poorly tolerated, and the combination remains an uncommon treatment strategy.

Rituximab and Cytotoxic Chemotherapy

The monoclonal antibody rituximab targets CD20, a nearly pan-B-cell marker that is retained on most PTLD B cells. Rituximab given in both a preemptive and initial treatment manner has become a mainstay of the treatment of CD20-positive PTLD in both HSCT and SOT recipients.

For clinical PTLD as opposed to asymptomatic viremia, initial therapy with rituximab either after or with RI (if possible) is a common and frequently effective treatment strategy. This has been addressed in multiple studies and can be curative in a proportion of patients, with most studies falling in the 20–40% CR and 20–70% objective response rate (ORR) range [267–269]. For example, in a study of 11 SOT recipients with CD20-positive PTLD, a regimen of 4 weekly doses of rituximab repeated every 6 months for 2 years led to a 64% ORR with 54% CR rate [270]. A prospective study of 43 SOT recipients treated with single-agent rituximab demonstrated an ORR of 44% and CR in 28% with an OS of 67% at 1 year [271]. Rituximab-related toxicity was minimal, and primary adverse effects include infusional reactions, prolonged immunosuppression due to B-cell suppression, and neutropenia.

Chemotherapy remains an option for patients with a suitable performance status when other therapies have failed or for non-CD20 or non-EBV types of PTLD. Cytotoxic chemotherapy is best studied in patients with CD20- and EBV-positive PTLD, usually of the DLBCL type. Although highly effective, chemotherapy in the transplant population can be markedly toxic and occasionally fatal. As such, numerous studies have examined up-front versus delayed chemotherapy, most commonly with rituximab plus CHOP (cyclophosphamide, doxorubicin, vincristine, prednisone). A study of sequential therapy with 4 weekly doses of rituximab followed by 4 cycles of CHOP-21 in 74 SOT recipients with CD20-positive PTLD led to an ORR of 90% with 68% CRs [272]. There was, however, a CHOP-associated mortality of 11%. Significant neutropenia and infections developed in 68% and 41% of patients, respectively. Overall CHOP-related mortality was lower in the patients treated with rituximab initially when compared to those who started CHOP earlier due to progression on rituximab, suggesting that sequential rather than concurrent therapy may lead to improved tolerability of CHOP. A smaller study of 11 SOT recipients with CD20-positive PTLD examined giving CHOP after failure of rituximab and RI alone [273]. Ten patients received CHOP, with an ORR of 70% and CR of 50%, most of which were durable. There was one possible CHOP-associated death, and two of the ten patients did not tolerate CHOP and had to be changed to less toxic therapy. Another study of 26 patients with late PTLD of both B- and T-cell types demonstrated a 50% CR and 15% PR rate, with a 5-year PFS of 43% [274].

Overall, rituximab monotherapy can be curative in some patients with CD20-positive neoplasms and is a reasonable initial option with low concomitant toxicity. Many patients who fail rituximab monotherapy can be salvaged with subsequent CHOP. Additionally, patients who receive sequential rather than concurrent R-CHOP may tolerate the CHOP portion better. For patients with unusual subtypes of PTLD such as Burkitt lymphoma, HL, or T-cell lymphomas, RI and, if needed, standard chemotherapy regimens are the standard of care. For example, patients not responding to RI with HL should in general receive ABVD (doxorubicin, bleomycin, vinblastine, and dacarbazine), patients with T-cell lymphomas CHOP, and patients with Burkitt lymphoma a Burkitt-type regimen if it can be tolerated or CHOP if it cannot [275].

Adoptive T-Cell Immunotherapy

Adoptive T-cell immunotherapy is an effective treatment option for select patients with EBV-driven PTLD when available. The principle of adoptive immunotherapy is to restore immunity by transferring T cells from an allogeneic donor to a recipient with PTLD. This was first attempted with unmanipulated donor T cells, which can be rapidly available in the HSCT population, if the donor is willing and available. Treatment with donor lymphocyte infusion (DLI) has efficacy rates of up to 70% for the treatment of PTLD, but at the substantial risk of severe or even fatal GVHD [276, 277], likely due to the fact that alloreactive T cells are often tenfold higher in number than viral reactive T cells in unmanipulated grafts [278].

Another option is EBV-specific T-cell transfer, which dramatically reduces the risk of GVHD. Polyclonal EBV-specific T-cell lines comprised of both CD8+ and CD4+ T cells can be expanded ex vivo from donor cells and infused into patients with PTLD. These cell lines can be either obtained directly from the original allograft donor, which is time-consuming and may not be an option for patients with rapidly progressive disease or unavailable donor, or obtained rapidly from previously banked ("off-the-shelf"), closely HLA-matched virus-specific T cells. A seminal study of 33 patients with refractory EBV-PTLD demonstrated high response rates to closely matched EBV-cytotoxic lymphocytes (CTL), with ongoing responses of 52% at 6 months, including 14 CRs [279]. Patients who had closer HLA matches and higher numbers of infused CTLs had better response rates. At a minimum of 5-year follow-up of the CR patients, 12 were still living, 1 died of relapsed disease, and 1 died of unrelated infection [280]. All patients with PR or no response received alternative PTLD therapy. A more recent study examined 49 HSCT recipients with EBV-PTLD who were either treatment naïve or had received only rituximab [281]. Patients were given either DLI or EBV-specific CTLs. The combined partial and complete response rate for DLI was 73% and for EBV-specific CTLs was 68%. Seventeen percent of DLI recipients developed reversible acute GVHD. Patients with multiorgan involvement of lymphoma were less likely to respond, as were patients with CTLs that did not expand in vivo.

Avoidance of toxicities associated with cytotoxic chemotherapy is one of the major advantages of EBV-specific adoptive T-cell immunotherapy. The chief limitation is availability of donor T cells, either because the initial graft donor is not available (cord blood, cadaveric solid organ, or unwilling/unavailable donor), because the time needed for ex vivo expansion of T-cell lines is too long, or because of the limited availability of preformed T-cell products. Thus, adoptive immunotherapy at this point is generally limited to recipients with living and available donors or to those in transplant centers with access to protocol-based T-cell grafts. Such cells are in practicality only available for HSCT recipients at this point, although there are some techniques for obtaining autologous EBV-specific T cells in SOT recipients with some short-term anti-EBV efficacy. The role of newer agents, including antibody drug conjugates or chimeric antigen receptor (CAR) T cells against antigens like CD19, in the treatment of PTLD remains to be determined.

EBV Vaccine Development

An EBV vaccine was originally proposed nearly 40 years ago by Epstein and Achong [282]. However, the EBV vaccine remains an elusive goal. A US National Institutes of Health (NIH) meeting noted challenges of EBV vaccine development but strongly endorsed ongoing vaccine efforts

[283]. While prevention of infection would be the ultimate endpoint, the biology of EBV may complicate this goal. For instance, in a murine model of the EBV-related gammaherpesvirus 68 infection, a single target cell infected by single viral particle was sufficient to establish persistent host infection [284]. Furthermore, an EBV vaccine would face a high regulatory hurdle – since EBV does not generally cause severe disease, an approvable EBV vaccine could only have minimal side effects. Additionally since EBV is an oncogenic virus, live-virus vaccines would raise safety concerns. Nonetheless, an EBV vaccine that protects against the complications of EBV infection, even without preventing lifelong EBV infection, could still have a substantial public health impact. The NIH study group recommended that an EBV vaccine should have two major goals: to prevent infectious mononucleosis and to prevent EBV-associated cancers [283]. Both of these goals may be attainable without achieving sterilizing immunity that prevents EBV infection. As an example, the attenuated varicella zoster virus (VZV) Oka strain vaccine has greatly reduced the burden of VZV-associated disease without necessarily preventing infection.

Even prevention of AIM alone would have a tremendous public health and economic impact. The major goal would be to limit the extent of lytic virus replication and the growth of latently infected B cells following primary EBV oropharyngeal transmission [7]. Encouragingly, asymptomatic primary EBV infection protects against subsequent AIM, and a vaccine may be able to capture this benefit. A vaccine-primed immune system might be able to better control primary EBV infection. For instance, elevated primary infection EBV viral loads correlate with AIM severity [101], and AIM is associated with a 3.4-fold increased risk for the development of EBV+ HL [285]. An EBV vaccine that reduces viral loads might also reduce the incidence of IM and HL. Likewise, reduction of EBV viral load may lessen the likelihood of PTLD development.

The major EBV envelope glycoprotein gp350 is the principal target of most EBV vaccines in development. EBV initiates B-cell infection via gp350 binding to CD21, the B-cell receptor for complement component C3d [286, 287]. Additional interactions between the EBV glycoprotein gp42 and the co-receptor HLA class II further promote viral entry [288]. EBV also infects CD21-negative cell types such as oropharyngeal epithelial cells, mesenchymal cells, and T cells, suggesting that additional unidentified receptor(s) must exist. Nonetheless, gp350 is an attractive target, since it is the most abundant glycoprotein on the surface of EBV and EBV-infected cells and is the dominant target of neutralizing antibody responses [92, 283, 289].

A recombinant VZV vaccine vector was developed to deliver gp350 nearly 25 years ago [290]. However, the first randomized, placebo-controlled, multicenter, double-blind trial of a gp350-based vaccine to prevent AIM was not reported until some 20 years later [291]. The recombinant gp350 and alum/monophosphoryl lipid adjuvant vaccine induced anti-gp350 antibodies in 98.7% of subjects for at least 18 months after administration of the third vaccine dose. The vaccine also reduced the proportion of symptomatic primary EBV infection over an 18-month observation period, from 10% in the control group to 2% in the vaccine group. Not surprisingly, the vaccine did not protect against asymptomatic EBV infection. An EBV-antibody-seropositive study participant developed an oligoarthritis syndrome, raising potential safety concerns. In a small Phase I trial in children with chronic kidney disease awaiting transplantation, vaccination with recombinant gp350 plus alum induced IgG responses in all 13 evaluable patients [292]. However, neutralizing antibodies were only detectable in four vaccine recipients, and anti-gp350 antibody levels rapidly diminished following completion of the vaccine cycles. More recently, the use of self-assembling nanoparticles to display gp350 domains elicited potent neutralizing antibody responses in mice and nonhuman primate models [293].

The gp350 vaccination can also stimulate cell-mediated immunity, a property that was important for prevention of EBV-associated lymphomas in an animal model [294]. Since many EBV-derived HLA class I epitopes are generated during primary infection, a second vaccine approach has been to stimulate a CD8+ T-cell response to EBV antigens. Indeed, in a small single-blind, randomized, placebo-controlled, single-center trial, an EBNA3 CD8+ T-cell peptide-based vaccine was administered to 9 HLA B*0801-positive individuals. Four individuals received a placebo vaccine. In follow-up, none of the four EBNA3 vaccine recipients experienced symptomatic AIM with primary EBV infection [295]. While exciting and potentially applicable to the prevention and/or treatment of EBV-associated malignancies, this approach is complicated by the diversity of HLA molecules across different human populations. Consequently, a CD8+ T-cell peptide-based vaccine would need to incorporate multiple appropriate EBV epitopes. This goal might be achievable with the use of recombinant polyepitope protein constructs that encode multiple distinct CTL peptide targets in tandem. Vaccines might also combine a gp350-based component with CD8+ T-cell antigens to further limit virus replication and spread [296].

Vaccines to treat EBV-associated malignancies are also being developed. Nasopharyngeal carcinoma (NPC) may be a particularly attractive candidate, as EBV epitopes are detected in most undifferentiated NPC cases. Furthermore, in NPC-endemic regions of Southern China, HLA alleles such as HLA-A11, A24, and B40 are common, potentially simplifying the cocktail of epitopes that may be needed [297]. In one promising approach, an adenoviral vector-based vaccine has been developed that delivers EBNA1, LMP1, and LMP2 epitopes suitable for these HLA alleles. In a preclinical study of patients with recurrent and metastatic NPC, the vaccine stimulated EBV-specific T-cell development in 72% of patients [297]. T cells were expanded ex vivo and then adoptively transferred back to the appropriate NPC patient. The median overall survival increased from 220 days, without T-cell transfusion, to 523 days with primed T-cell transfer.

References

1. Henle G, Henle W, Clifford P, Diehl V, Kafuko GW, Kirya BG, et al. Antibodies to Epstein-Barr virus in Burkitt's lymphoma and control groups. J Natl Cancer Inst. 1969;43(5):1147–57.
2. Kieff E, Rickinson AB. Epstein-Barr virus and its replication. In: Field BN, Knipe DM, Howley PM, editors. Field's virology. 5th ed. Philadelphia: Lippincott, Williams and Wilkins; 2007. p. 2603–54.
3. Cohen J. Virology and molecular biology of Epstein-Barr virus. In: Tselis A, Jenson HB, editors. Epstein-Barr Virus. New York: Taylor and Francis; 2006. p. 21–38.
4. Yao QY, Rickinson AB, Epstein MA. A re-examination of the Epstein-Barr virus carrier state in healthy seropositive individuals. Int J Cancer. 1985;35(1):35–42.
5. Hadinoto V, Shapiro M, Greenough TC, Sullivan JL, Luzuriaga K, Thorley-Lawson DA. On the dynamics of acute EBV infection and the pathogenesis of infectious mononucleosis. Blood. 2008;111(3):1420–7.
6. Straus SE, Cohen JI, Tosato G, Meier J. NIH conference. Epstein-Barr virus infections: biology, pathogenesis, and management. Ann Intern Med. 1993;118(1):45–58.
7. Rickinson AB, Kieff E. Epstein-Barr virus. In: Field BN, Knipe DM, Howley PM, editors. Field's virology. 5th ed. Philadelphia: Lippincott, Williams and Wilkins; 2007. p. 2655–700.
8. Luka J, Kallin B, Klein G. Induction of the Epstein-Barr virus (EBV) cycle in latently infected cells by n-butyrate. Virology. 1979;94(1):228–31.
9. Miller G, El-Guindy A, Countryman J, Ye J, Gradoville L. Lytic cycle switches of oncogenic human gammaherpesviruses. Adv Cancer Res. 2007;97:81–109.
10. Kalla M, Hammerschmidt W. Human B cells on their route to latent infection--early but transient expression of lytic genes of Epstein-Barr virus. Eur J Cell Biol. 2012;91(1):65–9.
11. Concha M, Wang X, Cao S, Baddoo M, Fewell C, Lin Z, et al. Identification of new viral genes and transcript isoforms during Epstein-Barr virus reactivation using RNA-Seq. J Virol. 2012;86(3):1458–67.
12. Babcock GJ, Decker LL, Volk M, Thorley-Lawson DA. EBV persistence in memory B cells in vivo. Immunity. 1998;9(3):395–404.
13. Wagner HJ, Bein G, Bitsch A, Kirchner H. Detection and quantification of latently infected B lymphocytes in Epstein-Barr virus-seropositive, healthy individuals by polymerase chain reaction. J Clin Microbiol. 1992;30(11):2826–9.
14. Hislop AD, Taylor GS, Sauce D, Rickinson AB. Cellular responses to viral infection in humans: lessons from Epstein-Barr virus. Annu Rev Immunol. 2007;25:587–617.
15. Babcock GJ, Thorley-Lawson DA. Tonsillar memory B cells, latently infected with Epstein-Barr virus, express the restricted pattern of latent genes previously found only in Epstein-Barr virus-associated tumors. Proc Natl Acad Sci U S A. 2000;97(22):12250–5.
16. Auwaerter PG. Infectious mononucleosis in middle age. JAMA. 1999;281(5):454–9.
17. Taylor GS, Long HM, Brooks JM, Rickinson AB, Hislop AD. The immunology of Epstein-Barr virus-induced disease. Annu Rev Immunol. 2015;33:787–821.
18. Kutok JL, Wang F. Spectrum of Epstein-Barr virus-associated diseases. Annu Rev Pathol. 2006;1:375–404.
19. Rickinson AB, Moss DJ. Human cytotoxic T lymphocyte responses to Epstein-Barr virus infection. Annu Rev Immunol. 1997;15:405–31.
20. Castillo JJ, Beltran BE, Miranda RN, Paydas S, Winer ES, Butera JN. Epstein-barr virus-positive diffuse large B-cell lymphoma of the elderly: what we know so far. Oncologist. 2011;16(1):87–96.
21. Casola S, Otipoby KL, Alimzhanov M, Humme S, Uyttersprot N, Kutok JL, et al. B cell receptor signal strength determines B cell fate. Nat Immunol. 2004;5(3):317–27.
22. Thorley-Lawson DA, Gross A. Persistence of the Epstein-Barr virus and the origins of associated lymphomas. N Engl J Med. 2004;350(13):1328–37.
23. Minamitani T, Yasui T, Ma Y, Zhou H, Okuzaki D, Tsai CY, et al. Evasion of affinity-based selection in germinal centers by Epstein-Barr virus LMP2A. Proc Natl Acad Sci U S A. 2015;112(37):11612–7.
24. Joseph AM, Babcock GJ, Thorley-Lawson DA. Cells expressing the Epstein-Barr virus growth program are present in and restricted to the naive B-cell subset of healthy tonsils. J Virol. 2000;74(21):9964–71.
25. Klein E. The complexity of the Epstein-Barr virus infection in humans. Pathol Oncol Res. 1998;4(1):3–7.
26. Hochberg D, Middeldorp JM, Catalina M, Sullivan JL, Luzuriaga K, Thorley-Lawson DA. Demonstration of the Burkitt's lymphoma Epstein-Barr virus phenotype in dividing latently infected memory cells in vivo. Proc Natl Acad Sci U S A. 2004;101(1):239–44.
27. Miyashita EM, Yang B, Babcock GJ, Thorley-Lawson DA. Identification of the site of Epstein-Barr virus persistence in vivo as a resting B cell. J Virol. 1997;71(7):4882–91.
28. Yin Y, Manoury B, Fahraeus R. Self-inhibition of synthesis and antigen presentation by Epstein-Barr virus-encoded EBNA1. Science. 2003;301(5638):1371–4.
29. Soni V, Cahir-McFarland E, Kieff E. LMP1 TRAFficking activates growth and survival pathways. Adv Exp Med Biol. 2007;597:173–87.
30. Ersing I, Bernhardt K, Gewurz BE. NF-kappaB and IRF7 pathway activation by Epstein-Barr virus latent membrane protein 1. Viruses. 2013;5(6):1587–606.
31. Kieser A, Sterz KR. The Latent Membrane Protein 1 (LMP1). Curr Top Microbiol Immunol. 2015;391:119–49.
32. Rastelli J, Homig-Holzel C, Seagal J, Muller W, Hermann AC, Rajewsky K, et al. LMP1 signaling can replace CD40 signaling in B cells in vivo and has unique features of inducing class-switch recombination to IgG1. Blood. 2008;111(3):1448–55.
33. Wang D, Liebowitz D, Kieff E. An EBV membrane protein expressed in immortalized lymphocytes transforms established rodent cells. Cell. 1985;43(3 Pt 2):831–40.
34. Uchida J, Yasui T, Takaoka-Shichijo Y, Muraoka M, Kulwichit W, Raab-Traub N, et al. Mimicry of CD40 signals by Epstein-Barr virus LMP1 in B lymphocyte responses. Science. 1999;286(5438):300–3.
35. Thornburg NJ, Kulwichit W, Edwards RH, Shair KH, Bendt KM, Raab-Traub N. LMP1 signaling and activation of NF-kappaB in LMP1 transgenic mice. Oncogene. 2006;25(2):288–97.
36. Zhang B, Kracker S, Yasuda T, Casola S, Vanneman M, Homig-Holzel C, et al. Immune surveillance and therapy of lymphomas driven by Epstein-Barr virus protein LMP1 in a mouse model. Cell. 2012;148(4):739–51.
37. Caldwell RG, Wilson JB, Anderson SJ, Longnecker R. Epstein-Barr virus LMP2A drives B cell development and survival in the absence of normal B cell receptor signals. Immunity. 1998;9(3):405–11.

38. Mancao C, Hammerschmidt W. Epstein-Barr virus latent membrane protein 2A is a B-cell receptor mimic and essential for B-cell survival. Blood. 2007;110(10):3715–21.
39. Miller CL, Burkhardt AL, Lee JH, Stealey B, Longnecker R, Bolen JB, et al. Integral membrane protein 2 of Epstein-Barr virus regulates reactivation from latency through dominant negative effects on protein-tyrosine kinases. Immunity. 1995;2(2):155–66.
40. Schmitz R, Hansmann ML, Bohle V, Martin-Subero JI, Hartmann S, Mechtersheimer G, et al. TNFAIP3 (A20) is a tumor suppressor gene in Hodgkin lymphoma and primary mediastinal B cell lymphoma. J Exp Med. 2009;206(5):981–9.
41. Shair KH, Bendt KM, Edwards RH, Nielsen JN, Moore DT, Raab-Traub N. Epstein-Barr virus-encoded latent membrane protein 1 (LMP1) and LMP2A function cooperatively to promote carcinoma development in a mouse carcinogenesis model. J Virol. 2012;86(9):5352–65.
42. Alfieri C, Birkenbach M, Kieff E. Early events in Epstein-Barr virus infection of human B lymphocytes. Virology. 1991;181(2):595–608.
43. Kaiser C, Laux G, Eick D, Jochner N, Bornkamm GW, Kempkes B. The proto-oncogene c-myc is a direct target gene of Epstein-Barr virus nuclear antigen 2. J Virol. 1999;73(5):4481–4.
44. Grossman SR, Johannsen E, Tong X, Yalamanchili R, Kieff E. The Epstein-Barr virus nuclear antigen 2 transactivator is directed to response elements by the J kappa recombination signal binding protein. Proc Natl Acad Sci U S A. 1994;91(16):7568–72.
45. Henkel T, Ling PD, Hayward SD, Peterson MG. Mediation of Epstein-Barr virus EBNA2 transactivation by recombination signal-binding protein J kappa. Science. 1994;265(5168):92–5.
46. Zhao B, Zou J, Wang H, Johannsen E, Peng CW, Quackenbush J, et al. Epstein-Barr virus exploits intrinsic B-lymphocyte transcription programs to achieve immortal cell growth. Proc Natl Acad Sci U S A. 2011;108(36):14902–7.
47. Maruo S, Zhao B, Johannsen E, Kieff E, Zou J, Takada K. Epstein-Barr virus nuclear antigens 3C and 3A maintain lymphoblastoid cell growth by repressing p16INK4A and p14ARF expression. Proc Natl Acad Sci U S A. 2011;108(5):1919–24.
48. Saha A, Bamidele A, Murakami M, Robertson ES. EBNA3C attenuates the function of p53 through interaction with inhibitor of growth family proteins 4 and 5. J Virol. 2011;85(5):2079–88.
49. Knight JS, Sharma N, Robertson ES. Epstein-Barr virus latent antigen 3C can mediate the degradation of the retinoblastoma protein through an SCF cellular ubiquitin ligase. Proc Natl Acad Sci U S A. 2005;102(51):18562–6.
50. Zhou H, Schmidt SC, Jiang S, Willox B, Bernhardt K, Liang J, et al. Epstein-Barr virus oncoprotein super-enhancers control B cell growth. Cell Host Microbe. 2015;17(2):205–16.
51. Altmann M, Hammerschmidt W. Epstein-Barr virus provides a new paradigm: a requirement for the immediate inhibition of apoptosis. PLoS Biol. 2005;3(12):e404.
52. Forte E, Luftig MA. The role of microRNAs in Epstein-Barr virus latency and lytic reactivation. Microbes Infect. 2011;13(14–15):1156–67.
53. Xia T, O'Hara A, Araujo I, Barreto J, Carvalho E, Sapucaia JB, et al. EBV microRNAs in primary lymphomas and targeting of CXCL-11 by ebv-mir-BHRF1-3. Cancer Res. 2008;68(5):1436–42.
54. Feederle R, Haar J, Bernhardt K, Linnstaedt SD, Bannert H, Lips H, et al. The members of an Epstein-Barr virus microRNA cluster cooperate to transform B lymphocytes. J Virol. 2011;85(19):9801–10.
55. Bernhardt K, Haar J, Tsai MH, Poirey R, Feederle R, Delecluse HJ. A viral microRNA cluster regulates the expression of PTEN, p27 and of a bcl-2 homolog. PLoS Pathog. 2016;12(1):e1005405.
56. McGeoch DJ, Rixon FJ, Davison AJ. Topics in herpesvirus genomics and evolution. Virus Res. 2006;117(1):90–104.
57. Ehlers B, Spiess K, Leendertz F, Peeters M, Boesch C, Gatherer D, et al. Lymphocryptovirus phylogeny and the origins of Epstein-Barr virus. J Gen Virol. 2010;91(Pt 3):630–42.
58. Azzi T, Lunemann A, Murer A, Ueda S, Beziat V, Malmberg KJ, et al. Role for early-differentiated natural killer cells in infectious mononucleosis. Blood. 2014;124(16):2533–43.
59. Williams H, McAulay K, Macsween KF, Gallacher NJ, Higgins CD, Harrison N, et al. The immune response to primary EBV infection: a role for natural killer cells. Br J Haematol. 2005;129(2):266–74.
60. Balfour HH Jr, Odumade OA, Schmeling DO, Mullan BD, Ed JA, Knight JA, et al. Behavioral, virologic, and immunologic factors associated with acquisition and severity of primary Epstein-Barr virus infection in university students. J Infect Dis. 2013;207(1):80–8.
61. Djaoud Z, Guethlein LA, Horowitz A, Azzi T, Nemat-Gorgani N, Olive D, et al. Two alternate strategies for innate immunity to Epstein-Barr virus: one using NK cells and the other NK cells and gammadelta T cells. J Exp Med. 2017;214(6):1827–41.
62. Chijioke O, Muller A, Feederle R, Barros MH, Krieg C, Emmel V, et al. Human natural killer cells prevent infectious mononucleosis features by targeting lytic Epstein-Barr virus infection. Cell Rep. 2013;5(6):1489–98.
63. Nachmani D, Stern-Ginossar N, Sarid R, Mandelboim O. Diverse herpesvirus microRNAs target the stress-induced immune ligand MICB to escape recognition by natural killer cells. Cell Host Microbe. 2009;5(4):376–85.
64. Rezaei N, Mahmoudi E, Aghamohammadi A, Das R, Nichols KE. X-linked lymphoproliferative syndrome: a genetic condition typified by the triad of infection, immunodeficiency and lymphoma. Br J Haematol. 2011;152(1):13–30.
65. Detre C, Keszei M, Garrido-Mesa N, Kis-Toth K, Castro W, Agyemang AF, et al. SAP expression in invariant NKT cells is required for cognate help to support B-cell responses. Blood. 2012;120(1):122–9.
66. Long HM, Taylor GS, Rickinson AB. Immune defence against EBV and EBV-associated disease. Curr Opin Immunol. 2011;23(2):258–64.
67. Meazza R, Falco M, Marcenaro S, Loiacono F, Canevali P, Bellora F, et al. Inhibitory 2B4 contributes to NK cell education and immunological derangements in XLP1 patients. Eur J Immunol. 2017;47(6):1051–61.
68. Grier JT, Forbes LR, Monaco-Shawver L, Oshinsky J, Atkinson TP, Moody C, et al. Human immunodeficiency-causing mutation defines CD16 in spontaneous NK cell cytotoxicity. J Clin Invest. 2012;122(10):3769–80.
69. Gineau L, Cognet C, Kara N, Lach FP, Dunne J, Veturi U, et al. Partial MCM4 deficiency in patients with growth retardation, adrenal insufficiency, and natural killer cell deficiency. J Clin Invest. 2012;122(3):821–32.
70. Bollard CM, Rooney CM, Heslop HE. T-cell therapy in the treatment of post-transplant lymphoproliferative disease. Nat Rev Clin Oncol. 2012;9(9):510–9.
71. Hislop AD. Early virological and immunological events in Epstein-Barr virus infection. Curr Opin Virol. 2015;15:75–9.
72. Silins SL, Sherritt MA, Silleri JM, Cross SM, Elliott SL, Bharadwaj M, et al. Asymptomatic primary Epstein-Barr virus infection occurs in the absence of blood T-cell repertoire perturbations despite high levels of systemic viral load. Blood. 2001;98(13):3739–44.
73. Hislop AD, Ressing ME, van Leeuwen D, Pudney VA, Horst D, Koppers-Lalic D, et al. A CD8+ T cell immune evasion protein specific to Epstein-Barr virus and its close relatives in Old World primates. J Exp Med. 2007;204(8):1863–73.
74. Horst D, van Leeuwen D, Croft NP, Garstka MA, Hislop AD, Kremmer E, et al. Specific targeting of the EBV lytic phase protein BNLF2a to the transporter associated with antigen processing results in impairment of HLA class I-restricted antigen presentation. J Immunol. 2009;182(4):2313–24.
75. Zuo J, Thomas W, van Leeuwen D, Middeldorp JM, Wiertz EJ, Ressing ME, et al. The DNase of gammaherpesviruses impairs rec-

ognition by virus-specific CD8+ T cells through an additional host shutoff function. J Virol. 2008;82(5):2385–93.
76. Zuo J, Quinn LL, Tamblyn J, Thomas WA, Feederle R, Delecluse HJ, et al. The Epstein-Barr virus-encoded BILF1 protein modulates immune recognition of endogenously processed antigen by targeting major histocompatibility complex class I molecules trafficking on both the exocytic and endocytic pathways. J Virol. 2011;85(4):1604–14.
77. Zuo J, Currin A, Griffin BD, Shannon-Lowe C, Thomas WA, Ressing ME, et al. The Epstein-Barr virus G-protein-coupled receptor contributes to immune evasion by targeting MHC class I molecules for degradation. PLoS Pathog. 2009;5(1):e1000255.
78. Albanese M, Tagawa T, Bouvet M, Maliqi L, Lutter D, Hoser J, et al. Epstein-Barr virus microRNAs reduce immune surveillance by virus-specific CD8+ T cells. Proc Natl Acad Sci U S A. 2016;113(42):E6467–E75.
79. Tagawa T, Albanese M, Bouvet M, Moosmann A, Mautner J, Heissmeyer V, et al. Epstein-Barr viral miRNAs inhibit antiviral CD4+ T cell responses targeting IL-12 and peptide processing. J Exp Med. 2016;213(10):2065–80.
80. Diekmann J, Adamopoulou E, Beck O, Rauser G, Lurati S, Tenzer S, et al. Processing of two latent membrane protein 1 MHC class I epitopes requires tripeptidyl peptidase II involvement. J Immunol. 2009;183(3):1587–97.
81. Levitskaya J, Sharipo A, Leonchiks A, Ciechanover A, Masucci MG. Inhibition of ubiquitin/proteasome-dependent protein degradation by the Gly-Ala repeat domain of the Epstein-Barr virus nuclear antigen 1. Proc Natl Acad Sci U S A. 1997;94(23):12616–21.
82. Levitskaya J, Coram M, Levitsky V, Imreh S, Steigerwald-Mullen PM, Klein G, et al. Inhibition of antigen processing by the internal repeat region of the Epstein-Barr virus nuclear antigen-1. Nature. 1995;375(6533):685–8.
83. Orlova N, Wang F, Fogg MH. Persistent infection drives the development of CD8+ T cells specific for late lytic infection antigens in lymphocryptovirus-infected macaques and Epstein-Barr virus-infected humans. J Virol. 2011;85(23):12821–4.
84. Long HM, Leese AM, Chagoury OL, Connerty SR, Quarcoopome J, Quinn LL, et al. Cytotoxic CD4+ T cell responses to EBV contrast with CD8 responses in breadth of lytic cycle antigen choice and in lytic cycle recognition. J Immunol. 2011;187(1): 92–101.
85. Nikiforow S, Bottomly K, Miller G, Munz C. Cytolytic CD4(+)-T-cell clones reactive to EBNA1 inhibit Epstein-Barr virus-induced B-cell proliferation. J Virol. 2003;77(22):12088–104.
86. Walter EA, Greenberg PD, Gilbert MJ, Finch RJ, Watanabe KS, Thomas ED, et al. Reconstitution of cellular immunity against cytomegalovirus in recipients of allogeneic bone marrow by transfer of T-cell clones from the donor. N Engl J Med. 1995;333(16): 1038–44.
87. Zuo J, Thomas WA, Haigh TA, Fitzsimmons L, Long HM, Hislop AD, et al. Epstein-Barr virus evades CD4+ T cell responses in lytic cycle through BZLF1-mediated downregulation of CD74 and the cooperation of vBcl-2. PLoS Pathog. 2011;7(12):e1002455.
88. Li D, Qian L, Chen C, Shi M, Yu M, Hu M, et al. Down-regulation of MHC class II expression through inhibition of CIITA transcription by lytic transactivator Zta during Epstein-Barr virus reactivation. J Immunol. 2009;182(4):1799–809.
89. Mullen MM, Haan KM, Longnecker R, Jardetzky TS. Structure of the Epstein-Barr virus gp42 protein bound to the MHC class II receptor HLA-DR1. Mol Cell. 2002;9(2):375–85.
90. Ressing ME, Horst D, Griffin BD, Tellam J, Zuo J, Khanna R, et al. Epstein-Barr virus evasion of CD8(+) and CD4(+) T cell immunity via concerted actions of multiple gene products. Semin Cancer Biol. 2008;18(6):397–408.
91. Garzelli C, Taub FE, Scharff JE, Prabhakar BS, Ginsberg-Fellner F, Notkins AL. Epstein-Barr virus-transformed lymphocytes produce monoclonal autoantibodies that react with antigens in multiple organs. J Virol. 1984;52(2):722–5.
92. Thorley-Lawson DA, Geilinger K. Monoclonal antibodies against the major glycoprotein (gp350/220) of Epstein-Barr virus neutralize infectivity. Proc Natl Acad Sci U S A. 1980;77(9):5307–11.
93. Tanner J, Whang Y, Sample J, Sears A, Kieff E. Soluble gp350/220 and deletion mutant glycoproteins block Epstein-Barr virus adsorption to lymphocytes. J Virol. 1988;62(12):4452–64.
94. Thorley-Lawson DA, Poodry CA. Identification and isolation of the main component (gp350-gp220) of Epstein-Barr virus responsible for generating neutralizing antibodies in vivo. J Virol. 1982;43(2):730–6.
95. Panikkar A, Smith C, Hislop A, Tellam N, Dasari V, Hogquist KA, et al. Impaired Epstein-Barr virus-specific neutralizing antibody response during acute infectious mononucleosis is coincident with global B-cell dysfunction. J Virol. 2015;89(17):9137–41.
96. Andiman WA. Epidemiology of primary Epstein-Barr virus infection and infectious mononucleosis. In: Tselis A, Jenson HB, editors. Epstein-Barr Virus. New York City: Taylor & Francis; 2006. p. 39–59.
97. Balfour HH Jr, Sifakis F, Sliman JA, Knight JA, Schmeling DO, Thomas W. Age-specific prevalence of Epstein-Barr virus infection among individuals aged 6-19 years in the United States and factors affecting its acquisition. J Infect Dis. 2013;208(8):1286–93.
98. Niederman JC, Evans AS, Subrahmanyan L, McCollum RW. Prevalence, incidence and persistence of EB virus antibody in young adults. N Engl J Med. 1970;282(7):361–5.
99. McKinnon GT, Pringle RC. A serological study of antibody to Epstein-Barr virus in an Australian population. Med J Aust. 1974;2(7):243–6.
100. Hallee TJ, Evans AS, Niederman JC, Brooks CM, Voegtly jH. Infectious mononucleosis at the United States Military Academy. A prospective study of a single class over four years. Yale J Biol Med. 1974;47(3):182–95.
101. Balfour HH Jr, Holman CJ, Hokanson KM, Lelonek MM, Giesbrecht JE, White DR, et al. A prospective clinical study of Epstein-Barr virus and host interactions during acute infectious mononucleosis. J Infect Dis. 2005;192(9):1505–12.
102. Glaser R, Strain EC, Tarr KL, Holliday JE, Donnerberg RL, Kiecolt-Glaser JK. Changes in Epstein-Barr virus antibody titers associated with aging. Proc Soc Exp Biol Med. 1985;179(3):352–5.
103. Sumaya CV, Henle W, Henle G, Smith MH, LeBlanc D. Seroepidemiologic study of Epstein-Barr virus infections in a rural community. J Infect Dis. 1975;131(4):403–8.
104. Henle G, Henle W. Observations on childhood infections with the Epstein-Barr virus. J Infect Dis. 1970;121(3):303–10.
105. Brodsky AL, Heath CW Jr. Infectious mononucleosis: epidemiologic patterns at United States colleges and universities. Am J Epidemiol. 1972;96(2):87–93.
106. Chang RS, Rosen L, Kapikian AZ. Epstein-Barr virus infections in a nursery. Am J Epidemiol. 1981;113(1):22–9.
107. Sixbey JW, Lemon SM, Pagano JS. A second site for Epstein-Barr virus shedding: the uterine cervix. Lancet. 1986;2(8516):1122–4.
108. Naher H, Gissmann L, Freese UK, Petzoldt D, Helfrich S. Subclinical Epstein-Barr virus infection of both the male and female genital tract--indication for sexual transmission. J Invest Dermatol. 1992;98(5):791–3.
109. Morris SR, Zhao M, Smith DM, Vargas MV, Little SJ, Gianella S. Longitudinal viral dynamics in Semen during early HIV infection. Clin Infect Dis. 2017;64(4):428–34.
110. Lisco A, Munawwar A, Introini A, Vanpouille C, Saba E, Feng X, et al. Semen of HIV-1-infected individuals: local shedding of herpesviruses and reprogrammed cytokine network. J Infect Dis. 2012;205(1):97–105.

111. Crawford DH, Swerdlow AJ, Higgins C, McAulay K, Harrison N, Williams H, et al. Sexual history and Epstein-Barr virus infection. J Infect Dis. 2002;186(6):731–6.
112. Alfieri C, Tanner J, Carpentier L, Perpete C, Savoie A, Paradis K, et al. Epstein-Barr virus transmission from a blood donor to an organ transplant recipient with recovery of the same virus strain from the recipient's blood and oropharynx. Blood. 1996;87(2):812–7.
113. Qu L, Xu S, Rowe D, Triulzi D. Efficacy of Epstein-Barr virus removal by leukoreduction of red blood cells. Transfusion. 2005;45(4):591–5.
114. Qu L, Triulzi DJ, Rowe DT, Griffin DL, Donnenberg AD. Stability of lymphocytes and Epstein-Barr virus during red blood cell storage. Vox Sang. 2007;92(2):125–9.
115. Trottier H, Delage G, Hu J, Robitaille N, Buteau C, Tucci M, et al. Detection of Epstein-Barr virus in leucoreduced blood products. Vox Sang. 2016;110(2):199–201.
116. Finn L, Reyes J, Bueno J, Yunis E. Epstein-Barr virus infections in children after transplantation of the small intestine. Am J Surg Pathol. 1998;22(3):299–309.
117. Correia S, Palser A, Elgueta Karstegl C, Middeldorp JM, Ramayanti O, Cohen JI, et al. Natural variation of Epstein-Barr virus genes, proteins, and primary MicroRNA. J Virol. 2017;91(15). pii: e00375–17.
118. Rickinson AB, Young LS, Rowe M. Influence of the Epstein-Barr virus nuclear antigen EBNA 2 on the growth phenotype of virus-transformed B cells. J Virol. 1987;61(5):1310–7.
119. Yao QY, Croom-Carter DS, Tierney RJ, Habeshaw G, Wilde JT, Hill FG, et al. Epidemiology of infection with Epstein-Barr virus types 1 and 2: lessons from the study of a T-cell-immunocompromised hemophilic cohort. J Virol. 1998;72(5):4352–63.
120. Sculley TB, Apolloni A, Hurren L, Moss DJ, Cooper DA. Coinfection with A- and B-type Epstein-Barr virus in human immunodeficiency virus-positive subjects. J Infect Dis. 1990;162(3):643–8.
121. Ibrahim HA, Menasce LP, Pomplun S, Burke M, Bower M, Naresh KN. Epstein-Barr virus (EBV) genotypes among human immunodeficiency virus (HIV)-related B-cell lymphomas and B-cell post-transplant lymphoproliferative disorders (B-PTLD)--late-onset lymphomas, especially in the HIV setting, are associated with type-B-EBV. Eur J Haematol. 2010;85(3):227–30.
122. Frank D, Cesarman E, Liu YF, Michler RE, Knowles DM. Posttransplantation lymphoproliferative disorders frequently contain type A and not type B Epstein-Barr virus. Blood. 1995;85(5):1396–403.
123. Jenson HB. Virologic diagnosis, viral monitoring, and treatment of Epstein-Barr virus infectious mononucleosis. Curr Infect Dis Rep. 2004;6(3):200–7.
124. Duverlie G, Driencourt M, Roussel C, Orfila J. Heterophile IgM, IgA, and IgE antibodies in infectious mononucleosis. J Med Virol. 1989;28(1):38–41.
125. Bruu AL, Hjetland R, Holter E, Mortensen L, Natas O, Petterson W, et al. Evaluation of 12 commercial tests for detection of Epstein-Barr virus-specific and heterophile antibodies. Clin Diagn Lab Immunol. 2000;7(3):451–6.
126. Luzuriaga K, Sullivan JL. Infectious mononucleosis. N Engl J Med. 2010;362(21):1993–2000.
127. Horwitz CA, Henle W, Henle G, Penn G, Hoffman N, Ward PC. Persistent falsely positive rapid tests for infectious mononucleosis. Report of five cases with four--six-year follow-up data. Am J Clin Pathol. 1979;72(5):807–11.
128. Evans AS, Niederman JC, Cenabre LC, West B, Richards VA. A prospective evaluation of heterophile and Epstein-Barr virus-specific IgM antibody tests in clinical and subclinical infectious mononucleosis: Specificity and sensitivity of the tests and persistence of antibody. J Infect Dis. 1975;132(5):546–54.
129. Pitetti RD, Laus S, Wadowsky RM. Clinical evaluation of a quantitative real time polymerase chain reaction assay for diagnosis of primary Epstein-Barr virus infection in children. Pediatr Infect Dis J. 2003;22(8):736–9.
130. Sumaya CV, Ench Y. Epstein-Barr virus infectious mononucleosis in children. II. Heterophile antibody and viral-specific responses. Pediatrics. 1985;75(6):1011–9.
131. van Essen GG, Lieverse AG, Sprenger HG, Schirm J, Weits J. False-positive Paul-Bunnell test in HIV seroconversion. Lancet. 1988;2(8613):747–8.
132. Hendry BM, Longmore JM. Systemic lupus erythematosus presenting as infectious mononucleosis with a false positive monospot test. Lancet. 1982;1(8269):455.
133. Schumacher HR, Austin RM, Stass SA. False-positive serology in infectious mononucleosis. Lancet. 1979;1(8118):722.
134. Fisher BA, Bhalara S. False-positive result provided by rapid heterophile antibody test in a case of acute infection with hepatitis E virus. J Clin Microbiol. 2004;42(9):4411.
135. Tselis A, Merline JR, Storch GA. Epstein-Barr virus disease - serologic and virologic diagnosis. In: Tselis A, Jenson HB, editors. Epstein-Barr virus. New York: Taylor and Francis, LLC; 2006. p. 125–46.
136. Horwitz CA, Henle W, Henle G, Rudnick H, Latts E. Long-term serological follow-up of patients for Epstein-Barr virus after recovery from infectious mononucleosis. J Infect Dis. 1985;151(6):1150–3.
137. Bauer G. Simplicity through complexity: immunoblot with recombinant antigens as the new gold standard in Epstein-Barr virus serology. Clin Lab. 2001;47(5–6):223–30.
138. Robertson P, Beynon S, Whybin R, Brennan C, Vollmer-Conna U, Hickie I, et al. Measurement of EBV-IgG anti-VCA avidity aids the early and reliable diagnosis of primary EBV infection. J Med Virol. 2003;70(4):617–23.
139. Semenova T, Lupo J, Alain S, Perrin-Confort G, Grossi L, Dimier J, et al. Multicenter evaluation of whole-blood Epstein-Barr viral load standardization using the WHO International Standard. J Clin Microbiol. 2016;54(7):1746–50.
140. Fryer JF, Heath AB, Wilkinson DE, Minor PD, Collaborative Study G. A collaborative study to establish the 1st WHO International Standard for Epstein-Barr virus for nucleic acid amplification techniques. Biologicals. 2016;44(5):423–33.
141. Fafi-Kremer S, Brengel-Pesce K, Bargues G, Bourgeat MJ, Genoulaz O, Seigneurin JM, et al. Assessment of automated DNA extraction coupled with real-time PCR for measuring Epstein-Barr virus load in whole blood, peripheral mononuclear cells and plasma. J Clin Virol. 2004;30(2):157–64.
142. Tsai DE, Douglas L, Andreadis C, Vogl DT, Arnoldi S, Kotloff R, et al. EBV PCR in the diagnosis and monitoring of posttransplant lymphoproliferative disorder: results of a two-arm prospective trial. Am J Transplant. 2008;8(5):1016–24.
143. Stevens SJ, Pronk I, Middeldorp JM. Toward standardization of Epstein-Barr virus DNA load monitoring: unfractionated whole blood as preferred clinical specimen. J Clin Microbiol. 2001;39(4):1211–6.
144. Wagner HJ, Wessel M, Jabs W, Smets F, Fischer L, Offner G, et al. Patients at risk for development of posttransplant lymphoproliferative disorder: plasma versus peripheral blood mononuclear cells as material for quantification of Epstein-Barr viral load by using real-time quantitative polymerase chain reaction. Transplantation. 2001;72(6):1012–9.
145. Kanakry JA, Hegde AM, Durand CM, Massie AB, Greer AE, Ambinder RF, et al. The clinical significance of EBV DNA in the plasma and peripheral blood mononuclear cells of patients with or without EBV diseases. Blood. 2016;127(16):2007–17.

146. Gulley ML, Tang W. Using Epstein-Barr viral load assays to diagnose, monitor, and prevent posttransplant lymphoproliferative disorder. Clin Microbiol Rev. 2010;23(2):350–66.
147. Ruf S, Behnke-Hall K, Gruhn B, Bauer J, Horn M, Beck J, et al. Comparison of six different specimen types for Epstein-Barr viral load quantification in peripheral blood of pediatric patients after heart transplantation or after allogeneic hematopoietic stem cell transplantation. J Clin Virol. 2012;53(3):186–94.
148. Stevens SJ, Verschuuren EA, Pronk I, van Der Bij W, Harmsen MC, The TH, et al. Frequent monitoring of Epstein-Barr virus DNA load in unfractionated whole blood is essential for early detection of posttransplant lymphoproliferative disease in high-risk patients. Blood. 2001;97(5):1165–71.
149. Bakker NA, Verschuuren EA, Veeger NJ, van der Bij W, van Imhoff GW, Kallenberg CG, et al. Quantification of Epstein-Barr virus-DNA load in lung transplant recipients: a comparison of plasma versus whole blood. J Heart Lung Transplant. 2008;27(1):7–10.
150. Fellner MD, Durand KA, Solernou V, Bosaleh A, Balbarrey Z, Garcia de Davila MT, et al. Epstein-Barr virus load in transplant patients: Early detection of post-transplant lymphoproliferative disorders. Rev Argent Microbiol. 2016;48(2):110–8.
151. Shimizu H, Saitoh T, Koya H, Yuzuriha A, Hoshino T, Hatsumi N, et al. Discrepancy in EBV-DNA load between peripheral blood and cerebrospinal fluid in a patient with isolated CNS post-transplant lymphoproliferative disorder. Int J Hematol. 2011;94(5):495–8.
152. Boersma MN, van der Zanden A, Laverman GD, Sanders JS, de Vries PA. Epstein-Barr virus-positive post-transplant lymphoproliferative disorder of the central nervous system, after renal transplantation with a discrepancy in viral load between peripheral blood and cerebrospinal fluid. Transpl Int. 2012;25(11):e113–6.
153. Sampaio MS, Cho YW, Qazi Y, Bunnapradist S, Hutchinson IV, Shah T. Posttransplant malignancies in solid organ adult recipients: an analysis of the U.S. National Transplant Database. Transplantation. 2012;94(10):990–8.
154. Hocker B, Fickenscher H, Delecluse HJ, Bohm S, Kusters U, Schnitzler P, et al. Epidemiology and morbidity of Epstein-Barr virus infection in pediatric renal transplant recipients: a multicenter, prospective study. Clin Infect Dis. 2013;56(1):84–92.
155. Cleper R, Ben Shalom E, Landau D, Weissman I, Krause I, Konen O, et al. Post-transplantation lymphoproliferative disorder in pediatric kidney-transplant recipients - a national study. Pediatr Transplant. 2012;16(6):619–26.
156. Pinho-Apezzato ML, Tannuri U, Tannuri AC, Mello ES, Lima F, Gibelli NE, et al. Multiple clinical presentations of lymphoproliferative disorders in pediatric liver transplant recipients: a single-center experience. Transplant Proc. 2010;42(5):1763–8.
157. Wiederkehr JC, Coelho IM, Avilla SG, e Silva EM, Schuller S, Ouno DD, et al. Prevalence of posttransplantation lymphoproliferative disease in pediatric liver transplant recipients. Transplant Proc. 2010;42(2):521–2.
158. Uribe M, Hunter B, Alba A, Calabran L, Flores L, Soto P, et al. Posttransplant lymphoproliferative disorder in pediatric liver transplantation. Transplant Proc. 2009;41(6):2679–81.
159. Chinnock R, Webber SA, Dipchand AI, Brown RN, George JF. A 16-year multi-institutional study of the role of age and EBV status on PTLD incidence among pediatric heart transplant recipients. Am J Transplant. 2012;12(11):3061–8.
160. Wilde GE, Moore DJ, Bellah RD. Posttransplantation lymphoproliferative disorder in pediatric recipients of solid organ transplants: timing and location of disease. AJR Am J Roentgenol. 2005;185(5):1335–41.
161. Curtis RE, Travis LB, Rowlings PA, Socie G, Kingma DW, Banks PM, et al. Risk of lymphoproliferative disorders after bone marrow transplantation: a multi-institutional study. Blood. 1999;94(7):2208–16.
162. van Esser JW, van der Holt B, Meijer E, Niesters HG, Trenschel R, Thijsen SF, et al. Epstein-Barr virus (EBV) reactivation is a frequent event after allogeneic stem cell transplantation (SCT) and quantitatively predicts EBV-lymphoproliferative disease following T-cell--depleted SCT. Blood. 2001;98(4):972–8.
163. Cohen JM, Cooper N, Chakrabarti S, Thomson K, Samarasinghe S, Cubitt D, et al. EBV-related disease following haematopoietic stem cell transplantation with reduced intensity conditioning. Leuk Lymphoma. 2007;48(2):256–69.
164. Blaes AH, Cao Q, Wagner JE, Young JA, Weisdorf DJ, Brunstein CG. Monitoring and preemptive rituximab therapy for Epstein-Barr virus reactivation after antithymocyte globulin containing nonmyeloablative conditioning for umbilical cord blood transplantation. Biol Blood Marrow Transplant. 2010;16(2):287–91.
165. Brunstein CG, Weisdorf DJ, DeFor T, Barker JN, Tolar J, van Burik JA, et al. Marked increased risk of Epstein-Barr virus-related complications with the addition of antithymocyte globulin to a nonmyeloablative conditioning prior to unrelated umbilical cord blood transplantation. Blood. 2006;108(8):2874–80.
166. Peric Z, Cahu X, Chevallier P, Brissot E, Malard F, Guillaume T, et al. Features of EBV reactivation after reduced intensity conditioning unrelated umbilical cord blood transplantation. Bone Marrow Transplant. 2012;47(2):251–7.
167. Gandhi MK. Epstein-Barr virus-associated lymphomas. Expert Rev Anti-Infect Ther. 2006;4(1):77–89.
168. Quinlan SC, Pfeiffer RM, Morton LM, Engels EA. Risk factors for early-onset and late-onset post-transplant lymphoproliferative disorder in kidney recipients in the United States. Am J Hematol. 2011;86(2):206–9.
169. Hatton O, Martinez OM, Esquivel CO. Emerging therapeutic strategies for Epstein-Barr virus+ post-transplant lymphoproliferative disorder. Pediatr Transplant. 2012;16(3):220–9.
170. Dotti G, Fiocchi R, Motta T, Mammana C, Gotti E, Riva S, et al. Lymphomas occurring late after solid-organ transplantation: influence of treatment on the clinical outcome. Transplantation. 2002;74(8):1095–102.
171. Moss DJ, Rickinson AB, Pope JH. Long-term T-cell-mediated immunity to Epstein-Barr virus in man. III. Activation of cytotoxic T cells in virus-infected leukocyte cultures. Int J Cancer. 1979;23(5):618–25.
172. Moss DJ, Rickinson AB, Pope JH. Long-term T-cell-mediated immunity to Epstein-Barr virus in man. I. Complete regression of virus-induced transformation in cultures of seropositive donor leukocytes. Int J Cancer. 1978;22(6):662–8.
173. Rickinson AB, Moss DJ, Pope JH, Ahlberg N. Long-term T-cell-mediated immunity to Epstein-Barr virus in man. IV. Development of T-cell memory in convalescent infectious mononucleosis patients. Int J Cancer. 1980;25(1):59–65.
174. Kuzushima K, Hoshino Y, Fujii K, Yokoyama N, Fujita M, Kiyono T, et al. Rapid determination of Epstein-Barr virus-specific CD8(+) T-cell frequencies by flow cytometry. Blood. 1999;94(9):3094–100.
175. Haque T, Crawford DH. Role of donor versus recipient type Epstein-Barr virus in post-transplant lymphoproliferative disorders. Springer Semin Immunopathol. 1998;20(3–4):375–87.
176. Young L, Alfieri C, Hennessy K, Evans H, O'Hara C, Anderson KC, et al. Expression of Epstein-Barr virus transformation-associated genes in tissues of patients with EBV lymphoproliferative disease. N Engl J Med. 1989;321(16):1080–5.
177. Gratama JW, Zutter MM, Minarovits J, Oosterveer MA, Thomas ED, Klein G, et al. Expression of Epstein-Barr virus-encoded growth-transformation-associated proteins in lymphoproliferations of bone-marrow transplant recipients. Int J Cancer. 1991;47(2):188–92.

178. Oudejans JJ, Jiwa M, van den Brule AJ, Grasser FA, Horstman A, Vos W, et al. Detection of heterogeneous Epstein-Barr virus gene expression patterns within individual post-transplantation lymphoproliferative disorders. Am J Pathol. 1995;147(4):923–33.
179. Olagne J, Caillard S, Gaub MP, Chenard MP, Moulin B. Post-transplant lymphoproliferative disorders: determination of donor/recipient origin in a large cohort of kidney recipients. Am J Transplant. 2011;11(6):1260–9.
180. Dharnidharka VR, Lamb KE, Gregg JA, Meier-Kriesche HU. Associations between EBV serostatus and organ transplant type in PTLD risk: an analysis of the SRTR National Registry Data in the United States. Am J Transplant. 2012;12(4):976–83.
181. Sturm-O'Brien AK, Hicks MJ, Giannoni CM, Sulek M, Friedman EM. Tonsillectomy in post-transplant lymphoproliferative disease in children. Laryngoscope. 2010;120(3):608–11.
182. Jain A, Nalesnik M, Reyes J, Pokharna R, Mazariegos G, Green M, et al. Posttransplant lymphoproliferative disorders in liver transplantation: a 20-year experience. Ann Surg. 2002;236(4):429–36; discussion 36-7.
183. Gao SZ, Chaparro SV, Perlroth M, Montoya JG, Miller JL, DiMiceli S, et al. Post-transplantation lymphoproliferative disease in heart and heart-lung transplant recipients: 30-year experience at Stanford University. J Heart Lung Transplant. 2003;22(5):505–14.
184. Gottschalk S, Rooney CM, Heslop HE. Post-transplant lymphoproliferative disorders. Annu Rev Med. 2005;56:29–44.
185. Swinnen LJ, Costanzo-Nordin MR, Fisher SG, O'Sullivan EJ, Johnson MR, Heroux AL, et al. Increased incidence of lymphoproliferative disorder after immunosuppression with the monoclonal antibody OKT3 in cardiac-transplant recipients. N Engl J Med. 1990;323(25):1723–8.
186. McDonald RA, Smith JM, Ho M, Lindblad R, Ikle D, Grimm P, et al. Incidence of PTLD in pediatric renal transplant recipients receiving basiliximab, calcineurin inhibitor, sirolimus and steroids. Am J Transplant. 2008;8(5):984–9.
187. Bustami RT, Ojo AO, Wolfe RA, Merion RM, Bennett WM, McDiarmid SV, et al. Immunosuppression and the risk of post-transplant malignancy among cadaveric first kidney transplant recipients. Am J Transplant. 2004;4(1):87–93.
188. Opelz G, Dohler B. Lymphomas after solid organ transplantation: a collaborative transplant study report. Am J Transplant. 2004;4(2):222–30.
189. Opelz G, Naujokat C, Daniel V, Terness P, Dohler B. Disassociation between risk of graft loss and risk of non-Hodgkin lymphoma with induction agents in renal transplant recipients. Transplantation. 2006;81(9):1227–33.
190. Grinyo J, Charpentier B, Pestana JM, Vanrenterghem Y, Vincenti F, Reyes-Acevedo R, et al. An integrated safety profile analysis of belatacept in kidney transplant recipients. Transplantation. 2010;90(12):1521–7.
191. Pestana JO, Grinyo JM, Vanrenterghem Y, Becker T, Campistol JM, Florman S, et al. Three-year outcomes from BENEFIT-EXT: a phase III study of belatacept versus cyclosporine in recipients of extended criteria donor kidneys. Am J Transplant. 2012;12(3):630–9.
192. Wekerle T, Grinyo JM. Belatacept: from rational design to clinical application. Transpl Int. 2012;25(2):139–50.
193. Cohen J, Gandhi M, Naik P, Cubitt D, Rao K, Thaker U, et al. Increased incidence of EBV-related disease following paediatric stem cell transplantation with reduced-intensity conditioning. Br J Haematol. 2005;129(2):229–39.
194. Hale G, Waldmann H. Risks of developing Epstein-Barr virus-related lymphoproliferative disorders after T-cell-depleted marrow transplants. CAMPATH Users. Blood. 1998;91(8):3079–83.
195. Barker JN, Martin PL, Coad JE, DeFor T, Trigg ME, Kurtzberg J, et al. Low incidence of Epstein-Barr virus-associated posttransplantation lymphoproliferative disorders in 272 unrelated-donor umbilical cord blood transplant recipients. Biol Blood Marrow Transplant. 2001;7(7):395–9.
196. Izadi M, Taheri S. Allograft involvement by lymphoproliferative disorders after lung transplantation: report from the PTLD. Int survey. Prog Transplant. 2011;21(4):353–9.
197. Bakker NA, van Imhoff GW, Verschuuren EA, van Son WJ. Presentation and early detection of post-transplant lymphoproliferative disorder after solid organ transplantation. Transpl Int. 2007;20(3):207–18.
198. Penn I, Porat G. Central nervous system lymphomas in organ allograft recipients. Transplantation. 1995;59(2):240–4.
199. Dolcetti R. B lymphocytes and Epstein-Barr virus: the lesson of post-transplant lymphoproliferative disorders. Autoimmun Rev. 2007;7(2):96–101.
200. Styczynski J, Reusser P, Einsele H, de la Camara R, Cordonnier C, Ward KN, et al. Management of HSV, VZV and EBV infections in patients with hematological malignancies and after SCT: guidelines from the Second European Conference on Infections in Leukemia. Bone Marrow Transplant. 2009;43(10):757–70.
201. European best practice guidelines for renal transplantation. Section IV: Long-term management of the transplant recipient. IV.6.3. Cancer risk after renal transplantation. Solid organ cancers: prevention and treatment. Nephrol Dial Transplant. 2002;17 Suppl 4:32, 4–6.
202. Center. CCsHM. Evidence based clinical practice guideline for management of EBV-associated post-transplant lymphoproliferative disease (PTLD) in solid organ transplant. 2011.
203. Costanzo MR, Dipchand A, Starling R, Anderson A, Chan M, Desai S, et al. The International Society of Heart and Lung Transplantation Guidelines for the care of heart transplant recipients. J Heart Lung Transplant. 2010;29(8):914–56.
204. Parker A, Bowles K, Bradley JA, Emery V, Featherstone C, Gupte G, et al. Diagnosis of post-transplant lymphoproliferative disorder in solid organ transplant recipients - BCSH and BTS Guidelines. Br J Haematol. 2010;149(5):675–92.
205. Chadban SJ, Barraclough KA, Campbell SB, Clark CJ, Coates PT, Cohney SJ, et al. KHA-CARI guideline: KHA-CARI adaptation of the KDIGO Clinical Practice Guideline for the Care of Kidney Transplant Recipients. Nephrology (Carlton). 2012;17(3):204–14.
206. Allen UD, Preiksaitis JK, Practice ASTIDCo. Epstein-Barr virus and posttransplant lymphoproliferative disorder in solid organ transplantation. Am J Transplant. 2013;13(Suppl 4):107–20.
207. Network NCC. NCCN Clinical Practice Guidelines in Oncology: B-Cell Lymphomas, V 1.2017 [Available from: https://www.nccn.org/professionals/physician_gls/pdf/b-cell.pdf.
208. Oertel S, Trappe RU, Zeidler K, Babel N, Reinke P, Hummel M, et al. Epstein-Barr viral load in whole blood of adults with post-transplant lymphoproliferative disorder after solid organ transplantation does not correlate with clinical course. Ann Hematol. 2006;85(7):478–84.
209. Benden C, Aurora P, Burch M, Cubitt D, Lloyd C, Whitmore P, et al. Monitoring of Epstein-Barr viral load in pediatric heart and lung transplant recipients by real-time polymerase chain reaction. J Heart Lung Transplant. 2005;24(12):2103–8.
210. Gartner BC, Fischinger J, Schafer H, Einsele H, Roemer K, Muller-Lantzsch N. Epstein-Barr viral load as a tool to diagnose and monitor post-transplant lymphoproliferative disease. Recent Results Cancer Res. 2002;159:49–54.
211. Omar H, Hagglund H, Gustafsson-Jernberg A, LeBlanc K, Mattsson J, Remberger M, et al. Targeted monitoring of patients at high risk of post-transplant lymphoproliferative disease by quantitative Epstein-Barr virus polymerase chain reaction. Transpl Infect Dis. 2009;11(5):393–9.
212. Aalto SM, Juvonen E, Tarkkanen J, Volin L, Ruutu T, Mattila PS, et al. Lymphoproliferative disease after allogeneic stem cell trans-

plantation--pre-emptive diagnosis by quantification of Epstein-Barr virus DNA in serum. J Clin Virol. 2003;28(3):275–83.
213. Wheless SA, Gulley ML, Raab-Traub N, McNeillie P, Neuringer IP, Ford HJ, et al. Post-transplantation lymphoproliferative disease: Epstein-Barr virus DNA levels, HLA-A3, and survival. Am J Respir Crit Care Med. 2008;178(10):1060–5.
214. D'Antiga L, Del Rizzo M, Mengoli C, Cillo U, Guariso G, Zancan L. Sustained Epstein-Barr virus detection in paediatric liver transplantation. Insights into the occurrence of late PTLD. Liver Transpl. 2007;13(3):343–8.
215. Bingler MA, Feingold B, Miller SA, Quivers E, Michaels MG, Green M, et al. Chronic high Epstein-Barr viral load state and risk for late-onset posttransplant lymphoproliferative disease/lymphoma in children. Am J Transplant. 2008;8(2):442–5.
216. Green M, Soltys K, Rowe DT, Webber SA, Mazareigos G. Chronic high Epstein-Barr viral load carriage in pediatric liver transplant recipients. Pediatr Transplant. 2009;13(3):319–23.
217. Wagner HJ, Cheng YC, Huls MH, Gee AP, Kuehnle I, Krance RA, et al. Prompt versus preemptive intervention for EBV lymphoproliferative disease. Blood. 2004;103(10):3979–81.
218. Kidney Disease: Improving Global Outcomes (KDIGO) Transplant Work Group. KDIGO clinical practice guideline for the care of kidney transplant recipients. Am J Transplant. 2009;9(Suppl 3):S1–155.
219. Imadome K, Fukuda A, Kawano F, Imai Y, Ichikawa S, Mochizuki M, et al. Effective control of Epstein-Barr virus infection following pediatric liver transplantation by monitoring of viral DNA load and lymphocyte surface markers. Pediatr Transplant. 2012;16(7):748–57.
220. Gotoh K, Ito Y, Ohta R, Iwata S, Nishiyama Y, Nakamura T, et al. Immunologic and virologic analyses in pediatric liver transplant recipients with chronic high Epstein-Barr virus loads. J Infect Dis. 2010;202(3):461–9.
221. Zawilinska B, Kosinska A, Lenart M, Kopec J, Piatkowska-Jakubas B, Skotnicki A, et al. Detection of specific lytic and latent transcripts can help to predict the status of Epstein-Barr virus infection in transplant recipients with high virus load. Acta Biochim Pol. 2008;55(4):693–9.
222. Lee TC, Goss JA, Rooney CM, Heslop HE, Barshes NR, Caldwell YM, et al. Quantification of a low cellular immune response to aid in identification of pediatric liver transplant recipients at high-risk for EBV infection. Clin Transpl. 2006;20(6):689–94.
223. Lee TC, Savoldo B, Barshes NR, Rooney CM, Heslop HE, Gee AP, et al. Use of cytokine polymorphisms and Epstein-Barr virus viral load to predict development of post-transplant lymphoproliferative disorder in paediatric liver transplant recipients. Clin Transpl. 2006;20(3):389–93.
224. D'Aveni M, Aissi-Rothe L, Venard V, Salmon A, Falenga A, Decot V, et al. The clinical value of concomitant Epstein Barr virus (EBV)-DNA load and specific immune reconstitution monitoring after allogeneic hematopoietic stem cell transplantation. Transpl Immunol. 2011;24(4):224–32.
225. Bhaduri-McIntosh S, Rotenberg MJ, Gardner B, Robert M, Miller G. Repertoire and frequency of immune cells reactive to Epstein-Barr virus-derived autologous lymphoblastoid cell lines. Blood. 2008;111(3):1334–43.
226. Faraci M, Caviglia I, Morreale G, Lanino E, Cuzzubbo D, Giardino S, et al. Viral-load and B-lymphocyte monitoring of EBV reactivation after allogeneic hemopoietic SCT in children. Bone Marrow Transplant. 2010;45(6):1052–5.
227. Macedo C, Webber SA, Donnenberg AD, Popescu I, Hua Y, Green M, et al. EBV-specific CD8+ T cells from asymptomatic pediatric thoracic transplant patients carrying chronic high EBV loads display contrasting features: activated phenotype and exhausted function. J Immunol. 2011;186(10):5854–62.
228. Hinrichs C, Wendland S, Zimmermann H, Eurich D, Neuhaus R, Schlattmann P, et al. IL-6 and IL-10 in post-transplant lymphoproliferative disorders development and maintenance: a longitudinal study of cytokine plasma levels and T-cell subsets in 38 patients undergoing treatment. Transpl Int. 2011;24(9):892–903.
229. Baiocchi OC, Colleoni GW, Caballero OL, Vettore AL, Bulgarelli A, Dalbone MA, et al. Epstein-Barr viral load, interleukin-6 and interleukin-10 levels in post-transplant lymphoproliferative disease: a nested case-control study in a renal transplant cohort. Leuk Lymphoma. 2005;46(4):533–9.
230. Barton M, Wasfy S, Hebert D, Dipchand A, Fecteau A, Grant D, et al. Exploring beyond viral load testing for EBV lymphoproliferation: role of serum IL-6 and IgE assays as adjunctive tests. Pediatr Transplant. 2010;14(7):852–8.
231. Clave E, Agbalika F, Bajzik V, Peffault de Latour R, Trillard M, Rabian C, et al. Epstein-Barr virus (EBV) reactivation in allogeneic stem-cell transplantation: relationship between viral load, EBV-specific T-cell reconstitution and rituximab therapy. Transplantation. 2004;77(1):76–84.
232. Annels NE, Kalpoe JS, Bredius RG, Claas EC, Kroes AC, Hislop AD, et al. Management of Epstein-Barr virus (EBV) reactivation after allogeneic stem cell transplantation by simultaneous analysis of EBV DNA load and EBV-specific T cell reconstitution. Clin Infect Dis. 2006;42(12):1743–8.
233. Sebelin-Wulf K, Nguyen TD, Oertel S, Papp-Vary M, Trappe RU, Schulzki A, et al. Quantitative analysis of EBV-specific CD4/CD8 T cell numbers, absolute CD4/CD8 T cell numbers and EBV load in solid organ transplant recipients with PLTD. Transpl Immunol. 2007;17(3):203–10.
234. Smets F, Latinne D, Bazin H, Reding R, Otte JB, Buts JP, et al. Ratio between Epstein-Barr viral load and anti-Epstein-Barr virus specific T-cell response as a predictive marker of posttransplant lymphoproliferative disease. Transplantation. 2002;73(10):1603–10.
235. Meij P, van Esser JW, Niesters HG, van Baarle D, Miedema F, Blake N, et al. Impaired recovery of Epstein-Barr virus (EBV)--specific CD8+ T lymphocytes after partially T-depleted allogeneic stem cell transplantation may identify patients at very high risk for progressive EBV reactivation and lymphoproliferative disease. Blood. 2003;101(11):4290–7.
236. Meng Q, Hagemeier SR, Fingeroth JD, Gershburg E, Pagano JS, Kenney SC. The Epstein-Barr virus (EBV)-encoded protein kinase, EBV-PK, but not the thymidine kinase (EBV-TK), is required for ganciclovir and acyclovir inhibition of lytic viral production. J Virol. 2010;84(9):4534–42.
237. Kuo PC, Dafoe DC, Alfrey EJ, Sibley RK, Scandling JD. Posttransplant lymphoproliferative disorders and Epstein-Barr virus prophylaxis. Transplantation. 1995;59(1):135–8.
238. Davis CL, Harrison KL, McVicar JP, Forg PJ, Bronner MP, Marsh CL. Antiviral prophylaxis and the Epstein Barr virus-related post-transplant lymphoproliferative disorder. Clin Transpl. 1995;9(1):53–9.
239. Darenkov IA, Marcarelli MA, Basadonna GP, Friedman AL, Lorber KM, Howe JG, et al. Reduced incidence of Epstein-Barr virus-associated posttransplant lymphoproliferative disorder using preemptive antiviral therapy. Transplantation. 1997;64(6):848–52.
240. McDiarmid SV, Jordan S, Kim GS, Toyoda M, Goss JA, Vargas JH, et al. Prevention and preemptive therapy of posttransplant lymphoproliferative disease in pediatric liver recipients. Transplantation. 1998;66(12):1604–11.
241. Birkeland SA, Andersen HK, Hamilton-Dutoit SJ. Preventing acute rejection, Epstein-Barr virus infection, and posttransplant lymphoproliferative disorders after kidney transplantation: use of aciclovir and mycophenolate mofetil in a steroid-free immunosuppressive protocol. Transplantation. 1999;67(9):1209–14.
242. Green M, Kaufmann M, Wilson J, Reyes J. Comparison of intravenous ganciclovir followed by oral acyclovir with

intravenous ganciclovir alone for prevention of cytomegalovirus and Epstein-Barr virus disease after liver transplantation in children. Clin Infect Dis. 1997;25(6):1344–9.
243. Funch DP, Walker AM, Schneider G, Ziyadeh NJ, Pescovitz MD. Ganciclovir and acyclovir reduce the risk of post-transplant lymphoproliferative disorder in renal transplant recipients. Am J Transplant. 2005;5(12):2894–900.
244. Schnute ME, Anderson DJ, Brideau RJ, Ciske FL, Collier SA, Cudahy MM, et al. 2-Aryl-2-hydroxyethylamine substituted 4-oxo-4,7-dihydrothieno[2,3-b]pyridines as broad-spectrum inhibitors of human herpesvirus polymerases. Bioorg Med Chem Lett. 2007;17(12):3349–53.
245. Matthews T, Boehme R. Antiviral activity and mechanism of action of ganciclovir. Rev Infect Dis. 1988;10(Suppl 3):S490–4.
246. Hocker B, Bohm S, Fickenscher H, Kusters U, Schnitzler P, Pohl M, et al. (Val-)Ganciclovir prophylaxis reduces Epstein-Barr virus primary infection in pediatric renal transplantation. Transpl Int. 2012;25(7):723–31.
247. AlDabbagh MA, Gitman MR, Kumar D, Humar A, Rotstein C, Husain S. The role of antiviral prophylaxis for the prevention of Epstein-Barr virus-associated posttransplant lymphoproliferative disease in solid organ transplant recipients: a systematic review. Am J Transplant. 2017;17(3):770–81.
248. van Esser JW, Niesters HG, van der Holt B, Meijer E, Osterhaus AD, Gratama JW, et al. Prevention of Epstein-Barr virus-lymphoproliferative disease by molecular monitoring and preemptive rituximab in high-risk patients after allogeneic stem cell transplantation. Blood. 2002;99(12):4364–9.
249. Worth A, Conyers R, Cohen J, Jagani M, Chiesa R, Rao K, et al. Pre-emptive rituximab based on viraemia and T cell reconstitution: a highly effective strategy for the prevention of Epstein-Barr virus-associated lymphoproliferative disease following stem cell transplantation. Br J Haematol. 2011;155(3):377–85.
250. Heslop HE, Slobod KS, Pule MA, Hale GA, Rousseau A, Smith CA, et al. Long-term outcome of EBV-specific T-cell infusions to prevent or treat EBV-related lymphoproliferative disease in transplant recipients. Blood. 2010;115(5):925–35.
251. Rooney CM, Smith CA, Ng CY, Loftin SK, Sixbey JW, Gan Y, et al. Infusion of cytotoxic T cells for the prevention and treatment of Epstein-Barr virus-induced lymphoma in allogeneic transplant recipients. Blood. 1998;92(5):1549–55.
252. Gustafsson A, Levitsky V, Zou JZ, Frisan T, Dalianis T, Ljungman P, et al. Epstein-Barr virus (EBV) load in bone marrow transplant recipients at risk to develop posttransplant lymphoproliferative disease: prophylactic infusion of EBV-specific cytotoxic T cells. Blood. 2000;95(3):807–14.
253. Comoli P, Basso S, Zecca M, Pagliara D, Baldanti F, Bernardo ME, et al. Preemptive therapy of EBV-related lymphoproliferative disease after pediatric haploidentical stem cell transplantation. Am J Transplant. 2007;7(6):1648–55.
254. Gulley ML, Tang W. Laboratory assays for Epstein-Barr virus-related disease. J Mol Diagn. 2008;10(4):279–92.
255. Swerdlow SH, Campo E, Harris NL, et al. World Health Organization classification of tumours of haematopoietic and lymphoid tissues. 4th ed. Lyon: IARC Press; 2008.
256. Dockrell DH, Strickler JG, Paya CV. Epstein-Barr virus-induced T cell lymphoma in solid organ transplant recipients. Clin Infect Dis. 1998;26(1):180–2.
257. Hoshida Y, Li T, Dong Z, Tomita Y, Yamauchi A, Hanai J, et al. Lymphoproliferative disorders in renal transplant patients in Japan. Int J Cancer. 2001;91(6):869–75.
258. Pitman SD, Huang Q, Zuppan CW, Rowsell EH, Cao JD, Berdeja JG, et al. Hodgkin lymphoma-like posttransplant lymphoproliferative disorder (HL-like PTLD) simulates monomorphic B-cell PTLD both clinically and pathologically. Am J Surg Pathol. 2006;30(4):470–6.
259. Vakiani E, Basso K, Klein U, Mansukhani MM, Narayan G, Smith PM, et al. Genetic and phenotypic analysis of B-cell post-transplant lymphoproliferative disorders provides insights into disease biology. Hematol Oncol. 2008;26(4):199–211.
260. Tsai DE, Hardy CL, Tomaszewski JE, Kotloff RM, Oltoff KM, Somer BG, et al. Reduction in immunosuppression as initial therapy for posttransplant lymphoproliferative disorder: analysis of prognostic variables and long-term follow-up of 42 adult patients. Transplantation. 2001;71(8):1076–88.
261. Paya CV, Fung JJ, Nalesnik MA, Kieff E, Green M, Gores G, et al. Epstein-Barr virus-induced posttransplant lymphoproliferative disorders. ASTS/ASTP EBV-PTLD Task Force and The Mayo Clinic Organized International Consensus Development Meeting. Transplantation. 1999;68(10):1517–25.
262. Reshef R, Vardhanabhuti S, Luskin MR, Heitjan DF, Hadjiliadis D, Goral S, et al. Reduction of immunosuppression as initial therapy for posttransplantation lymphoproliferative disorder(bigstar). Am J Transplant. 2011;11(2):336–47.
263. Swinnen LJ, LeBlanc M, Grogan TM, Gordon LI, Stiff PJ, Miller AM, et al. Prospective study of sequential reduction in immunosuppression, interferon alpha-2B, and chemotherapy for posttransplantation lymphoproliferative disorder. Transplantation. 2008;86(2):215–22.
264. Lin JC, Smith MC, Pagano JS. Activation of latent Epstein-Barr virus genomes: selective stimulation of synthesis of chromosomal proteins by a tumor promoter. J Virol. 1983;45(3):985–91.
265. Feng WH, Hong G, Delecluse HJ, Kenney SC. Lytic induction therapy for Epstein-Barr virus-positive B-cell lymphomas. J Virol. 2004;78(4):1893–902.
266. Perrine SP, Hermine O, Small T, Suarez F, O'Reilly R, Boulad F, et al. A phase 1/2 trial of arginine butyrate and ganciclovir in patients with Epstein-Barr virus-associated lymphoid malignancies. Blood. 2007;109(6):2571–8.
267. Oertel SH, Verschuuren E, Reinke P, Zeidler K, Papp-Vary M, Babel N, et al. Effect of anti-CD 20 antibody rituximab in patients with post-transplant lymphoproliferative disorder (PTLD). Am J Transplant. 2005;5(12):2901–6.
268. Jain AB, Marcos A, Pokharna R, Shapiro R, Fontes PA, Marsh W, et al. Rituximab (chimeric anti-CD20 antibody) for posttransplant lymphoproliferative disorder after solid organ transplantation in adults: long-term experience from a single center. Transplantation. 2005;80(12):1692–8.
269. Milpied N, Vasseur B, Parquet N, Garnier JL, Antoine C, Quartier P, et al. Humanized anti-CD20 monoclonal antibody (Rituximab) in post transplant B-lymphoproliferative disorder: a retrospective analysis on 32 patients. Ann Oncol. 2000;11(Suppl 1):113–6.
270. Blaes AH, Peterson BA, Bartlett N, Dunn DL, Morrison VA. Rituximab therapy is effective for posttransplant lymphoproliferative disorders after solid organ transplantation: results of a phase II trial. Cancer. 2005;104(8):1661–7.
271. Choquet S, Leblond V, Herbrecht R, Socie G, Stoppa AM, Vandenberghe P, et al. Efficacy and safety of rituximab in B-cell post-transplantation lymphoproliferative disorders: results of a prospective multicenter phase 2 study. Blood. 2006;107(8): 3053–7.
272. Trappe R, Oertel S, Leblond V, Mollee P, Sender M, Reinke P, et al. Sequential treatment with rituximab followed by CHOP chemotherapy in adult B-cell post-transplant lymphoproliferative disorder (PTLD): the prospective international multicentre phase 2 PTLD-1 trial. Lancet Oncol. 2012;13(2):196–206.
273. Trappe R, Riess H, Babel N, Hummel M, Lehmkuhl H, Jonas S, et al. Salvage chemotherapy for refractory and relapsed posttransplant lymphoproliferative disorders (PTLD) after treatment with single-agent rituximab. Transplantation. 2007;83(7):912–8.
274. Choquet S, Trappe R, Leblond V, Jager U, Davi F, Oertel S. CHOP-21 for the treatment of post-transplant lymphoprolif-

erative disorders (PTLD) following solid organ transplantation. Haematologica. 2007;92(2):273–4.
275. Zimmermann H, Reinke P, Neuhaus R, Lehmkuhl H, Oertel S, Atta J, et al. Burkitt post-transplantation lymphoma in adult solid organ transplant recipients: Sequential immunochemotherapy with rituximab (R) followed by cyclophosphamide, doxorubicin, vincristine, and prednisone (CHOP) or R-CHOP is safe and effective in an analysis of 8 patients. Cancer. 2012;118(19):4715–24.
276. Heslop HE, Brenner MK, Rooney CM. Donor T cells to treat EBV-associated lymphoma. N Engl J Med. 1994;331(10):679–80.
277. O'Reilly RJ, Small TN, Papadopoulos E, Lucas K, Lacerda J, Koulova L. Biology and adoptive cell therapy of Epstein-Barr virus-associated lymphoproliferative disorders in recipients of marrow allografts. Immunol Rev. 1997;157:195–216.
278. Heslop HE. How I treat EBV lymphoproliferation. Blood. 2009;114(19):4002–8.
279. Haque T, Wilkie GM, Jones MM, Higgins CD, Urquhart G, Wingate P, et al. Allogeneic cytotoxic T-cell therapy for EBV-positive posttransplantation lymphoproliferative disease: results of a phase 2 multicenter clinical trial. Blood. 2007;110(4):1123–31.
280. Haque T, McAulay KA, Kelly D, Crawford DH. Allogeneic T-cell therapy for Epstein-Barr virus-positive posttransplant lymphoproliferative disease: long-term follow-up. Transplantation. 2010;90(1):93–4.
281. Doubrovina E, Oflaz-Sozmen B, Prockop SE, Kernan NA, Abramson S, Teruya-Feldstein J, et al. Adoptive immunotherapy with unselected or EBV-specific T cells for biopsy-proven EBV+ lymphomas after allogeneic hematopoietic cell transplantation. Blood. 2012;119(11):2644–56.
282. Epstein MA, Achong BG. The EB virus. Annu Rev Microbiol. 1973;27:413–36.
283. Cohen JI, Fauci AS, Varmus H, Nabel GJ. Epstein-Barr virus: an important vaccine target for cancer prevention. Sci Transl Med. 2011;3(107):107fs7.
284. Tibbetts SA, Loh J, Van Berkel V, McClellan JS, Jacoby MA, Kapadia SB, et al. Establishment and maintenance of gammaherpesvirus latency are independent of infective dose and route of infection. J Virol. 2003;77(13):7696–701.
285. Hjalgrim H, Rostgaard K, Johnson PC, Lake A, Shield L, Little AM, et al. HLA-A alleles and infectious mononucleosis suggest a critical role for cytotoxic T-cell response in EBV-related Hodgkin lymphoma. Proc Natl Acad Sci U S A. 2010;107(14):6400–5.
286. Nemerow GR, Mold C, Schwend VK, Tollefson V, Cooper NR. Identification of gp350 as the viral glycoprotein mediating attachment of Epstein-Barr virus (EBV) to the EBV/C3d receptor of B cells: sequence homology of gp350 and C3 complement fragment C3d. J Virol. 1987;61(5):1416–20.
287. Tanner J, Weis J, Fearon D, Whang Y, Kieff E. Epstein-Barr virus gp350/220 binding to the B lymphocyte C3d receptor mediates adsorption, capping, and endocytosis. Cell. 1987;50(2):203–13.
288. Borza CM, Hutt-Fletcher LM. Alternate replication in B cells and epithelial cells switches tropism of Epstein-Barr virus. Nat Med. 2002;8(6):594–9.
289. Hoffman GJ, Lazarowitz SG, Hayward SD. Monoclonal antibody against a 250,000-dalton glycoprotein of Epstein-Barr virus identifies a membrane antigen and a neutralizing antigen. Proc Natl Acad Sci U S A. 1980;77(5):2979–83.
290. Lowe RS, Keller PM, Keech BJ, Davison AJ, Whang Y, Morgan AJ, et al. Varicella-zoster virus as a live vector for the expression of foreign genes. Proc Natl Acad Sci U S A. 1987;84(11): 3896–900.
291. Sokal EM, Hoppenbrouwers K, Vandermeulen C, Moutschen M, Leonard P, Moreels A, et al. Recombinant gp350 vaccine for infectious mononucleosis: a phase 2, randomized, double-blind, placebo-controlled trial to evaluate the safety, immunogenicity, and efficacy of an Epstein-Barr virus vaccine in healthy young adults. J Infect Dis. 2007;196(12):1749–53.
292. Rees L, Tizard EJ, Morgan AJ, Cubitt WD, Finerty S, Oyewole-Eletu TA, et al. A phase I trial of epstein-barr virus gp350 vaccine for children with chronic kidney disease awaiting transplantation. Transplantation. 2009;88(8):1025–9.
293. Kanekiyo M, Bu W, Joyce MG, Meng G, Whittle JR, Baxa U, et al. Rational design of an Epstein-Barr virus vaccine targeting the receptor-binding site. Cell. 2015;162(5):1090–100.
294. Wilson AD, Lovgren-Bengtsson K, Villacres-Ericsson M, Morein B, Morgan AJ. The major Epstein-Barr virus (EBV) envelope glycoprotein gp340 when incorporated into Iscoms primes cytotoxic T-cell responses directed against EBV lymphoblastoid cell lines. Vaccine. 1999;17(9–10):1282–90.
295. Elliott SL, Suhrbier A, Miles JJ, Lawrence G, Pye SJ, Le TT, et al. Phase I trial of a CD8+ T-cell peptide epitope-based vaccine for infectious mononucleosis. J Virol. 2008;82(3):1448–57.
296. Smith C, Cooper L, Burgess M, Rist M, Webb N, Lambley E, et al. Functional reversion of antigen-specific CD8+ T cells from patients with Hodgkin lymphoma following in vitro stimulation with recombinant polyepitope. J Immunol. 2006;177(7):4897–906.
297. Smith C, Tsang J, Beagley L, Chua D, Lee V, Li V, et al. Effective treatment of metastatic forms of Epstein-Barr virus-associated nasopharyngeal carcinoma with a novel adenovirus-based adoptive immunotherapy. Cancer Res. 2012;72(5):1116–25.

Herpes Simplex Viruses 1 and 2, Varicella Zoster Virus, and Human Herpes Viruses 6, 7, and 8 in Transplant Recipients

39

Raymund R. Razonable

Introduction

Human herpes viruses are a family of eight large double-stranded DNA viruses. They are subdivided into α-herpesviruses, herpes simplex viruses 1 and 2 (HSV-1 & HSV-2) and varicella zoster virus (VZV); β-herpes viruses include cytomegalovirus (CMV), human herpesviruses 6 and 7 (HHV-6 & HHV-7), and γ-herpes viruses are Epstein-Barr virus (EBV) and human herpesvirus 8 (HHV-8). All eight members share the characteristic property of establishing lifelong latency in the host. Latent herpes viruses may reactivate causing opportunistic diseases in individuals with compromised immunity such as transplant recipients. Control of herpes virus infection and its reactivation is a function of cell-mediated immunity. Hence, factors that impair cell-mediated immune responses predispose to a potentially severe illness caused by these herpes viruses.

All human herpesviruses have been implicated in various clinical diseases in solid organ transplant (SOT) and hematopoietic stem cell transplant (HSCT) recipients. This chapter will review the epidemiology, clinical diseases, diagnosis, prevention, and treatment of six of the eight members of the human herpesvirus family, including HSV-1, HSV-2, VZV, HHV-6A and HHV-6B, HHV-7, and HHV-8 (Table 39.1).

Herpes Simplex Viruses 1 and 2

Epidemiology

HSV-1 and HSV-2 are α-herpesviruses that most commonly cause mucocutaneous ulcers. HSV-1 infection, which manifests clinically as orolabial herpes, is usually acquired during early childhood through adulthood. HSV-1 seroprevalence rates in the United States range from 44% in 12–19-year-old individuals up to 80% among individuals older than 60 years [1]. Seroprevalence rates of HSV-2 infection, which manifests as genital ulcers, increase at the onset of sexual activity, from 1.6% among 14–19-year-old individuals to 26.3% among 40–49-year-old individuals in the United States [2]. After primary infection, HSV-1 and HSV-2 establish latency in nerve root ganglia. Periodic HSV reactivations occur throughout life, and this could be in the form of subclinical shedding or manifested as oral or genital ulcers [3, 4].

Seroprevalence rates of HSV-1 and HSV-2 in transplant recipients mirror that of the general population. Up to 80% of adult HSCT patients are HSV-seropositive [5]. Because most transplant recipients are HSV-seropositive, the majority of symptomatic HSV disease and asymptomatic HSV shedding after SOT and HSCT results from reactivation of latent virus. Compared with immunocompetent persons, transplant recipients shed HSV-1 and HSV-2 more frequently and they may have more severe clinical manifestations [6, 7]. The onset of HSV disease occurs during the first 4 weeks after SOT and HSCT [5, 8–12]. Without antiviral prophylaxis, the rate of HSV reactivation among HSV-seropositive HSCT recipients reaches up to 80% [13]. The risk of HSV disease increases during periods associated with intense immunosuppression, such as with the use of muromonab-CD3 and mycophenolate mofetil [14, 15]. Primary HSV-1 and HSV-2 infections may occur less commonly, when HSV-seronegative transplant recipients are exposed to virus shed in bodily secretions of HSV-seropositive individuals. Donor-derived HSV infection, transmitted through the allograft, has been reported rarely after kidney and liver transplantation [10, 16–18].

Clinical Disease

The most common clinical manifestation of HSV-1 and HSV-2 disease after transplantation, whether this is primary or reactivation infection, is orolabial, genital, or perianal

R. R. Razonable (✉)
Division of Infectious Diseases, Department of Medicine, and the William J. von Liebig Center for Transplantation and Clinical Regeneration, College of Medicine, Mayo Clinic, Rochester, MN, USA
e-mail: razonable.raymund@mayo.edu

A. Safdar (ed.), *Principles and Practice of Transplant Infectious Diseases*, https://doi.org/10.1007/978-1-4939-9034-4_39

Table 39.1 Human herpesvirus infections in transplant recipients

Virus	Clinical disease	Diagnosis	Prevention	Treatment
HSV-1 and HSV-2	Oral and genital herpes Visceral disease (hepatitis) Disseminated disease Encephalitis and meningitis Keratitis	Clinical diagnosis HSV NAT Tzanck smear Histopathology Viral culture	Acyclovir prophylaxis Alternatives: Valacyclovir Famciclovir Ganciclovir Valganciclovir	Acyclovir (IV or oral) Valacyclovir Famciclovir Foscarnet (resistant cases) Cidofovir (resistant cases)
VZV	Varicella Zoster (localized or disseminated)	Clinical diagnosis VZV NAT Viral culture	Avoid exposure Vaccination Postexposure prophylaxis Acyclovir prophylaxis	IV acyclovir Valacyclovir Famciclovir
HHV-6	Fever Rash Encephalitis Hepatitis Pneumonitis	HHV-6 NAT Histopathology	None	IV ganciclovir Valganciclovir Foscarnet Cidofovir
HHV-7	Not well defined Fever	HHV-7 NAT	None	Foscarnet Cidofovir
HHV-8	Kaposi's sarcoma Castleman's disease Primary effusion lymphoma Bone marrow failure	HHV-8 NAT Histopathology	None Role of valganciclovir is debated	Reduction in immunosuppression Role of antivirals debated Chemotherapy Surgical debulking Sirolimus

Notes: *HSV* herpes simplex virus, *VZV* varicella zoster virus, *HHV* human herpesvirus, *NAT* nucleic acid testing, *IV* intravenous

disease [4, 12]. In the HSCT population, HSV mucocutaneous disease occurs in the orofacial region in 85–90% of cases, while only 10–15% occurs in the anogenital region [13, 19]. Up to 10% of HSCT recipients with orolabial HSV disease may have esophageal involvement [20]. While orolabial disease is classically due to HSV-1 and anogenital disease is due to HSV-2, there may be an overlap since some cases of orolabial disease have been caused by HSV-2, while HSV-1 may also be associated with anogenital disease.

Mucocutaneous herpes infections are typically vesicular and/or ulcerative and are often localized. In severe cases, particularly among highly immunocompromised transplant patients, HSV infection may disseminate to visceral organs and cause hepatitis, encephalitis, and pneumonitis [12]. Fever, leukopenia, and hepatitis are the most common signs and symptoms of disseminated HSV disease [12]. Central nervous system (CNS) involvement may occur in the form of encephalitis and viral meningitis [21]. Ocular involvement may occur in the form of keratitis. Bone marrow suppression and damage to the transplanted stem cell graft have also been reported in association with HSV disease following HSCT.

Diagnosis

The diagnosis of mucocutaneous HSV disease in transplant recipients may be made on clinical grounds alone since the symptoms are often typical, with vesicles and ulcers. Occasionally, the clinical manifestations may be atypical, and other pathogens may be suspected. In HSCT recipient, severe mucositis may be due to a number of causes and often multifactorial in nature; this further complicates the diagnosis of HSV infection based only on clinical presentation. In such cases, laboratory confirmation of HSV infection is needed. Laboratory tests are also useful in the diagnosis of extra-mucocutaneous HSV disease such as CNS disease, fulminant hepatitis, and disseminated disease.

The laboratory methods available for the diagnosis of HSV infection are (1) direct fluorescent antibody (DFA) testing of mucocutaneous lesions, bronchoalveolar lavage, and other clinical samples, (2) histopathology of biopsy specimens, (3) viral culture, and (4) nucleic acid testing (NAT) by PCR. Serology is rarely useful for diagnosing HSV infections after transplantation since HSV seropositivity is common, and generation of HSV antibodies may be delayed due to underlying immunosuppression.

Detection of HSV antigens on scrapings of ulcerative lesions by immunofluorescence assay (IFA) is a useful test for diagnosis of HSV disease. Tzanck smear, which demonstrates viral cytopathic effects, can be performed on scraping obtained from herpetic ulcers, although this is not very specific for HSV. Histopathology with immunocytochemistry for HSV may be used to document tissue-invasive disease such as fulminant hepatitis [22]. Culture of the vesicular fluid is very specific for diagnosis of HSV disease, although this is now replaced by molecular HSV NAT by PCR assay as the diagnostic test of choice, especially for cerebrospinal fluid (CSF) [23].

HSV NAT provides high sensitivity, high specificity, and rapid turn-around time compared to culture and other diagnostic modalities [23]. The molecular assay can be optimized to distinguish HSV-1 from HSV-2 [24]. NAT is especially useful for identifying HSV in blood or other sterile fluids, as viral cultures have poor sensitivity in detecting HSV in these samples. If disseminated disease is suspected in transplant patients, detection of HSV NAT in the blood confirms the clinical suspicion [25]. Quantification of HSV viral load in a clinical sample such as CSF or blood may be used to assess infection severity and guide efficacy of antiviral therapies.

Prevention

HSV reactivation occurs most commonly during the first month after transplantation. Routine surveillance using viral culture or NAT to detect HSV is not recommended. Instead, it is standard clinical practice for transplant recipients to receive antiviral prophylaxis such as acyclovir during the first 4–6 weeks after undergoing SOT [5, 12]. The duration may be prolonged in certain situations such as HSCT, especially if being treated for GVHD, treatment of acute rejection, or recurrent infections [5]. In a placebo-controlled study in HSV-seropositive HSCT recipients, acyclovir abrogated HSV reactivation, while culture-proven HSV lesions were observed in seven of ten placebo-treated patients [26]. Oral acyclovir is preferred, but the intravenous formulation may be needed in HSCT patients with severe mucositis. Valacyclovir, famciclovir, ganciclovir, and valganciclovir are alternative agents. Many SOT recipients receive valganciclovir prophylaxis for CMV prevention after transplantation. Since valganciclovir (or ganciclovir) is also effective against HSV, no additional HSV prevention (such as acyclovir) is necessary in these patients.

Treatment

Antiviral therapy shortens the duration of HSV shedding and disease, facilitates healing, and prevents HSV dissemination to visceral sites. In addition to antiviral therapy, cautious reduction in immunosuppression should be considered, especially those with severe and life-threatening HSV diseases [12].

Limited or mild mucocutaneous HSV disease can be treated with oral acyclovir, valacyclovir, or famciclovir for a minimum of 5–7 days and until complete healing of the lesions. Mucocutaneous HSV disease can also be treated with intravenous acyclovir, especially in HSCT patients with severe mucositis. Intravenous acyclovir at a higher dose (5–10 mg/kg every 8 h) should be considered for disseminated, cerebral, visceral, or extensive mucocutaneous HSV disease. A minimum of 14 days of treatment is recommended for severe disease, and others have extended the duration to as long as 21 days in cases of pneumonia and encephalitis. Some have used HSV NAT to guide the duration of treatment of HSV meningoencephalitis [27].

Acyclovir-resistant HSV may occur in less than 5% of immunocompromised patients. The most common mechanism of resistance is a genetic mutation that results in diminished or absent activity thymidine kinase, an enzyme that is essential for the activation of acyclovir, valacyclovir, and famciclovir. The drug of choice for treatment of acyclovir-resistant HSV is foscarnet and cidofovir as the alternative agent. There is significant toxicity associated with the use of these drugs, most commonly nephrotoxicity. Topical formulations of cidofovir and imiquimod may be used for localized mucocutaneous disease [12].

Varicella Zoster Virus

Epidemiology and Clinical Disease

VZV is a highly infectious α-herpesvirus that causes varicella commonly known as chickenpox. Infection is acquired through direct contact with a skin lesion or airborne spread from respiratory droplets. Varicella is manifested by fever, constitutional symptoms, and vesicular, pruritic, widely disseminated rash. The distinctive feature of varicella is the concurrent appearance of papules, vesicles, and crusted lesions that typically spares the palms and soles. Varicella is generally a self-limited illness lasting 7–10 days in the immunocompetent patients, although it may infrequently lead to viral hepatitis, pneumonitis, encephalitis; retinal necrosis, and purpura fulminans are uncommon albeit, serious complication often noted in severely immunosuppressed individuals [28].

After primary infection, VZV establishes latency in cranial nerve and dorsal root ganglia. Reactivation of VZV later in life is manifested as zoster (shingles), which is characterized by grouped vesicular exanthem in 1–3 dermatomal distribution [29]. Some patients, especially those who are immunocompromised such as transplant patients, may develop disseminated zoster that mimics primary varicella infection. Others may have visceral involvement [29], with fulminant hepatitis as one of the severe forms of visceral zoster [30]. Zoster lesions may be secondarily infected with bacteria and, in the long term, may be associated with debilitating postherpetic neuralgia [29].

Since over 90% of adult transplant recipients are VZV-seropositive from prior primary varicella infection, the vast majority of VZV infection after transplantation presents as zoster. Reactivation VZV, which is manifested most commonly as single or multiple dermatomal zoster, occurs in approximately 8–11% of SOT recipients [29] and 10–68%

among patients undergoing HSCT [5]. The peak incidence of herpes zoster occurs during the first 12–14 months after SOT [29] or 3–12 months after HSCT with a median of 5 months after transplantation [5]. Risk factors after SOT are older age, use of mycophenolate mofetil, and recipients of heart and lung transplants [31–33]. Older age, severe immunosuppression, a myeloablative regimen, severe lymphopenia, receipt of cord blood transplant, and chronic GVHD are associated with increased risk of VZV after HSCT [5]. While the majority of herpes zoster remains localized to one or few adjacent dermatomes, severely immunocompromised transplant patients may have poly-dermatomal distribution or may have disseminated disease with visceral involvement [29], including fulminant VZV hepatitis [34]. Some cases of VZV disease may manifest without the classic herpes skin lesions and present only with severe pain such as abdominal pain in patients with VZV gastritis and hepatitis.

Since the majority of patients are VZV-immune prior to transplantation due to prior infection or immunization, primary varicella is rarely seen after transplantation. Chickenpox may still occur in non-vaccinated VZV-seronegative transplant recipients. The clinical manifestation of varicella in these patients is typical, with fever and a generalized pruritic vesicular rash. The illness may be very severe and devastating, sometimes with encephalitis, hepatitis, pneumonia, and other visceral involvement [29]. VZV-seronegative transplant candidates should therefore be vaccinated prior to transplantation.

Diagnosis

The diagnosis of varicella and zoster is made based on clinical grounds due to their classic presentations. However, transplant patients may present atypically (such as disseminated disease without skin rash) or may have disseminated herpes that can mimic other disease states. In these cases, laboratory testing for VZV is essential to establish the diagnosis.

Rapid diagnostic assays for VZV diagnosis are NAT by PCR and direct fluorescent assay (DFA) [5, 35]. DFA is performed on scraping taken from the base of the skin lesion. A PCR test to detect and amplify VZV DNA is currently the most sensitive test, and this may be used to detect VZV in the vesicle fluid, peripheral blood, CSF, and tissues [36]. VZV NAT in the blood is used to diagnose visceral zoster in the absence of skin manifestations. Most VZV NAT assays are qualitative, although many offer quantification [35, 36]. Quantitative VZV NAT may be used to assess the severity of disease such as higher viral load, which often reflects more severe disease, and to guide management strategies, for example, a persistently high viral load may require longer duration of treatment and a concern for drug-resistant viral strain.

Viral culture is a less sensitive assay with slower turnaround time [29]. Serologic testing is rarely helpful in the diagnosis of varicella and zoster due to high rates of seropositivity, and transplant patients have delayed ability to mount antibody response [29].

Prevention

Vaccination is the most effective method for the prevention of varicella in transplant recipients, but it should be given prior to transplantation. Since the varicella vaccine contains a live-attenuated virus, it is contraindicated after transplantation. Varicella vaccine should be given to VZV-susceptible transplant candidates at least 2–4 weeks prior to SOT [29] or >4 weeks prior to conditioning regimen for HSCT [5]. Giving the live-attenuated virus vaccine within a short-time period prior to immunosuppression may risk for clinical illness due to the vaccine strain. The role of recombinant zoster vaccine for VZV prevention in transplant recipients is under investigation.

VZV-seronegative transplant recipients should avoid exposure to individuals with varicella or zoster or those who recently received live virus vaccine. VZV-seronegative transplant recipients who have significant exposure to varicella and zoster are at high risk of developing severe primary infection and should receive postexposure prophylaxis using immunoglobulin within 10 days of exposure. Antiviral prophylaxis with oral acyclovir or valacyclovir may also be used for 3–21 days as an adjunct to VZV immunoglobulin prophylaxis or as the primary method for prevention in patients unable to receive VZV immunoglobulin [5, 29]. If used, antiviral prophylaxis should be given as soon as possible, and within 10 days of significant exposure. VZV-seronegative transplant recipients with significant exposure to varicella or herpes zoster could be considered contagious, and thus, airborne precautions should be instituted 7 days after and up to 21 days exposure or for 28 days after exposure for patients who received passive immunization against VZV.

Because of the high risk of zoster, antiviral prophylaxis is recommended for VZV-seropositive allogeneic HSCT recipients [5]. This can be in the form of oral acyclovir (800 mg PO twice daily) or valacyclovir (500 mg orally once or twice daily) for at least 1 year after allogeneic HSCT or longer for patients with severe immunosuppression and chronic GVHD [5]. Antiviral prophylaxis for autologous HSCT and SOT recipients is not currently recommended.

Treatment

Antiviral treatment for varicella and zoster halts disease progression, prevents visceral dissemination, reduces the duration of viral replication, and reduces postherpetic pain syndrome. Transplant patients who develop primary varicella infection should be treated as soon as possible with intravenous high-dose acyclovir, 10 mg/kg given every 8 h; the dose requires adjustment in patients with declining renal function. Reduction in immunosuppression should be considered, as these patients are at risk of developing severe and potentially fatal disease. The role of immunoglobulins as adjunct to antiviral therapy is debated [29]. Alternative drugs are valacyclovir and famciclovir. Intravenous therapy is indicated for severe disease, but this can be tapered to oral treatment once there is sufficient control of the infection [5, 29].

Localized or nonsevere forms of herpes zoster may be treated with oral famciclovir and valacyclovir. Treatment should be given for at least 7 days but should be continued until 2 days after the lesions have crusted. Localized disease involving vital organs such as herpes zoster ophthalmicus involving the trigeminal ganglion and herpes zoster oticus also known as Ramsay Hunt syndrome should be treated with intravenous acyclovir. Disseminated or organ invasive herpes zoster should be treated with intravenous acyclovir [5, 29].

Human Herpes Viruses 6A and 6B

Epidemiology

HHV-6A and HHV-6B are two distinct lymphotropic β-herpesviruses that infect the majority of humans [37, 38]. By age 5, the majority of humans are HHV-6 seropositive [38]. In immunocompetent individuals, primary HHV-6 infection is often asymptomatic, or it could be manifested clinically as a febrile illness associated with an exanthem, diarrhea, respiratory symptoms, or seizures [37–40]. The classic presentation of primary HHV-6 infection is roseola infantum also known as sixth disease or exanthem subitum. A disease in young children characterized by high fever that lasts for 3–5 days followed by erythematous blanching maculopapular rash that starts at the neck and trunk spreading to the extremities [39]. HHV-6B accounts for the majority of documented primary HHV-6 infections [38]. In contrast, the epidemiology of HHV-6A infection is less defined [41], although it is more neurotrophic and thus has been implicated in neurologic disorders.

After primary infection, HHV-6 establishes lifelong latency in hosts' mononuclear cells [39], and frequently reactivates later in life, especially in patients with severe adaptive immune dysfunction. HHV-6 is unique among human herpes viruses because of its ability to integrate into the human chromosome known as chromosomally integrated HHV-6 (CIHHV-6) [42–45]. Chromosomal integration by HHV-6A and HHV-6B occurs in 1% of individuals [42–45], and the integrated viral genome is passed to offspring in a Mendelian manner [42].

HHV-6 infection after SOT and HSCT occurs either as primary or as secondary infection due to reactivation of endogenous latent virus or reinfection from donor-transmitted HHV-6 virus [37, 46]. Since HHV-6 seroprevalence is over 90% in adults, most HHV-6 infections are believed to be due to reactivation or reinfection [37, 46]. For the minority of HHV-6 seronegative transplant recipients, primary HHV-6 infection may occur in the following manner: acquired from the donor allograft, blood and blood product transfusions, or natural transmission from close contacts [47, 48]. Pediatric transplant recipients, especially those younger than 2 years of age, are likely HHV-6 seronegative and at risk of primary infection [48].

The incidence of HHV-6 infections has been reported in 10–60% of SOT [37, 46] and approximately 50% of HSCT recipients [49]. The majority is due to HHV-6B and detected during the first 2–4 weeks after transplantation [37, 46]; in contrast, only 2–3% of HHV-6 infections after HSCT are due to HHV-6A. The vast majority of HHV-6 infections are transient subclinical reactivations with clinical consequences [37, 46]. In contrast, clinical disease directly due to HHV-6 occurs in <1% of transplant recipients [50, 51]. HHV-6B accounts for most cases of clinical disease [37, 46]; only a few cases have been associated with HHV-6A [47].

Clinical Disease

HHV-6 disease after transplantation is most commonly manifested as a febrile illness accompanied by bone marrow suppression [52]. HHV-6 encephalitis is one of the most severe clinical manifestations, often in the form of limbic encephalitis [53, 54]. Encephalitis is particularly seen in HSCT recipients, although it has been reported in SOT recipients [55, 56]. Clinical manifestations include confusion, depressed sensorium, seizures, disorientation, and short-term memory loss. HHV-6 is also known to infect hematopoietic progenitor cells, and may delay engraftment, especially of platelets, after HSCT [57]. HHV-6 has also been associated with fever and rash [58], hepatitis [47], gastritis and enteritis [59], colitis [60], pneumonitis [55], pancytopenia, hemophagocytosis syndrome, and disseminated infection [61].

HHV-6 has several indirect effects in SOT recipients, possibly as a result of its immunomodulatory effects [37, 46]. These indirect effects of HHV-6 infection include the increased risk of CMV disease after kidney and liver transplantation [62, 63], higher risk of fungal and other opportunistic infections [64], allograft rejection and dysfunction

[65], early fibrosis due to hepatitis C virus recurrence after liver transplantation [66], and a higher mortality rate after transplantation [67, 68].

The impact of CIHHV-6 in transplant recipients is not well defined. Because of the very high levels of HHV-6 DNA in the blood, patients with CIHHV-6 have been mistaken to have active infection and given unnecessary treatment. The clinical impact of CIHHV-6 was recently investigated in a cohort of liver and other transplant recipients and was found to be associated with a significantly higher risk of bacterial infections and allograft rejection [42–45].

Diagnosis

HHV-6 NAT by PCR is the most commonly used test for the diagnosis of HHV-6 infection after transplantation [37, 46, 69]. HHV-6 PCR is most commonly performed on blood samples [52, 70], although it has been used to detect HHV-6 DNA in CSF and BAL fluid [71, 72]. HHV-6 DNA is demonstrated in the CSF of patients with HHV-6 encephalitis, often accompanied by non-specific CSF findings. Only half of the patients may have CSF pleiocytosis and elevated protein. MRI of the brain is sensitive in demonstrating multiple non-enhancing low attenuation signals in the temporal lobe and the limbic system. Active HHV-6 infection is often indicated by high viral load compared to the low DNA level in some cases of latent infection. Quantitative HHV-6 PCR test is therefore preferred, as viral load is also used to differentiate severe from mild HHV-6 infection, assess antiviral treatment responses, and guide duration of treatment [37, 69].

In the interpretation of HHV-6 PCR assay results, it is critically important to consider the potential detection of CIHHV-6 [42–45]. In a consensus statement, detection of 5.5 logs of HHV-6 in the blood should raise suspicion for chromosomally integrated virus, and this can be confirmed by persistently elevated viral load over time and, if needed, cytogenetic analysis, hair follicle analysis, and testing of siblings and relatives [42–45].

Histopathology with or without immunohistochemistry is preferred for the diagnosis of tissue-invasive HHV-6 disease, such as hepatitis and pneumonitis [37]. The other tests for the diagnosis of HHV-6 are serology, viral culture, and antigenemia [37]. However, these are rarely used in clinical practice since they are not widely available.

Prevention

Ganciclovir, foscarnet, and cidofovir are active against HHV-6. There have been few observational studies to indicate that ganciclovir may reduce the incidence of HHV-6 infection in SOT [70] and HSCT recipients [73]. However, HHV-6 reactivation is common after HSCT and SOT, and clinical disease occurs very rarely [69]. Hence, antiviral prophylaxis and preemptive therapy are not recommended after SOT [37] and HSCT [49]. There is no clinical benefit in preventing HHV-6, since the majority is subclinical, self-limited, and transient [37].

Treatment

For established HHV-6 disease in SOT and HSCT, antiviral therapy with foscarnet and/or ganciclovir is recommended, and cidofovir is considered as alternative agent [37]. The doses recommended follow the guidelines for the treatment of CMV disease [37]. Antiviral treatment is especially indicated in the setting of HHV-6 encephalitis and other tissue-invasive diseases, and it should also be considered for other clinical syndromes attributable to HHV-6 [37]. In addition to antiviral therapies, SOT recipients with HHV-6 disease should have cautious reduction in their pharmacologic immunosuppression [37]. Antiviral treatment is generally guided by serial monitoring of HHV-6 viral load, and it is recommended to continue therapy until the virus is cleared from the blood or other sites of infection. It is recommended to rule out the existence of CIHHV-6 in the interpretation of HHV-6 PCR results [42–45].

Human Herpes Virus 7

Epidemiology

HHV-7 is a β-herpesvirus that infects humans during the first 5 years of life [74]. Primary HHV-7 infection occurs at a slightly later age compared to HHV-6 [75], and it presents most commonly as an asymptomatic infection or as a benign self-limited illness characterized most commonly by fever and seizures [76]. Upper respiratory symptoms, vomiting, diarrhea, seizures, encephalitis, or a Roseola-like illness have been reported in association with HHV-7 infection [74, 76].

Detection of HHV-7 DNA in blood samples of patients is common during the early period after transplantation. It has been reported in up to 40% of transplant recipients. Almost all of these are transient, low level, and not associated with any clinical manifestations [37]. Since over 95% of individuals are HHV-7 seropositive, the detection of HHV-7 DNA in transplant recipients is likely a reflection of viral reactivation [37]. HHV-7 reactivation occurs mostly during the first 2–4 weeks after transplantation [37, 77]. Reinfection with donor-transmitted virus may also occur, while primary HHV-7 infection is rare [37].

Clinical Disease

Clinical disease due to HHV-7 is rare after transplantation [37]. The true incidence of clinical disease is not known but likely less than 1% of patients [37, 78]. There have only been a few sporadic cases of HHV-7 disease reported. Fever, thrombocytopenia, and acute myelitis have been described as potentially caused by HHV-7 [52, 78, 79]. Most commonly, HHV-7 is detected in the blood of patients with CMV disease [52]. HHV-7 has been implicated to have indirect effects such as predisposition for CMV disease [63, 80] and acute rejection [81].

Diagnosis

There are no tests recommended for surveillance of HHV-7 in SOT recipients [37]. In patients with clinical suspicion for HHV-7 infection, nucleic acid testing, serology, culture, and histopathology are the tests for diagnosis [37]. The most commonly used test is HHV-7 NAT by PCR [37, 52, 82]. However, clinical correlation between HHV-7 load and clinical disease has not been established [52]. To document tissue-invasive HHV-7 disease, including encephalitis, histopathology is required. Demonstration of HHV-7 proteins is preferred over DNA detection in order to confirm the diagnosis of HHV-7 disease. A less invasive strategy to diagnose HHV-7 encephalitis would be to demonstrate HHV-7 nucleic acid in the CSF, although this should be interpreted with caution since latent virus may be amplified from reactive lymphocytes and other leukocytes present in the CSF.

Prevention and Treatment

Since HHV-7 is not a well-established common cause of clinical disease after transplantation, there is no recommendation for its prevention after HSCT [49] and SOT [37, 69]. For the rare occurrence of proven HHV-7 disease, treatment may be initiated with foscarnet or cidofovir [37]. Ganciclovir is not active against HHV-7. Data suggest that HHV-7 is resistant to ganciclovir in vitro and may not be inhibited with achievable concentrations of ganciclovir [70, 83, 84]. Antiviral treatment should be complemented by a reduction in the degree of pharmacologic immunosuppression [37].

Human Herpes Virus 8

Epidemiology

HHV-8 is a γ-herpesvirus that causes Kaposi's sarcoma [85]; hence, it is also known as Kaposi's sarcoma-associated herpes virus. Unlike other ubiquitous members of the human herpesvirus family, HHV-8 is a geographically restricted virus [86]. HHV-8 seropositivity is highest in Africa (up to 50%) [87] and the Mediterranean (up to 35%) [88] and intermediate in South America (up to 16%) [89] and Asia (up to 24%) [90]. Seroprevalence rates in North America and Northern Europe are comparatively lower [86].

Primary HHV-8 infection occurs commonly in children [91]. Transmission occurs during close contact, likely through transfer of body secretions such as saliva and genital secretions [92–94]. Primary HHV-8 infection is associated with mild non-specific symptoms of fever and rash [91], and it has also been associated with diarrhea, fatigue, and lymphadenopathy [95].

HHV-8 infection in transplant recipients may occur either as primary infection in HHV-8 seronegative patients who receive allograft from HHV-8 seropositive donors [96–101] or as secondary reactivation of latent virus [102]. Overall, KS and other HHV-8 disease are generally rare in HSCT [49] and SOT recipients, although the rates vary depending on the geographic area [86]. The reported incidences of KS in SOT recipients vary from as low as 0.5% among transplant recipients from North America, Asia, and Northern Europe to as high as 28% among HHV-8 seropositive transplant recipients from the Middle East [103–106]. In Saudi Arabia, KS was the most common malignancy in kidney recipients, representing 87.5% of all tumors in these patients [104]. The median time to the onset of KS is 30 months after transplantation, although it may occur as early as 3 months to as late as 124 months after transplantation [107].

Risk factors for HHV-8-associated disease, specifically KS, include older age, male gender, and residence or exposures in HHV-8 endemic area [37, 86]. Certain populations in areas of low endemicity may be at higher risk such as the men who have sex with men [37, 86]. Both pretransplant HHV-8 seronegativity and seropositivity have been associated with KS, suggesting that both primary HHV-8 infection and reactivation, respectively, can result in clinical disease [37, 86]. Because control of HHV-8 infection is mediated by T cells, the intensity of pharmacologic immunosuppression and the use of antilymphocyte agents have been suggested to play a role in HHV-8 pathogenesis after transplantation [108].

Clinical Disease

The most common clinical manifestation of HHV-8 infection is KS, a multicentric neoplasm of lymphatic endothelium-derived cells, which manifests as multifocal progressive mucocutaneous lesions with dissemination to visceral organs [109–112]. More than 95% of transplant patients with KS present with a skin lesion characterized by reddish-bluish or purplish discoloration, mainly in extremities. In 25% of cases, KS has visceral involvement and may involve the lymph node, lungs, gastrointestinal tract, and liver. The other malignancies associated with HHV-8 are body cavity lymphoma also known as primary effusion lymphoma (PEL) and Castleman's disease [96, 107, 113]. PEL is a form of non-Hodgkin lymphoma characterized by involvement of serosal surfaces such as the peritoneum, pericardium, and pleura. Castleman's disease is an angiofollicular lymphoproliferative disease characterized by high fever, night sweats, and other constitutional manifestations related to overexpression of IL-6. The prognosis of Castleman's disease and PEL is generally poorer compared to KS [86]. HHV-8 has also been reported as a cause of nonmalignant illnesses presenting with fever, hemophagocytosis, myelosuppression, and multiorgan failure in transplant recipients [88, 100, 114, 115].

Diagnosis

Histopathology is required for diagnosis of KS, Castleman's disease, and PEL [37, 86]. Demonstrating HHV-8 in the tissues can be done through immunohistochemistry using monoclonal antibodies against the virus [111].

Active HHV-8 infection may be indicated by seroconversion or IgM response [100, 116, 117]. However, serology has limited utility in immunocompromised transplant recipients [100, 116, 117]. Active HHV-8 infection can be diagnosed using NAT to quantitate HHV-8 load in clinical samples [37, 86]. Studies conducted using these PCR assays have demonstrated their potential clinical utility in the surveillance, diagnosis, and management of HHV-8 infection and malignant disease [37, 86]. HHV-8 quantification has been utilized for infection and disease risk surveillance [108, 117, 118] and has been used to monitor patients with KS and assess their response to therapy [108, 117, 118].

Prevention and Treatment

Treatment of HHV-8 and its associated malignant disease would potentially include (1) reduction in immunosuppression, (2) surgical debulking, (3) cytotoxic chemotherapy, and (4) antiviral therapies [37, 86]. The cornerstone and first-line therapy for KS and other malignant HHV-8-associated diseases is the cautious reduction or cessation of immunosuppression [37, 86, 119]. Reduction in immunosuppression has resulted in complete remission in 25–30% of patients with isolated cutaneous KS [86]. Another emerging strategy is to switch the immunosuppressive regimens from calcineurin inhibitors like cyclosporine to mTOR inhibitor such as sirolimus or rapamycin [96, 97, 101, 120, 121]. Sirolimus has antiproliferative properties that may be useful in the treatment of KS and other angiogenic proliferation diseases. Several studies have demonstrated that conversion to sirolimus has led to regression of KS lesions in some patients [96, 97, 101, 120, 121].

Patients whose lesions do no not regress despite reduction in immunosuppression may require surgical excision, radiation therapy, or cytotoxic chemotherapy. The standard treatment of Castleman's disease is surgical resection, which is highly curative if this is unicentric and localized [122]. The benefits of ganciclovir, foscarnet, and cidofovir therapy in transplant recipients with established KS or other manifestations of HHV-8 infection are not well defined [107].

References

1. Schillinger JA, Xu F, Sternberg MR, et al. National seroprevalence and trends in herpes simplex virus type 1 in the United States, 1976-1994. Sex Transm Dis. 2004;31(12):753.
2. Xu F, Sternberg MR, Kottiri BJ, et al. Trends in herpes simplex virus type 1 and type 2 seroprevalence in the United States. JAMA. 2006;296(8):964.
3. Wald A, Zeh JE, Selke SA, et al. Reactivation of genital herpes simplex virus type 2 infection in asymptomatic seropositive persons. N Engl J Med. 2000;342(12):844.
4. Zhu J, Peng T, Johnston C, Phasouk K, Kask AS, Klock A, Jet a. Immune surveillance by CD8αα+ skin-resident T cells in human herpes virus infection. Nature. 2013;497:494–7.
5. Styczynski J, Reusser P, Einsele H, et al. Management of HSV, VZV and EBV infections in patients with hematological malignancies and after SCT: guidelines from the second European conference on infections in leukemia. Bone Marrow Transplant. 2009;43(10):757.
6. Greenberg MS, Friedman H, Cohen SG, Oh SH, Laster L, Starr S. A comparative study of herpes simplex infections in renal transplant and leukemic patients. J Infect Dis. 1987;156(2):280.
7. Naraqi S, Jackson GG, Jonasson O, Yamashiroya HM. Prospective study of prevalence, incidence, and source of herpesvirus infections in patients with renal allografts. J Infect Dis. 1977;136(4):531.
8. Pettersson E, Hovi T, Ahonen J, et al. Prophylactic oral acyclovir after renal transplantation. Transplantation. 1985;39(3):279.
9. Seale L, Jones CJ, Kathpalia S, et al. Prevention of herpesvirus infections in renal allograft recipients by low-dose oral acyclovir. JAMA. 1985;254(24):3435.
10. Singh N, Dummer JS, Kusne S, et al. Infections with cytomegalovirus and other herpesviruses in 121 liver transplant recipients: transmission by donated organ and the effect of OKT3 antibodies. J Infect Dis. 1988;158(1):124.
11. Zuckerman RA, Limaye AP. Varicella zoster virus (VZV) and herpes simplex virus (HSV) in solid organ transplant patients. Am J Transplant. 2013;13(Suppl 3):55.
12. Wilck MB, Zuckerman RA. Herpes simplex virus in solid organ transplantation. Am J Transplant. 2013;13(Suppl 4):121.
13. Meyers JD, Flournoy N, Thomas ED. Infection with herpes simplex virus and cell-mediated immunity after marrow transplant. J Infect Dis. 1980;142(3):338.
14. Tang IY, Maddux MS, Veremis SA, Bauma WD, Pollak R, Mozes MF. Low-dose oral acyclovir for prevention of herpes simplex virus infection during OKT3 therapy. Transplant Proc. 1989;21(1 Pt 2):1758.
15. Singh N, Dummer JS, Kusne S, et al. Infections with cytomegalovirus and other herpesviruses in 121 liver transplant recipients:

transmission by donated organ and the effect of OKT3 antibodies. J Infect Dis. 1988;158(1):124.
16. Basse G, Mengelle C, Kamar N, et al. Disseminated herpes simplex type-2 (HSV-2) infection after solid-organ transplantation. Infection. 2008;36(1):62.
17. Dummer JS, Armstrong J, Somers J, et al. Transmission of infection with herpes simplex virus by renal transplantation. J Infect Dis. 1987;155(2):202.
18. Goodman JL. Possible transmission of herpes simplex virus by organ transplantation. Transplantation. 1989;47(4):609.
19. Meyers JD, Wade JC, Mitchell CD, et al. Multicenter collaborative trial of intravenous acyclovir for treatment of mucocutaneous herpes simplex virus infection in the immunocompromised host. Am J Med. 1982;73(1A):229.
20. Spencer GD, Hackman RC, McDonald GB, et al. A prospective study of unexplained nausea and vomiting after marrow transplantation. Transplantation. 1986;42(6):602.
21. Mommeja-Marin H, Lafaurie M, Scieux C, Galicier L, Oksenhendler E, Molina JM. Herpes simplex virus type 2 as a cause of severe meningitis in immunocompromised adults. Clin Infect Dis. 2003;37(11):1527.
22. Levitsky J, Duddempudi AT, Lakeman FD, et al. Detection and diagnosis of herpes simplex virus infection in adults with acute liver failure. Liver Transpl. 2008;1410:1498.
23. Strick LB, Wald A. Diagnostics for herpes simplex virus: is PCR the new gold standard? Mol Diagn Ther. 2006;10(1):17.
24. Issa NC, Espy MJ, Uhl JR, Smith TF. Sequencing and resolution of amplified herpes simplex virus DNA with intermediate melting curves as genotype 1 or 2 by LightCycler PCR assay. J Clin Microbiol. 2005;43(4):1843.
25. Roubalova K, Suchankova A, Vitek A, Sajdova J. Presence of herpes simplex virus (HSV) in peripheral leukocytes of patient who developed active HSV infection after bone marrow transplantation. J Clin Virol. 2000;17(1):37.
26. Saral R, Burns WH, Laskin OL, Santos GW, Lietman PS. Acyclovir prophylaxis of herpes-simplex-virus infections. N Engl J Med. 1981;305(2):63.
27. Mejias A, Bustos R, Ardura MI, Ramirez C, Sanchez PJ. Persistence of herpes simplex virus DNA in cerebrospinal fluid of neonates with herpes simplex virus encephalitis. J Perinatol. 2009;29(4):290.
28. Fluri S, Kaczala GW, Leibundgut K, Alberio L. Chickenpox is not always benign: postvaricella purpura fulminans requires prompt and aggressive treatment. Pediatr Emerg Care. 2010;26(12):932.
29. Pergam SA, Limaye AP. Varicella zoster virus in solid organ transplantation. Am J Transplant. 2013;13(Suppl 4):138.
30. Roque-Afonso AM, Bralet MP, Ichai P, et al. Chickenpox-associated fulminant hepatitis that led to liver transplantation in a 63-year-old woman. Liver Transpl. 2008;14(9):1309.
31. Arness T, Pedersen R, Dierkhising R, Kremers W, Patel R. Varicella zoster virus-associated disease in adult kidney transplant recipients: incidence and risk-factor analysis. Transpl Infect Dis. 2008;10(4):260.
32. Pergam SA, Forsberg CW, Boeckh MJ, et al. Herpes zoster incidence in a multicenter cohort of solid organ transplant recipients. Transpl Infect Dis. 2011;13(1):15.
33. Lauzurica R, Bayes B, Frias C, et al. Disseminated varicella infection in adult renal allograft recipients: role of mycophenolate mofetil. Transplant Proc. 2003;35(5):1758.
34. Alvite-Canosa M, Paniagua-Martin MJ, Quintela-Fandino J, Otero A, Crespo-Leiro MG. Fulminant hepatic failure due to varicella zoster in a heart transplant patient: successful liver transplant. J Heart Lung Transplant. 2009;28(11):1215.
35. Ishizaki Y, Tezuka J, Ohga S, et al. Quantification of circulating varicella zoster virus-DNA for the early diagnosis of visceral varicella. J Infect. 2003;47(2):133.
36. Watzinger F, Suda M, Preuner S, et al. Real-time quantitative PCR assays for detection and monitoring of pathogenic human viruses in immunosuppressed pediatric patients. J Clin Microbiol. 2004;42(11):5189.
37. Razonable RR, Zerr DM. HHV-6, HHV-7 and HHV-8 in solid organ transplant recipients. Am J Transplant. 2009;9. Suppl 4:S97.
38. Zerr DM, Meier AS, Selke SS, et al. A population-based study of primary human herpesvirus 6 infection. N Engl J Med. 2005;352(8):768.
39. Pruksananonda P, Hall CB, Insel RA, et al. Primary human herpesvirus 6 infection in young children. N Engl J Med. 1992;326(22):1445.
40. Caserta MT, Hall CB, Schnabel K, Long CE, D'Heron N. Primary human herpesvirus 7 infection: a comparison of human herpesvirus 7 and human herpesvirus 6 infections in children. J Pediatr. 1998;133(3):386.
41. Razonable RR, Fanning C, Brown RA, et al. Selective reactivation of human herpesvirus 6 variant a occurs in critically ill immunocompetent hosts. J Infect Dis. 2002;185(1):110.
42. Pellett PE, Ablashi DV, Ambros PF, et al. Chromosomally integrated human herpesvirus 6: questions and answers. Rev Med Virol. 2012;22(3):144–55. Epub 2011 Nov 4
43. Lee SO, Brown RA, Eid AJ, Razonable RR. Chromosomally integrated human herpesvirus-6 in kidney transplant recipients. Nephrol Dial Transplant. 2011;26(7):2391.
44. Lee SO, Brown RA, Razonable RR. Clinical significance of pretransplant chromosomally integrated human herpesvirus-6 in liver transplant recipients. Transplantation. 2011;92(2):224.
45. Lee SO, Brown RA, Razonable RR. Chromosomally integrated human herpesvirus-6 in transplant recipients. Transpl Infect Dis. 2012;14(4):346–54.
46. Lautenschlager I, Razonable RR. Human herpesvirus-6 infections in kidney, liver, lung, and heart transplantation: review. Transpl Int. 2012;25(5):493.
47. Potenza L, Luppi M, Barozzi P, et al. HHV-6A in syncytial giant-cell hepatitis. N Engl J Med. 2008;359(6):593.
48. Feldstein AE, Razonable RR, Boyce TG, et al. Prevalence and clinical significance of human herpesviruses 6 and 7 active infection in pediatric liver transplant patients. Pediatr Transplant. 2003;7(2):125.
49. Ljungman P, de la Camara R, Cordonnier C, et al. Management of CMV, HHV 6, HHV-7 and Kaposi-sarcoma herpesvirus (HHV-8) infections in patients with hematological malignancies and after SCT. Bone Marrow Transplant. 2008;42(4):227.
50. Cervera C, Marcos MA, Linares L, et al. A prospective survey of human herpesvirus-6 primary infection in solid organ transplant recipients. Transplantation. 2006;82(7):979.
51. Humar A, Kumar D, Caliendo AM, et al. Clinical impact of human herpesvirus 6 infection after liver transplantation. Transplantation. 2002;73(4):599.
52. Razonable RR, Rivero A, Brown RA, et al. Detection of simultaneous beta-herpesvirus infections in clinical syndromes due to defined cytomegalovirus infection. Clin Transplant. 2003;17(2):114.
53. Zerr DM, Gooley TA, Yeung L, et al. Human herpesvirus 6 reactivation and encephalitis in allogeneic bone marrow transplant recipients. Clin Infect Dis. 2001;33(6):763.
54. Wang FZ, Linde A, Hagglund H, Testa M, Locasciulli A, Ljungman P. Human herpesvirus 6 DNA in cerebrospinal fluid specimens from allogeneic bone marrow transplant patients: does it have clinical significance? Clin Infect Dis. 1999;28(3):562.
55. Nash PJ, Avery RK, Tang WH, Starling RC, Taege AJ, Yamani MH. Encephalitis owing to human herpesvirus-6 after cardiac transplant. Am J Transplant. 2004;4(7):1200.
56. Vinnard C, Barton T, Jerud E, Blumberg E. A report of human herpesvirus 6-associated encephalitis in a solid organ transplant

recipient and a review of previously published cases. Liver Transpl. 2009;15(10):1242.
57. Ljungman P, Wang FZ, Clark DA, et al. High levels of human herpesvirus 6 DNA in peripheral blood leucocytes are correlated to platelet engraftment and disease in allogeneic stem cell transplant patients. Br J Haematol. 2000;111(3):774.
58. Singh N, Carrigan DR, Gayowski T, Singh J, Marino IR. Variant B human herpesvirus-6 associated febrile dermatosis with thrombocytopenia and encephalopathy in a liver transplant recipient. Transplantation. 1995;60(11):1355.
59. Randhawa PS, Jenkins FJ, Nalesnik MA, et al. Herpesvirus 6 variant A infection after heart transplantation with giant cell transformation in bile ductular and gastroduodenal epithelium. Am J Surg Pathol. 1997;21(7):847.
60. Delbridge MS, Karim MS, Shrestha BM, McKane W. Colitis in a renal transplant patient with human herpesvirus-6 infection. Transpl Infect Dis. 2006;8(4):226.
61. Rossi C, Delforge ML, Jacobs F, et al. Fatal primary infection due to human herpesvirus 6 variant A in a renal transplant recipient. Transplantation. 2001;71(2):288.
62. Dockrell DH, Prada J, Jones MF, et al. Seroconversion to human herpesvirus 6 following liver transplantation is a marker of cytomegalovirus disease. J Infect Dis. 1997;176(5):1135.
63. Mendez JC, Dockrell DH, Espy MJ, et al. Human beta-herpesvirus interactions in solid organ transplant recipients. J Infect Dis. 2001;183(2):179.
64. Dockrell DH, Mendez JC, Jones M, et al. Human herpesvirus 6 seronegativity before transplantation predicts the occurrence of fungal infection in liver transplant recipients. Transplantation. 1999;67(3):399.
65. Lautenschlager I, Hockerstedt K, Linnavuori K, Taskinen E. Human herpesvirus-6 infection after liver transplantation. Clin Infect Dis. 1998;26(3):702.
66. Singh N, Husain S, Carrigan DR, et al. Impact of human herpesvirus-6 on the frequency and severity of recurrent hepatitis C virus hepatitis in liver transplant recipients. Clin Transpl. 2002;16(2):92.
67. Jacobs F, Knoop C, Brancart F, et al. Human herpesvirus-6 infection after lung and heart-lung transplantation: a prospective longitudinal study. Transplantation. 2003;75(12):1996.
68. Rogers J, Rohal S, Carrigan DR, et al. Human herpesvirus-6 in liver transplant recipients: role in pathogenesis of fungal infections, neurologic complications, and outcome. Transplantation. 2000;69(12):2566.
69. Razonable RR. Human herpesviruses 6, 7 and 8 in solid organ transplant recipients. Am J Transplant. 2013;13(Suppl 3):67.
70. Razonable RR, Brown RA, Humar A, Covington E, Alecock E, Paya CV. Herpesvirus infections in solid organ transplant patients at high risk of primary cytomegalovirus disease. J Infect Dis. 2005;192(8):1331.
71. Manuel O, Kumar D, Moussa G, et al. Lack of association between beta-herpesvirus infection and bronchiolitis obliterans syndrome in lung transplant recipients in the era of antiviral prophylaxis. Transplantation. 2009;87(5):719.
72. Neurohr C, Huppmann P, Leuchte H, et al. Human herpesvirus 6 in bronchalveolar lavage fluid after lung transplantation: a risk factor for bronchiolitis obliterans syndrome? Am J Transplant. 2005;5(12):2982.
73. Rapaport D, Engelhard D, Tagger G, Or R, Frenkel N. Antiviral prophylaxis may prevent human herpesvirus-6 reactivation in bone marrow transplant recipients. Transpl Infect Dis. 2002;4(1):10.
74. Tanaka K, Kondo T, Torigoe S, Okada S, Mukai T, Yamanishi K. Human herpesvirus 7: another causal agent for roseola (exanthem subitum). J Pediatr. 1994;125(1):1.
75. Wyatt LS, Rodriguez WJ, Balachandran N, Frenkel N. Human herpesvirus 7: antigenic properties and prevalence in children and adults. J Virol. 1991;65(11):6260.
76. Suga S, Yoshikawa T, Nagai T, Asano Y. Clinical features and virological findings in children with primary human herpesvirus 7 infection. Pediatrics. 1997;99(3):E4.
77. Yoshikawa T. Human herpesvirus-6 and -7 infections in transplantation. Pediatr Transplant. 2003;7(1):11.
78. Anton A, Cervera C, Pumarola T, et al. Human herpesvirus 7 primary infection in kidney transplant recipients. Transplantation. 2008;85(2):298.
79. Ward KN, White RP, Mackinnon S, Hanna M. Human herpesvirus-7 infection of the CNS with acute myelitis in an adult bone marrow recipient. Bone Marrow Transplant. 2002;30(12):983.
80. Tong CY, Bakran A, Williams H, Cheung CY, Peiris JS. Association of human herpesvirus 7 with cytomegalovirus disease in renal transplant recipients. Transplantation. 2000;70(1):213.
81. Griffiths PD, Ait-Khaled M, Bearcroft CP, et al. Human herpesviruses 6 and 7 as potential pathogens after liver transplant: prospective comparison with the effect of cytomegalovirus. J Med Virol. 1999;59(4):496.
82. Fernandez C, Boutolleau D, Manichanh C, Mangeney N, Agut H, Gautheret-Dejean A. Quantitation of HHV-7 genome by real-time polymerase chain reaction assay using MGB probe technology. J Virol Methods. 2002;106(1):11.
83. Yoshida M, Yamada M, Tsukazaki T, et al. Comparison of antiviral compounds against human herpesvirus 6 and 7. Antivir Res. 1998;40(1–2):73.
84. Brennan DC, Storch GA, Singer GG, Lee L, Rueda J, Schnitzler MA. The prevalence of human herpesvirus-7 in renal transplant recipients is unaffected by oral or intravenous ganciclovir. J Infect Dis. 2000;181(5):1557.
85. Chang Y, Cesarman E, Pessin MS, et al. Identification of herpesvirus-like DNA sequences in AIDS-associated Kaposi's sarcoma. Science. 1994;266(5192):1865.
86. Ariza-Heredia EJ, Razonable RR. Human herpes virus 8 in solid organ transplantation. Transplantation. 2011;92(8):837.
87. Butler LM, Were WA, Balinandi S, et al. Human herpesvirus 8 infection in children and adults in a population-based study in rural Uganda. J Infect Dis. 2011;203(5):625.
88. Luppi M, Barozzi P, Schulz TF, et al. Bone marrow failure associated with human herpesvirus 8 infection after transplantation. N Engl J Med. 2000;343(19):1378.
89. Freitas RB, Freitas MR, Linhares AC. Prevalence of human herpesvirus 8 antibodies in the population of Belem, Para, Brazil. Rev Inst Med Trop Sao Paulo. 2002;44(6):309.
90. Chen N, Nelson KE, Jenkins FJ, et al. Seroprevalence of human herpesvirus 8 infection in Northern Thailand. Clin Infect Dis. 2004;39(7):1052.
91. Andreoni M, Sarmati L, Nicastri E, et al. Primary human herpesvirus 8 infection in immunocompetent children. JAMA. 2002;287(10):1295.
92. Pauk J, Huang ML, Brodie SJ, et al. Mucosal shedding of human herpesvirus 8 in men. N Engl J Med. 2000;343(19):1369.
93. Vieira J, Huang ML, Koelle DM, Corey L. Transmissible Kaposi's sarcoma-associated herpesvirus (human herpesvirus 8) in saliva of men with a history of Kaposi's sarcoma. J Virol. 1997;71(9):7083.
94. Blackbourn DJ, Lennette ET, Ambroziak J, Mourich DV, Levy JA. Human herpesvirus 8 detection in nasal secretions and saliva. J Infect Dis. 1998;177(1):213.
95. Wang QJ, Jenkins FJ, Jacobson LP, et al. Primary human herpesvirus 8 infection generates a broadly specific CD8(+) T-cell response to viral lytic cycle proteins. Blood. 2001;97(8):2366.
96. Boulanger E, Afonso PV, Yahiaoui Y, Adle-Biassette H, Gabarre J, Agbalika F. Human herpesvirus-8 (HHV-8)-associated primary effusion lymphoma in two renal transplant recipients receiving rapamycin. Am J Transplant. 2008;8(3):707.
97. Di Benedetto F, Di Sandro S, De Ruvo N, et al. Kaposi's sarcoma after liver transplantation. J Cancer Res Clin Oncol. 2008;134(6):653.

98. Luppi M, Barozzi P, Santagostino G, et al. Molecular evidence of organ-related transmission of Kaposi sarcoma-associated herpesvirus or human herpesvirus-8 in transplant patients. Blood. 2000;96(9):3279.
99. Marcelin AG, Roque-Afonso AM, Hurtova M, et al. Fatal disseminated Kaposi's sarcoma following human herpesvirus 8 primary infections in liver-transplant recipients. Liver Transpl. 2004;10(2):295.
100. Regamey N, Tamm M, Wernli M, et al. Transmission of human herpesvirus 8 infection from renal-transplant donors to recipients. N Engl J Med. 1998;339(19):1358.
101. Wasywich CA, Croxson MC, van Doornum GJ, Coverdale HA, Ruygrok PN. Sirolimus for Kaposi's sarcoma. J Heart Lung Transplant. 2006;25(6):726.
102. Barozzi P, Luppi M, Facchetti F, et al. Post-transplant Kaposi sarcoma originates from the seeding of donor-derived progenitors. Nat Med. 2003;9(5):554.
103. Farge D. Kaposi's sarcoma in organ transplant recipients. The Collaborative Transplantation Research Group of Ile de France. Eur J Med. 1993;2(6):339.
104. Qunibi W, Akhtar M, Sheth K, et al. Kaposi's sarcoma: the most common tumor after renal transplantation in Saudi Arabia. Am J Med. 1988;84(2):225.
105. Ahmadpoor P, Ilkhanizadeh B, Sharifzadeh P, et al. Seroprevalence of human herpes virus-8 in renal transplant recipients: a single center study from Iran. Transplant Proc. 2007;39(4):1000.
106. Cattani P, Capuano M, Graffeo R, et al. Kaposi's sarcoma associated with previous human herpesvirus 8 infection in kidney transplant recipients. J Clin Microbiol. 2001;39(2):506.
107. Antman K, Chang Y. Kaposi's sarcoma. N Engl J Med. 2000;342(14):1027.
108. Farge D, Lebbe C, Marjanovic Z, et al. Human herpes virus-8 and other risk factors for Kaposi's sarcoma in kidney transplant recipients. Groupe Cooperatif de Transplantation d' Ile de France (GCIF). Transplantation. 1999;67(9):1236.
109. Babel N, Eibl N, Ulrich C, et al. Development of Kaposi's sarcoma under sirolimus-based immunosuppression and successful treatment with imiquimod. Transpl Infect Dis. 2008;10(1):59.
110. Dudderidge TJ, Khalifa M, Jeffery R, Amlot P, Al-Akraa M, Sweny P. Donor-derived human herpes virus 8 related Kaposi's sarcoma in renal allograft ureter. Transpl Infect Dis. 2008;10(3):221.
111. Lebbe C, Legendre C, Frances C. Kaposi sarcoma in transplantation. Transplant Rev. 2008;22(4):252.
112. Martinez S, McAdams HP, Youens KE. Kaposi sarcoma after bilateral lung transplantation. J Thoracic Imaging. 2008;23(1):50.
113. Dotti G, Fiocchi R, Motta T, et al. Primary effusion lymphoma after heart transplantation: a new entity associated with human herpesvirus-8. Leukemia. 1999;13(5):664.
114. Luppi M, Barozzi P, Rasini V, et al. Severe pancytopenia and hemophagocytosis after HHV-8 primary infection in a renal transplant patient successfully treated with foscarnet. Transplantation. 2002;74(1):131.
115. Regamey N, Hess V, Passweg J, et al. Infection with human herpesvirus 8 and transplant-associated gammopathy. Transplantation. 2004;77(10):1551.
116. Laney AS, Peters JS, Manzi SM, Kingsley LA, Chang Y, Moore PS. Use of a multiantigen detection algorithm for diagnosis of Kaposi's sarcoma-associated herpesvirus infection. J Clin Microbiol. 2006;44(10):3734.
117. Spira TJ, Lam L, Dollard SC, et al. Comparison of serologic assays and PCR for diagnosis of human herpesvirus 8 infection. J Clin Microbiol. 2000;38(6):2174.
118. Pellet C, Chevret S, Frances C, et al. Prognostic value of quantitative Kaposi sarcoma--associated herpesvirus load in posttransplantation Kaposi sarcoma. J Infect Dis. 2002;186(1):110.
119. Montagnino G, Bencini PL, Tarantino A, Caputo R, Ponticelli C. Clinical features and course of Kaposi's sarcoma in kidney transplant patients: report of 13 cases. Am J Nephrol. 1994;14(2):121.
120. Kolhe N, Mamode N, Van der Walt J, Pattison J. Regression of post-transplant Kaposi's sarcoma using sirolimus. Int J Clin Pract. 2006;60(11):1509.
121. Stallone G, Schena A, Infante B, et al. Sirolimus for Kaposi's sarcoma in renal-transplant recipients. N Engl J Med. 2005;352(13):1317.
122. Al Otaibi T, Al Sagheir A, Ludwin D, Meyer R. Post renal transplant Castleman's disease resolved after graft nephrectomy: a case report. Transplant Proc. 2007;39(4):1276.

Respiratory Viral Infections in Transplant Recipients

40

Catherine Liu, Dora Y. Ho, and Michael Boeckh

Introduction

Respiratory viral infections (RVIs) are common causes of illness in humans. While such infections tend to be mild and self-limiting in healthy individuals, severe or even life-threatening disease can be seen in immunocompromised hosts, as well as the very young and the elderly. In particular, RVIs are frequently associated with significant morbidity following hematopoietic stem cell transplantation (HSCT) or solid organ transplantation (SOT). A number of RNA and DNA viruses can cause respiratory tract infections. This chapter focuses on the epidemiology, clinical manifestations, diagnosis, treatment and prevention of respiratory syncytial virus (RSV), parainfluenza viruses (PIVs), human metapneumovirus (HMPV), influenza viruses, human coronaviruses (HCoV), and human rhinoviruses (HRV).

The respiratory viruses are associated with a wide range of clinical syndromes in the general population, including the common cold, pharyngitis, tracheobronchitis, laryngotracheobronchitis (croup), bronchiolitis, and pneumonia. For transplant recipients, disease spectrum similarly spans from asymptomatic or mild infections to life-threatening lower respiratory tract involvement, although severe complications tend to be more frequent. The severity and outcome of infection largely depend on the type of virus as well as host factors, including the type of transplantation and the degree of immunosuppression at the time of infection. Coinfections with other pulmonary pathogens including bacteria or fungi, e.g., *Aspergillus* species, *Pneumocystis jiroveci*, or other viruses like CMV or more than one respiratory viruses, are also common and can further complicate treatment and lead to poorer outcomes [1–3]. For HSCT recipients, most RVIs occur in 1–10% of the patients during the first 100 days post-transplantation [1, 4, 5], with cumulative incidence varying from a few percent (e.g., HMPV, influenza, RSV, PIVs) to 11–22% such as HCoV and HRV [5]. Infections with RSV, influenza, HMPV, PIVs, and adenovirus have a higher risk of progression from upper respiratory tract infection (URTI) to lower respiratory tract infection (LRTI) and tend to cause the most serious disease, with mortality rate of up to 40–60% among those with LRTI [6–9]; HRV and HCoV infections tend to be mild, but severe LRTI from these viruses can rarely occur [10]. Risk factors for disease progression to LRTI include pre-engraftment status, allogeneic transplant, myeloablative conditioning, graft-versus host disease, and lymphopenia [1, 2, 6, 11–15].

SOT recipients can also suffer from severe disease and complications from RVI. Risk factors for disease progression are not as well defined, but those with lung and heart-lung transplant are particularly vulnerable. Cumulative rates of RVIs in lung transplant recipients range from 8% to 21% in retrospective studies of 5–7 years [16, 17], and a high incidence of progression to LRTI up to 26% has been reported [18]. In contrast, the incidence of RVIs among heart, liver, and kidney transplant recipients is similar to that of the general population, although complications are more frequent [19].

In addition to direct effects from viral infection, RVIs may promote immunologically mediated lung injury in HSCT or lung transplant recipients, potentially leading to acute allograft rejection in the case of lung transplant recipients and/or the development of bronchiolitis obliterans syndrome (BOS), which is characterized by progressive circumferential fibrosis of the small terminal airways histopathologically, resulting in fixed airflow obstruction [20, 21]. BOS is the major limiting factor for long-term survival after lung transplantation [22–28]. The reported incidence of BOS associated with RVIs ranges from 6% to 42% [17, 23], while

C. Liu (✉) · M. Boeckh
Fred Hutchinson Cancer Research Center, University of Washington Medical Center, Seattle, Washington, USA
e-mail: catherine.liu@fredhutch.org; mboeckh@fredhutch.org

D. Y. Ho
Division of Infectious Diseases and Geographic Medicine, Stanford University School of Medicine, Stanford, CA, USA
e-mail: doraywho@stanford.edu

A. Safdar (ed.), *Principles and Practice of Transplant Infectious Diseases*, https://doi.org/10.1007/978-1-4939-9034-4_40

the incidence of acute rejection associated with RVIs varies from 16% to as high as 82% [25, 28–30]. For HSCT, BOS is often observed in the setting of chronic graft-versus-host disease, but it has also been associated with RVIs [31–34]. Among the respiratory viruses, RSV, PIV, HMPV, and influenza have all been associated with BOS [30, 35, 36], and mortality associated with these viruses can be up to 20% in lung transplant patients [37]. For heart, liver, or kidney transplantation, no relationship between RVI and rejection has been noted [19].

Paramyxoviruses

RSV, PIVs, and HMPV are members of the *Paramyxoviridae* family. The epidemiology, clinical manifestations, and treatment of each of these viruses are discussed separately.

Respiratory Syncytial Virus (RSV)

Epidemiology and Clinical Manifestations

RSV has two subtypes, A and B, with the former typically causing more severe disease. While both subtypes can simultaneously circulate during outbreaks, a few distinct genotypes of each subtype can predominate within a community. The dominant strains can also shift yearly. This shifting of viral strains, along with the waning protective immunity from natural infection, might account for frequent re-infections throughout life [38].

RSV usually causes mild and self-limited URTI in healthy older children and nonelderly adults, but certain patient populations are at risk for developing severe RSV infection, including premature or very young infants, elderly patients with comorbidities, or immunocompromised hosts [39–41]. RSV has been associated with apnea in young or preterm infants [42] and can cause severe LRTI in children including bronchiolitis, pneumonia, and acute respiratory failure [42]. Among adults infected with RSV, more than 80% are symptomatic, and lower respiratory tract signs and symptoms can occur in a quarter of the patients [43]. Signs of URTI include cough, rhinorrhea, and conjunctivitis, and compared to influenza, RSV is more frequently associated with nasal congestion, ear and sinus involvement, productive cough, and longer duration of illness [43].

RSV Infection in Transplantation

For transplant patients, RSV is a leading cause of viral respiratory tract infections [44, 45]. Among HSCT recipients, the incidence may be as high as 10% during winter months [6]. URTI precedes pneumonia in 80–90% of patients, and approximately 30–40% of patients with URTI progress to pneumonia after a median of 7 days [46]. Attributable mortality among HSCT patients ranges from 7% to 83% [47, 48], with more recent studies showing mortality rates of about 20–35% [49–54]. Risk factors for the development of LRTI include allogeneic transplant, mismatched or unrelated transplant, presence of graft versus host disease, myeloablative regimens, advanced age, prolonged lymphopenia, relapse of malignancy, and lack of engraftment [1, 6, 8, 9, 12, 13, 15, 55, 56].

For SOT recipients, RSV-associated mortality rate is significantly lower than that experienced in HSCT [57] although mortality rates among lung transplant patients of up to 20% have been reported [17, 37]. While there have been some reports of favorable outcomes in lung transplant recipients even in the absence of specific antiviral treatment [58], other studies suggest that up to 33% of RSV-infected patients develop long-term pulmonary dysfunction [23, 24, 37] and up to 60% have worsening of BOS stage [58].

Treatment of RSV

Available Agents for RSV Treatment

Treatment modalities for RSV are limited to ribavirin with or without the addition of immunomodulatory agents and/or corticosteroids. Currently, the only Food and Drug Administration (FDA)-approved therapy for RSV is aerosolized ribavirin (1-β-D-ribofuranosyl-1,2,4-triazole-3-carboximide), which was licensed in 1986 for the treatment of RSV LRTI in hospitalized high-risk infants and young children [59]. Ribavirin is a synthetic nucleoside analog with a broad spectrum of activities against many RNA and DNA viruses in vitro and in vivo. It competitively inhibits inosine monophosphate dehydrogenase and can be incorporated into the viral genome, leading to lethal mutagenesis [60]. The drug also has immunomodulatory properties that might contribute to its efficacy in vivo [61, 62].

The standard regimen of aerosolized ribavirin consists of a daily dose of 6 g delivered at a concentration of 20 mg/ml of sterile water for 18 h/day. Due to potential teratogenicity, the drug is usually administered to patients within a scavenging tent and preferably in a negative pressure room to prevent environmental contamination. After administration, the room needs to be cleaned to minimize secondary exposure to health care workers and visitors [48]. Women of childbearing potential should not care for or visit patients receiving aerosolized ribavirin. For ease of administration and improved compliance, the drug is often delivered with an intermittent dosing schedule at 2 g administered for 2–3 h every 8 h [63, 64]. In a randomized trial of 50 subjects, patients receiving intermittent vs continuous dosing had a lower incidence of progression from URTI to LRTI [65]. The reported duration of treatment is variable in the literature; the 4th European Conference on Infections in Leukaemia (ECIL-4) guidelines recommend a duration of 7–10 days [66].

Side effects of aerosolized ribavirin treatment include cough, dyspnea, bronchospasm, rash, nausea, headache, and conjunctival irritation. Patients can also experience claustrophobia and deterioration of pulmonary function. Ribavirin can also be administered intravenously or orally, with major side effects including hemolytic anemia, leukopenia, and hyperbilirubinemia [47].

Intravenous RSV-specific immunoglobulin (RSV-IVIG and palivizumab [PVZ]) were licensed initially for prevention of serious complications from RSV infection in high-risk children (refer to section "Immunoprophylaxis") [67], but they have also been employed for RSV treatment [68–72]. Intravenous immunoglobulin (IVIG) is also frequently used for the treatment of RSV and other severe viral infections in transplant recipients. The efficacy of these agents for prophylaxis or treatment among transplant patients has not been evaluated in randomized controlled trials although in an observational study of HSCT patients with RSV LRTI, multivariate analysis did not find any effect of antibody-based therapies on treatment outcomes [73].

Treatment of RSV in HSCT

The evaluation of any treatment modalities for RSV, or any other respiratory viruses, has been limited by the fact that most published studies are small observational studies which lack standardized definitions of URTI and LRTI, use different dosages and duration of therapy, and are subject to selection and publication bias. Among dozens of reports on the treatment of RSV in HSCT patients, there have only been two small randomized clinical trials. One study of aerosolized ribavirin was discontinued due to slow accrual, after enrollment of 14 patients in 5 years [69]. The other trial enrolled 50 patients and found that an intermittent dosing schedule of aerosolized ribavirin for treatment of RSV URTI was more effective than a continuous dosing schedule for prevention of progression to LRTI [64].

Two pooled analyses of published studies between 1980 and 2010 suggest that treatment of RSV URTI and LRTI with aerosolized ribavirin and IVIG reduces the risk of progression to LRTI in individuals with URTI and reduces mortality [47, 48]. When compared to no treatment, aerosolized ribavirin decreased the rate of progression to LRTI and mortality with the greatest impact observed when aerosolized ribavirin was given in combination with an immunomodulator. Specifically, when comparing aerosolized ribavirin treatment alone with no treatment, progression to LRTI was decreased from 47% to 25% and the mortality rate was reduced from 89% to 50% [47]. The addition of immunomodulators such as PVZ, IVIG, and/or RSV-IVIG to ribavirin compared to no treatment decreased progression to LTRI from 45% to 12% and mortality rate from 77% to 24%. There are paucity of reports on the use of intravenous or oral ribavirin, but the combined data suggest a benefit compared to no treatment. It is important to recognize that neither of these systematic reviews represented formal meta-analyses; there was no adjustment for confounders, and thus, results should be interpreted with caution. The only trial to date that evaluated PVZ as monotherapy for the treatment of RSV infection in HSCT recipients showed no benefit in prevention of progression to LRTI or mortality [74].

Overall, these analyses show a trend toward improved outcomes with regard to progression to LRTI and mortality among HSCT recipients treated with a combination of aerosolized ribavirin and immunomodulators than those treated with aerosolized ribavirin alone or with intravenous/oral ribavirin, or those given no treatment. However, the use of aerosolized ribavirin is cumbersome and very costly with the price increase in 2015 to $30,000 per day [75]. In addition, the aerosolized form of ribavirin is not available in all countries, and the intravenous form is not commercially available in the United States. The experience with oral ribavirin in HSCT is limited and warrants further evaluation, but some studies suggest that it may be a safe and effective alternative to aerosolized ribavirin for the treatment of RSV [51, 76–78]. In a retrospective study of 124 HSCT recipients with RSV infection, there was no difference in rates of progression to LRTI and mortality among patients receiving oral compared to aerosolized ribavirin [51]. The optimal dose of oral ribavirin for treatment of RSV is unclear and quite variable in the literature [79]. Commonly described dosing strategies include a fixed dose of 600–800 mg two or three times a day or a loading dose of 10 mg/kg followed by 20 mg/kg/day divided into three doses, adjusted for renal failure [51, 77, 79].

Treatment of RSV in SOT

Similar to the HSCT population, the mainstay of treatment for paramyxoviral infections in SOT populations has been aerosolized ribavirin [37, 80]. In an observational study, a combination of aerosolized ribavirin, IVIG, and corticosteroids was found to be safe and effective in preserving lung function in lung transplant recipients after RSV or PIV infections 29. Few studies have examined the role of oral ribavirin. Pelaez et al. [81] reported treatment of five lung transplant patients with RSV infection using oral ribavirin in combination with methylprednisolone and found this regimen well tolerated and effective with mean forced expiratory volume in 1 s (FEV1) returning to baseline with treatment. In a prospective observational study, oral ribavirin treatment in 38 patients with RSV, PIV, or HMPV infection was associated with earlier recovery of graft function and prevention of BOS as compared to 29 patients with only supportive care including corticosteroids [82]. In one study that evaluated lung transplant patients who received either aerosolized or oral ribavirin for RSV infection, no significant differences in 6-month outcomes were noted between the two groups, but variations in their adjunctive therapies, e.g., use of corticosteroids, IVIG, and/or montelukast, might have altered the patients' clinical response [83]. Intravenous ribavirin was also found to be a safe and cost-effective treatment among 18 patients with RSV after lung transplantation [84].

Overall, these studies support the use of ribavirin in treating RSV infection among SOT recipients although it is important to recognize that the evidence is limited to small, uncontrolled studies. There are significant variabilities among these studies regarding the dose and duration of treatment as well as the use of immunomodulating agents such as corticosteroids, IVIG, or PVZ as adjunctive measures.

More recently, a new agent presatovir (GS-5806), an orally bioavailable antiviral agent that inhibits fusion of RSV with host cell membranes, is being developed for treatment of RSV infection. Phase II clinical trials studying HSCT and lung transplant recipients were completed, and the data on lung transplant recipients has been published [85]. In this Phase 2b randomized controlled trial that enrolled a total of 61 lung transplant patients with RSV, presatovir was apparently well tolerated, but its use did not result in improved viral or clinical or outcomes.

Parainfluenza Viruses (PIVs)

Epidemiology and Clinical Manifestations

There are four distinct serotypes of PIVs, namely, PIV-1 to -4. These viruses can circulate throughout the year in most communities, although PIV-3, the dominant serotype affecting transplant populations, seems to have the highest prevalence during spring and summer seasons [38]. PIVs cause a spectrum of respiratory tract infections similar to RSV, but most are URTIs and result in fewer hospitalizations. PIV-1 and, to a lesser extent, PIV-2 are the principal causative agents of croup or laryngotracheobronchitis, primarily in children between the ages of 6 and 48 months. PIV-3 is most frequently associated with pneumonia and bronchiolitis; neonates, immunocompromised, and the elderly are at particular risk for severe disease. PIV-4 is infrequently detected and is thought to cause mostly asymptomatic or mild infections.

PIV Infection in Transplantation

Symptomatic PIV infection affects about 3–7% of HSCT recipients [2, 64, 86, 87] and approximately 3–5% of lung transplant recipients [28, 88]. LRTI can develop in up to 50% of PIV-infected HSCT patients, with associated mortality rate ranging from 12% to 57% [2, 8, 64, 86, 87, 89, 90]. Two large retrospective studies have evaluated PIV infections in HSCT and found that most patients (70–87%) presented with URTI, but 13–24% subsequently progressed to LRTI [2, 64]. Among those with LRTI, overall mortality at 30 days was 17–35% [2, 64]. Independent risk factors for progression to LRTI included receipt of corticosteroids at the time of URTI diagnosis, neutropenia, an APACHE II score >15, and respiratory coinfections. Independent predictors of death included relapsed or refractory underlying cancer, APACHE II score >15, and high-dose corticosteroid use considered in patients given cumulative dose of prednisolone >600 mg within 4 weeks of PIV diagnosis [2, 14]. Whether steroids are still important if adjusted for lymphopenia requires further study. While RSV infections are always symptomatic, asymptomatic shedding is present in about 1/3 of PIV-infected HSCT patients [91]. In a surveillance study of lung transplant recipients, asymptomatic PIV infection was present in 70% of patients [28].

PIV LRTI has also been associated with a significantly increased risk of severe airflow decline after HSCT when compared to RSV 31. For lung transplant patients, PIV has been associated with acute rejection and BOS [18, 28, 88, 92, 93].

Treatment of PIV

A number of studies reported treatment of PIV with ribavirin (see section "Treatment of RSV"), but most are limited to case reports or small series. For HSCT, both aerosolized [2, 86, 87, 94, 95] and oral ribavirin [96, 97] have been employed, although some patients received intravenous ribavirin when they did not respond to aerosolized or oral treatment [86, 98]. In a series that included 55 patients with PIV-3 LRTI, 31 were treated with aerosolized ribavirin with or without IVIG in a nonrandomized fashion. Such therapy did not appear to alter mortality from PIV-3 pneumonia or decrease the duration of viral shedding [2]. A more recent retrospective study evaluated 173 HSCT recipients with PIV infection [90]. Forty-one patients with LRTI were treated with aerosolized ribavirin with or without IVIG, but 100-day mortality of this group was similar to those with LRTI not treated with ribavirin. Overall, there is no convincing evidence that ribavirin is effective for treatment of PIV upper or lower tract disease in HCT recipients. Effective prophylaxis and treatment for PIV in HSCT population are desperately needed.

Successful treatment of PIV LRTI has been reported in heart transplant recipients with aerosolized ribavirin or with intravenous ribavirin plus methylprednisolone [99, 100] as well as in a kidney transplant recipients with aerosolized ribavirin and IVIG [101] although none of these studies included controls.

DAS181 is a novel sialidase fusion protein with activities against multiple strains of influenza and PIVs. It has been used for PIV treatment in a small number of HSCT and lung transplant recipients. The drug was found effective in most of these cases and was well tolerated [102–106]. A phase II, randomized, double-blind, placebo-controlled study to examine the effects of DAS181 in immunocompromised hosts with LRTI by PIV has been completed, but no results have been published to date.

Human Metapneumovirus (HMPV)

Epidemiology and Clinical Manifestations

HMPV was first described in 2001 among Dutch children with bronchitis [107], although serological studies indicate that it has been a cause of human infection since 1958 [108]. There are two subgroups of HMPV, A and B, and each with two clades, A1, A2, B1, and B2. All four subtypes co-circulate, while a single subtype tends to dominate each year [109]. HMPV has a worldwide distribution; it circulates in late winter to early spring in temperate climates and in late spring to summer in tropical regions [108].

HMPV may contribute to 12–20% of all previously virus-negative LRTI [110]. When compared to RSV, infection with HMPV tends to occur in slightly older children and cause milder symptoms, but severe disease can occur among small children, elderly, and those with immunosuppression or chronic medical conditions [111]. Clinical manifestations range from mild URTIs to severe pneumonia. Elderly patients are much more likely to experience dyspnea and wheezing than young adults, and hoarseness is a more common complaint when compared to other paramyxoviruses [112]. Among hospitalized patients and recipients of HSCT, wheezing is prominent and noted in up to 80–90% of patients [113, 114].

HMPV Infection in Transplantation

For patients with hematologic malignancies or HSCT, HMPV is responsible for approximately 3–14% of RVIs [114–117]. A systematic review of HMPV infections among HSCT recipients and hematologic malignancy patients found that despite lack of directed antiviral therapy, overall mortality rates are low (6%) unless patients progress to LRTI (27%) [118]. Approximately one-third of patients with HMPV URTI develop LRTI [119].

In lung transplant recipients, HMPV is responsible for 14–30% of RVIs with a similar morbidity when compared to other community-acquired respiratory viruses [3, 35, 36, 120]. Acute HPMV infection has been associated with allograft rejection [36]. In a study [120] of 89 lung transplant patients who presented with RVIs, HMPV and RSV were equally prevalent and had similar clinical manifestations, although severe bronchospasm was less common with HMPV. A significant number of patients with either HMPV or RSV infection developed graft dysfunction (63% and 72%, respectively), but onset or progression of BOS occurred only in patients with RSV (38%) at 6 months and in none with HMPV. Another study of 60 lung transplant patients also showed that HMPV infection increased the risk of acute graft rejection without associated chronic rejection or BOS [3, 120].

Treatment of HMPV

Treatment for HMPV is largely supportive, as there is currently no antiviral therapy licensed for this virus. Ribavirin is active against HMPV in vitro and in animal models [121, 122]. In clinical settings, there have been scattered reports in the literature describing HMPV cases treated successfully using aerosolized, oral, or intravenous ribavirin given with or without IVIG [3, 120, 123–126]. However, these studies did not include any untreated control groups, and the efficacy of these regimens cannot be determined. Some have suggested that ribavirin with IVIG may be considered as a treatment option for patients with severe disease [125], but this approach is not routinely used.

Several new approaches for treatment of HMPV are in development, including monoclonal antibodies against the fusion protein [127, 128] or synthetic peptides with antiviral activities [129]. Their efficacies against HMPV have been demonstrated in vitro and in animal models, but studies in human have not been reported.

Diagnosis of Paramyxoviruses

Radiographic Evaluation

LRTI by respiratory viruses produces a spectrum of imaging findings; with the most common high-resolution chest computed tomography (HRCT) scan, observations include small, poorly defined centrilobular nodules or tree-in-bud opacities, ground-glass opacities, bronchial wall thickening, and airspace consolidations, which may be difficult to differentiate from other causes of pulmonary consolidation [130–137]. There is considerable overlap in the imaging appearance of viral, bacterial, mycobacterial, and fungal respiratory tract infections in transplant population. The findings such as tree-in-bud opacities, bronchial wall thickening, and peribronchiolar consolidation may suggest a viral etiology [138]. HRCT findings between immunocompetent and immunocompromised patients are relatively similar [139], but infection with co-pathogens is common among transplant recipients, thus complicating interpretation of radiographic findings. Correlation with patient immune status, recent treatment, and exposure history, as well as epidemiologic factors, are essential to help narrow the list of possible etiologies both infectious and noninfectious and to guide diagnostic testing and appropriate therapy [130].

Laboratory Diagnosis of Paramyxoviruses

Laboratory diagnosis of respiratory viruses is usually made by analysis of respiratory secretions. Samples can be obtained as a nasal wash, nasopharyngeal or throat swab, bronchoalveolar lavage, or, for those incubated, tracheal aspirate. Detection of the virus in the respiratory samples can be performed by cell culture, antigen testing, and PCR.

Viral isolation by cell culture used to be the gold standard for diagnosis but has largely been replaced by molecular studies. Reverse transcriptase (RT)–PCR is now routinely used for respiratory viral diagnosis for the detection of RNA viruses in respiratory secretions [140] and has higher sensitivity than either viral culture or antigen detection assays, particularly in immunocompromised patients [91, 140]. Compared with culture, the sensitivity and specificity of RT-PCR techniques can reach 100% and 95–98%, respectively [141–143]. PCR-based tests for respiratory viral detection are often designed as part of a multiplex PCR assay that can allow detection of multiple respiratory pathogens simultaneously [144], and rapid point-of-care tests are being developed as well [145, 146].

Transmission and Prevention of Paramyxovirus Infection

The modes of transmission of PIVs and HMPV are not as well studied as RSV, but these respiratory viruses are mostly transmitted by direct person-to-person contact, through exposure to nasopharyngeal secretions from infected individuals such as respiratory droplets or by self-inoculation after touching contaminated surfaces has also been described [147, 148]. Outbreaks of RSV, PIVs, or HMPV have been reported in outpatient clinics, in long-term care facilities, and in hospitals, including hematology and HSCT units [94, 149–153]. To prevent transmission of respiratory viruses in health care setting, policies and procedures regarding patients with respiratory viruses should be formulated; in particular, compliance with proper hand hygiene and contact precautions are of paramount importance. Other infection control measures include isolating infected patients in private room, cohorting patients, and/or limiting transport of patients from their rooms. During a nosocomial outbreak, personnel caring for infected patients should be restricted from caring for uninfected high-risk patients if possible [154–156].

Immunoprophylaxis

PVZ is a RSV-specific humanized monoclonal antibody directed against the F glycoprotein of RSV and is FDA approved for immunoprophylaxis against RSV in high-risk children. Data for its use in immunocompromised adult patients are limited [48, 68], with only one uncontrolled study in the literature reporting the use of PVZ as immunoprophylaxis during an RSV outbreak in an adult HSCT unit [150]. RSV-IVIG prophylaxis has also been studied in high-risk adult HSCT recipients; an increase in antibody titers against RSV was demonstrated, but the study was underpowered to evaluate its efficacy [157]. There are several monoclonal antibodies against RSV under development.

Vaccines

Despite the major clinical importance of paramyxoviruses, there is currently no vaccine approved for these viruses in humans. Using various strategies for vaccine development, those tested in animal models include live-attenuated virus vaccines including chimeric and recombinant variety, inactivated virus vaccines, and subunit vaccines. A number of them are currently in phase I–II clinical trials [158–161].

Other Strategies

In a retrospective study of 37 HSCT patients with pretransplant RSV URTI, 34 patients had their transplant delayed or conditioning aborted [162]. Overall, RSV pneumonia occurred in 1 of 34 patients for whom HSCT was delayed, compared with two of three patients for whom there was no delay. This study suggested that for HSCT candidates with pretransplant RSV URTI, a delay of HSCT might reduce the risk of developing RSV pneumonia. Thus, the strategy of delaying transplantation to prevent progression of a viral URTI to LRTI is recommended unless precluded by progression of underlying malignancy. There are limited data for other respiratory viruses [66, 147] although some proposed guidance is available (Table 40.1) [163].

Orthomyxovirus: Influenza

Influenza belongs to the family *Orthomyxoviridae* with three types, influenza A, influenza, B, and influenza C virus. Influenza A viruses are further classified into subtypes based on their hemagglutinins (HA) and neuraminidases (NA). One of the unique features of influenza virus is the frequency by which antigenic variation occurs which is the reason that influenza continues to be a cause of major epidemics. Annual variation of the influenza virus is due to relatively minor antigenic changes within the HA and/or NA and is known as antigenic drift. Major changes in HA or NA through genetic reassortment or a major mutation are known as antigenic shift and occur once every 10–30 years. This results in an entirely novel strain to which the population has no immunity, leading to an unhindered global spread; the last pandemic occurred in 2009 with the emergence of a novel strain of influenza A/H1N1.

Table 40.1 Recommendations for respiratory viral infections prior to hematopoietic stem cell transplantation

Virus	Recommendation for URTI	Recommendation for LRTI
RSV	Delay transplant if possible If not possible to delay, consider oral ribavirin	Delay transplant; consider ribavirin if delay is not feasible (anecdotal data)
Influenza virus	Delay transplant if possible and treat If not possible to delay, treat	Delay transplant and treat
Parainfluenza virus	Delay transplant if possible If not possible to delay, supportive care	Delay transplant; consider ribavirin if delay is not feasible (anecdotal data)
Metapneumovirus	Delay transplant if possible	Delay transplant; no data on ribavirin
Rhinovirus	No delay needed for URTI	Delay transplant for allogeneic transplant if feasible
Coronavirus	No data	No data
Bocavirus	No data	No data

Adapted from Waghmare et al. [163]

Table 40.2 Role of corticosteroid treatment in progression of respiratory viral illnesses

	Progression				Mortality			
Virus	Steroid dose per day		HR (95% CI)	P-value	Steroid dose per day		HR (95% CI)	P-value
RSV	>2 mg/kg	+	1.4 (0.4–5.2)	0.19[3]	>2 mg/kg	+ + +	3.3 (1.7–6.3)	<0.001[11]
Influenza	≥1 mg/kg	+/–	0.8 (0.2–2.4)	0.60[46]	≥1 mg/kg	+/–	1.1 (0.3–3.5)	0.87[46]
PIV	>2 mg/kg	+ + +	4.6 (1.2–17.0)	0.02[74]	>2 mg/kg	+ + +	3.2 (1.5–7.2)	0.004[13]
HMPV or RSV	No data				Any steroid	+ + +	5.0 (1.8–14)	0.002[16]
					≥1 mg/kg	+ + + +	7.1 (2.3–22)	<0.001[16]

Adapted from Waghmare et al. [163]
RSV respiratory syncytial virus, *PIV* parainfluenza virus, *HMPV* human metapneumovirus, *HR* hazard ratio

Epidemiology

Influenza is a significant cause of morbidity and mortality in transplant patients. In recipients of solid organ transplantation, up to 42% of URTIs and 48% of LRTIs may be due to influenza infection and the annual between 1% and 4% [164]. During the 2009 H1N1 pandemic, mortality rates ranged from 0 to 8% in most case series [4] although one study reported a mortality rate of 21% among lung transplant recipients [165]. Of the organ transplants, lung transplant recipients appear to be at the highest risk; in one study, the incidence of influenza was 10–15 times higher in recipients of lung transplantation compared with recipients of other solid organs such as kidney or liver [166].

The incidence of influenza among HSCT ranges between 1% and 4% with 7–44% of such patients may develop LRTI. Death rates associated with influenza in HSCT recipients are higher than in SOT. Among patients with LRTI, mortality rates ranged from 15% to 28% and case fatality rates during the 2009 H1N1 pandemic ranged from 0 to 38% [4]. The main risk factor for disease progression to LRTI was lymphopenia; allogeneic HSCT, infection during early post-transplant period, presence of graft-versus-host disease, myeloablative preparatory regimen, and delayed initiation of antiviral therapy were other risk factors [1, 11, 12, 167]. Of interest, concomitant corticosteroid use has not been associated with an increased risk for progression to LRTI, a need for mechanical ventilation, or infection associated death; however, patients given systemic higher doses (≥1 mg/kg) of corticosteroids may be predisposed to prolonged viral shedding [11, 168]. The potential role of corticosteroids in influencing risk of progression to LRTI and mortality of influenza and other respiratory viral infections is summarized in Table 40.2 [163].

Clinical Manifestations

Clinical manifestations of influenza are similar to those in immunocompetent patients. In a multicenter cohort study of 242 organ transplant patients during the 2009 H1N1 pandemic, the most common presenting symptoms were cough (91%), fever (85%), myalgias (51%), gastrointestinal symptoms (44%), rhinorrhea (43%), and sore throat (43%) [169]. In a multicenter cohort study of 286 HSCT recipients during the 2009 H1N1 pandemic, the most common presenting symptoms were cough (85%), fever (81%), rhinorrhea (49%), myalgias (29%), and sore throat (23%) [170]. However, atypical presentations may occur in those with significant immunosuppression, which may include fever as the only presenting symptom or afebrile patient with rhinorrhea alone. It is speculated that corticosteroid use and blunting of the cytokine response associated with acute influenza infection in these patients may contribute to the reduction or absence of systemic symptoms in selected patients.

The primary complication of influenza infection in transplant patients is progression from URTI to LRTI which can lead to acute lung injury and death. Morbidity and mortality appear to be greatest among HSCT and lung transplant recipients. While diffuse or peribronchial ground-glass opacity is the typical radiographic appearance in patients with LRTI, centrilobular nodules and frank lower lobe consolidation can also be observed [171]. Coinfection with other viral, bacterial, or fungal pathogens may occur and was reported in 29% of patients in a multicenter study of SOT recipients with pandemic influenza A/H1N1 [172]. Compared to those with viral co-pathogens, patients with bacterial or fungal coinfections had worse outcomes [11, 172]. Although uncommon, influenza can also a cause a variety of extrapulmonary complications including myocarditis, myositis, encephalopathy, renal failure, severe diarrhea, and pneumomediastinum [166, 173, 174]. Virus-associated hemophagocytic syndrome has been reported as a severe complication of pandemic H1N1 leading to multiorgan failure [175]. As discussed previously, several studies suggest an association between RVIs including influenza and allograft rejection/BOS in the case of lung transplants, while others have not; a prospective study is needed to better characterize the impact of these infections on long-term sequelae [19, 44, 172, 176].

In healthy adults, seasonal influenza virus shedding ranges from 5 to 7 days and may extend beyond 1 week in hospitalized patients [177, 178] and even longer in transplant recipients. The median duration of viral shedding among allogeneic HSCT recipients was between 11 and 12 days compared to 1 week among recipients of autologous transplants [11, 179]. Prolonged viral shedding beyond 2 weeks and, in some cases, for months has been described in HSCT recipient. Risk factors for prolonged viral shedding include the use of corticosteroids at dosages ≥1 mg/kg per day and use of bone marrow and cord blood versus peripheral blood stem cell.

Diagnosis

There are several methods available for detection of influenza including rapid antigen, direct immunofluorescence antibody (DFA), viral culture, and PCR. As for other respiratory viruses, molecular tests have largely replaced these other testing modalities. In a study evaluating test characteristics of four different diagnostic assays during the 2009 H1N1 pandemic, PCR was found to have the greatest sensitivity and specificity. Given their improved sensitivity and specificity over other methods, PCR or other nucleic acid-based detection assays are preferred for the diagnosis of influenza infection in this susceptible patient population. Multiplex PCRs have the added advantage of identifying other causes of respiratory viral infections as well.

Treatment

Currently, there are two major classes of antiviral agents with activity against influenza: adamantanes which block the viral M2 protein ion channel, thereby preventing fusion of the virus with host cell membranes, and neuraminidase inhibitors which prevent the release of progeny virus from infected cells. While the adamantanes, amantadine, and rimantadine are only active against influenza A, the neuraminidase inhibitors oseltamivir and zanamivir are active against both influenza A and B viruses, although reduced effectiveness of oseltamivir has occasionally been reported for influenza B virus [180]. The development of resistance to the adamantanes among influenza A virus has substantially limited their utility in clinical practice. Although 2008–2009 seasonal H1N1 remained susceptible to the adamantanes, resistance emerged among seasonal H3N2 in 2003 and was widespread among 2009 pandemic H1N1 viruses. Oseltamivir resistance first emerged in 2007 among seasonal H1N1 viruses and was described during the 2009 H1N1 pandemic [181]. Oseltamivir resistance is primarily conferred by the H275Y mutation which does not result in cross-resistance to zanamivir. PCR testing is available for the detection of the H275Y mutation. In 2010, the S247 N mutation was detected in strains of 2009 pandemic H1N1 collected in Asia and was found to confer low to moderate oseltamivir and zanamivir resistance [182]. Otherwise, there has been very little zanamivir resistance reported to date, and thus, it is recommended for the treatment of oseltamivir-resistant influenza infection.

Because resistance patterns evolve over time, clinicians should become familiar with local patterns of influenza circulation in their communities throughout each influenza season and refer to the Centers for Disease Control and Prevention (CDC) influenza website (http://www.cdc.gov/flu) [183] for updated information regarding antiviral resistance and recommendations regarding antiviral use. In addition, antiviral resistance appears to occur more commonly among severely immunocompromised patients likely due to prolonged viral shedding [184, 185]. During the 2009 H1N1 pandemic, the majority of patients with oseltamivir-resistant virus reported to the CDC were HSCT recipients or patients who had a hematologic malignancy receiving chemo- or immunosuppressive therapy [186].

There have been no randomized clinical trials of antiviral therapy for influenza in transplant patients. All randomized trials have included healthy adult outpatients who were treated within 48 h after symptom onset and, in aggregate, demonstrate a reduction in duration of symptoms by ~1 day and time to return to normal activity [180]. Although further study is needed regarding the role of antiviral therapy >48 h of symptom onset, the 2009 IDSA guidelines for management of seasonal influenza suggest that antiviral therapy initiated >48 h after symptom onset may be beneficial in hospitalized patients based on a prospective cohort study [167, 180, 187]. Observational studies suggest that early antiviral therapy of HSCT recipients with influenza URTI is effective in preventing progression to LRTI [8, 11, 168, 179, 188]. Among SOT recipients, a multicenter study found that early antiviral therapy was associated with a lower incidence of hospitalization and likelihood of ICU admission as compared to delayed (>48 h after symptom onset) therapy [169]. Although antiviral therapy may have its greatest value when initiated early, it is felt that symptomatic transplant patients may benefit even beyond 48 h if they have evidence of viral replication, and in general, treatment of all symptomatic transplant patients is recommended regardless of the duration of symptoms [189–191].

The optimal dose and duration of antiviral therapy in transplant patients has not been established. Oseltamivir has been studied at doses of 75 mg or 150 mg twice daily in immunocompetent patients with seasonal influenza; there was no significant advantage of the higher dose although a slightly higher rate of adverse effects was observed [192, 193]. However, due to concerns over higher viral loads, prolonged viral shedding, and uncertain drug absorption particularly in those patients undergoing chemotherapy or with gastrointestinal graft-versus-host disease, some experts suggest using the higher dose in transplant patients particularly if absorption is uncertain, in those patients with severe LRTI or who are critically ill [189–191]. Based on clinical studies in healthy adults, the recommended duration of treatment of influenza in immunocompetent patients is 5 days [180]. However, transplant patients may need longer durations of therapy due to prolonged viral shedding. Some experts recommend treating all SOT recipients until viral replication has ceased; authors recommend checking PCR once a week and treat until negative [190, 191]. Others have suggested a 10-day course for HSCT recipients and extending treatment in those patients with pneumonia, ongoing symptoms, or viral shedding [189]. Resistance testing should be considered in those patients with persistent viral shedding or who progress despite antiviral therapy.

While most literature in transplant recipients has focused on oseltamivir, inhaled zanamivir appears to be a reasonable alternative. IV zanamivir is currently available for compassionate use, and there is limited published experience among transplant recipients where it has been used with some benefit among patients with oseltamivir-resistant influenza or severe disease [194].

Peramivir, a parenteral neuraminidase inhibitor, was FDA approved in 2014 for the treatment of uncomplicated influenza infection in adults who have been ill for ≤2 days. There are limited data regarding the use of peramivir in transplant recipients. Of note, the H275Y mutation which confers oseltamivir resistance also confers cross-resistance to peramivir.

There are currently no data that indicates a clear clinical benefit of combination antiviral therapy over single drug therapy. A randomized, double-blind, multicenter phase 2 trial found that combination antiviral therapy with oseltamivir, amantadine and ribavirin reduced day 3 viral shedding compared to oseltamivir monotherapy, but there was no difference in clinical outcomes including resolution of symptoms or fever or time to recovery after illness [195].

Table 40.3 summarizes antiviral options for treatment of influenza.

Table 40.3 Antiviral options for the treatment of influenza

Antiviral agent	Dose	Parenteral formulation?	Side effects	Remarks
Oseltamivir	75 mg PO twice daily	Yes, investigational	Gastrointestinal: nausea, vomiting, diarrhea Neurologic: confusion, delirium, depressed consciousness (mostly reported among Japanese adolescents and adults)	Some experts recommend higher doses (150 mg PO BID) in transplant patients who are critically ill with LRTI
Zanamivir	2 puffs (10 mg) inhaled twice daily	Yes, investigational	Bronchospasm, cough, headache, dizziness, sinusitis, nausea, diarrhea	Little cross-resistance with oseltamivir
Peramivir	600 mg IV once daily	Yes (only available as parenteral formulation)	Gastrointestinal: nausea, vomiting, diarrhea Neutropenia	Cross-resistance with oseltamivir exists.
Amantadine	100 mg PO twice daily	No	Neurologic: insomnia, lethargy, inability to concentrate, dizziness Gastrointestinal: nausea	No longer routinely recommended due to high incidence of resistant influenza unless circulating strain known to be susceptible
Rimantadine	100 mg PO twice daily	No	Gastrointestinal Neurologic (less common than amantadine): lightheadedness, insomnia, inability to concentrate, nervousness	No longer routinely recommended due to high incidence of resistant influenza unless circulating strain known to be susceptible

Prevention

Annual influenza vaccination is a key component of infection prevention among HSCT and SOT recipients. There are several types of influenza vaccines: standard-dose inactivated influenza vaccines (IIV), available either as a trivalent or quadrivalent injection, high-dose IIV (available as a trivalent injection), live attenuated influenza vaccine (LAIV), intradermal IIV, and recombinant egg-free IIV. All vaccines are modified annually based on the anticipated circulating strains during the upcoming influenza season. The LAIV is contraindicated in immunocompromised patients and should not be used in transplant recipients. The intradermal IIV has not been evaluated in transplant recipients.

For HSCT recipients, influenza vaccination is recommended ≥6 months post-transplant and beginning 4 months following transplant if there is a community influenza outbreak [196]. If the vaccine is administered earlier than 6 months after HSCT, a second dose should be considered. The timing of vaccine administration appears to predict response with one study demonstrating that influenza immunization at least 6 months after HCT was 80% effective in preventing influenza [197]. The high-dose trivalent IIV is FDA approved for individuals ≥65 years of age and was found in a multicenter randomized clinical trial to induce higher antibody responses and improved protection against influenza compared to standard dose IIV [198]. In a phase I trial, HSCT recipients randomized to receive high-dose trivalent IIV had evidence of greater immunogenicity when compared to those receiving standard-dose trivalent IIV [199]. There was a higher frequency of injection site reactions, but most were mild. There are ongoing studies to further evaluate the role of high-dose IIV in HSCT.

For SOT recipients, influenza vaccination is recommended 3–6 months after transplant [164]. The immunogenicity of influenza vaccine following SOT is variable depending on the type of transplant, time from transplant, and immunosuppressive regimens. Among SOT recipients, overall responses based on seroprotection or seroconversion have ranged from 15% to 93% with greater responses observed several years after kidney transplant and lower responses seen in lung transplant [164]. Although there is a theoretical concern that influenza immunization may be associated with early allograft rejection or allosensitization of patients after transplant, this has not been observed in clinical trials [200]. In a randomized, double-blind trial of 172 SOT recipients, high-dose influenza vaccine demonstrated significantly better immunogenicity than the standard-dose vaccine [201]; no increased risk of rejection was reported although the study was not powered to address this outcome.

Immunization of health care workers and household contacts of transplant recipients is a critical component of influenza prevention and is strongly recommended in published guidelines [147, 164]. A systematic review suggests that vaccination of healthcare workers reduces influenza-like illness and all-cause mortality in the elderly [202]. Due to the theoretical risk of transmission of LAIV, the CDC recommends that IIV not be used for household members and health care workers who have close contact with severely immunosuppressed patients such as recipient of hematopoietic stem cell allograft transplantation during those periods in which the patient requires care in a protective environment. Those persons who receive LAIV should avoid providing care for and contact with such patients for 7 days after vaccination.

Although influenza vaccination is the primary tool for influenza prevention, antiviral chemoprophylaxis may be considered as a prevention strategy in selected situations. The 2009 IDSA Guidelines for Management of Seasonal Influenza recommends consideration of antiviral chemoprophylaxis in high-risk patients during the 2 weeks after vaccination before an adequate immune response develops if influenza is circulating in the community [180]. It should also be considered among transplant recipients following exposure within the previous 48 h to an individual with influenza, particularly among those for whom the vaccine is contraindicated, unavailable, or expected to have low effectiveness such as patients with severe immune suppression. The choice of chemoprophylactic agent depends on the susceptibility pattern of the circulating influenza strain.

Human Coronaviruses (HCoV) and Human Rhinoviruses (HRV)

Epidemiology

HRVs and HCoVs are also common causes of RVIs in human, classified into the *Picornaviridiae* family (genus *Enterovirus*) and the *Coronaviriae* family, respectively. Approximately 100 serotypes of HRV have been identified. In comparison, HCoV-229E and HCoV-OC43 were the only two known HCoVs for >40 years. In 2004, a new HCoV was identified as the causative agent of the outbreak of Severe Acute Respiratory Syndrome (SARS) and was named SARS-CoV. Subsequently, two other new HCoVs, NL63 and HKU1, were discovered in 2004 and 2005, respectively. In the latter part of 2012, another novel CoV was identified as the cause of severe respiratory illness in two adults from the Middle East [203] and was termed Middle East respiratory syndrome coronavirus (MERS CoV). Similar to SARS-CoV, this virus can also cause severe, life-threatening disease. The ability of these emerging HCoVs to cause major outbreaks can be a potential threat to global public health and economy [204].

HCoV and HRV in Transplantation

In immunocompetent hosts, HRVs and HCoVs usually cause URTIs, but HCoVs can also cause croup, wheezing, as well as pneumonia, which can be severe with significant mortality, as in the case of SARS. The significance of HRV and HCoV in transplant populations has not been well established. According to a prospective study of HSCT recipients [5], infection with these viruses appears common in the first 100 days after allogeneic transplant, with day 100 cumulative incidence estimated as 22% for HRV and 11% for HCoV. HRV infection was associated with URTI signs and symptoms, but HCoV infection was asymptomatic. More than half of the infected patients had prolonged viral shedding for more than 3 weeks, and about 13% shed virus for more than 3 months [5]; only a few patients developed LRTI in that study. Fatal pneumonia associated with HRV and HCoV have been reported among HSCT recipients [205–207]. Recent studies suggested that HRV and HCoV LRTI with viral detection in the BAL are associated with mortality rates similar to those seen with RSV, PIV, or influenza viruses [10, 208].

For SOT, HRV and HCoV are frequently isolated among lung transplant patients [23, 25, 28], but a majority of these patients can be asymptomatic, according to a prospective surveillance study [28]. As discussed previously, RVI can increase the risk for developing acute rejection and/or BOS even with asymptomatic infections [23, 25, 28], but whether HRV or HCoV infection confer the same level of risk as compared to the paramyxoviruses or influenza cannot be delineated from these studies.

Currently, there are no specific agents licensed for the treatment of HRV and HCoV, but antiviral therapy for enteroviruses is under intense research.

Conclusions and Future Directions

Respiratory viral infections are common and associated with significant morbidity and mortality among patients undergoing hematopoietic stem cells and solid organ transplantation. The optimal management of these infections is limited by insufficient randomized treatment data as well as a limited new and novel antiviral drugs being investigated for potential clinical use. Large, preferably multicenter prospective, randomized trials are essential to (1) assess preferred therapy for life-threatening infections such as RSV, (2) define the role of combination antivirals for influenza virus infections, and (3) determine the use of adjunctive immunomodulatory therapy and/or corticosteroids in the management of these infections among the highly susceptible transplant population. The evaluation of novel long-lasting potent monoclonal antibodies for prevention may be warranted.

References

1. Schiffer JT, Kirby K, Sandmaier B, Storb R, Corey L, Boeckh M. Timing and severity of community acquired respiratory virus infections after myeloablative versus non-myeloablative hematopoietic stem cell transplantation. Haematologica. 2009;94:1101–8.
2. Nichols WG, Corey L, Gooley T, Davis C, Boeckh M. Parainfluenza virus infections after hematopoietic stem cell transplantation: risk factors, response to antiviral therapy, and effect on transplant outcome. Blood. 2001;98:573–8.
3. Weinberg A, Lyu DM, Li S, Marquesen J, Zamora MR. Incidence and morbidity of human metapneumovirus and other community-acquired respiratory viruses in lung transplant recipients. Transpl Infect Dis. 2010;12:330–5.
4. Renaud C, Campbell AP. Changing epidemiology of respiratory viral infections in hematopoietic cell transplant recipients and solid organ transplant recipients. Curr Opin Infect Dis. 2011;24: 333–43.
5. Milano F, Campbell AP, Guthrie KA, et al. Human rhinovirus and coronavirus detection among allogeneic hematopoietic stem cell transplantation recipients. Blood. 2010;115:2088–94.
6. Nichols WG, Gooley T, Boeckh M. Community-acquired respiratory syncytial virus and parainfluenza virus infections after hematopoietic stem cell transplantation: the Fred Hutchinson Cancer Research Center experience. Biol Blood Marrow Transplant. 2001;7(Suppl):11S–5S.
7. Champlin RE, Whimbey E. Community respiratory virus infections in bone marrow transplant recipients: the M.D. Anderson Cancer Center experience. Biol Blood Marrow Transplant. 2001;7(Suppl):8S–10S.
8. Chemaly RF, Ghosh S, Bodey GP, et al. Respiratory viral infections in adults with hematologic malignancies and human stem cell transplantation recipients: a retrospective study at a major cancer center. Medicine (Baltimore). 2006;85:278–87.
9. Whimbey E, Champlin RE, Couch RB, et al. Community respiratory virus infections among hospitalized adult bone marrow transplant recipients. Clin Infect Dis. 1996;22:778–82.
10. Seo S, Waghmare A, Scott EM, et al. Human rhinovirus detection in the lower respiratory tract of hematopoietic cell transplant recipients: association with mortality. Haematologica. 2017;102:1120–30.
11. Nichols WG, Guthrie KA, Corey L, Boeckh M. Influenza infections after hematopoietic stem cell transplantation: risk factors, mortality, and the effect of antiviral therapy. Clin Infect Dis. 2004;39: 1300–6.
12. Ljungman P, Ward KN, Crooks BN, et al. Respiratory virus infections after stem cell transplantation: a prospective study from the infectious diseases working party of the European Group for Blood and Marrow Transplantation. Bone Marrow Transplant. 2001;28:479–84.
13. Kim YJ, Guthrie KA, Waghmare A, et al. Respiratory syncytial virus in hematopoietic cell transplant recipients: factors determining progression to lower respiratory tract disease. J Infect Dis. 2014;209:1195–204.
14. Seo S, Xie H, Leisenring WM, et al. Risk factors for parainfluenza virus lower respiratory tract disease after hematopoietic cell transplantation. Biol Blood Marrow Transplant. 2019;25(1):163–71.
15. Shah DP, Ghantoji SS, Ariza-Heredia EJ, et al. Immunodeficiency scoring index to predict poor outcomes in hematopoietic cell transplant recipients with RSV infections. Blood. 2014;123:3263–8.
16. Billings JL, Hertz MI, Wendt CH. Community respiratory virus infections following lung transplantation. Transpl Infect Dis. 2001;3:138–48.
17. Palmer SM Jr, Henshaw NG, Howell DN, Miller SE, Davis RD, Tapson VF. Community respiratory viral infection in adult lung transplant recipients. Chest. 1998;113:944–50.

18. Vilchez R, McCurry K, Dauber J, et al. Influenza and parainfluenza respiratory viral infection requiring admission in adult lung transplant recipients. Transplantation. 2002;73:1075–8.
19. Lopez-Medrano F, Aguado JM, Lizasoain M, et al. Clinical implications of respiratory virus infections in solid organ transplant recipients: a prospective study. Transplantation. 2007;84:851–6.
20. Dudek AZ, Mahaseth H, DeFor TE, Weisdorf DJ. Bronchiolitis obliterans in chronic graft-versus-host disease: analysis of risk factors and treatment outcomes. Biol Blood Marrow Transplant. 2003;9:657–66.
21. Belperio JA, Lake K, Tazelaar H, Keane MP, Strieter RM, Lynch JP 3rd. Bronchiolitis obliterans syndrome complicating lung or heart-lung transplantation. Semin Respir Crit Care Med. 2003;24:499–530.
22. Fishman JA. Infection in solid-organ transplant recipients. N Engl J Med. 2007;357:2601–14.
23. Gottlieb J, Schulz TF, Welte T, et al. Community-acquired respiratory viral infections in lung transplant recipients: a single season cohort study. Transplantation. 2009;87:1530–7.
24. Khalifah AP, Hachem RR, Chakinala MM, et al. Respiratory viral infections are a distinct risk for bronchiolitis obliterans syndrome and death. Am J Respir Crit Care Med. 2004;170:181–7.
25. Kumar D, Erdman D, Keshavjee S, et al. Clinical impact of community-acquired respiratory viruses on bronchiolitis obliterans after lung transplant. Am J Transplant. 2005;5:2031–6.
26. Milstone AP, Brumble LM, Barnes J, et al. A single-season prospective study of respiratory viral infections in lung transplant recipients. Eur Respir J. 2006;28:131–7.
27. Husain S, Singh N. Bronchiolitis obliterans and lung transplantation: evidence for an infectious etiology. Semin Respir Infect. 2002;17:310–4.
28. Kumar D, Husain S, Chen MH, et al. A prospective molecular surveillance study evaluating the clinical impact of community-acquired respiratory viruses in lung transplant recipients. Transplantation. 2010;89:1028–33.
29. Liu V, Dhillon GS, Weill D. A multi-drug regimen for respiratory syncytial virus and parainfluenza virus infections in adult lung and heart-lung transplant recipients. Transpl Infect Dis. 2010;12:38–44.
30. Fisher CE, Preiksaitis CM, Lease ED, et al. Symptomatic respiratory virus infection and chronic lung allograft dysfunction. Clin Infect Dis. 2016;62:313–9.
31. Erard V, Chien JW, Kim HW, et al. Airflow decline after myeloablative allogeneic hematopoietic cell transplantation: the role of community respiratory viruses. J Infect Dis. 2006;193:1619–25.
32. Versluys AB, Rossen JW, van Ewijk B, Schuurman R, Bierings MB, Boelens JJ. Strong association between respiratory viral infection early after hematopoietic stem cell transplantation and the development of life-threatening acute and chronic alloimmune lung syndromes. Biol Blood Marrow Transplant. 2010;16:782–91.
33. Au BK, Au MA, Chien JW. Bronchiolitis obliterans syndrome epidemiology after allogeneic hematopoietic cell transplantation. Biol Blood Marrow Transplant. 2011;17:1072–8.
34. Chien JW, Duncan S, Williams KM, Pavletic SZ. Bronchiolitis obliterans syndrome after allogeneic hematopoietic stem cell transplantation-an increasingly recognized manifestation of chronic graft-versus-host disease. Biol Blood Marrow Transplant. 2010;16:S106–14.
35. Gerna G, Vitulo P, Rovida F, et al. Impact of human metapneumovirus and human cytomegalovirus versus other respiratory viruses on the lower respiratory tract infections of lung transplant recipients. J Med Virol. 2006;78:408–16.
36. Larcher C, Geltner C, Fischer H, Nachbaur D, Muller LC, Huemer HP. Human metapneumovirus infection in lung transplant recipients: clinical presentation and epidemiology. J Heart Lung Transplant. 2005;24:1891–901.
37. McCurdy LH, Milstone A, Dummer S. Clinical features and outcomes of paramyxoviral infection in lung transplant recipients treated with ribavirin. J Heart Lung Transplant. 2003;22:745–53.
38. Hall CB. Respiratory syncytial virus and parainfluenza virus. N Engl J Med. 2001;344:1917–28.
39. Boyce TG, Mellen BG, Mitchel EF Jr, Wright PF, Griffin MR. Rates of hospitalization for respiratory syncytial virus infection among children in medicaid. J Pediatr. 2000;137:865–70.
40. Duncan CB, Walsh EE, Peterson DR, Lee FE, Falsey AR. Risk factors for respiratory failure associated with respiratory syncytial virus infection in adults. J Infect Dis. 2009;200:1242–6.
41. Walsh EE, Peterson DR, Falsey AR. Risk factors for severe respiratory syncytial virus infection in elderly persons. J Infect Dis. 2004;189:233–8.
42. CDC. Respiratory syncytial virus activity – United States, July 2008-December 2009. MMWR Morb Mortal Wkly Rep. 2010;59:230–3.
43. Hall CB, Long CE, Schnabel KC. Respiratory syncytial virus infections in previously healthy working adults. Clin Infect Dis. 2001;33:792–6.
44. Kim YJ, Boeckh M, Englund JA. Community respiratory virus infections in immunocompromised patients: hematopoietic stem cell and solid organ transplant recipients, and individuals with human immunodeficiency virus infection. Semin Respir Crit Care Med. 2007;28:222–42.
45. Weigt SS, Gregson AL, Deng JC, Lynch JP 3rd, Belperio JA. Respiratory viral infections in hematopoietic stem cell and solid organ transplant recipients. Semin Respir Crit Care Med. 2011;32:471–93.
46. Boeckh M. The challenge of respiratory virus infections in hematopoietic cell transplant recipients. Br J Haematol. 2008;143:455–67.
47. Shah JN, Chemaly RF. Management of RSV infections in adult recipients of hematopoietic stem cell transplantation. Blood. 2011;117:2755–63.
48. Hynicka LM, Ensor CR. Prophylaxis and treatment of respiratory syncytial virus in adult immunocompromised patients. Ann Pharmacother. 2012;46:558–66.
49. Waghmare A, Xie H, Kimball L, et al. Supplemental oxygen-free days in hematopoietic cell transplant recipients with respiratory syncytial virus. J Infect Dis. 2017;216:1235–44.
50. Anderson NW, Binnicker MJ, Harris DM, et al. Morbidity and mortality among patients with respiratory syncytial virus infection: a 2-year retrospective review. Diagn Microbiol Infect Dis. 2016;85:367–71.
51. Foolad F, Aitken SL, Shigle TL, et al. Oral versus aerosolized ribavirin for the treatment of respiratory syncytial virus infections in hematopoietic cell transplantation recipients. Clin Infect Dis. 2018. https://doi.org/10.1093/cid/ciy760. [Epub ahead of print].
52. Pilie P, Werbel WA, Riddell J, Shu X, Schaubel D, Gregg KS. Adult patients with respiratory syncytial virus infection: impact of solid organ and hematopoietic stem cell transplantation on outcomes. Transpl Infect Dis. 2015;17:551–7.
53. Waghmare A, Campbell AP, Xie H, et al. Respiratory syncytial virus lower respiratory disease in hematopoietic cell transplant recipients: viral RNA detection in blood, antiviral treatment, and clinical outcomes. Clin Infect Dis. 2013;57:1731–41.
54. Shah DP, Ghantoji SS, Shah JN, et al. Impact of aerosolized ribavirin on mortality in 280 allogeneic haematopoietic stem cell transplant recipients with respiratory syncytial virus infections. J Antimicrob Chemother. 2013;68:1872–80.
55. Martino R, Porras RP, Rabella N, et al. Prospective study of the incidence, clinical features, and outcome of symptomatic upper and lower respiratory tract infections by respiratory viruses in adult recipients of hematopoietic stem cell transplants for hematologic malignancies. Biol Blood Marrow Transplant. 2005;11:781–96.

56. Ghosh S, Champlin RE, Englund J, et al. Respiratory syncytial virus upper respiratory tract illnesses in adult blood and marrow transplant recipients: combination therapy with aerosolized ribavirin and intravenous immunoglobulin. Bone Marrow Transplant. 2000;25:751–5.
57. Ariza-Heredia EJ, Fishman JE, Cleary T, Smith L, Razonable RR, Abbo L. Clinical and radiological features of respiratory syncytial virus in solid organ transplant recipients: a single-center experience. Transpl Infect Dis. 2012;14:64–71.
58. Uckay I, Gasche-Soccal PM, Kaiser L, et al. Low incidence of severe respiratory syncytial virus infections in lung transplant recipients despite the absence of specific therapy. J Heart Lung Transplant. 2010;29:299–305.
59. Hall CB, McBride JT, Walsh EE, et al. Aerosolized ribavirin treatment of infants with respiratory syncytial viral infection. A randomized double-blind study. N Engl J Med. 1983;308:1443–7.
60. Graci JD, Cameron CE. Quasispecies, error catastrophe, and the antiviral activity of ribavirin. Virology. 2002;298:175–80.
61. Tam RC, Lau JY, Hong Z. Mechanisms of action of ribavirin in antiviral therapies. Antivir Chem Chemother. 2001;12:261–72.
62. Sookoian S, Castano G, Flichman D, Cello J. Effects of ribavirin on cytokine production of recall antigens and phytohemaglutinin-stimulated peripheral blood mononuclear cells. (Inhibitory effects of ribavirin on cytokine production). Ann Hepatol. 2004;3: 104–7.
63. Englund JA, Piedra PA, Ahn YM, Gilbert BE, Hiatt P. High-dose, short-duration ribavirin aerosol therapy compared with standard ribavirin therapy in children with suspected respiratory syncytial virus infection. J Pediatr. 1994;125:635–41.
64. Chemaly RF, Hanmod SS, Rathod DB, et al. The characteristics and outcomes of parainfluenza virus infections in 200 patients with leukemia or recipients of hematopoietic stem cell transplantation. Blood. 2012;119:2738–45; quiz 969.
65. Chemaly RF, Torres HA, Munsell MF, et al. An adaptive randomized trial of an Intermittent Dosing Schedule of Aerosolized Ribavirin in patients with cancer and respiratory syncytial virus infection. J Infect Dis. 2012;206:1367–71.
66. Hirsch HH, Martino R, Ward KN, Boeckh M, Einsele H, Ljungman P. Fourth European Conference on Infections in Leukaemia (ECIL-4): guidelines for diagnosis and treatment of human respiratory syncytial virus, parainfluenza virus, metapneumovirus, rhinovirus, and coronavirus. Clin Infect Dis. 2013;56:258–66.
67. Newborn AAoPCoIDaCoFa. Prevention of respiratory syncytial virus infections: indications for the use of palivizumab and update on the use of RSV-IGIV. American Academy of Pediatrics Committee on Infectious Diseases and Committee of Fetus and Newborn. Pediatrics. 1998;102:1211–6.
68. Boeckh M, Berrey MM, Bowden RA, Crawford SW, Balsley J, Corey L. Phase 1 evaluation of the respiratory syncytial virus-specific monoclonal antibody palivizumab in recipients of hematopoietic stem cell transplants. J Infect Dis. 2001;184:350–4.
69. Boeckh M, Englund J, Li Y, et al. Randomized controlled multicenter trial of aerosolized ribavirin for respiratory syncytial virus upper respiratory tract infection in hematopoietic cell transplant recipients. Clin Infect Dis. 2007;44:245–9.
70. Small TN, Casson A, Malak SF, et al. Respiratory syncytial virus infection following hematopoietic stem cell transplantation. Bone Marrow Transplant. 2002;29:321–7.
71. McCoy D, Wong E, Kuyumjian AG, Wynd MA, Sebti R, Munk GB. Treatment of respiratory syncytial virus infection in adult patients with hematologic malignancies based on an institution-specific guideline. Transpl Infect Dis. 2011;13:117–21.
72. Tsitsikas DA, Oakervee H, Cavenagh JD, Gribben J, Agrawal SG, Mattes FM. Treatment of respiratory syncytial virus infection in haemopoietic stem cell transplant recipients with aerosolized ribavirin and the humanized monoclonal antibody palivizumab: a single centre experience. Br J Haematol. 2009;146:574–6.
73. Seo S, Campbell AP, Xie H, et al. Outcome of respiratory syncytial virus lower respiratory tract disease in hematopoietic cell transplant recipients receiving aerosolized ribavirin: significance of stem cell source and oxygen requirement. Biol Blood Marrow Transplant. 2013;19:589–96.
74. de Fontbrune FS, Robin M, Porcher R, et al. Palivizumab treatment of respiratory syncytial virus infection after allogeneic hematopoietic stem cell transplantation. Clin Infect Dis. 2007;45:1019–24.
75. Chemaly RF, Aitken SL, Wolfe CR, Jain R, Boeckh MJ. Aerosolized ribavirin: the most expensive drug for pneumonia. Transpl Infect Dis. 2016;18:634–6.
76. Khanna N, Widmer AF, Decker M, et al. Respiratory syncytial virus infection in patients with hematological diseases: single-center study and review of the literature. Clin Infect Dis. 2008;46: 402–12.
77. Marcelin JR, Wilson JW, Razonable RR, Mayo Clinic HO. Transplant Infectious Diseases S. Oral ribavirin therapy for respiratory syncytial virus infections in moderately to severely immunocompromised patients. Transpl Infect Dis. 2014;16:242–50.
78. Trang TP, Whalen M, Hilts-Horeczko A, Doernberg SB, Liu C. Comparative effectiveness of aerosolized versus oral ribavirin for the treatment of respiratory syncytial virus infections: a single-center retrospective cohort study and review of the literature. Transpl Infect Dis. 2018;20:e12844.
79. Beaird OE, Freifeld A, Ison MG, et al. Current practices for treatment of respiratory syncytial virus and other non-influenza respiratory viruses in high-risk patient populations: a survey of institutions in the Midwestern Respiratory Virus Collaborative. Transpl Infect Dis. 2016;18:210–5.
80. Luo YH, Huang CY, Yang KY, Lee YC. Inhaled ribavirin therapy in adult respiratory syncytial virus-induced acute respiratory distress syndrome. Arch Bronconeumol. 2011;47:315–7.
81. Pelaez A, Lyon GM, Force SD, et al. Efficacy of oral ribavirin in lung transplant patients with respiratory syncytial virus lower respiratory tract infection. J Heart Lung Transplant. 2009;28:67–71.
82. Fuehner T, Dierich M, Duesberg C, et al. Single-centre experience with oral ribavirin in lung transplant recipients with paramyxovirus infections. Antivir Ther. 2011;16:733–40.
83. Li L, Avery R, Budev M, Mossad S, Danziger-Isakov L. Oral versus inhaled ribavirin therapy for respiratory syncytial virus infection after lung transplantation. J Heart Lung Transplant. 2012;31(8):839–44.
84. Glanville AR, Scott AI, Morton JM, et al. Intravenous ribavirin is a safe and cost-effective treatment for respiratory syncytial virus infection after lung transplantation. J Heart Lung Transplant. 2005;24:2114–9.
85. Gottlieb J, Torres F, Haddad T, et al. Respiratory syncytial virus (RSV) in lung transplant (LT) recipients. J Heart Lung Transplant. 2018;37:S155.
86. Elizaga J, Olavarria E, Apperley J, Goldman J, Ward K. Parainfluenza virus 3 infection after stem cell transplant: relevance to outcome of rapid diagnosis and ribavirin treatment. Clin Infect Dis. 2001;32:413–8.
87. Lewis VA, Champlin R, Englund J, et al. Respiratory disease due to parainfluenza virus in adult bone marrow transplant recipients. Clin Infect Dis. 1996;23:1033–7.
88. Vilchez RA, Dauber J, McCurry K, Iacono A, Kusne S. Parainfluenza virus infection in adult lung transplant recipients: an emergent clinical syndrome with implications on allograft function. Am J Transplant. 2003;3:116–20.
89. Whimbey E, Vartivarian SE, Champlin RE, Elting LS, Luna M, Bodey GP. Parainfluenza virus infection in adult bone marrow transplant recipients. Eur J Clin Microbiol Infect Dis. 1993;12:699–701.

90. Ustun C, Slaby J, Shanley RM, et al. Human parainfluenza virus infection after hematopoietic stem cell transplantation: risk factors, management, mortality, and changes over time. Biol Blood Marrow Transplant. 2012;18:1580–8.
91. Peck AJ, Englund JA, Kuypers J, et al. Respiratory virus infection among hematopoietic cell transplant recipients: evidence for asymptomatic parainfluenza virus infection. Blood. 2007;110:1681–8.
92. Billings JL, Hertz MI, Savik K, Wendt CH. Respiratory viruses and chronic rejection in lung transplant recipients. J Heart Lung Transplant. 2002;21:559–66.
93. Garbino J, Gerbase MW, Wunderli W, et al. Respiratory viruses and severe lower respiratory tract complications in hospitalized patients. Chest. 2004;125:1033–9.
94. Maziarz RT, Sridharan P, Slater S, et al. Control of an outbreak of human parainfluenza virus 3 in hematopoietic stem cell transplant recipients. Biol Blood Marrow Transplant. 2010;16:192–8.
95. Wendt CH, Weisdorf DJ, Jordan MC, Balfour HH Jr, Hertz MI. Parainfluenza virus respiratory infection after bone marrow transplantation. N Engl J Med. 1992;326:921–6.
96. Chakrabarti S, Collingham KE, Holder K, Fegan CD, Osman H, Milligan DW. Pre-emptive oral ribavirin therapy of paramyxovirus infections after haematopoietic stem cell transplantation: a pilot study. Bone Marrow Transplant. 2001;28:759–63.
97. Shima T, Yoshimoto G, Nonami A, et al. Successful treatment of parainfluenza virus 3 pneumonia with oral ribavirin and methylprednisolone in a bone marrow transplant recipient. Int J Hematol. 2008;88:336–40.
98. Chakrabarti S, Collingham KE, Holder K, Oyaide S, Pillay D, Milligan DW. Parainfluenza virus type 3 infections in hematopoetic stem cell transplant recipients: response to ribavirin therapy. Clin Infect Dis. 2000;31:1516–8.
99. Cobian L, Houston S, Greene J, Sinnott JT. Parainfluenza virus respiratory infection after heart transplantation: successful treatment with ribavirin. Clin Infect Dis. 1995;21:1040–1.
100. Wright JJ, O'Driscoll G. Treatment of parainfluenza virus 3 pneumonia in a cardiac transplant recipient with intravenous ribavirin and methylprednisolone. J Heart Lung Transplant. 2005;24:343–6.
101. Park SY, Sung H, Park KT, et al. Parainfluenza virus 3 pneumonia in a kidney transplant recipient. Transpl Infect Dis. 2009;11:333–6.
102. Chen YB, Driscoll JP, McAfee SL, et al. Treatment of parainfluenza 3 infection with DAS181 in a patient after allogeneic stem cell transplantation. Clin Infect Dis. 2011;53:e77–80.
103. Guzman-Suarez BB, Buckley MW, Gilmore ET, et al. Clinical potential of DAS181 for treatment of parainfluenza-3 infections in transplant recipients. Transpl Infect Dis. 2012;14(4):427–33.
104. Drozd DR, Limaye AP, Moss RB, et al. DAS181 treatment of severe parainfluenza type 3 pneumonia in a lung transplant recipient. Transpl Infect Dis. 2013;15:E28–32.
105. Chalkias S, Mackenzie MR, Gay C, et al. DAS181 treatment of hematopoietic stem cell transplant patients with parainfluenza virus lung disease requiring mechanical ventilation. Transpl Infect Dis. 2014;16:141–4.
106. Salvatore M, Satlin MJ, Jacobs SE, et al. DAS181 for treatment of Parainfluenza virus infections in Hematopoietic stem cell transplant recipients at a single center. Biol Blood Marrow Transplant. 2016;22:965–70.
107. van den Hoogen BG, de Jong JC, Groen J, et al. A newly discovered human pneumovirus isolated from young children with respiratory tract disease. Nat Med. 2001;7:719–24.
108. Kroll JL, Weinberg A. Human metapneumovirus. Semin Respir Crit Care Med. 2011;32:447–53.
109. Biacchesi S, Skiadopoulos MH, Boivin G, et al. Genetic diversity between human metapneumovirus subgroups. Virology. 2003;315:1–9.
110. Williams JV, Harris PA, Tollefson SJ, et al. Human metapneumovirus and lower respiratory tract disease in otherwise healthy infants and children. N Engl J Med. 2004;350:443–50.
111. Falsey AR. Human metapneumovirus infection in adults. Pediatr Infect Dis J. 2008;27:S80–3.
112. Falsey AR, Erdman D, Anderson LJ, Walsh EE. Human metapneumovirus infections in young and elderly adults. J Infect Dis. 2003;187:785–90.
113. Walsh EE, Peterson DR, Falsey AR. Human metapneumovirus infections in adults: another piece of the puzzle. Arch Intern Med. 2008;168:2489–96.
114. Debur MC, Vidal LR, Stroparo E, et al. Human metapneumovirus infection in hematopoietic stem cell transplant recipients. Transpl Infect Dis. 2010;12:173–9.
115. Englund JA, Boeckh M, Kuypers J, et al. Brief communication: fatal human metapneumovirus infection in stem-cell transplant recipients. Ann Intern Med. 2006;144:344–9.
116. Williams JV, Martino R, Rabella N, et al. A prospective study comparing human metapneumovirus with other respiratory viruses in adults with hematologic malignancies and respiratory tract infections. J Infect Dis. 2005;192:1061–5.
117. Oliveira R, Machado A, Tateno A, Boas LV, Pannuti C, Machado C. Frequency of human metapneumovirus infection in hematopoietic SCT recipients during 3 consecutive years. Bone Marrow Transplant. 2008;42:265–9.
118. Shah DP, Shah PK, Azzi JM, El Chaer F, Chemaly RF. Human metapneumovirus infections in hematopoietic cell transplant recipients and hematologic malignancy patients: A systematic review. Cancer Lett. 2016;379:100–6.
119. Seo S, Gooley TA, Kuypers JM, et al. Human metapneumovirus infections following hematopoietic cell transplantation: Factors associated with disease progression. Clin Infect Dis. 2016;63:178–85.
120. Hopkins P, McNeil K, Kermeen F, et al. Human metapneumovirus in lung transplant recipients and comparison to respiratory syncytial virus. Am J Respir Crit Care Med. 2008;178:876–81.
121. Wyde PR, Chetty SN, Jewell AM, Boivin G, Piedra PA. Comparison of the inhibition of human metapneumovirus and respiratory syncytial virus by ribavirin and immune serum globulin in vitro. Antivir Res. 2003;60:51–9.
122. Hamelin ME, Prince GA, Boivin G. Effect of ribavirin and glucocorticoid treatment in a mouse model of human metapneumovirus infection. Antimicrob Agents Chemother. 2006;50:774–7.
123. Bonney D, Razali H, Turner A, Will A. Successful treatment of human metapneumovirus pneumonia using combination therapy with intravenous ribavirin and immune globulin. Br J Haematol. 2009;145:667–9.
124. Shachor-Meyouhas Y, Ben-Barak A, Kassis I. Treatment with oral ribavirin and IVIG of severe human metapneumovirus pneumonia (HMPV) in immune compromised child. Pediatr Blood Cancer. 2011;57:350–1.
125. Shahda S, Carlos WG, Kiel PJ, Khan BA, Hage CA. The human metapneumovirus: a case series and review of the literature. Transpl Infect Dis. 2011;13:324–8.
126. Raza K, Ismailjee SB, Crespo M, et al. Successful outcome of human metapneumovirus (hMPV) pneumonia in a lung transplant recipient treated with intravenous ribavirin. J Heart Lung Transplant. 2007;26:862–4.
127. Williams JV, Chen Z, Cseke G, et al. A recombinant human monoclonal antibody to human metapneumovirus fusion protein that neutralizes virus in vitro and is effective therapeutically in vivo. J Virol. 2007;81:8315–24.
128. Ulbrandt ND, Ji H, Patel NK, et al. Isolation and characterization of monoclonal antibodies which neutralize human metapneumovirus in vitro and in vivo. J Virol. 2006;80:7799–806.

129. Deffrasnes C, Hamelin ME, Prince GA, Boivin G. Identification and evaluation of a highly effective fusion inhibitor for human metapneumovirus. Antimicrob Agents Chemother. 2008;52:279–87.
130. Kanne JP, Godwin JD, Franquet T, Escuissato DL, Muller NL. Viral pneumonia after hematopoietic stem cell transplantation: high-resolution CT findings. J Thorac Imaging. 2007;22:292–9.
131. Ko JP, Shepard JA, Sproule MW, et al. CT manifestations of respiratory syncytial virus infection in lung transplant recipients. J Comput Assist Tomogr. 2000;24:235–41.
132. Ferguson PE, Sorrell TC, Bradstock KF, Carr P, Gilroy NM. Parainfluenza virus type 3 Pneumonia in bone marrow transplant recipients: multiple small nodules in high-resolution lung computed tomography scans provide a radiological clue to diagnosis. Clin Infect Dis. 2009;48(7):905–9.
133. Franquet T, Rodriguez S, Martino R, Salinas T, Gimenez A, Hidalgo A. Human metapneumovirus infection in hematopoietic stem cell transplant recipients: high-resolution computed tomography findings. J Comput Assist Tomogr. 2005;29:223–7.
134. Franquet T, Rodriguez S, Martino R, Gimenez A, Salinas T, Hidalgo A. Thin-section CT findings in hematopoietic stem cell transplantation recipients with respiratory virus pneumonia. AJR Am J Roentgenol. 2006;187:1085–90.
135. Escuissato DL, Gasparetto EL, Marchiori E, et al. Pulmonary infections after bone marrow transplantation: high-resolution CT findings in 111 patients. AJR Am J Roentgenol. 2005;185:608–15.
136. Gasparetto EL, Escuissato DL, Marchiori E, Ono S, Frare e Silva RL, Muller NL. High-resolution CT findings of respiratory syncytial virus pneumonia after bone marrow transplantation. AJR Am J Roentgenol. 2004;182:1133–7.
137. Kamboj M, Gerbin M, Huang CK, et al. Clinical characterization of human metapneumovirus infection among patients with cancer. J Infect. 2008;57:464–71.
138. Miller WT Jr, Barbosa E Jr, Mickus TJ, Mullin C, Van Deerlin VM, Shiley KT. Chest computed tomographic imaging characteristics of viral acute lower respiratory tract illnesses: a case-control study. J Comput Assist Tomogr. 2011;35:524–30.
139. Shiley KT, Van Deerlin VM, Miller WT Jr. Chest CT features of community-acquired respiratory viral infections in adult inpatients with lower respiratory tract infections. J Thorac Imaging. 2010;25:68–75.
140. Mahony JB. Detection of respiratory viruses by molecular methods. Clin Microbiol Rev. 2008;21:716–47.
141. Fan J, Henrickson KJ. Rapid diagnosis of human parainfluenza virus type 1 infection by quantitative reverse transcription-PCR-enzyme hybridization assay. J Clin Microbiol. 1996;34:1914–7.
142. Fan J, Henrickson KJ, Savatski LL. Rapid simultaneous diagnosis of infections with respiratory syncytial viruses A and B, influenza viruses A and B, and human parainfluenza virus types 1, 2, and 3 by multiplex quantitative reverse transcription-polymerase chain reaction-enzyme hybridization assay (Hexaplex). Clin Infect Dis. 1998;26:1397–402.
143. Kuypers J, Campbell AP, Cent A, Corey L, Boeckh M. Comparison of conventional and molecular detection of respiratory viruses in hematopoietic cell transplant recipients. Transpl Infect Dis. 2009;11:298–303.
144. Mahony JB, Petrich A, Smieja M. Molecular diagnosis of respiratory virus infections. Crit Rev Clin Lab Sci. 2011;48:217–49.
145. Hammond SP, Gagne LS, Stock SR, et al. Respiratory virus detection in immunocompromised patients with FilmArray respiratory panel compared to conventional methods. J Clin Microbiol. 2012;50:3216–21.
146. Poritz MA, Blaschke AJ, Byington CL, et al. FilmArray, an automated nested multiplex PCR system for multi-pathogen detection: development and application to respiratory tract infection. PLoS One. 2011;6:e26047.
147. Tomblyn M, Chiller T, Einsele H, et al. Guidelines for preventing infectious complications among hematopoietic cell transplant recipients: a global perspective. Preface. Bone Marrow Transplant. 2009;44:453–5.
148. Hall CB, Douglas RG Jr, Schnabel KC, Geiman JM. Infectivity of respiratory syncytial virus by various routes of inoculation. Infect Immun. 1981;33:779–83.
149. Jalal H, Bibby DF, Bennett J, et al. Molecular investigations of an outbreak of parainfluenza virus type 3 and respiratory syncytial virus infections in a hematology unit. J Clin Microbiol. 2007;45:1690–6.
150. Kassis C, Champlin RE, Hachem RY, et al. Detection and control of a nosocomial respiratory syncytial virus outbreak in a stem cell transplantation unit: the role of palivizumab. Biol Blood Marrow Transplant. 2010;16:1265–71.
151. Sydnor ER, Greer A, Budd AP, et al. An outbreak of human parainfluenza virus 3 infection in an outpatient hematopoietic stem cell transplantation clinic. Am J Infect Control. 2012;40(7):601–5.
152. Tu CC, Chen LK, Lee YS, et al. An outbreak of human metapneumovirus infection in hospitalized psychiatric adult patients in Taiwan. Scand J Infect Dis. 2009;41:363–7.
153. Nichols WG, Erdman DD, Han A, Zukerman C, Corey L, Boeckh M. Prolonged outbreak of human parainfluenza virus 3 infection in a stem cell transplant outpatient department: insights from molecular epidemiologic analysis. Biol Blood Marrow Transplant. 2004;10:58–64.
154. Tablan OC, Anderson LJ, Besser R, Bridges C, Hajjeh R. Guidelines for preventing health-care--associated pneumonia, 2003: recommendations of CDC and the Healthcare Infection Control Practices Advisory Committee. MMWR Recomm Rep. 2004;53:1–36.
155. Yokoe D, Casper C, Dubberke E, et al. Infection prevention and control in health-care facilities in which hematopoietic cell transplant recipients are treated. Bone Marrow Transplant. 2009;44:495–507.
156. http://www.cdc.gov/hicpac/pdf/isolation/Isolation2007.pdf. 2007.
157. Cortez K, Murphy BR, Almeida KN, et al. Immune-globulin prophylaxis of respiratory syncytial virus infection in patients undergoing stem-cell transplantation. J Infect Dis. 2002;186:834–8.
158. Le Bayon JC, Lina B, Rosa-Calatrava M, Boivin G. Recent developments with live-attenuated recombinant paramyxovirus vaccines. Rev Med Virol. 2013;23(1):15–34.
159. Graham BS. Vaccine development for respiratory syncytial virus. Curr Opin Virol. 2017;23:107–12.
160. Marquez-Escobar VA. Current developments and prospects on human metapneumovirus vaccines. Expert Rev Vaccines. 2017;16:419–31.
161. Pawelczyk M, Kowalski ML. The role of human Parainfluenza virus infections in the immunopathology of the respiratory tract. Curr Allergy Asthma Rep. 2017;17:16.
162. Peck AJ, Corey L, Boeckh M. Pretransplantation respiratory syncytial virus infection: impact of a strategy to delay transplantation. Clin Infect Dis. 2004;39:673–80.
163. Waghmare A, Englund JA, Boeckh M. How I treat respiratory viral infections in the setting of intensive chemotherapy or hematopoietic cell transplantation. Blood. 2016;127:2682–92.
164. Kumar D, Blumberg EA, Danziger-Isakov L, et al. Influenza vaccination in the organ transplant recipient: review and summary recommendations. Am J Transplant. 2011;11:2020–30.
165. Ng BJ, Glanville AR, Snell G, et al. The impact of pandemic influenza A H1N1 2009 on Australian lung transplant recipients. Am J Transplant. 2011;11:568–74.
166. Vilchez RA, McCurry K, Dauber J, et al. Influenza virus infection in adult solid organ transplant recipients. Am J Transplant. 2002;2:287–91.

167. Choi SM, Boudreault AA, Xie H, Englund JA, Corey L, Boeckh M. Differences in clinical outcomes after 2009 influenza A/H1N1 and seasonal influenza among hematopoietic cell transplant recipients. Blood. 2011;117:5050–6.
168. Boudreault AA, Xie H, Leisenring W, Englund J, Corey L, Boeckh M. Impact of corticosteroid treatment and antiviral therapy on clinical outcomes in hematopoietic cell transplant patients infected with influenza virus. Biol Blood Marrow Transplant. 2011;17:979–86.
169. Kumar D, Michaels MG, Morris MI, et al. Outcomes from pandemic influenza A H1N1 infection in recipients of solid-organ transplants: a multicentre cohort study. Lancet Infect Dis. 2010;10:521–6.
170. Ljungman P, de la Camara R, Perez-Bercoff L, et al. Outcome of pandemic H1N1 infections in hematopoietic stem cell transplant recipients. Haematologica. 2011;96:1231–5.
171. Elicker BM, Schwartz BS, Liu C, et al. Thoracic CT findings of novel influenza A (H1N1) infection in immunocompromised patients. Emerg Radiol. 2010;17:299–307.
172. Cordero E, Perez-Romero P, Moreno A, et al. Pandemic influenza A(H1N1) virus infection in solid organ transplant recipients: impact of viral and non-viral co-infection. Clin Microbiol Infect. 2012;18:67–73.
173. Lee N, Chan PK, Lui GC, et al. Complications and outcomes of pandemic 2009 Influenza A (H1N1) virus infection in hospitalized adults: how do they differ from those in seasonal influenza? J Infect Dis. 2011;203:1739–47.
174. Liu C, Schwartz BS, Vallabhaneni S, et al. Pandemic (H1N1) 2009 infection in patients with hematologic malignancy. Emerg Infect Dis. 2010;16:1910–7.
175. Beutel G, Wiesner O, Eder M, et al. Virus-associated hemophagocytic syndrome as a major contributor to death in patients with 2009 influenza A (H1N1) infection. Crit Care. 2011;15:R80.
176. Vu DL, Bridevaux PO, Aubert JD, Soccal PM, Kaiser L. Respiratory viruses in lung transplant recipients: a critical review and pooled analysis of clinical studies. Am J Transplant. 2011;11:1071–8.
177. Lee N, Chan PK, Hui DS, et al. Viral loads and duration of viral shedding in adult patients hospitalized with influenza. J Infect Dis. 2009;200:492–500.
178. Ng S, Cowling BJ, Fang VJ, et al. Effects of oseltamivir treatment on duration of clinical illness and viral shedding and household transmission of influenza virus. Clin Infect Dis. 2010;50:707–14.
179. Khanna N, Steffen I, Studt JD, et al. Outcome of influenza infections in outpatients after allogeneic hematopoietic stem cell transplantation. Transpl Infect Dis. 2009;11:100–5.
180. Harper SA, Bradley JS, Englund JA, et al. Seasonal influenza in adults and children--diagnosis, treatment, chemoprophylaxis, and institutional outbreak management: clinical practice guidelines of the Infectious Diseases Society of America. Clin Infect Dis. 2009;48:1003–32.
181. Moscona A. Global transmission of oseltamivir-resistant influenza. N Engl J Med. 2009;360:953–6.
182. Hurt AC, Lee RT, Leang SK, et al. Increased detection in Australia and Singapore of a novel influenza A(H1N1)2009 variant with reduced oseltamivir and zanamivir sensitivity due to a S247N neuraminidase mutation. Euro surveillance: bulletin europeen sur les maladies transmissibles = European communicable disease bulletin 2011;16.
183. Centers for Disease Control. Flu. www.cdc.gov/flu. Accessed Sept 2018.
184. Ison MG, Gubareva LV, Atmar RL, Treanor J, Hayden FG. Recovery of drug-resistant influenza virus from immunocompromised patients: a case series. J Infect Dis. 2006;193:760–4.
185. Weinstock DM, Gubareva LV, Zuccotti G. Prolonged shedding of multidrug-resistant influenza A virus in an immunocompromised patient. N Engl J Med. 2003;348:867–8.
186. Graitcer SB, Gubareva L, Kamimoto L, et al. Characteristics of patients with oseltamivir-resistant pandemic (H1N1) 2009, United States. Emerg Infect Dis. 2011;17:255–7.
187. McGeer A, Green KA, Plevneshi A, et al. Antiviral therapy and outcomes of influenza requiring hospitalization in Ontario, Canada. Clin Infect Dis. 2007;45:1568–75.
188. Machado CM. Influenza infections after hematopoietic stem cell transplantation. Clin Infect Dis. 2005;41:273–4.
189. Casper C, Englund J, Boeckh M. How I treat influenza in patients with hematologic malignancies. Blood. 2010;115:1331–42.
190. Ison MG, Michaels MG. RNA respiratory viral infections in solid organ transplant recipients. Am J Transplant. 2009;9(Suppl 4):S166–72.
191. Kumar D, Morris MI, Kotton CN, et al. Guidance on novel influenza A/H1N1 in solid organ transplant recipients. Am J Transplant. 2010;10:18–25.
192. Nicholson KG, Aoki FY, Osterhaus AD, et al. Efficacy and safety of oseltamivir in treatment of acute influenza: a randomised controlled trial. Neuraminidase Inhibitor Flu Treatment Investigator Group. Lancet. 2000;355:1845–50.
193. Treanor JJ, Hayden FG, Vrooman PS, et al. Efficacy and safety of the oral neuraminidase inhibitor oseltamivir in treating acute influenza: a randomized controlled trial. US Oral Neuraminidase Study Group. JAMA. 2000;283:1016–24.
194. Ison MG. Influenza prevention and treatment in transplant recipients and immunocompromised hosts. Influenza Other Respir Viruses. 2013;7(Suppl 3):60–6.
195. Beigel JH, Bao Y, Beeler J, et al. Oseltamivir, amantadine, and ribavirin combination antiviral therapy versus oseltamivir monotherapy for the treatment of influenza: a multicentre, double-blind, randomised phase 2 trial. Lancet Infect Dis. 2017;17:1255–65.
196. Rubin LG, Levin MJ, Ljungman P, et al. 2013 IDSA clinical practice guideline for vaccination of the immunocompromised host. Clin Infect Dis. 2014;58:e44–100.
197. Machado CM, Cardoso MR, da Rocha IF, Boas LS, Dulley FL, Pannuti CS. The benefit of influenza vaccination after bone marrow transplantation. Bone Marrow Transplant. 2005;36:897–900.
198. DiazGranados CA, Dunning AJ, Kimmel M, et al. Efficacy of high-dose versus standard-dose influenza vaccine in older adults. N Engl J Med. 2014;371:635–45.
199. Halasa NB, Savani BN, Asokan I, et al. Randomized double-blind study of the safety and immunogenicity of standard-dose trivalent inactivated influenza vaccine versus high-dose trivalent inactivated influenza vaccine in adult hematopoietic stem cell transplantation patients. Biol Blood Marrow Transplant. 2016;22:528–35.
200. Chong PP, Handler L, Weber DJ. A systematic review of safety and immunogenicity of influenza vaccination strategies in solid organ transplant recipients. Clin Infect Dis. 2018;66:1802–11.
201. Natori Y, Shiotsuka M, Slomovic J, et al. A double-blind, randomized trial of high-dose vs standard-dose influenza vaccine in adult solid-organ transplant recipients. Clin Infect Dis. 2018;66:1698–704.
202. Thomas RE, Jefferson T, Lasserson TJ. Influenza vaccination for healthcare workers who work with the elderly. Cochrane Database Syst Rev. 2010:CD005187.
203. Zaki AM, van Boheemen S, Bestebroer TM, Osterhaus AD, Fouchier RA. Isolation of a Novel Coronavirus from a man with Pneumonia in Saudi Arabia. N Engl J Med. 2012;367(19):1814–20.
204. de Wit E, van Doremalen N, Falzarano D, Munster VJ. SARS and MERS: recent insights into emerging coronaviruses. Nat Rev Microbiol. 2016;14:523–34.
205. Uhlenhaut C, Cohen JI, Pavletic S, et al. Use of a novel virus detection assay to identify coronavirus HKU1 in the lungs of a hematopoietic stem cell transplant recipient with fatal pneumonia. Transpl Infect Dis. 2012;14:79–85.

206. Oosterhof L, Christensen CB, Sengelov H. Fatal lower respiratory tract disease with human corona virus NL63 in an adult haematopoietic cell transplant recipient. Bone Marrow Transplant. 2010;45:1115–6.
207. Gutman JA, Peck AJ, Kuypers J, Boeckh M. Rhinovirus as a cause of fatal lower respiratory tract infection in adult stem cell transplantation patients: a report of two cases. Bone Marrow Transplant. 2007;40:809–11.
208. Ogimi C, Waghmare AA, Kuypers JM, et al. Clinical significance of human coronavirus in bronchoalveolar lavage samples from hematopoietic cell transplant recipients and patients with hematologic malignancies. Clin Infect Dis. 2017;64:1532–9.

Hepatitis A, B, and C

41

Jonathan Merola, Alexander Z. Jow, and Samuel H. Sigal

Introduction

Inflammation in the liver secondary to viral infection defines viral hepatitis. Infections may manifest with acute pathology but may also take on a more indolent, chronic form. The five most common hepatitis viral infections are unrelated and classified as hepatitis A, B, C, D, and E. The former three viruses are commonly considered and managed in transplant population and are the focus of this chapter. Hepatitis A is an RNA virus acquired enterally that often manifests as an acute, self-limited illness. It can be prevented with vaccination and is treated supportively. Hepatitis B is a DNA virus that directly integrates into the host genome following infection by blood or sexual transmission. In addition to an initial acute infection, it may result in an indolent, chronic inflammatory disease following an initial acute infection occurring by blood or sexual transmission. While preventable by vaccination, hepatitis B may be treated with direct antiviral therapy but confers a significant risk of developing hepatocellular carcinoma despite complete response to treatment. Hepatitis C, also acquired through blood-borne transmission, is an RNA virus that often results in a chronic, subclinical inflammation. Chronic infection may at times lead to cirrhosis, and new direct antiviral therapies have recently become available with high rates of cure. While the hepatotropic nature of these viruses unites these pathogens, prevention, treatment, and post-treatment surveillance vary widely between them and are described in this chapter.

J. Merola
Department of Surgery, Yale School of Medicine, Yale-New Haven Hospital, New Haven, CT, USA
e-mail: jonathan.merola@yale.edu

A. Z. Jow
Division of Gastroenterology, Mid-Atlantic Kaiser Permanente Medical Group, Springfield, VA, USA

S. H. Sigal (✉)
Division of Gastroenterology and Hepatology, Department of Medicine, Albert Einstein College of Medicine, Montefiore Medical Center, Bronx, NY, USA
e-mail: ssigal@montefiore.com

Hepatitis A

Hepatitis A virus (HAV) is an enteric picornavirus that harbors a single-stranded 7.5 kilobase RNA genome of positive-strand polarity. The genomic sequence encodes for multiple proteins that are processed to give rise to several viral proteins including VP-1, VP-2, and VP-3. Predominantly transmitted by the fecal-oral route, HAV is often acquired from contaminated food and water sources or close contact with infected individuals. Infection is most common in developing regions, with an annual 1.5 million cases reported worldwide, although reported cases likely underestimate the true incidence of global HAV infection [1].

In immunocompetent individuals, HAV typically causes a self-limited illness characterized by fever, anorexia, right upper quadrant abdominal pain, and jaundice that follows a 4-week viral incubation period [2]. The severity of acute illness is closely related to age, as symptomatic infection is more common in older adults while acute infection in children is typically asymptomatic [3]. Laboratory findings typically demonstrate the presence of anti-HAV IgM in patients' serum and detection of virus in stool prior to the onset of clinical illness, whereas elevation in serum hepatic transaminases appears to coincide with the development of clinical symptoms. In patients with recent HAV exposure, a single-antigen vaccine or immune globulin can be given within 2 weeks for prevention of symptomatic hepatitis [4]. Supportive care is the mainstay of treatment in most cases [5]. In patients with severe acute hepatitis A associated liver injury, early treatment with N-acetylcysteine has been shown to provide benefit and potential for recovery [6].

A subset of patients (1–12%) experience relapsing HAV cholestatic hepatitis. This is characterized by jaundice and cholestasis, 1–3 months after resolution of the initial

A. Safdar (ed.), *Principles and Practice of Transplant Infectious Diseases*, https://doi.org/10.1007/978-1-4939-9034-4_41

symptoms of acute hepatitis A infection [2]. In such cases, treatment is predominantly supportive, as the infection commonly spontaneously resolves within 6 months, although the use of oral corticosteroids may be considered in patients with severe cholestasis [7]. Additionally, treatment with ursodeoxycholic acid has been demonstrated to improve biochemical indices in cases of relapsing hepatitis [8].

In rare cases (~0.2%), HAV infection can lead to acute liver failure (ALF), particularly in elderly patients or those with chronic liver disease [9]. Mortality rates in such cases approaches 40–50%, leaving emergency liver transplantation as the only lifesaving measure for a considerable number of patients with HAV ALF [10]. Severe HAV infection is responsible for a small proportion (3%) of cases of fulminant acute hepatic failure requiring liver transplantation [11].

Transplant recipients on immunosuppressive medications are particularly susceptible to acute HAV infection [12]. Cases of intractable recurrent HAV infection requiring re-transplantation after initial liver transplantation procedure have been reported [13, 14]. All patients undergoing transplant evaluation should be screened for hepatitis A IgG and vaccinated if not immune. Two doses of the Hepatitis A vaccine, given 6 months apart, successfully induced seroconversion in 95% of patients with compensated liver disease [15]. The development of liver failure is closely associated with a lack of response to the HAV vaccine [16]. Due to pre-transplant screening and vaccination for susceptible individuals, post-transplant acute hepatitis A infection is rare. If there is suspicion for an acute infection, the patient should be tested for serum IgM antibodies [17].

Reinfection of allografts after liver transplantation in patients with fulminant hepatic failure associated with HAV hepatitis is rare. Recurrent hepatitis A infection presents as acute graft dysfunction and may be misinterpreted as an episode of allograft. Routine measurements of anti-HAV IgM and viral RNA in peripheral blood during the early post-transplant period in HAV-associated liver transplant recipients may differentiate reinfection from an episode of acute cellular rejection [14]. Detection of genomic HAV RNA by RT-PCR in serum and stool at the time of graft dysfunction is diagnostic of recurrent HAV infection [13].

Hepatitis A vaccination is less effective in patients after transplantation. In a retrospective review of children following liver transplantation, vaccine antibody responses developed in only 7 of 18 individuals (39%), and only 25% developed an antibody response after undergoing heart transplantation [18]. In addition, a significant proportion of patients with detectable protective antibodies before liver transplantation can lose immunity following transplantation: 18% and 29%, first and second year after undergoing transplantation, respectively [12]. In liver and kidney transplant recipients with satisfactory seroconversion rate after complete immunization, there is a rapid decline in antibody levels compared with controls; 59% of liver and 26% of renal transplant seroconverters showed titers above the cutoff level considered protective against HAV infection [19]. Based on the above observations, it is recommended that patients with chronic liver disease undergo vaccination early in the course of their disease and that patients on immunosuppressive antirejection therapy be re-immunized [19, 20].

Hepatitis B

Hepatitis B virus (HBV) is a DNA virus that integrates into the host genome and replicates by reverse transcription [21]. HBV infection is a major cause of hepatic cirrhosis and liver-related mortality evidenced by the roughly 250 million people chronically infected worldwide. HBV is attributable to over half of all hepatocellular cancers [22, 23]. In the United States, HBV represents the second most common viral infection after hepatitis C virus leading to liver transplantation. The proportion of liver transplants for HBV have been decreasing in the United States from 4% in 1994 to about 2% in 2009, primarily due to advances in treatment for infection and HBV-related liver disease [24, 25].

HBV is often acquired through intravenous drug use and sexual transmission in Western countries, while transmission in high-prevalence areas is often through perinatal transmission [26]. In the United States, vaccination is routinely performed in infancy. Screening is recommended in persons from high prevalence areas and those with high-risk exposures [27]. Testing includes serologic tests for Hepatitis B surface antigen as well as surface and core antibodies. The presence of core antigen or the presence of core antibody in the absence of surface antibody indicates HBV exposure, while the co-presence of core and surface antibodies occurs in those immune following vaccination.

Chronic HBV infection occurs in less than 5% of adults but in over 95% of infected infants [28, 29]. Such infections are often subclinical until advanced cirrhosis develops. An annual rate of 0.5–1% of hepatocellular carcinoma is estimated for non-cirrhotic HBV patients and 2–3% among those with cirrhosis [30].

Early results of liver transplantation in patients with chronic HBV infection showed recurrence rates of greater than 80% and 5-year survival rates of 40–60% [31]. Subsequently, HBV infection was initially viewed to be a contraindication to liver transplant. Liver transplantation in HBsAg positive patients remained controversial until 1993 when studies demonstrated that long-term passive immunoprophylaxis with hepatitis B immune globulin (HBIG) could be used to prevent graft reinfection and reduce the rate of recurrence from 75% to about 36%, thus improving patient survival [32]. The absence of HBV DNA in serum prior to transplantation was also found to be an independent predictor of lower risk of HBV recurrence after transplantation [32]. With the use of long-term HBIG prophylaxis, survival significantly improved from 53% in the period of 1987–1991, to 69% between 1992 and 1996, to 76% in the period of 1997–2002 [33]. The main limitations to long-term HBIG prophylaxis is its limited supply and its cost of up to $100,000 in the first year and $40,000–50,000 each year thereafter. The combination of HBIG and lamivudine achieves significantly lower HBV recurrence rates in comparison with HBIG or lamivudine monoprophylaxis, more potent nucleos(t)ide analogues may lead to substantial reduction in HBIG dosage or even eliminate the need for HBIG after the initial postoperative period [34, 35].

Nucleos(t)ide analogues (NUCs) inhibit viral replication by targeting the HBV reverse transcriptase in competitively incorporating into the viral DNA and preventing transcriptional elongation and are capable of altering the natural history of HBV pre-transplant and enabling most patients to safely undergo transplantation with outcomes similar, if not better, than those achieved for other liver transplant indications [36, 37]. Currently available drugs for the treatment of chronic HBV infection target HBV DNA polymerase and include the nucleoside antagonists lamivudine (LAM), entecavir (ETV), and telbivudine (TBV) and the nucleotide antagonists adefovir (ADV) and tenofovir (TDF). These antiviral medications have been shown to delay disease progression and even reverse hepatic decompensation, as well as reverse histologic changes such as hepatic inflammation and fibrosis [38, 39]. Until recently, tenofovir disoproxil fumarate and entecavir were used as first-line agents due to resistance profiles [40]. Although not yet studied in the transplant setting, tenofovir is now available as the prodrug tenofovir alafenamide, which is capable of delivery to target cells more efficiently at a lower dose and, as a result, is associated with a more favorable renal and bone safety profile [41].

Antiviral prophylaxis is also an important consideration for prevention of de novo HBV infection in hepatitis B surface antigen (HBsAg)-negative recipients receiving liver transplantation of hepatitis B core antibody (HBcAb)-positive donors. The use of HBcAb (+) grafts is associated with a 25–95% risk of de novo HBV transmission without the use of antiviral agents and immunoprophylaxis, which can lead to severe hepatitis and graft loss [42]. Both lamivudine monotherapy and HBIG + lamivudine have been shown to significantly decrease the risk of de novo infections to about 3%, with viral breakthrough infection frequently related to medication noncompliance. While risk of developing lamivudine resistance with long-term use is likely less in the population because of significantly less or undetectable viral loads, other new and more potent nucleos(t)ide analogues with lower resistance profiles such as tenofovir and entecavir are preferable over lamivudine [43].

Non-liver Transplant Recipients

Kidney Transplant Recipients

Kidney Transplant Recipients

The prevalence of HBV infection in dialyzed patients varies by regions; it is estimated to be between 0% and 10% in industrialized countries and 2–20% in the developing regions of the world [44]. Over the last 20 years, the prevalence of HBV infection has declined dramatically due to improved screening, hygiene, and preventative measures such as vaccination. Prior to the advent of effective antiviral agents, patients with chronic HBV infection were excluded from kidney and other organ transplantation due to the risk of severe viral recurrence and progression of disease. Fornairon et al. reported in a large cohort study of 151 HBsAg-positive renal transplant recipients a high rate of persistent viral replication (50%) and reactivation (30%) [45]. Histologic deterioration was observed in 85.3% of 101 patients who underwent serial liver biopsies, and liver disease was the leading cause of death. Among renal transplant recipients, reactivation was reported in patients with prior exposure and clearance of HBV infection [46]; with the widespread availability of new-generation antiviral drugs, it is important to note that renal transplantation can be safely performed in patients with chronic HBV kidney transplant recipient infection and end-stage kidney disease in need of long-term renal replacement therapy.

The impact on positive HbsAg on mortality and survival in renal transplant recipients has been controversial. Earlier studies failed to show a difference in 5-year survival between HBsAg-positive and HBsAg-negative patients [47, 48, 49]. However, subsequent studies of larger populations with longer follow-up indicated worse graft and patient survival [50, 51, 52]. A meta-analysis including 6050 patients performed by Fabrizi et al. found that HBsAg was an independent risk factor for death after transplantation [51]. However, the study included recipients transplanted between 1972 and 1999, prior to the widespread use of effective antiviral agents. In a more recent analysis of 1346 HBsAg-positive renal transplant recipients in the period between 2001 and 2007 in the United States, patient and graft survivals in HBsAg-positive recipients were comparable to HBV-negative recipients, even though HBsAg-positive recipients were at increased kidney transplant recipient risk of developing liver disease [53].

The rates of HCC were higher in renal transplant recipients prior to the use of antiviral therapy, likely secondary to antirejection drug-induced immunosuppression [50, 54]. The utilization of antiviral therapy has changed the clinical course of liver disease after transplantation, presumably by reducing the risk for development of HCC; however, further larger prospective trials are needed to investigate the long-term outcomes of transplant recipients receiving antiviral therapy. It is recommended that transplant recipients with HBV and/or HCV infection to kidney transplant recipients receive early screening for HCC with abdominal ultrasound every 3 months for patients with cirrhosis and every 6–12 months for those without evidence of cirrhosis [55].

The current recommendation is that all HBsAg-positive patients who are candidates for solid organ transplantation be treated with nucleos(t)ide analogues. While immunosuppressive therapy lasts, patients should receive preemptive therapy regardless of HBV DNA levels. Anti-HBc-positive HBsAg-negative patients with undetectable HBV DNA may also be at risk for reactivation and should be followed up closely with HBV DNA and serum ALT testing every 3 months and treated with antiviral therapy if reactivation occurs. The most experience has been with lamivudine, the first nucleos(t)ide agent approved in 1998. Studies have shown that HBsAg-positive renal transplant recipients treated with lamivudine have similar 10-year survival rates as HBsAg-negative patients (85% vs. 88%) [56, 57]. However, the high rate of developing drug resistance and subsequent breakthrough viral reactivation is a concern with the use of lamivudine. Althoug lamivudine improves short-term (50 month) reactivation-free survival, it is nor effective in preventing HBV reactivation or improving long-term survival after transplantation suggested that although the use of lamivudine improved reactivation-free survival in the short term (first 50 months), it was not effective in the prevention of HBV reactivation or improvement in long-term survival after transplantation [58]. Newer agents such as entecavir and tenofovir are preferable to lamivudine because of lower risk of development of post-exposure viral kidney transplant recipient mutation resulting in de novo drug resistance [59, 60].

Heart Transplant Recipients

Similar to renal transplantation, chronic HBV can often progress aggressively after heart transplantation.

In early studies among cardiac transplant recipients, chronic HBV after transplantation was seen frequently. Reports in 1980s had attributed this to iatrogenic acquisition of HBV infection during the post-transplant endomyocardial biopsies; sporadic standards for infection prevention and equipment contamination were regarded as a potential source for such infections [61]. In a study, 56% of patients with de novo HBV infection after heart transplantation developed severe fibrosis or cirrhosis within a mean duration of 7.4 years [62] . Long-term follow-up of HBsAg-positive patients also showed significantly reduced survival when compared with HBV non-infected controls, often as a result of liver-related deaths (32% vs. 62%, respectively) [62]. As with the experience in the recipients of renal transplants, long-term antiviral therapy has been shown to be well-tolerated and efficacious, preventing progression of liver disease and potential for hepatic decompensation [63]. Observational studies have also shown that HBsAg-positive donor hearts can be safely transplanted into HBsAb-positive recipients; however, HBsAg-positive donors should only be considered for high-risk situations [64].

Bone-Marrow Transplant Recipients

The risk of HBV reactivation is most significant among patients undergoing allogenic bone marrow transplantation and can often have serious, life-threatening consequences. Due to severity of hosts' immune dysregulation following myeloablative allogeneic HSCT preparatory conditioning regimens, reactivation of hepatitis B viral infection in HBsAg-positive patients is near-universal [65]. HBV reverse seroconversion in patients with serologic evidence of past HBV infection (HBsAg negative, HBcAb positive) has also been frequently reported [66, 67]. Because of fatal consequences of reverse seroconversion and viral reactivation, all potential bone marrow recipients are tested for HBV biomarkers and receive antiviral prophylaxis if there is evidence of past HBV infection. Reactivation often develops during late HSCT period, between 1 and 3 years after undergoing transplantation, so long-term, if not lifelong, antiviral treatment is often recommended [68, 69, 70].

Pre-transplant Evaluation

All patients undergoing a transplant evaluation should be evaluated for exposure and/or active infection with hepatitis B with HBsAg, HBsAb, and HBcAb. Level of viremia with HBV DNA viral load should be assessed in all patients. Occasionally, patients will have occult HBV infection (OBI), in which low viral replication is present without detection of HBsAg. The prevalence of OBI depends on both the sensitivity of testing available as well as the prevalence of HBV infection in the population. In low HBV prevalence countries such as the United States, OBI has been reported in 0.1–2.4% of HBsAg-negative, HBcAb-positive blood donors, with or without the evidence of HBsAb positivity. In the regions with high HBV endemicity, the risk of OBI may be as high as 15% [71, 72, 73]. The clinical significance of OBI is controversial, with some case reports describing HBV reactivation in allogeneic HSCT and solid organ transplant recipients with OBI receiving post-transplant immunosuppression [74, 75]. Other studies have found that OBIs have not been associated with increased risk of acute rejection or development of de novo hepatitis B virus infection [76]. There is, however, significant evidence that OBI is a risk factor for HCC development [77].

For patients without evidence of previous exposure, vaccination should be provided prior to transplantation due to suboptimum vaccine response noted after undergoing allogeneic transplantation. In prior nonresponders to hepatitis B virus vaccine, revaccination with a double dose may be more effective [78]. In hemodialysis patients, who have impaired response to hepatitis B vaccines, double dose revaccination and repeated booster doses are often necessary to achieve prolonged seroconversion [79]. There is also evidence that combined HAV/HBV vaccination may enhance vaccination response to HBV [80].

Hepatitis C

Hepatitis C virus (HCV) is a small 30–60-nm-diameter, enveloped, positive-sense, single-stranded RNA virus belonging to *Flaviviridae* family [81]. It possesses a 9.6 kb genome that encodes ten proteins as well as two glycoproteins, E1 and E2, which possess two hypervariable regions that are prone to extensive mutation and antigenic variability [82]. Six major HCV genotypes have been identified, differing in their nucleotide sequence by approximately 30% [83]. The major genotypes differ in geographic location and therapeutic options. Genotype 1a is most prevalent in the United States and Northern Europe [83].

There are approximately 160 million human carriers of HCV worldwide and over 4 million or 1.6% of the population in the United States [84, 85]. The highest prevalence of 15% is reported from Egypt's Nile Delta, whereas prevalence in Europe, the Americas, Southeast Asia, and Africa ranges from 1% to 5% [84]. HCV is predominantly transmitted through percutaneous exposure to infected blood and less commonly via unprotected sexual intercourse and vertical transmission [86, 87]. Populations at highest risk include intravenous drug users, tattoo recipients, and health care workers. Prior to 1992, recipients of blood and blood products and patients who underwent solid organ transplantation were at increased risk for HCV infection, due to less sensitive HCV screening assays [88].

HCV has historically carried a significant disease burden in industrialized countries as the leading cause for liver failure and the most frequent indication for liver transplantation [89]. The approval of direct antiviral agents in 2011 has dramatically altered the treatment landscape in providing a near-complete virologic response rate in most cases [90]. This stands in contrast to traditional treatment strategies based on pegylated interferon and ribavirin, which achieved virologic response rates of <50% in patients with HCV genotypes 1 and 4 infection and up to 80% in HCV genotypes 2 and 3 infection [90]. Direct-acting antivirals may also now be used safely in patients with advanced liver disease, who can be treated prior to undergoing liver transplantation, substantially reducing the risk for HCV recurrence during post-transplant period. HCV eradication in cirrhotic patients leads to improvements in MELD score and portal hypertension, albeit, such viral eradication may heighten the risk of progression of hepatocellular carcinoma. Patients with HCV infection who have received a liver transplant may also now be safely treated with the new effective direct anti-HCV drugs, although the choice of regimen should be tailored to minimize interactions with immunosuppressive medications. New areas of controversy have been ushered in by the use of direct antiviral agents, as the ability to utilize of HCV-positive organs and treat patients effectively following transplantation had led to careful consideration regarding timing of treatment that can on one hand hinder disease progression but may also limit access to HCV-positive organ grafts. Direct-acting antivirals can be utilized to eradicate HCV infection in non-liver transplant patients; however, despite effective anti-HCV therapy, the accompanying risks of cirrhosis and hepatocellular carcinoma remain.

Hepatitis C-Mediated Liver Disease

Acute Hepatitis C

The majority of acute HCV infections are asymptomatic and subclinical. Symptomatic HCV infection manifests with nonspecific flu-like symptoms, including fatigue, nausea, abdominal pain, loss of appetite, mild fever, and pruritus [91]. HCV RNA may be detected in the serum within 1–3 weeks following the initial exposure to the virus [92]. Viral detection is followed by a rise in bilirubin as well as an increase in serum transaminase levels frequently to values of more than ten times the upper limit of normal, indicating active hepatocellular injury [92]. HCV-induced fulminant hepatic failure (FHF) is uncommon, with occurrence in 10% of patients presenting with acute HCV infection [93]. Coinfection with hepatitis B virus is an important risk factor for developing HCV-induced FHF and carries a survival rate of 20–30% [93, 94].

Chronic Hepatitis C

Disease progression and risk of development of cirrhosis is variable in patients with HCV infection. End-stage liver cirrhosis develops in 4–24% of patients with chronic HCV infection within 20 years [95–97]. Host, viral, and external interactions influence the time frame between initial HCV infection and the development of cirrhosis. The progression of HCV-induced fibrosis is closely related to the age at the time of initial infection; older individuals appear to progress to cirrhosis at a much more rapid rate compared with those in whom the infection is acquired at a younger age [98].

Factors known to promote hepatic inflammation augment disease progression in HCV-infected patients. Increased hepatic iron promotes increased inflammation in the liver and fibrosis in patients with chronic HCV infection [99, 100]. Ongoing steatohepatitis is associated with more rapid progression in liver fibrosis and may increase the risk for HCC by nearly threefold [101]. Excessive alcohol consumption is an independent risk factor for the development of cirrhosis [98]. Alcohol intake of >50 g daily has been shown to markedly increase the progression of liver fibrosis [102]. Viral factors such as infection with HCV genotype 3 result in greater progression of liver disease and risk of death [103, 104].

HCV coinfection with HBV significantly enhances risk of death compared to patients with chronic HCV infection alone [105]. The frequency of hepatic failure appears to be eightfold higher among the 35 million people coinfected with HBV and HCV [93]. Nearly 30% of HIV-infected patients are coinfected with HCV in the United States [106]. Coinfection in this population is associated with greater risk of cirrhosis-related complications compared to HCV infection without HIV [106].

Complications associated with hepatic decompensation include ascites, variceal bleeding, and severe bacterial infections. The annual rate of these severe complications is approximately 2–9% among cirrhotic patients [107]. Following the first episode of hepatic decompensation, a 1-year mortality rate ranges between 15% and 20%; furthermore, a 10-year patient survival rate declines below 50% [108].

In patients with chronic HCV infection, hepatocellular carcinoma typically develops in the context of liver cirrhosis with an annual risk ranging between 2% and 4% [109]. Surveillance is not recommended for all HCV-infected patients, but it is recommended for all HCV-infected patients with cirrhosis [110]. Overall, hepatitis C virus is responsible for 25% of hepatocellular carcinomas worldwide [111].

Treatment of Hepatitis C in the Liver Transplant Setting

Effective antiviral treatment prevents the progression of liver disease at all stages and leads to improvement in hepatic histopathology and degree of fibrosis [112, 113]. Among cirrhotic patients who achieve a sustained virologic response, 64% of such patients demonstrate regression in hepatic cirrhosis [113]. Treatment with a sustained virologic response (SVR) in cirrhotic patients is associated with improvement in portal hypertension, prevention of varices, and hepatic decompensation. It is important to emphasize that SVR following interferon-based therapy was associated with a 10–20% rate of hepatocellular carcinoma [114].

Until the approval of direct antiviral, interferon-free therapy (DAA) in 2011, treatment of HCV infection in both the pre- and post-transplant periods was highly problematic due to low efficacy and high treatment-related toxicity [90]. Cirrhotic patients were often ineligible to receive pegylated-interferon and ribavirin-based regimen due to risk of further decompensation, development of bacterial sepsis, or the occurrence of potentially life-threatening myelosuppression evident by leukopenia and/or thrombocytopenia. Ribavirin-induced anemia posed a significant challenge in cirrhotic patients with preexisting spur cell hemolytic anemia and those with gastrointestinal bleeding. Psychiatric comorbidities may be intensified due to interferon-associated neuropsychiatric adverse events, particularly depression [115]. In the post-transplant setting, HCV recurrence after interferon-based therapy was associated with high morbidity, especially hematologic toxicity that may be accentuated in patients with renal insufficiency and concurrent treatment with antirejection drugs or anti-GVHD therapy; SVR rate ranged from 8% to 50%.

With the advent of DAA, the treatment of hepatitis C virus infection in the transplant setting was immediately transformed. In cirrhotic patients, effective therapy is associated with improvement in liver function as evidenced by a decline in MELD score as well as diminished in hepatic portal venous pressures and esophageal varices [116, 117]. With the population of HCV-positive patients diminishing due to successful antiviral treatment prior to liver transplantation, and the availability of effective post-transplant treatment (see below), the burden and clinical significance of post-transplant HCV recurrence have greatly diminished.

Timing of Direct-Acting Antiviral Therapy

Controversy exists as to the optimum timing and most clinical benefit of DAA during pre-transplant period. In contrast to patients with decompensated hepatitis B cirrhosis, in whom up to 60% demonstrate a dramatic clinical and biochemical response to effective anti-HBV therapy, patients treated for HCV cirrhosis frequently improve biochemically with decrease in MELD and CTP scores but may not exhibit clinical improvement [118]. Although pre-transplant treatment improves MELD score and diminishes the risk of death and need for transplantation, it may also render a patient with more advanced cirrhosis with a poor quality of life and nonprogressive liver disease with diminished priority for liver transplant. Opting for post-transplant treatment also enables access to HCV-positive allografts. Recently, this approach has been taken one step further with transplantation of HCV-positive allografts into HCV-negative recipients followed by DAA therapy given after transplantation [119]. As a result, there is currently a debate as to the optimal timing of DAA therapy. Although recent analyses have found pre-transplant treatment to be more cost-effective, both options are now commonly a focal point of patient-physician decision-making. Finally, DAA therapy has recently been reported to be possibly associated with the increased risk of aggressive and early recurrence of hepatocellular carcinoma. Protective anti-HCV endogenous interferon release, critical for maintaining effective tumor surveillance by hindering tumor proliferation and angiogenesis, may be downregulated following DAA therapy [120]. These observations have led some clinicians to monitor cirrhotic patients closely during and after treatment for malignancy and consider deferral of therapy in patients with active and recently treated hepatocellular cancer.

Direct-Acting Antiviral Therapy in the Pre-transplant Setting

Essentially all patients with advanced liver disease can be safely treated for HCV with a high degree of expectation and probability for achieving a durable SVR. Treatment of hepatitis C prior to liver transplantation is associated with rare post-transplant HCV recurrence, especially for those who are HCV RNA negative for at least 1 month prior to undergoing transplantation [121]. Fatty liver disease is common among HCV-positive patients, and progression of fibrosis in patients achieving an SVR may progress due to nonalcoholic steatohepatitis [122]. Moreover, the risk for hepatocellular carcinoma persists, particularly in patients with HCV genotype 3 [123].

Treatment options are based on the HCV genotype and involve combinations of agents directed at two or three specific viral targets, including the RNA polymerase, protease, and NS5a. Due to rapidly expanding options, the American Association for the Study of Liver Diseases (AASLD) maintains a web-based consensus statement that permits frequent updates [124]. As a result, specific therapies will not be discussed. As a general guideline, however, the patient with advanced cirrhosis who is commonly treatment experienced requires a longer duration of therapy and occasionally with the concomitant use of ribavirin to achieve comparable treatment results to those with less advanced disease. In addition, the use of protease inhibitors is usually avoided due to the risk of drug-induced hepatotoxicity with the potential for rapid and progressive liver failure leading to death.

Direct-Acting Antiviral Therapy in the Post-transplant Setting

The treatment options for post-transplant hepatitis C virus are, for the most part, similar to those applied during the pretransplant period with a minor difference in effectiveness despite the concomitant use of immunosuppression; the reader is referred to the AASLD guidelines that are regularly updated [124] Special considerations for patients after allograft transplantation include drug-drug interactions with tacrolimus and cyclosporine with several of the regimens requiring calcineurin inhibitor (CNI) dose adjustment or altogether CNI avoidance, with a possible need for prolonged therapy and/or concomitant use of ribavirin. Patients may also need an increased immunosuppressant dose after HCV virologic clearance and its potential adverse effect on hosts' antiviral immune surveillance.

Recurrent Hepatitis C After Liver Transplantation

Hepatitis C infection following transplantation is nearly universal for those with active viremia prior to transplantation [125]. Until recently, recurrent hepatitis C infection was a major cause of graft failure and risk of death. Recurrent HCV infection is associated with a more rapid rate of progression of liver fibrosis compared to immunocompetent patients, and up to 30% of patients develop cirrhosis within 5 years compared with cirrhosis that took 20–30 years to develop in the immunocompetent population [126]. Recurrence of HCV-related cirrhosis was until recently the main cause of allograft dysfunction or graft loss and significantly curtailed patient survival as compared to non-HCV controls undergoing liver transplantation [127, 128] In addition, approximately 5–10% of patients developed a severe form of recurrent HCV known as fibrosing cholestatic hepatitis, characterized by very high HCV RNA levels, cholestatic laboratory patterns with bilirubin levels >6 mg/dL, and alkaline phosphatase >5-fold normal values; ballooning hepatocytes, sinusoidal fibrosis, cholestasis, and a low level of tissue inflammation despite bile duct proliferation on liver biopsy were prominent histologic features of FCH in this setting [129, 130]. High viral load, older recipient age, non-Caucasian race, female gender, insulin resistance and diabetes mellitus, high-dose corticosteroid treatment for acute cellular graft rejection, donor age greater than 55 years, and HIV coinfection were significant risk factors for more severe HCV recurrence following liver transplantation.

Hepatitis C and Non-liver Transplantation

Kidney Transplantation

Hepatitis C and End-Stage Kidney Disease

Chronic hepatitis C is common in the kidney transplant population, with the prevalence of HCV seropositivity ranging from 7% to 40% in developed countries [131–133]. Several factors account for this high prevalence. Firstly, HCV is a possible factor in the development of the renal disease. Chronic HCV infection may induce a mixed cryoglobulinemia and a systemic vasculitis, leading to glomerulonephritis and renal failure [134–136]. Chronic HCV infection is also associated with a high rate of insulin resistance and type 2 diabetes mellitus [137]. In addition, de novo acquisition of hepatitis C among patients on hemodialysis occurs with high frequency. In patients receiving routine hemodialysis,

HCV seroprevalence (8–10%) and acquisition rate (1–3% annually) was higher compared to patients on peritoneal dialysis (3–5% and <1% annually, respectively) [138–140]. Nosocomial HCV transmission has been described in several reports and can be averted by strict adherence to standard HCV precautions [141, 142]. Mortality rates are higher in dialysis patients with HCV infection as compared to uninfected individuals [143]. While there is a higher incidence of liver disease in HCV-infected patients, cardiovascular causes are the most frequent cause of death, and the presence of diabetes mellitus and the duration of dialysis are the two factors associated most closely with mortality [144].

Hepatitis C and Kidney Transplantation

HCV-positive renal transplant recipients have better survival than matched HCV-positive patients awaiting transplant [145]. Although the presence of HCV infection is not a contraindication to kidney transplantation, a complete evaluation of the infection and its impact on liver function and presence of portal hypertension should be noted [146]. The natural progression of chronic hepatitis C in the kidney transplant patient and impact of accelerated liver fibrosis during the post-transplant periods were concerns historically, although are much less so now with the availability of effective post-transplant DAA therapy.

Evaluation of the Kidney Transplant Patient

Given the high incidence and a significant effect of HCV infection on survival in ESRD patients, screening is routinely recommended for patients undergoing routine hemodialysis [131]. Although traditional ELISA are a useful screening tool for the presence of HCV infection, it is important to note that HCV viremia in anti-HCV Ab-negative HD patients may occur and ranges between 1% and 15% [147, 148]. While it has been suggested that immunologic alterations in this population may account for negative anti-HCV antibodies, newly available commercial third-generation assays have been demonstrated to be more effective and sensitive as HCV PCR in detecting infection in this patient population [149, 150]. Additionally, in the HCV population, the presence of normal liver enzymes is more common among uremic patients compared to non-uremic patients, and normal aminotransferase levels do not exclude the presence of significant hepatic pathology [151]. Historically, staging of fibrosis with liver biopsy of elasticity was recommended in all HCV-positive patients undergoing pre-transplant screening, as aminotransferase levels are not reliable in determining HCV disease activity [152]. However, noninvasive elastography is now widely used during pre-transplant evaluation.

Natural History of Hepatitis C in the Kidney Transplant Patient

The natural history of the kidney transplant patient with chronic hepatitis C is highly variable. It has been reported that HCV-postive renal transplant recipients matched with individuals without renal failure have a significantly lower annual rate of fibrosis progression in the transplanted group (0.05–0.18) compared to patients without renal failure (0.13–0.26) observed on 37-month follow-up liver biopsy [153]. HCV infection after renal transplantation in most patients did not adversely affect liver histology in the extended follow-up. In fact, liver fibrosis might regress after transplantation in some patients, especially in those with an initial mild fibrosis score [154]. While the presence of cirrhosis on pre-transplant liver biopsy has been reported to be associated with a 26% 10-year survival, renal transplantation may still be considered in this population [153]. Acquisition of acute hepatitis C infection at the time of kidney transplantation or during the post-transplantation period, however, is characterized by a rapid progression of hepatic fibrosis, development of cholestatic syndrome, and high mortality rate [155].

Renal transplantation among HCV-infected individuals undergoing renal transplantation have decreased mortality and cardiovascular events and improved qualitiy of life compared to those maintained on long-term renal replacement therapy [145, 156]. Overall survival is improved following kidney transplantation for the HCV-infected individual; however, long-term patient and graft survivals are reduced in HCV-infected patients compared with uninfected transplanted controls, with a reported relative risk of 1.6 12 years after undergoing transplantation [157, 158]. Additionally, increased burden due to liver disease, new-onset diabetes mellitus, post-transplant glomerulonephritis, and sepsis was observed notably more frequently among HCV-positive patients [158, 159].

Successful treatment of HCV in patients with end-stage renal disease is associated with a lower incidence of HCV-related post-transplant glomerulonephritis [160]. Due to the potential for interferon treatment-induced acute allograft rejection, post-transplant HCV treatment was previously regarded as a contraindication. The strong efficacy of DAA now renders all HCV patients potential treatment candidates after kidney transplantation.

Source of Allograft

The use of HCV-positive donors in HCV-positive recipients is commonly employed to mitigate the shortage of organs in the face of increasing waitlist times. The prevalence of post-transplant liver disease and graft and patient survival in the HCV-positive population was similar after an average of 26–30-month follow-up regardless of donor HCV status [161]. A subsequent large retrospective study demonstrated that longer-term survival was favorable among HCV-negative donors, and in HCV-positive donor kidney transplant, survival improved compared with such patients who remained on hemodialysis [162]. Due to effectiveness of post-transplant treatment, a clinical trial of transplantation of HCV-positive allografts into HCV-negative recipients is currently underway [163].

Heart and Lung Transplantation

Among heart transplant recipients, the presence of HCV ranges from 7% to 18% [164, 165]. In a retrospective study of 96 patients with and without pre-existing HCV infection, no difference in mortality rates was observed, although liver-related deaths were more common among HCV infected patients (39%) compared with those without HCV infection (2%) [166]. Several subsequent studies with follow-up periods of 5 years have found a significantly higher mortality in HCV-seropositive individuals [167, 168].

Unlike liver and kidney allograft transplants, which are known viral reservoirs, the reported rate of HCV transmission from HCV-seropositive donor heart transplants has been lower, ranging between 25% and up to 82% [169, 170]. Although satisfactory outcomes of allocating HCV-positive hearts to elderly recipients have been reported, recent studies have reported an increased mortality in recipients of HCV-infected donor hearts [171].

Heart transplantation recipients should be carefully evaluated for antiviral treatment. Interferon may exacerbate heart failure or arrhythmias, and ribavirin-induced anemia may precipitate coronary ischemia and should be used with caution in such patients. Direct-acting antiviral treatments with improved side effect profiles have demonstrated successful eradication of HCV and may therefore become more widely utilized in this population [172].

The prevalence of HCV-seropositive lung transplant recipients in the period 2000–2007 was 1–2% [173]. Rapidly progressive hepatic fibrosis largely accounts for the high mortality rate following lung transplantation [174]. Most centers defer lung transplantation in HCV-seropositive patients. However, a survey report published in 2011 indicated that 19 centers that considered HCV-seropositive patients for lung transplantation had a 5-year post-transplant survival rate of 51% compared with 49% observed in HCV-Ab-negative recipients [173]. Although the study was encouraging, it had many important limitations as it did not distinguish the virologic status of HCV-seropositive lung transplant recipients by the level of HCV viremia and pre-transplant liver histopathology in HCV-seropositive candidates. Based on data from a few single-center reports with small numbers, guidelines from the American Society for Transplant Physicians and International Society for Heart and Lung Transplantation indicate that "Hepatitis C with biopsy-proven histologic evidence of liver disease" is a contraindication for lung transplantation [173–175]. Finally, combined liver/heart transplantation for patients with decompensated cirrhosis has been proposed [176].

Hepatitis C in Bone Marrow Transplantation

Hepatitis C is an important pathogen in patients undergoing HSCT. Recent epidemiologic and molecular observations have linked HCV to the development of mostly non-Hodgkin B-cell lymphomas following allogenic stem cell transplantation. Studies from Italy and Japan, where HCV prevalence in the general population ranges between 2% and 10%, demonstrated an increased risk for B-cell lymphoma (odds ratio from 2 to 4) in individuals with chronic HCV infection [177, 178, 179]. Although the precise molecular basis for HCV-induced B-cell proliferation remains to be determined, possible mechanisms include chronic antigen stimulation of B-cell subpopulation through B-cell surface receptors and complex cell immortalization and proliferation via a variety of pathways currently under investigation [180, 181, 182]. Antiviral therapy for the treatment of chronic HCV infection in patients with potential HCV-related B-cell neoplastic processes is without effect.

The prevalence of HCV infection was nearly 6% in HSCT recipients [183]. HCV infection poses unique challenges in this population during early and late post-transplant period. In the early transplant period, HCV infection has been associated with a higher risk for veno-occlusive disease and acute graft-versus-host disease involving the liver [184, 185]. Patients after HSCT may have five- to tenfold increase in the serum alanine aminotransferase level; distinguishing between acute hepatic GVHD vs. acute viral or drug-induced hepatitis becomes difficult [184]. In the late transplant period, patients with chronic HCV infection may have a higher rate of liver-related mortality. Eleven to twenty-four percent of long-term HSCT survivors (20 years) may develop cirrhosis of the liver [186, 187]. In one series, HCV genotype 3 was determined to be a risk factor for the development of cirrhosis, and the median time to cirrhosis in 96 HCV-seropositive allogeneic HSCT recipients was 18 years as compared with 40 years in 158 HCV-infected controls who did not receive transplants [187].

Because of the increased risk of complications, determination of the stage of HCV disease prior to stem cell transplantation is essential. Presence of severe hepatic fibrosis and cirrhosis increases the risk for fatal sinusoidal obstruction syndrome (SOS) following certain myeloablative preparatory regimens, and in such patients, highly immunosuppressive conditioning regimens are contraindicated. While the presence of hepatitis C infection is not an absolute contraindication to undergo allogeneic HSCT, patients should be selected based on the potential risk for complications during the post-transplant period. Liver biopsy may be considered in certain high-risk individuals before transplantation. There is limited literature describing the optimal approach to treatment of hepatitis C following blood and bone marrow stem cell transplantation. However, because of higher risk of earlier cirrhosis, it is recommended to repeat histological liver evaluation in all patients to evaluate the degree of fibrosis and grade of necrosis and inflammation. Interferon and ribavirin treatment in patients with hematologic malignancies posed a serious challenge due to the increased risk of drug toxicity [184]. Nearly 30% of patients cannot be treated because of contraindications [188]. In patients who can tolerate therapy, 20–40% may demonstrate a sustained virological response after bone marrow transplantation with combination treatment, reducing the risk for severe HCV-related complications [186, 187]. While direct-acting antivirals have prospects for improving treatment efficacy in this population, they have not to date been rigorously evaluated in the setting of allogeneic blood and bone marrow transplantation.

References

1. Franco E, Meleleo C, Serino L, Sorbara D, Zaratti L, Hepatitis A. Epidemiology and prevention in developing countries. World J Hepatol. 2012;4(3):68–73.
2. Cuthbert JA. Hepatitis A: old and new. Clin Microbiol Rev. 2001;14(1):38–58.
3. Trepo C, Zoulim F, Pradat P. Viral hepatitis. Curr Opin Infect Dis. 1999;12(5):481–90.
4. Victor JC, Monto AS, Surdina TY, Suleimenova SZ, Vaughan G, Nainan OV, et al. Hepatitis A vaccine versus immune globulin for postexposure prophylaxis. N Engl J Med. 2007;357(17):1685–94.
5. Matheny ME, Fitzhenry F, Speroff T, Green JK, Griffith ML, Vasilevskis EE, et al. Detection of infectious symptoms from VA emergency department and primary care clinical documentation. Int J Med Inform. 2012;81(3):143–56.
6. Ben-Ari Z, Vaknin H, Tur-Kaspa R. N-acetylcysteine in acute hepatic failure (non-paracetamol-induced). Hepato-Gastroenterology. 2000;47(33):786–9.
7. Yoon EL, Yim HJ, Kim SY, Kim JH, Lee JH, Lee YS, et al. Clinical courses after administration of oral corticosteroids in patients with severely cholestatic acute hepatitis A; three cases. Korean J Hepatol. 2010;16(3):329–33.
8. Attili AF, Rusticali A, Varriale M, Carli L, Repice AM, Callea F. The effect of ursodeoxycholic acid on serum enzymes and liver histology in patients with chronic active hepatitis. A 12-month double-blind, placebo-controlled trial. J Hepatol. 1994;20(3):315–20.
9. Keeffe EB. Hepatitis A and B superimposed on chronic liver disease: vaccine-preventable diseases. Trans Am Clin Climatol Assoc. 2006;117:227–37; discussion 37–8
10. Vento S, Garofano T, Renzini C, Cainelli F, Casali F, Ghironzi G, et al. Fulminant hepatitis associated with hepatitis A virus superinfection in patients with chronic hepatitis C. N Engl J Med. 1998;338(5):286–90.
11. Taylor RM, Davern T, Munoz S, Han SH, McGuire B, Larson AM, et al. Fulminant hepatitis A virus infection in the United States: Incidence, prognosis, and outcomes. Hepatology. 2006;44(6):1589–97.
12. Arslan M, Wiesner RH, Poterucha JJ, Gross JB Jr, Zein NN. Hepatitis A antibodies in liver transplant recipients: evidence for loss of immunity posttransplantation. Liver Transpl. 2000;6(2):191–5.
13. Eisenbach C, Longerich T, Fickenscher H, Schalasta G, Stremmel W, Encke J. Recurrence of clinically significant hepatitis A following liver transplantation for fulminant hepatitis A. J Clin Virol. 2006;35(1):109–12.
14. Park GC, Hwang S, Yu YD, Park PJ, Choi YI, Song GW, et al. Intractable recurrent hepatitis A virus infection requiring repeated liver transplantation: a case report. Transplant Proc. 2010;42(10):4658–60.
15. Keeffe EB, Iwarson S, McMahon BJ, Lindsay KL, Koff RS, Manns M, et al. Safety and immunogenicity of hepatitis A vaccine in patients with chronic liver disease. Hepatology. 1998;27(3):881–6.
16. Dumot JA, Barnes DS, Younossi Z, Gordon SM, Avery RK, Domen RE, et al. Immunogenicity of hepatitis A vaccine in decompensated liver disease. Am J Gastroenterol. 1999;94(6):1601–4.
17. Brundage SC, Fitzpatrick AN, Hepatitis A. Am Fam Physician. 2006;73(12):2162–8.
18. Martin K, Drabble A, Manlhiot C, Dipchand AI. Response to hepatitis A and B vaccination after pediatric heart transplant. Pediatr Transplant. 2012;16(7):699–703.
19. Gunther M, Stark K, Neuhaus R, Reinke P, Schroder K, Bienzle U. Rapid decline of antibodies after hepatitis A immunization in liver and renal transplant recipients. Transplantation. 2001;71(3):477–9.
20. Unal Ince E, Ertem M, Ileri T, Sayili A, Belgemen T, Uysal Z. Significant loss of hepatitis A Ab after allogeneic hematopoietic SCT in pediatric patients. Bone Marrow Transplant. 2010;45(1):171–5.
21. Karayiannis P. Hepatitis B virus: virology, molecular biology, life cycle and intrahepatic spread. Hepatol Int. 2017;11(6):500–8.
22. Ott JJ, Stevens GA, Groeger J, Wiersma ST. Global epidemiology of hepatitis B virus infection: new estimates of age-specific HBsAg seroprevalence and endemicity. Vaccine. 2012;30(12):2212–9.
23. Bosch FX, Ribes J, Cleries R, Diaz M. Epidemiology of hepatocellular carcinoma. Clin Liver Dis. 2005;9(2):191–211, v
24. Singal AK, Guturu P, Hmoud B, Kuo YF, Salameh H, Wiesner RH. Evolving frequency and outcomes of liver transplantation based on etiology of liver disease. Transplantation. 2013;95(5):755–60.
25. Kim WR. Epidemiology of hepatitis B in the United States. Hepatology. 2009;49(5 Suppl):S28–34.
26. Gust ID. Epidemiology of hepatitis B infection in the Western Pacific and South East Asia. Gut. 1996;38(Suppl 2):S18–23.
27. LeFevre ML, U.S. Preventive Services Task Force. Screening for hepatitis B virus infection in nonpregnant adolescents and adults: U.S. Preventive Services Task Force recommendation statement. Ann Intern Med. 2014;161(1):58–66.
28. Stevens CE, Beasley RP, Tsui J, Lee WC. Vertical transmission of hepatitis B antigen in Taiwan. N Engl J Med. 1975;292(15):771–4.
29. Tassopoulos NC, Papaevangelou GJ, Sjogren MH, Roumeliotou-Karayannis A, Gerin JL, Purcell RH. Natural history of acute hepatitis B surface antigen-positive hepatitis in Greek adults. Gastroenterology. 1987;92(6):1844–50.
30. Fattovich G, Giustina G, Schalm SW, Hadziyannis S, Sanchez-Tapias J, Almasio P, et al. Occurrence of hepatocellular carcinoma and decompensation in western European patients with cirrhosis type B. The EUROHEP Study Group on Hepatitis B Virus and Cirrhosis. Hepatology. 1995;21(1):77–82.
31. Terrault N, Roche B, Samuel D. Management of the hepatitis B virus in the liver transplantation setting: a European and an American perspective. Liver Transpl. 2005;11(7):716–32.
32. Samuel D, Muller R, Alexander G, Fassati L, Ducot B, Benhamou JP, et al. Liver transplantation in European patients with the hepatitis B surface antigen. N Engl J Med. 1993;329(25):1842–7.

33. Kim WR, Poterucha JJ, Kremers WK, Ishitani MB, Dickson ER. Outcome of liver transplantation for hepatitis B in the United States. Liver Transpl. 2004;10(8):968–74.
34. Fox AN, Terrault NA. The option of HBIG-free prophylaxis against recurrent HBV. J Hepatol. 2012;56(5):1189–97.
35. Han SH, Ofman J, Holt C, King K, Kunder G, Chen P, et al. An efficacy and cost-effectiveness analysis of combination hepatitis B immune globulin and lamivudine to prevent recurrent hepatitis B after orthotopic liver transplantation compared with hepatitis B immune globulin monotherapy. Liver Transpl. 2000;6(6):741–8.
36. Steinmuller T, Seehofer D, Rayes N, Muller AR, Settmacher U, Jonas S, et al. Increasing applicability of liver transplantation for patients with hepatitis B-related liver disease. Hepatology. 2002;35(6):1528–35.
37. Young K, Liu B, Bhuket T, Younossi Z, Saab S, Ahmed A, et al. Long-term trends in chronic hepatitis B virus infection associated liver transplantation outcomes in the United States. J Viral Hepat. 2017;24(9):789–96.
38. Marcellin P, Gane E, Buti M, Afdhal N, Sievert W, Jacobson IM, et al. Regression of cirrhosis during treatment with tenofovir disoproxil fumarate for chronic hepatitis B: a 5-year open-label follow-up study. Lancet. 2013;381(9865):468–75.
39. Chang TT, Liaw YF, Wu SS, Schiff E, Han KH, Lai CL, et al. Long-term entecavir therapy results in the reversal of fibrosis/cirrhosis and continued histological improvement in patients with chronic hepatitis B. Hepatology. 2010;52(3):886–93.
40. Buti M, Riveiro-Barciela M, Esteban R. Long-term safety and efficacy of nucleo(t)side analogue therapy in hepatitis B. Liver Int. 2018;38 Suppl 1:84–9.
41. Wong GL, Seto WK, Wong VW, Yuen MF, Chan HL. Review article: long-term safety of oral anti-viral treatment for chronic hepatitis B. Aliment Pharmacol Ther. 2018;47(6):730–7.
42. Skagen CL, Jou JH, Said A. Risk of de novo hepatitis in liver recipients from hepatitis-B core antibody-positive grafts – a systematic analysis. Clin Transpl. 2011;25(3):E243–9.
43. Chang MS, Olsen SK, Pichardo EM, Stiles JB, Rosenthal-Cogan L, Brubaker WD, et al. Prevention of de novo hepatitis B in recipients of core antibody-positive livers with lamivudine and other nucleos(t)ides: a 12-year experience. Transplantation. 2013;95(7):960–5.
44. Degott C, Degos F, Jungers P, Naret C, Courouce AM, Potet F, et al. Relationship between liver histopathological changes and HBsAg in 111 patients treated by long-term hemodialysis. Liver. 1983;3(6):377–84.
45. Fornairon S, Pol S, Legendre C, Carnot F, Mamzer-Bruneel MF, Brechot C, et al. The long-term virologic and pathologic impact of renal transplantation on chronic hepatitis B virus infection. Transplantation. 1996;62(2):297–9.
46. Raheem OA, Hickey DP. Treatment of hepatitis B virus reactivation in a cadaveric renal transplant recipient with entecavir. Arab J Nephrol Transplant. 2013;6(1):41–4.
47. Rivolta E, De Vecchi A, Tarantino A, Castelnovo C, Berardinelli L, Ponticelli C. Prognostic significance of hepatitis B surface antigenemia in cadaveric renal transplant patients. Transplant Proc. 1987;19(1 Pt 3):2153–4.
48. Flagg GL, Silberman H, Takamoto SK, Berne TV. The influence of hepatitis B infection on the outcome of renal allotransplantation. Transplant Proc. 1987;19(1 Pt 3):2155–8.
49. Huang CC, Lai MK, Fong MT. Hepatitis B liver disease in cyclosporine-treated renal allograft recipients. Transplantation. 1990;49(3):540–4.
50. Mathurin P, Mouquet C, Poynard T, Sylla C, Benalia H, Fretz C, et al. Impact of hepatitis B and C virus on kidney transplantation outcome. Hepatology. 1999;29(1):257–63.
51. Fabrizi F, Martin P, Dixit V, Kanwal F, Dulai G. HBsAg seropositive status and survival after renal transplantation: meta-analysis of observational studies. Am J Transplant. 2005;5(12):2913–21.
52. Lee WC, Shu KH, Cheng CH, Wu MJ, Chen CH, Lian JC. Long-term impact of hepatitis B, C virus infection on renal transplantation. Am J Nephrol. 2001;21(4):300–6.
53. Reddy PN, Sampaio MS, Kuo HT, Martin P, Bunnapradist S. Impact of pre-existing hepatitis B infection on the outcomes of kidney transplant recipients in the United States. Clin J Am Soc Nephrol. 2011;6(6):1481–7.
54. Breitenfeldt MK, Rasenack J, Berthold H, Olschewski M, Schroff J, Strey C, et al. Impact of hepatitis B and C on graft loss and mortality of patients after kidney transplantation. Clin Transpl. 2002;16(2):130–6.
55. Hoffmann CJ, Subramanian AK, Cameron AM, Engels EA. Incidence and risk factors for hepatocellular carcinoma after solid organ transplantation. Transplantation. 2008;86(6):784–90.
56. Chan TM, Fang GX, Tang CS, Cheng IK, Lai KN, Ho SK. Preemptive lamivudine therapy based on HBV DNA level in HBsAg-positive kidney allograft recipients. Hepatology. 2002;36(5):1246–52.
57. Ahn HJ, Kim MS, Kim YS, Kim SI, Huh KH, Ju MK, et al. Clinical outcome of renal transplantation in patients with positive pre-transplant hepatitis B surface antigen. J Med Virol. 2007;79(11):1655–63.
58. Park KS, Yang WS, Han DJ, Park JB, Park JS, Park SK. Long-term impact of prophylactic antiviral treatment in Hepatitis B surface antigen positive renal allograft recipients. Clin Nephrol. 2012;78(4):303–11.
59. Kidney Disease: Improving Global Outcomes Transplant Work Group. KDIGO clinical practice guideline for the care of kidney transplant recipients. Am J Transplant. 2009;9(Suppl 3):S1–155.
60. Daude M, Rostaing L, Saune K, Lavayssiere L, Basse G, Esposito L, et al. Tenofovir therapy in hepatitis B virus-positive solid-organ transplant recipients. Transplantation. 2011;91(8):916–20.
61. Drescher J, Wagner D, Haverich A, Flik J, Stachan-Kunstyr R, Verhagen W, et al. Nosocomial hepatitis B virus infections in cardiac transplant recipients transmitted during transvenous endomyocardial biopsy. J Hosp Infect. 1994;26(2):81–92.
62. Wedemeyer H, Pethig K, Manns MP, Boker KH. Hepatitis B infection in heart transplant patients. Gastroenterology. 2001;120(5):1311–3.
63. Potthoff A, Tillmann HL, Bara C, Deterding K, Pethig K, Meyer S, et al. Improved outcome of chronic hepatitis B after heart transplantation by long-term antiviral therapy. J Viral Hepat. 2006;13(11):734–41.
64. Wang SS, Chou NK, Ko WJ, Yu HY, Chen YS, Hsu RB, et al. Heart transplantation using donors positive for hepatitis. Transplant Proc. 2004;36(8):2371–3.
65. Lau GK, Liang R, Chiu EK, Lee CK, Lam SK. Hepatic events after bone marrow transplantation in patients with hepatitis B infection: a case controlled study. Bone Marrow Transplant. 1997;19(8):795–9.
66. Martin BA, Rowe JM, Kouides PA, DiPersio JF. Hepatitis B reactivation following allogeneic bone marrow transplantation: case report and review of the literature. Bone Marrow Transplant. 1995;15(1):145–8.
67. Webster A, Brenner MK, Prentice HG, Griffiths PD. Fatal hepatitis B reactivation after autologous bone marrow transplantation. Bone Marrow Transplant. 1989;4(2):207–8.
68. Hashino S, Nozawa A, Izumiyama K, Yonezumi M, Chiba K, Kondo T, et al. Lamivudine treatment for reverse seroconversion of hepatitis B 4 years after allogeneic bone marrow transplantation. Bone Marrow Transplant. 2002;29(4):361–3.
69. Hsiao LT, Chiou TJ, Liu JH, Chu CJ, Lin YC, Chao TC, et al. Extended lamivudine therapy against hepatitis B virus infection in hematopoietic stem cell transplant recipients. Biol Blood Marrow Transplant. 2006;12(1):84–94.
70. Myers RP, Swain MG, Urbanski SJ, Lee SS. Reactivation of hepatitis B e antigen-negative chronic hepatitis B in a bone marrow transplant recipient following lamivudine withdrawal. Can J Gastroenterol. 2001;15(9):599–603.

71. Hollinger FB. Hepatitis B virus infection and transfusion medicine: science and the occult. Transfusion. 2008;48(5):1001–26.
72. Hollinger FB, Sood G. Occult hepatitis B virus infection: a covert operation. J Viral Hepat. 2010;17(1):1–15.
73. Said ZN. An overview of occult hepatitis B virus infection. World J Gastroenterol. 2011;17(15):1927–38.
74. Giudice CL, Martinengo M, Pietrasanta P, Bocciardo L, Malavasi C, Rastelli S, et al. Occult hepatitis B virus infection: a case of reactivation in a patient receiving immunosuppressive treatment for allogeneic bone marrow transplantation. Blood Transfus. 2008;6(1):46–50.
75. Chen GD, Gu JL, Qiu J, Chen LZ. Outcomes and risk factors for hepatitis B virus (HBV) reactivation after kidney transplantation in occult HBV carriers. Transpl Infect Dis. 2013;15(3):300–5.
76. Ghisetti V, Marzano A, Zamboni F, Barbui A, Franchello A, Gaia S, et al. Occult hepatitis B virus infection in HBsAg negative patients undergoing liver transplantation: clinical significance. Liver Transpl. 2004;10(3):356–62.
77. Torbenson M, Thomas DL. Occult hepatitis B. Lancet Infect Dis. 2002;2(8):479–86.
78. Cardell K, Akerlind B, Sallberg M, Fryden A. Excellent response rate to a double dose of the combined hepatitis A and B vaccine in previous nonresponders to hepatitis B vaccine. J Infect Dis. 2008;198(3):299–304.
79. Pin M, Compte MT, Angelet P, Gallego C, Gutierrez C, Martinez Vea A. Long-term evaluation of immune response to hepatitis B vaccine in 136 patients undergoing hemodialysis. Nefrologia. 2009;29(5):415–20.
80. Kramer ES, Hofmann C, Smith PG, Shiffman ML, Sterling RK. Response to hepatitis A and B vaccine alone or in combination in patients with chronic hepatitis C virus and advanced fibrosis. Dig Dis Sci. 2009;54(9):2016–25.
81. Rosen HR. Clinical practice. Chronic hepatitis C infection. N Engl J Med. 2011;364(25):2429–38.
82. Murray PR, Rosenthal KS, Pfaller MA. Medical microbiology. 8th ed. Philadelphia, PA: Elsevier; 2016. x, 836 p
83. Smith DB, Simmonds P, International Committee on the Taxonomy of Viruses Hepeviridae Study Group, Jameel S, Emerson SU, Harrison TJ, et al. Consensus proposals for classification of the family Hepeviridae. J Gen Virol. 2015;96(Pt 5):1191–2.
84. Lavanchy D. Evolving epidemiology of hepatitis C virus. Clin Microbiol Infect. 2011;17(2):107–15.
85. Te HS, Jensen DM. Epidemiology of hepatitis B and C viruses: a global overview. Clin Liver Dis. 2010;14(1):1–21, vii
86. Grebely J, Prins M, Hellard M, Cox AL, Osburn WO, Lauer G, et al. Hepatitis C virus clearance, reinfection, and persistence, with insights from studies of injecting drug users: towards a vaccine. Lancet Infect Dis. 2012;12(5):408–14.
87. Lopez-Dieguez M, Montes ML, Pascual-Pareja JF, Quereda C, Von Wichmann MA, Berenguer J, et al. The natural history of liver cirrhosis in HIV-hepatitis C virus-coinfected patients. AIDS. 2011;25(7):899–904.
88. Williams JL, Cagle HH, Christensen CJ, Fox-Leyva LK, McMahon BJ. Results of a hepatitis C general transfusion lookback program for patients who received blood products before July 1992. Transfusion. 2005;45(6):1020–6.
89. Ly KN, Xing J, Klevens RM, Jiles RB, Ward JW, Holmberg SD. The increasing burden of mortality from viral hepatitis in the United States between 1999 and 2007. Ann Intern Med. 2012;156(4):271–8.
90. Gonzalez-Grande R, Jimenez-Perez M, Gonzalez Arjona C, Mostazo Torres J. New approaches in the treatment of hepatitis C. World J Gastroenterol. 2016;22(4):1421–32.
91. Maasoumy B, Wedemeyer H. Natural history of acute and chronic hepatitis C. Best Pract Res Clin Gastroenterol. 2012;26(4):401–12.
92. Mosley JW, Operskalski EA, Tobler LH, Andrews WW, Phelps B, Dockter J, et al. Viral and host factors in early hepatitis C virus infection. Hepatology. 2005;42(1):86–92.
93. Chu CM, Yeh CT, Liaw YF. Fulminant hepatic failure in acute hepatitis C: increased risk in chronic carriers of hepatitis B virus. Gut. 1999;45(4):613–7.
94. Hughes RD, Wendon J, Gimson AE. Acute liver failure. Gut. 1991;32(Suppl):S86–91.
95. Seeff LB. Natural history of chronic hepatitis C. Hepatology. 2002;36(5 Suppl 1):S35–46.
96. Thein HH, Yi Q, Dore GJ, Krahn MD. Estimation of stage-specific fibrosis progression rates in chronic hepatitis C virus infection: a meta-analysis and meta-regression. Hepatology. 2008;48(2):418–31.
97. Freeman AJ, Dore GJ, Law MG, Thorpe M, Von Overbeck J, Lloyd AR, et al. Estimating progression to cirrhosis in chronic hepatitis C virus infection. Hepatology. 2001;34(4 Pt 1):809–16.
98. Poynard T, Bedossa P, Opolon P. Natural history of liver fibrosis progression in patients with chronic hepatitis C. The OBSVIRC, METAVIR, CLINIVIR, and DOSVIRC groups. Lancet. 1997;349(9055):825–32.
99. Giannini E, Mastracci L, Botta F, Romagnoli P, Fasoli A, Risso D, et al. Liver iron accumulation in chronic hepatitis C patients without HFE mutations: relationships with histological damage, viral load and genotype and alpha-glutathione S-transferase levels. Eur J Gastroenterol Hepatol. 2001;13(11):1355–61.
100. Larson AM, Taylor SL, Bauermeister D, Rosoff L Jr, Kowdley KV. Pilot study of the relationship between histologic progression and hepatic iron concentration in chronic hepatitis C. J Clin Gastroenterol. 2003;37(5):406–11.
101. Poynard T, Ratziu V, McHutchison J, Manns M, Goodman Z, Zeuzem S, et al. Effect of treatment with peginterferon or interferon alfa-2b and ribavirin on steatosis in patients infected with hepatitis C. Hepatology. 2003;38(1):75–85.
102. Zarski JP, Mc Hutchison J, Bronowicki JP, Sturm N, Garcia-Kennedy R, Hodaj E, et al. Rate of natural disease progression in patients with chronic hepatitis C. J Hepatol. 2003;38(3):307–14.
103. Bochud PY, Cai T, Overbeck K, Bochud M, Dufour JF, Mullhaupt B, et al. Genotype 3 is associated with accelerated fibrosis progression in chronic hepatitis C. J Hepatol. 2009;51(4):655–66.
104. Probst A, Dang T, Bochud M, Egger M, Negro F, Bochud PY. Role of hepatitis C virus genotype 3 in liver fibrosis progression--a systematic review and meta-analysis. J Viral Hepat. 2011;18(11):745–59.
105. Cacciola I, Pollicino T, Squadrito G, Cerenzia G, Orlando ME, Raimondo G. Occult hepatitis B virus infection in patients with chronic hepatitis C liver disease. N Engl J Med. 1999;341(1):22–6.
106. Weber R, Sabin CA, Friis-Moller N, Reiss P, El-Sadr WM, Kirk O, et al. Liver-related deaths in persons infected with the human immunodeficiency virus: the D:A:D study. Arch Intern Med. 2006;166(15):1632–41.
107. Alazawi W, Cunningham M, Dearden J, Foster GR. Systematic review: outcome of compensated cirrhosis due to chronic hepatitis C infection. Aliment Pharmacol Ther. 2010;32(3):344–55.
108. Fattovich G, Giustina G, Degos F, Tremolada F, Diodati G, Almasio P, et al. Morbidity and mortality in compensated cirrhosis type C: a retrospective follow-up study of 384 patients. Gastroenterology. 1997;112(2):463–72.
109. Davila JA, Morgan RO, Shaib Y, McGlynn KA, El-Serag HB. Hepatitis C infection and the increasing incidence of hepatocellular carcinoma: a population-based study. Gastroenterology. 2004;127(5):1372–80.
110. El-Serag HB, Davila JA. Surveillance for hepatocellular carcinoma: in whom and how? Therap Adv Gastroenterol. 2011;4(1):5–10.
111. Tanaka Y, Kurbanov F, Mano S, Orito E, Vargas V, Esteban JI, et al. Molecular tracing of the global hepatitis C virus epidemic predicts regional patterns of hepatocellular carcinoma mortality. Gastroenterology. 2006;130(3):703–14.
112. George SL, Bacon BR, Brunt EM, Mihindukulasuriya KL, Hoffmann J, Di Bisceglie AM. Clinical, virologic, histologic, and

biochemical outcomes after successful HCV therapy: a 5-year follow-up of 150 patients. Hepatology. 2009;49(3):729–38.
113. Marcellin P, Boyer N, Gervais A, Martinot M, Pouteau M, Castelnau C, et al. Long-term histologic improvement and loss of detectable intrahepatic HCV RNA in patients with chronic hepatitis C and sustained response to interferon-alpha therapy. Ann Intern Med. 1997;127(10):875–81.
114. Davila JA, Morgan RO, Richardson PA, Du XL, McGlynn KA, El-Serag HB. Use of surveillance for hepatocellular carcinoma among patients with cirrhosis in the United States. Hepatology. 2010;52(1):132–41.
115. Ghany MG, Strader DB, Thomas DL, Seeff LB, American Association for the Study of Liver Diseases. Diagnosis, management, and treatment of hepatitis C: an update. Hepatology. 2009;49(4):1335–74.
116. Bruno S, Crosignani A, Facciotto C, Rossi S, Roffi L, Redaelli A, et al. Sustained virologic response prevents the development of esophageal varices in compensated, Child-Pugh class A hepatitis C virus-induced cirrhosis. A 12-year prospective follow-up study. Hepatology. 2010;51(6):2069–76.
117. Roberts S, Gordon A, McLean C, Pedersen J, Bowden S, Thomson K, et al. Effect of sustained viral response on hepatic venous pressure gradient in hepatitis C-related cirrhosis. Clin Gastroenterol Hepatol. 2007;5(8):932–7.
118. Chien RN, Lin CH, Liaw YF. The effect of lamivudine therapy in hepatic decompensation during acute exacerbation of chronic hepatitis B. J Hepatol. 2003;38(3):322–7.
119. Gonzalez SA, Trotter JF. The rise of the opioid epidemic and hepatitis C positive organs: a new era in liver transplantation. Hepatology. 2018;67(4):1600–8.
120. Conti F, Buonfiglioli F, Scuteri A, Crespi C, Bolondi L, Caraceni P, et al. Early occurrence and recurrence of hepatocellular carcinoma in HCV-related cirrhosis treated with direct-acting antivirals. J Hepatol. 2016;65(4):727–33.
121. Coilly A, Roche B, Duclos-Vallee JC, Samuel D. Management of post transplant hepatitis C in the direct antiviral agents era. Hepatol Int. 2015;9(2):192–201.
122. Hwang SJ, Lee SD. Hepatic steatosis and hepatitis C: Still unhappy bedfellows? J Gastroenterol Hepatol. 2011;26(Suppl 1):96–101.
123. Chan A, Patel K, Naggie S. Genotype 3 infection: the last stand of hepatitis C virus. Drugs. 2017,77(2).131–44.
124. AASLD/IDSA HCV Guidance Panel. Hepatitis C guidance: AASLD-IDSA recommendations for testing, managing, and treating adults infected with hepatitis C virus. Hepatology. 2015;62(3):932–54.
125. Grassi A, Ballardini G. Post-liver transplant hepatitis C virus recurrence: an unresolved thorny problem. World J Gastroenterol. 2014;20(32):11095–115.
126. Gane EJ, Naoumov NV, Qian KP, Mondelli MU, Maertens G, Portmann BC, et al. A longitudinal analysis of hepatitis C virus replication following liver transplantation. Gastroenterology. 1996;110(1):167–77.
127. Gane EJ, Portmann BC, Naoumov NV, Smith HM, Underhill JA, Donaldson PT, et al. Long-term outcome of hepatitis C infection after liver transplantation. N Engl J Med. 1996;334(13):815–20.
128. Neumann UP, Berg T, Bahra M, Seehofer D, Langrehr JM, Neuhaus R, et al. Fibrosis progression after liver transplantation in patients with recurrent hepatitis C. J Hepatol. 2004;41(5): 830–6.
129. Watt KD, Laryea MA. Recurrent disease following liver transplantation. In: Schiff ER, Maddrey WC, Sorrell MF, editors. Schiff's diseases of the liver. 11th ed. Philadelphia, PA: Wiley & Sons; 2012. p. 1152–66.
130. Dixon LR, Crawford JM. Early histologic changes in fibrosing cholestatic hepatitis C. Liver Transpl. 2007;13(2):219–26.
131. Jadoul M, Poignet JL, Geddes C, Locatelli F, Medin C, Krajewska M, et al. The changing epidemiology of hepatitis C virus (HCV) infection in haemodialysis: European multicentre study. Nephrol Dial Transplant. 2004;19(4):904–9.
132. Fissell RB, Bragg-Gresham JL, Woods JD, Jadoul M, Gillespie B, Hedderwick SA, et al. Patterns of hepatitis C prevalence and seroconversion in hemodialysis units from three continents: the DOPPS. Kidney Int. 2004;65(6):2335–42.
133. Finelli L, Miller JT, Tokars JI, Alter MJ, Arduino MJ. National surveillance of dialysis-associated diseases in the United States, 2002. Semin Dial. 2005;18(1):52–61.
134. Ferri C, Zignego AL, Pileri SA. Cryoglobulins. J Clin Pathol. 2002;55(1):4–13.
135. Sene D, Limal N, Cacoub P. Hepatitis C virus-associated extrahepatic manifestations: a review. Metab Brain Dis. 2004;19(3–4):357–81.
136. Pischke S, Cornberg M, Manns MP. Hepatitis associated cryoglobulinemia. Internist (Berl). 2008;49(3):297–304.
137. White DL, Ratziu V, El-Serag HB. Hepatitis C infection and risk of diabetes: a systematic review and meta-analysis. J Hepatol. 2008;49(5):831–44.
138. Meyers CM, Seeff LB, Stehman-Breen CO, Hoofnagle JH. Hepatitis C and renal disease: an update. Am J Kidney Dis. 2003;42(4):631–57.
139. Hardy NM, Sandroni S, Danielson S, Wilson WJ. Antibody to hepatitis C virus increases with time on hemodialysis. Clin Nephrol. 1992;38(1):44–8.
140. Chan TM, Lok AS, Cheng IK. Hepatitis C in renal transplant recipients. Transplantation. 1991;52(5):810–3.
141. Okuda K, Hayashi H, Kobayashi S, Irie Y. Mode of hepatitis C infection not associated with blood transfusion among chronic hemodialysis patients. J Hepatol. 1995;23(1):28–31.
142. Arenas MD, Sanchez-Paya J, Barril G, Garcia-Valdecasas J, Gorriz JL, Soriano A, et al. A multicentric survey of the practice of hand hygiene in haemodialysis units: factors affecting compliance. Nephrol Dial Transplant. 2005;20(6):1164–71.
143. Rahnavardi M, Hosseini Moghaddam SM, Alavian SM. Hepatitis C in hemodialysis patients: current global magnitude, natural history, diagnostic difficulties, and preventive measures. Am J Nephrol. 2008;28(4):628–40.
144. Fabrizi F, Martin P, Dixit V, Bunnapradist S, Dulai G. Meta-analysis: Effect of hepatitis C virus infection on mortality in dialysis. Aliment Pharmacol Ther. 2004;20(11–12):1271–7.
145. Bloom RD, Sayer G, Fa K, Constantinescu S, Abt P, Reddy KR. Outcome of hepatitis C virus-infected kidney transplant candidates who remain on the waiting list. Am J Transplant. 2005;5(1):139–44.
146. Pham T. Effect of hepatitis C infection and renal transplantation on survival in end-stage renal disease. CANNT J. 2001;11(3):46.
147. Patel PR, Thompson ND, Kallen AJ, Arduino MJ. Epidemiology, surveillance, and prevention of hepatitis C virus infections in hemodialysis patients. Am J Kidney Dis. 2010;56(2):371–8.
148. Bukh J, Wantzin P, Krogsgaard K, Knudsen F, Purcell RH, Miller RH. High prevalence of hepatitis C virus (HCV) RNA in dialysis patients: failure of commercially available antibody tests to identify a significant number of patients with HCV infection. Copenhagen Dialysis HCV Study Group. J Infect Dis. 1993;168(6): 1343–8.
149. Dalekos GN, Boumba DS, Katopodis K, Zervou E, Sferopoulos G, Elisaf M, et al. Absence of HCV viraemia in anti-HCV-negative haemodialysis patients. Nephrol Dial Transplant. 1998;13(7):1804–6.
150. Kelley VA, Everett-Kitchens J, Brannon LE, Connor K, Martinez EJ, Pearson TC, et al. Lack of seronegative hepatitis C virus infections in patients with chronic renal failure. Transplantation. 2002;74(10):1473–5.
151. Terrault NA, Adey DB. The kidney transplant recipient with hepatitis C infection: pre- and posttransplantation treatment. Clin J Am Soc Nephrol. 2007;2(3):563–75.
152. Kidney Disease: Improving Global Outcomes. KDIGO clinical practice guidelines for the prevention, diagnosis, evaluation, and treatment of hepatitis C in chronic kidney disease. Kidney Int Suppl. 2008;(109):S1–99.

153. Alric L, Di-Martino V, Selves J, Cacoub P, Charlotte F, Reynaud D, et al. Long-term impact of renal transplantation on liver fibrosis during hepatitis C virus infection. Gastroenterology. 2002;123(5):1494–9.
154. Kamar N, Rostaing L, Selves J, Sandres-Saune K, Alric L, Durand D, et al. Natural history of hepatitis C virus-related liver fibrosis after renal transplantation. Am J Transplant. 2005;5(7): 1704–12.
155. Delladetsima I, Psichogiou M, Sypsa V, Psimenou E, Kostakis A, Hatzakis A, et al. The course of hepatitis C virus infection in pretransplantation anti-hepatitis C virus-negative renal transplant recipients: a retrospective follow-up study. Am J Kidney Dis. 2006;47(2):309–16.
156. Knoll GA, Tankersley MR, Lee JY, Julian BA, Curtis JJ. The impact of renal transplantation on survival in hepatitis C-positive end-stage renal disease patients. Am J Kidney Dis. 1997;29(4):608–14.
157. Aroldi A, Lampertico P, Montagnino G, Passerini P, Villa M, Campise MR, et al. Natural history of hepatitis B and C in renal allograft recipients. Transplantation. 2005;79(9):1132–6.
158. Cosio FG, Pesavento TE, Osei K, Henry ML, Ferguson RM. Post-transplant diabetes mellitus: increasing incidence in renal allograft recipients transplanted in recent years. Kidney Int. 2001;59(2):732–7.
159. Roth D, Cirocco R, Zucker K, Ruiz P, Viciana A, Burke G, et al. De novo membranoproliferative glomerulonephritis in hepatitis C virus-infected renal allograft recipients. Transplantation. 1995;59(12):1676–82.
160. Papafragkakis H, Fabrizi F, Martin P. Viral hepatitis in renal transplantation. Clin Nephrol. 2011;76(1):29–39.
161. Morales JM, Campistol JM, Castellano G, Andres A, Colina F, Fuertes A, et al. Transplantation of kidneys from donors with hepatitis C antibody into recipients with pre-transplantation anti-HCV. Kidney Int. 1995;47(1):236–40.
162. Ali MK, Light JA, Barhyte DY, Sasaki TM, Currier CB Jr, Grandas O, et al. Donor hepatitis C virus status does not adversely affect short-term outcomes in HCV+ recipients in renal transplantation. Transplantation. 1998;66(12):1694–7.
163. Gupta G, Kang L, Yu JW, Limkemann AJ, Garcia V, Bandyopadhyay D, et al. Long-term outcomes and transmission rates in hepatitis C virus-positive donor to hepatitis C virus-negative kidney transplant recipients: analysis of United States national data. Clin Transpl. 2017;31(10)
164. Fagiuoli S, Minniti F, Pevere S, Farinati F, Burra P, Livi U, et al. HBV and HCV infections in heart transplant recipients. J Heart Lung Transplant. 2001;20(7):718–24.
165. Cadranel JF, Di Martino V, Dorent R, Bernard B, Hoang C, Myara A, et al. Effects of ursodeoxycholic acid (ursodiol) treatment on chronic viral hepatitis in heart transplant patients: results of a prospective, double-blind, placebo-randomized study. Transplantation. 2003;75(7):977–82.
166. Lake KD, Smith CI, Milfred-La Forest SK, Pritzker MR, Emery RW. Outcomes of hepatitis C positive (HCV+) heart transplant recipients. Transplant Proc. 1997;29(1–2):581–2.
167. Fong TL, Hou L, Hutchinson IV, Cicciarelli JC, Cho YW. Impact of hepatitis C infection on outcomes after heart transplantation. Transplantation. 2009;88(9):1137–41.
168. Lee I, Localio R, Brensinger CM, Blumberg EA, Lautenbach E, Gasink L, et al. Decreased post-transplant survival among heart transplant recipients with pre-transplant hepatitis C virus positivity. J Heart Lung Transplant. 2011;30(11):1266–74.
169. Marelli D, Bresson J, Laks H, Kubak B, Fonarow G, Tsai FC, et al. Hepatitis C-positive donors in heart transplantation. Am J Transplant. 2002;2(5):443–7.
170. Ong JP, Barnes DS, Younossi ZM, Gramlich T, Yen-Lieberman B, Goormastic M, et al. Outcome of de novo hepatitis C virus infection in heart transplant recipients. Hepatology. 1999;30(5):1293–8.
171. Gasink LB, Blumberg EA, Localio AR, Desai SS, Israni AK, Lautenbach E. Hepatitis C virus seropositivity in organ donors and survival in heart transplant recipients. JAMA. 2006;296(15):1843–50.
172. Trakroo S, Qureshi K. Successful treatment of chronic hepatitis C infection with direct-acting antivirals in a heart transplant recipient: a case report. Transplant Proc. 2015;47(7):2295–7.
173. Fong TL, Cho YW, Hou L, Hutchinson IV, Barbers RG, Herrington CS. Outcomes after lung transplantation and practices of lung transplant programs in the United States regarding hepatitis C seropositive recipients. Transplantation. 2011;91(11): 1293–6.
174. Carreno MC, Piedad UG, Maite L, Andres V, Francisca P, Cesar B, et al. Hepatitis C virus infection after lung transplantation: dim prognosis. J Heart Lung Transplant. 2001;20(2):224.
175. Orens JB, Estenne M, Arcasoy S, Conte JV, Corris P, Egan JJ, et al. International guidelines for the selection of lung transplant candidates: 2006 update--a consensus report from the Pulmonary Scientific Council of the International Society for Heart and Lung Transplantation. J Heart Lung Transplant. 2006;25(7): 745–55.
176. Carbone M, Lenci I, Baiocchi L. Prevention of hepatitis C recurrence after liver transplantation: an update. World J Gastrointest Pharmacol Ther. 2012;3(4):36–48.
177. Ferri C, Caracciolo F, Zignego AL, La Civita L, Monti M, Longombardo G, et al. Hepatitis C virus infection in patients with non-Hodgkin's lymphoma. Br J Haematol. 1994;88(2):392–4.
178. Silvestri F, Barillari G, Fanin R, Pipan C, Falasca E, Salmaso F, et al. Hepatitis C virus infection among cryoglobulinemic and non-cryoglobulinemic B-cell non-Hodgkin's lymphomas. Haematologica. 1997;82(3):314–7.
179. Viswanatha DS, Dogan A. Hepatitis C virus and lymphoma. J Clin Pathol. 2007;60(12):1378–83.
180. Hermine O, Lefrere F, Bronowicki JP, Mariette X, Jondeau K, Eclache-Saudreau V, et al. Regression of splenic lymphoma with villous lymphocytes after treatment of hepatitis C virus infection. N Engl J Med. 2002;347(2):89–94.
181. Levine AM, Shimodaira S, Lai MM. Treatment of HCV-related mantle-cell lymphoma with ribavirin and pegylated interferon Alfa. N Engl J Med. 2003;349(21):2078–9.
182. Takahashi K, Nishida N, Kawabata H, Haga H, Chiba T. Regression of Hodgkin lymphoma in response to antiviral therapy for hepatitis C virus infection. Intern Med. 2012;51(19):2745–7.
183. Locasciulli A, Testa M, Valsecchi MG, Bacigalupo A, Solinas S, Tomas JF, et al. The role of hepatitis C and B virus infections as risk factors for severe liver complications following allogeneic BMT: a prospective study by the Infectious Disease Working Party of the European Blood and Marrow Transplantation Group. Transplantation. 1999;68(10):1486–91.
184. Lyra AC, Brunt EM, Pincus S, Di Bisceglie AM. A 32-year-old man with hepatitis C who developed progressive liver failure after a bone marrow transplant. Semin Liver Dis. 2002;22(1): 103–8.
185. Hwang YY, Liang RH. Hepatitis C in haematological patients. Hepat Res Treat. 2010;2010:961359.
186. Ljungman P, Johansson N, Aschan J, Glaumann H, Lonnqvist B, Ringden O, et al. Long-term effects of hepatitis C virus infection in allogeneic bone marrow transplant recipients. Blood. 1995;86(4):1614–8.
187. Peffault de Latour R, Levy V, Asselah T, Marcellin P, Scieux C, Ades L, et al. Long-term outcome of hepatitis C infection after bone marrow transplantation. Blood. 2004;103(5):1618–24.
188. Peffault de Latour R, Asselah T, Levy V, Scieux C, Devergie A, Ribaud P, et al. Treatment of chronic hepatitis C virus in allogeneic bone marrow transplant recipients. Bone Marrow Transplant. 2005;36(8):709–13.

Enterovirus Infection in Immunocompromised Hosts

42

Joanna M. D. Schaenman, Dora Y. Ho, Lindsey R. Baden, and Amar Safdar

Introduction

Enteroviruses are single-stranded RNA viruses with a small genome that, as their name suggests, are typically spread by the fecal-oral route and replicate in the gastrointestinal (GI) tract. Most enteroviral infections are asymptomatic, but may spread to secondary sites outside of the GI tract. Such infections may present as mild upper respiratory tract illness; epidemic hand, foot, and mouth disease; or more serious diseases such as myocarditis, meningitis, and acute flaccid paralysis [1]. It is not unexpected that enteroviral infections lead to potentially more serious illness in the immunocompromised host.

Virology

The *Picornaviridae* family includes clinically significant genera like *Rhinovirus*, *Hepatovirus* (hepatitis A virus), and *Enterovirus*; viruses belonging to *Picornaviridae* are common cause of viral infection in humans [2]. Poliovirus, the best-studied member of the *Enterovirus* genus, was one of the first viruses to be completely sequenced, allowing for mapping of viral proteins and a better understanding of the viral replication process [3]. The non-enveloped enterovirus virion is small and consists of an icosahedral capsid of approximately 300 angstroms in diameter enclosing a positive strand of RNA of 7.4 kilobases [4]. The viral RNA codes for a 250 kD polyprotein which is then cleaved into P1, P2, and P3 proteins [5]. Protein P1 is processed by viral proteases into capsid proteins VP1, VP2, VP3, and VP4, while proteins P2 and P3 undergo subsequent processing to generate the viral RNA polymerase (protein 3D), viral protease (protein 3C), and other proteins necessary for viral replication [6, 7]. Like other RNA viruses, the high mutation rate during genome replication coupled with short replication times and a large number of daughter viruses per infected cell can give rise to heterogeneous viral populations in the course of a single infection [8].

The lack of a lipid envelope makes these viruses resistant to alcohol; *Enteroviridae* are stable at a wide range of pH [9]. They are vulnerable to drying, ultraviolet radiation, extreme heat, as well as sodium hypochlorite and glutaraldehyde [10].

Nomenclature

The nomenclature of the subgenera can be confusing, as it has changed over time based on enhanced genome sequencing data. The traditional classification divided the *Enteroviridae* into four main groups. Poliovirus (PV), the causative agent of poliomyelitis, was the first subgenera to be identified [11]. Subsequently coxsackievirus was isolated in 1948 from the stool of children in Coxsackie, New York, with evidence of myelitis or meningitis and no evidence of

J. M. D. Schaenman (✉)
Division of Infectious Diseases, David Geffen School of Medicine at UCLA, Los Angeles, CA, USA
e-mail: Jschaenman@mednet.ucla.edu

D. Y. Ho
Division of Infectious Diseases and Geographic Medicine, Stanford University School of Medicine, Stanford, CA, USA
e-mail: doraywho@stanford.edu

L. R. Baden
Division of Infectious Diseases, Brigham and Women's Hospital, Dana-Farber Cancer Institute, Harvard Medical School, Boston, MA, USA
e-mail: lbaden@bwh.harvard.edu

A. Safdar
Clinical Associate Professor of Medicine, Texas Tech University Health Sciences Center El Paso, Paul L. Foster School of Medicine, El Paso, TX, USA
e-mail: amar.safdar@cidimmunology.com

A. Safdar (ed.), *Principles and Practice of Transplant Infectious Diseases*, https://doi.org/10.1007/978-1-4939-9034-4_42

poliovirus [12]. Initial classification was based on the results in a newborn mouse model of neurologic disease, as injection of what came to be known as the group A coxsackieviruses (CVA) associated with milder disease with flaccid limb paralysis. Group B coxsackieviruses (CVB) caused spastic paralysis and widespread tissue destruction. The so-called echoviruses (enteric cytopathic human orphan viruses) were initially isolated from the stool of asymptomatic individuals and were initially thought to cause no discernable clinical disease [13]. Over 60 human serotypes were described that were distinguished by cross-reactivity of serum from clinical isolates and were given sequential notations, for example, CVA9 or CVB1. The newer enteroviruses (EV) were assigned numbers, for example, EV71 [3]. Some gaps in the numbering exist due to changes in classification because some serotypes were subsequently found to be identical to other viral subtype [14]. Limitations of this classification system include (1) difficulty in culturing some enteroviruses, (2) limited availability of antisera for serotyping, and (3) serotyping procedures which are technically challenging [15].

An alternate method for enterovirus typing based on molecular genetic techniques has been developed which relies on sequencing of the P1 region that encodes the capsid proteins. The current viral taxonomy divides the enteroviruses into groups A through D based on sequence homologies. There are data that suggest a stronger association with clinical syndromes when this typing method is used as compared with the previous classification [16]. The assignment of the classical subtypes and new genetic subtypes is shown in Table 42.1. Many members of species human enterovirus A and human enterovirus B have now been sequenced [2, 17].

An interesting insight from the mass sequencing of the enteroviruses has been the discovery of the frequent recombination events between genetic material outside of the capsid protein-encoding region [18]. Recombination typically occurs within species, and interestingly, sequence similarity between strains has been found to mirror previously described antigenic cross-reactivity [17].

Table 42.1 Classification of the enteroviruses [14]

Current taxonomy	Traditional taxonomy
HEV-A	CAV2–8, CAV10, CAV12, CAV14, CAV16; EV71, EV76, EV89, EV90, EV91
HEV-B	CAV9; CBV1–6; E1–7, E9, E11–21, E24–27, E29–33; EV69, EV73–75, EV77–78, EV79–88, EV100–101
HEV-C	CAV1, CAV11, CAV13, CAV17, CAV19–22, CAV24, PV1–3
HEV-D	EV68, EV70

Adapted from the CDC report on enterovirus surveillance Khetsuriani et al. [14]

HEV-A human enterovirus A, *HEV-B* human enterovirus B, *HEV-C* human enterovirus C, *HEV-D* human enterovirus D, *CAV* coxsackie A virus, *EV* enterovirus, *CBV* coxsackie B virus, *E* echovirus

Although there remains much overlap in clinical syndromes among the species classifications, in general human enterovirus A (HEV-A) has been associated with hand, foot, and mouth disease and CNS infections; human enterovirus B (HEV-B) with pleurodynia, myocarditis, meningitis, and encephalitis; human enterovirus C (HEV-C) with poliomyelitis, meningitis, and hemorrhagic conjunctivitis; and human enterovirus D (HEV-D) with respiratory tract infection [14, 16].

Enterovirus 71 (EV71) in the HEV-A species is also notable for its appearance in several epidemics in Asia, causing an especially large and severe outbreak in Sarawak, Malaysia, which was associated with high mortality [19]. Other countries in Asian such as Taiwan, Singapore, Malaysia, and Japan had reported similar infections [20]. Hand, foot, and mouth disease and herpangina are common illnesses due to this virus; EV71-related encephalitis and acute flaccid paralysis are a concerning complication noted with the emergence of this virus, mostly described in outbreaks in Asia [21]. Some studies have suggested that virologic differences may exist between strains isolated from patients with herpangina compared with neurotropic strains causing encephalitis [22].

Pathogenesis

The reservoirs for human enterovirus infection are humans; nonhuman primates may be experimentally infected with human enteroviruses; they are not the source of virus in naturally occurring infection [13]. The standard model for pathogenesis is that of the poliovirus, where the process begins with the initial infection of host cells in the oropharynx and/or intestinal mucosa. From there, the virus can gain access to the cervical and mesenteric lymph nodes resulting in transient viremia (Fig. 42.1) [11]. Although fecal-oral transmission is the most common, infection via the respiratory route may also occur. At this point infection may be asymptomatic or may cause nonspecific symptoms such as fever, malaise, and sore throat. One study showed that the presence of intestinal bacteria may promote replication of enteroviruses in the gut as mice treated with antibiotics had a 50% decrease in mortality compared with untreated mice, and the reintroduction of bacteria in this model enhanced poliovirus disease [23]. Central nervous system (CNS) access may be gained either directly from the blood or by axonal transport.

Enteroviruses gain entry into epithelial and lymphoid cells via binding to specific cell surface receptors, which varies by subtype. Poliovirus binds to the poliovirus receptor (CD155), a cell surface molecule whose physiologic function is still uncertain [24]. The coxsackievirus A group utilizes intercellular adhesion molecule 1 (ICAM-1 or CD54)

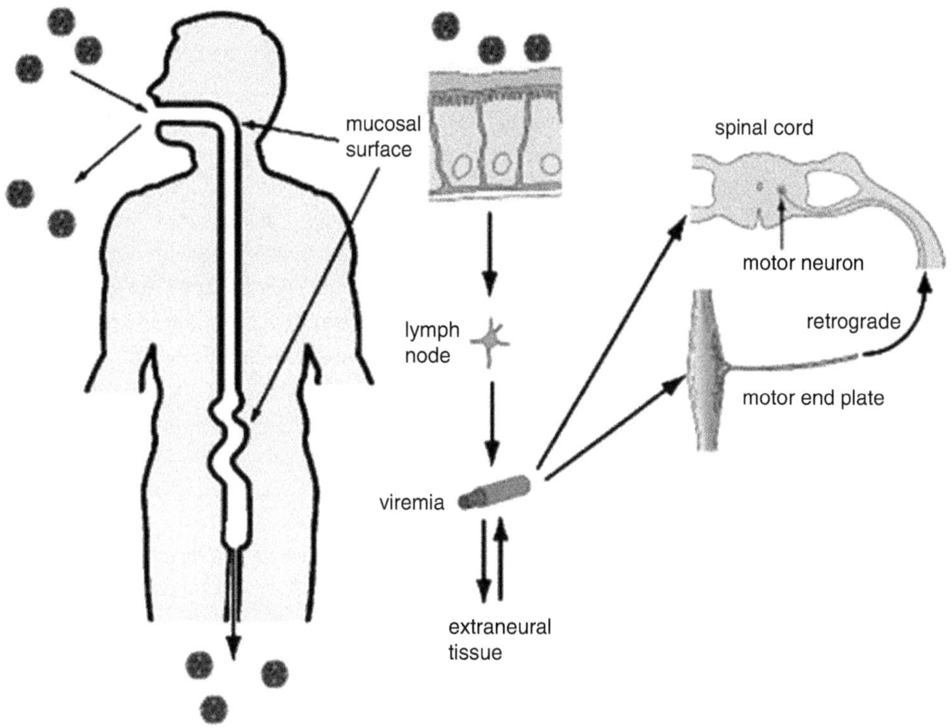

Fig. 42.1 Hypothetical scheme of poliovirus pathogenesis based on experimental findings in humans, monkeys, chimpanzees, and transgenic mice. Ingested virus initially replicates in the oropharyngeal and intestinal mucosa. Virus replication at these sites reaches the blood through the lymph nodes, resulting in a primary viremia. Invasion of virus into the central nervous system may occur either directly from the blood or by retrograde axonal transport when the virus enters the neuromuscular junction. It is believed that invasion of the brain or spinal cord must be preceded by viral multiplication in extraneural tissues, which leads to a sustained viremia. These extraneural tissues may include the skeletal muscle and brown fat. Virus is spread most frequently by the fecal-oral route. Shedding of virus from the nasopharynx may lead to transmission of infection by the respiratory route, which occurs in developed countries with high standards of sanitation [11]. (Reprinted from Virology, Vol. 344/Issue 1, Racaniello VR, One hundred years of poliovirus pathogenesis, pages 344:9–16, © 2006, https://www.sciencedirect.com/science/article/pii/S0042682205005830, with permission from Elsevier)

that functions as an integrin receptor to gain entry into host cells; rhinovirus also uses ICAM-1 for this purpose [25]. The coxsackievirus B group can bind to either decay-accelerating factor (DAF or CD55) or coxsackievirus-adenovirus receptor (CAR), another immunoglobulin superfamily member, with the latter thought to be the dominant receptor [26]. Many of the enterovirus and host receptor protein crystal structures are now known [27]. For some of these cell surface receptors, it has been postulated that the level of expression in the host may determine susceptibility to viral infection. For example, children have high levels of CAR expression in the heart and may exhibit a heightened susceptibility to myocarditis [28]. Other host factors that may play a role in susceptibility to enteroviral diseases such as poliomyelitis and myocarditis include malnutrition, pregnancy, and exhaustion from strenuous exercise [1, 28].

For specific disease entities, the details of pathogenesis vary by the organ type involved. For poliomyelitis, when the virus enters the CNS either via blood or via axonal transport, the replication in motor neurons within the spinal cord, brainstem, or motor cortex leads to cellular damage and muscle paralysis [11].

CNS disease due to EV71 reflects viruses' high propensity for neurotropism, with the brainstem being the major target of infection [29]. Axonal pathway spread similar to poliovirus has been suggested. In a study among children in Taiwan with this infection, there was correlation with the levels of cytokines IL-6 and interferon-gamma in the CNS with more severe cases of brainstem encephalitis presenting with autonomic system dysregulation and pulmonary edema [30].

In myocarditis, the pathogenesis of disease includes both direct cellular damage from the viral infection and secondary damage due to the elicit hosts' immune response. Coxsackievirus proteases can inhibit cell protein synthesis machinery by protease cleavage of eukaryotic initiation factor, and these proteases can also cleave dystrophin, affecting the integrity of the sarcolemma membrane [28]. The antiviral immune response can be beneficial in limiting the extent of viral replication but can also lead to increased cellular destruction and clinical disease [31]. Cellular damage is irreparable in organs such as the heart and brain with terminally differentiated cells. Persistence of enterovirus RNA in the heart after acute infection has also been associated with worsened clinical outcome in patients with enteroviral myocarditis [32].

Immune Response

The response to enterovirus infection involves both innate and adaptive immunity. One important experimental model has been transgenic mice expressing CD155, the poliovirus receptor. The use of this model has demonstrated the importance of type I interferons as mice deficient in the interferon-alpha receptor demonstrate viral replication in many tissues that are not normal targets of poliovirus such as the liver and spleen [33]. Not surprisingly, the Toll-like receptors (TLR) have also been shown to be important in the control of viral infection as TLR7 detects viral single-stranded RNA and TLR3 viral double-stranded RNA, which is an intermediate in the replication pathway. In a mouse model of poliovirus infection, knockout mice lacking TLR3 had much higher viral loads in nonneural tissues and high mortality [34]. The importance of TLR3 has also been shown in a myocarditis model of coxsackie B virus infection [35]. In addition, both NK cells and macrophages have been thought to play an important role in the control of infection [36].

It has been observed that both humoral and cellular immunity are important for the control of infection for all species of enteroviruses [37]. The crucial role of neutralizing antibodies for the control of viral infection is highlighted by the observation that patients with agammaglobulinemia are very vulnerable to chronic enterovirus infections [38]. This is further supported by the strong antibody response generated by poliovirus vaccination, which is also seen in mouse models of infection [37]. B cells, however, may also play a role in viral dissemination as mice deficient in B cells have lower viral titers on day 1 postinfection compared with normal mice [39]. It has also been postulated that the virus gains access to these immune cells by binding to cell surface proteins at tight junctions between epithelial cells, allowing for virus tagged along the migratory immune cells to sites of injury or inflammation. This may represent a mechanism for spread throughout the body as well as evading neutralizing antibody response [40].

Early studies in mice demonstrated the importance of T cells in the control of enterovirus replication as longer virus persistence was seen in athymic nude mice in the myocarditis model [41]. Similarly, in a mouse model of poliomyelitis, administration of antithymocyte globulin led to longer persistence of virus in the CNS with associated increased rates of CNS disease and death [42]. The effect of inflammatory cells such as T cells is important for clearance of infection but may cause additional cell-mediated injury and necrosis [28]. This CD8+ T-cell role, however, appears to be independent of perforin in the mouse model as perforin knockout mice were able to clear infection at similar rates to wild type but had less myocarditis and subsequent fibrosis [43]. CD4+ T cells are also thought to play a role in inflammation as transfer of naïve cells exacerbated myocarditis in a mouse model, while transfer of CD4 + CD25+ Tregs protected mice from early mortality with decreased viral load and inflammation [44].

The role of autoimmunity has also been posited in myocarditis, either through molecular mimicry where sequence similarities between viral and host antigens lead to autoimmunity, through the release of autoantigenic host cell proteins released from dying cells, or possibly via nonspecific upregulation of the immune system with increased CD40 expression and TLR stimulation creating a permissive atmosphere for autoimmunity to develop leading to cardiomyopathy [45]. A large volume of literature also exists exploring the likely connection between enterovirus infection of the pancreas and the development of type 1 diabetes [46]. Both the genetic predisposition of the host and the age at which one is exposed to enterovirus infection, with delayed exposure now common in the developed world due to improving standards of hygiene over the past 50 years, may play a role in the propensity to develop diabetes after infection.

Epidemiology

In the USA, enterovirus infections are tracked by the National Enterovirus Surveillance System as well as the National Respiratory and Enteric Virus Surveillance System, two laboratory surveillance systems that rely on voluntary reporting. The peak of enterovirus activity in temperate climates is in the summer and fall, with 70% of reported detections in the 2006–2008 period occurring between July and October [47]. The five most common serotypes in that period were CVA9, CVB1, E6, E9, and E18 and accounted for over 50% of total serotyped detection. In over 1600 cases reported, the mean age was 9 years and median age 2 years [47]. These findings regarding the time of onset, age range, and serotypes are similar to previous trends described in the USA [14]. Enterovirus is endemic worldwide; epidemics can also occur, observed in underdeveloped regions with suboptimum hygiene [46]. Viral spread has also been reported from recreational water exposure [48].

The epidemiology of poliovirus charts an incredible chronicle of public health response to infection, with a groundbreaking vaccination campaign launched in response to a surge of cases in the 1940s and 1950s in the USA [49] resulting in eradication of this public menace in the USA in 1979. A greater than 99% reduction in the incidence of new polio cases worldwide as of the year 2000 through the use of oral poliovirus vaccine (OPV) and inactivated poliovirus vaccine (IVP) was encouraging [50]. However, over the past decade, the struggles continue in preventing the remaining 1% of polio cases due to under-immunization in developing regions such as Africa, where vulnerable population remains susceptible to the reimportations of wild-type poliovirus in previously polio-free regions [50, 51]. As of 2013, there are three remaining countries where endemic wild-type poliovirus continues to exist; these include Pakistan, Afghanistan, and Nigeria [52].

In addition to naturally occurring poliovirus disease, the use of OPV, a live-attenuated virus, has led to circulation of vaccine-strain viruses, and in some instances, vaccine-derived polioviruses have acquired neurovirulence resulting in clinical disease even in immunocompetent hosts [53, 54]. Due to this concern, IPV has been exclusively used in the USA since the year 2000 [55]. Worldwide, new outbreaks of vaccine-derived poliovirus continue to occur with new outbreaks since 2009 in Afghanistan, Ethiopia, and India [56].

Clinical Syndromes

Poliovirus

Although poliovirus is best known for causing paralytic poliomyelitis, like other enteroviruses, it manifests a range of clinical entities ranging from asymptomatic illness to mild gastrointestinal disease to severe paralysis and death [49]. Nearly 5% of patients who do develop symptoms after exposure most experience "minor illness" or "abortive poliomyelitis" with fever, malaise, headache, sore throat, and GI complaints without neurologic findings [13]. Poliovirus can also cause an aseptic meningitis, known as "nonparalytic poliomyelitis."

Paralytic poliomyelitis can present initially similar to the aforementioned minor clinical illness; resolution of these nonspecific symptoms may be followed by meningitis with recurrence of fever, malaise, meningismus, and muscle pain followed by motor weakness and paralysis [13]. The so-called provocation poliomyelitis can be seen when an intramuscular injection is given after poliovirus exposure and paralysis begins or is most severe in the extremity where the injection occurred [49]. Patients can experience severity of illness ranging from weakness of a single muscle to complete quadriplegia, with an asymmetric distribution of flaccid paralysis, and rarely paralysis of muscles innervated by cranial nerves possibly leading to airway obstruction. The differential diagnosis would include other enteroviral infection including EV71 as well as West Nile virus. Guillain-Barré is more symmetrical in presentation and is associated with loss of sensation, which is very rarely described in poliomyelitis. Paralytic poliomyelitis leads to permanent weakness in two-thirds of patients [57].

Vaccine-derived poliovirus can also cause disease, especially in population with poor immune coverage. OPV recipients without previous poliovirus immunity can shed vaccine virus in their feces for 1–6 weeks and in the oropharynx for 1–3 weeks.

There are several different clinical scenarios that can occur with OPV vaccine strains. Rarely, OPV vaccinees can develop vaccine-associated paralytic poliomyelitis; frequency of this dreaded complication is estimated at one to two cases per million OPV immunizations [58]. Family members or other individuals in close contact with vaccinees are also exposed to the altered vaccine strain with disease-causing potential and at risk of such, albeit, exceedingly rare complications [58]. Finally, these reverted vaccine strains can enter the community; immunocompromised transplant recipients may rarely encounter these infections via casual person-to-person contact resulting in clinical disease and an unwitting reservoir for such infections due to prolonged periods of viral shedding [56].

Non-poliovirus

Most non-poliovirus enterovirus infections are asymptomatic; over 90% of patients are either asymptomatic or exhibit mild symptoms such as nonspecific fever or upper respiratory infection symptoms [13]. In every infection, there is an approximate 3- to 5-day incubation period during which viral shedding occurs without clinical symptoms.

Aseptic meningitis is one of the most common clinically diagnosed manifestations of enteroviruses, often seen with the HEV-B species such as CVB and echoviruses [14]. In review of cases with aseptic meningitis in whom CSF PCR testing was routinely performed, enteroviruses were identified in 20–40% of such cases reported from Sweden, Finland, Greece, and the USA [59–62]. Many patients initially presented with fever and upper respiratory infection-like symptoms, which temporarily abate followed by the appearance of headache and reappearance of fever.

Encephalitis or meningoencephalitis may be the primary clinical presentation of infection due to enteroviruses. Clinical presentation includes depressed or altered state of consciousness, presence of focal neurologic signs, and new-onset seizures [13]. In fact, enteroviruses make up a substantial portion of known causes of such illnesses; in a case series using PCR for viral diagnosis, enteroviruses were second in frequency to herpes simplex virus in patients with central nervous system viral infections [59]. EV71 can cause a severe form of brainstem encephalitis presenting with symptoms such as truncal ataxia, myoclonus, intention tremor, and altered mental status [29]. For enterovirus CNS infections in children, deaths are often due to pulmonary edema, which is hypothesized to have resulted from neurogenic sympathetic overactivation. Patients undergoing transplantation with severe immune dysregulation are considered at additional risk for enteroviral encephalitis or meningoencephalitis.

A syndrome of flaccid paralysis can also be seen secondary to the non-poliovirus enteroviruses that are often difficult to differentiate from poliovirus infection as well as other viral CNS infections due to flaviviruses and rabies [19]. Flaccid paralysis is described in patients with HEV-B, EV68, and EV71 infections [14, 29].

One of the best-known enterovirus manifestations is viral exanthem including hand, foot, and mouth disease (HFMD). In the USA, HEV-A species is the prominent cause of HFMD and CAV16 the most common serotype isolated with such infections [63]. Children are most commonly affected. The presentation includes mild fever with skin rash on palms and soles along with shallow ulcers in the oral cavity. The rash is classically vesicular-papular and can also involve the buttocks; less commonly it may be seen with a maculopapular rash on palms and soles with or without oral ulcers [64]. Herpangina is another relatively benign manifestation of enterovirus and presents with fever and painful ulcers over the tonsillar pillars [64]. HFMD and herpangina are caused by the HEV-A species including EV71 as well as the HEV-B species [14, 19]. It is unclear if such infections are more severe in transplant recipients.

Acute hemorrhagic conjunctivitis is another syndrome caused by enteroviruses that is highly contagious resulting in often large epidemics around the world, mostly in individuals residing in tropics and subtropical regions [65]. This syndrome is clinically indistinguishable from adenovirus-associated conjunctivitis and is typically caused by HEV-C, typically CAV24 [14]. To our understanding, transplant patients do not have high susceptibility for acute enteroviral hemorrhagic conjunctivitis compared with the general population.

Myositis can also be seen with enterovirus infection and most commonly manifests as pleurodynia, a syndrome characterized by fever and sharp, spasmodic chest or upper abdomen pain [66]. Although it is a benign disease, patients may experience severe anxiety due to splinting and resultant difficulty in breathing. It was originally reported as "acute rheumatism spread by contagion" in Norway; more recent epidemics are reported in Asia [66]. It is commonly associated with HEV-B species CVB1, whereas EV71 is associated with myositis [14, 19].

Myocarditis due to enteroviruses is a major cause of acute and chronic heart disease; its exact incidence in the general population is unknown; however, autopsies in children have reported a frequency of 2% [67], with an estimated range between 6% and 29% among children dying with idiopathic cardiomyopathy thought to be viral in origin [68]. Among the known causes of myocarditis, enteroviruses, notably CVB3 of HEV-B species, accounted for 50% of all cases [31, 69]. Other important viruses associated with myocarditis include adenovirus and cytomegalovirus infections and may be of concern in transplant recipients with severe adaptive T-cell dysfunction [70]. Presentation of viral myocarditis, which often involves myopericarditis, is sharp anterior chest pain, accompanied with cardiac arrhythmias, and dyspnea and acute pulmonary edema have been described and so are cases of unexplained sudden cardiac arrest [68]. In addition to causing acute-onset heart failure, enteroviral infections have also been implicated in playing a role in patients with chronic cardiomyopathy. PCR studies in autopsy cases and explanted hearts demonstrated persistence of enterovirus RNA and protein in such myocardial tissue [71].

Infections in Immunocompromised Hosts

The classic enterovirus disease associated with impaired immunity is chronic meningoencephalitis, a persistent CNS infection due to enteroviral infections. Patients with B-cell immunodeficiencies such as X-linked agammaglobulinemia are susceptible, and such infections are often fatal [38]. Patients typically present with symptoms of encephalitis, weakness, lethargy, depressed consciousness, ataxia, and seizures. Additional manifestations of clinical viral infection with a diffuse skin rash or acute viral hepatitis may also be present in some individuals. This syndrome is often due to echoviruses in HEV-B species, also seen in neonates [38]. Maintenance therapy with intravenous immunoglobulin (IVIG) has shown to reduce the risk for this complication in such patients [72]. This syndrome has also been described secondary to vaccine-derived poliovirus in patients with hypogammaglobulinemia or those with common variable immunodeficiency (CVID) syndrome; in one report viral persistence for 22 years despite treatment attempts underscores patients' vulnerability with profound defects in mounting a sustained and robust humoral antiviral response [73, 74].

There are many case reports of vaccine-derived poliomyelitis secondary to vaccination with OPV in patients with CVID and other causes of hypo- or agammaglobulinemia prior to the switch to IPV [75]. This disease has also been described in immunocompromised children who did not receive vaccine but reside in communities where OPV is in use. For example, a fatal case of meningoencephalitis was seen in Japan in an infant with hypogammaglobulinemia who had not been vaccinated; cultures grew a revertant neurovirulent strain of attenuated OPV [76]. Case reports as well as the fact that, even without causing clinical disease, OPV viral strains can replicate for years in patients with severe immune deficiency should alert caregivers for the transplant patients for this potential complication in these highly susceptible populations [56].

Although common in the community, the literature on enteroviral infections in immunocompromised hosts is relatively sparse with a limited number of case reports described in patients undergoing hematopoietic stem cell transplant (HSCT) or antineoplastic chemotherapy [77]. PCR-based studies of stool and oropharyngeal samples in recipients of T-cell-depleted HSCT in the UK revealed a 10% incidence of enteroviral infection, unrelated donor graft being the prominent risk factor for such infections [78]. Most infections in these patients were symptomatic; upper respiratory tract illness was common, although persistent pneumonia with CVB and CMV and protracted weakness, fatigue, and myalgia were observed in one patient each. A study in children receiving chemotherapy revealed a high incidence of enteroviral infection. Over 50% of children undergoing treatment for acute leukemia developed a symptomatic infection detected by PCR testing. It was not surprising that incidence and seasonal variation reflected those of the surrounding community [79]. These infections often lead to severe clinical disease, and 15% died from complications of such infections including encephalitis and myocarditis.

Typical enteroviral infections such as hand, foot, and mouth disease have also been reported in immunocompromised hosts, with case reports of patients with lymphopenia experiencing prolonged periods of new crops of rash appearing over a duration of several weeks [80]. There was an additional report of disseminated enterovirus infection resulting in conjunctivitis, nephritis, and persistent diarrhea in a patient with lymphopenia following alemtuzumab therapy [81]. Some investigators have hypothesized that increasing use of B-cell-depleting agents such as anti-CD20, rituximab, and anti-CD52, alemtuzumab, may lead to higher rates of enterovirus infections [82]. Finally, a fatal case of disseminated enterovirus infection was reported in autologous HSCT recipient with an extensive prior history of antineoplastic therapy for Hodgkin's disease; the virus was demonstrated to have involved the heart, lung, liver, and spleen in this patient [83].

Similar to non-immunosuppressed patients, enteroviral CNS infection in the immunocompromised patients includes encephalitis and myelitis. Two children following HSCT in Austria presented with fever, lethargy, and seizures, diagnosis of enterovirus infection was made, and both patients made full recovery [84]. Whereas a patient with heavily treated relapsed lymphoma and known stable chronic enterovirus meningitis underwent HSCT, 40 days after transplantation, a rapidly progressive enterovirus encephalitis was fatal [82]. Several cases of enterovirus meningoencephalitis in patients given rituximab have been described including those undergoing combination chemotherapy such as R-CHOP for non-Hodgkin's B-cell lymphoma [85]. Enterovirus 71 encephalitis has been observed to result in more severe disease in patients with primary immunodeficiency and those with agammaglobulinemia. Similarly, cancer patients with treatment-induced leukopenia and those undergoing treatment with rituximab have also demonstrated a high disease severity due to enterovirus 71 infection. In immunosuppressed patients, diagnostic workup should include PCR analysis of CSF and skin lesions, when present [77, 86]. A report from Italy described severe myelitis in a patient receiving interferon therapy for chronic HBV hepatitis; this patient presented with lower limb paraplegia, and diagnosis was confirmed by PCR on CSF sample [87].

Pneumonia and other respiratory tract infections due to enterovirus are well described in immunocompromised hosts. A case series from Spain in patients undergoing treatment and HSCT for hematologic malignancies showed 33% had enterovirus respiratory tract infections detected by immunofluorescence and viral culture [88]. Among these patients presence of lymphopenia was noted as an important risk factor for enterovirus infection compared with a comparable cohort of patients diagnosed with rhinovirus lower respiratory tract disease [88]. The mortality rate approached 30%, especially in patients with concurrent and/or superimposed infections due to bacteria, *Aspergillus* spp., or CMV. Others have reported 75% mortality in enteroviral lung infection among HSCT recipients, even in the absence of concurrent infection due to other pathogen(s) [89]. Fatal cases of enteroviral pneumonia have also been described in pediatric recipients of hematopoietic stem cell allografts [82]. Enteroviral respiratory infections have been described after lung transplantation; enterovirus was detected in respiratory secretions from symptomatic and asymptomatic lung transplant recipients in PCR screening studies for potential viral pathogens [90, 91].

Gastroenteritis in patients undergoing allograft hematopoietic stem cell transplantation showed approximately 10% of cases were due to enterovirus infection [92]. Another interesting study in HSCT recipients identified an increased frequency of enterovirus isolation in the recipients of unrelated donor grafts; such patients also tested positive for other intestinal pathogens [93].

Hemophagocytic syndrome secondary to enterovirus infection has also been described in children with malignancy. In a study from Greece, 5% of patients admitted to a hospital with enterovirus infection had evidence of infection-associated hemophagocytic syndrome; diagnosis was confirmed by PCR in bone marrow biopsy samples along with immune staining illustrating the presence of enteroviruses and exclusion of other potential pathogens [94].

Viral myocarditis is not well described in immunocompromised hosts, although it has a strong correlation with transplant-induced immune suppression and clinical presentation such as idiopathic cardiomyopathy. A study from Germany in heart transplant recipients reported 60%, of mostly young donors, had PCR presence of enteroviral nucleic acid in the heart tissue; not unexpected that CVB was the prominent viral strain identified [95]. This observation suggests a significant risk for graft-transmitted viral infection in patients undergoing heart transplantation, especially from a young donor. In fact, there have been suggestions that enterovirus or adenovirus infection of the transplanted cardiac graft in children attributed toward the subsequent risk for allograft loss [96].

Given the increased morbidity and mortality associated with enteroviral infections among the immunocompromised host, high prevalence of asymptomatic or mild clinical illness in the general population including household contacts of patients undergoing allograft hematopoietic stem cell or solid organ transplantation remains a cause for concern. Such patients should be instructed to take precautions regarding contact with any individual with a viral illness including diarrheal illness, especially in infants, children, and young adults. Table 42.2 shows some clinical syndromes caused by enteroviruses.

Table 42.2 Clinical syndromes caused by enteroviruses [14, 72, 94]

Clinical syndrome	Predominant enterovirus species (serotype(s))
Hand, foot, and mouth disease	HEV-A (CAV16, EV71), HEV-B (CVB5)
Herpangina	HEV-A (EV71), HEV-B (CVB3, CVB5, E30)
Gastroenteritis	HEV-B (E6, E7, E13)
Respiratory infections	HEV-A (EV71), HEV-B (E30), HEV-D (EV68)
Myositis/pleurodynia	HEV-B (CVB1)
Myocarditis	HEV-A (CAV16), HEV-B (CVB3, CVB5)
Acute hemorrhagic conjunctivitis	HEV-C (CAV24)
Aseptic meningitis	HEV-A (EV71), HEV-B (CVB5, E9, E30)
Encephalitis	HEV-A (EV71), HEV-B (CVB5, E9, E30)
Chronic meningoencephalitis	HEV-B (E3, E11, E24)
Myelitis/flaccid paralysis	HEV-A (EV71), HEV-B (CVB5, E7, E9)
Poliomyelitis	HEV-C (PV1, PV2, PV3)
Vaccine-derived poliovirus disease	OPV
Hemophagocytic syndrome	HEV-B (CVB3)
Systemic infection	HEV-B (CVB3, CVB5)

Adapted from the CDC report on enterovirus surveillance Khetsuriani et al. [14] plus other selected references [72, 94].

HEV-A human enterovirus A, *HEV-B* human enterovirus B, *HEV-C* human enterovirus C, *HEV-D* human enterovirus D, *CAV* coxsackie A virus, *EV* enterovirus, *CBV* coxsackie B virus, *E* echovirus, *OPV* oral poliovirus vaccine

The most common etiologies of each clinical syndrome are listed based primarily on US epidemiologic studies; the indicated species are not meant to be a complete list of possible enteroviral causes of each syndrome. Serotypes are listed alphabetically/numerically, not in the order of frequency

Diagnosis

As can be appreciated from the diverse clinical syndromes associated with enteroviruses that often present with a significant overlap in various disease manifestations, the key approach tends to be a presumption for such infections. For CNS disease including poliomyelitis, examination of the CSF includes pleocytosis, classically described as with a neutrophil predominance early in infection followed by prominent lymphocytes during the post-acute phase of infection. CSF proteins may be modestly elevated as seen with other cases of viral meningitis [49]. Enteroviral meningitis in children recently challenged the dogma of late appearance of lymphocytes in the course of such infections [97].

Cell culture is the traditional method for diagnosis. Enteroviruses grow ex vivo in a variety of commercially available cell lines. The observation of cytopathic effects, followed by evaluation of serotype either by testing with antisera or using commercially available monoclonal antibodies for florescent staining, is used for species and subtype confirmation [98]. Tissue samples, pericardial fluid, CSF, blood, and feces can be used for laboratory cell culture analysis.

RT-PCR which targets the conserved 5′ noncoding region of the enterovirus genome is a newer technique that allows for quicker and more sensitive test results compared with culture-based identification methods [98]. PCR assay on CSF samples now plays an important role in the accurate diagnosis of enteroviral meningitis in children presenting with nonspecific febrile illness [99]. CSF, throat swabs, stool, urine, serum, and endomyocardial biopsy material are suitable samples for PCR analysis. Newer methodologies aimed at EV71 utilize real-time RT-PCR allowing for a more rapid and accurate diagnosis of both enteroviral infection and diagnosis of specific EV71 viral strain [100]. Serology testing of the blood using neutralization type-specific immunoassays is often used for outbreak investigations and prevalence analysis of enteroviral infections [13].

In patients with CNS disease, MRI examination is now considered as the gold standard for evaluation of patients with flaccid paralysis due to enterovirus; characteristic lesions in the anterior horns of the spinal cord are considered highly suggestive for such infections [101]. A series of patients with enterovirus 71 encephalitis revealed hyperintensity in the posterior portion of the brainstem on T2-weighted and FLAIR images; however, less typical lesions including leptomeningeal enhancement have also been observed in other patients with EV71 encephalitis [102].

Prevention

Prevention against poliovirus infection and disease has a long history [1] and continues to be part of the CDC's Advisory Committee on Immunization Practices "Recommended

Immunization Schedule for Persons Aged 0 Through 18 Years." New developments in vaccines have spurred the rising frequency of reported enterovirus outbreaks, especially EV71, in many parts of Asia, leading to increasing calls for a public health vaccination approach [21, 103]. A multicenter, randomized trial conducted in China including more than 10,000 children demonstrated vaccine safety and efficacy of 90% in the prevention of hand, foot, and mouth disease and 80% efficacy in the prevention of EV71-associated herpangina and neurological complications [104]. Other EV71 vaccine trials have shown improved immunogenicity with higher vaccine doses that may persist for up to 12 months after vaccination [105].

Treatment

There is hope for significant future progress in the treatment of severe enteroviral disease although specific antiviral drug treatment is still not available. In the early days of poliomyelitis, strict bed rest was found to reduce the extension of paralysis [49]. For bulbar involvement, the "iron lung" was the supportive treatment of choice. In the modern era, patients presenting with hypoxia and inability to control secretions may require endotracheal intubation for airway protection. Once progression of paralysis has ceased, physical therapy can begin [49].

IVIG is considered as the mainstay of treatment for both enteroviral myocarditis and encephalitis. A Cochrane review of IVIG therapy for viral myocarditis illustrated favorable response with IVIG therapy in both adult and pediatric population; this treatment approach is also recommended for patients with suspected enteroviral disease [106]. In a randomized controlled trial, IVIG daily dose of 1 g per kg body weight given for 2 consecutive days was regarded as beneficial [107].

For CNS disease, a formal review of IVIG effectiveness has not been performed. Several case reports in patients with severe meningoencephalitis due to HEV-B and EV71 in children with hematologic and other neoplastic diseases had a favorable response to IVIG therapy [77, 108]. A more recent randomized controlled trial from India in children with severe enteroviral encephalitis, myocarditis, or both, showed a reduced mortality in patients given IVIG; mortality was 4% in the treatment group compared with 23% in patients in whom IVIG was not given [109]. In this study, daily IVIG dose was 400 mg per kg body weight given for 5 consecutive days. A study from Taiwan among children with severe EV71 brainstem encephalitis showed that plasma levels of interferon-gamma, IL-6, IL-8, IL-10, and IL-13 were significantly reduced after IVIG administration, which may reflect a potential mechanism for IVIG-mediated modification in enteroviral CNS disease via modulation of hosts' immune inflammatory response [110]. This is underscored by the observation that in patients with hypogammaglobulinemia and persistent vaccine-derived poliovirus infection, IVIG therapy has not been shown to successfully eradicate chronic enteroviral infection [74].

In cases of chronic meningoencephalitis, treatment with IVIG and intraventricular immunoglobulin administration via reservoir devices have resulted in favorable response [38]. However, this treatment is not universally successful, and patients have died with this disease despite salvage intraventricular immunoglobulin and ribavirin treatment in the setting of X-linked agammaglobulinemia [72].

Milrinone, a cyclic nucleotide phosphodiesterase typically used for heart failure, has also been used for treatment of severe EV71 infection presenting with severe encephalitis and pulmonary edema. The antiviral or disease-ameliorative mechanism for this drug in life-threatening enteroviral infection remains unknown [111].

Pleconaril is an antiviral compound which is thought to work by inhibiting the uncoating of the viral capsid in all enteroviruses, preventing the virus from undergoing RNA replication; it has antiviral activity against both enteroviruses and rhinoviruses [112]. The initial use of pleconaril on compassionate release for treatment of severe enteroviral infections was encouraging, yielding a favorable clinical response up to 80% [113]. Other case series also suggested efficacy in the treatment of viral myocarditis as well as systemic enteroviral infection in immunocompromised hosts [112]. However, as phase 1 and 2 studies in previously healthy adults and children with enteroviral encephalitis showed only marginal improvement in symptom duration compared with patients given placebo, this compound did not receive FDA licensing, and production was abandoned in 2003. Interest in pleconaril has rekindled after Schering-Plough acquired the compound from ViroPharma. A phase 2 clinical trial of pleconaril nasal spray for the treatment of rhinovirus cold symptoms and asthma exacerbations is now completed; results are pending [114]. Another trial of pleconaril for treatment of enteroviral sepsis syndrome in infants sponsored by NIAID is listed as "ongoing, but not recruiting participants" [115].

There are other capsid targeting antiviral compounds under development including pirodavir (BTA-798) and V-073 that are being targeted for human respiratory viruses and poliovirus, respectively [114]. One concern, however, with any single-drug approach is the ability of RNA viruses to develop mutations, increasing the chances for development of de novo drug resistance. With this in mind, for-profit and research laboratories are investigating compounds that target a variety of antiviral targets such as protease, helicase, and RNA polymerase [114].

Another therapeutic approach under development is RNA interference. This approach appears promising against a range of enteroviruses including poliovirus, coxsackievirus, and EV71 in in vitro models as well as in a murine model of myocarditis [116]. These and other new drugs under investigation are expected to provide much-needed treatment option for immunocompromised patients undergoing transplantation with severe, potentially life-threatening enteroviral infections.

Summary

As for all community-onset infections that are transmitted via casual person-to-person contact, enteroviral infections pose a risk to transplant recipients. The risk is further enhanced by the ease of infection transmission from an unsuspected, asymptomatic individual or those with clinically subtle disease, and infection may be transmitted by saliva, respiratory secretions, and fecal contamination. As most enteroviral infections are difficult to clinically differentiate from other viral illnesses, and present with a wide range of clinical presentations, a low threshold of suspicion should be maintained, especially during the summer and fall months when these viruses have high seasonal presence in most communities. Humoral immune defects and lymphopenia are known risk factors for potentially life-threatening systemic enteroviral disease including viral pneumonitis and encephalitis in recipients of allogeneic HSCT [89, 117]. OPV should never be given to transplant recipients. Furthermore, these patients are at risk for vaccine-derived disease for close contacts in countries where OPV vaccination is prevalent [58]. IVIG is important for prevention of serious enteroviral infections in individuals with hypogammaglobulinemia. IVIG therapy has been successful in some patients with serious lung, heart, and CNS acute enteroviral disease [72]. The future developments in (1) novel antiviral therapies, (2) advances in rapid and accurate diagnostic tests, and (3) better understanding of host susceptibility for such infections and proclivity for various end-organ diseases remain an encouraging prospect, especially in the care for highly susceptible transplant population.

References

1. Mueller S, Wimmer E, Cello J. Poliovirus and poliomyelitis: a tale of guts, brains, and an accidental event. Virus Res. 2005;111:175–93.
2. Oberste MS, Maher K, Flemister MR, Marchetti G, Kilpatrick DR, Pallansch MA. Comparison of classic and molecular approaches for the identification of untypeable enteroviruses. J Clin Microbiol. 2000;38:1170–4.
3. Oberste MS. Comparative genomics of the coxsackie B viruses and related enteroviruses. Curr Top Microbiol Immunol. 2008;323:33–47.
4. Hogle JM. Poliovirus cell entry: common structural themes in viral cell entry pathways. Annu Rev Microbiol. 2002;56:677–702.
5. Palmenberg A, Neubauer D, Skern T. Genome organization and encoded proteins. In: Ehrenfeld E, Domingo E, Roos RP, editors. The picornaviruses. Washington, DC: ASM Press; 2010. p. 3–17.
6. Wimmer E, Nomoto A. Molecular biology and cell-free synthesis of poliovirus. Biologicals. 1993;21:349–56.
7. Cameron CE, Suk OH, Moustafa IM. Expanding knowledge of P3 proteins in the poliovirus lifecycle. Future Microbiol. 2010;5:867–81.
8. Domingo E, Perales C, Agudo R, Arias A, Escarmis C, Ferrer-Orta C. Mutation, quasispecies, and lethal mutagenesis. In: Ehrenfeld E, Domingo E, Roos RP, editors. The picornaviruses. Washington, DC: ASM Press; 2010. p. 197–211.
9. Kadurugamuwa JL, Shaheen E. Inactivation of human enterovirus 71 and coxsackie virus A16 and hand, foot, and mouth disease. Am J Infect Control. 2011;39:788–9.
10. Maillard J-Y. Virus susceptibility to biocides: an understanding. Rev Med Microbiol. 2001;12:63–74.
11. Racaniello VR. One hundred years of poliovirus pathogenesis. Virology. 2006;344:9–16.
12. Mahy BWJ. Coxsackie B viruses: an introduction. Curr Top Microbiol Immunol. 2008;323:vii–xiii.
13. Pallansch M, Roos R. Enteroviruses: polioviruses, coxsackieviruses, echoviruses, and newer enteroviruses. In: Knipe DM, Howley PM, editors. Fields virology. Philadelphia: Lippincott Williams & Wilkins; 2007. p. 840–93.
14. Khetsuriani N, Lamonte-Fowlkes A, Oberst S, Pallansch MA, Centers for Disease Control and Prevention. Enterovirus surveillance--United States, 1970–2005. MMWR Surveill Summ. 2006;55:1–20.
15. Muir P, Kämmerer U, Korn K, et al. Molecular typing of enteroviruses: current status and future requirements. The European Union concerted action on virus meningitis and encephalitis. Clin Microbiol Rev. 1998;11:202–27.
16. Lo C-W, Wu K-G, Lin M-C, et al. Application of a molecular method for the classification of human enteroviruses and its correlation with clinical manifestations. J Microbiol Immunol Infect. 2010;43:354–9.
17. Oberste MS. Complete genome sequences of all members of the species human enterovirus A. J Gen Virol. 2004;85:1597–607.
18. Lukashev AN. Role of recombination in evolution of enteroviruses. Rev Med Virol. 2005;15:157–67.
19. Ooi MH, Wong SC, Lewthwaite P, Cardosa MJ, Solomon T. Clinical features, diagnosis, and management of enterovirus 71. Lancet Neurol. 2010;9:1097–105.
20. Solomon T, Lewthwaite P, Perera D, Cardosa MJ, McMinn P, Ooi MH. Virology, epidemiology, pathogenesis, and control of enterovirus 71. Lancet Infect Dis. 2010;10:778–90.
21. Xu J, Qian Y, Wang S, et al. EV71: an emerging infectious disease vaccine target in the Far East? Vaccine. 2010;28:3516–21.
22. Lee BE, Davies HD. Aseptic meningitis. Curr Opin Infect Dis. 2007;20:272–7.
23. Kuss SK, Best GT, Etheredge CA, et al. Intestinal microbiota promote enteric virus replication and systemic pathogenesis. Science. 2011;334:249–52.
24. He Y, Bowman VD, Mueller S, et al. Interaction of the poliovirus receptor with poliovirus. Proc Natl Acad Sci U S A. 2000;97:79–84.
25. Shafren DR, Dorahy DJ, Greive SJ, Burns GF, Barry RD. Mouse cells expressing human intercellular adhesion molecule-1 are susceptible to infection by coxsackievirus A21. J Virol. 1997;71:785–9.
26. Freimuth P, Philipson L, Carson SD. The coxsackievirus and adenovirus receptor. Curr Top Microbiol Immunol. 2008;323:67–87.

27. Xiao C, Bator CM, Bowman VD, et al. Interaction of coxsackievirus A21 with its cellular receptor, ICAM-1. J Virol. 2001;75:2444–51.
28. Yajima T, Knowlton KU. Viral myocarditis: from the perspective of the virus. Circulation. 2009;119:2615–24.
29. Lee T-C, Guo H-R, H-JJ S, Yang Y-C, Chang H-L, Chen K-T. Diseases caused by enterovirus 71 infection. Pediatr Infect Dis J. 2009;28:904–10.
30. Wang SM, Lei HY, Su LY, et al. Cerebrospinal fluid cytokines in enterovirus 71 brain stem encephalitis and echovirus meningitis infections of varying severity. Clin Microbiol Infect. 2007;13:677–82.
31. Knowlton KU. CVB infection and mechanisms of viral cardiomyopathy. Curr Top Microbiol Immunol. 2008;323:315–35.
32. Chapman NM, Kim KS. Persistent coxsackievirus infection: enterovirus persistence in chronic myocarditis and dilated cardiomyopathy. Curr Top Microbiol Immunol. 2008;323:275–92.
33. Ida-Hosonuma M, Iwasaki T, Yoshikawa T, et al. The alpha/beta interferon response controls tissue tropism and pathogenicity of poliovirus. J Virol. 2005;79:4460–9.
34. Abe Y, Fujii K, Nagata N, et al. The toll-like receptor 3-mediated antiviral response is important for protection against poliovirus infection in poliovirus receptor transgenic mice. J Virol. 2011;86:185–94.
35. Richer MJ, Lavallée DJ, Shanina I, Horwitz MS. Toll-like receptor 3 signaling on macrophages is required for survival following coxsackievirus B4 infection. PLoS One. 2009;4:e4127.
36. Huber S. Host immune responses to coxsackievirus B3. Curr Top Microbiol Immunol. 2008;323:199–221.
37. Kemball CC, Fujinami RS, Whitton JL. Adaptive immune responses. In: Ehrenfeld E, Domingo E, Roos RP, editors. The picornaviruses. Washington, DC: ASM Press; 2010. p. 303–19.
38. McKinney RE, Katz SL, Wilfert CM. Chronic enteroviral meningoencephalitis in agammaglobulinemic patients. Rev Infect Dis. 1987;9:334–56.
39. Mena I, Perry CM, Harkins S, Rodriguez F, Gebhard J, Whitton JL. The role of B lymphocytes in coxsackievirus B3 infection. Am J Pathol. 2010;155:1205–15.
40. Rhoades RE, Tabor-Godwin JM, Tsueng G, Feuer R. Enterovirus infections of the central nervous system. Virology. 2011;411:288–305.
41. Schnurr DP, Schmidt NJ. Coxsackievirus B3 persistence and myocarditis in NFR nu/nu and +/nu mice. Med Microbiol Immunol. 1984;173:1–7.
42. Jubelt B, Ropka SL, Goldfarb SJ, Janavs JL. Anti-thymocyte serum delays clearance of poliovirus from the mouse central nervous system. J Neuroimmunol. 1989;22:223–32.
43. Gebhard JR, Perry CM, Harkins S, et al. Coxsackievirus B3-induced myocarditis. Am J Pathol. 1998;153:417–28.
44. Shi Y, Fukuoka M, Li G, et al. Regulatory T cells protect mice against coxsackievirus-induced myocarditis through the transforming growth factor-coxsackie-adenovirus receptor pathway. Circulation. 2010;121:2624–34.
45. Tam PE. Coxsackievirus myocarditis: interplay between virus and host in the pathogenesis of heart disease. Viral Immunol. 2006;19:133–46.
46. Tracy S, Drescher KM, Jackson JD, Kim K, Kono K. Enteroviruses, type 1 diabetes and hygiene: a complex relationship. Rev Med Virol. 2010;20:106–16.
47. Centers for Disease Control and Prevention (CDC). Nonpolio enterovirus and human parechovirus surveillance – United States, 2006–2008. MMWR Morb Mortal Wkly Rep. 2010;59:1577–80.
48. Faustini A, Fano V, Muscillo M, et al. An outbreak of aseptic meningitis due to echovirus 30 associated with attending school and swimming in pools. Int J Infect Dis. 2006;10:291–7.
49. Mulder DW. Clinical observations on acute poliomyelitis. Ann N Y Acad Sci. 1995;753:1–10.
50. Kew O. Reaching the last one per cent: progress and challenges in global polio eradication. Curr Opin Virol. 2012;2:188–98.
51. World Health Organization. Resurgence of wild poliovirus type 1 transmission and effect of importation into polio-free countries, 2002–2005. Wkly Epidemiol Rec. 2006;81:63–8.
52. Gulland A. World could be declared free of polio by 2018. BMJ. 2011;346:f2373.
53. Kew O. Outbreak of poliomyelitis in Hispaniola associated with circulating type 1 vaccine-derived poliovirus. Science. 2002;296:356–9.
54. Wassilak S, Pate MA, Wannemuehler K, et al. Outbreak of type 2 vaccine-derived poliovirus in Nigeria: emergence and widespread circulation in an underimmunized population. J Infect Dis. 2011;203:898–909.
55. Committee on Infectious Diseases. Poliovirus. Pediatrics. 2011;128:805–8.
56. Centers for Disease Control and Prevention (CDC). Update on vaccine-derived polioviruses--worldwide, July 2009–March 2011. MMWR Morb Mortal Wkly Rep. 2011;60:846–50.
57. Modlin JF. Poliovirus. In: Mandell GL, Bennett JE, Dolin R, editors. Principle and practice of infectious diseases. Philadelphia: Elsevier Churchill Livingstone; 2005. p. 2141–8.
58. Nathanson N, Kew OM. From emergence to eradication: the epidemiology of poliomyelitis deconstructed. Am J Epidemiol. 2010;172:1213–29.
59. Huang C, Chatterjee NK, Grady LJ. Diagnosis of viral infections of the central nervous system. N Engl J Med. 1999;340:483–4.
60. Frantzidou F, Kamaria F, Dumaidi K, Skoura L, Antoniadis A, Papa A. Aseptic meningitis and encephalitis because of herpesviruses and enteroviruses in an immunocompetent adult population. Eur J Neurol. 2008;15:995–7.
61. Franzen-Röhl E, Larsson K, Skoog E, et al. High diagnostic yield by CSF-PCR for entero- and herpes simplex viruses and TBEV serology in adults with acute aseptic meningitis in Stockholm. Scand J Infect Dis. 2008;40:914–21.
62. Huttunen P, Lappalainen M, Salo E, et al. Differential diagnosis of acute central nervous system infections in children using modern microbiological methods. Acta Paediatr. 2009;98:1300–6.
63. Centers for Disease Control and Prevention (CDC). Notes from the field. severe hand, foot, and mouth disease associated with coxsackievirus A6 – Alabama, Connecticut, California, and Nevada, November 2011–February 2012. MMWR Morb Mortal Wkly Rep. 2012;61:213–4.
64. Chong C-Y, Chan K-P, Shah V, et al. Hand, foot and mouth disease in Singapore: a comparison of fatal and non-fatal cases. Acta Paediatr. 2007;92:1163–9.
65. Centers for Disease Control and Prevention (CDC). Notes from the field: acute hemorrhagic conjunctivitis outbreaks caused by coxsackievirus A24v – Uganda and southern Sudan, 2010. MMWR Morb Mortal Wkly Rep. 2010;59:1024.
66. Huang W-T, Lee P-I, Chang L-Y, et al. Epidemic pleurodynia caused by coxsackievirus B3 at a medical center in Northern Taiwan. J Microbiol Immunol Infect. 2010;43:515–8.
67. Weber MA, Ashworth MT, Risdon RA, Malone M, Burch M, Sebire NJ. Clinicopathological features of paediatric deaths due to myocarditis: an autopsy series. Arch Dis Child. 2008;93:594–8.
68. Kereiakes DJ, Parmley WW. Myocarditis and cardiomyopathy. Am Heart J. 1984;108:1318–26.
69. Friman G, Wesslén L, Fohlman J, Karjalainen J, Rolf C. The epidemiology of infectious myocarditis, lymphocytic myocarditis and dilated cardiomyopathy. Eur Heart J. 1995;16(Suppl O):36–41.
70. Bowles NE, Ni J, Kearney DL, et al. Detection of viruses in myocardial tissues by polymerase chain reaction. J Am Coll Cardiol. 2003;42:466–72.

71. Li Y, Bourlet T, Andreoletti L, et al. Enteroviral capsid protein VP1 is present in myocardial tissues from some patients with myocarditis or dilated cardiomyopathy. Circulation. 2000;101:231–4.
72. Misbah SA, Spickett GP, Ryba PC, et al. Chronic enteroviral meningoencephalitis in agammaglobulinemia: case report and literature review. J Clin Immunol. 1992;12:266–70.
73. Centers for Disease Control and Prevention (CDC). Prolonged poliovirus excretion in an immunodeficient person with vaccine-associated paralytic poliomyelitis. MMWR Morb Mortal Wkly Rep. 1997;46:641–3.
74. MacLennan C, Dunn G, Huissoon AP, et al. Failure to clear persistent vaccine-derived neurovirulent poliovirus infection in an immunodeficient man. Lancet. 2004;363:1509–13.
75. Kew OM, Sutter RW, Nottay BK, et al. Prolonged replication of a type 1 vaccine-derived poliovirus in an immunodeficient patient. J Clin Microbiol. 1998;36:2893–9.
76. Inaba H, Hori H, Ito M, et al. Polio vaccine virus-associated meningoencephalitis in an infant with transient hypogammaglobulinemia. Scand J Infect Dis. 2001;33:630–1.
77. Frange P, Michon J, Fromantin I, et al. Enterovirus 71 meningoencephalitis during chemotherapy in a child with metastatic osteosarcoma. J Pediatr Hematol Oncol. 2007;29:566–8.
78. Chakrabarti S, Osman H, Collingham KE, Fegan CD, Milligan DW. Enterovirus infections following T-cell depleted allogeneic transplants in adults. Bone Marrow Transplant. 2003;33:425–30.
79. Moschovi MA, Katsibardi K, Theodoridou M, et al. Enteroviral infections in children with malignant disease: a 5-year study in a single institution. J Infect. 2007;54:387–92.
80. Faulkner CF, Godbolt AM, DeAmbrosis B, Triscott J. Hand, foot and mouth disease in an immunocompromised adult treated with acyclovir. Australas J Dermatol. 2003;44:203–6.
81. Roch N, Salameire D, Gressin R, et al. Fatal adenoviral and enteroviral infections and an Epstein-Barr virus positive large B-cell lymphoma after alemtuzumab treatment in a patient with refractory Sézary syndrome. Scand J Infect Dis. 2008;40:343–6.
82. Tan P-L, Verneris MR, Charnas LR, Reck SJ, van Burik J-AH, Blazar BR. Outcome of CNS and pulmonary enteroviral infections after hematopoietic cell transplantation. Pediatr Blood Cancer. 2005;45:74–5.
83. Galama JM, de Leeuw N, Wittebol S, Peters H, Melchers WJ. Prolonged enteroviral infection in a patient who developed pericarditis and heart failure after bone marrow transplantation. Clin Infect Dis. 1996;22:1004–8.
84. Fischmeister G, Wiesbauer P, Holzmann HM, Peters C, Eibl M, Gadner H. Enteroviral meningoencephalitis in immunocompromised children after matched unrelated donor-bone marrow transplantation. Pediatr Hematol Oncol. 2000;17:393–9.
85. Servais S, Caers J, Warling O, et al. Enteroviral meningoencephalitis as complication of Rituximab therapy in a patient treated for diffuse large B-cell lymphoma. Br J Haematol. 2010;150:379–81.
86. Ahmed R, Buckland M, Davies L, et al. Enterovirus 71 meningoencephalitis complicating rituximab therapy. J Neurol Sci. 2011;305:149–51.
87. Polidori M, Tagliaferri E, Tascini C, Andreotti G, Flammini S, Menichetti F. Myelitis due to enterovirus in patient on interferon therapy for chronic hepatitis B: case report. Clin Immunol. 2010;137:176–7.
88. Parody R, Rabella N, Martino R, et al. Upper and lower respiratory tract infections by human enterovirus and rhinovirus in adult patients with hematological malignancies. Am J Hematol 2007;82:807–11.
89. González Y, Martino R, Badell I, et al. Pulmonary enterovirus infections in stem cell transplant recipients. Bone Marrow Transplant. 1999;23:511–3.
90. Liu M, Worley S, Arrigain S, et al. Respiratory viral infections within one year after pediatric lung transplant. Transpl Infect Dis. 2009;11:304–12.
91. Vu DL, Bridevaux PO, Aubert JD, Soccal PM, Kaiser L. Respiratory viruses in lung transplant recipients: a critical review and pooled analysis of clinical studies. Am J Transplant. 2011;11:1071–8.
92. Yolken RH, Bishop CA, Townsend TR, et al. Infectious gastroenteritis in bone-marrow-transplant recipients. N Engl J Med. 1982;306:1010–2.
93. Chakrabarti S, Collingham KE, Stevens RH, Pillay D, Fegan CD, Milligan DW. Isolation of viruses from stools in stem cell transplant recipients: a prospective surveillance study. Bone Marrow Transplant. 2000;25:277–82.
94. Katsibardi K, Moschovi MA, Theodoridou M, et al. Enterovirus-associated hemophagocytic syndrome in children with malignancy: report of three cases and review of the literature. Eur J Pediatr. 2007;167:97–102.
95. Donoso Mantke O, Meyer R, Prösch S, et al. High prevalence of cardiotropic viruses in myocardial tissue from explanted hearts of heart transplant recipients and heart donors: a 3-year retrospective study from a German patients' pool. J Heart Lung Transplant. 2005;24:1632–8.
96. Shirali GS, Ni J, Chinnock RE, et al. Association of viral genome with graft loss in children after cardiac transplantation. N Engl J Med. 2001;344:1498–503.
97. Shah SS, Hodinka RL, Turnquist JL, Elliott MR, Coffin SE. Cerebrospinal fluid mononuclear cell predominance is not related to symptom duration in children with enteroviral meningitis. J Pediatr. 2006;148:118–21.
98. Terletskaia-Ladwig E, Meier S, Hahn R, Leinmuller M, Schneider F, Enders M. A convenient rapid culture assay for the detection of enteroviruses in clinical samples: comparison with conventional cell culture and RT-PCR. J Med Microbiol. 2008;57:1000–6.
99. Stellrecht KA, Harding I, Woron AM, Lepow ML, Venezia RA. The impact of an enteroviral RT-PCR assay on the diagnosis of aseptic meningitis and patient management. J Clin Virol. 2002;25(Suppl 1):S19–26.
100. Hwang S, Kang B, Hong J, et al. Development of duplex real-time RT-PCR based on Taqman technology for detecting simultaneously the genome of pan-enterovirus and enterovirus 71. J Med Virol. 2013;85:1274–9.
101. Kornreich L, Dagan O, Grunebaum M. MRI in acute poliomyelitis. Neuroradiology. 1996;38:371–2.
102. Jang S, Suh S-I, Ha SM, et al. Enterovirus 71-related encephalomyelitis: usual and unusual magnetic resonance imaging findings. Neuroradiology. 2011;54:239–45.
103. Liang Z-L, Mao Q-Y, Wang Y-P, et al. Progress on the research and development of inactivated EV71 whole-virus vaccines. Hum Vaccin Immunother. 2013;9(8):1701–5.
104. Zhu F-C, Meng F-Y, Li J-X, et al. Efficacy, safety, and immunology of an inactivated alum-adjuvant enterovirus 71 vaccine in children in China: a multicentre, randomised, double-blind, placebo-controlled, phase 3 trial. Lancet. 2013;381:2024–32.
105. Li Y-P, Liang Z-L, Xia J-L, et al. Immunogenicity, safety, and immune persistence of a novel inactivated human enterovirus 71 (EV71) vaccine: a phase II, randomized, double-blind, placebo-controlled trial. J Infect Dis. 2014;209(1):46–55.
106. Robinson J, Hartling L, Vandermeer B, Klassen TP. Intravenous immunoglobulin for presumed viral myocarditis in children and adults. Cochrane Database Syst Rev. 2005;(1):CD004370; updated 2015 May 20;(5):CD004370.
107. McNamara DM, Holubkov R, Starling RC, et al. Controlled trial of intravenous immune globulin in recent-onset dilated cardiomyopathy. Circulation. 2001;103:2254–9.

108. Geller TJ, Condie D. A case of protracted coxsackie virus meningoencephalitis in a marginally immunodeficient child treated successfully with intravenous immunoglobulin. J Neurol Sci. 1995;129:131–3.
109. Bhatt GC, Sankar J, Kushwaha KP. Use of intravenous immunoglobulin compared with standard therapy is associated with improved clinical outcomes in children with acute encephalitis syndrome complicated by myocarditis. Pediatr Cardiol. 2012;33(8):1370–6.
110. Wang S-M, Lei H-Y, Huang M-C, et al. Modulation of cytokine production by intravenous immunoglobulin in patients with enterovirus 71-associated brainstem encephalitis. J Clin Virol. 2006;37:47–52.
111. Wang S-M, Lei H-Y, Huang M-C, et al. Therapeutic efficacy of milrinone in the management of enterovirus 71-induced pulmonary edema. Pediatr Pulmonol. 2005;39:219–23.
112. Webster ADB. Pleconaril – an advance in the treatment of enteroviral infection in immuno-compromised patients. J Clin Virol. 2005;32:1–6.
113. Rotbart HA, Webster AD, Pleconaril Treatment Registry Group. Treatment of potentially life-threatening enterovirus infections with pleconaril. Clin Infect Dis. 2001;32:228–35.
114. Thibaut HJ, De Palma AM, Neyts J. Combating enterovirus replication: state-of-the-art on antiviral research. Biochem Pharmacol. 2012;83:185–92.
115. National Institute of Allergy and Infectious Diseases. Pleconaril enteroviral sepsis syndrome. Available at: http://clinicaltrials.gov/ct2/show/NCT00031512?term=pleconaril&rank=1. Accessed 20 May 2012.
116. Schönhofer-Merl S, Wessely R. RNA interference to treat enteroviral disease: current status and clinical perspectives. Curr Mol Med. 2010;10:550–64.
117. Tan P-L, Verneris MR, Charnas LR, Reck SJ, van Burik J-AH, Blazar BR. Outcome of CNS and pulmonary enteroviral infections after hematopoietic cell transplantation. Pediatr Blood Cancer. 2005;45:74–5.

Parvovirus B19

43

Morgan Hakki and Lynne Strasfeld

Introduction

The family *Parvoviridae* encompasses two subfamilies, *Parvovirinae* and *Densovirinae* [1]. The *Parvovirinae* are further divided into five genera, of which parvovirus B19 (B19) is a member of the genus *Erythrovirus* [1]. Three distinct phylogenetic clusters (genotypes 1–3) of B19 are recognized based on 13–14% sequence divergence at the nucleotide level, with B19 representing the prototype of genotype 1 [2–5]. However, sequence variability does not account for the various clinical manifestations of B19 infection, as the clinical spectrum of illness caused by the three genotypes tends to overlap [6].

B19 was discovered in 1975 during screening of blood for the hepatitis B virus [7], and the first reports linking B19 infection to human disease appeared in 1981 with the description of cases of aplastic crisis in patients with sickle cell disease [8, 9]. The first published report of B19 infection after transplantation, in 1986, described persistent anemia in a renal transplant recipient [10]. Since then, B19 infection has come to be a recognized infectious complication of solid organ (SOT) and hematopoietic cell transplantation (HCT). While typically a benign, self-limited infection in immunocompetent hosts, B19 can have serious sequelae in SOT and HCT recipients.

The B19 Genome and Proteins

B19 is a relatively small (18–25 nm) unenveloped virus [1]. The genome consists of plus- or minus-sense single-stranded linear DNA of 5.6 kilobases (kb) characterized by an internal unique region flanked by inverted terminal hairpin repeats. It is thought that DNA replication initiates at the terminal hairpins, with the hairpin formed by the 3′ repeat serving as a primer for DNA synthesis [11]. A series of linear duplex monomeric and dimeric intermediate forms leads to a template for DNA synthesis, and the resulting plus- and minus-sense single-stranded DNA is packaged in the virion with equal frequency [1].

Five proteins are translated from nine mRNA forms transcribed from a single promoter, p6 [12, 13].

The 77 kilodalton (kD) nonstructural protein (NS1) is encoded by the single nonspliced transcript located near the 5′ end of the genome [14–16]. NS1 is a polyfunctional protein that is required for B19 replication [17]. NS1 regulates activity of the p6 promoter [18, 19], and sequence analysis has shown that NS1 contains motifs for nucleoside triphosphate (NTP) binding and hydrolysis [20] associated with helicase activity, suggesting a role of NS1 in B19 DNA replication. NS1 induces caspase-dependent apoptosis [21, 22] and regulates the activity of the E2F family of transcription factors to promote cell cycle arrest in G1 and G2 phases [23–25].

Two proteins, the 83 kD VP1 and the 58 kD VP2, make up the B19 capsid. Because the sequences of VP1 and VP2 are collinear, VP2 is identical to the carboxy-terminus of VP1, while the amino-terminal 227 amino acids of VP1 are unique (VP1u) [13]. VP2 is the major capsid protein, comprising 95% of the capsid [15]. VP2 functions in viral entry by binding directly to blood group P antigen (globoside), the cellular receptor of B19 virus [26]. VP1 is the minor capsid protein, accounting for the remaining 5% of the capsid protein content [15]. The main neutralizing epitopes of B19 are in VP1u, which is located on the outside of the capsid [27–29]. VP1u also contains a conserved phospholipase A2-like motif (HDXXY), and mutation of this motif attenuates the infectivity of B19, indicative of a role for VP1 phospholipase activity in the B19 life cycle [30, 31].

Two other smaller nonstructural proteins, 7.5 kD and 11 kD, have been detected during B19V infection [32, 33]. The 11 kDa protein has been shown to have a role in

M. Hakki (✉) · L. Strasfeld
Oregon Health and Science University,
Division of Infectious Diseases, Portland, OR, USA
e-mail: hakki@ohsu.edu; strasfel@ohsu.edu

A. Safdar (ed.), *Principles and Practice of Transplant Infectious Diseases*, https://doi.org/10.1007/978-1-4939-9034-4_43

virion production and trafficking in infected cells and induces apoptosis by activation of caspase-10 in primary erythroid progenitor cells (EPCs) [34, 35]. The role of the 7.5 kDa protein during B19 infection, if any, is unknown.

Infection and Pathogenesis

Humans are the only known host for B19 infection, and the consequent lack of animal models, coupled with the difficulty in culturing B19 in vitro, has posed obstacles to studies of B19 infection and pathogenesis. Culture systems utilizing bone marrow cells [36], megakaryoblastoid cells [24, 37], erythroid leukemia cells [38], and ex vivo expanded EPCs [22, 39, 40] have been developed, but each system is marked by limitations inherent to in vitro models. As a result, fundamental aspects of the virus-host interaction remain poorly understood, and more research is needed in this area.

During acute infection, viremia is typically detectable by 5–6 days post-infection, peaks at 6–12 days post-infection, and clears by days 15–20 [41]. However, using more sensitive modern diagnostic techniques such as polymerase chain reaction (PCR), it is now known that many immunocompetent persons exhibit low-level persistent viremia for months after initial detection [42].

The primary sites of B19 replication are erythroid progenitor cells (EPCs) found in bone marrow and peripheral blood, due in part to the limited expression of P antigen [26]. While P antigen expression is necessary for B19 infection [26, 43], it does not appear to be sufficient, as some cell lines are resistant to transduction by a B19 vector despite P antigen expression [44]. Thus, it is possible that a co-receptor(s), such as beta-integrins [45], may contribute to viral entry. P antigen is also expressed on other tissues, including placental villous trophoblast cells during the first and second trimesters of pregnancy [46], potentially accounting for B19 transmission during pregnancy.

Viral entry by endocytosis is followed by release of the viral capsid into the perinuclear cytoplasm, nuclear transport, and release of genomic DNA [1, 26]. The mechanisms governing the latter two processes are not precisely defined. Unlike *Parvoviridae* such as adeno-associated virus, B19 is autonomous in that it can replicate in the absence of a helper virus. However, since B19 does not encode a DNA polymerase, genome replication is dependent on host cell proteins, and efficient replication requires the infected cell to pass through S phase of the cell cycle [1].

Ultimately, induction of host cell apoptosis, particularly of primary EPCs and megakaryoblastoid cell lines, results in the severe disease manifestations (hydrops, aplastic crisis) of B19 infection [21, 22, 34, 47, 48].

Immunology

The development of IgM antibodies directed against conformational and linear epitopes of VP1 and VP2 occurs 7–10 days post-infection and correlates with virus clearance [41, 49, 50]. Symptoms of fifth disease, such as rash and arthralgias, as well as post-infectious polyarthropathies in adults with acute B19 infection, develop during this phase of illness, consistent with a role for immune complex deposition in the pathogenesis of these disease manifestations [41]. An IgG response, directed primarily against conformational epitopes of VP1 and VP2, develops soon thereafter and confers lifelong protection from reinfection [51–56]. The successful use of immune globulin to control viremia and the association of persistent B19 infection with a deficient antibody response support the role of antibodies in providing immunity to B19 [57–60]. Additionally, VP1 and VP2 can elicit neutralizing antibodies when administered together as a recombinant vaccine [61]. Antibodies directed against epitopes present on NS1 have been found and may be useful as a tool to diagnose recent (<6 weeks) infection [62–65].

B19-specific CD4+ and CD8+ T-cell responses have been detected against VP1, VP2, and NS1 [66–71], although the role that CD4+ and CD8+ responses play in B19 protective immunity or in the pathogenesis of post-infectious syndromes is not clear.

Epidemiology

The seroprevalence of B19 increases with age, and by adulthood approximately 70–90% of persons are seropositive [52, 72]. The annual seroconversion rate among women of childbearing age has been estimated to be 1.5% [73]. The primary mechanism of B19 transmission is incompletely understood. The finding of viral DNA in respiratory specimens during viremia indicates that community-acquired B19 infection may result from transmission of virus excreted in the nasopharynx and upper airway [41, 74, 75]. Whether transmission occurs by close contact, droplet, aerosol, or fomites is not clear. B19, like most parvoviruses, is relatively stable in the environment, suggesting that contaminated surfaces may contribute to transmission [76]. While secondary attack rates ranging from 20% to 50% during school outbreaks and at home [74, 75, 77] indicate efficient transmission, the precise probability of transmission via various routes (i.e., droplet, aerosol, fomite) has not been conclusively established.

Transmission via whole blood or blood products, such as factor VIII and factor IX concentrates, is a well-documented but rare event [78, 79]. The prevalence of B19 DNA varies from 0.003% to 1.07% in blood donor samples, the variability likely due to differences in the sensitivity of the assay being used as well as the population and seasonality [78,

80–83]. Screening of whole blood components intended for individual patient transfusions is not currently routinely performed in the United States [42]. However, plasma derivatives have been screened for B19 by PCR since 2002 [84].

Transmission of B19 from donor to recipient via solid organ transplant has been suspected on occasion due to factors such as time of onset of infection after transplant and the finding of B19 in non-transplanted donor tissue [85, 86]. However, these findings must be interpreted with caution, and B19 transmission in this manner has not been definitively proven by documenting the genetic relatedness of a B19 strain present in the donor and recipient.

Clinical Presentation

Manifestations in the Non-transplant Host

There are five well-established clinical syndromes associated with B19 infection that are largely dependent on host age and immune status (Table 43.1). Most seropositive, immunocompetent individuals do not recall specific symptoms of infection. Roughly 25% of infections will be entirely asymptomatic, 50% will have nonspecific flu-like symptoms, and the remaining 25% will present with more classic symptoms, including arthralgias and rash [87, 88]. B19 infection is self-limited in nonpregnant immunocompetent individuals, with severe or complicated disease a rare exception [89].

B19 infection in immunocompetent children manifests most commonly as erythema infectiosum, frequently referred to as "fifth disease" [90]. The illness is typified by a nonspecific viral prodrome, followed 2–5 days later by a characteristic erythematous malar rash ("slapped cheek rash") with circumoral pallor. The facial rash is often followed by a lacey rash involving the trunk and extremities. The characteristic rash is reported more often in children, whereas arthralgias and myalgia are seen more commonly in immunocompetent adults, particularly in women [88, 91, 92]. A nondestructive polyarthropathy, often symmetric and most frequently involving the small joints of the hands, wrists, knees, and feet, may occur. Both the rash and joint symptoms typically occur soon after B19 antibody response is detectable, suggesting these phenomena are immunologically mediated. In pregnancy, complications of infection include nonimmune hydrops fetalis, intrauterine fetal death, or miscarriage [93]. Transient aplastic crisis (TAC), characterized by severe anemia and a dramatic decrease or even absence of measurable reticulocytes, may occur with B19 infection in patients with chronic hemolytic disorders (e.g., sickle cell anemia) [8].

Table 43.1 Clinical presentation of parvovirus B19, based on host immune status and age

Patient population	Clinical presentation
Immunocompetent hosts	
Children	Erythema infectiosum ("fifth disease")
Pregnant women	Hydrops fetalis
Adults (women > men)	Polyarthropathy syndrome
Patients with red cell disorders	Transient aplastic crisis
Immunocompromised hosts	Pure red cell aplasia Other less common manifestations: rash, leukopenia, thrombocytopenia, hepatitis, myocarditis, pneumonitis, encephalitis Allograft dysfunction

Clinical Manifestations in the Transplant Recipient

The classic presentation of B19 infection in transplant recipients and other immunosuppressed hosts (HIV with advanced immunodeficiency, congenital immunodeficiencies, etc.) is chronic infection with pure red cell aplasia. Although most reported cases of B19-associated pure red cell aplasia have occurred within the first year posttransplant [85, 94–97], when immunosuppression is maximal, there are numerous reports of late-onset disease as well [98, 99]. B19 DNA was demonstrated in serum in 23% of 48 kidney transplant recipients presenting with anemia compared with 5% of the controls [95]. In a prospective single-center study of kidney transplant recipients with erythropoietin-resistant anemia over a 3-month period, three of eight (38%) patients screened had B19 infection [99]. Therefore, testing for B19 should be strongly considered in transplant recipients with otherwise unexplained anemia.

The largest published review to date of B19 infection after SOT or HCT summarized 98 cases, of which 7 were seen at the Mayo Clinic over a 16 year period and the remainder found by review of the medical literature [96]. In this study, the median time to diagnosis posttransplant was 7 weeks (range, 1 week to 96 months). Not surprising given the tropism of B19 for EPCs, anemia was present in the vast majority (99%). However, other cell lines were often affected as well, with leukopenia occurring in 38% and thrombocytopenia in 21%. Fever and flu-like symptoms occurred in 26%, and, perhaps due to impaired immune responses, rash (13%) and arthralgia (6%) were less common. Proven or suspected accompanying organ-invasive disease occurred in 11%, including myocarditis, pneumonitis, hepatitis, and glomerulonephritis. Allograft loss or dysfunction was observed at the time of B19 infection in 10%. Death attributable to B19 disease occurred in three patients, all a result of cardiogenic shock related to myocarditis.

While anemia is the hallmark of B19 infection, other manifestations have been described in transplant recipients.

Myocarditis is perhaps the most common, and the cardiotropism of B19 has been demonstrated in transplant as well as in immunocompetent patient populations [96, 100–103]. Hepatitis [96, 104], encephalitis [97], pneumonia [94, 96], rash [105], hemophagocytic lymphohistiocytosis with thrombotic microangiopathy [98], and multi-organ system failure [106] have also been reported.

There is evidence to suggest that B19 may play a role in chronic allograft injury. Numerous studies have reported on the association of allograft dysfunction with B19 infection, documented by detecting the presence of the viral genome in graft tissue [85, 100, 107]. In a study of 69 kidney transplant recipients with allograft dysfunction, B19 DNA was found in nearly two-thirds (35/57) of baseline biopsies, and intrarenal persistence of B19 DNA was a risk factor for the development of acute rejection [107]. B19 DNA was detected on endomyocardial biopsy in 35 of 99 consecutive pediatric cardiac transplant recipients, on 14% of 700 biopsies performed [100]. In this series, B19 was the most common viral genome amplified, more common than cytomegalovirus, Epstein-Barr virus, adenovirus, and enterovirus. While the presence of B19 DNA in the myocardium was not associated with cellular rejection, patients with chronic infection had significantly increased risk for early development of advanced transplant coronary artery disease (TCAD), the leading long-term cause of death in pediatric heart transplant recipients. It has been speculated that because virus is detected in endothelial cells of the vasculature [108], rather than in cardiomyocytes, that B19 may be involved in the endothelial cell dysfunction associated with TCAD.

Incidence of B19 Infection After SOT and HCT

The incidence of posttransplant B19 infection ranges widely in the literature and is generally poorly characterized. The variability is due in part to screening parameters (symptomatic vs. universal screening, serial vs. episodic screening), along with heterogeneity of host immune status and diagnostic test performance characteristics.

In a retrospective study of 137 SOT and 75 HCT recipients, the incidence of infection was 1.4% (3/212), with only 1 patient (<1%), a liver transplant recipient, presenting with clinically overt disease as manifested by anemia [109]. On molecular surveillance throughout the first year posttransplant in a mixed group with 47 transplant recipients (32 SOT and 15 allogeneic HCT recipients), none were found to be positive for B19 by PCR testing of serum [96]. Thus, serial screening for B19 by PCR in all-comers posttransplant is low yield. Risk factors for B19 infection and disease after transplant are not well described.

Diagnostics

Diagnosis of B19 infection typically rests on detection of viral DNA in clinical samples coupled with histopathologic assessment of bone marrow if cytopenias are present and/or serologic testing for B19-specific IgM and IgG. B19 is not easily cultured in vitro, and therefore culture-based methods are not routinely used to diagnose B19 infection. Classification of B19 disease entails diagnosis of infection, along with anemia and/or organ-specific findings.

The diagnostic test of choice depends on host immune status. In immunocompetent individuals, serology is the preferred methodology, with detection of B19-specific IgM consistent with acute or recent infection and IgG with previous infection. In a large study of B19 infection in transplant recipients, however, 29% had negative IgM at disease onset [96].

Given that serology is often unreliable in the immunosuppressed host [59], PCR testing to detect B19 DNA, or nucleic acid amplification testing (NAAT), is the recommended diagnostic approach. PCR testing is routinely performed on serum, plasma, and bone marrow [96, 110], with reports describing B19 DNA detection in various other body fluids [94, 106, 111, 112] and tissue specimens [94, 103, 107]. PCR-based B19 assays can provide a quantitative assessment of viral load in addition to a simple qualitative result. Although there is some evidence that higher viral loads are more likely to be associated with symptomatic infection in transplant recipients [113], it has yet to be determined what the clinically significant level of B19 DNA is. Given the lack of specificity for active or acute disease, PCR-based testing requires careful clinical interpretation. The value of following PCR to monitor response to treatment is unclear, noting that viremia can persist for months despite appropriate clinical response [114].

Bone marrow examination may reveal giant, multinucleated erythroblasts and pronormoblasts, with near-complete absence of late normoblasts [115]. Confirmation of B19 is provided by PCR testing for B19 DNA and in situ hybridization or immunohistochemical staining for B19.

Treatment

There are no antiviral drugs available for the treatment of B19 infection. As infection is chiefly self-limited in immunocompetent individuals, care is supportive. The cornerstone of therapy for symptomatic B19 infection in transplant recipients and other immunosuppressed hosts is intravenous immunoglobulin, based largely on the observation that specific antibodies neutralize the activity of virus in vitro [116]. Since the first description of the use of immune globulin for treatment of B19-associated red cell aplasia [58], there have been numerous reports on the application of such therapy in transplant recipients and other immunocompromised hosts [96, 99, 117–119]. Moreover, the observation that B19 disease is not seen in cohorts of HCT recipients who are receiving prophylactic immune globulin for other reasons is supportive of the utility of this therapy [120].

The optimal dosing regimen and duration of therapy with immune globulin are not well established. Based largely on expert opinion and accepted standard practice, 400 mg/kg/day of intravenous immune globulin for 5 days is the usual approach [99, 110]. Following treatment with immune globulin, relapse of infection, defined by the reappearance of signs and symptoms of infection after completion of treatment, was observed in 27.6% of SOT and 9.5% of HCT recipients in one study [96]. Interestingly, the rate of relapse did not differ significantly among patients according to the total dose of immune globulin (when stratified by >2 g/kg or <2 g/kg) [96]. Relapses can be treated with a second course of immune globulin [110]. However, it should be noted that immune globulin therapy was associated with nephrotoxicity in 11.6% of SOT recipients [96], and therefore this intervention should be undertaken with care, balancing the risk of treatment with the potential benefit to be derived.

While immune globulin is the accepted approach to B19 disease in transplant recipients, there are reports of patients who have cleared infection solely with reduction in immunosuppression [96]. Therefore, reduction of immunosuppression, as an adjunct to immune globulin therapy, should be considered at the time of diagnosis. The key role of host immune response in clearing infection is perhaps best exemplified by reports of HIV-positive patients with B19-associated chronic red cell aplasia who have had resolution of anemia following initiation of antiretroviral therapy alone [121–123].

Prevention

Vaccine Development

The ability of the capsid proteins VP1 and VP2 to elicit protective antibody responses during natural infection makes them natural proteins to include in vaccine development. A phase I study evaluated a recombinant B19 vaccine consisting of ~25% VP1 and ~75% VP2 conjugated to a surfactant-stabilized emulsion conjugate (MF59C.1) given to B19-seronegative adults at 0, 1, and 6 months [61]. Subjects received either 2.5 or 25 μg of vaccine, and all subjects in both groups developed virus-neutralizing antibodies that persisted for at least 6 months after the third dose, although titers were higher in the 25 μg group. A third trial comparing the safety and immunogenicity of three doses of a 25 μg dose of B19 recombinant capsid to 2.5 and 25 μg doses of the recombinant capsid plus MF59C.1 and saline placebo was then performed in healthy adults [124]. The study was halted before any subject could receive the third scheduled dose due to the occurrence of three unexplained cutaneous events. After two doses, neutralizing antibodies developed in 11.1%, 37.5%, and 42.9% of persons who received 2.5 μg + adjuvant, 25 μg + adjuvant, and 25 μg without adjuvant, respectively. Ultimately, it was decided by the Safety Monitoring Committee and the Food and Drug Administration that the potential benefits of the vaccine to those affected most severely by B19 infection would outweigh the adverse events encountered in the study, and therefore the study could be resumed [124]. By the time this decision was reached, re-enrollment of a new group of volunteers and preparation of new batches of vaccine and adjuvant were required [124]. Thus, efforts to develop and test a safe and effective B19 vaccine continue.

Hospital Infection Control

B19 is most commonly transmitted by the respiratory route, through close person-to-person contact, fomites, and respiratory secretions or saliva [41]. Contagion coincides with viremia, and so immunocompetent individuals are infectious before, but typically not after, the onset of B19-associated rash or arthritis. B19-viremic patients with TAC or red cell aplasia represent a potential risk for transmission in the healthcare setting, with reports of nosocomial transmission and infection among hospital staff associated with contact with TAC patients [125–127]. To prevent healthcare-associated infection, droplet and standard precautions should be implemented for patients with TAC and for immunosuppressed hosts with chronic infection [128].

Conclusions

B19 infection remains a relatively rare but potentially serious infection following SOT or HCT. Suspicion for B19 infection should be heightened in transplant recipients presenting with unexplained anemia, particularly red cell aplasia, with or without other cytopenias. Diagnosis depends primarily on detection of B19 DNA by PCR in serum and/or tissue, or the finding of characteristic bone marrow changes by histopathology, in the appropriate clinical setting. Treatment is largely supportive, although intravenous immune globulin may be beneficial in severe cases. Continued effort may lead to the development of a safe and effective vaccine for populations at risk for severe sequelae of B19 infection.

References

1. Berns K, Parrish CR. Parvoviridae. In: Knipe DM, Howley PM, editors. Fields virology. 5th ed. Philadelphia: Lippincott Williams & Wilkins; 2007. p. 2437–77.
2. Candotti D, Etiz N, Parsyan A, Allain JP. Identification and characterization of persistent human erythrovirus infection in blood donor samples. J Virol. 2004;78(22):12169–78.
3. Hokynar K, Soderlund-Venermo M, Pesonen M, Ranki A, Kiviluoto O, Partio EK, et al. A new parvovirus genotype persistent in human skin. Virology. 2002;302(2):224–8.
4. Nguyen QT, Wong S, Heegaard ED, Brown KE. Identification and characterization of a second novel human erythrovirus variant, A6. Virology. 2002;301(2):374–80.
5. Servant A, Laperche S, Lallemand F, Marinho V, De Saint Maur G, Meritet JF, et al. Genetic diversity within human erythroviruses: identification of three genotypes. J Virol. 2002;76(18):9124–34.
6. Gallinella G, Venturoli S, Manaresi E, Musiani M, Zerbini M. B19 virus genome diversity: epidemiological and clinical correlations. J Clin Virol. 2003;28(1):1–13.
7. Cossart YE, Field AM, Cant B, Widdows D. Parvovirus-like particles in human sera. Lancet. 1975;1(7898):72–3.
8. Pattison JR, Jones SE, Hodgson J, Davis LR, White JM, Stroud CE, et al. Parvovirus infections and hypoplastic crisis in sickle-cell anaemia. Lancet. 1981;1(8221):664–5.
9. Serjeant GR, Topley JM, Mason K, Serjeant BE, Pattison JR, Jones SE, et al. Outbreak of aplastic crises in sickle cell anaemia associated with parvovirus-like agent. Lancet. 1981;2(8247):595–7.
10. Neild G, Anderson M, Hawes S, Colvin BT. Parvovirus infection after renal transplant. Lancet. 1986;2(8517):1226–7.
11. Ozawa K, Kurtzman G, Young N. Replication of the B19 parvovirus in human bone marrow cell cultures. Science. 1986;233(4766):883–6.
12. Blundell MC, Beard C, Astell CR. In vitro identification of a B19 parvovirus promoter. Virology. 1987;157(2):534–8.
13. Ozawa K, Ayub J, Hao YS, Kurtzman G, Shimada T, Young N. Novel transcription map for the B19 (human) pathogenic parvovirus. J Virol. 1987;61(8):2395–406.
14. Cotmore SF, McKie VC, Anderson LJ, Astell CR, Tattersall P. Identification of the major structural and nonstructural proteins encoded by human parvovirus B19 and mapping of their genes by procaryotic expression of isolated genomic fragments. J Virol. 1986;60(2):548–57.
15. Ozawa K, Young N. Characterization of capsid and noncapsid proteins of B19 parvovirus propagated in human erythroid bone marrow cell cultures. J Virol. 1987;61(8):2627–30.
16. St Amand J, Beard C, Humphries K, Astell CR. Analysis of splice junctions and in vitro and in vivo translation potential of the small, abundant B19 parvovirus RNAs. Virology. 1991;183(1):133–42.
17. Brown KE, Young NS, Liu JM. Molecular, cellular and clinical aspects of parvovirus B19 infection. Crit Rev Oncol Hematol. 1994;16(1):1–31.
18. Doerig C, Hirt B, Antonietti JP, Beard P. Nonstructural protein of parvoviruses B19 and minute virus of mice controls transcription. J Virol. 1990;64(1):387–96.
19. Raab U, Beckenlehner K, Lowin T, Niller HH, Doyle S, Modrow S. NS1 protein of parvovirus B19 interacts directly with DNA sequences of the p6 promoter and with the cellular transcription factors Sp1/Sp3. Virology. 2002;293(1):86–93.
20. Momoeda M, Wong S, Kawase M, Young NS, Kajigaya S. A putative nucleoside triphosphate-binding domain in the nonstructural protein of B19 parvovirus is required for cytotoxicity. J Virol. 1994;68(12):8443–6.
21. Moffatt S, Yaegashi N, Tada K, Tanaka N, Sugamura K. Human parvovirus B19 nonstructural (NS1) protein induces apoptosis in erythroid lineage cells. J Virol. 1998;72(4):3018–28.
22. Sol N, Le Junter J, Vassias I, Freyssinier JM, Thomas A, Prigent AF, et al. Possible interactions between the NS-1 protein and tumor necrosis factor alpha pathways in erythroid cell apoptosis induced by human parvovirus B19. J Virol. 1999;73(10):8762–70.
23. Morita E, Nakashima A, Asao H, Sato H, Sugamura K. Human parvovirus B19 nonstructural protein (NS1) induces cell cycle arrest at G(1) phase. J Virol. 2003;77(5):2915–21.
24. Morita E, Tada K, Chisaka H, Asao H, Sato H, Yaegashi N, et al. Human parvovirus B19 induces cell cycle arrest at G(2) phase with accumulation of mitotic cyclins. J Virol. 2001;75(16):7555–63.
25. Wan Z, Zhi N, Wong S, Keyvanfar K, Liu D, Raghavachari N, et al. Human parvovirus B19 causes cell cycle arrest of human erythroid progenitors via deregulation of the E2F family of transcription factors. J Clin Invest. 2010;120(10):3530–44.
26. Brown KE, Anderson SM, Young NS. Erythrocyte P antigen: cellular receptor for B19 parvovirus. Science. 1993;262(5130):114–7.
27. Kawase M, Momoeda M, Young NS, Kajigaya S. Most of the VP1 unique region of B19 parvovirus is on the capsid surface. Virology. 1995;211(2):359–66.
28. Rosenfeld SJ, Yoshimoto K, Kajigaya S, Anderson S, Young NS, Field A, et al. Unique region of the minor capsid protein of human parvovirus B19 is exposed on the virion surface. J Clin Invest. 1992;89(6):2023–9.
29. Saikawa T, Anderson S, Momoeda M, Kajigaya S, Young NS. Neutralizing linear epitopes of B19 parvovirus cluster in the VP1 unique and VP1-VP2 junction regions. J Virol. 1993;67(6):3004–9.
30. Dorsch S, Liebisch G, Kaufmann B, von Landenberg P, Hoffmann JH, Drobnik W, et al. The VP1 unique region of parvovirus B19 and its constituent phospholipase A2-like activity. J Virol. 2002;76(4):2014–8.
31. Filippone C, Zhi N, Wong S, Lu J, Kajigaya S, Gallinella G, et al. VP1u phospholipase activity is critical for infectivity of full-length parvovirus B19 genomic clones. Virology. 2008;374(2):444–52.
32. Luo W, Astell CR. A novel protein encoded by small RNAs of parvovirus B19. Virology. 1993;195(2):448–55.
33. St Amand J, Astell CR. Identification and characterization of a family of 11-kDa proteins encoded by the human parvovirus B19. Virology. 1993;192(1):121–31.
34. Chen AY, Zhang EY, Guan W, Cheng F, Kleiboeker S, Yankee TM, et al. The small 11 kDa nonstructural protein of human parvovirus B19 plays a key role in inducing apoptosis during B19 virus infection of primary erythroid progenitor cells. Blood. 2010;115(5):1070–80.
35. Zhi N, Mills IP, Lu J, Wong S, Filippone C, Brown KE. Molecular and functional analyses of a human parvovirus B19 infectious clone demonstrates essential roles for NS1, VP1, and the 11-kilodalton protein in virus replication and infectivity. J Virol. 2006;80(12):5941–50.
36. Ozawa K, Kurtzman G, Young N. Productive infection by B19 parvovirus of human erythroid bone marrow cells in vitro. Blood. 1987;70(2):384–91.
37. Leruez M, Pallier C, Vassias I, Elouet JF, Romeo P, Morinet F. Differential transcription, without replication, of non-structural and structural genes of human parvovirus B19 in the UT7/EPO cell as demonstrated by in situ hybridization. J Gen Virol. 1994;75(Pt 6):1475–8.
38. Miyagawa E, Yoshida T, Takahashi H, Yamaguchi K, Nagano T, Kiriyama Y, et al. Infection of the erythroid cell line, KU812Ep6 with human parvovirus B19 and its application to titration of B19 infectivity. J Virol Methods. 1999;83(1–2):45–54.
39. Filippone C, Franssila R, Kumar A, Saikko L, Kovanen PE, Soderlund-Venermo M, et al. Erythroid progenitor cells expanded from peripheral blood without mobilization or preselection: molecular characteristics and functional competence. PLoS One. 2010;5(3):e9496.

40. Wong S, Zhi N, Filippone C, Keyvanfar K, Kajigaya S, Brown KE, et al. Ex vivo-generated CD36+ erythroid progenitors are highly permissive to human parvovirus B19 replication. J Virol. 2008;82(5):2470–6.
41. Anderson MJ, Higgins PG, Davis LR, Willman JS, Jones SE, Kidd IM, et al. Experimental parvoviral infection in humans. J Infect Dis. 1985;152(2):257–65.
42. Lee TH, Kleinman SH, Wen L, Montalvo L, Todd DS, Wright DJ, et al. Distribution of parvovirus B19 DNA in blood compartments and persistence of virus in blood donors. Transfusion. 2011;51(9):1896–908.
43. Chipman PR, Agbandje-McKenna M, Kajigaya S, Brown KE, Young NS, Baker TS, et al. Cryo-electron microscopy studies of empty capsids of human parvovirus B19 complexed with its cellular receptor. Proc Natl Acad Sci U S A. 1996;93(15):7502–6.
44. Weigel-Kelley KA, Yoder MC, Srivastava A. Recombinant human parvovirus B19 vectors: erythrocyte P antigen is necessary but not sufficient for successful transduction of human hematopoietic cells. J Virol. 2001;75(9):4110–6.
45. Weigel-Kelley KA, Yoder MC, Srivastava A. Alpha5beta1 integrin as a cellular coreceptor for human parvovirus B19: requirement of functional activation of beta1 integrin for viral entry. Blood. 2003;102(12):3927–33.
46. Jordan JA, DeLoia JA. Globoside expression within the human placenta. Placenta. 1999;20(1):103–8.
47. Morey AL, Ferguson DJ, Fleming KA. Ultrastructural features of fetal erythroid precursors infected with parvovirus B19 in vitro: evidence of cell death by apoptosis. J Pathol. 1993;169(2):213–20.
48. Brown KE, Young NS. Parvovirus B19 in human disease. Annu Rev Med. 1997;48:59–67.
49. Manaresi E, Zuffi E, Gallinella G, Gentilomi G, Zerbini M, Musiani M. Differential IgM response to conformational and linear epitopes of parvovirus B19 VP1 and VP2 structural proteins. J Med Virol. 2001;64(1):67–73.
50. Palmer P, Pallier C, Leruez-Ville M, Deplanche M, Morinet F. Antibody response to human parvovirus B19 in patients with primary infection by immunoblot assay with recombinant proteins. Clin Diagn Lab Immunol. 1996;3(2):236–8.
51. Kaikkonen L, Lankinen H, Harjunpaa I, Hokynar K, Soderlund-Venermo M, Oker-Blom C, et al. Acute-phase-specific heptapeptide epitope for diagnosis of parvovirus B19 infection. J Clin Microbiol. 1999;37(12):3952–6.
52. Kerr S, O'Keeffe G, Kilty C, Doyle S. Undenatured parvovirus B19 antigens are essential for the accurate detection of parvovirus B19 IgG. J Med Virol. 1999;57(2):179–85.
53. Manaresi E, Gallinella G, Zerbini M, Venturoli S, Gentilomi G, Musiani M. IgG immune response to B19 parvovirus VP1 and VP2 linear epitopes by immunoblot assay. J Med Virol. 1999;57(2):174–8.
54. Soderlund M, Brown CS, Spaan WJ, Hedman L, Hedman K. Epitope type-specific IgG responses to capsid proteins VP1 and VP2 of human parvovirus B19. J Infect Dis. 1995;172(6):1431–6.
55. Corcoran A, Doyle S. Advances in the biology, diagnosis and host-pathogen interactions of parvovirus B19. J Med Microbiol. 2004;53(Pt 6):459–75.
56. Young NS, Brown KE. Parvovirus B19. N Engl J Med. 2004;350(6):586–97.
57. Koduri PR, Kumapley R, Valladares J, Teter C. Chronic pure red cell aplasia caused by parvovirus B19 in AIDS: use of intravenous immunoglobulin--a report of eight patients. Am J Hematol. 1999;61(1):16–20.
58. Kurtzman G, Frickhofen N, Kimball J, Jenkins DW, Nienhuis AW, Young NS. Pure red-cell aplasia of 10 years' duration due to persistent parvovirus B19 infection and its cure with immunoglobulin therapy. N Engl J Med. 1989;321(8):519–23.
59. Kurtzman GJ, Cohen BJ, Field AM, Oseas R, Blaese RM, Young NS. Immune response to B19 parvovirus and an antibody defect in persistent viral infection. J Clin Invest. 1989;84(4):1114–23.
60. Schwarz TF, Roggendorf M, Hottentrager B, Modrow S, Deinhardt F, Middeldorp J. Immunoglobulins in the prophylaxis of parvovirus B19 infection. J Infect Dis. 1990;162(5):1214.
61. Ballou WR, Reed JL, Noble W, Young NS, Koenig S. Safety and immunogenicity of a recombinant parvovirus B19 vaccine formulated with MF59C.1. J Infect Dis. 2003;187(4):675–8.
62. Heegaard ED, Rasksen CJ, Christensen J. Detection of parvovirus B19 NS1-specific antibodies by ELISA and western blotting employing recombinant NS1 protein as antigen. J Med Virol. 2002;67(3):375–83.
63. Mitchell LA, Leong R, Rosenke KA. Lymphocyte recognition of human parvovirus B19 non-structural (NS1) protein: associations with occurrence of acute and chronic arthropathy? J Med Microbiol. 2001;50(7):627–35.
64. Tolfvenstam T, Lundqvist A, Levi M, Wahren B, Broliden K. Mapping of B-cell epitopes on human parvovirus B19 non-structural and structural proteins. Vaccine. 2000;19(7–8):758–63.
65. von Poblotzki A, Gigler A, Lang B, Wolf H, Modrow S. Antibodies to parvovirus B19 NS-1 protein in infected individuals. J Gen Virol. 1995;76(Pt 3):519–27.
66. Corcoran A, Doyle S, Waldron D, Nicholson A, Mahon BP. Impaired gamma interferon responses against parvovirus B19 by recently infected children. J Virol. 2000;74(21):9903–10.
67. Isa A, Kasprowicz V, Norbeck O, Loughry A, Jeffery K, Broliden K, et al. Prolonged activation of virus-specific CD8+T cells after acute B19 infection. PLoS Med. 2005;2(12):e343.
68. Kasprowicz V, Isa A, Tolfvenstam T, Jeffery K, Bowness P, Klenerman P. Tracking of peptide-specific CD4+ T-cell responses after an acute resolving viral infection: a study of parvovirus B19. J Virol. 2006;80(22):11209–17.
69. Norbeck O, Isa A, Pohlmann C, Broliden K, Kasprowicz V, Bowness P, et al. Sustained CD8+ T-cell responses induced after acute parvovirus B19 infection in humans. J Virol. 2005;79(18):12117–21.
70. Tolfvenstam T, Oxenius A, Price DA, Shacklett BL, Spiegel HM, Hedman K, et al. Direct ex vivo measurement of CD8(+) T-lymphocyte responses to human parvovirus B19. J Virol. 2001;75(1):540–3.
71. von Poblotzki A, Gerdes C, Reischl U, Wolf H, Modrow S. Lymphoproliferative responses after infection with human parvovirus B19. J Virol. 1996;70(10):7327–30.
72. Cohen BJ, Buckley MM. The prevalence of antibody to human parvovirus B19 in England and Wales. J Med Microbiol. 1988;25(2):151–3.
73. Koch WC, Adler SP. Human parvovirus B19 infections in women of childbearing age and within families. Pediatr Infect Dis J. 1989;8(2):83–7.
74. Chorba T, Coccia P, Holman RC, Tattersall P, Anderson LJ, Sudman J, et al. The role of parvovirus B19 in aplastic crisis and erythema infectiosum (fifth disease). J Infect Dis. 1986;154(3):383–93.
75. Plummer FA, Hammond GW, Forward K, Sekla L, Thompson LM, Jones SE, et al. An erythema infectiosum-like illness caused by human parvovirus infection. N Engl J Med. 1985;313(2):74–9.
76. Dowell SF, Torok TJ, Thorp JA, Hedrick J, Erdman DD, Zaki SR, et al. Parvovirus B19 infection in hospital workers: community or hospital acquisition? J Infect Dis. 1995;172(4):1076–9.
77. Gillespie SM, Cartter ML, Asch S, Rokos JB, Gary GW, Tsou CJ, et al. Occupational risk of human parvovirus B19 infection for school and day-care personnel during an outbreak of erythema infectiosum. JAMA. 1990;263(15):2061–5.
78. Azzi A, Morfini M, Mannucci PM. The transfusion-associated transmission of parvovirus B19. Transfus Med Rev. 1999;13(3):194–204.

79. Yu MY, Alter HJ, Virata-Theimer ML, Geng Y, Ma L, Schechterly CA, et al. Parvovirus B19 infection transmitted by transfusion of red blood cells confirmed by molecular analysis of linked donor and recipient samples. Transfusion. 2010;50(8):1712–21.
80. Aubin JT, Defer C, Vidaud M, Maniez Montreuil M, Flan B. Large-scale screening for human parvovirus B19 DNA by PCR: application to the quality control of plasma for fractionation. Vox Sang. 2000;78(1):7–12.
81. Jordan J, Tiangco B, Kiss J, Koch W. Human parvovirus B19: prevalence of viral DNA in volunteer blood donors and clinical outcomes of transfusion recipients. Vox Sang. 1998;75(2):97–102.
82. Kleinman SH, Glynn SA, Lee TH, Tobler L, Montalvo L, Todd D, et al. Prevalence and quantitation of parvovirus B19 DNA levels in blood donors with a sensitive polymerase chain reaction screening assay. Transfusion. 2007;47(10):1756–64.
83. Parsyan A, Candotti D. Human erythrovirus B19 and blood transfusion - an update. Transfus Med. 2007;17(4):263–78.
84. Brown KE, Young NS, Alving BM, Barbosa LH. Parvovirus B19: implications for transfusion medicine. Summary of a workshop. Transfusion. 2001;41(1):130–5.
85. Yango A Jr, Morrissey P, Gohh R, Wahbeh A. Donor-transmitted parvovirus infection in a kidney transplant recipient presenting as pancytopenia and allograft dysfunction. Transpl Infect Dis. 2002;4(3):163–6.
86. Zolnourian ZR, Curran MD, Rima BK, Coyle PV, O'Neill HJ, Middleton D. Parvovirus B19 in kidney transplant patients. Transplantation. 2000;69(10):2198–202.
87. Hayakawa H, Tara M, Niina K, Osame M. A clinical study of adult human parvovirus B19 infection. Intern Med. 2002;41(4):295–9.
88. Woolf AD, Campion GV, Chishick A, Wise S, Cohen BJ, Klouda PT, et al. Clinical manifestations of human parvovirus B19 in adults. Arch Intern Med. 1989;149(5):1153–6.
89. Krygier DS, Steinbrecher UP, Petric M, Erb SR, Chung SW, Scudamore CH, et al. Parvovirus B19 induced hepatic failure in an adult requiring liver transplantation. World J Gastroenterol. 2009;15(32):4067–9.
90. Anderson MJ, Jones SE, Fisher-Hoch SP, Lewis E, Hall SM, Bartlett CL, et al. Human parvovirus, the cause of erythema infectiosum (fifth disease)? Lancet. 1983;1(8338):1378.
91. Naides SJ. Rheumatic manifestations of parvovirus B19 infection. Rheum Dis Clin N Am. 1998;24(2):375–401.
92. Scroggie DA, Carpenter MT, Cooper RI, Higgs JB. Parvovirus arthropathy outbreak in southwestern United States. J Rheumatol. 2000;27(10):2444–8.
93. Anderson LJ, Hurwitz ES. Human parvovirus B19 and pregnancy. Clin Perinatol. 1988;15(2):273–86.
94. Beske F, Modrow S, Sorensen J, Schmidt H, Kriener S, Allwinn R, et al. Parvovirus B19 pneumonia in a child undergoing allogeneic hematopoietic stem cell transplantation. Bone Marrow Transplant. 2007;40(1):89–91.
95. Cavallo R, Merlino C, Re D, Bollero C, Bergallo M, Lembo D, et al. B19 virus infection in renal transplant recipients. J Clin Virol. 2003;26(3):361–8.
96. Eid AJ, Brown RA, Patel R, Razonable RR. Parvovirus B19 infection after transplantation: a review of 98 cases. Clin Infect Dis. 2006;43(1):40–8.
97. Laurenz M, Winkelmann B, Roigas J, Zimmering M, Querfeld U, Muller D. Severe parvovirus B19 encephalitis after renal transplantation. Pediatr Transplant. 2006;10(8):978–81.
98. Ardalan MR, Shoja MM, Tubbs RS, Esmaili H, Keyvani H. Postrenal transplant hemophagocytic lymphohistiocytosis and thrombotic microangiopathy associated with parvovirus b19 infection. Am J Transplant. 2008;8(6):1340–4.
99. Egbuna O, Zand MS, Arbini A, Menegus M, Taylor J. A cluster of parvovirus B19 infections in renal transplant recipients: a prospective case series and review of the literature. Am J Transplant. 2006;6(1):225–31.
100. Breinholt JP, Moulik M, Dreyer WJ, Denfield SW, Kim JJ, Jefferies JL, et al. Viral epidemiologic shift in inflammatory heart disease: the increasing involvement of parvovirus B19 in the myocardium of pediatric cardiac transplant patients. J Heart Lung Transplant. 2010;29(7):739–46.
101. Donoso Mantke O, Meyer R, Prosch S, Nitsche A, Leitmeyer K, Kallies R, et al. High prevalence of cardiotropic viruses in myocardial tissue from explanted hearts of heart transplant recipients and heart donors: a 3-year retrospective study from a German patients' pool. J Heart Lung Transplant. 2005;24(10):1632–8.
102. Kuhl U, Pauschinger M, Seeberg B, Lassner D, Noutsias M, Poller W, et al. Viral persistence in the myocardium is associated with progressive cardiac dysfunction. Circulation. 2005;112(13):1965–70.
103. Jonetzko P, Graziadei I, Nachbaur K, Vogel W, Pankuweit S, Zwick R, et al. Fatal course of parvovirus B19-associated myocarditis in a female liver transplant recipient. Liver Transpl. 2005;11(4):463–6.
104. Lee PC, Hung CJ, Lei HY, Chang TT, Wang JR, Jan MS. Parvovirus B19-related acute hepatitis in an immunosuppressed kidney transplant. Nephrol Dial Transplant. 2000;15(9):1486–8.
105. Muetherig A, Christopeit M, Muller LP, Grothe W, Weber T, Theurich S, et al. Human parvovirus B19 infection with GvHD-like erythema in two allogeneic stem cell transplant recipients. Bone Marrow Transplant. 2007;39(5):315–6.
106. Klumpen HJ, Petersen EJ, Verdonck LF. Severe multiorgan failure after parvovirus B19 infection in an allogeneic stem cell transplant recipient. Bone Marrow Transplant. 2004;34(5):469–70.
107. Barzon L, Murer L, Pacenti M, Biasolo MA, Della Vella M, Benetti E, et al. Investigation of intrarenal viral infections in kidney transplant recipients unveils an association between parvovirus B19 and chronic allograft injury. J Infect Dis. 2009;199(3):372–80.
108. Bultmann BD, Klingel K, Sotlar K, Bock CT, Baba HA, Sauter M, et al. Fatal parvovirus B19-associated myocarditis clinically mimicking ischemic heart disease: an endothelial cell-mediated disease. Hum Pathol. 2003;34(1):92–5.
109. Gallinella G, Manaresi E, Venturoli S, Grazi GL, Musiani M, Zerbini M. Occurrence and clinical role of active parvovirus B19 infection in transplant recipients. Eur J Clin Microbiol Infect Dis. 1999;18(11):811–3.
110. Eid AJ, Posfay-Barbe KM. Parvovirus B19 in solid organ transplant recipients. Am J Transplant. 2009;9(Suppl 4):S147–50.
111. Douvoyiannis M, Litman N, Goldman DL. Neurologic manifestations associated with parvovirus B19 infection. Clin Infect Dis. 2009;48(12):1713–23.
112. Koch WC, Adler SP. Detection of human parvovirus B19 DNA by using the polymerase chain reaction. J Clin Microbiol. 1990;28(1):65–9.
113. Park JB, Kim DJ, Woo SY, Choi GS, Chun JM, Jung GO, et al. Clinical implications of quantitative real time-polymerase chain reaction of parvovirus B19 in kidney transplant recipients - a prospective study. Transpl Int. 2009;22(4):455–62.
114. Kumar J, Shaver MJ, Abul-Ezz S. Long-term remission of recurrent parvovirus-B associated anemia in a renal transplant recipient induced by treatment with immunoglobulin and positive seroconversion. Transpl Infect Dis. 2005;7(1):30–3.
115. Florea AV, Ionescu DN, Melhem MF. Parvovirus B19 infection in the immunocompromised host. Arch Pathol Lab Med. 2007;131(5):799–804.
116. Mortimer PP, Humphries RK, Moore JG, Purcell RH, Young NS. A human parvovirus-like virus inhibits haematopoietic colony formation in vitro. Nature. 1983;302(5907):426–9.
117. Corbett TJ, Saw H, Popat U, MacMahon E, Cohen BJ, Knowles WA, et al. Successful treatment of parvovirus B19 infection and red cell aplasia occurring after an allogeneic bone marrow transplant. Bone Marrow Transplant. 1995;16(5):711–3.
118. Frickhofen N, Abkowitz JL, Safford M, Berry JM, Antunez-de-Mayolo J, Astrow A, et al. Persistent B19 parvovirus infection in patients infected with human immunodeficiency virus type 1

(HIV-1): a treatable cause of anemia in AIDS. Ann Intern Med. 1990;113(12):926–33.
119. Moudgil A, Shidban H, Nast CC, Bagga A, Aswad S, Graham SL, et al. Parvovirus B19 infection-related complications in renal transplant recipients: treatment with intravenous immunoglobulin. Transplantation. 1997;64(12):1847–50.
120. Azzi A, Fanci R, Ciappi S, Zakrzewska K, Bosi A. Human parvovirus B19 infection in bone marrow transplantation patients. Am J Hematol. 1993;44(3):207–9.
121. Arribas JR, Pena JM, Echevarria JE. Parvovirus B19-related anemia in an HIV-infected patient: rapid control after production of neutralizing antibodies during highly active antiretroviral therapy. Ann Intern Med. 2000;132(12):1011.
122. Chen MY, Hung CC, Fang CT, Hsieh SM. Reconstituted immunity against persistent parvovirus B19 infection in a patient with acquired immunodeficiency syndrome after highly active antiretroviral therapy. Clin Infect Dis. 2001;32(9):1361–5.
123. Ware AJ, Moore T. Resolution of chronic parvovirus b19-induced anemia, by use of highly active antiretroviral therapy, in a patient with acquired immunodeficiency syndrome. Clin Infect Dis. 2001;32(7):E122–3.
124. Bernstein DI, El Sahly HM, Keitel WA, Wolff M, Simone G, Segawa C, et al. Safety and immunogenicity of a candidate parvovirus B19 vaccine. Vaccine. 2011;29(43):7357–63.
125. Bell LM, Naides SJ, Stoffman P, Hodinka RL, Plotkin SA. Human parvovirus B19 infection among hospital staff members after contact with infected patients. N Engl J Med. 1989;321(8):485–91.
126. Lui SL, Luk WK, Cheung CY, Chan TM, Lai KN, Peiris JS. Nosocomial outbreak of parvovirus B19 infection in a renal transplant unit. Transplantation. 2001;71(1):59–64.
127. Seng C, Watkins P, Morse D, Barrett SP, Zambon M, Andrews N, et al. Parvovirus B19 outbreak on an adult ward. Epidemiol Infect. 1994;113(2):345–53.
128. Siegel JD, Rhinehart E, Jackson M, Chiarello L. 2007 Guideline for isolation precautions: preventing transmission of infectious agents in health care settings. Am J Infect Control. 2007;35(10 Suppl 2):S65–164.

West Nile Virus in Immunocompromised Hosts

44

Dora Y. Ho, Joanna M. D. Schaenman, and Lindsey R. Baden

Abbreviations

AFP	Acute flaccid paralysis
CDC	Center for Disease Control and Prevention
CNS	Central nervous system
CSF	Cerebrospinal fluid
ELISA	Enzyme-linked immunosorbent assay
HSCT	Hematopoietic stem cell transplantation
IFN	Interferon
IVIG	Intravenous immunoglobulin
MAC-ELISA	IgM antibody capture enzyme-linked immunosorbent assay
NAAT	Nucleic acid amplification testing
PRNT	Plaque reduction neutralization test
SOT	Solid organ transplantation
TLR	Toll-like receptor
WNE	West Nile encephalitis
WNF	West Nile fever
WNND	West Nile virus neuroinvasive disease
WNV	West Nile virus

Introduction

West Nile virus (WNV) is an emerging pathogen endemic in Africa and Europe. Recent events demonstrate the speed with which a vector-borne pathogen, such as WNV, can disseminate when introduced into a susceptible, pathogen-naïve population, where competent reservoir and vectors are present. Since the arrival of WNV to the North American continent in 1999, it is estimated that 2–4 million people have been infected in the USA alone [1, 2]. It has special relevance to the immunocompromised host populations because of the possibility of WNV transmission through organ transplantation and the increased risk of neuroinvasive disease in immunocompromised patients. Here we present epidemiology, clinical manifestations, as well as avenues for diagnosis, treatment, and prevention of this viral pathogen, with emphasis on transplant recipients.

D. Y. Ho (✉)
Division of Infectious Diseases and Geographic Medicine, Stanford University School of Medicine, Stanford, CA, USA
e-mail: doraywho@stanford.edu

J. M. D. Schaenman
Division of Infectious Diseases, David Geffen School of Medicine at UCLA, Los Angeles, CA, USA
e-mail: jschaenman@mednet.ucla.edu

L. R. Baden
Division of Infectious Diseases, Brigham and Women's Hospital, Dana-Farber Cancer Institute, Harvard Medical School, Boston, MA, USA
e-mail: lbaden@partners.org

Virus and Reservoir

WNV is a member of genus *Flavivirus* in the family *Flaviviridae*. The genus *Flavivirus* has >70 members and includes other important human pathogens such as dengue, yellow fever, Zika, St. Louis encephalitis, and Japanese encephalitis viruses. WNV is an enveloped, single-stranded, positive-sense RNA virus, of about 11 kilobase genome size. The single open reading frame is translated into a polyprotein, which is further cleaved into ten proteins by cellular and viral proteases. The three structural proteins include a capsid protein (C), an envelope protein (E), and a transmembrane protein (prM). The seven nonstructural proteins, i.e., NS1, NS2A, NS2B, NS3, NS4A, NS4B, and NS5, form the viral replication machinery and also modulate the host immune response [3, 4]. Natural transmission of WNV is mosquito-borne with the principal vectors being *Culex* spp., although at least 43 other mosquito species, including *Aedes* and *Anopheles*, have been found to harbor the virus [5–8]. Susceptible birds, especially corvids such as crows and jays, are principal vertebrate reservoirs, and humans appear to be incidental host. Many animal species, including humans, horses, squirrels, and even alligators, can become infected with WNV and present with clinical disease, but they do not develop sufficiently prolonged or high-level viremia to play

A. Safdar (ed.), *Principles and Practice of Transplant Infectious Diseases*, https://doi.org/10.1007/978-1-4939-9034-4_44

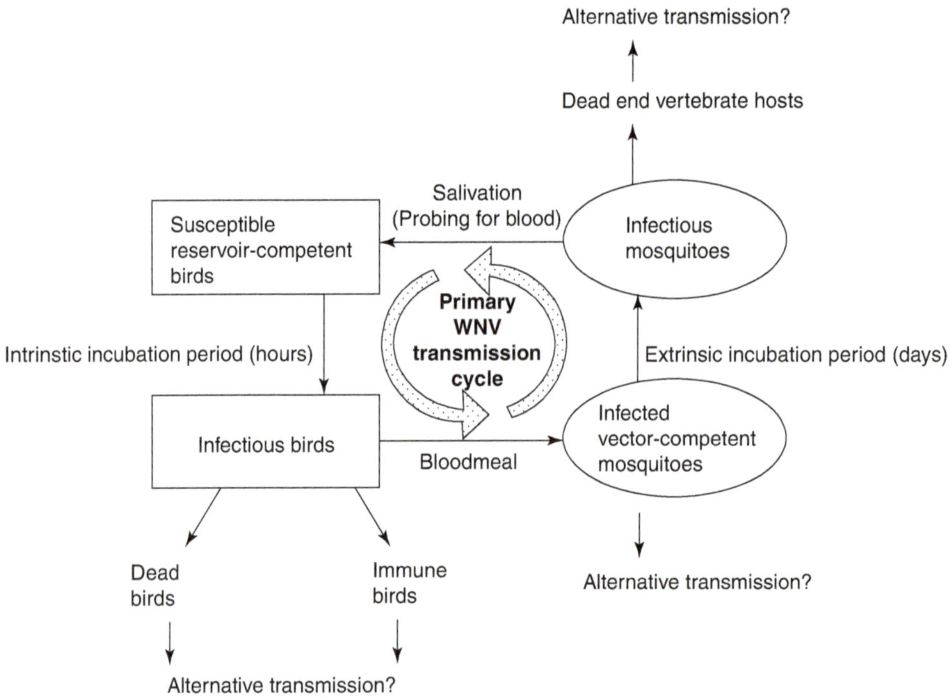

Fig. 44.1 The primary West Nile virus transmission cycle involves certain reservoir-competent birds that transmit virus to feeding mosquitoes during a brief period of elevated viremia that follows infection. Viremia is rapidly neutralized by development of antibodies. A portion of vector-competent mosquitoes that survive the extrinsic incubation period may transmit to susceptible birds to keep the cycle going. Alternative modes of transmission may exist at multiple points along the cycle. (Reprinted from Komar [7], © 2003; with permission from Elsevier)

a significant role in WNV amplification and transmission [7, 9–11] (Fig. 44.1).

Although WNV has a single serotype, it exhibits considerable genetic variation and a large variety of strains have been described worldwide. Based on their genetic differences, they are classified into at least eight lineages [12]. The two major lineages, 1 and 2, are responsible for outbreaks in humans and equines. Dramatic differences in the virulence and neuroinvasion properties have been observed between lineage 1 and lineage 2 strains [13]. Lineage 1 strains have been responsible for most human outbreaks since the 1950s. However, since the beginning of this century, lineage 2 strains have emerged to cause recent outbreaks in various European countries, including Greece (2013) and Italy (2014) [14, 15].

Epidemiology

WNV was first isolated in 1937 from a febrile patient in Uganda [6]. Prior to 1996, there were several documented epidemics in the Old World, but most cases were asymptomatic or mild, and severe neurological manifestations were rare. Since the mid-1990s, there was an increased frequency and scale of outbreaks in humans and horses, including large outbreaks in Romania (1996), Volgograd region of Russia (1999), Northeastern USA (1999), and Israel (2000) [6, 8, 16–19]. There was also worsened disease severity in humans, including neurological complications and death [20]. WNV entered the USA in August 1999 and was identified in an unusual cluster of cases of meningoencephalitis in New York City. Concurrent to these clinical cases were extensive mortality in crows as well as deaths of several exotic birds at a zoological park was noted in the same area. The initial epidemiologic and environmental investigations suggested an arboviral etiology [17], and sequence analyses of viral isolates from dead birds, mosquitoes, and two fatal human cases identified WNV as the causative agent [21, 22]. This outbreak represented the first time WNV was detected in the Western Hemisphere [17]. The WNV strain from the 1999 New York outbreak showed a close phylogenetic relationship to an isolate obtained from a goose in Israel in 1998 [21, 22]. Although the specifics of how WNV was introduced in the USA was not known, it is conceivable that infected mosquitoes or birds could have been carried to New York City on an incoming flight or ship [20]. Alternatively, a viremic person might have been the carrier.

Since the initial 1999 outbreak in New York, the virus has spread, like a slow wave, across the continental USA from East to West, likely representing movement between the mosquito and the presumed avian reservoir (Table 44.1) [20]. By 2006, WNV has spread to all 48 states of the US continent. A marked increase in the total number of cases was observed between 2002 and 2003 and was likely due to the request of Center for Disease Control and Prevention (CDC) to include West Nile Fever (WNF) cases as reportable to ArboNET (the national surveillance system for arboviral diseases in the USA) and wider availability of testing for suspected cases. From 1999 to December of 2017, more than 48,000 cases have been reported in the USA, including 22,999 cases of neuroinvasive disease and 2,163 deaths [23]. However, most WNV infections are

Table 44.1 1999–2017 West Nile virus human infections in the United States [23]

Year	Neuroinvasive cases	Non-neuroinvasive cases	Total cases	Total deaths
1999	59	3	62	7
2000	19	2	21	2
2001	64	2	66	10
2002	2946	1210	4156	284
2003[a]	2866	6996	9862	264
2004	1148	1391	2539	100
2005	1309	1691	3000	119
2006	1495	2774	4269	177
2007	1227	2403	3630	124
2008	689	667	1356	44
2009	386	334	720	32
2010	629	392	1021	57
2011	486	226	712	43
2012	2873	2801	5674	286
2013	1267	1202	2469	119
2014	1347	858	2205	97
2015	1455	720	2175	146
2016	1309	840	2149	106
2017	1425	672	2097	146
Cumulative	**22,999**	**25,184**	**48,183**	**2163**

[a]CDC requested WNV cases be reported to ArboNET in 2003, resulting in a change of case definition

Data adapted from CDC website https://www.cdc.gov/westnile/stats-maps/cummapsdata.html

asymptomatic and therefore, not reported. It is estimated that 2–4 million people in the USA have been infected by this virus, resulting in 0.4–1 million cases of viral illness [1]. Since its peak incidence of 1.02 cases/100,000 US population in 2003, the annual incidence rate up to 2011 was in a continued decline, with an incidence of 0.4/100,000 in 2004–2007, 0.2/100,000 in 2008, and down to 0.13/100,000 in 2009 [24]. However, after a period of low level activities from 2008 to 2011, a resurgence of WNV cases was noted in 2012, with a total of 5,674 human cases reported to the CDC, including 2,873 cases of neuroinvasive disease and 286 deaths. The fluctuation of WNV activities might be attributed to a number of factors including variation in population of vectors and susceptible vertebrate host, immunity or the lack of avian amplifying host, human behavior such as the use of insect repellents and protective clothing, community-level interventions, reporting practices, and environmental factors, such as warming temperature and rainfall [1, 25]. Importantly, the 2012 resurgence of WNV cases suggests that the USA can expect periodic epidemics of WNV infection and highlights the importance of continued research and preparedness for future outbreaks [26].

In the USA, about 85% of human infections occur in the late summer, peaking around August and September. This reflects the seasonal activity of its major vector *Culex* mosquitoes as well as the virus' amplification in the late spring and early summer in its avian hosts. In fact, the magnitude of birds dying from WNV in early summer often predicts the severity of subsequent human or equine disease in the area [7]. In warmer areas, transmission might be year-round. During an epidemic, the seroconversion rate in a human population is estimated at about 3–4% [19, 27].

Other than natural transmission through mosquito bites, WNV infections in human have also been acquired through transfusion of blood products [28, 29], breast-feeding [30], transplacental transmission [31], occupational exposure in laboratory workers [32], as well as infected solid organ allograft transplantation (SOT; see below). In 2002, 23 patients were confirmed to have acquired WNV infection through transfusion of blood products in the USA [33]. These cases led to the development and implementation of nucleic acid amplification testing (NAAT) of pooled or individual samples of blood products. Since then, transmission of WNV by transfusion has largely been prevented [34]. WNV transmission through tissue transplantation, e.g., cornea, is also theoretically possible as demonstrated in animal experiments [35, 36], although no human cases via this mechanism have been reported, thus far.

Pathogenesis and Immune Response

Much of our current knowledge on WNV pathogenesis and its host immune response has stemmed from experiments in animals [37]. After a mosquito bite, WNV first infects keratinocytes and Langerhans cells, which then migrate to regional lymph nodes [38]. Replication in these cells results in primary viremia and seeding of other visceral organs, such as the kidney and spleen. A second round of replication then ensues. The level of viremia appears to correlate with subsequent risk for central nervous system (CNS) disease, although the mechanisms by which WNV enters the CNS remain unclear. Several mechanisms have been proposed, including infection or passive transport through the endothelium or choroid plexus epithelial cells, infection of olfactory neurons and spread to the olfactory bulb, transport by infected immune cells trafficking to the CNS, as well as direct axonal retrograde transport from infected peripheral neurons [37–39]. A number of host proteins or cytokines, e.g., TNF-α, Drak2, ICAM-1, MIF, and MMP-9, have been implicated in altering blood-brain barrier permeability during WNV infection [3, 40] and might facilitate WNV entry into the CNS. However, the disruption of the blood-brain barrier may not be the primary mechanism of WNV invasion into the CNS. Instead, it is possibly a multistep process employing different mechanisms as the infection progresses [41].

Since most WNV human infections are asymptomatic and only about 1 in 150 develops CNS disease, it is thought that subclinical infection presumably reflects peripheral clearance of the virus by the immune response before neuroinvasion or before neuronal damage occurs. The innate immune system appears to be important for viral clearance [42]. For instance, type I interferons (IFNs) IFN-α and IFN-β inhibit WNV replication in vitro; IFN-α/β receptor-deficient mice infected with WNV showed uncontrolled viral replication, rapid dissemination to the CNS, as well as increased mortality [43]. Type II IFN (IFN-γ) can also prevent viral dissemination to the CNS; mice deficient in IFN-γ or its receptor had higher peripheral viral burden, earlier viral entry into CNS, and higher lethality [44].

The complement system also protects against WNV infection and limits viral infection by stimulating the adaptive immune response (reviewed in [45]). Complement activation augments antibody-mediated neutralization of viruses, including WNV [46]. Mice deficient in complement C3 or complement receptor 1 and 2 showed increased mortality after lethal WNV challenge [46]. Deficiencies in C1q, C4, factor B, or factor D also led to increased mortality in WNV-infected mice [47]. These observations suggest that many components of the complement activation pathways seem to orchestrate protection against WNV [47, 48]. The RIG-I-like receptors, Toll-like receptors especially TLR3 and TLR7, and Nod-like receptors have been implicated in modulating the innate immune response against WNV infection as well [49, 50]. γδ T cells and NK cells are also crucial components of the host innate immune system. However, while animal studies have demonstrated protective effects of γδ T cells against WNV infection, the role of NK cells remains controversial, with reports suggesting active suppression of the virus to no effect on viral replication at all [51]. Overall, the innate immune response plays a crucial role in orchestrating various arms of the immune system, including the humoral and cell-mediated immunities to control WNV replication and to limit the virus-induced pathology [37, 50].

For the adaptive immune response, WNV appears to be more susceptible to antibody-mediated than cell-mediated immunity [52, 53]. The humoral immune response plays a key role in the pathogenesis of WNV infection [54]. B-cell-deficient mice uniformly died after WNV infection but were protected by passive transfer of immune sera [51, 55]. In particular, induction of a specific, neutralizing IgM response early in the course of WNV infection is crucial in limiting viremia and dissemination into the CNS, as well as protecting against lethal infection [38, 56]. T cells are also essential [57] as the absence of functional CD4 or CD8 T cells results in the failure of clearing WNV from the CNS [51]. In rodent models, CD4 T cells provide help for antibody responses and sustain WNV-specific CD8 T-cell responses in the CNS, which then enable viral clearance [58, 59]. Regulatory T cells may also play a modulatory role during acute WNV infection. In one study, symptomatic patients were found to have fewer regulatory T cells than asymptomatic patients, suggesting that regulatory T-cell responses might exert a protective effect by dampening the WNV immune response and inflammation [60].

Chemokines have important roles in the host response to WNV infection. Early neutrophil recruitment to the infection site was associated with CXCR2, and leukocyte movement from the blood to brain was affected by CXCR 4, CXCR 3, CXCL10, and CCR5 [61]. In particular, individuals genetically deficient in CCR5 have increased risk of symptomatic disease once infected [62, 63]. Another human gene, OAS1 (2′-5′-oligoadenylate synthetase 1b), has also been implicated in playing a role in the susceptibility to WNV infection [64]. OAS1 is a member of the type I IFN-regulated OAS gene family involved in viral RNA degradation. A single nucleotide polymorphism in OAS1 was found associated with increased risk for WNV encephalitis and paralysis in human [65]. SNPs in IRF3 and MX1 have been identified as susceptibility loci to WNV infection as well [65].

While an intact immune system is essential for the control of WNV infection, the inflammatory response to infection may play a role in disease pathology. WNV infection can cause neuronal death directly by inducing apoptosis and the process appears to be caspase-3 dependent [66]. Pro-inflammatory markers IL-1β, IL-6, IL-8, and TNF-α also play a role in mediating neuronal death in response to WNV infection in vitro [67]. Both neurons and microglial cells are potential sources of such pro-inflammatory cytokines [68].

Collectively, in vitro and in vivo studies have demonstrated the importance of innate, humoral, and cellular immunity in controlling WNV infection, but the inflammatory response may contribute to the pathogenesis of the disease.

Clinical Syndromes

Incubation period from the initial exposure to WNV and onset of clinical illness is between 2 and 14 days. Among those infected, about 80% are asymptomatic [27, 69], while 20–30% develops a mild infection called WNF. WNF in most cases is self-limiting, but some cases might be severe. During the 2002 Illinois outbreak [70], 38% of patients with WNF required hospitalization, although there might be a bias toward diagnosing and reporting WNF in persons with more severe illness [70].

Common symptoms of WNF include fever, malaise, lymphadenopathy, periocular pain, gastrointestinal symptoms such as nausea, vomiting, and abdominal pain; myalgia, and headache. A maculopapular rash, when present is more frequently seen in younger patients [71]. While some symptoms, such as fever, typically resolve in a 1 week or so, others can persist for weeks. In a case series studying the symptoms and outcome of 98 patients with WNF in Illinois, 63% of respondents continued to have symptoms 30 days

Table 44.2 Clinical characteristics in patients reported with confirmed or probable West Nile virus meningitis and encephalitis and overall cases in Illinois in 2002

Characteristic	Total cases ($n = 884$) number/total number (%)	Total neurologic (aseptic meningitis and encephalitis) cases ($n = 543$) number/total number (%)	Aseptic meningitis ($n = 232$) number/total number (%)	Encephalitis ($n = 311$) number/total number (%)
Fever	764/816 (94)	495/521 (95)	212/220 (96)	283/301 (94)
Headache	636/764 (83)	390/473 (83)	205/217 (95)	185/256 (72)
Rash	301/654 (46)	151/390 (39)	83/174 (48)	68/216 (32)
Stiff neck	291/632 (49)	198/402 (49)	105/176 (60)	93/226 (41)
Altered mental status/ change in consciousness	264/627 (42)	249/424 (59)	0/142 (0)	249/282 (88)
Photophobia	155/583 (27)	101/369 (19)	57/165 (35)	44/204 (22)
Weakness[a]	201/884 (23)	120/543 (22)	30/232 (13)	90/311 (29)
Tremor	103/543 (19)	76/339 (22)	6/142 (4)	70/197 (36)
Vomiting[a]	154/884 (17)	124/543 (23)	65/232 (28)	59/311 (19)
Coma/stupor	78/550 (14)	74/356 (21)	0/141 (0)	74/215 (34)
Paresis/paralysis	56/572 (10)	46/361 (9)	3/144 (2)	43/217 (20)
Kernig/Brudzinski sign	31/496 (6)	25/302 (8)	12/130 (9)	13/172 (8)
Seizures	28/557 (5)	26/355 (7)	2/144 (1)	24/211 (11)
Cranial nerve palsies	18/519 (4)	14/327 (3)	2/139 (1)	12/188 (6)

[a]Written in as "other" symptom on case report form

after the onset of illness, and 96% had fatigue for a median of 36 days [72]. Non-neurologic manifestations of WNV infection include myocarditis, myositis, orchitis, and pancreatitis [73–76], but these complications are rare. In contrast, retinopathy associated with WNV has been noted in about one fourth of patients with a history of WNV infection and is more frequently observed among those with severe neurological complications [77].

For the general population, the risk for developing WNV neuroinvasive disease (WNND) was estimated to be less than 1% [27]. Clinical syndromes of WNND include meningitis, encephalitis, and acute flaccid paralysis (AFP). Risk factors for the development of WNND have been examined after several outbreaks [19, 78–80], and advanced age was noted as a major risk factor [70]. Other independent risk factors associated with developing WNND include male sex, hypertension, diabetes mellitus, immunosuppressing conditions, and cardiovascular disease [81, 82].

Similar to other forms of viral encephalitis, symptoms of WNV encephalitis (WNE) are non-specific, but most patients have fever (70–100%), headache (50–100%), and altered mental status (50–100%) [24]. Vomiting (30–75%), diarrhea (15–35%), and rash (5–50%) are also seen, but a prominent finding of WNE is muscle weakness with flaccid paralysis and hyporeflexia, in up to 30–50% patients. Other neurologic findings include cranial neuropathies, e.g., peripheral seventh nerve palsy, optic neuritis, and ataxia. Movement disorders including postural or kinetic tremor, myoclonus, and Parkinsonian features such as rigidity or postural instability are also common [24, 83]. Seizures, increased intracranial pressure and cerebral edema are infrequent events [83]. An example of clinical characteristics in patients with WNV meningitis and encephalitis during the 2002 Illinois outbreak is illustrated in Table 44.2 [70]. Among those with severe illness due to WNV, the overall case-fatality rates range from 3% to 15% and are highest among the elderly [84].

AFP occurs in 5–15% of patients with clinically apparent neuroinvasive disease and can present as a poliomyelitis or Guillain-Barré-like syndrome [20, 85]. The Guillain-Barré form is rare and likely results from a peripheral demyelinating polyneuropathy [86]. Saad et al. reviewed 56 cases of AFP from the literature and summarized the clinical characteristics of these patients [87]. Notably, the spectrum of clinical presentations ranged from single extremity paralysis to flaccid quadriplegia with cranial nerve involvement. Respiratory failure and bladder dysfunction were also common, observed in 54% and 22% of patients, respectively [87]. AFP was found more common in younger patients, but elderly patients had a higher mortality with an overall mortality up to 22%, and the survivors were left with persistent neurologic impairment [87, 88].

After symptomatic WNV infection, more than half of the patients experience persistent symptoms for more than 6 months [89]. While patients with WNND can be left with persistent cognitive or physical deficits, even those with mild WNF may have long-lasting subjective or somatic complaints [90], including tremor, abnormalities in motor skills, and executive functions [91]. For instance, Klee et al. studied the recovery of New York City residents infected during the 1999 WNV outbreak and reported that only 37% achieved a full recovery by 1 year [92]. Another study followed 56 cases of WNV, including 48 patients with meningitis or encephalitis, which occurred in Tennessee 2002. One year later, 12 of 22 (55%) persons still reported lack of complete recovery, with symptoms including fatigue, weakness, difficulty ambulating, and memory problems [93]. More recently, Weather et al. reported an observational study [94] which studied the long-term neurological outcomes of WNV-infected patients. Neurological examinations were conducted 1–2 and 8–11 years following acute WNV infection. Depending on the severity of their initial illness, e.g., WNF vs. WNE, 27–86% of patients had abnormal neurological exam at the first assessment at 1–2 years postinfection. Among those available for the second assessment at 8–11 years postinfection, many had persistent neurological deficits, and some were noted to have developed new neurological complications.

Other than physical symptoms, a significant proportion of patients may experience neuropsychiatric disturbances, with about one-thirds of patients reported new-onset depression in a study [95]. During the 1999 WNV outbreak in New York City, 38% of patients reported depression 1 year after the onset of infection. Similarly, a study conducted after a WNV outbreak in Louisiana reported that 23% of patient still had depression and anxiety at 1-year follow-up [96]. Thus, physicians should be aware of the neuropsychiatric consequences of WNV in patients.

The possibility of persistent WNV infection has been suggested. Several investigators have reported the persistence of WNV viral RNA for months or years in animal models as well as in human [20, 97–99]. In particular, WNV RNA was demonstrated in urine samples from convalescent patients up to >6 years after the initial infection, suggestive of a persistent renal infection [99]. The same group of researchers also linked WNV infection to the development of chronic kidney disease [100]. The association between WNV and chronic kidney disease remains inconclusive, but whether WNV can establish any significant chronic infections in human warrants further investigation.

In conclusion, other than acute morbidity and mortality, WNV infection can lead to significant long-term physical, cognitive, and functional sequelae, as reviewed systemically by Patel et al. [101]. An understanding of these complications and their risk factors can allow early diagnosis, preventive measures, and improved patient care.

Laboratory and Imaging Findings

For patients with WNV infection, total leukocyte counts in peripheral blood are mostly normal or elevated, but lymphocytopenia and anemia can also occur [17, 102]. Hyponatremia can be seen, especially in patients with encephalitis. Studies of cerebrospinal fluid (CSF) in general show pleocytosis with lymphocytic dominance generally <500 cells/μL, but a predominance of neutrophils has also been reported [103]. Protein levels are usually elevated (<150 mg/dL), while glucose levels remain normal.

The MR imaging findings of WNV encephalitis are nonspecific and share similarities with many other inflammatory and infectious processes, including those of St. Louis encephalitis and Japanese encephalitis. Patients with WNND can have normal neuroimaging studies, but abnormalities, when present, are primarily seen in areas of the basal ganglia, thalamus, cerebellum, and brainstem [104]. Some patients may also have involvement of the mesial temporal structures. For patients with extremity weakness, abnormalities can be seen in the gray matter of the spinal cord, more pronounced in the ventral horns, as well as the conus medullaris and the cauda equina. Abnormalities seen by MRI might be progressive, transient and/or migratory, and the transient nature of the imaging abnormalities might explain the negative studies in some patients [105]. Overall, although imaging results of WNV are non-specific, certain MRI findings, such as deep gray matter or mesial temporal lobe involvement, should prompt inclusion of WNV on the differential diagnosis, especially if the clinical picture, epidemiologic factors, and mosquito exposures are taken into account.

WNV Infection in Transplant Recipients

For transplant recipients, the most likely mode of transmission is still through mosquito bites, the natural route of WNV transmission. However, transmissions through blood transfusion and organ transplantation have also been well documented. In a review of 23 past reports of transfusion-transmitted infections in SOT [106], six reports described WNV transmission through blood transfusion, resulting in infection of nine organ recipients. All nine patients developed severe neurological complications, and two subsequently died. While most of these cases involved transfusion of infectious blood products into organ recipients, rarely, the organ donor was the one to receive the infectious unit just prior to transplantation resulting in graft-transmitted WNV infection the recipient [107].

Graft Transmitted WNV Infection

Transmission through SOT was first described in 2002 [107]. Fever and mental status changes developed in four organ recipients from a common donor. Subsequent investigation identified WNV infection in the organ donor and in all four organ recipients. Three recipients developed encephalitis with one death and one developed a febrile illness. The organ donor was thought to have required WNV through blood transfusion. In 2005, three cases of WNV infection were reported among four patients who received organs from a single donor. Two recipients developed WNE. The donor's infection was likely mosquito-borne [108]. In 2008, a patient developed WNE shortly after heart transplantation, and the donor was thought to be infected through blood transfusion [109].

In 2009, a patient developed fever and neurological symptoms approximately 2 weeks after undergoing liver allograft transplant surgery. CSF showed pleocytosis. The patient was treated empirically with intravenous immunoglobulin (IVIG) for possible WNV encephalitis, with prompt clinical improvement. Both CSF and serum of the recipient were positive for WNV IgM. The organ was procured from a 53-year-old man who died from brainstem herniation secondary to an intracranial hemorrhage during a hypertensive crisis. His blood was negative for WNV IgM but positive by NAAT. The route of WNV transmission to the donor was unclear, but presumably he may have acquired mosquito-borne WNV shortly before death, as he had not received blood transfusion [110]. There are two other clusters of WNV transmission in the USA that occurred in 2009 and 2010, and both resulted in encephalitis in one of the two kidney recipients, but the details of these cases were not reported (Table 44.3) [111].

The first case of WNV transmission through organ transplant in Europe was reported in 2010 [112]. The donor died from cerebral hemorrhage, and her liver was harvested and transplanted into a 25-year-old woman. As the local public health authority in the Emilia Romagna region, Italy, mandated NAAT for WNV in blood and organ donations from all subjects in WNV risk areas, the donor's blood sample was tested the day after the harvest and was found positive. On the third postoperative day, the recipient was tested positive for WNV by NAAT, before the development of any clinical evidence of WNV infection. Her immunosuppressive therapy was promptly reduced to a minimum, and she was treated with WNV hyperimmune plasma and gamma globulin. Her posttransplant course was complicated by two episodes of rejection, but she did not develop any clinical WNV disease.

Despite the mandate by the Italian National Transplant Network to perform NAAT within 72 h of donation on all donors living in the WNV endemic areas, four cases of WNV transmission from a single multi-organ donor was reported in August 2011 [113]. The donor's death was not related to a transmissible disease, and the donor's blood sample were tested negative by NAAT within 72 h of organ procurement. However, about 10 days after transplant, the two recipients of kidneys from this donor developed fever and symptoms of encephalitis. The liver and heart recipients remained in good health, while the lung recipient developed neurological symptoms, which was ascribed to immunosuppressive therapy toxicity. WNV transmission was confirmed in the recipients of kidney, liver, and lung, whereas, liver and lung recipients did not develop clinical WNV disease. Repeat testing of the donor materials confirmed a negative test result by NAAT, however, serological tests showed the presence of IgM and IgG. The donor likely had very low level of viremia, which was insufficient for detection by the NAAT technique.

The most recent known cluster of WNV transmission through organ transplantation occurred in the fall of 2011 and was reviewed by Winston et al. [114]. A patient with a recent kidney transplant from a deceased donor was diagnosed with WNV encephalitis, which led to an urgent investigation by the local Department of Public Health and CDC [115]. Three other organ recipients from the same donor were identified. The donor was a 56-year-old man with a history of cerebral palsy, developmental cognitive delay, blindness, and seizures [35, 114] and had outdoor exposure in a region of with known WNV activity. He presented to the emergency room of a local hospital with acute onset of fever, muscle weakness, and an altered mental status and was sent home on an antibiotic for a possible urinary tract infection. Three days later, he was found unresponsive at home and in cardiopulmonary arrest. After resuscitation and intubation, he was brought to another local hospital by paramedics and was admitted to the intensive care unit. However, he remained unresponsive and an electroencephalogram showed no cortical activity consistent with brain death. His death was initially attributed to culture negative sepsis, but his serum was subsequently found positive for WNV IgM. WNV RNA was detected in samples from his spleen/lymph node, skin, and fat associated with the tibia bone, as well as some of the muscle, tendon, and bone marrow specimens, but not in serum [35]. All four organ recipients had WNV RNA in serum and CSF. Three developed WNE, while the liver recipient had no neurological symptoms. The recipients were treated with various modalities, including IVIG, fresh frozen plasma containing WNV IgG, IFN, ribavirin, and/or reduced immunosuppression, with two deaths resulted.

Characteristics of WNV Infection in Transplant Recipients

Reports of WNND in transplant recipients including SOT or hematopoietic stem cell transplant (HSCT) suggest that prodrome and symptoms were similar to those reported in the immunocompetent patients, including fever, weakness, gastrointestinal complaints, and altered mental status. Laboratory findings, e.g., CSF profile, as well as imaging findings on MRI were also similar [116, 117], although the

Table 44.3 Cases of West Nile virus (WNV) transmission through solid organ transplantation [107–114,168]

Case # (reference) Donor/recipient	Age/ Sex	Year Location	Organ	Mode of donor WNV acquisition	WNV testing NAAT/PCR CSF	NAAT/PCR Serum	Serology CSF	Serology Serum	Others	Clinical diagnosis	Treatment	Outcome
Case 1 [107] Donor	20F	2002 Georgia, USA	/	Blood transfusion		(+)		(−)IgM	Serum (+) viral culture	/	/	/
Recipient 1	31F		Kidney				(+)IgM	Equivocal IgM		WNV encephalitis	Supportive	Alive, + neurologic deficit
Recipient 2	38M		Kidney				(−)IgM	(−)IgM	Brain at autopsy (+) PCR/IHC/ viral culture	WNV encephalitis	Supportive	Died
Recipient 3	63M		Heart			(+)	(+)IgM	(+)IgM		WNV encephalitis	Supportive	Alive
Recipient 4	71F		Liver					(+)IgM		WNV fever	Supportive	Alive
Case 2 [108] Donor	NA	2005 New York, USA	/	Mosquito-borne		(−)		(+)IgM/IgG		/	/	/
Recipient 1	NA		Liver		(+)		(+)IgM	(+)IgM		WNV encephalitis	Omr-IgG-am	Comatose
Recipient 2	NA		Lung		(−)		(+)IgM/ IgG	(+)IgM/IgG		WNV encephalitis	Omr-IgG-am	Comatose
Recipient 3	NA		Kidney			(+)		(−)IgM (+)IgG		Asymptomatic	Omr-IgG-am	Alive
Recipient 4	NA		Kidney			(−)		(−)IgM/IgG		Not infected	Omr-IgG-am	Alive
Case 3 [109] Donor	18M	2008 Louisiana, USA	/	Blood transfusion		(−)		(−)IgM/IgG	Blood donor to organ donor (+)IgM	/	/	/
Recipient 1	62M		Heart				(+)IgM	(+)IgM		WNV encephalitis	Supportive	Alive, + neurologic deficit
Case 4 [112] Donor	78F	2009 Italy	/	Mosquito-borne		(+)						
Recipient 1	25F		Liver			(+)		(+)IgM		Asymptomatic	FFP, Omr-IgG-am	Alive
Case 5 [110] Donor	53 M	2009 California, USA	/	Possibly mosquito-borne		(+)		(−)IgM		/	/	/
Recipient 1	55M		Liver			(−)	(+)IgM	(+)IgM		WNV encephalitis	IVIG	Alive
Case 6 [111] Donor	50M	2009 USA	/	Mosquito-borne		(+)		(+) IgM Equivocal IgG		/	/	/
Recipient 1	55M		Kidney							WNV encephalitis	NA	Alive
Recipient 2	54F		Kidney							Not infected	NA	Alive
Recipient 3	49M		Liver							Not infected	NA	Alive

Case 7 [111] Donor	55M	2010 USA	/	Mosquito-borne		(+)		(−)IgM (+)IgG		/	/	/
Recipient 1	NA		Kidney							WNV encephalitis	NA	Died
Recipient 2	NA		Kidney							Asymptomatic	NA	Alive
Recipient 3	NA		Liver							Not infected	NA	Alive
Case 8 [113] Donor	NA	2011 Italy	/	NA		(−)		(+)IgM/IgG		/	/	/
Recipient 1	NA		Kidney		(+)	(+)	(+)IgM/IgG	(+)IgM/IgG		WNV encephalitis	IVIG with high WN titer	Critically ill
Recipient 2	NA		Kidney		(+)	(+)	(+)IgM/IgG	(+)IgM/IgG		WNV encephalitis	NA	Critically ill
Recipient 3	NA		Heart			(−)		(−) IgM/IgG		Asymptomatic	NA	Alive and well
Recipient 4	NA		Liver			(−)		(+) IgM/IgG		Asymptomatic	NA	Alive and well
Recipient 5	NA		Lung			(+)		(+) IgM/IgG		Neurological symptoms thought due to immunosuppressive therapy toxicity		Neurological symptoms thought due to immunosuppressive therapy toxicity
Case 9 [114] Donor	56M	2011 California, USA	/	Mosquito-borne		(−)		(+)IgM/IgG	Tissues (+) PCR	/	/	/
Recipient 1	59M		Kidney		(+)	(+)	(−)	(−)		WNV encephalitis	IVIG, IFN,	Died
Recipient 2	51M		Kidney		(+)	(+)	(−)	(+)IgM		WNV encephalitis	IVIG, IFN, FFP	Alive, no residual neurologic deficits
Recipient 3	59M		Lung		(+)	(+)	(+)IgM/IgG	(−)[a]		WNV encephalitis	IVIG, IFN	Died
Recipient 4	63M		Liver		(+)	(−)	(−)	(−)IgM (+)IgG		Asymptomatic	IVIG, ribavirin	Alive and well

FFP fresh frozen plasma, *IFN* interferon alpha-2b, *IHC Flavivirus*-specific immunohistochemical staining, *IVIG* intravenous immunoglobulin, *NA* not available, *NAAT* nucleic acid amplification testing, *PCR* polymerase chain reaction

[a]Pre-transplant serum of the lung recipient was positive for WNV IgG, but sera posttransplant were negative

CSF WBC counts in transplant patients with WNE are minimally elevated as compared to immunocompetent patients (mean CSF WBC counts were 86 cells/mm^3 versus 227 cells/mm^3, respectively) [114]. Due to their immunocompromised status, transplant recipients might have longer incubation periods and prolonged phase of viremia [112]. The incubation period for WNV is generally thought to range from 2 to 14 days, but for the patients that acquired WNV through SOT, symptoms began 5–37 days after the transplantation, with a median of 13 days [114]. Studying 23 patients that acquired WNV through blood transfusion, Pealer et al. also reported a median incubation time of 13.5 days for transplant recipients versus 8 days for those without any immunosuppressing conditions [33]. The duration of viremia can last for about 4 weeks, as compared to approximately ≤2 weeks of viremia in immunocompetent hosts [112]. The development of antibody might also be delayed [116]. For instance, the liver recipient reported by Morelli et al. [112] developed a WNV IgM antibody response by day 26 posttransplant but did not develop IgG seroconversion to WNV for more than 4 months after transplantation. In comparison, IgM and IgG seroconversion was noted within the first 1–2 weeks in normal hosts [118].

A seroprevalence study previously reported that asymptomatic WNV infection is as common among immunocompromised SOT patients as in non-immunocompromised controls and the incidence of WNND is low in the SOT population, comparable to the <1% estimated rate in the general population [119]. However, most studies support an increased risk of neuroinvasive disease and suggest a higher mortality among immunocompromised patients. During the epidemic in Israel in 2000, immunocompromised patients were noted to have a mortality rate at 31%, as compared to 13% among those not immunocompromised [120]. A case series of 11 transplant patients with mosquito-borne WNV reported a mortality rate of 18% [116]. For the 2002 outbreak in Toronto, Canada, the risk of WNND in a transplant patient infected with WNV was estimated at 40% as compared to 1% in the general population [121]. These reports studied naturally transmitted WNV infection in transplant patients, in whom infection occurred months to years after transplantation. SOT patients that acquired WNV through donor-organ transmission might have even higher rates of morbidity and mortality, as the level of immunosuppression is likely higher during the immediately posttransplant period. Of the 26 transplant recipients exposed to WNV through SOT (Table 44.3), infection was confirmed in 22 patients and 14 (64%) developed WNV encephalitis, resulting in high morbidity and mortality. The high level of immunosuppression routinely given in posttransplant period may also alter the "expected" clinical and laboratory findings. For instance, Winslow et al. noted that although 70% of patients that acquired WNV through SOT eventually developed encephalitis, only 33% had neurological symptoms at the initial presentation [114]. For the case series of naturally acquired WNV encephalitis in transplant patients reported by Klenishcmidr-DeMasters [116], pleocytosis was present in all cases and ranged between 5 and 540 cells/mm^3 with a mean cell count of 89 ± 152 cells/mm^3. In contrast, among the 14 patients with organ graft-transmitted WNE, CSF data were available for nine patients, and three did not have any pleocytosis (Table 44.3). For HSCT recipients, morbidity and mortality are likely increased as well. Among seven such patients reported in the literature, five died shortly after presentation [122].

In summary, the diagnosis of WNV infection in transplant recipients requires a high index of clinical suspicions, when the patient presents with unexplained fever, with or without neurological manifestations, and, in particular, when there is known WNV activity in the region. Furthermore, the possibility of donor- or transfusion-derived WNV infection must be considered during the early posttransplant period.

Diagnosis

Laboratory diagnosis of WNV is typically made by detecting the presence of either antibodies specifically IgM against the virus or the viral nucleic acid in blood or CSF. The dynamics of viremia and IgM and IgG seroconversion during the early stages of WNV infection have been described (Fig. 44.2) [118]. WNV-specific IgM antibodies are usually detectable 3–8 days after disease onset [123]. WNV IgM in serum or CSF is routinely detected by IgM antibody capture enzyme-linked immunosorbent assay (MAC-ELISA). The test is available commercially but can also be obtained with the state or county public health departments. A lateral-flow rapid IgM strip assay, which has a 98.8% sensitivity and a 95.3% specificity as compared to two commercially available MAC-ELISA tests and two public health-developed WNV IgM tests, was also approved [124]. Since IgM does not cross the blood-brain barrier, its presence in CSF is indicative of CNS involvement. However, the finding of IgM in serum must be interpreted with caution, as IgM can persist for months or even >1 year [118, 125]. In those cases, correlation with clinical picture and exposure history would be crucial. IgG can also be detected by ELISA, but the presence of IgG alone may represent past infection only and is difficult to use in isolation to diagnosis acute infection. Past exposure to or vaccination against other flaviviruses can lead to false-positive serological results due to cross-reactivity. Thus, a careful assessment of the patient's prior travel, exposure, and vaccination history is important. Definitive serological diagnosis would require the use of different flaviviral antigens or a comparison of neutralization activity against related flaviviruses. Confirmation of WNV infection can be obtained using the

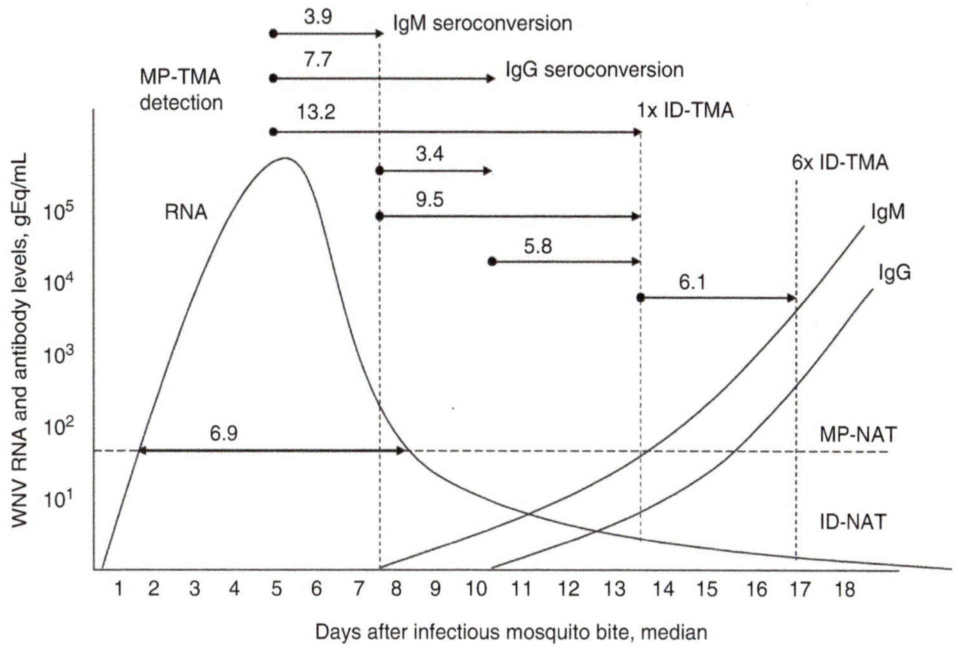

Fig. 44.2 Dynamics of West Nile virus (WNV) RNA and WNV-specific antibody positivity and negativity. Please refer to [118] for details. A total of 245 donors with WNV viremia were followed up weekly for 4 weeks and then monthly for up to 6 additional months or until seroconversion. Plasma samples were tested for WNV RNA by transcription-mediated amplification (TMA) and for WNV-specific IgM and IgG antibodies. The top three intervals represent window periods that start with the index donation (i.e., the donation that tested positive for WNV in minipools of 16 donor specimens [MP] by TMA [MP-TMA]). Although positive results of MP-TMA can occur anytime during the 6.9-day window period when results of MP nucleic acid amplification testing (NAT) are positive, for illustrative purposes, the first three window periods are depicted as beginning at the midpoint of this window period. The median time from RNA detection to IgM seroconversion was 3.9 days; to IgG seroconversion, 7.7 days; to RNA negativity by single-replicate (1x-ID) TMA, 13.2 days; and to RNA negativity by 6-replicate (6x-ID) TMA, 6.1 additional days after results of 1x ID-TMA are negative. (Reproduced from Busch et al. [118], © 2008, with modification of figure legend, by permission of Oxford University Press)

plaque reduction neutralization test (PRNT), which is more specific for WNV. A rising titer by PRNT can also be used to confirm an acute WNV infection, when the presence of IgM alone cannot provide any certainty of the diagnosis. However, this test usually takes several days to perform and is not routinely used to confirm all WNV cases.

NAAT can be used to detect WNV in CSF, tissues, or other body fluids. Although NAAT has high specificity, due to the transient nature of viremia lasting only 2–15 days [118], sensitivity is relatively low. However, NAAT may aid in diagnosis among immunocompromised patients, with whom viremia can be prolonged and antibody response to infections may be delayed or inadequate. Isolation of the virus by culture techniques or detection of viral antigen can also be performed, but these methods are less sensitive than NAAT and are not routinely employed for diagnostic purpose. Furthermore, isolation of the virus by culture requires a Biosafety Level 3 laboratory and is limited to facilities with this capability. It is important to note that transplant patients may be seronegative, especially early in the course of infection. Therefore, both serologic assays and NAAT should be considered in transplant recipients with the clinical suspicion of WNV infection [126].

Treatment

Treatment of WNV is mostly supportive, and there is no specific accepted antiviral therapy. However, several modalities of treatment have been tested or employed in animal studies and human cases [127].

IVIG

IVIG is a preparation of human IgG obtained from pooled plasma from thousands of healthy blood donors and contains antibodies directed against a broad spectrum of microbes. However, the activity against any specific pathogen depends on the prior exposure of the donors to the microbes in their environment as well as immunity obtained through vaccination. Different lots of IVIG from different areas or countries can have substantial variability in WNV neutralizing capacity [128], but overall, preparations from areas endemic for WNV show higher titers to WNV. Plasma obtained from blood donors with anti-WNV antibodies can be further pooled to develop preparations with greater potency than those from regular donors [129]. Besides the neutralizing activities against WNV, the non-specific anti-inflammatory and immunomodulating properties of IVIG may also play an important role in its protective effects against WNV infection [130].

The successful use of IVIG to treat WNV infection was first reported in 2001, when a woman with chronic lymphocytic leukemia became comatose from WNE and recovered with IVIG treatment [131]. Successful outcome associated with IVIG treatment for WNE has also been reported in organ transplant recipients, including those of lung [132], kidney [133], and liver [110] transplantation. In all these cases, the patients had severe neuroinvasive disease from WNV but recovered fully after prompt administration of IVIG. IVIG has also been used to treat AFP caused by WNV successfully [134]. However, there might be a reporting bias and cases of failure have been noted [135].

A phase I/II randomized, placebo-controlled trial that evaluated the safety and efficacy of hyperimmune IVIG (Omr-IgG-am) in the treatment of patients with or at high risk for progression to WNV encephalitis was completed in 2007 [ClinicalTrials.gov: NCT00069316]. The timing of IVIG administration appears to be critical, as most patients that responded to IVIG therapy had received treatment early in the course of infection, especially prior to developing neurological symptoms [108, 136]. In 2005, when four patients received organ transplantation from a WNV-infected donor, all four patients received Omr-IgG-am. While the two asymptomatic patients that received Omr-IgG-am as a prophylactic measure remained well, the other two patients received Omr-IgG-am 10 days after the development of neurological symptoms and did not respond [108]. Makhoul et al. also reported a case series of eight patients with WNE treated with high dose of hyperimmune IVIG; those patients who received early treatment showed significant improvement [136]. Together, these cases argue that the timing of IVIG administration may be critical to its efficacy [110].

Animal studies also support early treatment of WNV with IVIG. A number of animal models demonstrated clear protection by IVIG when the animals are treated during the viremic phase, before or shortly after inoculation with WNV [52, 137]. After infection by flaviviruses, invasion of the CNS may occur in a few days. Using a murine model, Roehrig et al. showed that the window for successful application of prophylactic antibody to prevent flaviviral encephalitis closes at about 4–6 days postinfection concomitant with viral invasion of the brain [138]. In fact, when most patients present, they are no longer viremic [139, 140] and, therefore, may not respond to IVIG treatment. Other than the timing of starting IVIG, the route of administration may be important as well [135]. IgG enters the blood-brain barrier at only low level and might explain the relative ineffectiveness of IVIG treatment when CNS involvement is already evident. Intraventricular or intrathecal administration can deliver higher levels of immunoglobulins into the CNS. This approach has been used successfully in a few cases of enterovirus encephalitis in children with hypogammaglobulinemia [141] although this approach has not been reported for treatment of *Flavivirus*-associated CNS disease. However, if CNS infection might have an immunopathological component, then administration of IVIG, especially via intraventricular or intrathecal route, could potentially exacerbate the clinical disease [142]. There is also a theoretical concern for "antibody-dependent enhancement" of infection, during which subneutralizing concentrations of antibodies bound to *Flavivirus* can enhance infection by facilitating uptake into Fc-receptor-bearing cells [143].

Humanized monoclonal antibodies against WNV were developed [127]. A humanized monoclonal antibody against WNV E protein (MGAWN1) was found to be safe and generally well-tolerated in healthy human subjects in a phase I clinical trial [144]. A phase II study to evaluate the safety and efficacy of MGAWN1 in patients with WNV infection was initiated in 2009, however the clinical trial was terminated due to inability to enroll study subjects [ClinicalTrials.gov: NCT000927953].

Interferon Therapy

IFN play important role in defense against viral infections. IFN-α was studied in several clinical trials against flaviviral disease. A small pilot study showed efficacy of IFN-α-2b against meningoencephalitis due to St. Louis encephalitis virus [145], but a larger randomized double-blind placebo-controlled trial of IFN-α-2a for Japanese encephalitis did not show an improved outcome [146]. For WNV, only case reports exist, and experiences of both success [147, 148] and failure [149]. Kalil et al. [147] reported two patients with WNE who showed significant improvement of neurological function with IFN-α treatment. Lewis and Amsden [148] also described successful treatment of an 83-year-old man with WNE, even though IFN was given 3 weeks after the onset of clinical disease. In contrast, Chan-Tack and Forrest [149] reported failure of IFN-α-2b in the treatment of a 72-year-old man with WNE and AFP. As pointed out by the authors, the failure of treatment in this case may be due to the patient's advanced age, severity of CNS disease, and delay in starting treatment, 17 days after the onset of symptoms. Similar to IVIG, failure of IFN in treatment of WNV CNS disease may also be under-reported due to potential for publication basis.

There are concerns that IFN therapy may induce an immunoreactive state and promote the risk of graft rejection in patients following solid organ allograft transplantation [150]. For instance, long-term use of IFN-α-2b has been associated with an increased risk of acute rejection in renal transplant recipients [151]. In contrast, four renal transplant recipients with WNE in a single cohort received short courses of IFN given between 4 and 17 days; none of these patients had demonstrated significant deterioration in renal graft function [116].

Ribavirin

Ribavirin (1-β-D-ribofuranosyl-1,2,4-triazole-3-carboximide) is a synthetic nucleoside analog with in vitro and in vivo activities against a number of DNA and RNA viruses. It competitively inhibits inosine monophosphate dehydrogenase and can be incorporated into the viral genome, leading to lethal mutagenesis [152]. It also has immunomodulatory properties that may contribute to its efficacy against viral infections [153, 154].

Ribavirin has inhibitory activity again WNV in cell culture, but only at high drug concentrations (EC50 of 60–100 μM) [127, 155]. To approximate the in vitro EC50, high ribavirin doses would need to be given intravenously, increasing the risk for drug toxicity [156]. Animal studies showed little effect of ribavirin on CNS viral infections; in fact, ribavirin treatment increased mortality in a hamsters with experimental WNV infection [157]. During the 2000 WNF outbreak in Israel, the use of enteral ribavirin was associated with increased mortality, although this was likely due to the fact that oral ribavirin was offered to the sicker patients and later in the course of illness [78]. Its lack of efficacy in treating CNS infections appears to be attributed to its low lipid solubility, resulting in ineffective drug passage through the blood brain barrier [155].

Other Strategies

RNA interference-based intervention were shown to protect mice against lethal encephalitis from WNV and Japanese encephalitis [158], but the experience with this strategy is limited to in vitro and animal models. Antisense technology has also been used to protect mice against WNV infection [159]. A phase I/II randomized-blinded study in human was initiated in 2004 to evaluate the safety and efficacy of an antisense compound, AVI-4020 targeting WNV [ClinicalTrials.gov: NCT00091845]. However, the study was terminated due to limited pool of eligible WNV patients.

In recent years, high-throughput screens with small molecule libraries have been used to identify potential therapeutic compounds against various pathogens. Several groups have identified small molecules that have anti-WNV activities in vitro, but there are only scant reports using these compounds in animal models [127].

As pointed out by Diamond [127], regardless of the type of treatment used, a major challenge is to effectively administer the drug before extensive and/or irreversible end organ (CNS) damage occurs. Ideally, the anti-WNV agent should be able to cross the blood-brain barrier, as intracranial drug administration might not be feasible in severely ill patients following allograft transplantation.

Prevention

For natural WNV infection through mosquitoes, preventive strategies, such as avoiding outside activities at dawn and dusk when it is prime mosquito feeding time, application of insect-repellents; (e.g., N,N-diethyl-m-toluamide, DEET), and elimination of stagnant waters as breeding sites, may reduce this route of transmission. Screening of blood donors can also help reduce acquisition of WNV through transfusion of blood products [160].

The Organ Procurement and Transplant Network in the USA currently does not require WNV laboratory testing of organ donors. Instead, organ procurement organizations are advised to exclude deceased donors with encephalitis, meningitis, or acute flaccid paralysis of undetermined etiology from regions with reported WNV activity [111]. The impact of this decision was examined in 2004 by Kiberd et al. [160]. It was concluded that since most positive test results would be false positive, annual screening could result in the loss of potentially 452.4 life years. However, this report was based on an assumption of WNV prevalence among donors at 0.024%. In the USA, the prevalence of WNV might be substantially higher in certain counties, especially during the peak seasons of transmission. Furthermore, this report assumed the baseline screening test specificity and sensitivity to be 99.5% and 95%, respectively. Current assays have improved performance, e.g., Procleix WNV assay reportedly has a specificity of >99.9%, although actual test performance might differ among various laboratories.

A 3-year experience of donor screening for WNV by NAAT in Alberta, Canada [161], showed no false-positive results and no solid organs lost due to WNV testing. It was concluded that such WNV screening can be implemented without compromising availability of donors. Of note, there were no confirmed positive donors in this study, and a direct benefit could not be demonstrated either, but screening of donors in highly endemic areas should be considered. Recommendations for identification of potentially WNV-infected SOT donors have been outlined by Singh and Levi (Table 44.4) [162].

As most people infected with WNV remain asymptomatic, prevention of WNV transmission through organ transplantation relies on the exclusion of donors with viremia. However, among the nine clusters of organ-transmitted WNV, screening by NAAT alone would have only identified five donors as acutely infected with WNV (Table 44.3). This certainly underscores the fact that current methodologies for donor screening for WNV are imperfect. Clinicians evaluat-

Table 44.4 Recommendations for identification of potentially WNV-infected SOT donors (Grade III – opinions of respected authorities, descriptive epidemiology)

1. Defer donors with meningitis, encephalitis, or flaccid paralysis of unknown etiology from regions with reported WNV activity
2. Live donor screening:
(a) Consider live donor screening with WNV NAAT as close to time of donation as possible
(b) Liver donors with positive WNV NAAT should be deferred for 120 days
(c) Live donors who report a post-donation febrile illness with headache, eye pain, body aches, generalized weakness, new skin rash, or swollen lymph nodes within 2 weeks of donation during WNV season should be tested with WNV IgM and NAAT
3. Obtain WNV IgM and NAAT for SOT recipients with febrile illnesses if WNV is suspected
4. Deceased donors who are WNV NAAT positive prior to organ harvesting:
(a) Consider transplantation only in emergent, life threatening situations
(b) Counsel patient and family with regard to risks of transplantation of potentially infected organ

Reproduced with permission from Singh and Levi [162], © 2013, with permission from John Wiley and Sons

ing donors for organ transplantation or taking care of transplant recipients need to carry a high index of suspicion for WNV infection when the patient presents with a febrile illness and neurological symptoms, especially during the peak season of transmission in endemic areas.

Vaccines

Currently, several WNV vaccines have been licensed for use in horses, but none is available for human use. Various strategies have been employed to develop WNV vaccines and several human vaccine candidates have entered or completed phase I and/or phase II clinical trials. For example, a live, attenuated chimeric vaccine, ChimeriVax-WN02, was tested in a phase II randomized, double-blind, placebo-controlled trial. This vaccine was produced by insertion of the WNV genes encoding proteins prM and E in a yellow fever vector and was found to be highly immunogenic and generally well-tolerated [163–165]. A DNA vaccine encoding prM and E was also tested in a phase I clinical trial. It was generally well-tolerated and able to elicit T-cell response in healthy human subjects [166]. Other than attenuated chimeric vaccines and DNA vaccines, other approaches include vector-based vaccines, such as canarypox or vesicular stomatitis virus vectors that express prM and E, as well as live-attenuated WNV vaccines [167]. Universal WNV vaccination in the USA is not likely to be cost-effective, given the sporadic nature of WNV infection. However, certain high-risk patients, such as those with immunodeficiency and/or residence in endemic areas, may benefit from a safe and effective WNV vaccine.

Conclusion

WNV remains an important threat to public health, whereas effective treatment and vaccines for this virus are currently not available. While sporadic cases and outbreaks of WNV disease features interplay of multiple factors that are often unpredictable, surveillance systems at national level such as ArboNET; state, and local levels are expected to play a vital role in monitoring WNV disease activity. This in turn heightens public awareness and allows appropriate public health responses to be administered in a timely manner. Physicians need to be aware of the local WNV activities and become familiar with the clinical syndromes of WNV disease, in particular, the lack of easily recognizable signs and symptoms of infection in the immunocompromised patients undergoing transplantation.

References

1. Petersen LR, Fischer M. Unpredictable and difficult to control – the adolescence of West Nile virus. N Engl J Med. 2012;367(14):1281–4.
2. Petersen LR, Brault AC, Nasci RS. West Nile virus: review of the literature. JAMA. 2013;310(3):308–15.
3. Rossi SL, Ross TM, Evans JD. West Nile virus. Clin Lab Med. 2010;30(1):47–65.
4. Lindenbach BD, Thiel H-J, Rice CM. *Flaviviridae*: the viruses and their replication. In: Fields BN, Knipe DM, Howley PM, editors. Fields virology. 5th ed. Philadelphia: Wolters Kluwer Health/Lippincott Williams & Wilkins; 2007.
5. Granwehr BP, Lillibridge KM, Higgs S, Mason PW, Aronson JF, Campbell GA, et al. West Nile virus: where are we now? Lancet Infect Dis. 2004;4(9):547–56.
6. Hayes CG. West Nile virus: Uganda, 1937, to New York City, 1999. Ann N Y Acad Sci. 2001;951:25–37.
7. Komar N. West Nile virus: epidemiology and ecology in North America. Adv Virus Res. 2003;61:185–234.
8. Petersen LR, Roehrig JT. West Nile virus: a reemerging global pathogen. Emerg Infect Dis. 2001;7(4):611–4.
9. Hardinger KL, Miller B, Storch GA, Desai NM, Brennan DC. West Nile virus-associated meningoencephalitis in two chronically immunosuppressed renal transplant recipients. Am J Transplant. 2003;3(10):1312–5.
10. Heinz-Taheny KM, Andrews JJ, Kinsel MJ, Pessier AP, Pinkerton ME, Lemberger KY, et al. West Nile virus infection in free-ranging squirrels in Illinois. J Vet Diagn Investig. 2004;16(3):186–90.
11. Miller DL, Mauel MJ, Baldwin C, Burtle G, Ingram D, Hines ME 2nd, et al. West Nile virus in farmed alligators. Emerg Infect Dis. 2003;9(7):794–9.
12. Donadieu E, Bahuon C, Lowenski S, Zientara S, Coulpier M, Lecollinet S. Differential virulence and pathogenesis of West Nile viruses. Viruses. 2013;5(11):2856–80.
13. Beasley DW, Li L, Suderman MT, Barrett AD. Mouse neuroinvasive phenotype of West Nile virus strains varies depending upon virus genotype. Virology. 2002;296(1):17–23.
14. Hernandez-Triana LM, Jeffries CL, Mansfield KL, Carnell G, Fooks AR, Johnson N. Emergence of west nile virus lineage 2 in Europe: a review on the introduction and spread of a mosquito-borne disease. Front Public Health. 2014;2:271.
15. Barzon L, Papa A, Lavezzo E, Franchin E, Pacenti M, Sinigaglia A, et al. Phylogenetic characterization of Central/Southern European lineage 2 West Nile virus: analysis of human outbreaks in Italy

and Greece, 2013–2014. Clin Microbiol Infect. 2015;21(12):1122. e1–10.
16. Cernescu C, Ruta SM, Tardei G, Grancea C, Moldoveanu L, Spulbar E, et al. A high number of severe neurologic clinical forms during an epidemic of West Nile virus infection. Rom J Virol. 1997;48(1–4):13–25.
17. Nash D, Mostashari F, Fine A, Miller J, O'Leary D, Murray K, et al. The outbreak of West Nile virus infection in the New York City area in 1999. N Engl J Med. 2001;344(24):1807–14.
18. Platonov AE, Shipulin GA, Shipulina OY, Tyutyunnik EN, Frolochkina TI, Lanciotti RS, et al. Outbreak of West Nile virus infection, Volgograd Region, Russia, 1999. Emerg Infect Dis. 2001;7(1):128–32.
19. Tsai TF, Popovici F, Cernescu C, Campbell GL, Nedelcu NI. West Nile encephalitis epidemic in southeastern Romania. Lancet. 1998;352(9130):767–71.
20. Murray KO, Walker C, Gould E. The virology, epidemiology, and clinical impact of West Nile virus: a decade of advancements in research since its introduction into the Western Hemisphere. Epidemiol Infect. 2011;139(6):807–17.
21. Jia XY, Briese T, Jordan I, Rambaut A, Chi HC, Mackenzie JS, et al. Genetic analysis of West Nile New York 1999 encephalitis virus. Lancet. 1999;354(9194):1971–2.
22. Lanciotti RS, Roehrig JT, Deubel V, Smith J, Parker M, Steele K, et al. Origin of the West Nile virus responsible for an outbreak of encephalitis in the northeastern United States. Science. 1999;286(5448):2333–7.
23. CDC. https://www.cdc.gov/westnile/statsmaps/cummapsdata.html.
24. Debiasi RL. West Nile virus neuroinvasive disease. Curr Infect Dis Rep. 2011;13(4):350–9.
25. Lindsey NP, Staples JE, Lehman JA, Fischer M. Surveillance for human West Nile virus disease - United States, 1999–2008. MMWR Surveill Summ. 2010;59(2):1–17.
26. Beasley DW, Barrett AD, Tesh RB. Resurgence of West Nile neurologic disease in the United States in 2012: what happened? What needs to be done? Antivir Res. 2013;99(1):1–5.
27. Mostashari F, Bunning ML, Kitsutani PT, Singer DA, Nash D, Cooper MJ, et al. Epidemic West Nile encephalitis, New York, 1999: results of a household-based seroepidemiological survey. Lancet. 2001;358(9278):261–4.
28. CDC. Investigation of West Nile virus infection in recipients of blood transfusion. MMWR. 2002;51:973–4.
29. Meny GM, Santos-Zabala L, Szallasi A, Stramer SL. West Nile virus infection transmitted by granulocyte transfusion. Blood. 2011;117(21):5778–9.
30. CDC. Possible West Nile virus transmission to an infant through breast-feeding: Michigan, 2002. MMWR. 2002;51:877–8.
31. CDC. Intrauterine West Nile virus infection: New York, 2002. MMWR. 2002;51:1135–6.
32. CDC. Laboratory-acquired West Nile virus infections – United States, 2002. MMWR. 2002;51(50):1133–5.
33. Pealer LN, Marfin AA, Petersen LR, Lanciotti RS, Page PL, Stramer SL, et al. Transmission of West Nile virus through blood transfusion in the United States in 2002. N Engl J Med. 2003;349(13):1236–45.
34. Dodd RY, Foster GA, Stramer SL. Keeping blood transfusion safe from West Nile virus: American Red Cross Experience, 2003 to 2012. Transfus Med Rev. 2015;29(3):153–61.
35. Blau DM, Rabe IB, Bhatnagar J, Civen R, Trivedi KK, Rollin D, et al. West Nile virus RNA in tissues from donor associated with transmission to organ transplant recipients. Emerg Infect Dis. 2013;19(9):1518–20.
36. Blitvich BJ, Wang T, Saxena V, Zeng S, Harmon KM, Raymond MD, et al. West Nile virus infection in human and mouse cornea tissue. Am J Trop Med Hyg. 2016;95(5):1185–91.
37. Suthar MS, Diamond MS, Gale M Jr. West Nile virus infection and immunity. Nat Rev Microbiol. 2013;11(2):115–28.
38. Lim SM, Koraka P, Osterhaus AD, Martina BE. West Nile virus: immunity and pathogenesis. Viruses. 2011;3(6):811–28.
39. Suen WW, Prow NA, Hall RA, Bielefeldt-Ohmann H. Mechanism of West Nile virus neuroinvasion: a critical appraisal. Viruses. 2014;6(7):2796–825.
40. Wang T, Town T, Alexopoulou L, Anderson JF, Fikrig E, Flavell RA. Toll-like receptor 3 mediates West Nile virus entry into the brain causing lethal encephalitis. Nat Med. 2004;10(12):1366–73.
41. Fredericksen BL. The neuroimmune response to West Nile virus. J Neurovirol. 2014;20(2):113–21.
42. Thomas SJ, Endy TP, Rothman AL, Barrett AD. Chapter 155: Flaviviruses. In: Bennett JE, Dolin R, Blaser MJ, editors. Mandell, Douglas, and Bennett's principles and practice of infectious diseases. 8th ed: 1600 John F. Kennedy Blvd: Elsevier; 2015. p. 1881–903.
43. Samuel MA, Diamond MS. Alpha/beta interferon protects against lethal West Nile virus infection by restricting cellular tropism and enhancing neuronal survival. J Virol. 2005;79(21):13350–61.
44. Shrestha B, Wang T, Samuel MA, Whitby K, Craft J, Fikrig E, et al. Gamma interferon plays a crucial early antiviral role in protection against West Nile virus infection. J Virol. 2006;80(11):5338–48.
45. Avirutnan P, Mehlhop E, Diamond MS. Complement and its role in protection and pathogenesis of flavivirus infections. Vaccine. 2008;26(Suppl 8):I100–7.
46. Mehlhop E, Whitby K, Oliphant T, Marri A, Engle M, Diamond MS. Complement activation is required for induction of a protective antibody response against West Nile virus infection. J Virol. 2005;79(12):7466–77.
47. Mehlhop E, Diamond MS. Protective immune responses against West Nile virus are primed by distinct complement activation pathways. J Exp Med. 2006;203(5):1371–81.
48. Mehlhop E, Fuchs A, Engle M, Diamond MS. Complement modulates pathogenesis and antibody-dependent neutralization of West Nile virus infection through a C5-independent mechanism. Virology. 2009;393(1):11–5.
49. Arjona A, Wang P, Montgomery RR, Fikrig E. Innate immune control of West Nile virus infection. Cell Microbiol. 2011;13(11):1648–58.
50. Quicke KM, Suthar MS. The innate immune playbook for restricting West Nile virus infection. Viruses. 2013;5(11):2643–58.
51. Diamond MS, Mehlhop E, Oliphant T, Samuel MA. The host immunologic response to West Nile encephalitis virus. Front Biosci. 2009;14:3024–34.
52. Agrawal AG, Petersen LR. Human immunoglobulin as a treatment for West Nile virus infection. J Infect Dis. 2003;188(1):1–4.
53. Diamond MS. Development of effective therapies against West Nile virus infection. Expert Rev Anti-Infect Ther. 2005;3(6):931–44.
54. Austin SK, Dowd KA. B cell response and mechanisms of antibody protection to West Nile virus. Viruses. 2014;6(3):1015–36.
55. Diamond MS, Shrestha B, Marri A, Mahan D, Engle M. B cells and antibody play critical roles in the immediate defense of disseminated infection by West Nile encephalitis virus. J Virol. 2003;77(4):2578–86.
56. Diamond MS, Sitati EM, Friend LD, Higgs S, Shrestha B, Engle M. A critical role for induced IgM in the protection against West Nile virus infection. J Exp Med. 2003;198(12):1853–62.
57. Netland J, Bevan MJ. CD8 and CD4 T cells in West Nile virus immunity and pathogenesis. Viruses. 2013;5(10):2573–84.
58. Sitati EM, Diamond MS. CD4+ T-cell responses are required for clearance of West Nile virus from the central nervous system. J Virol. 2006;80(24):12060–9.
59. Shrestha B, Diamond MS. Role of CD8+ T cells in control of West Nile virus infection. J Virol. 2004;78(15):8312–21.
60. Lanteri MC, O'Brien KM, Purtha WE, Cameron MJ, Lund JM, Owen RE, et al. Tregs control the development of symptomatic

West Nile virus infection in humans and mice. J Clin Invest. 2009;119(11):3266–77.

61. Lim JK, Murphy PM. Chemokine control of West Nile virus infection. Exp Cell Res. 2011;317(5):569–74.
62. Glass WG, McDermott DH, Lim JK, Lekhong S, Yu SF, Frank WA, et al. CCR5 deficiency increases risk of symptomatic West Nile virus infection. J Exp Med. 2006;203(1):35–40.
63. Lim JK, McDermott DH, Lisco A, Foster GA, Krysztof D, Follmann D, et al. CCR5 deficiency is a risk factor for early clinical manifestations of West Nile virus infection but not for viral transmission. J Infect Dis. 2010;201(2):178–85.
64. Lim JK, Lisco A, McDermott DH, Huynh L, Ward JM, Johnson B, et al. Genetic variation in OAS1 is a risk factor for initial infection with West Nile virus in man. PLoS Pathog. 2009;5(2):e1000321.
65. Bigham AW, Buckingham KJ, Husain S, Emond MJ, Bofferding KM, Gildersleeve H, et al. Host genetic risk factors for West Nile virus infection and disease progression. PLoS One. 2011;6(9):e24745.
66. Samuel MA, Morrey JD, Diamond MS. Caspase 3-dependent cell death of neurons contributes to the pathogenesis of West Nile virus encephalitis. J Virol. 2007;81(6):2614–23.
67. Kumar M, Verma S, Nerurkar VR. Pro-inflammatory cytokines derived from West Nile virus (WNV)-infected SK-N-SH cells mediate neuroinflammatory markers and neuronal death. J Neuroinflammation. 2010;7:73.
68. van Marle G, Antony J, Ostermann H, Dunham C, Hunt T, Halliday W, et al. West Nile virus-induced neuroinflammation: glial infection and capsid protein-mediated neurovirulence. J Virol. 2007;81(20):10933–49.
69. Zou S, Foster GA, Dodd RY, Petersen LR, Stramer SL. West Nile fever characteristics among viremic persons identified through blood donor screening. J Infect Dis. 2010;202(9):1354–61.
70. Huhn GD, Austin C, Langkop C, Kelly K, Lucht R, Lampman R, et al. The emergence of West Nile virus during a large outbreak in Illinois in 2002. Am J Trop Med Hyg. 2005;72(6):768–76.
71. Brilla R, Block M, Geremia G, Wichter M. Clinical and neuroradiologic features of 39 consecutive cases of West Nile Virus meningoencephalitis. J Neurol Sci. 2004;220(1–2):37–40.
72. Watson JT, Pertel PE, Jones RC, Siston AM, Paul WS, Austin CC, et al. Clinical characteristics and functional outcomes of West Nile Fever. Ann Intern Med. 2004;141(5):360–5.
73. Buber J, Fink N, Bin H, Mouallem M. West Nile virus-induced pancreatitis. Travel Med Infect Dis. 2008;6(6):373–5.
74. Khouzam RN. Significant cardiomyopathy secondary to West Nile virus infection. South Med J. 2009;102(5):527–8.
75. Pergam SA, DeLong CE, Echevarria L, Scully G, Goade DE. Myocarditis in West Nile virus infection. Am J Trop Med Hyg. 2006;75(6):1232–3.
76. Smith RD, Konoplev S, DeCourten-Myers G, Brown T. West Nile virus encephalitis with myositis and orchitis. Hum Pathol. 2004;35(2):254–8.
77. Hasbun R, Garcia MN, Kellaway J, Baker L, Salazar L, Woods SP, et al. West Nile virus retinopathy and associations with long term neurological and neurocognitive sequelae. PLoS One. 2016;11(3):e0148898.
78. Chowers MY, Lang R, Nassar F, Ben-David D, Giladi M, Rubinshtein E, et al. Clinical characteristics of the West Nile fever outbreak, Israel, 2000. Emerg Infect Dis. 2001;7(4):675–8.
79. Bode AV, Sejvar JJ, Pape WJ, Campbell GL, Marfin AA. West Nile virus disease: a descriptive study of 228 patients hospitalized in a 4-county region of Colorado in 2003. Clin Infect Dis. 2006;42(9):1234–40.
80. O'Leary DR, Marfin AA, Montgomery SP, Kipp AM, Lehman JA, Biggerstaff BJ, et al. The epidemic of West Nile virus in the United States, 2002. Vector Borne Zoonotic Dis. 2004;4(1):61–70.
81. Jean CM, Honarmand S, Louie JK, Glaser CA. Risk factors for West Nile virus neuroinvasive disease, California, 2005. Emerg Infect Dis. 2007;13(12):1918–20.
82. Murray KO, Koers E, Baraniuk S, Herrington E, Carter H, Sierra M, et al. Risk factors for encephalitis from West Nile Virus: a matched case-control study using hospitalized controls. Zoonoses Public Health. 2009;56(6–7):370–5.
83. Sejvar JJ, Marfin AA. Manifestations of West Nile neuroinvasive disease. Rev Med Virol. 2006;16(4):209–24.
84. CDC. https://www.cdc.gov/westnile/index.html.
85. Jeha LE, Sila CA, Lederman RJ, Prayson RA, Isada CM, Gordon SM. West Nile virus infection: a new acute paralytic illness. Neurology. 2003;61(1):55–9.
86. Ahmed S, Libman R, Wesson K, Ahmed F, Einberg K. Guillain-Barre syndrome: an unusual presentation of West Nile virus infection. Neurology. 2000;55(1):144–6.
87. Saad M, Youssef S, Kirschke D, Shubair M, Haddadin D, Myers J, et al. Acute flaccid paralysis: the spectrum of a newly recognized complication of West Nile virus infection. J Infect. 2005;51(2):120–7.
88. CDC. Acute flaccid paralysis syndrome associated with West Nile virus infection - Mississippi and Louisiana, July–August 2002. MMWR. 2002;51:862–28.
89. Cook RL, Xu X, Yablonsky EJ, Sakata N, Tripp JH, Hess R, et al. Demographic and clinical factors associated with persistent symptoms after West Nile virus infection. Am J Trop Med Hyg. 2010;83(5):1133–6.
90. Sejvar JJ. The long-term outcomes of human West Nile virus infection. Clin Infect Dis. 2007;44(12):1617–24.
91. Carson PJ, Konewko P, Wold KS, Mariani P, Goli S, Bergloff P, et al. Long-term clinical and neuropsychological outcomes of West Nile virus infection. Clin Infect Dis. 2006;43(6):723–30.
92. Klee AL, Maidin B, Edwin B, Poshni I, Mostashari F, Fine A, et al. Long-term prognosis for clinical West Nile virus infection. Emerg Infect Dis. 2004;10(8):1405–11.
93. Gottfried K, Quinn R, Jones T. Clinical description and follow-up investigation of human West Nile virus cases. South Med J. 2005;98(6):603–6.
94. Weatherhead JE, Miller VE, Garcia MN, Hasbun R, Salazar L, Dimachkie MM, et al. Long-term neurological outcomes in West Nile virus-infected patients: an observational study. Am J Trop Med Hyg. 2015;92(5):1006–12.
95. Murray KO, Resnick M, Miller V. Depression after infection with West Nile virus. Emerg Infect Dis. 2007;13(3):479–81.
96. Sejvar JJ, Haddad MB, Tierney BC, Campbell GL, Marfin AA, Van Gerpen JA, et al. Neurologic manifestations and outcome of West Nile virus infection. JAMA. 2003;290(4):511–5.
97. Penn RG, Guarner J, Sejvar JJ, Hartman H, McComb RD, Nevins DL, et al. Persistent neuroinvasive West Nile virus infection in an immunocompromised patient. Clin Infect Dis. 2006;42(5):680–3.
98. Tesh RB, Siirin M, Guzman H, Travassos da Rosa AP, Wu X, Duan T, et al. Persistent West Nile virus infection in the golden hamster: studies on its mechanism and possible implications for other flavivirus infections. J Infect Dis. 2005;192(2):287–95.
99. Murray K, Walker C, Herrington E, Lewis JA, McCormick J, Beasley DW, et al. Persistent infection with West Nile virus years after initial infection. J Infect Dis. 2010;201(1):2–4.
100. Nolan MS, Podoll AS, Hause AM, Akers KM, Finkel KW, Murray KO. Prevalence of chronic kidney disease and progression of disease over time among patients enrolled in the Houston West Nile virus cohort. PLoS One. 2012;7(7):e40374.
101. Patel H, Sander B, Nelder MP. Long-term sequelae of West Nile virus-related illness: a systematic review. Lancet Infect Dis. 2015;15(8):951–9.
102. Weiss D, Carr D, Kellachan J, Tan C, Phillips M, Bresnitz E, et al. Clinical findings of West Nile virus infection in hospital-

ized patients, New York and New Jersey, 2000. Emerg Infect Dis. 2001;7(4):654–8.
103. Crichlow R, Bailey J, Gardner C. Cerebrospinal fluid neutrophilic pleocytosis in hospitalized West Nile virus patients. J Am Board Fam Pract. 2004;17(6):470–2.
104. Davis LE, DeBiasi R, Goade DE, Haaland KY, Harrington JA, Harnar JB, et al. West Nile virus neuroinvasive disease. Ann Neurol. 2006;60(3):286–300.
105. Petropoulou KA, Gordon SM, Prayson RA, Ruggierri PM. West Nile virus meningoencephalitis: MR imaging findings. AJNR Am J Neuroradiol. 2005;26(8):1986–95.
106. Mezochow AK, Henry R, Blumberg EA, Kotton CN. Transfusion transmitted infections in solid organ transplantation. Am J Transplant. 2015;15(2):547–54.
107. Iwamoto M, Jernigan DB, Guasch A, Trepka MJ, Blackmore CG, Hellinger WC, et al. Transmission of West Nile virus from an organ donor to four transplant recipients. N Engl J Med. 2003;348(22):2196–203.
108. CDC. West Nile virus infections in organ transplant recipients – New York and Pennsylvania, August-September, 2005. MMWR. 2005;54(40):1021–3.
109. CDC. West Nile virus transmission via organ transplantation and blood transfusion - Louisiana, 2008. MMWR. 2009;58(45):1263–7.
110. Rhee C, Eaton EF, Concepcion W, Blackburn BG. West Nile virus encephalitis acquired via liver transplantation and clinical response to intravenous immunoglobulin: case report and review of the literature. Transpl Infect Dis. 2011;13(3):312–7.
111. Nett RJ, Kuehnert MJ, Ison MG, Orlowski JP, Fischer M, Staples JE. Current practices and evaluation of screening solid organ donors for West Nile virus. Transpl Infect Dis. 2012;14(3):268–77.
112. Morelli MC, Sambri V, Grazi GL, Gaibani P, Pierro A, Cescon M, et al. Absence of neuroinvasive disease in a liver transplant recipient who acquired West Nile virus (WNV) infection from the organ donor and who received WNV antibodies prophylactically. Clin Infect Dis. 2010;51(4):e34–7.
113. Costa AN, Capobianchi MR, Ippolito G, Palu G, Barzon L, Piccolo G, et al. West Nile virus: the Italian national transplant network reaction to an alert in the north-eastern region, Italy 2011. Euro Surveill. 2011;16(41).
114. Winston DJ, Vikram HR, Rabe IB, Dhillon G, Mulligan D, Hong JC, et al. Donor-derived West Nile virus infection in solid organ transplant recipients: report of four additional cases and review of clinical, diagnostic, and therapeutic features. Transplantation. 2014;97(9):881–9.
115. Vikram H, Weber I, Winston D, Honng J, Mulligan D, Dhillon G, et al. Investigation of donor-derived West Nile virus (WNV) infection in four recipients. Boston: American Transplant Congress; 2012.
116. Kleinschmidt-DeMasters BK, Marder BA, Levi ME, Laird SP, McNutt JT, Escott EJ, et al. Naturally acquired West Nile virus encephalomyelitis in transplant recipients: clinical, laboratory, diagnostic, and neuropathological features. Arch Neurol. 2004;61(8):1210–20.
117. DeSalvo D, Roy-Chaudhury P, Peddi R, Merchen T, Konijetti K, Gupta M, et al. West Nile virus encephalitis in organ transplant recipients: another high-risk group for meningoencephalitis and death. Transplantation. 2004;77(3):466–9.
118. Busch MP, Kleinman SH, Tobler LH, Kamel HT, Norris PJ, Walsh I, et al. Virus and antibody dynamics in acute west nile virus infection. J Infect Dis. 2008;198(7):984–93.
119. Freifeld AG, Meza J, Schweitzer B, Shafer L, Kalil AC, Sambol AR. Seroprevalence of West Nile virus infection in solid organ transplant recipients. Transpl Infect Dis. 2010;12(2):120–6.
120. Weinberger M, Pitlik SD, Gandacu D, Lang R, Nassar F, Ben David D, et al. West Nile fever outbreak, Israel, 2000: epidemiologic aspects. Emerg Infect Dis. 2001;7(4):686–91.
121. Kumar D, Drebot MA, Wong SJ, Lim G, Artsob H, Buck P, et al. A seroprevalence study of west nile virus infection in solid organ transplant recipients. Am J Transplant. 2004;4(11):1883–8.
122. Brenner W, Storch G, Buller R, Vij R, Devine S, DiPersio J. West Nile Virus encephalopathy in an allogeneic stem cell transplant recipient: use of quantitative PCR for diagnosis and assessment of viral clearance. Bone Marrow Transplant. 2005;36(4):369–70.
123. CDC. https://www.cdc.gov/westnile/healthcareproviders/healthcareproviders-diagnostic.html.
124. Sambol AR, Hinrichs SH. Evaluation of a new West Nile Virus lateral-flow rapid IgM assay. J Virol Methods. 2009;157(2):223–6.
125. Roehrig JT, Nash D, Maldin B, Labowitz A, Martin DA, Lanciotti RS, et al. Persistence of virus-reactive serum immunoglobulin m antibody in confirmed West Nile virus encephalitis cases. Emerg Infect Dis. 2003;9(3):376–9.
126. Koepsell SA, Freifeld AG, Sambol AR, McComb RD, Kazmi SA. Seronegative naturally acquired West Nile virus encephalitis in a renal and pancreas transplant recipient. Transpl Infect Dis. 2010;12(5):459–64.
127. Diamond MS. Progress on the development of therapeutics against West Nile virus. Antivir Res. 2009;83(3):214–27.
128. Planitzer CB, Modrof J, Kreil TR. West Nile virus neutralization by US plasma-derived immunoglobulin products. J Infect Dis. 2007;196(3):435–40.
129. Ben-Nathan D, Gershoni-Yahalom O, Samina I, Khinich Y, Nur I, Laub O, et al. Using high titer West Nile intravenous immunoglobulin from selected Israeli donors for treatment of West Nile virus infection. BMC Infect Dis. 2009;9:18.
130. Srivastava R, Ramakrishna C, Cantin E. Anti-inflammatory activity of intravenous immunoglobulins protects against West Nile virus encephalitis. J Gen Virol. 2015;96(Pt 6):1347–57.
131. Shimoni Z, Niven MJ, Pitlick S, Bulvik S. Treatment of West Nile virus encephalitis with intravenous immunoglobulin. Emerg Infect Dis. 2001;7(4):759.
132. Hamdan A, Green P, Mendelson E, Kramer MR, Pitlik S, Weinberger M. Possible benefit of intravenous immunoglobulin therapy in a lung transplant recipient with West Nile virus encephalitis. Transpl Infect Dis. 2002;4(3):160–2.
133. Saquib R, Randall H, Chandrakantan A, Spak CW, Barri YM. West Nile virus encephalitis in a renal transplant recipient: the role of intravenous immunoglobulin. Am J Kidney Dis. 2008;52(5):e19–21.
134. Walid MS, Mahmoud FA. Successful treatment with intravenous immunoglobulin of acute flaccid paralysis caused by West Nile virus. Perm J. 2009;13(3):43–6.
135. Haley M, Retter AS, Fowler D, Gea-Banacloche J, O'Grady NP. The role for intravenous immunoglobulin in the treatment of West Nile virus encephalitis. Clin Infect Dis. 2003;37(6):e88–90.
136. Makhoul B, Braun E, Herskovitz M, Ramadan R, Hadad S, Norberto K. Hyperimmune gammaglobulin for the treatment of West Nile virus encephalitis. Isr Med Assoc J. 2009;11(3):151–3.
137. Ben-Nathan D, Lustig S, Tam G, Robinzon S, Segal S, Rager-Zisman B. Prophylactic and therapeutic efficacy of human intravenous immunoglobulin in treating West Nile virus infection in mice. J Infect Dis. 2003;188(1):5–12.
138. Roehrig JT, Staudinger LA, Hunt AR, Mathews JH, Blair CD. Antibody prophylaxis and therapy for flavivirus encephalitis infections. Ann N Y Acad Sci. 2001;951:286–97.
139. Campbell GL, Marfin AA, Lanciotti RS, Gubler DJ. West Nile virus. Lancet Infect Dis. 2002;2(9):519–29.
140. Petersen LR, Marfin AA. West Nile virus: a primer for the clinician. Ann Intern Med. 2002;137(3):173–9.

141. Dwyer JM, Erlendsson K. Intraventricular gamma-globulin for the management of enterovirus encephalitis. Pediatr Infect Dis J. 1988;7(5 Suppl):S30–3.
142. Jackson AC. Therapy of West Nile virus infection. Can J Neurol Sci. 2004;31(2):131–4.
143. Beasley DW. Vaccines and immunotherapeutics for the prevention and treatment of infections with West Nile virus. Immunotherapy. 2011;3(2):269–85.
144. Beigel JH, Nordstrom JL, Pillemer SR, Roncal C, Goldwater DR, Li H, et al. Safety and pharmacokinetics of single intravenous dose of MGAWN1, a novel monoclonal antibody to West Nile virus. Antimicrob Agents Chemother. 2010;54(6):2431–6.
145. Rahal JJ, Anderson J, Rosenberg C, Reagan T, Thompson LL. Effect of interferon-alpha2b therapy on St. Louis viral meningoencephalitis: clinical and laboratory results of a pilot study. J Infect Dis. 2004;190(6):1084–7.
146. Solomon T, Dung NM, Wills B, Kneen R, Gainsborough M, Diet TV, et al. Interferon alfa-2a in Japanese encephalitis: a randomised double-blind placebo-controlled trial. Lancet. 2003;361(9360):821–6.
147. Kalil AC, Devetten MP, Singh S, Lesiak B, Poage DP, Bargenquast K, et al. Use of interferon-alpha in patients with West Nile encephalitis: report of 2 cases. Clin Infect Dis. 2005;40(5):764–6.
148. Lewis M, Amsden JR. Successful treatment of West Nile virus infection after approximately 3 weeks into the disease course. Pharmacotherapy. 2007;27(3):455–8.
149. Chan-Tack KM, Forrest G. Failure of interferon alpha-2b in a patient with West Nile virus meningoencephalitis and acute flaccid paralysis. Scand J Infect Dis. 2005;37(11–12):944–6.
150. O'Grady J. The immunoreactive patient: rejection and autoimmune disease. Liver Transpl. 2011;17(Suppl 3):S29–33.
151. Baid S, Tolkoff-Rubin N, Saidman S, Chung R, Williams WW, Auchincloss H, et al. Acute humoral rejection in hepatitis C-infected renal transplant recipients receiving antiviral therapy. Am J Transplant. 2003;3(1):74–8.
152. Graci JD, Cameron CE. Quasispecies, error catastrophe, and the antiviral activity of ribavirin. Virology. 2002;298(2):175–80.
153. Tam RC, Lau JY, Hong Z. Mechanisms of action of ribavirin in antiviral therapies. Antivir Chem Chemother. 2001;12(5):261–72.
154. Sookoian S, Castano G, Flichman D, Cello J. Effects of ribavirin on cytokine production of recall antigens and phytohemaglutinin-stimulated peripheral blood mononuclear cells. (Inhibitory effects of ribavirin on cytokine production). Ann Hepatol. 2004;3(3):104–7.
155. Morrey JD, Smee DF, Sidwell RW, Tseng C. Identification of active antiviral compounds against a New York isolate of West Nile virus. Antivir Res. 2002;55(1):107–16.
156. Jordan I, Briese T, Fischer N, Lau JY, Lipkin WI. Ribavirin inhibits West Nile virus replication and cytopathic effect in neural cells. J Infect Dis. 2000;182(4):1214–7.
157. Morrey JD, Day CW, Julander JG, Blatt LM, Smee DF, Sidwell RW. Effect of interferon-alpha and interferon-inducers on West Nile virus in mouse and hamster animal models. Antivir Chem Chemother. 2004;15(2):101–9.
158. Kumar P, Lee SK, Shankar P, Manjunath N. A single siRNA suppresses fatal encephalitis induced by two different flaviviruses. PLoS Med. 2006;3(4):e96.
159. Deas TS, Bennett CJ, Jones SA, Tilgner M, Ren P, Behr MJ, et al. In vitro resistance selection and in vivo efficacy of morpholino oligomers against West Nile virus. Antimicrob Agents Chemother. 2007;51(7):2470–82.
160. Kiberd BA, Forward K. Screening for West Nile virus in organ transplantation: a medical decision analysis. Am J Transplant. 2004;4(8):1296–301.
161. Tilley PA, Fox JD, Lee B, Chui L, Preiksaitis J. Screening of organ and tissue donors for West Nile virus by nucleic acid amplification – a three year experience in Alberta. Am J Transplant. 2008;8(10):2119–25.
162. Singh N, Levi ME. Arenavirus and West Nile virus in solid organ transplantation. Am J Transplant. 2013;13(Suppl 4):361–71.
163. Biedenbender R, Bevilacqua J, Gregg AM, Watson M, Dayan G. Phase II, randomized, double-blind, placebo-controlled, multicenter study to investigate the immunogenicity and safety of a West Nile virus vaccine in healthy adults. J Infect Dis. 2011;203(1):75–84.
164. Dayan GH, Bevilacqua J, Coleman D, Buldo A, Risi G. Phase II, dose ranging study of the safety and immunogenicity of single dose West Nile vaccine in healthy adults >/= 50 years of age. Vaccine. 2012;30(47):6656–64.
165. Dayan GH, Pugachev K, Bevilacqua J, Lang J, Monath TP. Preclinical and clinical development of a YFV 17 D-based chimeric vaccine against West Nile virus. Viruses. 2013;5(12):3048–70.
166. Ledgerwood JE, Pierson TC, Hubka SA, Desai N, Rucker S, Gordon IJ, et al. A West Nile virus DNA vaccine utilizing a modified promoter induces neutralizing antibody in younger and older healthy adults in a phase I clinical trial. J Infect Dis. 2011;203(10):1396–404.
167. Amanna IJ, Slifka MK. Current trends in West Nile virus vaccine development. Expert Rev Vaccines. 2014;13(5):589–608.
168. Robinson ML, Enriquez K, Ho DY. A tale of two flaviviruses: West Nile virus and Zika virus in solid organ transplantation. OBM Transplantation. 2019;3(1). e-published.

Rare and Emerging Viral Infections in the Transplant Population

45

Susanna K. Tan, Jesse J. Waggoner, and Stan Deresinski

List of Abbreviations

AIDS	Acquired immune deficiency syndrome
APMV-1	Avian paramyxovirus 1
ATL	Adult T-cell leukemia
CDC	US Centers for Disease Control and Prevention
cDNA	Complementary DNA
CHIKV	Chikungunya virus
CMV	Cytomegalovirus
CSF	Cerebrospinal fluid
DENV	Dengue virus
DF	Dengue fever
DFA	Direct fluorescent antibody
DHF	Dengue hemorrhagic fever
DNA	Deoxyribonucleic acid
DSS	Dengue shock syndrome
FLAIR	Fluid-attenuated inversion recovery
GVHD	Graft-versus-host disease
HAM	HTLV-associated myelopathy
HBoV	Human bocavirus
HCV	Hepatitis C virus
HEV	Hepatitis E virus
HFRS	Hemorrhagic fever with renal syndrome
HHV-8	Human herpes virus 8
HIV	Human immunodeficiency virus
hMPV	Human metapneumovirus
HPS	Hantavirus pulmonary syndrome
HSCT	Hematopoietic stem cell transplant
HTLV-1	Human T-cell leukemia virus 1
HYSV	Huaiyangshan virus
Ig	Immunoglobulin
IHC	Immunohistochemistry
IV	Intravenous
IVIG	Intravenous immunoglobulin
JEV	Japanese encephalitis virus
LCMV	Lymphocytic choriomeningitis virus
MDMA	3,4-methylenedioxymethamphetamine (ecstasy)
MMLV	Moloney murine leukemia virus
MMR	Measles, mumps, and rubella vaccine
NP	Nasopharyngeal
OPO	Organ procurement organization
OPTN	US Organ Procurement and Transplantation Network
PARV4	Parvovirus 4
PBMC	Peripheral blood mononuclear cell
PCMV	Porcine cytomegalovirus
PCR	Polymerase chain reaction
PEP	Postexposure prophylaxis
PERV	Porcine endogenous retrovirus
PLHV	Porcine lymphotropic herpesvirus
RDA	Representation difference analysis
RNA	Ribonucleic acid
RSV	Respiratory syncytial virus
RT-PCR	Reverse transcription polymerase chain reaction
RVFV	Rift Valley fever virus
SARS	Severe adult respiratory syndrome
SFTSV	Severe fever with thrombocytopenia syndrome virus
SISPA	Sequence-independent single-primer amplification
SME	Subacute measles encephalitis
SOT	Solid organ transplant
TBEV	Tick-borne encephalitis virus
TNF	Tumor necrosis factor
TTV	Torque teno virus
USUV	Usutu virus
WNV	West Nile virus
XMRV	Xenotropic murine leukemia virus-related virus
YFV	Yellow fever virus
ZIKV	Zika virus

S. K. Tan (✉) · S. Deresinski
Stanford University School of Medicine, Department of Medicine, Division of Infectious Diseases and Geographic Medicine, Stanford, CA, USA
e-mail: susietan@stanford.edu; stan@polishmd.com

J. J. Waggoner
Emory University School of Medicine, Department of Medicine, Division of Infectious Diseases, Atlanta, GA, USA
e-mail: jesse.j.waggoner@emory.edu

A. Safdar (ed.), *Principles and Practice of Transplant Infectious Diseases*, https://doi.org/10.1007/978-1-4939-9034-4_45

Introduction

An emerging infectious disease, as defined by the Institute of Medicine and adopted by the CDC, is an infectious disease whose incidence in the human population has increased in the preceding two decades or threatens to increase in the near future [1, 2]. Viral diseases account for a large proportion of such infections, and the emerging viruses are typically divided into two groups: (1) newly identified viruses and (2) previously recognized viruses with an apparent increase in disease incidence [3, 4]. When applied to the transplant population, this second category can include agents with no recognized pathogenicity in the immunocompetent patient and those that result in atypical, more frequent, or more severe disease presentations in the immunocompromised host [5].

In this chapter, we will begin by discussing viral diagnostics and the rapidly evolving field of viral discovery, which has increased the speed of virus identification but has brought along new challenges for clinicians and researchers. Our focus then shifts to discussing specific emerging and re-emerging viral pathogens in the transplant community (see Tables 45.1 and 45.2). A number of emerging viral pathogens in the transplant population are discussed in detail in other chapters throughout this text (human herpes virus 7, human metapneumovirus, hepatitis E virus (HEV), novel polyomaviruses, and non-SARS coronaviruses) and will not be covered further here. Recent reviews in the literature have also discussed the topics of emerging viral infections in transplant recipients generally [4–10], as well as in solid organ transplant (SOT) [11] and hematopoietic stem cell transplant (HSCT) recipients specifically [12].

Following the discussion of emerging viral pathogens identified in the transplant community, we will briefly discuss global emerging viral pathogens, including flaviviruses, alphaviruses, bunyaviruses, and filoviruses. Given the nature of many of these pathogens, including their endemic ranges or relatively recent identification, few, if any, reports exist on their presentation in transplant recipients. Finally, we discuss the special situation of xenotransplantation and the reporting of suspected emerging viral diseases.

Table 45.1 Rare and emerging viral infections in the transplant population: case series or multiple cases reported [10]

Species	Virus family	Transplant	Clinical manifestations	Comments
HTLV-1	*Retroviridae*	SOT and HSCT; donor-derived infections reported	Adult T-cell leukemia and HTLV-1 associated myelopathy	Associated with lower survival after HSCT from HTLV-1+ donor
Rabies	*Rhabdoviridae*	SOT, ileac artery graft, cornea transplants; all cases donor-derived	Fatal encephalitis; cornea transplants present with pain in eye with graft	Survivors reported: cornea transplant with immediate PEP; liver transplant 20 years after vaccination; two exposed cornea transplants, grafts negative by RT-PCR
LCMV and a novel arenavirus	*Arenaviridae*	SOT; all reported cases donor-derived	Fever, abdominal pain, nausea, vomiting, diarrhea, altered mental status; often peri-incisional rash and tenderness	14 of 17 patients died; ribavirin employed but effect unclear; three cornea transplants unaffected; evidence of LCMV in donor rarely found
Measles	*Paramyxoviridae*	SOT and HSCT	Occasional clinical measles; SME (afebrile, altered mental status, intractable seizures); interstitial pneumonia	SME fatal in 4/6 transplant patients; case series suggest severe measles represents minority of cases in transplant patients
Mumps	*Paramyxoviridae*	SOT and HSCT	Parotitis, orchitis, vestibular neuronitis, and renal allograft involvement (SOT); fatal encephalitis (HSCT)	Three cases in SOT, all renal transplant patients and all survived; single case in HSCT
Dengue	*Flaviviridae*	SOT and HSCT	Dengue fever, severe dengue including hemorrhagic fever and shock; single case of colitis reported	Dengue shock associated with high mortality; rates of severe dengue differ in case series
Orf	*Poxviridae*	SOT; infected from contact with infected sheep	Giant and recurrent skin lesions on hands and forearms	Often misdiagnosed and treated with excision or amputation; case reports document responses to cryotherapy, cidofovir cream, or imiquimod
Bocavirus	*Parvoviridae*	SOT and HSCT	Associated with LRTI in young children; disseminated infection in transplant patients documented	Clinical significance of infection or reactivation in the immunocompromised patient remains unclear; no treatment available
Parvovirus 4	*Parvoviridae*	SOT	Associated with "viral syndrome" or early HIV; detected in renal and lung transplant recipients	Clinical significance in the immunocompromised patient remains unclear, thus far not associated with disease

Reprinted from Waggoner et al. [10], by permission of Oxford University Press

HSCT hematopoietic stem cell transplant, *HTLV-1* human T-cell leukemia virus 1, *IVDU* intravenous drug users, *LCMV* lymphocytic choriomeningitis virus, *LRTI* lower respiratory tract infection, *PEP* postexposure prophylaxis, *SME* subacute measles encephalitis, *SOT* solid organ transplant

Table 45.2 Rare and emerging infections in the transplant population: single cases reported [10]

Species	Virus family	Transplant	Clinical manifestations	Comments
APMV-1	*Paramyxoviridae*	HSCT	Fatal pneumonia; no other pathogens identified	Known pathogen in birds; tested in virotherapy for certain malignancies
Chikungunya	*Togaviridae*	SOT	Fever, headache, abdominal pain; no arthritis or arthralgia; recovered fully	Identified in four corneal grafts during Reunion outbreak, no transplant cases reported
Monkeypox	*Poxviridae*	HSCT	Fever and headache followed by characteristic rash (similar to smallpox)	Clinical course not reported as severe, patient recovered, though full details not reported
Usutu virus	*Flaviviridae*	SOT	Fever and headache; recovered but required prolonged rehabilitation	Viremic prior to developing liver failure and receiving liver transplant
Hantavirus	*Bunyaviridae*	SOT	Fever, headache, arthralgia, oliguric renal failure	Dobrava-Belgrade virus isolated (mild HFRS), no cases of HPS reported

Reprinted from Waggoner et al. [10], by permission of Oxford University Press

APMV-1 avian paramyxovirus 1, *HFRS* hemorrhagic fever with renal syndrome, *HPS* hantavirus pulmonary syndrome, *HSCT* hematopoietic stem cell transplant, *SOT* solid organ transplant

Methods

The body of literature referenced in this chapter is no doubt fraught with bias as it is largely based on case reports and small case series. Our understanding of most of these emerging viral infections, including their incidence, clinical manifestations, diagnosis, and management, in the immunocompromised host is limited, and larger, prospective studies in endemic areas are necessary. With the increasing number of transplants, both SOT and HSCT, performed globally, any description of emerging viral infections in this population will require frequent monitoring and updating. For the purposes of this chapter, we performed searches of the medical literature in PubMed, limited to studies reported in English. Searches were performed through May of 2016, using the name of the virus family, genus, or species of interest matched with the search terms "transplant," "transplant*," and "immunocompromised." We also performed general searches for emerging viruses and transplant recipients to identify case reports of novel or rare pathogens causing disease in transplant recipients. Finally, we included pertinent references from the publications identified during our search. With rare exceptions, we excluded reports involving only patients with HIV or AIDS.

Viral Discovery and Disease Association

Clinical virology laboratories affiliated with transplant centers typically employ a range of techniques for the diagnosis of viral infections from patient samples as well as for the quantitation and resistance testing of certain viruses. These techniques include, but are not limited to, viral culture, serology, antigen detection, direct fluorescent antibody staining (DFA), polymerase chain reaction (PCR) and reverse-transcription PCR (RT-PCR), and sequencing of certain pathogens (particularly HIV). While viral diagnostics are discussed in detail elsewhere in the text, we will briefly discuss these tests in the context of emerging viral infections followed by a discussion of newer technologies employed in viral discovery.

Viral culture provides a semi-unbiased technique for virus identification from patient samples, though this is a labor-intensive process and often requires days to weeks to detect viral growth. Many viral pathogens do not grow well, or do not grow at all, in cell culture, and viral detection is limited by the range of cells on which a given virus will grow and the number of cell lines a given lab can maintain. Even when cytopathic effect develops in a cell monolayer, the virus has to be identified by other means (often DFA or PCR). The majority of the viruses discussed in this chapter are diagnosed by other means, though agents such as lymphocytic choriomeningitis virus (LCMV) and dengue can be grown in culture as well [13, 14].

The other testing modalities routinely offered in a clinical virology lab, or even specialized tests performed at state and national reference laboratories, utilize conserved sequences (in the case of PCR or RT-PCR) or specific antigens or antibodies to detect the causative virus in patient samples. Hence, pathogen detection is limited by the knowledge and judgment of the ordering clinician or the available tests. The increasing use of multiplex testing for clinical syndromes, particularly for respiratory tract infections, will allow for a less biased approach to viral diagnosis but still faces limitations in identifying rare or emerging pathogens [15]. It should be noted that in very rare situations, as in the case of Usutu virus (USUV) discussed below, an unusual or novel pathogen may be detected by testing for known pathogens. In this case, a woman presented with USUV viremia, which gave a low-positive result by WNV PCR and was eventually identified by sequencing [16].

Viral discovery has typically relied on the replication of a new virus in cell culture. Despite the aforementioned limitations of viral culture, this technique remains useful, as indicated by the identification of two novel bunyaviruses, Huaiyangshan virus (HYSV, also known as severe fever with thrombocytopenia syndrome virus, SFTSV) in China and Heartland virus [17, 18] A number of more rapid molecular methods are now being employed in viral discovery; however, these are typically categorized as sequence-dependent (such as the pan-viral microarray or PCR based on conserved sequences) or sequence-independent techniques [19]. The pan-viral microarray (Virochip) is an array spotted with oligonucleotide sequences representing all known viral pathogens. Novel viruses can also be identified if there is sufficient similarity between sequences in the new virus and those included on the array. Amplicons can be then be recovered from the array, cloned, and sequenced [20]. This technology has been used in the identification of the SARS coronavirus, XMRV, and was also tested as a means to rapidly identify the 2009 pandemic influenza strain (H1N1) [19, 21]. PCR based on conserved sequences is possible but generally has limited applicability in viral diagnostics, as viruses do not contain highly conserved sequences analogous to the 16s ribosomal sequences utilized in bacterial identification [22]. One example of this is the performance of PCR using primer sets that amplify members of a virus family followed by sequencing, as reported in the identification of USUV from patient samples using a pan-flavivirus RT-PCR [16, 23].

The sequence-independent amplification and sequencing of nucleic acids in biological fluids or environmental samples has been termed viral metagenomics [19, 24]. Sequence-independent approaches include subtractive hybridization or representation difference analysis (RDA), sequence-independent single–primer amplification (SISPA), rolling circle amplification, and next-generation sequencing. Subtractive hybridization or representational difference analysis (RDA) uses infected and uninfected samples from an individual patient. Viral nucleic acid is selectively concentrated by repeated rounds of hybridization and purification of the unhybridized, single-stranded nucleic acid molecules, which are then subcloned and sequenced. These techniques have been used in the identification of human herpes virus 8 (HHV-8) and the torque teno viruses (TTV), but they require large amounts of starting material as well as relatively high virus levels [19, 22, 25]. SISPA circumvents the need for large amounts of viral genomic material. This technique, introduced in 1991, and its derivations involve the attachment of a linker/primer to blunt-ended nucleic acid and the subsequent amplification of all nucleic acid present, followed by cDNA library creation and sequencing [26]. SISPA was utilized in the identification of HEV, Norwalk virus, and Parvovirus 4 [22, 27]. Rolling circle amplification involves the use of the PhiX29 polymerase primed with random primers to amplify circular viral genomes or cloned fragments. It was used in the identification of human bocavirus (HBoV) among others [19, 28].

Viral metagenomics has been aided in the last few years by the development of a number of new sequencing platforms. Termed "next-generation sequencing" or "deep-sequencing," such technologies allow for the rapid and parallel generation of one million to over one billion sequences per run. Most of the current technologies rely on the non-specific amplification of DNA or RNA molecules followed by sequencing by synthesis using different technologies to detect base incorporation [22, 24, 29, 30]. Recently, single-molecule sequencing has become available, and this technology continues to develop, resulting in a greater number of reads (i.e., deeper sequencing) and longer read lengths [30]. These technologies are able to detect viral copy numbers near the limit of detection for specific quantitative PCR assays and have been shown to be more sensitive than microarray analysis (2 per 10^6 versus 1 per 10^5 sequences in one study) [31, 32]. Next-generation sequencing has been utilized to identify novel viruses in patient samples (see arenaviruses below) and determine the cause of fevers of unknown origin [32–35]. The potential utility of direct sequencing in the outbreak setting has also been shown following the 2009 influenza pandemic [21].

Deep sequencing, to the extent that it is sensitive and sequence-independent, has a great ability to detect both known and previously unknown (divergent) viruses as well as provide phylogenetic information. What it cannot do, however, is demonstrate causation. For many of these viruses, classical Koch's postulates cannot be applied, and as recently demonstrated in the cases of TTV, GB virus C, and human bocavirus (HBoV), establishing a causative role for many of these agents can be difficult [22, 25, 36]. Mokili and colleagues have instead proposed an approach they call "Metagenomic Koch's Postulates," but whether they are sufficient remains a matter for discussion [22].

At this time (and for the near future), next-generation sequencing remains a tool for research purposes rather than clinical diagnostics. Sequencing reactions take a good deal of time to set up and perform, with run times between 12 h and 14 days [29]. These runs also generate massive amounts of data that must be filtered to remove human and low-complexity sequence prior to analysis using various alignment programs designed to handle the large numbers of short reads [29, 32]. Finally, results must be interpreted carefully, as contaminants from the laboratory and even from commercial reagents, such as Moloney murine leukemia virus (MMLV, from polymerase preparations), are often identified [21, 32]. Confirming the presence of a virus identified with small numbers of sequences can also be difficult. In the study of metagenomics following the 2009 influenza pandemic, one patient from British Columbia was found to have two sequences matching an Ebola Sudan isolate, and during the evaluation of children in Nicaragua with fevers of unknown origin, a child had sequence similar to African swine fever virus [21, 32]. Run-time and data management and analysis will need to be streamlined before such technology will be applicable for relatively routine use in a clinical laboratory.

Emerging and Re-emerging Pathogens

Human T-Cell Leukemia Virus Type 1

Human T-cell leukemia virus type 1 (HTLV-1) infection is endemic in Japan, West Africa, South America, the Middle East, and the Caribbean with seroprevalence ranging approximately from 3% to 30%, while in western countries <1% are infected [37]. Most of the millions who are affected acquired their infections vertically via breast milk, but this retrovirus may also be transmitted by blood transfusion, sharing of needles, and organ transplantation. A number of complications are associated with chronic HTLV-1 infection, most frequently adult T-cell leukemia (ATL) and HTLV-associated myelopathy (HAM), which occur in 5% or fewer of those infected. Immunosuppression administered to transplant recipients who are HTLV-1 carriers may trigger progression to these known complications of the infection (for a brief summary, see Table 45.1) [38–40]. Numerous reports document the devastating clinical impact of ATL and HAM from HTLV-1 infection in solid organ transplant recipients [38, 41, 42]. The majority of these cases are from Spain and Japan, though additional reports in the United States have surfaced in recent years involving donors and recipients with expected epidemiologic risk factors (i.e., residence in endemic regions) [43, 44].

Complications from HTLV-1 can be a result of reactivation disease in HTLV-1/2 seropositive recipients, de novo primary infection, and donor-derived infection in organ transplant recipients. In a nationwide survey in Japan, Yoshizumi et al. identified 82 living donor liver transplant recipients who were HTLV-1 positive prior to transplantation. ATL developed in 5 of these 26 (15.4%) after intervals of 181–1315 days after transplantation. All five died, four due to ATL and one due to rejection after reduction in immunosuppressive therapy. In a compelling case series of donor-derived HTLV-1 infection, liver and two kidney recipients from HTLV-1 seropositive donor were acutely infected with HTLV-1 with rapid dissemination early in the posttransplant period. HTLV-1 provirus was detected by PCR on days 16–23 and increased by 2–3 logs by day 38–45, after which steady state was reached. HTLV-1 antibodies were first detected between 16 and 39 days following transplantation. Alignment of the HTLV-1 5′ LTR of the donor and the three recipients showed 100% sequence identity consistent with a common viral source of infection. Though no cases of early onset or rapid progression of HAM were observed in this series, in another case series, all three HLTV-1-negative recipients of organs from a single HTLV-1-positive donor (two kidney transplants and a liver transplant) developed antibodies to the retrovirus and developed HAM within the 2 years of transplantation. HTLV-1 isolates from these three recipients were homologous to the donor isolate by DNA sequencing [45, 46]. Two case reports also document the occurrence of HAM in a heart transplant recipient and an HSCT recipient who both acquired HTLV-1 through blood transfusions [39, 47].

Despite these case examples, clinical disease due to HTLV-1 occurs infrequently after solid organ transplantation, even in endemic regions with high seroprevalence [38, 41, 42]. Shirai et al. reviewed the courses of nine HTLV-1-positive patients who underwent renal transplantation with basiliximab (anti-CD25) induction together with corticosteroids, mycophenolate mofetil, and cyclosporine or tacrolimus. No patient developed ATL or HAM during follow-up of approximately 5 years, although one patient died of aspiration pneumonia 17 days after transplantation [48]. A previous study also found no cases of ATL in 16 HTLV-1-positive kidney transplant recipients after up to 10 years of observation, at which point patient survival was 81%. Patient and graft survival were not significantly different from HTLV-1 negative patients [49]. Smaller reports from western Japan (10 patients with up to 17 years of follow-up) and Iran (10 patients with up to 6 years of follow-up) presented similar findings [50, 51].

While screening of donors may prevent the transmission of HTLV-1 to recipients, the demand for organs may override this concern, even in highly endemic areas such as certain regions of Japan. In regions with low rates of infection, screening of all donors generates many false positives, resulting in delays in transplantation or the loss of potential organs for donation. Following the three cases of donor-derived HTLV-1 infection in Spain, 2870 potential organ donors and recipients were screened for antibodies to HTLV-1, including 1079 immigrants. Only five patients tested positive (confirmed by Western blot), and all of them were immigrants from South America or Africa [52]. The practice of universal HTLV-1 screening is no longer recommended by the United States Organ Procurement and Transplantation Network (OPTN) [37, 53]. However, targeted screening for HTLV-1/2 seropositivity by organ procurement organizations (OPO) may be encouraged in high-risk living and deceased donors based on local prevalence data [43, 54].

HSCT has been used in the treatment of ATL in HTLV-1-positive patients, but since leukemia is a known complication of HTLV-1 infection, it can be asked if HSCT is safe and effective in such patients. Near relatives are the preferred sources of stem cells for transplantation, but in endemic areas, such individuals are also frequently infected with this retrovirus. The largest study addressing this question involved a retrospective analysis of data from three centers in Japan. In this study, 386 patients with ATL underwent allogeneic HSCT with a 3-year survival rate of 33%. Unfortunately, those who received their transplant from a related HTLV-1-positive donor had a higher risk of disease-associated mortality relative to those whose related donor was HTLV-1 negative. HSCT recipients in complete remission at the time of transplantation had a higher rate of survival compared to patients not in complete remission (51% versus 26%). These results likely account for the finding that patients who received an HSCT from matched unrelated donors did as well as those from matched related donors (3-year survival, 39% versus 41%) [55]. No proven effective therapy for HAM exists. Some experts suggest antiviral prophylaxis with zidovudine and raltegravir, but antiviral therapy drugs are generally believed to have little effect on HTLV-1 because it is a cell-associated virus and proviral load is predominantly maintained by cell division of infected cells rather than free viral replication. Furthermore, definitive long-term benefits of interferon and corticosteroids have yet to be established [43].

Rabies Virus

Rabies virus is a member of the *Rhabdoviridae* family of RNA viruses and is one of seven species belonging to the genus *Lyssavirus*. All of these viruses except for Lagos bat virus have resulted in fatal human disease, but at this time, only rabies has been reported in the transplant population [56]. Rabies virus is typically acquired in humans through the bite of an infected animal. It is estimated that over 55,000 cases occur annually, worldwide, and most result from the bite of an infected dog [56, 57]. In countries where canine vaccination is routine, bites from insectivorous bats have emerged as the most common source [57]. Rabies infection results in an encephalitis that is nearly universally fatal unless the patient has been vaccinated or receives postexposure prophylaxis (PEP). Limited data suggest that some individuals can survive rabies exposure without intervention, including a single case in the United States and serologic data from humans in the Peruvian Amazon, but these cases appear to be rare [58, 59].

Sixteen cases of rabies have been reported in transplant recipients, and to date, all of these cases have been transmitted through the transplanted tissue or organ (Table 45.1) [60–70]. Houff et al. first reported the transmission of rabies through a corneal graft in 1979 [66]. Since that time, eight other cases of rabies transmission have occurred through corneal transplantation. In seven of these nine cases, the cornea recipients presented with neurological symptoms within 40 days of their surgery and died soon after admission. Symptoms often included significant pain involving the eye that received the transplant [61, 62, 65–67]. In a case from France, reported in 1981, a patient exposed to rabies through corneal transplant survived after receiving PEP on the first postoperative day [70]. A second corneal transplant recipient, documented in a report from India, received partial PEP but then refused further treatment. He developed rabies 9 months after transplant and died shortly thereafter [67].

Three clusters of rabies cases have occurred following solid organ transplantation. The first four cases occurred in Texas in 2004 [63, 64, 69]. Rabies developed following the transplantation of the liver, both kidneys, and an iliac artery graft from an Arkansas man who died after being diagnosed with a subarachnoid hemorrhage. All four patients developed encephalitis within 30 days of transplantation and died between 7 and 23 days later. The diagnosis was confirmed by serology in the three recipients, immunohistochemistry (IHC) staining of pathological samples, and viral isolation in cell culture. During the follow-up investigation, it was determined that the donor had been bitten by a bat shortly before organ donation [69].

The second cluster of cases occurred in Germany in 2005 but was not widely published until 2010 [71–73]. Six patients were potentially exposed to rabies virus following the death of a 26-year-old woman, who died after presenting with altered mental status. She had reportedly consumed cocaine, amphetamines, and MDMA before her admission, developed cerebral edema, and was declared brain dead. During a contact investigation after the report of cases, it was discovered that she had been bitten by a dog on a recent trip to India. PEP was administered to all six transplant recipients (lung, liver, kidney, kidney-pancreas, and both corneas), though not until at least 45 days after transplantation. The recipients of lung, kidney, and kidney-pancreas transplants died of rabies. Antiviral treatment was administered (with ribavirin and interferon) in these three cases as well as in the case of the liver transplant recipient. The lung recipient died on posttransplantation day 49 despite the initiation of deep sedation with ketamine and midazolam. The kidney transplant recipient died on day 52 despite the addition of amantadine but not deep sedation. The kidney-pancreas recipient was also treated with deep sedation starting with midazolam followed by ketamine and phenobarbital. Brain death was declared after 9 weeks and supportive measures discontinued. The liver transplant recipient had been vaccinated against rabies over 20 years before transplantation and never developed disease [71, 72]. Both corneal grafts were explanted, but rabies virus was not detected in either cornea by RT-PCR. It has been suggested that the lack of rabies in these corneal grafts was the result of the limited excision procedure performed such as subcorneal complex excision rather than enucleation and the prolonged storage of the grafts prior to transplant for 5 days [72, 73].

In 2013, another case of transplant-transmitted rabies was identified in the United States. Signs and symptoms of rabies developed in a deceased-donor kidney recipient, a Maryland native, 17 months after transplantation, who ultimately died from rabies 3 weeks after hospitalization. Given lack of epidemiologic risk factors, an exploration of donor transmission was sought. In addition to a clinical presentation consistent with rabies in the organ donor, a raccoon rabies virus variant more than 99.9% identical across the entire N gene was identified in both the organ donor and the infected recipient. The genetic sequence was also closely associated with a raccoon variant circulating in North Carolina, the donor's state of residence [74]. Three unvaccinated recipients of organs (kidney, liver, and heart) from the same donor were asymptomatic when rabies was diagnosed in the donor. PEP with rabies vaccination and immunoglobulin was initiated in these asymptomatic organ transplant recipients, and protective neutralizing antibodies developed in all three [75].

As mentioned previously, the management of rabies focuses on prevention either with vaccination in high-risk patients or PEP following an animal bite. Three individuals have apparently recovered from rabies (diagnosed by antibody testing) without receiving either intervention. These have all been young women (aged 8, 15, and 17), and two patients received treatment with what is now called the Milwaukee protocol (named after Milwaukee, WI), which includes a prolonged therapeutic coma, antiviral therapy, management of vasospasm, and avoidance of prophylaxis [58, 76, 77]. To date, 30 patients have received the Milwaukee protocol, but only one other patient has survived to hospital discharge [78, 79]. This patient had received partial PEP, however [78]. In two reports (one case report and a case series of eight patients), transplant recipients who received rabies PEP appeared to mount an adequate response (antibody titers of 0.5 IU/mL), though titers were lower than those seen in immunocompetent patients [80–82]. Rodriguez-Romo et al. reported the case of a kidney transplant recipient who received two courses of PEP after being bitten by a rabid dog. Following the first course, adequate antibody titers developed but then declined. A second PEP course was administered along with a reduction in immunosuppression; he maintained an adequate antibody level and remained asymptomatic [81]. Taken together, these data indicate that rabies vaccination can be effective, even after transplantation, and PEP may be safe and effective in transplant recipients.

Lymphocytic Choriomeningitis Virus and the Arenaviridae

Lymphocytic choriomeningitis virus (LCMV) is a member of the Old World complex of *Arenaviridae*, a family of viruses that also contains important hemorrhagic fever pathogens endemic in Africa and South America. LCMV was the first isolated arenavirus, identified in 1933 during an outbreak of St. Louis encephalitis [83]. Infection with LCMV in the immunocompetent host is often mild or asymptomatic. Symptomatic infections present as aseptic meningitis, but the mortality in immunocompetent patients is <1%. In the largest recorded outbreak, 181 cases were documented in the United States associated with pet hamsters. While 46 patients were hospitalized, no one died [83–85].

In contrast to the clinical course of infection in immunocompetent patients, five clusters of cases following LCMV transmission through organ transplantation (including 17 cases and 12 deaths) document the ability of this pathogen to cause severe disease in transplant recipients (Table 45.1) [13, 33, 86–88]. Another cluster of cases involved the transmission of a newly identified arenavirus in Australia (three patients, all of whom died) [33]. As in rabies infections documented in transplant recipients, all of these cases resulted from human-to-human transmission through organ transplantation [13, 33, 86, 87]. At this time, cases acquired following transplant by exposure to rodents and their excreta have not been described. Also, cases have not been described in the HSCT population.

All five reported case clusters of LCMV infection occurred in SOT recipients in the United States (ten kidney, four liver, and three lung transplants). The first set of cases took place in 2003 in Wisconsin (four cases, four deaths), followed by clusters in 2005 in Massachusetts and Rhode Island (four cases, three deaths), 2008 in Massachusetts (two cases, two deaths), 2011 in Arkansas (four cases, two deaths), and 2013 in Iowa [13, 86–88]. Symptoms developed between 2 and 23 days posttransplant and included fever, abdominal pain, nausea, diarrhea, and altered mental status occasionally accompanied by seizures. A number of patients also developed a peri-incisional rash and tenderness. Laboratory findings included increased transaminases and creatinine. Both leucopenia and leukocytosis occurred. CSF findings included elevated protein (often marked), normal to low glucose, and a mild pleocytosis. The diagnosis of LCMV was confirmed in all patients using IHC on tissue samples or RT-PCR on tissue and serum samples. Serology was performed less frequently and was often negative. Bronchopneumonia or diffuse alveolar damage and hepatic inflammation or necrosis were the most common findings at autopsy [13, 86, 87, 89].

Five patients survived LCMV infection following SOT, including four kidney transplant recipients and a single liver recipient. One kidney transplant patient received treatment with ribavirin starting on posttransplant day 26 (2005 cluster) and survived, though a second kidney transplant recipient was treated with ribavirin (2008 cluster, starting 6 weeks posttransplant) and died [13, 86]. Similarly, in the 2013 cluster, all three recipients received ribavirin therapy, and two also received intravenous immunoglobulin starting 6 weeks posttransplant, with survival in the two kidney recipients and death in the liver transplant recipient [88]. The two other survivors (2011 cluster) recovered without antiviral therapy [87]. Ribavirin has been shown to be clinically effective in the early treatment of Lassa fever, a related Old World arenavirus, but data for efficacy in the treatment of LCMV is lacking [90]. Four corneal transplant recipients were also potentially exposed to LCMV in these clusters, though none of them developed symptoms or seroconverted (two recipients in 2005 and a single recipient in 2011). The second cornea removed from the 2011 donor was never transplanted. This tissue tested negative for LCMV by IHC and RT-PCR [13, 87].

Contact investigation following these cases revealed exposure to rodents for two of the donors: a pet hamster (2005 donor) and rodent infestation of the home (2011 donor) [13, 87]. No definitive evidence of rodent exposure was discovered for the 2013 donor, although he had spent substantial time outside along the Mississippi River. Three of the donors also had positive LCMV testing: detectable IgM and IgG in archived serum from the day before death (2008 donor), a positive RT-PCR from a single lymph node (2011 donor), and a positive RT-PCR from aortic endothelial cells (2013 donor) [86–88]. Investigation into the 2003 donor revealed no clear exposure history and serology, viral culture, and IHC performed on other tissues collected at the time of donation were all negative [13, 91]. Likewise, all diagnostic testing (including RT-PCR) performed on stored samples from the 2005 donor was negative, and all further testing performed on samples from the 2011 donor was negative (including other lymph nodes) [13, 87]. It has been advised that immunocompromised patients avoid contact with rodents, including pets [92, 93]. While this recommendation seems intuitive, this was not the mode of acquisition in these outbreaks, and it is unclear to what extent this will prevent future LCMV cases in transplant recipients.

An additional cluster of arenavirus cases occurred after the transplantation of the kidneys and liver from a single donor to three recipients in Australia in 2007. Patients developed fever, altered mental status, pulmonary infiltrates, and graft rejection soon after transplant, and they died between 29 and 36 days posttransplant. While their clinical course is not discussed in great detail, it sounds similar to that described for LCMV. The agent was identified by next-generation sequencing (Roche, 454 pyrosequencing) as Dandenong virus following random primer amplification. Sequences were consistent with an arenavirus, though certain segments were closest to LCMV and others more closely resembled Kodoko virus (isolated in African wild mice) [33].

It has been noted that the clinical disease caused by LCMV and this newly identified arenavirus are more similar to the severe illnesses caused by the other Old World arenaviruses, Lassa and Lujo viruses, and the New World arenaviruses such as Junin, Machupo, and Guanarito viruses [91]. Infection with any of these pathogens can result in a viral hemorrhagic fever with varying degrees of encephalopathy [83, 90]. Cases of Lassa, Lujo, and New World arenavirus infections have not been described in immunocompromised patients, however. This absence of reporting may result from the relatively defined areas of endemicity for each virus as well as the limited number of transplants that are performed in those regions. Another possible explanation may stem from the unusual mode of transmission that leads to severe LCMV infection after SOT.

Human Bocavirus and Parvovirus 4

Human bocavirus (HBoV) and Parvovirus 4 (PARV4) are newly identified members of the *Parvoviridae* family of DNA viruses, subfamily *Parvovirnae*. Prior to their discovery, the only parvovirus known to infect humans was parvovirus B19. Both of these agents were identified in 2005, though there is a greater amount of clinical information on HBoV currently than PARV4 [27, 28, 94].

HBoV was initially detected in the nasopharyngeal (NP) aspirates of children with respiratory tract infections. Allander et al. randomly amplified DNA and RNA from these samples, followed by cloning and sequencing. This identified sequences similar to members of the genus *Bocavirus*, named for the type species *bo*vine parvovirus and *ca*nine minute virus. They then showed that 17 pediatric patients (of 540 screened) had HBoV detectable by PCR, and in 14 of these patients, HBoV was the only pathogen detected. All patients had been admitted with respiratory distress and ten had fevers. The virus was also predominantly detected in the winter months (14 of 17) [28].

Since the original study, a number of reports have confirmed the association between HBoV detection and respiratory tract infections, along with the seasonality of detection [95–102]. The establishment of HBoV as a pathogen, however, has been complicated by the high rates of detection of co-pathogens along with HBoV (up to 90%), detection of the virus in asymptomatic patients (43% in one study from Canada), and significant difference in the study design of published reports, including different methods of sample collection (NP swab, NP aspirate, or bronchoalveolar lavage) and the extent to which other pathogens were excluded [36, 97, 100]. It does appear that HBoV causes a subset of respiratory tract infections, particularly among infants and young children (<2 years of age), and the use of quantitative PCR may be a means to identify these patients. A 5.7% prevalence of HBoV has been reported from testing over 1800 NP swabs from healthy children presenting with a respiratory illness over a 3-year period [103]. In a separate study by Allander et al., patients with high HBoV viral loads (>10^4 copies/mL) in NP aspirates were more likely to have an isolated HBoV infection (though 18 of 28 patients still had another pathogen detected) and often had concomitant viremia detectable by PCR [95]. One study also reported an association between high HBoV viral loads in NP aspirates with longer duration of hospitalization in healthy pediatric children presenting with a respiratory illness [103]. The detection of HBoV in the blood is not necessarily surprising as other parvoviruses (B19 and PARV4) are also detected in this compartment. HBoV DNA has also been detected from stool, though its potential as a gastrointestinal pathogen is unclear [102].

The incidence and clinical manifestations of HBoV infections in the immunocompromised host have not been established (Table 45.1). In 2007, Schenk et al. reported the case of an HSCT recipient with disseminated HBoV infection. The patient was a 4-year-old boy who underwent HSCT and had a complicated hospital course including persistent fevers, which improved but did not completely resolve upon neutrophil engraftment, a lower respiratory tract infection, and diarrhea. HBoV was detected repeatedly from NP aspirates, serum, and stool, though its role in this case is complicated by the co-detection of rhinovirus from an NP aspirate, CMV reactivation, and grade I GVHD of the skin (no mention of path from the GI tract) [104]. In 2011, the same group reported on three more cases of immunocompromised patients (along with the case from 2007) with repeatedly positive tests for HBoV. These patients had virus detectable after weeks of isolation, often during the summer months, which supports the hypothesis that HBoV may establish latency and reactivate in the setting of a coinfection or impaired immunity [105]. Severe diarrhea was also reported in a 9-year-old transplant recipient (both liver and HSCT) associated with detectable HBoV in plasma and stool [106]. Other studies evaluating the role of HBoV as a respiratory pathogen in immunocompromised adults have detected the virus at low levels (or not at all) and have not documented a difference in outcomes between immunocompromised patients and immunocompetent controls [107–109].

Many significant questions remain regarding the significance of HBoV in the transplant population, both pediatric and adult. One seroepidemiologic study out of Japan showed that between 94% and 100% of individuals have been exposed to HBoV by 6 years of age [110]. If this virus establishes latency, most transplant recipients will be at risk to develop reactivation, but whether that results in disease or is simply a marker of severe immune suppression has yet to be determined. The reporting of HBoV will no doubt increase. There are a number of published PCR assays to use for detection, and at least one platform for multiplex respiratory pathogen detection includes HBoV in a panel of 21 agents [36, 111]. There is no specific antiviral treatment for HBoV at this time.

Much less clinical information on PARV4 exists. This virus was originally identified by SISPA from the serum of 1 of 25 patients presenting with an unidentified "viral syndrome" [27]. The virus has since been detected in a high percentage of patients who use IV drugs (30%) and patients with HIV-HCV co-infection (95%) [112, 113]. The clinical significance of these infections is unclear, though PARV4 may be associated with symptomatic early HIV infection [113]. One report also documents two cases of encephalitis of unclear etiology in children (2 and 3 years of age) where PARV4 DNA was detected in the CSF [114]. Studies in transplant recipients have documented PARV4 in 5 of 164 renal transplant recipients and 14 of 104 lung transplant recipients (Table 45.1). No associations with clinical outcome have been identified [112, 115].

Enterovirus D-68

Enterovirus D-68 (EV-D68) belongs to the family *Picornaviridae* and is the causative agent of an outbreak of severe respiratory illness in 2014 that began in the United States and spread to several countries around the world. EV-D68 was first identified in 1962 in four children suffering from pneumonia and bronchiolitis and, prior to 2014, detected in only a small number of patients [116]. The 2014 outbreak began concurrently in Kansas City, MO, and Chicago, IL, where an increase in hospitalizations for severe respiratory illness was noted in pediatric patients. Multiplex PCR assays detected an increase in rhinovirus/enterovirus in nasopharyngeal specimens. Evaluation by the CDC found 19 of 22 specimens from Kansas City and 11 of 14 specimens from Chicago positive for EV-D68. Of these 30 patients, 29 (96.7%) were admitted to the ICU and 6 (20.0%) required mechanical ventilation [117]. By the end of 2014, over 1100 cases of respiratory illness caused by EV-D68 had been *reported* in the United States, predominantly among children. Subsequently, more than 2000 cases of respiratory illness were attributed to EV-D68 in 20 countries worldwide [118, 119].

Though the manifestations of EV-D68 can be severe, EV-D68 more commonly causes an upper respiratory tract infection that does not require hospitalization. Factors that predispose to milder disease are incompletely understood, though several studies report asthma as a risk factor for ICU admission and need for mechanical ventilation [118, 120]. Concurrent with the respiratory outbreak, clusters of children with acute flaccid paralysis and severe neurologic disease were observed in the United States and Europe and attributed to EV-D68 given the temporal relationship of symptoms and detection of the virus in pharyngeal swabs [121]. EV-D68 has since been linked with acute paralytic poliomyelitis, encephalitis, myelitis, encephalomyelitis, or acute transverse myelitis [119]. As no specific vaccine or antiviral for EV-D68 exists, treatment of children with EV-D68 is mainly supportive and focused on symptom relief for fever and respiratory support if needed.

Few studies have evaluated the extent of EV-D68 infection in immunocompromised patients. Eight cases of EV-D68 in hematologic malignancy or HSCT recipients were found in one study, which retrospectively tested for the presence of the virus in respiratory samples (n = 506) that had tested positive for human rhinovirus (HRV) or negative for all respiratory viruses in a multiplex panel collected over a 3-month period. Thirteen (11.5%) cases originally identified as HRV were subsequently characterized as EV-D68 with a specific PCR assay, highlighting the limited specificity of HRV primers and the potential for inaccurate diagnosis. Furthermore, of the 393 cases initially negative for all respiratory viruses, 8 (2%) were presumptive EV-D68. This has implications for infection control as patients with negative tests results would likely be removed from droplet isolation and theoretically could result in person-to-person transmission particularly among immunocompromised patients. The eight cases of EVD-68 in hematologic malignancy or HSCT recipients (51–1833 days from transplant) developed symptoms ranging from mild upper respiratory tract infection to respiratory failure [122]. Cases were not limited to children, as all were in immunocompromised adults aged 22–69 years old. At this time, cases of EV-D68 in solid organ transplants have yet to be reported in the literature.

Measles, Mumps, and the Paramyxoviridae

The family *Paramyxoviridae* contains a number of significant human pathogens and is divided into two subfamilies, *Paramyxovirinae* and *Pneumovirinae*. The major pathogens within the *Pneumonvirinae*, respiratory syncytial virus (RSV) and human metapneumovirus (hMPV), are discussed in detail elsewhere in this text. *Paramyxovirinae* contains five genera and includes measles (*Morbillivirus*) and mumps (*Rubulavirus*), the emerging pathogens nipah and hendra (*Henipavirus*), as well as the avian pathogen, avian paramyxovirus 1 (APMV-1, also known as Newcastle disease virus; *Avulavirus*). Measles and mumps are not typically considered emerging pathogens. However, the potential to cause severe disease in transplant recipients as well as the recent rise in incidence for both agents brings them into consideration here [123–131]. Nipah, hendra, and APMV-1 will also be discussed briefly.

Measles and mumps are both vaccine preventable illnesses and following the introduction of the MMR vaccine in 1967, there was a marked decrease in the incidence of these diseases in developed countries [125]. However, immunity can wane over time, even after the recommended two dose series in the immunocompetent patient. This decline in humoral immunity has been well documented in the transplant population, and even following repeat vaccination, response rates are suboptimal [132–135]. Repeat MMR vaccination posttransplant appears to be safe, and this topic will be covered in detail in a later chapter [133–135].

Severe disease in transplant recipients has more often been reported as a result of measles infection than mumps. The most significant manifestation of measles in this patient population is subacute measles encephalitis (SME, also reported as immunosuppressive measles encephalitis or measles inclusion body encephalitis), but severe cases of pneumonia and one case of liver transplant rejection possibly resulting from measles have also been reported (Table 45.1) [127, 129, 130, 136–142]. SME was originally documented in patients immunocompromised from chemotherapy or malignancy, and the disease was first reported in a renal transplant recipient in 1979 [127]. It has since been reported in other renal transplant recipients, though not always confirmed by IHC staining or RT-PCR, and a single patient following HSCT [129, 136, 141, 143]. Patients with SME may initially present with an illness compatible with measles, including fever, conjunctivitis, and a rash, though this is not consistent and typically is only recognized as measles in retrospect [127, 136, 139, 141]. Patients typically improve but then re-present with altered mental status and seizures between 2 weeks and 4 months after their initial illness. In a review of the literature, the range was 1–7 months, but this included predominantly nontransplant patients [129, 136, 139, 141]. At the time of admission for seizures, fevers are particularly uncommon, and CT imaging and CSF analysis are often normal. The first imaging changes are seen by MRI with increased signal intensity on FLAIR. The clinical course is one of deteriorating mental status and worsening seizures refractory to anti-epileptic drugs [127, 129, 136, 139]. Four of six transplant cases of SME died. The two survivors were reported in 2006 by Turner et al. Both cases occurred in pediatric renal transplant recipients, 6 and 11 years out from transplant. They both received one dose of IVIG and a course of IV ribavirin. Both of them survived, though both had significant neurological deficits [141]. A single case of SME occurred in a previously healthy boy following MMR vaccination, though during admission, he was found to have a primary immune deficiency [144].

The incidence of severe measles in transplant recipients is unclear as most of the data comes from case reports and reviews of the literature. In an attempt to answer this question, Machado et al. evaluated 156 HSCT recipients during the 1997 outbreak of measles in Sao Paolo. These investigators identified eight cases among 54 patients deemed to be susceptible (based on an IgG $\leq$ 100 mIU/mL), and notably, only one of them had severe disease, manifested as interstitial pneumonia. All eight patients survived [138]. It has been noted that the case definition, requiring a serological response (appearance of IgM or rise in IgG), may be too restrictive for HSCT recipients, resulting in a number of missed cases [145]. A second, short report by Lee et al. documented a fatal case of pneumonia in an HSCT recipient clinically diagnosed with measles during an outbreak in Korea from 2000 to 2001. At their center, they presumptively diagnosed 16 HSCT recipients with measles (methods not specified), with this as the only case of severe disease. The patient who died of pneumonia never developed detectable IgM or IgG [137]. The incidence of measles in SOT and HSCT recipients remains unclear, though given the 222 cases of measles in the United States and tens of thousands of cases in Europe in 2011, it is likely under reported [128, 131].

Five cases of posttransplant mumps infection have been documented, including three renal transplant recipients and two HSCT recipients (Table 45.1) [123, 124, 146–148]. The three renal transplant patients developed parotid gland swelling. Two patients showed involvement of their graft: one in a patient with a failed graft already on dialysis and the second with a previously functioning graft who developed tubulointerstitial nephritis and permanent graft failure. This second patient also developed orchitis and vestibular neuronitis with persistent vertigo after recovery. All three patients survived [123, 146, 147]. Both cases in the HSCT literature document fatal encephalitis in young patients with severe combined immunodeficiency treated with HSCT. The first patient was a 16-month-old infant who developed meningoencephalitis and seizures prior to HSCT and deteriorated rapidly after transplant. Mumps was isolated in culture from urine, blood, and CSF. The infant had been vaccinated for mumps several months prior, and the authors suggest the vaccine strain as the potential cause of infection [124]. The second patient was a 19-year-old who developed subacute encephalomyelitis from a wild-type mumps strain 2 years after HSCT. Infection occurred during an outbreak of mumps in England and Wales in 2004 and 2005 [148].

APMV-1 causes lethal infections in birds and has been tested as a potential agent for virotherapy in certain malignancies [149]. Cases in humans have rarely been documented and typically involve an acute, self-limited conjunctivitis, often in poultry workers. In 2007, Goebel et al. reported a case of pneumonia in a 42-year-old HSCT recipient where APMV-1 was isolated in culture from bronchoalveolar lavage fluid, a lung biopsy, stool, and urine (identity confirmed by sequencing; Table 45.2). The patient died after 24 days, and IHC was consistent with APMV-1 infection. No other pathogens were isolated, though the patient was on broad spectrum antibiotics at the time of bronchoscopy [150].

Nipah and hendra viruses (and the recently identified Cedar virus, which will not be discussed further) comprise the genus *Henipavirus* and were identified in the 1990s as causes of encephalitis [151–153]. Old World fruit bats serve as the natural host for nipah and hendra, but these pathogens are notable among the *Paramyxoviridae* for their ability to infect a wide range of hosts, including pigs, horses, and humans. Hendra has been transmitted from horses to their handlers, and nipah has been transmitted from pigs and bats to humans [152, 154]. Human-to-human spread of nipah has also been documented in recent outbreaks [154–156]. Infection resulting from either virus can result in severe respiratory tract disease, encephalitis, or both. In a series of 92 cases of encephalitis from Bangladesh, 69% of patients also had respiratory difficulty, though this rate was higher than that seen in a series from Malaysia (21%) [157, 158]. Mortality from encephalitis has ranged from 30% to 70% in different series, and residual neurological deficits can persist in survivors [157, 158]. An unusual feature of infection with either of these viruses is the occurrence of relapsing or late-onset encephalitis that has been documented to occur up to 22 months after initial presentation and still carries a high mortality [159]. Treatment remains supportive. In the large series reported to date, which involve nipah virus, there have not been documented cases involving transplant recipients or immunocompromised hosts, though the comorbid illnesses of patients included in these series have not been fully described [157, 158].

Poxviridae

Poxviridae is a family of large DNA viruses that includes four genera (among many) of viruses with the potential to infect humans: *Orthopoxvirus* (including variola), *Molluscipoxvirus* (including molluscum contagiosum virus), *Parapoxvirus*, and *Yatapoxvirus*. Molluscum contagiosum is widely recognized, and in the immunocompromised patient, molluscum contagiosum virus infection can cause an eruption of large and widespread skin lesions. We will not discuss this agent further in this chapter.

Orf virus, a *Parapoxvirus*, is a well-known pathogen in sheep, particularly young lambs, and causes papulovesicular lesions in the mouth and groin of affected animals [160, 161]. Orf lesions, also known as ecthyma contagiosum, also occur in humans. These lesions tend to be solitary and occur on the extremities of individuals who work with infected sheep. In the immunocompetent patient, these lesions are self-limited and tend to heal over 1–2 months [160, 161]. In transplant and immunocompromised patients, however, a number of cases of recurrent and giant orf lesions have been reported (Table 45.1) [160–164]. These lesions can be 5 cm or more in diameter and have been confined to the hand or forearm. All patients reported contact with sheep. Patients have undergone excision with skin grafting or even amputation when these lesions are not diagnosed correctly, but even with such aggressive treatment, lesions tend to recur after a few weeks to months [160, 162–164]. A single patient also developed a new lesion at the skin-graft donor site [164]. While no standard treatment exists, three case-reports document responses in renal transplant patients using cryotherapy, cidofovir cream, or imiquimod (a single case for each treatment) [161, 163, 164]. The patients treated with cryotherapy and cidofovir required a second course of treatment but again responded well [161, 163].

Cases of human monkeypox, an *Orthopoxvirus*, were first recognized in 1970 during the vaccination campaigns to eradicate smallpox, though earlier cases may have been diagnosed as the clinically similar smallpox [165, 166]. Outbreaks of disease continue in the Democratic Republic of the Congo and neighboring Sudan, and indeed, the incidence appears to be increasing after cessation of routine smallpox vaccination over 30 years ago [165–167]. In 2003, the first cases of monkeypox outside of Africa occurred in the Midwestern United States, with 37 confirmed cases associated with exposure to sick pet prairie dogs that in turn had been infected by rodents imported from West Africa [152, 166, 168]. Though fatal cases of monkeypox in Africa are well described, no fatalities were reported among these 37 patients [167–169]. Nine patients were described as having severe disease, including a single case each of encephalitis and respiratory distress, and five patients were hospitalized. One patient described in the series had received an HSCT, but they were not reported among the cases of severe disease and appear to have recovered fully (Table 45.2) [152, 166, 168].

A novel orthopoxvirus was recently identified to cause a rash illness in a renal transplant recipient who was 26 months posttransplantation. The patient developed a tender, erythematous, and indurated rash with development of vesiculopustular lesions on the right lateral chest wall. Multiple debridements failed to demonstrate the causative agent and were negative for HSV and VZV by IHC straining and acid-fast and fungal organisms by special staining. A dense inflammatory infiltrate composed of lymphocytes, histiocytes, and focal eosinophils extending into the subcutaneous adipose tissue was consistently demonstrated on multiple specimens. Culture on human epithelial type 2 cells and BSC40 cells demonstrated viral cytopathic effects, but could not be further identified with standard evaluation. Viral DNA was then sequenced by next-generation sequencing. De novo assembly of the viral genome and phylogenetic analysis revealed a novel poxvirus most closely related to Yoka poxvirus, which was isolated from mosquitoes in the Central African Republic in 1972 during an ecologic survey. The patient had no travel outside of his community in upper New York state. The epidemiology of this novel pox virus is not known at this time; however this case serves as reminder that immunocompromised patients are prone to novel infectious diseases [170].

Global Emerging Pathogens

SOT and HSCT have become the treatments of choice for a large number of disease processes. Advancements in immune suppression and improvements in the management of opportunistic infections have allowed a growing number of centers worldwide to perform such procedures. According to the Global Observatory on Donation and Transplantation, over 100,000 solid organ transplants were performed in 2013, including 80,000 kidney and 25,000 liver transplants. From 2000 to 2010, the number of countries performing kidney transplant increased from 33 to 84. While the number of kidney transplants performed annually in the United States and Canada stayed relatively stable from 2005 to 2015 (16,485–17,878 and 1049–1265, respectively), the total number performed in the Americas region nearly doubled (from 14,512 to 28,324). Countries that include endemic areas for many emerging infectious diseases are now performing a significant number of transplants (e.g. Brazil and India, which both performed around 5000 kidney transplants in 2010) [171]. In the following sections, we will briefly discuss a number of different emerging viral pathogens. To date, few of these have been documented in transplant recipients. With the marked increase in both SOT and HSCT, this will no doubt change, and we expect a corresponding increase in emerging viral infections in transplant hosts, both from known viruses and those yet to be identified.

Dengue Virus, Zika, and the Flaviviruses

Flaviviruses are single-stranded RNA viruses, and this genus contains a number of important human pathogens, including dengue virus (DENV), Zika virus (ZIKV), yellow fever virus (YFV), Japanese encephalitis virus (JEV), West Nile virus (WNV), St. Louis encephalitis virus, and tick-borne encephalitis virus (TBEV), among others. In this section, we will focus on DENV but also briefly discuss ZIKV, YFV, and case reports of USUV, an emerging avian pathogen in Africa and Europe [172]. Cases or case series of other flaviviruses have not been reported in the transplant literature, which may be partly explained by effective vaccines for both JEV and TBEV.

DENV is the most common vector-borne disease worldwide and has emerged as a significant pathogen in an increasing number of countries over the last 40 years [173]. Four serotypes of DENV exist (DENVs 1–4) and are transmitted by *Aedes aegypti* and *Aedes albopictus* mosquitoes. All have the potential to cause a range of clinical illness, from asymptomatic infection to classical dengue fever (DF) to severe dengue, including dengue hemorrhagic fever (DHF) and dengue shock syndrome (DSS). Infection with one serotype (primary infection) results in immunity to that serotype, but infection can occur with any of the remaining serotypes (secondary infection) [173]. Secondary infection has been shown to be a significant risk factor for the development of severe dengue, and this appears to result from both disadvantageous humoral and cellular immune responses (termed antibody-dependent enhancement and original antigenic sin, respectively) [174, 175]. Other factors are also important, such as the order of infection as well as the specific DENV strain [176, 177].

A number of reports have documented the occurrence of both DF and severe dengue in transplant recipients (Table 45.1) [178–187]. Two case series from Brazil (27 patients) and Singapore (6 cases) present a less severe picture of DENV infection in renal transplant patients [178, 182]. In the study from Brazil, eight patients had been hospitalized and one died of respiratory failure. Only a single patient developed DHF, and this person recovered [178]. The six patients in Singapore were identified on presentation to the hospital. Though all survived, the mean platelet count was 80,000 and 5 patients developed leucopenia. There were no cases of DHF or DSS [182]. All 33 patients in these 2 series had stable graft function.

Severe cases of dengue were reported from India in a series of eight renal transplant patients, who were diagnosed with DENV on admission to the hospital. Five patients developed DHF, and three patients developed DSS. All those in the latter group died [186]. Four other case reports in renal transplant recipients include three cases of DHF and a single, fatal case of DSS [179, 181, 184, 185]. Though these represent a small number of cases, it is notable that four of the patients with severe dengue developed disease within 1 month of transplantation (two during their initial hospitalization), while all of the patients in the series from Brazil and Singapore developed their illness 3 months or more after transplant. Reports also document a single fatal case of DSS occurring in a liver transplant recipient (date of transplant not reported) and a fatal case of severe dengue 4 days after HSCT [180, 183] Most patients were diagnosed using NS1 protein detection or rapid IgM and IgG, and RT-PCR was less commonly performed. The serotypes, when reported, included DENVs 1, 3, and 4 [180, 183 185].

Human-to-human transmission of DENV as a result of organ transplantation has been documented. In one case of DENV transmission from a living donor to liver transplant recipient in India, the donor developed fevers, thrombocytopenia, and transaminitis 2 days after liver donation. Donor blood was positive for DENV NS1 antigen. The recipient developed a similar clinical presentation 5 days after transplantation and was also positive for DENV NS1 antigen. Both recipient and donor were treated with supportive measures and discharged after their full recovery 2–3 weeks after transplantation [188]. A case of donor-derived DENV transmission in HSCT has also been reported. In this report from Germany, the donor similarly developed clinical symptoms of DENV days after donation of peripheral blood stem cells to a recipient with acute myeloblastic leukemia and was only later noted to have returned from a trip to Sri Lanka. DENV NS1 antigen and PCR were positive in the donor. The recipient was subsequently treated with IVIG; however, the recipient ultimately developed cardiopulmonary arrest and died 9 days posttransplant. Blood testing of the recipient also was positive by DENV NS1 antigen and PCR. Sequencing of virus showed genotype 1 infection with sequence similarity to circulating DEV 1 genotype 1 strains in Sri Lanka [189].

Emergence of ZIKV, another mosquito-borne flavivirus, was first reported in 2007 in the Federated States of Micronesia where an outbreak of febrile illness occurred that was characterized by rash, conjunctivitis, and arthralgias. By 2015, ZIKV spread throughout the Pacific Islands, continental South America and into Central America, the Caribbean, and Mexico. ZIKV is linked with outbreaks of Guillain-Barre syndrome and devastating birth defects, most notably fetal microcephaly, from infection during pregnancy. Given the recency of the epidemic, the effects of ZIKV infection in transplant recipients are currently not known. The potential impact of any major viral infection on transplant outcomes can be significant with increased morbidity and mortality in transplant recipients who develop disease [190]. The full influence of ZIKV on transplantation remains to be determined.

YFV is closely related to DENV, exists in sub-Saharan Africa and South America, and is transmitted by the bite of infected *Aedes* species mosquitoes. To date, no cases of YFV have been reported in the transplant literature [191]. The YFV vaccine is effective, but it is live-attenuated and not currently recommended for transplant recipients. In one small study, 19 SOT recipients received the YFV vaccine inadvertently during outbreaks in Brazil. No severe AEs were reported, and the mean posttransplant time at vaccination was over 5 years [192]. Similarly, a patient with AML who started chemotherapy just 7 days after receiving YFV vaccination did not develop AEs despite detection of the 17D attenuated viral strain by RT-PCR in plasma samples for 15 days after vaccination. Interestingly, protective neutralizing antibodies were detected 1 month after the vaccine, indicating that memory B lymphocytes may have been preserved despite ablative bone marrow suppression [193].

Two case reports exist, both from Italy in 2009, of USUV causing encephalitis in immunocompromised patients [16, 23, 172]. The first report was of a woman with diffuse large B-cell lymphoma who presented with fever and a resting tremor. CSF was sent for a pan-flavivirus RT-PCR, and sequencing was consistent with USUV [23]. The second patient had TTP and was admitted with fevers and a headache. She developed fulminant liver failure and received a liver transplant (Table 45.2). Plasma drawn just before transplant gave a weak positive signal in a WNV RT-PCR. Flavivirus RT-PCR was then performed, and sequencing was consistent with USUV [16]. Both patients recovered, though had some residual neurological deficits.

Alphaviruses

The alphaviruses are a genus of single-stranded, positive-sense RNA viruses (within the *Togaviridae* family) that cause either encephalitis such as eastern, western, and Venezuelan equine encephalitis viruses or a systemic febrile illness with a rash and arthritis including Semliki Forest, Sindbis, O'nyong-nyong, Mayaro, Ross River, and Chikungunya viruses. In 2004, Chikungunya virus (CHIKV) re-emerged in Kenya and spread to countries around the Indian Ocean, including Reunion, a French overseas district, and India, resulting in millions of cases [194, 195]. Autochthonous spread was even detected in Italy in 2007 [196]. Symptomatic CHIKV infections result in a severe arthritis, which can persist for months following resolution of the fever and rash [197, 198]. Cases of meningoencephalitis and fatalities have been reported [199, 200]. Two cases of severe CHIKV infections in immunocompromised patients were reported by Kee et al., in 2010, including one patient taking an herbal medicine felt to contain steroids and a liver transplant recipient (Table 45.2). The liver transplant recipient presented with fever, headache, and abdominal complaints. IgM was positive for CHIKV, but IgG and serum RT-PCR remained negative (lumbar puncture was not performed). He recovered fully. Neither patient developed arthritis or arthralgias during the course of their infections [201]. A subsequent case of CHIKV infection in an HIV-infected kidney transplant recipient who had traveled to the Dominican Republic 4 years of transplantation reported an episode of arthritis lasting 2 months, which ultimately self-resolved [202]. In a second study, investigators tested corneal grafts from patients living in La Reunion during the 2005–2006 CHIKV outbreak. Twelve of 69 asymptomatic, potential donors were found to be viremic (3 patients) or IgM positive (11 patients, including 2 patients with viremia), and corneal grafts from 4 of these patients (all 3 viremic patients) had detectable CHIKV RNA on RT-PCR. While no cases of transplant-associated CHIKV transmission have been documented, researchers did show that transmission can occur by the ocular route in mice [203].

Bunyaviridae

Bunyaviridae is a family of segmented RNA viruses that includes a number of emerging pathogens, including Rift Valley fever virus (RVFV), the hantaviruses, Crimean-Congo hemorrhagic fever virus, and two newly identified phleboviruses, HYSV and Heartland virus. Bunyaviruses are vector-borne viruses, except for the hantaviruses, which are transmitted through aerosols from infected rodents. RVFV is an important livestock pathogen in Africa and causes outbreaks of severe human disease, often following periods of heavy rain. Many human infections are asymptomatic or result in a self-limited febrile illness, though cases of encephalitis and hemorrhagic fever are reported. Disease severity tends to be greater during large outbreaks, and mortality rates of up to 30% in symptomatic patients have been seen. Recently, this infection was seen for the first time in countries outside of Africa, causing outbreaks in Saudi Arabia and Yemen [204, 205]. To date, there have not been reported cases within the transplant community.

HYSV and Heartland virus have been described in the last 2 years, and clinical experience remains limited. HYSV is a tick-borne bunyavirus and was identified in patients in China presenting with fevers and thrombocytopenia without an identified cause [17]. A recent publication on the clinical course of 49 inpatients with confirmed HYSV documented a mortality of 16%, which correlated with high viral loads on admission [206]. Heartland virus has been isolated from two patients in Missouri, United States, who were admitted with fevers, diarrhea, and thrombocytopenia. They both improved with supportive care [18]. Both of these viruses were initially isolated in cell culture before being further characterized by electron microscopy and sequencing, and they appear to be closely related members of the genus *Phlebovirus* [17, 18]. Given their recent identification, it is not unexpected that these infections have not been characterized in the transplant population.

The *Hantavirus* genus includes at least 23 related viruses that cause hemorrhagic fever with renal syndrome (HFRS) or hantavirus pulmonary syndrome (HPS). Three cases of hantavirus infection in immunocompromised patients, including a single case in a renal transplant recipient, have been reported (Table 45.2) [207–209]. All of these cases involved Old World hantaviruses that are associated with HFRS including Dobrava-Belgrade virus, one case, and Puumala virus, two cases. The renal transplant recipient, 18 months after transplantation, presented with 5 days of fevers, headache, and arthralgia. He developed oliguric renal failure and required 5 days of dialysis prior to return of normal urine output. He was treated with steroids for acute rejection, but given his presentation, he was also evaluated for other causes. IgM returned positive for Dobrava-Belgrade virus, and the patient made a full recovery [207]. The two cases of Puumala virus infection involved a patient with acute leukemia and one receiving anti-TNF therapy. Both patients did well, though interestingly, the patient with leukemia was felt to be infected through a platelet transfusion [208, 209]. The treatment of hantavirus infections remains largely supportive. There is limited data for the use of ribavirin, which decreased mortality in a study of HFRS in China, reported in 1991 [210]. A trial of ribavirin in HPS was terminated early due to slow patient accrual. This study showed no improvement in the patients given ribavirin, though it was underpowered [211]. No benefit was seen in the use of oral prednisone in HFRS [212].

Filoviridae

Marburg and Ebola viruses are the only members of the *Filoviridae* family and are two of the most virulent human pathogens, causing outbreaks of hemorrhagic fever with mortality rates of up to 90%. Except for the first identified outbreak of Marburg virus in 1967, when it was isolated from patients in Germany and Yugoslavia who had handled infected African green monkeys, these viruses have only caused hemorrhagic fever outbreaks in Africa. The largest Ebola outbreak recorded began in 2013 in West Africa (predominantly Liberia, Sierra Leone, and Guinea) and has resulted in over 28,000 cases and 11,000 deaths to date and include the transmission from individuals infected in West Africa to health-care workers in the United States and Europe [213–215].

The incubation period for these viruses is 3–13 days. Patients then become acutely ill, developing high fevers and other nonspecific complaints such as malaise, nausea, vomiting, and diarrhea. Most patients develop a maculopapular rash, and they often develop hemorrhagic manifestations from multiple mucosal sites. Laboratory abnormalities are not diagnostic but include initial leucopenia, often followed by a leukocytosis, thrombocytopenia, increased transaminases (typically AST more than ALT), and prolonged prothrombin time [213]. Virus is detectable, using RT-PCR, antigen detection, or culture, in the blood and other body fluids at the time of presentation [213, 216, 217]. Care at this time is supportive along with infection control procedures including patient isolation. The majority of patients who die as a result of Marburg or Ebola do so within the first 2 weeks, and convalescent time for survivors is often prolonged [213]. Many long-term complications have been reported in survivors, with rheumatologic and ocular complaints most predominant. 50–75% of survivors report symmetric, polyarthritic arthralgias. Eye pain, conjunctivitis, photophobia, hyperlacrimation, uveitis, and loss of visual acuity also seem to be common with reports in as much as half of survivors in certain regions during the West Africa outbreak.

Though Marburg and Ebola infections have not been reported in the transplant population, likely due to the barriers to the establishment of robust transplant program in these countries, recognition of risk factors for Ebola among potential donors during outbreak periods may be of importance. Symptomatic patients have virus disseminated in multiple organs and body fluids, and transmission occurs via contact with infected fluids. Donor-derived infection may involve a donor who died of unrecognized Ebola or an infected but not yet symptomatic donor. Donors who have traveled to areas with significant Ebola activity, health-care workers working directly with Ebola, and others with direct exposure to a patient with proven Ebola infection in the prior 21 days should raise caution for possible donor-derived Ebola transmission [217].

Xenotransplantation

Acellular xenografts have been in use for decades, and porcine islet cell transplantation recently entered clinical trials, but the xenotransplantation of organs remains experimental and beyond the realm of clinical medicine [218]. The scientific and ethical questions surrounding the transplantation of organs, cells, and tissues from nonhuman species have generated an independent body of literature. The handling of these questions is beyond the scope of this text, and we will only briefly discuss some of the concerns regarding the transmission of viral zoonoses to human xenograft recipients.

The porcine endogenous retroviruses (so called PERVs) are incorporated in swine DNA and genetically acquired [218, 219]. These viruses can be found in the genomes of all swine, and there is concern that they could infect transplant recipients, as human cells have been shown to be susceptible in vitro [219–224]. In a study using a pig-to-baboon model of SOT, PERV proviral DNA was found in the PBMCs of all ten animals, though viral RNA was not detected [223]. In studies of recipients of islet cell transplants, PERV transmission has not been documented, though in these studies, patients are rarely immunocompromised [224–226]. PERV transmission was not detected in liver allotransplant recipients who happened to be pig farmers [221]. If these infections do occur, their clinical significance still remains unclear.

Other viruses are also a concern in xenotransplantation. These include the porcine herpesviruses, porcine CMV (PCMV) and porcine lymphotropic herpesvirus (PLHV); HEV, particularly genotypes 3 and 4; and certain parvoviruses [218]. Many of these viral agents can be excluded from herds by careful breeding practices and frequent herd monitoring. A single study of islet cell transplant to human recipients did not detect PCMV or PLHV, which were also not detected in the herds prior to transplantation [225]. In the pig-to-baboon model of SOT, PCMV DNA was detected in two recipients and PLHV DNA was detected in six (of ten baboons). RNA was not detected for either of these viruses, supporting the conclusion that these were not productive infections. The outcome of these infections remains unclear, however, as the longest surviving recipient after transplantation was only 179 days [223].

Prevention and Reporting

The majority of viral infections discussed in this chapter appear to occur rarely in transplant recipients, though data are insufficient to determine the true incidence of disease. Measles, mumps, and yellow fever are vaccine-preventable illnesses, though these vaccines are all live-attenuated. Also, the response to vaccines in this patient population is lower than the response in immunocompetent patients. Donor-transmitted rabies carries a dire prognosis, and though limited data exists, the use of PEP in transplant recipients appears safe.

Given their apparent rarity, screening for many of these diseases in organ donors cannot be recommended at this time. The examples of HTLV-1 and LCMV are illustrative of some of the difficulties involved with donor screening. In low-prevalence settings, HTLV-1 testing generates a large number of false-positive tests, and confirmatory testing can delay transplantation [37, 53]. Hence, this is no longer required by the US OPTN [37, 53]. In the outbreak investigations for LCMV, only one of four donors had detectable antibodies. Indeed, RT-PCR from multiple samples failed to detect LCMV from one donor and yielded a positive result in a single lymph node (but not other samples) in another [13, 86, 87]. It seems prudent to obtain a comprehensive history of potential organ donors, including all recent exposures and travel, though it remains unclear how certain findings, such as rodent ownership, should affect one's status as an organ donor.

Reporting rare or unusual infections in transplant recipients, though retroactive, will help to identify agents for which more research is needed and screening may be warranted. At this time, expectations in the United States are for transplant centers to report unexpected potential or proven infections discovered after procurement of a donor organ to the OPTN Patient Safety System [227]. This remains a passive reporting system, however, and it is possible that events are missed if these infections are underdiagnosed or if symptoms are attributed to more common, and potentially coincident, posttransplant infections.

References

1. IOM. Executive summary. In: Lederberg JS, Shope RE, Oaks Jr SC, editors. Emerging infections: microbial threats to health in the United States. Washington, DC: National Academy Press; 1992.
2. Addressing emerging infectious disease threats: a prevention strategy for the United States. Executive summary. MMWR Recommendations and reports: Morb Mortal Wkly Rep Recommendations Reports / Centers for Disease Control 1994;43:1–18.
3. Woolhouse ME, Gowtage-Sequeria S. Host range and emerging and reemerging pathogens. Emerg Infect Dis. 2005;11:1842–7.
4. Kumar D. Emerging viruses in transplantation. Curr Opin Infect Dis. 2010;23:374–8.
5. Nishi SPE, Valentine VG, Duncan S. Emerging bacterial, fungal and viral respiratory infections in transplantation. Infect Dis Clin N Am. 2010;24:541–55.
6. Fischer SA. Emerging viruses in transplantation: there is more to infection after transplant than CMV and EBV. Transplantation. 2008;86:1327–39.
7. Boeckh M. The challenge of respiratory virus infections in hematopoietic cell transplant recipients. Br J Haematol. 2008;143:455–67.
8. Renaud C, Campbell AP. Changing epidemiology of respiratory viral infections in hematopoietic cell transplant recipients and solid organ transplant recipients. Curr Opin Infect Dis. 2011;24:333–43.
9. Kotton CN. Zoonoses in solid-organ and hematopoietic stem cell transplant recipients. Clin Infect Dis. 2007;44:857–66.
10. Waggoner JJ, Soda EA, Deresinski S. Rare and emerging viral infections in transplant recipients. Clin Infect Dis. 2013;57(8):1182–8.
11. Razonable RR. Rare, unusual, and less common virus infections after organ transplantation. Curr Opin Organ Transplant. 2011;16:580–7.
12. Chatzidimitriou D, Gavriilaki E, Diza E. Hematopoietic cell transplantation and emerging viral infections. J Med Virol. 2010;82:528–38.
13. Fischer SA, Graham MB, Kuehnert MJ, et al. Transmission of lymphocytic choriomeningitis virus by organ transplantation. N Engl J Med. 2006;354:2235–49.
14. Tesh RB. A method for the isolation and identification of dengue viruses, using mosquito cell cultures. Am J Trop Med Hyg. 1979;28:1053–9.
15. Caliendo AM. Multiplex PCR and emerging technologies for the detection of respiratory pathogens. Clin Infect Dis. 2011;52(Suppl 4):S326–30.
16. Cavrini F, Baibani P, Longo G, et al. Usutu virus infection in a patient who underwent orthotropic liver transplantation, Italy, August–September 2009. Euro Surveill. 2009;14:19448.
17. Yu XJ, Liang MF, Zhang SY, et al. Fever with thrombocytopenia associated with a novel bunyavirus in China. N Engl J Med. 2011;364:1523–32.
18. McMullan LK, Folk SM, Kelly AJ, et al. A new phlebovirus associated with severe febrile illness in Missouri. N Engl J Med. 2012;367:834–41.
19. Delwart EL. Viral metagenomics. Rev Med Virol. 2007;17:115–31.
20. Wang D, Urisman A, Liu Y, et al. Viral discovery and sequence recovery using DNA microarrays. PLoS Biol. 2003;1:257–60.
21. Greninger AL, Chen EC, Sittler T, et al. A metagenomic analysis of pandemic influenza A (2009 H1N1) infection in patients from North America. PLoS One. 2010;5:e13381.
22. Mokili JL, Rohwer F, Dutilh BE. Metagenomics and future perspectives in virus discovery. Curr Opin Virol. 2011;2:63–77.
23. Pecorari M, Longo G, Gennari W, et al. First human case of Usutu virus neuroinvasive infection, Italy, August–September 2009. Euro Surveill. 2009;14:pii: 19446.
24. Li L, Delwart E. From orphan virus to pathogen: the path to the clinical lab. Curr Opin Virol. 2011;1:282–8.
25. Okamoto H. History of discoveries and pathogenicity of TT viruses. Curr Top Microbiol Immunol. 2009;331:1–20.
26. Reyes GR, Kim JP. Sequence-independent, single-primer amplification (SISPA) of complex DNA populations. Mol Cell Probes. 1991;5:473–81.
27. Jones MS, Kapoor A, Lukashov VV, Simmonds P, Hecht F, Delwart E. New DNA viruses identified in patients with acute viral infection syndrome. J Virol. 2005;79:8230–6.
28. Allander T, Tammi MT, Eriksson M, Bjerkner A, Tiveljung-Lindell A, Andersson B. Cloning of a human parvovirus by molecular screening of respiratory tract samples. Proc Natl Acad Sci U S A. 2005;102:12891–6.
29. Su Z, Ning B, Fang H, Perkins R, Tong W, Shi L. Next-generation sequencing and its applications in molecular diagnostics. Expert Rev Mol Diagn. 2011;11:333–43.
30. Eid J, Fehr A, Gray J, et al. Real-time DNA sequencing from single polymerase molecules. Science. 2009;323:133–8.
31. Cheval J, Sauvage V, Frangeul L, et al. Evaluation of high-throughput sequencing for identifying known and unknown viruses in biological samples. J Clin Micobiol. 2011;49:3268–75.

32. Yozwiak NL, Skewes-Cox P, Stenglein MD, Balmaseda A, Harris E, DeRisi JL. Virus identification in unknown tropical febrile illness cases using deep sequencing. PLoS Negl Trop Dis. 2012;6:e1485.
33. Palacios G, Druce J, Du L, et al. A new arenavirus in a cluster of fatal transplant-associated diseases. N Engl J Med. 2008;358:991–8.
34. Sridhar S, To KK, Chan JF, Lau SK, Woo PC, Yuen KY. A systematic approach to novel virus discovery in emerging infectious disease outbreaks. J Mol Diagn. 2015;17:230–41.
35. Lipkin WI, Anthony SJ. Virus hunting. Virology. 2015;479–480:194–9.
36. Schildgen O, Muller A, Allander T, et al. Human bocavirus: passenger or pathogen in acute respiratory tract infections? Clin Microbiol Rev. 2008;21:291–304. table of contents
37. Network USOPaT. Guidance for HTLV-1 screening and confirmation in potential donors and reporting potential HTLV-1 infection, 2011 June 29. 2011.
38. Tsurumi H, Tani K, Tsuruta T, et al. Adult T-cell leukemia developing during immunosuppressive treatment in a renal transplant recipient. Am J Hematol. 1992;41:292–4.
39. Gout O, Baulac M, Gessain A, et al. Rapid development of myelopathy after HTLV-I infection acquired by transfusion during cardiac transplantation. N Engl J Med. 1990;322:383–8.
40. Yoshizumi T, Shirabe K, Ikegami T, et al. Impact of human T cell leukemia virus type 1 in living donor liver transplantation. Am J Transplant. 2012;12:1479–85.
41. Jenks PJ, Barrett WY, Raftery MJ, et al. Development of human T-cell lymphotropic virus type I-associated adult T-cell leukemia/lymphoma during immunosuppressive treatment following renal transplantation. Clin Infect Dis. 1995;21:992–3.
42. Zanke BW, Rush DN, Jeffery JR, Israels LG. HTLV-1 T cell lymphoma in a cyclosporine-treated renal transplant patient. Transplantation. 1989;48:695–7.
43. Ramanan P, Deziel PJ, Norby SM, Yao JD, Garza I, Razonable RR. Donor-transmitted HTLV-1-associated myelopathy in a kidney transplant recipient--case report and literature review. Am J Transplant. 2014;14:2417–21.
44. Ramanan P, Deziel PJ, Norby SM, Yao JD, Garza I, Razonable RR. Donor-derived HTLV-1 associated myelopathy after transplantation: a call for targeted screening. Am J Transplant. 2015;15:1125.
45. Cook LB, Melamed A, Demontis MA, et al. Rapid dissemination of human T-lymphotropic virus type 1 during primary infection in transplant recipients. Retrovirology. 2016;13:3.
46. Zarranz Imirizaldu JJ, Gomez Esteban JC, Rouco Axpe I, et al. Post-transplantation HTLV-1 myelopathy in three recipients from a single donor. J Neurol Neurosurg Psychiatry. 2003;74:1080–4.
47. Emmanouilides CE, Territo M. HTLV-I-associated myelopathy following allogeneic bone marrow transplantation. Bone Marrow Transplant. 1999;24:205–6.
48. Shirai H, Suzuki M, Tomita Y, et al. Renal transplantation in patients with human T-cell lymphotropic virus type 1. Transplant Proc. 2012;44:83–6.
49. Tanabe K, Kitani R, Takahashi K, et al. Long-term results in human T-cell leukemia virus type 1-positive renal transplant recipients. Transplant Proc. 1998;30:3168–70.
50. Naghibi O, Nazemian F, Naghibi M, Ali Javidi DB. Prognosis of HTLV-1 positive renal transplant recipients in Iran. Saudi J Kidney Dis Transpl Saudi Arabia. 2011;22:670–4.
51. Nakamura N, Tamaru S, Ohshima K, Tanaka M, Arakaki Y, Miyauchi T. Prognosis of HTLV-I-positive renal transplant recipients. Transplant Proc. 2005;37:1779–82.
52. Toro C, Benito R, Aguilera A, et al. Infection with human T lymphotropic virus type I in organ transplant donors and recipients in Spain. J Med Virol. 2005;76:268–70.
53. Network USOPaT. Policy 2: minimum procurement standards for an organ procurement organization (OPO). 2012:7.
54. Tedla F, Brar A, John D, Sumrani N. Risk of transmission of human T-lymphotropic virus through transplant. Am J Transplant. 2015;15:1123–4.
55. Hishizawa M, Kanda J, Utsunomiya A, et al. Transplantation of allogeneic hematopoietic stem cells for adult T-cell leukemia: a nationwide retrospective study. Blood. 2010;116:1369–76.
56. Warrell MJ. Emerging aspects of rabies infection: with a special emphasis on children. Curr Opin Infect Dis. 2008;21:251–7.
57. De Serres G, Dallaire F, Cote M, Skowronski DM. Bat rabies in the United States and Canada from 1950 through 2007: human cases with and without bat contact. Clin Infect Dis. 2008;46:1329–37.
58. Centers for Disease Control and Prevention. Presumptive abortive human rabies – Texas, 2009. MMWR Morb Mortal Wkly Rep. 2010;59:185–90.
59. Gilbert AT, Petersen BW, Recuenco S, et al. Evidence of rabies virus exposure among humans in the Peruvian Amazon. Am J Trop Med Hyg. 2012;87:206–15.
60. Bronnert J, Wilde H, Tepsumethanon V, Lumlertdacha B, Hemachudha T. Organ transplantations and rabies transmission. J Travel Med. 2007;14:177–80.
61. Centers for Disease Control. Human-to-human transmission of rabies via a corneal transplant – France. MMWR Morb Mortal Wkly Rep. 1980;29:25–6.
62. Centers for Disease Control. Human-to-human transmission of rabies via corneal transplant--Thailand. MMWR Morb Mortal Wkly Rep. 1981;30:473–4.
63. Centers for Disease Control and Prevention. Update: investigation of rabies infections in organ donor and transplant recipients--Alabama, Arkansas, Oklahoma, and Texas, 2004. MMWR Morb Mortal Wkly Rep. 2004;53:615–6.
64. Centers for Disease Control and Prevention. Investigation of rabies infections in organ donor and transplant recipients--Alabama, Arkansas, Oklahoma, and Texas, 2004. MMWR Morb Mortal Wkly Rep. 2004;53:586–9.
65. Gode GR, Bhide NK. Two rabies deaths after corneal grafts from one donor. Lancet. 1988;2:791.
66. Houff SA, Burton RC, Wilson RW, et al. Human-to-human transmission of rabies virus by corneal transplant. N Engl J Med. 1979;300:603–4.
67. Javadi MA, Fayaz A, Mirdehghan SA, Ainollahi B. Transmission of rabies by corneal graft. Cornea. 1996;15:431–3.
68. Manning SE, Rupprecht CE, Fishbein D, et al. Human rabies prevention--United States, 2008: recommendations of the Advisory Committee on Immunization Practices. MMWR Recomm Rep. 2008;57:1–28.
69. Srinivasan A, Burton EC, Kuehnert MJ, et al. Transmission of rabies virus from an organ donor to four transplant recipients. N Engl J Med. 2005;352:1103–11.
70. Sureau P, Portnoi D, Rollin P, Lapresle C, Chaouni-Barbich A. Prevention of inter-human rabies transmission after corneal graft. C R Seances Acad Sci III. 1981;293:4.
71. Hellenbrand W, Meyer C, Rasch G, Steffens I, Ammon A. Cases of rabies in Germany following organ transplantation. Euro Surveill. 2005;10:E050224 6.
72. Maier T, Schwarting A, Mauer D, et al. Management and outcomes after multiple corneal and solid organ transplantations from a donor infected with rabies virus. Clin Infect Dis. 2010;50:1112–9.
73. Vetter JM, Frisch L, Drosten C, et al. Survival after transplantation of corneas from a rabies-infected donor. Cornea. 2011;30:241–4.
74. Wallace RM, Stanek D, Griese S, et al. A large-scale, rapid public health response to rabies in an organ recipient and the previously undiagnosed organ donor. Zoonoses Public Health. 2014;61:560–70.

75. Vora NM, Basavaraju SV, Feldman KA, et al. Raccoon rabies virus variant transmission through solid organ transplantation. JAMA. 2013;310:398–407.
76. Centers for Disease Control and Prevention. Recovery of a patient from clinical rabies--California, 2011. MMWR Morb Mortal Wkly Rep. 2012;61:61–5.
77. Willoughby RE Jr, Tieves KS, Hoffman GM, et al. Survival after treatment of rabies with induction of coma. N Engl J Med. 2005;352:2508–14.
78. Aramburo A, Willoughby RE, Bollen AW, et al. Failure of the Milwaukee protocol in a child with rabies. Clin Infect. 2011;53:572–4.
79. Rabies registry home page. At http://www.chw.org/display/PPF/DocID/33223/router.asp.
80. Cramer CH 2nd, Shieck V, Thomas SE, Kershaw DB, Magee JC, Lopez MJ. Immune response to rabies vaccination in pediatric transplant patients. Pediatr Transplant. 2008;12:874–7.
81. Rodriguez-Romo R, Morales-Buenrostro LE, Lecuona L, et al. Immune response after rabies vaccine in a kidney transplant recipient. Transpl Infect Dis. 2011;13:492–5.
82. Vora NM, Orciari LA, Niezgoda M, et al. Clinical management and humoral immune responses to rabies post-exposure prophylaxis among three patients who received solid organs from a donor with rabies. Transpl Infect Dis. 2015;17:389–95.
83. Buchmeier MJ, de la Torres J, Peters CJ. Arenaviridae: the viruses and their replication. In: Knipe DM, Howley PM, editors. Field's virology. 5th ed. Philadelphia: Lippincott Williams & Wilkins. p. 2007.
84. Gregg MB. Recent outbreaks of lymphocytic choriomeningitis in the United States of America. Bull World Health Organ. 1975;52:549–53.
85. Hadler JL, Nelson R, Mshar P, Sosa LE. Survey of lymphocytic choriomeningitis virus diagnosis and testing – Connecticut, 2005. MMWR Morb Mortal Wkly Rep. 2006;55:398–9.
86. Barry A, Gunn J, Tormey P, et al. Lymphocytic choriomeningitis virus transmitted through solid organ transplantation – Massachusetts, 2008. MMWR Morb Mortal Wkly Rep. 2008;57:799–801.
87. MacNeil A, Stroher U, Farnon E, et al. Solid organ transplant-associated lymphocytic choriomeningitis, United States, 2011. Emerg Infect Dis. 2012;18:1256–62.
88. Schafer IJ, Miller R, Stroher U, Knust B, Nichol ST, Rollin PE. Notes from the field: a cluster of lymphocytic choriomeningitis virus infections transmitted through organ transplantation-Iowa, 2013. Am J Transplant. 2014;14:1459.
89. Centers for Disease Control and Prevention. Lymphocytic choriomeningitis virus infection in organ transplant recipients – Massachusetts, Rhode Island, 2005. MMWR Morb Mortal Wkly Rep. 2005;54:537–9.
90. McCormick JB, King IJ, Webb PA, et al. Lassa fever. Effective therapy with ribavirin. N Engl J Med. 1986;314:20–6.
91. Peters CJ. Lymphocytic Choriomeningitis virus – an old enemy up to new tricks. N Engl J Med. 2006;354:2208–11.
92. Centers for Disease Control and Prevention. Update: interim guidance for minimizing risk for human lymphocytic choriomeningitis virus infection associated with pet rodents. MMWR Morb Mortal Wkly Rep. 2005;54:799–801.
93. Amman BR, Pavlin BI, Albarino CG, et al. Pet rodents and fatal lymphocytic choriomeningitis in transplant patients. Emerg Infect Dis. 2007;13:719–25.
94. Lou S, Xu B, Huang Q, et al. Molecular characterization of the newly identified human parvovirus 4 in the family Parvoviridae. Virology. 2012;422:59–69.
95. Allander T, Jartti T, Gupta S, et al. Human bocavirus and acute wheezing in children. Clin Infect Dis. 2007;44:904–10.
96. Arnold JC, Singh KK, Spector SA, Sawyer MH. Human bocavirus: prevalence and clinical spectrum at a children's hospital. Clin Infect Dis. 2006;43:283–8.
97. Fry AM, Lu X, Chittaganpitch M, et al. Human bocavirus: a novel parvovirus epidemiologically associated with pneumonia requiring hospitalization in Thailand. J Infect Dis. 2007;195:1038–45.
98. Garbino J, Soccal PM, Aubert JD, et al. Respiratory viruses in bronchoalveolar lavage: a hospital-based cohort study in adults. Thorax. 2009;64:399–404.
99. Kesebir D, Vazquez M, Weibel C, et al. Human bocavirus infection in young children in the United States: molecular epidemiological profile and clinical characteristics of a newly emerging respiratory virus. J Infect Dis. 2006;194:1276–82.
100. Longtin J, Bastien M, Gilca R, et al. Human bocavirus infections in hospitalized children and adults. Emerg Infect Dis. 2008;14:217–21.
101. Manning A, Russell V, Eastick K, et al. Epidemiological profile and clinical associations of human bocavirus and other human parvoviruses. J Infect Dis. 2006;194:1283–90.
102. Tozer SJ, Lambert SB, Whiley DM, et al. Detection of human bocavirus in respiratory, fecal, and blood samples by real-time PCR. J Med Virol. 2009;81:488–93.
103. Principi N, Piralla A, Zampiero A, et al. Bocavirus infection in otherwise healthy children with respiratory disease. PLoS One. 2015;10:e0135640.
104. Schenk T, Strahm B, Kontny U, Hufnagel M, Neumann-Haefelin D, Falcone V. Disseminated bocavirus infection after stem cell transplant. Emerg Infect Dis. 2007;13:1425–7.
105. Schenk T, Maier B, Hufnagel M, et al. Persistence of human bocavirus DNA in immunocompromised children. Pediatr Infect Dis J. 2011;30:82–4.
106. de Vries JJ, Bredius RG, van Rheenen PF, et al. Human bocavirus in an immunocompromised child presenting with severe diarrhea. J Clin Microbiol. 2009;47:1241–3.
107. Costa C, Bergallo M, Cavallo R. Detection of human bocavirus in bronchoalveolar lavage from Italian adult patients. J Clin Virol. 2009;45:81–2.
108. Miyakis S, van Hal SJ, Barratt J, Stark D, Marriott D, Harkness J. Absence of human bocavirus in bronchoalveolar lavage fluid of lung transplant patients. J Clin Virol. 2009;44:179–80.
109. Muller A, Klinkenberg D, Vehreschild J, et al. Low prevalence of human metapneumovirus and human bocavirus in adult immunocompromised high risk patients suspected to suffer from Pneumocystis pneumonia. J Infect. 2009;58:227–31.
110. Endo R, Ishiguro N, Kikuta H, et al. Seroepidemiology of human bocavirus in Hokkaido prefecture, Japan. J Clin Microbiol. 2007;45:3218–23.
111. The FilmArray® Respiratory Panels. 2012. At http://www.biofiredx.com/FilmArray/RespiratoryTest.html. Accessed 20 Sept 2012.
112. Biagini P, Dussol B, Touinssi M, et al. Human parvovirus 4 in kidney transplant patients, France. Emerg Infect Dis. 2008;14:1811–2.
113. Simmons R, Sharp C, McClure CP, et al. Parvovirus 4 infection and clinical outcome in high-risk populations. J Infect Dis. 2012;205:1816–20.
114. Benjamin LA, Lewthwaite P, Vasanthapuram R, et al. Human parvovirus 4 as potential cause of encephalitis in children, India. Emerg Infect Dis. 2011;17:1484–7.
115. Touinssi M, Reynaud-Gaubert M, Gomez C, et al. Parvovirus 4 in French in-patients: a study of hemodialysis and lung transplant cohorts. J Med Virol. 2011;83:717–20.
116. Schieble JH, Fox VL, Lennette EH. A probable new human picornavirus associated with respiratory diseases. Am J Epidemiol. 1967;85:297–310.
117. Midgley CM, Jackson MA, Selvarangan R, et al. Severe respiratory illness associated with enterovirus D68 – Missouri and Illinois, 2014. MMWR Morb Mortal Wkly Rep. 2014;63:798–9.
118. Midgley CM, Watson JT, Nix WA, et al. Severe respiratory illness associated with a nationwide outbreak of enterovirus D68 in the

USA (2014): a descriptive epidemiological investigation. Lancet Respir Med. 2015;3:879–87.
119. Holm-Hansen CC, Midgley SE, Fischer TK. Global emergence of enterovirus D68: a systematic review. Lancet Infect Dis. 2016;16(5):e64–75.
120. Schuster JE, Miller JO, Selvarangan R, et al. Severe enterovirus 68 respiratory illness in children requiring intensive care management. J Clin Virol. 2015;70:77–82.
121. Greninger AL, Naccache SN, Messacar K, et al. A novel outbreak enterovirus D68 strain associated with acute flaccid myelitis cases in the USA (2012–14): a retrospective cohort study. Lancet Infect Dis. 2015;15:671–82.
122. Waghmare A, Pergam SA, Jerome KR, Englund JA, Boeckh M, Kuypers J. Clinical disease due to enterovirus D68 in adult hematologic malignancy patients and hematopoietic cell transplant recipients. Blood. 2015;125:1724–9.
123. Baas MC, van Donselaar KA, Florquin S, van Binnendijk RS, ten Berge IJ, Bemelman FJ. Mumps: not an innocent bystander in solid organ transplantation. Am J Transplant. 2009;9:2186–9.
124. Bakshi N, Lawson J, Hanson R, Ames C, Vinters HV. Fatal mumps meningoencephalitis in a child with severe combined immunodeficiency after bone marrow transplantation. J Child Neurol. 1996;11:159–62.
125. Dayan GH, Quinlisk MP, Parker AA, et al. Recent resurgence of mumps in the United States. N Engl J Med. 2008;358:1580–9.
126. Hatchette TF, Mahony JB, Chong S, LeBlanc JJ. Difficulty with mumps diagnosis: what is the contribution of mumps mimickers? J Clin Virol. 2009;46:381–3.
127. Agamanolis DP, Tan JS, Parker DL. Immunosuppressive measles encephalitis in a patient with a renal transplant. Arch Neurol. 1979;36:686–90.
128. Centers for Disease Control and Prevention. Increased transmission and outbreaks of measles--European Region, 2011. MMWR Morb Mortal Wkly Rep. 2011;60:1605–10.
129. Freeman AF, Jacobsohn DA, Shulman ST, et al. A new complication of stem cell transplantation: measles inclusion body encephalitis. Pediatrics. 2004;114:e657–60.
130. Kaplan LJ, Daum RS, Smaron M, McCarthy CA. Severe measles in immunocompromised patients. JAMA. 1992;267:1237–41.
131. Final 2011 reports of nationally notifiable infectious diseases. MMWR Morb Mortal Wkly Rep. 2012;61:624–37.
132. Ljungman P, Fridell E, Lonnqvist B, et al. Efficacy and safety of vaccination of marrow transplant recipients with a live attenuated measles, mumps, and rubella vaccine. J Infect Dis. 1989;159:610–5.
133. Ljungman P, Aschan J, Barkholt L, et al. Measles immunity after allogeneic stem cell transplantation; influence of donor type, graft type, intensity of conditioning, and graft-versus host disease. Bone Marrow Transplant. 2004;34:589–93.
134. Spoulou V, Giannaki M, Vounatsou M, Bakoula C, Grafakos S. Long-term immunity to measles, mumps and rubella after MMR vaccination among children with bone marrow transplants. Bone Marrow Transplant. 2004;33:1187–90.
135. Kano H, Mizuta K, Sakakihara Y, et al. Efficacy and safety of immunization for pre- and post- liver transplant children. Transplantation. 2002;74:543–50.
136. Kalman S, Bakkaloglu SA, Ozkaya O, Buyan N, Soylemezoglu O. Measles: a rare communicable disease in a child with renal transplantation. Pediatr Transplant. 2002;6:432–4.
137. Lee DG, Yoo JH, Choi JH, et al. A fatal case of measles pneumonia complicating an adult recipient of hemopoietic stem cell transplantation during the nationwide epidemic in Korea. Int J Infect Dis. 2006;10:410–1.
138. Machado CM, Goncalves FB, Pannuti CS, Dulley FL, de Souza VA. Measles in bone marrow transplant recipients during an outbreak in Sao Paulo, Brazil. Blood. 2002;99:83–7.
139. Mustafa MM, Weitman SD, Winick NJ, Bellini WJ, Timmons CF, Siegel JD. Subacute measles encephalitis in the young immunocompromised host: report of two cases diagnosed by polymerase chain reaction and treated with ribavirin and review of the literature. Clin Infect Dis. 1993;16:654–60.
140. Sternfeld T, Spori-Byrtus V, Riediger C, et al. Acute measles infection triggering an episode of liver transplant rejection. Int J Infect Dis. 2010;14:e528–30.
141. Turner A, Jeyaratnam D, Haworth F, et al. Measles-associated encephalopathy in children with renal transplants. Am J Transplant. 2006;6:1459–65.
142. Liu Y, Sun LY, Zhu ZJ, Lin W, Qu W, Zeng ZG. Measles virus infection in pediatric liver transplantation recipients. Transplant Proc. 2015;47:2715–8.
143. Klapper PE, Cleator GM, Clarke MC, Postlethwaite RJ. Measles immunisation. Arch Dis Child. 1991;66:369.
144. Bitnun A, Shannon P, Durward A, et al. Measles inclusion-body encephalitis caused by the vaccine strain of measles virus. Clin Infect Dis. 1999;29:855–61.
145. Storek J. Measles in bone marrow transplant recipients. Blood. 2002;99:3070.
146. Aiello FB, Calabrese F, Furian L, et al. Mumps-associated nephritis mimicking acute rejection in a patient under chronic dialysis treatment because of graft dysfunction. Transpl Int. 2002;15:523–4.
147. Park SB, Jin KB, Hwang EA, et al. Case of adult mumps infection after renal transplantation. Transplant Proc. 2008;40:2442–3.
148. Eyre TA, Pelosi E, McQuaid S, et al. Mumps virus encephalomyelitis in a 19-year old male patient with an undefined severe combined immunodeficiency post-haematopoietic bone marrow transplantation: a rare fatal complication. J Clin Virol. 2013;57:165–8.
149. Lam HY, Yeap SK, Rasoli M, et al. Safety and clinical usage of Newcastle disease virus in cancer therapy. J Biomed Biotechnol. 2011;2011:718710.
150. Goebel SJ, Taylor J, Barr BC, et al. Isolation of avian paramyxovirus 1 from a patient with a lethal case of pneumonia. J Virol. 2007;81:12709–14.
151. Woolhouse ME, Howey R, Gaunt E, Reilly L, Chase-Topping M, Savill N. Temporal trends in the discovery of human viruses. Proc Biol Sci. 2008;275:2111–5.
152. Tyler KL. Emerging viral infections of the central nervous system: part 2. Arch Neurol. 2009;66:1065–74.
153. Marsh GA, de Jong C, Barr JA, et al. Cedar virus: a novel Henipavirus isolated from Australian bats. PLoS Pathog. 2012;8:e1002836.
154. Eaton BT, Broder CC, Middleton D, Wang LF. Hendra and Nipah viruses: different and dangerous. Nat Rev Microbiol. 2006;4:23–35.
155. Chua KB, Lam SK, Goh KJ, et al. The presence of Nipah virus in respiratory secretions and urine of patients during an outbreak of Nipah virus encephalitis in Malaysia. J Infect. 2001;42:40–3.
156. Gurley ES, Montgomery JM, Hossain MJ, et al. Person-to-person transmission of Nipah virus in a Bangladeshi community. Emerg Infect Dis. 2007;13:1031–7.
157. Goh KJ, Tan CT, Chew NK, et al. Clinical features of Nipah virus encephalitis among pig farmers in Malaysia. N Engl J Med. 2000;342:1229–35.
158. Hossain MJ, Gurley ES, Montgomery JM, et al. Clinical presentation of nipah virus infection in Bangladesh. Clin Infect Dis. 2008;46:977–84.
159. Tan CT, Goh KJ, Wong KT, et al. Relapsed and late-onset Nipah encephalitis. Ann Neurol. 2002;51:703–8.
160. Tan ST, Blake GB, Chambers S. Recurrent orf in an immunocompromised host. Br J Plast Surg. 1991;44:465–7.

161. Geerninck K, Lukito G, Snoeck R, et al. A case of human orf in an immunocompromised patient treated successfully with cidofovir cream. J Med Virol. 2001;64:543–9.
162. Savage J, Black MM. Giant orf of finger in a patient with lymphoma. Proc R Soc Med. 1972;65:766.
163. Degraeve C, De Coninck A, Senneseael J, Rosseeuw D. Recurrent contagious ecthyma (orf) in an immunocompromised host successfully treated with cryotherapy. Dermatology. 1999;198:162–3.
164. Ara M, Zaballos P, Sanchez M, et al. Giant and recurrent orf virus infection in a renal transplant recipient treated with imiquimod. J Am Acad Dermatol. 2008;58:S39–40.
165. Rimoin AW, Mulembakani PM, Johnston SC, et al. Major increase in human monkeypox incidence 30 years after smallpox vaccination campaigns cease in the Democratic Republic of Congo. Proc Natl Acad Sci U S A. 2010;107:16262–7.
166. Reynolds MG, Damon IK. Outbreaks of human monkeypox after cessation of smallpox vaccination. Trends Microbiol. 2012;20:80–7.
167. Hutin YJ, Williams RJ, Malfait P, et al. Outbreak of human monkeypox, Democratic Republic of Congo, 1996 to 1997. Emerg Infect Dis. 2001;7:434–8.
168. Huhn GD, Bauer AM, Yorita K, et al. Clinical characteristics of human monkeypox, and risk factors for severe disease. Clin Infect Dis. 2005;41:1742–51.
169. Meyer H, Perrichot M, Stemmler M, et al. Outbreaks of disease suspected of being due to human monkeypox virus infection in the Democratic Republic of Congo in 2001. J Clin Microbiol. 2002;40:2919–21.
170. Lakis NS, Li Y, Abraham JL, et al. Novel poxvirus infection in an immune suppressed patient. Clin Infect Dis. 2015;61:1543–8.
171. 2012. At http://www.transplant-observatory.org/Pages/home.aspx. Accessed 13 Sept 2012.
172. Nikolay B, Diallo M, Boye CS, Sall AA. Usutu virus in Africa. Vector Borne Zoonotic Dis. 2011;11:1417–23.
173. WHO. Dengue: Guidelines for diagnosis, treatment, prevention and control. France: WHO Press; 2009.
174. Kliks SC, Nisalak A, Brandt WE, Wahl L, Burke DS. Antibody-dependent enhancement of dengue virus growth in human monocytes as a risk factor for dengue hemorrhagic fever. Am J Trop Med Hyg. 1989;40:444.
175. Martina BEE, Koraka P, Osterhaus ADME. Dengue virus pathogenesis: an integrated view. Clin Microbiol Rev. 2009;22:564.
176. Rico-Hesse R. Dengue virus evolution and virulence models. Clin Infect Dis. 2007;44:1462.
177. Sierra B, Perez AB, Alvarez M, et al. Variation in inflammatory/regulatory cytokines in secondary, tertiary, and quaternary challenges with dengue virus. Am J Trop Med Hyg. 2012;87(3):538–47.
178. Azevedo LS, Carvalho DBM, Matuck T, et al. Dengue in renal transplant patients: a retrospective analysis. Transplantation. 2007;84:792–4.
179. Chacko B, John GT, Jacob C. Dengue shock syndrome in a renal transplant recipient. Transplantation. 2004;77:634–5.
180. Garcia JHP, Rocha TDS, Viana CFG, et al. Dengue shock syndrome in a liver transplant recipient. Tranplantation. 2006;82:850–1.
181. Park SB, Ryu SY, Jin KB, et al. Acute colitis associated with dengue fever in a renal transplant recipient. Transplant Proc. 2008;40:2431–2.
182. Renaud CJ, Manjit K, Pary S. Dengue has a benign presentation in renal transplant patients: a case series. Nephrology. 2007;12:305–7.
183. Rigau-Perez JG, Vorndam V, Clark GG. The dengue and dengue hemorrhagic fever epidemic in Puerto Rico, 1994–1995. Am J Trop Med Hyg. 2001;64:67–74.
184. Tan FL, Loh DLSK, Prabhakaran K. Dengue haemorrhagic fever after living donor renal transplantation. Nephrol Dial Transplant. 2005;20:447–8.
185. Tangnararatchakit K, Tirapanich W, Tapaneya-Olarn W, et al. Severe nonfebrile dengue infection in an adolescent after postoperative kidney transplantation: a case report. Transplant Proc. 2012;44:303–6.
186. Prasad N, Bhadauria D, Sharma RK, Gupta A, Kaul A, Srivastava A. Dengue virus infection in renal allograft recipients: a case series during 2010 outbreak. Transpl Infect Dis. 2012;14:163–8.
187. Costa SD, da Silva GB Jr, Jacinto CN, et al. Dengue fever among renal transplant recipients: a series of 10 cases in a tropical country. Am J Trop Med Hyg. 2015;93:394–6.
188. Gupta RK, Gupta G, Chorasiya VK, et al. Dengue virus transmission from living donor to recipient in liver transplantation: a case report. J Clin Exp Hepatol. 2016;6:59–61.
189. Punzel M, Korukluoglu G, Caglayik DY, et al. Dengue virus transmission by blood stem cell donor after travel to Sri Lanka; Germany, 2013. Emerg Infect Dis. 2014;20:1366–9.
190. Kotton CN. Zika virus and solid organ transplantation: significant pathogen or harbinger of things to come? Transplantation. 2016;100:970–2.
191. Machado CM, Martins TC, Colturato I, et al. Epidemiology of neglected tropical diseases in transplant recipients. Review of the literature and experience of a Brazilian HSCT center. Rev Inst Med Trop Sao Paulo. 2009;51:309–24.
192. Azevedo LS, Lasmar EP, Contieri FLC, et al. Yellow fever vaccination in organ transplanted patients: is it safe? A multicenter study. Transpl Infect Dis. 2012;14:237–41.
193. Avelino-Silva VI, Leal FE, Sabino EC, et al. Yellow fever vaccine viremia following ablative BM suppression in AML. Bone Marrow Transplant. 2013;48:1008–9.
194. Charrel RN, de Lamballerie X, Raoult D. Chikungunya outbreaks--the globalization of vectorborne diseases. N Engl J Med. 2007;356:769–71.
195. Staples JE, Breiman RF, Powers AM. Chikungunya fever: an epidemiological review of a re-emerging infectious disease. Clin Infect Dis. 2009;49:942.
196. Bonilauri P, Bellini R, Calzolari M, et al. Chikungunya virus in Aedes albopictus, Italy. Emerg Infect Dis. 2008;14:852–4.
197. Borgherini G, Poubeau P, Jossaume A, et al. Persistent arthralgia associated with chikungunya virus: a study of 88 adult patients on Reunion island. Clin Infect Dis. 2008;47:469–75.
198. Simon F, Parola P, Grandadam M, et al. Chikungunya infection: an emerging rheumatism among travelers returned from Indian Ocean islands. Report of 47 cases. Medicine. 2007;86:123–37.
199. Borgherini G, Paubeau P, Staikowsky F, et al. Outbreak of chikungunya on Reunion island: early clinical and laboratory features in 157 adult patients. Clin Infect Dis. 2007;44:1401.
200. Chusri S, Siripaitoon P, Hirunpat S, Silpapojakul K. Case reports of neuro-chikungunya in southern Thailand. Am J Trop Med Hyg. 2011;85:386–9.
201. Kee AC, Yang S, Tambyah P. Atypical chikungunya virus infections in immunocompromised patients. Emerg Infect Dis. 2010;16:1038–40.
202. Dalla Gasperina D, Balsamo ML, Garavaglia SD, Rovida F, Baldanti F, Grossi PA. Chikungunya infection in a human immunodeficiency virus-infected kidney transplant recipient returning to Italy from the Dominican Republic. Transpl Infect Dis. 2015;17:876–9.
203. Couderc T, Gangneux N, Chretien F, et al. Chikungunya virus infection of corneal grafts. J Infect Dis. 2012;206:851–9.
204. Boshra H, Lorenzo G, Busquets N, Brun A. Rift valley fever: recent insights into pathogenesis and prevention. J Virol. 2011;85:6098–105.
205. Hassan OA, Ahlm C, Sang R, Evander M. The 2007 Rift Valley fever outbreak in Sudan. PLoS Negl Trop Dis. 2011;5:e1229.

206. Zhang YZ, He YW, Dai YA, et al. Hemorrhagic fever caused by a novel bunyavirus in China: pathogenesis and correlates of fatal outcome. Clin Infect Dis. 2012;54:527–33.
207. Meier M, Helmchen U, Fricke L, Ulrich R, Schutt M. Acute hantavirus infection or renal transplant rejection. Transpl Infect Dis. 2007;9:225–8.
208. Moutschen P, Bourhaba M, Frippiat F, et al. A pauci-symptomatic case of documented hantavirus (Puumala) infection in a patient under anti-TNF treatment. J Clin Virol. 2011;50:247–8.
209. Sinisalo M, Vapalahti O, Ekblom-Kullberg S, et al. Headache and low platelets in a patient with acute leukemia. J Clin Virol. 2010;48:159–61.
210. Huggins JW, Hsiang CM, Cosgriff TM, et al. Prospective, double-blind, concurrent, placebo-controlled clinical trial of intravenous ribavirin therapy of hemorrhagic fever with renal syndrome. J Infect Dis. 1991;164:1119–27.
211. Mertz GJ, Miedzinski L, Goade D, et al. Placebo-controlled, double-blind trial of intravenous ribavirin for the treatment of hantavirus cardiopulmonary syndrome in North America. Clin Infect Dis. 2004;39:1307–13.
212. Qian DY, Ding YS, Chen GF, et al. A placebo-controlled clinical trial of prednisone in the treatment of early hemorrhagic fever. J Infect Dis. 1990;162:1213–4.
213. Kortepeter MG, Bausch DG, Bray M. Basic clinical and laboratory features of filoviral hemorrhagic fever. J Infect Dis. 2011;204(Suppl 3):S810–6.
214. Leroy EM, Gonzalez JP, Baize S. Ebola and Marburg haemorrhagic fever viruses: major scientific advances, but a relatively minor public health threat for Africa. Clin Microbiol Infect. 2011;17:964–76.
215. 2014. Ebola outbreak in West Africa – outbreak distribution map, 2016. At http://www.cdc.gov/vhf/ebola/outbreaks/2014-west-africa/distribution-map.html. Accessed 28 May 2016.
216. Bausch DG, Towner JS, Dowell SF, et al. Assessment of the risk of Ebola virus transmission from bodily fluids and fomites. J Infect Dis. 2007;196(Suppl 2):S142–7.
217. Kaul DR, Mehta AK, Wolfe CR, Blumberg E, Green M. Ebola virus disease: implications for solid organ transplantation. Am J Transplant. 2015;15:5–6.
218. Mueller NJ, Takeuchi Y, Mattiuzzo G, Scobie L. Microbial safety in xenotransplantation. Curr Opin Organ Transplant. 2011;16:201–6.
219. Scobie L, Takeuchi Y. Porcine endogenous retrovirus and other viruses in xenotransplantation. Curr Opin Organ Transplant. 2009;14:175–9.
220. Patience C, Takeuchi Y, Weiss RA. Infection of human cells by an endogenous retrovirus of pigs. Nat Med. 1997;3:282–6.
221. Hermida-Prieto M, Domenech N, Moscoso I, et al. Lack of cross-species transmission of porcine endogenous retrovirus (PERV) to transplant recipients and abattoir workers in contact with pigs. Transplantation. 2007;84:548–50.
222. Gu C, Wei X, Wang Y, et al. No infection with porcine endogenous retrovirus in recipients of acellular porcine aortic valves: a two-year study. Xenotransplantation. 2008;15:121–8.
223. Issa NC, Wilkinson RA, Griesemer A, et al. Absence of replication of porcine endogenous retrovirus and porcine lymphotropic herpesvirus type 1 with prolonged pig cell microchimerism after pig-to-baboon xenotransplantation. J Virol. 2008;82:12441–8.
224. Valdes-Gonzalez R, Dorantes LM, Bracho-Blanchet E, Rodriguez-Ventura A, White DJ. No evidence of porcine endogenous retrovirus in patients with type 1 diabetes after long-term porcine islet xenotransplantation. J Med Virol. 2010;82:331–4.
225. Garkavenko O, Croxson MC, Irgang M, Karlas A, Denner J, Elliott RB. Monitoring for presence of potentially xenotic viruses in recipients of pig islet xenotransplantation. J Clin Microbiol. 2004;42:5353–6.
226. Garkavenko O, Dieckhoff B, Wynyard S, et al. Absence of transmission of potentially xenotic viruses in a prospective pig to primate islet xenotransplantation study. J Med Virol. 2008;80:2046–52.
227. Network USOPaT. Policy 4: identification of transmissible diseases in organ recipients. 2010:4.

Parasitic Infections in Transplant Recipients: Toxoplasmosis, Strongyloidiasis, and Other Parasites

46

Brian G. Blackburn and José G. Montoya

Toxoplasmosis

Toxoplasma gondii infects approximately one-third of the world's population and has the potential to cause significant morbidity and mortality in transplant recipients [1]. The term "toxoplasmosis" refers to symptomatic patients with ongoing clinical manifestations stemming from a recently acquired infection (primary infection) or reactivation of a previously acquired infection (chronic or latent infection). In contrast, the term "*T. gondii* infection" should be reserved for chronically infected patients without symptoms.

Immunocompromised individuals (including transplant recipients) are at higher risk of developing life-threatening toxoplasmosis. However, toxoplasmosis can be prevented and successfully treated if an early diagnosis is made. Toxoplasmosis in transplant patients can be the result of a primary infection (acquired orally or via the transplanted organ) or reactivation of a latent infection acquired prior to transplantation.

It is important to realize that toxoplasmosis should be suspected even in patients who do not appear to have conventional epidemiological risk factors such as cat ownership or ingestion of raw meat or history of an illness suggestive of toxoplasmosis. Approximately half of individuals infected with *T. gondii* do not recall traditional risk factors for infection with the parasite or experiencing a clinical illness consistent with toxoplasmosis. In order to determine whether an unexplained syndrome like pneumonia, fever, seizures, and/or brain abscesses in a transplant recipient can be attributed to toxoplasmosis, laboratory tests should be performed in the pretransplant period to establish the level of risk and need for empirical treatment including *Toxoplasma* serological screening in all transplant recipient candidates and all organ donors. In addition, testing should be performed in the posttransplant period in various body fluids or tissues according to the clinical scenario; this may include polymerase chain reaction in bronchoalveolar lavage, peripheral blood, cerebrospinal fluid, and immunohistochemistry in biopsy specimens.

B. G. Blackburn (✉)
Stanford University Medical Center, Stanford, CA, USA

Division of Infectious Diseases and Geographic Medicine, Stanford University School of Medicine, Stanford, CA, USA
e-mail: blackburn@stanford.edu

J. G. Montoya
Stanford University Medical Center, Stanford, CA, USA

Division of Infectious Diseases and Geographic Medicine, Stanford University School of Medicine, Stanford, CA, USA

Palo Alto Medical Foundation Toxoplasma Serology Laboratory, National Reference Center for the Study and Diagnosis of Toxoplasmosis, Palo Alto, CA, USA
e-mail: gilberto@stanford.edu

The Organism

The infectious forms of *T. gondii* include the tachyzoite, the tissue cyst containing bradyzoites, and the oocyst containing sporozoites (Fig. 46.1). The tachyzoite is semilunar in shape, is 2–3 μm wide and 5–7 μm long, and is responsible for the clinical manifestations observed in patients with toxoplasmosis.

The tissue cyst measures up to 100 μm in diameter; it is responsible for chronic infection believed to be mostly asymptomatic, and establishes latency in organs such as the heart, skeletal muscle, eye, brain, liver, and kidney. The tissue cyst can be transmitted to transplant recipients through consumption of infected meat or implantation of an infected allograft from an infected donor with acute or chronic infection. Bradyzoites have limited metabolic activity and do not replicate but can reactivate and transform into tachyzoites, especially when significant impairments in T-cell-mediated immunity occur.

Oocysts are shed in soil and water by wild or domestic felids, measure 10–12 μm in diameter in the unsporulated form, and are responsible for transmission to patients via inadvertent oral ingestion of items contaminated by infected

A. Safdar (ed.), *Principles and Practice of Transplant Infectious Diseases*, https://doi.org/10.1007/978-1-4939-9034-4_46

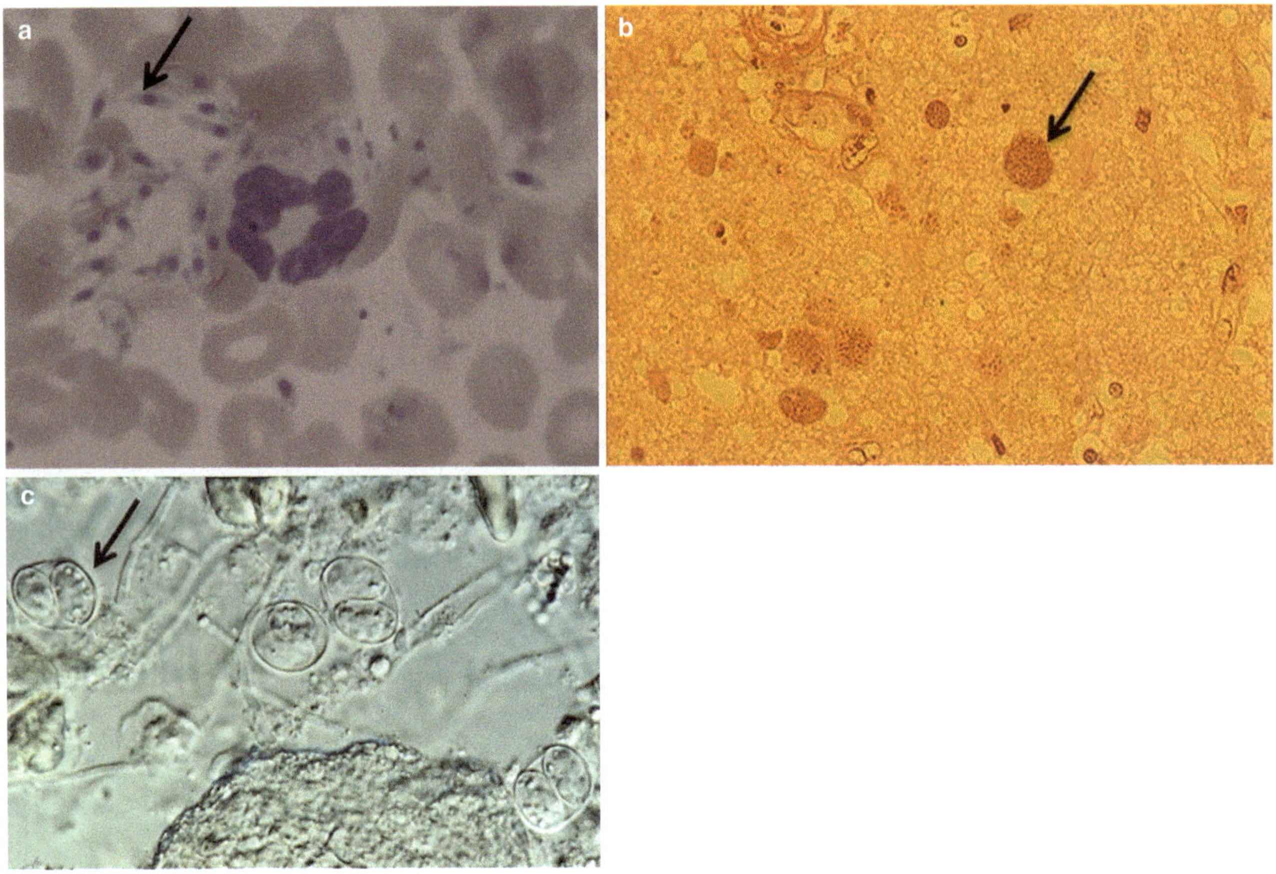

Fig. 46.1 (**a–c**). Main forms of *T. gondii* found in nature (see arrows). Tachyzoites (**a**), tissue cysts (**b**) containing bradyzoites, and oocysts (**c**) containing sporozoites

cat feces (e.g., water, vegetables, or other food; contact with infected soil or while gardening). As many as ten million oocysts can be shed by an infected cat in a single day. Sporulation is required for oocysts to become infectious and occurs outside the cat within 1–5 days depending on temperature and oxygen availability. Oocysts may remain viable for as long as 18 months in moist soil, resulting in an environmental reservoir from which incidental hosts may be infected.

Although toxoplasmosis is widely distributed across continents, a clonal expansion of few lineages appears to have occurred. *Toxoplasma* strains can be primarily classified as types I, II, III, and atypical. Type II strains appear to predominate in Europe and types I/III and atypical strains in South America. The United States appears to have both European-like type II and South American-like strains. In Latin America, for example, a more aggressive and lethal form of toxoplasmosis has been associated with atypical strains rarely found in Europe [2–4]. Pneumonia, disseminated disease, admission to intensive care units, and even death have been observed in immunocompetent individuals infected with these strains in South America. These emerging and more virulent strains have potentially serious implications for transplant patients who receive organs from individuals from those areas or travel to these places.

Life Cycle and Epidemiology

Humans are incidental hosts of the parasite and acquire infection primarily by the oral route. Two important additional routes of transmission to humans include vertical transmission from mother to unborn child and transmission via infected allografts during transplantation.

Domestic and feral cats are the definitive hosts of *T. gondii*. They can be infected with any of the primary infectious forms of the parasite including tachyzoites, tissue cysts, or oocysts. Once in their small intestine, the parasite undergoes asexual or sexual (gametogony) reproduction. Oocysts are subsequently excreted via their feces in soil or water.

Humans can acquire the parasite by ingestion of infected meat (containing tissue cysts) or other contaminated food or water (containing oocysts). Untreated water has been recognized as a major source of infection in community-acquired outbreaks of toxoplasmosis [5]. Exposure to contaminated cat feces, soil, or soil-related activities not limited to gardening can also result in primary infection. Novel routes of transmission to humans have been identified over the past few years. Ingestion of raw shellfish like oysters, mussels, and clams has been recently recognized as a potential means of *T. gondii* transmission [6].

An epidemiological study in the United States revealed that an elevated risk for recent *T. gondii* infection was associated with the following factors: eating raw ground beef; eating rare lamb; eating locally produced cured, dried, or smoked meat; eating raw oysters, clams, or mussels; working with meat; drinking unpasteurized goat milk; and having three or more kittens [6]. However, 48% of the infected individuals did not have an identified risk factor for *T. gondii* infection in this study. This is consistent with findings from previous epidemiological studies where many infected individuals did not have a known epidemiological risk factor [7]. It appears that infected individuals are often unaware of their exposure or may have difficulty recalling specific risk behaviors.

Donor-derived *Toxoplasma* infection is a well-known risk for recipients of solid organ transplants. *Toxoplasma* seronegative recipients (R−) are at greater risk of developing toxoplasmosis when they receive infected organs from seropositive donors (D+) and do not receive anti-*Toxoplasma* prophylaxis. In a study performed at Stanford University Medical Center, 25% of D+/R− heart transplant recipients developed or died from toxoplasmosis in the absence of prophylaxis, whereas none of the D+/R− patients who received prophylaxis developed toxoplasmosis [8].

Transmission of *T. gondii* through hematopoietic stem cell transplants (HSCT) or blood transfusion products appears to occur but is considered rare. HSCT patients who are *Toxoplasma* seronegative prior to transplantation (R−) are at low risk of developing posttransplant toxoplasmosis; this has occurred in only a few cases where the recipient was seronegative and the HSCT donor was seropositive (D+/R−). Most HSCT patients who develop toxoplasmosis do so from reactivation of a previously acquired infection in the recipient (i.e., seropositive prior to transplantation; R+) [9].

The risk of toxoplasmosis in a given transplant center varies by geographic region and the age of donors and recipients because the *T. gondii* seroprevalence varies considerably by locale and socioeconomic strata and increases with age [10].

For solid organ transplant programs, patients should be screened for *T. gondii* infection prior to transplant so that high risk patients (D+/R−) can be identified prior to transplantation. For instance, at Stanford University Medical Center, results of serological testing for *Toxoplasma* were available prior to heart transplant for 575 D/R pairs; of these, 454 (79%) were D−/R−, 84 (14.6%) D−/R+, 32 (5.6%) D+/R−, and 5 (0.8%) D+/R+ [8]. Similarly for HSCT programs, identification of R+ patients is highly recommended [9]. Serological testing following transplantation is often not helpful since serologies may rise or change posttransplant without necessarily indicating that patients have toxoplasmosis. In addition, serologies may not change, become negative, or remain negative (due to immunosuppression), even in the setting of toxoplasmosis [11].

Immune Response and Genetic Susceptibility of the Host

Coordinated innate, humoral, and cellular immune responses are required to prevent morbidity and mortality from primary infection and reactivation of latent *T. gondii* infection. A well-orchestrated and effective systemic immune response results in early disappearance of *T. gondii* from peripheral blood during the acute infection limiting parasite burden in target organs and successfully maintains latency in chronically infected individuals. Immunity in the immunocompetent individual is lifelong. Macrophages; dendritic cells; natural killer cells; CD4+ and CD8+ T cells; Th1 cytokines (e.g., IFN-γ, IL-12), tumor necrosis factor-α (TNF-α); co-stimulatory molecules, (e.g., CD28 and CD40 ligand); and, to a lesser degree, immunoglobulins, appear to be essential for the effective disappearance of tachyzoites from peripheral blood, their conversion to bradyzoites, and subsequent formation of tissue cysts.

Clinical Manifestations

T. gondii infection can result in symptoms and signs of toxoplasmosis in the setting of a primary infection or reactivation of a previously acquired latent infection. The parasite has coevolved with humans to the point of being capable of causing asymptomatic primary infections. Therefore, transplant donors and recipients may have been infected without their knowledge and without recognition of conventional risk factors for acute infection. The most effective approach for early diagnosis and treatment is for high clinical suspicion and appropriate laboratory testing.

Toxoplasmosis in the setting of heart transplantation is most likely to occur in D+/R− patients. In other solid organ transplant recipients, toxoplasmosis can occur as a result of D+/R− mismatch as well, or reactivation of a latent infection (R+). Toxoplasmosis in the setting of HSCT most commonly occurs as a result of reactivation of a chronic infection in the recipient (R+).

In autologous HSCT patients, reactivation is rare. In allogeneic HSCT patients, reactivation (R+) occurs more frequently in those who have developed graft-versus-host disease (GVHD); the median day of onset for toxoplasmosis is day 64 (range = 4–516 days) posttransplant. Although reactivation of latent *Toxoplasma* infection in allogeneic HSCT recipients most often occurs in the first six months posttransplant (most in the first 30–90 days), late reactivation has been observed and must be considered, especially in patients in whom late-onset (beyond six months posttransplant) GVHD occurs [9, 12, 13]. Conversely, an HSCT patient who is seronegative for *T. gondii* pretransplant has a very low risk of toxoplasmosis in the first 100 days after transplant [9, 12, 13].

Acute Toxoplasmosis

Although most individuals are asymptomatic, symptomatic primary infection may manifest as a painless, nonsuppurative lymphadenopathy. Lymphadenopathy develops more commonly in the cervical chain but can occur almost anywhere. A mononucleosis-like syndrome can be the presenting illness of the primary infection. Fever, headache, stiff neck, fatigue, arthralgia, myalgia, anorexia, skin rash, and visual symptoms (with retinal involvement) may also be present. When retinochoroiditis occurs, patients can develop blurred vision, eye pain, decreased visual acuity, floaters, scotoma, photophobia, or epiphora. Less frequently hepatitis, myositis, and myocarditis can occur. More aggressive disease including pneumonia, brain abscesses, and death has been observed in immunocompetent patients in Latin America [2]. Patients with these severe manifestations require admission to intensive care units and may have been infected with atypical strains of the parasite. Transplant patients may be at higher risk of developing severe toxoplasmosis if infected with these atypical strains. Acute toxoplasmosis has been reported when seropositive heart, liver, and kidney donors transmitted the parasite to seronegative recipients via the infected organ. In this setting, syndromes such as fever, sepsis, pneumonia, seizures, brain abscesses, and retinochoroiditis have occurred.

Reactivation of Latent Infection

In most individuals, primary infection is followed by chronic latency in which the parasite remains dormant for the life of the host. Aside from reactivation in the eye, which can also occur in immunocompetent hosts, overt reactivation including life-threatening clinical manifestations is only observed in patients with significantly impaired cell-mediated immunity. Reactivation in immunocompromised patients can present as pneumonia, fever, seizures, diffuse encephalitis, space-occupying brain lesions (Fig. 46.2), retinochoroiditis, myocarditis, hepatosplenomegaly, lymphadenopathy, and rash. Although multiple brain abscesses are commonly described in patients with toxoplasmic encephalitis, diffuse encephalitis without space-occupying lesions by MRI has been reported with a very high case-fatality rate. Fever and/or pneumonia can be the sole manifestation(s) of toxoplasmosis in immunocompromised patients including solid organ and HSCT recipients. Toxoplasmic pneumonitis can present with cough, dyspnea, hypoxia, and diffuse bilateral infiltrates, usually reported as ground glass opacities or localized lung infiltrates. Fever alone has frequently been described in allogeneic HSCT and liver transplant recipients.

Laboratory Diagnosis

Clinically available laboratory methods for the diagnosis of *Toxoplasma* infection and toxoplasmosis include serological tests, polymerase chain reaction (PCR), direct visualization of the parasite by Wright-Giemsa or immunoperoxidase stains, and parasite isolation (Table 46.1) [14]. It is critical to remember that symptoms and/or history of conventional epidemiological factors associated with acute *Toxoplasma* infection are often absent in patients with acute or chronic infection. Thus, all transplant recipients and donors should be serologically screened for toxoplasmosis before transplantation in order to establish their risk for primary infection (D+/R−) or reactivation (R+). It is important that screening be performed prior to transplantation because these results may not be reliable in the posttransplant period [11].

Diagnosis of Latent *T. gondii* Infection

Initial serological testing for *T. gondii*-specific IgG and IgM antibodies can be performed at non-reference commercial or hospital-based laboratories. Involvement of a reference laboratory, e.g., the Palo Alto Medical Foundation *Toxoplasma* Serology Laboratory (PAMF-TSL) in Palo Alto, CA (www.pamf.org/serology/ +1-650-853-4828; toxolab@pamf.org), is only required when positive or equivocal IgM test results are obtained or an equivocal IgG result is observed [15].

Transplant recipients and donors with negative IgG and IgM test results do not have serological evidence of prior exposure to *T. gondii* and are at low risk for developing toxoplasmosis. Transplant recipients who are *Toxoplasma* IgG positive and IgM negative have been infected for at least three months and are at risk for *Toxoplasma* reactivation if they are undergoing HSCT, liver, or kidney transplantation. Reactivation in heart, heart-lung, and lung transplant recipients occurs rarely in this setting. Donors who are seropositive for *T. gondii*, however, pose a serious risk to seronegative recipients (D+/R− mismatch) in the setting of heart, heart-lung, liver, kidney, and kidney-pancreas transplantation.

Diagnosis of Primary *T. gondii* Infection and Toxoplasmosis

Primary *T. gondii* infection should be suspected in a transplant candidate or donor with positive serum *Toxoplasma* IgG and IgM test results. However, this serum should be sent to a reference laboratory (e.g., PAMF_TSL) for confirmation, since

Table 46.1 Laboratory diagnosis of toxoplasmosis (acute infection or reactivation) in transplant patients

Serological tests
All transplant candidates and donors should undergo serological testing for *T. gondii*-specific IgG and IgM antibody tests before the transplant procedure or initiation of immunosuppression, whichever is first
Positive IgM test results should not be interpreted as necessarily indicative of a recently acquired infection. In these cases, serum should be sent for confirmatory testing to a reference laboratory specialized in the diagnosis of toxoplasmosis (e.g., the Palo Alto Medical Foundation *Toxoplasma* serology laboratory[a])
Serological test results confirmed by a reference laboratory as consistent with a recently acquired infection (e.g., within 6 months of sera sampling) should trigger consideration for treatment of the donor or recipient or postponing the transplant procedure
Serological tests performed posttransplant may not be accurate
Polymerase chain reaction (by PCR)
T. gondii DNA amplification by PCR can be performed on any body fluid including peripheral blood; cerebrospinal fluid; bronchoalveolar lavage fluid;vitreous fluid; aqueous humor; and peritoneal, pleural or ascitic fluids.
A positive PCR test result in any body fluid should be interpreted as laboratory confirmation of *Toxoplasma* reactivation or toxoplasmosis.
PCR can also be performed in tissues, but positive test results should be interpreted with caution since they may reflect chronic infection
Microscopy (direct visualization of the parasite)
Tachyzoite
Wright-Giemsa stain of any body fluid or "touch" preparation slides of any tissue. *T. gondii*-specific immunoperoxidase stains of biopsy specimens. Presence of tachyzoites in any fluid or tissue should be interpreted as laboratory confirmation of *Toxoplasma* reactivation or toxoplasmosis
Tissue cysts in histopathology samples
Hematoxylin and eosin or *T. gondii*-specific immunoperoxidase stains of any tissue or biopsy specimen. Numerous cysts or an associated strong inflammatory response is highly suggestive of toxoplasmosis and not simply *T. gondii* infection
Attempts to isolate the parasite
Attempts to isolate *T. gondii* can be performed in tissue culture or the peritoneal cavity of animals[a]
Establishing the strain of the parasite may have clinical and prognostic implications
Lymph node histology
Presence of a characteristic histologic triad in lymph node biopsy specimens can also be used for the diagnosis of toxoplasmosis (a reactive follicular hyperplasia; irregular clusters of epithelioid histiocytes encroaching on and blurring the margins of the germinal centers; and focal distention of sinuses with monocytoid cells)

[a]Palo Alto Medical Foundation Toxoplasmosis Serology Laboratory: http://www.pamf.org/serology/; telephone number (650) 853–4828; e-mail, toxolab@pamf.org

only 40% of such sera are confirmed to represent an acute infection when additional confirmatory testing is performed at a reference laboratory. Confirmatory testing of positive IgM test results at PAMF-TSL includes repeating the IgG and IgM tests, and performing IgA, IgE, differential agglutination (AC/HS), and IgG avidity assays [14]. If a primary infection is confirmed in a transplant candidate at PAMF-TSL, anti-*Toxoplasma* treatment should be promptly initiated in consultation with a transplant infectious diseases specialist. If a primary infection is confirmed in a potential donor following confirmatory testing, consultation with a transplant infectious diseases physician is strongly recommended since an evolving acute infection in the allograft may preclude utilization of these organs for transplantation purposes.

Toxoplasmosis from reactivation in transplant patients previously established as R+ is rarely diagnosed by serological tests alone. Additional laboratory methods are required including nucleic acid amplification such as PCR, stains to visualize the tachyzoite, histological methods to identify tissue cysts surrounded by inflammation or characteristic pathological findings, and parasite isolation (Table 46.1).

A positive *Toxoplasma* PCR test on any body fluid (e.g., peripheral blood, cerebrospinal fluid, bronchoalveolar lavage fluid, vitreous fluid, aqueous humor, and peritoneal, pleural, or ascitic fluids) is diagnostic of toxoplasmosis. PCR can

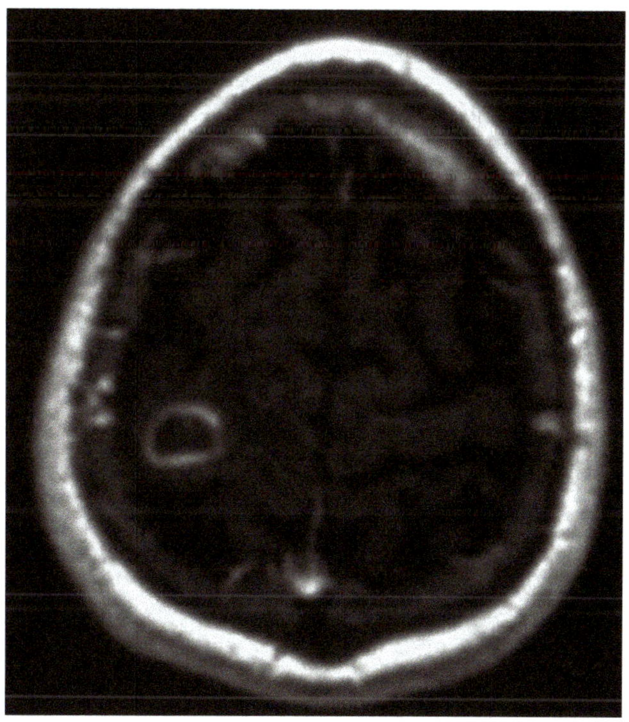

Fig. 46.2 Brain MRI depicting ring-enhancing brain lesion in an immunocompromised patient. *T. gondii*-specific immunoperoxidase staining of brain biopsy tissue was diagnostic of toxoplasmic encephalitis

Table 46.2 Treatment regimens for immunocompromised patients with toxoplasmosis[a]

Pyrimethamine (PO)	200 mg loading dose followed by 50 mg (for patient wt. <60 kg) to 75 mg (for patient wt. >60 kg)/day
[b]Folinic acid (PO)	10–20 mg daily (up to 50 mg/day) (during and for one week after completing therapy with pyrimethamine)
plus	
Sulfadiazine (PO)	1000 mg (for patient wt. <60 kg) to 1500 mg (for patient wt. >60 kg) every 6 h
or	
Clindamycin (PO or IV)	600 mg every 6 h (up to 1200 mg every 6 h)
or	
Atovaquone (PO)	1500 mg orally twice daily
Trimethoprim/sulfamethoxazole (PO or IV)	10 mg/kg/day (trimethoprim component) in two to three doses (doses as high as 15–20 mg/kg/day have been used)
Atovaquone (PO)	1500 mg orally twice daily
plus	
Sulfadiazine (PO)	1000 (for patient wt.<60 kg) to 1500 mg (for patient wt. >60 kg) every 6 h
Pyrimethamine	200 mg loading dose followed by 50 mg (for patient wt. <60 kg) to 75 mg (for patient wt. >60 kg)/day
[b]Folinic acid	10–20 mg daily (up to 50 mg/day) (during and for one week after completing therapy with pyrimethamine)
plus	
Clarithromycin (PO)	500 mg every 12 h
or	
Dapsone (PO)	100 mg/day
or	
Azithromycin (PO)	900–1200 mg/day

[a]Prefered regimens: pyrimethamine/sulfadiazine/folinic acid or trimethoprim/sulfamethoxazole. Assistance is available for the diagnosis and manag ement of patients with toxoplasmosis at the Palo Alto Medical Foundation *Toxoplasma* Serology Laboratory, PAMF-TSL; Palo Alto, CA; www.pamf. org/serology/; +1-650-853-4828; toxolab@pamf.org

[b]Folinic acid = leucovorin; folic acid must not be used as a substitute for folinic acid

[c]After the successful use of a combination regimen during the acute/primary therapy phase, the same agents at half doses are usually used for maintenance or secondary prophylaxis

also be performed on tissues, but this method has not been standardized, and a positive result cannot be necessarily interpreted as diagnostic of toxoplasmosis since the presence of tissue cysts in chronically infected individuals can also yield positive test results. The two most commonly used gene targets are the multi-copy *B-1* and 529 genes. For maximum reliability, clinical samples should be sent to reference laboratories experienced in performing this assay.

Visualization of the tachyzoite form in any body fluid or tissue is also diagnostic of toxoplasmosis in the setting of primary infection or reactivation of a latent infection. In contrast, the visualization of tissue cysts in biopsy specimens may simply represent chronic infection and does not necessarily indicate that toxoplasmosis is the cause of a symptomatic patient's clinical manifestations since cysts are typically present in chronically infected individuals. However, the presence of "numerous" cysts surrounded by a prominent inflammatory response is suggestive of toxoplasmosis.

Attempts to isolate the parasite from any body fluid or tissue, as clinically indicated, can be attempted at reference laboratories (e.g., PAMF-TSL). A positive isolation test from any body fluid is diagnostic of toxoplasmosis, but tissue specimens share the same limitation with regard to specificity as noted above for the PCR test. If positive, strain typing and genotyping can be used to further study the emerging data which correlates certain strains with more aggressive disease. Characteristic lymph node histology can also be used to diagnose toxoplasmosis [16].

Treatment

Anti-*Toxoplasma* therapy should be initiated immediately in any transplant recipient with acute *T. gondii* infection or reactivation of a latent infection regardless of symptoms (Table 46.2). High morbidity and mortality is observed in transplant recipients if treatment for toxoplasmosis is delayed. Treatment is also indicated for transplant candidates and donors with acute infection if transplantation is likely to occur within six months of the primary infection.

High doses of anti-*Toxoplasma* drugs are typically indicated for posttransplant immunocompromised patients with toxoplasmosis (Table 46.2). Folate antagonists are preferred; monotherapy should be avoided. Pyrimethamine is probably the most active drug against *T. gondii* and appears to have the most synergy when combined with sulfadiazine. Pyrimethamine in combination with clindamycin is an acceptable alternative regimen, as is trimethoprim/sulfamethoxazole (TMP/SMX).

Prevention

Primary Prophylaxis for Seropositive HSCT Recipients and D+/R− SOT Patients

Primary anti-*Toxoplasma* prophylaxis is indicated in allogeneic HSCT patients who are found to be *Toxoplasma* IgG positive before transplant (R+) as well as in solid organ transplant patients found to be D+/R−. Trimethoprim/sulfamethoxazole primarily used by transplant physicians to prevent *Pneumocystis jirovecii* pneumonia (PCP), has been successful in the prevention of toxoplasmosis in transplant patients. Effective regimens include one single-strength TMP/SMX tablet daily and one double-strength TMP/SMX tablet three times per week. For patients with allergy or intolerance to sulfa drugs, atovaquone 1500 mg daily is an alternative. Other drug regimens used to prevent PCP, e.g., pentamidine or dapsone alone, are not effective in preventing toxoplasmosis. Pyrimethamine 25 mg/day has also been reported to be effective *T. gondii* primary prophylaxis in D+/R- solid organ transplant patients [8, 17].

The use of TMP/SMX as primary prophylaxis for allogeneic or cord blood HSCT (R+) patients is usually delayed until after engraftment has been achieved due to the myelosuppressive potential of the drug. There are two strategies to address this window of vulnerability that can be implemented. Atovaquone prophylaxis can be used as the prophylactic drug until engraftment allows the use of TMP/SMX in these patients or screening for *Toxoplasma* reactivation can be done with the use of weekly PCR in peripheral blood for the first 100 days after transplant. PCR-positive patients should subsequently be treated with TMP/SMX or atovaquone at treatment doses plus an additional second drug. Of note, a negative blood PCR result does not rule out disease in a seropositive HSCT recipient who is symptomatic with clinical manifestations suggestive of toxoplasmosis [13].

Table 46.3 Measures suggested for the primary prevention of *T. gondii* infection in seronegative individuals[a]

Source	Measures
Meat and other edibles	Meat should be thoroughly cooked to 63 to 71 °C (74 °C for poultry) or to "well done"
	Meat should not be pink in the center
	Freezing and thawing meat can kill *T. gondii* tissue cysts, freeze meat to −20 °C for at least 48 h
	Infected meat that has been smoked, cured in brine, or dried may still be infectious
	Wash hands thoroughly following contact with raw meat
	Avoid mucous membrane contact when handling raw meat
	Wash (wearing gloves) kitchen surfaces and utensils that have come in contact with raw meat
	Abstain from skinning or butchering animals without gloves
	Avoid drinking unpasteurized goat milk
	Avoid eating raw oysters, clams, or mussels
	Thoroughly wash fruits, vegetables, or any organic edible
Cat feces and soil	Avoid contact with materials potentially contaminated exposure with cat feces
	Abstain from handling of cat litter or gardening
	Wearing gloves is recommended when these activities cannot be avoided
Untreated water	Avoid drinking untreated water including that from wells, ponds, or reservoirs that have not been secured from potential contamination with feces of infected felids

[a]Up to 50% of infected individuals are unable to recall behaviors known to be associated with *T. gondii* infection

Primary Prevention for Seronegative Transplant Candidates, Recipients, and Donors

Transplant candidates and recipients who do not have serological evidence of prior exposure to *T. gondii* should be aware of the risk factors for acute infection (Table 46.3). These same preventive measures also apply to seronegative donors prior to the transplant procedure.

Strongyloidiasis

Strongyloidiasis is caused by the intestinal nematode, *Strongyloides stercoralis*. Primarily transmitted in tropical areas, *S. stercoralis* usually causes a chronic gastrointestinal syndrome or can remain asymptomatic for decades [18]. The primary medical importance of this parasite in the developed world lies in its potential to cause the hyperinfection syndrome in immunocompromised patients, wherein larvae may disseminate throughout the body, with mortality rates of up to 70–80% [19–21].

The Organism

The life cycle of *S. stercoralis* is complex, alternating between free-living and parasitic cycles, and includes adult worms, two different larval stages, and eggs. These cycles form the basis for autoinfection and multiplication within the host, features relatively unique among helminths to *Strongyloides* [22, 23].

Soil-living adult worms produce eggs, which give rise to non-infective **rhabditiform larvae**. These either continue the free-living cycle by maturing into adults or become infective **filariform larvae**. Filariform larvae can penetrate intact human skin, after which they migrate to the lungs.

From there, they are expectorated, swallowed, and reach the small intestine; this journey takes about 3–4 weeks. In the intestine, *S. stercoralis* matures into adult worms, which are semitranslucent and about two millimeters long. These produce eggs, which hatch and become rhabditiform larvae. Although most of these larvae exit the gastrointestinal tract via the stool and subsequently develop into adult worms in the soil, a small number develop directly into infective (filariform) larvae within the gut and penetrate the intestinal mucosa or perianal skin, completing the life cycle without leaving the host. This is termed **autoinfection** and differentiates *S. stercoralis* from nearly all other helminths in several ways, including lifelong persistence in a host in the absence of treatment, multiplication in the absence of exogenous reinfection, and potential person-to-person transmission [24].

Epidemiology

Global estimates of strongyloidiasis prevalence vary widely, from 30 to 100 million people infected [21, 22, 25]. *S. stercoralis* is less common than other major intestinal nematodes such as *Ascaris*, *Trichuris*, and hookworms [18]. Strongyloidiasis is found throughout the tropics and subtropics and in limited foci of the United States (mostly Appalachia) and in Europe [25]. Transmission occurs via skin contact with fecal contaminated soil, so transmission is favored where poor hygienic conditions are combined with a warm, moist climate. Primary prevention involves improving social hygiene and universal use of footwear in endemic regions.

Studies based on stool examination in the 1960s and 1970s demonstrated prevalence rates of 0.5–4.0% in differing US cohorts, mostly in the Southeast and Appalachia [22, 25]. Although prevalence has subsequently decreased, infections are still seen in patients from those areas, especially those that are older than 50 years, institutionalized, of low socioeconomic status, or who have lived in rural areas [25]. In developing countries, strongyloidiasis prevalence rates can be striking in some cohorts, for example 25% in Thailand and Nigeria, 28% in Brazil, and 40% in Colombia [22, 25]. Because of the superior sensitivity of serology for diagnosis, seroepidemiology studies generally report higher prevalence rates than those based on parasite detection in stool samples; in one Peruvian cohort, 9% tested positive by stool examination for *S. stercoralis*, while 72% were seropositive [26]. Prevalence rates in resettled US refugees can also be high, where one recent study found 46% of a group of resettled Sudanese refugees to be seropositive for *S. stercoralis* [27]. Another study found that 39% of asymptomatic refugees in Boston with eosinophilia were *S. stercoralis* seropositive [28]. Given the high prevalence in many tropical and subtropical areas and the lifelong persistence of this parasite in the absence of treatment, physicians should consider strongyloidiasis both in persons with recent exposure to endemic areas and immigrant or refugee patients in developed countries even if they immigrated decades earlier.

Pathogenesis, Immunity, and the Hyperinfection Syndrome

Strongyloides infection is sustained over time in a given host by a small, stable number of intestinal adult worms. Although these die after a finite lifespan, autoinfection ensures the constant production of new worms, perpetuating the cycle even in the absence of reinfection [29]. In patients with chronic strongyloidiasis, autoinfection is normally well controlled by cell-mediated immunity, and the number of adult worms remains low and stable. With immunosuppression, more autoinfective larvae complete the cycle, and the population of parasitic adult worms increases, causing hyperinfection [29]. The large numbers of migrating larvae can disseminate, often associated with polymicrobial sepsis, pneumonia, and meningitis. Untreated, disseminated strongyloidiasis is usually fatal, and even with treatment, mortality approaches 25–30% [20, 30].

Both parasite and host factors affect regulation of this cycle. The population size of *S. stercoralis* in a host depends in part on secreted parasite hormones that regulate autoinfection [23, 31]. When the immune response is impaired, larger numbers of autoinfective parasites can develop, as reported in patients with hematologic malignancies, solid organ transplants (SOTs) and hematopoietic stem cell transplants (HSCTs), hypogammaglobulinemia, and those suffering from severe malnutrition [32–34]. Interestingly, there has been little association between cyclosporine use and hyperinfection syndrome; some evidence suggests cyclosporine may have an antihelminthic effect on *S. stercoralis* [35]. Conversely, tacrolimus does not appear to offer similar protection against *Strongyloides* [36].

Among HTLV-infected patients, there is a strong association with increased susceptibility to infection with *Strongyloides*, the hyperinfection syndrome, and poor response to treatment. Control of *S. stercoralis* in vivo is most dependent on the Th2 immune response, but the predominant immune response in HTLV-infected patients shifts from Th2 to Th1 [37–39]. There is some suggestion that *S. stercoralis* may hasten the development of leukemia among HTLV coinfected patients [40]. In contrast, there have been surprisingly few reports of hyperinfection among *S. stercoralis*-infected patients with AIDS. Although disseminated strongyloidiasis does occasionally occur in AIDS patients, this disease was removed from the list of AIDS-defining illness by the Centers for Disease Control and Prevention (CDC) in 1987 [41, 42].

Corticosteroid use carries a disproportionately high risk for disseminated strongyloidiasis compared to other forms of immunosuppression [43, 44]. Corticosteroids may upregulate growth of *S. stercoralis* and allow the parasite to develop preferentially into autoinfective filariform larvae, in addition to suppressing immunity [23, 45, 46]. They may also allow nonreproductive adult worms to regain reproductivity [31, 47]. Patients have developed hyperinfection after only a few days of corticosteroid administration [48].

Clinical Findings

Most patients infected with *S. stercoralis* are asymptomatic or have only mild symptoms. Shortly after infection, some patients develop a localized, erythematous, pruritic rash [30, 49–51]. Pulmonary symptoms and eosinophilia may appear several days later; diarrhea and abdominal pain may follow. Blood is occasionally detected in the stool, but over 50% of infected patients are asymptomatic. Chronic strongyloidiasis is not generally associated with pulmonary symptoms. Although about 75% of chronically infected patients have eosinophilia, it is usually low-grade [22, 52]. Migrating larvae may produce larva currens, a serpiginous, erythematous, track-like rash. Some chronically infected patients note epigastric pain, nausea, diarrhea, blood loss, and possibly malabsorption. Rarely, heavy infections can cause bowel obstruction. The majority of chronically infected patients are asymptomatic [43]. There has been an association between *S. stercoralis* infection and biliary cancer, but this observation requires confirmation [53].

With hyperinfection, the intestines and lungs harbor many larvae, and diarrhea is common (Fig. 46.3). When dissemination occurs, larvae are found widely, sometimes involving the central nervous system (CNS). Eosinophilia is usually absent during hyperinfection. Other gastrointestinal manifestations are common, including abdominal pain, vomiting, and intestinal obstruction. Hemorrhage, peritonitis, or bacteremia can occur. Pneumonitis is common, with cough, respiratory failure, and diffuse interstitial infiltrates or consolidation on radiographs; respiratory secretions often contain the parasite (Figs. 46.4a–b). CNS invasion may cause meningitis and brain abscesses, with larvae in the cerebrospinal fluid or tissue. An association with SIADH has been reported [54, 55].

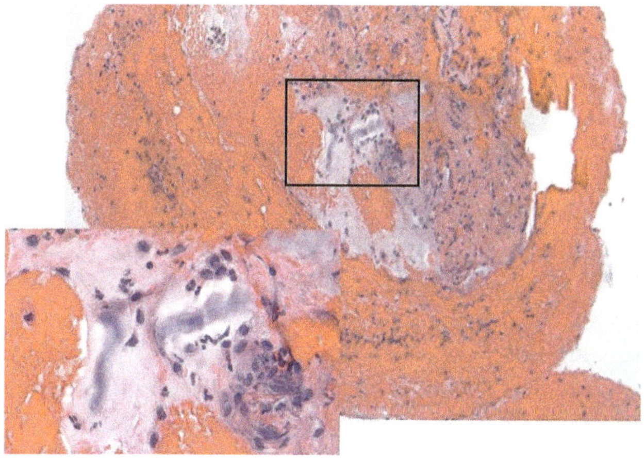

Fig. 46.3 Bronchoscopic biopsy in a patient with *Strongyloides* hyperinfection syndrome

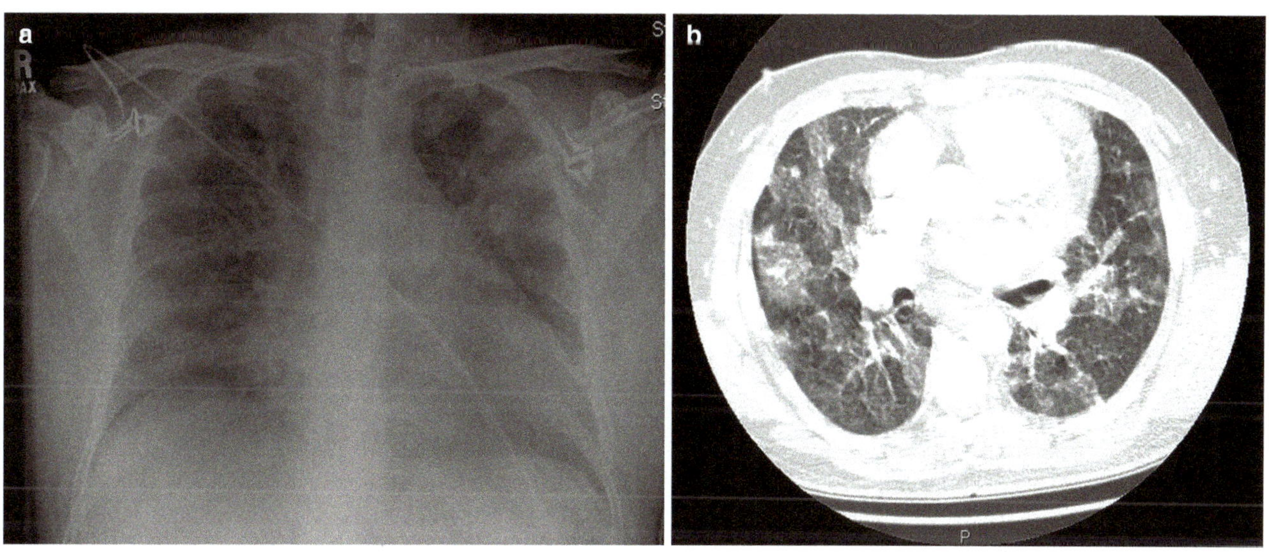

Fig. 46.4 (**a**) Chest radiograph in a patient with *Strongyloides* hyperinfection syndrome. (**b**) Chest computed tomographic examination in a patient with *Strongyloides* hyperinfection syndrome

Diagnosis

Uncomplicated strongyloidiasis can be diagnosed by finding rhabditiform larvae in microscopic stool examination; it is uncommon to find eggs in the stool. Because few larvae are shed, the sensitivity of a single stool examination is only about 30%; multiple samples should therefore be examined, preferably using concentration techniques. Examination of up to seven stool samples can significantly increase sensitivity [22, 56]. Sampling of duodenal fluid or a small bowel biopsy can increase sensitivity, but practical issues limit usefulness [57]. Placing stool samples on agar plates to observe tracks left by the motile larvae may be the most sensitive method among the stool examination techniques [58–60]. Although not yet in widespread use, PCR assays of stool samples for the diagnosis of intestinal strongyloidiasis have recently begun to show promise [61, 62].

Because of the difficulty with microscopic diagnosis, serologic tests (which are more sensitive) are often favored, such as the enzyme-linked immunoassay offered by CDC (Atlanta, GA). This assay is about 95% sensitive in stool-positive patients, although specificity is lower because of cross-reactivity with other helminths [26, 52]. The titer of *Strongyloides* antibodies in infected patients generally begins to decline 6–12 months after cure, as does the peripheral eosinophil count [52, 63, 64]. In contrast to chronic strongyloidiasis, hyperinfection and disseminated strongyloidiasis are easily diagnosed by microscopic stool examination (or other samples, such as sputum), which typically contain many filariform larvae (Figs. 46.5 and 46.6).

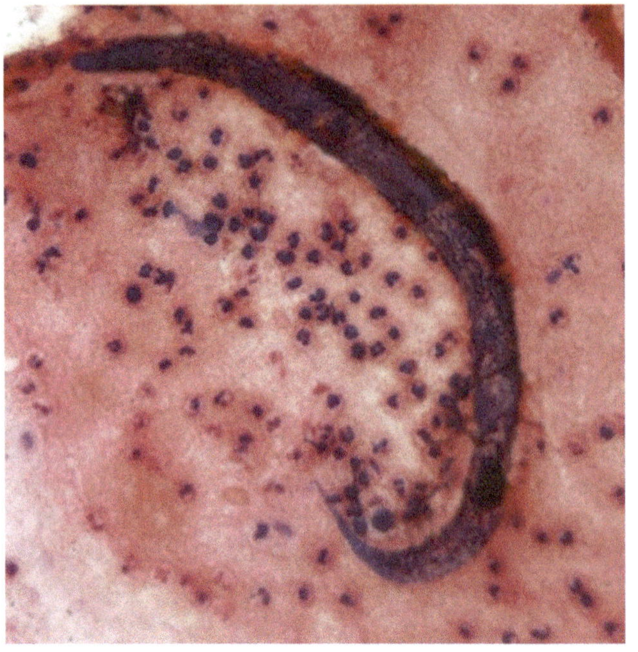

Fig. 46.5 Sputum sample from a patient with *Strongyloides* hyperinfection syndrome showing filariform larvae

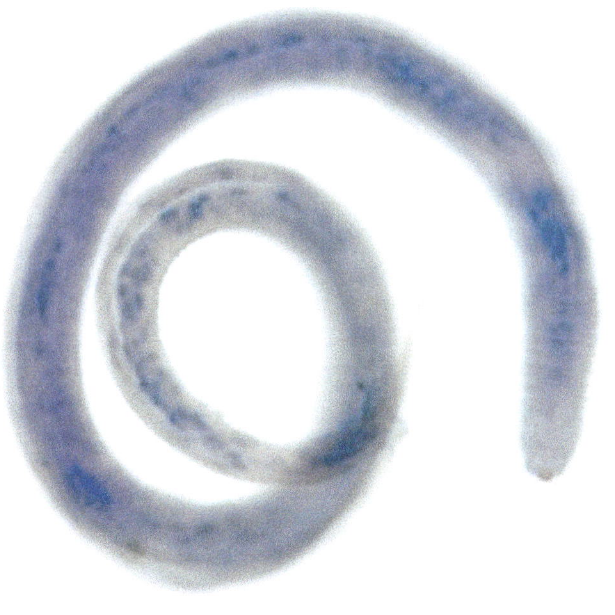

Fig. 46.6 Bronchoalveolar lavage sample showing filariform *S. stercoralis* larvae in a patient with hyperinfection syndrome

Strongyloidiasis in Transplant Patients

Given the risk of hyperinfection syndrome, identifying strongyloidiasis in transplant patients is critical. Although most common in endemic areas, this consideration is also paramount in non-endemic areas, given the global increase in travel and immigration. One retrospective review at a U.S. cancer center found 2.0 *S. stercoralis* infections per 10,000 leukemia patients and 0.8 infections per 10,000 cancer patients overall; however, systematic screening was not done, so these are likely underestimates. Among the infected patients, 48% had received systemic corticosteroids, and 36% had received anti-neoplastic therapy. Fifty-seven percent had diarrhea, 48% eosinophilia, and 24% developed the hyperinfection syndrome [65].

Strongyloidiasis has been well described in the posttransplant setting, and has been reported in scores of renal transplant recipients, most of whom developed the *Strongyloides* hyperinfection syndrome [66–68]; about 40% died as a result. These patients presented 18 days to over six months after their transplant, with most manifesting at least two months after transplant. Strongyloidiasis has also been reported in the recipients of over a dozen non-renal SOTs, including in heart, liver, lung, pancreas, pancreas-kidney, and intestinal transplant recipients [66, 69–71]. These patients presented 16 days to nine months after their transplant, with over half occurring at least one month posttransplant. Most of these patients developed the *Strongyloides* hyperinfection syndrome, and over half died as a result. The *Strongyloides* hyperinfection syndrome has also been reported in several HSCT recipients (both in autologous and allogeneic HSCT recipients) [66, 72–74]. These patients presented a mean of 87 days after undergoing transplantation (range 2–480 days), and almost 90% died.

Almost all of these patients had been to a *Strongyloides* endemic area at some point in their lives, including the southeastern United States in half of these cases. In about 15% of these cases, no exposure history was present and the transplanted allograft was therefore suspected to be the source of the *Strongyloides* infection in the recipient [66–74].

Only 18 (34%) of the 53 patients for whom data were available had eosinophilia prior to their transplant, while only 13 (25%) of 51 patients had reported symptoms possibly consistent with chronic strongyloidiasis prior to transplant. Despite the high prevalence of exposure to *Strongyloides*-endemic areas among the recipient population, only six (21%) patients among 29 for whom data were reported had been screened for *Strongyloides* infection prior to undergoing transplantation, all by stool ova and parasite (O&P) examination, and none by serology.

Treatment

All persons infected with *S. stercoralis* should be treated. The drug of choice for uncomplicated strongyloidiasis is oral ivermectin, 200 μg/kg per day for two days, which cures 70–85% of chronically infected patients. One study demonstrated a higher cure rate with two-dose ivermectin regimens compared to previously used single-dose regimens [75, 76]. Alternatives include thiabendazole or albendazole for 3–7 days, although ivermectin appears more effective; thiabendazole is poorly tolerated, and albendazole has the lowest cure rate among these drugs [76–80]. Ivermectin is also preferred for hyperinfection/disseminated strongyloidiasis. It should be administered daily until symptoms have resolved and larvae have not been detected for at least two weeks [21, 43]. Several patients with disseminated strongyloidiasis have received veterinary formulations of subcutaneous ivermectin. Although still experimental, this is an alternative for patients poorly tolerant of oral therapy and for those with severe infection [81–84]. Some patients have received a combination of ivermectin and albendazole with success [85]. If possible, immunosuppressive therapy should be stopped (particularly corticosteroids) or at least decreased. Some recommend monthly treatment subsequently for patients who require continued immunosuppression [19–21]. Follow-up stool examinations should be repeated frequently to document cure. For long-term follow-up, serology and eosinophil counts may offer stronger evidence of treatment efficacy. These findings generally begin to normalize 6–12 months after cure [52, 63].

Prevention of Hyperinfection

For all patients who are (or will soon become) immunosuppressed, examination of stool and preferably serologic evaluation for latent/occult *S. stercoralis* infestation should be undertaken for those who have lived in an endemic area or had other possible exposure to *S. stercoralis* at any time in their life, particularly those infected with HTLV-1 or receiving high-dose systemic corticosteroids [86]. Though most important for persons from highly endemic developing countries, this is also a consideration for patients with potential exposure in the southeastern United States, especially older persons who lived in these areas during childhood when the prevalence of *Strongyloides* was higher. Such screening would be particularly important for those with clinical symptoms of strongyloidiasis (e.g., eosinophilia, larva currens, and abdominal pain), although as noted above, screening should not be limited only to patients with these findings, as most infected individuals are asymptomatic. All infected patients should be treated promptly, preferably prior to the initiation of immunosuppressive therapy.

Although data regarding the cost-effectiveness of routine screening remain scarce, transplant programs should consider implementation of such a screening strategy as part of their pretransplant evaluation, to reduce the risk of *Strongyloides* hyperinfection syndrome and life-threatening dissemination post-transplant. In our opinion, screening solely by stool studies during the pretransplant workup is not adequate, and we recommend using at minimum the more sensitive serological assays for diagnosing of *Strongyloides* infection, with . stool studies added for patients who may not be producing antibodies normally. If a patient's condition requires immunosuppression before *S. stercoralis* diagnostics are available, the risks of empiric antiparasitic therapy for strongyloidiasis must be weighed against the risks of disseminated infection [87].

Other Parasitic Infections of Importance in Transplant Recipients

Although *T. gondii* and *S. stercoralis* are the most important parasitic infections in transplant recipients, others also warrant discussion given the increased risk of severe disease due to infection with these parasites in immunocompromised hosts.

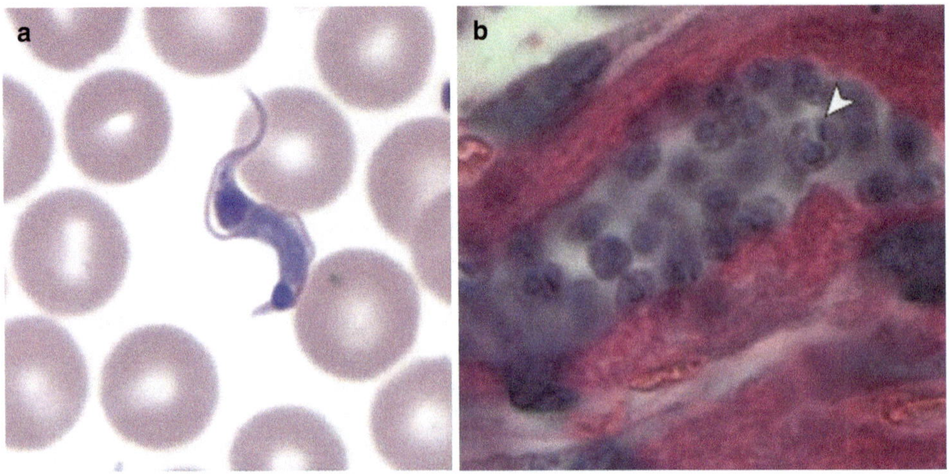

Fig. 46.7 (**a**) *Trypanosoma cruzi* trypomastigote in a thin blood smear. (**b**) *Trypanosoma cruzi* amastigotes in heart tissue [90]. (Courtesy Division of Parasitic Diseases and Malaria/Centers for Disease Control and Prevention, DPDx – Laboratory Identification of Parasites of Public Health Concern, https://www.cdc.gov/dpdx/trypanosomiasisAmerican/index.html)

Trypanosoma cruzi (Chagas Disease)

T. cruzi is a protozoan endemic to the American tropics and subtropics, where it is transmitted primarily by bloodsucking triatomine insects, and transmitted occasionally by blood transfusion, the oral route, or vertically from mother to unborn child [88]. About 8–10 million people are chronically infected, 300,000 of whom live in the United States (almost all of whom were infected in Latin America) [89]. Acute infection is often asymptomatic, but patients occasionally suffer systemic symptoms in the weeks following infection such as fever, lymphadenopathy, hepatosplenomegaly, myocarditis, or meningoencephalitis; the parasite is often detectable in the peripheral blood during this phase of infection (Fig. 46.7a). Most patients recover and subsequently enter an asymptomatic *indeterminate phase* of infection, during which patients usually have only subpatent parasitemia. *T. cruzi* then persists indefinitely, causing end-organ disease in 20–30%, years to decades later [88]. Chronic heart disease is most common (e.g., conduction disease and heart failure), with chronic gastrointestinal disease (megaesophagus or megacolon) also seen. Diagnosis of chronic infection can usually be made serologically, although in immunocompromised hosts seroconversion may not occur.

Infection can also be transmitted by transplantation, as has been observed in 18% of kidney transplants involving *T. cruzi*-infected donors and in 22–29% of two small liver transplant cohorts who had received their organs from *T. cruzi*-infected donors in the United States and Argentina [91, 92]. Transmission rates from infected heart donors appears to be higher, and known *T. cruzi* infection of a potential donor is a contraindication to heart transplant, although the use of other organs from *T. cruzi*-infected donors might be considered in some situations [93]. Importantly, acute infection in transplant patients is more likely to be severe and may follow a prolonged incubation period (mean onset 112 days after transplantation) [92]. Several cases of SOT-associated transmission of *T. cruzi* have been reported in the United States [92].

A common indication for heart transplantation is chronic Chagas heart disease; in Brazil, it is the third most common indication for heart transplant [92]. Immunocompromised hosts chronically infected with *T. cruzi* are at increased risk for reactivation; this syndrome resembles acute infection but can be more severe. It can also resemble rejection, especially in heart transplant recipients. In these patients, reactivation rates of 20–90% have been reported with cyclophosphamide, and corticosteroid-containing regimens have been associated with higher rates; mycophenolate mofetil also appears to increase the risk of *T. cruzi* reactivation [92]. Atypical manifestations can be seen, including *T. cruzi* brain abscesses, skin lesions, and mucosal involvement [94, 95]. Treatment is with either nifurtimox or benznidazole; these drugs are relatively toxic, require 2–3 months of therapy, and in the United States are available only through CDC.

No consensus exists regarding an approach for detecting *T. cruzi* infection in U.S. transplant programs, but some form of serologic screening should be considered in all centers. For programs in areas with high *T. cruzi* prevalence in the population, universal screening could be considered, whereas in other areas, selective screening could be done based on any history of the donor or recipient living in a *T. cruzi*-endemic area (or being born to a mother that had lived in an endemic area). Posttransplant, if either the donor or recipient is infected with *T. cruzi*, guidelines now favor prospective monitoring of blood by Giemsa-stained peripheral blood smears and PCR, even if treatment had occurred earlier in life. Initiation of antiparasitic therapy is then recommended if this screening becomes positive [92, 93]. This approach detects most reactivation before patients become symptomatic while obviating the need for prolonged, toxic antiparasitic treatment regimens that most transplant recipients would receive if a preemptive, prophylactic treatment approach were used universally.

Such monitoring is recommended weekly for two months, every two weeks for the third month, and then monthly until

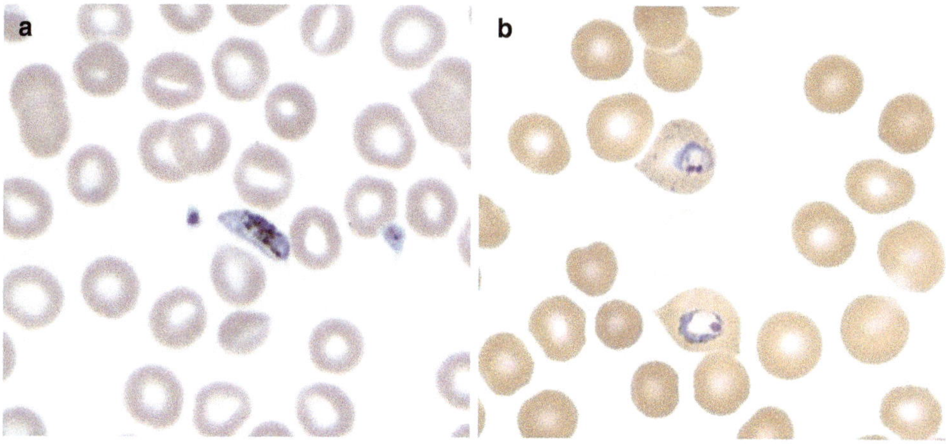

Fig. 46.8 (**a**) *Plasmodium falciparum* gametocyte in a thin blood smear. (**b**) *Plasmodium vivax* trophozoites (ring forms) in a thin blood smear

at least six months following transplantation [92]. Additional testing should accompany any febrile episodes or suspected rejection crises. In addition, endomyocardial biopsy specimens collected for routine monitoring or suspected rejection in heart transplant recipients should also be tested for *T. cruzi* by PCR and examined for the presence of the parasite and acute myocarditis [92, 96, 97] (Fig. 46.7b).

Malaria

Human malaria is caused by the mosquito-borne parasites *Plasmodium falciparum*, *P. vivax*, *P. ovale*, *P. malariae*, and *P. knowlesi*, which parasitize (and subsequently hemolyze) red blood cells (Fig. 46.8a and b). Malaria is the most important parasitic infection globally, killing over 400,000 people annually and causing over 200 million symptomatic illnesses annually, with most of this morbidity and mortality attributable to *P. falciparum* [98]. Malaria is endemic primarily to sub-Saharan Africa, Asia, Oceania, and Latin America, with most of the mortality occurring in young African children. Diagnosis centers on the identification of parasites in blood smears, as well as by newer methods such as antigen and PCR detection. Uncomplicated malaria can manifest as fever, anemia, thrombocytopenia, myalgia, cough, and diarrhea. Severe malaria is defined in part by respiratory distress, renal failure, altered mental status, seizures, intolerance of oral medications, metabolic acidosis, hypoglycemia, or parasitemia greater than 5%. The mortality rate of severe malaria is high.

In the United States, the preferred treatment for uncomplicated *P. falciparum* malaria acquired in areas with chloroquine resistance is artemether-lumefantrine; atovaquone-proguanil, or oral quinine plus doxycycline are alternatives. The preferred treatment is chloroquine if malaria is acquired in one of the few remaining areas where *P. falciparum* is not chloroquine resistant (such as most of Central America and the Caribbean). Severe malaria (usually caused by *P. falciparum*) should usually be treated with intravenous artesunate plus doxycycline or alternatively intravenous quinine (quinidine in the United States) plus doxycycline. Chloroquine plus primaquine (or tafenoquine) is effective for uncomplicated *P. vivax* and *P. ovale* malaria in most of the world, and *P. malariae* or *P. knowlesi* infections can be treated with chloroquine.

Although not a disease classically associated with the immunocompromised state, malaria-infected patients who are coinfected with HIV are more likely to be febrile, have detectable parasitemia, and develop severe malaria compared with malaria-infected patients without HIV infection. Moreover, the clinical severity of malaria appears to worsen with advanced immunosuppression [99]. Malaria has been reported in over 50 SOT recipients, about three-quarters of whom were kidney recipients [100]. In at least 30% of these cases, the mode of transmission appears to have been the transplanted organ [100]. Cases have occurred in malaria-endemic areas, where both the donor and recipient could have been the source of the infection, and in non-endemic areas where the donor had previously visited malaria-endemic area and probably transmitted infection to the recipient. The incubation period for posttransplant malaria has ranged from three days to several months, with the potential for incubation periods as brief as a few days in contrast to naturally acquired malaria, for which the minimum is six or seven days [100]. The case-fatality rate has varied widely, depending on the infecting species, host immune status, and promptness of diagnosis and treatment.

Although malaria transmission due to blood transfusion is well established, transmission in the context of HSCTs has been described only rarely, possibly because *Plasmodium* spp. do not parasitize hematopoietic progenitor cells as they do mature red blood cells (RBCs). The risk of transmission thus appears to be lower for HSCTs and may depend on the small number of RBCs that inevitably accompany these transplants. An allogeneic HSCT donor transmitted malaria to a recipient in the United Kingdom in the 1990s, and recently, a peripheral blood stem cell transplant donor transmitted malaria to the recipient [101–103].

Although malaria in the transplant setting has been rare, screening for malaria by thick and thin blood smear assessment should be considered if the donor or recipient has traveled to a malaria-endemic region in the three years preceding transplantation. In addition, malaria can also be acquired posttransplant by a mosquito bite in an endemic area, and it is particularly important that immunocompromised patients who travel to malaria-endemic areas be administered a chemoprophylaxis regimen appropriate for that region.

Leishmaniasis

Leishmania spp. are intracellular protozoans usually transmitted by sandflies. Although cutaneous and mucocutaneous leishmaniasis can occur posttransplantation, the syndrome seen in most transplant patients is visceral leishmaniasis (VL) due to reactivation of subclinical infection or latent disease. Ninety percent of visceral leishmaniasis (VL) infections are acquired in South Asia, East Africa, or Brazil, although transmission also occurs in the Mediterranean littoral. A wide clinical spectrum exists, with most infections subclinical. Although immunocompetent patients can progress to symptomatic disease, immunosuppression is an established precipitant of progression [104–107].

Over 100 cases of leishmaniasis have been reported in the posttransplant setting, with about 75% in kidney transplant recipients and 12% in liver transplant recipients. Two-thirds of these cases were reported from the Mediterranean basin (mainly Spain, Italy, and France) [107–109]. Only ten cases have been reported in HSCT recipients [110].

Even in apparently immunocompetent patients who develop symptomatic VL, clinical disease often presents months or years after initial infection. When VL has occurred in transplant recipients, the onset was a median of 18 months after transplantation [109]. VL is characterized by fever, hepatosplenomegaly, weight loss, skin changes, pancytopenia, and hyperglobulinemia. Diagnosis is by biopsy and microscopic examination or culture of involved tissues, although serology can be an adjunct; untreated, progressive VL is usually fatal (Fig. 46.9). Treatment options include pentavalent antimony compounds, miltefosine, and paromomycin, but liposomal amphotericin seems to be the most effective drug. After clinical cure, relapse is a concern (although less than in AIDS patients), so secondary anti-*Leishmania* prophylaxis with various agents has been used in a small number of patients.

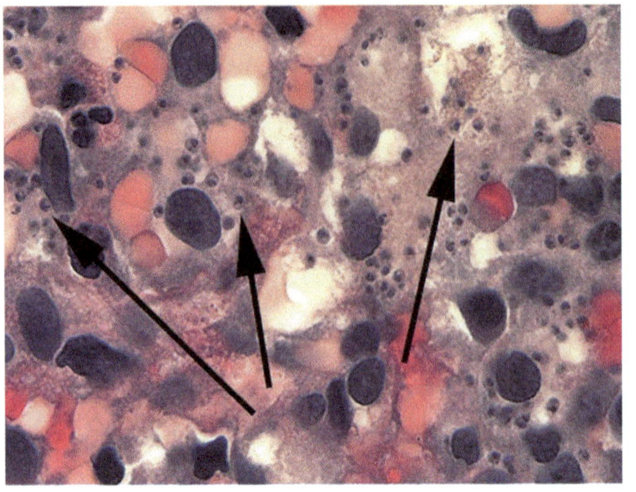

Fig. 46.9 *Leishmania* amastigotes in a bone marrow biopsy

Acanthamoeba and *Balamuthia*

Acanthamoeba spp. and *Balamuthia mandrillaris* are free-living, ubiquitous environmental amoebae. Although clinically apparent human infection with these organisms is rare, immunocompromised hosts can develop granulomatous amebic encephalitis, a subacute or chronic syndrome manifested by altered mental status, focal neurologic deficits, fever, headache, seizures, and CNS mass lesions [111]. Disseminated disease can involve the skin, sinuses, lungs, liver, and bones; typical progression is over weeks to months [112]. Cutaneous lesions can be an early sign which heralds imminent dissemination and CNS involvement. Affected patients have included recipients of kidney, liver, heart, lung, and hematopoietic stem cell transplants [113–117]. *Balamuthia* transmission has also been reported as a result of graft-transmitted infection in a liver, heart, iliac vessel, and two kidney transplant recipients from a common donor in 2011; in liver and kidney-pancreas transplant recipients from a common donor in Arizona in 2010; and in two recipients of kidney transplants from a common donor in Mississippi in 2009 [118, 119]. Diagnosis typically requires microscopic examination of infected tissues, although serologic and PCR tests exist [120]. Case-fatality rates are high, even with combination antimicrobial therapy. There is no consensus regarding the best drug regimen to treat these devastating infections, but such regimens often include many of the following agents: pentamidine, azoles, sulfonamides, macrolides, albendazole, miltefosine, and flucytosine.

Schistosomiasis

Schistosoma spp. are blood flukes acquired through skin contact with infested freshwater; 200 million people worldwide are infected. *Schistosoma mansoni* is found primarily in Africa, the Arabian Peninsula, and South America, while *S. japonicum* is mostly seen in China, the Philippines, Southeast Asia, and Indonesia; both are associated with gastrointestinal or hepatic disease. *Schistosoma haematobium* is endemic to Africa and parts of the Middle

East, and it causes primarily genitourinary disease. Patients are often asymptomatic but with chronic infection can develop eosinophilia, abdominal pain, diarrhea, and hepatosplenomegaly. A minority may also develop symptoms with acute infection. Chronic infection can cause hepatic fibrosis, portal hypertension, and intestinal disease (due to *S. mansoni* or *S. japonicum*) or hematuria, urinary obstruction, and bladder cancer (due to *S. haematobium*) [121]. Diagnosis is classically through stool or urine examinations, but serologic assays and pathologic examination of infected tissues are more sensitive. Treatment with praziquantel is usually curative.

Over a dozen cases of schistosomiasis have been reported due to a transplanted graft mostly in liver recipients [122–124]. The course of schistosomiasis does not appear to be impacted by the immunocompromised state, and treatment is effective in most cases. The presence of schistosomiasis did not impact graft outcomes among a cohort of 240 kidney transplant recipients [125].

Intestinal Protozoa

Intestinal protozoa such as *Cryptosporidium* spp., *Cystoisospora belli*, and *Cyclospora cayetanensis* are transmitted by contaminated food and water, and can cause severe diarrheal illness in immunocompromised transplant recipients. Diarrhea is generally watery, and diagnosis is by stool studies. All three parasites can be detected through modified acid fast stains, *Cryptosporidium* and *Cyclospora* can also be detected through sensitive real-time PCR assays (often as part of an enteric pathogen diagnostic PCR panel), and *Cryptosporidium* can also be detected through sensitive stool immunoassays. Treatment of *Cryptosporidium* is with nitazoxanide, while *Cystoisospora* and *Cyclospora* are treated with trimethoprim-sulfamethoxazole [75].

Microsporida are protozoans that are closely related to fungi and can cause diarrheal disease in the immunocompromised patients. Disseminated microsporidiosis may also occur in this population, and can involve the CNS, lungs, or other internal organs [126]. Diagnosis is by trichrome staining of the stool, and treatment is with albendazole or fumagillin, depending on the species [75].

References

1. Montoya JG, Liesenfeld O. Toxoplasmosis. Lancet. 2004;36:1965–76.
2. Demar M, Ajzenberg D, Maubon D, et al. Fatal outbreak of human toxoplasmosis along the Maroni River: epidemiological, clinical, and parasitological aspects. Clin Infect Dis. 2007;45:e88–95.
3. Elbez-Rubinstein A, Ajzenberg D, Darde ML, et al. Congenital toxoplasmosis and reinfection during pregnancy: case report, strain characterization, experimental model of reinfection, and review. J Infect Dis. 2009;199:280–5.
4. Gilbert RE, Freeman K, Lago EG, et al. Ocular sequelae of congenital toxoplasmosis in Brazil compared with Europe. PLoS Negl Trop Dis. 2008;2:e277.
5. Bowie WR, King AS, Werker DH, et al. Outbreak of toxoplasmosis associated with municipal drinking water. Lancet. 1997;350:173–7.
6. Jones JL, Dargelas V, Roberts J, Press C, Remington JS, Montoya JG. Risk factors for *Toxoplasma gondii* infection in the United States. Clin Infect Dis. 2009;49:878–84.
7. Cook AJ, Gilbert RE, Buffolano W, et al. Sources of *Toxoplasma* infection in pregnant women: European multicentre case-control study. On behalf of the European research network on congenital toxoplasmosis. BMJ. 2000;321:142–7.
8. Montoya JG, Giraldo LF, Efron B, et al. Infectious complications among 620 consecutive heart transplant patients at Stanford University Medical Center. Clin Infect Dis. 2001;33:629–40.
9. Martino R, Maertens J, Bretagne S, et al. Toxoplasmosis after hematopoietic stem cell transplantation. Clin Infect Dis. 2000;31:1188–95.
10. Rosso F, Les JT, Agudelo A, et al. Prevalence of infection with *Toxoplasma gondii* among pregnant women in Cali, Colombia, South America. Am J Trop Med Hyg. 2008;78:504–8.
11. Luft BJ, Naot Y, Araujo FG, Stinson EB, Remington JS. Primary and reactivated *Toxoplasma* infection in patients with cardiac transplants. Clinical spectrum and problems in diagnosis in a defined population. Ann Intern Med. 1983;99:27–31.
12. Martino R, Bretage S, Rovira M, et al. Toxoplasmosis after hematopoietic stem transplantation. Report of a 5-year survey from the Infectious Diseases Working Party of the European Group for Blood and Marrow Transplantation. Bone Marrow Transplant. 2000;25:1111–4.
13. Martino R, Bretagne S, Einsele H, et al. Early detection of *Toxoplasma* infection by molecular monitoring of *Toxoplasma gondii* in peripheral blood samples after allogeneic stem cell transplantation. Clin Infect Dis. 2005;40:67–78.
14. Montoya JG. Laboratory diagnosis of *Toxoplasma gondii* infection and toxoplasmosis. J Infect Dis. 2002;185(Suppl 1):S73–82.
15. Public. Health Service, Dept. of Health and Human Services (US) and Food and Drug Administration (FDA). FDA Public Health Advisory: limitations of *Toxoplasma* IgM commerical test kits. Rockville: Department of Health and Human Services, Food and Drug Administration, 1997 July 25, 1997.
16. Dorfman RF, Remington JS. Value of lymph-node biopsy in the diagnosis of acute acquired toxoplasmosis. N Engl J Med. 1973;289:878–81.
17. Wreghitt TG, Hakim M, Gray JJ, et al. Toxoplasmosis in heart and heart lung transplant recipients. J Clin Pathol. 1989;42:194–9.
18. Bethony J, Brooker S, Albonico M, et al. Soil-transmitted helminth infections: ascariasis, trichuriasis, and hookworm. Lancet. 2006;367:1521–32.
19. Lam CS, Tong MK, Chan KM, Siu YP. Disseminated strongyloidiasis: a retrospective study of clinical course and outcome. Eur J Clin Microbiol Infect Dis. 2006;25:14–8.
20. Marcosa LA, Terashimab A, DuPont HL, Gotuzzo E. *Strongyloides* hyperinfection syndrome: an emerging global infectious disease. Trans R Soc Trop Med Hyg. 2008;102:314–8.
21. Maguire JH. Intestinal nematodes (roundworms). In: Mandell GL, Bennett JE, Dolin R, editors. Principles and practices of infectious diseases. 7th ed. Philadelphia: Churchill Livingstone Elsevier; 2010. p. 3577–86.
22. Siddiqui AA, Berk SL. Diagnosis of *Strongyloides stercoralis* infection. Clin Infect Dis. 2001;33:1040–7.
23. Siddiqui AA, Genta RM, Maguilnik I, Berk SL. Strongyloidiasis. In: Guerrant RL, Walker DH, Weller PF, editors. Tropical infectious diseases, 3rd edition – principles, pathogens, & practice. Philadelphia: Elsevier Mosby Saunders; 2011. p. 805–12.
24. Schad GA. Morphology and life history of *Strongyloides stercoralis*. In: Grove DI, editor. Strongyloidiasis: a major round-

worm infection of man. London: Taylor & Francis; 1989. p. 85–104.
25. Genta RM. Global prevalence of strongyloidiasis: critical review with epidemiologic insights into the prevention of disseminated disease. Rev Infect Dis. 1989;11:755–67.
26. Yori PP, Kosek M, Gilman RH, et al. Seroepidemiology of strongyloidiasis in the Peruvian Amazon. Am J Trop Med Hyg. 2006;74:97–102.
27. Posey DL, Blackburn BG, Weinberg M, et al. High prevalence and presumptive treatment of schistosomiasis and strongyloidiasis among African refugees. Clin Infect Dis. 2007;45:1310–5.
28. Seybolt LM, Christiansen D, Barnett ED. Diagnostic evaluation of newly arrived asymptomatic refugees with eosinophilia. Clin Infect Dis. 2006;42:363–7.
29. Neva FA. Biology and immunology of human strongyloidiasis. J Infect Dis. 1986;153:397–406.
30. Grove DI. Human strongyloidiasis. Adv Parasitol. 1996;38:251–309.
31. Genta RM. Dysregulation of strongyloidiasis: a new hypothesis. Clin Microbiol Rev. 1992;5:345–55.
32. Schaeffer MW, Buell JF, Gupta M, Conway GD, Akhter SA, Wagoner LE. *Strongyloides* hyperinfection syndrome after heart transplantation: case report and review of the literature. J Heart Lung Transplant. 2004;23:905–11.
33. Seet RC, Lau LG, Tambyah PA. *Strongyloides* hyperinfection and hypogammaglobulinemia. Clin Diagn Lab Immunol. 2005;12:680–2.
34. Morgan JS, Schaffner W, Stone WJ. Opportunistic strongyloidiasis in renal transplant recipients. Transplantation. 1986;42:518–24.
35. Schad GA. Cyclosporine may eliminate the threat of overwhelming strongyloidiasis in immunosuppressed patients. J Infect Dis. 1986;153:178.
36. Nolan TJ, Schad GA. Tacrolimus allows autoinfective development of the parasitic nematode *Strongyloides stercoralis*. Transplantation. 1996;62:1038.
37. Carvalho EM, Da Fonseca Porto A. Epidemiological and clinical interaction between HTLV-1 and *Strongyloides stercoralis*. Parasite Immunol. 2004;26:487–97.
38. Gotuzzo E, Terashima A, Alvarez H, et al. *Strongyloides stercoralis* hyperinfection associated with human T cell lymphotropic virus type-1 infection in Peru. Am J Trop Med Hyg. 1999;60:146–9.
39. Hirata T, Uchima N, Kishimoto K, et al. Impairment of host immune response against *Strongyloides stercoralis* by human T cell lymphotropic virus type 1 infection. Am J Trop Med Hyg. 2006;74:246–9.
40. Plumelle Y, Gonin C, Edouard A, et al. Effect of *Strongyloides stercoralis* infection and eosinophilia on age at onset and prognosis of adult T-cell leukemia. Am J Clin Pathol. 1997;107:81–7.
41. Viney ME, Brown M, Omoding NE, et al. Why does HIV infection not lead to disseminated strongyloidiasis? J Infect Dis. 2004;190:2175–80.
42. Centers for Disease Control. Revision of the CDC surveillance case definition for acquired immunodeficiency syndrome. MMWR. 1997;36(Suppl):1–15.
43. Keiser PB, Nutman TB. *Strongyloides stercoralis* in the immunocompromised population. Clin Microbiol Rev. 2004;17:208–17.
44. Newberry AM, Williams DN, Stauffer WM, Boulware DR, Hendel-Paterson BR, Walker PF. *Strongyloides* hyperinfection presenting as acute respiratory failure and gram- negative Sepsis. Chest. 2005;128:3681–4.
45. Siddiqui AA, Stanley CS, Skelly PJ, et al. A cDNA encoding a nuclear hormone receptor of the steroid/thyroid hormone-receptor superfamily from the human parasitic nematode *Strongyloides stercoralis*. Parasitol Res. 2000;86:24–9.
46. Nolan TJ, Megyeri Z, Bhopale VM, et al. *Strongyloides stercoralis*: the first rodent model for uncomplicated and hyperinfective strongyloidiasis, the Mongolian gerbil (*Meriones unguiculatus*). J Infect Dis. 1993;168:1479–84.
47. Mansfield LS, Niamatali S, Bhopale V, et al. *Strongyloides stercoralis*: maintenance of exceedingly chronic infections. Am J Trop Med Hyg. 1996;55:617–24.
48. Fardet L, Généreau T, Poirot JL, Guidet B, Kettaneh A, Cabane J. Severe strongyloidiasis in corticosteroid-treated patients: case series and literature review. J Infect. 2007;54:18–27.
49. Segarra-Newnham M. Manifestations, diagnosis, and treatment of *Strongyloides stercoralis* infection. Ann Pharmacother. 2007;41:1992–2001.
50. Liu LX, Weller PF. Strongyloidiasis and other intestinal nematode infections. Infect Dis Clin N Am. 1993;7:655–82.
51. Berk SL, Verghese A, Alvarez S, Hall K, Smith B. Clinical and epidemiologic features of strongyloidiasis. A prospective study in rural Tennessee. Arch Intern Med. 1987;147:1257–61.
52. Loutfy MR, Wilson M, Keystone JS, Kain KC. Serology and eosinophil count in the diagnosis and management of strongyloidiasis in a non-endemic area. Am J Trop Med Hyg. 2002;66:749–52.
53. Hirata T, Kishimoto K, Kinjo N, Hokama A, Kinjo F, Fujita J. Association between *Strongyloides stercoralis* infection and biliary tract cancer. Parasitol Res. 2007;101:1345–8.
54. Reddy TS, Myers JW. Syndrome of inappropriate secretion of antidiuretic hormone and nonpalpable purpura in a woman with *Strongyloides stercoralis* hyperinfection. Am J Med Sci. 2003;325:288–91.
55. Hayashi E, Ohta N, Yamamoto H. Syndrome of inappropriate secretion of antidiuretic hormone associated with strongyloidiasis. Southeast Asian J Trop Med Public Health. 2007;38:239–46.
56. Nielsen PB, Mojon M. Improved diagnosis of *Strongyloides stercoralis* by seven consecutive stool specimens. Zentralbl Mikrobiol. 1987;263:616–8.
57. Agrawal V, Agarwal T, Ghoshal UC. Intestinal strongyloidiasis: a diagnosis frequently missed in the tropics. Trans R Soc Trop Med Hyg. 2009;103:242–6.
58. Sato Y, Kobayashi J, Toma H, Shiroma Y. Efficacy of stool examination for detection of *Strongyloides* infection. Am J Trop Med Hyg. 1995;53:248–50.
59. Hirata T, Nakamura H, Kinjo N, et al. Increased detection rate of *Strongyloides stercoralis* by repeated stool examinations using the agar plate culture method. Am J Trop Med Hyg. 2007;77:683–4.
60. de Kaminsky RG. Evaluation of three methods for laboratory diagnosis of *Strongyloides stercoralis* infection. J Parasitol. 1993;79:277–80.
61. Verweij JJ, Canales M, Polman K, et al. Molecular diagnosis of *Strongyloides stercoralis* in faecal samples using real-time PCR. Trans R Soc Trop Med Hyg. 2009;103:342–6.
62. Basuni M, Muhi J, Othman N, et al. A pentaplex real-time polymerase chain reaction assay for detection of four species of soil-transmitted helminths. Am J Trop Med Hyg. 2011;84:338–43.
63. Karunajeewa H, Kelly H, Leslie D, Leydon J, Saykao P, Biggs BA. Parasite-specific IgG response and peripheral blood eosinophil count following albendazole treatment for presumed chronic strongyloidiasis. J Travel Med. 2006;13:84–91.
64. Page WA, Dempsey K, McCarthy JS. Utility of serological follow-up of chronic strongyloidiasis after anthelminthic chemotherapy. Trans R Soc Trop Med Hyg. 2006;100:1056–62.
65. Safdar A, Malathum K, Rodriguez SJ, Husni R, Rolston KV. Strongyloidiasis in patients at a comprehensive cancer center in the United States. Cancer. 2004;100:1531–6.
66. Roxby AC, Gottlieb GS, Limaye AP. Strongyloidiasis in transplant patients. Clin Infect Dis. 2009;49:1411–23.
67. Issa H, Aljama MA, Al-Salem AH. *Strongyloides stercoralis* hyperinfection in a post-renal transplant patient. Clin Exp Gastroenterol. 2011;4:269–71.

68. Mokaddas EM, Shati S, Abdulla A, et al. Fatal strongyloidiasis in three kidney recipients in Kuwait. Med Princ Pract. 2009;18:414–7.
69. Vilela EG, Clemente WT, Mira RR, et al. *Strongyloides stercoralis* hyperinfection syndrome after liver transplantation: case report and literature review. Transpl Infect Dis. 2009;11:132–6.
70. Patel G, Arvelakis A, Sauter BV, Gondolesi GE, Caplivski D, Huprikar S. *Strongyloides* hyperinfection syndrome after intestinal transplantation. Transpl Infect Dis. 2008;10:137–41.
71. Mizuno S, Iida T, Zendejas I, Martin TD, Schain DC, Turner B, Fujita S. *Strongyloides* hyperinfection syndrome following simultaneous heart and kidney transplantation. Transpl Int. 2009;22:251–3.
72. Wirk B, Wingard JR. *Strongyloides stercoralis* hyperinfection in hematopoietic stem cell transplantation. Transpl Infect Dis. 2009;11:143–8.
73. Qazilbash MH, Ueno NT, Hosing C, et al. Strongyloidiasis after unrelated nonmyeloablative allogeneic stem cell transplantation. Bone Marrow Transplant. 2006;38:393–4.
74. Orlent H, Crawley C, Cwynarski K, Dina R, Apperley J. Strongyloidiasis pre and post autologous peripheral blood stem cell transplantation. Bone Marrow Transplant. 2003;32:115–7.
75. Treatment guidelines from the medical letter. Drugs for parasitic infections. Med Lett Drugs Ther. 2007;5(Suppl):e1–e15.
76. Igual-Adell R, Oltra-Alcaraz C, Soler-Company E, Sánchez-Sánchez P, Matogo-Oyana J, Rodríguez-Calabuig D. Efficacy and safety of ivermectin and thiabendazole in the treatment of strongyloidiasis. Expert Opin Pharmacother. 2004;5:2615–9.
77. Salazar SA, Berk SH, Howe D, Berk SL. Ivermectin vs thiabendazole in the treatment of strongyloidiasis. Inf Med. 1994;11:50–9.
78. Suputtamongkol Y, Kungpanichkul N, Silpasakorn S, Beeching NJ. Efficacy and safety of a single-dose veterinary preparation of ivermectin versus 7-day high-dose albendazole for chronic strongyloidiasis. Int J Antimicrob Agents. 2008;31:46–9.
79. Datry A, Hilmarsdottir I, Mayorga-Sagastume R, et al. Treatment of *Strongyloides stercoralis* infection with ivermectin compared with albendazole: results of an open study of 60 cases. Trans R Soc Trop Med Hyg. 1994;88:344–5.
80. Marti H, Haji HJ, Savioli L, et al. A comparative trial of a single-dose ivermectin versus three days of albendazole for treatment of *Strongyloides stercoralis* and other soil-transmitted helminth infections in children. Am J Trop Med Hyg. 1996;55:477–81.
81. Pacanowski J, Santos MD, Roux A, et al. Subcutaneous ivermectin as a safe salvage therapy in *Strongyloides stercoralis* hyperinfection syndrome: a case report. Am J Trop Med Hyg. 2005;73:122–4.
82. Chiodini PL, Reid AJ, Wiselka MJ, Firmin R, Foweraker J. Parenteral ivermectin in *Strongyloides* hyperinfection. Lancet. 2000;355:43–4.
83. Turner SA, Maclean JD, Fleckenstein L, Greenaway C. Parenteral administration of ivermectin in a patient with disseminated strongyloidiasis. Am J Trop Med Hyg. 2005;73:911–4.
84. Marty FM, Lowry CM, Rodriguez M, et al. Treatment of human disseminated strongyloidiasis with a parenteral veterinary formulation of ivermectin. Clin Infect Dis. 2005;41:e5–8.
85. Pornsuriyasak P, Niticharoenpong K, Sakapibunnan A. Disseminated strongyloidiasis successfully treated with extended duration ivermectin combined with albendazole: a case report of intractable strongyloidiasis. Southeast Asian J Trop Med Public Health. 2004;35:531–4.
86. Centers for Disease Control and Prevention. Guidelines for preventing opportunistic infections among hematopoietic stem cell transplant recipients. MMWR. 2000;49(RR-10):26–7.
87. Blackburn B. Strongyloidiasis. In: Pickering LK, Baker CJ, Long SS, JA MM, editors. (American Academy of Pediatrics). Red book: 2006 report of the committee on infectious diseases. 27th ed. Elk Grove Village: American Academy of Pediatrics; 2006. p. 629–31.
88. Barrett MP, Burchmore RJS, August Stich A, et al. The trypanosomiases. Lancet. 2003;362:1469–80.
89. Bern C, Kjos S, Yabsley MJ, Montgomery SP. *Trypanosoma cruzi* and Chagas' disease in the United States. Clin Microbiol Rev. 2011;24:655–81.
90. Centers for Disease Control and Prevention, DPDx – Laboratory Identification of Parasites of Public Health Concern, https://www.cdc.gov/dpdx/trypanosomiasisamerican/index.html.
91. McCormack L, Quiñónez E, Goldaracena N, et al. Liver transplantation using Chagas-infected donors in uninfected recipients: a single-center experience without prophylactic therapy. Am J Transplant. 2012;12:2832–7.
92. Bern C. Chagas disease in the immunosuppressed host. Curr Opin Infect Dis. 2012;25:450–7.
93. Chin-Hong PV, Schwartz BS, Bern C, et al. Screening and treatment of Chagas disease in organ transplant recipients in the United States: recommendations from the chagas in transplant working group. Am J Transplant. 2011;11:672–80.
94. Fontes Rezende RE, Lescano MA, Zambelli Ramalho LN, et al. Reactivation of Chagas' disease in a patient with non-Hodgkin's lymphoma: gastric, oesophageal and laryngeal involvement. Trans R Soc Trop Med Hyg. 2006;100:74–8.
95. Lury KM, Castillo M. Chagas' disease involving the brain and spinal cord: MRI findings. Am J Roentgenol. 2005;185:550–2.
96. Altclas J, Sinagra A, Dictar M, et al. Chagas disease in bone marrow transplantation: an approach to preemptive therapy. Bone Marrow Transplant. 2005;36:123–9.
97. Dictar M, Sinagra A, Verón MT, et al. Recipients and donors of bone marrow transplants suffering from Chagas' disease: management and preemptive therapy of parasitemia. Bone Marrow Transplant. 1998;21:391–3.
98. World Health Organization. World Malaria Report 2012 Geneva, Switzerland. 2012;pp. 53–62.
99. Walker M, Kublin JG, Zunt JR. Parasitic central nervous system infections in immunocompromised hosts: malaria, microsporidiosis, leishmaniasis, and African trypanosomiasis. Clin Infect Dis. 2006;42:115–25.
100. Martín-Dávila P, Fortún J, López-Vélez R, et al. Transmission of tropical and geographically restricted infections during solid-organ transplantation. Clin Microbiol Rev. 2008;21:60–96.
101. Mejia R, Booth GS, Fedorko DP, et al. Peripheral blood stem cell transplant-related *Plasmodium falciparum* infection in a patient with sickle cell disease. Transfusion. 2012;52:2677–82.
102. Salutari P, Sica S, Chiusolo P, et al. *Plasmodium vivax* malaria after autologous bone marrow transplantation: an unusual complication. Bone Marrow Transplant. 1996;18:805–6.
103. O'Donnell J, Goldman JM, Wagner K, et al. Donor-derived *Plasmodium vivax* infection following volunteer unrelated bone marrow transplantation. Bone Marrow Transplant. 1998;21:313–4.
104. Sah SP, Rijal S, Bhadani PP, Rani S, Koirala S. Visceral leishmaniasis in two cases of leukemia. Southeast Asian J Trop Med Public Health. 2002;33:25–7.
105. Fakhar M, Asgari Q, Motazedian MH, Monabati A. Mediterranean visceral leishmaniasis associated with acute lymphoblastic leukemia (ALL). Parasitol Res. 2008;103:473–5.
106. Sirvent-von Bueltzingsloewen A, Marty P, Rosenthal E. Visceral leishmaniasis: a new opportunistic infection in hematopoietic stem-cell transplanted patients. Bone Marrow Transplant. 2004;33:667–8.
107. Muñoz P, Valerio M, Eworo A, Bouza E. Parasitic infections in solid-organ transplant recipients. Curr Opin Organ Transplant. 2011;16:565–75.
108. Machado CM, Levi JE. Transplant-associated and blood transfusion-associated tropical and parasitic infections. Infect Dis Clin N Am. 2012;26:225–41.
109. Antinori S, Cascio A, Parravicini C, Bianchi R, Corbellino M. Leishmaniasis among organ transplant recipients. Lancet Infect Dis. 2008;8:191–9.

110. Bautista G, Ramos A, Gil S. Visceral leishmaniasis in hematopoietic stem cell transplantation. Transpl Int. 2012;25:e83–5.
111. Visvesvara GS, Moura H, Schuster FL. Pathogenic and opportunistic free-living amoebae: *Acanthamoeba* spp., *Balamuthia mandrillaris*, *Naegleria fowleri*, and *Sappinia diploidea*. FEMS Immunol Med Microbiol. 2007;50:1–26.
112. Kaul DR, Lowe L, Visvesvara GS, Farmen S, Khaled YA, Yanik GA. *Acanthamoeba* infection in a patient with chronic graft-versus-host disease occurring during treatment with voriconazole. Transpl Infect Dis. 2008;10:437–41.
113. Barete S, Combes A, de Jonckheere JF. Fatal disseminated *Acanthamoeba lenticulata* infection in a heart transplant patient. Emerg Infect Dis. 2007;13:736–8.
114. Walia R, Montoya JG, Visvesvera GS, Booton GC, Doyle RL. A case of successful treatment of cutaneous *Acanthamoeba* infection in a lung transplant recipient. Transpl Infect Dis. 2007;9:51–4.
115. Fung KT, Dhillon AP, McLaughlin JE, et al. Cure of *Acanthamoeba* cerebral abscess in a liver transplant patient. Liver Transpl. 2008;14:308–12.
116. Steinberg JP, Galindo RL, Kraus ES, Ghanem KG. Disseminated acanthamebiasis in a renal transplant recipient with osteomyelitis and cutaneous lesions: case report and literature review. Clin Infect Dis. 2002;35:e43–9.
117. Akpek G, Uslu A, Huebner T, et al. Granulomatous amebic encephalitis: an under-recognized cause of infectious mortality after hematopoietic stem cell transplantation. Transpl Infect Dis. 2011;13:366–73.
118. Centers for Disease Control and Prevention (CDC). Notes from the field: transplant-transmitted *Balamuthia mandrillaris* – Arizona, 2010. MMWR Morb Mortal Wkly Rep. 2010;59:1182.
119. Centers for Disease Control and Prevention. (CDC). *Balamuthia mandrillaris* transmitted through organ transplantation – Mississippi, 2009. MMWR Morb Mortal Wkly Rep. 2010;59:1165–70.
120. Visvesvara GS. Amebic meningoencephalitides and keratitis: challenges in diagnosis and treatment. Curr Opin Infect Dis. 2010;23:590–4.
121. Bedwani R, Renganathan E, El Kwhsky F. Schistosomiasis and the risk of bladder cancer in Alexandria, Egypt. Br J Cancer. 1998;77:1186–9.
122. Hoare M, Gelson WT, Davies SE, Curran M, Alexander GJ. Hepatic and intestinal schistosomiasis after orthotopic liver transplant. Liver Transpl. 2005;11:1603–7.
123. Ahmed K, Safdar K, Kemmer N, Atiq M, Wang J, Neff GW. Intestinal schistosomiasis following orthotopic liver transplantation: a case report. Transplant Proc. 2007;39:3502–4.
124. Vincenzi R, Neto JS, Fonseca EA, et al. *Schistosoma mansoni* infection in the liver graft: the impact on donor and recipient outcomes after transplantation. Liver Transpl. 2011;17:1299–303.
125. Muñoz P, Valerio M, Puga D, Bouza E. Parasitic infections in solid organ transplant recipients. Infect Dis Clin N Am. 2010;24:461–95.
126. Teachey DT, Russo P, Orenstein JM, Didier ES, Bowers C, Bunin N. Pulmonary infection with microsporidia after allogeneic bone marrow transplantation. Bone Marrow Transplant. 2004;33:299–302.

Part IV

Diagnosis of Infectious Diseases in Special Host

Impacts and Challenges of Advanced Diagnostic Assays for Transplant Infectious Diseases

47

N. Esther Babady, Yeon Joo Lee, Genovefa Papanicolaou, and Yi-Wei Tang

Introduction

The administration of immunosuppressive therapy to prevent rejection of allografts and graft-versus-host disease, although necessary, renders transplant recipients susceptible to opportunistic infections [1, 2]. As a group, transplant patients present a real challenge for initial diagnosis of infection partly due to lowered or absent markers of inflammation [2]. Traditionally, these infections have been diagnosed using bacterial, fungal, and viral culture as well as a variety of immunological assays. These methods still remain the standard of care for diagnosis of most infections. However, a series of advanced detection techniques led by nucleic acid amplification have now become prominent in most clinical microbiology laboratories, and novel proteomic assays are currently being added in the list of diagnostic tools available for infectious pathogen detection and identification.

The goal of this chapter is to review traditional and molecular methods used for the diagnosis of infectious diseases in transplants patients and discuss novel methodologies currently in development and their potential impact on clinical decisions.

Traditional Diagnostic Assays

Culture-Based Assays

Culture remains the gold standard for the diagnosis of most infectious diseases including those caused by bacteria, mycobacteria, and fungi [3, 4]. One of the advantages of culture is that it does not require a priori knowledge of the specific pathogen responsible for the infection as it casts a wide search net by using multiple growth media and incubation conditions. For example, diarrhea and vomiting are common symptoms in transplant patients, and determining the infectious cause for those symptoms can be challenging due to confounding factors such as intestinal graft-versus-host diseases (GVHD) in hematopoietic stem cell transplantation (HSCT) recipients, neutropenic enterocolitis, and immunosuppressive drugs [5]. A request for a bacterial stool culture will allow detection of the most common cause of bacterial gastroenteritis, namely, *Salmonella* species, *Shigella* species, *Campylobacter* species, and *E. coli* O157 with a recovery rate ranging from 0.2% to 2.4% [3, 6–8]. In addition, any other bacterial organisms growing on the culture media, with potential for causing gastrointestinal symptoms, will be detected and reported. However, culture of certain organisms, including *C. difficile*, the most common cause of bacterial diarrhea in hospitalized patients, requires special culture media and setup and has been replaced in most part by non-culture-based methods. Similarly, viral causes of diarrhea including cytomegalovirus (CMV), norovirus, adenovirus, rotavirus, and other small round viruses are better detected

N. E. Babady
Department of Laboratory Medicine, Clinical Microbiology Service, Memorial Sloan Kettering Cancer Center, New York, NY, USA

Y. J. Lee
Department of Internal Medicine, Infectious Diseases Service, Memorial Sloan Kettering Cancer Center, New York, NY, USA

Weill Cornell Medical College, Cornell University, New York, NY, USA
e-mail: leey1@mskcc.org

G. Papanicolaou
Department of Internal Medicine, Infectious Diseases Service, Memorial Sloan Kettering Cancer Center, New York, NY, USA

Weill Cornell Medical College, Cornell University, New York, NY, USA
e-mail: papanicg@mskcc.org

Y.-W. Tang (✉)
Department of Laboratory Medicine, Clinical Microbiology Service, Memorial Sloan-Kettering Cancer Center, New York, NY, USA

Weill Cornell Medical College, Cornell University, New York, NY, USA
e-mail: tangy@mskcc.org

A. Safdar (ed.), *Principles and Practice of Transplant Infectious Diseases*, https://doi.org/10.1007/978-1-4939-9034-4_47

by nucleic acid amplification tests (NAAT) and antigen tests [9–11].

The diagnostic yield of culture for various specimen types remains low. In one retrospective study, the yield of bronchoalveolar lavage (BAL) fluid culture for diagnosis of pneumonia in bone marrow transplant patients was reported at 2.2%, 3.0%, and 16.4% for bacteria, fungi, and viruses, respectively [4]. In contrast, the use of PCR tests and antigen testing increased the overall diagnostic yield to 22%, although the increased detection of CMV by PCR was not deemed clinically significance for all cases. The diagnostic yield of BAL in other studies was higher with one study reporting rates of 31%, 12.7%, and 23.6% for detection of bacteria, fungi, and viruses, respectively, in cancer patients [12]. For solid organ transplants (SOT), the overall recovery of pathogens by culture can be higher, up to 58.9% in lung transplants [13–15].

Blood culture is important for diagnosis of bacteremia and fungemia [16]. Unfortunately, the yield of blood culture remains low for both conditions [17–20]. Current blood culture systems are automated and set up to continuously monitor blood culture for the detection of microorganisms. An exception to continuous monitoring is the use of the isolator tube system, a manual lysis-centrifugation system (Wampole Laboratories, Cranbury, NJ). Performance of the isolator tube has been evaluated extensively against other automated blood culture systems designed to improve recovery of fungi such as the MYCO/F Lytic bottle (BD Diagnostics, Sparks, MD) with some studies showing increased recovery of *H. capsulatum* and *C. neoformans* [21, 22], while other concludes that the two systems performed equally well [23, 24]. A study by Creger et al. retrospectively analyzed the performance of the isolator tube system specifically in a cancer population and did not observed an advantage over conventional blood culture methods [25]. Even with the use of the isolator tube, the detection of fungi in blood culture is low, and in biopsy-proven candidiasis, only 50% of patients had a positive blood culture [26].

In transplant patients, the yield of blood culture varies with the type of transplant and the degree of immunosuppression. In lung transplant patients, the yield of blood culture can be as high as 25% with *S. aureus*, *P. aeruginosa*, and *Candida* species being the most common isolates recovered [27, 28], while in HSCT, the yield varies greatly from 4.9% to 8.7% and is dominated by Gram-positive bacteria [29–32].

The majority of fungal isolates from blood culture are *Candida* species, *with C. albicans* being the most common species isolated [18]. Although rare, other non-*Candida* yeasts including *Trichosporon* species, *Rhodotorula* species, and *Saccharomyces cerevisiae* are being recovered with increased frequency from blood cultures of immunocompromised patients [33, 34]. Fungemia caused by molds, including *Aspergillus* species, is rarely detected by blood culture [35–37]. In patients with indwelling devices, molds such as *Fusarium*, *Paecilomyces*, *Scedosporium*, and *Wangiella* have been recovered from blood culture [38–40].

A recent study by Limmathurotsakul et al. highlighted the limitation of culture as a diagnostic tools and an imperfect gold standard [41]. The authors applied Bayesian latent class models (LCM) to establish the true sensitivity of culture and the true specificity of four serological tests for detection of pathogens using *Burkholderia pseudomallei* and melioidosis as a model system. Using Bayesian LCM with either conditional independence (i.e., no single test considered gold standard and no correlation among tests) or conditional dependence (i.e., correlation among all tests), the sensitivity of culture was estimated to be 61% with a negative predictive value of 62.1% [41]. The specificity and positive predictive value of the four serological tests increased significantly using both Bayesian LCM models, emphasizing the limitation of using the culture as an imperfect gold standard.

Recent studies defining microbial populations of various organs using deep sequencing and high-density sequencing methods have now revealed the complexity of microbial organisms, many of them non-culturable, present in various tissues and the difference in composition for transplants versus healthy patients [42, 43]. The significance of detecting these non-culturable organisms for infectious diseases management remains to be established.

Antigens and Antibody Assays

Depending on the degree and type of immunosuppression, transplant patients may not be able to mount a sufficient antibody response to pathogens limiting the use of serological assays to detect antibodies [2]. On the other hand, antigen testing can be beneficial, especially for fungal infections where results of these tests are used as one of the mycological criteria to define invasive fungal disease (IFD) [44]. Some of the most commonly used antigen tests include the galactomannan (GM) antigen produced by members of the *Aspergillus* family and the (1,3) β-D (BD) glucans, present in the cell wall of *Aspergillus* and a variety of other molds and yeasts [45].

The serum GM assay (Platelia *Aspergillus* EIA, Bio-Rad Laboratories) was approved by the United States Food and Drugs Administration (FDA) in 2003. The assay is an enzyme immunoassay that uses rat monoclonal antibody EBA-2 to detect circulating GM antigen in serum. The GM assay has been evaluated extensively in various patient populations with sensitivity ranging from 30% to 100% and specificity ranging from 38% to 98% in serum with greater utility in HSCT patients than in SOT recipients [46]. In a study by Jathavedam and colleagues, the GM assay was shown to have limited utility within the first 100 days after auto-SCT and therefore not useful for patient management decision [47]. In another study conducted in patients with hematologic malignancies, the sensitivity of the GM assay was 49% for invasive fungal infections caused by *Aspergillus* species other than *A. fumigatus* and only 13% for IFD caused by *A. fumigatus* [48]. Results of these various studies suggested that the performance of the GM assay depends on several factors including the infecting species of *Aspergillus*, the type of transplant populations, the frequency of testing, and the duration of antifungal therapy [45, 49]. The sensitivity of the GM assay in BAL of HSCT recipients and patients with hematological malignancies is higher than that reported for serum and ranges between 88% and 100% using the same optical density cutoff value used for serum [45, 50, 51]. In solid-organ transplant patients, the sensitivity and specificity of the GM assay in BAL ranged from 60% to 100% and 84–98%, respectively, depending on the optical density cutoff value used [50, 52–56]. Thus, the GM assay in BAL is a useful additional test for diagnosing IFD. False-positive results were observed in patients receiving piperacillin, amoxicillin, or ticarcillin with or without a beta-lactamase inhibitor, in patients being administered electrolyte replacement fluids (i.e., PlasmaLyte), and in patients infected with molds other than *Aspergillus* for a low specificity and positive predictive value [45, 57]. However, a study by Vergidis et al. showed that the current formulation of piperacillin-tazobactam do not appear to be contaminated with galactomannan [58].

Four assays, the Fungitell (Associates of Cape Cod Inc., East Falmouth, MA, cutoff, 60–80 pg/mL), the Fungitec-G (Seikagaku, Tokyo, Japan, cutoff, 20 pg/mL), the Wako (Wako Pure Chemical Industries, Tokyo, Japan, cutoff, 11 pg/mL), and Maruha (Maruha-Nichiro Foods, Tokyo, Japan, cutoff, 11 pg/mL) are commercially available for the detection of (1,3)-β-D (BD) glucans, a cell wall antigen found in most fungal species cell wall excluding *Mucormycetes* and *Cryptococcus* species [59]. A recent meta-analysis review of studies conducted in adult hemato-oncology patients showed similar performance for all four assays in the diagnosis of IFD, a higher diagnostic yield for performance of two consecutive tests, and an overall low sensitivity (52%) and high specificity (99%) for proven or probable IFD [59]. In another meta-analysis study, which included reports with various patient populations, the sensitivity and specificity of the BD glucans test were 77% and 85%, respectively [60]. Both studies concluded that the BD glucans assay was a useful adjunct test, especially for diagnosis of IFD due to *Candida* and *Aspergillus*. However, a recent report of high-false positive in patients with hematologic malignancies puts in question the value of this test as a stand-alone test for diagnosis of IFD [61].

The sensitivity of BD glucans is highest (90–100%) for the diagnosis of *Pneumocystis jirovecii* pneumonia (PCP), although its specificity in non-HIV immunocompromised patients varies widely (42–98%); therefore, results of the test taken alone are not conclusive for making a diagnosis of PCP [62, 63]. However, studies have shown that serum BD glucan levels correlate well with *P. jirovecii* fungal load in BAL as determined by *Pneumocystis* PCR, supporting the use of the assay to monitor response to therapy [62, 63].

Other useful antigens tests used for diagnosis of fungal infections include the latex agglutination cryptococcal antigen, which has higher sensitivity for central nervous system infection than disseminated disease, and the urine and serum antigen for endemic mycoses (*Blastomyces dermatitidis* and *Histoplasma capsulatum* antigens), although some cross-reaction occurs among targets [64].

The diagnosis of viral infections has been replaced in most instances by nucleic acid-based tests. Antigens testing and serological assays by methods such as direct fluorescent antibody (DFA) staining and enzyme immunoassays (EIA) do still play a part in the diagnosis of certain infections including diagnosis of acute or chronic hepatitis, infectious mononucleosis, and HTLV-1-/HTLV-2-associated T-cell leukemia [65]. One of the most common viral antigens tested in transplant patients is the CMV pp65 antigen for monitoring of viral loads [66]. The reported sensitivity and specificity of the CMV antigenemia test varies greatly due to lack of standardization in protocols including specimen processing, monoclonal antibody used, slide processing, and quantification [67]. Advantages of the antigenemia assay include its low cost in terms of reagents and equipment, but due to its disadvantages including the need for rapid specimen processing, the labor-intensive nature of the assay, and the subjectivity in reading of the slides, the antigenemia test has been replaced in many institutions by molecular tests for monitoring of CMV viral loads [67–69].

Bacterial antigen tests of importance for transplant patients include the urinary antigen tests for *Legionella pneumophila* serotype 1 (Binax, Scarborough, Maine, USA) and *Streptococcus pneumoniae* (Binax, Scarborough, Maine, USA), which are rapid, noninvasive tests useful in the diagnosis of both community- and hospital-acquired pneumonia [70, 71].

New Generation Diagnostic Assays

Although the use of culture and serological assays provides important information, their shortcomings created a need to develop faster and more sensitive assays. The following sections will cover the more rapid methods currently in use in most laboratories for diagnosis of infection and the newer methods being developed and conclude with the impact of these methods on the diagnosis and management of transplant patients.

Genomic Assays

The first published polymerase chain reaction (PCR) report described the amplification of specific target sequences of the β-globin gene for diagnosis of sickle cell anemia [72, 73]. Several modifications and improvements have occurred since that first report, ultimately resulting in the transfer of PCR from research laboratories to clinical diagnostic laboratories [74, 75]. Alternative nucleic acid amplification formats have since been developed including ligase chain reaction (LCR), nucleic acid sequence-based amplification (NASBA), branched DNA (b-DNA) signal amplification, strand displacement amplification (SDA), helicase-dependent amplification (HDA), and loop-mediated amplification (LAMP) [76, 77]. Numerous commercial molecular assays have been approved by DFA for diagnosis of microbial infections in transplant patients (Table 47.1).

The development of real-time PCR, combining rapid thermal cycling and real-time monitoring of amplification

Table 47.1 List of US FDA-cleared commercial molecular tests

Manufacturer	Test name	Targets	Complexity level
BD diagnostics	BD MAX MRSA assay	MDRO surveillance	√
	BD GeneOhm MRSA ACP assay	MDRO surveillance	√
	BD GeneOhm StaphSR assay	Bacteremia	√
bioMérieux	BioFire FilmArray blood culture identification panel	Bacteremia	√
	NucleiSENS EasyQ MRSA assay	MDRO surveillance	√
Cepheid	Xpert MRSA	MDRO surveillance	√
	Xpert SA nasal complete	MDRO surveillance	√
	Xpert MRSA/SA SSTI	Skin and soft tissue infections	√
	Xpert MRSA/SA BC	Bacteremia	√
Nanosphere, Inc.	Verigene gram-positive blood culture test	Bacteremia	√
Roche molecular diagnostics	LightCycler MRSA advanced test	MDRO surveillance	√
AdvanDx, Inc.	*E. faecalis*/OE PNA FISH	Bacteremia	
	E. faecalis PNA FISH	Bacteremia	
BD diagnostics	BD GeneOhm VanR assay	MDRO surveillance	√
bioMérieux/BioFire	BioFire FilmArray blood culture identification panel	Bacteremia	√
Cepheid	Xpert vanA	MDRO surveillance	√
Intelligent medical devices, Inc.	IMDx VanR for Abbott m200	MDRO surveillance	√
Nanosphere, Inc.	Verigene gram-positive blood culture test	Bacteremia	√
BD diagnostics	BD MAX C. diff assay	*C. difficile* infection	
	BD GeneOhm C. diff assay	*C. difficile* infection	
bioMérieux/BioFire	FilmArray gastrointestinal panel	Gastrointestinal tract infection	
Cepheid	Xpert *C. difficile*	*C. difficile* infection	
	Xpert *C. difficile*/epi	*C. difficile* infection	
Focus diagnostics, Inc.	Simplexa *C. difficile* universal direct assay	*C. difficile* infection	
Great Basin scientific, Inc.	Portrait Toxigenic *C. difficile* assay	*C. difficile* infection	
Intelligent medical devices, Inc.	IMDx *C. difficile* for Abbott m200	*C. difficile* infection	
Luminex molecular diagnostics, Inc.	xTAG gastrointestinal pathogen panel (GPP)	Gastrointestinal tract infection	
Meridian biosciences, Inc.	Illumigene *C. difficile* DNA amplification	*C. difficile* infection	
Nanosphere, Inc.	Verigene *C. difficile* test	*C. difficile* infection	
PrimeraDx	ICEPlex *C. difficile* kit	*C. difficile* infection	
Prodesse, Inc.	ProGastro Cd assay	*C. difficile* infection	
Quidel Corp.	Quidel molecular Direct *C. difficile* assay	*C. difficile* infection	
AdvanDx, Inc.	GNR traffic light PNA FISH	Bacteremia	√
	E. coli/*P. aeruginosa* PNA FISH	Bacteremia	
	EK/*P. aeruginosa* PNA FISH	Bacteremia	
	E. coli PNA FISH	Bacteremia	
bioMérieux	BioFire FilmArray blood culture identification panel	Bacteremia	√
Nanosphere, Inc.	Verigene gram-negative blood culture test	Bacteremia	√
AdvanDx, Inc.	*C. albicans* PNA FISH	Bacteremia	√
	C. albicans/*C. glabrata* PNA FISH	Bacteremia	

Table 47.1 (continued)

Manufacturer	Test name	Targets	Complexity level
	Yeast traffic light PNA FISH	Bacteremia	
bioMérieux	BioFire FilmArray blood culture identification panel	Bacteremia	
Alere Scarborough, Inc.	Alere I influenza A and B	Pneumonia	
bioMérieux/BioFire	FilmArray respiratory panel	Pneumonia	
Cepheid	Xpert flu/RSV	Pneumonia	√
	Xpert flu	Pneumonia	
Focus diagnostics, Inc.	Simplexa flu A/B & RSV	Pneumonia	
	Simplexa influenza A H1N1	Pneumonia	
GenMark diagnostics, Inc.	eSensor respiratory viral panel	Pneumonia	
Intelligent medical devices, Inc.	IMDx flu A/B and RSV for Abbott m200	Pneumonia	
IQuum/Roche molecular Inc.	Liat influenza A/B assay	Pneumonia	
Luminex molecular diagnostics, Inc.	xTAG respiratory viral panel (RVP)	Pneumonia	
	xTAG respiratory viral panel FAST (RVP FAST)	Pneumonia	
Meridian biosciences, Inc.	Illumigene mycoplasma DNA amplification	Pneumonia	
Nanosphere, Inc.	Verigene respiratory virus + test	Pneumonia	
	Verigene respiratory pathogens flex nucleic acid test (RP flex)	Pneumonia	
Prodesse, Inc.	Pro hMPV assay	Pneumonia	
	ProFAST assay	Pneumonia	
	ProParaflu assay	Pneumonia	
	ProFlu+ assay	Pneumonia	√
QIAGEN GmbH	Artus Infl A/B RG RT-PCR kit	Pneumonia	
Quidel Corp.	Quidel molecular RSV + hMPV assay	Pneumonia	
	Quidel molecular hMPV assay	Pneumonia	
	Quidel molecular influenza A + B assay	Pneumonia	
BD diagnostics	BD MAX enteric parasite panel		
BD diagnostics	BD MAX enteric bacterial panel		
bioMérieux	BioFire FilmArray gastrointestinal panel	Gastrointestinal tract infection	
Cepheid	Xpert norovirus	Gastrointestinal tract infection	
Luminex molecular diagnostics, Inc.	xTAG gastrointestinal pathogen panel (GPP)	Gastrointestinal tract infection	
Luminex molecular diagnostics, Inc.	xTAG gastrointestinal pathogen panel (GPP)	Gastrointestinal tract infection	
Prodesse, Inc.	ProGastro SSCS assay	Gastrointestinal tract infection	
Prodesse, Inc.	ProAdeno+ assay	Gastrointestinal tract infection	
Nanosphere, Inc.	Verigene enteric test	Gastrointestinal tract infection	

products [78, 79], completely revolutionized the practice of clinical microbiology [80, 81]. Today, real-time nucleic acid amplification methods are mainstream in most sections of clinical microbiology, and their impact on care of transplant patients is significant.

Several real-time PCR laboratory-developed tests (LDT) as well as a few FDA-approved assays are used for the diagnosis of bacterial infections in transplant patients. Bacteria targeted for assays development have traditionally been those related to nosocomial infections. For example, until recently, most PCR assays for detection of *C. difficile* were LDT assays that resulted in an increased sensitivity and turnaround time for results [82–85]. At the time of this chapter preparation, the FDA had cleared over eight molecular assays for the diagnosis of *Clostridium difficile* infection (CDI). Similarly, rapid molecular assays have been developed for a variety of bacterial targets including difficult-to-culture or slow-growing organisms (i.e., *Mycoplasma pneumoniae*, *Chlamydophila pneumoniae*, *Borrelia burgdorferi*), targeted diagnosis (i.e., group A *Streptococcus* in throat swabs), and nosocomial pathogens (methicillin-resistant *S. aureus*, methicillin-sensitive *S. aureus*, and vancomycin-resistant *Enterococci*) [80].

The turnaround time and identification of the most common *Mycobacteria* species were greatly improved with the introduction of nucleic acid hybridization probes in the laboratory. Nucleic acid hybridization probes are single-stranded or double-stranded DNA/RNA fragments complementary to a sequence in the target organisms and most commonly labeled with a fluorescent or chemiluminescent marker for detection [86]. Probes for same-day identification of *M. tuberculosis* complex, *M. kansasii*, *M. avium* complex, and *M. gordonae* from either solid or liquid cultures have been commercially available since the early 1990s (Gen-Probes, San Diego, CA). These probes show excellent sensitivity and specificity, although cross-reaction has been reported between *M. tuberculosis* complex and *M. terrae* [87–90]. Similar probes are available for identification of medically important filament fungal species.

The current trend for molecular diagnosis is a move toward syndromic, highly multiplexed real-time PCR assays and newer technologies including various solid and liquid microarray formats. Currently, FDA-cleared molecular syndromic panels are available for the diagnosis of respiratory tract infections, bloodstream infections, gastrointestinal infections, and meningitis/encephalitis (Table 47.2). These panels differ on the numbers of pathogens they can detect (5–27 targets), the type of pathogens included (e.g., bacteria, viruses, or yeasts), the level of complexity (low versus high), and the turnaround time to results (from 1 h to 12 h). Performance characteristics, however, are comparable with sensitivity and specificity greater than 90% when compared to culture or bi-directional sequencing as the gold standard [91].

Other multiplexed bacterial assays are available outside of the United States, for example, the LightCycler Septi*Fast* (Roche Diagnostics GmbH, Wien/Austria), a multiplexed real-time PCR-based assay that can detect bacteria and yeasts directly from whole blood. An agreement of up to 83% between SeptiFast and blood culture results has been reported with the overall conclusion that in its current form, the assay can be used to supplement rather than replace blood culture methods [92–94]. The SeptiFast assay has been shown to be especially useful in providing additional information for immunocompromised patients including liver transplants, septic ICU patients, and neutropenic patients, for fungal infection and in cases of prior antibiotic administration [93–96].

Other potential molecular methods have been developed and evaluated for the diagnosis of bacterial infections including sequencing [97], quantitative loop-mediated isothermal amplification [98], PCR hybridization [99], and mass spectrometry [100].

As described in the previous section, the diagnosis of IFD currently relies on microscopic examination, recovery of molds or yeasts in culture, detection of fungal antigens including galactomannan and BD glucans, and various radiological findings of pulmonary infiltrates [45, 101]. Although useful, these methods can lack specificity, be time-consuming, or result in inconclusive findings. A study by Lin et al. [102] suggested that earlier diagnosis of fungal infection could result in decreased mortality in neutropenic and cancer patients. Molecular diagnosis of fungal infections has relied mostly on the identification of organisms growing in culture. Nucleic acid hybridization probes for identification of *Blastomyces dermatitidis*, *Histoplasma capsulatum*, and *Coccidioides immitis* from culture isolates have been available since the early 1990s (AccuProbes, Gen-Probe, San Diego, CA) with sensitivity ranging from 87.8 to 100% and specificity nearing 100% [103, 104]. The hybridization probes are rapid and demonstrate good sensitivity and specificity from culture, although some cross-reactivity with uncommon fungal organisms has been reported [104, 105]. More recently, peptide nucleic acid fluorescent in situ hybridization (PNA FISH) probes and syndromic panel for bloodstream infections (FilmArray Blood Culture ID panel) have become available for rapid identification of *C. albicans/Candida*

Table 47.2 US FDA-cleared syndromic molecular tests

Manufacturer	Test name	Syndrome	# targets	Date cleared
Luminex	xTAG respiratory viral panel (RVP)	Respiratory	12	01/2008
	NxTAG respiratory pathogen panel (RPP)	Respiratory	20	12/2015
	xTAG gastrointestinal pathogen panel (GPP)	GI tract	14	01/2013
Nanosphere	Verigene respiratory virus + test	Respiratory	8	01/2011
	Verigene gram-positive blood culture test	Bacteremia	15	06/2012
	Verigene enteric test	GI tract	9	06/2014
	Verigene gram-negative blood culture test	Bacteremia	14	11/2014
	Verigene respiratory pathogens flex NA test	Respiratory	16	09/2015
bioMérieux/BioFire	FilmArray respiratory panel	Respiratory	20	05/2011
	FilmArray blood culture identification panel	Bacteremia	27	06/2013
	FilmArray gastrointestinal panel	GI tract	22	05/2014
	FilmArray meningitis/encephalitis panel	CNS	14	10/2015
GenMark	eSensor respiratory viral panel	Respiratory	14	02/2012
Prodesse	ProGastro SSCS assay	GI tract	5	01/2013

parapsilosis, *C. glabrata/Candida krusei*, and *Candida tropicalis* from positive blood cultures [91, 106–108].

Several real-time PCR assays have been developed over the last few years with varied level of sensitivity and specificity and often with limited range, only targeting a few *Candida* or mold species [109–113]. A recent shift toward development of pan-fungal assay can be observed in the literature and reflect the need for tools that detect most of the clinically relevant fungal pathogens in patient specimens [114–117].

More recently, a few commercial assays and reagents have become available for the detection of mold directly from specimens. Several MycArray™ assays (Myconostica Ltd., UK) targeting yeasts, *Aspergillus* species, and *Pneumocystis jirovecii* are commercially available outside of the United States and demonstrates high sensitivity and specificity compared to culture or LDT assays [118–120]. Other molecular methods used for fungal diagnosis include sequence-based identification using the ITS1 and ITS2 regions between the 18S and 28S rRNA subunits and the D1/D2 region of the 25–28S large ribosomal subunit [121]. Several studies have been published showing the utility of sequencing for fungal identification, and in some laboratories, sequencing has completely replaced the use of phenotypic methods to identify fungi growing in culture [122–126].

Unlike bacteria and fungi, molecular methods for detection of viruses are well established and for most pathogens are considered the gold standard. As such, there is extensive literature on the development and applications of molecular assays for the detection of viruses of importance to transplant patients including herpesviruses (*Cytomegalovirus* and Epstein-Barr viruses), polyomavirus (BK and JC virus), hepatitis viruses, and respiratory viruses [80, 127].

One of the first application of molecular assays in virology included qualitative and quantitative real-time PCR assays for the diagnosis and monitoring of human immunodeficiency virus (HIV), hepatitis B virus (HBV), and hepatitis C virus (HCV). These assays have been extensively evaluated and shown to be useful for the management and monitoring of patients with these infections [128–132]. A variety of commercial tests based on PCR (or RT-PCR) combined with sequencing (i.e., TRUGENE HIV-1 Genotyping Kit and ViroSeq genotyping system) or hybridization (i.e., INNO-LiPA HBV DR v2) are available for genotypic resistance testing of HIV [133, 134], HBV [135, 136], and HCV [137, 138].

Similarly, quantitative viral load testing has been developed for monitoring of viruses of importance to various transplant groups including cytomegalovirus (CMV), Epstein-Barr virus (EBV), BK virus, JC virus, and adenoviruses [80]. However, the biggest challenge associated with the use of these laboratory-developed quantitative assays is the inability to compare viral load results obtained across laboratories due to differences in genomic target (single vs multi-copy genes), extraction methods (manual vs automated), detection platforms, and lack of international standards and calibrators [139]. These limitations of quantitative assays have made the establishment of useful quantitative threshold for treatment difficult to establish [140–145]. The recent introduction of the first World Health Organization (WHO) international standards for cytomegalovirus [146] and Epstein-Barr viruses [147] as well as the availability of the first FDA-approved commercial real-time quantitative assay for monitoring of CMV viral loads was aimed at decreasing the variability in viral loads measured across methods, but a recent study by Hayden et al. showed that although improved, the standardization challenge remains in the field [148].

Other useful molecular assays for transplant patients include genotypic assays for drug resistance testing. Because transplant patients are often on prolonged antiviral therapy, these patients tend to develop mutations. These mutations can be detected by real-time PCR assays targeting known existing mutations that confer resistance to certain drugs, i.e., CMV UL97 mutations for ganciclovir or sequencing assay to detect all wild-type variants [149].

Several molecular assays have received FDA clearance for detection of respiratory viruses (Tables 47.1 and 47.2). The configuration of these assays varies from single target to highly multiplexed assays. The first FDA-cleared multiplexed molecular assay for respiratory viruses, the xTAG® Respiratory Viral Panel (RVP) (Luminex Molecular Diagnostics, Toronto, Canada), targets 12 viruses and subtypes (respiratory syncytial viruses A and B; influenza A (H1 subtype, H3 subtype, and untypeable), influenza B; parainfluenza 1, 2, and 3; human metapneumovirus; adenovirus; and enterovirus/rhinovirus). This assay provided a significant improvement in the diagnosis of respiratory viral infections compared to conventional method and was instrumental in the rapid diagnosis of influenza A H1N1 during the 2009 outbreak in New York City [150, 151]. Additional multiplex molecular assays have since been approved including the FilmArray Respiratory Viral Panel (FA RVP) (BioFire Diagnostic Inc., Salt Lake City, Utah) FDA cleared for the detection of 17 viruses and subtypes including the virus targets in xTAG RVP plus human coronaviruses (NL63, HKU1, 229E, and OC43) and parainfluenza 4 as well as three bacterial targets: *Bordetella pertussis*, *Chlamydia pneumoniae*, and *Mycoplasma pneumoniae*. Multiple studies have been published comparing these highly multiplexed assays against each other, against monoplexed assays, and against traditional methods in various patient populations [152–157]. Results have shown comparable performance with overall sensitivity and specificity between 90% and 100%, although differences were detected for specific targets including adenoviruses, which are detected with higher sensitivity by single target assays than by highly multiplexed PCR [156]. Other molecular devices for detection and identification of a panel of respiratory viral pathogens are also commercially available from several manufacturers including Gen-Probes (Prodesse assays), Focus Diagnostics (Simplexa assays), and Nanosphere, Inc. (Verigene assays) [158, 159].

A parasite of interest for transplant patients, especially those undergoing heart transplantation, is *Toxoplasma gondii*, which can be due to either reactivation of latent infection or acquisition of parasites from transplanted organs [160]. Unlike immunocompetent hosts, the diagnosis of toxoplasmosis in immunocompromised patients, including transplant recipients, is most effectively done using PCR on the appropriate specimens [160, 161].

Transcriptomic Assays

Genomic assays detect microbial organism-specific nucleic acids; therefore, a positive result can occur with both alive and dead microorganisms, which is particularly true for those pathogens that have protective cell wall. The best example of this is the detection of *Mycobacterium tuberculosis* DNA in sputum where the dead microbial pathogen DNA can remain un-degraded due to the fatty acid-rich cell walls [162, 163]. Unlike the results of a function-based testing method, such as mycobacterial cultures, in the clinical setting, a positive PCR result after antituberculosis therapy does not necessarily mean treatment failure. Therefore, DNA-targeted molecular assays are usually not considered to be tests of cure. This is also true for sexually transmitted pathogens such as *Chlamydia trachomatis* and *Neisseria gonorrhoeae* [164]. A positive result may reflect treatment failure with persistent infection but may also reflect resolved infection by detecting the mere presence of ribosomal RNA debris and nonviable *C. trachomatis* DNA [165].

To overcome this disadvantage, transcriptomic assays have been explored. The ability of mRNA-based assays to distinguish viable from nonviable organisms suggests that such assays should be useful in monitoring the efficacy of antituberculosis therapy [166–170]. For monitoring efficacy of therapy, mRNA RT-PCR results paralleled well with those of culture at the follow-up time points [163]. Another study further demonstrated sputum *M. tuberculosis* mRNA is a reliable marker of bacteriologic clearance in response to several mono or combined antituberculosis therapies [162]. Nucleic acid amplification assays targeting microbial mRNA have also been used for diagnosis and assessment of human papillomavirus (HPV) infections. Several reports have shown not only the ubiquitous presence of E6 and E7 mRNA in cervical cancer but also a quantitative difference in the overexpression of E6/E7 depending on the severity of the cervical lesion [171]. Several E6 and E7 mRNA qualitative assays including Aptima (Gen-Probe), NucliSENS EasyQ HPV (bioMérieux), and PreTect HPV-Proofer (NorChip) have been reported to improve the low specificity and positive predictive value of HPV DNA assays [172].

Advances in molecular biology technologies, especially the real-time quantitative PCR formats, have made the implementation of mRNA-based assay relevant and accurate. Another novel approach known as RNA-seq, which uses next-generation sequencing technologies to generate transcriptome profiling [173], is starting to come into the diagnostic microbiology field [174, 175]. Using dual-species transcriptional profiling in a murine model of systemic candidiasis, Hebecker et al. observed a delayed transcriptional immune response accompanied by late induction of fungal stress response genes in the kidneys. In contrast, early upregulation of the proinflammatory response in the liver was associated with a fungal transcriptome resembling response to phagocytosis, suggesting that phagocytes contribute significantly to fungal control in the liver [176]. Rasmussen et al. combined longitudinal, dimensionality reduction and categorical analysis of the transcriptome from 111 liver biopsy specimens taken from 57 HCV-infected patients over time and identified alterations in gene expression that occur before histologic evidence of liver disease progression, suggesting that events that occur during the acute phase of infection influence patient outcome [177].

In contrast to these "fancy" and advanced technologies, transcriptomic assays face basic specimen source-related challenges. Currently, there are limited methods which can be used to differentiate and overcome the DNA contamination when mRNA targets are tested. Theoretically, specimens can be pre-treated with DNAase prior to the mRNA amplification and detection [178, 179]. However, absolutely RNase-free DNAase is rarely available to actually do the job. Designing primers/probes to cover RNA splicing sites has been demonstrated efficient if relevant RNA splicing sites are available in targeted bacteria and viruses [180, 181]. Indirect methods have been reported to determine antimicrobial susceptibility by selectively detecting viable microorganisms. This assay uses a DNA-binding dye that penetrates damaged bacterial cells and renders DNA un-amplifiable, thereby decreasing background amplification from killed organisms [182, 183].

Proteomic Assays

One leading proteomic technology, matrix-assisted laser desorption ionization-time of flight mass spectrometry (MALDI-TOF MS), has emerged as a rapid and powerful tool for microbial species identification [100]. The analyte molecules embedded within the saturated matrix on the target plate are irradiated by a laser of special wavelength and intensity, inducing desorption and ionization; the charged analytes then are accelerated by an electric field in a flight tube to a detector, where they are captured. The separation of various molecules depends on the time of flight, which is reversely proportional to the mass of molecules. After detection signals are processed and interpreted into the mass spectra, the characteristic mass peaks are used to characterize and eventually identify the microorganisms. By measuring the exact sizes of peptides and small proteins, which are assumed to be characteristic for each bacterial species, it is possible to determine the species within a few minutes of when the analysis is started with whole cells, cell lysates, or crude bacterial extracts [184–186].

Numerous reports have shown that MALDI-TOF MS has revolutionized the routine identification of microorganisms in clinical microbiology laboratories by introducing an easy, rapid, high-throughput, low-cost, and efficient identification technique [187–190]. Two such systems, the Bruker Biotyper (Bruker Daltonics Inc., Billerica, MA) and Vitek MS (bioMérieux Inc., Durham, NC), have been successfully used in the routine clinical microbiology laboratory [191, 192]. A recent comparative study was performed on five methods for differentiation of coagulase-negative staphylococci (CoNS), i.e., Vitek2 (Gram-positive card REF 21342; bioMérieux), the ID 32 Staph strip (bioMérieux), partial 16S rRNA gene sequencing (MicroSeq; Applied Biosystems), partial *tuf* gene sequencing (in-house), and MALDI-TOF MS (Bruker Daltonics), on 142 CoNS clinical isolates. MALDI-TOF MS showed the best results for rapid and accurate CoNS differentiation with 99.3% of strains correctly identified [193]. In addition to microbial identification from purified colonies, the MALDI-TOF MS has been successfully used directly from urine and positive liquid culture media [194–197].

In addition to rapid identification of microorganisms, MALDI-TOF MS has been explored for determining epidemic relatedness and antibiotic resistance of microbial isolates. The utility of MALDI-TOF MS for microbial typing was investigated in *Staphylococcus aureus* in two recent studies. The composition correlation index analysis of the MALDI-TOF MS data demonstrated the similar inter-strain relatedness found with the standard typing methods used to confirm the outbreak [198, 199]. These data indicated that this technology is a potential rapid screening tool for nosocomial infection investigations. The MALDI-TOF MS was capable of rapidly and accurately identifying *mecA*-positive *S. aureus* and *vanB*-positive *Enterococcus faecium* from susceptible isolates [200, 201]. The MALDI-TOF MS has been directly used to determine mechanisms of antibiotic resistance [202]. Bittar et al. described the use of a MALDI-TOF MS profile and a ClinPro Tools software to detect and identify staphylococcal Panton-Valentine leukocidin [203]. The detection and identification of a series of β-lactamases from Gram-negative bacilli by MALDI-TOF MS seem to be a powerful, quick, and cost-effective method for clinical microbiology laboratories [204–207]. These studies represented a proof of concept for the use of MALDI-TOF MS technology as a rapid method to timely monitoring microbial infections.

Numerous proteomic biomarkers have been used to diagnosis and monitoring of microbial infections. One of the most promising biomarkers in recent years is procalcitonin (PCT). PCT has many favorable properties as it is rapidly induced during infections and has a long half-life with capacity to differentiate bacterial from viral etiologies [208]. For the use and value of procalcitonin in SOT transplantation, the existing literature suggests reasonable sensitivity and specificity for the PCT test in identifying infection complications among patients undergoing transplantation. Monitoring PCT in the early posttransplant period seems to be a promising method for early detection of infectious complications; however, given the imperfect sensitivity and specificity of the PCT test, medical decisions should be based on both PCT test results and clinical findings [209, 210]. Recently, van Houten et al. reported the use of a three-host protein (TRAIL, IP-10, and CRP)-based assay to differentiate between bacterial and viral infections in children with lower respiratory tract infection or fever without source [211].

Metabolic Assays

Diagnosing bacterial infections by smell has been practiced for millennia. Volatile organic compounds (VOCs), produced by bacteria as metabolites, may be produced in different quantities and combinations by each bacterial species or serovar, generating characteristic odors. These compounds, in combination with other VOCs, could be used as a volatile fingerprint of each bacterium. Recently, fast and sensitive techniques, led by a variety of mass spectrometry platforms, have been developed and implemented to detect and characterize microbial pathogens based on microbial metabolite analysis [212]. In addition, metabolic analysis can be used for functional characterization including virulence and resistance determination. Gilreel et al. recently examined the metabolic potential of multidrug-resistant uropathogenic *Escherichia coli* and demonstrate metabolic activity of members of the ST131 lineage correlated with antibiotic susceptibility profiles [213].

Direct detection of exogenous fungal metabolites in breath may be used as a novel, noninvasive, species-specific approach to identify patients with invasive aspergillosis (IA), potentially allowing more precise targeting of antifungal therapy and fewer invasive diagnostic procedures. Gas chromatography coupled with mass spectrometry (GC-MS) has been the mainstay for the detection and characterization of VOCs produced by a panel of Gram-negative bacilli [214–216]. Unique GC-MS VOCs were found to be produced by five *Aspergillus* species such as *A. fumigatus*, *A. versicolor*, *A. sydowii*, *A. flavus*, *and A. niger* cultivated on malt extract agar and gypsum board [217]. In another study, 2-Pentylfuran (2PF) was consistently detected in the media of *A. fumigatus*, *Fusarium* spp., *A. terreus*, and *A. flavus* and to a lesser extent by *A. niger*. 2PF was detected in breath samples from 4/4 patients with cystic fibrosis and *A. fumigatus* colonization, 3/7 patients with cystic fibrosis but no microbiological evidence of *A. fumigatus*, and none of the 10 healthy controls [218]. Using thermal desorption-GC-MS, Koo et al. characterized the in vitro volatile metabolite profile of *A. fumigatus*. A pathogen-specific metabolic signature combined with β-trans-bergamotene, α-trans-bergamotene, a β-vatirenene-like sesquiterpene, and trans-geranylacetone accurately discriminated patients with IA from patients with other pneumonia [219]. Besides *Aspergillus* species, VOCs such as nicotinic acid have been found to be promising biomarkers for *Mycobacterium tuberculosis* infections [220].

Clinical Perspective

During the last 10 years, mortality related to infection after HSCT has declined substantially [221]. Nonetheless infection remains a substantial cause of non-relapse mortality. Use of alternative donors such as cord blood and haploidentical donors, older age at transplant, and increased comorbidities continue to increase [222, 223]. These transplant characteristics have been associated with increased infection risk. Furthermore neutropenia, T-cell depletion, GVHD, and immunosuppressive agents continue to shape the spectrum and period of risk for specific infections. Our expanding knowledge of the role of the human microbiome in the outcomes of transplantation provides new challenges and opportunities for clinical interventions.

Management of infections in the immunocompromised host poses several challenges. Inflammatory host responses are usually reduced or absent. Patients with life-threatening infections may present with minimal signs and symptoms and deteriorate rapidly often developing disseminated disease. Organisms of little or no pathogenicity for healthy individuals may cause life-threatening infections, and multiple pathogens may coexist in the same patient. Invasive procedures needed to maximize diagnostic accuracy may be not feasible due to thrombocytopenia or other conditions. Timely institution of broad empiric therapy is essential to improved outcomes; yet polypharmacy may lead to substantial toxicities and serious drug interactions.

The increasing implementation of nucleic acid-based assays in clinical practice has enabled rapid and often quantifiable diagnosis of an expanding list of organisms. Clinical decision-making is complex as quantification enables real-time monitoring of pathogen replication dynamics.

Table 47.3 Clinical applications of diagnostic assays in immunocompromised patients

Level	Goal
Prevention	Risk assessment
Preemptive	Testing asymptomatic patients at risk for disease
Diagnostic	Testing patients with clinical signs and symptoms of infection for specific pathogens
Therapeutic	Testing patients with established infection to direct treatment, assess response to therapy, and evaluate prognosis
Prognostic	Test patients at risk for recurrence of disease

Diagnostic assays are used by the clinicians to predict risk of infection in asymptomatic patients, monitor patients at risk for disease, diagnose disease in symptomatic patients, or monitor response to therapy or predict outcomes in patients with established disease (Table 47.3).

Prediction of Risk for Infection

The pretransplant evaluation of donors and recipients of HSCT includes serology to determine prior exposure to pathogens. The Federation for Accreditation of Cellular Therapies (FACT) requires donors and recipients to be tested for antibodies to HIV, human T-cell lymphotropic viruses I and II, HBV, HCV, and herpes viruses (HSV, VZV, CMV, EBV). Donors and recipients are tested for exposure to West Nile virus and *Trypanosoma cruzi*. Donors should be tested within 30 days prior to collection. Emergence of pathogens with potential for transmission through cellular products requires development of new diagnostic assays. A recent example is Zika virus. A non- FDA approved test is currently used to screen blood donors (https://www.cdc.gov/zika/transmission/blood-transfusion.html). However the current CDC recommendations to reduce transmission of Zika through human cells and cellular-based products are based on epidemiologic history (https://www.fda.gov/downloads/BiologicsBloodVaccines/GuidanceComplianceRegulatoryInformation/Guidances/Tissue/UCM488582.pdf).

Based on the results of the pretransplant tests, clinicians assess risks, benefits, and alternatives to HSCT or implement preventive treatment. For example, recipients with positive IgG antibody for hepatitis B (HBV) core antigen (with negative HBV surface Ag and negative HBV PCR) are treated with entecavir to prevent reactivation of HBV posttransplant.

CMV serology of the donor and recipient has major implications. For recipients with acute CMV infection indicated by positive CMV IgM (negative IgG), transplant may be delayed, and treatment may be required. The CMV serostatus of the recipient is the most important predictor for development of CMV infection posttransplant. Combined results of donor and recipient serology is used to optimize donor selection [224] . Given the availability several donors with similar degree of HLA match, preference is given to donor matching the CMV serostatus of the recipient. For CMV-seronegative patients, the use of a CMV-seronegative donor alleviates the risk of CMV transmission through the allograft [225]. CMV-seropositive recipients who receive conventional allografts from CMV-seropositive donors are receiving CMV-specific cytotoxic T lymphocytes (CTL) contained in the allograft. Lymphocytes from CMV-seropositive donors can also be used to generate ex vivo CMV CTL for adoptive immunotherapy posttransplant [226]. The CMV serostatus of donor and recipient also determines the need for posttransplant serial monitoring for CMV. Recipients who are CMV positive or receive grafts of CMV-seropositive donors are monitored by CMV PCR, and preemptive therapy is initiated, if CMV infection occurs [227]. Another approach is antiviral prophylaxis for CMV for high-risk groups such as recipients of mismatched or T-cell-depleted allografts [228]. It will be interesting to assess whether CMV monitoring by the PCR will eliminate survival differences between CMV-seropositive and CMV-seronegative recipients.

Additional screening may be indicated for donors and recipients of T-cell-depleted grafts. Toxoplasma serology is not required by FACT and is tested per institutional practices. Patients receiving T-cell-depleted allografts are at higher risk of toxoplasmosis compared to patients who receive conventional allografts. Thus recipients of T-cell-depleted allografts may be candidates for prophylaxis against toxoplasma posttransplant. At present the interpretation of serology is qualitative (positive vs negative). Recent studies suggest that the magnitude of titers may be relevant in predicting disease risk. Meers et al. reported that high titers of toxoplasma IgG pretransplant were associated with increased risk of toxoplasmosis after HSCT [229]. Given the low frequency of toxoplasmosis in HSCT, a multicenter study would be required to confirm these findings.

The notion that the magnitude of IgG titers may be useful as a predictor for infection posttransplant was also supported by a pilot study assessing pretransplant antibodies to adenovirus (ADV). In that study, patients with high pretransplant IgG titers to a specific ADV serotype were more likely to develop ADV infection with the same ADV serotype after HSCT [230].

Patient exposures may also indicate the need for additional testing. For example, QuantiFERON Gold ™ testing for detection of latent tuberculous infection is pertinent for transplant candidates from endemic areas for *M. tuberculosis* [231, 232]. Patients with latent tuberculous infection pretransplant will require treatment posttransplant. Pretransplant stool examination for ova and parasites for transplant candidates coming for endemic areas of *Strongyloides stercoralis* or empiric treatment for *Strongyloides stercoralis* pretransplant could be employed for such individuals [233].

PCR Assays for Detection of Double-Stranded (ds) DNA Viruses

The availability of commercially available quantitative PCR assays for many dsDNA viruses has enabled the detection of these viruses in body compartments such as blood, urine, stool, bronchoalveolar lavage (BAL), or cerebrospinal fluid. While PCR assays provide accurate and rapid identification and quantification, several challenges remain regarding their optimal use and interpretation of results.

Cytomegalovirus (CMV)

CMV is an important cause of morbidity and mortality in transplantation. The biologic properties and natural history of CMV are well defined [234]. CMV viremia occurs frequently after HSCT and in most instances precedes development of end-organ CMV disease. Effective antiviral treatment is available, and preemptive treatment of CMV infection has been shown to be effective in preventing end-organ disease [235]. Routine monitoring is recommended for patients at risk for CMV disease [236, 237]. Currently PCR-based assays for CMV have replaced pp65 antigenemia assay in most centers. Green et al. reported that transition of preemptive therapy strategy from antigenemia to PCR-based monitoring and host risk factors successfully prevented CMV disease without increasing the proportion of patients receiving preemptive therapy and attributable toxicity [238]. The performance characteristics of individual CMV PCR assays vary; thus cutoff values and thresholds for treatment are not comparable among laboratories [145]. The availability of the World Health Organization (WHO) International Standard (IS) for CMV for nucleic acid amplification techniques is an important development for decreases variance between laboratories and enables to develop international clinical practice guideline [227]. Even with the WHO standardized assay, there is considerable variability (up to 1.5 $\log_{10}$ IU/mL) in different determinations of viral load from the same specimen [239].

Other Double-Stranded (ds) DNA Viruses

BK polyomavirus (BKV), adenovirus (ADV), and human herpesvirus 6 (HHV-6) are detected with variable frequencies in HSCT patients, yet their natural history is not fully understood. All these viruses have been associated with potentially serious end-organ disease and adverse transplantation outcomes. Yet the utility of routine monitoring and preemptive intervention have not been evaluated in prospective clinical trials. Because of the relatively low frequency of end-organ disease caused by these viruses, multicenter studies would be better suited to address such questions. Differences in diagnostic assays and clinical practices among institution and lack of approved treatments for these pathogens pose logistical difficulties.

BK Polyomavirus (BKV)

BK polyomavirus (BKV) is identified as a cause of allograft nephropathy in kidney transplants (BKVAN) and a cause of hemorrhagic cystitis in HSCT recipients [233, 240]. In renal transplant recipients, several studies have directly linked BKV replication to BKV nephropathy (BKVN), and BKV viremia is a predictor of BKVN in renal allografts [241]. Furthermore an association between the magnitude of BKV viral load in the blood and development of BKVN has been well described, and appropriate cutoffs have been established for the clinical significance of BKV viremia. BKVN cases have been reported in HSCT recipients [242–244]. The diagnosis for BKVN in HSCT recipients is challenging as kidney biopsy is oftentimes not feasible due to thrombocytopenia and bleeding risk.

The exact biologic relationship between BKV and hemorrhagic cystitis in HCT recipients is not well understood [245–252]. Some studies have shown a relationship between the magnitude of urine BKV viral load and development of hemorrhagic cystitis [253–255]. However the concentrations of virus vary widely and often overlap with patients who do not develop hemorrhagic cystitis. Unfortunately, no effective therapy is currently available for the prevention or treatment of symptoms associated with BKV, in large part due to a lack of understanding about its etiology and pathogenesis [256–261]. It is likely that the pathophysiology of cystitis in this setting is multifactorial with BKV reactivation as a contributing factor. The level of BKV viruria in HSCT exceeds by several logs the levels observed in renal transplants [250, 251, 254, 262]. Reduction of immunosuppression, the mainstay for management in renal transplantation, is not an option in the allogeneic HSCT due to the risk of triggering or exacerbating graft-versus-host disease. Despite the lack of established guidelines for the interpretation of BKV PCR results in HSCT and paucity of therapeutic measures for BKV in HSCT, BKV PCR is frequently ordered in symptomatic patients.

At our institution we prospectively monitored in 100 adult HSCT recipients for BKV in the urine by Q-PCR every 2 weeks from beginning of conditioning until week +15 posttransplant [252]. We found that 50% of patients had BKV viruria by day +30, and the rate remained stable for the duration of the study. Ten (10%) patients developed hemorrhagic cystitis (grade ≥2 by Bedi et al. [245]. Seven (70%) patients with hemorrhagic cystitis had BKV in the urine (two with concomitant adenovirus). In univariate analyses, high BKV viral load ($\geq 1.0 \times 10^7$ copies/mL) and older age were predictors of hemorrhagic cystitis. During the study period, 36 patients died and 8 patients had autopsies performed. One patient was found to have BKVN at autopsy. Our findings suggest that factors in addition to BKV are likely involved in the pathogenesis of hemorrhagic cystitis posttransplant. At present, we do not recommend monitoring asymptomatic patients for BKV in urine. In patients with symptoms of cystitis and no other identified etiology, we suggest checking BKV PCR once. We discourage monitoring of BKV viral load in the urine in patients with known BKV viruria. BKV nephropathy should be considered as a cause of renal dysfunction in severely immunosuppressed HSCT patients without any other obvious etiology.

Adenovirus (ADV)

Adenovirus infection occurs in <5–20% of HCT recipients depending on patient age, type of transplant, and degree of immunosuppression [263–265]. ADV-associated hepatitis, pneumonitis, and encephalitis are frequently fatal, while colitis and hemorrhagic cystitis cause substantial morbidity and may contribute to mortality [266–268]. More than 50 ADV serotypes are identified and differ in terms of frequency, tropism, and potential for disease severity [269]. ADV viremia has been associated with decreased overall survival after HSCT [270, 271].

Quantitative PCR assays for ADV have replaced for most part culture or antigen assays. Routine surveillance for ADV is suggested for high-risk patients such as recipients of T-cell-depleted transplant (TCD), cord blood transplant, or haploidentical transplant or for patients with refractory GVHD [272–274]. The American Society of Bone Marrow Transplant recommends serial monitoring for ADV by PCR during the first 6 months after HSCT or for the duration of severe immunosuppression and/or lymphopenia for patients at highest risk [275]. These recommendations are based on single-center experience and expert opinion but not validated in controlled trials. Ohrmalm et al. found little utility in serial monitoring of plasma ADV PCR in a cohort of 97 HSCT comprised of 64% T-cell-depleted allografts [276]. High level or rising ADV viremia has been reported to predict disseminated ADV disease and death [277–280]. Rising ADV viral load in the stool has also been reported as a useful predictor of ADV disease [279]. T-cell depletion, younger age, and GVHD have been associated with invasive ADV disease [266, 277–279]. Cidofovir has been used in established ADV disease and ADV viremia, yet its efficacy is based on small noncontrolled studies and case series [272–274]. Brincidofovir, a novel, orally administered, broad-spectrum antiviral active against ADV, has shown promising results in case reports [277, 281, 282]. A small randomized placebo-controlled clinical trial of preemptive treatment of ADV viremia with brincidofovir confirmed the antiviral activity in HCT patients however [283]. A subsequent open-label phase III study evaluated brincidofovir treatment for localized or disseminated ADV infection in adult and pediatric HSCT recipients. Virologic response was correlated with lower ADV viral load at start of treatment and earlier start of brincidofovir after ADV diagnosis. Gastrointestinal-related (abdominal pain, diarrhea, nausea, vomiting) symptoms were most common adverse events and led to treatment discontinuation especially in adult HCT.

Since 2012, we have implemented routine blood PCR monitoring from day+14 until day+100 posttransplant in TCD and cord blood HSCT recipients. The rate of ADV viremia was 8%, and 33% of viremic patients developed ADV disease in TCD HSCT recipients. ADV disease was diagnosed within 60 days posttransplant, and 85% of patients with ADV diseases died. The benefit of preemptive therapy for ADV for prevention of ADV disease in recipients of TCD grafts should be evaluated in prospective clinical trials.

Human Herpesvirus 6 (HHV-6)

HHV-6 infects over 90% of individuals in the first 18 months of life. After resolution of the primary infection, the virus establishes latency mainly in CD34+ cells including monocytes and macrophages. An alternative form of HHV-6 persistence is integration of viral sequences into host cell chromosomes [284]. Approximately 40% of all HSCT recipients develop HHV-6 reactivation, and the cords rates may be >90% [285]. At our Institution 61% CD34+ selected HCT and 94% cord blood recipients (without ATG) developed early HHV6 viremia. Rates of HHV6 encephalitis were low in our patients, 0.7% and 1.6% in Cd34+ and cord blood, respectively [286].

HHV6 has been associated with a host of indirect consequences such as acute GVHD, CMV reactivation, and mortality after HSCT [287]. Zerr et al. suggest HHV-6 reactivation is associated with delirium and neurocognitive decline after HSCT [288]. The most recognized and severe form of HHV-6 is posttransplant acute limbic encephalitis (PALE). Hill et al. examined a cohort of 1243 adult donor HSCT and 101 umbilical cord transplants to identify risk factors for PALE. In multivariate analyses cord blood transplant, grade II-IV GVHD and adult mismatched donor were significant. While viral loads for HHV-6 were higher in patients with PALE, values greatly overlapped. Furthermore, peak values were detected a median 1 day to 9 days form symptom onset [289]. Foscarnet, cidofovir, and ganciclovir are available antiviral agents that demonstrated in vitro activity against HHV-6, but there are no controlled trials to study these agents for HHV-6 therapy. A few studies evaluating the efficacy of preemptive or prophylactic therapy to prevent PALE have been disappointing [290–292].

Diagnostic Evaluation of Specific Syndromes

Challenges

Infectious complications in transplant patients are often extremely complex to assess since there is a wide array of pathogens that can cause infections, including bacteria, viruses, fungi, and parasites. Further, patterns of pathogen infectivity vary tremendously, particularly in the setting of HSCT in which immune recovery plays a major role in defining the type and clinical presentation of many infections. Infections may occur as acute events such as a pneumonia or bloodstream infection, reactivation of latent organisms as in the case of herpesvirus infections, and colonization without true invasive infection or as recurrent, nonresponding, or resistant infections. Furthermore, sites of infections may be localized to a single body area or tissue or may be disseminated. HSCT recipients may be suffering from immune incompetence that can last for years.

Multiplex assays offer the advantages when the quantity of sample is limited as they provide information on multiple pathogens. Combination of multiple diagnostic platforms in the same sample and testing of several body compartments cast a wider net and expand diagnostic capabilities. We present specific challenges in clinical evaluation of pulmonary syndromes in HSCT patients.

Evaluation of Pulmonary Syndromes

Viral Infections

The use of PCR to analyze samples from HSCT recipients may facilitate early detection of respiratory viruses, even prior to onset of symptoms when viral loads are likely to be low. For symptomatic patients, PCR testing provides a sensitive diagnostic approach to identify the etiology of respiratory symptoms and an appropriate isolation of the ill patient. Additionally, quantitative RT-PCR assays can be used to initiate appropriate treatment and monitor changes in viral load during therapy.

Some respiratory viruses such as RSV, parainfluenza viruses, adenovirus, and influenza viruses are known to cause low respiratory infections associated with substantial morbidity and mortality in immunosuppressed patients. In contrast the correlation of the presence of rhinovirus or coronavirus in the upper respiratory tract with development of lower respiratory infection in HSCT is not clear [293]. The correlation between magnitude of viral load in bronchoalveolar lavage fluid and pneumonia or transplant outcomes is currently being investigated for a variety of viruses [294, 295].

The use of nucleic acid assays may contribute to identification of organisms not previously associated with pulmonary disease. Enterovirus D68 was recently associated with acute respiratory distress syndrome in infants and HSCT [293, 296]. Human metapneumovirus (hMPV) and human bocavirus have been reported as a cause of severe lower respiratory tract infection [297–299]. Two new human polyomaviruses, KI polyomavirus (KiPyV) and WU polyomavirus (WUPyV), are found in one third of allogeneic HSCT recipient's respiratory specimens during the first year posttransplant, but the associations with respiratory symptoms are unclear [300].

Invasive Fungal Infections

Diagnosing invasive pulmonary aspergillosis (IPA) remains a challenge. Tissue diagnosis is ideal, yet invasive procedures may not be feasible in critically ill patients especially those with cytopenia. Isolation of *Aspergillus* species from BAL may represent colonization or invasive infection depending on species and clinical context. For example, *Aspergillus versicolor* and *Aspergillus niger* are often not associated with disease when they were isolated from BAL specimens [301, 302]. Cytology in combination with traditional culture techniques may improve diagnostic yield. In a retrospective study comparing diagnostic yield of cytology and culture for septate, mold infections (cytology of BAL and bronchial wash specimens) had higher yield compared to culture of tissue (autopsy and biopsy) samples (58% vs 30%, $P < 0.03$) [303].

Noninvasive sensitive tests are needed for the diagnosis of mold infections. Detection of an *Aspergillus* secondary metabolite signature in a simple breath test showed 94% sensitivity and 93% specificity in diagnosis of IPA in a small preliminary study [219]. Such tests offer promising alternatives for patients that cannot undergo bronchoscopy.

Molecular-based assays are expected to allow a rapid diagnosis of *Aspergillus* and non-*Aspergillus* invasive fungal infections with a high sensitivity. In a recent multicenter prospective study evaluation, addition of PCR to GM in BAL sampling improved the diagnosis of invasive aspergillosis [51]. Initial validation studies of the serum GM assay reported 61% sensitivity and 93% specificity in probable and proven IPA; however, the sensitivity of serum GM is considerably lower in setting of mold-active azole prophylaxis [304, 305]. Determination of GM in the BAL fluid may improve the diagnostic utility of this assay. In a prospective cohort study including 530 patients with hematologic malignancy, the sensitivity and specificity of BAL GM was 50% and 73% for detecting probable and proven IPA [306]. Further prospective studies are needed for the combination of these two diagnostic modalities for the diagnosis of proven and probable aspergillosis.

Fungal PCR has been useful in confirming diagnosis of invasive fungal infections when traditional cultures are negative especially in patients previously treated with antifungal agents. At our institution among 46 patients participating in a randomized trial for antifungal prophylaxis of fungal infection in neutropenic patients undergoing induction or re-induction chemotherapy, six patients underwent bronchoscopy for evaluation of pulmonary infiltrates. BAL was tested by cytology, traditional fungal cultures, GM, and universal fungal PCR. None of the patients had positive fungal cultures or positive GM in the BAL. Fungal PCR identified *Rhodotorula nogopathi* and *Cryptococcus saitoi* in one patient each. While these fungi are not recognized previously as pathogens in humans, our patients responded clinically when antifungal therapy was adjusted to target these organisms.

Traditional culture techniques are routinely used for diagnosis of candidemia. The clinical relevance of non-*Candida* species isolated from blood has to be interpreted with caution. In a retrospective study of non-*Candida* fungemia episodes in allogenic HSCT recipients, 42% of patients did not have clinically significant fungemia [307].

Therapeutic Monitoring

Viral PCR

Monitoring of the viral load to assess response to treatment is a well-established practice for CMV. CMV viral replication in the blood usually correlates with disease activity. Depending on CMV viral load, clinicians may continue treatment, change dose or type of antiviral, or discontinue treatment. Less evidence exist on the correlation of ADV or HHV-6 viral loads with disease activity, yet clinicians routinely use viral loads as an aid to treatment decisions.

Monitoring of viral load of respiratory viruses as a prognostic indicator of lower respiratory tract infection in HSCT patients is not a routine clinical practice at present. Recent studies suggest that this approach may be of value [294, 308].

Genotypic Assays for Mutations Conferring Resistance to Antivirals

Genotypic assays for antiviral resistance may offer clinical guidance in a timely fashion. Commercially available assays are available for cytomegalovirus. Resistance usually emerges after prolonged or subtherapeutic exposure to antivirals in the setting of immunosuppression [309]. CMV resistance to current antiviral agents is mediated by alterations in either the UL97 kinase or DNA polymerase, encoded by the UL97 and UL54 genes, respectively. UL97 mutations are capable of conferring resistance to ganciclovir, while UL54 mutations can impart resistance to ganciclovir, cidofovir, and foscarnet [310].

Studies correlating CMV genotypes and drug susceptibility phenotypes may further guide treatment decisions. This will improve the interpretation of sequence-based assays currently used for clinical diagnosis and guide the development of new antiviral drugs [311].

Resistance of influenza virus to antiviral agents is a concern in immunocompromised HSCT patients due to high grade and prolonged viral replication and prolonged exposure to antivirals. Rapid identification of emerging resistance during treatment would be helpful in modifying treatment [312, 313].

Serial Monitoring of Fungal Burden Markers

In patients with invasive aspergillosis and positive serum GM at baseline, serial monitoring of serum GM provides useful information on response to treatment and prognosis. Koo et al.

reported that the combination of GM at baseline and at 1 week was predictive of all-cause mortality independent of other traditional risk factors for mortality and antifungal exposure [314]. In a prospective study, Bergeron et al. showed that (i) a poor day 45 outcome was strongly associated with a high baseline serum GM index; (ii) a consistently negative serum GM index during the follow-up was associated with a good outcome, in contrast to either a steady or an emerging positive GM index; and (iii) the day 14 clinical evaluation was predictive of the day 45 outcome [315]. In patients with treated *Aspergillosis*, rising GM levels after initial normalization raise concern for breakthrough infection and inadequate exposure of development of resistance to ongoing antifungal therapy.

Summary

In the last decade, nucleic acid-based assays have enhanced diagnostic sensitivity and specificity, shortened test turnaround time, provided automatic and high-throughput processing, and enabled quantification of microbial pathogens. A positive molecular test result indicates that targeted pathogen-specific nucleic acids are detected. For opportunistic pathogens in particular, clinical interpretation is crucial in determining the clinical significance of a positive test. Evolving genomics, transcriptomic, proteomic, and metabolomic technologies are being translated into clinical applications at a fast pace. Collaboration between laboratory and clinical medicine is paramount to ensuring optimal utilization and interpretation of diagnostic modalities.

References

1. Sayer HG, Longton G, Bowden R, Pepe M, Storb R. Increased risk of infection in marrow transplant patients receiving methylprednisolone for graft-versus-host disease prevention. Blood. 1994;84(4):1328–32.
2. Patel R, Paya CV. Infections in solid-organ transplant recipients. Clin Microbiol Rev. 1997;10(1):86–124.
3. Guerrant RL, Van Gilder T, Steiner TS, Thielman NM, Slutsker L, Tauxe RV, et al. Practice guidelines for the management of infectious diarrhea. Clin Infect Dis. 2001;32(3):331–51.
4. Hohenthal U, Itala M, Salonen J, Sipila J, Rantakokko-Jalava K, Meurman O, et al. Bronchoalveolar lavage in immunocompromised patients with haematological malignancy--value of new microbiological methods. Eur J Haematol. 2005;74(3):203–11.
5. Krones E, Hogenauer C. Diarrhea in the immunocompromised patient. Gastroenterol Clin N Am. 2012;41(3):677–701.
6. Kamboj M, Mihu CN, Sepkowitz K, Kernan NA, Papanicolaou GA. Work-up for infectious diarrhea after allogeneic hematopoietic stem cell transplantation: single specimen testing results in cost savings without compromising diagnostic yield. Transplant Infect Dis. 2007;9(4):265–9.
7. Zaidi AK, Macone A, Goldmann AD. Impact of simple screening criteria on utilization of low-yield bacterial stool cultures in a Children's hospital. Pediatrics. 1999;103(6 Pt 1):1189–92.
8. Ginsburg PM, Thuluvath PJ. Diarrhea in liver transplant recipients: etiology and management. Liver Transplant. 2005;11(8):881–90.
9. Glass RI, Parashar UD, Estes MK. Norovirus gastroenteritis. N Engl J Med. 2009;361(18):1776–85.
10. Logan C, O'Leary JJ, O'Sullivan N. Real-time reverse transcription PCR detection of norovirus, sapovirus and astrovirus as causative agents of acute viral gastroenteritis. J Virol Methods. 2007;146(1–2):36–44.
11. Wolffs PF, Bruggeman CA, van Well GT, van Loo IH. Replacing traditional diagnostics of fecal viral pathogens by a comprehensive panel of real-time PCRs. J Clin Microbiol. 2011;49(5):1926–31.
12. Sampsonas F, Kontoyiannis DP, Dickey BF, Evans SE. Performance of a standardized bronchoalveolar lavage protocol in a comprehensive cancer center: a prospective 2-year study. Cancer. 2011;117(15):3424–33.
13. Chan CC, Abi-Saleh WJ, Arroliga AC, Stillwell PC, Kirby TJ, Gordon SM, et al. Diagnostic yield and therapeutic impact of flexible bronchoscopy in lung transplant recipients. J Heart Lung Transplant. 1996;15(2):196–205.
14. Lehto JT, Anttila VJ, Lommi J, Nieminen MS, Harjula A, Taskinen E, et al. Clinical usefulness of bronchoalveolar lavage in heart transplant recipients with suspected lower respiratory tract infection. J Heart Lung Transplant. 2004;23(5):570–6.
15. Lehto JT, Koskinen PK, Anttila VJ, Lautenschlager I, Lemstrom K, Sipponen J, et al. Bronchoscopy in the diagnosis and surveillance of respiratory infections in lung and heart-lung transplant recipients. Transpl Int. 2005;18(5):562–71.
16. Palmer SM, Alexander BD, Sanders LL, Edwards LJ, Reller LB, Davis RD, et al. Significance of blood stream infection after lung transplantation: analysis in 176 consecutive patients. Transplantation. 2000;69(11):2360–6.
17. Roth A, Wiklund AE, Palsson AS, Melander EZ, Wullt M, Cronqvist J, et al. Reducing blood culture contamination by a simple informational intervention. J Clin Microbiol. 2010;48(12):4552–8.
18. Kosmin AR, Fekete T. Use of fungal blood cultures in an academic medical center. J Clin Microbiol. 2008;46(11):3800–1.
19. Bates DW, Cook EF, Goldman L, Lee TH. Predicting bacteremia in hospitalized patients. A prospectively validated model. Ann Int Med. 1990;113(7):495–500.
20. Ramanujam P, Rathlev NK. Blood cultures do not change management in hospitalized patients with community-acquired pneumonia. Acad Emerg Med. 2006;13(7):740–5.
21. Vetter E, Torgerson C, Feuker A, Hughes J, Harmsen S, Schleck C, et al. Comparison of the BACTEC MYCO/F Lytic bottle to the isolator tube, BACTEC Plus Aerobic F/bottle, and BACTEC Anaerobic Lytic/10 bottle and comparison of the BACTEC Plus Aerobic F/bottle to the Isolator tube for recovery of bacteria, mycobacteria, and fungi from blood. J Clin Microbiol. 2001;39(12):4380–6.
22. Waite RT, Woods GL. Evaluation of BACTEC MYCO/F lytic medium for recovery of mycobacteria and fungi from blood. J Clin Microbiol. 1998;36(5):1176–9.
23. Fuller DD, Davis TE Jr, Denys GA, York MK. Evaluation of BACTEC MYCO/F Lytic medium for recovery of mycobacteria, fungi, and bacteria from blood. J Clin Microbiol. 2001;39(8):2933–6.
24. Archibald LK, McDonald LC, Addison RM, McKnight C, Byrne T, Dobbie H, et al. Comparison of BACTEC MYCO/F LYTIC and WAMPOLE ISOLATOR 10 (lysis-centrifugation) systems for detection of bacteremia, mycobacteremia, and fungemia in a developing country. J Clin Microbiol. 2000;38(8):2994–7.
25. Creger RJ, Weeman KE, Jacobs MR, Morrissey A, Parker P, Fox RM, et al. Lack of utility of the lysis-centrifugation blood culture method for detection of fungemia in immunocompromised cancer patients. J Clin Microbiol. 1998;36(1):290–3.
26. Berenguer J, Buck M, Witebsky F, Stock F, Pizzo PA, Walsh TJ. Lysis-centrifugation blood cultures in the detection of tissue-proven

invasive candidiasis. Disseminated versus single-organ infection. Diagn Microbiol Infect Dis. 1993;17(2):103–9.
27. Speich R, van der Bij W. Epidemiology and management of infections after lung transplantation. Clin Infect Dis. 2001;33(Suppl 1):S58–65.
28. Hsu RB, Chang CI, Fang CT, Chang SC, Wang SS, Chu SH. Bloodstream infection in heart transplant recipients: 12-year experience at a university hospital in Taiwan. Eur J Cardiothorac Surg. 2011;40(6):1362–7.
29. Joosten A, Maertens J, Verhaegen J, Lodewyck T, Vermeulen E, Lagrou K. High incidence of bloodstream infection detected by surveillance blood cultures in hematology patients on corticosteroid therapy. Support Care Cancer. 2012;20(11):3013–7.
30. Rodriguez L, Ethier MC, Phillips B, Lehrnbecher T, Doyle J, Sung L. Utility of peripheral blood cultures in patients with cancer and suspected blood stream infections: a systematic review. Support Care Cancer. 2012;20(12):3261–7.
31. Hummel M, Warga C, Hof H, Hehlmann R, Buchheidt D. Diagnostic yield of blood cultures from antibiotic-naive and antibiotically treated patients with haematological malignancies and high-risk neutropenia. Scand J Infect Dis. 2009;41(9):650–5.
32. Rubio M, Palau L, Vivas JR, del Potro E, Diaz-Mediavilla J, Alvarez A, et al. Predominance of gram-positive microorganisms as a cause of septicemia in patients with hematological malignancies. Infect Control Hosp Epidemiol. 1994;15(2):101–4.
33. Chitasombat MN, Kofteridis DP, Jiang Y, Tarrand J, Lewis RE, Kontoyiannis DP. Rare opportunistic (non-Candida, non-Cryptococcus) yeast bloodstream infections in patients with cancer. J Infect. 2012;64(1):68–75.
34. Miceli MH, Diaz JA, Lee SA. Emerging opportunistic yeast infections. Lancet Infect Dis. 2011;11(2):142–51.
35. Duthie R, Denning DW. Aspergillus fungemia: report of two cases and review. Clin Infect Dis. 1995;20(3):598–605.
36. Reimer LG, Wilson ML, Weinstein MP. Update on detection of bacteremia and fungemia. Clin Microbiol Rev. 1997;10(3):444–65.
37. Geha DJ, Roberts GD. Laboratory detection of fungemia. Clin Lab Med. 1994;14(1):83–97.
38. Park BJ, Pappas PG, Wannemuehler KA, Alexander BD, Anaissie EJ, Andes DR, et al. Invasive non-aspergillus mold infections in transplant recipients, United States, 2001-2006. Emerg Infect Dis. 2011;17(10):1855–64.
39. Campo M, Lewis RE, Kontoyiannis DP. Invasive fusariosis in patients with hematologic malignancies at a cancer center: 1998–2009. J Infect. 2010;60(5):331–7.
40. Petti CA, Hassan H, Reller LB. Bloodstream infections. In: Hayden RT, Carroll KC, Tang Y-W, Wolk DM, editors. Diagnostic microbiology of the immunocompromised host. Washington, DC: ASM Press; 2009. p. 409–18.
41. Limmathurotsakul D, Jamsen K, Arayawichanont A, Simpson JA, White LJ, Lee SJ, et al. Defining the true sensitivity of culture for the diagnosis of melioidosis using Bayesian latent class models. PLoS One. 2010;5(8):e12485.
42. Charlson ES, Diamond JM, Bittinger K, Fitzgerald AS, Yadav A, Haas AR, et al. Lung-enriched organisms and aberrant bacterial and fungal respiratory microbiota following lung transplant. Am J Respir Crit Care Med. 2012;186(6):536–45.
43. Taur Y, Xavier JB, Lipuma L, Ubeda C, Goldberg J, Gobourne A, et al. Intestinal domination and the risk of bacteremia in patients undergoing allogeneic hematopoietic stem cell transplantation. Clin Infect Dis. 2012;55(7):905–14.
44. De Pauw B, Walsh TJ, Donnelly JP, Stevens DA, Edwards JE, Calandra T, et al. Revised definitions of invasive fungal disease from the European Organization for Research and Treatment of Cancer/Invasive Fungal Infections Cooperative Group and the National Institute of Allergy and Infectious Diseases Mycoses Study Group (EORTC/MSG) consensus group. Clin Infect Dis. 2008;46(12):1813–21.
45. Wheat LJ. Approach to the diagnosis of invasive aspergillosis and candidiasis. Clin Chest Med. 2009;30(2):367–77. viii.
46. Pfeiffer CD, Fine JP, Safdar N. Diagnosis of invasive aspergillosis using a galactomannan assay: a meta-analysis. Clin Infect Dis. 2006;42(10):1417–27.
47. Jathavedam A, Dure DC, Taur Y, Weinstock DM. Limited utility of serum galactomannan assay after auto-SCT. Bone Marrow Transplant. 2009;44(1):59–61.
48. Hachem RY, Kontoyiannis DP, Chemaly RF, Jiang Y, Reitzel R, Raad I. Utility of galactomannan enzyme immunoassay and (1,3) beta-D-glucan in diagnosis of invasive fungal infections: low sensitivity for Aspergillus fumigatus infection in hematologic malignancy patients. J Clin Microbiol. 2009;47(1):129–33.
49. Marr KA, Balajee SA, McLaughlin L, Tabouret M, Bentsen C, Walsh TJ. Detection of galactomannan antigenemia by enzyme immunoassay for the diagnosis of invasive aspergillosis: variables that affect performance. J Infect Dis. 2004;190(3):641–9.
50. Nguyen MH, Leather H, Clancy CJ, Cline C, Jantz MA, Kulkarni V, et al. Galactomannan testing in bronchoalveolar lavage fluid facilitates the diagnosis of invasive pulmonary aspergillosis in patients with hematologic malignancies and stem cell transplant recipients. Biol Blood Marrow Transplant. 2011;17(7):1043–50.
51. Reinwald M, Spiess B, Heinz WJ, Vehreschild JJ, Lass-Florl C, Kiehl M, et al. Diagnosing pulmonary aspergillosis in patients with hematological malignancies: a multicenter prospective evaluation of an Aspergillus PCR assay and a galactomannan ELISA in bronchoalveolar lavage samples. Eur J Haematol. 2012;89(2):120–7.
52. Husain S, Clancy CJ, Nguyen MH, Swartzentruber S, Leather H, LeMonte AM, et al. Performance characteristics of the platelia Aspergillus enzyme immunoassay for detection of Aspergillus galactomannan antigen in bronchoalveolar lavage fluid. Clin Vaccine Immunol. 2008;15(12):1760–3. PubMed.
53. Husain S, Paterson DL, Studer SM, Crespo M, Pilewski J, Durkin M, et al. Aspergillus galactomannan antigen in the bronchoalveolar lavage fluid for the diagnosis of invasive aspergillosis in lung transplant recipients. Transplantation. 2007;83(10):1330–6.
54. Nguyen MH, Jaber R, Leather HL, Wingard JR, Staley B, Wheat LJ, et al. Use of bronchoalveolar lavage to detect galactomannan for diagnosis of pulmonary aspergillosis among nonimmunocompromised hosts. J Clin Microbiol. 2007;45(9):2787–92.
55. Clancy CJ, Jaber RA, Leather HL, Wingard JR, Staley B, Wheat LJ, et al. Bronchoalveolar lavage galactomannan in diagnosis of invasive pulmonary aspergillosis among solid-organ transplant recipients. J Clin Microbiol. 2007;45(6):1759–65.
56. D'Haese J, Theunissen K, Vermeulen E, Schoemans H, De Vlieger G, Lammertijn L, et al. Detection of galactomannan in bronchoalveolar lavage fluid samples of patients at risk for invasive pulmonary aspergillosis: analytical and clinical validity. J Clin Microbiol. 2012;50(4):1258–63.
57. Tortorano AM, Esposto MC, Prigitano A, Grancini A, Ossi C, Cavanna C, et al. Cross-reactivity of Fusarium spp. in the Aspergillus Galactomannan enzyme-linked immunosorbent assay. J Clin Microbiol. 2012;50(3):1051–3.
58. Vergidis P, Razonable RR, Wheat LJ, Estes L, Caliendo AM, Baden LR, et al. Reduction in false-positive Aspergillus serum galactomannan enzyme immunoassay results associated with use of piperacillin-tazobactam in the United States. J Clin Microbiol. 2014;52(6):2199–201.
59. Lamoth F, Cruciani M, Mengoli C, Castagnola E, Lortholary O, Richardson M, et al. beta-Glucan antigenemia assay for the diagnosis of invasive fungal infections in patients with hematological malignancies: a systematic review and meta-analysis of cohort studies from the Third European Conference on Infections in Leukemia (ECIL-3). Clin Infect Dis. 2012;54(5):633–43.
60. Karageorgopoulos DE, Vouloumanou EK, Ntziora F, Michalopoulos A, Rafailidis PI, Falagas ME. beta-D-glucan assay for the diagno-

sis of invasive fungal infections: a meta-analysis. Clin Infect Dis. 2011;52(6):750–70.

61. Racil Z, Kocmanova I, Lengerova M, Weinbergerova B, Buresova L, Toskova M, et al. Difficulties in using 1,3-{beta}-D-glucan as the screening test for the early diagnosis of invasive fungal infections in patients with haematological malignancies--high frequency of false-positive results and their analysis. J Med Microbiol. 2010;59(Pt 9):1016–22.
62. Costa JM, Botterel F, Cabaret O, Foulet F, Cordonnier C, Bretagne S. Association between circulating DNA, serum (1->3)-beta-D-glucan, and pulmonary fungal burden in pneumocystis pneumonia. Clin Infect Dis. 2012;55(2):e5–8.
63. de Boer MG, Gelinck LB, van Zelst BD, van de Sande WW, Willems LN, van Dissel JT, et al. beta-D-glucan and S-adenosylmethionine serum levels for the diagnosis of pneumocystis pneumonia in HIV-negative patients: a prospective study. J Infect. 2011;62(1):93–100.
64. Smith JA, Kauffman CA. Pulmonary fungal infections. Respirology. 2012;17(6):913–26.
65. Specter S, Hodinka RL, Wiedbrauk DL, Young SA. Diagnosis of viral infections. In: Richman DD, Whitley RJ, Hayden FG, editors. Clinical virology. Washington, DC: ASM Press; 2002. p. 243–72.
66. Boeckh M, Bowden RA, Goodrich JM, Pettinger M, Meyers JD. Cytomegalovirus antigen detection in peripheral blood leukocytes after allogeneic marrow transplantation. Blood. 1992;80(5):1358–64.
67. Boeckh M, Boivin G. Quantitation of cytomegalovirus: methodologic aspects and clinical applications. Clin Microbiol Rev. 1998;11(3):533–54.
68. Razonable RR, Paya CV, Smith TF. Role of the laboratory in diagnosis and management of cytomegalovirus infection in hematopoietic stem cell and solid-organ transplant recipients. J Clin Microbiol. 2002;40(3):746–52.
69. Pang XL, Chui L, Fenton J, LeBlanc B, Preiksaitis JK. Comparison of LightCycler-based PCR, COBAS amplicor CMV monitor, and pp65 antigenemia assays for quantitative measurement of cytomegalovirus viral load in peripheral blood specimens from patients after solid organ transplantation. J Clin Microbiol. 2003;41(7):3167–74.
70. Gudiol C, Garcia-Vidal C, Fernandez-Sabe N, Verdaguer R, Llado L, Roca J, et al. Clinical features and outcomes of legionnaires' disease in solid organ transplant recipients. Transpl Infect Dis. 2009;11(1):78–82.
71. Sousa D, Justo I, Dominguez A, Manzur A, Izquierdo C, Ruiz L, et al. Community-acquired pneumonia in immunocompromised older patients: incidence, causative organisms and outcome. Clin Microbiol Infect. 2013;19(2):187–92.
72. Saiki RK, Scharf S, Faloona F, Mullis KB, Horn GT, Erlich HA, et al. Enzymatic amplification of beta-globin genomic sequences and restriction site analysis for diagnosis of sickle cell anemia. Science. 1985;230(4732):1350–4.
73. Mullis KB, Faloona FA. Specific synthesis of DNA in vitro via a polymerase-catalyzed chain reaction. Methods Enzymol. 1987;155:335–50.
74. Lisby G. Application of nucleic acid amplification in clinical microbiology. Mol Biotechnol. 1999;12(1):75–99.
75. Persing DH. Diagnostic molecular microbiology. Current challenges and future directions. Diagn Microbiol Infect Dis. 1993;16(2):159–63.
76. Datta VaH RT. In vitro nucleic acid amplification. In: Persing DH, Tenover FC, Tang YW, Nolte FS, Hayden RT, Van Belkum A, editors. Molecular Microbiology. Washington, DC: ASM Press; 2011. p. 33–62.
77. Sidoti F, Bergallo M, Costa C, Cavallo R. Alternative molecular tests for virological diagnosis. Mol Biotechnol. 2013;53(3):352–62.
78. Higuchi R, Fockler C, Dollinger G, Watson R. Kinetic PCR analysis: real-time monitoring of DNA amplification reactions. Biotechnology (N Y). 1993;11(9):1026–30.
79. Higuchi R, Dollinger G, Walsh PS, Griffith R. Simultaneous amplification and detection of specific DNA sequences. Biotechnology (N Y). 1992;10(4):413–7.
80. Espy MJ, Uhl JR, Sloan LM, Buckwalter SP, Jones MF, Vetter EA, et al. Real-time PCR in clinical microbiology: applications for routine laboratory testing. Clin Microbiol Rev. 2006;19(1):165–256.
81. Cockerill FR 3rd. Application of rapid-cycle real-time polymerase chain reaction for diagnostic testing in the clinical microbiology laboratory. Arch Pathol Lab Med. 2003;127(9):1112–20.
82. Belanger SD, Boissinot M, Clairoux N, Picard FJ, Bergeron MG. Rapid detection of Clostridium difficile in feces by real-time PCR. J Clin Microbiol. 2003;41(2):730–4.
83. van den Berg RJ, Bruijnesteijn van Coppenraet LS, Gerritsen HJ, Endtz HP, van der Vorm ER, Kuijper EJ. Prospective multicenter evaluation of a new immunoassay and real-time PCR for rapid diagnosis of Clostridium difficile-associated diarrhea in hospitalized patients. J Clin Microbiol. 2005;43(10):5338–40.
84. Peterson LR, Manson RU, Paule SM, Hacek DM, Robicsek A, Thomson RB Jr, et al. Detection of toxigenic Clostridium difficile in stool samples by real-time polymerase chain reaction for the diagnosis of C. difficile-associated diarrhea. Clin Infect Dis. 2007;45(9):1152–60.
85. Sloan LM, Duresko BJ, Gustafson DR, Rosenblatt JE. Comparison of real-time PCR for detection of the tcdC gene with four toxin immunoassays and culture in diagnosis of Clostridium difficile infection. J Clin Microbiol. 2008;46(6):1996–2001.
86. Wetmur JG. DNA probes: applications of the principles of nucleic acid hybridization. Crit Rev Biochem Mol Biol. 1991;26(3–4):227–59.
87. Reisner BS, Gatson AM, Woods GL. Use of Gen-Probe AccuProbes to identify Mycobacterium avium complex, Mycobacterium tuberculosis complex, Mycobacterium kansasii, and Mycobacterium gordonae directly from BACTEC TB broth cultures. J Clin Microbiol. 1994;32(12):2995–8.
88. Peterson EM, Lu R, Floyd C, Nakasone A, Friedly G, de la Maza LM. Direct identification of Mycobacterium tuberculosis, Mycobacterium avium, and Mycobacterium intracellulare from amplified primary cultures in BACTEC media using DNA probes. J Clin Microbiol. 1989;27(7):1543–7.
89. Ford EG, Snead SJ, Todd J, Warren NG. Strains of Mycobacterium terrae complex which react with DNA probes for M. tuberculosis complex. J Clin Microbiol. 1993;31(10):2805–6.
90. Lim SD, Todd J, Lopez J, Ford E, Janda JM. Genotypic identification of pathogenic Mycobacterium species by using a nonradioactive oligonucleotide probe. J Clin Microbiol. 1991;29(6):1276–8.
91. Buchan BW, Ledeboer NA. Emerging technologies for the clinical microbiology laboratory. Clin Microbiol Rev. 2014;27(4):783–822.
92. von Lilienfeld-Toal M, Lehmann LE, Raadts AD, Hahn-Ast C, Orlopp KS, Marklein G, et al. Utility of a commercially available multiplex real-time PCR assay to detect bacterial and fungal pathogens in febrile neutropenia. J Clin Microbiol. 2009;47(8):2405–10.
93. Lamoth F, Jaton K, Prod'hom G, Senn L, Bille J, Calandra T, et al. Multiplex blood PCR in combination with blood cultures for improvement of microbiological documentation of infection in febrile neutropenia. J Clin Microbiol. 2010;48(10):3510–6.
94. Rath PM, Saner F, Paul A, Lehmann N, Steinmann E, Buer J, et al. Multiplex PCR for rapid and improved diagnosis of bloodstream infections in liver transplant recipients. J Clin Microbiol. 2012;50(6):2069–71.
95. Mauro MV, Cavalcanti P, Perugini D, Noto A, Sperli D, Giraldi C. Diagnostic utility of LightCycler SeptiFast and procalcitonin assays in the diagnosis of bloodstream infection in immunocompromised patients. Diagn Microbiol Infect Dis. 2012;73(4):308–11.
96. Mancini N, Clerici D, Diotti R, Perotti M, Ghidoli N, De Marco D, et al. Molecular diagnosis of sepsis in neutropenic patients with haematological malignancies. J Med Microbiol. 2008;57(Pt 5):601–4.

97. Janda JM, Abbott SL. 16S rRNA gene sequencing for bacterial identification in the diagnostic laboratory: pluses, perils, and pitfalls. J Clin Microbiol. 2007;45(9):2761–4.
98. Kang Y, Deng R, Wang C, Deng T, Peng P, Cheng X, et al. Etiologic diagnosis of lower respiratory tract bacterial infections using sputum samples and quantitative loop-mediated isothermal amplification. PLoS One. 2012;7(6):e38743.
99. Esteban J, Alonso-Rodriguez N, del-Prado G, Ortiz-Perez A, Molina-Manso D, Cordero-Ampuero J, et al. PCR-hybridization after sonication improves diagnosis of implant-related infection. Acta Orthop. 2012;83(3):299–304.
100. Welker M. Proteomics for routine identification of microorganisms. Proteomics. 2011;11(15):3143–53.
101. Cuenca-Estrella M, Bassetti M, Lass-Florl C, Racil Z, Richardson M, Rogers TR. Detection and investigation of invasive mould disease. J Antimicrob Chemother. 2011;66(Suppl 1):i15–24.
102. Lin MT, Lu HC, Chen WL. Improving efficacy of antifungal therapy by polymerase chain reaction-based strategy among febrile patients with neutropenia and cancer. Clin Infect Dis. 2001;33(10):1621–7.
103. Stockman L, Clark KA, Hunt JM, Roberts GD. Evaluation of commercially available acridinium ester-labeled chemiluminescent DNA probes for culture identification of Blastomyces dermatitidis, Coccidioides immitis, Cryptococcus neoformans, and Histoplasma capsulatum. J Clin Microbiol. 1993;31(4):845–50.
104. Padhye AA, Smith G, Standard PG, McLaughlin D, Kaufman L. Comparative evaluation of chemiluminescent DNA probe assays and exoantigen tests for rapid identification of Blastomyces dermatitidis and Coccidioides immitis. J Clin Microbiol. 1994;32(4):867–70.
105. Brandt ME, Gaunt D, Iqbal N, McClinton S, Hambleton S, Sigler L. False-positive Histoplasma capsulatum Gen-Probe chemiluminescent test result caused by a Chrysosporium species. J Clin Microbiol. 2005;43(3):1456–8.
106. Hall L, Le Febre KM, Deml SM, Wohlfiel SL, Wengenack NL. Evaluation of the yeast traffic light PNA FISH probes for identification of Candida species from positive blood cultures. J Clin Microbiol. 2012;50(4):1446–8.
107. Shepard JR, Addison RM, Alexander BD, Della-Latta P, Gherna M, Haase G, et al. Multicenter evaluation of the Candida albicans/Candida glabrata peptide nucleic acid fluorescent in situ hybridization method for simultaneous dual-color identification of C. albicans and C. glabrata directly from blood culture bottles. J Clin Microbiol. 2008;46(1):50–5.
108. Reller ME, Mallonee AB, Kwiatkowski NP, Merz WG. Use of peptide nucleic acid-fluorescence in situ hybridization for definitive, rapid identification of five common Candida species. J Clin Microbiol. 2007;45(11):3802–3.
109. Hata DJ, Buckwalter SP, Pritt BS, Roberts GD, Wengenack NL. Real-time PCR method for detection of zygomycetes. J Clin Microbiol. 2008;46(7):2353–8.
110. Innings A, Ullberg M, Johansson A, Rubin CJ, Noreus N, Isaksson M, et al. Multiplex real-time PCR targeting the RNase P RNA gene for detection and identification of Candida species in blood. J Clin Microbiol. 2007;45(3):874–80.
111. Maaroufi Y, Heymans C, De Bruyne JM, Duchateau V, Rodriguez-Villalobos H, Aoun M, et al. Rapid detection of Candida albicans in clinical blood samples by using a TaqMan-based PCR assay. J Clin Microbiol. 2003;41(7):3293–8.
112. Spiess B, Buchheidt D, Baust C, Skladny H, Seifarth W, Zeilfelder U, et al. Development of a LightCycler PCR assay for detection and quantification of Aspergillus fumigatus DNA in clinical samples from neutropenic patients. J Clin Microbiol. 2003;41(5):1811–8.
113. Suarez F, Lortholary O, Buland S, Rubio MT, Ghez D, Mahe V, et al. Detection of circulating Aspergillus fumigatus DNA by real-time PCR assay of large serum volumes improves early diagnosis of invasive aspergillosis in high-risk adult patients under hematologic surveillance. J Clin Microbiol. 2008;46(11):3772–7.
114. Landlinger C, Preuner S, Willinger B, Haberpursch B, Racil Z, Mayer J, et al. Species-specific identification of a wide range of clinically relevant fungal pathogens by use of Luminex xMAP technology. J Clin Microbiol. 2009;47(4):1063–73.
115. Mandviwala T, Shinde R, Kalra A, Sobel JD, Akins RA. High-throughput identification and quantification of Candida species using high resolution derivative melt analysis of panfungal amplicons. J Mol Diagn. 2010;12(1):91–101.
116. Schabereiter-Gurtner C, Selitsch B, Rotter ML, Hirschl AM, Willinger B. Development of novel real-time PCR assays for detection and differentiation of eleven medically important Aspergillus and Candida species in clinical specimens. J Clin Microbiol. 2007;45(3):906–14.
117. Baskova L, Landlinger C, Preuner S, Lion T. The Pan-AC assay: a single-reaction real-time PCR test for quantitative detection of a broad range of Aspergillus and Candida species. J Med Microbiol. 2007;56(Pt 9):1167–73.
118. McTaggart LR, Wengenack NL, Richardson SE. Validation of the MycAssay pneumocystis kit for detection of pneumocystis jirovecii in bronchoalveolar lavage specimens by comparison to a laboratory standard of direct immunofluorescence microscopy, real-time PCR, or conventional PCR. J Clin Microbiol. 2012;50(6):1856–9.
119. White PL, Perry MD, Moody A, Follett SA, Morgan G, Barnes RA. Evaluation of analytical and preliminary clinical performance of Myconostica MycAssay Aspergillus when testing serum specimens for diagnosis of invasive Aspergillosis. J Clin Microbiol. 2011;49(6):2169–74.
120. Farina C, Russello G, Andreoni S, Bonetti C, Conte M, Fazi P, et al. Microarray technology for yeast identification directly from positive blood cultures. A multicenter Italian experience. Med Mycol. 2012;50(5):549–55.
121. Wengenack NL, Binnicker MJ. Fungal molecular diagnostics. Clin Chest Med. 2009;30(2):391–408. viii.
122. Hall L, Wohlfiel S, Roberts GD. Experience with the MicroSeq D2 large-subunit ribosomal DNA sequencing kit for identification of commonly encountered, clinically important yeast species. J Clin Microbiol. 2003;41(11):5099–102.
123. Hall L, Doerr KA, Wohlfiel SL, Roberts GD. Evaluation of the MicroSeq system for identification of mycobacteria by 16S ribosomal DNA sequencing and its integration into a routine clinical mycobacteriology laboratory. J Clin Microbiol. 2003;41(4):1447–53.
124. Hall L, Wohlfiel S, Roberts GD. Experience with the MicroSeq D2 large-subunit ribosomal DNA sequencing kit for identification of filamentous fungi encountered in the clinical laboratory. J Clin Microbiol. 2004;42(2):622–6.
125. Hinrikson HP, Hurst SF, Lott TJ, Warnock DW, Morrison CJ. Assessment of ribosomal large-subunit D1-D2, internal transcribed spacer 1, and internal transcribed spacer 2 regions as targets for molecular identification of medically important Aspergillus species. J Clin Microbiol. 2005;43(5):2092–103.
126. Linton CJ, Borman AM, Cheung G, Holmes AD, Szekely A, Palmer MD, et al. Molecular identification of unusual pathogenic yeast isolates by large ribosomal subunit gene sequencing: 2 years of experience at the United Kingdom mycology reference laboratory. J Clin Microbiol. 2007;45(4):1152–8.
127. Razonable RR, Eid AJ. Viral infections in transplant recipients. Minerva Med. 2009;100(6):479–501.
128. Caliendo AM, Valsamakis A, Bremer JW, Ferreira-Gonzalez A, Granger S, Sabatini L, et al. Multilaboratory evaluation of real-time PCR tests for hepatitis B virus DNA quantification. J Clin Microbiol. 2011;49(8):2854–8.

129. Caliendo AM, Valsamakis A, Zhou Y, Yen-Lieberman B, Andersen J, Young S, et al. Multilaboratory comparison of hepatitis C virus viral load assays. J Clin Microbiol. 2006;44(5):1726–32.
130. Forman MS, Valsamakis A. Performance characteristics of a quantitative hepatitis C virus RNA assay using COBAS AmpliPrep total nucleic acid isolation and COBAS taqman hepatitis C virus analyte-specific reagent. J Mol Diagn. 2008;10(2):147–53.
131. Sloma CR, Germer JJ, Gerads TM, Mandrekar JN, Mitchell PS, Yao JD. Comparison of the Abbott realtime human immunodeficiency virus type 1 (HIV-1) assay to the Cobas AmpliPrep/Cobas TaqMan HIV-1 test: workflow, reliability, and direct costs. J Clin Microbiol. 2009;47(4):889–95.
132. Pas S, Rossen JW, Schoener D, Thamke D, Pettersson A, Babiel R, et al. Performance evaluation of the new Roche Cobas AmpliPrep/Cobas TaqMan HIV-1 test version 2.0 for quantification of human immunodeficiency virus type 1 RNA. J Clin Microbiol. 2010;48(4):1195–200.
133. Baxter JD, Mayers DL, Wentworth DN, Neaton JD, Hoover ML, Winters MA, et al. A randomized study of antiretroviral management based on plasma genotypic antiretroviral resistance testing in patients failing therapy. CPCRA 046 study team for the Terry Beirn community programs for clinical research on AIDS. AIDS. 2000;14(9):F83–93.
134. Sturmer M, Reinheimer C. Description of two commercially available assays for genotyping of HIV-1. Intervirology. 2012;55(2):134–7.
135. Niesters HG, Zoulim F, Pichoud C, Buti M, Shapiro F, D'Heuvaert N, et al. Validation of the INNO-LiPA HBV DR assay (version 2) in monitoring hepatitis B virus-infected patients receiving nucleoside analog treatment. Antimicrob Agents Chemother. 2010;54(3):1283–9.
136. Gintowt AA, Germer JJ, Mitchell PS, Yao JD. Evaluation of the MagNA pure LC used with the TRUGENE HBV genotyping kit. J Clin Virol. 2005;34(2):155–7.
137. Germer JJ, Majewski DW, Rosser M, Thompson A, Mitchell PS, Smith TF, et al. Evaluation of the TRUGENE HCV 5'NC genotyping kit with the new GeneLibrarian module 3.1.2 for genotyping of hepatitis C virus from clinical specimens. J Clin Microbiol. 2003;41(10):4855–7.
138. Zekri AR, El-Din HM, Bahnassy AA, El-Shehabi AM, El-Leethy H, Omar A, et al. TRUGENE sequencing versus INNO-LiPA for sub-genotyping of HCV genotype-4. J Med Virol. 2005;75(3):412–20.
139. Caliendo AM, Shahbazian MD, Schaper C, Ingersoll J, Abdul-Ali D, Boonyaratanakornkit J, et al. A commutable cytomegalovirus calibrator is required to improve the agreement of viral load values between laboratories. Clin Chem. 2009;55(9):1701–10.
140. Hayden RT, Hokanson KM, Pounds SB, Bankowski MJ, Belzer SW, Carr J, et al. Multicenter comparison of different real-time PCR assays for quantitative detection of Epstein-Barr virus. J Clin Microbiol. 2008;46(1):157–63.
141. Hoffman NG, Cook L, Atienza EE, Limaye AP, Jerome KR. Marked variability of BK virus load measurement using quantitative real-time PCR among commonly used assays. J Clin Microbiol. 2008;46(8):2671–80.
142. Wolff DJ, Heaney DL, Neuwald PD, Stellrecht KA, Press RD. Multi-site PCR-based CMV viral load assessment-assays demonstrate linearity and precision, but lack numeric standardization: a report of the association for molecular pathology. J Mol Diagn. 2009;11(2):87–92.
143. Pang XL, Fox JD, Fenton JM, Miller GG, Caliendo AM, Preiksaitis JK. Interlaboratory comparison of cytomegalovirus viral load assays. Am J Transplant. 2009;9(2):258–68.
144. Preiksaitis JK, Pang XL, Fox JD, Fenton JM, Caliendo AM, Miller GG. Interlaboratory comparison of epstein-barr virus viral load assays. Am J Transplant. 2009;9(2):269–79.
145. Kraft CS, Armstrong WS, Caliendo AM. Interpreting quantitative cytomegalovirus DNA testing: understanding the laboratory perspective. Clin Infect Dis. 2012;54(12):1793–7.
146. Fryer JF, Heath AB AR, Minor PD and the collaborative study group. Collaborative study to evaluate the proposed 1st WHO International Standard for human cytomegalovirus (HCMV) for nucleic acid amplification (NAT)-based assays. 2010 Contract No.: WHO/BS/10.2138.
147. Fryer JF HA, Wilkinson DE, Minor PD and the collaborative study group. Collaborative study to evaluate the proposed 1st WHO International Standard for Epstein-Barr virus (EBV) for nucleic acid amplification (NAT)-based assays. 2011 Contract No.: WHO/BS/11.2172.
148. Hayden RT, Sun Y, Tang L, Procop GW, Hillyard DR, Pinsky BA, et al. Progress in quantitative viral load testing: variability and impact of the WHO quantitative international standards. J Clin Microbiol. 2017;55(2):423–30.
149. Drew WL. Cytomegalovirus resistance testing: pitfalls and problems for the clinician. Clin Infect Dis. 2010;50(5):733–6.
150. Ginocchio CC, Zhang F, Manji R, Arora S, Bornfreund M, Falk L, et al. Evaluation of multiple test methods for the detection of the novel 2009 influenza A (H1N1) during the New York City outbreak. J Clin Virol. 2009;45(3):191–5.
151. Ginocchio CC, St George K. Likelihood that an unsubtypeable influenza A virus result obtained with the Luminex xTAG respiratory virus panel is indicative of infection with novel A/H1N1 (swine-like) influenza virus. J Clin Microbiol. 2009;47(7):2347–8.
152. Hayden RT, Gu Z, Rodriguez A, Tanioka L, Ying C, Morgenstern M, et al. Comparison of two broadly multiplexed PCR systems for viral detection in clinical respiratory tract specimens from immunocompromised children. J Clin Virol. 2012;53(4):308–13.
153. Babady NE, Mead P, Stiles J, Brennan C, Li H, Shuptar S, et al. Comparison of the Luminex xTAG RVP fast assay and the Idaho technology FilmArray RP assay for detection of respiratory viruses in pediatric patients at a cancer hospital. J Clin Microbiol. 2012;50(7):2282–8.
154. Sanghavi SK, Bullotta A, Husain S, Rinaldo CR. Clinical evaluation of multiplex real-time PCR panels for rapid detection of respiratory viral infections. J Med Virol. 2012;84(1):162–9.
155. Gadsby NJ, Hardie A, Claas EC, Templeton KE. Comparison of the Luminex respiratory virus panel fast assay with in-house real-time PCR for respiratory viral infection diagnosis. J Clin Microbiol. 2010;48(6):2213–6.
156. Loeffelholz MJ, Pong DL, Pyles RB, Xiong Y, Miller AL, Bufton KK, et al. Comparison of the FilmArray respiratory panel and Prodesse real-time PCR assays for detection of respiratory pathogens. J Clin Microbiol. 2011;49(12):4083–8.
157. Murali S, Langston AA, Nolte FS, Banks G, Martin R, Caliendo AM. Detection of respiratory viruses with a multiplex polymerase chain reaction assay (MultiCode-PLx respiratory virus panel) in patients with hematologic malignancies. Leuk Lymphoma. 2009;50(4):619–24.
158. Alby K, Popowitch EB, Miller MB. Comparative evaluation of the Nanosphere Verigene RV+ assay with the Simplexa Flu A/B & RSV kit for the detection of influenza and respiratory syncytial viruses. J Clin Microbiol. 2013;51(1):352–3. Epub 2012 Nov 14.
159. Selvaraju SB, Selvarangan R. Evaluation of three influenza A and B real-time reverse transcription-PCR assays and a new 2009 H1N1 assay for detection of influenza viruses. J Clin Microbiol. 2010;48(11):3870–5.
160. Robert-Gangneux F, Darde ML. Epidemiology of and diagnostic strategies for toxoplasmosis. Clin Microbiol Rev. 2012;25(2):264–96.
161. Patrat-Delon S, Gangneux JP, Lavoue S, Lelong B, Guiguen C, le Tulzo Y, et al. Correlation of parasite load determined by quantitative

PCR to clinical outcome in a heart transplant patient with disseminated toxoplasmosis. J Clin Microbiol. 2010;48(7):2541–5.

162. Li L, Mahan CS, Palaci M, Horter L, Loeffelholz L, Johnson JL, et al. Sputum *Mycobacterium tuberculosis* mRNA as a marker of bacteriologic clearance in response to antituberculosis therapy. J Clin Microbiol. 2010;48(1):46–51.
163. Mdivani N, Li H, Akhalaia M, Gegia M, Goginashvili L, Kernodle DS, et al. Monitoring therapeutic efficacy by real-time detection of *Mycobacterium tuberculosis* mRNA in sputum. Clin Chem. 2009;55(9):1694–700.
164. Gaydos CA, Howell MR, Quinn TC, Gaydos JC, McKee KT Jr. Use of ligase chain reaction with urine versus cervical culture for detection of *Chlamydia trachomatis* in an asymptomatic military population of pregnant and nonpregnant females attending Papanicolaou smear clinics. J Clin Microbiol. 1998;36(5):1300–4.
165. Morre SA, Sillekens PT, Jacobs MV, de Blok S, Ossewaarde JM, van Aarle P, et al. Monitoring of *Chlamydia trachomatis* infections after antibiotic treatment using RNA detection by nucleic acid sequence based amplification. Mol Pathol. 1998;51(3):149–54.
166. Aellen S, Que YA, Guignard B, Haenni M, Moreillon P. Detection of live and antibiotic-killed bacteria by quantitative real-time PCR of specific fragments of rRNA. Antimicrob Agents Chemother. 2006;50(6):1913–20.
167. Desjardin LE, Perkins MD, Wolski K, Haun S, Teixeira L, Chen Y, et al. Measurement of sputum *Mycobacterium tuberculosis* messenger RNA as a surrogate for response to chemotherapy. Am J Resp Crit Care Med. 1999;160(1):203–10.
168. Eltringham IJ, Drobniewski FA, Mangan JA, Butcher PD, Wilson SM. Evaluation of reverse transcription-PCR and a bacteriophage-based assay for rapid phenotypic detection of rifampin resistance in clinical isolates of *Mycobacterium tuberculosis*. J Clin Microbiol. 1999;37(11):3524–7.
169. Hu Y, Mangan JA, Dhillon J, Sole KM, Mitchison DA, Butcher PD, et al. Detection of mRNA transcripts and active transcription in persistent *Mycobacterium tuberculosis* induced by exposure to rifampin or pyrazinamide. J Bacteriol. 2000;182(22):6358–65.
170. Jou NT, Yoshimori RB, Mason GR, Louie JS, Liebling MR. Single-tube, nested, reverse transcriptase PCR for detection of viable *Mycobacterium tuberculosis*. J Clin Microbiol. 1997;35(5):1161–5.
171. Sotlar K, Stubner A, Diemer D, Menton S, Menton M, Dietz K, et al. Detection of high-risk human papillomavirus E6 and E7 oncogene transcripts in cervical scrapes by nested RT-polymerase chain reaction. J Med Virol. 2004;74(1):107–16.
172. Szarewski A, Ambroisine L, Cadman L, Austin J, Ho L, Terry G, et al. Comparison of predictors for high-grade cervical intraepithelial neoplasia in women with abnormal smears. Cancer Epidemiol Biomark Prev. 2008;17(11):3033–42.
173. Nagalakshmi U, Wang Z, Waern K, Shou C, Raha D, Gerstein M, et al. The transcriptional landscape of the yeast genome defined by RNA sequencing. Science. 2008;320(5881):1344–9.
174. Phattarasukol S, Radey MC, Lappala CR, Oda Y, Hirakawa H, Brittnacher MJ, et al. Identification of a p-coumarate degradation regulon in *Rhodopseudomonas palustris* using Xpression, an integrated tool for prokaryotic RNA-seq data processing. Appl Environ Microbiol. 2012;13:13.
175. Law GL, Korth MJ, Benecke AG, Katze MG. Systems virology: host-directed approaches to viral pathogenesis and drug targeting. Nat Rev Microbiol. 2013;11(7):455–66.
176. Hebecker B, Vlaic S, Conrad T, Bauer M, Brunke S, Kapitan M, et al. Dual species transcriptional profiling during systemic candidiasis reveals organ-specific host-pathogen interactions. Sci Rep. 2016;6:36055.
177. Rasmussen AL, Tchitchek N, Susnow NJ, Krasnoselsky AL, Diamond DL, Yeh MM, et al. Early transcriptional programming links progression to hepatitis C virus-induced severe liver disease in transplant patients. Hepatology (Baltimore, Md). 2012;56(1):17–27.
178. Ko G, Cromeans TL, Sobsey MD. Detection of infectious adenovirus in cell culture by mRNA reverse transcription-PCR. Appl Environ Microbiol. 2003;69(12):7377–84.
179. Wang G, Barton C, Rodgers FG. Bacterial DNA decontamination for reverse transcription polymerase chain reaction (RT-PCR). J Microbiol Methods. 2002;51(1):119–21.
180. Chen Y, Klein JR, McKay LL, Dunny GM. Quantitative analysis of group II intron expression and splicing in *Lactococcus lactis*. Appl Environ Microbiol. 2005;71(5):2576–86.
181. Cricca M, Venturoli S, Leo E, Costa S, Musiani M, Zerbini M. Molecular analysis of HPV 16 E6I/E6II spliced mRNAs and correlation with the viral physical state and the grade of the cervical lesion. J Med Virol. 2009;81(7):1276–82.
182. Parshionikar S, Laseke I, Fout GS. Use of propidium monoazide in reverse transcriptase PCR to distinguish between infectious and noninfectious enteric viruses in water samples. Appl Environ Microbiol. 2010;76(13):4318–26.
183. Pholwat S, Heysell S, Stroup S, Foongladda S, Houpt E. Rapid first- and second-line drug susceptibility assay for *Mycobacterium tuberculosis* isolates by use of quantitative PCR. J Clin Microbiol. 2011;49(1):69–75.
184. Fenselau C, Demirev PA. Characterization of intact microorganisms by MALDI mass spectrometry. Mass Spectrom Rev. 2001;20(4):157–71.
185. Holland RD, Wilkes JG, Rafii F, Sutherland JB, Persons CC, Voorhees KJ, et al. Rapid identification of intact whole bacteria based on spectral patterns using matrix-assisted laser desorption/ionization with time-of-flight mass spectrometry. Rapid Commun Mass Spectrom. 1996;10(10):1227–32.
186. Krishnamurthy T, Ross PL, Rajamani U. Detection of pathogenic and non-pathogenic bacteria by matrix-assisted laser desorption/ionization time-of-flight mass spectrometry. Rapid Commun Mass Spectrom. 1996;10(8):883–8.
187. Bizzini A, Greub G. Matrix-assisted laser desorption ionization time-of-flight mass spectrometry, a revolution in clinical microbial identification. Clin Microbiol Infect. 2010;16(11):1614–9.
188. Croxatto A, Prod'hom G, Greub G. Applications of MALDI-TOF mass spectrometry in clinical diagnostic microbiology. FEMS Microbiol Rev. 2012;36(2):380–407.
189. Seng P, Drancourt M, Gouriet F, La Scola B, Fournier PE, Rolain JM, et al. Ongoing revolution in bacteriology: routine identification of bacteria by matrix-assisted laser desorption ionization time-of-flight mass spectrometry. Clin Infect Dis. 2009;49(4):543–51.
190. He Y, Li H, Lu X, Stratton CW, Tang YW. Mass spectrometry biotyper system identifies enteric bacterial pathogens directly from colonies grown on selective stool culture media. J Clin Microbiol. 2010;48(11):3888–92.
191. Cherkaoui A, Hibbs J, Emonet S, Tangomo M, Girard M, Francois P, et al. Comparison of two matrix-assisted laser desorption ionization-time of flight mass spectrometry methods with conventional phenotypic identification for routine identification of bacteria to the species level. J Clin Microbiol. 2010;48(4):1169–75.
192. Marko DC, Saffert RT, Cunningham SA, Hyman J, Walsh J, Arbefeville S, et al. Evaluation of the Bruker Biotyper and Vitek MS matrix-assisted laser desorption ionization-time of flight mass spectrometry systems for identification of nonfermenting gram-negative bacilli isolated from cultures from cystic fibrosis patients. J Clin Microbiol. 2012;50(6):2034–9.
193. Loonen AJ, Jansz AR, Bergland JN, Valkenburg M, Wolffs PF, van den Brule AJ. Comparative study using phenotypic, genotypic, and proteomics methods for identification of coagulase-negative staphylococci. J Clin Microbiol. 2012;50(4):1437–9.
194. Ferreira L, Sanchez-Juanes F, Guerra IP, Garcia Garcia MI, Sanchez JE, Gonzalez-Buitrago JM, et al. Microorganisms direct

identification from blood culture by Maldi-Tof mass spectrometry. Clin Microbiol Infect. 2011;17(4):546–51.

195. Ferroni A, Suarez S, Beretti JL, Dauphin B, Bille E, Meyer J, et al. Real-time identification of bacteria and *Candida* species in positive blood culture broths by matrix-assisted laser desorption ionization-time of flight mass spectrometry. J Clin Microbiol. 2010;48(5):1542–8.
196. La Scola B, Raoult D. Direct identification of bacteria in positive blood culture bottles by matrix-assisted laser desorption ionisation time-of-flight mass spectrometry. PLoS One. 2009;4(11):e8041.
197. Yan Y, He Y, Maier T, Quinn C, Shi G, Li H, et al. Improved identification of yeast species directly from positive blood culture media by combining Sepsityper specimen processing and microflex analysis with the matrix-assisted laser desorption ionization Biotyper system. J Clin Microbiol. 2011;49(7):2528–32.
198. Schlebusch S, Price GR, Hinds S, Nourse C, Schooneveldt JM, Tilse MH, et al. First outbreak of PVL-positive nonmultiresistant MRSA in a neonatal ICU in Australia: comparison of MALDI-TOF and SNP-plus-binary gene typing. Eur J Clin Microbiol Infect Dis. 2010;29(10):1311–4.
199. Wolters M, Rohde H, Maier T, Belmar-Campos C, Franke G, Scherpe S, et al. MALDI-TOF MS fingerprinting allows for discrimination of major methicillin-resistant *Staphylococcus aureus* lineages. Int J Med Microbiol. 2011;301(1):64–8.
200. Du Z, Yang R, Guo Z, Song Y, Wang J. Identification of *Staphylococcus aureus* and determination of its methicillin resistance by matrix-assisted laser desorption/ionization time-of-flight mass spectrometry. Anal Chem. 2002;74(21):5487–91.
201. Griffin PM, Price GR, Schooneveldt JM, Schlebusch S, Tilse MH, Urbanski T, et al. The use of MALDI-TOF MS to identify vancomycin resistant enterococci and investigate the epidemiology of an outbreak. J Clin Microbiol. 2012;27:27.
202. Hrabak J, Walkova R, Studentova V, Chudackova E, Bergerova T. Carbapenemase activity detection by matrix-assisted laser desorption ionization-time of flight mass spectrometry. J Clin Microbiol. 2011;49(9):3222–7.
203. Bittar F, Ouchenane Z, Smati F, Raoult D, Rolain JM. MALDI-TOF-MS for rapid detection of staphylococcal Panton-valentine leukocidin. Int J Antimicrob Agents. 2009;34(5):467–70.
204. Burckhardt I, Zimmermann S. Using matrix-assisted laser desorption ionization-time of flight mass spectrometry to detect carbapenem resistance within 1 to 2.5 hours. J Clin Microbiol. 2011;49(9):3321–4.
205. Hrabak J, Studentova V, Walkova R, Zemlickova H, Jakubu V, Chudackova E, et al. Detection of NDM-1, VIM-1, KPC, OXA-48, and OXA-162 carbapenemases by matrix-assisted laser desorption ionization-time of flight mass spectrometry. J Clin Microbiol. 2012;50(7):2441–3.
206. Kempf M, Bakour S, Flaudrops C, Berrazeg M, Brunel JM, Drissi M, et al. Rapid detection of carbapenem resistance in Acinetobacter baumannii using matrix-assisted laser desorption ionization-time of flight mass spectrometry. PLoS One. 2012;7(2):e31676.
207. Sparbier K, Schubert S, Weller U, Boogen C, Kostrzewa M. Matrix-assisted laser desorption ionization-time of flight mass spectrometry-based functional assay for rapid detection of resistance against beta-lactam antibiotics. J Clin Microbiol. 2012;50(3):927–37.
208. Simon L, Gauvin F, Amre DK, Saint-Louis P, Lacroix J. Serum procalcitonin and C-reactive protein levels as markers of bacterial infection: a systematic review and meta-analysis. Clin Infect Dis. 2004;39(2):206–17.
209. Sandkovsky U, Kalil AC, Florescu DF. The use and value of procalcitonin in solid organ transplantation. Clin Transpl. 2015;29(8):689–96.
210. Yu XY, Wang Y, Zhong H, Dou QL, Song YL, Wen H. Diagnostic value of serum procalcitonin in solid organ transplant recipients: a systematic review and meta-analysis. Transplant Proc. 2014;46(1):26–32.
211. van Houten CB, de Groot JA, Klein A, Srugo I, Chistyakov I, de Waal W, et al. A host-protein based assay to differentiate between bacterial and viral infections in preschool children (OPPORTUNITY): a double-blind, multicentre, validation study. Lancet Infect Dis. 2017;17(4):431–40.
212. Kaluzna-Czaplinska J. Current medical research with the application of coupled techniques with mass spectrometry. Med Sci Monit. 2011;17(5):RA117–23.
213. Gibreel TM, Dodgson AR, Cheesbrough J, Bolton FJ, Fox AJ, Upton M. High metabolic potential may contribute to the success of ST131uropathogenicEscherichia coli. J Clin Microbiol. 2012;18:18.
214. Chambers ST, Bhandari S, Scott-Thomas A, Syhre M. Novel diagnostics: progress toward a breath test for invasive Aspergillus fumigatus. Med Mycol. 2011;49(Suppl 1):S54–61. Epub 2010 Aug 26.
215. Zechman JM, Aldinger S, Labows JN Jr. Characterization of pathogenic bacteria by automated headspace concentration-gas chromatography. J Chromatogr. 1986;377:49–57.
216. Labows JN, McGinley KJ, Webster GF, Leyden JJ. Headspace analysis of volatile metabolites of *Pseudomonas aeruginosa* and related species by gas chromatography-mass spectrometry. J Clin Microbiol. 1980;12(4):521–6.
217. Gao P, Korley F, Martin J, Chen BT. Determination of unique microbial volatile organic compounds produced by five Aspergillus species commonly found in problem buildings. AIHA J (Fairfax, Va). 2002;63(2):135–40.
218. Syhre M, Scotter JM, Chambers ST. Investigation into the production of 2-Pentylfuran by *Aspergillus fumigatus* and other respiratory pathogens in vitro and human breath samples. Med Mycol. 2008;46(3):209–15.
219. Koo S, Thomas HR, Daniels SD, Lynch RC, Fortier SM, Shea MM, et al. A breath fungal secondary metabolite signature to diagnose invasive aspergillosis. Clin Infect Dis. 2014;59(12):1733–40.
220. Syhre M, Manning L, Phuanukoonnon S, Harino P, Chambers ST. The scent of *Mycobacterium tuberculosis*--part II breath. Tuberculosis (Edinb). 2009;89(4):263–6.
221. Gooley TA, Chien JW, Pergam SA, Hingorani S, Sorror ML, Boeckh M, et al. Reduced mortality after allogeneic hematopoietic-cell transplantation. N Engl J Med. 2010;363(22):2091–101.
222. Slavin S, Nagler A, Naparstek E, Kapelushnik Y, Aker M, Cividalli G, et al. Nonmyeloablative stem cell transplantation and cell therapy as an alternative to conventional bone marrow transplantation with lethal cytoreduction for the treatment of malignant and nonmalignant hematologic diseases. Blood. 1998;91(3):756–63.
223. Ponce DM, Zheng J, Gonzales AM, Lubin M, Heller G, Castro-Malaspina H, et al. Reduced late mortality risk contributes to similar survival after double-unit cord blood transplantation compared with related and unrelated donor hematopoietic stem cell transplantation. Biol Blood Marrow Transplant. 2011;17(9):1316–26.
224. Confer DL, Abress LK, Navarro W, Madrigal A. Selection of adult unrelated hematopoietic stem cell donors: beyond HLA. Biol Blood Marrow Transplant. 2010;16(1 Suppl):S8–S11.
225. Pergam SA, Xie H, Sandhu R, Pollack M, Smith J, Stevens-Ayers T, et al. Efficiency and risk factors for CMV transmission in seronegative hematopoietic stem cell recipients. Biol Blood Marrow Transplant. 2012;18(9):1391–400.
226. Meij P, Jedema I, Zandvliet ML, van der Heiden PL, van de Meent M, van Egmond HM, et al. Effective treatment of refractory CMV reactivation after allogeneic stem cell transplantation with in vitro-generated CMV pp65-specific CD8+ T-cell lines. J Immunother. 2012;35(8):621–8.
227. Boeckh M, Ljungman P. How we treat cytomegalovirus in hematopoietic cell transplant recipients. Blood. 2009;113(23):5711–9.

228. Milano F, Pergam SA, Xie H, Leisenring WM, Gutman JA, Riffkin I, et al. Intensive strategy to prevent CMV disease in seropositive umbilical cord blood transplant recipients. Blood. 2011;118(20):5689–96.
229. Meers S, Lagrou K, Theunissen K, Dierickx D, Delforge M, Devos T, et al. Myeloablative conditioning predisposes patients for toxoplasma gondii reactivation after allogeneic stem cell transplantation. Clin Infect Dis. 2010;50(8):1127–34.
230. Veltrop-Duits LA, van Vreeswijk T, Heemskerk B, Thijssen JC, El Seady R, Jol-van der Zijde EM, et al. High titers of pre-existing adenovirus serotype-specific neutralizing antibodies in the host predict viral reactivation after allogeneic stem cell transplantation in children. Clin Infect Dis. 2011;52(12):1405–13.
231. Moon SM, Lee SO, Choi SH, Kim YS, Woo JH, Yoon DH, et al. Comparison of the QuantiFERON-TB gold in-tube test with the tuberculin skin test for detecting latent tuberculosis infection prior to hematopoietic stem cell transplantation. Transpl Infect Dis. 2013;15:104–9. Epub 2012 Jul 23.
232. Wirk B, Wingard JR. Strongyloides stercoralis hyperinfection in hematopoietic stem cell transplantation. Transpl Infect Dis. 2009;11(2):143–8.
233. Bogdanovic G, Ljungman P, Wang F, Dalianis T. Presence of human polyomavirus DNA in the peripheral circulation of bone marrow transplant patients with and without hemorrhagic cystitis. Bone Marrow Transplant. 1996;17(4):573–6.
234. Boeckh M, Geballe AP. Cytomegalovirus: pathogen, paradigm, and puzzle. J Clin Invest. 2011;121(5):1673–80.
235. Boeckh M. Complications, diagnosis, management, and prevention of CMV infections: current and future. ASH Education Program Book. 2011;2011:305–9.
236. Kotton CN, Kumar D, Caliendo AM, Asberg A, Chou S, Danziger-Isakov L, et al. Updated international consensus guidelines on the management of cytomegalovirus in solid-organ transplantation. Transplantation. 2013;96(4):333–60.
237. Tomblyn M, Chiller T, Einsele H, Gress R, Sepkowitz K, Storek J, et al. Guidelines for preventing infectious complications among hematopoietic cell transplantation recipients: a global perspective. Biol Blood Marrow Transplant. 2009;15(10):1143–238.
238. Green ML, Leisenring W, Stachel D, Pergam SA, Sandmaier BM, Wald A, et al. Efficacy of a viral load-based, risk-adapted, preemptive treatment strategy for prevention of cytomegalovirus disease after hematopoietic cell transplantation. Biol Blood Marrow Transplant. 2012;18(11):1687–99.
239. Hayden RT, Preiksaitis J, Tong Y, Pang X, Sun Y, Tang L, et al. Commutability of the first World Health Organization international standard for human cytomegalovirus. J Clin Microbiol. 2015;53(10):3325–33.
240. Cottler-Fox M, Lynch M, Deeg HJ, Koss LG. Human polyomavirus: lack of relationship of viruria to prolonged or severe hemorrhagic cystitis after bone marrow transplant. Bone Marrow Transplant. 1989;4(3):279–82.
241. Hirsch HH. BK virus: opportunity makes a pathogen. Clin Infect Dis. 2005;41(3):354–60.
242. Burbach M, Birsen R, Denis B, Munier AL, Verine J, de Fontbrune FS, et al. A case of BK virus nephropathy without hemorrhagic cystitis after hematopoietic stem cell transplantation. Ann Hematol. 2016;95(9):1567–8.
243. Papanicolaou GA, Lee YJ, Young JW, Seshan SV, Boruchov AM, Chittick G, et al. Brincidofovir for polyomavirus-associated nephropathy after allogeneic hematopoietic stem cell transplantation. Am J Kidney Dis. 2015;65(5):780–4.
244. Raval M, Gulbis A, Bollard C, Leen A, Chemaly R, Shpall E, et al. Evaluation and management of BK virus-associated nephropathy following allogeneic hematopoietic cell transplantation. Biol Blood Marrow Transplant. 2011;17(11):1589–93.
245. Bedi A, Miller CB, Hanson JL, Goodman S, Ambinder RF, Charache P, et al. Association of BK virus with failure of prophylaxis against hemorrhagic cystitis following bone marrow transplantation. J Clin Oncol. 1995;13(5):1103–9.
246. Cesaro S, Facchin C, Tridello G, Messina C, Calore E, Biasolo MA, et al. A prospective study of BK-virus-associated haemorrhagic cystitis in paediatric patients undergoing allogeneic haematopoietic stem cell transplantation. Bone Marrow Transplant. 2008;41(4):363–70.
247. Imperiale MJ. The human polyomaviruses, BKV and JCV: molecular pathogenesis of acute disease and potential role in cancer. Virology. 2000;267(1):1–7.
248. Rabenau HF, Preiser W, Franck S, Schwerdtfeger S, Doerr HW. Polyomavirus viruria in bone marrow transplant recipients: lack of correlation with clinical symptoms. Infection. 2002;30(2):91–3.
249. Tomonari A, Takahashi S, Ooi J, Fukuno K, Takasugi K, Tsukada N, et al. Hemorrhagic cystitis in adults after unrelated cord blood transplantation: a single-institution experience in Japan. Int J Hematol. 2006;84(3):268–71.
250. Erard V, Kim HW, Corey L, Limaye A, Huang ML, Myerson D, et al. BK DNA viral load in plasma: evidence for an association with hemorrhagic cystitis in allogeneic hematopoietic cell transplant recipients. Blood. 2005;106(3):1130–2.
251. Erard V, Storer B, Corey L, Nollkamper J, Huang ML, Limaye A, et al. BK virus infection in hematopoietic stem cell transplant recipients: frequency, risk factors, and association with postengraftment hemorrhagic cystitis. Clin Infect Dis. 2004;39(12):1861–5.
252. Lee YJ, Zheng J, Kolitsopoulos Y, Chung D, Amigues I, Son T, et al. Relationship of BK polyoma virus (BKV) in the urine with hemorrhagic cystitis and renal function in recipients of T cell-depleted peripheral blood and cord blood stem cell transplantations. Biol Blood Marrow Transplant. 2014;20(8):1204–10.
253. Leung AY, Chan MT, Yuen KY, Cheng VC, Chan KH, Wong CL, et al. Ciprofloxacin decreased polyoma BK virus load in patients who underwent allogeneic hematopoietic stem cell transplantation. Clin Infect Dis. 2005;40(4):528–37.
254. Leung AY, Suen CK, Lie AK, Liang RH, Yuen KY, Kwong YL. Quantification of polyoma BK viruria in hemorrhagic cystitis complicating bone marrow transplantation. Blood. 2001;98(6):1971–8.
255. Randhawa PS, Popescu I, Macedo C, Zeevi A, Shapiro R, Vats AN, et al. Detection of CD8+ T cells sensitized to BK virus large T antigen in healthy volunteers and kidney transplant recipients. Hum Immunol. 2006;67(4–5):298–302.
256. Andrei G, Snoeck R, Vandeputte M, De Clercq E. Activities of various compounds against murine and primate polyomaviruses. Antimicrob Agents Chemother. 1997;41(3):587–93.
257. Bridges B, Donegan S, Badros A. Cidofovir bladder instillation for the treatment of BK hemorrhagic cystitis after allogeneic stem cell transplantation. Am J Hematol. 2006;81(7):535–7.
258. Ferrazzi E, Peracchi M, Biasolo MA, Faggionato O, Stefanelli S, Palu G. Antiviral activity of gyrase inhibitors norfloxacin, coumermycin A1 and nalidixic acid. Biochem Pharmacol. 1988;37(9):1885–6.
259. Portolani M, Pietrosemoli P, Cermelli C, Mannini-Palenzona A, Grossi MP, Paolini L, et al. Suppression of BK virus replication and cytopathic effect by inhibitors of prokaryotic DNA gyrase. Antivir Res. 1988;9(3):205–18.
260. Savona MR, Newton D, Frame D, Levine JE, Mineishi S, Kaul DR. Low-dose cidofovir treatment of BK virus-associated hemorrhagic cystitis in recipients of hematopoietic stem cell transplant. Bone Marrow Transplant. 2007;39(12):783–7.
261. Walden O, Hartel C, Doehn C, Jocham D. Intravesical cidofovir--instillation therapy for polyomavirus-associated hemorrhagic cystitis after bone marrow transplantation. Urologe A.

2007;46(5):535–7. Intravesikale Cidofovir--Instillationstherapie bei Polyomavirus-assoziierter hamorrhagischer Zystitis nach Knochenmarktransplantation. ger.
262. Wong AS, Chan KH, Cheng VC, Yuen KY, Kwong YL, Leung AY. Relationship of pretransplantation polyoma BK virus serologic findings and BK viral reactivation after hematopoietic stem cell transplantation. Clin Infect Dis. 2007;44(6):830–7.
263. Lee YJ, Palomino-Guilen P, Babady NE, Lamson DM, St George K, Tang YW, et al. Disseminated adenovirus infection in cancer patients presenting with focal pulmonary consolidation. J Clin Microbiol. 2014;52(1):350–3.
264. Rustia E, Violago L, Jin Z, Foca MD, Kahn JM, Arnold S, et al. Risk factors and utility of a risk-based algorithm for monitoring cytomegalovirus, Epstein-Barr virus, and adenovirus infections in pediatric recipients after allogeneic hematopoietic cell transplantation. Biol Blood Marrow Transplant. 2016;22(9):1646–53.
265. Sive JI, Thomson KJ, Morris EC, Ward KN, Peggs KS. Adenoviremia has limited clinical impact in the majority of patients following alemtuzumab-based allogeneic stem cell transplantation in adults. Clin Infect Dis. 2012;55(10):1362–70.
266. Flomenberg P, Babbitt J, Drobyski WR, Ash RC, Carrigan DR, Sedmak GV, et al. Increasing incidence of adenovirus disease in bone marrow transplant recipients. J Infect Dis. 1994;169(4):775–81.
267. Symeonidis N, Jakubowski A, Pierre-Louis S, Jaffe D, Pamer E, Sepkowitz K, et al. Invasive adenoviral infections in T-cell-depleted allogeneic hematopoietic stem cell transplantation: high mortality in the era of cidofovir. Transpl Infect Dis. 2007;9(2):108–13.
268. Howard DS, Phillips IG, Reece DE, Munn RK, Henslee-Downey J, Pittard M, et al. Adenovirus infections in hematopoietic stem cell transplant recipients. Clin Infect Dis. 1999;29(6):1494–501.
269. Lynch JP 3rd, Kajon AE. Adenovirus: epidemiology, global spread of novel serotypes, and advances in treatment and prevention. Sem Resp Crit Care Med. 2016;37(4):586–602.
270. Boeckh M, Gooley TA, Myerson D, Cunningham T, Schoch G, Bowden RA. Cytomegalovirus pp65 antigenemia-guided early treatment with ganciclovir versus ganciclovir at engraftment after allogeneic marrow transplantation: a randomized double-blind study. Blood. 1996;88(10):4063–71.
271. Zaia JA. Prevention of cytomegalovirus disease in hematopoietic stem cell transplantation. Clin Infect Dis. 2002;35(8):999–1004.
272. Lindemans CA, Leen AM, Boelens JJ. How I treat adenovirus in hematopoietic stem cell transplant recipients. Blood. 2010;116(25):5476–85.
273. Matthes-Martin S, Feuchtinger T, Shaw PJ, Engelhard D, Hirsch HH, Cordonnier C, Ljungman P, Fourth European Conference on Infections in Leukemia. European guidelines for diagnosis and treatment of adenovirus infection in leukemia and stem cell transplantation: summary of ECIL-4 (2011). Transpl Infect Dis. 2012;14(6):555–63.
274. Williams KM, Agwu AL, Dabb AA, Higman MA, Loeb DM, Valsamakis A, et al. A clinical algorithm identifies high risk pediatric oncology and bone marrow transplant patients likely to benefit from treatment of adenoviral infection. J Pediatr Hematol Oncol. 2009;31(11):825–31.
275. Zaia J, Baden L, Boeckh MJ, Chakrabarti S, Einsele H, Ljungman P, et al. Viral disease prevention after hematopoietic cell transplantation. Bone Marrow Transplant. 2009;44(8):471–82.
276. Ohrmalm L, Lindblom A, Omar H, Norbeck O, Gustafson I, Lewensohn-Fuchs I, et al. Evaluation of a surveillance strategy for early detection of adenovirus by PCR of peripheral blood in hematopoietic SCT recipients: incidence and outcome. Bone Marrow Transplant. 2011;46(2):267–72.
277. Ganzenmueller T, Buchholz S, Harste G, Dammann E, Trenschel R, Heim A. High lethality of human adenovirus disease in adult allogeneic stem cell transplant recipients with high adenoviral blood load. J Clin Virol. 2011;52(1):55–9.
278. Walls T, Hawrami K, Ushiro-Lumb I, Shingadia D, Saha V, Shankar AG. Adenovirus infection after pediatric bone marrow transplantation: is treatment always necessary? Clin Infect Dis. 2005;40(9):1244–9.
279. Lion T, Kosulin K, Landlinger C, Rauch M, Preuner S, Jugovic D, et al. Monitoring of adenovirus load in stool by real-time PCR permits early detection of impending invasive infection in patients after allogeneic stem cell transplantation. Leukemia. 2010;24(4):706–14.
280. Schilham MW, Claas EC, van Zaane W, Heemskerk B, Vossen JM, Lankester AC, et al. High levels of adenovirus DNA in serum correlate with fatal outcome of adenovirus infection in children after allogeneic stem-cell transplantation. Clin Infect Dis. 2002;35(5):526–32.
281. Grimley MS, Marsh RA, Bleesing JJ, Mehta PA, Jodele SA, Myers KM, et al. Cmx001 as therapy for severe adenovirus infections in immunocompromised pediatric patients: single experience in 5 patients. Biol Blood Marrow Transplant. 2012;18(2):S315.
282. Florescu DF, Pergam SA, Neely MN, Qiu F, Johnston C, Way S, et al. Safety and efficacy of CMX001 as salvage therapy for severe adenovirus infections in immunocompromised patients. Biol Blood Marrow Transplant. 2012;18(5):731–8.
283. Grimley MS, Chemaly RF, Englund JA, Kurtzberg J, Chittick G, Brundage TM, et al. Brincidofovir for asymptomatic adenovirus viremia in pediatric and adult allogeneic hematopoietic cell transplant recipients: a randomized placebo-controlled phase II trial. Biol Blood Marrow Transplant. 2017;23(3):512–21.
284. Caserta MT, Dewhurst S. Dazed and confused by HHV-6. Blood. 2011;117(19):5016–8.
285. Yamane A, Mori T, Suzuki S, Mihara A, Yamazaki R, Aisa Y, et al. Risk factors for developing human herpesvirus 6 (HHV-6) reactivation after allogeneic hematopoietic stem cell transplantation and its association with central nervous system disorders. Biol Blood Marrow Transplant. 2007;13(1):100–6.
286. Olson AL, Dahi PB, Zheng J, Devlin SM, Lubin M, Gonzales AM, et al. Frequent human herpesvirus-6 viremia but low incidence of encephalitis in double-unit cord blood recipients transplanted without antithymocyte globulin. Biol Blood Marrow Transplant. 2014;20(6):787–93.
287. Zerr DM, Boeckh M, Delaney C, Martin PJ, Xie H, Adler AL, et al. HHV-6 reactivation and associated sequelae after hematopoietic cell transplantation. Biol Blood Marrow Transplant 2012;18(11):1700–8.
288. Zerr DM, Fann JR, Breiger D, Boeckh M, Adler AL, Xie H, et al. HHV-6 reactivation and its effect on delirium and cognitive functioning in hematopoietic cell transplantation recipients. Blood. 2011;117(19):5243–9.
289. Hill JA, Koo S, Guzman Suarez BB, Ho VT, Cutler C, Koreth J, et al. Cord-blood hematopoietic stem cell transplant confers an increased risk for human Herpesvirus-6-associated acute limbic encephalitis: a cohort analysis. Biol Blood Marrow Transplant. 2012;18(11):1638–48.
290. Betts BC, Young JA, Ustun C, Cao Q, Weisdorf DJ. Human herpesvirus 6 infection after hematopoietic cell transplantation: is routine surveillance necessary? Biol Blood Marrow Transplant. 2011;17(10):1562–8.
291. Ogata M, Satou T, Kawano R, Goto K, Ikewaki J, Kohno K, et al. Plasma HHV-6 viral load-guided preemptive therapy against HHV-6 encephalopathy after allogeneic stem cell transplantation: a prospective evaluation. Bone Marrow Transplant. 2008;41(3):279–85.
292. Ishiyama K, Katagiri T, Hoshino T, Yoshida T, Yamaguchi M, Nakao S. Preemptive therapy of human herpesvirus-6 encephalitis

with foscarnet sodium for high-risk patients after hematopoietic SCT. Bone Marrow Transplant. 2011;46(6):863–9.

293. Milano F, Campbell AP, Guthrie KA, Kuypers J, Englund JA, Corey L, et al. Human rhinovirus and coronavirus detection among allogeneic hematopoietic stem cell transplantation recipients. Blood. 2010;115(10):2088–94.
294. Campbell AP, Chien JW, Kuypers J, Englund JA, Wald A, Guthrie KA, et al. Respiratory virus pneumonia after hematopoietic cell transplantation (HCT): associations between viral load in bronchoalveolar lavage samples, viral RNA detection in serum samples, and clinical outcomes of HCT. J Infect Dis. 2010;201(9):1404–13.
295. Seo S, Renaud C, Kuypers JM, Chiu CY, Huang ML, Samayoa E, et al. Idiopathic pneumonia syndrome after hematopoietic cell transplantation: evidence of occult infectious etiologies. Blood. 2015;125(24):3789–97.
296. Waghmare A, Pergam SA, Jerome KR, Englund JA, Boeckh M, Kuypers J. Clinical disease due to enterovirus D68 in adult hematologic malignancy patients and hematopoietic cell transplant recipients. Blood. 2015;125(11):1724–9.
297. Dokos C, Masjosthusmann K, Rellensmann G, Werner C, Schuler-Luttmann S, Muller KM, et al. Fatal human metapneumovirus infection following allogeneic hematopoietic stem cell transplantation. Transpl Infect Dis. 2013;15(3):E97–E101.
298. Englund JA, Boeckh M, Kuypers J, Nichols WG, Hackman RC, Morrow RA, et al. Brief communication: fatal human metapneumovirus infection in stem-cell transplant recipients. Ann Int Med. 2006;144(5):344–9.
299. Schenk T, Strahm B, Kontny U, Hufnagel M, Neumann-Haefelin D, Falcone V. Disseminated bocavirus infection after stem cell transplant. Emerg Infect Dis. 2007;13(9):1425–7.
300. Kuypers J, Campbell AP, Guthrie KA, Wright NL, Englund JA, Corey L, et al. WU and KI polyomaviruses in respiratory samples from allogeneic hematopoietic cell transplant recipients. Emerg Infect Dis. 2012;18(10):1580–8.
301. Perfect JR, Cox GM, Lee JY, Kauffman CA, de Repentigny L, Chapman SW, et al. The impact of culture isolation of aspergillus species: a hospital-based survey of aspergillosis. Clin Infect Dis. 2001;33(11):1824–33.
302. Wald A, Leisenring W, van Burik JA, Bowden RA. Epidemiology of aspergillus infections in a large cohort of patients undergoing bone marrow transplantation. J Infect Dis. 1997;175(6):1459–66.
303. Tarrand JJ, Lichterfeld M, Warraich I, Luna M, Han XY, May GS, et al. Diagnosis of invasive septate mold infections. A correlation of microbiological culture and histologic or cytologic examination. Am J Clin Pathol. 2003;119(6):854–8.
304. Cornely OA. Galactomannan testing during mold-active prophylaxis. Clin Infect Dis. 2014;59(12):1703–4.
305. Duarte RF, Sanchez-Ortega I, Cuesta I, Arnan M, Patino B, Fernandez de Sevilla A, et al. Serum galactomannan-based early detection of invasive aspergillosis in hematology patients receiving effective antimold prophylaxis. Clin Infect Dis. 2014;59(12):1696–702.
306. Affolter K, Tamm M, Jahn K, Halter J, Passweg J, Hirsch HH, et al. Galactomannan in bronchoalveolar lavage for diagnosing invasive fungal disease. Am J Resp Crit Care Med. 2014;190(3):309–17.
307. Safdar A, Singhal S, Mehta J. Clinical significance of non-Candida fungal blood isolation in patients undergoing high-risk allogeneic hematopoietic stem cell transplantation (1993–2001). Cancer. 2004;100(11):2456–61.
308. Choi SM, Xie H, Campbell AP, Kuypers J, Leisenring W, Boudreault AA, et al. Influenza viral RNA detection in blood as a marker to predict disease severity in hematopoietic cell transplant recipients. J Infect Dis. 2012;206(12):1872–7.
309. El Chaer F, Shah DP, Chemaly RF. How I treat resistant cytomegalovirus infection in hematopoietic cell transplantation recipients. Blood. 2016;128(23):2624–36.
310. Chou S. Approach to drug-resistant cytomegalovirus in transplant recipients. Curr Opin Infect Dis. 2015;28(4):293–9.
311. Hakki M, Chou S. The biology of cytomegalovirus drug resistance. Curr Opin Infect Dis. 2011;24(6):605–11.
312. Iioka F, Sada R, Maesako Y, Nakamura F, Ohno H. Outbreak of pandemic 2009 influenza a/H1N1 infection in the hematology ward: fatal clinical outcome of hematopoietic stem cell transplant recipients and emergence of the H275Y neuraminidase mutation. Int J Hematol. 2012;96(3):364–9.
313. Renaud C, Pergam SA, Polyak C, Jain R, Kuypers J, Englund JA, et al. Early emergence of an H275Y mutation in a hematopoietic cell transplant recipient treated with intravenous peramivir. Transpl Infect Dis. 2010;12(6):513–7.
314. Koo S, Bryar JM, Baden LR, Marty FM. Prognostic features of galactomannan antigenemia in galactomannan-positive invasive aspergillosis. J Clin Microbiol. 2010;48(4):1255–60.
315. Bergeron A, Porcher R, Menotti J, Poirot JL, Chagnon K, Vekhoff A, et al. Prospective evaluation of clinical and biological markers to predict the outcome of invasive pulmonary aspergillosis in hematological patients. J Clin Microbiol. 2012;50(3):823–30.

Diagnosis of Systemic Fungal Diseases

48

Simon Frédéric Dufresne, Kieren A. Marr, and Shmuel Shoham

Introduction

Rapid and accurate diagnosis of invasive fungal infections (IFI) is critical to the care of solid organ transplant (SOT) and hematopoietic stem cell transplant (HSCT) recipients. Such infections are a by-product of immunosuppression and carry substantial morbidity and mortality. Improved diagnostic approaches and new and safer broad-spectrum antifungal agents have revolutionized treatment in these patients. This chapter will review the major diagnostic tools and their role in patients with suspected fungal infections. Diagnosis will be approached from the laboratory perspective, with an overview of methods used in clinical laboratories. Major organisms will then be presented separately, incorporating relevant clinical aspects that guide diagnostic approach.

Overview of Diagnostic Laboratory Methods in Clinical Mycology

General Principles

Until recently diagnosis centered upon detection of fungi from clinical samples using traditional staining and culture techniques, with nucleic acid and antibody-based assays playing a supportive role. The testing paradigm is shifting, with nonculture tests moving to the fore. Such assays are increasingly used as primary methods of diagnosis in a variety of invasive mycoses, including aspergillosis, candidiasis, cryptococcosis, and histoplasmosis [1–3]. Traditional and newer diagnostic approaches are complementary, and multiple tests are frequently employed simultaneously.

The major diagnostic modalities are (A) microscopic examination of biological specimens, including direct microscopy, cytopathology and histopathology; (B) culture followed by speciation using morphological, biochemical, and/or molecular methods and antifungal susceptibility testing; (C) serodiagnosis, antigen or antibody detection; and (D) nucleic acid amplification techniques (NAAT). The relative contributions of these methods for diagnosis of systemic fungal diseases are presented in Table 48.1.

Histopathology

Microscopic examination of thin-sectioned formalin-fixed paraffin-embedded tissue (histopathology) is generally sensitive and can provide definitive proof of infection when tissue invasion is seen. Major limitations are the requirement for an invasive procedure and the effort required for specimen preparation and processing. As for direct microscopy and cytopathology, unique morphological features can be used to differentiate hyalohyphomycosis (hyaline, septate, acute-angle branching hyphae), phaeohyphomycosis (darkly pigmented, septate hyphae), and mucormycosis (hyaline, non-septate, large ribbon-like, right-angle branching hyphae) and to identify *Cryptococcus neoformans/gattii*, *Pneumocystis jiroveci*, and the endemic fungi to the genus or species level. In addition, histopathology can demonstrate host responses, such as patterns of inflammation and tissue damage. For example, the asteroid bodies (Splendore-Hoeppli reaction) are associated with several fungal infections, including sporotrichosis [4].

S. F. Dufresne (✉)
University of Montreal, Maisonneuve-Rosemont Hospital, Department of Medicine, Division of Infectious Diseases and Clinical Microbiology, Montréal, QC, Canada
e-mail: sf.dufresne@umontreal.ca

K. A. Marr · S. Shoham
Johns Hopkins University School of Medicine, Department of Medicine, Division of Infectious Diseases, Baltimore, MD, USA
e-mail: kmarr4@jhmi.edu; sshoham1@jhmi.edu

A. Safdar (ed.), *Principles and Practice of Transplant Infectious Diseases*, https://doi.org/10.1007/978-1-4939-9034-4_48

Table 48.1 Relative contribution of different diagnostic modalities for detection of invasive fungi

						Host immune response	
Organisms	Histopathology	Direct microscopy/cytopathology	Culture	Antigen detection	NAAT	Humoral	Cellular
Aspergillus	++	++	++	+++	++	–	+
Other filamentous fungi[a]	++	++	++	–	+	–	+
Candida	+	++	+++	+	+	+	–
Cryptococcus	+	++	+++	+++	+	–	–
Pneumocystis	+	+++	–	++	++	–	–
Endemic	+++	++	+++	+++	+	++	–

–: not useful or available
+: rarely contributive; important limitations with regard to safety, availability, or performance (including lack of clinical data)
++: sometimes contributive; some limitations with regard to safety, availability, or performance
+++: often contributive; considered standard method for diagnosis
[a]Includes *Fusarium* species, *Scedosporium* species, *Mucorales*, dematiaceous fungi, and others

Modern histopathology relies on a combination of dyes with immunological and molecular techniques. Most fungi can be observed with hematoxylin-eosin (H&E), but specialized stains such as GMS and periodic acid-Schiff (PAS) are preferred and facilitate visualization of certain fungal structures. Certain stains are useful for specific fungi. For example, Giemsa is helpful for identifying *P. jiroveci* trophic forms, mucicarmine for *Cryptococcus* spp. (stains capsule), and Fontana-Masson for dematiaceous molds (stains melanin). When fungal structures are observed in tissue, formalin-fixed paraffin-embedded specimens can be analyzed further with immunohistochemistry [5] and in situ hybridization [6–8] to facilitate identification. Furthermore, DNA can be extracted from paraffin-embedded tissue, allowing nucleic acid amplification and sequencing [9–11]. This procedure may prove extremely useful when fungal elements are visualized in tissue, but concomitant culture is negative or not available.

Direct Microscopy and cytopathology

Microscopic examination of clinical samples is an extremely valuable tool. Despite lacking sensitivity, it is relatively simple, rapid, and reasonably specific. Visualization of fungal structures by direct microscopy serves three main purposes: 1) primary detection of a fungal pathogen in the sampled body site, 2) identification of the fungal pathogen based on morphological features (it reliably distinguishes major fungal groups such as yeasts, hyphomycetes and Mucorales, and even various species including Pneumocystis jirovecii, Coccidioides immitis/posadasii, Blastomyces dermatitidis and Paracoccidioidesbrasiliensis), and 3) interpretation of positive cultures, by helping determine whether growth from non-sterile specimens is clinically significant. Direct microscopy involves fresh specimens, which can be either directly mounted using saline alone (plain preparation), or stained with a dye that facilitates fungal visualization (with or without prior smear fixation). Common stains are the chitin-binding fluorescent dye calcofluor white (CFW), India ink, toluidine blue and immunofluorescent stains using P. jirovecii-directed antibodies. Cytopathology refers to examination of fixed free cells, usually obtained from liquid specimens such as bronchoalveolar lavage and pleural fluid. Solid tissues may also be sampled using fine-needle aspiration. Several stains are then used to visualize fungal elements, including Grocott-Gomori's methenamine silver (GMS) and Giemsa. Accurate microscopic examination relies on the experience and skills of the operator.

Culture

Culture is a cornerstone of fungal diagnostics. It is generally more sensitive than microscopy alone and facilitates fungal identification and antimicrobial susceptibility testing. Major limitations include suboptimal sensitivity, prolonged turnaround time, and biosafety issues. The significance of a positive culture depends upon the site from which the specimen was obtained, the organism isolated, and the clinical scenario. Growth from a normally sterile site is indicative of invasive infection. Isolation of certain pathogens (e.g., *Cryptococcus neoformans*, *C. gattii*, the endemic fungi) from any body site is virtually synonymous with disease. Conversely, recovery of *Candida*, *Aspergillus*, *Scedosporium*, *Mucorales*, and dematiaceous fungi from sites that are not normally sterile does not necessarily indicate infection and requires careful consideration of both the host and clinical context.

The initial steps involved in fungal culture are specimen collection and inoculation on media. Specimen quality is critical for optimal fungal recovery and to minimize contamination. Table 48.2 summarizes adequate specimens for recovery of different fungi.

Table 48.2 Adequate specimens for culture of pathogenic fungi

Organisms	Blood	Bone marrow	CSF	Respiratory secretions	Urine	Skin
Aspergillus	+	–	+	++	–	++
Other filamentous fungi	+[a]	–	+	++	–	++
Candida	+++	–	++	+	++	++
Cryptococcus	+++	–	+++	++	+++	++
Endemic	+++[b]	+++	++	++	++	++

CSF cerebrospinal fluid
–: virtually never recovered from this site
+: may be recovered, but generally considered colonization or contamination, or yield is very low
++: may be recovered only if site is clinically infected
+++: may be recovered in invasive disease and can be done even if site is not clinically infected or infection is not apparently disseminated
[a]Except for *Fusarium* spp. (+++)
[b]For *H. capsulatum*, using lysis-centrifugation methods or mycological media blood culture bottles for continuous monitoring blood culture systems; low yield for *Coccidioides* spp. (+)

In general, tissue and fluids are preferred over swabs. Volume should be ≥2 ml for cerebrospinal fluid and as much as possible for other sterile fluids. Most specimens should be transported to the laboratory as soon as possible, and some (e.g., corneal scrapings, prostatic fluids) require direct inoculation. Fungal culture media such as Sabouraud dextrose agar (SDA), inhibitory mold agar (IMA), brain heart infusion (BHI) agar, and malt extract agar usually contain antimicrobial agents to prevent overgrowth by competing microbiota [12–14]. Many fungi grow within a few days, but some, including *Histoplasma capsulatum*, may need up to 6 weeks. Few studies have directly compared the yield of different media in a clinical setting. IMA was recently shown to recover more isolates than SDA in cultures of specimens from various sites, including yeasts and hyaline hyphomycetes and *Mucorales* [15]. For recovery from the blood, modern aerobic bottles in continuously monitored blood culture systems are adequate for yeasts and *Fusarium*. Special lytic mycological media bottles or the lysis-centrifugation procedure may be preferable for fastidious fungi such as *Histoplasma capsulatum* [16, 17].

Once an isolate is grown, identification is typically achieved using standard procedures. Macroscopic and microscopic morphology remain the mainstay of mold identification. Several vegetable-based or poor media (e.g., potato dextrose agar, Czapek-Dox agar, tap water agar) enhance conidiation and/or pigment production of some fungi and facilitate identification. Simple biochemical tests are also commonly used for yeasts. Other techniques include thermotolerance, nutritional requirements, and conversion assays for thermally dimorphic fungi [12, 18]. Molecular methods, such as simple hybridization [19] and genomic DNA sequencing [20], are increasingly used, especially when a higher taxonomic resolution is needed. Matrix-assisted laser desorption ionization-time of flight (MALDI-TOF) mass spectrometry is emerging as a powerful tool for identification [21–24]. With the exception of some saprophytic filamentous fungi, identification should be made to the species level. Because many species have well established and predictable susceptibility patterns, identifying the species can have important prognostic and treatment implications.

Biosafety of laboratory personnel is a concern when culturing fungi, especially the thermally dimorphic fungi. Biosafety level 3 (BSL-3) practices, containment equipment, and appropriate facilities are required for handling sporulating mold-form cultures of *B. dermatitidis*, *C. immitis/posadasii*, and *H. capsulatum* [25]. *Coccidioides* poses a particular threat to laboratory workers [26]. This fungus can grow rapidly on bacterial primary isolation plates, and clinicians should alert the microbiology laboratory when infection with one of these organisms is suspected.

Antigen Detection

Assays that detect fungal antigens now assume an important role in the evaluation of patients with suspected invasive mycoses and are indispensible aids for diagnosing cryptococcosis, histoplasmosis, and aspergillosis. Their role in candidiasis, pneumocystosis, and other fungal infections is evolving. Favorable aspects of antigen detection assays include rapidity, ease of performance, and potential for diagnosing infections early in the disease course. Sensitivity and specificity remain a concern. Considerations of their pros and cons are important in developing preemptive strategies and point-of-care fungal antigen testing.

Various commercially available assays detect polysaccharides released from the cryptococcal capsule and cell walls of *Histoplasma* and *Aspergillus* and *Candida*. Suitable samples include serum, cerebrospinal fluid (CSF), bronchoalveolar lavage (BAL) fluid, urine, and other body fluids. Methodologies include latex agglutination (LA), enzyme immunoassays (EIA), and lateral-flow immunochromatographic assays (LFIA). Performance characteristics vary by kit, organism, specimen, clinical context, and cutoff used. A summary of commercially available assays is presented in Table 48.3.

(1-->3) β-D-glucan (BG) is an important fungal marker. This polysaccharide cell wall component is found in many fungi, with the notable exceptions of *Cryptococcus* spp. and the *Mucorales*, making it an almost "panfungal" marker.

Table 48.3 Commercial assays for detection of fungal antigens

Assay (manufacturer)	Method	Antigen detected	FDA-approved kit	Approved or most studied specimens (other specimens with clinical data)
Cryptococcus neoformans/gattii				
CALAS®: Cryptococcal antigen latex agglutination system (Meridian Bioscience Inc.)	LA	GXM	Yes	Serum, CSF
Latex-*Cryptococcus* antigen detection system (Immuno-Mycologics Inc.)	LA	GXM	Yes	Serum, CSF
Remel™ Cryptococcal antigen test kit (Thermo Fisher Scientific, Inc.)	LA	GXM	Yes	Serum, CSF
ALPHA cryptococcal antigen EIA (Immuno-Mycologics, Inc.)	ELISA	GXM	Yes	Serum, CSF
Premier® Cryptococcal antigen (Meridian Bioscience Inc.)	ELISA	GXM	Yes	Serum, CSF
CrAg lateral-flow assay (Immuno-Mycologics Inc.)	LFIA	GXM	Yes	Serum, plasma, CSF (urine)
Histoplasma capsulatum				
ALPHA *Histoplasma* antigen EIA (Immuno-Mycologics Inc.)	ELISA	N/A	Yes	Urine
MVista® *Histoplasma capsulatum* quantitative antigen EIA (MiraVista Diagnostics)	ELISA	GM	No	Urine, Serum (BALF, CSF)
Blastomyces dermatitidis				
MVista® *Blastomyces dermatitidis* quantitative antigen EIA (MiraVista Diagnostics)	ELISA	GM	No	Urine, serum (BALF, CSF)
Coccidioides immitis/posadasii				
MVista® *Coccidioides* quantitative antigen EIA (MiraVista Diagnostics)	ELISA	GM	No	Urine, serum (BALF, CSF)
Candida albicans				
Platelia™ *Candida* Ag Plus	ELISA	M	No	Serum
Aspergillus fumigatus				
Platelia™ *Aspergillus* Ag	ELISA	GM	Yes	Serum, BALF (urine, CSF)

LA latex agglutination, *ELISA* enzyme-linked immunosorbent assay, *LFIA* lateral-flow immunochromatographic assay, *GXM* glucuronoxylomannan, *GM* galactomannan, *M* mannan, *CSF* cerebrospinal fluid, *BALF* bronchoalveolar lavage fluid, normally sterile body fluids

Serum BG measurement has been mostly studied for diagnosis of aspergillosis, candidiasis, and, more recently, pneumocystosis. Four commercial assays are currently marketed, but only Fungitell® (Associates of Cape Cod) is available in the United States and Canada.

Nucleic Acid Amplification Techniques

NAATs are characterized by high analytical sensitivity and specificity and may allow reliable fungal identification directly from clinical samples, independently of culture. These assays are rapid (especially real-time PCR) and amenable to automation. However, discriminating infection from colonization or environmental contamination, especially when analyzing specimens from non-normally sterile sites, can be difficult. The reliability of these tests is impacted by fungal concentration, ease of DNA extraction (typically difficult for fungi), specimen type, and clinical scenario.

Most effort has focused on *Aspergillus* spp., *Candida* spp., and *Pneumocystis jirovecii*, but NAATs have been developed for most pathogenic fungi. Some target specific genera or species, while others are "panfungal," targeting universal sequences in the fungal genome [27]. Suitable samples include whole blood, serum, plasma, BALF, sputum, CSF, and tissue. Techniques include PCR, semi-nested PCR, nested PCR, PCR-ELISA, nucleic acid sequence-based amplification (NASBA), and real-time PCR. Novel technologies include PCR coupled with electrospray ionization mass spectrometry (PCR/ESI-MS) [28–30], PCR coupled with surface-enhanced Raman scattering (PCR-SERS) [31], and PCR with magnetic resonance [32].

For now, NAATs are not part of standard diagnostic definitions of IFI [33], although many experts advocate for their inclusion [34]. Many centers use "home-brewed" fungal NAATs, and standardization and reproducibility of the assays are areas of ongoing efforts. The recent development of commercial assays will likely pave the way to wider availability and routine use.

Host Response

Another approach to fungal diagnosis is by measurement of antifungal host responses. This includes serology for detection of specific antibodies (humoral immunity) and detection of specific cell-mediated immunity. Serological methods include immunoprecipitation, complement fixation (CF), immunodiffusion (ID), counterimmunoelectrophoresis (CIE), and EIA. Cell-mediated immunity can be tested in vivo or ex vivo, with hypersensitivity skin testing and enzyme-linked immunoblot (ELISPOT) assay, respectively. While providing useful information, limitations of host response assays are that they may lack sensitivity in immunocompromised patients and may not be able to differentiate from active, quiescent, or past infection. Clinically, serology is most commonly used for coccidioidomycosis and histoplasmosis, and the tests are generally performed at reference laboratories.

Diagnosis by Organisms

Aspergillus

Clinical Syndromes and Diagnostic Approach

Invasive aspergillosis (IA) is a disease of immunocompromised patients. At highest risk are patients with profound quantitative and/or qualitative neutrophil abnormalities. Major risk factors include hematological malignancies and their treatment, allogeneic hematopoietic stem cell transplantation (HSCT), receipt of corticosteroid-based therapy (e.g., solid organ transplant recipients and patients with graft-versus-host disease), advanced HIV, and chronic granulomatous disease. *Aspergillus fumigatus* is the leading species involved, followed by *A. flavus*, *A. niger*, and *A. terreus* [35–40].

The most common sites of infection are the respiratory tract and sinuses. However, almost any organ can be involved with hematogenous seeding and continuous spread or due to inoculation at non-respiratory sites (e.g., skin, ears). The most common presentations include airway and sinus disease, which may manifest as antibacterial-refractory undifferentiated fever in the setting of prolonged and profound neutropenia. Given the wide spectrum of clinical disease, IA is included in the differential diagnosis of many pathogenic processes in susceptible hosts [40, 41].

The typical diagnostic approach includes pulmonary imaging followed by microbiological testing. For example, an HSCT recipient with fever, neutropenia, and lung abnormalities on computed tomography (CT) scan may have respiratory samples evaluated by direct microscopy, culture, galactomannan antigen detection, and possibly NAAT while simultaneously having blood tested for circulating biomarkers (GM, BG, DNA). With regard to respiratory sample, fiber-optic bronchoscopy with BAL is generally helpful and safe [42]. In HSCT recipients, the procedure may have a higher diagnostic yield and improve outcome when performed early after presentation [43]. Transbronchial biopsies are riskier, thereby limiting their utility in HSCT recipients [44].

In some high-risk populations, a preemptive approach is favored. In this setting, surveillance assays are performed regularly and trigger antifungal treatment upon positivity. Among allogeneic HSCT recipients (along with other high-risk hematologic patients), this strategy reduces antifungal consumption without affecting survival [45–49]. A recent meta-analysis suggested that a combination of GM and NAATs provides optimal performance, and aspergillosis is extremely unlikely when both biomarkers are negative [50]. Importantly, surveillance GM and PCR testing is not recommended for patients receiving anti-mold prophylaxis, in which context the very low prevalence of IA leads to a poor positive predictive value [51, 52]. In lung transplant recipients, limited data suggest that a culture-based preemptive strategy may reduce the occurrence of IA [53].

Laboratory Detection

Visualization of fungal structures by microscopy provides rapid and definitive evidence of infection when the sample is obtained from a normally sterile site. When the source is from a non-sterile site (e.g., respiratory secretions), results should be interpreted more cautiously. *Aspergillus* species appear in vivo as narrow (3–6 μm), septate hyphae with dichotomous 45° branching. The hyphae are hyaline after staining and usually indistinguishable from other hyalohyphomycetes [18]. Conidia are not typically seen in vivo, except in lesions with air-tissue interface, and in infections caused by *A. terreus*, in which vegetative conidia (aleurioconidia) can be observed along the hyphae [54, 55].

Culture is an important diagnostic modality but may remain negative even with positive stains. This may be due to disruption of delicate fungal structures during acquisition, transport, and processing of the specimen prior to inoculation onto fungal media. Moreover, host-adapted hyphae growing in a microaerophilic environment may not be fit for usual laboratory conditions [56]. It is extremely rare to grow *Aspergillus* from blood cultures and such growth often represents a laboratory contaminant [57, 58]. *Aspergillus* isolates that do grow in culture can generally be identified further by simple phenotypic characteristics such as macroscopic and microscopic morphology (morphotyping) and thermotolerance. Occasionally, dysgonic isolates may grow as nonsporulating molds (i.e., sterile mycelium), which prevent identification through morphotyping. Such isolates may be mistaken as environmental contaminants or colonizers [59–61], but simple laboratory procedures can avoid such misidentification [62]. Some species (e.g., *A. fumigatus*, *A. terreus*, and *A. calidoustus*) are now recognized as complexes (sections) comprising groups of genetically and biologically distinct species [63], which may have differing susceptibility patterns and clinical presentations [64–67]. Species-level identification is best achieved by molecular methods (e.g., PCR-RFLP [68] and sequencing [69]), although thermotolerance at 50 °C allows definitive identification of *A. fumigatus* sensu stricto within the section Fumigati [70]. Internal transcribed spacer (ITS), beta-tubulin (*BenA*), and calmodulin (*CaM*) are standard gene targets for sequence-based identification.

Galactomannan (GM) testing has assumed an increasingly important role. This antigen is released by the growing *Aspergillus* hyphae and detected using the FDA-cleared double-sandwich ELISA Platelia™ *Aspergillus* Ag (Bio-Rad Laboratories Inc., Marnes-la-Coquette, France) [71–73]. An Optical Density Index (ODI) value of ≥0.5 is considered positive for serum [74]. With this cutoff, overall sensitivity and specificity for probable and proven IA are approximately 70–80% and 80–90%, respectively [75, 76], but vary according to clinical setting (diagnosis of active disease versus surveillance), use of concomitant anti-mold prophylaxis, number of tests performed, and patient population. Cross-reactivity can be seen with *Penicillium* spp., *Fusarium* spp., and *Histoplasma capsulatum* [77–80]. Treatment with piperacillin-tazobactam was a cause of false positivity [81–86], but this problem has almost disappeared [87–89]. GM can be used on a range of fluids including BALF, urine, and CSF [90]. When using an ODI cutoff of ≥0.5, the sensitivity and specificity of BALF GM are ~90% [91, 92], although some have reported much lower performances and GM alone cannot distinguish airway colonization from invasive disease [93]. Baseline GM indices and GM dynamics can be used as prognostic and treatment response markers [94, 95]. Assays targeting other antigens and using the lateral-flow technology are in development and could be useful as point-of-care tests [96–100].

Serum BG testing is another important diagnostic approach. The sensitivity and specificity of serum BG for aspergillosis are in the mid 70–80% range, although data from transplant recipient populations are very limited [101–105]. Of note, circulating BG is not specific for *Aspergillus* and false positives due to a range of non-fungal causes are not uncommon.

Tests of antifungal host immune responses have a limited role for diagnosis of IA. In immunocompromised hosts anti-*Aspergillus* antibody titers do not correlate well with invasive infection [35], but may be useful for identifying patients at higher risk for developing invasive infection following HSCT [106–108].

Multiple NAATs have been developed for *A. fumigatus* and are used at some centers. Earlier generation assays were largely "home brewed," lacked standardization, and exhibited variable performance characteristics [109–116]. Efforts at standardizing NAATs have been made [52, 117–120] and several commercially available assays have emerged. The LightCycler® Septi*Fast* (Roche Diagnostics) test detects 25 bacterial and fungal pathogens from whole blood samples, including *A. fumigatus*. Limited clinical data is available for hematological and solid organ transplant patients [121–124]. The MycAssay™ *Aspergillus* (Trinity Biotech) is a real-time PCR assay targeting the 18S rRNA gene and that evaluated for BALF, serum, and tissue samples [125–130]. The AsperGenius® (PathoNostics) is a multiplex real-time PCR assay detecting multiple *Aspergillus* species (*A. fumigatus*, *A. terreus*, and other *Aspergillus* species) along with major *cyp51a* mutations associated with azole resistance (TR34/L98H, T289A, and Y121F) and has been studied in both BALF and serum samples [34, 131–133]. The RenDx Fungiplex assay (Renishaw Diagnostics) uses the PCR-surface-enhanced Raman scattering (PCR-SERS) technology and detects four *Aspergillus* species (*A. fumigatus*, *A. flavus*, *A. niger*, and *A. terreus*) [31]. Finally, the MycoGENIE® *Aspergillus fumigatus* kit (Ademtech) is designed to detect *A. fumigatus* and the TR34/L98H mutation from various clinical samples (biopsies, respiratory tract samples, and sera), although no clinical performance data is available to this date. None of these assays have FDA clearance for use as in vitro diagnostics. Overall, clinical data on commercial *Aspergillus* NAATs remain scarce, but available studies have yielded encouraging results. Collectively, NAATs are thought to perform at least as well as the galactomannan antigen and many advocate for their inclusion within standard definitions [34].

Non-*Aspergillus* Opportunistic Molds

Clinical Syndromes and Diagnostic Approach

The *Mucorales*, *Fusarium*, *Scedosporium/Pseudallescheria*, and to a lesser extent the dematiaceous molds are the most important non-*Aspergillus* filamentous pathogens in organ transplant recipients [36, 37, 134, 135]. Infections may be limited to the lung or skin or involve multiple sites including the CNS, bones and joints, and the eyes [136]. They are usually included with *Aspergillus* species in differential diagnosis of relevant clinical syndromes, and the diagnostic approach is similar, albeit with less reliance on circulating biomarkers and more on traditional diagnostic methods.

Laboratory Detection

In stained specimens, the hyphae of *Mucorales* fungi appear as broad, ribbon-like, and twisted with rare septa and irregular branching. Dematiaceous fungi appear darker on H&E and generally show moniliform (bead-like) hyphae along with large vesicular swellings. The dematiaceous molds are highlighted by the melanin-specific Fontana-Masson stain. *Fusarium*, *Scedosporium*, and *Aspergillus* appear very similar on microscopy of stained tissue and are difficult to differentiate from each other (collectively referred to as hyalohyphomycetes) [18].

Tissue should not be homogenized aggressively (with a mechanical tissue homogenizer or using a mortar and pestle) prior to culturing, as this may reduce the organism's viability. This is particularly critical for *Mucorales*. *Mucorales* are inhibited by cycloheximide contained in some selective media. Malt extract agar may increase primary isolation of the *Mucorales* from clinical samples [12]. *Fusarium* and to a lesser extent *Scedosporium* species may grow in blood cultures [137]. Growth from a non-sterile site does not necessarily indicate infection and must be evaluated in the context of the clinical scenario and direct staining results [138]. Identification to the species level and susceptibility testing can be very helpful for many non-*Aspergillus* molds.

There is only a limited role for serologic and NAAT-based techniques in non-*Aspergillus* mold infections. With the exception of the *Mucorales*, serum BG may be detected in such infections. Some *Fusarium* antigens cross-react with the GM-EIA [78]. Detection of *Mucorales*-specific T cells has shown promise as an adjunct to diagnosis of mucormycosis [139]. Innovative NAATs, including panfungal assays, have been developed but are limited to specialized laboratories [27, 140]. There are currently no commercial NAAT assays targeting those pathogens.

Candida

Clinical Syndromes and Diagnostic Approach

Candida species are normal commensals of the gut, skin, and female genital tract. Clinical manifestations can range from benign superficial infections to life-threatening deep-seated disease. The most common species are *C. albicans*, *C. glabrata*, *C. krusei*, *C. parapsilosis*, and *C. tropicalis*. Manifestations of superficial infection include thrush, esophagitis, intertrigo, and vulvovaginitis. Invasive candidiasis (IC) occurs when *Candida* gain access to deeper tissues, usually from an enteric or cutaneous source, with possible hematogenous dissemination to distant organs such as the liver, spleen, kidneys, lungs, heart, eyes, and skin. Candidemia is the most recognized form of IC and occurs with or without clinical evidence of deep-seated candidiasis. Conversely, deep-seated candidiasis is often not associated with candidemia [141].

It the SOT population, IC is mostly seen as a typical nosocomial infection, related to postoperative care, occurring during the weeks following transplantation in non-neutropenic hosts. Infection of the allograft itself, or at the site of surgery, is often found with concomitant bacterial infection [37, 39]. Conversely, most IC episodes after HSCT arise during or shortly after neutropenia, and the gut is the main source [38, 142].

Laboratory Detection

Microscopic examination may be useful for diagnosis of IC. Suitable stains include Gram stain, CFW, GMS, and PAS. Microscopically, most *Candida* species appear as oval-shaped 3–6 μm budding yeast cells with pseudohyphae and hyphae when invading tissue. Distinctively, *C. glabrata* produce smaller blastoconidia (2–5 μm) and do not form hyphae [18]. Results from non-normally sterile sites need to be interpreted cautiously, and histopathology is critical for distinguishing invasive disease from colonization.

Growth from a sterile body site, including blood, remains the principal means for diagnosis. *Candida* spp. are non-fastidious, fast-growing organisms that can be recovered on most routine media. Traditionally, *Candida* spp. were best cultured from blood by using a lysis-centrifugation method [143–147], but continuous monitoring blood culture systems (mycological media bottles or regular aerobic bottles) are as effective [16, 148, 149]. Regardless of the method, blood cultures are relatively insensitive because many IC forms do not have circulating viable organisms (candidemia) [141]. For instance, only about 10% of patients with candida endophthalmitis or chronic disseminated candidiasis (also called hepatosplenic candidiasis) have positive blood cultures [150, 151].

Identification of *Candida* to the species level following growth on primary culture is important for invasive infection. Methods include microscopic morphology (germ tube test and Dalmau method), biochemical tests, chromogenic media, and peptide nucleic acid fluorescence in situ hybridization (PNA FISH) [152–154]. MALDI-TOF is routinely used in many laboratories [23, 155–157] and can be performed directly from positive blood culture bottles [158].

Nonculture-based techniques are important adjuncts. The most developed of these is serum BG measurement. Many fungi including *Candida* produce BG. A cutoff of 60–80 pg/ml suggests invasive disease. Sensitivity and specificity are typically in the ~80% range [102]. False-positive results may be seen in a variety of circumstances including severe burns, extensive gauze packing, various blood products, renal replacement therapy with cellulose containing membranes, and infection with

Pseudomonas aeruginosa [159–161]. Accuracy is highest with candidemia, as compared to other forms of invasive candidiasis. The role of serial BG to guide early antifungal therapy in high-risk patients is unclear. There is a paucity of data evaluating BG-based preemptive therapy in the transplant population [104]. Controlled studies in high-risk intensive care unit patients have failed to demonstrate benefits over prophylaxis or empiric strategies [162–164]. Other biomarkers include mannan antigen (Platelia™ *Candida* Ag Plus, Bio-Rad Laboratories), anti-mannan antibody (Platelia™ Candida Ab Plus, Bio-Rad Laboratories), and the *Candida albicans* germ tube antibody (CAGTA) (invasive candidiasis (CAGTA) VirClia® IgG Monotest, Vircell), but clinical data are limited and the assays are not commercialized in North America [165–171].

Numerous NAATs have been developed for detection of *Candida* spp. directly from clinical specimens [172]. Until recently, standardization and clinical data was insufficient to support widespread use. A few commercial NAAT assays are currently available. The LightCycler® Septi*Fast* (Roche Diagnostics) detects five different *Candida* species (*C. albicans*, *C. tropicalis*, *C. parapsilosis*, *C. krusei*, *and C. glabrata)*, while the RenDx Fungiplex assay (Renishaw Diagnostics) targets three additional species (*C. guilliermondii*, *C. lusitaniae*, and *C. dubliniensis*) [31], from blood samples. Neither is currently available in North America and the data from transplant recipients is scanty [31, 123, 173].

The T2Candida® Panel (T2 Biosystems) uses a novel approach for diagnosis of invasive candidiasis from whole blood samples. This FDA-cleared test uses the T2Dx® instrument to extract and amplify *Candida* DNA (internal transcribed spacer 2) and then detects it via agglomeration of supermagnetic particles (attached to species-specific probes) and T2 magnetic resonance (T2MR) measurement. This technology exhibits high analytical sensitivity with limit of detection of 1 CFU/mL for *C. tropicalis* and *C. krusei*, 2 CFU/mL for *C. albicans* and *C. glabrata*, and 3 CFU/mL for *C. parapsilosis* [32]. The assay has a specificity of 99.4%, sensitivity of 91.1%, and negative predictive value reaching 99.5% (in a population with 5% prevalence of candidemia) [174]. Because of this high negative predictive value, the assay may serve to limit antifungal therapy in a low-to-moderate risk population, especially if coupled with an antimicrobial stewardship program. The cost-effectiveness of the test remains unclear based on model-derived analyses and should be assessed in prospective comparative trials [175, 176].

Cryptococcus

Clinical Syndromes and Diagnostic Approach

Cryptococcosis is caused by the ubiquitous *Cryptococcus neoformans* (serotypes A, D, and AD) and the more geographically confined *C. gattii* (serotypes B and C). Both encompass multiple phylogenetically distinct species, and some propose renaming them as "*C. neoformans* species complex" and "*C. gattii* species complex" [177]. Cryptococcosis is a major problem in patients with advanced HIV/AIDS but also affects other immunocompromised hosts such as SOT recipients. It is rare in HSCT recipients [36, 38, 39, 135, 178–180]. Primary infection occurs in the lungs, but CNS and disseminated diseases are common [181]. Virtually any organ can become infected including the skin, eyes, lymph nodes, and prostate. The latter can serve as a sanctuary for this yeast.

It is important to maintain a high clinical suspicion for cryptococcosis in immunocompromised patients. CNS, pulmonary, cutaneous, and lymph node abnormalities in an appropriate host should raise the possibility of this infection. Sometimes subtle neuropsychiatric symptoms or fever alone may be the only clues. Therefore, cryptococcal antigen testing is frequently done in transplant patients when an infection is considered. When cryptococcal infection is confirmed at any site in a transplant recipient, investigation of the CNS is recommended [182, 183].

Laboratory Detection

Cryptococcus can be observed directly in infected tissue and body fluids, including CSF, lung tissue, lower respiratory secretions, skin, and urine. Histopathology is sometimes required and is most helpful for skin biopsies. In clinical specimens, microscopic examination reveals GMS-positive round to oval yeasts, with a single narrow-base budding. Size may vary significantly (2–20 um for regular cells; up to 50–100 um for Titan cells), even within a microscopic field. The organism can be visualized with GMS, H&E, and even Gram staining. The thick polysaccharide capsule is a major feature and can be visualized with mucicarmine dye (for FFPE tissue). Occasionally, acapsular strains are encountered. Fontana-Masson, which stains melanin, is useful in such situations [18]. Visualization of the yeast cells in CSF with the India ink preparation is rapid but lacks sensitivity, especially in non-HIV/AIDS patients in whom the organism burden is lower [184].

Growth in culture is an important part of the diagnostic evaluation. *Cryptococcus* spp. can grow on most primary isolation media in 36–72 h but sometimes require longer incubation. Blood, CSF, respiratory specimens, and urine [185, 186] are all appropriate materials for culture. Identification is straightforward using standard biochemical tests. Differentiating between *C. neoformans* and *C. gattii* may have important clinical and therapeutic implications. This can be achieved using L-canavanine glycine bromothymol blue (CGB) agar, MALDI-TOF, or molecular methods [187–192], but most clinical laboratories do not currently distinguish between the two species.

The importance of the capsular polysaccharide antigen (glucuronoxylomannan, GXM) for diagnosis cannot be overstated. It has been used for diagnosis of cryptococcosis for more than half a century [193]. Suitable fluids include serum, CSF, BALF, and urine. Various immunoassays (e.g., LA, ELISA, lateral flow) have been developed and commercialized for this purpose [194–200]. Pretreatment of serum samples with pronase improves sensitivity and specificity of the LA-based tests [201]. Cross-reactivity with *Trichosporon* has been reported, but this is uncommon [202]. Conversely, serum antigen may not be detected in primary pulmonary cryptococcosis [203, 204]. A next-generation lateral-flow immunoassay for point-of-care diagnosis is now available. This test can be applied to a range of specimens including CSF, serum, and urine and compares favorably to other assays [200, 205–207]. Probably because of the high performance of antigen detection, NAATs for *Cryptococcus* detection directly from clinical specimens contribute only marginally to the diagnostic arsenal [208, 209].

Pneumocystis

Clinical Syndromes and Diagnostic Approach

Pneumocystis jirovecii is a human-specific fungal pathogen that colonizes both immunocompetent and immunocompromised hosts. In patients with defects in cell-mediated immunity, mostly in the context of advanced HIV/AIDS or transplantation, it can cause severe pneumonia. Mortality is especially high among non-HIV-infected patients. Extrapulmonary sites are rarely involved (e.g., lymph nodes, liver, spleen, bone marrow) [210, 211]. When *Pneumocystis* pneumonia (PCP) is suspected, respiratory tract specimens (e.g., sputum, induced sputum, BALF, lung tissue) should be obtained for microbiological testing. Serum beta-D-glucan (BG) is increasingly used as a noninvasive diagnostic test for PCP.

Laboratory Detection

Pneumocystis jirovecii is not routinely cultivatable (achieved by one laboratory using a complex cellular culture system [212]); hence diagnosis is via culture-independent methods including microscopy, BG, and NAATs.

Definitive diagnosis is achieved by microscopic evidence of infection. In vivo, two different forms can be observed: cystic and trophic. This nomenclature is a relic of its former (obsolete) classification as a parasite. Giemsa stains the trophic form, while CFW, GMS, and toluidine blue are useful for visualization of the cyst form. The cysts are 4–7 μm and display one or two dark dots on their surface. The cysts have an oval (intact) or crescent (collapsed) shape and often form aggregates in a foamy substance [18]. Monoclonal antibodies are available in commercial kits for direct or indirect immunofluorescence [213–215]. The sensitivity of immunofluorescence-aided microscopy is superior to other stains [215, 216]. For microscopic methods, sensitivity of BALF is superior to that of less invasive specimens [216–221]. Generally, microscopy lacks sensitivity when compared to other methods. Immunofluorescence was reported to detect as few as a third of positive samples as determined by PCR [222]. However, as discussed below, some PCR-positive/microscopy-negative samples represent *Pneumocystis* colonization; sensitivity of microscopy for actual *Pneumocystis* pneumonia is estimated at 55–60% [223, 224]. This is particularly relevant for non-AIDS patients, in whom the fungal burden is generally lower [224, 225]. Consequently, in transplant recipients with suspected PCP, negative microscopic examination of BALF cannot rule out PCP.

Polysaccharide detection (BG) is an important adjunct for PCP diagnosis. BG serum levels correlate well with fungal burden [223, 226, 227]. Most studies have reported serum BG detection to be >90% sensitive [102, 228]. In contrast with microscopic methods, BG accuracy for PCP is not affected by HIV status [102, 228]. BG results must be interpreted with caution as the assay is not specific, but in the appropriate context, it is a good screening test, and a negative result is reassuring for absence of PCP.

Multiple NAATs using respiratory samples have been developed. Many are "in-house" assays, but several commercial kits are available, including the *Pneumocystis jirovecii* PCR kit (Bio-Evolution) [229–231], the AmpliSens® *Pneumocystis jirovecii* (*carinii*)-FRT PCR kit (InterLabService) [229], the PneumoGenius® (PathoNostics) [231], and the MycAssay™ *Pneumocystis* (Trinity Biotech) [126, 222, 229, 232]. The latter has been the most extensively studied. None are FDA-cleared. Most *P. jirovecii* NAATs are real-time PCR assays targeting the multicopy mitochondrial large subunit ribosomal RNA gene (mtLSU). The PneumoGenius® allows detection of two mutations in the dihydropteroate synthase (DHPS) domain of the FAS gene that confer resistance to sulfa drugs. As a general rule, PCR assays are extremely sensitive with a limit of detection 100 times lower than microscopic methods [233]. This difference is due to the methods' intrinsic analytical sensitivities and because NAATs detect both trophozoites and cysts, while microscopic methods are unreliable for trophozoites [233]. Sensitivity is virtually 100%, but the assay cannot clearly distinguish between infection and colonization with clinical false positivity ranging from 6% to 17% [126, 229, 232]. Efforts to establish a fungal load cutoff that would discriminate pneumonia from colonization have proved difficult [223, 230, 231, 234, 235]. Compared with microscopy, NAATs' sensitivity is more homogenous across different types of respiratory samples [229]. Serum DNA level correlates with pulmonary fungal burden [227], but is detectable only in high-burden infections and hence adds little to other diagnostic methods. NAAT testing can be applied to nasopharyngeal aspirates where sensitivity is slightly better than BALF microscopy, but less than BALF NAAT [236, 237].

Overall, microscopic methods suffer from a low sensitivity in transplant recipients, while NAATs are very sensitive but also detect colonization. Blood BG testing could offer the best trade-off between sensitivity and specificity and is noninvasive. NAAT performed on a noninvasive respiratory sample such as nasopharyngeal aspirate may also become a useful tool for PCP diagnosis, but more data is needed.

Geographically Limited/Endemic Fungi

Histoplasmosis

Clinical Syndromes and Diagnostic Approach

Histoplasma capsulatum is associated with a range of clinical manifestations including asymptomatic infection (most common), acute and chronic pulmonary histoplasmosis, and progressive disseminated histoplasmosis (PDH). Disease may be due to reactivation or new infection [238]. Immunocompromised patients, such as SOT recipients, are particularly prone to PDH, which can take on a chronic-subacute to fulminant course [239]. Most infections become clinically apparent within 12–18 months after transplantation but may sometimes present much later [240, 241]. Typical sites of infection are organs of the reticuloendothelial system (RES) and the lungs. Other sites include the gastrointestinal tract (mucosa), genitourinary tract, adrenal glands, and skin. CNS disease is uncommon, even with disseminated infection [239]. Because of its protean manifestations, histoplasmosis is often part of the differential diagnosis of many clinical syndromes in SOT recipients, including various respiratory, hepatic, and febrile illnesses. When PDH is suspected in a transplant recipient, noninvasive assays such as antigen detection and blood culture are usually performed first. Additionally, samples from almost any clinically infected sites can be used for histopathology, culture, and/or antigen detection.

Laboratory Detection

Blood, bone marrow, lymph nodes, BALF, lung tissue, and occasionally CSF are important sources of specimens for staining and culture. On microscopy, the organism appears as small (2–4 μm) yeast cells with single narrow-base budding and a pseudocapsule. *Histoplasma capsulatum* var. *duboisii* is much larger (8–15 μm) with thick-walled budding. Yeast forms can be visualized extracellularly or within monocytes [18]. The latter can sometimes be seen in peripheral blood smear or a buffy coat preparation with Wright or Giemsa staining [242].

H. capsulatum can be grown using rich media such as brain-heart infusion (BHI) agar and incubated for at least 4 weeks [14]. Recovery in blood cultures is facilitated when a lysis-centrifugation system or an automated system with mycological blood culture bottles is used [16, 17, 148, 149]. In ambient temperature *H. capsulatum* grows as a mold on solid media. Once grown in this form, any manipulation of the fungus should be done in strict adherence to biosafety requirements [25]. Confirmation of *H. capsulatum* can be attained by the exoantigens method and by nucleic acid probes (AccuProbe® *Histoplasma capsulatum* Culture Identification Test, Gen-Probe®) [243] and PCR followed by sequencing [244].

Antigen testing is important for evaluation of disseminated histoplasmosis. For histoplasmosis after solid organ transplantation, antigenuria is the most common positive test (93% of cases in one study) [245]. The *Histoplasma* polysaccharide antigen (HPA), which is a galactomannan [246], is found in serum, urine, and BALF during infection. Detection of HPA is achieved mainly via the MVista® *Histoplasma capsulatum* quantitative antigen EIA (MiraVista Diagnostics, MVD). This test was first developed as a radioimmunoassay [247] and subsequently evolved over four generations of ELISAs [246, 248–250]. In certain circumstances, sensitivity can exceed 90% and tends to be highest with disseminated disease and when the test is performed on urine [239, 245, 246, 251–253]. Addition of EDTA-heat pretreatment for dissociation of immune complexes has further improved sensitivity [250]. The level of antigenuria correlates with severity of disease [254], and low-positive HPA results should be interpreted carefully considering the host, clinical presentation, and complementary tests [255–257]. Detection of HPA on BALF may complement antigenemia and antigenuria [258]. Cross-reactivity may be seen with other endemic mycoses, particularly blastomycosis and paracoccidioidomycosis [246]. The ALPHA *Histoplasma* antigen EIA (Immuno-Mycologics) was approved by the FDA in 2011 and remains the only commercially available kit for HPA detection. Similar to the MVD test, it is a sandwich ELISA utilizing polyclonal rabbit antibodies. This assay may be less sensitive than the MVD test, albeit proper clinical evaluation and comparison by independent laboratories have not been performed [259–265]. More sensitive second-generation reagents, based on a monoclonal antibody, are still less sensitive than the MVD test and are neither commercially available nor FDA-cleared at this time [266–268]. Of note, the HPA can be detected by the Platelia™ *Aspergillus* EIA, but at a lower magnitude [80, 269]. This can be particularly useful in areas where specific HPA assays are unavailable [79, 270]. While BG may be detectable during histoplasmosis [271, 272], it is not routinely used in this setting.

Serology is mainly performed using either CF or ID [1, 238]. Generally, serology lacks both sensitivity and specificity. Low sensitivity is particularly problematic in immunocompromised hosts. The two tests are complementary with ID being less sensitive, but more specific than CF. Combining both techniques may increase sensitivity. In CF, antigen extracts from the yeast and mold phases of the organism are used separately (the culture filtrate of the mold phase is histoplasmin). Results are reported as antibody titers against each of the antigen preparations. A titer ≥1:32 is suggestive of infection (recent of remote), while a fourfold increase in titers between acute and convalescent sera is diagnostic for recent infection. ID is a qualitative method that detects two antibodies, the H- and M-precipitins, which bind the H and M antigens, respectively (both are glycoproteins contained in histoplasmin). In the ID test an M band in seen in both acute and chronic forms, whereas the H band is encountered less commonly, usually in chronic or severe infections. The M band may persist for years even after complete resolution of the infection. Serology is best for mild-to-moderate acute pulmonary histoplasmosis, chronic pulmonary histoplasmosis, pericarditis, and acute rheumatologic forms. It is less useful for progressive disseminated histoplasmosis [238].

Several in-house NAATs have been developed for detection of *H. capsulatum* from clinical samples [209, 273–278], but their use remains marginal.

Coccidioidomycosis

Clinical Syndromes and Diagnostic Approach

Coccidioidomycosis is caused by *C. immitis* and *C. posadasii*. The majority of infections are either asymptomatic or mild and self-limited. The lungs are the most commonly affected organs. Disseminated disease can involve extrapulmonary sites including bones, joints, skin, and CNS [279]. Organ transplant recipients are at increased risk for more severe and disseminated disease [280]. Microbial investigation for coccidioidomycosis can be undertaken in the context of compatible clinical disease or as part of pre-immunosuppression serology-based preemptive strategy [281, 282].

Laboratory Detection

Suitable samples for testing include respiratory secretions, CSF, and material from almost any site of infection (e.g., bones, joints, skin, bone marrow, and urine). On microscopy, spherules that range from 10 to 100 μm and typically contain 2–5 μm endoconidia (endospores) can be seen [18]. Visualization of spherules filled with endoconidia is diagnostic, while empty spherules are strongly suggestive of coccidioidomycosis [283]. Endoconidia-containing spherules may resemble *Prototheca* or *Rhinosporidium* sporangia, but size helps distinguish between those organisms. Endoconidia can also be seen alone, in which case they may be confused with *Histoplasma*, *Cryptococcus*, or *Candida* yeast cells. Tissue preparations, stained with fungi-specific dyes (e.g., CFW, GMS, PAS), facilitate detection of the fungal structures.

Coccidioides grows well on a variety of fungal and bacterial media (e.g., sheep blood agar and BCYE) [283]. The incubation period for initial growth is 3–5 days (range 2–16 days), at which point another ~10 days are needed for the colonies to reach maturity. Yield from CSF is poor but can be improved with a large volume sample (>10 mL) [284]. Growth in blood culture is uncommon and more likely to be detected with lysis-centrifugation and the continuously monitored blood culture systems [285, 286]. In culture, *Coccidioides* grows as a filamentous fungus with arthroconidia, which appear as alternating barrel-shaped structures and are highly infectious. Because this appearance can be mistaken for the nonpathogenic environmental mold *Malbranchea*, at least one confirmatory test is required for definitive identification [18]. This is usually accomplished with the exoantigen assay, DNA-rRNA hybridization using commercial probes (AccuProbe® *Coccidioides immitis* Culture Identification Test, Gen-Probe®) [19], or with in-house PCR-based methods [287]. Older confirmatory tests such as the conversion assay (to yeast form) and animal inoculation for in vivo production of spherules are too cumbersome for widespread use. Because the arthroconidia are highly infectious, any manipulation of suspected or confirmed isolates should be done in strict adherence to biosafety regulations [25, 288].

Detection of specific anti-*Coccidioides* antibodies is helpful for diagnosis. Suitable specimens include serum and CSF. The traditional methods are tube precipitation and complement fixation. The former detects mainly an IgM antibody directed against a heat-stable antigen, often referred to as "TP" antibody or "precipitin" and "TP" antigen, respectively. The latter involves predominantly an IgG antibody specific to a heat-labile antigen, respectively, called "CF" antibody and "CF" or "F" antigen [1, 283, 289]. Both assays have been adapted to the immunodiffusion format. Because they could detect the same antibodies as TP and CF, they were named "immunodiffusion TP" (IDTP) and "immunodiffusion CF" (IDCF), a nomenclature that might be confusing [289]. These assays use heated or unheated coccidioidin (mycelial-phase broth culture filtrate) as antigen, although purified or recombinant antigens have also been studied [1]. EIAs detecting both IgM and IgG have been developed for serum and CSF [290–294]. The Premier® *Coccidioides* EIA test has been the most extensively studied. The CF assay is quantitative (titers), while ID and EIA are qualitative or semiquantitative. TP antibody (IgM) is detected early during acute infection and disappears after a few months, while the CF antibody (IgG) appears later and lasts for a longer time. IgM antibody may persist in chronic pulmonary forms, while IgG titers correlate with the extent of disease. As seen for *Histoplasma* serology, traditional methods (CF and ID) may lack sensitivity in immunocompromised hosts [289]. However, they are considered highly specific [293]. EIA is considered more sensitive but less specific than traditional methods (especially for IgM); hence many still recommend confirmation of EIA-positive results with ID or CF [283, 284]. From a limited number of cases, sen-

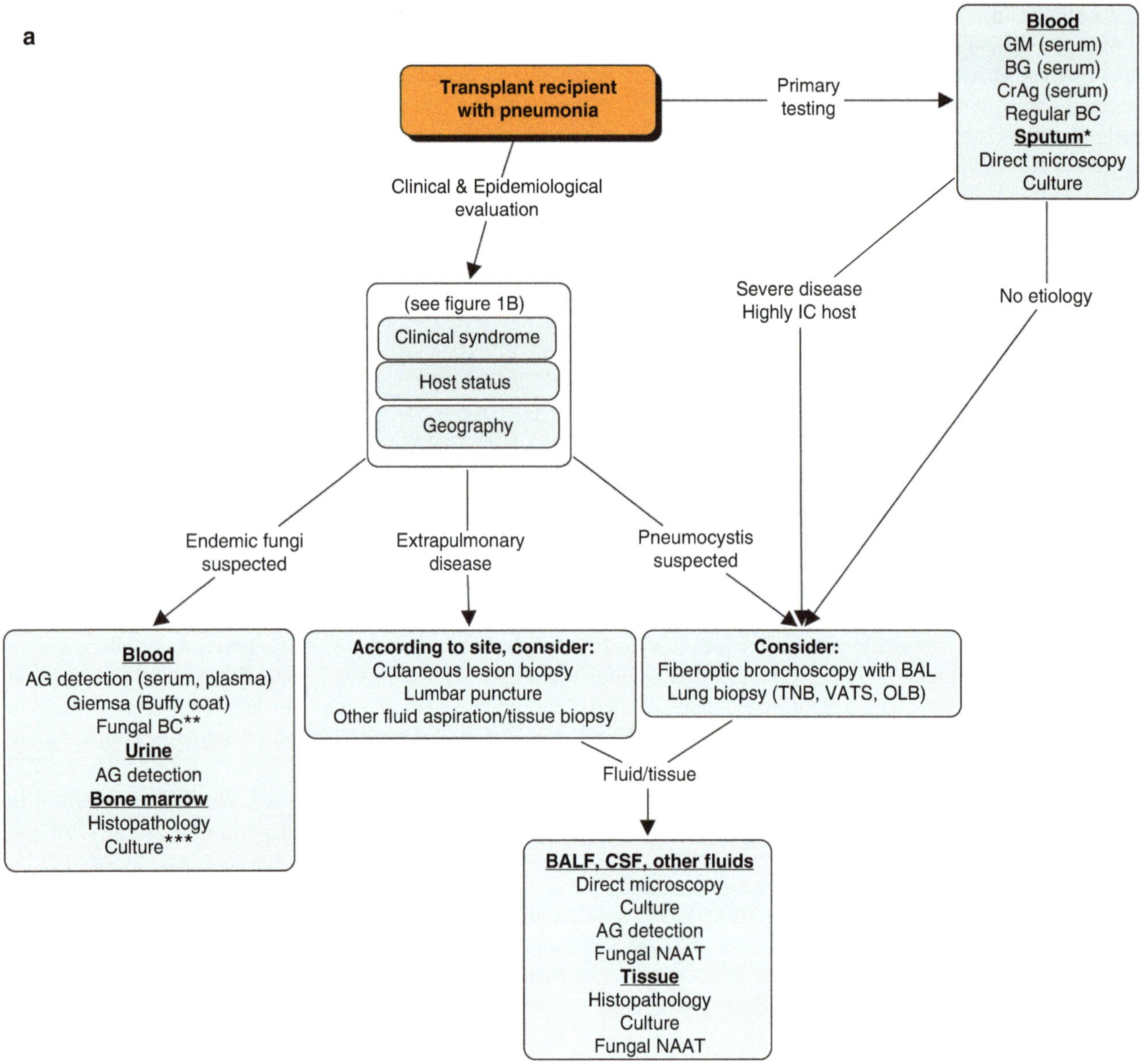

Fig. 48.1 (**a**) Diagnostic approach to suspected fungal pneumonia in transplant recipients. *Only if productive cough. **Mycological media bottles for continuous monitoring systems or lysis-centrifugation method. ***Using the same mycological media bottles as for blood. Legends: GM = galactomannane (Aspergillus); BG = beta-D-glucan; CrAg = cryptococcal antigen; BC = blood culture; IC = immunocompromised; AG = antigen; BALF = bronchoalveolar lavage fluid; TNB = transthoracic needle biopsy; VATS = video-assisted thoracoscopy; OLB = open lung biopsy; NAAT = nucleic acid amplification test. (**b**) Clinical and epidemiological clues for etiology of fungal pneumonia[a]. [a]List not exhaustive. *Includes organ donor origin for SOT recipients. Legend: BMT = bone marrow transplant; SOT = solid organ transplant; RES = reticuloendothelial system; CNS = central nervous system

sitivity of the recently developed MVista® *Coccidioides* Antibody IgG IgM EIA was reported to be unaffected by the immune status of the host [294].

Antigen and NAAT assays for *Coccidioides* are in various stages of development. These include a *Coccidioides* antigen that may be detected in serum or urine, which showed a sensitivity of 50–70% in severe disease [295, 296]. PCR-based methods for detection of *Coccidioides* DNA directly from clinical samples have also been described, but more work is needed before these can be widely used in clinical practice [297–299].

In Practice: The Clinician Perspective

From the practitioner standpoint, clinical presentation usually drives investigation, and hence a syndromic approach prevails. Figure 48.1 illustrates a stepwise diagnostic process for the investigation of fungal etiologies in a transplant recipient presenting with pulmonary infiltrates, a very common encounter in this population. This schematic representation is not meant as a formal guideline, but as an example of how different diagnostic tools might be used in a particular clinical context.

b

Clinical syndrome			
RES	**CNS**	**Skin**	**Diffuse lung infiltrate**
Histoplasma	*Cryptococcus* *Aspergillus* *Coccidioides*	*Fusarium, Aspergillus* *Blastomyces, Histoplasma* *Cryptococcus*	*Pneumocystis* *Histoplasma, Blastomyces*

Host		
BMT (early)	**BMT (late)**	**SOT**
Aspergillus Other molds (*Fusarium*)	*Aspergillus* Other molds (*Mucorales*) *Pneumocystis*	*Aspergillus* *Other molds* *Crytococcus* *Endemic fungi*

Geography*		
Southwest	**Ohio & Mississipi River Valleys**	**Pacific Northwest**
Coccidioides	*Histoplasma* *Blastomyces*	*Cryptococcus gattii*

Fig. 48.1 (continued)

Conclusion

The epidemiology of fungal infections has changed rapidly over the last decades, an evolution largely driven by advances in transplantation. In response, the growing threat posed by fungi has led to a dramatic improvement in the antifungal arsenal. Equally important has been the ongoing development of powerful tools that facilitate early and accurate diagnosis of fungal infections.

While tremendous progress has been made with regard to assay technology and analytical performance, major challenges remain. Widespread use of promising diagnostic tests has been limited by the complexity of the assays, costs related to infrastructure and reagents, and lack of standardization. Therefore, important future avenues in assay development include further advances in point-of-care technologies and automation, as well as commercialization. Finally, assays are commonly compared with one another using banked samples, but there is relative paucity of prospective data defining real clinical performance and usefulness. Further clinical evaluation of assays is needed, and this will be eased by standardization and accessibility, essential attributes for conducting large multicenter efforts.

Acknowledgments This work was partly supported by the National Institute of Health grant K24 (AI085118, to K.A.M.).

References

1. Yeo SF, Wong B. Current status of nonculture methods for diagnosis of invasive fungal infections. Clin Microbiol Rev 2002;15(3):465–84.
2. Wheat LJ. Antigen detection, serology, and molecular diagnosis of invasive mycoses in the immunocompromised host. Transpl Infect Dis. 2006;8(3):128–39.
3. Lau A, Chen S, Sleiman S, Sorrell T. Current status and future perspectives on molecular and serological methods in diagnostic mycology. Future Microbiol. 2009;4(9):1185–222.
4. Hussein MR. Mucocutaneous Splendore-Hoeppli phenomenon. J Cutan Pathol. 2008;35(11):979–88.
5. Schuetz AN, Cohen C. Aspergillus immunohistochemistry of culture-proven fungal tissue isolates shows high cross-reactivity. Appl Immunohistochem Mol Morphol. 2009;17(6):524–9.
6. Kobayashi M, Urata T, Ikezoe T, Hakoda E, Uemura Y, Sonobe H, et al. Simple detection of the 5S ribosomal RNA of pneumocystis carinii using in situ hybridisation. J Clin Pathol. 1996;49(9):712–6.
7. Kobayashi M, Sonobe H, Ikezoe T, Hakoda E, Ohtsuki Y, Taguchi H. In situ detection of aspergillus 18S ribosomal RNA in invasive pulmonary aspergillosis. Intern Med. 1999;38(7):563–9.
8. Rickerts V, Khot PD, Myerson D, Ko DL, Lambrecht E, Fredricks DN. Comparison of quantitative real time PCR with sequencing and ribosomal RNA-FISH for the identification of fungi in formalin fixed, paraffin-embedded tissue specimens. BMC Infect Dis. 2011;11:202.
9. Munoz-Cadavid C, Rudd S, Zaki SR, Patel M, Moser SA, Brandt ME, et al. Improving molecular detection of fungal DNA in formalin-fixed paraffin-embedded tissues: comparison of five tissue DNA extraction methods using panfungal PCR. J Clin Microbiol. 2010;48(6):2147–53.

10. Salehi E, Hedayati MT, Zoll J, Rafati H, Ghasemi M, Doroudinia A, et al. Discrimination of aspergillosis, mucormycosis, fusariosis, and scedosporiosis in formalin-fixed paraffin-embedded tissue specimens by use of multiple real-time quantitative PCR assays. J Clin Microbiol. 2016;54(11):2798–803.
11. Rickerts V. Identification of fungal pathogens in formalin-fixed, paraffin-embedded tissue samples by molecular methods. Fungal Biol. 2016;120(2):279–87.
12. Shea YR, Witebsky FG, Walsh TJ. Specimen selection, collection and transport. In: Hazen KC, Howell SA, Garcia LS, editors. Mycology and antifungal susceptibility testing, clinical microbiology procedures handbook. Volume 2. Washington, DC: ASM Press; 2010.
13. LaRocco M. Processing specimens for fungal cultures. In: Hazen KC, Howell SA, Garcia LS, editors. Mycology and antifungal susceptibility testing, clinical microbiology procedures handbook. Volume 2. Washington, DC: ASM Press; 2010.
14. CLSI. Principles and procedures for detection of fungi in clinical specimens -direct examination and culture; approved guidelines. CLSI Document M54-A. Wayne, PA: Clinical and Laboratory Standards Institute 2012.
15. Scognamiglio T, Zinchuk R, Gumpeni P, Larone DH. Comparison of inhibitory mold agar to Sabouraud dextrose agar as a primary medium for isolation of fungi. J Clin Microbiol. 2010;48(5):1924–5.
16. Cockerill FR 3rd, Reed GS, Hughes JG, Torgerson CA, Vetter EA, Harmsen WS, et al. Clinical comparison of BACTEC 9240 plus aerobic/F resin bottles and the isolator aerobic culture system for detection of bloodstream infections. J Clin Microbiol. 1997;35(6):1469–72.
17. Waite RT, Woods GL. Evaluation of BACTEC MYCO/F lytic medium for recovery of mycobacteria and fungi from blood. J Clin Microbiol. 1998;36(5):1176–9.
18. Larone DH. Medically important fungi. A guide to identification. Fifth ed. Washington, DC: ASM Press; 2011.
19. Padhye AA, Smith G, Standard PG, McLaughlin D, Kaufman L. Comparative evaluation of chemiluminescent DNA probe assays and exoantigen tests for rapid identification of Blastomyces dermatitidis and Coccidioides immitis. J Clin Microbiol. 1994;32(4):867–70.
20. Balajee SA, Borman AM, Brandt ME, Cano J, Cuenca-Estrella M, Dannaoui E, et al. Sequence-based identification of aspergillus, fusarium, and mucorales species in the clinical mycology laboratory: where are we and where should we go from here? J Clin Microbiol. 2009;47(4):877–84.
21. Sanguinetti M, Posteraro B. Identification of molds by matrix-assisted laser desorption ionizationt-time of flight mass spectrometry. J Clin Microbiol. 2017;55(2):369–79.
22. Cassagne C, Ranque S, Normand AC, Fourquet P, Thiebault S, Planard C, et al. Mould routine identification in the clinical laboratory by matrix-assisted laser desorption ionization time-of-flight mass spectrometry. PLoS One. 2011;6(12):e28425.
23. Buchan BW, Ledeboer NA. Advances in the identification of clinical yeast isolates using matrix-assisted laser desorption ionization-time of flight mass spectrometry. J Clin Microbiol. 2013;51:1359–66.
24. Posteraro B, Efremov L, Leoncini E, Amore R, Posteraro P, Ricciardi W, et al. Are the conventional commercial yeast identification methods still helpful in the era of new clinical microbiology diagnostics? A meta-analysis of their accuracy. J Clin Microbiol. 2015;53(8):2439–50.
25. Biosafety in Microbiological and Biomedical Laboratories, 5th Edition. U.S. Department of Health and Human Services, Public Health Service, Center for Disease Control and Prevention, National Institutes of Health; HHS Publication No. (CDC) 21-1112; Revised December 2009.
26. Singh K. Laboratory-acquired infections. Clin Infect Dis. 2009;49(1):142–7.
27. Van Burik JA, Myerson D, Schreckhise RW, Bowden RA. Panfungal PCR assay for detection of fungal infection in human blood specimens. J Clin Microbiol. 1998;36(5):1169–75.
28. Alanio A, Garcia-Hermoso D, Mercier-Delarue S, Lanternier F, Gits-Muselli M, Menotti J, et al. Molecular identification of Mucorales in human tissues: contribution of PCR electrospray-ionization mass spectrometry. Clin Microbiol Infect. 2015;21(6):594.e1–5.
29. Massire C, Buelow DR, Zhang SX, Lovari R, Matthews HE, Toleno DM, et al. PCR followed by electrospray ionization mass spectrometry for broad-range identification of fungal pathogens. J Clin Microbiol. 2013;51(3):959–66.
30. Shin JH, Ranken R, Sefers SE, Lovari R, Quinn CD, Meng S, et al. Detection, identification, and distribution of fungi in bronchoalveolar lavage specimens by use of multilocus PCR coupled with electrospray ionization/mass spectrometry. J Clin Microbiol. 2013;51(1):136–41.
31. White PL, Hibbitts SJ, Perry MD, Green J, Stirling E, Woodford L, et al. Evaluation of a commercially developed semiautomated PCR-surface-enhanced raman scattering assay for diagnosis of invasive fungal disease. J Clin Microbiol. 2014;52(10):3536–43.
32. Neely LA, Audeh M, Phung NA, Min M, Suchocki A, Plourde D, et al. T2 magnetic resonance enables nanoparticle-mediated rapid detection of candidemia in whole blood. Sci Transl Med. 2013;5(182):182ra54.
33. De Pauw B, Walsh TJ, Donnelly JP, Stevens DA, Edwards JE, Calandra T, et al. Revised definitions of invasive fungal disease from the European Organization for Research and Treatment of Cancer/Invasive Fungal Infections Cooperative Group and the National Institute of Allergy and Infectious Diseases Mycoses Study Group (EORTC/MSG) Consensus Group. Clin Infect Dis. 2008;46(12):1813–21.
34. White PL, Wingard JR, Bretagne S, Loffler J, Patterson TF, Slavin MA, et al. Aspergillus polymerase chain reaction: systematic review of evidence for clinical use in comparison with antigen testing. Clin Infect Dis. 2015;61(8):1293–303.
35. Latge JP. Aspergillus fumigatus and aspergillosis. Clin Microbiol Rev. 1999;12(2):310–50.
36. Neofytos D, Horn D, Anaissie E, Steinbach W, Olyaei A, Fishman J, et al. Epidemiology and outcome of invasive fungal infection in adult hematopoietic stem cell transplant recipients: analysis of Multicenter Prospective Antifungal Therapy (PATH) Alliance registry. Clin Infect Dis. 2009;48(3):265–73.
37. Neofytos D, Fishman JA, Horn D, Anaissie E, Chang CH, Olyaei A, et al. Epidemiology and outcome of invasive fungal infections in solid organ transplant recipients. Transpl Infect Dis. 2010;12(3):220–9.
38. Kontoyiannis DP, Marr KA, Park BJ, Alexander BD, Anaissie EJ, Walsh TJ, et al. Prospective surveillance for invasive fungal infections in hematopoietic stem cell transplant recipients, 2001-2006: overview of the Transplant-Associated Infection Surveillance Network (TRANSNET) Database. Clin Infect Dis. 2010;50(8):1091–100.
39. Pappas PG, Alexander BD, Andes DR, Hadley S, Kauffman CA, Freifeld A, et al. Invasive fungal infections among organ transplant recipients: results of the Transplant-Associated Infection Surveillance Network (TRANSNET). Clin Infect Dis. 2010;50(8):1101–11.
40. Steinbach WJ, Marr KA, Anaissie EJ, Azie N, Quan SP, Meier-Kriesche HU, et al. Clinical epidemiology of 960 patients with invasive aspergillosis from the PATH Alliance registry. J Infect. 2012;65(5):453–64.
41. Hope WW, Walsh TJ, Denning DW. The invasive and saprophytic syndromes due to aspergillus spp. Med Mycol. 2005;43(Suppl 1):S207–38.

42. Forslow U, Remberger M, Nordlander A, Mattsson J. The clinical importance of bronchoalveolar lavage in allogeneic SCT patients with pneumonia. Bone Marrow Transplant. 2010;45(5):945–50.
43. Shannon VR, Andersson BS, Lei X, Champlin RE, Kontoyiannis DP. Utility of early versus late fiberoptic bronchoscopy in the evaluation of new pulmonary infiltrates following hematopoietic stem cell transplantation. Bone Marrow Transplant. 2010;45(4):647–55.
44. Hofmeister CC, Czerlanis C, Forsythe S, Stiff PJ. Retrospective utility of bronchoscopy after hematopoietic stem cell transplant. Bone Marrow Transplant. 2006;38(10):693–8.
45. Maertens J, Theunissen K, Verhoef G, Verschakelen J, Lagrou K, Verbeken E, et al. Galactomannan and computed tomography-based preemptive antifungal therapy in neutropenic patients at high risk for invasive fungal infection: a prospective feasibility study. Clin Infect Dis. 2005;41(9):1242–50.
46. Hebart H, Klingspor L, Klingebiel T, Loeffler J, Tollemar J, Ljungman P, et al. A prospective randomized controlled trial comparing PCR-based and empirical treatment with liposomal amphotericin B in patients after allo-SCT. Bone Marrow Transplant. 2009;43(7):553–61.
47. Cordonnier C, Pautas C, Maury S, Vekhoff A, Farhat H, Suarez F, et al. Empirical versus preemptive antifungal therapy for high-risk, febrile, neutropenic patients: a randomized, controlled trial. Clin Infect Dis. 2009;48(8):1042–51.
48. Tan BH, Low JG, Chlebicka NL, Kurup A, Cheah FK, Lin RT, et al. Galactomannan-guided preemptive vs. empirical antifungals in the persistently febrile neutropenic patient: a prospective randomized study. Int J Infect Dis. 2011;15(5):e350–6.
49. Aguado JM, Vazquez L, Fernandez-Ruiz M, Villaescusa T, Ruiz-Camps I, Barba P, et al. Serum galactomannan versus a combination of galactomannan and polymerase chain reaction-based aspergillus DNA detection for early therapy of invasive aspergillosis in high-risk hematological patients: a randomized controlled trial. Clin Infect Dis. 2015;60(3):405–14.
50. Arvanitis M, Anagnostou T, Mylonakis E. Galactomannan and polymerase chain reaction-based screening for invasive aspergillosis among high-risk hematology patients: a diagnostic meta-analysis. Clin Infect Dis. 2015;61(8):1263–72.
51. Duarte RF, Sanchez-Ortega I, Cuesta I, Arnan M, Patino B, Fernandez de Sevilla A, et al. Serum galactomannan-based early detection of invasive aspergillosis in hematology patients receiving effective anti-mold prophylaxis. Clin Infect Dis. 2014;59(12):1696–702.
52. Springer J, Lackner M, Nachbaur D, Girschikofsky M, Risslegger B, Mutschlechner W, et al. Prospective multicentre PCR-based aspergillus DNA screening in high-risk patients with and without primary antifungal mould prophylaxis. Clin Microbiol Infect. 2016;22(1):80–6.
53. Hosseini-Moghaddam SM, Chaparro C, Luong ML, Azad S, Singer LG, Mazzulli T, et al. The effectiveness of culture-directed preemptive anti-aspergillus treatment in lung transplant recipients at one year after transplant. Transplantation. 2015;99(11):2387–93.
54. Seligsohn R, Rippon JW, Lerner SA. Aspergillus terreus osteomyelitis. Arch Intern Med. 1977;137(7):918–20.
55. Walsh TJ, Petraitis V, Petraitiene R, Field-Ridley A, Sutton D, Ghannoum M, et al. Experimental pulmonary aspergillosis due to aspergillus terreus: pathogenesis and treatment of an emerging fungal pathogen resistant to amphotericin B. J Infect Dis. 2003;188(2):305–19.
56. Tarrand JJ, Han XY, Kontoyiannis DP, May GS. Aspergillus hyphae in infected tissue: evidence of physiologic adaptation and effect on culture recovery. J Clin Microbiol. 2005;43(1):382–6.
57. Kontoyiannis DP, Sumoza D, Tarrand J, Bodey GP, Storey R, Raad II. Significance of aspergillemia in patients with cancer: a 10-year study. Clin Infect Dis. 2000;31(1):188–9.
58. Simoneau E, Kelly M, Labbe AC, Roy J, Laverdiere M. What is the clinical significance of positive blood cultures with aspergillus sp in hematopoietic stem cell transplant recipients? A 23 year experience. Bone Marrow Transplant. 2005;35(3):303–6.
59. Callister ME, Griffiths MJ, Nicholson AG, Leonard A, Johnson EM, Polkey MI, et al. A fatal case of disseminated aspergillosis caused by a non-sporulating strain of aspergillus fumigatus. J Clin Pathol. 2004;57(9):991–2.
60. Balajee SA, Lindsley MD, Iqbal N, Ito J, Pappas PG, Brandt ME. Nonsporulating clinical isolate identified as Petromyces alliaceus (anamorph aspergillus alliaceus) by morphological and sequence-based methods. J Clin Microbiol. 2007;45(8):2701–3.
61. Zhang C, Kong Q, Cai Z, Liu F, Chen P, Song J, et al. The newly nonsporulated characterization of an aspergillus fumigatus isolate from an immunocompetent patient and its clinic indication. Fungal Genet Biol. 2015;81:250–60.
62. Dufresne PJ, Moonjely SS, Ozaki K, Tremblay C, Laverdiere M, Dufresne SF. High frequency of pathogenic aspergillus species among nonsporulating moulds from respiratory tract samples. Med Mycol. 2017;55(2):233–6.
63. Samson RA, Visagie CM, Houbraken J, Hong SB, Hubka V, Klaassen CH, et al. Phylogeny, identification and nomenclature of the genus aspergillus. Stud Mycol. 2014;78:141–73.
64. Balajee SA, Weaver M, Imhof A, Gribskov J, Marr KA. Aspergillus fumigatus variant with decreased susceptibility to multiple antifungals. Antimicrob Agents Chemother. 2004;48(4):1197–203.
65. Alcazar-Fuoli L, Mellado E, Alastruey-Izquierdo A, Cuenca-Estrella M, Rodriguez-Tudela JL. Aspergillus section Fumigati: antifungal susceptibility patterns and sequence-based identification. Antimicrob Agents Chemother. 2008;52(4):1244–51.
66. Sugui JA, Vinh DC, Nardone G, Shea YR, Chang YC, Zelazny AM, et al. Neosartorya udagawae (aspergillus udagawae), an emerging agent of aspergillosis: how different is it from aspergillus fumigatus? J Clin Microbiol. 2010;48(1):220–8.
67. Vinh DC, Shea YR, Sugui JA, Parrilla-Castellar ER, Freeman AF, Campbell JW, et al. Invasive aspergillosis due to Neosartorya udagawae. Clin Infect Dis. 2009;49(1):102–11.
68. Staab JF, Balajee SA, Marr KA. Aspergillus section Fumigati typing by PCR-restriction fragment polymorphism. J Clin Microbiol. 2009;47(7):2079–83.
69. Balajee SA, Kano R, Baddley JW, Moser SA, Marr KA, Alexander BD, et al. Molecular identification of aspergillus species collected for the transplant-associated infection surveillance network. J Clin Microbiol. 2009;47(10):3138–41.
70. Etienne KA, Gade L, Lockhart SR, Diekema DJ, Messer SA, Pfaller MA, et al. Screening of a large global aspergillus fumigatus species complex collection by using a species-specific microsphere-based Luminex assay. J Clin Microbiol. 2009;47(12):4171–2.
71. Stynen D, Goris A, Sarfati J, Latge JP. A new sensitive sandwich enzyme-linked immunosorbent assay to detect galactofuran in patients with invasive aspergillosis. J Clin Microbiol. 1995;33(2):497–500.
72. Machetti M, Feasi M, Mordini N, Van Lint MT, Bacigalupo A, Latge JP, et al. Comparison of an enzyme immunoassay and a latex agglutination system for the diagnosis of invasive aspergillosis in bone marrow transplant recipients. Bone Marrow Transplant. 1998;21(9):917–21.
73. Mennink-Kersten MA, Donnelly JP, Verweij PE. Detection of circulating galactomannan for the diagnosis and management of invasive aspergillosis. Lancet Infect Dis. 2004;4(6):349–57.
74. Marr KA, Balajee SA, McLaughlin L, Tabouret M, Bentsen C, Walsh TJ. Detection of galactomannan antigenemia by enzyme immunoassay for the diagnosis of invasive aspergillosis: variables that affect performance. J Infect Dis. 2004;190(3):641–9.

75. Leeflang MM, Debets-Ossenkopp YJ, Visser CE, Scholten RJ, Hooft L, Bijlmer HA, et al. Galactomannan detection for invasive aspergillosis in immunocompromized patients. Cochrane Database Syst Rev. 2008;4:CD007394.
76. Pfeiffer CD, Fine JP, Safdar N. Diagnosis of invasive aspergillosis using a galactomannan assay: a meta-analysis. Clin Infect Dis. 2006;42(10):1417–27.
77. Stynen D, Sarfati J, Goris A, Prevost MC, Lesourd M, Kamphuis H, et al. Rat monoclonal antibodies against aspergillus galactomannan. Infect Immun. 1992;60(6):2237–45.
78. Tortorano AM, Esposto MC, Prigitano A, Grancini A, Ossi C, Cavanna C, et al. Cross-reactivity of Fusarium spp. in the aspergillus galactomannan enzyme-linked immunosorbent assay. J Clin Microbiol. 2012;50(3):1051–3.
79. Riviere S, Denis B, Bougnoux ME, Lanternier F, Lecuit M, Lortholary O. Serum aspergillus galactomannan for the management of disseminated histoplasmosis in AIDS. Am J Trop Med Hyg. 2012;87(2):303–5.
80. Vergidis P, Walker RC, Kaul DR, Kauffman CA, Freifeld AG, Slagle DC, et al. False-positive aspergillus galactomannan assay in solid organ transplant recipients with histoplasmosis. Transpl Infect Dis. 2012;14(2):213–7.
81. Adam O, Auperin A, Wilquin F, Bourhis JH, Gachot B, Chachaty E. Treatment with piperacillin-tazobactam and false-positive aspergillus galactomannan antigen test results for patients with hematological malignancies. Clin Infect Dis. 2004;38(6):917–20.
82. Maertens J, Theunissen K, Verhoef G, Van Eldere J. False-positive aspergillus galactomannan antigen test results. Clin Infect Dis. 2004;39(2):289–90.
83. Singh N, Obman A, Husain S, Aspinall S, Mietzner S, Stout JE. Reactivity of platelia aspergillus galactomannan antigen with piperacillin-tazobactam: clinical implications based on achievable concentrations in serum. Antimicrob Agents Chemother. 2004;48(6):1989–92.
84. Viscoli C, Machetti M, Cappellano P, Bucci B, Bruzzi P, Van Lint MT, et al. False-positive galactomannan platelia aspergillus test results for patients receiving piperacillin-tazobactam. Clin Infect Dis. 2004;38(6):913–6.
85. Walsh TJ, Shoham S, Petraitiene R, Sein T, Schaufele R, Kelaher A, et al. Detection of galactomannan antigenemia in patients receiving piperacillin-tazobactam and correlations between in vitro, in vivo, and clinical properties of the drug-antigen interaction. J Clin Microbiol. 2004;42(10):4744–8.
86. Machetti M, Furfaro E, Viscoli C. Galactomannan in piperacillin-tazobactam: how much and to what extent? Antimicrob Agents Chemother. 2005;49(9):3984–5.
87. Metan G. The interaction between piperacillin-tazobactam and aspergillus galactomannan antigenemia assay: is the story over? Infection. 2013;41(1):293–4.
88. Vergidis P, Razonable RR, Wheat LJ, Estes L, Caliendo AM, Baden LR, et al. Reduction in false-positive aspergillus serum galactomannan enzyme immunoassay results associated with use of piperacillin-tazobactam in the United States. J Clin Microbiol. 2014;52(6):2199–201.
89. Ko JH, Peck KR, Lee WJ, Lee JY, Cho SY, Ha YE, et al. Generic piperacillin/tazobactam is not associated with galactomannan false-positivity in adult patients with cancer: a case-control study. Eur J Clin Microbiol Infect Dis. 2015;34(7):1437–41.
90. Klont RR, Mennink-Kersten MA, Verweij PE. Utility of aspergillus antigen detection in specimens other than serum specimens. Clin Infect Dis. 2004;39(10):1467–74.
91. Guo YL, Chen YQ, Wang K, Qin SM, Wu C, Kong JL. Accuracy of BAL galactomannan in diagnosing invasive aspergillosis: a bivariate metaanalysis and systematic review. Chest. 2010;138(4):817–24.
92. Zou M, Tang L, Zhao S, Zhao Z, Chen L, Chen P, et al. Systematic review and meta-analysis of detecting galactomannan in bronchoalveolar lavage fluid for diagnosing invasive aspergillosis. PLoS One. 2012;7(8):e43347.
93. Affolter K, Tamm M, Jahn K, Halter J, Passweg J, Hirsch HH, et al. Galactomannan in bronchoalveolar lavage for diagnosing invasive fungal disease. Am J Respir Crit Care Med. 2014;190(3):309–17.
94. Bergeron A, Porcher R, Menotti J, Poirot JL, Chagnon K, Vekhoff A, et al. Prospective evaluation of clinical and biological markers to predict the outcome of invasive pulmonary aspergillosis in hematological patients. J Clin Microbiol. 2012;50(3):823–30.
95. Neofytos D, Railkar R, Mullane KM, Fredricks DN, Granwehr B, Marr KA, et al. Correlation between circulating fungal biomarkers and clinical outcome in invasive aspergillosis. PLoS One. 2015;10(6):e0129022.
96. Thornton CR. Development of an immunochromatographic lateral-flow device for rapid serodiagnosis of invasive aspergillosis. Clin Vaccine Immunol. 2008;15(7):1095–105.
97. Wiederhold NP, Thornton CR, Najvar LK, Kirkpatrick WR, Bocanegra R, Patterson TF. Comparison of lateral flow technology and galactomannan and (1->3)-beta-D-glucan assays for detection of invasive pulmonary aspergillosis. Clin Vaccine Immunol. 2009;16(12):1844–6.
98. Hoenigl M, Prattes J, Spiess B, Wagner J, Prueller F, Raggam RB, et al. Performance of galactomannan, beta-d-glucan, aspergillus lateral-flow device, conventional culture, and PCR tests with bronchoalveolar lavage fluid for diagnosis of invasive pulmonary aspergillosis. J Clin Microbiol. 2014;52(6):2039–45.
99. Willinger B, Lackner M, Lass-Florl C, Prattes J, Posch V, Selitsch B, et al. Bronchoalveolar lavage lateral-flow device test for invasive pulmonary aspergillosis in solid organ transplant patients: a semiprospective multicenter study. Transplantation. 2014;98(8):898–902.
100. Dufresne SF, Datta K, Li X, Dadachova E, Staab JF, Patterson TF, et al. Detection of urinary excreted fungal galactomannan-like antigens for diagnosis of invasive aspergillosis. PLoS One. 2012;7(8):e42736.
101. Karageorgopoulos DE, Vouloumanou EK, Ntziora F, Michalopoulos A, Rafailidis PI, Falagas ME. Beta-D-glucan assay for the diagnosis of invasive fungal infections: a meta-analysis. Clin Infect Dis. 2011;52(6):750–70.
102. Onishi A, Sugiyama D, Kogata Y, Saegusa J, Sugimoto T, Kawano S, et al. Diagnostic accuracy of serum 1,3-beta-D-glucan for pneumocystis jiroveci pneumonia, invasive candidiasis, and invasive aspergillosis: systematic review and meta-analysis. J Clin Microbiol. 2012;50(1):7–15.
103. Alexander BD, Smith PB, Davis RD, Perfect JR, Reller LB. The (1,3){beta}-D-glucan test as an aid to early diagnosis of invasive fungal infections following lung transplantation. J Clin Microbiol. 2010;48(11):4083–8.
104. Akamatsu N, Sugawara Y, Kaneko J, Tamura S, Makuuchi M. Preemptive treatment of fungal infection based on plasma (1 --> 3)beta-D-glucan levels after liver transplantation. Infection. 2007;35(5):346–51.
105. Duffner U, Abdel-Mageed A, Dahl K, Fogg G, Hester J. Serum (1 --> 3)-beta-D-glucan levels (Fungitell assay) is not useful as a screening test for recipients of an allogeneic HSCT while on immunoglobulin replacement. Bone Marrow Transplant. 2012;47(1):151–2.
106. Sarfati J, Monod M, Recco P, Sulahian A, Pinel C, Candolfi E, et al. Recombinant antigens as diagnostic markers for aspergillosis. Diagn Microbiol Infect Dis. 2006;55(4):279–91.
107. Du C, Wingard JR, Cheng S, Nguyen MH, Clancy CJ. Serum IgG responses against aspergillus proteins before hematopoietic

stem cell transplantation or chemotherapy identify patients who develop invasive aspergillosis. Biol Blood Marrow Transplant. 2012;18(12):1927–34.
108. Erdmann JH, Graf B, Blau IW, Fischer F, Timm G, Hemmati P, et al. Anti-aspergillus immunoglobulin-G testing in serum of hematopoietic stem cell transplant recipients. Transpl Infect Dis. 2016;18(3):354–60.
109. Hebart H, Loffler J, Meisner C, Serey F, Schmidt D, Bohme A, et al. Early detection of aspergillus infection after allogeneic stem cell transplantation by polymerase chain reaction screening. J Infect Dis. 2000;181(5):1713–9.
110. Hebart H, Loffler J, Reitze H, Engel A, Schumacher U, Klingebiel T, et al. Prospective screening by a panfungal polymerase chain reaction assay in patients at risk for fungal infections: implications for the management of febrile neutropenia. Br J Haematol. 2000;111(2):635–40.
111. Kawazu M, Kanda Y, Nannya Y, Aoki K, Kurokawa M, Chiba S, et al. Prospective comparison of the diagnostic potential of real-time PCR, double-sandwich enzyme-linked immunosorbent assay for galactomannan, and a (1-->3)-beta-D-glucan test in weekly screening for invasive aspergillosis in patients with hematological disorders. J Clin Microbiol. 2004;42(6):2733–41.
112. Buchheidt D, Hummel M, Schleiermacher D, Spiess B, Schwerdtfeger R, Cornely OA, et al. Prospective clinical evaluation of a LightCycler-mediated polymerase chain reaction assay, a nested-PCR assay and a galactomannan enzyme-linked immunosorbent assay for detection of invasive aspergillosis in neutropenic cancer patients and haematological stem cell transplant recipients. Br J Haematol. 2004;125(2):196–202.
113. Suarez F, Lortholary O, Buland S, Rubio MT, Ghez D, Mahe V, et al. Detection of circulating aspergillus fumigatus DNA by real-time PCR assay of large serum volumes improves early diagnosis of invasive aspergillosis in high-risk adult patients under hematologic surveillance. J Clin Microbiol. 2008;46(11):3772–7.
114. Florent M, Katsahian S, Vekhoff A, Levy V, Rio B, Marie JP, et al. Prospective evaluation of a polymerase chain reaction-ELISA targeted to aspergillus fumigatus and aspergillus flavus for the early diagnosis of invasive aspergillosis in patients with hematological malignancies. J Infect Dis. 2006;193(5):741–7.
115. Halliday C, Hoile R, Sorrell T, James G, Yadav S, Shaw P, et al. Role of prospective screening of blood for invasive aspergillosis by polymerase chain reaction in febrile neutropenic recipients of haematopoietic stem cell transplants and patients with acute leukaemia. Br J Haematol. 2006;132(4):478–86.
116. Blennow O, Remberger M, Klingspor L, Omazic B, Fransson K, Ljungman P, et al. Randomized PCR-based therapy and risk factors for invasive fungal infection following reduced-intensity conditioning and hematopoietic SCT. Bone Marrow Transplant. 2010;45(12):1710–8.
117. White PL, Perry MD, Loeffler J, Melchers W, Klingspor L, Bretagne S, et al. Critical stages of extracting DNA from aspergillus fumigatus in whole-blood specimens. J Clin Microbiol. 2010;48(10):3753–5.
118. White PL, Mengoli C, Bretagne S, Cuenca-Estrella M, Finnstrom N, Klingspor L, et al. Evaluation of aspergillus PCR protocols for testing serum specimens. J Clin Microbiol. 2011;49(11):3842–8.
119. Johnson GL, Bibby DF, Wong S, Agrawal SG, Bustin SA. A MIQE-compliant real-time PCR assay for aspergillus detection. PLoS One. 2012;7(7):e40022.
120. White PL, Barnes RA, Springer J, Klingspor L, Cuenca-Estrella M, Morton CO, et al. Clinical performance of aspergillus PCR for testing serum and plasma: a study by the European aspergillus PCR initiative. J Clin Microbiol. 2015;53(9):2832–7.
121. Steinmann J, Buer J, Rath PM, Paul A, Saner F. Invasive aspergillosis in two liver transplant recipients: diagnosis by SeptiFast. Transpl Infect Dis. 2009;11(2):175–8.
122. von Lilienfeld-Toal M, Lehmann LE, Raadts AD, Hahn-Ast C, Orlopp KS, Marklein G, et al. Utility of a commercially available multiplex real-time PCR assay to detect bacterial and fungal pathogens in febrile neutropenia. J Clin Microbiol. 2009;47(8):2405–10.
123. Lamoth F, Jaton K, Prod'hom G, Senn L, Bille J, Calandra T, et al. Multiplex blood PCR in combination with blood cultures for improvement of microbiological documentation of infection in febrile neutropenia. J Clin Microbiol. 2010;48(10):3510–6.
124. Steinmann J, Buer J, Rath PM. Detection of aspergillus fumigatus in blood samples from critically ill patients in intensive care units by use of the SeptiFast assay. J Clin Microbiol. 2016;54(7):1918–21.
125. Torelli R, Sanguinetti M, Moody A, Pagano L, Caira M, De Carolis E, et al. Diagnosis of invasive aspergillosis by a commercial real-time PCR assay for aspergillus DNA in bronchoalveolar lavage fluid samples from high-risk patients compared to a galactomannan enzyme immunoassay. J Clin Microbiol. 2011;49(12):4273–8.
126. Orsi CF, Bettua C, Pini P, Venturelli C, La Regina A, Morace G, et al. Detection of pneumocystis jirovecii and aspergillus spp. DNa in bronchoalveolar lavage fluids by commercial real-time PCr assays: comparison with conventional diagnostic tests. New Microbiol. 2015;38(1):75–84.
127. White PL, Perry MD, Moody A, Follett SA, Morgan G, Barnes RA. Evaluation of analytical and preliminary clinical performance of Myconostica MycAssay aspergillus when testing serum specimens for diagnosis of invasive Aspergillosis. J Clin Microbiol. 2011;49(6):2169–74.
128. Danylo A, Courtemanche C, Pelletier R, Boudreault AA. Performance of MycAssay aspergillus DNA real-time PCR assay compared with the galactomannan detection assay for the diagnosis of invasive aspergillosis from serum samples. Med Mycol. 2014;52(6):577–83.
129. Pini P, Bettua C, Orsi CF, Venturelli C, Faglioni L, Forghieri F, et al. Clinical performance of a commercial real-time PCR assay for aspergillus DNA detection in serum samples from high-risk patients: comparison with a galactomannan enzyme immunoassay. Eur J Clin Microbiol Infect Dis. 2015;34(1):131–6.
130. Lass-Florl C, Follett SA, Moody A, Denning DW. Detection of aspergillus in lung and other tissue samples using the MycAssay aspergillus real-time PCR kit. Can J Microbiol. 2011;57(9):765–8.
131. Chong GL, van de Sande WW, Dingemans GJ, Gaajetaan GR, Vonk AG, Hayette MP, et al. Validation of a new aspergillus real-time PCR assay for direct detection of aspergillus and azole resistance of aspergillus fumigatus on bronchoalveolar lavage fluid. J Clin Microbiol. 2015;53(3):868–74.
132. White PL, Posso RB, Barnes RA. Analytical and clinical evaluation of the PathoNostics AsperGenius Assay for detection of invasive Aspergillosis and resistance to azole antifungal drugs during testing of serum samples. J Clin Microbiol. 2015;53(7):2115–21.
133. Chong GM, van der Beek MT, von dem Borne PA, Boelens J, Steel E, Kampinga GA, et al. PCR-based detection of aspergillus fumigatus Cyp51A mutations on bronchoalveolar lavage: a multicentre validation of the AsperGenius assay(R) in 201 patients with haematological disease suspected for invasive aspergillosis. J Antimicrob Chemother. 2016;71(12):3528–35.
134. Park BJ, Pappas PG, Wannemuehler KA, Alexander BD, Anaissie EJ, Andes DR, et al. Invasive non-aspergillus mold infections in transplant recipients, United States, 2001-2006. Emerg Infect Dis. 2011;17(10):1855–64.

135. Azie N, Neofytos D, Pfaller M, Meier-Kriesche HU, Quan SP, Horn D. The PATH (Prospective Antifungal Therapy) Alliance(R) registry and invasive fungal infections: update 2012. Diagn Microbiol Infect Dis. 2012;73(4):293–300.
136. Nucci M. Emerging moulds: Fusarium, Scedosporium and Zygomycetes in transplant recipients. Curr Opin Infect Dis. 2003;16(6):607–12.
137. Lionakis MS, Bodey GP, Tarrand JJ, Raad II, Kontoyiannis DP. The significance of blood cultures positive for emerging saprophytic moulds in cancer patients. Clin Microbiol Infect. 2004;10(10):922–5.
138. Lionakis MS, Kontoyiannis DP. The significance of isolation of saprophytic molds from the lower respiratory tract in patients with cancer. Cancer. 2004;100(1):165–72.
139. Potenza L, Vallerini D, Barozzi P, Riva G, Forghieri F, Zanetti E, et al. Mucorales-specific T cells emerge in the course of invasive mucormycosis and may be used as a surrogate diagnostic marker in high-risk patients. Blood. 2011;118(20):5416–9.
140. Millon L, Larosa F, Lepiller Q, Legrand F, Rocchi S, Daguindau E, et al. Quantitative polymerase chain reaction detection of circulating DNA in serum for early diagnosis of mucormycosis in immunocompromised patients. Clin Infect Dis. 2013;56:e95–101.
141. Clancy CJ, Nguyen MH. Finding the "missing 50%" of invasive candidiasis: how nonculture diagnostics will improve understanding of disease spectrum and transform patient care. Clin Infect Dis. 2013;56(9):1284–92.
142. Marr KA, Bowden RA. Fungal infections in patients undergoing blood and marrow transplantation. Transpl Infect Dis. 1999;1(4):237–46.
143. Bille J, Stockman L, Roberts GD, Horstmeier CD, Ilstrup DM. Evaluation of a lysis-centrifugation system for recovery of yeasts and filamentous fungi from blood. J Clin Microbiol. 1983;18(3):469–71.
144. Guerra-Romero L, Edson RS, Cockerill FR 3rd, Horstmeier CD, Roberts GD. Comparison of Du Pont isolator and Roche Septi-Chek for detection of fungemia. J Clin Microbiol. 1987;25(9):1623–5.
145. Cockerill FR 3rd, Torgerson CA, Reed GS, Vetter EA, Weaver AL, Dale JC, et al. Clinical comparison of difco ESP, Wampole isolator, and Becton Dickinson Septi-Chek aerobic blood culturing systems. J Clin Microbiol. 1996;34(1):20–4.
146. Hellinger WC, Cawley JJ, Alvarez S, Hogan SF, Harmsen WS, Ilstrup DM, et al. Clinical comparison of the isolator and BacT/alert aerobic blood culture systems. J Clin Microbiol. 1995;33(7):1787–90.
147. Lyon R, Woods G. Comparison of the BacT/alert and isolator blood culture systems for recovery of fungi. Am J Clin Pathol. 1995;103(5):660–2.
148. Fuller DD, Davis TE Jr, Denys GA, York MK. Evaluation of BACTEC MYCO/F Lytic medium for recovery of mycobacteria, fungi, and bacteria from blood. J Clin Microbiol. 2001;39(8):2933–6.
149. Vetter E, Torgerson C, Feuker A, Hughes J, Harmsen S, Schleck C, et al. Comparison of the BACTEC MYCO/F Lytic bottle to the isolator tube, BACTEC Plus Aerobic F/bottle, and BACTEC Anaerobic Lytic/10 bottle and comparison of the BACTEC Plus Aerobic F/bottle to the Isolator tube for recovery of bacteria, mycobacteria, and fungi from blood. J Clin Microbiol. 2001;39(12):4380–6.
150. Essman TF, Flynn HW Jr, Smiddy WE, Brod RD, Murray TG, Davis JL, et al. Treatment outcomes in a 10-year study of endogenous fungal endophthalmitis. Ophthalmic Surg Lasers. 1997;28(3):185–94.
151. Thaler M, Pastakia B, Shawker TH, O'Leary T, Pizzo PA. Hepatic candidiasis in cancer patients: the evolving picture of the syndrome. Ann Intern Med. 1988;108(1):88–100.
152. Shepard JR, Addison RM, Alexander BD, Della-Latta P, Gherna M, Haase G, et al. Multicenter evaluation of the Candida albicans/Candida glabrata peptide nucleic acid fluorescent in situ hybridization method for simultaneous dual-color identification of C. albicans and C. glabrata directly from blood culture bottles. J Clin Microbiol. 2008;46(1):50–5.
153. Hall L, Le Febre KM, Deml SM, Wohlfiel SL, Wengenack NL. Evaluation of the yeast traffic light PNA FISH probes for identification of Candida species from positive blood cultures. J Clin Microbiol. 2012;50(4):1446–8.
154. Stone NR, Gorton RL, Barker K, Ramnarain P, Kibbler CC. Evaluation of PNA-FISH yeast traffic light for rapid identification of yeast directly from positive blood cultures and assessment of clinical impact. J Clin Microbiol. 2013;51(4):1301–2.
155. Deak E, Charlton CL, Bobenchik AM, Miller SA, Pollett S, McHardy IH, et al. Comparison of the Vitek MS and Bruker Microflex LT MALDI-TOF MS platforms for routine identification of commonly isolated bacteria and yeast in the clinical microbiology laboratory. Diagn Microbiol Infect Dis. 2015;81(1):27–33.
156. Levesque S, Dufresne PJ, Soualhine H, Domingo MC, Bekal S, Lefebvre B, et al. A side by side comparison of Bruker Biotyper and VITEK MS: utility of MALDI-TOF MS technology for microorganism identification in a public health reference laboratory. PLoS One. 2015;10(12):e0144878.
157. Wattal C, Oberoi JK, Goel N, Raveendran R, Khanna S. Matrix-assisted laser desorption ionization time of flight mass spectrometry (MALDI-TOF MS) for rapid identification of micro-organisms in the routine clinical microbiology laboratory. Eur J Clin Microbiol Infect Dis. 2017;36:807–12.
158. Spanu T, Posteraro B, Fiori B, D'Inzeo T, Campoli S, Ruggeri A, et al. Direct maldi-tof mass spectrometry assay of blood culture broths for rapid identification of Candida species causing bloodstream infections: an observational study in two large microbiology laboratories. J Clin Microbiol. 2012;50(1):176–9.
159. Usami M, Ohata A, Horiuchi T, Nagasawa K, Wakabayashi T, Tanaka S. Positive (1-->3)-beta-D-glucan in blood components and release of (1-->3)-beta-D-glucan from depth-type membrane filters for blood processing. Transfusion. 2002;42(9):1189–95.
160. Pickering JW, Sant HW, Bowles CA, Roberts WL, Woods GL. Evaluation of a (1->3)-beta-D-glucan assay for diagnosis of invasive fungal infections. J Clin Microbiol. 2005;43(12):5957–62.
161. Prattes J, Schilcher G, Krause R. Reliability of serum 1,3-beta-D-glucan assay in patients undergoing renal replacement therapy: a review of the literature. Mycoses. 2015;58(1):4–9.
162. Ostrosky-Zeichner L, Shoham S, Vazquez J, Reboli A, Betts R, Barron MA, et al. MSG-01: a randomized, double-blind, placebo-controlled trial of caspofungin prophylaxis followed by preemptive therapy for invasive candidiasis in high-risk adults in the critical care setting. Clin Infect Dis. 2014;58(9):1219–26.
163. Hanson KE, Pfeiffer CD, Lease ED, Balch AH, Zaas AK, Perfect JR, et al. Beta-D-glucan surveillance with preemptive anidulafungin for invasive candidiasis in intensive care unit patients: a randomized pilot study. PLoS One. 2012;7(8):e42282.
164. Knitsch W, Vincent JL, Utzolino S, Francois B, Dinya T, Dimopoulos G, et al. A randomized, placebo-controlled trial of preemptive antifungal therapy for the prevention of invasive candidiasis following gastrointestinal surgery for intra-abdominal infections. Clin Infect Dis. 2015;61(11):1671–8.
165. Rimek D, Singh J, Kappe R. Cross-reactivity of the PLATELIA CANDIDA antigen detection enzyme immunoassay with fungal antigen extracts. J Clin Microbiol. 2003;41(7):3395–8.
166. Ellis M, Al-Ramadi B, Bernsen R, Kristensen J, Alizadeh H, Hedstrom U. Prospective evaluation of mannan and anti-mannan antibodies for diagnosis of invasive Candida infections in patients with neutropenic fever. J Med Microbiol. 2009;58(Pt 5):606–15.

167. Lunel FM, Mennink-Kersten MA, Ruegebrink D, van der Lee HA, Donnelly JP, Blijlevens NM, et al. Value of Candida serum markers in patients with invasive candidiasis after myeloablative chemotherapy. Diagn Microbiol Infect Dis. 2009;64(4):408–15.
168. Mikulska M, Calandra T, Sanguinetti M, Poulain D, Viscoli C. The use of mannan antigen and anti-mannan antibodies in the diagnosis of invasive candidiasis: recommendations from the Third European Conference on infections in leukemia. Crit Care. 2010;14(6):R222.
169. Lunel FM, Donnelly JP, van der Lee HA, Blijlevens NM, Verweij PE. Performance of the new Platelia Candida Plus assays for the diagnosis of invasive Candida infection in patients undergoing myeloablative therapy. Med Mycol. 2011;49(8):848–55.
170. Nihtinen A, Anttila VJ, Richardson M, Ruutu T, Juvonen E, Meri T, et al. Factors influencing the performance level of Candida mannan antigen testing in allogeneic stem cell transplant recipients not receiving fluconazole prophylaxis. Transpl Infect Dis. 2011;13(3):266–72.
171. Leon C, Ruiz-Santana S, Saavedra P, Castro C, Ubeda A, Loza A, et al. Value of beta-D-glucan and Candida albicans germ tube antibody for discriminating between Candida colonization and invasive candidiasis in patients with severe abdominal conditions. Intensive Care Med. 2012;38(8):1315–25.
172. Avni T, Leibovici L, Paul M. PCR diagnosis of invasive candidiasis: systematic review and meta-analysis. J Clin Microbiol. 2011;49(2):665–70.
173. Mauro MV, Cavalcanti P, Perugini D, Noto A, Sperli D, Giraldi C. Diagnostic utility of LightCycler SeptiFast and procalcitonin assays in the diagnosis of bloodstream infection in immunocompromised patients. Diagn Microbiol Infect Dis. 2012;73(4):308–11.
174. Mylonakis E, Clancy CJ, Ostrosky-Zeichner L, Garey KW, Alangaden GJ, Vazquez JA, et al. T2 magnetic resonance assay for the rapid diagnosis of candidemia in whole blood: a clinical trial. Clin Infect Dis. 2015;60(6):892–9.
175. Bilir SP, Ferrufino CP, Pfaller MA, Munakata J. The economic impact of rapid Candida species identification by T2Candida among high-risk patients. Future Microbiol. 2015;10(7):1133–44.
176. Walker B, Powers-Fletcher MV, Schmidt RL, Hanson KE. Cost-effectiveness analysis of multiplex PCR with magnetic resonance detection versus empiric or blood culture-directed therapy for management of suspected candidemia. J Clin Microbiol. 2016;54(3):718–26.
177. Kwon-Chung KJ, Bennett JE, Wickes BL, Meyer W, Cuomo CA, Wollenburg KR, et al. The case for adopting the "species complex" nomenclature for the etiologic agents of cryptococcosis. mSphere. 2017;2(1):e00357–16.
178. Mendpara SD, Ustun C, Kallab AM, Mazzella FM, Bilodeau PA, Jillella AP. Cryptococcal meningitis following autologous stem cell transplantation in a patient with multiple myeloma. Bone Marrow Transplant. 2002;30(4):259–60.
179. Warkentien T, Crum-Cianflone NF. An update on Cryptococcus among HIV-infected patients. Int J STD AIDS. 2010;21(10):679–84.
180. Sun HY, Wagener MM, Singh N. Cryptococcosis in solid-organ, hematopoietic stem cell, and tissue transplant recipients: evidence-based evolving trends. Clin Infect Dis. 2009;48(11):1566–76.
181. Davis JA, Horn DL, Marr KA, Fishman JA. Central nervous system involvement in cryptococcal infection in individuals after solid organ transplantation or with AIDS. Transpl Infect Dis. 2009;11(5):432–7.
182. Perfect JR, Dismukes WE, Dromer F, Goldman DL, Graybill JR, Hamill RJ, et al. Clinical practice guidelines for the management of cryptococcal disease: 2010 update by the infectious diseases society of america. Clin Infect Dis. 2010;50(3):291–322.
183. Singh N, Forrest G. Cryptococcosis in solid organ transplant recipients. Am J Transplant. 2009;9(Suppl 4):S192–8.
184. Liao CH, Chi CY, Wang YJ, Tseng SW, Chou CH, Ho CM, et al. Different presentations and outcomes between HIV-infected and HIV-uninfected patients with Cryptococcal meningitis. J Microbiol Immunol Infect. 2012;45(4):296–304.
185. Severo CB, Pinto GL, Sotilli J, Garcia MR, Gazzoni AF, Oliveira FM, et al. Cryptococcuria as manifestation of disseminated cryptococcosis: Staib agar as a selective identification medium. Mycoses. 2011;54(6):e760–6.
186. Kiertiburanakul S, Sungkanuparph S, Buabut B, Pracharktam R. Cryptococcuria as a manifestation of disseminated cryptococcosis and isolated urinary tract infection. Jpn J Infect Dis. 2004;57(5):203–5.
187. Klein KR, Hall L, Deml SM, Rysavy JM, Wohlfiel SL, Wengenack NL. Identification of Cryptococcus gattii by use of L-canavanine glycine bromothymol blue medium and DNA sequencing. J Clin Microbiol. 2009;47(11):3669–72.
188. McTaggart L, Richardson SE, Seah C, Hoang L, Fothergill A, Zhang SX. Rapid identification of Cryptococcus neoformans var. grubii, C. neoformans var. neoformans, and C. gattii by use of rapid biochemical tests, differential media, and DNA sequencing. J Clin Microbiol. 2011;49(7):2522–7.
189. Posteraro B, Vella A, Cogliati M, De Carolis E, Florio AR, Posteraro P, et al. Matrix-assisted laser desorption ionization-time of flight mass spectrometry-based method for discrimination between molecular types of Cryptococcus neoformans and Cryptococcus gattii. J Clin Microbiol. 2012;50(7):2472–6.
190. McTaggart LR, Lei E, Richardson SE, Hoang L, Fothergill A, Zhang SX. Rapid identification of Cryptococcus neoformans and Cryptococcus gattii by matrix-assisted laser desorption ionization-time of flight mass spectrometry. J Clin Microbiol. 2011;49(8):3050–3.
191. Enache-Angoulvant A, Chandenier J, Symoens F, Lacube P, Bolognini J, Douchet C, et al. Molecular identification of Cryptococcus neoformans serotypes. J Clin Microbiol. 2007;45(4):1261–5.
192. Bovers M, Diaz MR, Hagen F, Spanjaard L, Duim B, Visser CE, et al. Identification of genotypically diverse Cryptococcus neoformans and Cryptococcus gattii isolates by Luminex xMAP technology. J Clin Microbiol. 2007;45(6):1874–83.
193. Bloomfield N, Gordon MA, Elmendorf DF Jr. Detection of Cryptococcus neoformans antigen in body fluids by latex particle agglutination. Proc Soc Exp Biol Med. 1963;114:64–7.
194. Scott EN, Muchmore HG, Felton FG. Comparison of enzyme immunoassay and latex agglutination methods for detection of Cryptococcus neoformans antigen. Am J Clin Pathol. 1980;73(6):790–4.
195. Gade W, Hinnefeld SW, Babcock LS, Gilligan P, Kelly W, Wait K, et al. Comparison of the PREMIER cryptococcal antigen enzyme immunoassay and the latex agglutination assay for detection of cryptococcal antigens. J Clin Microbiol. 1991;29(8):1616–9.
196. Temstet A, Roux P, Poirot JL, Ronin O, Dromer F. Evaluation of a monoclonal antibody-based latex agglutination test for diagnosis of cryptococcosis: comparison with two tests using polyclonal antibodies. J Clin Microbiol. 1992;30(10):2544–50.
197. Sekhon AS, Garg AK, Kaufman L, Kobayashi GS, Hamir Z, Jalbert M, et al. Evaluation of a commercial enzyme immunoassay for the detection of cryptococcal antigen. Mycoses. 1993;36(1–2):31–4.
198. Frank UK, Nishimura SL, Li NC, Sugai K, Yajko DM, Hadley WK, et al. Evaluation of an enzyme immunoassay for detection of cryptococcal capsular polysaccharide antigen in serum and cerebrospinal fluid. J Clin Microbiol. 1993;31(1):97–101.
199. Jaye DL, Waites KB, Parker B, Bragg SL, Moser SA. Comparison of two rapid latex agglutination tests for detection of cryptococcal capsular polysaccharide. Am J Clin Pathol. 1998;109(5):634–41.

200. Lindsley MD, Mekha N, Baggett HC, Surinthong Y, Autthateinchai R, Sawatwong P, et al. Evaluation of a newly developed lateral flow immunoassay for the diagnosis of cryptococcosis. Clin Infect Dis. 2011;53(4):321–5.
201. Tanner DC, Weinstein MP, Fedorciw B, Joho KL, Thorpe JJ, Reller L. Comparison of commercial kits for detection of cryptococcal antigen. J Clin Microbiol. 1994;32(7):1680–4.
202. Lyman CA, Devi SJ, Nathanson J, Frasch CE, Pizzo PA, Walsh TJ. Detection and quantitation of the glucuronoxylomannan-like polysaccharide antigen from clinical and nonclinical isolates of Trichosporon beigelii and implications for pathogenicity. J Clin Microbiol. 1995;33(1):126–30.
203. Taelman H, Bogaerts J, Batungwanayo J, Van de Perre P, Lucas S, Allen S. Failure of the cryptococcal serum antigen test to detect primary pulmonary cryptococcosis in patients infected with human immunodeficiency virus. Clin Infect Dis. 1994;18(1):119–20.
204. Singh N, Alexander BD, Lortholary O, Dromer F, Gupta KL, John GT, et al. Pulmonary cryptococcosis in solid organ transplant recipients: clinical relevance of serum cryptococcal antigen. Clin Infect Dis. 2008;46(2):e12–8.
205. Jarvis JN, Percival A, Bauman S, Pelfrey J, Meintjes G, Williams GN, et al. Evaluation of a novel point-of-care cryptococcal antigen test on serum, plasma, and urine from patients with HIV-associated cryptococcal meningitis. Clin Infect Dis. 2011;53(10):1019–23.
206. Binnicker MJ, Jespersen DJ, Bestrom JE, Rollins LO. Comparison of four assays for the detection of cryptococcal antigen. Clin Vaccine Immunol. 2012;19(12):1988–90.
207. Hansen J, Slechta ES, Gates-Hollingsworth MA, Neary B, Barker AP, Bauman S, et al. Large-scale evaluation of the immuno-mycologics lateral flow and enzyme-linked immunoassays for detection of cryptococcal antigen in serum and cerebrospinal fluid. Clin Vaccine Immunol. 2013;20(1):52–5.
208. Veron V, Simon S, Blanchet D, Aznar C. Real-time polymerase chain reaction detection of Cryptococcus neoformans and Cryptococcus gattii in human samples. Diagn Microbiol Infect Dis. 2009;65(1):69–72.
209. Gago S, Esteban C, Valero C, Zaragoza O, Puig de la Bellacasa J, Buitrago MJ. A multiplex real-time PCR assay for identification of Pneumocystis jirovecii, Histoplasma capsulatum, and Cryptococcus neoformans/Cryptococcus gattii in samples from AIDS patients with opportunistic pneumonia. J Clin Microbiol. 2014;52(4):1168–76.
210. Bartlett MS, Smith JW. Pneumocystis carinii, an opportunist in immunocompromised patients. Clin Microbiol Rev. 1991;4(2):137–49.
211. Bartlett JA, Hulette C. Central nervous system pneumocystosis in a patient with AIDS. Clin Infect Dis. 1997;25(1):82–5.
212. Schildgen V, Mai S, Khalfaoui S, Lusebrink J, Pieper M, Tillmann RL, et al. Pneumocystis jirovecii can be productively cultured in differentiated CuFi-8 airway cells. MBio. 2014;5(3):e01186–14.
213. Nato F, Contini C, Zamora-Zavala C, Viscardi P, Delia S, Mojon M, et al. Production and characterization of monoclonal antibodies to human Pneumocystis carinii for the diagnosis of P. carinii pneumonia. Eur J Med. 1992;1(3):132–8.
214. Stager CE, Fraire AE, Kim HS, Estrada R, Davis JR, Greenberg D, et al. Modification of the fungi-fluor and the genetic systems fluorescent antibody methods for detection of Pneumocystis carinii in bronchoalveolar lavage specimens. Arch Pathol Lab Med. 1995;119(2):142–7.
215. Procop GW, Haddad S, Quinn J, Wilson ML, Henshaw NG, Reller LB, et al. Detection of Pneumocystis jiroveci in respiratory specimens by four staining methods. J Clin Microbiol. 2004;42(7):3333–5.
216. Fortun J, Navas E, Marti-Belda P, Montilla P, Hermida JM, Perez-Elias MJ, et al. Pneumocystis carinii pneumonia in HIV-infected patients: diagnostic yield of induced sputum and immunofluorescent stain with monoclonal antibodies. Eur Respir J. 1992;5(6):665–9.
217. Cruciani M, Marcati P, Malena M, Bosco O, Serpelloni G, Mengoli C. Meta-analysis of diagnostic procedures for Pneumocystis carinii pneumonia in HIV-1-infected patients. Eur Respir J. 2002;20(4):982–9.
218. Silva RM, Bazzo ML, Borges AA. Induced sputum versus bronchoalveolar lavage in the diagnosis of pneumocystis jiroveci pneumonia in human immunodeficiency virus-positive patients. Braz J Infect Dis. 2007;11(6):549–53.
219. Wang Y, Doucette S, Qian Q, Kirby JE. Yield of primary and repeat induced sputum testing for Pneumocystis jiroveci in human immunodeficiency virus-positive and -negative patients. Arch Pathol Lab Med. 2007;131(10):1582–4.
220. Aderaye G, Woldeamanuel Y, Asrat D, Lebbad M, Beser J, Worku A, et al. Evaluation of Toluidine Blue O staining for the diagnosis of Pneumocystis jiroveci in expectorated sputum sample and bronchoalveolar lavage from HIV-infected patients in a tertiary care referral center in Ethiopia. Infection. 2008;36(3):237–43.
221. Jiancheng W, Minjun H, Yi-jun A, Lan S, Zengzhu G, Jianrong S, et al. Screening Pneumocystis carinii pneumonia in non-HIV-infected immunocompromised patients using polymerase chain reaction. Diagn Microbiol Infect Dis. 2009;64(4):396–401.
222. McTaggart LR, Wengenack NL, Richardson SE. Validation of the MycAssay Pneumocystis kit for detection of Pneumocystis jirovecii in bronchoalveolar lavage specimens by comparison to a laboratory standard of direct immunofluorescence microscopy, real-time PCR, or conventional PCR. J Clin Microbiol. 2012;50(6):1856–9.
223. Damiani C, Le Gal S, Da Costa C, Virmaux M, Nevez G, Totet A. Combined quantification of pulmonary Pneumocystis jirovecii DNA and serum (1->3)-beta-D-glucan for differential diagnosis of pneumocystis pneumonia and Pneumocystis colonization. J Clin Microbiol. 2013;51(10):3380–8.
224. Robert-Gangneux F, Belaz S, Revest M, Tattevin P, Jouneau S, Decaux O, et al. Diagnosis of Pneumocystis jirovecii pneumonia in immunocompromised patients by real-time PCR: a 4-year prospective study. J Clin Microbiol. 2014;52(9):3370–6.
225. Limper AH, Offord KP, Smith TF, Martin WJ 2nd. Pneumocystis carinii pneumonia. Differences in lung parasite number and inflammation in patients with and without AIDS. Am Rev Respir Dis. 1989;140(5):1204–9.
226. de Boer MG, Gelinck LB, van Zelst BD, van de Sande WW, Willems LN, van Dissel JT, et al. Beta-D-glucan and S-adenosylmethionine serum levels for the diagnosis of Pneumocystis pneumonia in HIV-negative patients: a prospective study. J Infect. 2011;62(1):93–100.
227. Costa JM, Botterel F, Cabaret O, Foulet F, Cordonnier C, Bretagne S. Association between circulating DNA, serum (1->3)-beta-D-glucan, and pulmonary fungal burden in Pneumocystis pneumonia. Clin Infect Dis. 2012;55(2):e5–8.
228. Karageorgopoulos DE, Qu JM, Korbila IP, Zhu YG, Vasileiou VA, Falagas ME. Accuracy of beta-D-glucan for the diagnosis of Pneumocystis jirovecii pneumonia: a meta-analysis. Clin Microbiol Infect. 2013;19(1):39–49.
229. Sasso M, Chastang-Dumas E, Bastide S, Alonso S, Lechiche C, Bourgeois N, et al. Performances of four real-time PCR assays for diagnosis of Pneumocystis jirovecii pneumonia. J Clin Microbiol. 2016;54(3):625–30.
230. Montesinos I, Brancart F, Schepers K, Jacobs F, Denis O, Delforge ML. Comparison of 2 real-time PCR assays for diagnosis of Pneumocystis jirovecii pneumonia in human immunodeficiency virus (HIV) and non-HIV immunocompromised patients. Diagn Microbiol Infect Dis. 2015;82(2):143–7.
231. Montesinos I, Delforge ML, Ajjaham F, Brancart F, Hites M, Jacobs F, et al. Evaluation of a new commercial real-time PCR

assay for diagnosis of Pneumocystis jirovecii pneumonia and identification of dihydropteroate synthase (DHPS) mutations. Diagn Microbiol Infect Dis. 2017;87(1):32–6.
232. Hauser PM, Bille J, Lass-Florl C, Geltner C, Feldmesser M, Levi M, et al. Multicenter, prospective clinical evaluation of respiratory samples from subjects at risk for Pneumocystis jirovecii infection by use of a commercial real-time PCR assay. J Clin Microbiol. 2011;49(5):1872–8.
233. Ribes JA, Limper AH, Espy MJ, Smith TF. PCR detection of Pneumocystis carinii in bronchoalveolar lavage specimens: analysis of sensitivity and specificity. J Clin Microbiol. 1997;35(4):830–5.
234. Alanio A, Desoubeaux G, Sarfati C, Hamane S, Bergeron A, Azoulay E, et al. Real-time PCR assay-based strategy for differentiation between active Pneumocystis jirovecii pneumonia and colonization in immunocompromised patients. Clin Microbiol Infect. 2011;17(10):1531–7.
235. Botterel F, Cabaret O, Foulet F, Cordonnier C, Costa JM, Bretagne S. Clinical significance of quantifying Pneumocystis jirovecii DNA by using real-time PCR in bronchoalveolar lavage fluid from immunocompromised patients. J Clin Microbiol. 2012;50(2):227–31.
236. To KK, Wong SC, Xu T, Poon RW, Mok KY, Chan JF, et al. Use of nasopharyngeal aspirate for diagnosis of pneumocystis pneumonia. J Clin Microbiol. 2013;51(5):1570–4.
237. Guigue N, Alanio A, Menotti J, Castro ND, Hamane S, Peyrony O, et al. Utility of adding Pneumocystis jirovecii DNA detection in nasopharyngeal aspirates in immunocompromised adult patients with febrile pneumonia. Med Mycol. 2015;53(3):241–7.
238. Kauffman CA. Histoplasmosis: a clinical and laboratory update. Clin Microbiol Rev. 2007;20(1):115–32.
239. Freifeld AG, Wheat LJ, Kaul DR. Histoplasmosis in solid organ transplant recipients: early diagnosis and treatment. Curr Opin Organ Transplant. 2009;14(6):601–5.
240. Jha V, Sree Krishna V, Varma N, Varma S, Chakrabarti A, Kohli HS, et al. Disseminated histoplasmosis 19 years after renal transplantation. Clin Nephrol. 1999;51(6):373–8.
241. Dufresne SF, Leblanc RE, Zhang SX, Marr KA, Neofytos D. Histoplasmosis and subcutaneous nodules in a kidney transplant recipient: erythema nodosum versus fungal panniculitis. Transpl Infect Dis. 2013;15:E58–63.
242. Kurtin PJ, McKinsey DS, Gupta MR, Driks M. Histoplasmosis in patients with acquired immunodeficiency syndrome. Hematologic and bone marrow manifestations. Am J Clin Pathol. 1990;93(3):367–72.
243. Padhye AA, Smith G, McLaughlin D, Standard PG, Kaufman L. Comparative evaluation of a chemiluminescent DNA probe and an exoantigen test for rapid identification of Histoplasma capsulatum. J Clin Microbiol. 1992;30(12):3108–11.
244. Martagon-Villamil J, Shrestha N, Sholtis M, Isada CM, Hall GS, Bryne T, et al. Identification of Histoplasma capsulatum from culture extracts by real-time PCR. J Clin Microbiol. 2003;41(3):1295–8.
245. Assi M, Martin S, Wheat LJ, Hage C, Freifeld A, Avery R, et al. Histoplasmosis after solid organ transplant. Clin Infect Dis. 2013;57(11):1542–9.
246. Connolly PA, Durkin MM, Lemonte AM, Hackett EJ, Wheat LJ. Detection of histoplasma antigen by a quantitative enzyme immunoassay. Clin Vaccine Immunol. 2007;14(12):1587–91.
247. Wheat LJ, Kohler RB, Tewari RP. Diagnosis of disseminated histoplasmosis by detection of Histoplasma capsulatum antigen in serum and urine specimens. N Engl J Med. 1986;314(2):83–8.
248. Durkin MM, Connolly PA, Wheat LJ. Comparison of radioimmunoassay and enzyme-linked immunoassay methods for detection of Histoplasma capsulatum var. capsulatum antigen. J Clin Microbiol. 1997;35(9):2252–5.
249. Wheat LJ, Connolly P, Durkin M, Book BK, Pescovitz MD. Elimination of false-positive Histoplasma antigenemia caused by human anti-rabbit antibodies in the second-generation Histoplasma antigen assay. Transpl Infect Dis. 2006;8(4):219–21.
250. Swartzentruber S, LeMonte A, Witt J, Fuller D, Davis T, Hage C, et al. Improved detection of Histoplasma antigenemia following dissociation of immune complexes. Clin Vaccine Immunol. 2009;16(3):320–2.
251. Cuellar-Rodriguez J, Avery RK, Lard M, Budev M, Gordon SM, Shrestha NK, et al. Histoplasmosis in solid organ transplant recipients: 10 years of experience at a large transplant center in an endemic area. Clin Infect Dis. 2009;49(5):710–6.
252. Hage C, Kleiman MB, Wheat LJ. Histoplasmosis in solid organ transplant recipients. Clin Infect Dis. 2010;50(1):122–3; author reply 3–4.
253. Hage CA, Ribes JA, Wengenack NL, Baddour LM, Assi M, McKinsey DS, et al. A multicenter evaluation of tests for diagnosis of histoplasmosis. Clin Infect Dis. 2011;53(5):448–54.
254. Grim SA, Proia L, Miller R, Alhyraba M, Costas-Chavarri A, Oberholzer J, et al. A multicenter study of histoplasmosis and blastomycosis after solid organ transplantation. Transpl Infect Dis. 2012;14(1):17–23.
255. Theel ES. Reply to "low-positive histoplasma antigen results in the MVista assay should not be assumed to be false positive". J Clin Microbiol. 2014;52(12):4446.
256. Hage CA, Wheat LJ. Low-positive histoplasma antigen results in the MVista assay should not be assumed to be false positive. J Clin Microbiol. 2014;52(12):4445.
257. Theel ES, Ramanan P. Clinical significance of low-positive histoplasma urine antigen results. J Clin Microbiol. 2014;52(9):3444–6.
258. Hage CA, Davis TE, Fuller D, Egan L, Witt JR 3rd, Wheat LJ, et al. Diagnosis of histoplasmosis by antigen detection in BAL fluid. Chest. 2010;137(3):623–8.
259. Cloud JL, Bauman SK, Neary BP, Ludwig KG, Ashwood ER. Performance characteristics of a polyclonal enzyme immunoassay for the quantitation of Histoplasma antigen in human urine samples. Am J Clin Pathol. 2007;128(1):18–22.
260. Wheat LJ. Invalid comparison of the IMMY Histoplasma antigen assay with the "gold standard". Am J Clin Pathol. 2008;129(4):661–3; author reply 3–5.
261. LeMonte A, Egan L, Connolly P, Durkin M, Wheat LJ. Evaluation of the IMMY ALPHA Histoplasma antigen enzyme immunoassay for diagnosis of histoplasmosis marked by antigenuria. Clin Vaccine Immunol. 2007;14(6):802–3.
262. Cloud JL, Bauman SK, Pelfrey JM, Ashwood ER. Biased report on the IMMY ALPHA Histoplasma antigen enzyme immunoassay for diagnosis of histoplasmosis. Clin Vaccine Immunol. 2007;14(10):1389–90; author reply 90–1.
263. McKinsey DS, McKinsey JP, Northcutt N, Sarria JC. Interlaboratory discrepancy of antigenuria results in 2 patients with AIDS and histoplasmosis. Diagn Microbiol Infect Dis. 2009;63(1):111–4.
264. Cloud JL, Hanson KE, Bauman SK, Ashwood ER. Extent of interlaboratory discrepancies for polyclonal Histoplasma antigen enzyme immunoassay cannot be determined without a large split-sample study. Diagn Microbiol Infect Dis. 2010;66(2):233–4.
265. McKinsey DS, McKinsey J, Northcutt N, Sarria J. Extent of Interlaboratory discrepancies for polyclonal Histoplasma antigen enzyme imunoassay (EIA) cannot be determined without a large split-sample study (reply). Diagn Microbiol Infect Dis. 2010;66(3):339–40.
266. Theel ES, Harring JA, Dababneh AS, Rollins LO, Bestrom JE, Jespersen DJ. Reevaluation of commercial reagents for detection of Histoplasma capsulatum antigen in urine. J Clin Microbiol. 2015;53(4):1198–203.

267. Theel ES, Jespersen DJ, Harring J, Mandrekar J, Binnicker MJ. Evaluation of an enzyme immunoassay for detection of Histoplasma capsulatum antigen from urine specimens. J Clin Microbiol. 2013;51(11):3555–9.
268. Zhang C, Lei GS, Lee CH, Hage CA. Evaluation of two new enzyme immunoassay reagents for diagnosis of histoplasmosis in a cohort of clinically characterized patients. Med Mycol. 2015;53(8):868–73.
269. Wheat LJ, Hackett E, Durkin M, Connolly P, Petraitiene R, Walsh TJ, et al. Histoplasmosis-associated cross-reactivity in the BioRad Platelia Aspergillus enzyme immunoassay. Clin Vaccine Immunol. 2007;14(5):638–40.
270. Ranque S, Pelletier R, Michel-Nguyen A, Dromer F. Platelia aspergillus assay for diagnosis of disseminated histoplasmosis. Eur J Clin Microbiol Infect Dis. 2007;26(12):941-3.
271. Girouard G, Lachance C, Pelletier R. Observations on (1-3)-beta-D-glucan detection as a diagnostic tool in endemic mycosis caused by Histoplasma or Blastomyces. J Med Microbiol. 2007;56(Pt 7):1001-2.
272. Egan L, Connolly P, Wheat LJ, Fuller D, Dais TE, Knox KS, et al. Histoplasmosis as a cause for a positive Fungitell (1 --> 3)-beta-D-glucan test. Med Mycol. 2008;46(1):93–5.
273. Bracca A, Tosello ME, Girardini JE, Amigot SL, Gomez C, Serra E. Molecular detection of Histoplasma capsulatum var. capsulatum in human clinical samples. J Clin Microbiol. 2003;41(4):1753–5.
274. Ohno H, Tanabe K, Umeyama T, Kaneko Y, Yamagoe S, Miyazaki Y. Application of nested PCR for diagnosis of histoplasmosis. J Infect Chemother. 2013;19(5):999–1003.
275. Simon S, Veron V, Boukhari R, Blanchet D, Aznar C. Detection of Histoplasma capsulatum DNA in human samples by real-time polymerase chain reaction. Diagn Microbiol Infect Dis. 2010;66(3):268–73.
276. Munoz C, Gomez BL, Tobon A, Arango K, Restrepo A, Correa MM, et al. Validation and clinical application of a molecular method for identification of Histoplasma capsulatum in human specimens in Colombia, South America. Clin Vaccine Immunol. 2010;17(1):62–7.
277. Qualtieri J, Stratton CW, Head DR, Tang YW. PCR detection of Histoplasma capsulatum var. capsulatum in whole blood of a renal transplant patient with disseminated histoplasmosis. Ann Clin Lab Sci. 2009;39(4):409–12.
278. Muraosa Y, Toyotome T, Yahiro M, Watanabe A, Shikanai-Yasuda MA, Kamei K. Detection of Histoplasma capsulatum from clinical specimens by cycling probe-based real-time PCR and nested real-time PCR. Med Mycol. 2016;54(4):433–8.
279. Saubolle MA, McKellar PP, Sussland D. Epidemiologic, clinical, and diagnostic aspects of coccidioidomycosis. J Clin Microbiol. 2007;45(1):26–30.
280. Blair JE. Coccidioidomycosis in patients who have undergone transplantation. Ann N Y Acad Sci. 2007;1111:365–76.
281. Galgiani JN, Ampel NM, Blair JE, Catanzaro A, Geertsma F, Hoover SE, et al. Executive summary: 2016 Infectious Diseases Society of America (IDSA) clinical practice guideline for the treatment of coccidioidomycosis. Clin Infect Dis. 2016;63(6):717–22.
282. Mendoza N, Noel P, Blair JE. Diagnosis, treatment, and outcomes of coccidioidomycosis in allogeneic stem cell transplantation. Transpl Infect Dis. 2015;17(3):380–8.
283. Saubolle MA. Laboratory aspects in the diagnosis of coccidioidomycosis. Ann N Y Acad Sci. 2007;1111:301–14.
284. Brandt ME, Gomez BL, Warnock DW. *Histoplasma, Blastomyces, Coccidioides*, and other dimorphic fungi causing systemic mycoses. In: Versalovic J, editor. Manual of clinical microbiology. 2. 10th ed. Washington, DC: ASM Press; 2011. p. 1902–18.
285. Rempe S, Sachdev MS, Bhakta R, Pineda-Roman M, Vaz A, Carlson RW. Coccidioides immitis fungemia: clinical features and survival in 33 adult patients. Heart Lung. 2007;36(1):64–71.
286. Keckich DW, Blair JE, Vikram HR. Coccidioides fungemia in six patients, with a review of the literature. Mycopathologia. 2010;170(2):107–15.
287. Sheff KW, York ER, Driebe EM, Barker BM, Rounsley SD, Waddell VG, et al. Development of a rapid, cost-effective TaqMan Real-Time PCR Assay for identification and differentiation of Coccidioides immitis and Coccidioides posadasii. Med Mycol. 2010;48(3):466–9.
288. Warnock DW. Coccidioides species as potential agents of bioterrorism. Future Microbiol. 2007;2(3):277–83.
289. Pappagianis D, Zimmer BL. Serology of coccidioidomycosis. Clin Microbiol Rev. 1990;3(3):247–68.
290. Kaufman L, Sekhon AS, Moledina N, Jalbert M, Pappagianis D. Comparative evaluation of commercial Premier EIA and microimmunodiffusion and complement fixation tests for Coccidioides immitis antibodies. J Clin Microbiol. 1995;33(3):618–9.
291. Martins TB, Jaskowski TD, Mouritsen CL, Hill HR. Comparison of commercially available enzyme immunoassay with traditional serological tests for detection of antibodies to Coccidioides immitis. J Clin Microbiol. 1995;33(4):940–3.
292. Zartarian M, Peterson EM, de la Maza LM. Detection of antibodies to Coccidioides immitis by enzyme immunoassay. Am J Clin Pathol. 1997;107(2):148–53.
293. Lindsley MD, Ahn Y, McCotter O, Gade L, Hurst SF, Brandt ME, et al. Evaluation of the specificity of two enzyme immunoassays for Coccidioidomycosis by using Sera from a region of Endemicity and a region of Nonendemicity. Clin Vaccine Immunol. 2015;22(10):1090–5.
294. Malo J, Holbrook E, Zangeneh T, Strawter C, Oren E, Robey I, et al. Enhanced antibody detection and diagnosis of Coccidioidomycosis with the MiraVista IgG and IgM detection enzyme immunoassay. J Clin Microbiol. 2017;55(3):893–901.
295. Durkin M, Connolly P, Kuberski T, Myers R, Kubak BM, Bruckner D, et al. Diagnosis of coccidioidomycosis with use of the Coccidioides antigen enzyme immunoassay. Clin Infect Dis. 2008;47(8):e69–73.
296. Durkin M, Estok L, Hospenthal D, Crum-Cianflone N, Swartzentruber S, Hackett E, et al. Detection of Coccidioides antigenemia following dissociation of immune complexes. Clin Vaccine Immunol. 2009;16(10):1453–6.
297. Binnicker MJ, Buckwalter SP, Eisberner JJ, Stewart RA, McCullough AE, Wohlfiel SL, et al. Detection of Coccidioides species in clinical specimens by real-time PCR. J Clin Microbiol. 2007;45(1):173–8.
298. de Aguiar CR, Nogueira Brilhante RS, Gadelha Rocha MF, Araujo Moura FE, Pires de Camargo Z, Costa Sidrim JJ. Rapid diagnosis of coccidioidomycosis by nested PCR assay of sputum. Clin Microbiol Infect. 2007;13(4):449–51.
299. Vucicevic D, Blair JE, Binnicker MJ, McCullough AE, Kusne S, Vikram HR, et al. The utility of Coccidioides polymerase chain reaction testing in the clinical setting. Mycopathologia. 2010;170(5):345–51.

Viral Diagnostics

49

Robin K. Avery and Belinda Yen-Lieberman

Background and Introduction

Advances in diagnostic testing for transplant-related infections, particularly molecular viral diagnostic assays, constitute one of the most notable changes in transplant infectious disease over the last two decades [1, 2]. This chapter discusses recent developments in diagnostics for cytomegalovirus (CMV), Epstein-Barr virus (EBV), BK virus (BKV), community respiratory viruses (CRVs), parvovirus, hepatitis viruses, HIV, and other viral agents of importance in solid organ and hematopoietic stem cell transplantation. The recent debate regarding the extent of nucleic acid amplification (NAT) testing for HIV, HBV, and HCV in proposed transplant donors is reviewed [3]. Different uses for molecular viral tests in the transplant recipient are discussed, ranging from facilitation of antiviral preventive strategies to determination of length of therapy for active infections. The advantages and disadvantages of single vs. multiplex assays are explored [2]. Challenges in this field include interlaboratory variation [4], management of false-positive and discordant test results, and need for consensus on which patients should receive which testing, at what intervals, and for what period of time. Despite these challenges, molecular viral diagnostics have clearly contributed significantly to the reduction of infectious morbidity, by enabling early diagnosis and intervention, resulting in such notable examples as the reduction in severe CMV disease [5, 6] and in kidney allograft loss due to BKV [7]. Future clinical trials in the field of transplantation should incorporate accepted definitions of infection and practices of viral monitoring for transplant-associated viruses [8].

R. K. Avery (✉)
Division of Infectious Disease, Johns Hopkins,
Baltimore, MD, USA
e-mail: ravery4@jhmi.edu

B. Yen-Lieberman
Pathology and Laboratory Medicine Institute, Cleveland Clinic,
Department of Laboratory Medicine, Cleveland, OH, USA
e-mail: yenb@ccf.org

General Considerations, Definitions, and Uses of Viral Diagnostic Tests

The term "serology" or "serologic test" refers in general to an assay which detects an antibody to a specific pathogen, usually IgG or IgM. A panel of serologic tests is performed on both donor and recipient prior to transplantation. The results may be used to disqualify a prospective donor or to restrict the use of the donor to a specific subgroup of recipients or more commonly may be used for risk stratification and posttransplant management for particular infections (e.g., the donor-seropositive, recipient-seronegative or D+/R- group which is the subgroup at the highest risk for both CMV and EBV, respectively, in solid organ transplantation) [9]. Serologies are of limited value in diagnosing active infections in the posttransplant patient, since immunosuppressed patients may not mount an IgM response even in the setting of an active infection and some recipients with de novo posttransplant hypogammaglobulinemia have globally low IgG levels [10]. IgG serology remains positive for life, and pathogen-specific IgG titers do not usually correlate with the activity of infection, so obtaining an IgG level (for CMV or EBV, among others) is not generally helpful in diagnosing an acute illness in a transplant recipient (an exception is when the clinician wants to know if a previously seronegative patient has seroconverted, which might have prognostic value, for example, in predicting ongoing risk for recurrences of CMV viremia) [11].

Antigen-based testing, such as the pp65 antigenemia test for CMV, does have a potential role in posttransplant recipients, as this is a direct detection of the virus and not a reflection of the patient's immune response to the virus [12, 13]. However, in most cases, antigen detection is semiquantitative and does not provide an exact viral load to follow over time. In addition, some antigen tests (such as the pp65 antigenemia test for CMV) decay with time, and thus lose sensitivity, if the sample is mailed into a central laboratory or if there is a delay between obtaining the blood sample and laboratory performance of the test.

A. Safdar (ed.), *Principles and Practice of Transplant Infectious Diseases*, https://doi.org/10.1007/978-1-4939-9034-4_49

Table 49.1 Molecular tests for selected transplant-related viruses

Test Name	Method	Dynamic range at Copies/ml	Sensitivity	Specificity	Test Status
Qiagen Artus CMV RGQ	Real-time PCR	159 IU/ml–1.0 × 10^7 IU/ml	96.6%	100%	IVD
Abbott RealTime CMV	Real-time PCR	31.21 IU/ml–156 × 10^6 IU/ml	95–97%	99%	IVD
Roche CMV [19]	Real-time PCR; CAP/CTM	137 IU/ml–1 × 10^6 IU/ml	97.5–98.0%	100%	IVD
RealStar qCMV (Altona) CMV	Real-time PCR	150 IU/ml–1 × 10^6 IU/ml	100%	100%	ASR
Qiagen Artus EBV	Real-time PCR	500–5.0 × 10^6 IU/ml	95–97%	99%	ASR
RealStar EBV qPCR (Altona)___	Real-time PCR	500–10,000,000 copies/ml	94.5%	98.1%	ASR
Qiagen BKV	Real-time PCR	500–5.0 × 10^6 copies/ml	95–97%	99%	ASR
RealStar BKV (Altona)	Real-time PCR	300–100,000,000 copies/ml	100%	100%	ASR

ASR analyte-specific reagents, *IVD* in vitro diagnostic test (FDA-cleared)

Molecular testing has revolutionized viral diagnosis in transplantation [14–16]. Molecular diagnostic tests are generally highly sensitive assays that directly detect the virus' genetic material such as DNA or RNA (depending on the type of virus) and can be qualitative or quantitative. There are a variety of methodologies, including polymerase chain reaction (PCR) technologies, hybrid capture assay, nucleic acid sequence-based amplification (NASBA), transcription-mediated amplification (TMA), and others [1, 2, 17, 18]. Performance characteristics of some of these tests in comparative studies are shown in Table 49.1. Testing may be *monoplex* (a single pathogen tested at one time) or *multiplex* (which refers to several or many pathogens tested in one sample).

The advantages and disadvantages of each strategy are discussed below. The uses of molecular diagnostic assays are many. Most commonly these tests are performed on whole blood or plasma (and may be referred to as the blood "viral load") when quantifying the virus, although other relevant samples may be tested, such as urine in the case of BK virus or a nasopharyngeal swab or bronchoalveolar lavage fluid in the case of respiratory viruses. A list of potential uses for quantitative molecular diagnostic tests is shown in Table 49.2. The most common uses are in preemptive therapy or screening for viral infection prior to symptoms, in diagnosis of an acute infectious syndrome, and in monitoring for blood viral clearance to help determine the duration of therapy for an infection episode.

An even newer set of diagnostic tests is currently under development, namely, pathogen-specific assays of cellular immune function. Of these, the one in widest use so far is the interferon-gamma release assay (IGRA) for tuberculosis (QuantiFERON-TB Gold in-tube, Cellestis/Qiagen Inc., Germantown, Maryland) [20]. This assay is specific for *Mycobacterium tuberculosis* and avoids false-positive results due to BCG vaccination, as with the tuberculin skin test [20]. Similar assays for CMV and BKV have been an area of intense research interest. Recent results suggest that measurement of CMV-specific immune function is useful in risk stratification of high-risk organ transplant recipients [21] and in hematopoietic stem cell transplant recipients [22]. It is likely that these tests will be more commonly used in the future in transplant virology, with an eye to devising personalized prevention programs using assessments of individual patients' pathogen-specific immunity. However, testing for virus-specific cell-mediated immunity has not yet become widely performed at the time of this writing, so the current chapter will focus mainly on molecular diagnostic testing.

Table 49.2 Potential uses for quantitative molecular diagnostic tests

Screening of living or deceased prospective organ donors
Diagnosis of an acute infectious syndrome
Preemptive therapy or monitoring/screening for viral infection
Prediction of severity of disease (quantitative viral load)
Monitoring for resolution of infection and guidance for duration of therapy
Monitoring for recurrence of infection after completion of therapy
Determining the success of viral suppression or secondary prophylaxis
Clues to the presence of antiviral resistance (rise in viral load or failure to decrease on therapy)
Genotypic antiviral resistance testing (e.g., UL97 or UL54 mutations in CMV)

Cytomegalovirus

CMV remains one of the most common viruses to reactivate in the posttransplant patient. In the early years of transplantation, diagnosis of CMV infection relied on detection of viral growth in tissue culture, which was laborious and could take several weeks for a positive result to be obtained, particularly if the samples have low viral load. The advent of shell-vial centrifugation culture methodology shortened the turnaround time from 4–5 days to 48 h, but this test was less sensitive at lower viral loads and did not provide quantitative results [13]. The pp65 antigenemia test was then devised, and multiple studies have validated its utility in posttransplant monitoring and as a basis for preemptive therapy [12, 13, 23]. The pp65 antigenemia test detects CMV-infected white blood cells in peripheral blood using a fluorescent assay which requires the laboratory technician to visually scan the slide and to report the number of positive (infected) cells per unit of area. It is thus a semiquantitative test. Although this does give some idea of the magnitude of the viral load, it is not as definitive in viral load measurement as quantitative molecular tests, which are usually expressed as DNA copies/ml or, most recently, in international units. The pp65 antigenemia assay is labor-intensive for the laboratory and thus may be problematic for transplant centers with very high volumes of tests. In addition, the results decay after obtaining the blood sample, so it is less suitable for mailing in to a central laboratory from patients who live a long distance away from the transplant center.

Molecular diagnostic tests for CMV have largely supplanted previous tests at many centers. Their quantification of the blood viral load, ease of handling high volumes of samples, and lack of decay with time if properly handled make the CMV DNA by PCR a useful choice for a transplant center with high volumes of samples and/or patients outside the immediate area. Quantitative viral loads often correspond to severity of disease, although interlaboratory variation has hampered the attempt to describe universal cutoff values for clinical categories and decision-making [4, 24, 25]. In solid organ transplant recipients, tissue-invasive CMV episodes generally have the highest viral loads (e.g., >50,000–100,000 copies/ml); asymptomatic viremia has the lowest viral loads (e.g., <5000 copies/ml); and the intermediate category of "CMV syndrome" has viral loads in between the other two categories, although exceptions may occur. However, widespread adoption of the WHO standard should allow for more reliable, shared correlations between viral loads and clinical manifestations, after the initial period of clinician adjustment to a new scale [25]. The quantification of the viral load also allows for following levels over time, so that treatment decisions, including when to initiate antiviral therapy, when to discontinue antiviral therapy, or when to switch from full-dose therapy to secondary suppressive dose prophylaxis, can be based on serial results of these quantitative tests (Table 49.2). A notable example of the use of sequential viral load measurements is the use of a risk-adapted, CMV viral load-based preemptive therapy program for CMV prevention in hematopoietic stem cell transplant recipients, utilized at the Fred Hutchinson Cancer Research Center [26].

Molecular tests are not without problems, however. PCR is a highly sensitive test, and false positives can occur, leading to unnecessary therapy or unnecessary concern on the part of patients and clinicians; such false-positive tests, however, are usually low level and may be subjected to repeat analysis or verified by obtaining a new sample. The risks of false-positive testing in disqualification of potential donors have been a topic of discussion regarding the revised solid organ transplant donor guidelines [3].

Other potential problems with molecular testing include logistics. A highly developed system must be in place, particularly for preemptive therapy, for the loss of even one sample or failure to act upon one sample result might lead to full-blown symptomatic infection. But perhaps the most problematic aspect is that of interlaboratory variation [4, 24, 25], depending on the use of whole blood versus plasma; commercial versus individually developed assays, different reagents, and primers; and a host of other factors. The American Society of Transplantation (AST)'s Infectious Disease Community of Practice, together with the Canadian Society of Transplantation, published an interlaboratory comparison of CMV PCR testing involving 33 laboratories, showing wide variation in results (between a 2- and 4-$\log_{10}$ copies/ml difference in some cases) and need for more standardization [4]. The World Health Organization (WHO)'s standardization initiative should help to ameliorate this situation and to improve the comparability of viral loads obtained in different laboratories. As of 2010, the WHO announced an international standard for CMV molecular testing, which enables laboratories to calibrate their assays and which involves reporting in international units per mL [25]. Another recent development, in 2012, was the first FDA approval of a quantitative CMV PCR test (the COBAS AmpliPrep/COBAS TaqMan CMV test or CAP/CTM CMV test) which is a fully automated test, and the one copy of CMV DNA (as defined by the COBAS® AmpliPrep/COBAS® TaqMan® CMV test) is equivalent to 0.91 international unit (IU) on the First WHO International Standard for Human Cytomegalovirus for Nucleic Acid Amplification Techniques (NIBSC 09/162) [19, 25]. An international multicenter comparison of the CAP/CTM CMV test in five laboratories at transplant centers compared the performance of this test with local assays, using blinded samples and clinical specimens [19]. This study showed high interlaboratory agreement of the CAP/CTM test and quantification differences using local assays [19]. It has been suggested that this test might serve as the basis for more widely accepted cutoffs for prediction of CMV disease and thresholds for preemptive therapy [25].

A final category of molecular diagnostic tests for CMV is those used to determine genotypic resistance, on analogy to HIV. CMV antiviral resistance commonly occurs in two sites, known as UL97 and UL54 [27, 28]. UL97 relates to the ability of a viral-encoded thymidine kinase to initiate triphosphorylation of ganciclovir to its active form, and thus UL97 mutations confer resistance to ganciclovir but not to foscarnet or cidofovir. UL54 mutations, on the other hand, affect the viral DNA polymerase and so may confer resistance to ganciclovir, foscarnet, or cidofovir or more than one of these [27, 28]. Phenotypic resistance testing is less commonly used now, as it is time-consuming and labor-intensive. Genotypic resistance testing should be obtained in any clinical situation where resistance is suspected, such as a persistently high CMV viral load, failure of the viral load to decrease on therapy, or clinical lack of response to therapy after sufficient time has elapsed.

Epstein-Barr Virus

The utility of EBV serologic testing such as EBV VCA-IgG is principally in the pretransplant period, establishing whether or not the donor and the recipient have ever been infected with EBV. Most adults, 90% or greater, are EBV-seropositive, although pediatric transplant recipients are more likely to be seronegative [29]. As with CMV, the donor and recipient serogroups carry differential risks for the development of serious infections. In the case of EBV, the main issue is risk for EBV-related posttransplant lymphoproliferative disorder (PTLD). The highest-risk category in solid organ transplantation is the EBV D+/R- category; as similar to the case of CMV, there is no antecedent immunity in the recipient, but a viral load is acquired from the donor at the time of transplantation [29]. Knowledge of this D+/R- status may allow for closer surveillance, modulation of immunosuppression, and, at some centers, serial monitoring of the EBV DNA viral load [30, 31]. There are several different EBV serologies that are commonly performed: the Epstein-Barr nuclear antibody (EBNA), Epstein-Barr early antigen (EA), viral capsid antigen (VCA) IgG, and VCA-IgM. Of these, the VCA-IgG is the most reliable test for assessing whether or not the patient is seropositive (i.e., whether they have ever had EBV infection), while the VCA-IgM correlates better with current or recent disease although IgM response may be blunted in an immunocompromised host, so there is limited utility in ordering EBV serologies in patients following transplantation. For the diagnosis of active EBV infection and the assessment of PTLD risk, obtaining quantitative blood PCR testing is more helpful than serologies [29, 30]. EBV DNA viral loads may be performed on plasma or on whole blood. As in the case of CMV, interlaboratory variation also exists with respect to EBV DNAemia measurement [24]. EBV DNA viral loads may be followed over time in high-risk patients and may be useful as a gauge of the degree of success of interventions such as reduction of immunosuppression, which should be followed by a corresponding decrease in the EBV DNA blood viral load, unless the patient has active PTLD. Green et al. have demonstrated the predictive value of this monitoring [30], and McDiarmid has shown the utility of EBV DNA monitoring, coupled with reduction of immunosuppression and ganciclovir therapy, in the reduction of PTLD risk (from 10% to 5%) in a cohort of pediatric liver transplant recipients [31]. Successful therapy of PTLD with rituximab or rituximab plus combination chemotherapy is often associated with a rapid fall of the EBV DNA blood viral load to undetectable levels. However, later rebounds of EBV DNAemia may occur and do not necessarily portend recurrences of PTLD [30].

BK Virus

BK virus (BKV) is a member of the polyomavirus family, along with JC virus, SV40, and others. Acquisition of BKV is common in the general population and may occur early in life in asymptomatic form. BKV has a predilection for cells of the urinary tract including the bladder, ureters, and kidneys. BKV can cause hemorrhagic cystitis in HSCT recipients. In kidney recipients, its effects can be devastating [7]. After kidney transplant, BKV can silently reactivate and can cause a type of allograft nephropathy (BKVAN) that begins with interstitial nephritis and progresses to fibrosis and nonfunctioning allograft tissue. If no prevention program is in place, between 4% and 8% of all kidney allografts may be lost to BKV.

Screening and early intervention for BKV have been a major advance over the last 10 years and have led to an approximately eightfold reduction in kidney graft loss due to BKV. Most kidney transplant centers now employ BKV screening of asymptomatic patients using one of several available tests on blood or urine [7]. Serial screening for BKV allows for early reduction of immunosuppression, which is the most established therapy for BKV, and may reduce viral load by allowing for a more vigorous host immune response to BKV [7, 32, 33].

The tests available for BKV screening include urine cytology for the evidence of polyomavirus-related changes in the form of inclusion-containing "decoy cells," quantitative or qualitative BKV DNA performed on urine or blood, and BKV VP1 mRNA [34]. If urine is screened, a positive test might trigger testing of blood for the BKV DNA viral load. Blood BKV DNA viral loads correlate more with the presence of BKV in renal allograft tissue, as urine may frequently be positive for lower levels of BKV DNA without active involvement of renal tissue. Urine BKV DNA viral loads are typically several logs higher than blood viral loads. International consensus guidelines have established the blood viral load of 10,000 copies/ml as a common threshold for intervention in kidney recipients [35]. By contrast, BKV blood viral load has not traditionally been considered as predictive of symptomatic disease in HSCT recipients, although recent results by Gilis et al. suggest that BKV viremia is correlated with severity of disease in HSCT also [36].

BKV DNA testing is also useful for monitoring responses to interventions such as reduction of immunosuppression. If reduction of immunosuppression appears not to have produced the desired reduction in viral load, some centers employ off-label antiviral therapies for BKV [37] such as cidofovir, quinolones, intravenous immune globulin (IVIg), and leflunomide. There are no randomized trials to date comparing these therapies, and reduction of immunosuppression remains the cornerstone of management. Thus, BKV DNA quantitative monitoring can serve as a guide to institution of interventions and as a guide to resumption of full-dose immunosuppression after an episode has resolved.

Routine serial monitoring of BKV DNA is not currently recommended in solid organ transplant recipients other than kidney or kidney-pancreas recipients. In liver, lung, and heart transplant recipients, reactivation of BKV may also occur, but the clinical significance is less certain. In hematopoietic stem cell transplant recipients, routine serial BKV viral load monitoring has not been standard in the past, but may emerge as a strategy in the future based on recent results [36].

Community-Acquired Respiratory Viruses

Community-acquired respiratory viruses (CRVs) pose a threat to transplant recipients in two ways: the risk of severe respiratory involvement during an infection episode and the late risk in lung transplant recipients for transient or permanent decreases in lung allograft function after a CRV infection has resolved [38]. Early diagnosis is crucial in allowing for rapid treatment; a multicenter study of pandemic H1N1 influenza in SOT recipients demonstrated that early treatment, within 2 days of onset of symptoms, was associated with lower risk of ICU admission and respiratory failure [39]. Early and rapid influenza diagnosis is particularly important, as antiviral medications effective against influenza are available. The CDC and Advisory Committee on Immunization Practices (ACIP) publish an annual guide to prevention and treatment of influenza which contains antiviral resistance information pertinent to the particular strains that are circulating in any given influenza season [40]. For other respiratory viruses, there is less agreement on treatment protocols, but many transplant centers use ribavirin (inhaled or oral) for treatment of respiratory syncytial virus (RSV) [41] and sometimes parainfluenza virus and human metapneumovirus (hMP) infections as well [42].

Diagnosis of CRV infections is also very important for infection control programs, as such viruses can spread rapidly through transplant wards and may have devastating effects particularly in patients with recent transplants or active rejection. Different respiratory viruses have different modes of transmission, so droplet precautions, contact precautions, or both may be appropriate. In any case, rapid application of appropriate precautions can prevent harm to other vulnerable hospitalized patients.

Diagnosis of CRVs has traditionally been performed on respiratory samples, most commonly nasopharyngeal (NP) swabs or washes or BAL fluid. Diagnosis may be accomplished by direct fluorescent antibody testing (DFA), by PCR, or by culture in tissue culture. Since culture-based diagnostics take at least several days, these are not suitable for rapid diagnosis and are now utilized primarily for determination of viral viability in a patient who is persistently PCR-positive, for example.

The choice of DFA or PCR for initial testing depends upon the virus(es) being detected. Some multiplex assays are wholly PCR-based and some are a combination of DFA and PCR tests. Since respiratory viruses have considerable overlap in their clinical presenting symptoms, and coinfections may occur, it makes sense to perform a multiplex assay incorporating the most likely agents, rather than testing for a single virus at a time. Common combinations of tests include influenza/RSV, influenza/RSV/parainfluenza/adenovirus/human metapneumovirus, and other more extensive combinations including rhinovirus and coronaviruses. Even rhinovirus infection (the "common cold") may have severe consequences in immunocompromised patients [43], so expanded multiplex testing is increasingly of interest.

In addition to initial diagnosis of an infection episode, repeat testing may be used for assessment of viral clearance in patients with ongoing symptoms or for infection control purposes in determination of the length of isolation precautions. It should be noted, however, that testing which does not rely on viral viability may be detecting residual fragments of nonviable virus.

There are special considerations for lung transplant recipients with regard to respiratory viruses, since long-lasting allograft dysfunction may result some months after resolution of the viral illness [38]. This may be true even for such common viruses as rhinoviruses and also for asymptomatic or minimally symptomatic infection episodes. At such times, viruses are not usually detectable, but progression to bronchiolitis obliterans syndrome (BOS), a chronic progressive form of lung allograft dysfunction, may occur due to cytokine release and injury and repair processes that are the subject of current research. It is thus of particular importance to test lung transplant recipients early, even if they are only minimally symptomatic, as viral detection might lead to therapy that can lessen the risk of this later allograft dysfunction. Obtaining a nasopharyngeal swab on all lung transplant recipients with new-onset respiratory symptoms is reasonable (Table 49.3).

Parvovirus

Parvovirus B19 is an under-recognized cause of anemia in transplant recipients [44]. While many centers test for parvovirus in patients who present with anemia without other

Table 49.3 Respiratory viruses (FDA cleared and commercially available)

Test name	Methods	Sample	Sensitivity/specificity	Status
xTAG Respiratory Viral Panel (12 viruses); Luminex NxTAG RPP (Luminex) ARIES FluA/B &RSV (Luminex)	PCR and Luminex; detection (9 h) MAGPIX RPP (12 viruses; 3 h) MultiCode PCR, WalkAway system	NP swabs NP swabs NP swabs	78.3–100%/91.3–100%; depends on which virus 97%/99% 97%/99%	IVD IVD IVD
ProFlu+ (FluA/FluB and RSV); Hologic	Real-time PCR; sample to results system – Panther	NP swabs/throat swabs	Sen/Spe 95–100%/ 92.6–98.6%	IVD
Simplexa FluA/B, RSV Focus (DiaSorin)	Real-time PCR (3.5 h)	NP swabs; tracheal aspirates	98–100%/93–99%	IVD
Verigene Respiratory Panel(FluA/B/RS) Luminex Nanosphere Luminex	Real-time PCR on Verigene SP system (3 h)	NP swabs/viral cultured samples	89.8–99.2%	IVD
ProFAST+ (Flu A/H1, A/H3); A/H1N1.2009; Hologic	Real-time PCR smart cycler (5.5 h)	NP swabs	95.4–100%/99.0–100%	IVD
RP FILMARRAY (22 viruses and bacteria), BioFire (BioMerieux)	Nested PCR; rapid test (70 min) WalkAway system	NP swabs, throat swab, and BAL	97% sensitivity 99.7% specificity	IVD
eSensor RVP (GenMark dx) XT-8. Tat 5.5 hrs NP swabs & throat swabs 99.2%/ 99.7% IVD	XT-8 System Detection; TAT 6.0 hrs (12 viruses)	NP swabs and throat swabs	99.2%/99.7%	IVD

explanations, it has only recently been recognized that parvovirus can also cause milder degrees of anemia in a larger number of patients [45]. Diagnosis by serology is less useful, as the majority of adults are IgG-seropositive and transplant recipients may not mount an IgM response even during active infections. Bone marrow examination may reveal disordered erythroid progenitors including giant erythroblasts. Parvovirus PCR testing on blood is the most useful noninvasive test for diagnosing active parvovirus infection in a transplant recipient. This testing is important both as a basis for therapy with IVIg and reduction of immunosuppression and also for infection control and isolation purposes. Molecular testing has also led to the suggestion that viral loads of parvovirus from the donated organ, detected in graft preservation solution, may correlate with increased risk for posttransplant parvovirus infection in the recipient [46].

Agents of Viral Hepatitis

Viral hepatitis agents include hepatitis A, hepatitis B, hepatitis C, hepatitis D, and hepatitis E abbreviated as HAV, HBV, HCV, HDV, HEV, respectively. Of these, HBV and HCV are most commonly found in transplant recipients, although recently detection of hepatitis E has been on the rise [47]. HBV or HCV may be pre-existing in the recipient or may be acquired de novo posttransplant, either from the donor or from transfusions [48]. In the pre-existing category, HBV or HCV may be the reason for performing a liver transplant or may be a comorbidity in a patient receiving a non-liver transplant.

Hepatitis B

Serologic testing for HBV is complex and relies on an understanding of the timing of detection of several different HBV antigens and antibodies. Active infection is characterized by a rise in the hepatitis B surface antigen (HBsAg), which then falls to undetectable in about 90% of patients; then subsequently there is a rise in the anti-HBs (hepatitis B surface antibody) titer. Between the time that HBsAg becomes undetectable and anti-HBs appears, there is a "window period" during which time neither is detectable, but the HBV core IgM antibody (anti-HBc IgM) and HBV DNA are detectable. After natural infection, the anti-HBc IgM disappears and the anti-HBc IgG appears, so persons in whom HBV infection has been successfully controlled by the immune system generally are positive for both anti-HBc and anti-HBs, but negative for HBsAg. In about 10% of infected individuals, antibody seroconversion does not occur and the HBsAg is persistently positive in chronic infection. Such individuals may progress to cirrhosis and/or hepatocellular carcinoma and may require a liver transplant with the goal of eradicating HBV infection, utilizing posttransplant prophylaxis with hepatitis B immune globulin (HBIg) and an anti-HBV antiviral agent such as entecavir. In such individuals the blood HBV DNA is also commonly positive pretransplant and may be serially followed posttransplant to detect any recurrence early.

Pretransplant screening of the recipient commonly includes HBsAg, anti-HBc, and anti-HBs. A positive HBsAg is indicative of current infection which may represent either recent infection or chronic carriage. An isolated positive anti-HBs is usually the result of HBV vaccination, as the vaccine is produced from recombinant HBsAg. A positive anti-HBc and anti-HBs are indicative of natural infection which has been controlled by the immune system. An isolated positive anti-HBc may either be a sign of recent or ongoing infection during the window period with positive IgM antibodies or past resolved infection if IgG antibodies are positive, where the anti-HBs titer has waned below the level of detectability. Alternatively, an isolated positive core antibody may be a false-positive test.

Occasional potential organ donors may be identified as "core-positive" donors, that is to say, the HBsAg is negative but anti-HBc is positive. Often only the total core antibody result is available and not whether it is IgM or IgG; also donor anti-HBs information may not be available. Although such donors may be in the "window period" between disappearance of HBsAg and appearance of anti-HBs, the risk of transmission of HBV to non-liver recipients is low ranging from 1:30 to 1:60 [49, 50] and can be further reduced by immunization of the recipient prior to transplantation; in some cases, antiviral prophylaxis is also given [48, 51]. The risk of transmission to a liver recipient from an HBV core-positive donor is higher, about 1:2 [49], but also can be minimized by use of pretransplant immunization and intensive posttransplant prophylaxis with hepatitis B immune globulin and an antiviral agent such as lamivudine or entecavir [48].

For any patient who is at risk for posttransplant HBV, either as a recurrence of their own previous infection or through donor-derived transmission, it is recommended to include serial posttransplant monitoring of the HBV DNA since posttransplant patients may not seroconvert but would still have viral DNA detectable if reactivation or transmission had occurred [48].

Hepatitis C

Hepatitis C is one of the most common indications for liver transplantation. In the past, HCV recurrence posttransplant was frequent and could be either early and aggressive or later and more slowly progressive [48]. Until recently there were no prophylactic antiviral protocols available for prevention of posttransplant HCV recurrence, although this has rapidly changed in the era of new and more effective HCV drugs.

In both liver and non-liver solid organ transplantation, donor-derived de novo HCV is a clinical concern because of poorer graft and patient outcomes in some settings in patients who are hepatitis C seronegative but experience HCV transmission from the donor [52], although a large study by Abbott et al. of kidney transplant candidates and recipients demonstrated improved survival with transplantation with HCV+ donors compared with the remaining on the waiting list [53]. The risk of transmission of HCV from a seropositive donor to a naïve recipient varies in different series, but has been reported to be as high as 75% in some studies [48]. An HCV-seropositive, HCV RNA-negative donor appears to be less likely to transmit HCV than a donor with detectable HCV RNA, but further data are awaited. Unlike the HBV core-positive donor, until recently the risk could be mitigated by prior immunization since there is no vaccine for HCV. Thus, transplantation from an HCV-seropositive donor to an HCV-seronegative recipient (HCV D+/R-) was usually reserved for situations where other donor offers were unlikely, with stringent informed consent [9]. However, the advent of effective HCV therapy is expected to change practice rapidly.

By contrast, the transplantation of a solid organ like a kidney from an HCV-positive donor to an HCV-positive recipient (HCV D+/R+) has been an accepted practice [53, 54]. Multiple studies have suggested that outcomes for transplantation are superior to those remaining on dialysis for an HCV+ transplant candidate [55], even if the donor is HCV+ [53, 54]. Since the waiting list is long and deceased-donor kidney transplants may not occur for years, it makes sense for the HCV-seropositive kidney transplant candidate to consider accepting an organ from an HCV-seropositive donor [53, 54].

In any of the above cases, where either the donor or the recipient (or both) is seropositive for, or at risk for, HCV, monitoring posttransplant for HCV reactivation in the recipient is important [48]. However, antibody seroconversion may be delayed or absent in the immunocompromised patient, even though HCV serology testing has undergone considerable evolution and improvement over time. Since HCV seroconversion may be delayed or absent in posttransplant patients experiencing transmission of HCV from the donor, molecular testing of HCV RNA is important in serial monitoring of the posttransplant patient at risk of HCV acquisition.

HIV

In the early years of transplantation, HIV seropositivity in the donor or the recipient was held to be an absolute contraindication. However, in recent years, a multicenter study of outcomes of solid organ transplants in selected HIV-positive recipients has been found to be comparable to those of HIV-negative recipients for kidney and liver transplantation [56, 57]; although the incidence of acute rejection in 150 HIV-positive kidney recipients was higher than expected, patient and graft survival were high [56]. These recipients are chosen because their kidney or liver disease is more clinically significant than their HIV-related illness, they have not had certain HIV-related opportunistic infections, and their HIV viral loads are well controlled except in the case of some liver candidates who could not tolerate antiviral therapy in the setting of end-stage liver disease. Careful monitoring of the drug interactions between calcineurin inhibitors and protease inhibitors by an experienced pharmacist is necessary, but excellent outcomes can be achieved in certain patients in this category.

Until recently, HIV-seropositive donors were not accepted for donation in the United States, but data from South Africa suggested that HIV-seropositive donors can be associated with acceptable outcomes in selected HIV-seropositive recipients [58]. This is an evolving field, spurred by the shortage of deceased donors and restricted availability of dialysis in resource-limited settings, and further data are awaited. In the United States, the HIV Organ Policy Equity (HOPE) Act was passed in 2015 [59], which allows for research into transplantation from HIV-positive donors to HIV-positive recipients; and the first such transplants in the United States were performed at Johns Hopkins in 2016 [60].

As with HBV and HCV, HIV antibody seroconversion may be delayed or absent in the transplant recipient, and serial monitoring with HIV molecular testing is suggested for any patient at risk for HIV acquisition or reactivation posttransplant [61]. Patients who are HIV-seropositive pretransplant should have HIV RNA viral loads and CD4 counts serially monitored in addition to drug levels and posttransplant lab testing.

NAT of Donors and CDC/PHS High-Risk Donors

For many years, until the development of rapid molecular tests that could be performed in the deceased donor testing time frame, testing of prospective deceased donors relied on antibody serologies for HIV, HBV, and HCV, which are performed as part of a serologic panel by the organ procurement organization (OPO). However, the window period prior to seroconversion that can occur for each of these viruses resulted in infection transmissions from apparently seronegative donors, yielding for a search for more accurate laboratory tests. For example, a donor transmitted HIV and HCV to multiple organ transplant recipients after testing negative for antibody serology for both of these viruses [62]. In addition, a case was reported of a living donor that transmitted HIV after initially testing negative but then continuing risky behavior between the time of initial donor evaluation and the time the transplant was performed [63].

Nucleic acid amplification testing (NAT) is a technology for rapid molecular testing that is highly sensitive and has been used in blood banking. In recent years it has become possible to perform this testing in the rapid time frame needed for making decisions about whether or not to accept a deceased donor, including nights and weekends. The availability of NAT has spurred a national debate in the United States regarding whether all potential deceased donors should be subjected to NAT for HIV/HBV/HCV or just those in the CDC-specified high-risk categories including sexual promiscuity, injection drug use, incarceration, and other categories of behavioral risk. A survey of OPOs revealed a heterogeneity of practices in this regard, with some OPOs performing NAT on all donors, some on a subset of donors, and some not at all [64]. In 2010, an expert consensus panel recommended restricting NAT to donors in the above risk categories, citing concerns about false-positive testing that could lead to discarding otherwise potentially acceptable donors and thus leading to increased deaths on the waiting list for transplantation [3]. Then in the fall of 2011, the Centers for Disease Control and Prevention (CDC) and the US Public Health Service (USPHS) published a comprehensive guideline which recommended NAT of all deceased donors and also retesting of potential living donors shortly before intended donation. After discussion within the transplant community, these recommendations were revised, and the current guidelines call for HCV NAT testing of all donors, with HIV NAT testing only of PHS/CDC high-risk donors, and with a revised list of risk categories [65]. All parties in this discussion are interested in protecting potential organ recipients from harm; the differences in opinion arose in balancing the risks of donor-derived transmission versus the risks of disqualifying donors through false-positive testing.

Multiplex Versus Single-Virus Testing

The fact that there are multiple transplant-associated viral infections, which are amenable to serial monitoring, has given rise to the development of multiplex assays that allow for the detection of more than one virus at any given time point from a single blood sample [2]. Viruses which are frequently serially monitored posttransplant, such as CMV, EBV, and BKV in kidney recipients and adenovirus particularly in pediatric HSCT recipients, would be candidates for inclusion in a blood multiplex viral molecular detection panel. In addition, the existence of a large number of respiratory viruses that produce similar symptomatology makes the use of a respiratory virus multiplex a natural one [2]. Potential advantages of a multiplex assay on blood or plasma would include the following: less blood drawn from the recipient for blood assays, detection of unsuspected coinfections, and rapid and sometimes quantitative results to facilitate preemptive strategies. The cost-effectiveness of multiplex testing has been evaluated in a study by Mahony et al., in which four strategies were compared for diagnosis of respiratory viral infections in pediatric patients (direct fluorescent antibody or DFA alone, DFA plus shell-vial culture, the xTAG RVP test alone, or the xTAG RVP test plus DFA) [66]. These authors reported that the least costly strategy was the xTAG RVP multiplex test alone when the prevalence was >11% and was DFA alone when the prevalence was <11% [66].

Disadvantages of some multiplex tests have included occasional lower sensitivity for one or more individual viruses on the panel, although that finding has led to alterations of the multiplex test such as the RespPlex test vis-à-vis adenovirus testing [2]. Potential disadvantages of multiplex testing of disparate viruses, for example, a panel that includes CMV, EBV, and BK virus and others, also include the clinical quandary of what to do with low-level positive results or results in a subgroup of patients in whom a particular virus is of less clinical importance like BKV in non-kidney organ transplant recipients. For certain subgroups of patients, all of the assays on a multiplex test might provide valuable information; but for others, the clinicians may be interested in only one or two viruses. In that situation, should the information on detection of the other viruses be routinely provided in laboratory reports? These and other questions remain to be fully addressed. The issue of cost also needs careful scrutiny. Costs could potentially decrease because of ordering fewer tests if the clinicians intended originally to monitor more than one virus, but costs could also increase if the cost of the multiplex assay exceeds that of the single-virus assay for clinicians who intended to monitor only one virus. Mahony et al. reported the cost-effectiveness may also depend on the prevalence of the viral infections being tested and so may vary from one region to another or one season to another [66].

Conclusion

Molecular testing for transplant-related viruses has revolutionized posttransplant care and is having a significant impact on pretransplant testing of donors. Serial monitoring for CMV, EBV, and BKV has become a cornerstone of management, as this monitoring allows for early detection and intervention in appropriate subsets of transplant recipients. The utility of quantitative molecular testing is supported by a variety of studies and facilitates the timing of starting and stopping antiviral therapy, assessing the effectiveness of therapy, monitoring for recurrences of viremia, and deciding when to test for antiviral resistance. Multiplex testing for panels of respiratory viruses has demonstrated utility and cost-effectiveness in certain scenarios. The use of NAT in potential deceased and living donors is promising for reduction of donor-derived transmission from donors in the window period of HIV, HBV, and HCV infection, but the recent vigorous national debate, regarding whether all or a subset of potential donors should be subjected to NAT, reflects the complexity of the issues involved. Finally, the availability of both multiplex and single-virus molecular tests will present challenges to the clinician as to how best to utilize the additional information provided by these tests.

References

1. Emmadi R, Boonyaratanakornkit JB, Selvarangan R, Shyamala V, Zimmer BL, Williams L, et al. Molecular methods and platforms for infectious diseases testing a review of FDA-approved and cleared assays. J Mol Diagn. 2011;13(6):583–604.
2. Caliendo AM. Multiplex PCR and emerging technologies for the detection of respiratory pathogens. Clin Infect Dis. 2011;52(Suppl 4):S326–30.
3. Humar A, Morris M, Blumberg E, Freeman R, Preiksaitis J, Kiberd B, et al. Nucleic acid testing (NAT) of organ donors: is the 'best' test the right test? A consensus conference report. Am J Transplant. 2010;10(4):889–99.
4. Pang XL, Fox JD, Fenton JM, Miller GG, Caliendo AM, Preiksaitis JK. Interlaboratory comparison of cytomegalovirus viral load assays. Am J Transplant. 2009;9(2):258–68.
5. Kotton CN, Kumar D, Caliendo AM, Asberg A, Chou S, Snydman DR, et al. International consensus guidelines on the management of cytomegalovirus in solid organ transplantation. Transplantation. 2010;89(7):779–95.
6. Razonable RR, Humar A, The AST Infectious Diseases Community of Practice. Cytomegalovirus in solid organ transplantation. Am J Transplant. 2013;13:93–106.
7. Hirsch HH, Randhawa P, the AST Infectious Diseases Community of Practice. BK virus in solid organ transplantation. Am J Transplant. 2013;13:179–88.
8. Humar A, Michaels M. American Society of Transplantation recommendations for screening, monitoring and reporting of infectious complications in immunosuppression trials in recipients of organ transplantation. Am J Transplant. 2006;6(2):262–74.
9. Fischer SA, Lu K, the AST Infectious Diseases Community of Practice. Screening of donor and recipient in solid organ transplantation. Am J Transplant. 2013;13:9–21.
10. Mawhorter S, Yamani MH. Hypogammaglobulinemia and infection risk in solid organ transplant recipients. Curr Opin Organ Transplant. 2008;13(6):581–5.
11. Humar A, Mazzulli T, Moussa G, Razonable RR, Paya CV, Pescovitz MD, et al. Clinical utility of cytomegalovirus (CMV) serology testing in high-risk CMV D+/R- transplant recipients. Am J Transplant. 2005;5(5):1065–70.
12. Caliendo AM, St George K, Kao SY, Allega J, Tan BH, LaFontaine R, et al. Comparison of quantitative cytomegalovirus (CMV) PCR in plasma and CMV antigenemia assay: clinical utility of the prototype AMPLICOR CMV MONITOR test in transplant recipients. J Clin Microbiol. 2000;38(6):2122–7.
13. Mazzulli T, Drew LW, Yen-Lieberman B, Jekic-McMullen D, Kohn DJ, Isada C, et al. Multicenter comparison of the Digene hybrid capture CMV DNA assay (version 2.0), the pp65 antigenemia assay, and cell culture for detection of cytomegalovirus viremia. J Clin Microbiol. 1999;37(4):958–63.
14. Humar A, Gregson D, Caliendo AM, McGeer A, Malkan G, Krajden M, et al. Clinical utility of quantitative cytomegalovirus viral load determination for predicting cytomegalovirus disease in liver transplant recipients. Transplantation. 1999;68(9):1305–11.
15. Humar A, Kumar D, Boivin G, Caliendo AM. Cytomegalovirus (CMV) virus load kinetics to predict recurrent disease in solid-organ transplant patients with CMV disease. J Infect Dis. 2002;186(6):829–33.
16. Emery VC, Cope AV, Bowen EF, Gor D, Griffiths PD. The dynamics of human cytomegalovirus replication in vivo. J Exp Med. 1999;190(2):177–82.
17. Caliendo AM, Yen-Lieberman B, Baptista J, Andersen J, Crumpacker C, Schuurman R, et al. Comparison of molecular tests for detection and quantification of cell-associated cytomegalovirus DNA. J Clin Microbiol. 2003;41(8):3509–13.

18. Caliendo AM, Ingersoll J, Fox-Canale AM, Pargman S, Bythwood T, Hayden MK, et al. Evaluation of real-time PCR laboratory-developed tests using analyte-specific reagents for cytomegalovirus quantification. J Clin Microbiol. 2007;45(6):1723–7.
19. Hirsch HH, Lautenschlager I, Pinsky BA, Cardenoso L, Aslam S, Cobb B, et al. An international multicenter performance analysis of cytomegalovirus load tests. Clin Infect Dis. 2013;56(3):367–73.
20. Casas S, Munoz L, Moure R, Castellote J, Guerra MR, Gonzalez L, et al. Comparison of the 2-step tuberculin skin test and the quantiFERON-TB Gold In-Tube Test for the screening of tuberculosis infection before liver transplantation. Liver Transpl. 2011;17(10):1205–11.
21. Manuel O, Husain S, Kumar D, Zayas C, Mawhorter S, Levi ME, et al. Assessment of cytomegalovirus-specific cell-mediated immunity for the prediction of cytomegalovirus disease in high-risk solid-organ transplant recipients: a multicenter cohort study. Clin Infect Dis. 2013;56(6):817–24.
22. Nesher L, Shah DP, Ariza-Heredia EJ, et al. Utility of the enzyme-linked immunospot interferon-gamma release assay to predict the risk of cytomegalovirus infection in hematopoietic stem cell transplant recipients. J Infect Dis. 2016;213:1701–7.
23. Singh N, Wannstedt C, Keyes L, Gayowski T, Wagener MM, Cacciarelli TV. Efficacy of valganciclovir administered as preemptive therapy for cytomegalovirus disease in liver transplant recipients: impact on viral load and late-onset cytomegalovirus disease. Transplantation. 2005;79(1):85–90.
24. Preiksaitis JK, Pang XL, Fox JD, Fenton JM, Caliendo AM, Miller GG. Interlaboratory comparison of epstein-barr virus viral load assays. Am J Transplant. 2009;9(2):269–79.
25. Caliendo AM. The long road toward standardization of viral load testing for cytomegalovirus. Editorial commentary. Clin Infect Dis. 2013;56:374–5.
26. Green ML, Leisenring W, Stachel D, et al. Efficacy of a viral load-based, risk-adapted, pre-emptive treatment strategy for prevention of cytomegalovirus disease after hematopoietic stem cell transplantation. Biol Blood Marrow Transplant. 2012;18:1687–99.
27. Lurain NS, Bhorade SM, Pursell KJ, Avery RK, Yeldandi VV, Isada CM, et al. Analysis and characterization of antiviral drug-resistant cytomegalovirus isolates from solid organ transplant recipients. J Infect Dis. 2002;186(6):760–8.
28. Limaye AP. Ganciclovir-resistant cytomegalovirus in organ transplant recipients. Clin Infect Dis. 2002;35(7):866–72.
29. Allen U, Preiksaitis J. Epstein-barr virus and posttransplant lymphoproliferative disorder in solid organ transplant recipients. Am J Transplant. 2009;9(Suppl 4):S87–96.
30. Green M, Cacciarelli TV, Mazariegos GV, Sigurdsson L, Qu L, Rowe DT, et al. Serial measurement of Epstein-Barr viral load in peripheral blood in pediatric liver transplant recipients during treatment for posttransplant lymphoproliferative disease. Transplantation. 1998;66(12):1641–4.
31. McDiarmid SV, Jordan S, Kim GS, Toyoda M, Goss JA, Vargas JH, et al. Prevention and preemptive therapy of postransplant lymphoproliferative disease in pediatric liver recipients. Transplantation. 1998;66(12):1604–11.
32. Almeras C, Vetromile F, Garrigue V, Szwarc I, Foulongne V, Mourad G. Monthly screening for BK viremia is an effective strategy to prevent BK virus nephropathy in renal transplant recipients. Transpl Infect Dis. 2011;13(2):101–8.
33. Comoli P, Hirsch HH, Ginevri F. Cellular immune responses to BK virus. Curr Opin Organ Transplant. 2008;13(6):569–74.
34. Bergallo M, Astegiano S, Sidoti F, Mantovani S, Segoloni GP, Cavallo R, et al. Real-time RT-PCR assay for the quantitation of polyomavirus BK VP1 mRNA levels in urine. Mol Biotechnol. 2010;45(1):82–6.
35. Hirsch HH, Brennan DC, Drachenberg CB, Ginevri F, Gordon J, Limaye AP, et al. Polyomavirus-associated nephropathy in renal transplantation: interdisciplinary analyses and recommendations. Transplantation. 2005;79(10):1277–86.
36. Gilis L, Morisset S, Billaud G, et al. High burden of BK virus-associated hemorrhagic cystitis in patients undergoing allogeneic hematopoietic stem cell transplantation. Bone Marrow Transplant. 2014;49:664–70.
37. Josephson MA, Williams JW, Chandraker A, Randhawa PS. Polyomavirus-associated nephropathy: update on antiviral strategies. Transpl Infect Dis. 2006;8(2):95–101.
38. Kumar D, Husain S, Chen MH, Moussa G, Himsworth D, Manuel O, et al. A prospective molecular surveillance study evaluating the clinical impact of community-acquired respiratory viruses in lung transplant recipients. Transplantation. 2010;89(8):1028–33.
39. Kumar D, Michaels MG, Morris MI, Green M, Avery RK, Liu C, et al. Outcomes from pandemic influenza A H1N1 infection in recipients of solid-organ transplants: a multicentre cohort study. Lancet Infect Dis. 2010;10(8):521–6.
40. Grohskopf LA, Sokolow LZ, Broder KR, et al. Prevention and control of seasonal influenza with vaccines. MMWR Recomm Rep. 2016;65(5):1–54.
41. Shah JN, Chemaly RF. Management of RSV infections in adult recipients of hematopoietic stem cell transplantation. Blood. 2011;117(10):2755–63.
42. Raza K, Ismailjee SB, Crespo M, Studer SM, Sanghavi S, Paterson DL, et al. Successful outcome of human metapneumovirus (hMPV) pneumonia in a lung transplant recipient treated with intravenous ribavirin. J Heart Lung Transplant. 2007;26(8):862–4.
43. Kraft CS, Jacob JT, Sears MH, Burd EM, Caliendo AM, Lyon GM. Severity of human rhinovirus infection in immunocompromised adults is similar to that of 2009 H1N1 influenza. J Clin Microbiol. 2012;50(3):1061–3.
44. Eid AJ, Chen SF. and the AST Infectious Diseases Community of Practice. Human parvovirus B19 in solid organ transplantation. Am J Transplant. 2013;13:201–5.
45. Ki CS, Kim IS, Kim JW, Lee NY, Kim SH, Lee KW, et al. Incidence and clinical significance of human parvovirus B19 infection in kidney transplant recipients. Clin Transplant. 2005;19(6): 751–5.
46. Barzon L, Murer L, Pacenti M, Biasolo MA, Vella MD, Ghirardo G, et al. Detection of viral DNA in kidney graft preservation and washing solutions is predictive of posttransplant infections in pediatric recipients. J Infect Dis. 2009;200(9):1425–33.
47. Moal V, Legris T, Burtey S, Morange S, Purgus R, Dussol B, et al. Infection with hepatitis E virus in kidney transplant recipients in southeastern France. J Med Virol. 2013;85:462–71.
48. Levitsky J, Doucette K. Viral hepatitis in solid organ transplantation. Am J Transplant. 2013;13:147–68.
49. Wachs ME, Amend WJ, Ascher NL, Bretan PN, Emond J, Lake JR, et al. The risk of transmission of hepatitis B from HBsAg(-), HBcAb(+), HBIgM(-) organ donors. Transplantation. 1995;59(2):230–4.
50. Pinney SP, Cheema FH, Hammond K, Chen JM, Edwards NM, Mancini D. Acceptable recipient outcomes with the use of hearts from donors with hepatitis-B core antibodies. J Heart Lung Transplant. 2005;24(1):34–7.
51. Chung RT, Feng S, Delmonico FL. Approach to the management of allograft recipients following the detection of hepatitis B virus in the prospective organ donor. Am J Transplant. 2001;1(2):185–91.
52. Gasink LB, Blumberg EA, Localio AR, Desai SS, Israni AK, Lautenbach E. Hepatitis C virus seropositivity in organ donors and survival in heart transplant recipients. JAMA. 2006;296(15):1843–50.
53. Abbott KC, Lentine KL, Bucci JR, Agodoa LY, Peters TG, Schnitzler MA. The impact of transplantation with deceased donor hepatitis c-positive kidneys on survival in wait-listed long-term dialysis patients. Am J Transplant. 2004;4(12):2032–7.

54. Kucirka LM, Peters TG, Segev DL. Impact of donor hepatitis C virus infection status on death and need for liver transplant in hepatitis C virus-positive kidney transplant recipients. Am J Kidney Dis. 2012;60(1):112–20.
55. Pereira BJ, Natov SN, Bouthot BA, Murthy BV, Ruthazer R, Schmid CH, et al. Effects of hepatitis C infection and renal transplantation on survival in end-stage renal disease. The New England Organ Bank Hepatitis C Study Group. Kidney Int. 1998;53(5):1374–81.
56. Stock PG, Barin B, Murphy B, Hanto D, Diego JM, Light J, et al. Outcomes of kidney transplantation in HIV-infected recipients. N Engl J Med. 2010;363(21):2004–14.
57. Roland ME, Barin B, Carlson L, Frassetto LA, Terrault NA, Hirose R, et al. HIV-infected liver and kidney transplant recipients: 1- and 3-year outcomes. Am J Transplant. 2008;8(2):355–65.
58. Muller E, Barday Z, Mendelson M, Kahn D. Renal transplantation between HIV-positive donors and recipients justified. S Afr Med J. 2012;102(6):497–8.
59. https://optn.transplant.hrsa.gov/learn/professional-education/hope-act/.
60. http://hub.jhu.edu/2016/03/31/first-kidney-liver-transplant-hiv-positive/.
61. Blumberg EA, Rogers CC, the AST Infectious Diseases Community of Practice. Human immunodeficiency virus in solid organ transplantation. Am J Transplant. 2013;13:169–78.
62. Ison MG, Llata E, Conover CS, Friedewald JJ, Gerber SI, Grigoryan A, et al. Transmission of human immunodeficiency virus and hepatitis C virus from an organ donor to four transplant recipients. Am J Transplant. 2011;11(6):1218–25.
63. HIV transmitted from a living organ donor--New York City, 2009. MMWR Morb Mortal Wkly Rep. 2011;60(10):297–301.
64. Ison MG, Stosor V. Transplantation of high-risk donor organs: a survey of US solid organ transplant center practices as reported by transplant infectious diseases physicians. Clin Transplant. 2009;23(6):866–73.
65. Seem DL, Lee I, Umscheid CA, Kuehnert MJ, United States Public Health Service. PHS Guideline for Reducing Human Immunodeficiency Virus, Hepatitis B Virus, and Hepatitis C Virus Transmission Through Organ Transplantation. Public Health Rep. 2013;128:247–343.
66. Mahony JB, Blackhouse G, Babwah J, Smieja M, Buracond S, Chong S, et al. Cost analysis of multiplex PCR testing for diagnosing respiratory virus infections. J Clin Microbiol. 2009;47(9):2812–7.

Part V

Therapeutics and Management of Patients Undergoing Transplantation

50 Antibiotic Consideration in Transplant Recipients

Jerry Altshuler, Samuel L. Aitken, Melanie Maslow, John Papadopoulos, and Amar Safdar

Introduction

Transplant patients are uniquely predisposed to infections. Severe iatrogenic immune suppression following allogeneic hematopoietic stem cell or solid organ transplantation predisposes such patients not only to increased risk of infection with conventional pathogens, but organisms with inherently low virulence and pathogenicity may result in devastating systemic disease. The severity of compromised hosts' immune defenses and patients' extensive exposure to the healthcare environment promote colonization and invasive systemic disease due to multidrug-resistant bacteria during the early and late phases after transplantation. Similarly, recipients of stem cell or solid organ allografts are also susceptibile to drug-resistant bacterial infections upon returning to their community and home environment.

Bacterial infections seen during the pretransplant period reflect upon the complications resulting from the treatment of underlying neoplastic processes in patient being considered for hematopoietic stem cell transplantation (HSCT). In patients awaiting solid organ transplantation, a series of complications arising from the end-stage organ disease predisposes them to a host of locally invasive and systemic bacterial infections.

Major risk factors for bacterial infections in patients undergoing transplantation procedures include prolonged and recurring hospitalization, prior exposure to a variety of broad-spectrum antibiotics, pre-engraftment neutropenia, extensive surgical procedures, need for critical care unit stay, assisted ventilatory support, and presence of indwelling intravascular catheters and other body cavity or organ system drains and devices. Antibiotic regimens are often more complex compared with general population and in a vast number of transplant recipients antimicrobials are given empirically or preemptively. Drug-drug interactions with immunosuppressive medications and serious, treatment-limiting adverse reactions further complicate management of infectious diseases in such high-risk individuals. Use of prophylactic antibiotics also contributes to selection of antibiotic resistance organisms. Furthermore, newly acquired drug resistance or more importantly, selection of less drug susceptible pathogens under the unsettling external influence(s) resulting in tandem of permutations in the composition of hosts' external microbiome and orointestional microbiota is an emerging area of research.

Bacterial infections in a variety of transplant population that places patients at a greater risk for higher morbidity and risk of death include *Pseudomonas aeruginosa*, *Stenotrophomonas maltophilia*, *Burkholderia cepacia*, *Acinetobacter baumannii*, MDR *Enterobacteriaceae*, methicillin-resistant *S. aureus*, and vancomycin-resistant enterococci [1–5]. This chapter provides a detailed review of major classes of antibiotics including conventional drugs and new antimicrobials in development, mechanisms of resistance, and the indications for use in the transplant population.

Beta-Lactams

Mechanism of Action

All β-lactam antibiotics share a common structure of a four-membered β-lactam ring. The penicillins have a thiazolidine

J. Altshuler (✉)
The Mount Sinai Hospital, Department of Pharmacy, New York, NY, USA
e-mail: jerry.altshuler@mountsinai.org

S. L. Aitken
Infectious Diseases, The University of Texas MD Anderson Cancer Center, Division of Pharmacy, Houston, TX, USA
e-mail: slaitken@mdanderson.org

M. Maslow
New York University School of Medicine, New York, NY, USA

J. Papadopoulos
Department of Pharmacy, Division of Pharmacotherapy, NYU Langone Medical Center, New York, NY, USA
e-mail: john.papadopoulos@nyumc.org

A. Safdar
Clinical Associate Professor of Medicine, Texas Tech University Health Sciences Center El Paso, Paul L. Foster School of Medicine, El Paso, TX, USA
e-mail: amar.safdar@cidimmunology.com

A. Safdar (ed.), *Principles and Practice of Transplant Infectious Diseases*, https://doi.org/10.1007/978-1-4939-9034-4_50

ring as a side chain, and the cephalosporins have a dihydrothiazine ring as a side chain. Carbapenems differ from penicillins and cephalosporins in two ways: first, a methylene group replaces a sulfur atom and double-bond in the five-membered ring, and, second, a hydroxyethyl side chain in the *trans*-configuration is attached to the β-lactam ring instead of the *cis*-configuration acylamino chain found in the penicillins and cephalosporins. This structural configuration allows binding to high molecular weight penicillin-binding proteins (PBPs), stability to β-lactamases, and rapid transit through the outer membrane of Gram-negative bacteria (GNB). Monobactams have a monocyclic β-lactam ring. β-Lactamase inhibitors are weak β-lactams that bind to select β-lactamases hydrolytic enzymes and restore activity of the parent β-lactam drug [6, 7].

β-Lactams are bactericidal antibiotics that act via time-dependent killing by inhibiting bacterial growth by covalent binding with and inactivation of serine protease enzymes located in the bacterial cell membrane (PBPs). β-Lactams bind to PBPs in the bacterial cell membrane involved in the transpeptidation step of peptidoglycan synthesis, conferring osmotic stability to the bacterium by cross-linking the peptidoglycan strands. There are between three and five different PBPs in Gram-positive organisms and seven to twelve in Gram-negative bacilli. Each PBP is responsible for distinct reactions in cell wall synthesis. Different β-lactam antibiotics may bind preferentially to and inhibit certain PBPs, producing characteristic effects on bacterial morphology such as cell lysis, elongation, and cell division and different efficacies in inhibiting bacterial growth or cell death. PBPs are divided according to high and low molecular weight [8]. The high molecular weight PBPs are responsible for peptidoglycan polymerization and insertion into a preexisting cell wall. The seven low molecular weight proteins found in *E. coli* are responsible for cell separation, peptidoglycan maturation, or recycling. The final common pathway of β-lactam killing involves autolysin release; these enzymes are present in the bacterial cell membrane that mediate autolysis of peptidoglycan to allow breakdown of peptidoglycan for remodeling at the points of bacterial growth. β-Lactam inhibition of cell wall synthesis leads to activation of the autolytic system, which initiates cell death, which is a two-component VncR system [9, 10].

Mechanisms of Resistance

The most common mechanism of resistance to this class is mediated by β-lactamases enzymes that covalently bind and hydrolyze the critical β-lactam ring. Other mechanisms include production of low-affinity PBPs, changes in membrane permeability involving downregulation of porin channels, and increased expression or upregulation of complex drug efflux pumps as seen with strains of multidrug-resistant *Pseudomonas aeruginosa* [11].

β-Lactamases can be encoded chromosomally or on plasmids, with either constitutive or inducible expression. The evolution of a number of novel β-lactamases has paralleled the development of new β-lactam antibiotics. Differences in Gram-positive and Gram-negative bacterial cellular structure greatly influence the action of β-lactamases. In GNB, β-lactamases may be trapped in the periplasmic space leading to an increased enzyme concentrations and more efficient hydrolysis of the β-lactam ring, whereas in Gram-positive bacteria (GPB) the outer cell membrane is lacking and antibiotics can more readily access PBPs without the exposure to high localized concentration of the enzyme-assisted hydrolysis. There are two main classification systems for β-lactamases, Ambler classes A through D, which are based on molecular structure, and the Bush-Jacoby-Medeiros classification which is based on functional similarities (Table 50.1). With over 900 known enzymes, classification is difficult [12–14]. Due to their ability to facilitate rapid dissemination of resistance, plasmid-mediated β-lactamases pose the greatest challenge to clinicians.

The TEM-1 and TEM-2 enzymes were the earliest β-lactamases observed in *E. coli* and SHV-1 enzyme in *K. pneumoniae*. These are considered narrow-spectrum β-lactamases and confer resistance to penicillins and early-generation cephalosporins. As more extended spectrum β-lactam drugs were introduced, the extended-spectrum β-lactamases (ESBLs) evolved, primarily from mutations in the TEM and SHV enzymes. ESBLs are a heterogeneous group of enzymes that confer resistance to some or all of the β-lactams with the exception of the cephamycins and carbapenems. ESBLs, when found in combination with mutations, lead to increased gene expression and downregulation of porins resulting in high-level resistance to third-generation cephalosporins and monobactams as well as low-level resistance to the carbapenems [12, 15]. β-Lactamase inhibitor combinations may still be active against certain ESBL producers. ESBLs are found exclusively in GNB, such as *Klebsiella* spp. and *E. coli* and in clinical isolates of *Acinetobacter*, *Burkholderia*, *Citrobacter*, *Enterobacter*, *Morganella*, *Proteus*, *Pseudomonas*, *Salmonella*, *Serratia*, *Shigella*, *H. influenzae*, and *N. gonorrhea*. There are currently over 200 enzymes of this type [12, 16].

The CTX-M family of β-lactamases has recently emerged and is now the predominant ESBL enzymes worldwide [17]. Natural CTX-M enzymes are found on the chromosome of *Kluyvera* and have since spread to the *Enterobacteriaceae*, including *K. pneumoniae*, pathogenic *E. coli*, and *Salmonella* spp. [12]. More than 120 CTX-M enzymes have been described, with CTX-M-15 and CTX-M-14 as the most frequently encountered members [18].

The latest β-lactamases to emerge are the carbapenemases, which have the widest spectrum of activity and can hydrolyze most beta-lactams. These include the *K. pneumoniae* carbapenemases (KPCs) which are encoded on transposons and are now seen in a wide variety of GNB. Metalloenzymes

Table 50.1 Classification of beta-lactamases

Ambler class	Bush-Jacoby-Medeiros group	Major subtypes	Substrate	Model organisms	Genetic location	Potential antibiotic alternatives
A	2a	Gram-positive	Penicillins	Ampicillin-R *E. coli* *H. influenzae*	Chromosomal or plasmid, inducible	Clavulanate
	2b	Gram-negative (TEM-1 and SHV-1)	Penicillins, some cephalosporins	*E. coli* *K. pneumoniae*	Plasmid or chromosomal	Clavulanate
	2be	Extended spectrum (TEM, SHV, CTX-M)	Penicillins, 3rd-generation cephalosporins, monobactams	*Enterobacteriaceae*	Plasmid	Carbapenems Tigecycline Piperacillin-tazobactam[a] Fluoroquinolones[a] Colistin
	2br	Inhibitor-resistant TEM (complex mutant TEMS)	Penicillins	*Klebsiella*, *Proteus*, *Citrobacter*, *Shigella* species	Plasmid	Carbapenems Cefepime[a]
	2e	Cephalosporin hydrolyzing	Extended spectrum cephalosporins	*Proteus* species	Chromosomal, inducible	Piperacillin-tazobactam
	2f	Carbapenem hydrolyzing β-lactamase (KPC, GES, SME)	Penicillins, cephalosporins, carbapenems	*Klebsiella*, *E. coli*, *Enterobacter*, *Pseudomonas*	Plasmid Transposons, chromosomal	Tigecycline Colistin[a] Polymyxin[a]
B	3	Metallo-β-lactamase 3 (VIM, IMP)	All β-lactams except monobactams	*Acinetobacter*, *Pseudomonas*, *Stenotrophomonas maltophilia*	Chromosomal Transposon	Monobactam Piperacillin-tazobactam[a] Ampicillin-sulbactam[a] Tigecycline[a]
C	2d	AmpC-type cephalosporinase 1	Cephalosporins, penicillins	*Enterobacter* *Citrobacter* *Serratia* *P. aeruginosa* *Providencia* Indole-positive *Proteus*	Chromosomal (inducible); constitutive, plasmid	Cefepime[a] Carbapenems
D	2df	Oxacillin-hydrolyzing carbapenemases (OXA)		*Acinetobacter* *Pseudomonas*	Chromosome	Cefepime Monobactam Polymyxin Aminoglycoside Fluoroquinolone

[a]In vitro confirmation by additional testing is necessary to confirm susceptibility

such as VIM-1 and NDM-1 are another class of carbapenemases that require metallic cations as cofactors and are carried on plasmids, integrons, and transposons. These enzymes hydrolyze aztreonam poorly, leaving this monobactam as a potential treatment option in cases where other classes of β-lactamase are not present. OXA β-lactamases are a diverse group of enzymes classically associated with *Acinetobacter* species but have widely disseminated among clinically important GNB [19]. Detection of carbapenemases may be difficult using common automated identification systems, which often report these organisms as falsely susceptible. The significance of infection with either carbapenem-resistant and ESBL *K. pneumonia* was studied in lung transplant recipients and found to be an independent risk factor for mortality compared with carbapenem-sensitive or ESBL-negative bacterial strains [20]. The chromosomal enzymes, predominantly class C cephalosporinases such as AmpC, are mostly inducible and are found in *Enterobacter* species, indole-positive bacteria like *Proteus*, *Serratia*, *Citrobacter*, and *Pseudomonas* species, among others.

Resistance in GPB occurs predominantly through mutations in PBPs that result in decreased binding affinity. Methicillin resistance in staphylococci including MRSA is mediated by a mobile chromosomal element known as staphylococcal chromosomal cassette mec (SCC*mec*) [21]. SCC*mec* encodes for the low-affinity PBP2a, which in turn results in complete resistance to most β-lactam antibiotics. The classical community-acquired strains of MRSA contain a smaller SCC*mec* than hospital-acquired strains. Methicillin resistance may also involve other mutations known as factors for methicillin resistance or auxiliary factors that encode functions involved in cell wall precursors [12].

Ampicillin resistance in *E. faecium* is due to expression of a low-affinity PBP-5. Penicillin-resistant *S. pneumoniae* has low-affinity PBPs that use genes referred to as "mosaic" [12] derived from recombination between *S. pneumoniae* and less susceptible viridans-group streptococcal genes. Penicillin resistance in *S. pneumoniae* is typically of low level, with the greatest clinical impact on the treatment of pneumococcal meningitis. Certain GNB such as *Neisseria* species may also contain mosaic resistance genes. A strain of *N. gonorrhea* containing a novel penA mosaic allele was recently identified with high-level resistance to ceftriaxone [22].

Penicillins

The penicillins are divided into five classes based on the bacterial spectrum: the natural penicillins, the penicillinase-resistant penicillins, the aminopenicillins, the carboxypenicillins, and the ureidopenicillins. The representative antibiotics and spectrum of activity are outlined in Table 50.2. Penicillins have short half-lives of <60 min and are administered every 4–6 h in patients with normal renal function. Most penicillins are excreted unchanged by renal tubular cells and require dose adjustment in patients with renal insufficiency. The antistaphylococcal penicillins and extended spectrum penicillins undergo considerable biliary excretion. Piperacillin has the longest half-life and can be administered every 6 h and requires dose adjustment only in patients with severe renal dysfunction. With most penicillins, therapeutic levels are achieved in most organs, including the central nervous system even in the absence of meningeal inflammation and compromised blood-brain barrier [23].

Beta-Lactamase Inhibitors

β-lactamase inhibitors are weak β-lactam drugs that are potent inhibitors of many class A serine β-lactamases. These drugs react with the serine enzymes to form a covalent acyl-enzyme intermediate. After opening of the β-lactam ring, the intermediate can undergo additional rearrangements or be hydrolyzed to regenerate the active β-lactamase enzyme. When combined with a β-lactam, they prevent hydrolysis of the parent antibiotic and preserve activity. The major bacteria producing class A enzymes include *S. aureus*, *H. influenzae*, *M. catarrhalis*, *Bacteroides* spp., and some *Enterobacteriaceae*. Some ESBL produced by *E. coli* and *Klebsiella* spp. may be inhibited in vitro by these inhibitors. The chromosomal β-lactamases, such as those produced by *Pseudomonas*, are generally not inhibited by these compounds with the occasional exception of tazobactam [24, 25].

The β-lactamase inhibitors in clinical use are clavulanic acid combined with amoxicillin for oral use and ticarcillin for parenteral use, sulbactam combined with ampicillin for parenteral use, and tazobactam combined with piperacillin for parenteral use. The main β-lactam generally determines the antimicrobial spectrum, with the β-lactamase inhibitor enhancing activity through inhibition of acquired or intrinsic β-lactamases. Sulbactam has a broader spectrum of activity but is less potent than clavulanic acid and tazobactam. The combination of amoxicillin and clavulanic acid has activity against most penicillinase-producing *S. aureus* (MSSA), β-lactamase-producing strains of *H. influenzae*, and some *Enterobacteriaceae*. It is used predominantly for respiratory tract and soft tissue infections when MRSA is not suspected. Ampicillin plus sulbactam has a similar spectrum of activity, including *B. fragilis*, and is used for

Table 50.2 Penicillin classes and spectrum

Class	Representative drugs	Gram-positive spectrum	Gram-negative spectrum	Atypical spectrum	Anaerobic spectrum
Natural penicillins	Penicillin G, Penicillin V	Streptococci including *E. faecalis* (static), Penicillinase negative *S., aureus, Listeria* spp., *C. diphtheriae*	*Neisseria* spp., *H. influenza, Pasteurella multocida*	*T. pallidum*	Peptostreptococci *Clostridium* spp. *Fusobacterium*
Penicillinase-resistant penicillins	Nafcillin, oxacillin, dicloxacillin	PCN-R *S. aureus*, CoNS, PCN-S streptococci (lacks *Enterococcus*)	None	None	Most anaerobic Gram-positive cocci
Aminopenicillins	Ampicillin, amoxicillin	Same as PCN G	PCN G plus β-lactamase-negative *H. influenzae, E. coli, P. mirabilis, Salmonella, Shigella, H. pylori*	*B. burgdorferi*	Same as PCN G
Ureidopenicillins	Piperacillin	PCN G including *E. faecalis*; less active against CNS	AMP-R Gram-negatives including *Pseudomonas, Serratia, Klebsiella, Enterobacter, Providencia* spp.	None	Similar to ampicillin

Abbreviations: *CoNS* coagulase-negative staphylococci, *PCN-S* penicillin susceptible, *PCR-R* penicillin resistance, *AMP-R* ampicillin resistant skin and soft tissue infections, community-acquired, intra-abdominal, and pelvic infections. Tazobactam enhances the piperacillin spectrum to include some *Enterobacteriaceae* and *B. fragilis* [26, 27].

Sulbactam is a unique β-lactamase inhibitor because it has activity against metallo-β-lactamase-producing strains of *Acinetobacter baumannii* [28]. A single-entity product is currently not available in the United States; therefore sulbactam is still clinically used in combination with ampicillin. Variable dosing regimens of sulbactam have been used against *A. baumannii* including 1 gram every 8 h in moderate infections and 1 gram every 6 h in serious infection with cure rates of 93% and 76.9%, respectively [29]. Lower cure rates seen with more aggressive dosing were likely due to the severity of infection. Higher sulbactam doses up to 12 grams a day have been reported for the treatment of MDR *Acinetobacter* ventilator-associated pneumonia (VAP) [30]. Paralleling the escalating carbapenem resistance, sulbactam-resistant *Acinetobacter* strains have been reported [31, 32].

The emergence of enzymes that are not inhibited by approved inhibitors has prompted research into new drugs. Avibactam, previously known as NXL-104, is a novel, non-β-lactam β-lactamase inhibitor that was recently approved in the United States in combination with ceftazidime. Avibactam is a structural class of inhibitor without a β-lactam core and retains capacity to covalently acylate β-lactamase targets. Deacylation of the enzyme occurs through regeneration of intact avibactam rather than the hydrolysis seen with other β-lactamase inhibitors [33]. Avibactam can inhibit β-lactamase enzymes in molecular classes A, C, and to a lesser extent D. Notably, avibactam does not have inhibitory activity against Class B metallo β-lactamases. In vitro data demonstrates that avibactam potentiates the activity of aztreonam against a broad array of *Enterobacteriaceae*, including metallo β-lactamase-producing strains [34, 35]. Other novel β-lactamase inhibitors, including relebactam combined with imipenem was accepted by FDA for regulatory review and vaborbactam paired with meropenem was recently approved by FDA for clinical use in treatment for carbapenemase-producing GNB [36, 37].

Cephalosporins

Since the first cephalosporin was introduced in the 1960s, cephalosporins have become one of the most widely prescribed classes of antibiotics. Most are semisynthetic derivatives of cephalosporin C and consist of a β-lactam ring attached to a six-membered dihydrothiazine ring containing a sulfur moiety. The cephamycins, which have a methoxy group at C-7, are included in this class due to the structural similarity. Cephalosporins have two variable side chains, R1 (C-7) and R2 (C-3); modifications in the R1 side chains usually result in β-lactamase stability and improved spectrum, whereas modification at R2 results in altered pharmacokinetics. The fourth-generation drug, cefepime, has a positively charged quaternary ammonium in the C-3 position which creates a zwitterion, enhancing penetration through the outer membrane of GNB [38].

There are five "generations" of cephalosporins, based predominantly on microbial spectrum (Table 50.3). Most cephalosporins are excreted unchanged in the urine and require dose adjustment in patients with renal insufficiency or renal failure. Ceftriaxone has dual hepatic and renal clearance and the longest half-life of 8–9 h among the cephalosporin class. Cefoperazone is eliminated through biliary clearance. Cefotaxime is metabolized to a weakly active deacetyl metabolite in the liver [39].

Cefepime, a zwitterion, has enhanced activity against *Enterobacter*, *Citrobacter*, and *Serratia* species compared to other cephalosporins. Cefepime is less susceptible to AmpC β-lactamase inactivation and may be active in vitro against some ESBL-producing *Klebsiella* and *E. coli*, although it is inactive against organisms producing the predominant CTX-M-type enzymes. Cefepime in combination with tazobactam is in clinical development, expanding the natural spectrum of cefepime to include a wider variety of ESBL-producing organisms [40]. Cha et al. observed bactericidal activity against ESBL *K. pneumoniae* and *E. coli* in 50% of isolates compared to 100% with imipenem [41]. Lee and colleagues noted increased mortality with bacteremia caused by ESBL-producing pathogens treated with cefepime compared to carbapenems [42]. Additionally, Chopra and colleagues found a trend toward increased mortality risk with cefepime versus a carbapenem in bloodstream infections caused by ESBL *K. pneumoniae* and *E. coli* [16] suggesting that transplant patients should receive a carbapenem for serious ESBL infections.

The recent addition of another zwitterionic compound, ceftolozane, in combination with tazobactam adds to the anti-pseudomonal armamentarium. Ceftolozane is highly resistant to hydrolysis via AmpC β-lactamases and is less affected by porin and efflux pump mutations than other cephalosporins. These characteristics make ceftolozane a potential option in the treatment of multidrug-resistant *Pseudomonas aeruginosa* [43–45]. The addition of tazobactam grants some protection to ceftolozane against class A ESBLs (2be); however, the clinical significance of this additional activity remains unclear [46]. A novel siderophore cephalosporin in clinical development, cefiderocol, utilizes bacterial iron transport systems to gain active transport into GNB and demonstrates potent in vitro activity against most GNB, including metallo β-lactamase producers, *S. maltophilia* and *A. baumannii* [47, 48].

Table 50.3 Classification of cephalosporins and spectrum

Class	Representative drugs	Gram-positive spectrum	Gram-negative spectrum	Atypical spectrum	Anaerobic spectrum
First generation	Cefazolin, cephalothin, cephalexin, cefadroxil	PNS-S streptococci except enterococci, MSSA	Some *E. coli*, *Salmonella*, *Shigella*	None	Gram-positive cocci
Second generation Cephamycins	Cefotetan, cefuroxime Cefoxitin, cefotetan	PNS-S streptococci except enterococci, MSSA	*H. influenzae*, *Neisseria* spp., *E. coli*, *Klebsiella*, some *Proteus* spp.	None	*B. fragilis*
Third Generation Pseudomonas	Cefotaxime, ceftriaxone, cefixime Cefoperazone, Ceftazidime	PNS-S and R *S. pneumoniae* (outside CoNS), streptococci MSSA	*H. influenzae*, *M. catarrhalis*, *Neisseria* spp., *Salmonella*, *Shigella* *Pseudomonas*	*B. burgdorferi* (ceftriaxone)	*Peptostreptococcus*, *Clostridium* spp. (excluding *C. difficile*), *Porphyromonas*, *B. melaninogenicus*
Fourth Generation	Cefepime	PCS-S streptococci except enterococci, MSSA	Third generation plus *Pseudomonas*, *Enterobacter*, *Citrobacter*, *Serratia*, *Enterobacteriaceae*		*Peptostreptococcus*
Fifth Generation	Ceftaroline	PCN-S and PCR streptococci, MSSA, and MRSA	*H. influenzae*, *M. catarrhalis*, *Neisseria* spp., *Salmonella*, *Shigella*		

Abbreviations: *CoNS* coagulase negative staphylococci, *PCN-S* penicillin susceptible, *PCR-R* penicillin resistance

Carbapenems and Monobactams

Carbapenems are among the smallest of the β-lactam antibiotics and exist as zwitterions, a compound with overall no electric charge, albeit containing separate positive and negatively charged parts. These antibiotics require channels created by porin proteins such as OprD that are open water-filled channels spanning the outer membrane of GNB and allow passive penetration of hydrophilic compounds into the periplasmic space. The *trans*-configuration of the hydroxyethyl side chain on the β-lactam ring confers resistance to cleavage by most plasmid and chromosomal β-lactamases including class A and C enzymes. Carbapenems have the broadest spectrum of the β-lactam class which is attributed to improve ability to penetrate the cell membrane of GNB, high affinity for critical PBPs, and resistance to multiple β-lactamases [49]. Increasing resistance has been seen with *P. aeruginosa* due to altered permeability secondary to mutations and downregulation of the OprD membrane proteins or both [50]. Carbapenem-hydrolyzing β-lactamases of the class B metalloenzymes have been increasingly isolated from Gram-negative bacteria and may limit therapy with these agents. Gram-positive resistance in MRSA and *E. faecium* is caused by production of low-affinity PBPs [7].

The GNB activity of carbapenems includes ESBL-producing *Enterobacteriaceae*, *P. aeruginosa*, anaerobes such as *B. fragilis*, MSSA, MSSE, *E. faecalis*, *Listeria monocytogenes*, *Bacillus* spp., and *Nocardia* spp. among the GPB. The gaps in coverage include *Stenotrophomonas maltophilia*, *Burkholderia cepacia*, *Enterococcus faecium*, MRSA, and JK diphtheroids. Ertapenem differs from the other marketed carbapenems in that it lacks significant activity against *P. aeruginosa* and *Acinetobacter* and is only approved for complicated skin and soft tissue infections, intra-abdominal infections, and community-acquired pneumonia [51].

Imipenem is readily cleaved by the renal dehydropeptidase 1 (DHP-1) and is combined with cilastatin, a DHP-1 inhibitor, to prolong the imipenem half-life and increase serum drug concentration. The other carbapenems such as meropenem, ertapenem, and doripenem are more stable in the presence of DHP-1 and do not require combination with DHP-1 inhibitor. All carbapenems require adjustment in patients with renal insufficiency. Imipenem, meropenem, and doripenem have half-lives of about 1 h and are dosed every 6–8 h. Ertapenem has a longer half-life of approximately 4 h and can be dosed once daily. Imipenem has the greatest potential to cause seizures compared to the other carbapenems, especially at higher doses and in individuals with impaired renal function [52].

Doripenem is the newest carbapenem, approved in 2007 for the treatment of complicated urinary tract and intra-abdominal infections [53]. Doripenem is more active against MSSA and methicillin-sensitive coagulase-negative staphylococci than meropenem and ertapenem. It tends to be less active against *E. faecalis* compared with imipenem. The Gram-negative activity is similar to meropenem with greater activity against *P. aeruginosa*. One study showed that doripenem retained activity against 29.4% of *P. aeruginosa* strains [54] that were resistant to imipenem and 20.8% of carbapenem-resistant *Acinetobacter* spp. [55]. Similar mechanisms of resistance are seen with doripenem, including metallo-β-lactamases, OprD outer membrane porin protein mutations, and upregulation of multidrug efflux pumps.

Some studies suggest that doripenem may have a higher threshold for the development of resistance, requiring more than one resistance mechanism [56]. The adverse reactions seen with doripenem are similar to meropenem, including gastrointestinal disturbances, rash, transaminase elevations, and, to a lesser extent, seizure activity. The clinical efficacy of doripenem in transplant recipients is very limited.

Aztreonam, the only marketed monobactam, has a sulfonic acid group on the nitrogen at the N-1 position of the β-lactam ring. Aztreonam penetrates quickly through the outer membrane of GNB and is resistant to hydrolysis by B class enzymes, many class C β-lactamases, but not ESBLs. The drug has a half-life of 2 h and undergoes renal excretion; therefore dose adjustment is necessary in patients with renal insufficiency. Aztreonam has a spectrum of activity similar to the aminoglycosides, including *Pseudomonas*. Most *S. maltophilia*, *B. cepacia*, and many *Acinetobacter* spp. are resistant; *Enterobacter* spp. and *C. freundii* demonstrate variable susceptibility. It lacks Gram-positive and anaerobic activity and is often used with another antibiotic-like clindamycin or vancomycin for additional Gram-positive coverage [57, 58]. A new aerosolized formulation of aztreonam lysine is approved for the treatment of respiratory infections in patients with cystic fibrosis [59]; its role in other patient populations remains to be explored.

Aztreonam is a weakly immunogenic compound which can be safely administered to penicillin-allergic patients. The site of antibody recognition against aztreonam differs from the bicyclic β-lactams. Hypersensitivity is secondary to antibodies against the side chain and occurs in under 1% of patients allergic to penicillin [60]. Other nonimmune adverse reactions include rash, diarrhea, nausea, vomiting, and local injection reactions (Table 50.4).

Beta-Lactams with MRSA Activity

Ceftaroline is a broad-spectrum cephalosporin developed with enhanced activity against GPB. Ceftaroline fosamil, the prodrug, was approved in 2010 for the treatment of complicated skin and skin-structure infections and community-acquired pneumonia. Ceftaroline binds to PBP2a, a PBP found in staphylococci with reduced affinity for other β-lactam compounds. The high-affinity binding of ceftaroline to PBP2a leads to rapid bactericidal activity against methicillin-resistant staphylococci, including MRSA. Ceftaroline is also active against heteroresistant vancomycin-intermediate *S. aureus*, vancomycin-resistant *S. aureus*, penicillin-resistant *S. pneumoniae*, certain strains of vancomycin-resistant *E. faecalis*, and common respiratory pathogens such as *H. influenzae*. Non-ESBL *Enterobacteriaceae* are susceptible, but ESBL-producing strains are resistant. Ceftaroline has minimal activity against *P. aeruginosa* and *A. baumannii* and has limited activity against anaerobic GNB. It also lacks activity against *E. faecium*. Of 12,000 isolates of MSSA, MRSA, and *S. pneumoniae* tested in vitro, both the MIC_{50} and MIC_{90} against MRSA were 1 μg/mL, and the drug was active against 95.6% of multidrug-resistant *S. pneumoniae* [61].

In two large phase III trials for patients with community-acquired pneumonia (CAP) and acute skin and skin structure infections (ASSSI), ceftaroline was shown to be noninferior to ceftriaxone in patients with CAP and vancomycin plus aztreonam in ASSSI treatment group. Clinical cure rates for ceftaroline were higher than ceftriaxone, particularly when the penicillin-resistant *S. pneumoniae* serotype 19A was the primary pathogen. The clinical cure rate in microbiologically evaluable patients with MRSA was similar to vancomycin plus aztreonam, and the drug was well-tolerated [62]. Dose adjustments are required in patients with moderate renal insufficiency. Further clinical studies are needed to determine the efficacy and safety of ceftaroline and to define its role in treating immunocompromised patients undergoing allograft transplantation.

Beta-Lactam Allergy and Other Adverse Reactions

The beta-lactams are reported to cause allergic events in 1 to 10% of patients, with life-threatening allergies observed in 0.01 and 0.05% of cases. Penicillins are quickly metabolized into benzylpenicilloyl, also known as the major antigenic determinant, by opening of the β-lactam ring [63]. This sta-

Table 50.4 Carbapenems and monobactams

Class	Representative drugs	Gram-positive spectrum	Gram-negative spectrum	Atypical spectrum	Anaerobic spectrum
Carbapenems	Imipenem-cilastatin meropenem, ertapenem, doripenem	MSSA, CoNS, streptococci, *B. anthracis*, *Listeria*, *Corynebacterium* spp., PCN-S *E. faecalis* (imipenem)	*H, influenzae*, *Neisseria* spp., *Klebsiella*, *Enterobacter* spp., *E. coli*, *Serratia*, *Citrobacter*, *Acinetobacter*, *Proteus* spp., *Pseudomonas*	*Nocardia*, rapidly growing Mycobacterium spp. (imipenem)	*B. fragilis*, *Prevotella* spp., *Clostridium* spp., Gram-positive cocci, *Actinomyces*
Monobactams	Aztreonam	None	*Pseudomonas*, *Enterobacteriaceae*, *Neisseria*	None	None

Abbreviations: *CoNS* coagulase negative staphylococci, *PCN-S* penicillin susceptible

ble metabolite can bind to protein conjugates through amide linkages in solution or with human proteins after administration, forming potentially immunogenic haptens. The minor determinants include penilloate, penicilloate, and benzylpenicillin that account for a minority of allergic reactions. Both can cause either anaphylaxis or urticarial reactions mediated by IgE antibodies. The β-lactam and dihydrothiazine rings of cephalosporins rapidly fragment into unstable compounds that are usually not similar in structure to the penicillin allergic determinants. Fragments of the cephem nucleus and parts of the cephalosporin side chains can act as haptens and lead to sensitization [63].

Type I immediate hypersensitivity reactions are mediated by IgE antibodies and result in anaphylaxis, urticaria, laryngeal edema, angioedema, and hypotension within minutes to hours through release of histamine and mediators such as vasoactive amines, cytokines, and proteases from mast cell degranulation. Type II reactions are mediated by complement and result in hemolytic anemia, thrombocytopenia, and neutropenia. Type III reactions occur later after exposure due to precipitation of immune complexes and activation of the complement system manifesting as serum sickness with fever, rash, and arthritis and allergic vasculitis. Type IV, or delayed type hypersensitivity, causes maculopapular and morbilliform rashes thought to be T cell-mediated. Exfoliative dermatitis, Stevens-Johnson syndrome, erythema multiforme, and drug reaction with eosinophilia and systemic symptoms (DRESS) fall under the idiopathic hypersensitivity reactions [63].

The rate of cross-allergy in penicillin allergic patients receiving a cephalosporin ranges from 1% to 5.5% with first-generation cephalosporins [64, 65]. Cross-reactivity between cephalosporins and penicillins is thought to be mediated as a result of similarities in the structural side chains as opposed to the β-lactam ring [63]. The carbapenem primary metabolite, a stable carbapenoyl, is structurally similar to benzylpenicilloyl, accounting for the higher rate of cross-reactivity seen with carbapenems [66]. Monobactam allergy is mediated by allergy to the sidechains acting as haptens which are the major determinants of allergy [60].

Other beta-lactam adverse reactions include reversible neutropenia, Coombs-positive hemolytic anemia, and platelet dysfunction with the extended spectrum penicillins; central nervous system toxicity consisting of seizures, myoclonus, and hyperreflexia is associated with extremely high doses of β-lactams and in patients with preexisting neurologic disorders and/or those with acute renal insufficiency. Elevations in transaminase levels are seen mostly with penicillinase-resistant penicillins. Antistaphylococcal penicillins are associated with interstitial nephritis. Gastrointestinal disturbances and *C. difficile* colitis may occur with the use of any beta-lactam antibiotic. Pulmonary infiltrates with eosinophilia syndrome have been described. Ceftriaxone-calcium complex may precipitate in the gallbladder leading to the development of stones consisting of ceftriaxone crystals, more commonly in children or patients in whom prolonged high-dose therapy is given [67]. Hypoprothrombinemia and a disulfiram reaction can occur with cephalosporins that possess an N-methylthiotetrazole substitution including cefamandole, moxalactam, cefotetan, and cefoperazone [68]. However, only cefoperazone and cefotetan are currently available for use in the United States, and moxalactam was withdrawn from the US market.

Vancomycin

Isolated from *Streptomyces orientalis* in 1952, vancomycin was originally utilized in penicillin-allergic patients or those infected with penicillin-resistant *Staphylococcus* [69]. The FDA originally approved vancomycin in 1958. Early on, serious drug toxicity reflected difficulties with the antibiotic purification methods, yielding to high rates of nephrotoxicity and concentration-related ototoxicity, in addition to a distinct brown color noted in infusion apparatus invoking the moniker "Mississippi mud." These early difficulties, in combination with the approval of methicillin in the same year, vancomycin use fell out of favor. With the emergence of MRSA in the 1980s as an important nosocomial pathogen, more recently, community-acquired pathogen saw a resurgence of vancomycin use [70–72]. Vancomycin continues to remain an important component of the antibiotic armamentarium.

Vancomycin is the representative agent of the glycopeptide class of antimicrobials. Teicoplanin, oritavancin, dalbavancin, and telavancin are the other agents that belong to the glycopeptide group. Vancomycin exhibits antimicrobial activity through disruption of peptidoglycan synthesis via high-affinity binding to the D-alanyl-D-alanine terminus of the N-acetylglucosamine (NAG) and N-acetylmuramic acid (NAM), leading to interruption in transglycosylation and further polymerization of peptidoglycan precursors. The bactericidal effects in replicating organisms are due to expression of autolytic enzymes that destroy damaged and incomplete cell walls [73].

Spectrum of Activity

The spectrum of activity of vancomycin includes most GPB such as staphylococci, streptococci, and enterococci. As with other cell wall active agents, minimum bactericidal concentrations of vancomycin are higher against enterococci (>32 mcg/ml) due to reduced expression of autolytic proteins [74]. Vancomycin is also active against *Bacillus* spp., *Corynebacterium* spp., and *Rhodococcus equi*. *Lactobacillus acidophilus* is the only susceptible member of this genus. *Erysipelothrix rhusiopathiae*, *Leuconostoc* spp., and *Pediococcus* spp. are inherently resistant to vancomycin. Anaerobes susceptible to vancomycin include most strains of *Clostridium* spp., *Actinomyces* spp., *Peptostreptococcus* spp., and *Propionibacterium* spp. With the exception of certain strains of *Neisseria*, GNB are uniformly resistant to vancomycin [75]. *Listeria monocytogenes* frequently show in vitro susceptibility to vancomycin although discouraging clinical response with vancomycin therapy to treat invasive listeriosis cautions against its use.

Resistance and Reduced Susceptibility

In 1988, European researchers identified the first vancomycin-resistant *Enterococcus* [76, 77]. Almost a decade later, *S. aureus* isolates with reduced vancomycin susceptibility were isolated in Japan [78]. In 2002, the first vancomycin-resistant *S. aureus* (VRSA) was isolated from patients in Detroit, Michigan [79]. Fortunately, VRSA has been isolated only rarely since 2002. As transplant patients are exposed to vancomycin frequently, understanding the mechanism of resistance among the GPB is essential for appropriate treatment selection.

Vancomycin resistance in *Enterococcus* spp. is attributed to specific gene clusters, specifically VanA, VanB, VanC, VanD, VanE, and VanG [80]. VanA is a prominent resistance genotype; it is plasmid bound and inducible. VanA and VanB are the only nonchromosomal resistance types. VanC and VanD are the non-inducible clusters. VanC confers intrinsic, albeit low-level vancomycin resistance in *E. gallinarum* and *E. casseliflavus–E. flavescens* [77, 81]. Vancomycin-resistant enterococcal clusters modify the terminal d-alanyl-d-alanine to either d-alanyl-d-lactate (VanA, VanB, VanD) or d-alanyl-d-serine (VanC, VanG, VanE) [82]. These amino acid alterations significantly decrease the affinity of the terminal NAG and NAM polymers for vancomycin. Interestingly, some strains of *E. faecalis* and *E. faecium* require vancomycin for growth. These isolates, known as vancomycin-dependent enterococcus (VDE), do not constitutively express d-alanyl-d-alanine ligase, necessary to produce d-alanyl-d-alanine. Instead, VDE strains produce inducible d-alanyl-d-lactate ligase present on VanA/VanB operons [83, 84]. As a result of this mutation, VDE will only grow in the presence of vancomycin. VDE has been isolated from liver transplant patients [83]. Discontinuation of vancomycin is occasionally insufficient for bacterial eradication as reverting mutants have been reported [85].

Vancomycin resistance in staphylococci was induced in laboratory experiments shortly after the drug was introduced. Clinical vancomycin-resistant isolates were not isolated, leading to speculation that vancomycin was intrinsically resilient in *Staphylococcus* [86, 87]. In the late 1970s however, cases of *S. epidermidis* with increased minimum inhibitory concentrations (MIC) to vancomycin were observed [88]. Diminished susceptibility of the more virulent *S. aureus* was first seen in 1997 [78]. Transference of the VanA gene from *E. faecalis* to *S. aureus* was experimentally accomplished by Nobre and colleagues in 1992. However, clinical isolates of vancomycin-resistant strains with this mechanism of resistance were not identified until 2003 in Michigan [79, 89]. Despite several documented cases of vancomycin-resistant *S. aureus* (VRSA), the majority of *S. aureus* strains with reduced susceptibility to vancomycin are identified as vancomycin-intermediate *S. aureus* (VISA) [90] or glycopeptide-intermediate *S. aureus* (GISA) [91]. VISA strains have an MIC of 4–8 mcg/ml based on the most recent recommendations from Clinical & Laboratory Standards Institute (CLSI) [92]. Increased cell wall thickness, decreased peptidoglycan cross-linking, and disorganized cell wall structure are salient mechanisms for reduced vancomycin activity among the VISA strains [93–95]. The irregularly thick peptidoglycan wall in VISA sequesters vancomycin away from the cell membrane where the drug would normally bind cell wall precursors. Colonies of VISA can coexist with vancomycin-susceptible colonies; these isolates known as heterogeneous vancomycin-intermediate *S. aureus* (hVISA) may have elevated MICs and are antecedent to VISA. While hVISA will usually maintain MICs in the CLSI susceptible range, infections due to hVISA, especially in the immunosuppressed patients, may result in failure to vancomycin therapy and should be approached with caution [96].

In recent years, investigators have noted an MIC creep in *S. aureus* isolates [97, 98]. The increased prevalence of hVISA strains may play an important role in this phenomenon. Additionally, the occurrence of vancomycin tolerance, where bactericidal activity is lost and physiologically unobtainable minimum bactericidal concentrations are observed while MICs appear to be in the susceptible range (MBC/MIC ≥32), is a concern [99, 100]. Loss of bactericidal activity may be the result of a downregulation of autolytic enzymes due to loss of function of the accessory gene regulator (*agr*) [101, 102]. Given this phenomenon, it is be prudent to select alternative drug to treat MRSA infection, especially in the severely immunocompromised patients following transplantation (Table 50.5).

Adverse Reactions

Much of the early toxicity noted with vancomycin use is attributed to suboptimum purification methods at the time. The adoption of an ion-exchange resin method of purification resulted in a significant decline in the frequency of drug-

Table 50.5 Agents with activity against MRSA/VRE

Drug	Usual dose	Route	VRE active	Prominent toxicity	Comments
Vancomycin	15 mg/kg q12h-q8h	*IV, PO/PR**	*N*	*Nephrotoxic at high doses, especially with concomitant nephrotoxins* *Ototoxicity with high peaks*	*First-line therapy for MRSA, efficacy may be decreasing with MIC creep* *Dose adjustment for renal impairment required* **PO/PR route for C. difficile*
Daptomycin	4–10 mg/kg q24	*IV (IVP over 2 min is an acceptable route)*	*Y*	*Myopathy, less prevalent now with once-daily dosing*	*Ineffective for pneumonia due to inactivation by surfactant* *Dose adjustment for renal impairment required*
Telavancin	10 mg/kg q24h	*IV*	*Y*	*Nephrotoxicity*	*Dose adjustment for renal impairment required*
Oritavancin	1200 mg once	*IV*	*Y*	*Nausea*	*Half-life approximately 250 h*
Dalbavancin	1500 mg once or 1000 mg followed by 500 mg in 1 week	*IV*	*Y*		*Half-life approximately 350 h* *Dose adjustment for renal impairment required*
Linezolid	600 mg q12h	*IV, PO*	*Y*	*Myelosuppression with thrombocytopenia predominance with prolonged use due to mitochondrial toxicity*	*Bacteriostatic agent* *May inhibit toxin production in toxic shock syndrome/ necrotizing fasciitis*
Tedizolid	200 mg q24h	*IV, PO*	*Y*	*Myelosuppression*	
Quinupristin/ dalfopristin	7.5 mg/kg q8–q12h	*IV*	*Y*	*Thrombophlebitis*	Only active against *E. faecium*
Ceftaroline	*600 mg/kg q12h*	*IV*	*N*	*Similar to other cephalosporins*	*Dose adjustment for renal impairment*
Tigecycline	*100 mg loading dose, then 50 mg q12h*	*IV*	*Y*	*Dose dependent, transient, nausea/ vomiting*	*Significant volume of distribution, primarily to bile results in low serum levels*
Sulfamethoxazole/ trimethoprim (SMX/ TMP)	*8–20 mg/kg/day, div q6–12 h*	*IV, PO*	*N*	*Hyperkalemia* *Myelosuppression* *Stevens-Johnson syndrome/TEN* *Hepatotoxicity*	*Dose adjustment required in renal impairment* *Dose dependent hyperkalemia due to inhibition of the ENaC in the cortical collecting ducts* *Antifolate effects can delay bone marrow engraftment* *Active only against certain community-acquired strains*
Tetracyclines Tetracycline Doxycycline Minocycline	 *250–500 mg q6h* *100 mg q12h* *200 mg loading dose, 100 mg q12h*	*IV, PO*	*N*	*Fanconi syndrome with outdated tetracyclines* *Tooth discoloration with pediatric use*	*Active only against certain community-acquired strains*

induced renal failure and ototoxicity [70]. Drug-attributable nephrotoxicity caused by current formulations of vancomycin is a matter of some controversy. Early retrospective data suggested that rates of renal failure in patients using vancomycin were approximately 5% although concurrent use of other nephrotoxic drugs may be a potential confounding factor in these analyses [103]. Concomitant vancomycin and aminoglycoside therapy has been recognized to heighten the risk for renal failure, especially with serum trough concentrations greater than 10 mcg/ml [104]. More recent clinical data suggests that nephrotoxicity associated with vancomycin may be more common in patients treated concomitantly with piperacillin-tazobactam in comparison to other β-lactam agents, although the mechanism by which this synergistic nephrotoxicity may occur remains unclear [105, 106]. In light of recent recommendations to target vancomycin trough concentrations between 15 and 20 mcg/ml range, vancomycin-related nephrotoxicity has become a greater concern [107]. Vancomycin has also been associated with acute interstitial nephritis [108].

Vancomycin-related ototoxicity is rare, generally reversible and observed with peak serum concentrations of greater than 50 μg/ml [109, 110]. Neutropenia and thrombocytopenia have been rarely seen and occur after a prolonged treatment course [103, 111, 112]. Thrombocytopenia is rare, immunologically mediated, but may not be readily appreciated

[113]. Infusion-related adverse reactions are not uncommon in patients receiving intravenous vancomycin. The non-IgE, histamine-related reaction known as the red man syndrome is associated with a pruritic erythematous rash from the head to the trunk which is occasionally accompanied by an anaphylactic picture [114]. Red man syndrome is related to the infusion rate of vancomycin. Infusing the drug at 500 mg/h greatly reduces the incidence of red man syndrome, and premedication with a histamine-1 receptor antagonist may be useful [115].

Vancomycin Use in the Transplant Patient

Vancomycin is commonly used in transplant patients. In a study of GPB infection in patients following liver transplantation, vancomycin-susceptible *S. aureus* and *Enterococcus* spp. were the predominant pathogens with MICs <2 μg/ml. Risk factors for infection included perioperative antibiotics, increased intraoperative blood transfusion, and renal failure after transplant surgery [116]. In a retrospective study among lung transplant recipients, vancomycin prophylaxis for transplant candidates with nasal MRSA carriage was continued for 7 days. MRSA infection increased over the first 90 days and was associated with a 7 and 12% mortality 30 and 90 days later, respectively. *S aureus* infection within the first 90 days after transplant was associated with an increased rate of acute and chronic rejection [117]. There is considerable literature about treatment of *C. difficile* infection (CDI) with oral vancomycin in transplant patients. One study showed a rate of CDI of 13% in stem cell transplant recipients. There was no increase in mortality, but recurrence was noted in 11% of patients; 2/3 of these patients were given vancomycin for CDI [118].

Aminoglycosides

Streptomycin was isolated from *Streptomyces griseus* in 1944. This first aminoglycoside was followed by neomycin and kanamycin in 1949 and 1957, respectively [119]. In 1963 gentamicin was isolated, "micin" ending to designate its origin from the *Micromonospora* genus as opposed to "mycin" for aminoglycosides isolated from *Streptomyces* spp. [120]. Additional aminoglycosides became available for clinical use, including sisomicin, netilmicin, tobramycin, and amikacin. To date, gentamicin, tobramycin, and amikacin have remained clinically useful agents against many bacteria, while streptomycin is used in the treatment of drug-resistant tuberculosis. A novel aminoglycoside, plazomicin, is in clinical development and has retained in vitro activity against bacteria resistant to earlier-generation aminoglycosides [121]. Aminoglycosides have maintained their clinical utility in the face of many multidrug-resistant GNB that poses a daunting management challenge for patients undergoing allograft transplantation.

Aminoglycosides are rapidly bactericidal poly-cationic sugars that exhibit concentration-dependent killing. The primary mechanism of action is through inhibition of protein translation. Aminoglycosides bind to the A site on the 16 s subunit of the prokaryotic ribosome and interfere with tRNA-mediated translocation [122]. Subsequently, incomplete protein products are inserted into the bacterial cell membrane causing leakage of cellular contents from the porous cell [123]. The rapid bacterial killing seen after aminoglycoside administration is not easily explained by this mechanism. A more rapid mode of killing displayed shortly after administration is binding to lipopolysaccharides (LPS) and disruption of adjoining calcium and magnesium bridges [124]. Disruption of bacterial membrane integrity precedes increased permeability and loss of intracellular content. This mechanism is similar to that seen with the cationic polymyxin class. The binding of aminoglycosides to LPS before their subsequent cytoplasmic infiltration is the first of three phases of drug transport, the latter two being energy dependent [125, 126]. The first energy-dependent phase (EDP1) is the slower of the two and relies on a sufficient negative membrane potential generated by proton motive force for drug entry [127]. Since aminoglycosides are positively charged in a physiological pH range, an acidic extracellular environment severely limits cellular entry due to a loss of electrochemical potential. In addition to low pH, anaerobic conditions and site-competitive Mg^{2+} and Ca^{2+} are antagonistic to aminoglycoside entry during EDP1 [128]. Anaerobic bacteria, lacking oxidative aerobic metabolism to establish a sufficient electronegative intracellular space, are intrinsically resistant to aminoglycosides. The final phase of cellular entry, known as EDP2 or energy-dependent phase II, is manifested as the ribosomal-binding phase and is initiated when sufficient porosity has been attained on the cell membrane.

Spectrum of Activity

The aminoglycosides in clinical use have consistent activity against the non-lactose-fermenting *P. aeruginosa* and *Acinetobacter* spp. while lacking activity against *S. maltophilia* and *B. cepacia*. All *Enterobacteriaceae* species are susceptible. Certain intracellular pathogens are susceptible, including *Bartonella* spp., *Brucella* spp., *Yersinia* spp., and *Francisella tularensis*. Amikacin is active against *Mycobacterium avium-intracellulare*. Select aminoglycosides display synergistic bacterial killing when combined with cell wall active agents due to enhanced cell entry [129] against GPB such as *Staphylococcus* spp., β-hemolytic *Streptococcus*, *S. viridans*, enterococci, and *Listeria mono-*

cytogenes. Aminoglycosides also exhibit synergistic properties against *P. aeruginosa* and *Enterobacteriaceae*.

Mechanisms of Resistance

A desirable attribute of the aminoglycosides is the preserved spectrum of activity against multidrug resistant bacteria that are often encountered in the transplant population. The predominant mechanisms of resistance to aminoglycosides are enzymatic drug alterations, ribosomal alterations, efflux pumps, and diminished cellular entry through porin mutations [130–133]. Resistance mechanisms in GNB can be chromosomal or acquired via plasmids or transposons. Mobile resistance elements often travel with genes for multidrug resistance and can be especially problematic [134].

Enzymatic modification of aminoglycosides is the most common and clinically important mechanism for acquired drug resistance. Drug modification is accomplished by three major classes of enzymes: acetyltransferases (AAC), adenylyltransferases (ANT), and phosphotransferases (APH). Numerous enzymes in each family have been identified, and a systematic nomenclature has been implemented to delineate the drug-inactivating proteins [134]. AAC enzymes target amino groups on the aminoglycoside molecule and are dependent on acetyl CoA, while ANT and APH enzymes are specific for hydroxyl groups and rely on ATP for activity. After enzymatic modification, the antibiotic has significantly less affinity for the ribosomal binding site. Compared to gentamicin and tobramycin, amikacin is susceptible to fewer modifying enzymes and may be more likely to retain activity against pathogenic isolates resistant to other aminoglycosides [135, 136]. Clinical strains may still possess modifying enzymes allowing susceptibility to one or more aminoglycosides. A detailed table of aminoglycoside modifying enzymes can be found in Shaw's review [134]. Reduced membrane permeability and drug efflux pumps are two additional resistance modalities. Alterations in the LPS structure from a smooth to a more rough form may be responsible for certain cases of low-level resistance [137]. The aminoglycoside efflux pump, designated MexXY-OprM, has been implicated in the transient loss of bactericidal activity of aminoglycosides in the time frame spanning between initial drug administration and several hours afterward [138]. This phenomenon, known as adaptive resistance, has been demonstrated in clinical isolates of *P. aeruginosa* [132, 139].

Adverse Reactions

Aminoglycosides are some of the most commonly used nephrotoxins in clinical practice of infectious diseases. The incidence of nephrotoxicity with aminoglycosides has been reported to be as high as 25% [140, 141]. Newer, extended-interval dosing regimens have resulted in reduced potential for nephrotoxicity, but risk still exists [142]. Data suggest that the nephrotoxic potential among the various aminoglycosides is not equivalent. Gentamicin is likely accompanied with a greater risk for nephrotoxicity than amikacin and tobramycin [140, 143–145]. The proposed pathogenesis for aminoglycoside-induced kidney injury comes mostly from animal data [146, 147]. After filtration in the glomerulus, approximately 5% of the aminoglycoside dose is reabsorbed in the proximal tubule via endocytosis by megalin receptors where they are sequestered in lysosomal vacuoles and the Golgi apparatus [148–150]. Gentamicin experiences the greatest cortical concentrations which may explain the perceived enhanced nephrotoxicity with this agent [147]. Altered cellular protein synthesis and mitochondrial toxicity after aminoglycoside exposure lead to necrosis of the tubules, manifested by loss of K^+, Mg^{2+}, and Ca^{2+} cations, HCO_3^-, glucose, and findings of proteinuria and cast in the urine [151–153]. Patients usually experience non-oliguric or polyuric renal failure with reduced glomerular filtration rate and elevations in blood urea nitrogen and serum creatinine; rarely, Fanconi's syndrome may be observed [154]. Aminoglycoside-induced acute tubular necrosis is generally reversible. Tubular regeneration begins to restore kidney function despite continued exposure to aminoglycosides [155, 156]. Administration of aminoglycosides with concomitant nephrotoxic drugs such as vancomycin, amphotericin B, and calcineurin inhibitors increases the risk for kidney injury. Sparse data suggests that penicillins with significant sodium content may reduce the risk for aminoglycoside-induced nephrotoxicity [157, 158].

Ototoxicity from aminoglycosides can present as cochlear toxicity and vestibular toxicity or both. Ototoxicity may occur in as many as 14% of patients, but asymptomatic loss of high-frequency sound perception has been reported more often when audiometric assessment is undertaken [159, 160]. While vestibular damage is usually reversible, injury to cochlear cells is generally not. The pathophysiology of ototoxicity is similar to the cellular changes occurring in the proximal renal tubule with uptake and accumulation occurring in type 1 hair cell lysosomes [161, 162]. The greatest risk factors are duration of exposure to aminoglycoside, renal failure, and concurrent therapy with other ototoxic agents such as loop diuretics and vancomycin [163–165]. Additionally, several mitochondrial rRNA mutations at the 12S ribosome subunit place patients at an increased risk for ototoxicity [166].

Neuromuscular blockade is a rare side effect of aminoglycosides and caused by prevention of postsynaptic and presynaptic acetylcholine release by interfering with the preceding calcium signal [167]. Major risk factors are predisposing conditions that impair neuromuscular junction activity such as co-administration of depolarizing or non-depolarizing neuromuscular blockers and potentially myasthenia gravis [168]. Additional risk factors include elevated aminoglycoside concentrations, hypomagnesemia, hypocalcemia [169], and use of calcium channel blockers [170]. The effects are not effectively reversible by acetylcholinesterase inhibitors like neostigmine; infusion of intravenous calcium restores neuromuscular function quickly and reliably [171].

Use in the Transplant Patient

An important potential use of aminoglycosides, especially amikacin, would be expected in the transplant patient with multidrug-resistant *Acinetobacter* and *Pseudomonas* infections. In a study of renal transplant patients, amikacin was used in 12% of patients, second to carbapenems. *Enterococcal* infection was associated with the highest mortality. No mention was made of renal toxicity from amikacin [172]. In another review of KPC infections in renal transplant recipients, gentamicin was used in one patient for 43 days along with polymyxin; the patient died 84 days after transplantation [173].

Oxazolidinones

The oxazolidinones are a class of synthetic antimicrobials discovered in the 1970s, with earnest clinical development in the late 1980s [174]. Due to favorable toxicology and pharmacokinetics, linezolid became the first marketed member of this novel class, with tedizolid as a more recent addition [175, 176]. The oxazolidinones inhibit bacterial protein synthesis through binding to the 50s ribosome at a site close to that of clindamycin and chloramphenicol, although the molecules have a distinct mechanism of action [177]. Crystal structure analysis of the linezolid-ribosome complex shows that linezolid binds to the A-site of the peptidyl transferase center, the universally conserved U2585 nucleotide of the 23S ribosomal subunit, interfering with proper tRNA positioning and leading to gross translational inaccuracy through frameshift mutations [178]. Early studies pointed toward inhibition of the ribosomal initiation complex as the primary mechanism of action; however, subsequent research has shown that while this may be an effect of linezolid, the drug concentrations at the ribosome required are higher than may be achievable in vivo [179]. Various oxazolidinone structures induce unique conformational changes at their binding sites, providing a starting point for the development of compounds that may overcome mutational resistance. Furthermore, oxazolidinones have been shown to serve as a cross-link between LepA and the ribosome, inhibiting a crucial cellular quality-control mechanism [180].

Spectrum of Activity

Linezolid is active against a broad variety of GPB, with MIC90 values of 1 μg/mL for most clinically relevant isolates, including MRSA and vancomycin-resistant enterococci. Linezolid is active against other less common Gram-positive organisms such as *Rhodococcus*, *Listeria*, and *Erysipelothrix* [181], although clinical experience is limited. *Nocardia* spp. also exhibit in vitro susceptibility to linezolid with an MIC of 4 mcg/mL for most clinical isolates [182]. Due to active efflux pumps and poor membrane penetrability, linezolid is inactive against most Gram-negative bacteria, with variable activity against *Moraxella* and *Haemophilus* spp. Linezolid has in vitro activity against anaerobes, including *C. difficile*, *Fusobacterium*, and *B. fragilis* although there is little clinical information and sporadic resistance may be noted among some anaerobes [183].

Linezolid has variable activity against acid-fast bacilli. Among isolates of rapidly growing *Mycobacteria*, linezolid inhibited most *M. fortuitum* isolates, whereas other rapid growers such as *M. abscessus* and *M. chelonae* demonstrated higher MICs to linezolid than that are physiologically achievable to treat an infection. Due to this high variability in susceptibility, determination of MICs to linezolid in rapidly growing *Mycobacteria* should be confirmed [184]. Against non-tuberculous slow-growing *Mycobacteria*, linezolid demonstrates good activity against *M. marinum*, *M. gordonae*, *M. szulgai*, and *M. kansasii*; however, less than half of *M. avium* complex strains tested showed in vitro susceptibility [185]. Linezolid is also active against clinical isolates of *M. tuberculosis* and has demonstrated utility as salvage therapy for MDR and XDR strains of *M. tuberculosis* [186]. Tedizolid has a similar spectrum of activity as linezolid, although with enhanced activity against certain linezolid-resistant strains [187].

Resistance

As synthetic antimicrobials, it was hoped that the development of resistance to oxazolidinones would be hindered by lack of a natural reservoir of resistance that has evolved in bacteria through the millennia [188]. Despite this theoretical advantage, a naturally occurring resistance gene was identified in a veterinary *Staphylococcus* isolate the same year that linezolid was marketed and was linked to an outbreak of linezolid-resistant *Staphylococcus* in Spain less than a decade later [189]. Single nucleotide polymorphisms near the target site of linezolid on the 23S ribosome may confer clinical resistance [190]. The first report of clinical resistance to linezolid came from two isolates of *E. faecium* identified in a compassionate-use trial that demonstrated a G2576T mutation in the 23S ribosome, with reduced susceptibility correlating to a greater amount of mutant ribosome. This mutation and numerous other single-nucleotide polymorphisms on the 23S bacterial ribosome have also been selected for in vitro in *Staphylococcus* spp. and enterococci [191]. While the risk for selection of de novo-resistant mutants appears to be low, with an estimated frequency of 10^{-10}, however, nosocomial spread of such mutant strains may potentially become a clinical problem [192]. In an early case control study of linezolid-resistant *Enterococcus* spp., prior exposure to and prolonged treatment with linezolid were identified as major risk factors for presence of linezolid resistance [193]. In subsequent analyses, solid organ transplantation, peripheral vascular disease, total parenteral nutrition, and exposure to a variety of antimicrobials were identified as risk factor for linezolid resistance [194]. Interestingly, this study failed to demonstrate an association between prior linezolid exposure and subsequent development of drug resistance; horizontal spread of the drug-resistant organism(s) is presently supported by epidemiologic data [195]. Mutational resistance to linezolid may also occur through alteration of the ribosomal L3 and L4 proteins, which facilitate the process of ribosomal translation and elongation [196]. The exact mechanism behind reduced susceptibility conferred by mutations in these proteins has yet to be elucidated fully, although they often coexist with and may facilitate subsequent development of ribosomal mutations [197].

Resistance to linezolid may also occur via enzymatic modification of the ribosomal target. Various modifications of nucleotides known to confer resistance to other protein synthesis inhibitors binding at sites near the peptidyl transferase center have also been shown to confer resistance to the oxazolidinones [198]. The *cfr* gene, encoding for an rRNA methyltransferase, is the most prominent mechanism, conferring resistance to a group of antimicrobials known as $PhLOPS_A$ (for phenicols, lincosamides, oxazolidinones, pleuromutilins, and streptogramin A) [199]. First identified in 2005 in livestock, a transposon bearing this gene in addition to *ermB* was identified in a clinical isolate of *S. aureus* [200]. This gene has subsequently been shown to be responsible for resistance in clinical isolates of *S. aureus*, *S. epidermidis*, and *E. faecalis* [201–203]. Based on US surveillance data, overall resistance rates to linezolid are stable at 0.3–1.48%, depending on the organism. However, local resistance rates may be as high as 7% in *E. faecalis* [204]. Linezolid resistance has recently been described in *S. pneumoniae* [204], warranting continued susceptibility surveillance among pneumococcal clinical isolates.

Adverse Reactions

Brief courses of linezolid are well-tolerated. Common adverse events include diarrhea, nausea, and vomiting. Serious adverse events may emerge with extended duration of therapy. Myelosuppression occurs in a dose- and duration-dependent manner, primarily causing thrombocytopenia, although trilineage suppression of hematopoiesis has been observed [205]. This effect becomes prominent if treatment is extended beyond 2 weeks and may be predicted on the basis of overall exposure to the drug and baseline hematologic parameters [206]. The mechanism for anemia appears similar to that of chloramphenicol, namely, inhibition of mitochondrial protein synthesis [207], and is likely a class effect of the oxazolidinones [208]. Thrombocytopenia is likely an immunologically mediated phenomenon [207]. Myelosuppression is generally reversible; however, use in hematopoietic stem cell transplant recipients may lead to prolonged pancytopenia and rarely permanent graft loss [209]. Prolonged use of linezolid may predispose to peripheral and optic neuropathy [210, 211] secondary to mitochondrial protein synthesis inhibition and may be irreversible [212]. Mitochondrial inhibition may also lead to lactic acidosis and the posterior reversible leukoencephalopathy syndrome [213, 214]. As an inhibitor of monoamine oxidase (MAO), linezolid has been associated with the serotonin syndrome when used with other serotonergic drugs in the general population and in patients undergoing HSCT [215]. An analysis of phase III and IV trials failed to support this association when compared to non-serotonergic antimicrobials [216], and clinical data supports the rarity of this event [217]. Tedizolid appears to have a diminished capacity to inhibit MAO and potentiate serotonin toxicity when compared to linezolid, although clinical trials have notably excluded recipients of MAO inhibitors [176].

Use in Transplant Patients

Linezolid has been studied in 25 HSCT recipients who received at least 3 days of linezolid versus 24 controls. There was no difference in the duration of thrombocytopenia or neutropenia but a trend toward difference in time to engraftment. In patients treated with 10 days or less of linezolid, duration of thrombocytopenia, time to engraftment, and need for platelet transfusions were not greater compared with controls. The conclusion from this review was that linezolid can be used safely for greater than 10 days with close monitoring of platelet counts and time to engraftment [209].

Daptomycin

Daptomycin is a cyclic lipopeptide antibiotic discovered in the early 1980s. Daptomycin exerts rapid bactericidal activity in a concentration-dependent manner by insertion of daptomycin's lipophilic decanoyl side chain into the bacterial cell membrane, forming an efflux channel that extrudes potassium ions down their concentration gradient. While the initial binding occurs independently, deeper membrane insertion and channel formation require the presence of calcium ions [218]. The depolarization that follows daptomycin binding destroys bacterial cells without inducing lysis and subsequent release of intracellular contents [219]. Due to its unique mode of killing, daptomycin continues to display bacterial killing in the presence of nondividing organisms [220]. Daptomycin binds to lung surfactant which inactivates the drug and renders it ineffective in treating lung infections: however effectiveness may still be sufficient in hematogenous lung infections such as septic emboli; however, no rigorous clinical data supports such use [221].

Spectrum of Activity

Daptomycin has activity against *Streptococcus* spp., *Enterococcus* including VRE, *Staphylococcus* spp. including VISA and VRSA, and specific Gram-positive anaerobes such as *Peptococcus* spp., *Peptostreptococcus* spp., and *C. perfringens* [222]. Daptomycin also has activity against *Bacillus* spp., *Corynebacterium* spp., and *Propionibacterium* spp.

Resistance and Reduced Susceptibility

Daptomycin is often used when vancomycin resistance and therapeutic failure are present and the potential for resistance is a concern. The overall incidence of daptomycin remains low, although a number of resistance mechanisms have been delineated. Investigators noted the relationship between increased daptomycin MICs during the course of treatment for *S. aureus* systemic infection. This was probably in part due to daptomycin membrane binding site interference resulting from thickened peptidoglycan wall among some VISA isolates [223, 224]. This has not been noted with the rare VRSA isolates due to a different resistance mechanism. Multiple additional distinct membrane alterations have been described as resistance mechanisms among *S. aureus* isolates [225] including decreased membrane fluidity, increased positive membrane surface charge, reduced sensitivity to permeability changes, decreased autolysis, reduced affinity to daptomycin, decreased membrane surface acidity, and finally diminished susceptibility to human neutrophil peptide-1 and thrombin-induced platelet microbicidal protein [226, 227]. It is likely that more than one of these mechanisms may be present in concert among resistant isolates as each individual mode of resistance generally causes a minor increase in daptomycin MIC. The *mprF* gene plays a major role in *S. aureus*. The product of *mprF* is an enzyme that couples phosphatidylglycerol to a lysine residue and subsequently mobilizes the lysyl-phosphatidylglycerol (LPG) to the outer cell membrane. Decreased acidity and increased positive charge due to the presence of LPG compromise calcium-mediated daptomycin binding to the deeper bacterial cell membrane. A distinct mechanism is responsible for daptomycin resistance in enterococci, and clinical resistance is increasingly observed in these organisms [228–230]. Gene mutations involving *liaF* and *gdpD* were identified in daptomycin-resistant *Enterococcus* strains, which appear to regulate cell membrane stability and phospholipid production. Recent data suggest that enterococci with an MIC of 3–4 mcg/mL harbor mutations in the *liaF* gene [231, 232]. Certain β-lactam antibiotics may potentiate daptomycin activity against *S. aureus* and enterococci [233, 234].

Adverse Reactions

Skeletal muscle toxicity is a relatively common adverse event seen in patients given prolonged courses of daptomycin. Initial trials utilizing 4 mg per kg twice daily dosing noted an unacceptable rate of creatinine kinase (CK) elevations [235]. Daptomycin was approved by the FDA after once-daily dosing was shown to cause significantly less muscle toxicity than seen with more frequent drug administration. The mechanism responsible for daptomycin-related CK elevations involves degeneration and regenerations of myofibers [236]. Clinical trials have shown that CK elevations occur in up to 6.7% of patients on once-daily dosing. The CK elevation is reversible and often returns to baseline in several weeks. Despite the relative safety of daptomycin, cases of rhabdomyolysis with subsequent renal failure have been reported [237–239]. Renal impairment without proper dose adjustment and concomitant administration of HMG-CoA reductase inhibitors have been considered as a potential risk for this toxicity. Additional adverse effects reported with daptomycin use are gastrointestinal disturbances and injection site reaction.

Daptomycin in Transplant Patients

Daptomycin is used in the transplant population to treat vancomycin-resistant enterococcal infections and as initial or salvage therapy for serious MRSA infections [240, 241]. In 72 patients with VRE bacteremia, including HSCT recipients and patients with acute myeloid leukemia, 43 received daptomycin and 29 received linezolid. The 30-day success rate was 76.7% with daptomycin and 75.9% with linezolid. Three patients in daptomycin treatment group developed CK elevations, which was mild in two but 28 times the upper limit of normal in one patient who complained of muscle weakness. This patient was switched to linezolid with resolution of symptoms and return of CK to baseline [240]. A retrospective review of stem cell transplant recipients from 2007 to 2010 revealed eight daptomycin non-susceptible *E. faecium*. Close to 90% had received daptomycin previously for a mean duration of 19 days. Interestingly, two of eight daptomycin non-susceptible enterococci were susceptible to vancomycin, and all eight retained susceptibility to linezolid [242]. Clinicians should be aware of potential emergence of daptomycin non-susceptibility enterococci and monitor daptomycin MICs during the course treatment, especially for patients with severe immune suppression with persistent and recurrent bcteremia. Synergistic combination of daptomycin with β-lactams such as ampicillin and ceftaroline has resulted in markedly reduced daptomycin MICs among *S. aureus* and enterococcal clinical isolates [243, 244].

Tetracyclines: Focus on Tigecycline

Tetracyclines bind reversibly to the 30S ribosomal subunit, inhibiting protein synthesis by preventing incorporation of amino acid residues into elongating peptide chains. The reversible binding renders this class bacteriostatic. Among GNB, tetracyclines diffuse through the outer membrane porin channels to gain access in the periplasmic space; however, it requires an energy-dependent mechanism to cross through cytoplasmic inner membrane to reach bacterial cytosol. Resistance is mediated by active efflux transport protein pumps, inhibition of binding to the ribosomal site by cytoplasmic protective proteins, and enzymatic inactivation. The most significant mechanism of resistance is active efflux [245].

Tigecycline is the first of the glycyclcyclines to be approved by the FDA for treatment of complicated skin and soft tissue infections, complicated intra-abdominal infections, and community-acquired pneumonia. Tigecycline is a structural analogue of minocycline that binds with fivefold higher affinity to the ribosome than tetracyclines [246]. The structural modifications and enhanced binding overcome the ribosomal and efflux pump mechanisms of resistance to the tetracycline class and extend the antimicrobial spectrum. Tigecycline is a poor substrate for the tetracycline efflux pumps and can still attach to ribosomes with the Tet(M) protein modification [247]. Resistance can develop in GNB due to the overexpression of multidrug efflux pumps. *P. aeruginosa* naturally expresses these multidrug efflux pumps, which explain the intrinsic resistance to tigecycline.

Spectrum of Activity

The spectrum of activity includes multidrug-resistant organisms such as MRSA, CoNS, *E. faecalis*, VREF, ESBL- and carbapenemase-producing GNB including *Acinetobacter* spp., *Enterobacteriaceae*, penicillin-resistant *S. pneumoniae*, β-lactamase-producing *H. influenzae*, and anaerobes, including *C. difficile*. *Pseudomonas* and *Proteus*, *Providencia*, and *Morganella* species are intrinsically resistant to tigecycline [247, 248]. Cases of tigecycline resistance developing after treatment were reported by Spanu et al., in ESBL-*Klebsiella* and a carbapenemase *E. coli* [249]. Emergence of tigecycline resistance during therapy has been described in *A. baumannii* [250]. A recent in vitro surveillance report of GPB in the United States showed that tigecycline maintained high rates of susceptibility to MRSA and enterococci, with susceptibility to *S. pneumoniae* varying by geographical region from 80.9% to 95.2% [251].

Use of Tigecycline in Transplant Recipients

The pharmacokinetics of tigecycline show a large volume of distribution of 7–10 L/kg and a half-life of 42 h after multiple doses [246], which was long enough to allow once-daily dosing. With standard intravenous dosing of an initial loading dose of 100 mg followed by 50 mg twice daily, the C_{max} was 1.45 mg/L after a 30-min infusion and 0.63 mg/L after a 60-minute infusion. The serum levels are low with an area under the curve at 12 h following a 50 mg dose of 3.07 ± 0.6 μg × h/mL. Concentrations in alveolar macrophages were 78 times higher than serum, and concentrations in neutrophils are 20–30 times higher than serum; penetration into skin blister fluid was 74% of serum concentration. Tigecycline has time-dependent killing mechanism and exhibits a postantibiotic effect for *K. pneumonia*, *E. cloacae*, and *E. coli* [247]. Tigecycline has been shown to be bactericidal against MRSA and MSSA in animal models and primarily bacteriostatic against experimental *E. faecalis* infections. The primary route of elimination is via biliary tract; 33% of the drug is excreted unchanged or as metabolites. Therefore, no drug modification is required in patients with renal insufficiency. Tigecycline is only available in an intravenous formulation.

The major adverse reactions include nausea, vomiting, elevated liver enzymes, and few case reports of pancreatitis [252]. It is labeled as a class D drug during pregnancy. The low serum concentrations of tigecycline have called into question the efficacy of drug for the treatment of bacteremia. Case series of bloodstream infections have been reported with varying results. In a study by Gardiner et al., patients with secondary bacteremia from biliary and urinary sources, tigecycline demonstrated cure rates comparable to conventional antibiotic therapy of 81% vs. 78%, respectively [253]. In September of 2010, the FDA released a warning for increased mortality in patients treated with tigecycline compared with other conventional antibiotics. Prasad and colleagues performed a meta-analysis of 13 trials of tigecycline including approved and off-label indications [254]. Tigecycline use was associated with 30% relative risk mortality and a 12% relative increase in non-cure rates. This result was independent of infection type and use in FDA approved and non-approved indications. The conclusion of these authors is that tigecycline should be used only when there are few or no alternatives. More prospective studies are needed to determine the cause for the higher mortality with tigecycline.

Tigecycline has been used in the transplant population to treat MDR GNB infections. Bergamasco and colleagues describe an outbreak of KPC-producing *Klebsiella* infections in solid organ transplant unit, including four patients with bacteremia [255]. Three patients were treated with tigecycline plus polymyxin and one with tigecycline plus imipenem-cilastatin. All four patients survived as did the single patient treated with polymyxin plus imipenem-cilastatin and two with polymyxin alone. Another study [256] used combination therapy with tigecycline, amikacin, and colistin. Emergence of tigecycline resistance during therapy for MDR *K. pneumoniae* and *E. coli* has been reported [249]. A case of recurrent renal graft infection and bacteremia due to ESBL *K. pneumoniae* was recently reported. The patient had a mixed population of carbapenem- and tigecycline-resistant isolates that emerged during antibiotic therapy. Tigecycline MIC increased from 0.5 to 8 μg/mL during therapy. The patient eventually required removal of the transplanted kidney due to severe graft rejection [257].

Macrolides and Streptogramins

Erythromycin is the prototype of the macrolide class, which includes clarithromycin and azithromycin, an azalide. Erythromycin is a 14-membered macrocyclic lactone ring attached to two sugar moieties. Macrolides and azalides insert into a pocket of the 23S subunit of the 50S ribosome, by attaching at domain V of the peptidyl transferase loop and blocking protein assembly by inhibiting the translocation step. Gram-positive bacteria accumulate about 100 times more erythromycin than GNB; *Pseudomonas* and *Acinetobacter* spp. are intrinsically resistant to this class of drugs. These drugs are generally regarded as bacteriostatic; high concentrations against susceptible organisms such as *S. pneumoniae* may be bactericidal [258].

Erythromycin use has been limited due to gastrointestinal intolerance, cholestatic hepatitis with the estolate form, and increasing drug resistance. It is still frequently used in colonic surgery bowel preps and topical dermatologic preparations. The newer macrolides, clarithromycin, and azithromycin were specifically developed to improve bioavailability, pharmacodynamics, pharmacokinetics, and antimicrobial spectrum of activity.

Azithromycin is an azalide because it has a methyl-substituted nitrogen in the 15-member lactone ring. Azithromycin has a half-life in many tissues that extends to 2–4 days and an average terminal half-life of 68 h. Clarithromycin has the 14-member lactone with modification of the C6 site with a methoxy ring. The major metabolite, 14-hydroxy-clarithromycin, has antibacterial activity. The mechanism of action and resistance of the newer macrolides are similar to erythromycin, and cross-resistance exists among the drugs within the class. Azithromycin has better penetration through the outer membrane envelope of GNB, especially *M. catarrhalis* and *H. influenzae*. Although the entire class is considered bacteriostatic, these agents are bactericidal against *S. pneumoniae*, *H. influenzae*, and *S. pyogenes* [259]. The newer macrolides also have the anti-inflammatory properties as described with erythromycin. These include suppression of proinflammatory cytokine release from endothelial cells, acceleration of neutrophil apoptosis, and inhibition of nuclear factor kappa B and activation protein-1, which regulate the chemoattractant chemokine, interleukin-8 [260, 261].

Resistance

Resistance to macrolides occurs through four mechanisms. Drug efflux by active drug efflux pumps is encoded by *mrs*A, *mef*A, or *mefE* in staphylococci, *S. pyogenes*, and *S. pneumoniae*. *MefA* encodes an efflux pump that extrudes macrolides at a lower level (<16 mcg/mL); high antibiotic concentrations might overcome the pump, forcing enough antibiotic into the bacterial cytosol to exert a measurable antibacterial effect. Clarithromycin and azithromycin are more active against pneumococci than erythromycin; however the level of resistance in *Mef*A-containing strains is on the rise [262]. Inducible or constitutive production of methylase enzymes is mediated through expression of *ermA*, *ermB*, and *ermC* that decrease binding of drug to the ribosomal target. *ErmB* encodes methylation of a base in domain V of the 23S rRNA altering the site of attachment and resulting in high-level resistance with MIC >64 mcg/mL [259]. Since the macrolides, lincosamides, and streptogramins share the same binding site, the MLS_B phenotype conferred by *erm* genes causes cross-resistance in all three classes. *Enterobacteriaceae* may produce esterases that hydrolyze the macrolide. The fourth mechanism of resistance is through chromosomal mutations that alter the 50S ribosomal protein, leading to resistance to macrolides and azalides. This mechanism can be found in *B. subtilis*, *Campylobacter* spp., mycobacteria, and Gram-positive cocci.

Spectrum of Activity

The spectrum of the newer macrolides includes GPB such as *S. pneumoniae*, *S. pyogenes*, *S. agalactiae*, *S. viridans*, *B. pertussis*, *Listeria monocytogenes*, *Corynebacterium diphtheria*, and some strains of MSSA although resistance among clinical MSSA and *S. pneumoniae* isolates is emerging. The Gram-negative activity includes *H. influenzae*, *M. catarrhalis*, *H. pylori*, *B. pertussis*, *Neisseria* spp., *P. multocida*, and some clinical strains of *Salmonella* and *Shigella*. Atypical activity includes *Legionella* spp., *Chlamydia trachomatis*, *Chlamydophila pneumoniae*, *Borrelia burgdorferi*, *H. pylori*, *Mycoplasma pneumoniae*, *Bartonella henselae*, *C. jejuni*, and *M. avium* complex. Anaerobic activity includes *C. perfringens* and *Propionibacterium* spp. Azithromycin and clarithromycin may differ in their activities against specific pathogens.

Adverse Reactions

Adverse reactions seen with the newer macrolides are predominantly gastrointestinal. Allergy has been reported with azithromycin. Higher doses can cause dizziness, tinnitus, and reversible hearing loss. Torsades de pointes have been reported in older patients, especially with concomitant use with cisapride. Clarithromycin can have cytochrome P450 interactions with drugs metabolized by CYP3A.

The emergence of erythromycin resistance in clinical *S. pneumoniae* and *S. pyogenes* isolates had an impact on susceptibility trends for the newer macrolides. Streptococci and staphylococci that are resistant to erythromycin are often resistant to clarithromycin and azithromycin. In Canada, over the past 20 years, pneumococcal surveillance studies have shown a steady rise in macrolide resistance correlated with declining prescriptions for erythromycin and higher clarithromycin and azithromycin use. In cities in the United States where pneumococcal vaccination of children has been widely used, a distinct reduction in the overall prevalence of macrolide resistance among invasive isolates was an encouraging trend. The explanation is that the serotypes most likely to express resistance are also the ones included in the pediatric vaccines and disease caused by these serotypes has declined dramatically as a result of strict adherence to childhood vaccination protocols.

Streptogramins

The streptogramins are a family of compounds divided into two groups based on structure. Dalfopristin (group A) and quinupristin (group B) are combined in a ratio of 30:70 and available for intravenous use. The combination of both drugs produces increased in vitro bactericidal activity. Quinupristin and dalfopristin bind to sequential sites on the 50S ribosomal subunit. Dalfopristin binding results in a conformational change in the ribosome that increases quinupristin binding. Inhibition of protein synthesis occurs through preventing peptide chain formation. Resistance occurs through several mechanisms including enzymatic inactivation by a hydrolase for quinupristin and acetyltransferase for dalfopristin, efflux or active transport, and alteration in ribosomal binding sites, which is the most common resistance mechanism. The combination of the two drugs requires multiple mutations targeting both components. Staphylococci can develop resistance to quinupristin by the *erm*A (MSL_B) mutation. A comparative study of linezolid and quinupristin-dalfopristin in VREF infection showed no difference in 30-day mortality; however, 11% of blood isolates developed resistance to quinupristin-dalfopristin compared with 0% in the linezolid arm [263].

Quinupristin-dalfopristin was approved by FDA in 1999 for the treatment of bloodstream infections due to vancomycin-resistant *Enterococcus faecium* (VREF) and skin and skin structure infections (SSSI) caused by MSSA and *S. pyogenes*. It was the first antibiotic to be indicated for the treatment of patients with serious or life-threatening infections associated with VREF bacteremia. Quinupristin-dalfopristin is bactericidal against most susceptible organisms and demonstrates a postantibiotic effect against *B. anthracis* for 7–8 h, longer than the other classes of antibiotics tested [264]. The recommended dose is 7.5 mg/kg every 8 h and produces plasma concentrations of 11–12 μg/ml. Both drugs undergo hepatic metabolism with most metabolites eliminated by fecal excretion (75%), and a smaller amount is via kidneys.

Quinupristin-dalfopristin is active against *E. faecium*, including VRE, but not *E. faecalis* due to intrinsic resistance. Other susceptible GPB include *S. aureus* including MRSA and CoNS and streptococci, except for *S. pneumoniae*. The susceptible MIC is <1 μg/ml. The combination has activity against most Van A and Van B strains of *E. faecium*. The anaerobic activity is mostly against *Lactobacillus* spp., *P. acnes*, *C. difficile*, and *C. perfringens*. It has some activity against upper respiratory pathogens except for *Haemophilus* species. It has no activity against *Enterobacteriaceae*, *Pseudomonas*, and *Acinetobacter* due to inability to enter the inside of the bacterial cell.

Adverse reactions include a high incidence of infusion irritation (30%), arthralgias, myalgias, gastrointestinal disturbances, and elevated liver enzymes and bilirubin. In vitro drug interaction studies have demonstrated that quinupristin-dalfopristin significantly inhibits cytochrome P450 3A4 metabolism of cyclosporin, tacrolimus, and other medication. Therapeutic level monitoring of cyclosporine should be performed when cyclosporine must be used concomitantly with quinupristin-dalfopristin. A kidney transplant recipient on both drugs had a threefold increase in the cyclosporine blood concentration 3 days after starting quinupristin-dalfopristin, reinforcing the need for frequent monitoring of cyclosporine levels in such patients [265]. The hyperbilirubinemia during quinupristin-dalfopristin in liver transplant recipients was found on liver biopsy to be multifactorial, including graft rejection, cholestasis, and periportal inflammation without specific drug-related hepatocyte injury [266].

Use in Transplant Patients

Despite the potentially serious interactions with cyclosporine and tacrolimus, quinupristin-dalfopristin has been used in the transplant population, mostly to treat VRE infections. In a study of mostly liver transplant recipients with VRE infections, including 19 with bacteremia, the clinical response was 80% using standard drug dose. Two of four treatment failures were associated with a decrease in in vitro susceptibility, myalgias and arthralgia occurred in 33%, and the mortality from VRE infection was 17% [267]. In another study of 28 VRE infections in 19 patients, 8 patients received quinupristin-dalfopristin for 9 infection episodes; only 2 of the patients survived [268]. In this report, linezolid therapy showed a trend toward improved survival. Quinupristin-dalfopristin has been used in pediatric stem cell transplant recipients with resolution of bacteremia in all five patients [269]. One case of successful treatment of VRE meningitis with quinupristin-dalfopristin combined with daptomycin has been reported [270]. The safety of quinupristin-dalfopristin was evaluated in 19 pediatric liver transplant recipients with VRE infection; infection resolution occurred in 74% of these patients. Adverse reactions were reversible elevation of the alkaline phosphatase, rash, itching, nausea, and vomiting; none of these adverse reactions necessitated discontinuation of therapy [271].

Clindamycin

Clindamycin is a lincosamide antibiotic developed by modification of lincomycin. Clindamycin binds to the 50S ribosomal subunit, disrupting protein synthesis by interfering with the transpeptidation reaction. The lincosamides may also stimulate dissociation of peptidyl-tRNA from ribosomes, similar to the macrolides. The lincosamide-binding site is in close proximity to that of the macrolides, so binding of one antibiotic may reduce binding of the other. Clindamycin is considered bacteriostatic, although bactericidal activity for some strains of staphylococci, streptococci, and anaerobes may exist. It may also exhibit a postantibiotic effect against some bacterial strains [264]. An attractive feature of clindamycin is that it promotes opsonization and phagocytosis of bacteria at a subinhibitory concentrations. Clindamycin causes changes in the cell wall surface, which decreases the adherence of bacteria to host cells and augments intracellular bacterial killing. Another quality of clindamycin is the ability to inhibit production of intracellular toxins, particularly those of *S. aureus* and *S. pyogenes* [272, 273].

Resistance

Resistance occurs through four mechanisms and may be plasmid and chromosomally mediated. The most common mechanism is alteration in the 23 rRNA of the 50S subunit by methylation of adenine. Plasmid-mediated resistance via MLS_B is present in some strains of *S. aureus*, *S. pyogenes*, and *B. fragilis*. In *S. aureus*, the *ermA* or *ermC* gene encodes this type of resistance. Mutations in the bacterial rRNA may confer resistance to clindamycin as do alterations in specific 50S ribosomal proteins at the receptor site. The fourth type of resistance is inactivation through adenylation, which affects lincomycin more than clindamycin; however this can reduce bactericidal activity of clindamycin. GNB are intrinsically resistant to clindamycin due to poor permeability of the outer membrane envelope, similar to what was seen with macrolide antibiotics [259].

Spectrum of Activity

Clindamycin has similar activity to the macrolides against *S. pneumoniae*, *S. pyogenes*, *S. viridans*, and MSSA. It continues to be active against over 90% of the USA300 strain of MRSA [274]. Clindamycin is most active against anaerobes, especially *B. fragilis*, *Fusobacterium* spp., *Peptostreptococcus*, *Peptococcus*, and *C. perfringens*. *C. difficile* is resistant to clindamycin. Atypical bacteria such as *Actinomyces israelii* and *Nocardia asteroides* are sensitive. Clindamycin is also active against parasitic organisms including *Toxoplasma gondii*, *Babesia*, and some strains of *P. falciparum* and *vivax*. Increasing resistance to clindamycin has been reported to *S. pneumoniae*, *S. aureus*, and *S. pyogenes*. Erythromycin-resistant bacteria may develop rapid resistance when exposed to clindamycin. Increasing resistance among *Bacteroides* species has been observed from 3% in 1987 to 26% in a study between 1997 and 2004 [275].

Adverse Reactions

Toxicity is mainly gastrointestinal and hypersensitivity reactions. Antibiotic-associated diarrhea has been reported in 2–20% of patients. *C. difficile* colitis has been reported to occur in up to 10% of clindamycin-treated patients. The current epidemic BI/NAP1/027 strain of *C. difficile* is more strongly associated with the use of broad-spectrum cephalosporins and fluoroquinolones [276, 277]. Allergic reactions may clinically present as fever, skin rash, and rarely as erythema multiforme. Other adverse reactions include elevation of hepatic transaminases and neutropenia, which is often reversible after discontinuation of therapy.

Use in Transplantation

Clindamycin is available in oral and intravenous formulations and has excellent oral bioavailability. The half-life is 2.4 h, and the drug is metabolized in the liver to active and inactive metabolites which are excreted in bile and urine. Dosage adjustments are not necessary in patients with kidney or liver disease. Clindamycin penetrates well into the bone and achieves high intracellular drug concentration. It achieves suboptimum drug concentration in CSF following parenteral, intravenous administration.

Clindamycin traditionally has been used predominantly to treat *B. fragilis* in polymicrobial intra-abdominal and pelvic infections, as second line to penicillins in anaerobic bronchopulmonary infections, and may be considered first line in serious skin and soft tissue necrotizing infections. The poor CSF penetration limits its use for treatment of meningitis and other intracranial infections. The emergence of the USA300 clone of MRSA has provided an additional role for clindamycin, especially in the outpatient setting. Studies have shown an incidence of MRSA cultured from 67% of skin and soft tissue infections, requiring empiric coverage for CA-MRSA in addition to beta-hemolytic streptococci [278]. A study of clindamycin resistance in CA-MRSA demonstrated that exposure to clindamycin or macrolides within the prior 3 months was an independent predictor for clindamycin-resistant MRSA. Other risk factors were infection or colonization with MRSA within the previous 12 months, surgery, and presence of intravenous catheter [279]. Cases have been reported of clindamycin-susceptible/erythromycin-resistant MRSA that did not respond to clindamycin. The double-disk diffusion test using clindamycin and erythromycin disks (D test) confirms the presence of in vitro inducible macrolide-lincosamide-streptogramin B resistance (iMLS) due to presence of *erm* genes. Additional testing in pediatric and adult isolates demonstrated that 56% had the iMLS phenotype, 50% among MRSA isolates and 63% in MSSA isolates. There was a higher rate in isolates from pediatric patients amounting to 77% in MSSA. It is therefore suggested that in patients with erythromycin-resistance/clindamycin-susceptible *S. aureus*, D test should be performed prior to commencing clindamycin therapy [280]. A multiresistance conjugative plasmid, pUSA03, has recently been isolated from men who have sex with men in San Francisco and Boston [281]. This isolate is resistant to β-lactams, clindamycin, fluoroquinolones, tetracycline, macrolides, and mupirocin. Both *ermC* and *mupA* genes are carried on this plasmid. Of note, 23% of the USA300 isolates without this plasmid were resistant to clindamycin in this population.

Hospital-acquired MRSA is a major cause of morbidity during the early period after transplantation [282, 283]. These infections are treated with parenteral agents such as vancomycin and daptomycin since these isolates, usually belonging to USA 100PFGE profile, are associated with a lower clindamycin susceptibility of nearly 54% [284]. Colonization of MRSA postoperatively has been shown to increase the risk for MRSA infection [285]. Limited data exists on the USA300 clone except for failed renal transplant patients followed in hemodialysis center who had higher risk for USA300 MRSA colonization. Clindamycin should be used with caution in this population; it may still be a valuable agent for anaerobic and parasitic infections.

The Quinolones

Derived from nalidixic acid and originally developed in the 1960s as a by-product of chloroquine synthesis, the fluoroquinolones share a common two-ring core structure, with a side-chain-bearing nitrogen located at position 1, carbon at position 8, and fluorine substituent at position 6. Addition of a halide group at position 8 enhanced activity against anaerobes and improved oral bioavailability. A methoxy group at position 8 enhances anaerobic activity; addition of a piperazinyl or methylated piperazinyl ring at position 7 enhances activity against GPB. A cyclopropyl group at position 1 greatly enhances activity against GNB [286].

Fluoroquinolones exert their antimicrobial activity through two distinct, yet related and overlapping drug targets: DNA gyrase and topoisomerase IV (Top IV). Both enzymes facilitate the highly regulated coiling necessary to fit the entirety of a bacterial chromosome into a relatively small area, and both serve unique functions [287]. DNA gyrase is a tetramer of two subunits A_2B_2, encoded by *gyrA* and *gyrB*, respectively [288]. The two subunits wrap around a DNA strand and introduce a negative supercoil into bacterial DNA, first through the formation of a positive supercoil and then passing one DNA region through another. Through an ATP-dependent process, DNA gyrase accomplishes this via a series of DNA strand breakages and rejoining [289]. Together, these functions serve a vital purpose in the facilitation of migration of fork through the DNA strand. Top IV, homologous to DNA gyrase, is encoded by the *parC* and *parE* genes and is primarily involved in the process of separating daughter chromosomes, known as decantation. In some cases, DNA gyrase is able to fulfill the functionality of topoisomerase IV at a reduced efficiency; however, Top IV is unable to introduce negative supercoils into bacterial DNA [290, 291]. Top IV functions by direct binding to sections of DNA crossover, rather than through wrapping around the target portion of the DNA strand. Through binding to topoisomerase IV and DNA gyrase with Top IV as the primary target in GPB and DNA gyrase in GNB, the quinolones inhibit bacterial DNA synthesis and lead to rapid bacterial cell death [292, 293]. The mechanism of this rapid bactericidal action has not yet been fully characterized. Prior to the introduction of a DNA break, the quinolones bind to the DNA-enzyme complex after which DNA cleavage occurs, with the quinolone-enzyme complex "locking" the cleaved complex in place [294, 295]. The formation of this cleaved complex causes rapid inhibition of DNA synthesis, which occurs more quickly when DNA gyrase is the target [296, 297]. The inhibition of DNA replication leads to several downstream effects ultimately responsible for rapid bacterial killing or slow cell death. The formation of multiple cleaved complexes throughout the bacterial chromosome leads to fragmentation and rapid cell death through induction of apoptosis [298]. This mechanism is unlikely the only explanation for rapid bacterial killing, as rapid cell death still occurs in the absence of the protein synthesis required for the induction of apoptosis [299]. Further investigation into the mechanism of rapid bacterial killing by quinolones is ongoing.

In a dose-dependent manner, exposure to quinolones induces bacterial expression of the SOS regulon, a global stress-response mediator carrying over 40 genes and controlled by the *lexA* gene [300]. This stress response is a characteristic shared by all bactericidal antibiotics [301]. Included in the SOS regulon is the gene *sfiA*, which codes an inhibitor of cell division in *E. coli* and leads to a change in bacterial morphology to an elongated, filamentous structure [302]. Low-level quinolone exposure and subsequent induction of the SOS response contribute to the dissemination of antibiotic resistance elements and bacterial virulence factors [303, 304].

Spectrum of Activity

The fluoroquinolones are active against a broad variety of enteric GN bacilli and cocci. Ciprofloxacin and levofloxacin retain sufficient in vitro potency for use against *Pseudomonas* species, with ciprofloxacin generally being more potent than levofloxacin against GNB. The activity of ciprofloxacin is limited against GPB, whereas moxifloxacin, levofloxacin, and gemifloxacin are highly active against most clinical strain of *Streptococcus* species. Moxifloxacin may retain activity against *S. aureus* isolates with low-level resistance to ciprofloxacin, while the use of levofloxacin is associated with the rapid selection of mutant colonies [305].

The next-generation fluoroquinolone, delafloxacin, demonstrated potent in vitro activity against *S. aureus* including MRSA and MSSA strains that exhibit high-level resistance to the currently marketed fluoroquinolones [306]. This agent demonstrates a low propensity for the development of resistant mutants as compared to other fluoroquinolones. All currently marketed fluoroquinolones have in vitro activity against the atypical respiratory pathogens such as *L. pneumophilia*, *C. pneumoniae*, and *Mycoplasma pneumoniae*. Other intracellular pathogens, including *C. trachomatis* and *U. urealyticum*, are also inhibited. *Ehrlichia* species show variable sensitivity due to the presence of natural mutations in the QRDR [307], with similar variability displayed by *Bartonella*, *Rickettsia*, and *Coxiella* species [308]. The fluoroquinolones are also active against a variety of *Mycobacteria*, including *M. tuberculosis*, *M. kansasii*, *M. xenopi*, *M. marinum*, and *M. leprae*, with members of the *M. avium* complex and *M. chelonae* displaying little to no susceptibility to these agents [309].

Resistance

Multiple mechanisms for quinolone resistance exist. Reduced susceptibility may arise through spontaneous chromosomal mutations particularly in regions that code for DNA gyrase and Top IV or through recently discovered plasmid-mediated resistance mechanisms [310, 311]. Plasmid-transferrable resistance mechanisms generally do not lead to MICs above the CLSI breakpoint for resistance but facilitate the acquisition of additional resistance factors that may further elevate MICs [312]. Point mutations in the vital *gyrA* may lead to high levels of quinolone resistance [293]. Due to the structural homology between DNA gyrase and Top IV, mutations conferring reduced susceptibility to quinolones occur at homologous points in the respective enzymes, known as the "quinolone-resistance determining region" (QRDR) [313–315]. Numerous point mutations throughout the QRDR contribute to reduced susceptibility; however proximity to the enzyme-DNA binding site is a common feature to many of the known mutations [316]. The primary target of a quinolone in a bacterial species is determined by genetic testing, in which the primary target is presumed to be that with the highest degree of inhibition [317]. Due to this structural preference, the relative overall decrease in quinolone susceptibility as mutations accumulate may be a result of declining inhibitory potential against the preferred target or a reflection of the inhibitory capacity of the quinolone against the wild-type secondary target [296].

Single-step mutations that reduce quinolone-binding affinity arise in an exposure-related manner, at a rate of 10^{-6}

to 10^{-11} as quinolone concentrations increase relative to the MIC of the organism. These mutations confer different degrees of reduced susceptibility dependent upon the quinolone agent studied, with point mutations in *S. aureus* conferring a 32-fold rise in MICs to ciprofloxacin and MICs to gemifloxacin demonstrating only a fourfold rise [318]. These mutations facilitate the development of additional mutations in both *gyrA* and *parC*, leading to high-level quinolone resistance [310]. Spontaneous double mutations, affecting both DNA gyrase and Top IV, are uncommon, occurring at a frequency of 10^{-14} to 10^{-16}. Interestingly, the accumulation of multiple mutations throughout these crucial enzymes does not appear to impact the fitness of the bacteria due to accumulation of a variety of compensatory mechanisms [319].

Active drug efflux by MDR efflux pumps also plays an important role in resistance. Drug efflux pumps are broadly categorized into five families of ancient evolutionary origin in bacteria that have evolved to facilitate intracellular communication and extrude environmental toxins in addition to contributing to resistance [320, 321]. The presence of one or more drug efflux pumps may promote resistance to multiple classes of antimicrobials. Efflux-mediated resistance to quinolones is most commonly mediated by chromosomally encoded RND pumps [322]. In *P. aeruginosa*, an example of this type is the MexAB-OprM pump, a tripartite pump composed of an outer membrane spanning domain, inner membrane efflux pump, and a membrane fusion protein [323]. *Enterobacteriaceae* can use the AcrAB-TolC efflux pump [324]. When co-expressed with other efflux pumps or *gyrA* mutations, GNB exhibits higher levels of drug resistance. The concomitant downregulation of outer membrane porins and overexpression of efflux pumps may also contribute to quinolone resistance among the GNB [325]. In *S. aureus*, low-level quinolone resistance is constitutively expressed by the norA pump [314], and, in *S. pneumoniae* by an efflux pump homologous to norA, pmrA conforms drug resistance [326].

Enzymatic modification of quinolones was first described in 2003, a variant of the aminoglycoside AAC which acetylates the piperazinyl group on ciprofloxacin and decreases binding affinity to its intracellular target [327]. This mutation does not produce MIC values above the CLSI breakpoint, but its presence increases the frequency of selection for chromosomal mutants [328]. Plasmid-mediated fluoroquinolone resistance was first described in a clinical isolate in 1998, encoded by the *qnr* genes, that generates a Qnr protein belonging to the pentapeptide repeat family [329, 330]. In addition to the unique Qnr proteins, both the AAC and two novel efflux pumps have been described on transmissible plasmids [331]. The prevalence of the pentapeptide Qnr proteins appears to be relatively low, among clinical isolates of *Enterobacteriaceae*, ranging from approximately 1.5% to 4.6%. Plasmid-mediated pumps are even less common. The AAC is more prevalent in clinical isolates, in nearly 10% of such isolates, and importantly, often coexists with genes encoding ESBLs [329].

Central to this progressive rise in quinolone resistance is the tendency of bacteria to evolve in a stepwise fashion. Mutations arise or plasmids are acquired in discrete steps, with one final step often a mutation in DNA gyrase or Top IV creating frank resistance [332]. Since these spontaneous mutations occur infrequently, a concept in quinolone dosing, referred to as the "mutant prevention concentration" (MPC), was proposed by Xiao and Drlica in 2001, which advocates for the use of doses that achieve drug concentrations above the level at which no resistant mutants will be selected, an inoculum of 10^{10} organisms rather than traditional dosing which focuses on MICs [333]. While this concept has not been tested clinically, it provides insight as to how low doses of quinolones contribute to high-level resistance, as well as potential pathways for development of future quinolone agents.

Adverse Reactions

The fluoroquinolones have a rate of adverse reactions similar to those of comparator agents in clinical trials. Gastrointestinal disturbances are the prominent adverse effects. Central nervous system toxicities are the second most common adverse effects, occurring in 1–2% of patients. CNS toxicities are thought to result from competitive inhibition of γ-aminobutyric acid ($GABA_A$) receptor and commonly manifested as headache and nausea, although grand mal seizures may occur [334]. Fluoroquinolones with a piperazinyl side chain at the 7-position have the highest potential for epileptogenesis. Levofloxacin, moxifloxacin, and gemifloxacin lack the structure-toxicity relationship associated with the development of seizures; however, caution should still be exercised in patients with history of seizure disorders. Through an unknown mechanism, the fluoroquinolones may cause exacerbation of myasthenia gravis and now carry an FDA "black box" warning for this occurrence [335].

The fluoroquinolones have been associated with prolongation of the QTc interval and risk for Torsades de pointes, although the causal link remains unclear [336]. Numerous case reports described the potential for fluoroquinolone-induced cardiac arrhythmias, and in vitro data showed that the fluoroquinolones have the potential to block delayed rectifier K+ current (I_{Kr}) through blockade of the human ether-a-go-go (hERG) K+ channel [337], although only moxifloxacin achieves this blockade at physiologic concentrations after standard treatment dose. A recent population-based, case-control study demonstrated a 3.3-fold greater risk for moxifloxacin, twofold higher risk with ciprofloxacin, and no such increased risk for levofloxacin [338]. Gatifloxacin, a quinolone that was shown to be associated with serious dysglycemic events, showed a fourfold greater risk for the development of arrhythmias. Based on these data, fluoroquinolones should be used with caution in patients at risk for the development of cardiac arrhythmias.

Quinolone-induced phototoxicity manifests shortly following exposure to UVA light in a dose-dependent manner and is believed to result from free radical generation, cellular toxicity, and local inflammation [339]. Moxifloxacin contains a protective 8-methoxy group and has not been associated with the development of phototoxicity, whereas levofloxacin and ciprofloxacin lack this group and are associated with phototoxicity. Patients should be warned to limit exposure to sources of UV light when using fluoroquinolones agents with known phototoxic potential.

Like all antimicrobial agents, the fluoroquinolones are associated with the development of *C. difficile* infection (CDI). The fluoroquinolones were historically thought to be agents that would result in less perturbation of the hosts' resident microbiota, therefore having a low risk for promoting CDI. Recent epidemiologic studies have shown that fluoroquinolone is a substantial risk factor for the development of CDI [340, 341]. This has been associated with the spread of the epidemic BI/NAP1/ribotype 027 strain, which is frequently resistant to the fluoroquinolones [342, 343].

Role of Fluoroquinolones in Transplantation

Fluoroquinolones are used in a variety of setting including treatment and prevention of bacterial infections. In 1 study, *S. viridans* bacteremia developed in 6 of 37 patients receiving levofloxacin neutropenic prophylaxis following autologous HSCT. The mean duration of neutropenia was 4.5 days; and three patients developed septic shock. All *S. viridans* isolates exhibited reduced levofloxacin susceptibility due to GYRA mutations and ParC mutation in one patient [344]. In 48 patients given gatifloxacin or moxifloxacin prophylaxis while undergoing HSCT, organisms showing fluoroquinolone class resistance were recovered from the oropharynx in greater frequency revealing gyrA and/or parC mutations among the resistant isolates [345].

Therriault and colleagues undertook a retrospective analysis of HSCT recipients given levofloxacin with penicillin or doxycycline combination prophylaxis through stem cell engraftment. Over time, GPB infections declined; however, it was noted that fluoroquinolone-resistant GNB emerged. Of note, resistance due to ESBL did not change. In this study, an increased colonization with VRE was an alarming finding [346]. Another study looked at bloodstream infections after allogeneic HSCT and found that among GNB only half were susceptible to fluoroquinolone [347]. Vehreschild and colleagues used moxifloxacin versus placebo in patients on high-dose chemotherapy followed by autologous HSCT for chemoprevention of bacteremia. Breakthrough bloodstream infections occurred in three prophylaxis group (8.8%) whereas 28% among patients given no antibiotic prophylaxis. In this study, moxifloxacin was effective in preventing bacteremia and shortened length of febrile episodes. Two of the isolates, *E. coli* and MSSA, were susceptible to moxifloxacin. The third episode occurred due to *P. aeruginosa* which was susceptible to ciprofloxacin and levofloxacin and as expected, resistant to moxifloxacin that is known to have limited activity against this pathogen [348].

An unusual use of fluoroquinolones is to reduce the incidence of BK virus-associated hemorrhagic cystitis in allogeneic HSCT recipients. Fluoroquinolones have been shown to inhibit polyoma virus BK replication through inhibition of viral-encoded DNA gyrase. A retrospective analysis of 48 patients received ciprofloxacin from day 0 through 60 following transplantation, versus a control group of similar patients given fluoroquinolone prophylaxis. The cumulative rate of hemorrhagic cystitis was significantly reduced from 20.9% to 2.6% in the patients given ciprofloxacin. Patients on ciprofloxacin did not experience an increased rate of CDI and were also less likely to develop bacteremia [349].

Yoon and colleagues investigated rifampin versus an oral fluoroquinolone in 109 renal transplant patients with latent tuberculosis. The incidence of adverse reactions was higher in the rifampin group, and the quinolone group showed a significantly higher 10-year graft survival compared with the rifampin group. In addition to being safe in this population, fluoroquinolones may lower the risk for graft failure [350].

Unusual toxicities are also seen in this population. A high incidence (5.8%) of Achilles tendinitis or rupture was seen in heart transplant patients. Independent risk factors were renal failure and increased time between transplantation and treatment with a fluoroquinolone advising providers to consider alternative therapy for such patients [351]. A case was reported in a HSCT recipient who developed a lymphomatoid hypersensitivity reaction to levofloxacin, an illness difficult to differentiate from recurrent or de novo lymphoid malignancy [352].

Metronidazole

Metronidazole is a synthetic drug discovered in the 1950s. Originally recognized for its activity against *Trichomonas vaginalis*, *Giardia*, and *Entamoeba*, a decade later, it was recognized as highly effective against anaerobes. Metronidazole remains a useful drug for the treatment of anaerobic, polymicrobial infections, *H. pylori*, and protozoa and as first-line treatment for patients with mild to moderate *C. difficile* infection (CDI).

Metronidazole enters the cell through passive diffusion as a prodrug, activated in the cytoplasm of susceptible bacteria and in specific organelles in protozoa. It is cytotoxic through production of free radicals. The molecule is converted by intracellular reduction to a short-lived nitroso free radical by intracellular reduction, which involves the transfer of an electron to the nitro group of the drug [353], a reaction that is catalyzed by a nitroreductase such as pyruvate. Reduction of the prodrug creates a concentration gradient, increasing uptake of metronidazole and leading to free radical formation [354]. The free radicals are highly unstable and interact with nucleic acids prior to decaying, resulting in breakage and destabilization of nucleic acids and proteins eventually leading to bacterial cell death [355]. The mechanism of action differs in facultative anaerobes such as *G. vaginalis* and *H. pylori*, where metronidazole reduction to active metabolite can occur by a one electron-transfer step; metabolites are re-oxidized with formation of toxic oxygen radicals that are then neutralized by an active scavenger system [356]. More recently, activation by a two electron transfer step in *H. pylori* was documented, allowing for activation in a microaerophilic environment. In parasites, the enzyme pyruvate/ferredoxin oxidoreductase activates metronidazole with energy provided by glycolysis of glucose in an organelle called the hydrogenosome [357].

Spectrum of Activity

Metronidazole is active against a broad array of anaerobes, protozoa, and microaerophilic bacteria. Metronidazole exerts rapid bactericidal effects against anaerobic bacteria and is rapidly bactericidal [358]. Metronidazole exhibits concentration-dependent kinetics in susceptible anaerobes, *Entamoeba histolytica* and *T. vaginalis* [358–360]. Metronidazole is potent against *B. fragilis*, *Fusobacterium* spp., *Prevotella*, and *Porphyromonas* spp. [361]. *Clostridium* species are susceptible, although *C. difficile* and *C. perfringens* are susceptible at slightly higher concentrations than Gram-negative anaerobes. The activity against Gram-positive cocci is variable, and most strains of *Actinomyces*, *Lactobacillus*, and *Propionibacterium* are resistant [362]. *Treponema pallidum*, oral spirochetes, *Campylobacter fetus*, *Gardnerella vaginalis*, and *H. pylori* are sensitive, although *H. pylori* resistance is increasing [363]. Anaerobic cocci such as *Peptostreptococcus* and *Veillonella* spp. are also inhibited. *Capnocytophaga* spp. are usually sensitive. Metronidazole also demonstrates concentration-dependent killing against *Entamoeba histolytica* and *Trichomonas vaginalis* [360] and is active against other protozoa including *Giardia lamblia*, *Blastocystis hominis*, and *Balantidium coli*.

Resistance

Several mechanisms of resistance to metronidazole have been observed that differ among organisms. The primary mechanisms of resistance are decreased uptake of the prodrug and/or altered efficiency of intracellular reduction. These mechanisms may act together with reduced activity of nitroreductase resulting in decreased uptake of metronidazole [364]. The level of susceptibility and rate of drug uptake vary with the level of pyruvate/ferredoxin oxidoreductase activity. Resistant bacteria compensate for reduced action of pyruvate/ferredoxin oxidoreductase by increasing pyruvate dehydrogenase activity [364]. It has been suggested that more than one mechanism may be required to confer clinical drug resistance [365]. Other resistance mechanisms include active efflux, drug inactivation, and heightened bacterial DNA damage repair [364]. Resistance genes, called *nim*, encode an alternative reductase that converts nitroimidazole to a nontoxic compound [366]. Transfer of these genes on plasmids can confer metronidazole resistance in *B. fragilis* [367].

In one large study over a 4-year period, overall resistance rates varied between 1.8% and 2.5% [368]. Studies have shown that more than 95% of anaerobic isolates in the United States remain susceptible to metronidazole [369]. Among *Bacteroides* spp., a large multicenter study over a 7-year period revealed no resistance to metronidazole among greater than 4000 clinical isolates tested [370]. In Canada, rates of resistance to metronidazole remained unchanged in *Bacteroides* spp. over a 6-year period, while resistance to clindamycin had increased [371]. In *Bacteroides* species, resistance is conferred by both plasmid- and chromosomally mediated mechanisms, although plasmid-mediated transfer of resistance to susceptible strains is rare. Multiple steps appeared to be necessary for development of resistance, which may explain why resistance is rare and infrequent in the absence of long-term therapy [365].

Although metronidazole resistance among anaerobic bacteria is rare, it has been reported more frequently with *H. pylori*. A large multinational, multicenter randomized clinical trial tested 516 clinical isolates and found resistance to metronidazole (>8 μ/ml) in 27% of strains by agar dilution method [372]. The mechanism of resistance to metronidazole is not well understood; resistant *H. pylori* strains may accumulate lesser amounts of metronidazole and at a slower rate [373]. The acquisition of resistance is associated with a mutation, resulting in inactivation of the *rdzA* gene that encodes an oxygen-insensitive NADPH nitroreductase [374].

Metronidazole-resistant *T. vaginalis* strains have been isolated from patients with refractory infections. Resistance is associated with reduced transcription activity of the ferredoxin gene, which results in decreased intracellular levels of ferredoxin and reduced pyruvate/ferredoxin oxidoreductase activity. In addition, oxidation of pyruvate to lactate within hydrogenosomes stops and occurs in the cytosol via lactate dehydrogenase [375, 376]. Resistance to metronidazole has also been found in *Giardia* [377]. In amebae, an increase in iron superoxide dismutase has been described as a mechanism of resistance [357].

Metronidazole is rapidly absorbed by the oral route, and serum levels are similar to intravenous doses. Metronidazole reaches all tissues and body fluids [378] including the central nervous system. Patients with meningitis achieve similar cerebrospinal fluid and serum concentrations. Metronidazole also penetrates into brain abscesses and is considered the most effective therapy for *B. fragilis* meningitis. [379]. Metronidazole has a mean plasma half-life of 8.3 h and a systemic oral bioavailability of 98.9%. Metronidazole is metabolized in the liver to glucuronide and oxidative products, including an active hydroxy metabolite [380]. Unchanged drug and the metabolites are excreted in the urine. The half-life of the drug may be as high as 20 h in patients with hepatic failure, and decreased doses are recommended for such patients.

Adverse Reactions

Nausea, vomiting, diarrhea, and metallic taste are common adverse events. *Candida* overgrowth may result in glossitis and stomatitis. More serious events involve the central and peripheral nervous systems that are usually associated with prolonged therapy and high doses or both. These can manifest as seizures, ataxia, dysarthria, cerebellar dysfunction, and often reversible peripheral neuropathy [381, 382]. Pancreatitis is an unusual complication of therapy [383]. Although the drug is active against *C. difficile*, paradoxically, cases of CDI have rarely been reported in patients on metronidazole [384]. Hypersensitivity reactions have been reported including urticaria, erythematous rash, flushing, bronchospasm, and serum sickness [385]. Genitourinary reactions include transient darkening of the urine to a deep red-brown color and dysuria. Patients should abstain from alcohol while taking the drug since a disulfiram-like reaction may occur characterized by flushing, tachycardia, palpitations, nausea, and vomiting [386]. Intravenous trimethoprim-sulfamethoxazole and over-the-counter cold syrups containing alcohol can also lead to a disulfiram-like reactions when taken along with metronidazole. Sudden deaths have been attributed to the metronidazole-ethanol disulfiram-like reaction [387]. Metronidazole is classified by the US Food and Drug Administration as category B during pregnancy.

Drug interactions can occur with phenytoin, carbamazepine, and lithium [388]. Metronidazole can increase the anticoagulant effect of warfarin, and preemptive dose reduction has been successful [389]. A potential interaction between metronidazole and amiodarone was reported resulting in QTc prolongation and torsades de pointes [390]. Of particular importance to transplant patients, metronidazole inhibits metabolic clearance of busulfan, and concomitant use may dramatically increase toxicity in HSCT patients receiving busulfan-containing conditioning regimens [391].

Use in Transplant Recipients

A few investigators have reported significant rise in cyclosporine and tacrolimus serum concentrations after patients were commenced on metronidazole therapy [392–394]. In one patient, cyclosporine increased 97% during concomitant metronidazole treatment and then returned to baseline after metronidazole was discontinued. In another patient, tacrolimus increased 99% and then returned to baseline levels after cessation of metronidazole. These reports suggest that caution should be used when dosing these agents concomitantly, with dose adjustments of cyclosporine and tacrolimus made as necessary. Another small study reported a significant interaction between metronidazole and busulfan. HSCT recipients given metronidazole for GVHD prophylaxis had significantly higher levels of busulfan than controls who received busulfan alone [391]. More adverse events were noted in the group of subjects receiving metronidazole and busulfan together such as multiorgan failure, veno-occlusive disease, and hemorrhagic cystitis; therefore, authors recommended avoiding these agents together in patients undergoing HSCT [395].

A sizable literature concerns treatment of CDI in the transplant population. One study identified over 49,000 cases following SOT among which 2.7% had CDI. Univariate comparisons of transplant cases with and without CDI revealed that CDI cases were independently associated with greater mortality, longer length of hospitalization, more complications for the transplanted solid organ graft, and increased need for colectomy [396]. Patients following liver transplantation were found to be at particularly high risk of developing CDI. The prevalence of CDI in this population was 2.7% versus 0.9% in other SOT recipients and a higher CDI mortality of 5.5% in liver vs. 3.2% in non-liver-transplant patients. CDI was an independent risk factor for death in this population [396].

In another study of CDI in SOT, *C. difficile* was the most common cause of diarrheal illness accounting for 2.7%. They also reported higher deaths, longer hospital stay, more complications for the transplanted organ, and increased need for colectomy in SOT recipients with CDI [395]. In children after lung transplantation, the incidence of CDI was 5.4%. One patient required a diverting ileostomy; another developed renal failure and expired. Overall 75% survival was encouraging; however, a significant morbidity and mortality in these children with CDI were for serious concern [397]. In recipient of SOT with CDI, metronidazole and vancomycin were equally effective for the treatment of mild to moderate disease, whereas vancomycin demonstrated superiority in patients with severe disease [398], an observation echoed among non-transplant population with CDI.

Rifamycins

The rifamycins were discovered in 1957 as a fermentation product of *Streptomyces mediterranei* and named after a popular French crime film Rififi [399]. There are four currently marketed rifamycins: rifampin, rifabutin, rifapentine, and rifaximin. Rifamycin B was the first marketed agent. Through binding to DNA-dependent RNA polymerase, rifamycins exert a potent antibacterial effect against a broad array of prokaryotes [400]. Crystal structure analysis of the rifampin-RNA polymerase complex in *Thermus aquaticus* shows that rifampin binds to the β-subunit of RNA polymerase at a site far from the active site of the DNA/RNA channel and physically blocks the elongation of RNA once the transcript is 2–3 nucleotides in length [401]. Rifabutin inhibits transcription between the first and second nucleotides, indicating that steric hindrance may not completely explain the mechanism behind the blockade of RNA polymerase. Further modeling of the rifabutin-RNA polymerase complex demonstrates an allosteric signal leading to unfavorable binding of the crucial Mg^{2+} catalytic ion at the active site resulting in a slowed biochemical reaction and dissociation of unstable nucleotide hybrids [402].

Spectrum of Activity

Rifampin, rifabutin, and rifapentine are all highly active against *M. tuberculosis* and other organisms in the *M. tuberculosis* complex. Rifabutin MIC values against wild-type *M. tuberculosis* are generally narrowly distributed, with most values ≤0.06 mcg/mL, and MIC values between 0.25 and 0.5 mcg/mL against isolates with low-level rifampin resistance. Isolates with high-level resistance to rifampin demonstrate cross-resistance with rifabutin [403, 404]. These MIC values are approximately two- to fourfold higher than those observed for rifampin among *M. tuberculosis* strains. For MAC, the differential MIC values are more pronounced, with MIC values for rifampin ranging from 2- to 16-fold higher than those of rifabutin. Rifapentine demonstrates similar in vitro activity to rifabutin against members of the *M. tuberculosis* family; however, rifampin-resistant isolates are often resistant to rifapentine [405]. Due to the highly conserved structure of RNA polymerase across bacteria, the rifamycins are highly active against a wide variety of Gram-positive, Gram-negative, and intracellular bacteria. A summary can be found in an excellent review by Thornsberry [406]. Rifaximin demonstrates a similarly broad spectrum of activity, but due to poor systemic absorption, its use is limited to the treatment of localized gastrointestinal infections [407].

Resistance and Decreased Susceptibility

Approximately 95% of the cases of resistance to rifampin may be mapped to the enzyme-coding RNA polymerase, *rpoB*, with the majority of these mutations in region I of the gene [408]. Most are single-point mutations; however, insertions and deletions are possible. Each mutation confers a different spectrum and level of resistance; however, due to decreased bacterial fitness, many of the possible mutations are not propagated in a clinical environment [408]. These mutations alter the binding affinity of rifamycins to the target enzyme. Resistance to rifampin due to spontaneous mutations in the *rpoB* gene occurs at a frequency of approximately 10^{-8} in staphylococci and 10^{-9} in *Mycobacterium tuberculosis*, with combination therapy effectively decreasing the development of resistance in clinical isolates [409]. Due to the rapid development of resistance when used as monotherapy, rifampin is used in combination with other antibiotics in the treatment of serious infections [410].

In addition to target-site alterations, other mechanisms of resistance or reduced susceptibility may arise. A rifamycin derivative, CGP 4832, is highly active against rifampin-resistant strains of *E. coli*, due to increased cellular uptake via the FhuA-TonB active transport system [411], indicating that decreased cell permeability may be responsible for the reduced rifamycin susceptibility among the GNB. However, this does not seem to be a factor in mycobacterial resistance including *M. tuberculosis*, *M. avium-intracellulare* complex (MAC), and *M. smegmatis* [412, 413]. Enzymatic modification of rifampin was identified in *Rhodococcus* and *M. smegmatis*, with the *arr* gene leading to inactive ribosylated derivatives of rifampin [414]. Variant *arr* genes with similar functionality have been found on plasmids in *P. aeruginosa*, *K. pneumoniae*, *E. coli*, and other *Enterobacteriaceae*; notably, these plasmids also contained mutations conferring mutations to other classes of antimicrobials [415–417].

Adverse Reactions

Rifampin is generally well-tolerated, with a surveillance population of patients receiving rifampin for the treatment of tuberculosis discontinuing therapy only 1.9% of the time, with over half of these discontinuations being inappropriate

[418]. A well-known side effect of rifampin is red-orange discoloration of body fluids as a result of distribution of the brightly colored drug into these fluids. This is most often a harmless cosmetic disturbance; however, it may lead to permanent discoloration of contact lenses or, in cases of overdose, cutaneous discoloration and periorbital edema, and intense pruritus may occur [419]. Hepatotoxicity from rifampin may manifest as hyperbilirubinemia, elevated liver enzymes or drug-induced hepatitis. Elevations in both conjugated and unconjugated bilirubin occur predictably shortly following the administration of the drug, and are thought to the result of impaired biliary excretion [420]. Elevations in transaminases are infrequent in patients treated for latent tuberculosis or brucellosis [421, 422], although combination with isoniazid leads to more frequent elevation than expected with either agent alone [423]. There are few case reports of fulminant hepatitis resulting in liver failure due to rifampin monotherapy, occurring mostly in patients with preexisting liver disease [424]. Mild suppression of all marrow lines may occur during rifampin therapy, leading to granulocytopenia, thrombocytopenia, and anemia. True hemolytic anemia and immune-mediated thrombocytopenia may rarely occur during treatment with rifampin as a result of immune complexes and during re-exposure to the drug [425, 426]. Through similar immunologic mechanisms, rifampin has been associated with the development of acute renal failure [427]. Manifestations of renal failure are predominantly oligoanuric acute tubular necrosis associated with systemic symptoms; however, recovery is slow and may occur during renal replacement dialysis. Other causes of renal failure, such as glomerulonephropathy, acute interstitial nephritis, and light-chain proteinuria, may occur; these are not associated with the development of antibodies to rifampin [428]. Increased levels of rifabutin in patients receiving clarithromycin or fluconazole during treatment of MAC infections have been reported and are probably due to inhibition of the CYP450. Patients with AIDS receiving rifabutin therapy at 600 mg daily dose are at risk for uveitis, risk adjusted with total body weight (TBW) of the patient, ranging from 64% in <55 kg TBW to 14% in patients with >65 kg TBW. Additionally, reduction in the dose to the currently recommended 300 mg/day, the risk dropped dramatically to 13% overall, with two of the three cases occurring in patients weighing <55 kg.

Use in Transplant Patients

Several interactions are particularly relevant in transplant population through induction of CYP-450 enzyme system [429, 430]. The use of rifampin with cyclosporine has been associated with numerous reported acute allograft rejections due to sub-therapeutic concentration of antirejection medicine, as well as acute GVHD for the same reason in pediatric and adult HSCT recipients [431, 432]. In a case series of four patients receiving cyclosporine and rifampin, the AUC of cyclosporine was found to be reduced by approximately two-fold, with a dose increase of 2.5–3 times baseline required to maintain adequate levels of immune suppression [433]. Similar potential for interactions with tacrolimus, sirolimus, everolimus, and, to a lesser extent, mycophenolate mofetil exists [433, 434]. A consensus statement on the use of rifamycins in the treatment of tuberculosis in patients undergoing SOT was published by the Spanish Society of Infectious Diseases and Clinical Microbiology, supporting the need for careful therapeutic drug monitoring of these agents and avoidance of rifamycins, when possible [435].

Rifaximin was evaluated in liver transplant recipients with *C. difficile* infection that was refractory to both metronidazole and vancomycin. Rifaximin at a dose of 400 mg TID for 28 days was initiated in three patients after oral vancomycin was discontinued; diarrhea resolved in all patients treated with rifaximin. Patients remained symptom-free for 155–250 day afterward [436]. Favorable observation in this very limited study needs to be assessed in a larger cohort of transplant patients with difficult-to-treat CDI diarrheal illness.

Sulfonamides

The sulfonamides were the first effective antimicrobials used to treat and cure infections in humans [437]. In 1932 the first sulfonamide, sulfachrysoidine, was found to be active against *Streptococcus*. The drug was marketed in Germany as prontosil. Sulfanilamide was introduced into the United States in the 1930s, and trimethoprim was synthesized several decades later. The combination of trimethoprim-sulfamethoxazole (TMP-SMX), also known as co-trimoxazole, was introduced in the 1970s and continues to be one of the most widely used compound for bacterial and parasitic infections. This section will concentrate on TMP-SMX, which is most commonly used sulfonamide and more relevant to the transplant patient population.

The sulfonamides are bacteriostatic antibiotics similar in structure to para-aminobenzoic acid (PABA) which is required for folic acid synthesis. The sulfonamides are competitive inhibitors of dihydropteroate synthase, the bacterial enzyme that incorporates PABA into dihydropteroic acid, the immediate precursor of folic acid. Sulfonamides have a higher affinity for the microbial enzyme tetrahydropteroic acid synthetase than PABA. Only bacteria that synthesize folic acid are susceptible; those that used preformed folic acid are resistant. Mammalian cells are comparable to resistant bacteria in requiring preformed folic acid; approximately 100,000 times more drug is required to inhibit the human enzyme than the bacteria enzyme [438]. TMP and

SMX work sequentially to inhibit enzymes involved in the bacterial synthesis of tetrahydrofolic acid (THF) and act synergistically in vitro and in vivo [439]. SMX competes with PABA to inhibit the synthesis of dihydrofolic acid, an intermediate step in the formation of THF, and TMP binds to bacterial dihydrofolate reductase also preventing the formation of THF [440]. The final results in decreased folic acid synthesis, reduced bacterial nucleotides, and inhibition of bacterial growth.

Spectrum of Activity

TMP-SMX is effective against a wide variety of aerobic Gram-positive and Gram-negative bacteria including *S. pneumoniae* and other streptococci, staphylococci including CA-MRSA, *H. influenzae*, *Enterobacteriaceae*, *Salmonella*, *Shigella*, *Listeria*, and *Nocardia* spp. It is active against *P. jirovecii*, *M. marinum*, and some protozoa including *Plasmodium*, *Cyclospora*, and *Toxoplasma* spp. [441]. Other nosocomial pathogens are susceptible, such as *B. cepacia*, *S. maltophilia*, and *S. marcescens*. Pathogens resistant to TMP-SMX include *P. aeruginosa*, most anaerobes, *M. tuberculosis*, *T. pallidum*, *Campylobacter*, and PCN-R S. *pneumoniae*. MRSA is variably susceptible, dependent upon whether the isolate is community or hospital acquired, as discussed in the sections on clindamycin and vancomycin.

Resistance

Different mechanisms mediate resistance to the two components and can be transferable on transposons of the *Tn*21 family [442]. Resistance to TMP-SMX is widespread and has developed in most bacterial species [443–445]. Multiple mechanisms have been described including permeability barriers and/or efflux pumps, bacteria with target enzymes that are not susceptible, regulational changes in target enzymes, mutations in target enzymes, and drug-resistant target enzymes. *P. aeruginosa* is one of the organisms known to have an active efflux pump, overexpressing the MexA-MexB-OprM system to eliminate the drug from the cell [446]. Naturally insensitive dihydrofolate reductase enzymes are found in *Bacteroides* spp., *Clostridium* spp., *Neisseria* spp., and *M. catarrhalis* [442].

Organisms can develop overproduction of PABA such as *N. gonorrhoeae* and *S. aureus* or altered dihydropteroate synthetase in the case of *E. coli*. Transferable resistance of approximately 20 genes conferring TMP resistance through mutations in dihydrofolate reductase genes has been reported over the past 40 years. Plasmid transfer can occur in the gastrointestinal tracts among various bacteria belonging to *Enterobacteriaceae*. Mutations in the chromosomal *dhps* gene of *E. coli* confer resistance to the sulfonamide component. These mutations may also mediate resistance in *S. aureus*, *S. haemolyticus*, *C. jejuni*, and *H. pylori* [442]. *S. pyogenes* is thought to have a change in the gene via transformational mutations [447] and *N. meningiditis* through recombination of mutations in the *folP* and *dhps* genes [448].

Plasmid-mediated SMX and TMP resistance is increasing worldwide. Studies have shown rates of resistance to *Salmonella* of 37% [449] and 76% in *Shigella* spp. [450]. A study of college student with urinary tract infections showed that *E. coli* resistance to TMP-SMX was 29.6% [451]. *S. pneumoniae* resistance to TMP-SMX varies geographically and may be as high as greater than 40% [452]. Resistance to *S. maltophilia* is also on the rise; a recent study reported 30.4% TMP-SMX-resistant isolates demonstrating a novel gene cassettes embedded in class 1 integrons [453].

Pneumocystis jirovecii resistance has been correlated with dihydropteroate synthase gene mutations [454], while dihydrofolate reductase gene mutations can account for high-level resistance in other organisms such as *E. faecalis* and *C. jejuni* [455, 456]. Naturally resistant bacteria to SMX such as *E. faecalis* are typically auxotrophic for folic acid. Maximal synergy occurs when organisms are susceptible to both drugs. However, bacteria naturally resistant to one of the drug component at a low level and susceptible to the other compound may still remain susceptible to the drug combination.

Adverse Reactions

TMP-SMX is generally well tolerated in non-HIV-infected patients, where HIV patients have a much greater rate of adverse reactions [457]. These include severe and life-threatening hypersensitivity reactions. Sulfamethoxazole hypersensitivity may involve the increased formation and decreased detoxification of reactive metabolites. The adverse reaction rate is as high as 50% in HIV-infected patients, with many of the reactions being severe [458]. The more common adverse reactions to TMP-SMX involve the gastrointestinal tract such as nausea and vomiting; skin rash and pruritus are also not uncommon. Life-threatening effects, more likely to occur in HIV-infected patients and older adults, include neutropenia and severe dermatologic reactions such as Steven-Johnson syndrome, exfoliative dermatitis, and toxic epidermal necrolysis [459]. TMP-SMX desensitization can be performed successfully in as many as 75% of HIV patients [460, 461].

There is data supporting an elevated risk of hypersensitivity to non-antibiotic sulfonamides such as loop and thiazide diuretics and sulfonylureas in patients with sulfonamide allergy. TMP-SMX should not be given to patients who have folic acid deficiency or who are pregnant. As a weak inhibitor of dihydrofolate reductase in high doses, it has been implicated in megaloblastic pancytopenia [462]. Co-administration of folinic acid may prevent or reduce the antifolate activity of TMP-SMX without affecting its antimicrobial activity; such results are controversial [463, 464]. TMP-SMX should be given with caution to patients with glucose-6-phosphate dehydrogenase deficiency; however, convincing data regarding drug-induced hemolysis in patients with heterozygous G6PD deficiency is rare [465]. Other adverse effects such as anaphylaxis, hepatitis [466], hyperkalemia [467], aseptic meningitis [468], and hypoglycemia have been reported [469].

Nephrotoxicity associated with TMP-SMX is uncommon. TMP can lead to decline in renal tubular secretion of creatinine resulting in higher serum creatinine levels through interference with certain assays that is not reflective of a true reduction in glomerular filtration rate [470]. Adequate hydration should be maintained in order to minimize the risk for urinary tract crystal formation. Patients with low urine output and low urinary pH are at an increased risk for SMX crystalluria [471]. The older sulfonamides are less soluble and can precipitate in the tubules when used in high doses. Patients in whom TMP-SMX were previously discontinued due to skin reactions, especially in HIV-infected patients, a successful desensitization attempt should be considered when treatment resumption is being contemplated [472]. TMP-SMX can interact with a variety of drugs including warfarin, cyclosporin, rifampin, dapsone, and phenytoin [473–475]. Hyperkalemia has been described in elderly patients on spironolactone [474, 476].

Use in Transplant Patients

The combination of TMP and SMX is highly bactericidal with maximum synergy at a ratio of 1:20. The optimal ratio is calculated by the ratio of the MICs of the drugs acting alone. Because TMP is more lipid soluble than SMX, resulting in a larger volume of distribution, the drug is formulated to achieve a SMX concentration in vivo that is 20 times greater than TMP. The drug is available in a fixed ratio of 1:5 for oral/intravenous use [441, 477]. Bioavailability of TMP-SMX is approximately 85%. The peak TMP concentration is achieved in 2 h, whereas the peak SMX concentration is achieved in 4 h [438]. The drug is widely distributed in the body with tissue concentrations usually less than serum concentrations. Peak concentrations of TMP and SMX in the CSF are 1 μg/ml and 13.8 μg/ml, respectively, and penetration was 18% for TMP and 12% for SMX [478]. The half-life of TMP is 8–10 h and SMX is 10 h [441].

TMP-SMX is excreted in the urine, 50% of the drug eliminated in the first 24 h. SMX is approximately 70% protein bound; it is acetylated and glucuronide-conjugated in the liver. TMP is excreted in the urine unchanged. There are four major TMP metabolites with little antibacterial activity. Renal dysfunction results in prolongation of the half-lives of each drug; necessitating dose adjustment creatinine clearance is less than 30 mL/min. Dosing of TMP-SMX is based on the TMP dose and expressed as mg/kg per day of TMP. Oral doses of TMP-SMX are usually given as a single strength or more commonly a double-strength (DS) tablet once to four times daily depending upon the indication and renal function [479]. Intravenous TMP-SMX is usually dosed at a concentration of 5 mL which contains 80 mg of TMP. TMP-SMX dosing should be altered for patients with renal insufficiency with a creatinine clearance ≤30 mL/ min. Dose adjustment guidelines are available for patients with a creatinine clearance ≤15 mL/min [480].

TMP-SMX is commonly used to treat *P. jirovecii* pneumonia (PCP) which remains an important opportunistic fungal infection in patients undergoing allograft transplantation. Outbreaks of PCP have occurred in renal transplant centers secondary to person-to-person transmission resulting in loss of allograft and high mortality. For this reason, TMP-SMX prophylaxis is routinely used after transplantation and continued for 4–12 months after transplantation procedure [481]. Prophylaxis reduced the incidence of PCP infection to less than 1% in renal transplant recipients and considered favorable for reducing risk for toxoplasmosis, listeriosis, and urinary tract infections in such patients. The most common side effects include hemolytic anemia and methemoglobinemia, which are less common with the lower prophylaxis TMP-SMX dose. Breakthrough PCP is exceedingly rare in patients compliant to TMP-SMX prophylaxis.

Nocardia infection is an opportunistic pathogen in transplant patients, especially in lung transplants due to the mode of acquisition. *Nocardia* infection occurs in 2.1–3.5% of lung transplant patients [482–484]. TMP-SMX remains a mainstay of treatment, sometimes combined with imipenem, amikacin, and ciprofloxacin. Most isolates are susceptible to TMP-SMX despite breakthrough infections. Patients experience a high rate of adverse effects including gastrointestinal, renal failure, and cytopenias. Adverse effects may also occur with imipenem when given in combination, albeit most patients tolerate TMP-SMX induction and maintenance therapy for invasive nocardiosis well.

Community-acquired MRSA retained susceptibility to TMP-SMX despite frequent use of the drug in outpatient settings [485]. Susceptibility to *E. coli* and *Proteus* spp. decreased slightly, whereas susceptibility among clinical *K. pneumonia* isolates improved. Continued surveillance is ongoing; TMP-SMX remains a first-line drug in all populations for treatment of infections due to CA-MRSA.

The Polymyxins

The polymyxins are a group of closely related cyclic, positively charged peptide antibiotics discovered in the 1940s [486]. Only polymyxin B and colistimethate, the prodrug of colistin, are available in the United States. These two drugs differ by one amino acid which changes the potency and pharmacokinetics [487]. The intravenous formulations available are polymyxin B and E; polymyxin E is also known as colistin. Polymyxins were largely abandoned secondary to the nephrotoxicity toxicities manifested as proteinuria, oliguria, and acute renal failure and neurotoxicity presenting as paresthesias, neuromuscular blockade, and ataxia. The emergence of MDR GNB, especially *Pseudomonas* and *Acinetobacter* spp., has created a need to form clinical revival of these agents.

The polymyxins are bactericidal agents classified as cationic detergents. The polymyxins interact with phospholipids in the cell membrane by competitively displacing divalent cations from the phosphate groups of the membrane lipids, causing an immediate permeability change, membrane disruption, and leakage of cellular content. Polymyxin B binds to the lipid A portion of endotoxin and can displace magnesium and calcium from cationic-binding sites [488]. This inactivation has been shown in animal models to prevent the effects of endotoxin [489]. Neither polymyxin B nor colistin is absorbed by the oral route. The serum half-life of polymyxin B is approximately 6 h; the majority of the drug is reabsorbed via the proximal tubules. Colistin is tightly bound to lipid membranes of many organs and is excreted in the urine. Pharmacokinetic studies are difficult to interpret since colistimethate assays do not measure the active drug colistin; one study showed a half-life of 4.2 h. Penetration into cerebrospinal fluid, pleural cavity, lung, and biliary tract is low. Polymyxins are rapidly bactericidal with concentration-dependent kinetics. A postantibiotic effect has been reported against *P. aeruginosa* in patients with cystic fibrosis [490].

The spectrum of polymyxin activity includes *P. aeruginosa* and *A. baumannii*, especially relevant for transplant population. Additionally, rising frequency of MDR *Enterobacteriaceae* and *Stenotrophomonas maltophilia* further enhances their appeal. These bacteria have their LPS molecules bridged and stabilized by divalent cations such as magnesium. Many nosocomial pathogens are inherently resistant to these drugs by virtue of replacement of the divalent cation by a positively charged H1 protein resulting in altered lipid A binding. These include *Providencia* spp., *Proteus* spp., most *Serratia* spp., *B. cepacia*, and *Morganella morganii*. The polymyxins have no activity against GPB. Resistance mechanisms to the polymyxins include overexpression of outer membrane proteins and reduction in the net negative charge of lipid A secondary to substitution of phosphate groups and esterification.

The culture medium can alter susceptibility results since cation concentration can affect the MICs, and the automated microdilution assays may not give reliable information. Comparison of disk diffusion, E-test, and broth microdilution to determine resistance to colistin and polymyxin B were found to be concordant in one analysis [491], and E-test was superior to disk diffusion method for *K. pneumoniae*, especially for isolates with disk zone diameters of 12–13 mm [492].

There are several dosing guidelines for these drugs. Conventional dosing for colistin used in the United States for a 70 kg person is 300 mg of drug base per day or 720 mg of colistimethate or 5 mg/kg colistin base daily with either ideal or actual body weight. For polymyxin B the dose is approximately 2 mg/kg/day given in two divided doses or 15,000–25,000 units/kg/day in two divided doses.

Retrospective toxicity studies showed neurotoxicity between 7% and 27% and nephrotoxicity approaching in 43% of patients [493]. Neurotoxicity has ranged from none to 5% in recent studies. Nephrotoxicity from polymyxin B ranges from 6% to 14% and is higher in patients with preexisting kidney disease and compromised renal function. Kubin et al. [487] performed a retrospective review of acute kidney injury (AKI) in 73 patients in whom polymyxin B was given for at least 3 days. The dose was adjusted by total body weight, and using creatinine clearance a daily dose of 1–1.5 mg/kg/day was given to patients with CrCl <80 mL/min and 2.5–3 mg/kg/day in patients with CrCl >80 mL/min. AKI occurred in 60% of patients with more severe elevations in creatinine constituting injury or renal failure in 33%. At the end of therapy, 49% of patients had AKI. Hospital mortality was not influenced by development of AKI. This study found that obese patients may be at an increased risk for AKI, and concurrent vancomycin therapy might potentiate nephrotoxicity.

At one center, in a new dosing protocol, patients were given a loading dose of 25,000 units/kg of polymyxin B with subsequent doses adjusted for creatinine clearance; the dose for CrCl >80 mL/min was 25,000 units/kg every 24 h [494]. The newer dosing trended in improved microbiological success; however, an increased albeit, reversible renal toxicity was also observed. Optimum dosing for patients with and without renal dysfunction remains uncertain. Yahav et al. reviewed recent studies of colistin and concluded that the drug was administered to sicker patients with carbapenem-resistant bacteria. Overall, nephrotoxicity rates were not higher with colistin in these studies, and colistin-induced nephrotoxicity was reversible in most patients [495].

Use in Transplant Infections

Kalpoe et al. [173] reviewed the mortality associated with carbapenemase-producing *K. pneumonia* in liver transplant patients. Fourteen patients had carbapenem-resistant isolates with a 30-day mortality of 71%. Ten patients received polymyxin B monotherapy and had 60% mortality rate. Polymyxin was combined with tigecycline in four patients with a 75% mortality and with cefepime and gentamicin in one patient who also died. Tigecycline monotherapy was given in three patients, in whom one patient survived. The patients who survived had surgical site infections and abdominal abscesses. Some in vitro studies have shown synergy between colistin and carbapenems for GNB that were resistant to carbapenems and susceptible to colistin [495]. Inhaled polymyxin has been added to systemic therapy to improve response; however, Kofteridis found that adding aerosolized colistin to intravenous colistin did not improve outcomes in patients with GNB VAP; there were only eight cases of *P. aeruginosa* in this group [496]. Another study compared three patient groups as follows: parenteral colistin, inhaled colistin, and inhaled and parenteral colistin in 20 ICU patients with pneumonia due to MDR *P. aeruginosa*. A clinical response was observed in all patients on inhaled, 40% given parenteral, and 78% in the inhaled-parenteral combined colistin treatment group. However, no patient achieved microbiological eradication, and mortality was lowest in the inhaled group suggesting that inhaled colistin may be useful as adjunctive therapy for the treatment of these daunting lung infections [497].

Fosfomycin

Fosfomycin is an antimicrobial that was first isolated in 1969 and approved in the United States in the form of a sachet containing 5.61 grams of fosfomycin tromethamine. Fosfomycin is a bactericidal agent that inhibits uridine diphosphate-GlcNAc enoyl-pyruvyltransferase, thereby inhibiting bacterial cell wall synthesis. An active bacterial transport system is necessary. Fosfomycin also decreases the adherence of bacteria to epithelial cells of the urinary tract. The original compound has a low bioavailability of 37%; the soluble salt is available for single-dose use with improved oral bioavailability.

Spectrum of Activity

Fosfomycin is approved in the United States for treatment of uncomplicated urinary tract infections due to *E. coli* and *E. faecalis*. The drug has broad in vitro activity against *K. pneumoniae*, *Proteus* spp., *Enterobacter* spp., and *S. marcescens*. *Pseudomonas* is known to develop resistance, and *Acinetobacter* isolates are inherently resistant. Fosfomycin also has activity against *S. pneumoniae*, *S. aureus*, and *S. epidermidis* and lacks anaerobic activity. Falagas et al. report fosfomycin activity against ESBL-producing *E. coli* adding fosfomycin to the list of antibiotics that may be used to treat urinary tract infections due to such pathogens. Falagas review of 17 studies in the treatment of drug-resistant *Enterobacteriaceae* demonstrated a good level of antimicrobial activity, especially against ESBL-producing *E. coli*. Of note, some of the studies involved sites outside the urinary tract such as decubitus ulcers, bloodstream infection, and other unspecified body sites. *E. coli* was the most common isolate, followed by *K. pneumonia* and *Enterobacter* spp. ESBL isolates accounted for 88% of the organisms with 91.3% showing in vitro susceptibility to fosfomycin. Efficacy of oral therapy in lower urinary tract infections was 94% in all studies and ranged between 78.8% and 93%.

An intravenous preparation of fosfomycin is available outside the United States, where it has been used for the treatment of various maladies such as respiratory tract, bone, obstetrical, joint, and bloodstream infections; furthermore, patients with meningitis and typhoid fever have also been treated with parenteral fosfomycin-based regimen [498]. A review of 31 studies had an overall cure rate of 81.2%. The intravenous formulation was well tolerated, and gastrointestinal, skin rash, and phlebitis at the IV site were prominent adverse events. Clinical trials to allow for eventual marketing of the intravenous formulation in the United States are underway. Resistance to fosfomycin has been observed, although the specific mechanisms are varied. Of note, Tullio et al. reported that fosfomycin mitigated depressed phagocytic response of neutrophils isolated from kidney allograft recipient even in the setting of uremia. This restoration of neutrophil functions against ESBL-producing *E. coli* in ex vivo experiments, although intriguing, needs thorough clinical validation.

Use of Fosfomycin in Transplant Patients

Fosfomycin tromethamine appears to have in vitro immunomodulating properties that may be desirable in the transplant population. When used in subinhibitory concentrations, exposure to fosfomycin was shown to induce ex vivo enhancement of depressed phagocytic neutrophil response against ESBL-producing *E.coli* isolated from patients on long-term hemodialysis and from recipients of renal allograft transplantation [499]. Fosfomycin has been used in the renal transplant population to treat urinary tract infections and is considered a therapeutic alternative for MDR GNB infection including graft pyelonephritis [500, 501]. Combination of fosfomycin with sulbactam was tested against eight clinical isolates of carbapenem-resistant *A. baumannii* using checkerboard assays; a synergy was demonstrated in 75% of these isolates. This in vitro study suggests that combined use of fosfomycin and sulbactam needs further clinical evaluation [502].

Fusidic Acid

Fusidic acid has a unique mechanism of action through binding to elongation factor G (EF-G) which prevents release from the ribosome and inhibition of protein synthesis. The structure is "steroid-like," but the stereochemistry at the ring junctions results in a boat-like structure [503], and the agent has no corticosteroid activity. Fusidic acid has been available in Europe for over 40 years and currently not FDA-approved for use in the United States. The "traditional" spectrum of activity includes MSSA, MRSA, *S. epidermidis*, some beta-hemolytic streptococci, *Corynebacterium* spp., *N. meningitidis*, and most Gram-positive anaerobes. It lacks activity against Gram-negative aerobes and has variable activity against Gram-negative anaerobes. Clinical efficacy has been demonstrated in cSSTIs, osteomyelitis, and other MRSA infections.

Fusidic acid is available by the oral and parenteral routes and is metabolized in the liver by CYP450. Fusidic acid penetrates well into phagocytes and has enhanced antimicrobial activity at low pH [504]. High and sustained serum concentrations are usually achieved. Intravenous preparations have been associated with a high rate of infusion-related phlebitis, and since the oral bioavailability is high, oral route of administration is preferred. Oral fusidic acid has a good safety profile. Kraus et al. reviewed over 1200 citations from the literature worldwide; the most common adverse reactions were gastrointestinal, reversible jaundice, neurologic, hematologic, and cytochrome P450 drug-drug interactions. There is a potential for rhabdomyolysis when given with statins and suggestion that fusidic acid combination may be antagonistic. Concerns about selection of resistance during therapy have contributed to the reluctance to approve this drug in the United States. Resistance is thought to be caused by mutations in the gene coding for EF-G. Chromosomal- or plasmid-mediated mutations, *fus A-E*, have been identified resulting in staphylococcal resistance expressed in vitro MIC ≥2 μg/ml. Resistance is readily acquired when fusidic acid is used as monotherapy and may develop during the course of therapy. The question remains as to whether fusidic acid should be used in combination with other agents.

Jones et al. summarized a fusidic acid (CEM-102) surveillance study (US SENTRY) in the United States in 2008 and 2009 as well as global resistance surveillance data [505]. Fusidic acid $MIC_{50/90}$ was 0.12/0.25 μg/ml against 99.65% of *S. aureus* strains tested. Approximately 53% of these were MRSA that had a trend toward MIC ≥2ug/ml. When compared with oral antibiotics, sulfamethoxazole-trimethoprim inhibited 98.6% of the isolates. Linezolid was eight times less potent than fusidic acid. Fusidic acid was active against 97.6% of MS CNS vs. 90.2% of MR CNS. Fusidic acid resistance was rare, and high-level resistance MIC >32 μg/ml was not seen in the US strains, probably reflecting, in most part, a lack of clinical exposure to this agent in the United States. Jones et al. proposed a staphylococcal breakpoint of ≤1 μg/mL based upon the pharmacodynamics of the drug and low frequency of resistance. Craft et al. published a phase II trial of CEM-102 compared with linezolid in GPB SSTIs using a loading-dose regimen of fusidic acid [506]. Fusidic acid safety, tolerability, and efficacy were comparable to linezolid in this study. Oral fusidic acid is in clinical development in the United States by Cempra Pharmaceuticals as monotherapy with a new dosing regimen. Phase II and III clinical trials are underway. If approved, FA may offer an additional oral agent for treatment of MRSA SSTIs and possibly osteomyelitis.

Fidaxomicin

Discovered in the fermentation broth of an isolate of *Dactylosporangium aurantiacum* subspecies *hamdenensis*, fidaxomicin also known as tiacumicin B and OPT-80 represents the only currently marketed member of the macrocyclic class of antibiotics [507]. Fidaxomicin inhibits bacterial RNA synthesis through blocking the activity of DNA-dependent RNA polymerase via a mechanism distinct from that of the rifamycins and other known inhibitors of RNA polymerase [508]. Specifically, fidaxomicin inhibits melting of the DNA promoter complexes around the start site for transcription through altering the conformation of the DNA in the structure around the complexes [509].

Spectrum of Activity

Fidaxomicin is active in vitro against a number of GPB including *S. aureus* and *E. faecalis*, with no activity demonstrated against most clinically relevant Gram-negative organisms [510]. *Bacteroides* species are not inhibited by fidaxomicin, whereas *C. difficile* is highly sensitive, with a MIC90 of 0.25mcg/mL, and no reports of wild-type isolates with MIC greater than 1mcg/ml have been demonstrated.

Resistance

Reduced susceptibility to fidaxomicin has been identified in one clinical isolate of *Clostridium difficile* resulting from β and β' subunits of RNA polymerase mutation [511]. In vitro studies have determined that serial passage of fidaxomicin may result in a number of single nucleotide polymorphisms in the *rpoB* and *rpoC* genes encoding RNA polymerase, with the Val1143Asp mutation in the β subunit resulting in reduced susceptibility among the clinical isolates [512].

Adverse Events

Due to negligible absorption from the gastrointestinal tract, it is not expected that oral administration of fidaxomicin would result in serious systemic adverse events [513]. Analysis of the clinical trials leading to marketing approval for fidaxomicin demonstrated no differences in the rates of toxicities experienced by patients receiving fidaxomicin as compared to those receiving the comparator agent such as oral vancomycin [514].

Fidaxomicin in Transplant Patients

CDI is associated with an overall significantly worse outcomes in hospitalized patients undergoing solid organ transplantation [395]. Treatment with vancomycin and/or metronidazole is associated with high rates of CDI recurrences in these severely immunosuppressed patients. Fidaxomicin has been shown in clinical trials to be noninferior when compared with oral vancomycin and favorably associated with a significantly lower rate of early CDI recurrence in the 4 weeks following cessation of therapy follow-up. It must be noted, however, that improved sustained response was not seen in the subgroup of patients with NAP1/B1/027 *C. difficile* strain. There is little data about the incidence of this strain in transplant population. It can be concluded that fidaxomicin is an option for the treatment of CDI in patients with an increased risk for infection recurrence and those with severe CDI [511, 515].

Summary

Infections in transplant recipients are more frequently due to multidrug-resistant organisms such as MRSA, VRE; ESBL and carbapenemase producing GNB. Infections with drug-resistant organisms in patients with severe immune dysfunction pose a serious management challenge, especially in planning empiric and preemptive therapy. Resurgence of old drug like polymyxins and fosfomycin, novel drug combinations, and the much-needed new antimicrobials with innovative mechanism of antimicrobial activity supplemented with structural and mechanistic resilience for evading microbial drug-resistance is the encouragement that current and future research provides. It is essential to recognize the clinical significance of potential drug-drug interactions in this patient population. Prudent antibiotic use is predicted upon careful selection and judicious use of antibiotics for infection prophylaxis, preemptive and empiric therapy, and, most importantly, ongoing surveillance to assess prevalence of causative bacterial pathogens and drug susceptibility profiles in an institution, transplant units, regions of temporary or permanent residence of transplant patients. Furthermore, travel-related exposure to bacteria with unique drug resistance profile; emergence, and distribution of drug resistance among common pathogens forms the core principles for optimized anti-infective treatment approach in caring for the highly susceptible patients undergoing transplantation procedures.

References

1. Shields RK, Kwak EJ, Potoski BA, Doi Y, Adams-Haduch JM, Silviera FP, et al. High mortality rates among solid organ transplant recipients infected with extensively drug-resistant Acinetobacter baumannii: using in vitro antibiotic combination testing to identify the combination of a carbapenem and colistin as an effective treatment regimen. Diagn Microbiol Infect Dis. 2011;70(2):246–52.
2. Nunley DR, Bauldoff GS, Mangino JE, Pope-Harman AL. Mortality associated with Acinetobacter baumannii infections experienced by lung transplant recipients. Lung. 2010;188(5):381–5.
3. Dobbin C, Maley M, Harkness J, Benn R, Malouf M, Glanville A, et al. The impact of pan-resistant bacterial pathogens on survival after lung transplantation in cystic fibrosis: results from a single large referral centre. J Hosp Infect. 2004;56(4):277–82.
4. Linares L, Garcia-Goez JF, Cervera C, Almela M, Sanclemente G, Cofan F, et al. Early bacteremia after solid organ transplantation. Transplant Proc. 2009;41(6):2262–4.
5. Hafkin J, Blumberg E. Infections in lung transplantation: new insights. Curr Opin Organ Transplant. 2009;14(5):483–7.
6. Chambers HF. In: Mandell Gerald L, Bennett JE, Raphael D, editors. Penicillins and Beta-lactam inhibitors. Philadelphia, PA: Churchill Livingstone, 2010.
7. Chambers HF. Penicillin-binding protein-mediated resistance in pneumococci and staphylococci. J Infect Dis. 1999;179(Suppl 2):S353–9.
8. Sauvage E, Kerff F, Terrak M, Ayala JA, Charlier P. The penicillin-binding proteins: structure and role in peptidoglycan biosynthesis. FEMS Microbiol Rev. 2008;32(2):234–58.
9. Tomasz A, Waks S. Mechanism of action of penicillin: triggering of the pneumococcal autolytic enzyme by inhibitors of cell wall synthesis. Proc Natl Acad Sci U S A. 1975;72(10):4162–6.
10. Novak R, Charpentier E, Braun JS, Tuomanen E. Signal transduction by a death signal peptide: uncovering the mechanism of bacterial killing by penicillin. Mol Cell. 2000;5(1):49–57.
11. Wolter DJ, Lister PD. Mechanisms of beta-lactam resistance among Pseudomonas aeruginosa. Curr Pharma Des. 2013;19(2):209–22.
12. Rice LB. Mechanisms of resistance and clinical relevance of resistance to beta-lactams, glycopeptides, and fluoroquinolones. Mayo Clin Proc Mayo Clin. 2012;87(2):198–208.
13. Bush K, Jacoby GA. Updated functional classification of beta-lactamases. Antimicrob Agents Chemother. 2010;54(3):969–76.
14. Hall BG, Barlow M. Revised ambler classification of {beta}-lactamases. J Antimicrob Chemother. 2005;55(6):1050–1.
15. Tangden T, Adler M, Cars O, Sandegren L, Lowdin E. Frequent emergence of porin-deficient subpopulations with reduced carbapenem susceptibility in ESBL-producing Escherichia coli during exposure to ertapenem in an in vitro pharmacokinetic model. J Antimicrob Chemother. 2013;68(6):1319–26.

16. Chopra T, Marchaim D, Veltman J, Johnson P, Zhao JJ, Tansek R, et al. Impact of cefepime therapy on mortality among patients with bloodstream infections caused by extended-spectrum-beta-lactamase-producing Klebsiella pneumoniae and Escherichia coli. Antimicrob Agents Chemother. 2012;56(7):3936–42.
17. Rossolini GM, D'Andrea MM, Mugnaioli C. The spread of CTX-M-type extended-spectrum beta-lactamases. Clin Microbiol Infect. 2008;14(Suppl 1):33–41.
18. Johnson JR, Urban C, Weissman SJ, Jorgensen JH, Lewis JS 2nd, Hansen G, et al. Molecular epidemiological analysis of Escherichia coli sequence type ST131 (O25:H4) and blaCTX-M-15 among extended-spectrum-beta-lactamase-producing E. coli from the United States, 2000 to 2009. Antimicrob Agents Chemother. 2012;56(5):2364–70.
19. Heritier C, Poirel L, Lambert T, Nordmann P. Contribution of acquired carbapenem-hydrolyzing oxacillinases to carbapenem resistance in Acinetobacter baumannii. Antimicrob Agents Chemother. 2005;49(8):3198–202.
20. Raviv Y, Shitrit D, Amital A, Fox B, Bakal I, Tauber R, et al. Multidrug-resistant Klebsiella pneumoniae acquisition in lung transplant recipients. Clin Transpl. 2012;26(4):E388–94.
21. Wang L, Archer GL. Roles of CcrA and CcrB in excision and integration of staphylococcal cassette chromosome mec, a Staphylococcus aureus genomic island. J Bacteriol. 2010;192(12):3204–12.
22. Ohnishi M, Golparian D, Shimuta K, Saika T, Hoshina S, Iwasaku K, et al. Is Neisseria gonorrhoeae initiating a future era of untreatable gonorrhea?: detailed characterization of the first strain with high-level resistance to ceftriaxone. Antimicrob Agents Chemother. 2011;55(7):3538–45.
23. Wright AJ. The penicillins. Mayo Clin Proc Mayo Clin. 1999;74(3):290–307.
24. Drawz SM, Bonomo RA. Three decades of beta-lactamase inhibitors. Clin Microbiol Rev. 2010;23(1):160–201.
25. Williams JD. Beta-lactamases and beta-lactamase inhibitors. Int J Antimicrob Agents. 1999;12(Suppl 1):S3–7. discussion S26–7.
26. Shahid M, Sobia F, Singh A, Malik A, Khan HM, Jonas D, et al. Beta-lactams and beta-lactamase-inhibitors in current- or potential-clinical practice: a comprehensive update. Crit Rev Microbiol. 2009;35(2):81–108.
27. Biondi S, Long S, Panunzio M, Qin WL. Current trends in beta-lactam based beta-lactamases inhibitors. Curr Med Chem. 2011;18(27):4223–36.
28. Poirel L, Nordmann P. Carbapenem resistance in Acinetobacter baumannii: mechanisms and epidemiology. Clin Microbiol Infect. 2006;12(9):826–36.
29. Vila J, Pachon J. Therapeutic options for Acinetobacter baumannii infections: an update. Expert Opin Pharmacother. 2012;13(16):2319–36.
30. Betrosian AP, Frantzeskaki F, Xanthaki A, Georgiadis G. High-dose ampicillin-sulbactam as an alternative treatment of late-onset VAP from multidrug-resistant Acinetobacter baumannii. Scand J Infect Dis. 2007;39(1):38–43.
31. Papp-Wallace KM, Senkfor B, Gatta J, Chai W, Taracila MA, Shanmugasundaram V, et al. Early insights into the interactions of different beta-lactam antibiotics and beta-lactamase inhibitors against soluble forms of Acinetobacter baumannii PBP1a and PBP3. Antimicrob Agents Chemother. 2012;56(11):5687–92.
32. Durante-Mangoni E, Zarrilli R. Global spread of drug-resistant Acinetobacter baumannii: molecular epidemiology and management of antimicrobial resistance. Future Microbiol. 2011;6(4):407–22.
33. Ehmann DE, Jahic H, Ross PL, Gu RF, Hu J, Kern G, et al. Avibactam is a covalent, reversible, non-beta-lactam beta-lactamase inhibitor. Proc Natl Acad Sci U S A. 2012;109(29):11663–8.
34. Kazmierczak KM, Biedenbach DJ, Hackel M, Rabine S, de Jonge BL, Bouchillon SK, et al. Global dissemination of blaKPC into bacterial species beyond Klebsiella pneumoniae and in vitro susceptibility to Ceftazidime-avibactam and Aztreonam-avibactam. Antimicrob Agents Chemother. 2016;60(8):4490–500.
35. Marshall S, Hujer AM, Rojas LJ, Papp-Wallace KM, Humphries RM, Spellberg B, et al. Can ceftazidime/avibactam and aztreonam overcome β-lactam resistance conferred by metallo-β-lactamases in Enterobacteriaceae? Antimicrob Agents Chemother. 2017;61(4). pii: e02243–16.
36. Castanheira M, Rhomberg PR, Flamm RK, Jones RN. Effect of the beta-lactamase inhibitor Vaborbactam combined with Meropenem against serine Carbapenemase-producing Enterobacteriaceae. Antimicrob Agents Chemother. 2016;60(9):5454–8.
37. Lob SH, Hackel MA, Kazmierczak KM, Young K, Motyl MR, Karlowsky JA, et al. In vitro activity of Imipenem-Relebactam against gram-negative ESKAPE pathogens isolated by clinical Laboratories in the United States in 2015 – results from the SMART global surveillance program. Antimicrob Agents Chemother. 2017;61(6):e02209–16.
38. Marshall WF, Blair JE. The cephalosporins. Mayo Clin Proc Mayo Clin. 1999;74(2):187–95.
39. Patel KB, Nicolau DP, Nightingale CH, Quintiliani R. Pharmacokinetics of cefotaxime in healthy volunteers and patients. Diagn Microbiol Infect Dis. 1995;22(1–2):49–55.
40. Sader HS, Castanheira M, Mendes RE, Flamm RK, Antimicrobial JRN. Activity of High-Proportion Cefepime-Tazobactam (WCK 4282) against a Large Number of Gram-Negative Isolates Collected Worldwide in 2014. Antimicrob Agents Chemother. 2017;61(4):e02409–16.
41. Cha R. In vitro activity of cefepime, imipenem, tigecycline, and gentamicin, alone and in combination, against extended-spectrum beta-lactamase-producing Klebsiella pneumoniae and Escherichia coli. Pharmacotherapy. 2008;28(3):295–300.
42. Lee NY, Lee CC, Huang WH, Tsui KC, Hsueh PR, Ko WC. Cefepime therapy for monomicrobial bacteremia caused by cefepime-susceptible extended-spectrum beta-lactamase-producing Enterobacteriaceae: MIC matters. Clin Infect Dis. 2013;56(4):488–95.
43. Arizpe A, Reveles KR, Patel SD, Aitken SL. Updates in the management of cephalosporin-resistant gram-negative bacteria. Curr Infect Dis Rep. 2016;18(12):39.
44. Cabot G, Bruchmann S, Mulet X, Zamorano L, Moyà B, Juan C, et al. Pseudomonas aeruginosa Ceftolozane-Tazobactam resistance development requires multiple mutations leading to overexpression and structural modification of AmpC. Antimicrob Agents Chemother. 2014;58(6):3091–9.
45. Munita JM, Aitken SL, Miller WR, Perez F, Rosa R, Shimose LA, et al. Multicenter evaluation of Ceftolozane/Tazobactam for Serious Infections Caused by Carbapenem-Resistant Pseudomonas aeruginosa. Clin Infect Dis. 2017;65(1):158–61.
46. Farrell DJ, Flamm RK, Sader HS, Jones RN. Antimicrobial activity of Ceftolozane-Tazobactam tested against Enterobacteriaceae and Pseudomonas aeruginosa with various resistance patterns isolated in U.S. hospitals (2011-2012). Antimicrob Agents Chemother. 2013;57(12):6305–10.
47. Ito A, Nishikawa T, Matsumoto S, Yoshizawa H, Sato T, Nakamura R, et al. Siderophore cephalosporin Cefiderocol utilizes ferric Iron transporter Systems for Antibacterial Activity against Pseudomonas aeruginosa. Antimicrob Agents Chemother. 2016;60(12):7396–401.
48. Falagas ME, Skalidis T, Vardakas KZ, Legakis NJ. Activity of cefiderocol (S-649266) against carbapenem-resistant gram-negative bacteria collected from inpatients in Greek hospitals. J Antimicrob Chemother. 2017;72(6):1704–8.
49. Li H, Luo YF, Williams BJ, Blackwell TS, Xie CM. Structure and function of OprD protein in Pseudomonas aeruginosa: from antibiotic resistance to novel therapies. Int J Med Microbiol. 2012;302(2):63–8.

50. Muller C, Plesiat P, Jeannot K. A two-component regulatory system interconnects resistance to polymyxins, aminoglycosides, fluoroquinolones, and beta-lactams in Pseudomonas aeruginosa. Antimicrob Agents Chemother. 2011;55(3):1211–21.
51. Zhanel GG, Wiebe R, Dilay L, Thomson K, Rubinstein E, Hoban DJ, et al. Comparative review of the carbapenems. Drugs. 2007;67(7):1027–52.
52. Norrby SR. Neurotoxicity of carbapenem antibacterials. Drug Safety. 1996;15(2):87–90.
53. Bazan JA, Martin SI, Kaye KM. Newer beta-lactam antibiotics: doripenem, ceftobiprole, ceftaroline, and cefepime. Med Clin N Am. 2011;95(4):743–60. viii
54. Jones RN, Huynh HK, Biedenbach DJ. Activities of doripenem (S-4661) against drug-resistant clinical pathogens. Antimicrob Agents Chemother. 2004;48(8):3136–40.
55. Fritsche TR, Stilwell MG, Jones RN. Antimicrobial activity of doripenem (S-4661): a global surveillance report (2003). Clin Microbiol Infect. 2005;11(12):974–84.
56. Mushtaq S, Ge Y, Livermore DM. Doripenem versus Pseudomonas aeruginosa in vitro: activity against characterized isolates, mutants, and transconjugants and resistance selection potential. Antimicrob Agents Chemother. 2004;48(8):3086–92.
57. Barry AL, Thornsberry C, Jones RN, Gavan TL. Aztreonam: antibacterial activity, beta-lactamase stability, and interpretive standards and quality control guidelines for disk-diffusion susceptibility tests. Rev Infect Dis. 1985;7(Suppl 4):S594–604.
58. Swabb EA. Review of the clinical pharmacology of the monobactam antibiotic aztreonam. Am J Med. 1985;78(2A):11–8.
59. Zeitler K, Salvas B, Stevens V, Brown J. Aztreonam lysine for inhalation: new formulation of an old antibiotic. Am J Health-Syst Pharm. 2012;69(2):107–15.
60. Buonomo A, Nucera E, De Pasquale T, Pecora V, Lombardo C, Sabato V, et al. Tolerability of aztreonam in patients with cell-mediated allergy to beta-lactams. Int Arch Allergy Immunol. 2011;155(2):155–9.
61. Farrell DJ, Castanheira M, Mendes RE, Sader HS, Jones RN. In vitro activity of Ceftaroline against multidrug-resistant Staphylococcus aureus and Streptococcus pneumoniae: a review of published studies and the AWARE surveillance program (2008-2010). Clin Infect Dis. 2012;55(Suppl 3):S206–14.
62. File TM Jr, Wilcox MH, Stein GE. Summary of ceftaroline fosamil clinical trial studies and clinical safety. Clin Infect Dis. 2012;55(Suppl 3):S173–80.
63. Lagace-Wiens P, Rubinstein E. Adverse reactions to beta-lactam antimicrobials. Expert Opin Drug Safety. 2012;11(3):381–99.
64. Romano A, Gaeta F, Valluzzi RL, Caruso C, Rumi G, Bousquet PJ. IgE-mediated hypersensitivity to cephalosporins: cross-reactivity and tolerability of penicillins, monobactams, and carbapenems. J Allergy Clin Immunol. 2010;126(5):994–9.
65. Chang C, Mahmood MM, Teuber SS, Gershwin ME. Overview of penicillin allergy. Clin Rev Allergy Immunol. 2012;43(1–2):84–97.
66. Prescott WA Jr, Kusmierski KA. Clinical importance of carbapenem hypersensitivity in patients with self-reported and documented penicillin allergy. Pharmacotherapy. 2007;27(1):137–42.
67. Bickford CL, Spencer AP. Biliary sludge and hyperbilirubinemia associated with ceftriaxone in an adult: case report and review of the literature. Pharmacotherapy. 2005;25(10):1389–95.
68. Alitalo R, Ruutu M, Valtonen V, Lehtonen T, Pentikainen PJ. Hypoprothrombinaemia and bleeding during administration of cefamandole and cefoperazone. Report of three cases. Ann Clin Res. 1985;17(3):116–9.
69. Levine DP. Vancomycin: a history. Clin Infect Dis. 2006;42(Suppl 1):S5–12.
70. Kirst HA, Thompson DG, Nicas TI. Historical yearly usage of vancomycin. Antimicrob Agents Chemother. 1998;42(5):1303–4.
71. Peacock JJE, Marsik FJ, Wenzel RP. Methicillin-resistant Staphylococcus aureus: introduction and spread within a hospital. Ann Intern Med. 1998;93(4):526–32.
72. Saravolatz LD, Pohlod DJ, Arking LM. Community-acquired methicillin-resistant Staphylococcus aureus infections: a new source for nosocomial outbreaks. Ann Intern Med. 1982;97(3):325–9.
73. Rogers HJ, Forsberg CW. Role of autolysins in the killing of bacteria by some bactericidal antibiotics. J Bacteriol. 1971;108(3):1235–43.
74. Krogstad DJ, Pargwette AR. Defective killing of enterococci: a common property of antimicrobial agents acting on the cell wall. Antimicrob Agents Chemother. 1980;17(6):965–8.
75. Geraci JE, Wilson WR. Vancomycin therapy for infective endocarditis. Rev Infect Dis. 1981;3(Suppl):S250–8.
76. Uttley AH, Collins CH, Naidoo J, George RC. Vancomycin-resistant enterococci. Lancet. 1988;1(8575–6):57–8.
77. Leclercq R, Derlot E, Duval J, Courvalin P. Plasmid-mediated resistance to vancomycin and teicoplanin in enterococcus faecium. N Engl J Med. 1988;319(3):157–61.
78. Hiramatsu K, Hanaki H, Ino T, Yabuta K, Oguri T, Tenover FC. Methicillin-resistant Staphylococcus aureus clinical strain with reduced vancomycin susceptibility. J Antimicrob Chemother. 1997;40(1):135–6.
79. Chang S, Sievert DM, Hageman JC, Boulton ML, Tenover FC, Downes FP, et al. Infection with vancomycin-resistant Staphylococcus aureus containing the vanA resistance gene. N Engl J Med. 2003;348(14):1342–7.
80. Courvalin P. Vancomycin resistance in gram-positive cocci. Clin Infect Dis. 2006;42(Suppl 1):S25–34.
81. Navarro F, Courvalin P. Analysis of genes encoding D-alanine-D-alanine ligase-related enzymes in enterococcus casseliflavus and enterococcus flavescens. Antimicrob Agents Chemother. 1994;38(8):1788–93.
82. Arthur M, Reynolds P, Courvalin P. Glycopeptide resistance in enterococci. Trends Microbiol. 1996;4(10):401–7.
83. Green M, Shlaes JH, Barbadora K, Shlaes DM. Bacteremia due to vancomycin-dependent Enterococcus faecium. Clin Infect Dis. 1995;20(3):712–4.
84. Farrag N, Eltringham I, Liddy H. Vancomycin-dependent Enterococcus faecalis. Lancet. 1996;348(9041):1581–2.
85. Van Bambeke F, Chauvel M, Reynolds PE, Fraimow HS, Courvalin P. Vancomycin-dependent enterococcus faecalis clinical isolates and revertant mutants. Antimicrob Agents Chemother. 1999;43(1):41–7.
86. Geraci JEHF, Nichols DR, Ross GT, Wellman WE. Some laboratory and clinical experiences with a new antibiotic, vancomycin. Proc Staff Meet Mayo Clin. 1956;31(21):564–82.
87. Moellering RC Jr. The specter of glycopeptide resistance: current trends and future considerations. Am J Med. 1998;104(5A):3S–6S.
88. Siebert WT, Moreland N, Williams TW Jr. Synergy of vancomycin plus cefazolin or cephalothin against methicillin-resistance Staphylococcus epidermidis. J Infect Dis. 1979;139(4):452–7.
89. Noble WC, Virani Z, Cree RG. Co-transfer of vancomycin and other resistance genes from enterococcus faecalis NCTC 12201 to Staphylococcus aureus. FEMS Microbiol Lett. 1992;72(2):195–8.
90. Srinivasan A, Dick JD, Perl TM. Vancomycin resistance in staphylococci. Clin Microbiol Rev. 2002;15(3):430–8.
91. Sievert DM, Rudrik JT, Patel JB, McDonald LC, Wilkins MJ, Hageman JC. Vancomycin-resistant Staphylococcus aureus in the United States, 2002-2006. Clin Infect Dis. 2008;46(5):668–74.
92. Tenover FC, Moellering RC Jr. The rationale for revising the clinical and laboratory standards institute vancomycin minimal inhibitory concentration interpretive criteria for Staphylococcus aureus. Clin Infect Dis. 2007;44(9):1208–15.
93. Daum RS, Gupta S, Sabbagh R, Milewski WM. Characterization of Staphylococcus aureus isolates with decreased susceptibility to vancomycin and teicoplanin: isolation and purification of a consti-

tutively produced protein associated with decreased susceptibility. J Infect Dis. 1992;166(5):1066–72.
94. Hanaki H, Kuwahara-Arai K, Boyle-Vavra S, Daum RS, Labischinski H, Hiramatsu K. Activated cell-wall synthesis is associated with vancomycin resistance in methicillin-resistant Staphylococcus aureus clinical strains Mu3 and Mu50. J Antimicrob Chemother. 1998;42(2):199–209.
95. Sieradzki K, Tomasz A. Gradual alterations in cell wall structure and metabolism in vancomycin-resistant mutants of Staphylococcus aureus. J Bacteriol. 1999;181(24):7566–70.
96. Charles PG, Ward PB, Johnson PD, Howden BP, Grayson ML. Clinical features associated with bacteremia due to heterogeneous vancomycin-intermediate Staphylococcus aureus. Clin Infect Dis. 2004;38(3):448–51.
97. Yeh YC, Yeh KM, Lin TY, Chiu SK, Yang YS, Wang YC, et al. Impact of vancomycin MIC creep on patients with methicillin-resistant Staphylococcus aureus bacteremia. J Microbiol Immunol Infect. 2012;45(3):214–20.
98. Steinkraus G, White R, Friedrich L. Vancomycin MIC Creep in non-vancomycin-intermediate Staphylococcus aureus (VISA), vancomycin-susceptible clinical methicillin-resistant S. aureus (MRSA) blood isolates from 2001-05. J Antimicrob Chemother. 2007;60(4):788–94.
99. Sherris JC. Problems in in vitro determination of antibiotic tolerance in clinical isolates. Antimicrob Agents Chemother. 1986;30(5):633–7.
100. Jones RN. Microbiological features of vancomycin in the 21st century: minimum inhibitory concentration creep, bactericidal/static activity, and applied breakpoints to predict clinical outcomes or detect resistant strains. Clin Infect Dis. 2006;42(Suppl 1):S13–24.
101. Sakoulas G, Eliopoulos GM, Moellering RC Jr, Wennersten C, Venkataraman L, Novick RP, et al. Accessory gene regulator (agr) locus in geographically diverse Staphylococcus aureus isolates with reduced susceptibility to vancomycin. Antimicrob Agents Chemother. 2002;46(5):1492–502.
102. Verdier I, Reverdy ME, Etienne J, Lina G, Bes M, Vandenesch F. Staphylococcus aureus isolates with reduced susceptibility to glycopeptides belong to accessory gene regulator group I or II. Antimicrob Agents Chemother. 2004;48(3):1024–7.
103. Farber BF, Moellering RC Jr. Retrospective study of the toxicity of preparations of vancomycin from 1974 to 1981. Antimicrob Agents Chemother. 1983;23(1):138–41.
104. Rybak MJ, Albrecht LM, Boike SC, Chandrasekar PH. Nephrotoxicity of vancomycin, alone and with an aminoglycoside. J Antimicrob Chemother. 1990;25(4):679–87.
105. Hammond DA, Smith MN, Li C, Hayes SM, Lusardi K, Bookstaver PB. Systematic review and meta-analysis of acute kidney injury associated with Concomitant Vancomycin and Piperacillin/tazobactam. Clin Infect Dis. 2017;64(5):666–74.
106. Navalkele B, Pogue JM, Karino S, Nishan B, Salim M, Solanki S, et al. Risk of acute kidney injury in patients on concomitant Vancomycin and Piperacillin-Tazobactam compared to those on Vancomycin and Cefepime. Clin Infect Dis. 2017;64(2):116–23.
107. Rybak MJ, Lomaestro BM, Rotschafer JC, Moellering RC Jr, Craig WA, Billeter M, et al. Therapeutic monitoring of vancomycin in adults summary of consensus recommendations from the American Society of Health-System Pharmacists, the Infectious Diseases Society of America, and the Society of Infectious Diseases Pharmacists. Pharmacotherapy. 2009;29(11):1275–9.
108. Bergman MM, Glew RH, Ebert TH. Acute interstitial nephritis associated with vancomycin therapy. Arch Int Med. 1988;148(10):2139–40.
109. Brummett RE. Ototoxicity of vancomycin and analogues. Otolaryngol Clin N Am. 1993;26(5):821–8.
110. Traber PG, Levine DP. Vancomycin ototoxicity in patient with normal renal function. Ann Intern Med. 1981;95(4):458–60.
111. Pai MP, Mercier RC, Koster SA. Epidemiology of vancomycin-induced neutropenia in patients receiving home intravenous infusion therapy. Ann Pharmacother. 2006;40(2):224–8.
112. Black E, Lau TT, Ensom MH. Vancomycin-induced neutropenia: is it dose- or duration-related? Ann Pharmacother. 2011;45(5):629–38.
113. Von Drygalski A, Curtis BR, Bougie DW, McFarland JG, Ahl S, Limbu I, et al. Vancomycin-induced immune thrombocytopenia. N Engl J Med. 2007;356(9):904–10.
114. O'Sullivan TL, Ruffing MJ, Lamp KC, Warbasse LH, Rybak MJ. Prospective evaluation of red man syndrome in patients receiving vancomycin. J Infect Dis. 1993;168(3):773–6.
115. Sahai J, Healy DP, Garris R, Berry A, Polk RE. Influence of antihistamine pretreatment on vancomycin-induced red-man syndrome. J Infect Dis. 1989;160(5):876–81.
116. Li H, Yu DL, Ren L, Zhong L, Peng ZH, Teng MJ. Analysis of gram-positive bacterial infection in patients following liver transplantation. Chin Med J. 2012;125(14):2417–21.
117. Shields RK, Clancy CJ, Minces LR, Kwak EJ, Silveira FP, Abdel Massih RC, et al. Staphylococcus aureus infections in the early period after lung transplantation: epidemiol risk factors outcomes. J Heart Lung Transplant. 2012;31(11):1199–206.
118. Willems L, Porcher R, Lafaurie M, Casin I, Robin M, Xhaard A, et al. Clostridium difficile infection after allogeneic hematopoietic stem cell transplantation: incidence, risk factors, and outcome. Biol Blood Marrow Transplant. 2012;18(8):1295–301.
119. Begg EJ, Barclay ML. Aminoglycosides--50 years on. Br J Clin Pharmacol. 1995;39(6):597–603.
120. Weinstein MJ, Luedemann GM, Oden EM, Wagman GH, Rosselet JP, Marquez JA, et al. Gentamicin, a new antibiotic complex from MICROMONOSPORA. J Med Chem. 1963;6:463–4.
121. Haidar G, Alkroud A, Cheng S, Churilla TM, Churilla BM, Shields RK, et al. Association between the presence of aminoglycoside-modifying enzymes and in vitro activity of gentamicin, tobramycin, Amikacin, and Plazomicin against Klebsiella pneumoniae Carbapenemase- and extended-Spectrum-beta-lactamase-producing Enterobacter species. Antimicrob Agents Chemother. 2016;60(9):5208–14.
122. Noller HF. Ribosomal RNA and translation. Annu Rev Biochem. 1991;60:191–227.
123. Davis BD, Chen LL, Tai PC. Misread protein creates membrane channels: an essential step in the bactericidal action of aminoglycosides. Proc Natl Acad Sci U S A. 1986;83(16):6164–8.
124. Peterson AA, Hancock RE, McGroarty EJ. Binding of polycationic antibiotics and polyamines to lipopolysaccharides of Pseudomonas aeruginosa. J Bacteriol. 1985;164(3):1256–61.
125. Bryan LE, Kwan S. Roles of ribosomal binding, membrane potential, and electron transport in bacterial uptake of streptomycin and gentamicin. Antimicrob Agents Chemother. 1983;23(6):835–45.
126. Taber HW, Mueller JP, Miller PF, Arrow AS. Bacterial uptake of aminoglycoside antibiotics. Microbiol Rev. 1987;51(4):439–57.
127. Damper PD, Epstein W. Role of the membrane potential in bacterial resistance to aminoglycoside antibiotics. Antimicrob Agents Chemother. 1981;20(6):803–8.
128. Zimelis VM, Jackson GG. Activity of aminoglycoside antibiotics against Pseudomonas aeruginosa: specificity and site of calcium and magnesium antagonism. J Infect Dis. 1973;127(6):663–9.
129. Fantin B, Carbon C. In vivo antibiotic synergism: contribution of animal models. Antimicrob Agents Chemother. 1992;36(5):907–12.
130. Magnet S, Blanchard JS. Molecular insights into aminoglycoside action and resistance. Chem Rev. 2005;105(2):477–98.
131. Miller GH, Sabatelli FJ, Hare RS, Glupczynski Y, Mackey P, Shlaes D, et al. The most frequent aminoglycoside resistance

mechanisms--changes with time and geographic area: a reflection of aminoglycoside usage patterns? Aminoglycoside resistance study groups. Clin Infect Dis. 1997;24(Suppl 1):S46–62.
132. Hocquet D, Vogne C, El Garch F, Vejux A, Gotoh N, Lee A, et al. MexXY-OprM efflux pump is necessary for a adaptive resistance of Pseudomonas aeruginosa to aminoglycosides. Antimicrob Agents Chemother. 2003;47(4):1371–5.
133. Benveniste R, Davies J. Mechanisms of antibiotic resistance in bacteria. Annu Rev Biochem. 1973;42:471–506.
134. Shaw KJ, Rather PN, Hare RS, Miller GH. Molecular genetics of aminoglycoside resistance genes and familial relationships of the aminoglycoside-modifying enzymes. Microbiol Rev. 1993;57(1):138–63.
135. Acar JF, Witchitz JL, Goldstein F, Talbot JN, Le Goffic F. Susceptibility of aminoglycoside-resistant gram-negative bacilli to amikacin: delineation of individual resistance patterns. J Infect Dis. 1976;134(SUPPL):S280–5.
136. Damaso D, Moreno-Lopez M, Martinez-Beltran J, Garcia-Iglesias MC. Susceptibility of current clinical isolates of Pseudomonas aeruginosa and enteric gram-negative bacilli to amikacin and other aminoglycoside antibiotics. J Infect Dis. 1976;134(SUPPL):S394–0.
137. Bryan LE, O'Hara K, Wong S. Lipopolysaccharide changes in impermeability-type aminoglycoside resistance in Pseudomonas aeruginosa. Antimicrob Agents Chemother. 1984;26(2):250–5.
138. Vogne C, Aires JR, Bailly C, Hocquet D, Plésiat P. Role of the multidrug efflux system MexXY in the emergence of moderate resistance to aminoglycosides among Pseudomonas aeruginosa isolates from patients with cystic fibrosis. Antimicrob Agents Chemother. 2004;48(5):1676–80.
139. Daikos GL, Jackson GG, Lolans VT, Livermore DM. Adaptive resistance to aminoglycoside antibiotics from first-exposure down-regulation. J Infect Dis. 1990;162(2):414–20.
140. Smith CR, Lipsky JJ, Laskin OL, Hellmann DB, Mellits ED, Longstreth J, et al. Double-blind comparison of the nephrotoxic ity and auditory toxicity of gentamicin and tobramycin. N Engl J Med. 1980;302(20):1106–9.
141. Bertino JS Jr, Booker LA, Franck PA, Jenkins PL, Franck KR, Nafziger AN. Incidence of and significant risk factors for aminoglycoside-associated nephrotoxicity in patients dosed by using individualized pharmacokinetic monitoring. J Infect Dis. 1993;167(1):173–9.
142. Prins JM, Weverling GJ, de Blok K, van Ketel RJ, Speelman P. Validation and nephrotoxicity of a simplified once-daily aminoglycoside dosing schedule and guidelines for monitoring therapy. Antimicrob Agents Chemother. 1996;40(11):2494–9.
143. Schentag JJ, Plaut ME, Cerra FB. Comparative nephrotoxicity of gentamicin and tobramycin: pharmacokinetic and clinical studies in 201 patients. Antimicrob Agents Chemother. 1981;19(5):859–66.
144. Gilbert DN, Plamp C, Starr P, Bennet WM, Houghton DC, Porter G. Comparative nephrotoxicity of gentamicin and tobramycin in rats. Antimicrob Agents Chemother. 1978;13(1):34–40.
145. Luft FC, Bloch R, Sloan RS, Yum MN, Costello R, Maxwell DR. Comparative nephrotoxicity of aminoglycoside antibiotics in rats. J Infect Dis. 1978;138(4):541–5.
146. Cohen L, Lapkin R, Kaloyanides GJ. Effect of gentamicin on renal function in the rat. J Pharmacol Exp Ther. 1975;193(1):264–73.
147. Kaloyanides GJ, Pastoriza-Munoz E. Aminoglycoside nephrotoxicity. Kidney Int. 1980;18(5):571–82.
148. Fabre J, Rudhardt M, Blanchard P, Regamey C. Persistence of sisomicin and gentamicin in renal cortex and medulla compared with other organs and serum of rats. Kidney Int. 1976;10(6):444–9.
149. Sandoval R, Leiser J, Molitoris BA. Aminoglycoside antibiotics traffic to the Golgi complex in LLC-PK1 cells. J Am Soc Nephrol. 1998;9(2):167–74.
150. Verroust PJ, Birn H, Nielsen R, Kozyraki R, Christensen EI. The tandem endocytic receptors megalin and cubilin are important proteins in renal pathology. Kidney Int. 2002;62(3):745–56.
151. Somermeyer MG, Knauss TC, Weinberg JM, Humes HD. Characterization of Ca2+ transport in rat renal brush-border membranes and its modulation by phosphatidic acid. Biochem J. 1983;214(1):37–46.
152. Klotman PE, Yarger WE. Reduction of renal blood flow and proximal bicarbonate reabsorption in rats by gentamicin. Kidney Int. 1983;24(5):638–43.
153. Tulkens PM. Experimental studies on nephrotoxicity of aminoglycosides at low doses. Mechanisms and perspectives. Am J Med. 1986;80(6B):105–14.
154. Russo JC, Adelman RD. Gentamicin-induced Fanconi syndrome. J Pediatr. 1980;96(1):151–3.
155. Gilbert DN, Houghton DC, Bennett WM, Plamp CE, Reger K, Porter GA. Reversibility of gentamicin nephrotoxicity in rats: recovery during continuous drug administration. Proc Soc Exp Biol Med. 1979;160(1):99–103.
156. Nonclercq D, Wrona S, Toubeau G, Zanen J, Heuson-Stiennon JA, Schaudies RP, et al. Tubular injury and regeneration in the rat kidney following acute exposure to gentamicin: a time-course study. Ren Fail. 1992;14(4):507–21.
157. Klastersky J, Hensgens C, Debusscher L. Empiric therapy for cancer patients: comparative study of ticarcillin-tobramycin, ticarcillin-cephalothin, and cephalothin-tobramycin. Antimicrob Agents Chemother. 1975;7(5):640–5.
158. Ohnishi A, Bryant TD, Branch KR, Sabra R, Branch RA. Role of sodium in the protective effect of ticarcillin on gentamicin nephrotoxicity in rats. Antimicrob Agents Chemother. 1989;33(6):928–32.
159. Fausti SA, Helt WJ, Phillips DS, Gordon JS, Bratt GW, Sugiura KM, et al. Early detection of ototoxicity using 1/6th-octave steps. J Am Acad Audiol. 2003;14(8):444–50.
160. Govaerts PJ, Claes J, van de Heyning PH, Jorens PG, Marquet J, De Broe ME. Aminoglycoside-induced ototoxicity. Toxicol Lett. 1990;52(3):227–51.
161. Lyford-Pike S, Vogelheim C, Chu E, Della Santina CC, Carey JP. Gentamicin is primarily localized in vestibular type I hair cells after intratympanic administration. J Assoc Res Otolaryngol. 2007;8(4):497–508.
162. Hashino E, Shero M, Salvi RJ. Lysosomal targeting and accumulation of aminoglycoside antibiotics in sensory hair cells. Brain Res. 1997;777(1–2):75–85.
163. Manian FA, Stone WJ, Alford RH. Adverse antibiotic effects associated with renal insufficiency. Rev Infect Dis. 1990;12(2): 236–49.
164. Brummett RE, Fox KE. Aminoglycoside-induced hearing loss in humans. Antimicrob Agents Chemother. 1989;33(6):797–800.
165. Moore RD, Smith CR, Lietman PS. Risk factors for the development of auditory toxicity in patients receiving aminoglycosides. J Infect Dis. 1984;149(1):23–30.
166. Fischel-Ghodsian N. Genetic factors in aminoglycoside toxicity. Pharmacogenomics. 2005;6(1):27–36.
167. Yamada S, Kuno Y, Iwanaga H. Effects of aminoglycoside antibiotics on the neuromuscular junction: part I. Int J Clin Pharmacol Ther Toxicol. 1986;24(3):130–8.
168. Barrons RW. Drug-induced neuromuscular blockade and myasthenia gravis. Pharmacotherapy. 1997;17(6):1220–32.
169. Snavely SR, Hodges GR. The neurotoxicity of antibacterial agents. Ann Intern Med. 1984;101(1):92–104.
170. Del Pozo E, Baeyens JM. Effects of calcium channel blockers on neuromuscular blockade induced by aminoglycoside antibiotics. Eur J Pharmacol. 1986;128(1–2):49–54.
171. Singh YN, Harvey AL, Marshall IG. Antibiotic-induced paralysis of the mouse phrenic nerve-hemidiaphragm preparation, and

reversibility by calcium and by neostigmine. Anesthesiology. 1978;48(6):418–24.

172. Linares L, Cervera C, Cofan F, Ricart MJ, Esforzado N, Torregrosa V, et al. Epidemiology and outcomes of multiple antibiotic-resistant bacterial infection in renal transplantation. Transplant Proc. 2007;39(7):2222–4.
173. Kalpoe JS, Sonnenberg E, Factor SH, del Rio MJ, Schiano T, Patel G, et al. Mortality associated with carbapenem-resistant Klebsiella pneumoniae infections in liver transplant recipients. Liver Transplant. 2012;18(4):468–74.
174. Slee AM, Wuonola MA, McRipley RJ, Zajac I, Zawada MJ, Bartholomew PT, et al. Oxazolidinones, a new class of synthetic antibacterial agents: in vitro and in vivo activities of DuP 105 and DuP 721. Antimicrob Agents Chemother. 1987;31(11): 1791–7.
175. Ford CW, Zurenko GE, Barbachyn MR. The discovery of linezolid, the first oxazolidinone antibacterial agent. Curr Drug Targets Infect Disord. 2001;1(2):181–99.
176. Das D, Tulkens PM, Mehra P, Fang E, Prokocimer P. tedizolid phosphate for the management of acute bacterial skin and skin structure infections: safety summary. Clin Infect Dis. 2014;58(suppl_1):S51–S7.
177. Lin AH, Murray RW, Vidmar TJ, Marotti KR. The oxazolidinone eperezolid binds to the 50S ribosomal subunit and competes with binding of chloramphenicol and lincomycin. Antimicrob Agents Chemother. 1997;41(10):2127–31.
178. Ippolito JA, Kanyo ZF, Wang D, Franceschi FJ, Moore PB, Steitz TA, et al. Crystal structure of the oxazolidinone antibiotic linezolid bound to the 50S ribosomal subunit. J Med Chem. 2008;51(12):3353–6.
179. Thompson J, O'Connor M, Mills JA, Dahlberg AE. The protein synthesis inhibitors, oxazolidinones and chloramphenicol, cause extensive translational inaccuracy in vivo. J Mol Biol. 2002;322(2):273–9.
180. Qin Y, Polacek N, Vesper O, Staub E, Einfeldt E, Wilson DN, et al. The highly conserved LepA is a ribosomal elongation factor that back-translocates the ribosome. Cell. 2006;127(4):721–33.
181. Bowersock TL, Salmon SA, Portis ES, Prescott JF, Robison DA, Ford CW, et al. MICs of oxazolidinones for Rhodococcus equi strains isolated from humans and animals. Antimicrob Agents Chemother. 2000;44(5):1367–9.
182. Brown-Elliott BA, Ward SC, Crist CJ, Mann LB, Wilson RW, Wallace RJ Jr. In vitro activities of linezolid against multiple Nocardia species. Antimicrob Agents Chemother. 2001;45(4):1295–7.
183. Behra-Miellet J, Calvet L, Dubreuil L. Activity of linezolid against anaerobic bacteria. Int J Antimicrob Agents. 2003;22(1):28–34.
184. Wallace RJ Jr, Brown-Elliott BA, Ward SC, Crist CJ, Mann LB, Wilson RW. Activities of linezolid against rapidly growing mycobacteria. Antimicrob Agents Chemother. 2001;45(3):764–7.
185. Brown-Elliott BA, Crist CJ, Mann LB, Wilson RW, Wallace RJ Jr. In vitro activity of linezolid against slowly growing nontuberculous mycobacteria. Antimicrob Agents Chemother. 2003;47(5):1736–8.
186. Condos R, Hadgiangelis N, Leibert E, Jacquette G, Harkin T, Rom WN. Case series report of a linezolid-containing regimen for extensively drug-resistant tuberculosis. Chest. 2008;134(1):187–92.
187. Barber KE, Smith JR, Raut A, Rybak MJ. Evaluation of tedizolid against Staphylococcus aureus and enterococci with reduced susceptibility to vancomycin, daptomycin or linezolid. J Antimicrob Chemother. 2016;71(1):152–5.
188. D'Costa VM, King CE, Kalan L, Morar M, Sung WW, Schwarz C, et al. Antibiotic resistance is ancient. Nature. 2011;477(7365):457–61.
189. Morales G, Picazo JJ, Baos E, Candel FJ, Arribi A, Pelaez B, et al. Resistance to linezolid is mediated by the cfr gene in the first report of an outbreak of linezolid-resistant Staphylococcus aureus. Clin Infect Dis. 2010;50(6):821–5.
190. Meka VG, Gold HS. Antimicrobial resistance to linezolid. Clin Infect Dis. 2004;39(7):1010–5.
191. Prystowsky J, Siddiqui F, Chosay J, Shinabarger DL, Millichap J, Peterson LR, et al. Resistance to linezolid: characterization of mutations in rRNA and comparison of their occurrences in vancomycin-resistant enterococci. Antimicrob Agents Chemother. 2001;45(7):2154–6.
192. Herrero IA, Issa NC, Patel R. Nosocomial spread of linezolid-resistant, vancomycin-resistant enterococcus faecium. N Engl J Med. 2002;346(11):867–9.
193. Pai MP, Rodvold KA, Schreckenberger PC, Gonzales RD, Petrolatti JM, Quinn JP. Risk factors associated with the development of infection with linezolid- and vancomycin-resistant enterococcus faecium. Clin Infect Dis. 2002;35(10):1269–72.
194. Pogue JM, Paterson DL, Pasculle AW, Potoski BA. Determination of risk factors associated with isolation of linezolid-resistant strains of vancomycin-resistant enterococcus. Infect Control Hosp Epidemiol. 2007;28(12):1382–8.
195. Dobbs TE, Patel M, Waites KB, Moser SA, Stamm AM, Hoesley CJ. Nosocomial spread of enterococcus faecium resistant to vancomycin and linezolid in a tertiary care medical center. J Clin Microbiol. 2006;44(9):3368–70.
196. Meskauskas A, Dinman JD. Ribosomal protein L3 functions as a 'rocker switch' to aid in coordinating of large subunit-associated functions in eukaryotes and archaea. Nucleic Acids Res. 2008;36(19):6175–86.
197. Long KS, Vester B. Resistance to linezolid caused by modifications at its binding site on the ribosome. Antimicrob Agents Chemother. 2012;56(2):603–12.
198. Davidovich C, Bashan A, Yonath A. Structural basis for cross-resistance to ribosomal PTC antibiotics. Proc Natl Acad Sci U S A. 2008;105(52):20665–70.
199. Long KS, Poehlsgaard J, Kehrenberg C, Schwarz S, Vester B. The Cfr rRNA methyltransferase confers resistance to Phenicols, Lincosamides, Oxazolidinones, Pleuromutilins, and Streptogramin a antibiotics. Antimicrob Agents Chemother. 2006;50(7):2500–5.
200. Mendes RE, Deshpande LM, Castanheira M, DiPersio J, Saubolle MA, Jones RN. First report of cfr-mediated resistance to linezolid in human staphylococcal clinical isolates recovered in the United States. Antimicrob Agents Chemother. 2008;52(6):2244–6.
201. Arias CA, Vallejo M, Reyes J, Panesso D, Moreno J, Castaneda E, et al. Clinical and microbiological aspects of linezolid resistance mediated by the cfr gene encoding a 23S rRNA methyltransferase. J Clin Microbiol. 2008;46(3):892–6.
202. Liu Y, Wang Y, Wu C, Shen Z, Schwarz S, Du XD, et al. First report of the multidrug resistance gene cfr in enterococcus faecalis of animal origin. Antimicrob Agents Chemother. 2012;56(3):1650–4.
203. Diaz L, Kiratisin P, Mendes RE, Panesso D, Singh KV, Arias CA. Transferable plasmid-mediated resistance to linezolid due to cfr in a human clinical isolate of enterococcus faecalis. Antimicrob Agents Chemother. 2012;56(7):3917–22.
204. Flamm RK, Farrell DJ, Mendes RE, Ross JE, Sader HS, Jones RN. LEADER surveillance program results for 2010: an activity and spectrum analysis of linezolid using 6801 clinical isolates from the United States (61 medical centers). Diagn Microbiol Infect Dis. 2012;74(1):54–61.
205. Gerson SL, Kaplan SL, Bruss JB, Le V, Arellano FM, Hafkin B, et al. Hematologic effects of linezolid: summary of clinical experience. Antimicrob Agents Chemother. 2002;46(8):2723–6.
206. Sasaki T, Takane H, Ogawa K, Isagawa S, Hirota T, Higuchi S, et al. Population pharmacokinetic and pharmacodynamic analysis of linezolid and a hematologic side effect, thrombocytopenia, in Japanese patients. Antimicrob Agents Chemother. 2011;55(5):1867–73.

207. Bernstein WB, Trotta RF, Rector JT, Tjaden JA, Barile AJ. Mechanisms for linezolid-induced anemia and thrombocytopenia. Ann Pharmacother. 2003;37(4):517–20.
208. McKee EE, Ferguson M, Bentley AT, Marks TA. Inhibition of mammalian mitochondrial protein synthesis by oxazolidinones. Antimicrob Agents Chemother. 2006;50(6):2042–9.
209. Hogan HL, Hachem RY, Neuhauser M, Raad II, Coyle E. Clinical experience of linezolid in bone marrow transplantation patients. J Pharm Pract. 2010;23(4):352–7.
210. Nambiar S, Rellosa N, Wassel RT, Borders-Hemphill V, Bradley JS. Linezolid-associated peripheral and optic neuropathy in children. Pediatrics. 2011;127(6):e1528–32.
211. Bressler AM, Zimmer SM, Gilmore JL, Somani J. Peripheral neuropathy associated with prolonged use of linezolid. Lancet Infect Dis. 2004;4(8):528–31.
212. Legout L, Senneville E, Gomel JJ, Yazdanpanah Y, Mouton Y. Linezolid-induced neuropathy. Clin Infect Dis. 2004;38(5):767–8.
213. Narita M, Tsuji BT, Yu VL. Linezolid-associated peripheral and optic neuropathy, lactic acidosis, and serotonin syndrome. Pharmacotherapy. 2007;27(8):1189–97.
214. Nagel S, Kohrmann M, Huttner HB, Storch-Hagenlocher B, Schwab S. Linezolid-induced posterior reversible leukoencephalopathy syndrome. Arch Neurol. 2007;64(5):746–8.
215. Hachem RY, Hicks K, Huen A, Raad I. Myelosuppression and serotonin syndrome associated with concurrent use of linezolid and selective serotonin reuptake inhibitors in bone marrow transplant recipients. Clin Infect Dis. 2003;37(1):e8–11.
216. Butterfield JM, Lawrence KR, Reisman A, Huang DB, Thompson CA, Lodise TP. Comparison of serotonin toxicity with concomitant use of either linezolid or comparators and serotonergic agents: an analysis of phase III and IV randomized clinical trial data. J Antimicrob Chemother. 2012;67(2):494–502.
217. Taylor JJ, Estes LL, Wilson JW. Linezolid and serotonergic drug interactions. Clin Infect Dis. 2006;43(10):1371.
218. Lakey JH, Ptak M. Fluorescence indicates a calcium-dependent interaction between the lipopeptide antibiotic LY146032 and phospholipid membranes. Biochemistry. 1988;27(13):4639–45.
219. Silverman JA, Perlmutter NG, Shapiro HM. Correlation of daptomycin bactericidal activity and membrane depolarization in Staphylococcus aureus. Antimicrob Agents Chemother. 2003;47(8):2538–44.
220. Mascio CT, Alder JD, Silverman JA. Bactericidal action of daptomycin against stationary-phase and nondividing Staphylococcus aureus cells. Antimicrob Agents Chemother. 2007;51(12):4255–60.
221. Silverman JA, Mortin LI, Vanpraagh AD, Li T, Alder J. Inhibition of daptomycin by pulmonary surfactant: in vitro modeling and clinical impact. J Infect Dis. 2005;191(12):2149–52.
222. Greenwood D, Palfreyman J. Comparative activity of LY146032 against anaerobic cocci. Eur J Clin Microbiol. 1987;6(6):682–4.
223. Cui L, Tominaga E, Neoh HM, Hiramatsu K. Correlation between reduced Daptomycin susceptibility and Vancomycin resistance in Vancomycin-intermediate Staphylococcus aureus. Antimicrob Agents Chemother. 2006;50(3):1079–82.
224. Patel JB, Jevitt LA, Hageman J, McDonald LC, Tenover FC. An association between reduced susceptibility to daptomycin and reduced susceptibility to vancomycin in Staphylococcus aureus. Clin Infect Dis. 2006;42(11):1652–3.
225. Jones T, Yeaman MR, Sakoulas G, Yang SJ, Proctor RA, Sahl HG, et al. Failures in clinical treatment of Staphylococcus aureus infection with daptomycin are associated with alterations in surface charge, membrane phospholipid asymmetry, and drug binding. Antimicrob Agents Chemother. 2008;52(1):269–78.
226. Baltz RH. Daptomycin: mechanisms of action and resistance, and biosynthetic engineering. Curr Opin Chem Biol. 2009;13(2):144–51.
227. Jones T, Yeaman MR, Sakoulas G, Yang S-J, Proctor RA, Sahl H-G, et al. Failures in clinical treatment of Staphylococcus aureus infection with Daptomycin are associated with alterations in surface charge, membrane phospholipid asymmetry, and drug binding. Antimicrob Agents Chemother. 2008;52(1):269–78.
228. Egli A, Schmid H, Kuenzli E, Widmer AF, Battegay M, Plagge H, et al. Association of daptomycin use with resistance development in Enterococcus faecium bacteraemia-a 7-year individual and population-based analysis. Clin Microbiol Infect. 2017;23(2):118.e1–7.
229. DiPippo AJ, Tverdek FP, Tarrand JJ, Munita JM, Tran TT, Arias CA, et al. Daptomycin non-susceptible enterococcus faecium in leukemia patients: role of prior daptomycin exposure. J Infect. 2017;74(3):243–7.
230. Arias CA, Panesso D, McGrath DM, Qin X, Mojica MF, Miller C, et al. Genetic basis for in vivo daptomycin resistance in enterococci. N Engl J Med. 2011;365(10):892–900.
231. Shukla BS, Shelburne S, Reyes K, Kamboj M, Lewis JD, Rincon SL, et al. Influence of minimum inhibitory concentration in clinical outcomes of enterococcus faecium bacteremia treated with Daptomycin: is it time to change the breakpoint? Clin Infect Dis. 2016;62(12):1514–20.
232. Moise PA, Sakoulas G, McKinnell JA, Lamp KC, DePestel DD, Yoon MJ, et al. Clinical outcomes of Daptomycin for Vancomycin-resistant Enterococcus Bacteremia. Clin Therapeut. 2015;37(7):1443–53.e2.
233. Smith JR, Barber KE, Raut A, Aboutaleb M, Sakoulas G, Rybak MJ. Beta-lactam combinations with daptomycin provide synergy against vancomycin-resistant enterococcus faecalis and enterococcus faecium. J Antimicrob Chemother. 2015;70(6):1738–43.
234. Henson KE, Yim J, Smith JR, Sakoulas G, Rybak MJ. Beta-Lactamase Inhibitors Enhance the Synergy between beta-Lactam Antibiotics and Daptomycin against Methicillin-Resistant Staphylococcus aureus. Antimicrob Agents Chemother. 2017;61(1):e01564–16.
235. Tally FP, DeBruin MF. Development of daptomycin for gram-positive infections. J Antimicrob Chemother. 2000;46(4):523–6.
236. Oleson FB Jr, Berman CL, Kirkpatrick JB, Regan KS, Lai JJ, Tally FP. Once-daily dosing in dogs optimizes daptomycin safety. Antimicrob Agents Chemother. 2000;44(11):2948–53.
237. Patel SJ, Samo TC, Suki WN. Early-onset rhabdomyolysis related to daptomycin use. Int J Antimicrob Agents. 2007;30(5):472–4.
238. Papadopoulos S, Ball AM, Liewer SE, Martin CA, Winstead PS, Murphy BS. Rhabdomyolysis during therapy with daptomycin. Clin Infect Dis. 2006;42(12):e108–10.
239. Kazory A, Dibadj K, Weiner ID. Rhabdomyolysis and acute renal failure in a patient treated with daptomycin. J Antimicrob Chemother. 2006;57(3):578–9.
240. Kraft S, Mackler E, Schlickman P, Welch K, DePestel DD. Outcomes of therapy: vancomycin-resistant enterococcal bacteremia in hematology and bone marrow transplant patients. Support Care Cancer. 2011;19(12):1969–74.
241. Vernadakis S, Saner FH, Rath PM, Kaiser GM, Mathe Z, Treckmann J, et al. Successful salvage therapy with daptomycin after linezolid and vancomycin failure in a liver transplant recipient with methicillin-resistant Staphylococcus aureus endocarditis. Transplant Infect Dis. 2009;11(4):346–8.
242. Wudhikarn K, Gingrich RD, de Magalhaes Silverman M. Daptomycin nonsusceptible enterococci in hematologic malignancy and hematopoictic stem cell transplant patients: an emerging threat. Ann Hematol. 2013;92(1):129–31.
243. Sakoulas G, Bayer AS, Pogliano J, Tsuji BT, Yang SJ, Mishra NN, et al. Ampicillin enhances daptomycin- and cationic host

defense peptide-mediated killing of ampicillin- and vancomycin-resistant enterococcus faecium. Antimicrob Agents Chemother. 2012;56(2):838–44.
244. Rose WE, Schulz LT, Andes D, Striker R, Berti AD, Hutson PR, et al. Addition of ceftaroline to daptomycin after emergence of daptomycin-nonsusceptible Staphylococcus aureus during therapy improves antibacterial activity. Antimicrob Agents Chemother. 2012;56(10):5296–302.
245. Roberts MC. Tetracycline therapy: update. Clin Infect Dis. 2003;36(4):462–7.
246. Zuckerman JM, Qamar F, Bono BR. Review of macrolides (azithromycin, clarithromycin), ketolids (telithromycin) and glycylcyclines (tigecycline). Med Clin N Am. 2011;95(4):761–91. viii
247. Stein GE, Craig WA. Tigecycline: a critical analysis. Clin Infect Dis. 2006;43(4):518–24.
248. Doan TL, Fung HB, Mehta D, Riska PF. Tigecycline: a glycylcycline antimicrobial agent. Clin Therapeut. 2006;28(8):1079–106.
249. Spanu T, De Angelis G, Cipriani M, Pedruzzi B, D'Inzeo T, Cataldo MA, et al. In vivo emergence of tigecycline resistance in multidrug-resistant Klebsiella pneumoniae and Escherichia coli. Antimicrob Agents Chemother. 2012;56(8):4516–8.
250. Boso-Ribelles V, Roma-Sanchez E, Carmena J, Caceres C, Bautista D. Tigecycline: a new treatment choice against Acinetobacter baumannii. Recent Pat Antiinfect Drug Discov. 2008;3(2):117–22.
251. Dowzicky MJ. Susceptibility to tigecycline and linezolid among gram-positive isolates collected in the United States as part of the tigecycline evaluation and surveillance trial (TEST) between 2004 and 2009. Clin Therapeut. 2011;33(12):1964–73.
252. Marot JC, Jonckheere S, Munyentwali H, Belkhir L, Vandercam B, Yombi JC. Tigecycline-induced acute pancreatitis: about two cases and review of the literature. Acta Clin Belg. 2012;67(3):229–32.
253. Gardiner D, Dukart G, Cooper A, Babinchak T. Safety and efficacy of intravenous tigecycline in subjects with secondary bacteremia: pooled results from 8 phase III clinical trials. Clin Infect Dis. 2010;50(2):229–38.
254. Prasad P, Sun J, Danner RL, Natanson C. Excess deaths associated with tigecycline after approval based on noninferiority trials. Clin Infect Dis. 2012;54(12):1699–709.
255. Bergamasco MD, Barroso Barbosa M, de Oliveira GD, Cipullo R, Moreira JC, Baia C, et al. Infection with Klebsiella pneumoniae carbapenemase (KPC)-producing K. pneumoniae in solid organ transplantation. Transplant Infect Dis. 2012;14(2):198–205.
256. Mlynarczyk G, Kosykowska E, de Walthoffen SW, Szymanek-Majchrzak K, Sawicka-Grzelak A, Baczkowska T, et al. A threat of the Klebsiella pneumoniae carbapenemase-producing strains among transplant recipients. Transplant Proc. 2011;43(8):3135–6.
257. Rodriguez-Avial C, Rodriguez-Avial I, Merino P, Picazo JJ. Klebsiella pneumoniae: development of a mixed population of carbapenem and tigecycline resistance during antimicrobial therapy in a kidney transplant patient. Clin Microbiol Infect. 2012;18(1):61–6.
258. Sevillano D, Alou L, Aguilar L, Echevarria O, Gimenez MJ, Prieto J. Azithromycin iv pharmacodynamic parameters predicting Streptococcus pneumoniae killing in epithelial lining fluid versus serum: an in vitro pharmacodynamic simulation. J Antimicrob Chemother. 2006;57(6):1128–33.
259. Sivapalasingam SASN. Macrolides, clindamycin, and ketolides. In: Gerald M, editor. Principles and practice of infectious diseases. Philadelphia: Elsevier Churchill Livingstone; 2005. p. 396–417.
260. Desaki M, Takizawa H, Ohtoshi T, Kasama T, Kobayashi K, Sunazuka T, et al. Erythromycin suppresses nuclear factor-kappaB and activator protein-1 activation in human bronchial epithelial cells. Biochem Biophys Res Commun. 2000;267(1):124–8.
261. Ianaro A, Ialenti A, Maffia P, Sautebin L, Rombola L, Carnuccio R, et al. Anti-inflammatory activity of macrolide antibiotics. J Pharmacol Exp Therapeut. 2000;292(1):156–63.
262. Doern GV. Macrolide and ketolide resistance with Streptococcus pneumoniae. Med Clin N Am. 2006;90(6):1109–24.
263. Chong YP, Lee SO, Song EH, Lee EJ, Jang EY, Kim SH, et al. Quinupristin-dalfopristin versus linezolid for the treatment of vancomycin-resistant enterococcus faecium bacteraemia: efficacy and development of resistance. Scand J Infect Dis. 2010;42(6–7):491–9.
264. Athamna A, Athamna M, Medlej B, Bast DJ, Rubinstein E. In vitro post-antibiotic effect of fluoroquinolones, macrolides, beta-lactams, tetracyclines, vancomycin, clindamycin, linezolid, chloramphenicol, quinupristin/dalfopristin and rifampicin on Bacillus anthracis. J Antimicrob Chemother. 2004;53(4):609–15.
265. Stamatakis MK, Richards JG. Interaction between quinupristin/dalfopristin and cyclosporine. Ann Pharmacother. 1997;31(5):576–8.
266. Linden PK, Bompart F, Gray S, Talbot GH. Hyperbilirubinemia during quinupristin-dalfopristin therapy in liver transplant recipients: correlation with available liver biopsy results. Pharmacotherapy. 2001;21(6):661–8.
267. Winston DJ, Emmanouilides C, Kroeber A, Hindler J, Bruckner DA, Territo MC, et al. Quinupristin/Dalfopristin therapy for infections due to vancomycin-resistant enterococcus faecium. Clin Infect Dis. 2000;30(5):790–7.
268. Gearhart M, Martin J, Rudich S, Thomas M, Wetzel D, Solomkin J, et al. Consequences of vancomycin-resistant enterococcus in liver transplant recipients: a matched control study. Clin Transpl. 2005;19(6):711–6.
269. Tsiatis AC, Manes B, Calder C, Billheimer D, Wilkerson KS, Frangoul H. Incidence and clinical complications of vancomycin-resistant enterococcus in pediatric stem cell transplant patients. Bone Marrow Transplant. 2004;33(9):937–41.
270. Knoll BM, Hellmann M, Kotton CN. Vancomycin-resistant enterococcus faecium meningitis in adults: case series and review of the literature. Scand J Infect Dis. 2013;45(2):131–9.
271. Verma A, Dhawan A, Philpott-Howard J, Rela M, Heaton N, Vergani GM, et al. Glycopeptide-resistant enterococcus faecium infections in paediatric liver transplant recipients: safety and clinical efficacy of quinupristin/dalfopristin. J Antimicrob Chemother. 2001;47(1):105–8.
272. Lappin E, Ferguson AJ. Gram-positive toxic shock syndromes. Lancet Infect Dis. 2009;9(5):281–90.
273. Holmstrom B, Grimsley EW. Necrotizing fasciitis and toxic shock-like syndrome caused by group B streptococcus. South Med J. 2000;93(11):1096–8.
274. McDougal LK, Fosheim GE, Nicholson A, Bulens SN, Limbago BM, Shearer JE, et al. Emergence of resistance among USA300 methicillin-resistant Staphylococcus aureus isolates causing invasive disease in the United States. Antimicrob Agents Chemother. 2010;54(9):3804–11.
275. Hedberg M, Nord CE. Antimicrobial susceptibility of Bacteroides fragilis group isolates in Europe. Clin Microbiol Infect. 2003;9(6):475–88.
276. Vardakas KZ, Konstantelias AA, Loizidis G, Rafailidis PI, Falagas ME. Risk factors for development of Clostridium difficile infection due to BI/NAP1/027 strain: a meta-analysis. Int J Infect Dis. 2012;16(11):e768–73.
277. O'Connor JR, Johnson S, Gerding DN. Clostridium difficile infection caused by the epidemic BI/NAP1/027 strain. Gastroenterology. 2009;136(6):1913–24.
278. Parchman ML, Munoz A. Risk factors for methicillin-resistant staphylococcal aureus skin and soft tissue infections presenting in primary care: a South Texas ambulatory research network (STARNet) study. J Am Board Fam Med. 2009;22(4):375–9.

279. Cadena J, Sreeramoju P, Nair S, Henao-Martinez A, Jorgensen J, Patterson JE. Clindamycin-resistant methicillin-resistant Staphylococcus aureus: epidemiologic and molecular characteristics and associated clinical factors. Diagn Microbiol Infect Dis. 2012;74(1):16–21.
280. Siberry GK, Tekle T, Carroll K, Dick J. Failure of clindamycin treatment of methicillin-resistant Staphylococcus aureus expressing inducible clindamycin resistance in vitro. Clin Infect Dis. 2003;37(9):1257–60.
281. Diep BA, Chambers HF, Graber CJ, Szumowski JD, Miller LG, Han LL, et al. Emergence of multidrug-resistant, community-associated, methicillin-resistant Staphylococcus aureus clone USA300 in men who have sex with men. Ann Intern Med. 2008;148(4):249–57.
282. Hashimoto M, Sugawara Y, Tamura S, Kaneko J, Matsui Y, Togashi J, et al. Acquisition of methicillin-resistant Staphylococcus aureus after living donor liver transplantation: a retrospective cohort study. BMC Infect Dis. 2008;8:155.
283. Florescu DF, McCartney AM, Qiu F, Langnas AN, Botha J, Mercer DF, et al. Staphylococcus aureus infections after liver transplantation. Infection. 2012;40(3):263–9.
284. Tsuji BT, Rybak MJ, Cheung CM, Amjad M, Kaatz GW. Community- and health care-associated methicillin-resistant Staphylococcus aureus: a comparison of molecular epidemiology and antimicrobial activities of various agents. Diagn Microbiol Infect Dis. 2007;58(1):41–7.
285. Hashimoto M, Sugawara Y, Tamura S, Kaneko J, Matsui Y, Moriya K, et al. Impact of new methicillin-resistant Staphylococcus aureus carriage postoperatively after living donor liver transplantation. Transplant Proc. 2007;39(10):3271–5.
286. Domagala JM. Structure-activity and structure-side-effect relationships for the quinolone antibacterials. J Antimicrob Chemother. 1994;33(4):685–706.
287. Hawkey PM. Mechanisms of quinolone action and microbial response. J Antimicrob Chemother. 2003;51(Suppl 1):29–35.
288. Gellert M, Mizuuchi K, O'Dea MH, Nash HA. DNA gyrase: an enzyme that introduces superhelical turns into DNA. Proc Natl Acad Sci U S A. 1976;73(11):3872–6.
289. Fisher LM, Austin CA, Hopewell R, Margerrison EE, Oram M, Patel S, et al. DNA supercoiling and relaxation by ATP-dependent DNA topoisomerases. Philos Trans R Soc Lond Ser B Biol Sci. 1992;336(1276):83–91.
290. Kato J, Nishimura Y, Imamura R, Niki H, Hiraga S, Suzuki H. New topoisomerase essential for chromosome segregation in E. coli. Cell. 1990;63(2):393–404.
291. Ullsperger C, Cozzarelli NR. Contrasting enzymatic activities of topoisomerase IV and DNA gyrase from Escherichia coli. J Biol Chem. 1996;271(49):31549–55.
292. Gonzalez I, Georgiou M, Alcaide F, Balas D, Linares J, de la Campa AG. Fluoroquinolone resistance mutations in the parC, parE, and gyrA genes of clinical isolates of viridans group streptococci. Antimicrob Agents Chemother. 1998;42(11):2792–8.
293. Weigel LM, Steward CD, Tenover FC. gyrA mutations associated with fluoroquinolone resistance in eight species of Enterobacteriaceae. Antimicrob Agents Chemother. 1998;42(10):2661–7.
294. Kampranis SC, Maxwell A. The DNA Gyrase-quinolone complex. ATP hydrolysis and the mechanism of DNA cleavage. J Biol Chem. 1998;273(35):22615–26.
295. Drlica K, Malik M, Kerns RJ, Zhao X. Quinolone-mediated bacterial death. Antimicrob Agents Chemother. 2008;52(2):385–92.
296. Khodursky AB, Zechiedrich EL, Cozzarelli NR. Topoisomerase IV is a target of quinolones in Escherichia coli. Proc Natl Acad Sci U S A. 1995;92(25):11801–5.
297. Heddle JG, Barnard FM, Wentzell LM, Maxwell A. The interaction of drugs with DNA gyrase: a model for the molecular basis of quinolone action. Nucleosides Nucleotides Nucleic Acids. 2000;19(8):1249–64.
298. Malik M, Zhao X, Drlica K. Lethal fragmentation of bacterial chromosomes mediated by DNA gyrase and quinolones. Mol Microbiol. 2006;61(3):810–25.
299. Chen CR, Malik M, Snyder M, Drlica K. DNA gyrase and topoisomerase IV on the bacterial chromosome: quinolone-induced DNA cleavage. J Mol Biol. 1996;258(4):627–37.
300. Schlacher K, Goodman MF. Lessons from 50 years of SOS DNA-damage-induced mutagenesis. Nat Rev Mol Cell Biol. 2007;8(7):587–94.
301. Kohanski MA, Dwyer DJ, Hayete B, Lawrence CA, Collins JJ. A common mechanism of cellular death induced by bactericidal antibiotics. Cell. 2007;130(5):797–810.
302. Diver JM, Wise R. Morphological and biochemical changes in Escherichia coli after exposure to ciprofloxacin. J Antimicrob Chemother. 1986;18(Suppl D):31–41.
303. Dorr T, Lewis K, Vulic M. SOS response induces persistence to fluoroquinolones in Escherichia coli. PLoS Genet. 2009;5(12):e1000760.
304. Beaber JW, Hochhut B, Waldor MK. SOS response promotes horizontal dissemination of antibiotic resistance genes. Nature. 2004;427(6969):72–4.
305. Lister PD. Pharmacodynamics of moxifloxacin and levofloxacin against Staphylococcus aureus and Staphylococcus epidermidis in an in vitro pharmacodynamic model. Clin Infect Dis. 2001;32(Suppl 1):S33–8.
306. Remy JM, Tow-Keogh CA, McConnell TS, Dalton JM, Devito JA. Activity of delafloxacin against methicillin-resistant Staphylococcus aureus: resistance selection and characterization. J Antimicrob Chemother. 2012;67(12):2814–20.
307. Maurin M, Abergel C, Raoult D. DNA gyrase-mediated natural resistance to fluoroquinolones in Ehrlichia spp. Antimicrob Agents Chemother. 2001;45(7):2098–105.
308. Angelakis E, Biswas S, Taylor C, Raoult D, Rolain JM. Heterogeneity of susceptibility to fluoroquinolones in Bartonella isolates from Australia reveals a natural mutation in gyrA. J Antimicrob Chemother. 2008;61(6):1252–5.
309. Jacobs MR. Activity of quinolones against mycobacteria. Drugs. 1999;58(Suppl 2):19–22.
310. Hooper DC, Wolfson JS, Souza KS, Tung C, McHugh GL, Swartz MN. Genetic and biochemical characterization of norfloxacin resistance in Escherichia coli. Antimicrob Agents Chemother. 1986;29(4):639–44.
311. Martinez-Martinez L, Pascual A, Jacoby GA. Quinolone resistance from a transferable plasmid. Lancet. 1998;351(9105):797–9.
312. Jacoby GA. Mechanisms of resistance to quinolones. Clin Infect Dis. 2005;41(Suppl 2):S120–6.
313. Yoshida H, Bogaki M, Nakamura M, Nakamura S. Quinolone resistance-determining region in the DNA gyrase gyrA gene of Escherichia coli. Antimicrob Agents Chemother. 1990;34(6):1271–2.
314. Belland RJ, Morrison SG, Ison C, Huang WM. Neisseria gonorrhoeae acquires mutations in analogous regions of gyrA and parC in fluoroquinolone-resistant isolates. Mol Microbiol. 1994;14(2):371–80.
315. Morais Cabral JH, Jackson AP, Smith CV, Shikotra N, Maxwell A, Liddington RC. Crystal structure of the breakage-Reunion domain of DNA gyrase. Nature. 1997;388(6645):903–6.
316. Yoshida H, Kojima T, Yamagishi J, Nakamura S. Quinolone-resistant mutations of the gyrA gene of Escherichia coli. Mol Gen Genet. 1988;211(1):1–7.
317. Takei M, Fukuda H, Kishii R, Hosaka M. Target preference of 15 quinolones against Staphylococcus aureus, based on antibacterial activities and target inhibition. Antimicrob Agents Chemother. 2001;45(12):3544–7.

318. Strahilevitz J, Hooper DC. Dual targeting of topoisomerase IV and gyrase to reduce mutant selection: direct testing of the paradigm by using WCK-1734, a new fluoroquinolone, and ciprofloxacin. Antimicrob Agents Chemother. 2005;49(5):1949–56.
319. Kugelberg E, Lofmark S, Wretlind B, Andersson DI. Reduction of the fitness burden of quinolone resistance in Pseudomonas aeruginosa. J Antimicrob Chemother. 2005;55(1):22–30.
320. Webber MA, Piddock LJ. The importance of efflux pumps in bacterial antibiotic resistance. J Antimicrob Chemother. 2003;51(1):9–11.
321. Saier MH Jr, Paulsen IT, Sliwinski MK, Pao SS, Skurray RA, Nikaido H. Evolutionary origins of multidrug and drug-specific efflux pumps in bacteria. FASEB J. 1998;12(3):265–74.
322. Poole K. Efflux-mediated resistance to fluoroquinolones in gram-positive bacteria and the mycobacteria. Antimicrob Agents Chemother. 2000;44(10):2595–9.
323. Akama H, Kanemaki M, Yoshimura M, Tsukihara T, Kashiwagi T, Yoneyama H, et al. Crystal structure of the drug discharge outer membrane protein, OprM, of Pseudomonas aeruginosa: dual modes of membrane anchoring and occluded cavity end. J Biol Chem. 2004;279(51):52816–9.
324. Pradel E, Pages JM. The AcrAB-TolC efflux pump contributes to multidrug resistance in the nosocomial pathogen Enterobacter aerogenes. Antimicrob Agents Chemother. 2002;46(8):2640–3.
325. Neves P, Berkane E, Gameiro P, Winterhalter M, de Castro B. Interaction between quinolones antibiotics and bacterial outer membrane porin OmpF. Biophys Chem. 2005;113(2):123–8.
326. Gill MJ, Brenwald NP, Wise R. Identification of an efflux pump gene, pmrA, associated with fluoroquinolone resistance in Streptococcus pneumoniae. Antimicrob Agents Chemother. 1999;43(1):187–9.
327. Vetting MW, Park CH, Hegde SS, Jacoby GA, Hooper DC, Blanchard JS. Mechanistic and structural analysis of aminoglycoside N-acetyltransferase AAC(6′)-Ib and its bifunctional, fluoroquinolone-active AAC(6′)-Ib-cr variant. Biochemistry. 2008;47(37):9825–35.
328. Park CH, Robicsek A, Jacoby GA, Sahm D, Hooper DC. Prevalence in the United States of aac(6′)-Ib-cr encoding a ciprofloxacin-modifying enzyme. Antimicrob Agents Chemother. 2006;50(11):3953–5.
329. Strahilevitz J, Jacoby GA, Hooper DC, Robicsek A. Plasmid-mediated quinolone resistance: a multifaceted threat. Clin Microbiol Rev. 2009;22(4):664–89.
330. Tran JH, Jacoby GA. Mechanism of plasmid-mediated quinolone resistance. Proc Natl Acad Sci U S A. 2002;99(8):5638–42.
331. Yamane K, Wachino J, Suzuki S, Kimura K, Shibata N, Kato H, et al. New plasmid-mediated fluoroquinolone efflux pump, QepA, found in an Escherichia coli clinical isolate. Antimicrob Agents Chemother. 2007;51(9):3354–60.
332. Singh R, Swick MC, Ledesma KR, Yang Z, Hu M, Zechiedrich L, et al. Temporal interplay between efflux pumps and target mutations in development of antibiotic resistance in Escherichia coli. Antimicrob Agents Chemother. 2012;56(4):1680–5.
333. Zhao X, Drlica K. Restricting the selection of antibiotic-resistant mutants: a general strategy derived from fluoroquinolone studies. Clin Infect Dis. 2001;33(Suppl 3):S147–56.
334. Kawakami J, Yamamoto K, Asanuma A, Yanagisawa K, Sawada Y, Iga T. Inhibitory effect of new quinolones on GABA(a) receptor-mediated response and its potentiation with felbinac in Xenopus oocytes injected with mouse-brain mRNA: correlation with convulsive potency in vivo. Toxicol Appl Pharmacol. 1997;145(2):246–54.
335. Jones SC, Sorbello A, Boucher RM. Fluoroquinolone-associated myasthenia gravis exacerbation: evaluation of postmarketing reports from the US FDA adverse event reporting system and a literature review. Drug Saf. 2011;34(10):839–47.
336. Owens RC Jr, Ambrose PG. Torsades de pointes associated with fluoroquinolones. Pharmacotherapy. 2002;22(5):663–8. discussion 8-72
337. Alexandrou AJ, Duncan RS, Sullivan A, Hancox JC, Leishman DJ, Witchel HJ, et al. Mechanism of hERG K+ channel blockade by the fluoroquinolone antibiotic moxifloxacin. Br J Pharmacol. 2006;147(8):905–16.
338. Lapi F, Wilchesky M, Kezouh A, Benisty JI, Ernst P, Suissa S. Fluoroquinolones and the risk of serious arrhythmia: a population-based study. Clin Infect Dis. 2012;55(11):1457–65.
339. Man I, Traynor NJ, Ferguson J. Recent developments in fluoroquinolone phototoxicity. Photodermatol Photoimmunol Photomed. 1999;15(1):32–3.
340. McCusker ME, Harris AD, Perencevich E, Roghmann MC. Fluoroquinolone use and Clostridium difficile-associated diarrhea. Emerg Infect Dis. 2003;9(6):730–3.
341. Muto CA, Pokrywka M, Shutt K, Mendelsohn AB, Nouri K, Posey K, et al. A large outbreak of Clostridium difficile-associated disease with an unexpected proportion of deaths and colectomies at a teaching hospital following increased fluoroquinolone use. Infect Control Hosp Epidemiol. 2005;26(3):273–80.
342. Zaiss NH, Witte W, Nubel U. Fluoroquinolone resistance and Clostridium difficile. Germany Emerg Infect Dis. 2010;16(4):675–7.
343. Pepin J, Saheb N, Coulombe MA, Alary ME, Corriveau MP, Authier S, et al. Emergence of fluoroquinolones as the predominant risk factor for Clostridium difficile-associated diarrhea: a cohort study during an epidemic in Quebec. Clin Infect Dis. 2005;41(9):1254–60.
344. Razonable RR, Litzow MR, Khaliq Y, Piper KE, Rouse MS, Patel R. Bacteremia due to viridans group streptococci with diminished susceptibility to levofloxacin among neutropenic patients receiving levofloxacin prophylaxis. Clin Infect Dis. 2002;34(11):1469–74.
345. Prabhu RM, Piper KE, Litzow MR, Steckelberg JM, Patel R. Emergence of quinolone resistance among viridans group streptococci isolated from the oropharynx of neutropenic peripheral blood stem cell transplant patients receiving quinolone antimicrobial prophylaxis. Eur J Clin Microbiol Infect Dis. 2005;24(12):832–8.
346. Therriault BL, Wilson JW, Barreto JN, Estes LL. Characterization of bacterial infections in allogeneic hematopoietic stem cell transplant recipients who received prophylactic levofloxacin with either penicillin or doxycycline. Mayo Clin Proc Mayo Clin. 2010;85(8):711–8.
347. Busca A, Cavecchia I, Locatelli F, D'Ardia S, De Rosa FG, Marmont F, et al. Blood stream infections after allogeneic stem cell transplantation: a single-center experience with the use of levofloxacin prophylaxis. Transplant Infect Dis. 2012;14(1):40–8.
348. Vehreschild JJ, Moritz G, Vehreschild MJ, Arenz D, Mahne M, Bredenfeld H, et al. Efficacy and safety of moxifloxacin as antibacterial prophylaxis for patients receiving autologous haematopoietic stem cell transplantation: a randomised trial. Int J Antimicrob Agents. 2012;39(2):130–4.
349. Miller AN, Glode A, Hogan KR, Schaub C, Kramer C, Stuart RK, et al. Efficacy and safety of ciprofloxacin for prophylaxis of polyomavirus BK virus-associated hemorrhagic cystitis in allogeneic hematopoietic stem cell transplantation recipients. Biol Blood Marrow Transplant. 2011;17(8):1176–81.
350. Yoon HE, Jeon YJ, Chung HW, Shin SJ, Hwang HS, Lee SJ, et al. Safety and efficacy of a quinolone-based regimen for treatment of tuberculosis in renal transplant recipients. Transplant Proc. 2012;44(3):730–3.
351. Barge-Caballero E, Crespo-Leiro MG, Paniagua-Martin MJ, Muniz J, Naya C, Bouzas-Mosquera A, et al. Quinolone-related Achilles tendinopathy in heart transplant patients: incidence and risk factors. J Heart Lung Transplant. 2008;27(1):46–51.

352. Esparza EM, Takeshita J, George E. Lymphomatoid hypersensitivity reaction to levofloxacin during autologous stem cell transplantation: a potential diagnostic pitfall in patients treated for lymphoma or leukemia. J Cutan Pathol. 2011;38(1):33–7.
353. Lofmark S, Edlund C, Nord CE. Metronidazole is still the drug of choice for treatment of anaerobic infections. Clin Infect Dis. 2010;50(Suppl 1):S16–23.
354. Edwards DI. Reduction of nitroimidazoles in vitro and DNA damage. Biochem Pharmacol. 1986;35(1):53–8.
355. Tocher JH, Edwards DI. Evidence for the direct interaction of reduced metronidazole derivatives with DNA bases. Biochem Pharmacol. 1994;48(6):1089–94.
356. van der Wouden EJ, Thijs JC, Kusters JG, van Zwet AA, Kleibeuker JH. Mechanism and clinical significance of metronidazole resistance in helicobacter pylori. Scand J Gastroenterol Suppl. 2001;234:10–4.
357. Upcroft P, Upcroft JA. Drug targets and mechanisms of resistance in the anaerobic protozoa. Clin Microbiol Rev. 2001;14(1):150–64.
358. Stratton CW, Weeks LS, Aldridge KE. Comparison of the bactericidal activity of clindamycin and metronidazole against cefoxitin-susceptible and cefoxitin-resistant isolates of the Bacteroides fragilis group. Diagn Microbiol Infect Dis. 1991;14(5):377–82.
359. Stratton CW, Weeks LS, Aldridge KE. Inhibitory and bactericidal activity of selected beta-lactam agents alone and in combination with beta-lactamase inhibitors compared with that of cefoxitin and metronidazole against cefoxitin-susceptible and cefoxitin-resistant isolates of the Bacteroides fragilis group. Diagn Microbiol Infect Dis. 1992;15(4):321–30.
360. Nix DE, Tyrrell R, Muller M. Pharmacodynamics of metronidazole determined by a time-kill assay for Trichomonas vaginalis. Antimicrob Agents Chemother. 1995;39(8):1848–52.
361. Schaumann R, Funke M, Janssen E, Rodloff AC. In vitro activities of clindamycin, imipenem, metronidazole, and piperacillin-tazobactam against susceptible and resistant isolates of Bacteroides fragilis evaluated by kill kinetics. Antimicrob Agents Chemother. 2012;56(6):3413–6.
362. Goldstein EJ, Citron DM, Cherubin CE, Hillier SL. Comparative susceptibility of the Bacteroides fragilis group species and other anaerobic bacteria to meropenem, imipenem, piperacillin, cefoxitin, ampicillin/sulbactam, clindamycin and metronidazole. J Antimicrob Chemother. 1993;31(3):363–72.
363. Teare L, Peters T, Saverymuttu S, Owen R, Tiwari I. Antibiotic resistance in helicobacter pylori. Lancet. 1999;353(9148):242.
364. Land KM, Johnson PJ. Molecular basis of metronidazole resistance in pathogenic bacteria and protozoa. Drug Resist Updat. 1999;2(5):289–94.
365. Rasmussen BA, Bush K, Tally FP. Antimicrobial resistance in Bacteroides. Clin Infect Dis. 1993;16(Suppl 4):S390–400.
366. Leiros HK, Kozielski-Stuhrmann S, Kapp U, Terradot L, Leonard GA, McSweeney SM. Structural basis of 5-nitroimidazole antibiotic resistance: the crystal structure of NimA from Deinococcus radiodurans. J Biol Chem. 2004;279(53):55840–9.
367. Lofmark S, Fang H, Hedberg M, Edlund C. Inducible metronidazole resistance and nim genes in clinical Bacteroides fragilis group isolates. Antimicrob Agents Chemother. 2005;49(3):1253–6.
368. Erwin ME, Fix AM, Jones RN. Three independent yearly analyses of the spectrum and potency of metronidazole: a multicenter study of 1,108 contemporary anaerobic clinical isolates. Diagn Microbiol Infect Dis. 2001;39(2):129–32.
369. Snydman DR, Jacobus NV, McDermott LA, Supran S, Cuchural GJ Jr, Finegold S, et al. Multicenter study of in vitro susceptibility of the Bacteroides fragilis group, 1995 to 1996, with comparison of resistance trends from 1990 to 1996. Antimicrob Agents Chemother. 1999;43(10):2417–22.
370. Aldridge KE, Ashcraft D, O'Brien M, Sanders CV. Bacteremia due to Bacteroides fragilis group: distribution of species, beta-lactamase production, and antimicrobial susceptibility patterns. Antimicrob Agents Chemother. 2003;47(1):148–53.
371. Labbe AC, Bourgault AM, Vincelette J, Turgeon PL, Lamothe F. Trends in antimicrobial resistance among clinical isolates of the Bacteroides fragilis group from 1992 to 1997 in Montreal, Canada. Antimicrob Agents Chemother. 1999;43(10):2517–9.
372. Megraud F, Lehn N, Lind T, Bayerdorffer E, O'Morain C, Spiller R, et al. Antimicrobial susceptibility testing of helicobacter pylori in a large multicenter trial: the MACH 2 study. Antimicrob Agents Chemother. 1999;43(11):2747–52.
373. Lacey SL, Moss SF, Taylor GW. Metronidazole uptake by sensitive and resistant isolates of helicobacter pylori. J Antimicrob Chemother. 1993;32(3):393–400.
374. Tankovic J, Lamarque D, Delchier JC, Soussy CJ, Labigne A, Jenks PJ. Frequent association between alteration of the rdxA gene and metronidazole resistance in French and north African isolates of helicobacter pylori. Antimicrob Agents Chemother. 2000;44(3):608–13.
375. Krajden S, Lossick JG, Wilk E, Yang J, Keystone JS, Elliott K. Persistent Trichomonas vaginalis infection due to a metronidazole-resistant strain. CMAJ. 1986;134(12):1373–4.
376. Quon DV, d'Oliveira CE, Johnson PJ. Reduced transcription of the ferredoxin gene in metronidazole-resistant Trichomonas vaginalis. Proc Nat Acad Sci USA. 1992;89(10):4402–6.
377. Liu SM, Brown DM, O'Donoghue P, Upcroft P, Upcroft JA. Ferredoxin involvement in metronidazole resistance of Giardia duodenalis. Mol Biochem Parasitol. 2000;108(1):137–40.
378. Finegold SM. Metronidazole. Ann Intern Med. 1980;93(4):585–7.
379. Feder HM Jr. Bacteroides fragilis meningitis. Rev Infect Dis. 1987;9(4):783–6.
380. Jensen JC, Gugler R. Single- and multiple-dose metronidazole kinetics. Clin Pharmacol Therapeut. 1983;34(4):481–7.
381. Gupta AK, Agarwal MP, Avasthi R, Bhadoria DP, Rohatgi N. Metronidazole-induced neurotoxicity. J Assoc Physicians India. 2003;51:617–8.
382. Tan CH, Chen YF, Chen CC, Chao CC, Liou HH, Hsieh ST. Painful neuropathy due to skin denervation after metronidazole-induced neurotoxicity. J Neurol Neurosurg Psychiatry. 2011;82(4):462–5.
383. Nigwekar SU, Casey KJ. Metronidazole-induced pancreatitis. A case report and review of literature. JOP. 2004;5(6):516–9.
384. Saginur R, Hawley CR, Bartlett JG. Colitis associated with metronidazole therapy. J Infect Dis. 1980;141(6):772–4.
385. Knowles S, Choudhury T, Shear NH. Metronidazole hypersensitivity. Ann Pharmacother. 1994;28(3):325–6.
386. Edwards DL, Fink PC, Van Dyke PO. Disulfiram-like reaction associated with intravenous trimethoprim-sulfamethoxazole and metronidazole. Clin Pharm. 1986;5(12):999–1000.
387. Cina SJ, Russell RA, Conradi SE. Sudden death due to metronidazole/ethanol interaction. Am J Forensic Med Pathol. 1996;17(4):343–6.
388. Teicher MH, Altesman RI, Cole JO, Schatzberg AF. Possible nephrotoxic interaction of lithium and metronidazole. JAMA. 1987;257(24):3365–6.
389. Holt RK, Anderson EA, Cantrell MA, Shaw RF, Egge JA. Preemptive dose reduction of warfarin in patients initiating metronidazole. Drug Metabol Drug Interact. 2010;25(1–4):35–9.
390. Kounas SP, Letsas KP, Sideris A, Efraimidis M, Kardaras F. QT interval prolongation and torsades de pointes due to a coadministration of metronidazole and amiodarone. Pacing Clin Electrophysiol. 2005;28(5):472–3.
391. Gulbis AM, Culotta KS, Jones RB, Andersson BS. Busulfan and metronidazole: an often forgotten but significant drug interaction. Ann Pharmacother. 2011;45(7–8):e39.
392. Page RL 2nd, Klem PM, Rogers C. Potential elevation of tacrolimus trough concentrations with concomitant metronidazole therapy. Ann Pharmacother. 2005;39(6):1109–13.

393. Montebugnoli L, Servidio D, Prati C. Effectiveness of metronidazole gel on cyclosporine-induced gingival overgrowth in heart transplant patients. Clin Oral Investig. 2002;6(1):24–7.
394. Aufricht C, Hogan EL, Ettenger RB. Oral metronidazole does not improve cyclosporine A-induced gingival hyperplasia. Pediatr Nephrol (Berlin, Germany). 1997;11(5):552–5.
395. Pant C, Anderson MP, O'Connor JA, Marshall CM, Deshpande A, Sferra TJ. Association of Clostridium difficile infection with outcomes of hospitalized solid organ transplant recipients: results from the 2009 Nationwide inpatient sample database. Transplant Infect Dis. 2012;14(5):540–7.
396. Ali M, Ananthakrishnan AN, Ahmad S, Kumar N, Kumar G, Saeian K. Clostridium difficile infection in hospitalized liver transplant patients: a nationwide analysis. Liver Transplant. 2012;18(8):972–8.
397. Rosen JB, Schecter MG, Heinle JS, McKenzie ED, Morales DL, Dishop MK, et al. Clostridium difficile colitis in children following lung transplantation. Pediatr Transplant. 2010;14(5):651–6.
398. Riddle DJ, Dubberke ER. Clostridium difficile infection in solid organ transplant recipients. Curr Opin Organ Transplant. 2008;13(6):592–600.
399. Sensi P. History of the development of rifampin. Rev Infect Dis. 1983;5(Suppl 3):S402–6.
400. Floss HG, Yu TW. Rifamycin-mode of action, resistance, and biosynthesis. Chem Rev. 2005;105(2):621–32.
401. Artsimovitch I, Vassylyeva MN, Svetlov D, Svetlov V, Perederina A, Igarashi N, et al. Allosteric modulation of the RNA polymerase catalytic reaction is an essential component of transcription control by rifamycins. Cell. 2005;122(3):351–63.
402. Campbell EA, Korzheva N, Mustaev A, Murakami K, Nair S, Goldfarb A, et al. Structural mechanism for rifampicin inhibition of bacterial rna polymerase. Cell. 2001;104(6):901–12.
403. Kunin CM. Antimicrobial activity of rifabutin. Clin Infect Dis. 1996;22(Suppl 1):S3–13. discussion S-4.
404. Cavusoglu C, Karaca-Derici Y, Bilgic A. In-vitro activity of rifabutin against rifampicin-resistant Mycobacterium tuberculosis isolates with known rpoB mutations. Clin Microbiol Infect. 2004;10(7):662–5.
405. Rastogi N, Goh KS, Berchel M, Bryskier A. Activity of rifapentine and its metabolite 25-O-desacetylrifapentine compared with rifampicin and rifabutin against Mycobacterium tuberculosis, Mycobacterium africanum, Mycobacterium bovis and M. bovis BCG. J Antimicrob Chemother. 2000;46(4):565–70.
406. Thornsberry C, Hill BC, Swenson JM, McDougal LK. Rifampin: spectrum of antibacterial activity. Rev Infect Dis. 1983;5(Suppl 3):S412–7.
407. Hoover WW, Gerlach EH, Hoban DJ, Eliopoulos GM, Pfaller MA, Jones RN. Antimicrobial activity and spectrum of rifaximin, a new topical rifamycin derivative. Diagn Microbiol Infect Dis. 1993;16(2):111–8.
408. Gillespie SH. Evolution of drug resistance in Mycobacterium tuberculosis: clinical and molecular perspective. Antimicrob Agents Chemother. 2002;46(2):267–74.
409. O'Neill AJ, Cove JH, Chopra I. Mutation frequencies for resistance to fusidic acid and rifampicin in Staphylococcus aureus. J Antimicrob Chemother. 2001;47(5):647–50.
410. Forrest GN, Tamura K. Rifampin combination therapy for nonmycobacterial infections. Clin Microbiol Rev. 2010;23(1):14–34.
411. Pugsley AP, Zimmerman W, Wehrli W. Highly efficient uptake of a rifamycin derivative via the FhuA-TonB-dependent uptake route in Escherichia coli. J Gen Microbiol. 1987;133(12):3505–11.
412. Telenti A, Imboden P, Marchesi F, Lowrie D, Cole S, Colston MJ, et al. Detection of rifampicin-resistance mutations in Mycobacterium tuberculosis. Lancet. 1993;341(8846):647–50.
413. Hui J, Gordon N, Kajioka R. Permeability barrier to rifampin in mycobacteria. Antimicrob Agents Chemother. 1977;11(5):773–9.
414. Dabbs ER, Yazawa K, Mikami Y, Miyaji M, Morisaki N, Iwasaki S, et al. Ribosylation by mycobacterial strains as a new mechanism of rifampin inactivation. Antimicrob Agents Chemother. 1995;39(4):1007–9.
415. Tribuddharat C, Fennewald M. Integron-mediated rifampin resistance in Pseudomonas aeruginosa. Antimicrob Agents Chemother. 1999;43(4):960–2.
416. Arlet G, Nadjar D, Herrmann JL, Donay JL, Lagrange PH, Philippon A. Plasmid-mediated rifampin resistance encoded by an arr-2-like gene cassette in Klebsiella pneumoniae producing an ACC-1 class C beta-lactamase. Antimicrob Agents Chemother. 2001;45(10):2971–2.
417. Naas T, Mikami Y, Imai T, Poirel L, Nordmann P. Characterization of In53, a class 1 plasmid- and composite transposon-located integron of Escherichia coli which carries an unusual array of gene cassettes. J Bacteriol. 2001;183(1):235–49.
418. Cook SV, Fujiwara PI, Frieden TR. Rates and risk factors for discontinuation of rifampicin. Int J Tuberc Lung Dis. 2000;4(2):118–22.
419. Holdiness MR. A review of the Redman syndrome and rifampicin overdosage. Med Toxicol Adverse Drug Exp. 1989;4(6):444–51.
420. Capelle P, Dhumeaux D, Mora M, Feldmann G, Berthelot P. Effect of rifampicin on liver function in man. Gut. 1972;13(5):366–71.
421. Cascio A, Scarlata F, Giordano S, Antinori S, Colomba C, Titone L. Treatment of human brucellosis with rifampin plus minocycline. J Chemother. 2003;15(3):248–52.
422. Menzies D, Dion MJ, Rabinovitch B, Mannix S, Brassard P, Schwartzman K. Treatment completion and costs of a randomized trial of rifampin for 4 months versus isoniazid for 9 months. Am J Respir Crit Care Med. 2004;170(4):445–9.
423. Steele MA, Burk RF, DesPrez RM. Toxic hepatitis with isoniazid and rifampin. A meta-analysis. Chest. 1991;99(2):465–71.
424. Prince MI, Burt AD, Jones DE. Hepatitis and liver dysfunction with rifampicin therapy for pruritus in primary biliary cirrhosis. Gut. 2002;50(3):436–9.
425. Hadfield JW. Rifampicin-induced thrombocytopenia. Postgrad Med J. 1980;56(651):59–60.
426. Pereira J, Hidalgo P, Ocqueteau M, Blacutt M, Marchesse M, Nien Y, et al. Glycoprotein Ib/IX complex is the target in rifampicin-induced immune thrombocytopenia. Br J Haematol. 2000;110(4):907–10.
427. De Vriese AS, Robbrecht DL, Vanholder RC, Vogelaers DP, Lameire NH. Rifampicin-associated acute renal failure: pathophysiologic, immunologic, and clinical features. Am J Kidney Dis. 1998;31(1):108–15.
428. Shafran SD, Singer J, Zarowny DP, Deschenes J, Phillips P, Turgeon F, et al. Determinants of rifabutin-associated uveitis in patients treated with rifabutin, clarithromycin, and ethambutol for Mycobacterium avium complex bacteremia: a multivariate analysis. Canadian HIV trials network protocol 010 study group. J Infect Dis. 1998;177(1):252–5.
429. Chen J, Raymond K. Roles of rifampicin in drug-drug interactions: underlying molecular mechanisms involving the nuclear pregnane X receptor. Ann Clin Microbiol Antimicrob. 2006;5:3.
430. Baciewicz AM, Chrisman CR, Finch CK, Self TH. Update on rifampin and rifabutin drug interactions. Am J Med Sci. 2008;335(2):126–36.
431. Koselj M, Bren A, Kandus A, Kovac D. Drug interactions between cyclosporine and rifampicin, erythromycin, and azoles in kidney recipients with opportunistic infections. Transplant Proc. 1994;26(5):2823–4.
432. Zelunka EJ. Intravenous cyclosporine-rifampin interaction in a pediatric bone marrow transplant recipient. Pharmacotherapy. 2002;22(3):387–90.

433. Kim YH, Yoon YR, Kim YW, Shin JG, Cha IJ. Effects of rifampin on cyclosporine disposition in kidney recipients with tuberculosis. Transplant Proc. 1998;30(7):3570–2.
434. Finch CK, Chrisman CR, Baciewicz AM, Self TH. Rifampin and rifabutin drug interactions: an update. Arch Int Med. 2002;162(9):985–92.
435. Aguado JM, Torre-Cisneros J, Fortun J, Benito N, Meije Y, Doblas A, et al. Tuberculosis in solid-organ transplant recipients: consensus statement of the group for the study of infection in transplant recipients (GESITRA) of the Spanish Society of Infectious Diseases and Clinical Microbiology. Clin Infect Dis. 2009;48(9):1276–84.
436. Neff G, Zacharias V, Kaiser TE, Gaddis A, Kemmer N. Rifaximin for the treatment of recurrent Clostridium difficile infection after liver transplantation: a case series. Liver Transplant. 2010;16(8):960–3.
437. Carithers HA. The first use of an antibiotic in America. Am J Dis Children (1960). 1974;128(2):207–11.
438. Petri W. Sulfonamides, trimethoprim-Sulfamethoxazole, quinolones, and agents for urinary tract infections. New York: McGraw Hill; 2011.
439. Kalkut G. Sulfonamides and trimethoprim. Cancer Investig. 1998;16(8):612–5.
440. Hong YL, Hossler PA, Calhoun DH, Meshnick SR. Inhibition of recombinant pneumocystis carinii dihydropteroate synthetase by sulfa drugs. Antimicrob Agents Chemother. 1995;39(8):1756–63.
441. Smilack JD. Trimethoprim-sulfamethoxazole. Mayo Clin Proc Mayo Clin. 1999;74(7):730–4.
442. Huovinen P. Resistance to trimethoprim-sulfamethoxazole. Clin Infect Dis. 2001;32(11):1608–14.
443. Martin JN, Rose DA, Hadley WK, Perdreau-Remington F, Lam PK, Gerberding JL. Emergence of trimethoprim-sulfamethoxazole resistance in the AIDS era. J Infect Dis. 1999;180(6):1809–18.
444. Karlowsky JA, Jones ME, Thornsberry C, Critchley I, Kelly LJ, Sahm DF. Prevalence of antimicrobial resistance among urinary tract pathogens isolated from female outpatients across the US in 1999. Int J Antimicrob Agents. 2001;18(2):121–7.
445. Jesudason MV, John TJ. Plasmid mediated multidrug resistance in Salmonella typhi. Indian J Med Res. 1992;95:66–7.
446. Ziha-Zarifi I, Llanes C, Kohler T, Pechere JC, Plesiat P. In vivo emergence of multidrug-resistant mutants of Pseudomonas aeruginosa overexpressing the active efflux system MexA-MexB-OprM. Antimicrob Agents Chemother. 1999;43(2):287–91.
447. Swedberg G, Ringertz S, Skold O. Sulfonamide resistance in Streptococcus pyogenes is associated with differences in the amino acid sequence of its chromosomal dihydropteroate synthase. Antimicrob Agents Chemother. 1998;42(5):1062–7.
448. Skold O. Sulfonamide resistance: mechanisms and trends. Drug Resist Updat. 2000;3(3):155–60.
449. Gallardo F, Ruiz J, Marco F, Towner KJ, Vila J. Increase in incidence of resistance to ampicillin, chloramphenicol and trimethoprim in clinical isolates of Salmonella serotype Typhimurium with investigation of molecular epidemiology and mechanisms of resistance. J Med Microbiol. 1999;48(4):367–74.
450. Prats G, Mirelis B, Llovet T, Munoz C, Miro E, Navarro F. Antibiotic resistance trends in enteropathogenic bacteria isolated in 1985-1987 and 1995-1998 in Barcelona. Antimicrob Agents Chemother. 2000;44(5):1140–5.
451. Olson RP, Harrell LJ, Kaye KS. Antibiotic resistance in urinary isolates of Escherichia coli from college women with urinary tract infections. Antimicrob Agents Chemother. 2009;53(3):1285–6.
452. Miranda Novales MG, Solorzano Santos F, Guiscafre Gallardo H, Leanos Miranda B, Echaniz Aviles G, Carnalla Barajas MN, et al. Streptococcus pneumoniae: low frequency of penicillin resistance and high resistance to trimethoprim-sulfamethoxazole in nasopharyngeal isolates from children in a rural area in Mexico. Arch Med Res. 1997;28(4):559–63.
453. Hu LF, Chang X, Ye Y, Wang ZX, Shao YB, Shi W, et al. Stenotrophomonas maltophilia resistance to trimethoprim/sulfamethoxazole mediated by acquisition of sul and dfrA genes in a plasmid-mediated class 1 integron. Int J Antimicrob Agents. 2011;37(3):230–4.
454. Ma L, Borio L, Masur H, Kovacs JA. Pneumocystis carinii dihydropteroate synthase but not dihydrofolate reductase gene mutations correlate with prior trimethoprim-sulfamethoxazole or dapsone use. J Infect Dis. 1999;180(6):1969–78.
455. Gibreel A, Skold O. High-level resistance to trimethoprim in clinical isolates of campylobacter jejuni by acquisition of foreign genes (dfr1 and dfr9) expressing drug-insensitive dihydrofolate reductases. Antimicrob Agents Chemother. 1998;42(12):3059–64.
456. Coque TM, Singh KV, Weinstock GM, Murray BE. Characterization of dihydrofolate reductase genes from trimethoprim-susceptible and trimethoprim-resistant strains of enterococcus faecalis. Antimicrob Agents Chemother. 1999;43(1):141–7.
457. Lin D, Tucker MJ, Rieder MJ. Increased adverse drug reactions to antimicrobials and anticonvulsants in patients with HIV infection. Ann Pharmacother. 2006;40(9):1594–601.
458. Floris-Moore MA, Amodio-Groton MI, Catalano MT. Adverse reactions to trimethoprim/sulfamethoxazole in AIDS. Ann Pharmacother. 2003;37(12):1810–3.
459. Mittmann N, Knowles SR, Koo M, Shear NH, Rachlis A, Rourke SB. Incidence of toxic epidermal necrolysis and Stevens-Johnson syndrome in an HIV cohort: an observational, retrospective case series study. Am J Clin Dermatol. 2012;13(1):49–54.
460. Leoung GS, Stanford JF, Giordano MF, Stein A, Torres RA, Giffen CA, et al. Trimethoprim-sulfamethoxazole (TMP-SMZ) dose escalation versus direct rechallenge for pneumocystis Carinii pneumonia prophylaxis in human immunodeficiency virus-infected patients with previous adverse reaction to TMP-SMZ. J Infect Dis. 2001;184(8):992–7.
461. Gluckstein D, Ruskin J. Rapid oral desensitization to trimethoprim-sulfamethoxazole (TMP-SMZ): use in prophylaxis for pneumocystis carinii pneumonia in patients with AIDS who were previously intolerant to TMP-SMZ. Clin Infect Dis. 1995;20(4):849–53.
462. Kocak Z, Hatipoglu CA, Ertem G, Kinikli S, Tufan A, Irmak H, et al. Trimethoprim-sulfamethoxazole induced rash and fatal hematologic disorders. J Infect. 2006;52(2):e49–52.
463. Bygbjerg IC, Lund JT, Hording M. Effect of folic and folinic acid on cytopenia occurring during co-trimoxazole treatment of pneumocystis carinii pneumonia. Scand J Infect Dis. 1988;20(6):685–6.
464. D'Antonio RG, Johnson DB, Winn RE, van Dellen AF, Evans ME. Effect of folinic acid on the capacity of trimethoprim-sulfamethoxazole to prevent and treat pneumocystis carinii pneumonia in rats. Antimicrob Agents Chemother. 1986;29(2):327–9.
465. Markowitz N, Saravolatz LD. Use of trimethoprim-sulfamethoxazole in a glucose-6-phosphate dehydrogenase-deficient population. Rev Infect Dis. 1987;9(Suppl 2):S218–29.
466. Kouklakis G, Mpoumponaris A, Zezos P, Moschos J, Koulaouzidis A, Nakos A, et al. Cholestatic hepatitis with severe systemic reactions induced by trimethoprim-sulfamethoxazole. Ann Hepatol. 2007;6(1):63–5.
467. Perazella MA, Mahnensmith RL. Trimethoprim-sulfamethoxazole: hyperkalemia is an important complication regardless of dose. Clin Nephrol. 1996;46(3):187–92.
468. Capra C, Monza GM, Meazza G, Ramella G. Trimethoprim-sulfamethoxazole-induced aseptic meningitis: case report and literature review. Intensive Care Med. 2000;26(2):212–4.
469. Rosini JM, Martinez E, Jain R. Severe hypoglycemia associated with use of trimethoprim/sulfamethoxazole in a patient with chronic renal insufficiency. Ann Pharmacother. 2008;42(4):593–4.

470. Delanaye P, Mariat C, Cavalier E, Maillard N, Krzesinski JM, White CA. Trimethoprim, creatinine and creatinine-based equations. Nephron Clin Pract. 2011;119(3):c187–93. discussion c93–4
471. Shrishrimal K, Wesson J. Sulfamethoxazole crystalluria. Am J Kidney Dis. 2011;58(3):492–3.
472. Ryan C, Madalon M, Wortham DW, Graziano FM. Sulfa hypersensitivity in patients with HIV infection: onset, treatment, critical review of the literature. WMJ. 1998;97(5):23–7.
473. Antoniou T, Gomes T, Mamdani MM, Juurlink DN. Trimethoprim/sulfamethoxazole-induced phenytoin toxicity in the elderly: a population-based study. Br J Clin Pharmacol. 2011;71(4):544–9.
474. Guastaldi RB, Reis AM, Figueras A, Secoli SR. Prevalence of potential drug-drug interactions in bone marrow transplant patients. Int J Clin Pharm. 2011;33(6):1002–9.
475. Macingwana L, Baker B, Ngwane AH, Harper C, Cotton MF, Hesseling A, et al. Sulfamethoxazole enhances the antimycobacterial activity of rifampicin. J Antimicrob Chemother. 2012;67(12):2908–11.
476. Antoniou T, Gomes T, Mamdani MM, Yao Z, Hellings C, Garg AX, et al. Trimethoprim-sulfamethoxazole induced hyperkalaemia in elderly patients receiving spironolactone: nested case-control study. BMJ. 2011;343:d5228.
477. Gleckman R, Gantz NM, Joubert DW. Intravenous sulfamethoxazole-trimethoprim: pharmacokinetics, therapeutic indications, and adverse reactions. Pharmacotherapy. 1981;1(3):206–11.
478. Dudley MN, Levitz RE, Quintiliani R, Hickingbotham JM, Nightingale CH. Pharmacokinetics of trimethoprim and sulfamethoxazole in serum and cerebrospinal fluid of adult patients with normal meninges. Antimicrob Agents Chemother. 1984;26(6):811–4.
479. Siber GR, Gorham CC, Ericson JF, Smith AL. Pharmacokinetics of intravenous trimethoprim-sulfamethoxazole in children and adults with normal and impaired renal function. Rev Infect Dis. 1982;4(2):566–78.
480. Nissenson AR, Wilson C, Holazo A. Pharmacokinetics of intravenous trimethoprim-sulfamethoxazole during hemodialysis. Am J Nephrol. 1987;7(4):270–4.
481. Goto N, Oka S. Pneumocystis jirovecii pneumonia in kidney transplantation. Transplant Infect Dis. 2011;13(6):551–8.
482. Husain S, McCurry K, Dauber J, Singh N, Kusne S. Nocardia infection in lung transplant recipients. J Heart Lung Transplant. 2002;21(3):354–9.
483. Peleg AY, Husain S, Qureshi ZA, Silveira FP, Sarumi M, Shutt KA, et al. Risk factors, clinical characteristics, and outcome of Nocardia infection in organ transplant recipients: a matched case-control study. Clin Infect Dis. 2007;44(10):1307–14.
484. Poonyagariyagorn HK, Gershman A, Avery R, Minai O, Blazey H, Asamoto K, et al. Challenges in the diagnosis and management of Nocardia infections in lung transplant recipients. Transplant Infect Dis. 2008;10(6):403–8.
485. Wood JB, Smith DB, Baker EH, Brecher SM, Gupta K. Has emergence of community-associated MRSA increased trimethoprim-Sulfamethoxazole use and resistance? A 10 year time series analysis. Antimicrob Agents Chemother. 2012;56(11): 5655–60.
486. Landman D, Georgescu C, Martin DA, Quale J. Polymyxins revisited. Clin Microbiol Rev. 2008;21(3):449–65.
487. Kubin CJ, Ellman TM, Phadke V, Haynes LJ, Calfee DP, Yin MT. Incidence and predictors of acute kidney injury associated with intravenous polymyxin B therapy. J Infect. 2012;65(1): 80–7.
488. Morrison DC, Jacobs DM. Binding of polymyxin B to the lipid a portion of bacterial lipopolysaccharides. Immunochemistry. 1976;13(10):813–8.
489. Warner SJ, Mitchell D, Savage N, McClain E. Dose-dependent reduction of lipopolysaccharide pyrogenicity by polymyxin B. Biochem Pharmacol. 1985;34(22):3995–8.
490. Bozkurt-Guzel C, Gerceker AA. Post-antibiotic effect of colistin, alone and in combination with amikacin, on Pseudomonas aeruginosa strains isolated from cystic fibrosis patients. J Antibiot. 2012;65(2):83–6.
491. Akin FE, Bayram A, Balci I. Comparison of disc diffusion, E-test, and broth microdilution methods for the determination of resistance to colistin, polymyxin B, and tigecycline in multi-resistant Acinetobacter baumannii isolates. Mikrobiyoloji Bulteni. 2010;44(2):203–10.
492. Galani I, Kontopidou F, Souli M, Rekatsina PD, Koratzanis E, Deliolanis J, et al. Colistin susceptibility testing by Etest and disk diffusion methods. Int J Antimicrob Agents. 2008;31(5):434–9.
493. Pogue JM, Lee J, Marchaim D, Yee V, Zhao JJ, Chopra T, et al. Incidence of and risk factors for colistin-associated nephrotoxicity in a large academic health system. Clin Infect Dis. 2011;53(9):879–84.
494. Esaian D, Dubrovskaya Y, Phillips M, Papadopoulos J. Effectiveness and tolerability of a polymyxin B dosing protocol. Ann Pharmacother. 2012;46(3):455–6.
495. Yahav D, Farbman L, Leibovici L, Paul M. Colistin: new lessons on an old antibiotic. Clin Microbiol Infect. 2012;18(1):18–29.
496. Kofteridis DP, Alexopoulou C, Valachis A, Maraki S, Dimopoulou D, Georgopoulos D, et al. Aerosolized plus intravenous colistin versus intravenous colistin alone for the treatment of ventilator-associated pneumonia: a matched case-control study. Clin Infect Dis. 2010;51(11):1238–44.
497. Naesens R, Vlieghe E, Verbrugghe W, Jorens P, Ieven M. A retrospective observational study on the efficacy of colistin by inhalation as compared to parenteral administration for the treatment of nosocomial pneumonia associated with multidrug-resistant Pseudomonas aeruginosa. BMC Infect Dis. 2011;11:317.
498. Falagas ME, Giannopoulou KP, Kokolakis GN, Rafailidis PI. Fosfomycin: use beyond urinary tract and gastrointestinal infections. Clin Infect Dis. 2008;46(7):1069–77.
499. Tullio V, Cuffini AM, Banche G, Mandras N, Allizond V, Roana J, et al. Role of fosfomycin tromethamine in modulating non-specific defence mechanisms in chronic uremic patients towards ESBL-producing Escherichia coli. Int J Immunopathol Pharmacol. 2008;21(1):153–60.
500. de Souza RM, Olsburgh J. Urinary tract infection in the renal transplant patient. Nat Clin Pract Nephrol. 2008;4(5):252–64.
501. Rivera-Sanchez R, Delgado-Ochoa D, Flores-Paz RR, Garcia-Jimenez EE, Espinosa-Hernandez R, Bazan-Borges AA, et al. Prospective study of urinary tract infection surveillance after kidney transplantation. BMC Infect Dis. 2010;10:245.
502. Santimaleeworagun W, Wongpoowarak P, Chayakul P, Pattharachayakul S, Tansakul P, Garey KW. In vitro activity of colistin or sulbactam in combination with fosfomycin or imipenem against clinical isolates of carbapenem-resistant Acinetobacter baumannii producing OXA-23 carbapenemases. Southeast Asian J Trop Med Public Health. 2011;42(4):890–900.
503. Fernandes P, Pereira D. Efforts to support the development of fusidic acid in the United States. Clin Infect Dis. 2011;52(Suppl 7):S542–6.
504. Moellering RC Jr, Corey GR, Grayson ML. Introduction: fusidic acid enters the United States. Clin Infect Dis. 2011;52(Suppl 7):S467–8.
505. Jones RN, Mendes RE, Sader HS, Castanheira M. In vitro antimicrobial findings for fusidic acid tested against contemporary (2008-2009) gram-positive organisms collected in the United States. Clin Infect Dis. 2011;52(Suppl 7):S477–86.
506. Craft JC, Moriarty SR, Clark K, Scott D, Degenhardt TP, Still JG, et al. A randomized, double-blind phase 2 study compar-

ing the efficacy and safety of an oral fusidic acid loading-dose regimen to oral linezolid for the treatment of acute bacterial skin and skin structure infections. Clin Infect Dis. 2011;52(Suppl 7): S520–6.

507. Theriault RJ, Karwowski JP, Jackson M, Girolami RL, Sunga GN, Vojtko CM, et al. Tiacumicins, a novel complex of 18-membered macrolide antibiotics. I. Taxonomy, fermentation and antibacterial activity. J Antibiot. 1987;40(5):567–74.
508. Artsimovitch I, Seddon J, Sears P. Fidaxomicin is an inhibitor of the initiation of bacterial RNA synthesis. Clin Infect Dis. 2012;55(Suppl 2):S127–31.
509. Tupin A, Gualtieri M, Leonetti JP, Brodolin K. The transcription inhibitor lipiarmycin blocks DNA fitting into the RNA polymerase catalytic site. EMBO J. 2010;29(15):2527–37.
510. Goldstein EJ, Babakhani F, Citron DM. Antimicrobial activities of fidaxomicin. Clin Infect Dis. 2012;55(Suppl 2):S143–8.
511. Louie TJ, Miller MA, Mullane KM, Weiss K, Lentnek A, Golan Y, et al. Fidaxomicin versus vancomycin for Clostridium difficile infection. N Engl J Med. 2011;364(5):422–31.
512. Seddon J BF, Sears P. Mutant prevention concentration of fidaxomicin for *Clostridium difficile.* Fifty-second Interscience Conference on Antimicrobial Agents and Chemotherapy 2012.
513. Sears P, Crook DW, Louie TJ, Miller MA, Weiss K. Fidaxomicin attains high fecal concentrations with minimal plasma concentrations following oral administration in patients with Clostridium difficile infection. Clin Infect Dis. 2012;55(Suppl 2):S116–20.
514. Weiss K, Allgren RL, Sellers S. Safety analysis of fidaxomicin in comparison with oral vancomycin for Clostridium difficile infections. Clin Infect Dis. 2012;55(Suppl 2):S110–5.
515. Johnson AP, Wilcox MH. Fidaxomicin: a new option for the treatment of Clostridium difficile infection. J Antimicrob Chemother. 2012;

Pharmacokinetics and Pharmacodynamics of Antibiotics in Transplant Patients

51

Kelly E. Schoeppler, Scott W. Mueller, and Gerard R. Barber

Introduction

Infection remains a major cause of morbidity and mortality among solid organ transplant (SOT) and hematopoietic stem cell transplant (HSCT) recipients. Within the first 30 days following organ transplantation, the most frequently encountered sites of bacterial infection are the surgical site, vascular access device, and the lungs. Since the introduction of azathioprine in the 1960s and especially cyclosporine in the mid-1980s, several new potent immunosuppressive manifesting activities through an array of efficient mechanisms have recently arrived to market. While becoming mainstays of immunosuppressive maintenance therapies, they place patients at a markedly increased risk of infection. Challenges placed to clinicians are maintaining a delicate, if not brittle, balance of desirable and sustained immunosuppression while successfully preventing or, if needed, treating acute bacterial or opportunistic infections.

There is a muted response of transplant recipients to infection when compared to the immunocompetent host. Thus, clinicians charged with the management of transplant recipients must seek and closely examine subjective patient findings in concert with the receipt of objective results when available. While serum levels of immunosuppressive agents are available, a definitive marker for true depth of immunosuppression is still not available for clinicians to assess a patient's risk of frequency and severity of infection. Though not within the scope of this chapter, the issue of nosocomial infection among organ donors and donor-derived infections should also be noted.

Presenting further challenge to the maintenance of medications for the more acute issues of immunosuppression and bacterial infection is that organ transplant recipients often take several other medications for comorbidities that may be associated with immunosuppressive drugs. Disease states such as hyperlipidemia, hyperglycemia, hypertension, osteoporosis, and arrhythmia are not infrequent, particularly as organ transplants are increasingly performed in aging populations. Other commonly encountered conditions in this high-risk population such as depression and psychoses can be chronic and particularly challenging to manage with medications [1].

The management of concomitant medical conditions in the transplant recipients often requires the use of a large number of medications, at best constituting a necessary form of polypharmacy. Medication use leading to adverse events is noted to increase the rate of hospitalization and mortality [2, 3] and with strong statistical methodology has been demonstrated to be among the leading causes of adverse events in the hospitalized patient. In Leape's landmark study of 1133 patients sustaining disabling injuries due to medical treatment, the leading causes of operative and nonoperative adverse events were wound infection and drug-related mishaps, respectively [4].

This chapter will focus on antibacterial agents and dosing in special patient populations as well as aerosol and other novel routes of drug administration. Drug-induced immune modulation will also be discussed as will drug-drug interactions, categorized by pharmacokinetic and pharmacodynamic interactions as well as special population parameters within P-glycoprotein and cytochrome P-450 enzyme systems related to the transplant recipient. Consideration of these factors in the presence of potent immunosuppressive agents dictates that close therapeutic

K. E. Schoeppler
Department of Pharmacy Services, University of Colorado Health, University of Colorado, Skaggs School of Pharmacy and Pharmaceutical Sciences, Aurora, CO, USA
e-mail: kelly.schoeppler@uchealth.org

S. W. Mueller
Department of Clinical Pharmacy, University of Colorado, Skaggs School of Pharmacy and Pharmaceutical Sciences, University of Colorado Health, Aurora, CO, USA
e-mail: scott.mueller@ucdenver.edu

G. R. Barber (✉)
Department of Pharmacy Services, University of Colorado Hospital, University of Colorado, Skaggs School of Pharmacy and Pharmaceutical Sciences, Aurora, CO, USA
e-mail: gerard.barber@uchealth.org

A. Safdar (ed.), *Principles and Practice of Transplant Infectious Diseases*, https://doi.org/10.1007/978-1-4939-9034-4_51

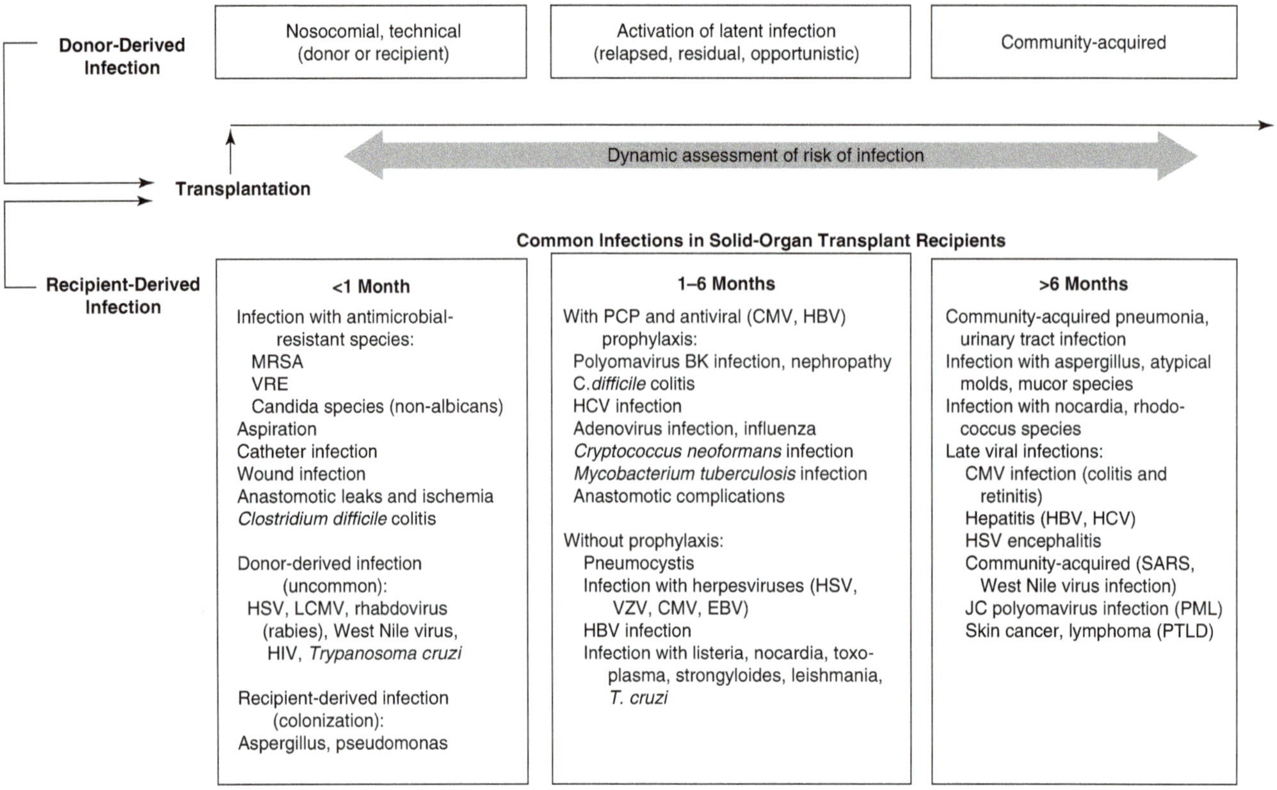

Fig. 51.1 A timeline of posttransplant infections [5]. (From Fishman [5]. © 2007 Massachusetts Medical Society. Reprinted with permission from Massachusetts Medical Society)

drug monitoring (TDM) be performed. This is especially important as these agents often have narrow therapeutic windows and the risk of infection is strongly influenced by the dose, duration, and sequence of immunosuppressive therapies.

Temporal relationships of the risk of infection and potential etiologic agent have long been noted (see Fig. 51.1), but it is also recognized that changes to therapeutics, such as corticosteroid-sparing immunosuppressive regimens and antimicrobial prophylaxis, have influenced changes to patient presentation and implicated pathogens among SOT recipients [5]. Similar relationships exist among HCST recipients.

The clinician caring for the transplant recipient will also be reminded to maintain a heightened index of suspicion for even the subtlest changes to drug product formulations and new market entries. These may directly or indirectly influence clinical events such as the occurrence of graft rejection.

Stewardship of antimicrobial and immunosuppressive regimens and optimization of the ensuing pharmacokinetic and pharmacodynamic interactions are crucial.

Pharmacokinetics/Pharmacodynamics Primer

Simply, pharmacokinetics is defined by what the body does to a drug molecule. Pharmacokinetic (PK) measures include drug absorption, distribution, metabolism, and excretion (ADME), and these parameters vary based on the chemical properties of the drug. The PK profile, metabolism, and disposition of immunosuppressive medications can be quite complex relying on the cytochrome P450 (CYP450) pathway and adenosine triphosphate binding cassette (ABC) transporters such as P-glycoprotein (P-gp or MDR1) and multidrug resistance-associated protein 2 (MRP2). Both CYP450 enzymes and P-gp are susceptible to enzyme inhibition, competition, and induction by various medications. Conversely, pharmacodynamics (PD) is defined by the effect of a drug on the body. These can be additive or inhibitory dynamic effects on the body, manifesting as therapeutic as well as adverse drug effects [6, 7]. The following indices are important determinants of a drug's PK/PD properties:

- Bioavailability (F): The fraction of drug absorbed into systemic circulation. Bioavailability is determined by the physiologic properties of the drug and dosage form, as well as the physiologic barriers at the site of absorption.

- Plasma protein binding (PPB): The percentage of circulating drug that is bound to plasma proteins. Only the unbound fraction of drug is able to exert a pharmacodynamic effect;
- Volume of distribution (Vd): A proportionality factor that relates the total amount of drug in the body to the concentration of drug measured in the plasma.
- Maximum concentration (Cmax): The peak concentration a drug achieves after administration.
- Minimum concentration (Cmin): The minimum or trough plasma concentration of a drug.
- Area under the concentration curve (AUC): The area under the plasma drug concentration-time curve, or AUC, reflects the actual total body exposure to drug. It is determined by the total amount of drug administered and the rate of elimination of the drug from the body.
- Clearance (CL): The volume of blood which is completely cleared of drug in a unit of time.
- Half-life ($t_{1/2}$): The amount of time required for the concentration of drug in the plasma to be reduce by 50%.

The minimum inhibitory concentration (MIC) of an antimicrobial is defined as the lowest concentration of the antimicrobial necessary to inhibit bacterial growth during incubation for 24 h in a growth medium. Furthermore, the effectiveness of an antibiotic against a susceptible microbe is typically governed by one of the following pharmacodynamic indices:

- T > MIC—The percentage of the dosage interval in which the concentration of the antimicrobial exceeds the MIC of the organism determines bacterial inhibition. This is also referred to as time-dependent activity in select antimicrobials.
- Cmax:MIC ratio—Bacterial inhibition is related to high concentrations of antimicrobial at the site of action. This is also referred to as concentration-dependent activity in select antimicrobials.
- AUC:MIC ratio—The total amount of drug exposure determines bacterial inhibition. This is a combination of time-dependent and concentration-dependent activity.

Not to be lost among an array of PK/PD characteristics of multiple medications is critical attention to the transplant patient. History is important and a thorough assessment of current patient status even more so. The state of vital organ function can strongly influence the disposition of many medications. Laboratory tests in conjunction with measurement and assessment of vital signs for renal, hepatic, pulmonary, gastrointestinal, and neurologic function should help aid the clinician charged with dosing antimicrobials as well as other medications.

Special Populations

Critical Illness

Despite recent advances leading to improved short-term survival rates in the SOT population, this patient population is at high risk for critical illness. In both the early post-surgery phase and long-term maintenance phase, sepsis and related septic shock are common causes of death [8]. Long-term immunosuppression may modify or mask clinical features of systemic inflammatory response syndrome in patients with sepsis. What is clear is the benefit of early effective antibiotics in SOT recipients with septic shock [9, 10]. The choice of antibiotics used should relate to the local patterns of bacterial susceptibility, patients' clinical presentation, and risk probability of infection, not to mention that patients with severe immune dysfunction are prone to multiple infections that may occur concurrently. Appropriate dosing of antibiotics in critical illness requires knowledge of the pathophysiology of sepsis; understanding of the patient's clinical status and current therapies such as fluid resuscitation status and renal replacement therapy, among others; as well as the PK/PD of the antibiotic being given.

Septic shock initially causes circulatory disruption due to vasodilatation and increased permeability of the microvascular endothelium [11]. Coupled with fluid resuscitation, these factors relate to an increased Vd of antibiotics, particularly hydrophilic antibiotics since the extracellular water compartment expands. Lipophilic antibiotics may be affected but to a lesser magnitude since adipose tissue remains unchanged. Beta-lactams, for example, are generally considered hydrophilic. A brief summary of the hydrophilic and lipophilic tendencies of antibiotics can be found in Table 51.1. A systematic review of beta-lactam pharmacokinetics in critical illness revealed an increased Vd for all studied beta-lactams compared to healthy volunteers [12]. Although this difference may be in part related to increased total body weight, it is important to note that standard renal dose adjustments may not result in effective concentrations of antibiotic after the first dose. Therefore, a full or loading dose should be given prior to dose adjustment for changes in clearance [13, 14].

Increased Vd typically causes a prolonged half-life, and renal dysfunction is common in septic shock; however, some critically ill populations show increased renal blood flow,

Table 51.1 General classification of hydrophilic and lipophilic antibiotics [14, 16]

Hydrophilic	Lipophilic
β-Lactams	Fluoroquinolones (levofloxacin, ciprofloxacin)
Aminoglycosides	Macrolides (azithromycin, clarithromycin)
Glycopeptides (vancomycin)	Lincosamide (clindamycin)
Lipopeptide (daptomycin)	Tetracyclines (including doxycycline, minocycline, tigecycline)
Lipoglycopeptide (telavancin)	Rifamycin (rifampin)
Oxazolidinone (linezolid)	
Polymyxin (colistin)	

and calculations of creatinine clearance may underestimate predicted drug clearance [15]. In the case of time-dependent killing bactericidal agents such as beta-lactams, the percentage of time the drug concentration is above the minimum inhibitory concentration (MIC) of the bacteria is crucial. Target ranges from 40% to 100% of the time above MIC for effective drug dosing and depends upon the beta-lactam drug used [14]. Given the wide therapeutic index of most beta-lactams and lack of available therapeutic drug monitoring, authors' preference is to dose at the higher or more frequent range whenever possible or reasonable to avoid marginally therapeutic underdosing. Continuous and extended infusions of beta-lactams may have benefit as they optimize the pharmacokinetic and pharmacodynamics by virtue of lower peak and higher trough concentrations. At this time, data on clinical outcomes is mixed and lacks rigorous prospective trials. Although intriguing, routine use of continuous or extended infusion beta-lactam antibiotics should be weighed against potential intravenous line access issues, and care should be taken to ensure delays in initial adequate systemic concentrations are not introduced by implementing a protocol for continuous or extended drug infusion.

Aminoglycosides are also considered hydrophilic. Unlike beta-lactams, the bactericidal activity of aminoglycosides is related to peak concentrations such as Cmax:MIC or AUC:MIC ratio. With once-daily dosing, an optimal peak to MIC ratio of 8–10:1 is often targeted [17]. Changes in Vd are again important to consider. Initial doses of 7 mg/kg of gentamicin or tobramycin [18] and 15–20 mg/kg of amikacin are typically recommended for once-daily dosing regimens; however, the patient populations used to validate these dosing regimens often excluded critically ill patients with altered Vd. Furthermore, higher doses of concentration-dependent antibiotics may be required to reach optimum peak concentrations in the critically ill patients [19–21]. Therapeutic drug monitoring is recommended and doses are adjusted to maintain adequate peak concentrations while extending the dosing interval to minimize trough concentrations. Renal toxicity with aminoglycosides is well-described. In an attempt to minimize renal injury, trough concentrations of undetectable or < 1 mg/L for gentamicin and tobramycin or < 5 mg/L for amikacin are recommended, whenever possible [13, 14]. This is especially important in transplant recipients taking concurrent nephrotoxins such as calcineurin inhibitors.

Vancomycin is a cell wall inhibitor, similar to beta-lactam antibiotics, but with a distinctly different binding mechanism. Unlike beta-lactam antibiotics, clinical effectiveness targets for vancomycin relate to an AUC:MIC value >400 [22]. This target is usually attained by using a weight-based dose of 15–20 mg/kg and adjusted frequency for renal function to attain a trough concentration between 15 and 20 mg/L. Because time to a steady-state trough concentration is variable in the critically ill patient and may not be realized for 24–48 h in many patients, a 25–30 mg/kg loading dose can be considered as an initial dose among the critically ill patients undergoing transplantation [22, 23].

Similar themes for the dosing of antibiotics in critically ill patients will be found throughout the literature. Namely, initial aggressive loading doses of intravenous antibiotics are important, and a dosing strategy without available TDM requires a balance between risks of under-treating a severe infection and the potential for drug toxicity. Although dose adjustments of hydrophilic antibiotics in the critically ill often dominate the literature, consideration should be given to all antibiotics to avoid underdosing with initial prescribed regimens when timely administration is of importance. Extracorporeal membrane oxygenation (ECMO) and renal replacement modalities add another layer of complexity. Dosing considerations and recommendations may vary depending on renal replacement machinery, modality, and prescribed utilization. We refer the reader to current reviews discussing dose considerations in continuous renal replacement [24, 25]. Antibiotic removal during ECMO requires further study before recommendations can be made; however, we refer the reader to a review of general dosing considerations [26].

Hematopoietic Stem Cell Transplantation and Neutropenia

HSCT has evolved as a life-saving therapy for many patients with lymphoproliferative disorders, leukemias, and non-malignant disorders including immune deficiencies and bone marrow failure syndrome [27]. Patients requiring HSCT are often at risk of infection prior to receiving their conditioning regimen due to their underlying illness. Further, profound and protracted neutropenia may occur with conditioning. The selection and use of myeloablative and non-myeloablative conditioning regimens given for the preparation for allogeneic or autologous stem cell transplantation are beyond the scope of this chapter. However, it is important to consider the conditioning regimen, expected engraftment time, use of immunosuppression for graft-versus-host disease after allogeneic transplantation, and complications including oral intestinal mucositis and veno-occlusive disease when selecting antibiotics. For example, drug-drug interactions should be considered when patients are given cyclophosphamide, busulfan, and etoposide as they utilize CYP450 for activation and/or elimination [28]. Methotrexate elimination may be reduced when given with beta-lactam antibiotics; notably penicillin. Other immunosuppressants used in patients with graft-versus-host disease and graft rejection in SOT recipients and their interaction(s) with antibiotics are discussed below. Patient status can often influence the selection of antimicrobial agent and dose as there are important PK/PD considerations in the HSCT and neutropenic populations in general. For example, the development of severe mucositis may preclude the use of oral agents, hepatic veno-occlusive disease may result in severe liver injury leading to decreased elimination of antibiotics metabolized by the liver or excreted through biliary mechanisms, and fluid retention and increased Vd may result in patients with ascites or renal injury. Antibiotics are indicated at the onset of fever and, in some specific populations, for prophylaxis from infection following HSCT conditioning [28].

During the pre-engraftment phase, patients are profoundly neutropenic. Despite a normal or even elevated neutrophil count prior to HSCT or after engraftment, qualitative defects in circulating neutrophils tend to exist. This "functional neutropenia" places the HSCT patient at high risk of infection even before myeloablative therapy is given. Neutropenia also occurs in SOT recipients, although it is less severe and often of brief duration compared with patients undergoing conventional high-risk allogeneic stem cell transplantation. The cause of neutropenia in SOT recipients is multifactorial and mostly attributed to the use of myelosuppressive drugs like azathioprine, mycophenolic acid, tacrolimus, sirolimus, ganciclovir, valganciclovir, antithymocyte globulin, rituximab, and sulfamethoxazole/trimethoprim, among others [28–34]. Peripheral blood neutrophil counts serve as a proxy for the host immune response against bacterial invasion as neutropenic patients are at an increased risk of systemic bacterial infections [29, 35]. Furthermore, in cancer patients with neutropenia, at least one-fifth of those with an absolute neutrophil count (ANC) less than 100 cells/μL may develop bacteremia [28]. As expected, antibiotics are commonly prescribed for such patients for infection prevention and treatment of febrile illnesses, even in the absence of a positive blood culture.

Studies of antimicrobials in HSCT and solid tumor cancer patients with febrile neutropenia have demonstrated significant PK changes for many agents; however, PK changes have not been confirmed in SOT populations with neutropenia. Nonetheless, pertinent antimicrobial PK changes will be reviewed here, as they should be given consideration in all neutropenic patients while identifying the optimal antimicrobial regimen.

Changes in PK indices, as well as a greater variability of these indices, have been demonstrated for many of the beta-lactam antibiotics in patients with febrile neutropenia. In two studies of febrile neutropenic cancer patients compared to healthy volunteers, an increased Vd was observed for both imipenem and meropenem. Imipenem also displayed an increased $t_{1/2}$, whereas the opposite was true for meropenem [36, 37]. A study of ceftazidime showed patients with febrile neutropenia had a reduced AUC and shorter $t_{1/2}$ compared to elderly, healthy subjects [38]. Many studies of the aminoglycosides have shown that these agents have an increased Vd in patients with febrile neutropenia [39–43]. Adequate initial dosing and TDM are essential in order to ensure appropriate aminoglycoside drug concentrations are achieved. Importantly, studies have demonstrated that once-daily aminoglycosides are likely as safe and efficacious as conventional three-times-daily administration in patients with neutropenia [44, 45]. In studies of vancomycin PK, a decreased CL, increased Vd, and slight reduction in AUC were observed in patients with febrile neutropenia [46, 47]. An increase in the variability of these PK parameters was also noted; therefore, careful monitoring of serum trough concentration is warranted. Increased variability along with a small decrease in AUC was also observed in cancer patients with neutropenic fever treated with daptomycin [48, 49]. In a study of compassionate-use linezolid, the PK profile of the drug in neutropenic patients with cancer did not differ significantly from that of the rest of the study population [50]. There is a paucity of data evaluating potential PK changes of fluoroquinolones in patients with neutropenia.

In patients undergoing treatment for hematologic malignancies, HSCT, solid tumors, and SOT, various medication regimens including antimicrobials may be expected to impart some increased risk of neutropenia. However, medication-related neutropenia from non-chemotherapeutic agents is uncommon [51–53]. Trimethoprim/sulfamethoxazole and linezolid are often cited as a potential cause of dose- and duration-related bone marrow suppression although the true incidence remains uncertain [54]. Vancomycin is known to suppress bone marrow function in vitro and observed in vivo [55]. Beta-lactam antibiotics, especially prolonged treatment courses, have been observed to cause leukopenia via an immune-mediated mechanism [51, 56]. Often it is difficult to discern antibiotic-associated myelosuppression from other causes of bone marrow suppression in these complex patients following transplantation. Table 51.2 provides a select list of antibiotics associated with blood cell line disturbances such as neutropenia, thrombocytopenia, or anemia and literature-guided relative risk of such occurrences. It should be noted that antibiotic-associated bone

Table 51.2 Selected antibiotics associated with neutropenia, thrombocytopenia, or anemia [51–53]

Antibiotic	Estimated relative risk of bone marrow suppression	Comment
Trimethoprim/sulfamethoxazole	+++	Potentially all cell line
Beta-lactams	++	Thrombocytopenia and neutropenia
Linezolid	++	Thrombocytopenia and neutropenia
Vancomycin	+/++	Thrombocytopenia and neutropenia
Dapsone	++	Hemolytic anemia with G6PD deficiency, reports of neutropenia and thrombocytopenia
Tetracyclines	+	
Macrolides	0/+	
Clindamycin	0/+	
Fluoroquinolones	0/+	

marrow suppression is relatively uncommon compared with myelotoxicity noted with other classes of medications, and such diagnosis requires a broad differential of possibilities and needs to be considered within the appropriate clinical context.

Elderly

Solid organ transplantation is being performed in an older population with increasing frequency [57]. In general, elderly patients are more likely to have comorbidities managed with multiple medications and subsequently can be subject to a higher risk for adverse drug events when prescribed additional antimicrobial therapy [58]. Because the number of medications most patients are prescribed increases substantially after undergoing SOT, it can be deduced this population of elderly patients is at an even higher risk for adverse drug events. Furthermore, age-related PK/PD changes have been linked with the risk for drug-related toxicity [59]. Anticipating these changes can help avoid or minimize adverse medication outcomes in this special population.

Differences in drug absorption are possible in elderly patients due to reduced gastric acid secretion, weakened peristalsis, and delayed gastric emptying [60–62]. It is unclear if these changes are of clinical significance; they are unlikely to affect a drug's AUC; however, lower Cmax may occur [62]. Vd for lipophilic antimicrobials in elderly patients is typically increased secondary to an increase in adipose tissue and reduced lean body mass compared to younger individuals [63, 64]. Conversely, the Vd for hydrophilic antibiotics will likely be decreased in elderly patients (see Table 51.1). Many elderly patients have a slightly decreased serum albumin concentration and an increased alpha1-acid glycoprotein [62]. While these changes potentially impact PPB and free fraction of highly protein-bound drugs, PPB alterations, however, have not been shown to significantly affect clinical response to antimicrobial agents [65]. Decreased hepatocyte mass and blood flow to the liver contribute to reduced first-pass hepatic metabolism and CL of some drugs [62, 66–68]. Glomerular filtration and tubular function decrease with increasing age, and concentrations of renal drug elimination are subsequently increased, including for several antimicrobial agents. Because muscle mass is often decreased in elderly patients, these patients will frequently present with a normal serum creatinine despite significant renal impairment [69]. Therefore, estimation of creatinine clearance (CrCl) with a predictive equation and clinical judgment is required when determining dosing regimens for renally eliminated antimicrobials in the elderly [70, 71]. The six-variable MDRD equation has been suggested as the most accurate predictor of renal function in this population [62].

Further complicating antimicrobial dosing in the elderly is the fact that elderly patients, especially those with comorbid conditions, are often excluded from clinical trials. Therefore, age-related dose adjustments derived from pharmacokinetic evaluations are not available for a large number of drugs used in this population. Monitoring for signs of clinical improvement or deterioration and drug toxicity and, when available, obtaining serum drug concentrations may assist in guiding dosing strategies among the elderly transplant recipients. The general rule for many classes of medications in the elderly, to start with lower doses and titrate up to an effective dose, should not be applied to antimicrobial therapy. Initial doses should be sufficiently high to rapidly achieve adequate concentrations, especially for antimicrobials dependent upon a high Cmax for efficacy. The subsequent dosage or interval can then be adjusted to maintain serum concentrations comparable to younger patients. In general, the dose should remain unchanged and the interval lengthened for concentration-dependent antimicrobials; conversely, doses can be adjusted for antimicrobials which depend on T > MIC for efficacy.

Cystic Fibrosis

Cystic fibrosis (CF) is the third most common diagnosis category leading to lung transplant in the USA [57]. When infection and inflammation lead to bronchiectasis and, ultimately, end-stage pulmonary disease in patients with CF, lung transplantation offers a survival benefit for most patients [72]. With few exception, the presence of multidrug-resistant pathogens pretransplant is generally not considered a contraindication to lung transplantation [73]. However, in the setting of posttransplant immunosuppression, infections remain a major source of complications and declining pulmonary graft function following lung transplantation. Additionally, the transplanted lung lacks innervation, resulting in suboptimum cough reflex and adequate clearance of respiratory secretions [74]. Patients with CF undergoing lung transplantation require perioperative antibiotics with a special attention paid to selecting antimicrobials active against the organism(s) the patient may be colonized with or had infectious episodes with prior to transplant. Frequent courses of antibiotics are also likely to be necessary during the posttransplant period. Consideration of antimicrobial PK/PD parameters is paramount for achieving optimum drug concentrations, especially at the infection site(s), and improved drug efficacy to treat often serious and life-threatening infections in this unique patient population.

The extent of drug absorption may be diminished in patients with CF secondary to reduced gastric acid secretion and bile acid malabsorption [75, 76]. While studies in patients with CF have failed to consistently demonstrate a clinically significant decrease in the AUC of orally administered antimicrobials, a reduced Cmax has been observed for some antimicrobial agents [77–82]. There are no PK studies to date which evaluate the impact of CF on the rate and extent of antimicrobial absorption following lung transplantation, although studies of antirejection medications have demonstrated higher oral dosage requirements in the CF population when compared to those without CF [83, 84].

In general, CF patients prior to transplantation have an increased Vd secondary to higher lean muscle mass per kilogram of body weight [85–87]. Hepatic dysfunction is a common complication of CF, but despite this, the CF population appears to have enhanced metabolism of many drugs [88]. Some of the CYP enzymes have demonstrated increased activity in patients with CF such as CYP1A2 and CYP2C8, whereas others like CYP2C9 and CYP3A4 appear to be unaffected [87–91]. The renal clearance of many drugs is also enhanced in patients with CF, although the mechanism for this enhancement is unclear [73, 92, 93].

Data for Vd, CL, $t_{1/2}$, and AUC of antimicrobials in CF patients following lung transplantation is less than adequate [94, 95]. In one retrospective study, tobramycin PK was evaluated in eight patients with CF before and after bilateral lung transplantation [95]. The investigators found no difference in AUC or Vd pretransplant versus posttransplant. CL decreased and $t_{1/2}$ increased from pretransplant values during the immediate postoperative period; however, only a significant difference in $t_{1/2}$ remained in the patients who received tobramycin ≥6 weeks posttransplant. The investigators noted a large interpatient variability in these PK parameters and recommended that they be reexamined during each tobramycin course following lung transplantation.

Taken together, these data suggest that antimicrobial dose requirements in patients with CF may not only differ from non-CF counterparts but may also diverge from pretransplant parameters after patients have undergone lung transplantation. Some potential explanations for these alterations include medication-associated organ dysfunction, drug interactions and changes in fluid, and patients' nutritional status. An individualized approach to antimicrobial dosing is required, one that takes into account the patient's organ function, body composition, and overall severity of illness; TDM should also be utilized when available.

Obesity

Historically, obesity has been considered a relative contraindication for SOT due to increased perioperative morbidity and mortality. While it does appear that obese patients are at an increased risk of surgical site infection, the benefits of transplantation outweigh the risks of surgical complications in many clinical situations among patients with obesity and end-organ disease [96–100]. Moreover, a survival benefit has been demonstrated in obese patients in whom kidney and liver transplants were undertaken compared with similar patients in whom transplantation was deferred due to obesity [101, 102]. Organ transplants are being performed in increasing numbers in such patients, and this trend is likely to continue given the continued rise in the prevalence of obesity nationally [103]. Moreover, the prevalence of obesity after undergoing organ transplantation is also on the rise. Nearly one-third of liver transplant recipients with a normal pretransplant body mass index (BMI) were noted to have BMI in obesity range after undergoing orthotropic liver transplantation [104, 105]. The development of posttransplant obesity has been linked to universal prednisone use and near-universal use of calcineurin inhibitors (CNIs), especially cyclosporine for prevention and treatment of allograft rejection [106, 107]. When treating infections in such patients, consideration for changes in the antimicrobial PK is critical for achieving adequate serum concentrations while minimizing drug toxicity.

Absorption of drugs remains essentially unchanged; however, an increased volume of adipose tissue results in an increased Vd and CL for many antimicrobial agents [108, 109]. The impact of obesity on a drug's Vd will vary based on the characteristics of the drug molecule; for example, hydrophilic molecules are less likely to be distributed into the adipose tissue (Table 51.1). The effect of obesity on hepatic metabolism is largely unknown; obese patients are known to have an increased GFR. This phenomenon has been attributed to the enlarged glomeruli observed in obese versus nonobese patients [110]. In fact, organs from obese kidney donors demonstrate a significantly higher GFR compared to renal grafts harvested from nonobese donors [110]. Estimating CrCl in obese patients presents a challenge to clinicians; transplant care teams should include experienced PharmDs. CrCl based on total body weight (TBW) in obese patients results in an overestimated renal clearance, whereas ideal body weight (IBW) tends to underestimate CrCl [111, 112]. Adjusted body weight (ABW) appears to closely correlate with CrCl in this population (ABW = IBW + correction factor x [TBW – IBW]). A correction factor of 0.4 is commonly used. The modification of diet in renal disease (MDRD) equation is an attractive option because it does not include body weight as a variable; it should be noted that this formula has not been rigorously tested for drug dose adjustments in obese patients [113]. It is interesting to note that Vd and CL differences have not significantly influenced antimicrobial drug elimination rates, possibly because elimination rate constant (ke) = Vd/Cl, which offset one another. Nonetheless, TDM should be used to help guide therapy in this patient population when possible.

The majority of studies for evaluating vancomycin PK in obese subjects suggest that Vd is increased compared to nonobese patients. It is generally recommended that vancomycin be dosed at 15–20 mg/kg using TBW [114, 115]. Vancomycin CL is also increased in obese patients; TDM of serum vancomycin trough levels should be monitored [114, 115]. For highly hydrophilic drugs, such as the aminoglycosides, it is generally recommended that doses be based on an ABW. For the aminoglycosides, a correction factor of 0.4 is generally recommended [116, 117]. Studies of the fluoroquinolones have produced variable results precluding any specific dosage recommendations; dosing at the higher end of the therapeutic range has been suggested [109]. Beta-lactam antibiotics display hydrophilic properties and have limited distribution into adipose tissue [109]. Nonetheless, higher doses of beta-lactam antibiotics may be required to achieve adequate concentrations, especially in adult transplant patients with extreme obesity. In a study, 2 g of cefazolin was required in obese patients undergoing bariatric surgery to obtain comparable tissue concentrations to 1 g cefazolin dose in nonobese patients [118]. This is reflected in the current antibiotic surgical prophylaxis guidelines as 3 g of cefazolin dose is recommended for patients weighing greater than 120 kg [119]. Authors recommend TBW be used to determine daptomycin dose [120], and for linezolid, IBW can be considered [121–123]. Further studies are required to assess and validate optimum antibiotic dosing in this patient population.

Antibiotic Drug Interactions in Solid Organ Transplantation

Pharmacokinetic Alterations of Calcineurin Inhibitors and Proliferation Signal Inhibitors by Antibiotics

The majority of recognized pharmacokinetic drug interactions with antimicrobial medications in SOT occur with CNIs such as cyclosporine, tacrolimus, and proliferation signal inhibitors (PSIs) like everolimus and sirolimus. This is mainly due to their reliance on CYP450 isoenzymes and transport proteins for clearance and due to TDM is routinely performed for these drugs in transplant recipients. It is important to note that pharmacokinetic alterations via CYP450 and ABC transporters do not only relate to changes in drug clearance, but also impact oral drug bioavailability. Differences in the magnitude of pharmacokinetic alterations due to concomitant use of antibiotic and CNIs or PSIs are a common occurrence in this population with specific treatment requirements. In general, TDM is strongly recommended when patients receiving CNIs or PSIs are initiated on or discontinued from medications with either inhibitory and/or induction effects on CYP3A and/or ABC transporters (such as P-gp) [124, 125]. Tables 51.3 and 51.4 provide a summary of interactions between antibiotics and antirejection agents. It should be noted that inherent variability among patients makes prediction for the extent of these interactions difficult; therefore, close TDM is required. In the event of difficult-to-manage drug-drug interactions, an alternative agent should be used.

Specific interactions requiring empiric dose adjustment are important to recognize. For example, when initiating the CYP3A inhibitors erythromycin or clarithromycin, CNI trough concentrations would be expected to increase 1.6- to sixfold necessitating an empiric dose reduction of 35–50% of the original dose and potentially more based on TDM [126, 127]. Accordingly, dose reductions of 50% for sirolimus and 25% for everolimus should be considered when initiating erythromycin or clarithromycin [128–130]. Once the offending agent is discontinued, dose increases are warranted based on TDM as enzyme and protein inhibition wanes. For the more commonly used azalide, azithromycin, recommendations are less clear. TDM is warranted as reports of increased CNI and, to a lesser extent, PSI concentrations with azithromycin have been reported, but not to the magnitude of the aforementioned macrolides [125, 131–133].

In contrast to enzyme inhibition, the antituberculosis agent rifampin is a potent enzyme inducer responsible for decreasing CNI concentrations by 6- to 15-fold and decreased PSI concentrations by two to fivefold due to reduced bioavailability and heightened enzymatic clearance [134–137]. Whenever possible, an alternative to rifampin should be used as it has been implicated in graft rejection resulting in irreparable graft damage due to subtherapeutic CNI levels. If the combination cannot be avoided, cyclosporine doses may be increased by 1–2 mg/kg/day with three-times-daily dosing and adjusted according to TDM [135]. Specific recommendations for the management of tacrolimus, sirolimus, and everolimus are lacking, but dose adjustments should be expected based on TDM [125]. Rifabutin, a possible substitute for rifampin, may also interact with CNIs and PSIs, albeit to a lesser magnitude [138, 139].

Table 51.3 Definitions of onset of action, magnitude of effect, and relative strength of evidence for immunosuppressant drug interactions [124]

Onset of action	
Rapid	PCK effect is demonstrated within 24 h of co-administration
Delayed	PCK effect will not be demonstrated until the interacting drug is administered for a period of days or weeks
Magnitude of effect	
Major	Effects are life-threatening, capable of permanent damage, or rejection
Moderate	May cause a detriment in clinical status, additional treatment, hospitalization, or extension of stay
Minor	Effects may be mild; consequences may be bothersome or noticeable; additional treatment not required; no sign of effect upon therapeutic outcomes
Relative strength of evidence	
Established	Proven to occur in well-controlled studies Altered pharmacologic effect has been demonstrated in well-controlled trials *OR* PCK effect has been demonstrated in well-controlled human studies. An altered pharmacologic response is expected based upon the magnitude of the kinetic effect, or clinical observations support the occurrence of the interaction
Probable	Very likely, but not proven clinically A PCK interaction has been demonstrated in well-controlled studies. Based on the magnitude of the kinetic changes and the known plasma level-response relationship of the affected drug, an altered pharmacologic response will probably occur *OR* When controlled human experimentation is impractical, well-designed animal experiments confirm an interaction which is suggested by multiple case reports or uncontrolled studies
Suspected	May occur; some good data, but needs further study A PCK interaction has been demonstrated in well-controlled studies Although an altered pharmacologic response might be expected to occur based on the magnitude of the kinetic change, no firm conclusion can be drawn since a plasma level-response relationship has not been established for the affected drug *OR* An altered pharmacologic response has been reported in multiple case reports or repeated uncontrolled clinical studies
Possible	Could occur, but data are very limited Although a PCK interaction has been demonstrated, the kinetic changes are of such magnitude that it is not possible to predict if an altered response will occur *OR* The evidence is divided as to whether an interaction exists *OR* An altered pharmacologic response is suggested by limited data

Used with permission from Page et al. [124]; http://circ.ahajournals.org/content/111/2/230; https://doi.org/10.1161/01.CIR.0000151805.86933.35, with permission from Wolters Kluwer Health, Inc.
PCK pharmacokinetic

Noteworthy is the fact that cyclosporine and, to a lesser extent, tacrolimus also inhibit the CYP450 isoenzymes and P-gp. However, there is a paucity of published data implicating elevated antibiotic concentrations due to decreased elimination or increased bioavailability with cyclosporine. Cyclosporine has been shown to increase serum concentrations of tacrolimus, everolimus, and sirolimus when given together. Midazolam and statins eliminated via the liver follow similarly metabolized medications resulting in higher drug exposures, although the significance will vary depending on the therapeutic index of the medication [7, 140, 141].

Pharmacokinetic Alterations of Antimetabolites by Antibiotics

Antibiotic pharmacokinetic interactions have been described for the antimetabolites as well. For example, mycophenolic acid (MPA) has a complex metabolic pathway. Briefly, MPA systemic clearance predominately involves glucuronidation via uridine diphosphate-glucuronosyltransferase (UGT) 1A9 in the liver to its major metabolite, 7-*O*-glucuronide MPA (MPAG). MPAG is a substrate for multidrug resistance-associated protein 2 (MRP2), which is responsible for biliary excretion of MPAG into the intestinal tract. Once in the colon, MPAG is de-glucuronidated by ß-glucuronidase-producing bacteria and reabsorbed as MPA. This enterohepatic recirculation is significant and can account for 10–60% of total MPA exposure, often noted in pharmacokinetic monitoring as a second peak of MPA concentration between 6 and 12 h of mycophenolic mofetil (MMF) administration. In addition, UGT 2B7 is responsible for a minor but active metabolite acyl-glucuronide MPA (AcMPAG). Urinary excretion of glucuronidated metabolites eventually accounts for the ultimate elimination of MPA, where MRP2 may play a role in active tubular secretion [7, 142, 143]. Pharmacokinetic analysis of MPA is assessed by calculating an area under the curve (AUC) profile to account for the total drug exposure and enterohepatic recirculation. Antibiotics such as metronidazole, norfloxacin, and the combination of metronidazole and norfloxacin have

Table 51.4 Documented pharmacokinetic interactions between antibiotic agents with calcineurin inhibitors and proliferation signal inhibitors [125]

Drug	Interaction drug (specific CNI studied)	Effect	Onset	Magnitude	Level of evidence	Management #
CSA/TAC	*Beta-lactams*					
	Cephalosporins					
	Ceftriaxone (CSA)	Increased CSA exposure	Delayed	Moderate	Possible	Monitor CSA/TAC concentrations closely for 1–2 weeks
	Carbapenems					
	Imipenem-cilastatin (CSA)	Increased/decreased CSA exposure	Delayed	Moderate	Possible	Monitor CSA/TAC concentrations closely for 1–2 weeks
	Penicillins					
	Ticarcillin (CSA)	Increased CSA exposure	Delayed	Moderate	Possible	Monitor CSA/TAC concentrations closely for 1–2 weeks
	Nafcillin (CSA)	Decreased CSA exposure	Delayed	Moderate	Possible	Monitor CSA/TAC concentrations closely for 1–2 weeks
	Fluoroquinolones					
	Ciprofloxacin (CSA)	Increased CSA exposure	Delayed	Moderate	Possible	Monitor CSA/TAC concentrations closely for 1–2 weeks; consider alternative fluoroquinolone
	Levofloxacin (CSA, TAC)	Increased CSA/TAC exposure	Delayed	Minimal	Possible	Not clinically significant
	Macrolides/azolides					
	Macrolides					
	Erythromycin (CSA, TAC)	Increase CSA/TAC exposure with subsequent renal, hepatic, and neurologic toxicity	Rapid	Moderate	Probable	Monitor CSA/TAC concentrations closely for 3 weeks and decrease CSA/TAC dose to 50–65% of original dose
	Clarithromycin (CSA, TAC)		Rapid	Moderate	Probable	
	Erythromycin (EVER, SIR)	Increased EVER/SIR exposure	Rapid	Moderate	Established	Reduce dose of SIR to 50% and EVER to 75% of original dose. Monitor SIR/EVER concentrations closely
	Clarithromycin (SIR)	Increased SIR	Rapid	Moderate	Established	Reduce dose of SIR to 50% of original dose. Monitor SIR/EVER concentrations closely
	Azalides					
	Azithromycin (CSA, TAC)	Increased CSA/TAC exposure	Delayed	Moderate	Possible	Monitor CSA/TAC concentrations closely for 1–2 weeks
	Azithromycin (EVER)	Increased EVER exposure	?	Minimal	Possible	Monitor SIR/EVER concentrations closely
	Antianerobic/antiparasitic agents					
	Metronidazole (CSA, TAC)	Increased CSA/TAC exposure	Delayed	Moderate	Possible	Monitor CSA/TAC concentrations closely for 1–2 weeks
	Rifamycins					
	Rifampin (CSA, TAC)	Decreased CSA/TAC exposure	Rapid	Major	Established	Monitor CSA/TAC concentrations closely for 2 weeks; consider use of alternative antimycobacterial agent^, for TAC increase dose accordingly, for CSA increase dose 1–2 mg/kg/day with three times a day dosing
	Rifabutin (CSA, TAC)		Delayed	Moderate	Possible	Monitor CSA/TAC concentration for up to 25 days after beginning rifabutin therapy and after discontinuation
	Rifampin (SIR, EVER)	Decreased SIR/EVER exposure	Rapid	Major	Established	Avoid combination; consider use of alternative antimycobacterial agent^. If unavoidable, monitor SIR/EVER concentrations closely for 1–2 weeks, and adjust dose accordingly
	Sulfonamides/sulfonamide combinations					
	Sulfadimidine/trimethoprim (CSA)	Decreased CSA exposure	Delayed	Major	Possible	Monitor CSA/TAC concentrations closely for the first 4 days
	Sulfadiazine (CSA, TAC)		?	Moderate	Possible	
	Miscellaneous agents					
	Quinupristin/dalfopristin (CSA)	Increased CSA exposure	Delayed	Moderate	Possible	Monitor CSA/TAC concentrations closely for the first 2–3 days; consider linezolid, daptomycin, or telavancin as an alternative
	Chloramphenicol (CSA, TAC)	Increased CSA/TAC exposure	Rapid	Moderate	Suspected	Monitor CSA/TAC concentrations daily for the first week; reduce initial CSA/TAC dose to 75% of original dose
	Clindamycin (CSA)	Reduced CSA exposure	Delayed	Moderate	Possible	Monitor CSA/TAC concentrations closely for the first 4 weeks
	Telithromycin	Increase CSA/TAC exposure	?	Moderate	Possible	Monitor CSA/TAC concentrations closely
	Tigecycline (CSA)	Increased CSA	Rapid	Moderate	Possible	Monitor CSA/TAC concentrations for the first 1–2 days; may need to reduce CSA dose to 50%

CSA cyclosporine, (*CSA*) reported with CSA, *EVER* everolimus, (*EVER*) reported with EVER, *SIR* sirolimus, (*SIR*), reported with SIR, *TAC* tacrolimus, (*TAC*) reported with TAC, ? unknown, ^ includes pyrazinamide, streptomycin, amikacin, ofloxacin, # the frequency in obtaining immunosuppressant concentrations may vary depending on a patient's clinical stability, time from transplant, or rejection history. Recommendations are based on published literature and varied magnitude of interactions frequently occurs; therefore, individualizing a monitoring plan is always appropriate been shown to decrease MPA 48-h AUC on average 10, 19, and 33%, respectively. To a similar magnitude, they decrease MPAG 48-h AUC [144]. The disruption of colonic and intestinal Gram-negative aerobic and anaerobic flora that produce ß-glucuronidase likely decreases enterohepatic recirculation leading to reduced drug and metabolite exposure. Similarly, pre-dose or trough MPA levels were significantly reduced from baseline in a group of renal transplant recipients that received either ciprofloxacin or amoxicillin/clavulanic acid on average by 47% between days 3 and 7 of therapy and trended to recover near baseline trough levels after 3 days following discontinuation of the antibiotics [145]. Given the complex pharmacokinetic profile, the utility of a single pre-dose MPA level is questionable, and the extent of reduced MPA AUC is not known, but the proof of an altered pharmacokinetic profile remains. It is likely that other antibiotics with the potential to disrupt the colonic normal flora may reduce enterohepatic recirculation, although this has not been specifically studied.

Rifampin has also been shown to decrease MPA exposure by both increased clearance via UGT induction and possibly inhibition of enterohepatic recirculation. A pharmacokinetic trial assessing the effect of rifampin on MPA concentrations after MMF administration showed a 17.5% reduced average 12-h MPA AUC from the baseline. Metabolite exposure measured by 12-h AUC increased by 34.4 and 193% for MPAG and AcMPAG, respectively [146]. This study showed a much lower magnitude of interaction compared to the reported MPA dose-adjusted 221% increase in 12-h AUC following rifampin discontinuation and a washout period first described by the same investigators [147]. Similarly, in pediatric liver transplant patients, 2 receiving rifampin with MMF had a four- to fivefold higher total clearance of drug from plasma ratio (CL/F) as assessed by 12-h AUC compared to 13 who did not receive rifampin. In this study, target 12-h AUCs were not attained despite dose adjustments [148].

As a whole, literature supports the existence of significant antibiotic-MPA interactions, but with a wide magnitude of variability. Further, MPA TDM is controversial and resource-intensive. At this time, it is unclear how such interactions should be monitored and managed. Broad-spectrum Gram-negative aerobic and anaerobic antimicrobials need judicious use, early de-escalation, or discontinuation when feasible, especially in the SOT recipients. In high-risk individuals, MPA AUCs may be calculated and monitored; however, evidence of improved outcomes with such an approach is currently lacking [7].

Pharmacokinetic Alterations of Corticosteroids by Antibiotics

Prednisone and methylprednisolone are two structurally similar and commonly used synthetic corticosteroids. However, these compounds differ greatly from a pharmacological perspective. Prednisone is an inactive prodrug that must be converted to the active moiety, prednisolone. Methylprednisolone is active but more susceptible to pharmacokinetic drug-drug interactions due to a methyl group at the 6α position. Corticosteroids undergo CYP3A-dependent 6β-hydroxylation which puts them at risk of interactions with other drugs [149]. Corticosteroids have also been shown to change MRP2 and P-gp activity [140]. Despite ubiquitous use in early transplantation and throughout medicine, data describing pharmacokinetic drug interactions with antibiotics are rare. Macrolides have long been considered to be "steroid-sparing" perhaps due to P-gp and CYP3A4 inhibition in addition to their anti-inflammatory effects. In asthmatics, erythromycin was shown to decrease intravenous methylprednisolone clearance by 46% [150]. Similarly, clarithromycin was shown to decrease oral methylprednisolone clearance by 65%. Interestingly, prednisolone pharmacokinetics following oral prednisone was not significantly altered by clarithromycin [151]. Thus, using an equivalent dose of prednisone or prednisolone may obviate the potential interaction with CYP3A4 inhibitors including some azole antifungal agents [125].

Rifampin has been shown to increase cortisol and prednisolone metabolism resulting in therapeutic failure of the anti-inflammatory effect when added to methylprednisolone. Prednisolone AUC was reduced by 66%, clearance increased by more than 200%, and half life decreased by 40 60% in the presence of rifampin, reported in various clinical scenarios [152]. Although not specifically studied, a similar if not greater pharmacokinetic interaction would be expected with methylprednisolone. A doubling of the prednisolone dose may be needed to retain therapeutic efficacy. This interaction should be avoided, or rifabutin, a less potent enzyme inducer, may be substituted when possible [125, 153].

Pharmacodynamic Interactions of Immunosuppressive Agents with Antibiotics

Pharmacodynamic interactions between CNIs, PSIs, antimetabolites, corticosteroids, and antibiotics may also occur. Due to the nature of these interactions and lack of reporting, the magnitude and incidence frequently go under-recognized. For example, tacrolimus has been reported to prolong the cardiac QT interval in a concentration-dependent manner and has been associated with torsades de pointes, usually when given with other drugs with the potential for QT interval prolongation [154, 155]. It would be expected that antibiotics that also prolong the QT interval would have an additive effect on QT interval aberration. Some of these drugs include, but are not limited to, the antimalarial chloroquine, macrolides, the fluoroquinolones, and trimethoprim/sulfamethoxazole (TMP/

SMX) [156]. Often, these interactions go unrecognized and frequently may be accompanied by the addition of other drugs that have the potential for QT prolongation before a cardiac arrhythmia is noticed. Therefore, the true incidence and clinical significance of such interactions are not known. If the combination is given in a hospital setting, QT monitoring may be employed to assess for severity of cardiac toxicity. However, it is controversial whether monitoring needs to routinely take place. The use of these medications with tacrolimus should be weighed against potential risks and alternatives on a per patient basis. For example, TMP/SMX should not be withheld in transplant patients receiving tacrolimus given the weak evidence and risk of torsades de pointes compared to the benefit for the prevention and treatment of *Pneumocystis jirovecii* pneumonia. In contrast, treatment alternatives to TMP/SMX or linezolid may be considered for cancer patients with severe neutropenia or for those undergoing HSCT if clinical equipoise with an alternative exists to minimize the potential drug-induced myelosuppression.

Similarly, the addition of an aminoglycoside to a CNI may result in a higher incidence of acute kidney injury due to additive nephrotoxic effects. As with most pharmacodynamics interactions, the true prevalence and impact of nephrotoxicity are not well established; however, such interactions with cyclosporine are well-described [157]. This is of particular concern given the increased incidence of resistant Gram-negative bacterial infections and increasing limited treatment options for transplant patients with multidrug-resistant bacteria infections. The use of this combination will primarily be in hospitalized patients; therefore, close monitoring of renal function as well as any needed adjustments to CNI and aminoglycoside concentrations may minimize the potential for toxicity. Nonsteroidal anti-inflammatory drugs (NSAIDs) should be avoided whenever possible with patients being treated with CNI. Renal toxicity due to afferent arterial constriction with CNIs may be potentiated further with repeated NSAID use.

Another example of a potential PD interaction is the use of imipenem/cilastatin with a CNI. Both CNIs and imipenem have been associated with seizures. However, clinical data describing an increased risk of seizure with the often-used combination compared to monotherapy of either drugs is lacking [158]. Nevertheless, whenever using this combination, an assessment of seizure risk should be considered.

In summary, pharmacokinetic interactions with antibiotics and CNIs or PSIs are frequently made apparent by TDM and can be managed by dose adjustments when the interaction is unavoidable. For immunosuppressive agents without readily identifiable target ranges or available TDM, empiric dose adjustments and heightened awareness of monitoring for toxicities and keen assessment of the allograft rejection are the only available strategies that clinicians can use to manage drug interactions with these agents. Further studies are needed to elucidate the role of dose-adjusted AUC monitoring in such patients. Pharmacokinetic interactions with corticosteroids are more often than not ignored and any resultant side effects treated palliatively.

Overlapping drug effects of various immunosuppressive agents such as CNIs, PSIs, antimetabolites, or corticosteroids and antibiotics may indicate a pharmacodynamic interaction. Often dynamic interactions are a result of additive side effects and may lead to unanticipated toxicities. Because of the complexity of the interaction, patient variability, and inability to measure biochemical indicators of the interaction, the true incidence, magnitude, and clinical significance for many PD interactions remain elusive. However, they are important to consider within a clinical context when developing an antimicrobial therapeutic plan for patients undergoing transplantation. Frequently, these potential PD interactions are appropriately managed if considered and carefully monitored without requiring antibiotic substitutions.

Aerosolized Delivery of Antimicrobials

Direct delivery of antibiotics via aerosolization is an appealing method of drug delivery in transplant recipients with tracheobronchial and lung infections. This method of drug delivery avoids delays in drug delivery to the site of infection and also bypasses first-pass metabolism in the liver. Systemic exposure to the drug is minimized, which helps limit systemic drug toxicity. Aerosolized delivery of antibiotics avoids PD drug interactions associated with systemic antibiotic therapy, including the additive nephrotoxicity of aminoglycosides in combinations with the CNIs. Still, this method of drug delivery is associated with significant increases in time for drug administration, cost, and adverse respiratory effects. Furthermore, distribution of inhaled antibiotic in the lungs is not necessarily homogenous; careful consideration of PK factors affecting aerosolized medication delivery is warranted.

The partial size of the molecule delivered via inhalation is the mass aerodynamic diameter (MMAD). The MMAD is important for ensuring delivery to the lower respiratory tract; the ideal MMAD of a particle undergoing aerosolization is 1–5 um [159–161]. Drug particles having MMAD >5 um are more likely to be deposited in the oropharynx and swallowed. Particles with an MMAD <1 um are more likely to be exhaled instead of deposited in the lung [159–162]. Once delivered to the lung, antimicrobials must avoid removal by mucociliary transport in the upper lung or uptake by macrophages in the alveolar region of the lung.

The dissolution rate, which is determined primarily by the lipophilicity of the molecule, is an important factor in this process. A balance between lipophilicity and hydrophilicity is required; while lipophilicity facilitates diffusion across cell membranes to the site of action, it also expedites diffusion out of pulmonary cells into systemic circulation. Conversely, highly hydrophilic compounds may not be absorbed quickly enough to avoid mucociliary clearance and uptake by macrophages [159–162]. The proportion of drug delivered by aerosolization will also differ by the type of nebulizer used. There are three basic types of nebulizers: the jet pneumatic, ultrasonic, and the vibrating mesh (MESH) nebulizer. The jet nebulizer is most common in the hospital setting and there are many different models of the jet nebulizer [162–165]. Although generally considered equivalent, the accuracy of drug delivery, time required for drug delivery, and the amount of drug wasted can vary between jet nebulizer models. Further, the newer breath-actuated and breath-enhanced jet nebulizers, which preferentially deliver medication during inhalation and minimize it during exhalation, improve the speed of medication delivery and reduce medication waste compared to traditional jet nebulizers. Ultrasonic nebulizers lack data regarding antimicrobial delivery; therefore, this nebulizer type is infrequently utilized for this indication. MESH nebulizers use a newer technology, which generates a higher fraction of fine-particles and offers a faster, more efficient method of aerosolization [162, 164]. In general, a lower dose of antimicrobial is required when using a MESH nebulizer compared to jet or ultrasonic nebulizers. The ultrasonic and MESH nebulizers require careful cleaning after each treatment, while jet nebulizers use disposable parts.

A patient's breathing pattern will also impact the deposition of drug particles in the respiratory tract [159, 161, 166]. This consideration is especially important in lung transplant recipients. Clinical studies of single lung transplant recipients have demonstrated that the drug is preferentially delivered to the transplanted, more ventilated, lung [167, 168]. Therefore, aerosolized medication delivery may not result in antimicrobial concentrations in the native lung necessary to eradicate the offending pathogen.

Some systemic absorption will occur following the aerosolized delivery of any drug. Medications gain access to the system circulation through the highly vascularized pulmonary tissue and through intestinal absorption of the swallowed drug. Pharmacokinetic factors determine the extent of the systemic absorption and toxicity following aerosolization of an antimicrobial compound. As mentioned above, a higher degree of lipophilicity equates to a propensity for quick diffusion into systemic circulation through the pulmonary vasculature. Also, the greater the MMAD of an aerosolize particle, the more likely it is to be swallowed and available for intestinal absorption. Once an aerosolized medication is swallowed, the bioavailability of the drug molecule is important for determining systemic exposure [159–162]. A lower bioavailability means less drug is absorbed through the gut into the systemic circulation. Furthermore, the higher the total body CL of a drug, the lower the total systemic drug exposure will be. Therefore, drugs characterized by a low bioavailability and high systemic CL will be less likely to reach high systemic concentrations and potential for systemic drug toxicity.

Aerosolized Delivery of Antimicrobials: Aminoglycosides

The aminoglycosides are highly hydrophilic, polar, compounds that penetrate poorly into lung tissue following intravenous administrations. High serum concentrations are required to ensure adequate drug concentrations at the site of action, thereby increasing the potential for systemic toxicity. Local administration of aminoglycosides via aerosolized delivery is an attractive alternative to intravenous therapy, offering high concentrations at the desired location while reducing systemic exposure.

A preservative-free formulation of tobramycin (TOBI®) was developed to minimize adverse effects associated with inhalation of the molecule. This formulation is the best studied of the aminoglycosides for aerosolized administration, with most clinical data derived from studies in the CF population [169–172]. In 2013, tobramycin inhalation powder (TIP) received FDA approval; the advantage of this powder formulation is the ease of administration via simple inhaler versus a nebulizer. Aerosolized gentamicin and amikacin have also been studied, but these compounds do not have formulations specifically indicated for inhalation [173–176].

Adverse effects commonly associated with aerosolized aminoglycosides include mild, transient voice alteration, wheezing, cough, and dyspnea [177, 178]. Nephrotoxicity from inhaled aminoglycosides has been reported, including several reports involving recipients of SOT [176, 179, 180]. Clinicians should be aware of the potential for systemic adverse effects secondary to aerosolized aminoglycosides in all patients, and especially cognizant of those patients with reduced systemic drug clearance due to renal dysfunction. The potential for development of drug resistance is also a concern; however, clinical trials to date have not demonstrated this to be a significant hindrance to aerosolized therapy [171, 181].

Aerosolized Delivery of Antimicrobials: Colistin

The polymyxin antibiotic colistin causes bacterial cell death by binding and damaging the cell membranes of Gram-negative bacteria, including *Pseudomonas aeruginosa*. Colistimethate sodium and colistin sulfate are the commercially available formulations that are hydrolyzed to colistin in vivo. The use of these agents fell out of favor because of the significant nephrotoxicity and neurotoxicity associated with conventional intravenous administration. Despite these toxicities, interest in colistin has been renewed because it maintained activity against many emerging multidrug-resistant (MDR) Gram-negative bacteria. Furthermore, in an effort to avoid colistin-induced systemic toxicities, the use of aerosolized colistin has been explored. The literature evaluating colistin for hospital acquired pneumonia (HAP) and ventilator associated pneumonia (VAP) is mounting, although much of the published clinical experience to date with aerosolized colistin remains in the CF population [182–186]. Both colistimethate sodium and colistin sulfate can be aerosolized, but neither has been formulated specifically for inhalation.

Bronchospasm following inhalation of either form of colistin is relatively common, although colistimethate sodium appears to be associated with a lower incidence compared to colistin sulfate [187, 188]. When compared to aerosolized tobramycin, aerosolized colistin is associated with an increased incidence of pulmonary adverse effects [189, 190]. Once mixed with a diluent for aerosolization, both colistimethate sodium and colistin sulfate are quickly hydrolyzed to active drug and a metabolite that is toxic to lung tissue [162, 191]. Therefore, these drugs must be administered immediately after reconstitution to minimize adverse effects.

Aerosolized Delivery of Antimicrobials: Aztreonam and Other Beta-Lactams

Aztreonam, a monobactam antipseudomonal antibiotic, has been formulated as a lysine salt specifically for aerosolized administration. Aztreonam lysine (Cayston®) was developed because aerosolization of the intravenous formulation of aztreonam induces airway inflammation. Aztreonam lysine is generally well-tolerated, and the most commonly reported side effects include cough, nasal congestion, and wheezing [192]. Amoxicillin, ceftazidime, and cefotaxime have also been given via the aerosolized route [174, 193, 194]. These treatments were generally well-tolerated, although the small sample sizes of patients evaluated in published reports preclude any conclusions regarding the efficacy or safety of these drugs given via aerosolized route.

Aerosolized Delivery of Antimicrobials: Chronic Suppressive Therapy

Airway colonization with *P. aeruginosa* is linked to an increased risk for bronchiolitis obliterans syndrome (BOS) after lung transplant [195]. Clinical studies in the CF population have demonstrated that chronic suppressive therapy in patients with mild to severe disease severity results in a reduction in the frequency of pulmonary exacerbations, improved FEV1, and/or a reduced requirement for intravenous antipseudomonal antibiotics [169–171, 189, 196–198]. A retrospective, single-center study compared outcomes of lung transplant patients with CF who were prescribed inhaled colistin at one million international units twice daily with posttransplant CF counterpart in whom inhaled colistin was not given. [199]. Groups were stratified based on the presence or absence of bacterial colonization prior to colistin initiation. There were no standardized criteria for colistin initiation in either group. The investigators found that aerosolized colistin was associated with a reduced number of hospitalizations due to infections in the group without previous bacterial colonization; however, this favorable association was not found in patients with prior bacterial colonization. These results suggest a potential role for inhaled colistin as prophylaxis against infection-related hospitalization in CF patients following lung transplantation; additional studies are needed. No published study to date has specifically evaluated the use of inhaled tobramycin or aztreonam in CF patients after undergoing lung transplantation. However, based on data in the pretransplant CF population, it seems reasonable to consider inhaled tobramycin or aztreonam (as well as to inhaled colistin) in patients with chronic, recurring *P. aeruginosa* lung infection after lung transplantation.

Aerosolized Delivery of Antimicrobials for Hospital-Acquired Pneumonia

Due to chronic immunosuppression and impaired host defenses in the lower respiratory tract, transplant recipients are at high risk of hospital acquired pneumonia (HAP), including ventilator associated pneumonia (VAP) [200]. Furthermore, recipients of allograft transplants are at a higher risk of infection due to MDR organism(s) resulting from extensive prior exposure to broad-spectrum antibiotics and underlying immune suppression. The American Thoracic Society and Infectious Diseases Society of America Guidelines now recommend the use of both inhaled and systemic antibiotics in patients with VAP due to certain MDR organisms [200].

Much of the evidence for aerosolized therapy in MDR HAP and VAP is with aerosolized colistin. In observational case reports of patients with MDR organisms, aerosolized colistin in combination with systemic antibiotics has been associated with increased response rates. One randomized trial demonstrated that the addition of aerosolized colistin to standard therapy conferred a higher likelihood of either confirmed or presumed MDR bacterial eradication, but a beneficial effect on clinical outcome was not demonstrated [188]. In a retrospective multicenter cohort analysis of critically ill patients with MDR Gram-negative pneumonia, an increased clinical cure rate was observed in patients receiving IV colistin plus inhaled colistin versus those who received IV colistin alone [201]. The authors of a recent meta-analysis concluded there was a positive albeit low-quality evidence, demonstrating the addition of aerosolized colistin to systemic antibiotics for VAP is associated with improved outcomes [202].

Although aerosolization of aminoglycosides is an attractive treatment option for patients with HAP for reasons already discussed, there is a paucity of data assessing such practice in a large prospective randomized clinical trial. Small trials have shown that inhaled tobramycin and gentamicin were associated with some positive outcomes in patients with pulmonary infections [178, 202, 203]. In one trial of 37 patients with VAP, intravenous amikacin plus ceftazidime was compared to inhaled amikacin and ceftazidime [193]. Although the trial found no statistically significant differences in clinical outcomes between the groups, the aerosolized group had a numerically higher rate of bacterial eradication and clinical success. Three patients in the intravenous therapy group demonstrated resistance to ceftazidime following treatment initiation compared to no patients with de novo ceftazidime resistant bacteria in the aerosolized group.

Aerosolized Delivery of Antimicrobials for Nontuberculous Mycobacterial Infection

Aerosolized amikacin has been used clinically in combination with other agents for the treatment of nontuberculous mycobacterial infections [175, 204]. Reasons for aerosolized delivery of amikacin in this patient population include pulmonary infections refractory to traditional treatment, drug interactions, and intolerance to oral agents and intravenous amikacin or both. While aerosolized delivery of amikacin was associated with therapeutic success in the aforementioned reports, routine administration of aerosolized amikacin is not recommended due to a relative lack of published data evaluating this practice.

Aerosolized Delivery of Antimicrobials: Other Investigational Therapies for Inhalation

Numerous clinical trials investigating aerosolized antibiotics are currently underway. Fosfomycin, a phosphonic acid antibiotic with a broad spectrum of action, has been formulated in combination with tobramycin for inhalation. In a Phase II trial of 119 patients with CF, fosfomycin plus tobramycin for inhalation (FTI) was compared with placebo in a randomized, double-blinded study following a 28-day course of inhaled aztreonam [205]. Relative improvements in FEV1 achieved during aztreonam therapy were better maintained in patients receiving FTI compared to placebo. The common adverse effects of FTI were cough, dyspnea, fever and wheezing.

Inhaled levofloxacin (Aeroquin™) in a Phase III study did not significantly reduce the time to next pulmonary exacerbation in CF patients when compared with CF patients given placebo [206]. A Phase III study of the new liposomal formulation of amikacin (Arikace™) for the treatment of Nontuberculous mycobacterial (NTM) infection is currently recruiting subjects [207]. A formulation of vancomycin for aerosolization (Aerovanc™) was evaluated in a Phase II trial for Methicillin resistant staphylococcus aureus (MRSA) in CF patients; however, the results of this trial are not available at the time of this publication [208].

Immunomodulation

As previously mentioned, the macrolide antibiotics—including the azalide, azithromycin—have been considered "steroid sparing" in part due to their anti-inflammatory effects. These anti-inflammatory and immunomodulating effects are not surprising given that tacrolimus, sirolimus, and everolimus are non-antibiotic macrolide chemicals. However, the mechanism of immunomodulation for the macrolide antibiotics is less clear and seems to be multifactorial. Several recent reviews of the immunomodulatory properties of macrolide and other antibiotics have been published [209–213], warranting a brief review of the anti-inflammatory and immunomodulatory effects of macrolide, tetracycline, fluoroquinolone, sulfone, and sulfonamide antibiotics. The impact of antibiotics on the hosts' microbiome and subsequent immunomodulation is a rapidly expanding area of research that is beyond the scope of this chapter.

Macrolide Antibiotics

Interest in the anti-inflammatory effects of macrolide antibiotics was ignited with the successful use of erythromycin in the treatment of diffuse panbronchiolitis (DPB), an inflammatory lung disease. Follow-up studies showed both erythromycin and roxithromycin reduced IL-8, IL-1β, and neutrophils in bronchoalveolar fluid of patients with DPB [209, 214]. The clinical effects of macrolides in DPB have been replicated for clarithromycin and azithromycin, and these effects are likely due to similar immunomodulating properties [215].

Since then, macrolides have been extensively researched for their non-antibacterial effects. Although exact mechanisms are not always clear, drug-mediated decrease inflammation through inhibiting proinflammatory cytokines and chemokines, such as IL-1, IL-2, IL-5, IL-6, TNFα, GM-GCSF, and IL-8, and various chemokine ligands, and they may also promote a milieu favoring anti-inflammatory cytokines [209–211, 216]. Studies also suggest macrolides inhibit phagocyte oxidative burst, promote phagocytosis of apoptotic cells by alveolar macrophages, stimulate neutrophil exocytosis, and reduce adhesion molecule I in bronchial epithelial cell, thereby potentially reducing leukocyte adhesion [210, 216]. Overall, macrolide antibiotics have shown anti-inflammatory effects on cytokine production and distinct immunomodulation of neutrophils. A common unifying mechanism for the immunomodulatory effect of macrolide antibiotics on the host immune system is unknown but likely related to high intracellular accumulation. Regardless, the immunomodulatory properties of macrolides are broad, and their use beyond antibiosis has increased considerably.

More recently, a complementary immunomodulatory effect of solithromycin, a late generation fluoroketolide receiving US Food and Drug Administration "Qualified Infectious Disease Product" status, has been investigated in concert with its antibacterial activity. In very late 2016, the drug is awaiting FDA approval to the US market for community-acquired bacterial pneumonia (CABP). An anti-inflammatory effect of solithromycin shows a decreased response of macrophages to produce lipopolysaccharide (LPS)-induced TNFα and IL-8. In a study of 132 adult ambulatory patients presenting with chest radiograph consolidation and having signs and symptoms of CABP, 5 days of oral solithromycin or levofloxacin was compared. The efficacy rates determined by early clinical response (ECR) and overall success at end of treatment and test of cure visits were considered comparable. The investigators attributed the comparable ECR rates of the slow-kill fluoroketolide to the rapidly bactericidal quinolone to solithromycin's immunomodulatory effects [217].

A study of an ovine (sheep) model of intrauterine infection with *Ureaplasma parvum* compared the administration of maternal intravenous azithromycin (AZ) or solithromycin (SOLI) or placebo. At 120-day gestational age (GA), sheep received a single regimen among five distinct regimens which included either IV AZ or SOLI, or placebo or IV + intra-amniotic AZ or SOLI, or placebo. Baby lambs were surgically delivered at 125-day GA. While the amniotic fluid (AF) of all control animals contained culturable *U. parvum*, the AF, lung, and chorioamnion from all AZ- or SOLI-treated animals were culture-negative. Compared to controls, the levels of expression of IL-1β, IL-6, IL-8, and monocyte chemoattractant protein 2 (MCP-2) in fetal skin were significantly decreased in the IV SOLI cohort, and the MCP-1 protein concentration in AF was significantly increased in the IV + IA SOLI cohort. No significant differences in histological inflammation scoring of the lung or chorioamnion were noted among the five active and placebo treatment groups. As intrauterine inflammation is thought to be a major influence to infection-associated preterm birth (PTB), the anti-inflammatory properties of these macrolides may be of value in stunting infections leading to PTB [218].

Tetracycline Antibiotics

Tetracycline antibiotics also exhibit non-antibacterial effects. Most notably is the effect of doxycycline on matrix metalloproteinases (MMPs). Doxycycline is reported to inhibit MMPs to a greater extent than tetracycline or minocycline due to its increased affinity for zinc ions; however, anti-inflammatory effects of both doxycycline and minocycline have been reported [212]. Doxycycline has been studied and shown to be beneficial for gastric ulceration and oxidative stress in rats and ischemia-reperfusion injury in rat hearts by modulating MMP activity [212, 219]. Tetracyclines also scavenge reactive oxygen species, a driver for ischemia-reperfusion injury, which may partially explain its benefit. In addition, minocycline and doxycycline have been shown to have anti-apoptotic effects following global brain ischemia in gerbils. Minocycline, having greater penetration across the blood-brain barrier, has been studied for its neuroprotective anti-apoptotic effects in models of traumatic brain injury, Huntington's disease, and Parkinson's disease. Protective mechanisms are thought to involve reduced caspase-1 and/or caspase-3 expression and inhibition of cytochrome c release from the mitochondria [212, 220]. Finally, doxycycline has been shown to reduce cytokines IL-1α, IL-1β, IL-6, IL-8, and TNFα while increasing IL-10 and IL-12 after human monocytes were challenged with an oral pathogen [221].

Fluoroquinolone Antibiotics

The fluoroquinolone antibiotics have shown conflicting effects on the immune system in vitro ranging from anti-inflammatory to neutral to proinflammatory depending on the experiment methods, cell type, fluoroquinolone, and concentration used. Most in vivo data, however, suggest fluoroquinolone antibiotics modulate the immune system by decreasing proinflammatory cytokines. Ciprofloxacin was shown to reduce TNFα and IL-12 and increase IL-10 during a lipopolysaccharide challenge in mice. Although conflicting data on the immunomodulatory effects of fluoroquinolones exist, the balance of data suggests an anti-inflammatory effect. The mechanism for these actions is still unclear but thought to be possibly mediated by increasing cyclic AMP and acting on cellular transcription factors [213].

Dapsone and Sulfonamides

Compared to newer antibiotics, little data exist evaluating the anti-inflammatory effects of dapsone and sulfonamides, such as sulfamethoxazole. Dapsone has been used to treat urticaria in rare cases [222] and likely has immunomodulatory effects on neutrophils by inhibiting chemotaxis and oxidant production. The exact mechanism is unknown, although dapsone has been shown to inhibit myeloperoxidase [210].

Sulfonamide antibiotics, namely, sulfamethoxazole, used commonly in combination with trimethoprim, inhibit dihydropteroate synthase decreasing tetrahydrofolate synthesis in bacteria. The sulfonamide class of chemicals has a wide range of clinical applications including inflammatory conditions such as Crohn's disease and ulcerative colitis. Sulfamethoxazole's hydroxylamine metabolite has been implicated in inhibiting peripheral blood monocytes in vitro, reducing antibody production, and interfering with T lymphocyte signaling and proliferation [223–225]. Synergistic immunosuppression between tacrolimus and cyclosporine with the hydroxylamine metabolite was shown in mononuclear leukocytes [226].

In summary, a variety of immunomodulating effects from many antibiotics have been reported. Macrolide antibiotics are currently used in respiratory disease partially for their anti-inflammatory properties. The tetracyclines are used in mouthwashes for periodontal diseases and under investigation for various neurologic disorders. The sulfonamides are used for a wide variety of indications outside of antibiosis including inflammatory disorders. With exceptions for macrolides in respiratory diseases, the overall impact of antibiotic immunomodulation antibiotics is largely unknown and requires further research.

Conclusion

Placebo-controlled, pharmacokinetic drug interaction trials are lacking for most commonly used antibiotics. Consequently, evidence supporting suspected, possible, or probable interactions is often presented in the form of case reports and case series-literature. Although currently not well defined, pharmacogenomic factors such as CYP3A, MRP, and P-gp expression may help better predict relevant drug interactions at an individual level and become clinically useful. Advancements within pharmacogenomics beyond our present understanding someday in the near future may result in minimizing the impact of these interactions. For now, among recipients of SOT and HSCT, the drug classes of antimicrobials and immunosuppressives are inextricably woven, each very much contributing to prolonged survival of these patients. The current state of aggressive nosocomial infection, especially regarding virulence and antibiotic resistance characteristics, strenuously support antibiotic optimization principles [227]. Still, whether in the newly transplanted solid organ allograft recipient or the bone marrow transplant recipient long past engraftment, the successful concomitant use of antimicrobials and immunosuppressives demands for clinical vigilance to monitor efficacy and consideration for potential drug interactions and, notably, constant reassessment regarding adverse effects of antimicrobial therapy in this highly susceptible transplant population.

References

1. Bernardo JF, McCauley L. Drug therapy in transplant recipients: special considerations in the elderly with comorbid conditions. Drugs Aging. 2004;5:323–48.
2. Einarsen TR. Drug-related hospital admissions. Ann Pharmacother. 1993;27:832–40.
3. Strand LM, Morley PC, Cipolle RJ, Ramsey R, Lamsam GB. Drug-related problems: their structure and function. Ann Pharmacother. 1990;24:1093–7.
4. Leape LL, Brennan TA, Laird N, Lawthers AG, Localio AR, Barnes BA, et al. The nature of adverse events in hospitalized patients – results of the Harvard Medical Practice study II. N Engl J Med. 1991;324:377–84.
5. Fishman JA. Infection in solid organ transplant recipients. N Engl J Med. 2007;357:2601–14.
6. Srinivas TR, Meier-Kriesche HU, Kaplan B. Pharmacokinetic principles of immunosuppressive drugs. Am J Transplant. 2005;5:207–17.
7. de Jonge H, Naesens M, Kuypers DRJ. New insights into the pharmacokinetics and pharmacodynamics of the calcineurin inhibitors and mycophenolic acid: possible consequences for therapeutic drug monitoring in solid organ transplantation. Ther Drug Monit. 2009;31:416–35.
8. Cervera C, Fernández-Ruiz M, Valledor A, et al. Epidemiology and risk factors for late infection in solid organ transplant recipients. Transpl Infect Dis. 2011;13:598–607.
9. Hamandi B, Holbrook AM, Humar A, Brunton J, Papadimitropoulos EA, Wong GG, Thabane L. Delay of adequate empiric antibiotic therapy is associated with increased mortality among solid-organ transplant patients. Am J Transplant. 2009;9:1657–65.
10. Dellinger RP, Levy MM, Rhodes A, et al. Surviving Sepsis campaign: international guidelines for management of severe sepsis and septic shock: 2012. Crit Care Med. 2013;41:580–637.
11. Elbers PWG, Ince C. Bench-to-bedside review: mechanisms of critical illness – classifying microcirculatory flow abnormalities in distributive shock. Crit Care. 2006;10:221.
12. Gonçalves-Pereira J, Póvoa P. Antibiotics in critically ill patients: a systematic review of the pharmacokinetics of β-lactams. Crit Care. 2011;15:R206.
13. McKenzie C. Antibiotic dosing in critical illness. J Antimicrob Chemother. 2011;66(suppl 2):ii25–31.
14. Roberts JA, Lipman J. Pharmacokinetic issues for antibiotics in the critically ill patient. Crit Care Med. 2009;37:840–51.
15. Baptista JP, Udy AA, Sousa E, Pimentel J, Wang L, Roberts JA, Lipman J. A comparison of estimates of glomerular filtration in critically ill patients with augmented renal clearance. Crit Care. 2011;15:R139.
16. Vincent JL, Bassetti M, Francois B, et al. Advances in antibiotic therapy in the critically ill. Crit Care. 2016;20:133.

17. Moore RD, Lietman PS, Smith CR. Clinical response to aminoglycoside therapy: importance of the ratio of peak concentration to minimal inhibitory concentration. J Infect Dis. 1987;155:93–9.
18. Nicolau DP, Freeman CD, Belliveau PP, Nightingale CH, Ross JW, Quintillani R. Experience with a once-daily aminoglycoside program administered to 2,184 adult patients. Antimicrob Agents Chemother. 1995;39:650–5.
19. Rea RS, Capitano B, Dies R, Bigos KL, Smith R, Lee H. Suboptimal aminoglycoside dosing in critically ill patients. Ther Drug Monit. 2008;30:674–81.
20. Taccone FS, Laterre PF, Spapen H, et al. Revisiting the loading dose of amikacin for patients with severe sepsis and septic shock. Crit Care. 2010;14:R53.
21. Roger C, Nucci B, Louart B, et al. Impact of 30 mg/kg amikacin and 8 mg/kg gentamicin on serum concentrations in critically ill patients with severe sepsis. J Antimicrob Chemother. 2016;71:208–12.
22. Rybak M, Lomaestro B, Rotschafer JC, et al. Therapeutic monitoring of vancomycin in adult patients: a consensus review of the American society of health-system pharmacists, the infectious disease society of America, and the society of infectious disease pharmacists. Am J Health Syst Pharm. 2009;66:82–98.
23. Roberts JA, Taccone FS, Udy AA, Vincent JL, Frédérique J, Lipman J. Vancomycin dosing in critically ill patients: robust methods for improved continuous-infusion regimens. Antimicrob Agents Chemother. 2011;55:2704–9.
24. Pea F, Viale P, Pavan F, Furlanut M. Pharmacokinetic considerations for antimicrobial therapy in patients receiving renal replacement therapy. Clin Pharmacokinet. 2007;46:997–1038.
25. Li AMMY, Gomersall CD, Choi G, Tian Q, Joynt GM, Lipman J. A systematic review of antibiotic dosing regimens for septic patients receiving continuous renal replacement therapy: do current studies supply sufficient data? J Antimicrob Chemother. 2009;64:929–37.
26. Shekar K, Fraser JF, Smith MR, Roberts JA. Pharmacokinetic changes in patients receiving extracorporeal membrane oxygenation. J Crit Care. 2012;27(6):741.e9–18.
27. Gratwohl A, Baldomero H, Aljurf M, et al. Hematopoietic stem cell transplantation: a global perspective. JAMA. 2010;303:1617–24.
28. National Comprehensive Cancer Network. Prevention and treatment of cancer-related infections. Clinical Practice Guidelines in Oncology (NCCN Guidelines®), v.2.2016. May 20, 2016. http://www.nccn.org/professionals/physician_gls/pdf/infections.pdf
29. Zafrani L, Truffaut L, Kreis H, Etienne D, Rafat C, Lechaton S. Incidence, risk factors and clinical consequence of neutropenia following kidney transplantation: a retrospective study. Am J Transplant. 2009;9:1816–25.
30. Brum S, Nolasco F, Sousa J, Ferreira A, Possante M, Pinto JR, et al. Leukopenia in kidney transplant patients with the association of valganciclovir and mycophenolate mofetil. Transplant Proc. 2008;40:752–4.
31. Brennan DC, Daller JA, Lake KD, Cibrik D, Del Castillo D. Thymoglobulin induction study group. N Engl J Med. 2006;355:1967–77.
32. Hong JC, Kahan BD. Sirolimus-induced thrombocytopenia and leukopenia in renal transplant recipients: risk factors, incidence, progression, and management. Transplantation. 2000;69:2085–90.
33. Keisu M, Wiholm BE, Palmblad J. Trimethoprim-sulphamethoxazole-associated blood dyscrasias. Ten years' experience of the Swedish spontaneous reporting system. J Intern Med. 1990;228:353–60.
34. Mitsuhata N, Fujita R, Ito S, Mannami M, Keimei K. Delayed-onset neutropenia in a patient receiving rituximab as treatment for refractory kidney transplantation. Transplantation. 2005;80:1355.
35. Lortholary O, Lefort A, Tod M, Chomat AM, Darras-Joly C, Cordonnier C. Pharmacodyamics and pharmacokinetics of antibacterial drugs in the management of febrile neutropenia. Lancet Infect Dis. 2008;8:612–20.
36. Nyhlen A, Ljunberg B, Nilsson-Ehle I. Pharmacokinetics of meropenem in febrile neutropenic patients. Swedish study group. Eur J Clin Microbiol Infect Dis. 1997;16:797–802.
37. Drusano GL, Plaisance KI, Forrest A, Bustamante C, Devlin A, Standiford HC, et al. Steady-state pharmacokinetics of imipenem in febrile neutropenic cancer patients. Antimicrob Agents Chemother. 1987;31:1420–2.
38. Nyhlen A, Ljunberg B, Nilsson-Ehle I. Pharmacokinetics of ceftazidime in febrile neutropenic patients. Scand J Infect Dis. 2001;33:222–6.
39. Davis RL, Lehmann D, Stidley CA, Neidhart J. Amikacin pharmacokinetics in patients receiving high-dose cancer chemotherapy. Antimicrob Agents Chemother. 1991;35:944–7.
40. Hary L, Andrejak M, Bernaert F, Desablens B. Pharmacokinetics of amikacin in neutropenic patients. Curr Ther Res. 1989;46:821–7.
41. Kaojarern S, Maoleekoonpairoj S, Atichartakarn V. Pharmacokinetics of amikacin in hematologic malignancies. Antimicrob Agents Chemother. 1989;33:1406–8.
42. Phillips JK, Spearing RL, Crome DJ, Davies JM. Gentamicin volumes of distribution in patients with hematologic disorders. N Engl J Med. 1988;319:1290.
43. Higa GM, Murray WE. Alterations in aminoglycoside pharmacokinetics in patients with cancer. Clin Pharm. 1987;6:963–6.
44. Anon. Efficacy and toxicity of single daily doses of amikacin and ceftriaxone versus multiple daily doses of amikacin and ceftazidime for infection in patients with cancer and granulocytopenia. The International Antimicrobial Therapy Cooperative Group of the European Organization for Research and Treatment of Cancer. Ann Intern Med. 1993;119(7 Pt 1):584–93.
45. Sung L, Dupuis LL, Bliss B, Taddio A, Abdolell M, Allen U, et al. Randomized controlled trial of once- versus thrice-daily tobramycin in febrile neutropenic children undergoing stem cell transplantation. J Natl Cancer Inst. 2003;95:1869–77.
46. Fernandez de Gatta MM, Fruns I, Hernandez JM, Caballero D, San Migues JF, Martinex Lanao J, et al. Vancomycin pharmacokinetics and dosage requirements in hematologic malignancies. Clin Pharm. 1993;12:515–20.
47. Le Normand Y, Milpied N, Kergueris MF, Harousseau JL. Pharmacokinetic parameters of vancomycin for therapeutic regimens in neutropenic adult patients. Int J Biomed Comput. 1994;36:121–5.
48. Bubalo JS, Munar MY, Cherala G, Hayes-Lattin B, Maziarz R. Daptomycin pharmacokinetics in adult oncology patients with neutropenic fever. Antimicrob Agents Chemother. 2009;53:428–34.
49. Benvenuto M, Benziger DP, Yankelev S, Vigliani G. Pharmacokinetics and tolerability of daptomycin at does up to 12 milligrams per kilogram of body weight once daily in healthy volunteers. Antimicrob Agents Chemother. 2006;50:3245–9.
50. Smith PF, Birmingham MC, Noskin GA, Meagher AK, Forrest A, Rayner CR, et al. Safety, efficacy and pharmacokinetics of linezolid for treatment of resistant Gram-positive infections in cancer patients with neutropenia. Ann Oncol. 2003;14:795–801.
51. Andersohn F, Konzen C, Garbe E. Systematic review: agranulocytosis induced by nonchemotherapy drugs. Ann Intern Med. 2007;146:657–65.
52. Reagan JL, Castillo JJ. Why is my patient neutropenic? Hematol Oncol Clin N Am. 2012;26:253–66.
53. Andres E, Kurtz JE, Maloisel F. Nonchemotherapy drug-induced agranulocytosis: experience of the Strasbourg teaching hospital (1985–2000) and review of the literature. Clin Lab Haematol. 2002;24:99–106.
54. Monson T, Schichman SA, Zent CS. Linezolid induced pure red blood cell aplasia. Clin Infect Dis. 2002;35:e29–31.
55. Meehan KR, Verma UN, Esteva-Lorenzo F, Mazumder A. Suppression of progenitor cell growth by vancomycin following autologous stem cell transplantation. Bone Marrow Transplant. 1997;10:1029–32.

56. Singh N, Yu VL, Mieles LA, Wagener M. Beta-lactam antibiotic-induced leucopenia in severe hepatic dysfunction: risk factors and implications for dosing patients with liver disease. Am J Med. 1996;94:251–6.
57. Organ Procurement and Transplantation Network (OPTN) and Scientific Registry of Transplant Recipients (SRTR). OPTN / SRTR 2010 Annual Data Report. Rockville: Department of Health and Human Services, Health Resources and Services Administration, Healthcare Systems Bureau, Division of Transplantation; 2011.
58. Field TS, Gurwitz JH, Avorn J, McCormick D, Jain S, Eckler M, et al. Risk factors for adverse drug events among nursing home residents. Arch Intern Med. 2001;161:1629–34.
59. Shi S, Morike K, Klotz U. The clinical implications of ageing for rational drug therapy. Eur J Clin Pharmacol. 2008;64:183–99.
60. Feldman M. The mature stomach. Still pumping out acid? JAMA. 1997;278:681–2.
61. Orr WC, Chen CL. Aging and neural control of the GI tract: IV. Clinical and physiological aspects of gastrointestinal motility and aging. Am J Physiol Gastrointest Liver Physiol. 2002;283:G1226–31.
62. Corsonello A, Pedone C, Incalzi RA. Age-related pharmacokinetic and pharmacodynamic changes and related risk of adverse drug reactions. Curr Med Chem. 2010;17:571–84.
63. Forbes GB, Reina JC. Adult lean body mass declines with age: some longitudinal observations. Metabolism. 1970;19:653–63.
64. Anderson S, Brenner BM. Effects of aging on the renal glomerulus. Am J Med. 1986;80:435–42.
65. Benet LZ, Hoener BA. Changes in plasma protein binding have little clinical relevance. Clin Pharmacol Ther. 2002;71:115–21.
66. Le Couteur DG, McLean AJ. The aging liver. Drug clearance and an oxygen diffusion barrier hypothesis. Clin Pharmacokinet. 1998;34:230–2.
67. Le Couteur DG, Fraser R, Hilmer S, Rivory LP, McLean AJ. The hepatic sinusoid in aging and cirrhosis: effect on hepatic substrate disposition and drug clearance. Clin Pharmacokinet. 2005;44:187–200.
68. McLean AJ, Le Couteur DG. Aging biology and geriatric clinical pharmacology. Pharmacol Rev. 2004;56:163–84.
69. Corsonello A, Pedone C, Corica F, Mussi C, Carbonin P, Antonelli Incalzi R. Concealed renal insufficiency and adverse reactions in elderly hospitalize patients. Arch Intern Med. 2005;165:790–5.
70. Cockcroft DW, Gault MH. Prediction of creatinine clearance from serum creatinine. Nephron. 1976;16:31–41.
71. Levey AS, Bosch JP, Lewis JB, Greene T, Rogers N, Roth D. A more accurate method to estimate glomerular filtration rate from serum creatinine: a new prediction equation. Ann Intern Med. 1999;130:461–70.
72. Liou TG, Adler FR, Cahill BC, et al. Survival effect of lung transplantation among patients with cystic fibrosis. JAMA. 2001;286:2683–9.
73. Alexander BD, Petzold EW, Reller LB. Survival after lung transplantation of cystic fibrosis patients infected with Burkholderia cepacia complex. Am J Tranplant. 2008;8:1025–30.
74. Rosenblatt RL. Lung transplantation in cystic fibrosis. Respir Care. 2009;54:777–87.
75. Cox KL, Isenberg JN, Ament ME. Gastric acid hypersecretion in cystic fibrosis. J Pediatr Gastroenterol Nutr. 1982;1:559–65.
76. Fondacaro JD, Heubi JE, Kellogg FW. Intestinal bile acid malabsorption in cystic fibrosis: a primary mucosal cell defect. Pediatr Res. 1982;16:494–8.
77. Goldfarb J, Wormser GP, Inchiosa MA, et al. Ciprofloxacin pharmacokinetics in patients with cystic fibrosis. J Clin Pharmacol. 1986;26:222–6.
78. Reed MD, Stern RC, Myers CM, et al. Lack of unique ciprofloxacin pharmacokinetic characteristics in patients with cystic fibrosis. J Clin Pharmacol. 1988;28:691–9.
79. Christensson BA, Nilsson-Ehle I, Ljungberg B, et al. Increased oral bioavailability of ciprofloxacin in cystic fibrosis patients. Antimicrob Agents Chemother. 1992;28:691–9.
80. Lebel M, Bergeron MG, Vallee F, et al. Ciprofloxacin pharmacokinetics in patients with cystic fibrosis. Infection. 1986;14:17–21.
81. Davis RL, Koup JR, Williams-Warren J, et al. Pharmacokinetics of ciprofloxacin in cystic fibrosis. Antimicrob Agents Chemother. 1987;21:915–9.
82. Spino M, Chai RP, Isles AF, et al. Cloxacillin absorption and disposition in cystic fibrosis. J Pediatr. 1984;105:829–35.
83. Walker S, Habib S, Rose M, Yacoub M, Banner N. Clinical use and bioavailability of tacrolimus in heart-lung and double lung transplant recipients with cystic fibrosis. Transplant Proc. 1998;30:1519–20.
84. Gerbase MW, Fathi M, Spiliopoulos A, Rochat T, Nicod LP. Pharmacokinetics of mycophenolic acid associated with calcineurin inhibitors: long-term monitoring in stable lung transplant recipients with and without cystic fibrosis. J Heart Lung Transplant. 2003;22:587–90.
85. Levy J, Smith AL, Koup JR, et al. Disposition of tobramycin in patients with cystic fibrosis: a prospective controlled study. J Pediatr. 1984;105:117–24.
86. De Groot R, Hack BD, Weber A, Chaffin D, Ramsey B, Smith AL. Pharmacokinetics of ticarcillin in patients with cystic fibrosis: a controlled prospective study. Clin Pharmacol Ther. 1990;47:73–8.
87. Kearns GL, Hilman BC, Wilson JT. Dosing implications of altered gentamicin disposition in patients with cystic fibrosis. J Pediatr. 1982;100:312–8.
88. Rey E, Treluyer J, Gerard P. Drug disposition in cystic fibrosis. Clin Pharmacokinet. 1998;35:313–29.
89. O'Sullivan T, Wang JP, Unadkat JD, et al. Disposition of drugs in cystic fibrosis: V. in vivo CYP2C9 activity as probed by (S)-warfarin is not enhanced in cystic fibrosis. Clin Pharmacol Ther. 1993;54:323–8.
90. Parker AC, Pritchard P, Preston T, et al. Enhanced drug metabolism in young children with cystic fibrosis. Arch Dis Child. 1997;77:239–41.
91. Wang JP, Unadkat JD, McNamara S, et al. Disposition of drugs in cystic fibrosis: VI. In vivo activity of cytochrome P450 isoforms involved in the metabolism of (R)-warfarin (including P450 3A4) is not enhanced in cystic fibrosis. Clin Pharmacol Ther. 1993;55:528–34.
92. Jusko WJ, Mosovich LL, Gerbracht LM, Mattar ME, Yaffe SJ. Enhanced renal excretion of dicloxacillin in patients with cystic fibrosis. Pediatrics. 1975;56:1038–44.
93. Reed MD, Stern RC, Bertino JS, et al. Dosing implications of rapid elimination of trimethoprim-sulfamethoxazole in patients with cystic fibrosis. J Pediatr. 1984;104:303–7.
94. Walsh KA, Davis GA, Hayes D, Kuhn RJ, Weant KA, Flynn JD. Tobramycin pharmacokinetics in patients with cystic fibrosis before and after bilateral lung transplantation. Transpl Infect Dis. 2011;13:616–21.
95. Dupuis RE, Sredzienski EJ. Tobramycin pharmacokinetics in patients with cystic fibrosis preceding and following lung transplantation. Ther Drug Monit. 1999;21:161–5.
96. Bennett WM, McEvoy KM, Henell KR, Valente JF, Douzkjian V. Morbid obesity does not preclude successful renal transplantation. Clin Transpl. 2004;18:89–93.
97. Singh D, Lawen J, Alkhudair W. Does pretransplant obesity affect the outcome in kidney transplant recipients? Transplant Proc. 2005;37:717–20.
98. Sawyer RG, Pelletier SJ, Pruett TL. Increased early morbidity and mortality with acceptable long-term function in severely obese patients undergoing liver transplantation. Clin Transpl. 1999;13:126–30.

99. Hanish SI, Petersen RP, Collins BH, et al. Obesity predicts increased overall complications following pancreas transplantation. Transplant Proc. 2005;37:3564–6.
100. Kocher AA, Ankersmit J, Khazen C, et al. Effect of obesity on outcome after cardiac transplantation. Transplant Proc. 1999;31:3187–9.
101. Gill JS, Lan J, Dong J, Rose C, Hendren E, Johnston O, Gill J. The survival benefit of kidney transplantation in obese patients. Am J Transplant. 2013;13:2083–90.
102. Leonard J, Heimbach JK, Malinchoc M, Watt K, Charlton M. The impact of obesity on long-term outcomes in liver transplant recipients – results of the NIDDK liver transplant database. Am J Transplant. 2008;8:667–72.
103. Ogden CL, Carroll MD, Kit BK, Flegal, KM. Prevalence of obesity in the United States, 2009–2010. NCHS data brief, no 82. Hyattsville: National Center for Health Statistics; 2012.
104. Bianchi G, Marchesini G, Marzocchi R, Pinna AD, Zoli M. Metabolic syndrome in liver transplantation: relation to etiology and immunosuppression. Liver Transpl. 2008;14:1648–54.
105. Stegall MD, Everson G, Schroter G, Bilir B, Karrer F, Kam I. Metabolic complications after liver transplantation. Diabetes, hypercholesterolemia, hypertension, and obesity. Transplantation. 1995;60:1057–60.
106. Everhart JE, Lombardero M, Lake JR, Wiesner RH, Zetterman RK, Hoofnagle J. Weight change and obesity after liver transplantation: incidence and risk factors. J Liver Transpl Surg. 1998;4:285–96.
107. Canzanello VJ, Schwartz L, Taler SJ, Textor SC, Wiesner RH, Porayko MK, Krom RA. Evolution of cardiovascular risk after liver transplantation: a comparison of cyclosporine A and tacrolimus (FK506). Liver Transpl Surg. 1997;3:1–9.
108. Abernethy DR, Greenblatt DJ. Drug disposition in obese humans: an update. Clin Pharmacokinet. 1986;11:199–213.
109. Pai MP, Bearden DT. Antimicrobial dosing considerations in obese patients. Pharmacotherapy. 2007;27:1081–91.
110. Rea DJ, Heimbach JK, Grande JP, et al. Glomerular volume and renal histology in obese and non-obese living kidney donors. Kidney Int. 2006;70:1636–41.
111. Verhave JC, Fesler P, Ribstein J, du Cailar G, Mimran A. Estimation of renal function in subjects with normal serum creatinine levels: influence of age and body mass index. Am J Kidney Dis. 2005;46:233–41.
112. Dionne RE, Bauer LA, Gibson GA, Griffen WO Jr, Blouin RA. Estimating creatinine clearance in morbidly obese patients. Am J Hosp Pharm. 1981;38:841–4.
113. Levey AS, Coresh J, Greene T, et al. Expressing the MDRD study equation for estimating GFR with IDMS traceable (gold standard) serum creatinine values. J Am Soc Nephrol. 2005;16:69A.
114. Bauer LA, Black DJ, Lill JS. Vancomycin dosing in morbidly obese patients. Eur J Clin Pharmacol. 1998;54:621–5.
115. Hall RG, Kenna D, Payne BAM, et al. Multicenter evaluation of vancomycin dosing: emphasis on obesity. Am J Med. 2008;121:515–8.
116. Bauer LA, Edward WA, Dellinger EP, Simonowitz DA. Influence of weight on aminoglycoside pharmacokinetics in normal weight and morbidly obese patients. Eur J Clin Pharmacol. 1983;24:643–7.
117. Traynor AM, Nafziger AN, Bertino JS Jr. Aminoglycoside dosing weight correction factors for patients of various body sizes. Antimicrob Agents Chemother. 1995;39:545–8.
118. Forse RA, Karam B, MacLean LD, Christou NV. Antibiotic prophylaxis for surgery in morbidly obese patients. Surgery 1989;106:750–6.
119. Bratzler DW, Dellinger EP, Olsen KM, et al. Clinical practice guidelines for antimicrobial prophylaxis in surgery. Am J Health Syst Pharm. 2013;70:195–283.
120. Dvorchik BH, Damphousse D. The pharmacokinetics of daptomycin in moderately obese, morbidly obese, and matched nonobese subjects. J Clin Pharmacol. 2005;45:48–56.
121. Mersfelder TL, Smith CL. Linezolid pharmacokinetics in an obese patient. Am J Health Syst Pharm. 2005;62:464–7.
122. Meagher AK, Forrest A, Rayner CR, Birmingham MC, Schentag JJ. Population pharmacokinetics of linezolid in patients treated in a compassionate-use program. Antimicrob Agents Chemother. 2003;47:548–53.
123. Stein GE, Schooley SL, Peloquin CA, et al. Pharmacokinetics and pharmacodynamics of linezolid in obese patients with cellulitis. Ann Pharmacother. 2005;39:427–32.
124. Page RL II, Miller GG, Lindenfeld J. Drug therapy in the heart transplant recipient: part IV: drug-drug interactions. Circulation. 2005;111:230–9.
125. Page RL II, Mueller SW, Levi ME, Lindenfeld J. Pharmacokinetic drug- drug interactions between calcineurin inhibitors and proliferation signal inhibitors with anti-microbial agents: implications for therapeutic drug monitoring. J Heart Lung Transplant. 2011;30:124–35.
126. Padhi ID, Long P, Basha M, et al. Interaction between tacrolimus and erythromycin. Ther Drug Monit. 1997;19:120–2.
127. Periti P, Mazzei T, Mini E, et al. Pharmacokinetic drug interactions of macrolides. Clin Pharmacokinet. 1992;23:106–31.
128. Capone D, Palmiero G, Gentile A, et al. A pharmacokinetic interaction between clarithromycin and sirolimus in kidney transplant recipient. Curr Drug Metab. 2007;8:379–81.
129. Kovarik JM, Beyer D, Bizot MN, et al. Effect of multiple-dose erythromycin on everolimus pharmacokinetics. Eur J Clin Pharmacol. 2005;61:35–8.
130. Claesson K, Brattstrom C, Burke JT. Sirolimus and erythromycin interaction: two cases. Transplant Proc. 2001;33:2136.
131. Page RL II, Ruscin JM, Fish D, et al. Possible interaction between intravenous azithromycin and oral cyclosporine. Pharmacotherapy. 2001;21:1436–43.
132. Mori T, Aisa Y, Nakazato T, et al. Tacrolimus-azithromycin interaction in a recipient of allogeneic bone marrow transplantation. Transplant Int. 2005;18:757–8.
133. Kovarik JM, Hsu CH, McMahon L, et al. Population pharmacokinetics of everolimus in de novo renal transplant patients: impact of ethnicity and comedications. Clin Pharmacol Ther. 2001;70:247–54.
134. Finch CK, Chrisman CR, Baciewicz AM, et al. Rifampin and rifabutin drug interactions: an update. Arch Intern Med. 2002;162:985–92.
135. Freitag VL, Skifton RD, Lake KD. Effect of short-term rifampin on stable cyclosporine concentrations. Ann Pharmacother. 1999;333:871–2.
136. Rapamune [package insert]. Philadelphia: Wyeth-Ayerst; April 2010.
137. Kovarik JM, Hartmann S, Figueiredo J, et al. Effect of rifampin on apparent clearance of everolimus. Ann Pharmacother. 2002;36:981–5.
138. Vandevelde C, Chang A, Andrews D, et al. Rifampin and ansamycin interactions with cyclosporine after renal transplantation. Pharmacotherapy. 1991;11:88–9.
139. Lopez-Montes A, Gallego E, Lopez E, et al. Treatment of tuberculosis with rifabutin in a renal transplant recipient. Am J Kidney Dis. 2004;44:e59–63.
140. Christians U, Strom T, Hang YL, et al. Active drug transport of immunosuppressants: new insights for pharmacokinetics and pharmacodynamics. Ther Drug Monit. 2006;28:39–44.
141. Amundsen R, Asberg A, Ohm IK, Christensen H. Cyclosporin A- and tacrolimus-medicated inhibition of CYP3A4 and CYP3A5 in vitro. Drug Metab Dispos. 2012;40:655–61.

142. Bullingham R, Monroe S, Nicholls A, et al. Pharmacokinetics and bioavailability of mycophenolate mofetil in healthy subjects after single-dose oral and intravenous administration. J Clin Pharmacol. 1996;36:315–24.
143. Picard N, Ratanasavanh D, Premaud A, et al. Identification of the UDP-glucuronosyltransferase isoforms involved in mycophenolic acid phase II metabolism. Drug Metab Dispos. 2005;33:139–46.
144. Naderer OJ, Dupuis RE, Heinzen EL, et al. Ther influence of norfloxacin and metronidazole on the disposition of mycophenolat mofetil. J Clin Pharmacol. 2005;45:219–26.
145. Borrows R, Chusney G, Loucaidou M, et al. The magnitude and time course of changes in mycophenolic acid 12-hour predose levels during antibiotic therapy in mycophenolate mofetil-based renal transplantation. Ther Drug Monit. 2007;29:122–6.
146. Naesens M, Kuypers DRJ, Streit F, et al. Rifampin induces alterations in mycophenolic acid glucuronidation and elimination: implications for drug exposure in renal allograft recipients. Clin Pharmacol Ther. 2006;80:509–21.
147. Kuypers DRJ, Verleden G, Naesens M, Vanrenterghem Y. Drug interaction between mycophenolate mofetil and rifampin: possible induction of uridine diphosphate-glucuronosyltransferase. Clin Pharmacol Ther. 2005;78:81–8.
148. Barau C, Barrail-Tran A, Hemerziu B, et al. Optimization of the dosing regimen of mycophenolate mofetil in pediatric liver transplant recipients. Liver Transpl. 2011;17:1152–8.
149. Czock D, Keller F, Rasche FM, Häussler U. Pharmacokinetics and pharmacodynamics of systemically administered glucocorticoids. Clin Pharmacokinet. 2005;44:61–98.
150. LaForce CF, Szefler SJ, Miller MF, Ebling W, Brenner M. Inhibition of methylprednisolone elimination in the presence of erythromycin therapy. J Allergy Clin Immunol. 1983;72:34–9.
151. Fost DA, Leung DY, Martin RJ, Brown EE, Szefler SJ, Spahn JD. Inhibition of methylprednisolone elimination in the presence of clarithromycin therapy. J Allergy Clin Immunol. 1999;103:1031–5.
152. McAllister WA, Thompson PJ, Al-Habet SM, Rogers HJ. Rifampicin reduces effectiveness and bioavailability of prednisolone. Br Med J (Clin Res Ed). 1983;286:923–5.
153. Carrie F, Roblot P, Bouquet S, Delon A, Roblot F, Becq-Giraudon B. Rifampin induced nonresponsiveness of giant cell arteritis to prednisone treatment. Arch Intern Med. 1994;154:1521–4.
154. Hodak SP, Moubarak JB, Rodriguez I, Gelfand MC, Mohammad AR, Tracy CM. QT prolongation and near fatal cardiac arrhythmia after intravenous tacrolimus administration: a case report. Transplantation. 1998;66:535–7.
155. Akers WS, Flynn JD, Davis GA, Green AE, Winstead PS, Strobel G. Prolonged cardiac repolarization after tacrolimus and haloperidol administration in the critically ill patient. Pharmacotherapy. 2004;24:404–8.
156. Arizona CERT. QT drug list by risk groups. Available at: www.QTdrugs.org. Accessed 12 Mar 2012.
157. Sands M, Brown RB. Interactions of cyclosporine with antimicrobial agents. Rev Infect Dis. 1989;11:691–7.
158. Turhal NS. Cyclosporin A and imipenem associated seizure activity in allogeneic bone marrow transplantation patients. J Chemother. 1999;11:410–3.
159. Dudley MN, Loutit J, Griffith DC. Aerosol antibiotics: considerations in pharmacological and clinical evaluation. Curr Opin Biotechnol. 2008;19:637–43.
160. Kuhn RJ. Pharmaceutical considerations in aerosol drug delivery. Pharmacotherapy. 2002;22(3 Pt 2):80S–5S.
161. Tayab ZR, Gunther H. Pharmacokinetic/pharmacodynamics evaluation of inhalation drugs: application to targeted pulmonary delivery systems. Expert Opin Drug Deliv. 2005;2:519–32.
162. Le J, Ashley ED, Neuhauser MM, et al. Consensus summary of aerosolized antimicrobial agents: application of guideline criteria. Insights from the Society of Infectious Diseases Pharmacists. Pharmacotherapy. 2010;30:562–84.
163. Shirk MB, Donahue KR, Shirvani J. Unlabeled uses of nebulized medications. Am J Health Syst Pharm. 2006;63:1704–16.
164. Kesser KC, Geller DE. New aerosol delivery devices for cystic fibrosis. Respir Care. 2009;54:754–67.
165. Dolovich MB, Ahrens RC, Hess DR, et al. Device selection and outcomes of aerosol therapy: evidence-based guidelines: American College of Chest Physicians/ American College of Asthma, Allergy, and Immunology. Chest. 2005;127:335–71.
166. Corcoran TE. Aerosol drug delivery in lung transplant recipients. Expert Opin Drug Deliv. 2009;6:139–48.
167. Corcoran TE, Smaldone GC, Dauber JH. Preservation of post-transplant lung function with aerosol cyclosporine. Eur Respir J. 2004;23:378–83.
168. Corcoran TE, Venkataramanan R, Mihelc KM. Aerosol deposition of lipid complex amphotericin-B (Abelcet) in lung transplant recipients. Am J Transplant. 2006;11:2765–73.
169. Ramsey BW, Pepe MS, Quan JM, et al. Intermittent administration of inhaled tobramycin in patients with cystic fibrosis. Cystic Fibrosis Inhaled Tobramycin Study Group. N Engl J Med. 1999;340:23–30.
170. Moss RB. Long-term benefits of inhaled tobramycin in adolescent patients with cystic fibrosis. Chest. 2002;121:55–63.
171. Burns JL, Van Dalfsen JM, Shawar RM, et al. Effect of chronic intermittent administration of inhaled tobramycin on respiratory microbial flora in patients with cystic fibrosis. J Infect Dis. 1999;179:1190–6.
172. Bowman CM. The long-term use of inhaled tobramycin in patients with cystic fibrosis. J Cyst Fibros. 2002;1(Suppl 2):194–8.
173. Lu Q, Yang J, Liu Z, Gutierrez C, Aymard G, Rouby JJ, Nebulized Antibiotics Study Group. Nebulized ceftazidime and amikacin in ventilator associated pneumonia caused by Pseudomonas aeruginosa. Am J Respir Crit Care Med. 2011;184:106–15.
174. Stead RJ, Hodson ME, Batten JC. Inhaled ceftazidime compared with gentamicin and carbenicillin in older patients with cystic fibrosis infected with Pseudomonas aeruginosa. Br J Dis Chest. 1987;81:272–9.
175. Safdar A. Aerosolized amikacin in patients with difficult to-treat pulmonary nontuberculous mycobacteriosis. Eur J Clin Microbiol Infect Dis. 2012;31(8):1883–7.
176. Ghannam DE, Rodriguez GH, Raad II, Safdar A. Inhaled aminoglycosides in cancer patients with ventilator-associated Gram-negative bacterial pneumonia: safety and feasibility in the era of escalating drug resistance. Eur J Clin Microbiol Infect Dis. 2009;28:253–9.
177. TOBI (tobramycin inhalation solution) [package insert]. East Hanover: Novartis Pharmaceuticals Corporation; November 2009.
178. Rubin BK. Aerosolized antibiotics for non-cystic fibrosis bronchiectasis. J Aerosol Med Pulm Drug Deliv. 2008;21:71–6.
179. Ahya VN, Doyle AM, Mendez JD, et al. Renal and vestibular toxicity due to inhaled tobramycin in a lung transplant recipient. J Heart Lung Transplant. 2005;24:932–5.
180. Laporta R, Ussetti P, Carreño MC. Renal toxicity due to inhaled tobramycin in lung transplant recipients. J Heart Lung Transplant. 2006;25:608.
181. Falagas ME, Siempos II, Bliziotis IA, Michalopoulos A. Administration of antibiotics via the respiratory tract for the prevention of ICU-acquired pneumonia: a meta-analysis of comparative results. Crit Care. 2006;10:R123.
182. Safdar A, Shelburne SA, Evans SE, Dickey BF. Inhaled therapeutics for prevention and treatment of pneumonia. Expert Opin Drug Saf. 2009;8:435–49.

183. Safdar A. Feasibility of aerosolized colistin in the era of escalating drug-resistant Pseudomonas pneumonia: pressing need for validation clinical trials. Intensive Care Med. 2010;36:1110–1.
184. Kwa AL, Loh C, Low JG, Kurup A, Tam VH. Nebulized colistin in the treatment of pneumonia due to multidrug-resistant Acinetobacter baumannii and Pseudomonas aeruginosa. Clin Infect Dis. 2005;41:754–7.
185. Michalopoulos A, Fotakis D, Virtzili S, et al. Aerosolized colistin as adjunctive treatment of ventilator-associated pneumonia due to multidrug-resistant Gram-negative bacteria: a prospective study. Respir Med. 2008;102:407–12.
186. Rattanaumpawan P, Lorsutthitham J, Ungprasert P, Angkasekwinai N, Thamlikitkul V. Randomized controlled trial of nebulized colistimethate sodium as adjunctive therapy of ventilator-associated pneumonia caused by Gram-negative bacteria. J Antimicrob Chemother. 2010;65:2645–9.
187. Alothman GA, Ho B, Alsaadi MM, Ho SL, O'Drowsky L, Louca E, Coates AL. Bronchial constriction and inhaled colistin in cystic fibrosis. Chest. 2005;127:522–9.
188. Falagas ME, Kasiakou SK. Colistin: the revival of polymyxins for the management of multidrug-resistant gram-negative bacterial infections. Clin Infect Dis. 2005;40:1333–41.
189. Hodson ME, Gallagher CG, Govan JR. A randomised clinical trial of nebulised tobramycin or colistin in cystic fibrosis. Eur Respir J. 2002;20:658–64.
190. Adeboyeku D, Scott S, Hodson ME. Open follow-up study of tobramycin nebuliser solution and colistin in patients with cystic fibrosis. J Cyst Fibros. 2006;5:261–3.
191. U.S Food and Drug Administration. Information for healthcare professionals on colistimethate. http://www.fda.gov/Drugs/DrugSafety/PostmarketDrugSafetyInformation forPatientsandProviders/ucm124896.htm. Accessed 19 June 2012.
192. Cayston (aztreonam lysine for inhalation) [package insert]. Foster City: Gilead Sciences, Inc; February 2010.
193. Lu Q, Yang J, Liu Z, et al. Nebulized ceftazidime and amikacin in ventilator-associated pneumonia caused by Pseudomonas aeruginosa. Am J Respir Crit Care Med. 2011;184:106–15.
194. Stockley RA, Hill SL, Burnett D. Nebulized amoxicillin in chronic purulent bronchiectasis. Clin Ther. 1985;7:593–9.
195. Botha P, Archer L, Anderson R, et al. Pseudomonas aeruginosa colonization of the allograft after lung transplantation and the risk of bronchiolitis obliterans syndrome. Transplantation. 2008;85:771–4.
196. Retsch-Bogart GZ, Quittner AL, Gibson RL. Efficacy and safety of inhaled aztreonam lysine for airway pseudomonas in cystic fibrosis. Chest. 2009;135:1223–32.
197. McCoy KS, Quittner AL, Oermann CM, Gibson RL, Retsch-Bogart GZ, Montgomery AB. Inhaled aztreonam lysine for chronic airway Pseudomonas aeruginosa in cystic fibrosis. Am J Respir Crit Care Med. 2008;178:921–8.
198. Wainwright CE, Quittner AL, Geller DE, et al. Aztreonam for inhalation solution (AZLI) in patients with cystic fibrosis, mild lung impairment, and P. aeruginosa. J Cyst Fibros. 2011;10:234–42.
199. Suhling H, Rademacher J, Greer M, Haverich A, Warnecke G, Gottlieb J, Welte T. Inhaled colistin following lung transplantation in colonized cystic fibrosis patients. Eur Respir J. 2013;42(2):542–4.
200. Kalil AC, Metersky ML, Klompas M, et al. Management of Adults with Hospital-acquired and Ventilator-associated Pneumonia: 2016 clinical practice guidelines by the Infectious Diseases Society of America and the American Thoracic Society. Clin Infect Dis. 2016;63(5):e61–e111.
201. Doshi NM, Cook CH, Mount KL, et al. Adjunctive aerosolized colistin for multi- drug resistant gram-negative pneumonia in the critically ill: a retrospective study. BMC Anesthesiol. 2013;13:45.
202. Valachis A, Samonis G, Kofteridis DP. The role of aerosolized colistin in the treatment of ventilator-associated pneumonia: a systematic review and metaanalysis. Crit Care Med. 2015;43:527–33.
203. Hallal A, Cohn SM, Namias N, et al. Aerosolized tobramycin in the treatment of ventilator-associated pneumonia: a pilot study. Surg Infect. 2007;8:73–82.
204. Davis KK, Kao PN, Jacobs SS, Ruoss SJ. Aerosolized amikacin for treatment of pulmonary Mycobacterium avium infections: an observational case series. BMC Pulm Med. 2007;7:2–6.
205. Trapnell BC, McColley SA, Kissner DG, et al. Fosfomycin/tobramycin for inhalation in patients with cystic fibrosis with Pseudomonas airway infection. Am J Respir Crit Care Med. 2012;185:171–8.
206. Flume PA, VanDevanter DR, Morgan EE, et al. A phase 3, multicenter, multinational, randomized, double-blind, placebo-controlled study to evaluate the efficacy and safety of levofloxacin inhalation solution (APT-1026) in stable cystic fibrosis patients. J Cyst Fibros. 2016;15(4):495–502.
207. Eagle G. Study to evaluate efficacy of LAI when added to multidrug regimen compared to multi-drug regimen alone (CONVERT). In: Clinical Trials.gov 20161116. Available from: https://clinicaltrials.gov/ct2/show/NCT02344004
208. Dasenbrook E. Efficacy and safety of AeroVanc for the treatment of persistent MRSA lung infection in cystic fibrosis patients. In: Clinical Trials.gov [Internet]. Bethesda: National Library of Medicine (US). 2000-20161116. Available from: http://clinicaltrials.gov/show/NCT01746095
209. Altenburg J, de Graaff CS, van der Werf TS, Boersma WG. Immunomodulatory effects of macrolide antibiotics – part 1: biologic mechanisms. Respiration. 2011;81:67–74.
210. Labro MT. Interference of antibacterial agents with phagocyte functions: immunomodulation or "immune-fairy tales?". Clin Microbiol Rev. 2000;13:615–50.
211. Zarogoulidis P, Papanas N, Kioumis I, Chatzaki E, Maltezos E, Zarogoulidis K. Macrolides: from in vitro anti-inflammatory and immunomodulatory properties to clinical practice in respiratory disease. Eur J Clin Pharmacol. 2012;68:479–503.
212. Griffin MO, Fricovsky E, Ceballos G, Villarreal F. Tetracyclines: a pleotropic family of compounds with promising therapeutic properties. Review of the literature. Am J Physiol Cell Physiol. 2010;299:C539–48.
213. Dalhoff A. Immunomodulatory activities of fluoroquinolones. Infection. 2005;33(suppl 2):55–70.
214. Sakito O, Kadota J, Kohno S, Abe K, Shirai R, Hara K. Interleukin 1 beta, tumor necrosis factor alpha, and interleukin 8 in bronchoalveolar lavage fluid of patients with diffuse panbronchiolitis: a potential mechanism of macrolide therapy. Respiration. 1996;63:42–8.
215. Sharma S, Jaffe A, Dixon G. Immunomodulatory effects of macrolide antibiotics in respiratory disease: therapeutic implications for asthma and cystic fibrosis. Pediatr Drugs. 2007;9:107–18.
216. Labro MT. Anti-inflammatory activity of macrolides: a new therapeutic potential? J Antimicrob Chemother. 1998;41(suppl. B):37–46.
217. Jamieson B, Oldach DW, Clark K, et al. Solithromycin, a novel IV and oral fluoroketolide, with enhanced antibacterial and immunomodulatory activity for CABP. Am J Respir Crit Care Med. 2013;187:A1697. [Abstract].
218. Muira Y, Payne MS, Keelan JA, et al. Maternal intravenous treatment with either azithromycin or solithromycin clears Ureaplasma parvum from the amniotic fluid in an ovine model of intrauterine infection. Antimicrob Agents Chemother. 2014;58:5413–20.
219. Singh LP, Mishra A, saha D, Swarnakar S. Doxycycline blocks gastric ulcer by regulating matrix metalloproteinase-2 activity and oxidative stress. World J Gastroenterol. 2011;17:3310–21.

220. Leite LM, Carvalho AGG, Ferreira PLFT, et al. Anti-inflammatory properties of doxycycline and minocycline in experimental models: an in vivo and in vitro comparative study. Inflammopharmacology. 2011;19:99–110.
221. Bostanci N, Akgül B, Tsakanika V, Allaker RP, Hughes FJ, McKay IJ. Effects of low-dose doxycycline on cytokine secretion in human monocytes stimulated with Aggregatibacter actinomycetemcomitans. Cytokine. 2011;56:656–61.
222. Weller K, Schoepke N, Krause K, Ardelean E, Bräutigam M, Maurer M. Selected urticarial patients benefit from a referral to tertiary care centres – results of an expert survey. J Eur Acad Dermatol Venereol. 2013 Jan;27(1):e8–16.
223. Rieder MJ, Sisson E, Bird IA, Almawi WY. Suppression of t-lymphocyte proliferation by sulphonamide hydroxylamines. Int J Immunopharmacol. 1992;14:1175–80.
224. Sisson ME, Rieder MJ, Bird IA, Almawi WY. Suppression of pokeweed mitogen-driven human IgM and IgG responses by the hydroxylamine of sulfamethoxazole. Int J Immunopharmacol. 1997;19:299–304.
225. Hess DA, Rieder MJ. Interference in IL-2 receptor mediated janus kinase activation by the hydroxylamine of sulfamethoxazole. Clin Pharmacol Ther. 1998;63:138. (abstract PI-3).
226. Hess DA, Bird IA, Almawi WY, Rieder MJ. The hydroxylamine of sulfamethoxazole synergizes with FK506 and cyclosporine A, inhibiting T-cell proliferation. J Pharmacol Exp Ther. 1997;281:540–8.
227. Roberts JA, Kruger P, Paterson DL, Lipman J. Antibiotic resistance – What's dosing got to do with it? Crit Care Med. 2008;36:2433–40.

Antifungal Consideration for Transplant Recipients

52

Yanina Dubrovskaya, Man Yee Merl, David S. Perlin, and Amar Safdar

Introduction

Due to recent advances in hematopoietic stem cell and solid organ transplantation (HSCT and SOT, respectively), the disease-free survival among transplant recipients continues to improve. Prolonged immunosuppression, conditioning preparatory chemotherapy, extended duration of pre-HSCT engraftment neutropenia, drug given to suppress adaptive cellular immune response for prevention and treatment of GVHD, and for preservation of visceral allograft predisposes transplant recipients to opportunistic fungal disease. These infections increase morbidity and risk of death among patients undergoing at risk transplantation procedures [1, 2].

Antifungal Classes

Three main classes of antifungal agents are available for systemic prophylaxis and treatment of invasive fungal infections (IFIs). These include polyenes, triazoles, and echinocandins.

Polyenes such as nystatin and amphotericin B (AmB) were the first drugs to be approved for clinical use in the United States; AmB deoxycholate became available for human use in 1957. AmB is a polyene macrolide antibiotic derived from the actinomycete *Streptomyces nodosus*. AmB is approved for the treatment of aspergillosis, cryptococcosis, blastomycosis, systemic candidiasis, coccidioidomycosis, histoplasmosis, and mucormycosis. AmB is named for its amphoteric behavior. It forms relatively soluble salts in basic or acidic aqueous media; however at the physiologic pH, it becomes insoluble in aqueous solutions. AmB is formulated for intravenous (IV) administration as a colloidal suspension by using the bile salt deoxycholate and sodium phosphate buffer. During the 1990s, lipid formulations, amphotericin B lipid complex (Abelcet®, ABLC), amphotericin B colloidal dispersion (Amphotec®, ABCD), and liposomal amphotericin B (AmBisome®, L-AmB) were developed to mitigate nephrotoxicity common with exposure to AmB deoxycholate. ABLC was approved for second-line treatment of IFIs in patients with refractory infections or those who were intolerant to AmB therapy. L-AmB was approved by the Food and Drug Administration (FDA) for empirical therapy in patients with febrile neutropenia, for the treatment of cryptococcal meningitis in human immunodeficiency virus (HIV) patients, for treatment of visceral leishmaniasis, and second-line treatment of aspergillosis, candidiasis, or cryptococcosis refractory to AmB deoxycholate or in patients, in whom renal impairment or unacceptable drug toxicity precluded the use of AmB deoxycholate. Lipid formulations of AmB are generally considered interchangeable with AmB but with considerably improved safety profiles [3–7].

The discovery of azole-based antifungal drugs was a notable step forward given the safety, efficacy, and oral bioavailability of these agents. The azoles are characterized by their core five-member azole ring, which contains two nitrogen (imidazoles) or three nitrogen molecules (triazoles). Triazole-based antifungals include fluconazole, itraconazole, voriconazole, posaconazole, and isavuconazonium sulfate. Favorable safety profile, fungal enzyme-specific target without crossover damage to mammalian cells unlike

Y. Dubrovskaya
NYU Langone Medical Center, NYU Langone Health, Department of Pharmacy, New York, NY, USA
e-mail: yanina.dubrovskaya@nyumc.org

M. Y. Merl
Smilow Cancer Hospital at Yale-New Haven Health, Department of Pharmacy, New Haven, CT, USA
e-mail: manyee.merl@ynhh.org

D. S. Perlin
Public Health Research Institute, Rutgers Biomedical and Health Sciences, Rutgers New Jersey Medical School, Newark, NJ, USA
e-mail: perlinds@njms.rutgers.edu

A. Safdar (✉)
Clinical Associate Professor of Medicine, Texas Tech University Health Sciences Center El Paso, Paul L. Foster School of Medicine, El Paso, TX, USA
e-mail: amar.safdar@cidimmunology.com

A. Safdar (ed.), *Principles and Practice of Transplant Infectious Diseases*, https://doi.org/10.1007/978-1-4939-9034-4_52

AmB make them preferred agents to treat IFIs. The newer triazoles known for their mold-active potency such as voriconazole, posaconazole, and isavuconazonium sulfate are synthetic derivatives of fluconazole and itraconazole with an improved spectrum of activity against filamentous fungi. Fluconazole was approved for treatment of candidiasis, cryptococcal meningitis, and antifungal prophylaxis in patients undergoing HSCT. Voriconazole was licensed in the United States in 2003 as a first-line agent to treat patients with invasive aspergillosis (IA) and invasive candidiasis in the non-neutropenic host and as a second-line therapy for IFIs due to *Scedosporium* and *Fusarium* species. Posaconazole was initially approved in 2006 for IFI prophylaxis in severely immunocompromised patients undergoing HSCT with GVHD and for the treatment of oropharyngeal candidiasis [3, 4, 8–11].

The echinocandin drugs caspofungin, micafungin, and anidulafungin are semisynthetic derivatives of a separate class of antifungals known as pneumocandins. These are large lipopeptide molecules with amphiphilic cyclic hexapeptide and *N*-linked acyl lipid side chain and can only be administered via IV route. The differences in composition of the side chain make each echinocandin structurally unique. Caspofungin acetate was first in this class to become available for clinical use (approved in 2001) as an agent for patients with conventional AmB treatment-refractory IA. This was soon followed by an expanded label indication including empiric therapy for presumed fungal infections in patients with febrile neutropenia and treatment of invasive candidiasis. Subsequently, micafungin and anidulafungin were added. Micafungin was approved by the FDA in 2005 for treatment of invasive candidiasis and prophylaxis of invasive candidiasis in HSCT recipients. Anidulafungin was approved in 2006 for the treatment of invasive candidiasis [3, 4, 12–14].

Mechanism of Action

Polyenes target the fungal cytoplasmic membrane by specific interaction with ergosterol in the fungal cell membrane by creating nonaqueous and aqueous channels. Efflux of potassium through the pores results in the loss of membrane potential and subsequent physiologic collapse and cell death. At low concentrations of AmB, the channels are permeable only to monovalent cations such as potassium. At high concentrations of AmB, the nonaqueous channels interact with cholesterol in the mammalian host cell membrane to form aqueous pores that are permeable to chloride and potassium. This results in increased permeability to H^+/OH^-, intracellular acidification, and subsequent membrane damage. AmB has higher affinity for ergosterol than mammalian cholestrol; ergosterol being the primary sterol constituent of fungal cell membrane. However, binding of AmB to cholesterol in mammalian cells results in drug-induced cellular toxicity as evident in common and often serious adverse events associated with its use. Other potential antifungal mechanisms of polyenes include (a) damage to the fungal cell wall at lower (below minimum inhibitory concentration [MIC]) concentrations, (b) modulation of hosts' immune and inflammatory response, and (c) promoting oxidative damage [3–7].

Azoles exert antifungal action on fungal cell membranes by blocking the biosynthesis of ergosterol. Azole-mediated inhibition of cytochrome P450 (CYP)-dependent 14-α-demethylase (CYP51) interferes with the conversion of lanosterol to ergosterol resulting in accumulation of methyl sterols, which cause disruption of fungal cellular function, impede fungal growth and replication. Inhibition of fungal ergosterol synthesis by triazoles results in cross-inhibition of some CYP-dependent enzymes in humans, an important mechanism for drug toxicity and drug-drug interactions associated with these agents [3, 4, 8–11]. The azole compounds exhibit varying degree of affinities for CYP-dependent 14-α-demethylase, which in return reflect upon their differential antifungal activity, adverse events, and extent of drug-drug interaction [15].

Echinocandins act through the inhibition of glucan synthase, an enzyme responsible for synthesis of β-1,3-D-glucan, which is an integral component of fungal cell wall. Decreased β-(1,3)-D-glucan cell wall content results in cell dysmorphia, weakened cell wall due to loss of cell integrity promoting cell lysis. Because mammalian cells do not contain glucan synthase or a cell wall, the echinocandins do not affect the integrity of human cells. The genes that encode β-(1,3)-D-glucan synthase complex are *FKS1*, *FKS2*, and *FKS3*, although *FKS3* is expressed at a very low level. Transcription of fungal cell wall proteins in some yeasts like *Candida glabrata* is regulated by *FKS2* and dependent on the enzyme calcineurin, whereas *FKS1*-linked proteins are regulated by fungal cell turnover [16].

Spectrum of Activity

AmB is a broad-spectrum antifungal agent, with activity against many clinically relevant yeasts and molds. It has demonstrated clinical activity against nearly all *Candida* species except certain isolates of *Candida lusitaniae, Candida guilliermondii*, and many strains of *Candida auris*. AmB is active against dimorphic fungi such as *Blastomyces*, *Histoplasma*, *Coccidioides*, and *Cryptococcus* spp. It is also active against filamentous molds, such as *Aspergillus* spp. and organisms associated with mucormycosis among other rare molds.

Important limitation of AmB coverage includes *Aspergillus terreus*, *Scedosporium apiospermum*, *Fusarium* spp., *Paecilomyces* spp., *Sporothrix schenckii,* and mostly pan-drug-resistant *Scedosporium prolificans* [3–7, 17]. Azoles are active against *Candida* spp., dimorphic endemic fungi, and *C. neoformans*. Among non-*albicans Candida* spp., azoles have variable dose-dependent activity against *C. glabrata.* Fluconazole is not active against *C. krusei, C. auris*, and filamentous fungi, whereas itraconazole has activity against *Aspergillus* spp. and some rarer molds. Voriconazole has activity against *Aspergillus* and *Fusarium* spp.; posaconazole and isavuconazonium sulfate is active against *Aspergillus, Fusarium*, most *Zygomycetes* species among other rarer molds [3, 4, 8–11, 17].

Echinocandins are broadly active against all *Candida* spp. including isolates resistant to other antifungal agents. Echinocandins have reduced in vitro activity against isolates of *C. parapsilosis* and *C. guilliermondii*, but this lesser activity does not appear to correlate with clinical treatment failure. These agents are not active against *C. neoformans*, *Fusarium*, and most *Zygomycetes* spp. In addition, *A. lentulus* is an emerging *Aspergillus* species associated with IA in patients undergoing allogeneic HSCT, heart, kidney, and liver allograft transplantation; this organism tends to be resistant to echinocandins [3, 4, 12–14, 17].

Resistance

Mechanisms of antifungal resistance are either primary or secondary and are related to intrinsic or acquired fungal characteristics [18]. Intrinsic resistance is defined as resistance to all or almost all isolates of a species to a antifungal drug, which does not involve an acquired resistance often seen following exposure to such a drug. Primary resistance occurs in organisms that have not been exposed to a specific antimicrobial agent in clinical practice. It is a significant factor contributing drug resistance among patients with invasive fungal disease resulting in a selection of inherently less susceptible fungal species. In contrast, secondary or acquired drug resistance arises after treatment with an antimicrobial agent; this is less prevalent and alludes to de novo mechanism(s) that confer reduced susceptibility for an organism, to which it was previously susceptible[19].

Poor therapeutic response to polyenes is generally relegated to inherently resistant molds such as *A. lentulus*, *A. terreus*, *Pseudallescheria boydii, Scedosporium apiospermum*, *Scedosporium prolificans*, *Paecilomyces lilanicus*, and *Fusarium* spp. and to some yeasts with varying degree of susceptibility such as *C. lusitaniae* and *C. auris***.** Mutation in genes involved in ergosterol biosynthesis pathway have the abilty to foist lack of susceptibility to AmB in such fungal strains, whereas, molecular mechanism(s) involved in inherent resistance remain elusive for a variety of fungal pathogens [19]. Secondary resistance to AmB is rare, even in patients with clinical failure to AmB; in contrast, resistant mutants may be selected in vitro experiments after exposure to AmB [20]. Prior exposure to azoles, such as itraconazole that acts by lowering fungal cell membrane sterol concentration, may unwittingly confer subsequent reduced susceptibility to polyenes [21]. Acquired resistance to AmB has been most extensively evaluated in yeasts and is associated with mutations in sterol biosynthesis genes like *ERG1*, *ERG2*, *ERG3*, *ERG4*, *ERG6*, and *ERG11*. For example, mutations in *erg3* encoding for C-5 sterol desaturase lead to qualitative and quantitative alterations of membrane lipids and an absence of ergosterol [22]. It should be noted that deletion of *erg3* genes in *A. fumigatus* did not change AmB susceptibility despite such mutants exhibited a marked alteration of cell membrane sterol composition including reduced ergosterol content [23]. This may reflect a more complex biosynthesis pathway for sterols in *Aspergillus* spp. Finally, *A. terreus* compared with *A. fumigatus* exhibits high catalase production, which has been suggested to undermine AmB-associated oxidative fungal damage, thereby resulting in ineffective drug-induced cell death [24].

The molecular mechanisms responsible for triazole resistance are common to most yeasts and molds [25, 26]. Three major mechanisms have been elucidated in recent years. First, mutations in the drug target, CYP450 14-α-demethylase, encoded by *erg11* among yeasts and *cyp51A* among the filamentous fungi, alter the apparent drug-binding domain [27, 28]. Second, overexpression of drug efflux transporters belonging to the adenosine triphosphate (ATP) binding cassette (ABC) and major facilitator system (MFS) classes reduces the intracellular steady-state drug levels [29]. Finally, azole resistance resulting from upregulation of demethylation target [25]. The evolution of drug resistance in susceptible yeast involves either a single-step mechanism or a progressive accumulation of mutations resulting in changes in target site affinity and induction of various drug efflux transporters or both. Many of these mechanisms are induced by changes in major transcriptional regulators such as Tac1, Pdr1, which are influenced by gain-of-function mutations and changes in copy number due to genomic modifications resulting in loss of heterozygosity and isochromosome formation [30–32]. This multifactorial basis of azole resistance in clinical isolates is widely observed [25, 33, 34]. For molds like *A. fumigatus*, target site modification is the principal mechanism of clinical resistance. Mutations in *cyp51A* gene result in structural alteration to the enzyme, which in turn inhibit binding to the drugs. Prominent mutational hotspots confirmed to cause multiazole resistance that have been characterized at amino acid positions Gly54, Met220, and Leu 98 [35, 36]. Other mutations in the *cyp51A* gene have been reported, and additional resistance mechanisms are postulated [35]. In Europe, nearly all resistance is due to tandem repeat mutations in the promoter region of *cyp51A* along with specific mutations in the coding region with the mechanisms TR34/L98H, TR46/Y121F/T289A [37, 38]. These prominent resistant isolates have been observed globally in more than 22 countries [39] and appear to arise as consequence of azole use in the agricultural industry and are selected out as primary resistance [40]. This specific resistance mechanism has rarely been observed in patients with fungal infections, in whom resistance develops during antifungal therapy. Azole resistance to *cyp51A* mutations is a growing phenomenon worldwide, and its magnitude may be overestimated, as chronic *Aspergillus* infection is often cryptic and can only be detected through molecular techniques [41, 42]. Overexpression of ABC and MFS drug transporters is a common mechanism in *Candida* species, but their role in *Aspergillus* is still not clear [43, 44]. Finally, in a small percentage of fungal isolates, the mechanism of triazole resistance remains uncertain.

Echinocandin resistance in *C. albicans* and most other *Candida* spp. occurs in two highly conserved "hotspot" regions of *FKS1* [45–48]. These limited regions encompass residues Phe641-Pro649 and Arg1361. In *C. glabrata*, the comparable mutations are found in either *FKS1* or *FKS2* [46, 49]. Mutations in *FKS* genes induce elevated MIC values 0.5–2 logs and reduce the sensitivity of glucan synthase IC_{50} or K_i to drug by 50- to 3000-fold [45, 49, 50]. Most clinical breakthrough infections were observed due to *C. albicans* and *C. glabrata*, which are the two common *Candida* spp. associated with yeast invasive disease in the immunocompromised patients. For *C. albicans*, amino acid changes at Ser645 (S645P, F, Y) are the most abundant and cause the most pronounced resistance phenotype; other substitutions at F641, L642, T643, L644, A645, L646, R647, and D648 account for remaining resistance [48–53]. In *C. glabrata* mutations, conferring resistance occurs in both *FKS1* and *FKS2*. S663P in *FKS2* is the most prominent amino acid substitution in more than half of the cases [49, 52]. Other substitutions in *FKS2* include F569S, F559V, Y, L664R, D666G, E, and P667T in hotspot 2, W1375L. In *C. glabrata*, some isolates contain nonsense mutation in either *FKS1* or *FKS2* and a *fks* mutation in the corresponding allele [46, 49]. Not all *FKS* mutations confer the same strong resistance phenotype and are less likely to result in breakthrough disease. On the basis of MIC testing of clinical isolates, pharmacokinetic-pharmacodynamic (PK-PD) studies, and kinetic inhibition of glucan synthase, an order for strength of resistance associated with substitutions at *fks* residues was proposed: S645, F641> > L642, T643, L644, L646, R647, and D648 > P649 [51]. In PK-PD studies involving Fks1-Ser645 substitutions, micafungin even in high doses was insufficient to elicit an antifungal response, suggesting that conventional dose therapy with micafungin would not be effective in treating infections due to such organisms [54]. However, yeast's behavior with the most prominent *FKS2* mutation Fks2p-S663F unlike *FKS1* mutant, Fks1p-S629P, in *C. glabrata* has responded to elevated drug dosing [53]. Furthermore, *C. glabrata* strains harboring the mutation Fks2p-P667T and Fks2p-D666F also differentially responded in a dose-dependent fashion to the three echinocandin drugs [54]. Drug-response relationships for high MIC mutant *Candida* strains may provide an approach to stratify resistance and assess dosing solutions to overcome potential lack of clinical response to therapy without the need to change drug class [55].

Toxicities

Systemic toxicity with AmB is well known. Nephrotoxicity is associated with dose-dependent reduction in glomerular filtration rate. Other effects on renal function include potassium, magnesium, and bicarbonate wasting and decreased erythropoietin production. Azotemia caused by AmB is often worse in patients taking other nephrotoxic drugs. Presence of hypotension, renal allograft transplantation, and preexisting chronic kidney disease increases the probability for AmB drug-induced azotemia. In infusion-related reactions such as fever, chills, rigors, tachypnea, and worsened hypoxemia in patients with preexisting cardiac or pulmonary disease. It is important to note that infusion-related adverse events tend to improve in severity as treatment with AmB is continued [3–5, 56]. The infusion toxicities are most prominent with AmB deoxycholate, whereas AmB lipid formulations are better tolerated [6, 7, 57]. Renal preservation was comparable for ABLC and L-AmB either given as prophylaxis or for treatment of invasive fungal disease [57].

Generally, azoles are well-tolerated drugs. Fluconazole has an excellent safety profile. Most adverse effects associated with fluconazole are minor and usually gastrointestinal in nature. Fluconazole carries modest risk of QTc (corrected QT interval)-interval prolongation rarely resulting in torsades de pointes. Elevation of hepatic transaminase levels is seldom seen even in patients treated with high-dose fluconazole given for an extended duration. These events typically occur in patients with a higher susceptibility for such events. Reversible alopecia is not uncommon with fluconazole [3, 4, 9, 58].

Posaconazole is associated with mild to moderate gastrointestinal symptoms including altered taste and reduced appetite; mild nausea is not uncommon in transplant patients receiving posaconazole. Liver toxicity is however, a serious concern with this agent, especially in the transplant population, and often due to concurrent use of other agents with hepatotoxicity risk profile [3, 4, 11]. Two unique adverse events were noted with voriconazole use: (1) dose-related reversible disturbance of vision or photopsia that may present as photophobia, changes in color vision, increased or decreased visual acuity and light perception, or blurred vision and (2) cutaneous phototoxicity. Visual disturbances are usually mild and transient and abate as treatment is continued beyond first week. Similarly, cutaneous phototoxicity is reversible after discontinuation of therapy. An elevation in serum transaminases levels, skin rash reported in nearly 8% of patients, and visual hallucinations in up to 4% of patients receiving voriconazole therapy have been reported. The cyclodextrin vehicle in IV formulation of voriconazole can accumulate in patients with insufficient renal clearance [3, 4, 10].

Itraconazole carries less favorable toxicity profile among the azole-based drugs. A negative inotropic effect that may precipitate congestive heart failure is a unique cardiotoxicity associated with itraconazole. The US federal registration and labeling guideline recommends avoidance of itraconazole in patients with heart failure. Oral itraconazole solution contains a cyclodextrin carrier which can cause gastrointestinal toxicity such as nausea, vomiting, diarrhea, and abdominal pain; these adverse events, if severe, may necessitate discontinuation of therapy. Like other azoles, itraconazole use may result in hepatic toxicity ranging from mild, transient elevations of hepatic enzymes to rare cases of life-threatening liver failure [3, 4, 8]. Close monitoring of liver function is recommended with all members of the azole-based drugs, especially in the at risk transplant population.

Overall, the echinocandin class has the most favorable safety profile. Echinocandin may infrequently lead to hepatic dysfunction, whereas, acute liver failure is an exceedingly rare complication. In clinical trials, all three currently licensed echinocandins show a comparable increase in liver enzymes, when compared with patients treated with polyene or triazole drugs. Monitoring liver enzymes is recommended during echinocandin therapy. A histamine-mediated, infusion-related reaction was seen in some patients; slowing the rate of infusion and pre-infusion antihistamines are effective [3, 4, 12–14].

Clinical Efficacy

Primary Antifungal Prophylaxis in HSCT Recipients

Primary antifungal prophylaxis with fluconazole has become the standard for patients undergoing HSCT since the early 1990s. The studies compared fluconazole with placebo or oral nonabsorbable agents and demonstrated significant 8–14% reduction in the cases of proven IFIs among patients following transplantation [16, 59–64]. Furthermore, fewer IFI-related deaths in fluconazole prophylaxis arm was encouraging [16, 60–62, 64, 65]. A significant reduction in overall mortality and probability of death up to 3 months after stem cell transplantation was an important finding (31 vs. 52 deaths in fluconazole and placebo groups, respectively [$p = 0.004$]) [16, 60]. The limitations for the prophylaxis studies are reflected in the variability among (a) the distribution of autologous vs. allogeneic HSCT recipients, (b) duration of antifungal prophylaxis after transplantation, and (c) dose of fluconazole used [16, 60–62, 64, 65]. In addition, breakthrough IFIs with *C. glabrata*, *C. krusei*, *Aspergillus* spp., and mucormycosis have occurred in patients given fluconazole prophylaxis [16, 60–62, 64]. Old age, concurrent use of antibacterial chemoprophylaxis, cytarabine plus anthracycline-based chemotherapy, and high *Candida* colonization index were identified as independent risk factors for fluconazole failure [64].

Routine use of recombinant myeloid growth factors, a decline in conventional myeloablative preparatory transplant conditioning regimens have favorably shortened the duration of pre-engraftment neutropenia. In addition, selective and less toxic conditioning regimens such as non-myeloablative stem cell transplantation and lower risk of orointestinal mucosal disruption have also favorably reduced invasive candidiasis risk during early transplant period. Despite these important improvements, risk for invasive mold infections continue to remain a serious concern for high-risk allogeneic HSCT recipients. The incidence of mold infection including IA in autologous stem cell transplant recipients is low, with a few following exceptions: (1) heavily pretreated patients with multiple myeloma and (2) those with fludarabine therapy for lymphoproliferative disorders [65].

The current National Comprehensive Cancer Network (NCCN) guidelines on prevention and treatment of cancer-related infections recommend fluconazole 400 mg daily among other antifungal agents for antifungal prophylaxis in autologous HSCT recipients until engraftment; for allogeneic HSCT recipients, it is recommended that prophylaxis should be continued for a minimum of 75 days after transplantation [66]. Lack of protection against infections caused by *C. krusei* and *Aspergillus* with fluconazole prophylaxis is important to note. Mold-active drug prophylaxis should be considered based on the assessment of patients' risk profile; furthermore taking into account the regional and local rates for such infections including seasonal variability for IFIs, where applicable [16]. Prophylaxis with a mold-active triazole drug like voriconazole or posaconazole is considered in select patients in whom treatment of acute or chronic GVHD requires accelerated immunosuppression. These drugs are also considered in patients undergoing high-risk transplant procedures with an anticipated delay in restitution of myeloid hematopoiesis. Anti-mold secondary prophylaxis is routinely introduced for patients with a history of successfully treated IFI prior to HSCT procedure.

Voriconazole has extended spectrum of activity against medically important yeasts and filamentous fungi such as *Aspergillus* spp. and most black molds. In high-risk HSCT patients, voriconazole prophylaxis is an appealing alternative to fluconazole. A randomized, double-blind study compared voriconazole 200 mg twice daily with fluconazole 400 mg once daily given for first 100 days after transplantation. Patients underwent assessment of serum galactomannan twice weekly for 60 days, then weekly until day 100; empiric antifungal therapy was therefore given for individuals with probable breakthrough IFI. Patients with prior systemic candidiasis in 2 months and mold IFIs in 4 months prior were excluded from participation in this study. There was no significant difference in the incidence of IFIs or fungus-free survival [67]. However, in patients with acute myeloid leukemia (AML) who underwent allogeneic HSCT, fewer IFIs (8.5 vs. 21%; $p = 0.04$) and improved fungus-free survival in voriconazole vs. fluconazole prophylaxis group was encouraging (78% vs. 61%, respectively; $p = 0.04$). There was no difference in overall survival in any of the subgroups including patients with AML [67]. Based on this data, specific patients such as those with AML undergoing allogeneic HSCT, in whom the risk of IA and invasive candidiasis due to fluconazole nonsusceptible organisms is high, may be suitable candidates for prophylaxis with voriconazole.

Micafungin is another agent recommended for prophylaxis in patients undergoing autologous or allogeneic HSCT. The multi-institutional, randomized trial included 882 adult and pediatric autologous or allogeneic HSCT recipients who were given 50 mg of micafungin ($n = 425$) or 400 mg of fluconazole ($n = 457$) once daily and continued through stem cell engraftment. Successful prophylaxis was defined as the absence of suspected, proven, or probable IFIs through the end of therapy and no evidence of proven or probable IFIs 4 weeks after prophylaxis was completed. The overall efficacy of micafungin was 80% vs. 73.5% in fluconazole group ($p = 0.03$). In patients given micafungin prophylaxis, a trend toward lower rates of aspergillosis was also encouraging. There was no difference in mortality between the two groups. Breakthrough infections in this study included four cases of candidemia and one case of probable aspergillosis in the micafungin group, whereas two cases of candidemia and seven cases of aspergillosis (four proven, three probable) in the HSCT recipients given fluconazole prophylaxis. A major limitation of this study was the short duration of prophylaxis (until engraftment), which did not allow assessment of efficacy of micafungin prophylaxis in patients at continued risk for IFI during other at risk postengraftment period that coincide with acute GVHD [16, 68–70]. A small prospective, randomized, open-labeled trial included 104 HSCT recipients given antifungal prophylaxis with 150 mg daily micafungin compared with 400 mg a day of fluconazole. There were no differences in the rate of breakthrough IFI in this small study [68, 70]. The duration of prophylaxis in this study was 5 days after engraftment or 42 days after HSCT. Currently, micafungin 50 mg daily is approved in the United States for prophylaxis in patients undergoing HSCT [13].

In stem cell transplant recipients with severe GVHD, an expanded antifungal coverage against mold infections is desirable. The role of posaconazole was assessed in a trial involving 600 patients, and the overall frequency of breakthrough IFIs within 16 weeks of randomization was 5.3% in posaconazole group given 600 mg in three divided doses vs. 9% in patients who were given 400 mg fluconazole daily ($p = 0.07$). Furthermore, frequency of proven or probable aspergillosis in posaconazole treatment cohort was 2.3% compared with 7% noted in patients, in whom fluconazole prophylaxis was given ($p = 0.006$). The rate of breakthrough invasive candidiasis was not significantly different between the two groups. The overall mortality in patients given posaconazole and fluconazole prophylaxis was 25% and 28%, respectively [16, 71].

The newer antifungal agents such as voriconazole, micafungin, posaconazole and isavuconazonium sulfate (presently only approved for the treatment of invasive aspergillosis and invasive mucormycosis) have made prophylactic itraconazole use obsolete due to higher rates of adverse events and drug-drug interactions [65, 66, 72, 73]. Efficacy and safety of voriconazole and itraconazole was evaluated in 234 patients undergoing allogeneic HSCT. In this study, the primary composite endpoints were success of prophylaxis, ability to tolerate study drug for more than 100 days, and survival past 180 days after HSCT without proven or probable IFI. Superiority of voriconazole in the composite primary endpoint was that patients given voriconazole prophylaxis were able to tolerate prophylaxis for 100 plus days with minimal treatment interruption [73]. Based on the toxicity profile of AmB deoxycholate, its use for antifungal prophylaxis in transplant patients is very limited.

Selection of antifungal agent for primary prophylaxis in transplant population should include the following considerations: (a) identify the type of HSCT procedure that portends greater risk for IFI such as T cell-depleted grafts, cord blood stem cell grafts, and mismatched allografts; (b) identify patients for high IFI vulnerability like heavily treated individuals with recurrent or treatment-refractory hematologic malignancy, high yeast colonization index, and evolving understating in disruptions in hosts' microbiota and various genetic polymorphisms in innate and adaptive immune pathways that may eccentuate post-transplant proclivity for fungal infections; the last two parameters are not routinely monitored. In addition, drug-related factors such as (1) oral bioavailability, (2) spectrum of antifungal activity, (3) voids in the antifungal coverage such as voriconazole's lack of efficacy against agents of human mucormycosis, (4) safety and tolerability, and (5) importantly, potential for drug-drug interaction. The optimum duration of antifungal prophylaxis in HSCT recipients is not certain; most experts surmise that antifungal prophylaxis be continued beyond pre-engraftment neutropenic period [66]. A gathering consensus is for prophylaxis to be continued through the period(s) of moderate to severe GVHD. Since death in HSCT recipients in most cases, is cumulation of a number of factors, both infectious (i.e., CMV, IFIs, bacterial sepsis) and noninfections (i.e., GVHD, cancer recurrence, graft failure) complications, it is, therefore, perhaps unwise to assess efficacy of IFI prophylaxis on the impact on overall mortality in this highly vulnerable complex population.

Primary Antifungal Prophylaxis in SOT Recipients

Among SOT population, recipients of orthotopic liver transplantation (OLT) are at an increase risk for locally invasive or systemic yeasts infections, whereas those undergoing lung and heart-lung transplantation have higher susceptibility for invasive mold disease [74–77]. Risk factors for invasive candidiasis in OLT recipients include (1) retransplantation, (2) serum creatinine >2.0 mg/dL, (3) choledochojejunostomy, (4) intraoperative use of >40 units of blood products, (5) prolonged intraoperative time > 1 h, and (6) demonstration of fungal colonization 2 days prior and 3 days following transplant surgery [77, 78]. In a randomized, placebo-controlled trial, fluconazole 400 mg given daily for 70 days after transplant surgery was associated with fungal infection rate of 6% compared with 23% in no prophylaxis group ($p < 0.001$). A significantly lower IFI-related deaths in patients given fluconazole prophylaxis compared with no antifungal prophylaxis were encouraging (2% vs. 13%, respectively; $p = 0.003$); however, the overall mortality was similar in both groups [76].

In a retrospective review of 445 consecutive pancreas transplant recipients, overall rate of intra-abdominal fungal infections (IAFIs) was 9.2%. In patients who received fluconazole 400 mg daily for 7 days after transplantation had 6% vs. 10% IAFIs in patients without prophylaxis. Donor age was noted as a significant risk factor. However, it was important to note that 1-year graft survival rate in recipients with IAFI was 17%, compared with 65% in patients without such infections ($p = 0.0001$) [79].

In a prospective review of 19 small bowel transplant recipients, 28% had at least 1 episode of fungal infections during the 524 days post-transplant follow-up [80]. There are no randomized trials of antifungal prophylaxis in this at risk visceral allograft group. According to Clinical Practice Guideline for the Management of Candidiasis, 200–400 mg (3–6 mg/kg) fluconazole for 7–14 days is recommended as postoperative prophylaxis for liver transplant recipients who have at least two key risk factors, whereas prophylaxis is recommended for all patients undergoing pancreas and small bowel transplantation surgery [81]. The risk of invasive candidiasis in kidney, heart, and lung transplant recipients is low and has significantly declined over the past 25 years [81, 82]. A detailed review on SOT antifungal prophylaxis is provided elsewhere in this volume.

Treatment of IFIs in HSCT and SOT

Despite the standard use of antifungal prophylaxis in patients undergoing HSCT and SOT, IFIs continue to be a significant cause of morbidity and mortality. Transplant-Associated Infection Surveillance Network (TRANSNET) is a network of 23 US transplant centers performing HSCT and SOT, or both. TRANSNET reported 983 proven (56%) and probable (44%) IFIs in 875 HSCT recipients between 2001 and 2006. IA was common (43%), followed by invasive candidiasis (28%), zygomycosis (8%), and invasive *Fusarium* spp. infection (3%). The incidence of IFIs was nearly 8% in the recipients of mismatched-related and matched-unrelated allogeneic HSCT; for matched-related allogeneic SCT, the incidence was marginally lower (5.8%), and as expected, IFI complication was reported in only 1% of patients undergoing autologous stem cell transplantation. Overall 1-year survival after infections was 6% for patients with fusariosis, 25% for aspergillosis, 28% for zygomycosis, and 34% for transplant recipients with invasive candidiasis [83]. This database received reports of 1,208 proven (42%) and probable (58%) IFIs among 1,063 SOT recipients during the same period. Invasive candidiasis was common (53%), followed by aspergillosis (19%), cryptococcosis (8%), non-*Aspergillus* molds (8%), endemic fungi (5%), and zygomycosis (2%). The 12-month cumulative incidence of first IFI was 12% for small bowel, 9% in lung, 5% in liver, 4% in heart, 3% in pancreas, and 1% in recipients of renal allograft transplantation. The 1-year survival after the diagnosis of IA was 59%; 61% for non-*Aspergillus* mold infections, 66% in patients with invasive candidiasis, and 73% among SOT recipients with cryptococcal infection [84].

fluconazole prophylaxis in patients undergoing HSCT has resulted in a noteworthy decline in cases of invasive candidiasis. The widespread use of systemic antifungal agent given for infection prevention, as expected, has influenced epidemiology of *Candida* spp. infection as drug-resistant or inherently nonsusceptible yeast stains and species become more common in clinical practice. It is important to recognize that IA is the most common fungal infection in HSCT recipients, whereas locally invasive or systemic candidiasis is more frequently encountered in patients undergoing SOT.

In this section, we discuss the current literature support for primary and salvage therapy for primary and breakthrough invasive candidiasis, IA, zygomycosis, and other non-*Aspergillus* mold infections.

Invasive Candidiasis

A randomized study comparing IV fluconazole 400 mg daily with AmB deoxycholate for the treatment of candidemia in non-neutropenic patients found both regimens were comparable [85]. Therefore, fluconazole and AmB were considered as standard-of-care treatment for candidemia in patients with intact peripheral blood neutrophil counts. Clinical efficacy and safety of echinocandins including caspofungin, micafungin, and anidulafungin as the initial treatment for invasive candidiasis has been established in four randomized multicenter trials. The first trial compared caspofungin 70 mg dose followed by 50 mg daily dose vs. AmB given (0.6–1.0 mg/kg daily) in 224 patients, which also included 14 patients with severe neutropenia and 7 SOT recipients. Successful outcomes following caspofungin and AmB therapy were 73 vs. 62%, respectively (95% confidence interval [CI]; −0.7–26.0) [86]. A double-blind, randomized, multinational trial included 531 patients with invasive candidiasis given either micafungin 100 mg daily or L-AmB given 3 mg/kg daily [87]. In this study, 62 patients had neutropenia and 32 had undergone SOT. Micafungin was as effective as L-AmB, resulting in nearly 90% successful outcome in either group. Anidulafungin 200 mg followed by 100 mg daily dose was compared with 800 mg of fluconazole followed by 400 mg daily for treatment of invasive candidiasis in a double-blind, noninferiority trial [88]. The study included 12 SOT recipients. Efficacy analysis in 245 patients showed anidulafungin therapy was associated with higher response rates of 76% vs. 60% in patients given fluconazole (95% CI; 3.9–27.0). Another large multicenter trial assessed efficacy and safety of micafungin vs. caspofungin for the treatment of invasive candidiasis [89]. The results of these trials consistently have shown superior efficacy and safety of echinocandins for the treatment of invasive candidiasis. There is insufficient clinical data to favor one echinocandin over the another. It is worth pointing out that HSCT and SOT recipients are underrepresented in these trials. Breakthrough infections in patients receiving azoles are most likely due to fluconazole-resistant *Candida* spp., especially *C. glabrata* and *C. krusei*; echinocandins or L-AmB as first-line therapy in patients undergoing hematopoietic or visceral allograft transplantation is strongly recommended.

In the 2016 Infectious Diseases Society of America (IDSA) guidelines for the treatment of candidiasis, an echinocandin is recommended as initial therapy in (a) patients with neutropenia, (b) critically ill patients, (c) those with recent triazole drug exposure, or (d) patients with suspected or proven *C. glabrata* and *C. krusei* infection [90]. If an organism is identified as fluconazole susceptible and patient is hemodynamically stable and no longer neutropenic, with sterile blood cultures, and has no prior exposure to azole prophylaxis, in such situations treatment with fluconazole at 6–12 mg/kg daily may be considered. NCCN and IDSA do not recommend using AmB products routinely for candidemia, patients with *Candida* spp. meningitis or endocarditis being an exception [66, 81]. Patients who fail to respond to echinocandins or those intolerant to these agents, treatment with L-AmB may thereupon commenced. There is no clinical trial-based experience for voriconazole use as first-line treatment in neutropenic patients with invasive candidiasis, it is often used as transition to oral therapy or given as second-line agent.

Most *C. glabrata* and *C. krusei* clinical isolates retain susceptibility to the mold-active triazoles like voriconazole, posaconazole and isavuconazonium sulfate [91]. The recommended duration of treatment for patients with uncomplicated candidemia is 2 weeks after the first sterile blood culture and resolution of signs and symptoms associated with these infections [81]. In patients with *Candida* retinal or other ophthalmic involvement, treatment is given for an extended duration. Those with candidemia associated with an infected intravascular devise, infected devices should be removed expeditiously. In patients with persistent neutropenia and candidemia without secondary complication, treatment may also be discontinued after 2 weeks of therapy.

Invasive Aspergillosis

For decades, AmB deoxycholate was the only treatment option for patients with IA. Voriconazole has replaced amphotericin as the first-line drug for the treatment of IA. The open-label, multicenter randomized trial in severely immunocompromised patients included 67 HSCT and 14 SOT recipients with probable or proven IA who were randomized to receive either voriconazole 6 mg/kg two doses followed by 4 mg/kg twice daily (n = 144) or AmB deoxycholate given as 1 to 1.5 mg/kg daily dose (n = 133) [92]. Twelve weeks after treatment commenced, voriconazole resulted in a significantly higher rate of complete and partial response compared with patients treated with AmB deoxycholate (53% vs. 32%, respectively; 95% CI, 10.4–32.9). Additionally, treatment with voriconazole also resulted in improved survival after 12 weeks of therapy (71% vs. 58% in patients given AmB deoxycholate; hazard ratio = 0.59; 95% CI, 0.40–0.88). In 67 HSCT recipients, 32% had a response to voriconazole compared with a dismal response of 13% in patients treated with AmB deoxycholate. In a retrospective study of 192 patients, 137 with proven and 55 with probable central nervous system (CNS) aspergillosis, 48% responded to treatment with voriconazole [93].

L-AmB is an alternative option for initial therapy in patients with IA. The AmBiLoad trial was a double-blind dose comparison trial of L-AmB 3 or 10 mg/kg/day given for the first 2 weeks, followed by 3 mg/kg daily maintenance dose as primary treatment of IFI [94]. Of 201 patients with confirmed invasive mold infection, 107 patients received the lower dose and 94 patients received 10 mg/kg daily dose. IA accounted for 97% of all IFIs in this study. Severe neutropenia was noted in 73% of patients at the start of therapy. The trial included 35 HSCT patients, and one patient after SOT. No significant difference in efficacy between the two groups was an unexpected finding. A 50% response in patients initially given low dose vs. 46% in those treated with 10 mg/kg dose during the first 2 weeks along with an improved survival at 12 weeks favored patients initially given 3 mg/kg dose (72% vs. 59% in high-dose treatment group; 95% CI, −0.2–26%). These results demonstrated efficacy of L-AmB 3 mg/kg daily dose, whereas no benefit could be seen in patients given initial 2 weeks of high-dose L-AmB therapy. L-AmB has been used as an alternative agent for the treatment of IA in transplant patients intolerant to voriconazole or those with concerns for drug toxicity and potential drug-drug interactions.

The optimum therapy for breakthrough IA in patients receiving mold-active prophylaxis is not clear. A switch in the class of antifungals is suggested, and for patients with treatment of refractory IA, salvage combination therapy may be entertained, albeit, stellar prospective large cohort data to support such combination antifungal drug treatment regimens is currently lacking.

Posaconazole has not been evaluated for primary therapy of IA. It was effective as salvage therapy given 800 mg daily in three to four divided doses for patients with IA and underlying hematologic malignancies, HSCT, and SOT [95–97]. In Europe, posaconazole is approved as salvage therapy for IA and other IFIs refractory to standard antifungal agents. In the United States, posaconazole is approved as prophylaxis for IA in high-risk patient.

Isavuconazonium sulfate is the newest triazole mold-active drug to be introduced for clinical use. A phase III, double-blind, global comparative study in 527 adults assessed safety and efficacy of isavuconazonium sulfate 372 mg prodrug, which is equivalent to 200 mg isavuconazole given three times daily for first 2 days followed by 372 mg prodrug taken once daily compared with standard IA dose voriconazole therapy. The primary efficacy endpoint was all-cause mortality after the first dose through 42 days after the treatment commenced. Safety was assessed in patients who received even a single dose of the study drugs. All-cause mortality was 19% and 20% in patients given isavuconazole or voriconazole, respectively. Drug-related adverse events were 42% in patients treated with isavuconazole compared with 60% in the voriconazole treatment group ($p < 0.001$). It is important to note that patients given isavuconazole had significantly lower hepatobiliary dysfunction, 9% vs. 16% in voriconazole treatment arm ($p = 0.016$). Similarly, eye disorders, 15% vs. 27% ($p = 0.002$), and skin and skin structure disorders, 33% vs. 42% ($p = 0.037$), favored isavuconazole vs. voriconazole, respectively [98]. This drug may be utilized as an alternative first-line therapy for transplant patients with IA, with a potential benefit in significantly less ocular and hepatotoxicity.

Caspofungin 70 mg single dose followed by 50 mg daily was evaluated as first-line IA therapy in patients with hematologic malignancy, autologous and allogeneic HSCT [99, 100]. The results from these two noncomparative trials showed a modest complete or partial response assessed as 12 week survival was 33% and 50–53%. Caspofungin was evaluated in 90 patients with IA who were refractory to or intolerant of amphotericin products or triazoles and showed success rate of 45% [101]. Caspofungin is approved by FDA as salvage therapy in patients with IA. A noncomparative study for micafungin alone or in combination with other antifungal agents as primary or salvage therapy for IA in HSCT recipient did not permit definitive conclusion regarding drug efficacy and clinical utility [102, 103].

A potential synergist antifungal effect of echinocandin in combination with a triazole agent was observed in vitro experiments [104]. The rationale is that echinocandins target the fungal cell wall, which is distinct from the polyenes and azoles that target the fungal cell membrane. The clinical database is limited, combination antifungal therapy may be considered with due caution in management of difficult-to-treat IA, especially in severely immunosuppressed transplant patients with a greater risk of failure to conventional single drug antifungal therapy. Its role remains to be formally defined by prospective, randomized comparative studies. A retrospective study reported an improved 3-month survival of 78% in SOT recipients treated with voriconazole plus caspofungin compared with voriconazole alone as salvage therapy for IA [103]. Combination of voriconazole plus caspofungin as primary therapy for IA also showed potential promise in SOT recipients in a prospective observational study [104].

Both NCCN and the 2008/2016 [105] IDSA guidelines for treatment of IA recommend IV or oral voriconazole as first-line therapy in patients with IA [66, 106]. A combination of antifungal drugs from different classes other than initial regimen or an additional antifungal agent to current therapy may be used as salvage therapy. Patients who have responded to initial IV therapy and are clinically stable may be switched to appropriate oral agents. The duration of therapy for IA is defined by the resolution of all clinical and radiographic features associated with IA; in patients with persistent immune defect(s), a secondary suppressive antifungal therapy is often needed to prevent infection recurrence.

Zygomycosis

Zygomycosis is now referred as mucormycosis. Mucormycosis typically manifests as invasive sino-orbital and pulmonary disease [107]. Voriconazole and echinocandins have no activity against the agents of mucormycosis. Mucormycosis is an uncommon infection even in the severely immunosuppressed transplant recipients. It may become marginally more prominent in patient presenting with sino-orbital or intracranial fungal disease, patients who may develop voriconazole-breakthrough IFIs, and patients with heavy metal overload conditions. There are no randomized studies to assess selection of ideal therapy for patients with this rare fungal disease. Most data regarding therapy is in patients with poorly controlled diabetes mellitus with or without ketoacidosis. High-dose lipid AmB preparations such as L-AmB or ABLC (5 mg/kg/day) are considered treatment of choice. Surgical debridement of necrotic devitalized tissue should be approached with a sense of urgency, when feasible, aggressive surgical debridement forms the cornerstone of comprehensive care for patients with this life-threatening fungal disease [107]. Posaconazole and isavuconazole show in vitro activity against the agents of mucormycosis. Posaconazole was given as 800 mg divided daily dose with a mixed result as salvage therapy in patients of AmB refractory disease or patients who were intolerant to AmB formulations [108, 109]. Rates of treatment success including partial or complete response or disease stabilization were between 60% and 80%. Posaconazole has also been used for prolonged infection suppression after an initial response with amphotericin and surgical debridement [66].

In a single-arm open-label trial (VITAL study), adult patients from 34 centers worldwide with rare mold disease including mucormycosis between 2008 and 2013 were given isavuconazole 200 mg three times daily for six doses, followed by 200 mg daily until infection resolved, or treatment failed, or for 180 days or more after treatment commenced. The primary endpoint was complete or partial response, which was regarded as treatment success; or treatment failure in patients with stable or progressive disease. In 37 patients with mucormycosis, isavuconazole was given for a median of 84 days and ranged between 2 and 882 days. Forty-two days after treatment began, 54% of patients had a partial or complete response, and in 43% disease became stable, whereas only one patient exhibited progression of fungal disease. Crude all-cause mortality was 33% after 42 days of isavuconazole therapy comparable to 39% in AmB-treated matched controls [110].

Free iron availability in fungal microenvironment supplements mucormycete growth and plays a fundamental role in the disease pathogenesis. Conventional iron chelators such as deferoxamine when given to patients with iron overload conditions promote iron ion-rich environment in which, agents of mucormycosis flourish and thrive. Whereas, the new-generation chelating agents like deferiprone and deferasirox reduce the concentration of free iron ions, thereby creating a nutritionally truncated milieu that impedes fungal growth and propagation. Iron chelation with deferasirox had encouraging results in experimental mucormycosis models. In a small phase II study, however, patients with mucormycosis treated with deferasirox plus L-AmB had a higher mortality rate at 90 days. Population imbalances may have contributed to this unexpected result. However, at present adjunctive deferasirox therapy for mucormycosis cannot be recommended [111, 112].

Other Invasive Mold Diseases

Fusarium spp. and *Scedosporium* spp. are uncommon causes of IFIs in the transplant population. However, these infections are on a gradual rise among all cause IFIs in certain geographic regions. These pathogens are associated with life-threatening disease that often fails to respond to conventional antifungal drug therapy [112, 113]. Therapy for invasive fusariosis generally involves drugs like voriconazole, posaconazole, and isavuconazole and lipid formulations of AmB [115–118]. *Scedosporium* species are resistant to AmB, although itraconazole, voriconazole, posaconazole, and isovuconazole retains activity against clinical *Scedosporium* isolates [118, 119].

Cryptococcus spp. infection typically manifest as CNS or lung infection, with proclivity for disseminated infection. The first-line therapy for cryptococcal meningoencephalitis is the combination of liposomal L-AmB (3–4 mg/kg/day) or ABLC (5 mg/kg/day) plus flucytosine (100 mg/kg/day orally in four divided doses) for the first 2 weeks, followed by fluconazole (400–800 mg, 4–6 mg/kg/day) for 8 weeks, then 200–400 mg/day orally fluconazole for another 6–12 months for secondary infection suppression. If flucytosine is not available, consider L-AmB or ABLC for at least 4 to 6 weeks of induction therapy L-AmB (6 mg/kg/day) might be considered in patients with relapsed infection or infection associated with high fungal burden. For mild-to-moderate pulmonary cryptococcosis, fluconazole 400 mg daily is given for 6–12 months. Patients with severe lung disease should be treated as those with CNS infection. For cryptococcemia or disseminated disease, consider fluconazole 400 mg or 6 mg/kg daily dose for 6–12 months [120].

Summary

Selection of antifungal agent for prophylaxis or treatment of IFIs in transplant recipients should be based on criteria outlined in this chapter. Status of hosts' immune response, local fungal epidemiology, drug pharmacology, spectrum of antifungal activity, drug toxicity, and importantly, potential for drug-drug interaction should all play an important part in such decision making. Management of IFIs requires optimization of immune function, which in most high-risk allograft transplant recipients remains unattainable. To abrogate this critical limitation, a number of ancillary immune boosting measures are currently under consideration including the evolving understanding of potential immune modulatory effects of the antifungal drugs. In the future, this may be an additional feature to consider in the selection of best possible, pathogen-targeted drug regimen for the highly vulnerable patients undergoing lifesaving transplantation procedures.

References

1. Kriengkauykiat J, Ito JI, Dadwal SS. Epidemiology and treatment approaches in management of invasive fungal infections. Clin Epidemiol. 2011;3:175–91. Epub 2011/07/14.
2. Tomblyn M, Chiller T, Einsele H, Gress R, Sepkowitz K, Storek J, et al. Guidelines for preventing infectious complications among hematopoietic cell transplantation recipients: a global perspective. Biol Blood Marrow Transplant. 2009;15(10):1143–238. Epub 2009/09/15.
3. Mohr J, Johnson M, Cooper T, Lewis JS, Ostrosky-Zeichner L. Current options in antifungal pharmacotherapy. Pharmacotherapy. 2008;28(5):614–45.
4. Ashley ESD, Lewis R, Lewis JS, Martin C, Andes D. Pharmacology of systemic antifungal agents. Clin Infect Dis. 2006;43(Supplement 1):S28–39.
5. Amphotercin B for Injection [package insert]. Big Flats: X-Gen Pharmaceuticals Inc; 2010.
6. Sigma-Tau PharmaSourse I. Abelcet (Amphotericin B Lipid Complex) [package insert]. Indianapolis; 2010.
7. AmBisome (Amphotericin B Liposomal) [package insert]. Deefield: Astellas Pharma US, Inc.; 2012.
8. Sporanox (itraconazole)[package insert]. Raritan: Pricara; 2009.
9. Diflucan (fluconazole)[package insert]. New York: Pfizer; 2011.
10. VFEND (voriconazole)[package insert]. New York: Pfizer; 2011.
11. Noxafil (posaconazole)[package insert]. Whitehouse Station: Merck & Co., Inc; 2011.
12. Cancidas (caspofungin acetate) [package insert]. Whitehouse Station: Merck & Co., Inc; 2010.
13. Mycamine (micafungin sodium) [package insert]. Deefield: Astellas Pharma US, Inc.; 2011.
14. Eraxis (anidulafungin) [package insert]. New York: Pfizer; 2010.
15. Lass-Florl C. Triazole antifungal agents in invasive fungal infections: a comparative review. Drugs. 2011;71(18):2405–19.
16. Perlin DS. Echinocandin resistance in Candida. Clin Infect Dis. 2015;61(Suppl 6):S612–7.
17. McCoy D, DePestel DD, Carver PL. Primary antifungal prophylaxis in adult hematopoietic stem cell transplant recipients: current therapeutic concepts. Pharmacotherapy. 2009;29(11):1306–25.
18. Pfaller MA. Antifungal drug resistance: mechanisms, epidemiology, and consequences for treatment. Am J Med. 2012;125(1 Suppl):S3–13. Epub 2012/01/04.
19. Loeffler J, Stevens DA. Antifungal drug resistance. Clin Infect Dis. 2003;36(Suppl 1):S31–41. Epub 2003/01/08.
20. Manavathu EK, Cutright JL, Chandrasekar PH. In vivo resistance of a laboratory-selected aspergillus fumigatus isolate to amphotericin B. Antimicrob Agents Chemother. 2005;49(1):428–30.
21. Schaffner A, Böhler A. Amphotericin B refractory aspergillosis after itraconazole: evidence for significant antagonism. Mycoses. 1993;36(11–12):421–4.
22. Kelly SL, Lamb DC, Kelly DE, Manning NJ, Loeffler J, Hebart H, et al. Resistance to fluconazole and cross-resistance to amphotericin B in Candida albicans from AIDS patients caused by defective sterol delta5,6-desaturation. FEBS Lett. 1997;400(1):80–2.
23. Alcazar-Fuoli L, Mellado E, Alastruey-Izquierdo A, Cuenca-Estrella M, Rodriguez-Tudela JL. Aspergillus section Fumigati: antifungal susceptibility patterns and sequence-based identification. Antimicrob Agents Chemother. 2008;52(4):1244–51.
24. Blum G, Perkhofer S, Haas H, Schrettl M, Würzner R, Dierich MP, et al. Potential basis for amphotericin B resistance in aspergillus terreus. Antimicrob Agents Chemother. 2008;52(4):1553–5.
25. Perea S, López-Ribot JL, Kirkpatrick WR, McAtee RK, Santillán RA, Martínez M, et al. Prevalence of molecular mechanisms of resistance to azole antifungal agents in Candida albicans strains displaying high-level fluconazole resistance isolated from human immunodeficiency virus-infected patients. Antimicrob Agents Chemother. 2001;45(10):2676–84.
26. Espinel-Ingroff A. Mechanisms of resistance to antifungal agents: yeasts and filamentous fungi. Rev Iberoam Micol. 2008;25(2):101–6.
27. Snelders E, Karawajczyk A, Schaftenaar G, Verweij PE, Melchers WJ. Azole resistance profile of amino acid changes in aspergillus fumigatus CYP51A based on protein homology modeling. Antimicrob Agents Chemother. 2010;54(6):2425–30.
28. Marichal P, Koymans L, Willemsens S, Bellens D, Verhasselt P, Luyten W, et al. Contribution of mutations in the cytochrome P450 14alpha-demethylase (Erg11p, Cyp51p) to azole resistance in Candida albicans. Microbiology. 1999;145(Pt 10):2701–13.
29. Sanglard D, Odds FC. Resistance of Candida species to antifungal agents: molecular mechanisms and clinical consequences. Lancet Infect Dis. 2002;2(2):73–85.
30. Coste A, Turner V, Ischer F, et al. A mutation in Tac1p, a transcription factor regulating CDR1 and CDR2, is coupled with loss of heterozygosity at chromosome 5 to mediate antifungal resistance in Candida albicans. Genetics. 2006;172(4):2139–56.
31. Vermitsky J-P, Earhart KD, Smith WL, Homayouni R, Edlind TD, Rogers PD. Pdr1 regulates multidrug resistance in Candida glabrata: gene disruption and genome-wide expression studies. Mol Microbiol. 2006;61(3):704–22.
32. Selmecki A, Forche A, Berman J. Aneuploidy and isochromosome formation in drug-resistant Candida albicans. Science. 2006;313(5785):367–70.
33. Camps SM, van der Linden JW, Li Y, Kuijper EJ, van Dissel JT, Verweij PE, et al. Rapid induction of multiple resistance mechanisms in aspergillus fumigatus during azole therapy: a case study and review of the literature. Antimicrob Agents Chemother. 2012;56(1):10–6.
34. White TC, Holleman S, Dy F, Mirels LF, Stevens DA. Resistance mechanisms in clinical isolates of Candida albicans. Antimicrob Agents Chemother. 2002;46(6):1704–13.
35. Howard SJ, Cerar D, Anderson MJ, Albarrag A, Fisher MC, Pasqualotto AC, et al. Frequency and evolution of azole resistance in aspergillus fumigatus associated with treatment failure. Emerg Infect Dis. 2009;15(7):1068–76.
36. Verweij PE, Howard SJ, Melchers WJ, Denning DW. Azole-resistance in aspergillus: proposed nomenclature and breakpoints. Drug Resist Updat. 2009;12(6):141–7.
37. Camps SM, Rijs AJ, Klaassen CH, Meis JF, O'Gorman CM, Dyer PS, et al. Molecular epidemiology of aspergillus fumigatus isolates harboring the TR34/L998H azole resistance mechanism. J Clin Microbiol. 2012;50(8):2674–80.
38. van der Linden JW, Snelders E, Kampinga GA, Rijnders BJ, Mattsson E, Debets-Ossenkopp YJ, et al. Clinical implications of azole resistance in aspergillus fumigatus, the Netherlands, 2007–2009. Emerg Infect Dis. 2011;17(10):1846–54.
39. Verweij PE, Chowdhary A, Melchers WJ, Meis JF. Azole resistance in aspergillus fumigatus: can we retain the clinical use of mold-active antifungal azoles? Clin Infect Dis. 2016;62(3):362–8.
40. Verweij PE, Snelders E, Kema GH, Mellado E, Melchers WJ. Azole resistance in aspergillus fumigatus: a side-effect of environmental fungicide use? Lancet Infect Dis. 2009;9(12):789–95.

41. Denning DW, Perlin DS. Azole resistance in aspergillus: a growing public health menace. Future Microbiol. 2011;6(11):1229–32.
42. Denning DW, Park S, Lass-Florl C, Fraczek MG, Kirwan M, Gore R, et al. High-frequency triazole resistance found in nonculturable aspergillus fumigatus from lungs of patients with chronic fungal disease. Clin Infect Dis. 2011;52(9):1123–9.
43. da Silva Ferreira ME, Capellaro JL, dos Reis Marques E, Malavazi I, Perlin D, Park S, et al. In vitro evolution of itraconazole resistance in aspergillus fumigatus involves multiple mechanisms of resistance. Antimicrob Agents Chemother. 2004;48(11):4405–13.
44. Rajendran R, Mowat E, McCulloch E, Lappin DF, Jones B, Lang S, et al. Azole resistance of aspergillus fumigatus biofilms is partly associated with efflux pump activity. Antimicrob Agents Chemother. 2011;55(5):2092–7.
45. Park S, Kelly R, Kahn JN, Robles J, Hsu MJ, Register E, et al. Specific substitutions in the echinocandin target Fks1p account for reduced susceptibility of rare laboratory and clinical Candida sp. isolates. Antimicrob Agents Chemother. 2005;49(8):3264–73.
46. Katiyar S, Pfaller M, Edlind T. Candida albicans and Candida glabrata clinical isolates exhibiting reduced echinocandin susceptibility. Antimicrob Agents Chemother. 2006;50(8):2892–4.
47. Perlin DS. Resistance to echinocandin-class antifungal drugs. Drug Resist Updat. 2007;10(3):121–30.
48. Perlin DS. Current perspectives on echinocandin class drugs. Future Microbiol. 2011;6(4):441–57.
49. Garcia-Effron G, Lee S, Park S, Cleary JD, Perlin DS. Effect of Candida glabrata FKS1 and FKS2 mutations on echinocandin sensitivity and kinetics of 1,3-beta-D-glucan synthase: implication for the existing susceptibility breakpoint. Antimicrob Agents Chemother. 2009;53(9):3690–9.
50. Garcia-Effron G, Park S, Perlin DS. Correlating echinocandin MIC and kinetic inhibition of fks1 mutant glucan synthases for Candida albicans: implications for interpretive breakpoints. Antimicrob Agents Chemother. 2009;53(1):112–22.
51. Perlin D. Echinocandin-resistant Candida: molecular methods and phenotypes. Curr Fungal Infect Rep. 2011;5:113–9.
52. Arendrup MC, Perlin DS. Echinocandin resistance: an emerging clinical problem? Curr Opin Infect Dis. 2014;27:484–92.
53. Arendrup MC, Perlin DS, Jensen RH, Howard SJ, Goodwin J, Hope W. Differential in vivo activities of anidulafungin, caspofungin, and micafungin against Candida glabrata isolates with and without FKS resistance mutations. Antimicrob Agents Chemother. 2012;56(5):2435–42.
54. Andes D, Ambrose PG, Hammel JP, Van Wart SA, Iyer V, Reynolds DK, et al. Use of pharmacokinetic-pharmacodynamic analyses to optimize therapy with the systemic antifungal micafungin for invasive candidiasis or candidemia. Antimicrob Agents Chemother. 2011;55(5):2113–21.
55. Mandell GL, Bennett JE, Dolin R. Principles and practice of infectious deaseses. Philadelphia: Churchill Livingstone; 2009.
56. Chandrasekar P. Management of invasive fungal infections: a role for polyenes. J Antimicrob Chemother. 2011;66(3):457–65.
57. Safdar A, Ma J, Saliba F, Dupont B, Wingard JR, Hachem RY, et al. Drug-induced nephrotoxicity caused by amphotericin B lipid complex and liposomal amphotericin B: a review and meta-analysis. Medicine (Baltimore). 2010;89(4):236–44. Epub 2010/07/10.
58. Pappas PG, Kauffman CA, Perfect J, et al. Alopecia associated with fluconazole therapy. Ann Intern Med. 1995;123:354–7.
59. Slavin MA, Osborne B, Adams R, Levenstein MJ, Schoch HG, Feldman AR. Efficacy and safety of fluconazole prophylaxis for fungal infections after marrow transplantation: a prospective, randomized, double-blind study. J Infect Dis. 1995;171:1545–52.
60. Ellis ME, Clink H, Ernst P, Halim MA, Padmos A, Spence D, et al. Controlled study of fluconazole in the prevention of fungal infections in neutropenic patients with haematological malignancies and bone marrow transplant recipients. Eur J Clin Microbiol Infect Dis. 1994;13(1):3–11.
61. Goodman JL, Winston DJ, Greenfield RA, Chandrasekar PH, Fox B, Kaizer H, et al. A controlled trial of fluconazole to prevent fungal infections in patients undergoing bone marrow transplantation. N Engl J Med. 1992;326(13):845–51.
62. Philpott-Howard JN, Wade JJ, Mufti GJ, Brammer KW, Ehninger G. Randomized comparison of oral fluconazole versus oral polyenes for the prevention of fungal infection in patients at risk of neutropenia. Multicentre Study Group. J Antimicrob Chemother. 1993;31(6):973–84.
63. Rotstein C, Bow EJ, Laverdiere M, Ioannou S, Carr D, Moghaddam N, et al. Randomized placebo-controlled trial of fluconazole prophylaxis for neutropenic cancer patients: benefit based on purpose and intensity of cytotoxic therapy. Clin Infect Dis. 1999;28(2):331–40.
64. Egger T, Gratwohl A, Tichelli A, Uhr M, Stebler Gysi C, Passweg J, et al. Comparison of fluconazole with oral polyenes in the prevention of fungal infections in neutropenic patients. A prospective, randomized, single-center study. Support Care Cancer. 1995;3(2):139–46.
65. Rogers TR, Slavin MA, Donnelly JP. Antifungal prophylaxis during treatment for haematological malignancies: are we there yet? Br J Haematol. 2011;153(6):681–97.
66. National Comprehensive Cancer Network. Clinical practice guidelines in oncology. Prevention and treatment of cancer related infections. V.2.2009. Available from http://www.nccn.org. Accessed 19 Mar 2012.
67. Wingard JR, Carter SL, Walsh TJ, Kurtzberg J, Small TN, Baden LR, et al. Randomized, double-blind trial of fluconazole versus voriconazole for prevention of invasive fungal infection after allogeneic hematopoietic cell transplantation. Blood. 2010;116(24):5111–8.
68. Chen SCA, Slavin MA, Sorrell TC. Echinocandin antifungal drugs in fungal infections: a comparison. Drugs. 2011;71(1):11–41.
69. van Burik JA, Ratanatharathorn V, Stepan DE, Miller CB, Lipton JH, Vesole DH, et al. Micafungin versus fluconazole for prophylaxis against invasive fungal infections during neutropenia in patients undergoing hematopoietic stem cell transplantation. Clin Infect Dis. 2004;39(10):1407–16.
70. Hiramatsu Y, Maeda Y, Fujii N, Saito T, Nawa Y, Hara M, et al. Use of micafungin versus fluconazole for antifungal prophylaxis in neutropenic patients receiving hematopoietic stem cell transplantation. Int J Hematol. 2008;88(5):588–95.
71. Ullmann AJ, Lipton JH, Vesole DH, Chandrasekar P, Langston A, Tarantolo SR, et al. Posaconazole or fluconazole for prophylaxis in severe graft-versus-host disease. N Engl J Med. 2007;356(4):335–47.
72. Marr KA. Primary antifungal prophylaxis in hematopoietic stem cell transplant recipients: clinical implications of recent studies. Curr Opin Infect Dis. 2008;21(4):409–14.
73. Marks DI, Pagliuca A, Kibbler CC, Glasmacher A, Heussel CP, Kantecki M, et al. Voriconazole versus itraconazole for antifungal prophylaxis following allogeneic haematopoietic stem-cell transplantation. Br J Haematol. 2011;155(3):318–27.
74. Paya CV. Fungal infections in solid-organ transplantation. Clin Infect Dis. 1993;16(5):677–88.
75. Winston DJ, Emmanouilides C, Busuttil RW. Infections in liver transplant recipients. Clin Infect Dis. 1995;21(5):1077–89. quiz 90-1.
76. Winston DJ, Pakrasi A, Busuttil RW. Prophylactic fluconazole in liver transplant recipients. A randomized, double-blind, placebo-controlled trial. Ann Intern Med. 1999;131(10):729–37.
77. Hadley S, Samore MH, Lewis WD, Jenkins RL, Karchmer AW, Hammer SM. Major infectious complications after orthotopic liver transplantation and comparison of outcomes in patients

receiving cyclosporine or FK506 as primary immunosuppression. Transplantation. 1995;59(6):851–9.

78. Karchmer AW, Samore MH, Hadley S, Collins LA, Jenkins RL, Lewis WD. Fungal infections complicating orthotopic liver transplantation. Trans Am Clin Climatol Assoc. 1995;106:38–47. discussion-8.
79. Benedetti E, Gruessner AC, Troppmann C, Papalois BE, Sutherland DE, Dunn DL, et al. Intra-abdominal fungal infections after pancreatic transplantation: incidence, treatment, and outcome. J Am Coll Surg. 1996;183(4):307–16.
80. Guaraldi G, Cocchi S, Codeluppi M, Di Benedetto F, De Ruvo N, Masetti M, et al. Outcome, incidence, and timing of infectious complications in small bowel and multivisceral organ transplantation patients. Transplantation. 2005;80(12):1742–8.
81. Pappas PG, Kauffman CA, Andes DR, Clancy CJ, Marr KA, Ostrosky-Zeichner L, Reboli AC, Schuster MG, Vazquez JA, Walsh TJ, Zaoutis TE, Sobel JD. Clinical practice guideline for the management of candidiasis: 2016 update by the Infectious Diseases Society of America. Clin Infect Dis. 2016;62(4):e1–50.
82. Schaenman JM, Rosso F, Austin JM, Baron EJ, Gamberg P, Miller J, et al. Trends in invasive disease due to Candida species following heart and lung transplantation. Transpl Infect Dis. 2009;11(2):112–21.
83. Kontoyiannis DP, Marr KA, Park BJ, Alexander BD, Anaissie EJ, Walsh TJ, et al. Prospective surveillance for invasive fungal infections in hematopoietic stem cell transplant recipients, 2001–2006: overview of the transplant-associated infection surveillance network (TRANSNET) database. Clin Infect Dis. 2010;50(8):1091–100.
84. Pappas PG, Alexander BD, Andes DR, Hadley S, Kauffman CA, Freifeld A, et al. Invasive fungal infections among organ transplant recipients: results of the transplant-associated infection surveillance network (TRANSNET). Clin Infect Dis. 2010;50(8):1101–11.
85. Rex JH, Bennett JE, Sugar AM, Pappas PG, van der Horst CM, Edwards JE, et al. A randomized trial comparing fluconazole with amphotericin B for the treatment of candidemia in patients without neutropenia. Candidemia Study Group and the National Institute. N Engl J Med. 1994;331(20):1325–30.
86. Mora-Duarte J, Betts R, Rotstein C, Colombo AL, Thompson-Moya L, Smietana J, et al. Comparison of caspofungin and amphotericin B for invasive candidiasis. N Engl J Med. 2002;347(25):2020–9.
87. Kuse ER, Chetchotisakd P, da Cunha CA, Ruhnke M, Barrios C, Raghunadharao D, et al. Micafungin versus liposomal amphotericin B for candidaemia and invasive candidosis: a phase III randomised double-blind trial. Lancet. 2007;369(9572):1519–27.
88. Reboli AC, Rotstein C, Pappas PG, Chapman SW, Kett DH, Kumar D, et al. Anidulafungin versus fluconazole for invasive candidiasis. N Engl J Med. 2007;356(24):2472–82.
89. Pappas PG, Rotstein CM, Betts RF, Nucci M, Talwar D, De Waele JJ, et al. Micafungin versus caspofungin for treatment of candidemia and other forms of invasive candidiasis. Clin Infect Dis. 2007;45(7):883–93.
90. Pappas PG, Kauffman CA, Andes DR, et al. Clinical practice guideline for the management of candidiasis: 2016 update by the Infectious Diseases Society of America. Clin Infect Dis. 2016;62(4):e1–e50.
91. Almyroudis NG, Segal BH. Antifungal prophylaxis and therapy in patients with hematological malignancies and hematopoietic stem cell transplant recipients. Expert Rev Anti-Infect Ther. 2010;8(12):1451–66.
92. Herbrecht R, Denning DW, Patterson TF, Bennett JE, Greene RE, Oestmann JW, et al. Voriconazole versus amphotericin B for primary therapy of invasive aspergillosis. N Engl J Med. 2002;347(6):408–15.
93. Schwartz S, Reisman A, Troke PF. The efficacy of voriconazole in the treatment of 192 fungal central nervous system infections: a retrospective analysis. Infection. 2011;39(3):201–10.
94. Cornely OA, Maertens J, Bresnik M, Ebrahimi R, Ullmann AJ, Bouza E, et al. Liposomal amphotericin B as initial therapy for invasive mold infection: a randomized trial comparing a high-loading dose regimen with standard dosing (AmBiLoad trial). Clin Infect Dis. 2007;44(10):1289–97.
95. Walsh TJ, Raad I, Patterson TF, Chandrasekar P, Donowitz GR, Graybill R, et al. Treatment of invasive aspergillosis with posaconazole in patients who are refractory to or intolerant of conventional therapy: an externally controlled trial. Clin Infect Dis. 2007;44(1):2–12.
96. Raad II, Hanna HA, Boktour M, Jiang Y, Torres HA, Afif C, et al. Novel antifungal agents as salvage therapy for invasive aspergillosis in patients with hematologic malignancies: posaconazole compared with high-dose lipid formulations of amphotericin B alone or in combination with caspofungin. Leukemia. 2008;22(3):496–503.
97. Alexander BD, Perfect JR, Daly JS, Restrepo A, Tobon AM, Patino H, et al. Posaconazole as salvage therapy in patients with invasive fungal infections after solid organ transplant. Transplantation. 2008;86(6):791–6.
98. Maertens JA, Raad II, Marr KA, Patterson TF, Kontoyiannis DP, Cornely OA, et al. Isavuconazole versus voriconazole for primary treatment of invasive mould disease caused by aspergillus and other filamentous fungi (SECURE): a phase 3, randomised-controlled, non-inferiority trial. Lancet. 2016;387:760–9.
99. Viscoli C, Herbrecht R, Akan H, Baila L, Sonet A, Gallamini A, et al. An EORTC phase II study of caspofungin as first-line therapy of invasive aspergillosis in haematological patients. J Antimicrob Chemother. 2009;64(6):1274–81.
100. Herbrecht R, Maertens J, Baila L, Aoun M, Heinz W, Martino R, et al. Caspofungin first-line therapy for invasive aspergillosis in allogeneic hematopoietic stem cell transplant patients: an European Organisation for Research and Treatment of Cancer study. Bone Marrow Transplant. 2010;45(7):1227–33.
101. Maertens J, Raad I, Petrikkos G, Boogaerts M, Selleslag D, Petersen FB, et al. Efficacy and safety of caspofungin for treatment of invasive aspergillosis in patients refractory to or intolerant of conventional antifungal therapy. Clin Infect Dis. 2004;39(11):1563–71.
102. Denning DW, Marr KA, Lau WM, Facklam DP, Ratanatharathorn V, Becker C, et al. Micafungin (FK463), alone or in combination with other systemic antifungal agents, for the treatment of acute invasive aspergillosis. J Infect. 2006;53(5):337–49.
103. Petraitis V, Petraitiene R, Sarafandi AA, Kelaher AM, Lyman CA, Casler HE, et al. Combination therapy in treatment of experimental pulmonary aspergillosis: synergistic interaction between an antifungal triazole and an echinocandin. J Infect Dis. 2003;187(12):1834–43.
104. Marr KA, Boeckh M, Carter RA, Kim HW, Corey L. Combination antifungal therapy for invasive aspergillosis. Clin Infect Dis. 2004;39(6):797–802.
105. Singh N, Limaye AP, Forrest G, Safdar N, Munoz P, Pursell K, et al. Combination of voriconazole and caspofungin as primary therapy for invasive aspergillosis in solid organ transplant recipients: a prospective, multicenter, observational study. Transplantation. 2006;81(3):320–6.
106. Patterson TF, Thompson GR 3rd, Denning DW, Fishman JA, Hadley S, Herbrecht R, Kontoyiannis DP, Marr KA, Morrison VA, Nguyen MH, Segal BH, Steinbach WJ, Stevens DA, Walsh TJ, Wingard JR, Young JA, Bennett JE. Practice guidelines for the diagnosis and Management of Aspergillosis: 2016 update by the Infectious Diseases Society of America. Clin Infect Dis. 2016;63(4):e1–e60.

107. Walsh TJ, Anaissie EJ, Denning DW, Herbrecht R, Kontoyiannis DP, Marr KA, et al. Treatment of aspergillosis: clinical practice guidelines of the Infectious Diseases Society of America. Clin Infect Dis. 2008;46(3):327–60.
108. Roden MM, Zaoutis TE, Buchanan WL, Knudsen TA, Sarkisova TA, Schaufele RL, et al. Epidemiology and outcome of zygomycosis: a review of 929 reported cases. Clin Infect Dis. 2005;41(5):634–53.
109. Greenberg RN, Mullane K, van Burik JA, Raad I, Abzug MJ, Anstead G, et al. Posaconazole as salvage therapy for zygomycosis. Antimicrob Agents Chemother. 2006;50(1):126–33.
110. van Burik JA, Hare RS, Solomon HF, Corrado ML, Kontoyiannis DP. Posaconazole is effective as salvage therapy in zygomycosis: a retrospective summary of 91 cases. Clin Infect Dis. 2006;42(7):e61–5.
111. Marty FM, Ostrosky-Zeichner L, Cornely OA, Mullane KM, Perfect JR, Thompson GR III, et al. Isavuconazole treatment for mucormycosis: a single-arm open-label trial and case-control analysis. Lancet Infect Dis. 2016;16:828–37.
112. Spellberg B, Ibrahim AS, Chin-Hong PV, Kontoyiannis DP, Morris MI, Perfect JR, et al. The Deferasirox-AmBisome therapy for Mucormycosis (DEFEAT Mucor) study: a randomized, double-blinded, placebo-controlled trial. J Antimicrob Chemother. 2012;67(3):715–22.
113. Nucci M, Marr KA, Queiroz-Telles F, Martins CA, Trabasso P, Costa S, et al. Fusarium infection in hematopoietic stem cell transplant recipients. Clin Infect Dis. 2004;38(9):1237–42.
114. Park BJ, Pappas PG, Wannemuehler KA, Alexander BD, Anaissie EJ, Andes DR, et al. Invasive non-aspergillus mold infections in transplant recipients, United States, 2001–2006. Emerg Infect Dis. 2011;17(10):1855–64.
115. Perfect JR, Marr KA, Walsh TJ, Greenberg RN, DuPont B, de la Torre-Cisneros J, et al. Voriconazole treatment for less-common, emerging, or refractory fungal infections. Clin Infect Dis. 2003;36(9):1122–31.
116. Raad II, Hachem RY, Herbrecht R, Graybill JR, Hare R, Corcoran G, et al. Posaconazole as salvage treatment for invasive fusariosis in patients with underlying hematologic malignancy and other conditions. Clin Infect Dis. 2006;42(10):1398–403.
117. Perfect JR. Treatment of non-aspergillus moulds in immunocompromised patients, with amphotericin B lipid complex. Clin Infect Dis. 2005;40(Suppl 6):S401–8.
118. Cuenca-Estrella M, Gomez-Lopez A, Mellado E, Buitrago MJ, Monzon A, Rodriguez-Tudela JL. Head-to-head comparison of the activities of currently available antifungal agents against 3,378 Spanish clinical isolates of yeasts and filamentous fungi. Antimicrob Agents Chemother. 2006;50(3):917–21.
119. Espinel-Ingroff A, Johnson E, Hockey H, Troke P. Activities of voriconazole, itraconazole and amphotericin B in vitro against 590 moulds from 323 patients in the voriconazole phase III clinical studies. J Antimicrob Chemother. 2008;61(3):616–20.
120. Perfect JR, Dismukes WE, Dromer F, Goldman DL, Graybill JR, Hamill RJ, et al. Clinical practice guidelines for the management of cryptococcal disease: 2010 update by the infectious diseases society of america. Clin Infect Dis. 2010;50(3):291–322.

Immunomodulatory Properties of Antifungal Agents on Immune Functions of the Host

53

Maria Simitsopoulou and Emmanuel Roilides

Introduction

During the past two to three decades, an increasing incidence of invasive fungal diseases among immunocompromised patients has been witnessed [1, 2]. The rising number of patients undergoing allogeneic hematopoietic stem cell transplantation and solid organ allograft transplantation receiving immunosuppressive drug regimens is in part responsible for this epidemiologic trend. The overall immunosuppressed status of these patients makes them highly susceptible to viral, bacterial, fungal, and protozoal opportunistic pathogens [3]. Fungi are a significant cause of morbidity and mortality in patients undergoing allogeneic graft transplantation [4, 5]. While *Candida* and *Aspergillus* species are the cause for most of the post-transplant invasive fungal diseases, a number of other less frequent pathogens, such as Zygomycetes, *Fusarium*, and *Scedosporium* species may sporadically cause serious disease [5–8].

These recent epidemiologic trends coupled with emergence and spread of drug-resistant fungal pathogens, i.e., multidrug-resistant *Candida* spp. like *Candida auris;* azole and polyene-resistant *Aspergillus* spp. such as *Aspergillus terreus* [9, 10]. Furthermore, antifungal drug toxicity, and drug-drug interaction have foster interest in exploring pharmacodynamic properties of antifungal drugs with emphasis on the potential immune modifying aspect on host-fungus interplay.

In this chapter the main in vitro and in vivo immunomodulatory effects of antifungal drugs on phagocytic cells in response to fungal stimulation with reference to their interaction with phagocyte functions is presented. When applicable, the underlying mechanism(s) and potential clinical relevance of such antifungal effects are given.

Host-Fungal Pathogen Interplay

The innate immune system is based not only on barrier and chemical defense mechanisms to combat infection, but also on various immune cells that recognize invading pathogens and activate a series of antimicrobial immune responses. Upon fungal invasion, ciliated respiratory epithelium and gastrointestinal and vaginal mucosa secrete antimicrobial compounds to neutralize or kill invading organisms. Similarly, resident or recruited phagocytic macrophages, polymorphonuclear leukocytes (PMNs), or dendritic cells (DCs), the cellular components of innate immunity, play a central role in cytokine production and T cell-mediated immunity.

Phagocytic cells recognize fungal particles through specific cell-surface pattern recognition receptors (PRRs), leading to the activation of phagocytosis, production of inflammatory molecules for the recruitment of additional Th1 and Th2 cell adaptive immune response, and production of microbicidal products. Pathogen detection involves recognition of conserved pathogen-associated molecular patterns (PAMPs), either secreted by or located on the surface of fungal particles, by the well-known Toll-like receptors (TLRs) like dectin-1, dectin-2, mannose receptors (MR), dendritic cell-specific ICAM3-grabbing non-integrin (DC-SIGN), and the nucleotide-binding domain and leucine-rich repeat containing (NLR) family of cytosolic receptors that mediate both inflammatory and cell death pathways [11, 12]. Most TLRs transduce the signal received from the surface to the nucleus via a signaling pathway that depends on the adaptor myeloid differentiation factor 88 (MyD88) and its downstream mediators interleukin-receptor-associated kinase 4 (IRAK-4) and tumor necrosis factor receptor-associated factor 6 (TRAF-6) that activate nuclear factor (NF)-κB in

M. Simitsopoulou
Research Infectious Disease Laboratory, 3rd Department Pediatrics, Aristotle University School of Medicine, Hippokration Hospital, Thessaloniki, Greece
e-mail: simitsop@med.auth.gr

E. Roilides (✉)
3rd Department of Pediatrics, Hippokration Hospital, School of Health Sciences, Aristotle University of Thessaloniki, Thessaloniki, Greece
e-mail: roilides@med.auth.gr

A. Safdar (ed.), *Principles and Practice of Transplant Infectious Diseases*, https://doi.org/10.1007/978-1-4939-9034-4_53

order for the appropriate cellular responses needed to be initiated [13–15]. The final effector response profile in the target cell depends on the cell type. For example, activation of TLR2 or dectin-1 in macrophages results in the production of several pro-inflammatory cytokines and chemokines, such as IL-1α/β, IL-6, TNF-α, IL-8, and RANTES, that initiate a protective immune response against fungal invasion. Upregulation of epithelial TLR4 is involved in mediating a secondary protective effect against *Candida albicans* invasion in the presence of PMNs [16]. Recognition of *Aspergillus fumigatus* and activation of PMNs occur through the involvement of other TLRs. Signaling through TLR2 promotes the oxidative fungicidal pathway of PMNs with the participation of pro-inflammatory cytokines and results in killing fungal microconidia. TLR4 signaling on the other hand, is essential for the induction of nonoxidative mechanisms mediated by the release of PMN azurophilic granule constituents and IL-10 upregulation, important for fungal hyphal damage. Both pathways are affected to various degrees by TLR3, TLR5, TLR6, TLR7, TLR8, and TLR9 signaling [17]. As PMNs are important for pathogen elimination in the early stages of fungal invasion, an excessive release of toxic reactive species may also result in tissue injury and SIRS vs. sepsis like syndrome. Therefore, PMNs through TLR cross talk mount a robust antifungal response which, however, is tightly regulated in order to balance between protection and inflammation. The specificity of immune host response is dictated not only by the different PAMP structures present in the fungal cell wall, but also by the complex interactions between the PRR pathways demonstrated in a number of studies [18].

Fungal conidia are damaged through a phagocytic process effected primarily by the incoming mononuclear cells (MNCs) or resident tissue macrophages; by comparison, hyphae are damaged through the extracellular release of fungicidal products of the oxidative burst and nonoxidative mechanisms of PMNs. During the oxidative burst, phagocytic cells generate reactive oxygen species (ROS), such as superoxide anion, hydrogen peroxide, and nitrogen intermediates; this microbicidal system employed primarily by PMNs is catalyzed by the nicotinamide adenine dinucleotide phosphate (NADPH) oxidase, a multisubunit enzyme complex embedded in the plasma membrane of the cells. Patients with chronic granulomatous disease (CGD), in which superoxide anion is not produced due to mutations in the NADPH oxidase, these patients are predisposed to severe systemic bacterial and fungal infections. Despite the absence of ROS production, the CGD neutrophil phagosome is able to kill significant microbial load by microbicidal molecules that are independent of the respiratory burst [19]. The oxygen-independent system, which relies on the microbicidal properties of proteases, cationic peptides, defensins, lactoferrin, or lysozyme stored in azurophilic granules, is essential for the optimal antifungal activity of phagocytes [20]. Myeloperoxidase (MPO), a granular enzyme released into the phagosome, catalyzes the conversion of superoxide into several reactive oxygen molecules such as hypochlorous acid, chloramines, hydroxyl radicals, and singlet oxygen. A study conducted with MPO−/− and X-linked CGD mice demonstrated that both MPO and NADPH oxidase are equally important for host defense against a large fungal inoculum [21]. Recently, PMN extracellular traps (NETs) consisting of decondensed chromatin and antimicrobial proteins released from dying PMNs have also been added to the protective mechanisms employed by the host against fungal invaders [22, 23].

While PMNs and macrophages are important effectors of innate immunity involved in the immediate killing of pathogens, DCs by being potent antigen-presenting cells needed for T-cell activation via appropriate signals are regarded as the principle communication between the innate and adaptive immune responses. Depending on the fungal morphotype ingested by DCs, different downstream signaling programs are activated: conidial ingestion leads to the production of pro-inflammatory cytokines and activation of protective Th1-cell responses; in contrast, hyphal ingestion results in production of IL-4 and/or IL-10 and activation of Th2/T_{reg} cells [24–26].

Antifungal Drug-Induced Effects on Host-Fungus Interplay

The main antifungal agents currently used for treatment of invasive fungal diseases belong to the following three categories: (1) polyenes represented by deoxycholate and lipid formulations of amphotericin B; (2) azoles most importantly fluconazole, voriconazole, posaconazole and isavuconazonium sulfate; and (3) echinocandins class consists of caspofungin, micafungin, and anidulafungin. Amphotericin B binds to ergosterol in the fungal cell membrane forming transmembrane channels, through which intracellular molecules leak out; azoles act by inhibiting synthesis of ergosterol; whereas echinocandins are cell-wall active drugs inhibiting 1,3-β-D-glucan synthesis. Members of each category exert various modulatory effects on host-pathogen interactions. In addition, certain antibacterial agents have interactions with antifungals and hosts' cytokine response.

In the phagocyte-fungus-antifungal drug interplay, drugs may directly interact with the immune effector cells through cell receptors, leading to altered antifungal activities. Following cellular uptake and intracellular accumulation, antifungals may modify immune responses by release of pro- or anti-inflammatory cytokines and influence production of reactive oxygen species or affect enzymatic pathways, such products are shown to possess antifungal properties [27–29]. In addition, antifungal agents at subinhibitory concentrations may indirectly affect phagocyte activities by alteration of fungal morphology, resulting in increased pathogen susceptibility to phagocyte actions, and by acting upon the fungal organisms either by fungistatic or fungicidal effect reduce fungal burden, thereby providing time for host to mount a robust and durable antifungal response needed to eradicate the invading pathogen, while keeping excessive unconstrained inflammation in check. Modulation of phagocyte behavior has also been observed after priming of phagocytes with cytokines, increasing the intracellular antifungal effect of drugs [30, 31].

The following drug-fungus or drug-host or drug-fungus-host interactions are described in the following parts of the chapter as:

1. Drug-phagocyte communication through cellular receptors
2. Antifungal drug-induced cytokine and chemokine expression profiles in human phagocytes
3. Modulation of phagocytes' activity by antifungal agents
4. Modulation of phagocytes' activity by the combined effect of cytokines and antifungal agents

Immunomodulatory Effects of Amphotericin B Formulations

During the past several years, studies have suggested that antifungal agents may alter phagocytes' immune responses against fungi by affecting specific PRRs. Amphotericin B is a broad-spectrum polyene antifungal agent. Deoxycholate compound is the oldest amphotericin B formulation and remains among the most useful agents against invasive fungal diseases especially in resource-limited countries. Its use is wide, despite the infusion-related reactions and risk for dose-dependent nephrotoxicity; the drug induced kidney injury is postulated to originate from a potent pro-inflammatory response by innate immune cells elicited by its affinity for cholesterol binding in mammalian cell membrane[32]. Two complementary studies have demonstrated that amphotericin B is probably perceived as a PAMP by CD14, TLR1, and TLR2 receptors, which are coactivated through a reorganization of lipid raft proteins in the microdomains of cell membrane serving as centers for assembly of signaling molecules, which promotes secretion of pro-inflammatory cytokines and chemokines [33, 34] (Table 53.1). A detailed investigation of the intracellular signaling induced by amphotericin B in a monocytic cell line has shown that pro-inflammatory cytokine production is mediated by B-cell progenitor tyrosine kinase (Btk), phospholipase C (PLC), protein kinase C (PKC), cellular tyrosine kinase (c-Src), and NF-κB signaling molecules [35]. These studies provide a molecular basis for the recognized inflammatory adverse effects associated with amphotericin B in patients and identify potential targets for agents that could minimize such effects.

Table 53.1 Effects of antifungal agents on pattern recognition receptors of phagocytes

Antifungal agent	Recognition receptors	Fungus studied
Fluconazole	Up-regulation of TLR9 in PMNs	*C. albicans*
Voriconazole	Up-regulation of TLR2, 4, 9 in PMNs	*A. fumigatus*
	Up-regulation of TLR2 in MNCs	*A. fumigatus*
Deoxycholate amphotericin B	Up-regulation of TLR1, TLR2, CD14 in MNCs	*A. fumigatus*
Liposomal Amphotercin B	Up-regulation of TLR4 in PMNs	*A. fumigatus, C. albicans*
Caspofungin	Up-regulation of TLR2, 4, 9, in PMNs dectin-1 in MNCs, PMNs	*A. fumigatus, C. albicans A. fumigatus*

Lipid formulations of amphotericin B were developed in order to avoid or minimize toxicity and contribute to the overall improvement of therapeutic index. Exposure of murine and human PMNs to *A. fumigatus* in the presence of liposomal amphotericin B (LAMB) involves different TLR-activation pathways as compared to deoxycholate amphotericin B (DAMB). While DAMB activates the oxidative antifungal response leading to an increased pro-inflammatory state through TLR2 signal transduction, LAMB by diverting signaling from TLR2 to TLR4, induces more IL-10 and less TNF-α or superoxide anion production in PMNs stimulated with *A. fumigatus* conidia (Table 53.1). In addition, LAMB augments the conidiocidal activity of both murine and human PMNs suggesting that it either has an immunomodulatory role on PMN antifungal functions or increases conidial susceptibility to PMN conidiocidal activity altering fungal membrane [36] (Table 53.2).

As stated above, infusion-related adverse drug reactions observed in patients treated with amphotericin B are associated with the ability of DAMB to induce the release of pro-inflammatory cytokines after activation of immune cells via TLRs and CD14 with the subsequent activation of MyD88 and NF-κB signal transducer molecules. In an attempt to understand the molecular mechanisms by which lipid amphotericin B formulations induce a specific gene expression profile as compared to DAMB, studies using human MNCs have identified a number of immune molecules that are induced and released following exposure to different amphotericin B formulations [37–45] or after challenge with *A. fumigatus* hyphae [46, 47] (Table 53.3). These studies indicated that DAMB and amphotericin B colloidal dispersion (ABCD) upregulate gene expression and production of pro-inflammatory cytokines and chemokines. By comparison, LAMB and ABLC generally downregulate or do not affect gene expression of pro-inflammatory cytokines and chemokines, which may explain the relatively lower frequency of adverse infusion-related reactions of these agents reported in clinical trials.

Table 53.2 Effects of antifungal agents on the antifungal activities of phagocytes

Immunomodulatory agent	Phagocyte function	Fungus/animal model studied
FLC	Moderate anticonidial activity in PMNs	*C. albicans*
FLC + G-CSF	Enhanced survival	Disseminated candidiasis
FLC + sIL-4R or FLC + rIL-12	Synergistic effect on survival	*C. albicans*; immunosuppressed murine model
VRC	Unaffected anticonidial activity in PMNs	*C. albicans*
VRC	Drug- and time-dependent anticonidial activity in MNCs	*Candida* spp.
VRC	Additive antihyphal activity in PMNs	*R. microsporus*
VRC + GM-CSF or G-CSF	Increased anticandidal activity in MNCs and PMNs	*Candida* spp., *Cryptococcus neoformans*
VRC + GM-CSF	No effect on antihyphal activity in MNCs; increased antihyphal activity in PMNs	*A. fumigatus*
PSC	Modest efficacy	*R. microsporus*; immunosuppressed murine model
PSC + GM-CSF	Increased hyphal damage	*S. prolificans*; ex vivo
PSC + G-CSF	Modest survival or antagonistic effect	*A. fumigatus*, *R. microsporus*; immunosuppressed murine model
DAMB	Increased anticonidial activity in MNCs	*A. fumigatus*, *C. albicans*
DAMB	Increased antihyphal activity in MNCs, PMNs	*A. fumigatus*, *F. solani*
DAMB	Reduction in fungal load, induction of Th1 immune response	disseminated aspergillosis
DAMB + sIL-4R or rIL-12	Synergistic effect on survival	*C. albicans*; immunosuppressed murine model
DAMB + IFN-γ	Additive inhibitory effect	*C. neoformans*
LAMB	Increased antihyphal activity in MNCs, PMNs	*A. fumigatus*, *F. solani*
ABLC	Increased antihyphal activity in MNCs, PMNs	*A. fumigatus*, *F. solani*
ABLC	Additive antihyphal activity in PMNs	*S. prolificans*, *S. apiospermum*
ABCD	Increased antihyphal activity in MNCs, PMNs	*A. fumigatus*, *F. solani*
CAS	Increased intracellular killing; unaffected phagocytosis	*C. albicans*
CAS	Augmented antihyphal activity in PMNs	*A. fumigatus*
CAS + GM-CSF	Increased anticandidal activity	*C. glabrata*
MICA	Augmented antihyphal activity in PMNs, MNCs	*A. fumigatus*
AND	Increased intracellular killing, unaffected phagocytosis	*C. albicans*
AND	Additive antifungal activity in PMNs	*C. parapsilosis* biofilms
AND	Additive antifungal activity in MNCs	*C. albicans* biofilms
AND	Augmented antihyphal activity in PMNs	*A. fumigatus*
CIP + AMB	Synergistic anticonidial activity in PMNs	*A. fumigatus*

FLC fluconazole, *VRC* voriconazole, *PSC* posaconazole, *DAMB* deoxycholate amphotericin B, *LAMB* liposomal amphotericin B, *ABLC* amphotericin B lipid complex, *ABCD* amphotericin B colloidal dispersion, *CAS* caspofungin, *MICA* micafungin, *AND* anidulafungin, *AMB* amphotericin B, *CIP* ciprofloxacin, *G-CSF* granulocyte colony stimulating factor, *sIL4R* soluble IL-4 receptor, *rIL12* recombinant IL-12, *GM-CSF* granulocyte macrophage colony stimulating factor, *IFN-g* interferon gamma

Table 53.3 Effects of antifungal agents on phagocytes' immune gene expression

Antifungal agents	MNCs function	Fungal morphotype
Voriconazole	Down-regulation of TNF-α Pro-inflammatory response	*A. fumigatus* conidia *A. fumigatus* hyphae
Deoxycholate amphotericin B	Pro-inflammatory response, signal transduction, cell differentiation, complement activation	*A. fumigatus* hyphae
Amphotericin B colloidal dispersion Liposomal amphotericin B	Substantial pro-inflammatory cytokine release Decreased Th1 immune response	*A. fumigatus* hyphae *A. fumigatus* hyphae
Amphotericin B lipid complex	Decreased Th1 immune response	*A. fumigatus* hyphae
Caspofungin	Up-regulation of TNF-α Down-regulation of TNF-α	*A. fumigatus* hyphae *A. fumigatus* conidia
Micafungin	Up-regulation of TNF-α Down-regulation of TNF-α	*A. fumigatus* hyphae *A. fumigatus* conidia

VRC voriconazole, *DAMB* deoxycholate amphotericin B, *LAMB* liposomal amphotericin B, *ABLC* amphotericin B lipid complex, *ABCD* amphotericin B colloidal dispersion, *CAS* caspofungin, *MICA* micafungin

Membrane cation channel formation measured in model cholesterol-containing large unilamellar vesicles showed that only DAMB and ABCD induce significant ion currents, providing an additional rationale for the different cytokine-mediated adverse effects observed with amphotericin B formulations [40]. Moreover, these studies demonstrated that DAMB and lipid formulations affect gene expression and release of IL-1β, IL-1Ra, MCP-1, MIP-1β, and TNF-α variably, which may further modulate host response to invasive fungal infections.

Microarray studies have expanded the previous observations on the effects of amphotericin B formulations in MNCs and identified new immunomodulatory proteins that are responsive to amphotericin B. In particular, DAMB induces the expression of IL-1α and the chemokines IL-8, MIP-1α, the signal transduction proteins nuclear factor of κ light polypeptide gene enhancer in B-cell inhibitor α (NFKBIA), COX2, and G6PD. The ability of IL-8 and MIP-1α to recruit MNCs and PMNs could mediate the pulmonary toxicity occasionally observed with amphotericin B formulations. COX2 regulates prostaglandin production and release believed to mediate fever and chills observed during amphotericin B administration. G6PD has a key role in the production of NADPH, which is required for the respiratory burst in PMNs; therefore, upregulation of G6PD could explain the stimulatory effects the drug has on PMNs [44].

Another microarray study evaluated the effects of DAMB and ABLC on gene expression of immune molecules by MNCs exposed to *A. fumigatus* hyphae; considerably fewer genes associated with inflammatory and chemotactic activity were induced in MNCs exposed to the combination treatments of *A. fumigatus*-DAMB or *A. fumigatus*-ABLC as compared to each component alone, suggesting that both antifungal agents act by damaging *Aspergillus* hyphae rather than by activating phagocytes for cell recruitment and enhancement of antihyphal activity [47].

The potential impact that antifungal agents, primarily directed against fungal organisms, could also have on modifying immune cell functions through intracellular drug accumulation was readily recognized. This occurred after initial observations on the influence of amphotericin B to augment the fungicidal activity of human MNCs against ingested *C. albicans* and *A. fumigatus* conidia [48, 49]. Similar enhancement of killing was demonstrated to occur with fluconazole, voriconazole, caspofungin, and anidulafungin on phagocytized *C. albicans*, *Candida glabrata*, and *Candida krusei* [50–55]. Results of these studies indicate the impact of drug accumulation and on intracellular antifungal activity.

Amphotericin B has direct antifungal activity against *Cryptococcus neoformans*, and it also possesses an immunomodulating activity by augmenting the anticryptococcal response of murine peritoneal macrophages via upregulation of nitric oxide synthesis mediated by either TNF-α or IL-1 [56]. Furthermore, DAMB and lipid amphotericin B formulations enhance fungicidal activity of human or rabbit phagocytes against hyphae or conidia of *A. fumigatus* and *Fusarium solani*. This upregulatory activity of amphotericin B formulations is associated with supplement production of H_2O_2 and H_2O_2-dependent intracellular intermediates [57–59] (Table 53.2). In addition, while LAMB exhibits synergistic activity with PMNs in inducing hyphal damage to *Rhizopus microsporus*, ABLC has synergistic or additive activity with PMNs against all three Zygomycetes tested, *Rhizopus oryzae*, *Rhizopus microsporus*, and *Absidia corymbifera* [60]. Similarly, both LAMB and ABLC interacted with phagocytes and produced additive antifungal activity against *A. fumigatus* and *Scedosporium* spp. selectively [61, 62] (Table 53.2). The mechanism(s) underlying these combinational activities may be related to the structure of the compounds and their molecular interaction with the fungal organisms. The ribbon-like structure of ABLC may have more hydrolysis sites exposed to the action of fungal or host cell-derived phospholipases than the lipid bilayer structure of LAMB, thus amphotericin B could be released more readily and in greater amounts from ABLC than from LAMB [63].

Immunomodulatory Effects of Azoles

Among azoles, voriconazole and fluconazole have been shown to interact with phagocytes through TLR receptors in response to *A. fumigatus* or *C. albicans* as stimuli [64, 65]. Specifically, voriconazole enhances pro-inflammatory phagocyte programs by signaling an upregulation of TLR2, this effect is mediated by NF-κB activation and nuclear translocation, resulting in increased MNC fungicidal activity following challenge with *A. fumigatus* hyphae [64]. In addition, interaction of voriconazole or fluconazole with PMNs stimulated with *A. fumigatus* or *C. albicans* induces upregulation of TLR9 receptor, whereas caspofungin induces PMNs to increase expression of TLR2 in response to *A. fumigatus* and TLR4 and TLR9 following *C. albicans* exposure [65] (Table 53.1). These findings indicate that host response to antifungal agents are mediated through different PRRs elicited via fungal stimuli.

Reduction of TNF-α mRNA expression was observed upon evaluation of the immunomodulatory effects of amphotericin B, voriconazole, and micafungin on human MNCs stimulated with *A. fumigatus* conidia [66]. A hypothesis provided is that intracellular accumulation of these drugs may have influenced conidial metabolism, which in turn changed fungal-cell interactions causing a reduced TNF-α production. In contrast, incubation of voriconazole with MNCs in the presence of *A. fumigatus* hyphae upregulates inflammation-related genes such as IFN-γ, IL-1R1, and TNF-α potentially leading to a more efficient host resistance to *A. fumigatus* [64] (Table 53.3).

Immunomodulatory Effects of Echinocandins

Echinocandins modify dectin-1-dependent inflammatory response against *A. fumigatus* through modulation of the surface β-glucan content. The immune modulating effects of β-glucans, a major fungal cell wall component, are attributed to the ability to bind PRRs including dectin-1 receptor. This receptor, primarily expressed by PMNs, macrophages, and DCs, mediate activation of various cellular functions from fungal binding, uptake, and fungal neutralization to cytokine and chemokine production [67, 68].

Preincubating *A. fumigatus* conidia with subinhibitory concentrations of caspofungin results in diminished TNF-α and CXCL2 release by macrophages; this molecular response is associated with diminished dectin-1 signaling, reflecting the minimal amounts of dectin-1 molecules present on the surface of conidia. In contrast, caspofungin or micafungin-treated *A. fumigatus* hyphae trigger enhanced inflammatory response, which is also highly associated with increased dectin-1 signaling [69] (Table 53.3). A complementary study [70] has confirmed that exposure to subinhibitory concentrations of caspofungin increases β-glucan exposure on the surface of *A. fumigatus*, *A. terreus*, *Fusarium solanii*, *F. oxysporum*, and *Scedosporium apiospermum* and augments PMN antihyphal activity. Similarly, in an in vivo animal model of disseminated candidiasis, subtherapeutic doses of caspofungin administered to mice resulted in exposure of the pro-inflammatory β-glucan epitope and augmentation of binding to dectin-1, leading to activation of innate immunity. In this study, direct measurement of morphotype-specific β-glucan exposure in mouse tissues during infection has shown that caspofungin causes hyphal-specific exposure of β-glucans with very few yeast-form cells to have exposed β-glucan molecules on their surface. These findings suggest that, during the normal course of infection, echinocandin-mediated unmasking and fungicidal activities are filament-biased. Such morphotype bias may be due to intrinsic structural differences between hyphal and yeast walls [71–73]. Of note, a recent report demonstrated that caspofungin-treated *C. albicans* is able to suppress ROS production in phagocytes, suggesting that suppression of ROS is independent of β-glucan exposure. Since phagocyte-generated ROS have microbicidal activity against many pathogenic microorganisms, suppression of ROS production may represent an evasion mechanism for *Candida* blastoconidia to escape phagocytic killing [74].

Modulation of phagocyte functions seems to be drug-specific as well as time- and organism-dependent. In particular, caspofungin significantly influences oxidative burst metabolism and improves intracellular killing rates of *C. albicans*, but has no effect on phagocytosis. Caspofungin used in clinically relevant concentrations synergizes with PMNs for intracellular killing of ingested *C. albicans* blastoconidia, providing indirect evidence of the drug's ability to pass through the cell membrane and remain in a biologically active form to clear intracellular proliferating *C. albicans* blastoconidia [75].

Infectious complications in renal transplant recipients, especially in the early post-transplant period, are mainly due to *C. albicans* [5]. A study evaluating the immunomodulating influence of caspofungin on PMNs isolated from such patients, in response to *C. albicans* echinocandin exerted antifungal activity by interacting with both the PMNs and the yeast. The drug interacted with the PMNs by entering cells and killing proliferating blastoconidia, and it also unmasked a virulence factor on *C. albicans* outer cell wall, rendering the fungus susceptible to PMNs lytic mechanisms [76].

Furthermore, when *A. fumigatus* hyphae are generated in the presence of sub-MIC values of micafungin and they are subsequently cultured with PMNs or MNCs, their metabolic activity is inhibited by >80% or > 60%, respectively. These findings support the hypothesis that the greater efficacy of micafungin could be due to the combined effect of phagocytic cells and anti-mold activity [77]. Similarly, anidulafungin was noted to significantly improve intracellular killing rates of *C. albicans* after 2 h of incubation [51] (Table 53.2). The encouraging data on the immunomodulating properties of echinocandins and particularly caspofungin come to reinforce their favorable pharmacodynamic and pharmacokinetic characteristics and clinical efficacy, supporting their use as empiric treatment in high-risk populations with impaired immune functions [78–80].

Candida, the most frequent pathogen isolated in bloodstream infections, form biofilm , a characteristic that increasesits disease causing potential and morbidity, especially among immunocompromised patients [81–83]. Biofilms are formed after single *Candida* cells attach to a suitable substrate i.e., vascular or urinary catheters, stents, pacemakers, or artificial joints; they then proliferate and grow into microcolonies forming well-organized cellular communities held together by pseudohyphae and a carbohydrate-rich extracellular matrix. Biofilms show increased resistance to antifungals compared to their planktonically grown forms and can withstand hosts' antifungal immune response [84–86]. In vitro biofilm models designed to evaluate MNC-mediated phagocytosis show that immune cells are unable to inhibit *C. albicans* to form biofilm and respond to the fungal form by differentially expressing several pro- and anti-inflammatory cytokines [87]. Although activities [this 'activity'] of voriconazole in combination with human MNCs have shown indifferent results in suppressing the metabolic activity of *C. albicans* within biofilms, the combined treatment of anidulafungin with MNCs have demonstrated additive interactions against the biofilm forms [88]. Similarly, anidulafungin in combination with PMNs also exert additive activity against *C. parapsilosis* biofilms [89].

Immunomodulatory Effects of Antibacterial Agents on Antifungal Activity

Immunocompromised patients are at high risk for *Candida* and *Aspergillus* infections, but they are also at high risk for bacterial infections. For this reason, antibacterial and antifungal agents may be administered simultaneously for prevention and treatement of an established infection. Fluoroquinolones, such as ciprofloxacin, moxifloxacin, or levofloxacin, when combined with antifungal agents show improved antifungal effect. In drug combination studies, where fluoroquinolones were combined with amphotericin B, voriconazole, or caspofungin, a synergistic pharmacodynamic interaction was observed against *C. albicans* and for *A. fumigatus* resulting in altered growth inhibitory activity. Fluoroquinolones, by binding to fungal topoisomerases, may interfere with DNA replication and inhibit fungal proliferation; since fluoroquinolones are unable to gain intracellular access due to lack of fungal cell membrane permeability, it has been hypothesized that antifungal agents may increase intracellular concentrations of fluoroquinolones [90, 91]. More importantly, the effectiveness of the combined action of ciprofloxacin and amphotericin B in modulating the antifungal activity of PMNs against *A. fumigatus* has recently been shown, suggesting that both antimicrobial agents exert a beneficial effect on the oxidative mechanisms of PMNs thereby optimizing antifungal effect [92].

Modulation of Phagocytes' Activity by the Combined Effect of Cytokines and Antifungal Agents

Indirect modulation of phagocyte behavior was demonstrated after pretreatment with cytokines and exposure to antifungal drugs. In vitro and in vivo preclinical studies of the combined effect of cytokines with antifungal agents on the antifungal activity of phagocytes have promised a better outcome for combined drug-cytokine therapy in treating life-threatening invasive fungal disease. Activation of phagocytes with granulocyte-macrophage colony-stimulating factor (GM-CSF) or IFN-γ enhances the intracellular anticandidal activity of voriconazole against fluconazole-resistant *Candida* spp. or *C. neoformans* [52, 93]. Caspofungin and the voriconazole-caspofungin combination enhances activity of GM-CSF-primed monocytes in both time- and dose-dependent manner [53]. In another in vitro study G-CSF- or GM-CSF-activated PMNs were shown to enhance collaboration with voriconazole against *A. fumigatus* hyphae [94] (Table 53.2). Pretreatment of murine macrophages with IFN-γ and subsequent amphotericin B exposure was able to activate the synthesis of nitrogen reactive intermediates inhibiting replication of ingested *C. neoformans* [95]. Most in vivo studies using hematopoietic growth factors or recombinant interleukins as adjunctive agents in antifungal therapy have reported either a beneficial response [96–99] or no significant difference [100, 101] (Table 53.2) in the survival of infected mice.

An important issue raised by these experimental models of invasive fungal infections is the impact of the host predisposing factors on the outcome of combined therapies with antifungal agents and cytokines. Early in infection, neutralization of the protective Th1 pro-inflammatory cytokines like IFN-γ, TNF-α, or IL-12 leads to the development of Th2 rather than Th1 cellular response, which promotes progressive fungal disease, whereas neutralization of IL-4 and IL-10 upregulates the desirable Th1 rather than Th2 response [102, 103]. In immunocompetent mice with lethal disseminated candidiasis, treatment with amphotericin B or fluconazole is associated with Th1 immune response. Leukopenic or neutropenic mice respond differently to the therapeutic efficacy of antifungal agents combined with cytokines. In particular, the efficacy of combined therapy with soluble IL-4 receptor and amphotericin B is higher in leukopenic than in neutropenic mice, whereas coadministration of recombinant IL-12 and fluconazole is higher in neutropenic than in leukopenic mice. The synergistic effect of the combination treatments is retained in immunocompromised mice [97]. Corticosteroids, another major predisposing factor for invasive fungal infections, maintain the number of dysfunctional PMNs, which are unable to restrict fungal growth; administration of G-CSF to corticosteroid-treated mice with disseminated aspergillosis contributes to the development of progressive disease by increasing the number of dysfunctional PMNs and antagonizing the therapeutic effect of posaconazole [100]. These data indicate that the host immune reactivity influences the efficacy of antifungal drugs given in combination with certain cytokines. The immune modulatory role that combined treatment of antifungal agents and cytokines play in promoting defenses against fungal pathogens; preclinical and limited clinical data for adjunct combination therapy with antifungals is periodically reviewed and perhaps such combination regimens may improve antifungal activity of neutrophils and monocytes/macrophages as well as upregulate protective T helper type 1 adaptive immune response, however at present, such combinations are not routinely recommneded in the management of IFIs even in severely immunosuppressed patients undergoing allogeneic transplantation [104–109].

Conclusions

In addition to their capacity to affect the development and proliferation of fungi, antifungal agents directly interact with the hosts' immune system. Immunomodulatory effects of antifungals include alteration of phagocytosis, augmentation of oxidative and nonoxidative mechanisms of first line immune defense cells, chemotaxis, and pro-inflammatory or anti-inflammatory cytokine production.

DAMB interacts with CD14, TLR1, and TLR2 receptors, inducing a MyD88-dependent intracellular signaling cascade that culminates in the activation of NF-κB transcription factor and the subsequent upregulation of pro-inflammatory cytokines and chemokines. By diverting signaling from

TLR2 to TLR4, LAMB augments antifungal activity of phagocytes while attenuating the pro-inflammatory effects observed with DAMB. Similarly, ABLC downregulates the pro-inflammatory response and increases the antihyphal activity of phagocytes, whereas ABCD shows similar gene expression and antifungal profiles noted with DAMB. These observations offer a putative molecular basis for optimization of LAMB/ABLC therapeutic efficacy for invasive fungal diseases as opposed to the cytokine-mediated adverse effects in response to DAMB/ABCD drug formulations.

Among azoles, voriconazole interact with TLR2, TLR4, or TLR9 thereby enhancing pro-inflammatory programs of phagocytes and augment their antifungal activity, a feature that is maintained after activation of phagocytes with GM-CSF or G-CSF. In contrast, fluconazole by interacting with TLR9 induces a moderate antifungal phagocytic activity; however, pretreatment of immune cells with G-CSF and subsequent exposure to fluconazole appears to synergistically effect in confronting fungal infections.

Among echinocandins, the immunomodulatory role of caspofungin was mediated via cross talk between TLR2, TLR4, TLR9, and dectin 1 receptor leading to the induction of Th1 pro-inflammatory program in activation of antifungal host defense. Similarly, anidulafungin and micafungin have a favorable effect on intracellular killing, especially for yeasts in biofilm. Antibacterial agents, such as ciprofloxacin, when combined with amphotericin B exert a positive effect on the oxidative antifungal mechanisms of phagocytes.

Considerable information has been accumulated on immunomodulatory properties of antifungal agents on hosts' immune response, there is still much to be deciphered regarding the potential interference between pathogen-targeting drugs and the phagocytic effector cell response, especially among allograft transplant recipients. Powerful new technology platforms for data acquisition and processing are urgently needed to perform genome-wide association studies comparing various treatment regimens in the context of antifungal-host-pathogen interaction. Presently, limited clinical data exist to conclude clinical feasibility and potential benefit from immunomodulatory therapy. The possible synergistic role of new antifungal agents on hosts' cytokines response offers an opportunity to optimize treatment for life-threatening fungal disease in the at risk transplant population.

Disclosure of Potential Conflict of Interest None of the authors of this manuscript have potential conflict of interest.

References

1. Walsh TJ, Groll A, Hiemenz J, Fleming R, Roilides E, Anaissie E. Infections due to emerging and uncommon medically important fungal pathogens. Clin Microbiol Infect. 2004;10(Suppl 1):48–66.
2. Miceli MH, Lee SA. Emerging moulds: epidemiological trends and antifungal resistance. Mycoses. 2011;54(6):e666–78.
3. Munoz P, Fernandez NS, Farinas MC. Epidemiology and risk factors of infections after solid organ transplantation. Enferm Infecc Microbiol Clin. 2012;30(Suppl 2):10–8.
4. Neofytos D, Fishman JA, Horn D, Anaissie E, Chang CH, Olyaei A, et al. Epidemiology and outcome of invasive fungal infections in solid organ transplant recipients. Transpl Infect Dis. 2012;12(3):220–9.
5. Pappas PG, Alexander BD, Andes DR, Hadley S, Kauffman CA, Freifeld A, et al. Invasive fungal infections among organ transplant recipients: results of the Transplant-Associated Infection Surveillance Network (TRANSNET). Clin Infect Dis. 2010;50(8):1101–11.
6. Lanternier F, Sun HY, Ribaud P, Singh N, Kontoyiannis DP, Lortholary O. Mucormycosis in organ and stem cell transplant recipients. Clin Infect Dis. 2012;54(11):1629–36.
7. Quan C, Spellberg B. Mucormycosis, pseudallescheriasis, and other uncommon mold infections. Proc Am Thorac Soc. 2010;7(3):210–5.
8. Pagano L, Akova M, Dimopoulos G, Herbrecht R, Drgona L, Blijlevens N. Risk assessment and prognostic factors for mould-related diseases in immunocompromised patients. J Antimicrob Chemother. 2011;66(Suppl 1):i5–14.
9. Anderson JB. Evolution of antifungal-drug resistance: mechanisms and pathogen fitness. Nat Rev Microbiol. 2005;3(7):547–56.
10. Morschhauser J. Regulation of multidrug resistance in pathogenic fungi. Fungal Genet Biol. 2010;47(2):94–106.
11. Joly S, Sutterwala FS. Fungal pathogen recognition by the NLRP3 inflammasome. Virulence. 2010;1(4):276–80.
12. Yamamoto M, Takeda K. Current views of toll-like receptor signaling pathways. Gastroenterol Res Pract. 2010;2010:240365.
13. Netea MG, Van der Meer JW, Kullberg BJ. Role of the dual interaction of fungal pathogens with pattern recognition receptors in the activation and modulation of host defence. Clin Microbiol Infect. 2006;12(5):404–9.
14. Willment JA, Brown GD. C-type lectin receptors in antifungal immunity. Trends Microbiol. 2008;16(1):27–32.
15. Vautier S, Sousa Mda G, Brown GD. C-type lectins, fungi and Th17 responses. Cytokine Growth Factor Rev. 2010;21(6):405–12.
16. Naglik JR, Moyes D. Epithelial cell innate response to Candida albicans. Adv Dent Res. 2011;23(1):50–5.
17. Bellocchio S, Moretti S, Perruccio K, Fallarino F, Bozza S, Montagnoli C, et al. TLRs govern neutrophil activity in aspergillosis. J Immunol. 2004;173(12):7406–15.
18. van de Veerdonk FL, Kullberg BJ, van der Meer JW, Gow NA, Netea MG. Host-microbe interactions: innate pattern recognition of fungal pathogens. Curr Opin Microbiol. 2008;11(4):305–12.
19. Gallin JI, Zarember K. Lessons about the pathogenesis and management of aspergillosis from studies in chronic granulomatous disease. Trans Am Clin Climatol Assoc. 2007;118:175–85.
20. Odell EW, Segal AW. Killing of pathogens associated with chronic granulomatous disease by the non-oxidative microbicidal mechanisms of human neutrophils. J Med Microbiol. 1991;34(3): 129–35.
21. Aratani Y, Kura F, Watanabe H, Akagawa H, Takano Y, Suzuki K, et al. Relative contributions of myeloperoxidase and NADPH-oxidase to the early host defense against pulmonary infections with Candida albicans and Aspergillus fumigatus. Med Mycol. 2002;40(6):557–63.
22. Hasenberg M, Behnsen J, Krappmann S, Brakhage A, Gunzer M. Phagocyte responses towards Aspergillus fumigatus. Int J Med Microbiol. 2011;301(5):436–44.
23. Fournier BM, Parkos CA. The role of neutrophils during intestinal inflammation. Mucosal Immunol. 2012;5(4):354–66.
24. Savina A, Amigorena S. Phagocytosis and antigen presentation in dendritic cells. Immunol Rev. 2007;219:143–56.

25. van Vliet SJ, den Dunnen J, Gringhuis SI, Geijtenbeek TB, van Kooyk Y. Innate signaling and regulation of Dendritic cell immunity. Curr Opin Immunol. 2007;19(4):435–40.
26. Zelante T, Bozza S, De Luca A, D'Angelo C, Bonifazi P, Moretti S, et al. Th17 cells in the setting of Aspergillus infection and pathology. Med Mycol. 2009;47(Suppl 1):S162–9.
27. Villar CC, Dongari-Bagtzoglou A. Immune defence mechanisms and immunoenhancement strategies in oropharyngeal candidiasis. Expert Rev Mol Med. 2008;10:e29.
28. Janes MR, Fruman DA. Immune regulation by rapamycin: moving beyond T cells. Sci Signal. 2009;2(67):pe25.
29. Yamaguchi H, Abe S, Tokuda Y. Immunomodulating activity of antifungal drugs. Ann N Y Acad Sci. 1993;685:447–57.
30. Stevens DA, Kullberg BJ, Brummer E, Casadevall A, Netea MG, Sugar AM. Combined treatment: antifungal drugs with antibodies, cytokines or drugs. Med Mycol. 2000;38(Suppl 1):305–15.
31. Hamad M. Antifungal immunotherapy and immunomodulation: a double-hitter approach to deal with invasive fungal infections. Scand J Immunol. 2008;67(6):533–43.
32. Laniado-Laborin R, Cabrales-Vargas MN. Amphotericin B: side effects and toxicity. Rev Iberoam Micol. 2009;26(4):223–7.
33. Sau K, Mambula SS, Latz E, Henneke P, Golenbock DT, Levitz SM. The antifungal drug amphotericin B promotes inflammatory cytokine release by a Toll-like receptor- and CD14-dependent mechanism. J Biol Chem. 2003;278(39):37561–8.
34. Razonable RR, Henault M, Lee LN, Laethem C, Johnston PA, Watson HL, et al. Secretion of proinflammatory cytokines and chemokines during amphotericin B exposure is mediated by coactivation of toll-like receptors 1 and 2. Antimicrob Agents Chemother. 2005;49(4):1617–21.
35. Matsuo K, Hotokezaka H, Ohara N, Fujimura Y, Yoshimura A, Okada Y, et al. Analysis of amphotericin B-induced cell signaling with chemical inhibitors of signaling molecules. Microbiol Immunol. 2006;50(4):337–47.
36. Bellocchio S, Gaziano R, Bozza S, Rossi G, Montagnoli C, Perruccio K, et al. Liposomal amphotericin B activates antifungal resistance with reduced toxicity by diverting Toll-like receptor signalling from TLR-2 to TLR-4. J Antimicrob Chemother. 2005;55(2):214–22.
37. Cleary JD, Rogers PD, Chapman SW. Differential transcription factor expression in human mononuclear cells in response to amphotericin B: identification with complementary DNA microarray technology. Pharmacotherapy. 2001;21(9):1046–54.
38. Turtinen LW, Bremer LA, Prall DN, Schwartzhoff J, Hartsel SC. Distinct cytokine release profiles from human endothelial and THP-1 macrophage-like cells exposed to different amphotericin B formulations. Immunopharmacol Immunotoxicol. 2005;27(1):85–93.
39. Turtinen LW, Croswell A, Obr A. Microarray analysis of amphotericin B-treated THP-1 monocytic cells identifies unique gene expression profiles among lipid and non-lipid drug formulations. J Chemother. 2008;20(3):327–35.
40. Turtinen LW, Prall DN, Bremer LA, Nauss RE, Hartsel SC. Antibody array-generated profiles of cytokine release from THP-1 leukemic monocytes exposed to different amphotericin B formulations. Antimicrob Agents Chemother. 2004;48(2):396–403.
41. Simitsopoulou M, Roilides E, Dotis J, Dalakiouridou M, Dudkova F, Andreadou E, et al. Differential expression of cytokines and chemokines in human monocytes induced by lipid formulations of amphotericin B. Antimicrob Agents Chemother. 2005;49(4):1397–403.
42. Rogers PD, Jenkins JK, Chapman SW, Ndebele K, Chapman BA, Cleary JD. Amphotericin B activation of human genes encoding for cytokines. J Infect Dis. 1998;178(6):1726–33.
43. Rogers PD, Kramer RE, Chapman SW, Cleary JD. Amphotericin B-induced interleukin-1beta expression in human monocytic cells is calcium and calmodulin dependent. J Infect Dis. 1999;180(4):1259–66.
44. Rogers PD, Pearson MM, Cleary JD, Sullivan DC, Chapman SW. Differential expression of genes encoding immunomodulatory proteins in response to amphotericin B in human mononuclear cells identified by cDNA microarray analysis. J Antimicrob Chemother. 2002;50(6):811–7.
45. Rogers PD, Stiles JK, Chapman SW, Cleary JD. Amphotericin B induces expression of genes encoding chemokines and cell adhesion molecules in the human monocytic cell line THP-1. J Infect Dis. 2000;182(4):1280–3.
46. Saxena S, Bhatnagar PK, Ghosh PC, Sarma PU. Effect of amphotericin B lipid formulation on immune response in aspergillosis. Int J Pharm. 1999;188(1):19–30.
47. Simitsopoulou M, Roilides E, Georgiadou E, Paliogianni F, Walsh TJ. Differential transcriptional profiles induced by amphotericin B formulations on human monocytes during response to hyphae of Aspergillus fumigatus. Med Mycol. 2011;49(2):176–85.
48. Martin E, Stuben A, Gorz A, Weller U, Bhakdi S. Novel aspect of amphotericin B action: accumulation in human monocytes potentiates killing of phagocytosed Candida albicans. Antimicrob Agents Chemother. 1994;38(1):13–22.
49. Jahn B, Rampp A, Dick C, Jahn A, Palmer M, Bhakdi S. Accumulation of amphotericin B in human macrophages enhances activity against Aspergillus fumigatus conidia: quantification of conidial kill at the single-cell level. Antimicrob Agents Chemother. 1998;42(10):2569–75.
50. Pascual A, Garcia I, Conejo C, Perea EJ. Uptake and intracellular activity of fluconazole in human polymorphonuclear leukocytes. Antimicrob Agents Chemother. 1993;37(2):187–90.
51. Frank U, Greiner M, Engels I, Daschner FD. Effects of caspofungin (MK-0991) and anidulafungin (LY303366) on phagocytosis, oxidative burst and killing of Candida albicans by human phagocytes. Eur J Clin Microbiol Infect Dis. 2004;23(9):729–31.
52. Baltch AL, Bopp LH, Smith RP, Ritz WJ, Carlyn CJ, Michelsen PB. Effects of voriconazole, granulocyte-macrophage colony-stimulating factor, and interferon gamma on intracellular fluconazole-resistant Candida glabrata and Candida krusei in human monocyte-derived macrophages. Diagn Microbiol Infect Dis. 2005;52(4):299–304.
53. Baltch AL, Bopp LH, Smith RP, Ritz WJ, Michelsen PB. Anticandidal effects of voriconazole and caspofungin, singly and in combination, against Candida glabrata, extracellularly and intracellularly in granulocyte-macrophage colony stimulating factor (GM-CSF)-activated human monocytes. J Antimicrob Chemother. 2008;62(6):1285–90.
54. Ballesta S, Garcia I, Perea EJ, Pascual A. Uptake and intracellular activity of voriconazole in human polymorphonuclear leucocytes. J Antimicrob Chemother. 2005;55(5):785–7.
55. Bopp LH, Baltch AL, Ritz WJ, Michelsen PB, Smith RP. Antifungal effect of voriconazole on intracellular Candida glabrata, Candida krusei and Candida parapsilosis in human monocyte-derived macrophages. J Med Microbiol. 2006;55(Pt 7):865–70.
56. Tohyama M, Kawakami K, Saito A. Anticryptococcal effect of amphotericin B is mediated through macrophage production of nitric oxide. Antimicrob Agents Chemother. 1996;40(8):1919–23.
57. Dotis J, Simitsopoulou M, Dalakiouridou M, Konstantinou T, Panteliadis C, Walsh TJ, et al. Amphotericin B formulations variably enhance antifungal activity of human neutrophils and monocytes against Fusarium solani: comparison with Aspergillus fumigatus. J Antimicrob Chemother. 2008;61(4):810–7.
58. Dotis J, Simitsopoulou M, Dalakiouridou M, Konstantinou T, Taparkou A, Kanakoudi-Tsakalidou F, et al. Effects of lipid formulations of amphotericin B on activity of human monocytes against Aspergillus fumigatus. Antimicrob Agents Chemother. 2006;50(3):868–73.

59. Roilides E, Lyman CA, Armstrong D, Stergiopoulou T, Petraitiene R, Walsh TJ. Deoxycholate amphotericin B and amphotericin B lipid complex exert additive antifungal activity in combination with pulmonary alveolar macrophages against Fusarium solani. Mycoses. 2006;49(2):109–13.
60. Simitsopoulou M, Roilides E, Maloukou A, Gil-Lamaignere C, Walsh TJ. Interaction of amphotericin B lipid formulations and triazoles with human polymorphonuclear leucocytes for antifungal activity against Zygomycetes. Mycoses. 2008;51(2):147–54.
61. Roilides E, Lyman CA, Filioti J, Akpogheneta O, Sein T, Lamaignere CG, et al. Amphotericin B formulations exert additive antifungal activity in combination with pulmonary alveolar macrophages and polymorphonuclear leukocytes against Aspergillus fumigatus. Antimicrob Agents Chemother. 2002;46(6):1974–6.
62. Gil-Lamaignere C, Roilides E, Maloukou A, Georgopoulou I, Petrikkos G, Walsh TJ. Amphotericin B lipid complex exerts additive antifungal activity in combination with polymorphonuclear leucocytes against Scedosporium prolificans and Scedosporium apiospermum. J Antimicrob Chemother. 2002;50(6):1027–30.
63. Swenson CE, Perkins WR, Roberts P, Ahmad I, Stevens R, Stevens DA, et al. In vitro and in vivo antifungal activity of amphotericin B lipid complex: are phospholipases important? Antimicrob Agents Chemother. 1998;42(4):767–71.
64. Simitsopoulou M, Roilides E, Paliogianni F, Likartsis C, Ioannidis J, Kanellou K, et al. Immunomodulatory effects of voriconazole on monocytes challenged with Aspergillus fumigatus: differential role of Toll-like receptors. Antimicrob Agents Chemother. 2008;52(9):3301–6.
65. Salvenmoser S, Seidler MJ, Dalpke A, Muller FM. Effects of caspofungin, Candida albicans and Aspergillus fumigatus on toll-like receptor 9 of GM-CSF-stimulated PMNs. FEMS Immunol Med Microbiol. 2010;60(1):74–7.
66. Choi JH, Kwon EY, Park CM, Choi SM, Lee DG, Yoo JH, et al. Immunomodulatory effects of antifungal agents on the response of human monocytic cells to Aspergillus fumigatus conidia. Med Mycol. 2010;48(5):704–9.
67. Kimberg M, Brown GD. Dectin-1 and its role in antifungal immunity. Med Mycol. 2008;46(7):631–6.
68. Murphy EA, Davis JM, Carmichael MD. Immune modulating effects of beta-glucan. Curr Opin Clin Nutr Metab Care. 2010;13(6):656–61.
69. Hohl TM, Feldmesser M, Perlin DS, Pamer EG. Caspofungin modulates inflammatory responses to Aspergillus fumigatus through stage-specific effects on fungal beta-glucan exposure. J Infect Dis. 2008;198(2):176–85.
70. Lamaris GA, Lewis RE, Chamilos G, May GS, Safdar A, Walsh TJ, et al. Caspofungin-mediated beta-glucan unmasking and enhancement of human polymorphonuclear neutrophil activity against Aspergillus and non-Aspergillus hyphae. J Infect Dis. 2008;198(2):186–92.
71. Wheeler RT, Kombe D, Agarwala SD, Fink GR. Dynamic, morphotype-specific Candida albicans beta-glucan exposure during infection and drug treatment. PLoS Pathog. 2008;4(12):e1000227.
72. Ruiz-Herrera J, Elorza MV, Valentin E, Sentandreu R. Molecular organization of the cell wall of Candida albicans and its relation to pathogenicity. FEMS Yeast Res. 2006;6(1):14–29.
73. Shibata N, Suzuki A, Kobayashi H, Okawa Y. Chemical structure of the cell-wall mannan of Candida albicans serotype A and its difference in yeast and hyphal forms. Biochem J. 2007;404(3):365–72.
74. Wellington M, Dolan K, Krysan DJ. Live Candida albicans suppresses production of reactive oxygen species in phagocytes. Infect Immun. 2009;77(1):405–13.
75. Tullio V, Mandras N, Scalas D, Allizond V, Banche G, Roana J, et al. Synergy of caspofungin with human polymorphonuclear granulocytes for killing Candida albicans. Antimicrob Agents Chemother. 2010;54(9):3964–6.
76. Allizond V, Banche G, Giacchino F, Merlino C, Scalas D, Tullio V, et al. Candida albicans infections in renal transplant recipients: effect of caspofungin on polymorphonuclear cells. Antimicrob Agents Chemother. 2011;55(12):5936–8.
77. Choi JH, Brummer E, Stevens DA. Combined action of micafungin, a new echinocandin, and human phagocytes for antifungal activity against Aspergillus fumigatus. Microbes Infect. 2004;6(4):383–9.
78. Anaissie EJ. Diagnosis and therapy of fungal infection in patients with leukemia--new drugs and immunotherapy. Best Pract Res Clin Haematol. 2008;21(4):683–90.
79. Gullo A. Invasive fungal infections: the challenge continues. Drugs. 2009;69(Suppl 1):65–73.
80. Walsh TJ, Teppler H, Donowitz GR, Maertens JA, Baden LR, Dmoszynska A, et al. Caspofungin versus liposomal amphotericin B for empirical antifungal therapy in patients with persistent fever and neutropenia. N Engl J Med. 2004;351(14):1391–402.
81. Mavor AL, Thewes S, Hube B. Systemic fungal infections caused by Candida species: epidemiology, infection process and virulence attributes. Curr Drug Targets. 2005;6(8):863–74.
82. Ramage G, Saville SP, Thomas DP, Lopez-Ribot JL. Candida biofilms: an update. Eukaryot Cell. 2005;4(4):633–8.
83. Mikulska M, Bassetti M, Ratto S, Viscoli C. Invasive candidiasis in non-hematological patients. Mediterr J Hematol Infect Dis. 2011;3(1):e2011007.
84. Kuhn DM, George T, Chandra J, Mukherjee PK, Ghannoum MA. Antifungal susceptibility of Candida biofilms: unique efficacy of amphotericin B lipid formulations and echinocandins. Antimicrob Agents Chemother. 2002;46(6):1773–80.
85. Shuford JA, Piper KE, Steckelberg JM, Patel R. In vitro biofilm characterization and activity of antifungal agents alone and in combination against sessile and planktonic clinical Candida albicans isolates. Diagn Microbiol Infect Dis. 2007;57(3):277–81.
86. Tobudic S, Kratzer C, Lassnigg A, Presterl E. Antifungal susceptibility of Candida albicans in biofilms. Mycoses. 2012;55(3):199–204.
87. Chandra J, McCormick TS, Imamura Y, Mukherjee PK, Ghannoum MA. Interaction of Candida albicans with adherent human peripheral blood mononuclear cells increases C. albicans biofilm formation and results in differential expression of pro- and anti-inflammatory cytokines. Infect Immun. 2007;75(5):2612–20.
88. Katragkou A, Kruhlak MJ, Simitsopoulou M, Chatzimoschou A, Taparkou A, Cotten CJ, et al. Interactions between human phagocytes and Candida albicans biofilms alone and in combination with antifungal agents. J Infect Dis. 2010;201(12):1941–9.
89. Katragkou A, Chatzimoschou A, Simitsopoulou M, Georgiadou E, Roilides E. Additive antifungal activity of anidulafungin and human neutrophils against Candida parapsilosis biofilms. J Antimicrob Chemother. 2011;66(3):588–91.
90. Stergiopoulou T, Meletiadis J, Sein T, Papaioannidou P, Tsiouris I, Roilides E, et al. Isobolographic analysis of pharmacodynamic interactions between antifungal agents and ciprofloxacin against Candida albicans and Aspergillus fumigatus. Antimicrob Agents Chemother. 2008;52(6):2196–204.
91. Stergiopoulou T, Meletiadis J, Sein T, Papaioannidou P, Tsiouris I, Roilides E, et al. Comparative pharmacodynamic interaction analysis between ciprofloxacin, moxifloxacin and levofloxacin and antifungal agents against Candida albicans and Aspergillus fumigatus. J Antimicrob Chemother. 2009;63(2):343–8.
92. Stergiopoulou T, Meletiadis J, Sein T, Papaioannidou P, Walsh TJ, Roilides E. Synergistic interaction of the triple combination of amphotericin B, ciprofloxacin, and polymorphonuclear neutrophils against Aspergillus fumigatus. Antimicrob Agents Chemother. 2011;55(12):5923–9.
93. Chiller T, Farrokhshad K, Brummer E, Stevens DA. Effect of granulocyte colony-stimulating factor and granulocyte-macrophage colony-stimulating factor on polymorphonuclear neutrophils, monocytes or monocyte-derived macrophages combined with

voriconazole against Cryptococcus neoformans. Med Mycol. 2002;40(1):21–6.
94. Vora S, Chauhan S, Brummer E, Stevens DA. Activity of voriconazole combined with neutrophils or monocytes against Aspergillus fumigatus: effects of granulocyte colony-stimulating factor and granulocyte-macrophage colony-stimulating factor. Antimicrob Agents Chemother. 1998;42(9):2299–303.
95. Herrmann JL, Dubois N, Fourgeaud M, Basset D, Lagrange PH. Synergic inhibitory activity of amphotericin-B and gamma interferon against intracellular Cryptococcus neoformans in murine macrophages. J Antimicrob Chemother. 1994;34(6):1051–8.
96. Graybill JR, Bocanegra R, Luther M. Antifungal combination therapy with granulocyte colony-stimulating factor and fluconazole in experimental disseminated candidiasis. Eur J Clin Microbiol Infect Dis. 1995;14(8):700–3.
97. Mencacci A, Cenci E, Bacci A, Bistoni F, Romani L. Host immune reactivity determines the efficacy of combination immunotherapy and antifungal chemotherapy in candidiasis. J Infect Dis. 2000;181(2):686–94.
98. Patera AC, Menzel F, Jackson C, Brieland JK, Halpern J, Hare R, et al. Effect of granulocyte colony-stimulating factor combination therapy on efficacy of posaconazole (SCH56592) in an inhalation model of murine pulmonary aspergillosis. Antimicrob Agents Chemother. 2004;48(8):3154–8.
99. Rodriguez MM, Pastor FJ, Calvo E, Salas V, Sutton DA, Guarro J. Correlation of in vitro activity, serum levels, and in vivo efficacy of posaconazole against Rhizopus microsporus in a murine disseminated infection. Antimicrob Agents Chemother. 2009;53(12):5022–5.
100. Graybill JR, Bocanegra R, Najvar LK, Loebenberg D, Luther MF. Granulocyte colony-stimulating factor and azole antifungal therapy in murine aspergillosis: role of immune suppression. Antimicrob Agents Chemother. 1998;42(10):2467–73.
101. Simitsopoulou M, Gil-Lamaignere C, Avramidis N, Maloukou A, Lekkas S, Havlova E, et al. Antifungal activities of posaconazole and granulocyte-macrophage colony-stimulating factor ex vivo and in mice with disseminated infection due to Scedosporium prolificans. Antimicrob Agents Chemother. 2004;48(10):3801–5.
102. Romani L. Immunity to fungal infections. Nat Rev Immunol. 2004;4(1):1–23.
103. Blanco JL, Garcia ME. Immune response to fungal infections. Vet Immunol Immunopathol. 2008;125(1-2):47–70.
104. Roilides E, Lyman CA, Panagopoulou P, Chanock S. Immunomodulation of invasive fungal infections. Infect Dis Clin North Am. 2003;17(1):193–219.
105. Roilides E, Walsh T. Recombinant cytokines in augmentation and immunomodulation of host defenses against Candida spp. Med Mycol. 2004;42(1):1–13.
106. Steinbach WJ, Stevens DA. Review of newer antifungal and immunomodulatory strategies for invasive aspergillosis. Clin Infect Dis. 2003;37(Suppl 3):S157–87.
107. Antachopoulos C, Roilides E. Cytokines and fungal infections. Br J Haematol. 2005;129(5):583–96.
108. Safdar A, Shelburne SA, Evans SE, Dickey BF. Inhaled therapeutics for prevention and treatment of pneumonia. Expert Opin Drug Saf. 2009;8(4):435–49.
109. Sorrell TC, Chen SC. Fungal-derived immune modulating molecules. Adv Exp Med Biol. 2009;666:108–20.

Antiviral Consideration for Transplantation Including Drug Resistance

54

Sunwen Chou and Nell S. Lurain

Introduction

Antiviral therapy is routinely used in transplant recipients for the prevention and treatment of herpesvirus infections and influenza, as well as treatment of chronic viral hepatitis and HIV. In addition, therapy is often considered for respiratory, gastrointestinal, and disseminated viral syndromes, for which in many cases no FDA-approved treatments are currently available. Where proven therapy is available for acute viral infections, a good outcome requires prompt treatment facilitated by rapid molecular viral diagnostic testing.

Active post-transplant viral infections arise from preexisting latent and persistent infections in the recipient and/or donor, and from nosocomial or community sources reflecting current epidemiology. Assessment of the timing and probabilities of these sources of infection enables a preventive or prophylactic antiviral approach that is more likely to be successful than the treatment of viral disease that has caused end-organ damage.

Host factors strongly influence the selection, duration, and expected outcome of antiviral treatment. Critical factors include prior host immunity to the infecting virus and the extent of post-transplant immunosuppression. Approved uses and benefits of antiviral treatment that are based on clinical trials in normal hosts or other patient populations do not necessarily apply to transplant recipients, leaving many unresolved questions on optimal use of current antivirals.

Natural history and treatment responsiveness of acute and chronic infections may depend on baseline genetic differences of infecting strains of viruses such as herpes simplex, influenza, and hepatitis C. Prolonged exposure to antiviral drugs may lead to the selection of drug-resistant mutants and a need for laboratory confirmation and/or alternative treatment.

Antiviral drug development requires multiple testing stages to evaluate potential benefits for various indications and patient populations, in relation to toxicity, pharmacological complexity, and cost. At each stage, candidate compounds are eliminated, or controlled trials may not be done. It is important to refrain from a presumption of efficacy based on promising preliminary uncontrolled findings. Case reports are problematic because the outcome of viral infection is highly dependent on host defenses. Favorable individual outcomes coincidental with unproven treatments may lead to complicated and costly recommended practices that should not be mistaken as evidence-based treatments.

In this chapter, we review antiviral drug therapy other than for HIV infection from the standpoint of mechanisms of action, clinical applications, and antiviral drug resistance. Recommendations for antiviral therapy of specific conditions and patient subsets are discussed in chapters dealing with the individual viruses.

Herpesvirus Antivirals

Several licensed herpesvirus antiviral drugs (see Table 54.1) are available, which target the viral DNA polymerase that is essential for viral replication. Herpesvirus genomes encode many other important gene products that are attractive targets for antiviral therapy. Issues of toxicity and emerging antiviral resistance associated with the longstanding approved drugs have led to clinical trials of promising experimental compounds.

S. Chou (✉)
Oregon Health and Science University, Division of Infectious Diseases, Portland, OR, USA
e-mail: chous@ohsu.edu

N. S. Lurain
Rush University Medical Center, Department of Microbial Pathogens and Immunity, Chicago, IL, USA
e-mail: nlurain@rush.edu

A. Safdar (ed.), *Principles and Practice of Transplant Infectious Diseases*, https://doi.org/10.1007/978-1-4939-9034-4_54

Table 54.1 Antiviral agents approved for therapy of herpesviruses (mid-2017)

Antiviral agent (abbreviation)	Structure and mechanism of action	Therapeutic uses and doses (see important cautions)[a]	Adverse effects	Resistance mechanisms
Acyclovir (ACV)	Acyclic guanosine nucleoside analog. Inactive until converted to monophosphate by viral thymidine kinase and then converted to triphosphate by cellular kinases. ACV triphosphate inhibits viral DNA polymerase; obligate DNA chain terminator when incorporated into growing DNA strands	Treatment of active disease: Mucocutaneous (oral, genital, skin) HSV infection PO, 400 mg 3×/day IV, 5 mg/kg every 8 h Visceral and disseminated HSV infection IV, 10 mg/kg every 8 h VZV infection: localized zoster PO, 800 mg 5×/day (VACV or FCV preferred) IV, 5 mg/kg every 8 h VZV infection, primary or disseminated IV, 10 mg/kg every 8 h Prevention of HSV and VZV reactivation PO, 400–800 mg 2×/day (not needed if receiving GCV or VGCV for CMV)	Nephrotoxicity: crystalluria with rapid IV infusion or renal dysfunction Neurotoxicity: headache, encephalopathy, seizures with drug accumulation resulting from high doses and/or renal dysfunction	Viral thymidine kinase mutations resulting in deficient, altered or partial activity; DNA polymerase mutations less common Cross-resistance with penciclovir and ganciclovir expected because resistant mutants are usually thymidine kinase deficient
Valacyclovir (VACV)	L-valyl ester prodrug of ACV. Metabolically converted to ACV in intestinal and liver cells and then same action as acyclovir	Treatment of active disease: Mucocutaneous HSV infection PO, 1000 mg 2×/day VZV infection: localized zoster PO, 1000 mg 3×/day Prevention of HSV and VZV reactivation PO, 500 mg 2×/day (not needed if receiving GCV or VGCV for CMV)	Same as ACV; GI[b] Thrombotic angiopathy at high doses (8 g/day) in AIDS	Same as ACV
Famciclovir (FCV)	Diacetyl ester prodrug of penciclovir (PCV), an acyclic guanosine analog. PCV is phosphorylated by viral thymidine kinase and cellular enzymes, as with acyclovir. PCV triphosphate inhibits DNA polymerase although not obligate DNA chain terminator	Treatment of active disease: Mucocutaneous HSV infection PO, 500 mg 2×/day VZV infection: localized zoster PO, 500 mg 3×/day Prevention of HSV and VZV reactivation PO, 500 mg 2×/day (if not receiving CMV prophylaxis; see below)	Headache, GI[b]	Thymidine kinase mutation more common than DNA polymerase mutations. Cross-resistance with ACV expected
Ganciclovir (GCV)	Acyclic guanosine nucleoside analog. Converted to monophosphate by viral kinase (HSV TK, CMV UL97), then to triphosphate by cellular kinases. GCV triphosphate inhibits viral DNA polymerase although not obligate DNA chain terminator	Treatment of active CMV disease: IV 5 mg/kg every 12 h Preemptive treatment of CMV reactivation: IV 5 mg/kg every 12 h Prophylaxis of CMV infection: IV 5 mg/kg per day Oral ganciclovir no longer marketed	Bone marrow suppression: Granulocytopenia, anemia, thrombocytopenia, GI[b] Avoid coadministration of GCV with imipenem-cilastatin; may cause seizures	Mutations in UL97 kinase, commonly M460V/I, H520Q, C592G, A594V, L595S, and C603W. Others mostly at codons 590–607 Less common DNA polymerase mutations, usually confer cross-resistance to CDV and less often to FOS

Table 54.1 (continued)

Antiviral agent (abbreviation)	Structure and mechanism of action	Therapeutic uses and doses (see important cautions)[a]	Adverse effects	Resistance mechanisms
Valganciclovir (VGCV)	L-valyl ester prodrug of GCV. Metabolically converted to GCV in intestinal and liver cells. Then same antiviral action as GCV	Treatment of mild-moderate CMV disease: PO 900 mg 2×/day Preemptive treatment of CMV reactivation: PO 900 mg 2×/day Prophylaxis of CMV infection: PO 900 mg per day for 100–200 days after solid organ transplantation (see text)	Same as GCV; GI[b]	Same as GCV
Foscarnet (FOS)	Trisodium phosphonoformate; pyrophosphate analog. Noncompetitive inhibitor of DNA polymerase pyrophosphate binding site	Treatment of tissue-invasive CMV disease when intolerant, resistant or refractory to GCV; IV, 90 mg/kg over 1.5–2 h every 12 h with prehydration; can be reduced to 90 mg/kg daily for maintenance therapy Treatment of ACV-resistant VZV disease: same dose as above Treatment of ACV-resistant HSV disease IV 40 mg/kg over 1 h every 8 or 12 h	Nephrotoxicity (25%), metabolic and electrolyte abnormalities, seizures; fluid load from saline prehydration. Must carefully monitor and replete multiple electrolytes as needed Avoid other nephrotoxic drugs	DNA polymerase mutations For CMV, some low-grade cross-resistance with GCV, rarely CDV For HSV and VZV, some cross-resistance with ACV
Cidofovir (CDV)	Cytosine monophosphate nucleotide analog. Phosphorylated by cellular kinases to cidofovir diphosphate (nucleoside triphosphate analog). Viral kinase not needed for antiviral activity	Treatment of CMV, HSV or VZV disease when intolerant, resistant, or refractory to GCV and FOS: IV, 5 mg/kg 1×/week for 2 weeks, then 5 mg/kg every 2 weeks, with saline pre- and post-hydration and oral probenecid 2 g, 3 h before dose, then 1 g 2 and 8 h after dose Treatment of disseminated adenovirus infection (same dosing)	Nephrotoxicity (25%); monitor closely and stop CDV if present Probenecid-related toxicity: GI[b], rash, drug interactions (e.g., decreased GCV renal clearance) Avoid other nephrotoxic drugs	DNA polymerase mutations For CMV, cross-resistance with GCV, rarely with FOS

[a]Recommended uses for adult transplant recipients with normal renal function. Doses of all drugs must be adjusted for renal function. Many of the listed uses are not FDA-approved; see text. See package insert for FDA-approved indications and doses. Abbreviations: *IV* intravenously, *PO* orally
[b]GI (gastrointestinal) symptoms include diarrhea, nausea, and vomiting

Acyclovir, Valacyclovir, Penciclovir, and Famciclovir

All of these drugs are structurally related guanosine nucleoside analogs that are selectively phosphorylated by a viral kinase during conversion to the active triphosphate form that inhibits the viral DNA polymerase (see Table 54.1). Valacyclovir is an oral prodrug of acyclovir, and famciclovir is the oral prodrug of penciclovir.

Acyclovir is active against herpes simplex (HSV-1 and HSV-2) and varicella-zoster (VZV) viruses, which all encode a thymidine kinase (TK) that phosphorylates acyclovir. Acyclovir is not a good substrate for the Epstein-Barr virus (EBV) TK [1]. However, EBV and cytomegalovirus (CMV) encode other kinases (BGLF4 and UL97, respectively), which can phosphorylate acyclovir to some extent [1, 2].

Traditionally, the drug concentration required to reduce viral growth by 50% (EC50) in a cell culture plaque reduction assay is used to assess HSV, VZV, and CMV susceptibility in vitro. Acyclovir is most active in vitro against HSV-1 (EC50 about 1 μM) and HSV-2 (EC50 about 2 μM), and VZV and EBV are less susceptible with EC50 about 4–6 μM [1], while CMV is relatively resistant with EC50 ≥40 μM [2]. The in vitro activity of penciclovir against herpesviruses is comparable to acyclovir. Penciclovir is more effectively phosphorylated in HSV-infected cells than is acyclovir, and the triphosphate persists within infected cells longer than acyclovir triphosphate, but the latter is a more potent inhibitor of the viral DNA polymerase than penciclovir triphosphate [3].

Pharmacology

Acyclovir is available for intravenous (IV) use, with peak plasma concentrations of 30–60 μM and elimination half-life by renal secretion and glomerular filtration of about 3 h [4]. Dose adjustment is required for impaired renal function. CSF levels of acyclovir are about 25% of plasma levels [5]. The oral bioavailability of acyclovir is poor (15–20%), but low cost and adequate achievable plasma concentrations (3–7 μM) resulted in widespread use for less severe HSV and VZV disease (Table 54.1) before the advent of generic valacyclovir.

The acyclovir prodrug valacyclovir has much better bioavailability [6] and achieves circulating levels comparable to IV therapy, which is useful for the prophylaxis and treatment of mild to moderate HSV and VZV disease (Table 54.1). Penciclovir itself is marketed only as a topical cream, but its oral prodrug famciclovir has bioavailability and therapeutic indications similar to valacyclovir.

Acyclovir, valacyclovir, and famciclovir are relatively well tolerated, with lack of bone marrow toxicity being a significant advantage. Problems may arise when high doses are used, infused too quickly, or where renal impairment is present. Good hydration and monitoring for renal function are essential during high-dose IV therapy. Excessive acyclovir doses may cause crystalluria and encephalopathy. Very high oral doses of valacyclovir (8 grams per day) have been associated with thrombotic microangiopathy and hemolytic uremic syndrome and should be avoided [7].

Clinical Indications

The routine use of acyclovir in transplantation is for the prevention of mucocutaneous HSV disease and herpes zoster (Table 54.1). For hematopoietic cell transplantation, current guidelines [8, 9] recommend acyclovir or valacyclovir prophylaxis for HSV and VZV starting at the beginning of conditioning therapy and continuing until engraftment or until mucositis resolves, usually about 1 month of prophylaxis. Prophylaxis can be extended beyond the early post-transplant period in patients with a history of recurrent symptomatic disease. Adequate doses are suggested to reduce the incidence of incomplete suppression and drug resistance, including recommendation for twice daily dosing of valacyclovir. Analogous recommendations apply in solid organ transplantation: if ganciclovir or valganciclovir is not being used to prevent CMV disease, acyclovir-based prophylaxis may be given for at least 1 month [10, 11].

Active post-transplant HSV and VZV infection can be treated with IV acyclovir (Table 54.1). Although oral acyclovir, valacyclovir, and famciclovir are not specifically FDA-approved for these indications in transplant recipients, they are widely used for less severe infections [10, 11]. Disseminated or visceral disease in transplant recipients should be treated with IV acyclovir until progressive disease has resolved, and then considered for conversion to oral therapy for several additional weeks. HSV encephalitis is rare in the transplant population, but disseminated HSV infection may present as pneumonia, severe hepatitis, and gastrointestinal disease and requires timely diagnosis to enable prompt initiation of IV acyclovir. Despite controlled clinical trials demonstrating a benefit of acyclovir or valacyclovir prophylaxis in reducing post-transplant CMV disease [12], ganciclovir and valganciclovir are currently preferred, as discussed below.

Drug Resistance Mechanisms

In over 90% of cases, HSV or VZV resistance to acyclovir results from a mutation in the TK gene [13, 14]. Because this gene is nonessential for viral replication, any mutation that prevents the translation of a functional kinase can confer resistance to both acyclovir and famciclovir. Frameshift mutations at homopolymer tracts (3–7 repeats of the same nucleotide) in the TK gene, resulting in a truncated molecule, are collectively the most common genetic basis for drug resistance in HSV and VZV. Premature stop mutations are also relatively frequent in VZV. Mutations causing single amino acid substitutions, clustering in the adenosine triphosphate (ATP) and nucleoside binding domains, can result in a functionally deficient kinase or one with decreased affinity for the antiviral nucleoside analog [13, 15]. The latter class of mutations may confer resistance to a specific drug, but acyclovir and famciclovir cross-resistance is the rule for TK mutants [16]. TK-defective HSV strains have been reported to be less pathogenic or less neurovirulent in animal models [17] but in clinical practice progressive disease due to acyclovir-resistant HSV is well described [13].

Mutations in the viral DNA polymerase gene (*pol*) can also confer resistance to nucleoside analogs and have the potential for cross-resistance to other drugs with the same target [18], but are far less common than TK mutations after acyclovir treatment. HSV *pol* mutations conferring acyclovir resistance have been mapped to conserved functional domains in herpesviruses DNA polymerases, with clustering in the palm and finger structure domains for both HSV and VZV [13, 18]. Available data suggest that such mutations frequently confer acyclovir-foscarnet cross-resistance.

Ganciclovir and Valganciclovir

Ganciclovir is structurally related to acyclovir and is also initially phosphorylated by a viral kinase, but unlike acyclovir its triphosphate is not an obligate chain terminator. Valganciclovir is the oral prodrug (Table 54.1). CMV does not encode a thymidine kinase, but the CMV UL97 protein kinase incidentally phosphorylates ganciclovir. Ganciclovir has much greater in vitro potency against CMV than acyclovir and is FDA-approved solely for this virus [19], although it has strong in vitro activity against HSV-1, HSV-2, and VZV as well [20].

Pharmacology

Ganciclovir is available for IV use (Table 54.1), with expected peak plasma concentrations of 30–40 μM and elimination half-life of about 3.5 hours primarily by renal clearance. After monophosphorylation by a virally encoded kinase and then by cellular enzymes, the resulting intracellular ganciclovir triphosphate has a prolonged half-life estimated at >24 h [21]. This probably accounts for the slower resumption of CMV growth after removal of ganciclovir from culture media, in comparison with some other CMV antivirals [22]. Oral ganciclovir has poor bioavailability [23] and is no longer marketed despite FDA approval for prevention of CMV disease in transplantation and AIDS. Valganciclovir has better oral bioavailability of about 60% and is the preferred oral formulation. Ganciclovir and valganciclovir toxicity manifests primarily as bone marrow suppression, which can become dose limiting [24, 25]. Granulocyte colony-stimulating factors may help with marrow recovery.

Clinical Indications

The introduction of ganciclovir did little to alter the fatal outcome of advanced CMV pneumonia [26]. Thus, the prevention of serious CMV disease became the main antiviral goal in transplant recipients. Two approaches to prevention were formulated: early identification of CMV viremia prior to end-organ disease by regular monitoring, followed by prompt "preemptive" treatment; or antiviral prophylaxis for planned durations after transplantation. Clinical trials showed that either approach using IV or oral ganciclovir was effective, more so than acyclovir-based regimens [12, 27].

Randomized clinical trials resulted in the current FDA-approved indications for valganciclovir in transplantation (Table 54.1). A trial of 100 days of valganciclovir vs. oral ganciclovir in high-risk solid organ recipients (mainly liver and kidney) showed comparable efficacy at preventing CMV disease when assessed at 6 and 12 months post-transplant [28]. FDA approval of valganciclovir was withheld for liver transplant recipients because of a higher incidence of invasive CMV disease, but valganciclovir therapy for this recipient subset is widely used and recommended [29]. Another trial concluded that valganciclovir prophylaxis for 200 days was superior to 100 days in preventing CMV disease at 12 months in high-risk kidney recipients [30], resulting in FDA approval for extended prophylaxis in this patient subset.

For treatment of overt CMV disease, ranging from an undifferentiated febrile syndrome to invasive disease such as colitis or pneumonia, IV ganciclovir remains a standard option. A controlled trial showed noninferiority of oral valganciclovir when compared to IV ganciclovir for the treatment of nonthreatening CMV disease in solid organ recipients [31], but this use of valganciclovir is not FDA-approved. Duration of therapy is dependent on clinical response but is typically several weeks followed by oral maintenance therapy until viremia is cleared.

Drug Resistance Mechanisms

Over 90% of ganciclovir-resistant clinical isolates contain a mutation in the UL97 kinase gene [32]. The most relevant mutations reduce the phosphorylation of ganciclovir while preserving biologically important UL97 kinase activity and near-normal viral growth. One of seven UL97 amino acid substitutions (Table 54.1) is found in about 80% of ganciclovir-resistant clinical isolates [32]. These substitutions generally confer five- to tenfold increases in ganciclovir EC50, except for C592G which confers only a threefold increase. In the UL97 codon range 590–607, less common sequence variants include point mutations and in-frame codon deletions, which confer degrees of ganciclovir resistance ranging from none to 15-fold [33].

Many CMV DNA polymerase (UL54 *pol*) mutations found in clinical specimens have been analyzed for their drug resistance phenotype [32, 34]. Such mutations may confer resistance to one or more of the currently approved CMV drugs ganciclovir, foscarnet and cidofovir, and in the case of ganciclovir may combine with a preexisting UL97 mutation to increase the overall level of drug resistance several fold. Rarely, ganciclovir may select for a *pol* resistance mutation before a UL97 mutation is detected. In general, ganciclovir and cidofovir dual resistance without foscarnet cross-resistance results from mutation in the exonuclease domains or codon 987 in the thumb domain.

Foscarnet

Foscarnet is trisodium phosphonoformate, a pyrophosphate analog, which inhibits the viral DNA polymerase by interfering with the release of pyrophosphate from the incoming nucleotide during DNA replication. The antiviral spectrum of foscarnet in vitro includes all herpesviruses, HIV, and hepatitis B virus [35], but it is FDA-approved only for treatment of HSV and CMV.

Pharmacology

Foscarnet is available as a solution containing 24 mg/mL for IV use [35]. To reduce toxicity, saline prehydration of up to a liter is recommended. Foscarnet is not further metabolized but is renally excreted by glomerular filtration and secretion, and is significantly deposited in bone. Variable uptake in bone may explain the great variation in plasma pharmacokinetics of foscarnet, with peak concentrations expected around 500 μM and a plasma elimination half-life of about 4.5 h. There is a prolonged phase of slow clearance of accumulated drug from bone.

Foscarnet therapy is frequently limited by nephrotoxicity and metabolic disturbances, such as hypocalcemia, hypophosphatemia, hypomagnesemia, and hypokalemia, all of which can become symptomatic (including tetany, seizures, and arrhythmias) and always require close monitoring and electrolyte repletion as needed. The infusion rate must be controlled to avoid acute impact on electrolyte concentrations. The need for prolonged IV infusions and access devices complicates treatment planning. The fluid and salt load of the saline prehydration may be poorly tolerated. Concentration of foscarnet in the urine may cause uroepithelial cytotoxicity and genital ulceration.

Clinical Indications

For treatment of overt CMV disease, FDA approval of foscarnet remains limited to retinitis, because there have been no controlled treatment trials for other tissue-invasive disease. There are, however, case series on the use of foscarnet especially in stem cell transplant recipients to avoid the dose-limiting hematologic toxicity of ganciclovir [36], and for treatment of ganciclovir-resistant infection [37]. Overall data suggest similar virologic efficacy as ganciclovir, but with a different set of major toxicities as outlined above. Comparison of 14 days of preemptive therapy with IV ganciclovir or foscarnet after allogeneic stem cell transplantation [38] showed similar efficacy in preventing CMV disease, with the expected toxicities for each drug.

Foscarnet is FDA-approved for treatment of acyclovir-resistant mucocutaneous HSV infection in immunocompromised hosts [13]. Although unapproved, this indication is in practice extended to the treatment of acyclovir-resistant herpes zoster.

Drug Resistance Mechanisms

Foscarnet resistance mutations in HSV, VZV, and CMV are clustered in the palm and finger structure domains of their corresponding DNA polymerases [13, 18, 32]. However, some mutations map to locations well outside these domains. Acyclovir and foscarnet cross-resistance of HSV and VZV may result from mutations that cluster in the same polymerase domains for both drugs [13]. CMV foscarnet resistance mutations may show variable low-grade or borderline ganciclovir and/or cidofovir cross-resistance. A few specific mutations such as A834P or deletion of codons 981–982 confer moderate triple drug resistance. The level of ganciclovir or foscarnet resistance conferred by CMV *pol* mutations is usually in the two- to fivefold range [32].

Cidofovir

Cidofovir is an acyclic nucleoside phosphonate nucleotide analog. It does not require initial phosphorylation by a viral kinase. Instead, cellular enzymes convert cidofovir to its active diphosphate form, which is a nonobligate DNA chain terminator. Cidofovir was FDA-approved in 1996 for treatment of CMV retinitis in AIDS. This narrow approved usage is in contrast with its wide in vitro antiviral spectrum which includes herpesviruses, adenoviruses, poxviruses, and even papovaviruses that do not encode their own DNA polymerase [39]. Cidofovir has good in vitro potency against HSV, VZV, and CMV.

Pharmacology

The specified cidofovir dosing protocol (see Table 54.1) includes extensive pre- and post-hydration and three doses of probenecid in an attempt to reduce nephrotoxicity. Cidofovir is renally cleared and renal function must be closely monitored both to guide dosing and to discontinue use for deteriorated renal function or proteinuria. The medication is given at long intervals, in part to avoid the rapid development of nephrotoxicity, and because the cidofovir diphosphate has a long intracellular half-life. In clinical trials, about a quarter of subjects developed nephrotoxicity, a similar fraction as foscarnet therapy despite the use of hydration and probenecid [40]. Ophthalmologists using cidofovir as systemic or intravitreal therapy have reported uveitis and intraocular hypotony as distinctive complications [41]. Intolerance of cidofovir therapy may also result from adverse reactions to the significant saline hydration and probenecid that accompanies each dose.

Clinical Indications

No controlled trials have established the efficacy of cidofovir for treating any tissue-invasive CMV disease in the transplant setting, whether as initial therapy or for salvage. In the stem cell transplant population, a retrospective series was collected of cidofovir use as salvage or preemptive therapy for CMV disease [40]. Such uncontrolled studies carry a risk of reporting bias. As salvage therapy, there was apparent benefit in 9 of 16 cases of CMV pneumonia, and the efficacy of cidofovir as preemptive therapy was estimated at about 65%. Nephrotoxicity was noted in 26% and was persistent in more than half of the cases where it occurred. Cidofovir is generally regarded as a third line treatment for resistant or refractory CMV disease in transplant populations. Efficacy is poorly documented, with both optimistic reports and those indicating only a transient virologic benefit followed by emergence of cidofovir resistance.

An orally bioavailable lipid conjugate of cidofovir, hexadecyloxypropyl-cidofovir or brincidofovir (CMX001), has undergone clinical trial. Nephrotoxicity is reduced with this formulation because cidofovir is not concentrated in renal tubular cells [42]. The in vitro antiviral potency of brincidofovir is orders of magnitude greater than the parent compound, but this did not allow a corresponding decrease in the prophylactic dose in a Phase II dose ranging trial in stem cell recipients [43]. At the selected dose, severe diarrhea and associated increased mortality caused the failure of a Phase III CMV prophylaxis trial in stem cell recipients (clinicaltrials.gov NCT01769170). Use of brincidofovir may possibly be revisited if an improved risk-benefit profile is established by use of new formulations or careful selection of treatment candidates.

There is interest in the antiviral activity of cidofovir against adenoviruses and polyomaviruses (BK, JC), which are significant pathogens in transplant recipients [39]. Use of cidofovir has been suggested for adenovirus infections in allogeneic stem cell transplantation [44]. More recently, 9 of 13 subjects with adenovirus disease appeared to have a virologic response to brincidofovir [45]. An expanded access protocol (clinicaltrials.gov NCT02596997) was registered in late 2015 to provide brincidofovir for treatment of serious adenovirus infection or disease.

Drug Resistance Mechanisms

Mutations conferring drug resistance to cidofovir in the CMV DNA polymerase gene are clustered in the exonuclease and thumb domains [32], and cross-resistance with ganciclovir is expected. In some cases, a relatively large increase in cidofovir EC50 (10–20-fold) is conferred by these mutations. There is little information on resistance mutations of HSV and VZV that develop after cidofovir treatment.

Incidence and Clinical Diagnosis of Herpesvirus Drug Resistance

The risk of drug resistance increases with the duration and intensity of active viral replication while under treatment. Contributory host factors include severe immunosuppression and lack of preexisting immunity. Resistance usually emerges after weeks to months of drug exposure, and is suspected when there is active viral replication or progressive disease despite adequate antiviral drug delivery.

The prevalence of acyclovir- and penciclovir-resistant HSV isolates among immunocompetent populations is generally <1% [13, 14, 17], except that those repeatedly treated for herpes keratitis may have a higher frequency of acyclovir resistance, reported at 6.4% [46]. In immunocompromised transplant recipients, prevalence of acyclovir-resistant HSV can reach 7–10% and higher in allogeneic marrow recipients [17, 47]. Limited data appear similar for VZV [48].

CMV-seronegative recipients of a CMV-seropositive transplanted solid organ (D+/R-subset) are at the highest risk of drug resistance because of prolonged prophylaxis or therapy for post-transplant primary CMV infection and disease [32]. Incidence of ganciclovir resistance in this subset is 5–12% and higher among lung recipients. Transplant recipients who have profound and prolonged T-cell depletion resulting from anti-CD52 alemtuzumab therapy, are also a high-risk population. Drug-resistant CMV disease is associated with increased morbidity and mortality, probably reflecting underlying conditions that predisposed the host to the development of resistant virus [49].

In high-risk populations, treated subjects should be monitored regularly for a virologic and clinical response. Rising plasma viral loads or progressive disease after more than 2 weeks of full treatment doses may be an early indicator of emerging drug resistance. The rapidity of development of resistance depends on the intensity of viral replication while under treatment, but is rarely detectable until after at least 6 weeks and usually a few months of drug exposure.

An unsatisfactory response to antiviral therapy may result from adverse host factors, inadequate drug potency at tissue sites of infection, or development of antiviral drug resistance. Laboratory confirmation of drug resistance is desirable to evaluate alternative therapeutic options.

For HSV, phenotypic testing of a patient's viral isolate against drug in cell culture to determine an EC50 value is recommended, because HSV grows easily and rapidly [13], whereas slow growth makes this assay less feasible for VZV. Genotypic assays for HSV and VZV involve polymerase chain reaction (PCR) amplification and sequencing of the viral TK and *pol* genes. TK deficiency can be inferred, if a TK frameshift or stop mutation is detected, but uncertainty can arise from the many uncharacterized TK and *pol* amino acid substitutions in HSV [13]. VZV has fewer TK sequence polymorphisms and strong clustering of *pol* mutations, which may facilitate interpretation [13, 15, 18]. TK deficient strains can be expected to be highly resistant to acyclovir while *pol* mutants would typically show more moderate resistance [15].

CMV drug resistance testing relies mainly on genotypic assays of viral sequences directly amplified from clinical specimens, usually the same plasma specimens used for viral load determinations. It is inadvisable to attempt genotyping on plasma loads of less than 1000 genome copies/mL because of the risk of nonrepresentative PCR amplification [50]. Assays are available from academic and commercial reference laboratories.

Interpretation of the results is straightforward if a known UL97 or *pol* resistance mutation is reported [32]. Uncharacterized UL54 *pol* sequence variants can be difficult to interpret because of significant baseline sequence polymorphisms, mostly outside conserved functional domains and technical artifacts that can arise during genotypic testing [51]. Newly recognized mutations can be tested for relevance to drug resistance after transferring them into baseline laboratory CMV strains. This recombinant phenotyping procedure is too slow to resolve a current diagnostic uncertainty [32].

Management of Herpesvirus Drug Resistance

Clinical guidelines have been developed that take into account a lack of prospective data to address the natural history of drug-resistant infection, the efficacy of alternative therapy, and criteria for their use [13, 29]. Proposed management algorithms require individual interpretation, given the great variability in host factors and prior antiviral drug exposure. At the outset, it is important to improve host antiviral defenses as much as possible, such as by minimizing immunosuppressive therapy. Another concern is for adequate antiviral drug delivery, including dosage, formulation, duration, and patient adherence.

The urgency with which antiviral treatment must be switched depends on the severity of the current infection as judged by measured viral loads and symptomatic disease. Severe disease in a seriously immunocompromised host may warrant empiric foscarnet therapy. Otherwise, full doses of IV acyclovir for HSV or VZV infection, or higher doses of IV ganciclovir for CMV infection, up to 10 mg/kg twice daily in patients with normal renal function can be continued, pending genotypic testing; high-dose ganciclovir is not FDA-approved [13, 29].

For confirmed acyclovir-resistant HSV or VZV, foscarnet is the main alternative therapy because resistance usually results from TK mutations [13]. However, acyclovir-foscarnet cross-resistance is typical for the uncommon *pol* mutants of HSV and VZV that may emerge [18]. In these instances, cidofovir may be an option [13].

Full- or high-dose IV ganciclovir may retain meaningful anti-CMV activity in the presence of mutations that confer lower-grade resistance to ganciclovir [33]. Foscarnet is the usual alternative therapy for ganciclovir-resistant CMV as it has less cross-resistance than cidofovir. Cidofovir should not be chosen for ganciclovir-resistant CMV infection without genotypic testing for a *pol* mutation conferring cross-resistance. Even if one is not detected, there is concern that undetected resistant *pol* mutant subpopulations may emerge relatively rapidly [52].

Other Herpesvirus Antivirals

Antiviral compounds that do not target the viral DNA polymerase are being developed with objectives of oral bioavailability, improved safety profile and lack of cross-resistance with existing drugs. The potential benefit of combination therapy directed at multiple viral targets is appealing in immunocompromised hosts.

Pritelivir and Amenamevir

Pritelivir and amenamevir are orally dosed helicase/primase inhibitors. They target enzymes other than DNA polymerase that are essential for viral DNA replication [53, 54]. The in vitro spectrum of activity of pritelivir includes HSV-1 and HSV-2, while amenamevir is active against HSV and VZV. A Phase II study showed amenamevir and valacyclovir to have similar efficacy in treating episodes of genital herpes [55]. Pritelivir has undergone two Phase II trials for suppression of recurrent HSV-2 in normal hosts. When compared with placebo, daily or weekly doses of pritelivir for 4 weeks reduced the incidence and quantity of genital lesions and HSV shedding [56]. In a crossover trial, pritelivir 100 mg daily was superior to valacyclovir 500 mg daily as measured by HSV detection in frequently sampled genital swabs [57]. After clinical trials were placed on hold pending review of primate toxicity data, a new trial was listed in 2017 to compare pritelivir with foscarnet for the treatment of acyclovir-resistant mucocutaneous herpes simplex infections in immunocompromised adults (clinicaltrials.gov NCT03073967). Mutations in the HSV helicase gene UL5 and to a lesser extent in the primase gene UL52 have been described that confer pritelivir and amenamevir cross-resistance, including high-level resistance conferred by UL5 K356N (HSV-1 codon numbering) with retained in vitro viral growth fitness [58, 59]. As expected, no pritelivir resistance was observed after short-term, 4-week exposure to pritelivir for prevention of genital herpes [60].

Maribavir

Maribavir is a benzimidazole L-riboside CMV UL97 kinase inhibitor [61] that has good anti-CMV activity in vitro depending on cell culture conditions [62]. CMV replication is greatly reduced but not entirely prevented in the absence of the UL97 kinase. After early studies showing low host toxicity and indications of antiviral efficacy, two randomized Phase III clinical trials of low-dose oral maribavir at 100 mg twice daily failed as prophylaxis for CMV reactivation after stem cell [63] or liver transplantation [64]. Open-label use of higher doses suggested a possible benefit as salvage therapy for refractory or resistant CMV disease [65] but resulted in the first documented instance of maribavir resistance in a clinical CMV isolate [66]. Additional Phase II trials were conducted in 2012 through 2015 to explore the use of maribavir as treatment of CMV viremia without end-organ disease (EudraCT 2010-024247-32) or for salvage treatment of resistant or refractory disease. Preliminary data suggested that oral doses ranging from 400 to 1200 mg twice daily all showed anti-CMV activity (clinicaltrials.gov NCT01611974), and corresponding Phase III trials were launched (clinicaltrials.gov NCT02927067 and NCT02931539). Major maribavir resistance mutations map to the UL97 kinase target, commonly T409 M and H411Y/N located at the ATP binding domain that is the presumed site of competitive binding of maribavir [67]. These specific mutations increase the maribavir EC50 by ~80-fold (T409 M) or 9- to −12-fold (H411 mutants) without significant ganciclovir cross-resistance. Unusual UL97 p-loop mutations, for example, at codon 342, can confer dual ganciclovir-maribavir resistance without knocking out biological kinase activity [68]. Diverse UL27 gene mutations confer low-grade maribavir resistance probably by modulating cell cycle conditions to compensate partially for the effects of UL97 kinase inhibition [69, 70].

Letermovir

Letermovir is an orally bioavailable CMV terminase inhibitor [71] with potent in vitro antiviral potency (low nanomolar EC50). The terminase complex includes components encoded by CMV genes UL56, UL89, and UL51 [72] and performs essential functions including cleavage of replicated viral DNA into unit length genomes and their translocation across the portal protein (UL104) into newly formed viral capsids. Phase II and III clinical trials for prophylaxis of CMV infection in stem cell transplant recipients were successful [73] (clinicaltrials.gov NCT02137772), and letermovir was FDA-approved for this indication in late 2017. Lack of hematologic toxicity is a distinct advantage over ganciclovir or valganciclovir, and is expected to be most useful in the period immediately following stem cell transplantation, as studied in the clinical trials. There are insufficient data to assess the efficacy of letermovir as therapy for active CMV disease, including cases resistant or refractory to treatment with standard DNA polymerase inhibitors. CMV UL56 gene mutants are readily selected in cell culture to confer letermovir resistance [74, 75], but no meaningful clinical correlation yet exists. In a letermovir prophylaxis trial, UL56 amino acid substitution V236M emerged to confer ~40-fold increased letermovir EC50 [76]. Amino acid substitutions at the C325 residue of UL56 confer absolute letermovir resistance in vitro and are a locus of interest for diagnostic testing. Cross-resistance with DNA polymerase inhibitors or maribavir is not expected given the different antiviral drug targets.

Antivirals for RNA Respiratory Viruses

Influenza, parainfluenza, respiratory syncytial virus (RSV), and other RNA viruses cause diffuse pneumonias often resulting in respiratory failure and death, especially in hematopoietic cell and lung transplant recipients. The role of antiviral therapy in reducing mortality and lung damage has not been proven by controlled trials, leaving many controversies regarding the proper application of available therapies (Table 54.2). Approved antiviral drugs include the neuraminidase inhibitors (NAIs) oseltamivir, peramivir, and zanamivir for influenza A and B, M2 ion channel blockers amantadine and rimantadine for influenza A only, and ribavirin, which is FDA-approved for aerosol use only in pediatric RSV infection. When considering antiviral therapy for these infections, attention should simultaneously be paid to infection control measures to prevent nosocomial spread, pending diagnostic confirmation.

Oseltamivir, Peramivir, and Zanamivir

Influenza types A and B are major human pathogens. Subtypes within type A are grouped by the antigenicity of the hemagglutinin (H) and neuraminidase (N) proteins. Currently circulating influenza A strains are subtypes H3N2 and to a lesser extent H1N1 2009 pandemic strain, with occasional human cases related to avian influenza strains H5, H7, and H9. Neuraminidase cleaves the sialic acid containing cell surface receptor that binds viral hemagglutinin, thus enabling the release of newly formed virions from infected cells. Oseltamivir and zanamivir are sialic acid analog neuraminidase inhibitors (NAIs) initially marketed in 1999 [77], with the former modified for oral bioavailability and the latter delivered by inhalation. Peramivir is an intravenously administered transition-state analog NAI approved by the FDA in 2014. Influenza A and B neuraminidases are susceptible to inhibition as long as they have not developed resistance mutations, although there may be strain variation in the degree of susceptibility.

Pharmacology

Oseltamivir phosphate in oral capsules is metabolized by hepatic esterases to the active drug oseltamivir carboxylate (Table 54.2) that has a bioavailability of at least 75% and plasma elimination half-life of 6–10 h. It is renally cleared and the dosing interval is doubled for creatinine clearance <30 mL/min. The drug is generally well toler-

Table 54.2 Antiviral agents approved for respiratory viral infections (2017)

Antiviral agent	Structure and mechanism of action	Therapeutic use[a]	Route and adult dose[b]	Side effects Adverse interactions	Resistance
Oseltamivir	Ethyl ester prodrug converted in liver to a cyclohexene carboxylic acid derivative Sialic acid analog competitive neuraminidase (NA) inhibitor targeting release of virus particles from host cells	Influenza A and B: treatment and prophylaxis Prompt initiation needed for best outcome. Some benefit possible with delayed treatment Pandemic 2009 H1N1 flu A: most strains initially susceptible. May become resistant after drug exposure and transmission Seasonal H1N1 (2008) flu A: almost all strains resistant	Oral Treatment: Standard dose: 75 mg 2×/day for 5 days, longer if severely ill Prophylaxis: 75 mg/day for at least 10 days (until 1 week after last case during influenza outbreaks in health care facilities; 10 days after household exposure) Not approved for age <1 year	GI[c], headache, rare neuropsychiatric symptoms	Most common NA mutations[d] some are cross-resistant to zanamivir (*) *H1N1*: H275Y *pH1/N1*: N294S, H275Y, E119V*, I222V, *H3N2*: N294S, R292K*, E119V/I, I222V *H5N1*: N294S, H275Y *Influenza B*: R152K*, D198N*, R371K*
Peramivir	Cyclopentane carboxylic acid derivative Transition state analog NA inhibitor	Influenza A and B	Intravenous infusion Treatment: 18 years and older One 600 mg dose by infusion for 15–30 minutes	GI[c], hypersensitivity	NA mutations[d] with some cross-resistance to oseltamivir (*) *H1N1*: H275Y *H3N2*: R292K*, *Influenza B*: R152K*, H275Y HA mutation K189E
Zanamivir	Dihydropyran carboxylic acid derivative Sialic acid analog NA inhibitor	Influenza A and B: treatment and prophylaxis Marketed as powder for inhalation. Intravenous form is experimental	Powder for inhalation: Treatment: 10 mg (2 puffs) 2 times/day for 5 days Not approved for age < 7 year Prophylaxis: 10 mg/day for durations as described for oseltamivir Not approved for age < 5 year or with underlying lung disease	Allergic reactions oropharyngeal or facial Cough, nasal and throat discomfort, bronchospasm GI[c], headache	NA mutations[d] with occasional cross-resistance to oseltamivir (*) *H1N1*: E119G, E119V*, Q136K *H3N2*: R292K*, Q136K, D151A/D *H5N1*: E119G, D198G *Influenza B*: R152K, D198N*, R371K*
Amantadine	1-aminoadamantane Blocks viral M2 protein, prevents internalization and uncoating of virus	Influenza A: treatment and prophylaxis (susceptible strains only) No activity against influenza B	Oral Treatment: 200 mg/day for 3–5 days Prophylaxis: 200 mg/day for 2–4 week	GI[c], CNS symptoms[e] Avoid use with anticholinergics and antihistamines	M2 mutations at residues 26, 27, 30, 31, 34, most commonly S31 N H3N2 and pandemic H1N1 > 90% resistant Cross-resistance to rimantadine
Rimantadine	(*RS*)-1-(1-adamantyl) ethanamine Mechanism same as amantadine	Same as amantadine	Oral Treatment: 100 mg 2 times/day for 7 days	Side effects similar to amantadine but less severe	M2 mutations at residues 26, 27, 30, 31, 34 Cross-resistance to amantadine

Table 54.2 (continued)

Antiviral agent	Structure and mechanism of action	Therapeutic use[a]	Route and adult dose[b]	Side effects Adverse interactions	Resistance
Ribavirin	1-β-D-ribofuranosyl-1,2,4-triazole-3-carboxamide Single antiviral mechanism not established Proposed mechanisms: 1. Depletion of guanosine triphosphate by inhibition of inosine monophosphate dehydrogenase 2. Inhibition of viral polymerase or induction of error-prone replication 3. Inhibition of RNA capping 4. Immunomodulatory or cell signaling effects	Respiratory syncytial virus (RSV) No FDA-approved indications in adult respiratory viral infections Treatment: lower respiratory tract infection Preventive treatment: to reduce lower respiratory tract extension of nasopharyngeal infection detected by PCR Ribavirin also proposed for parainfluenza, influenza (as adjunct), metapneumovirus	Inhaled aerosol 20 mg/mL: Treatment of RSV: 6 g by aerosol over 18 h/day for 7 days using a small particle aerosol generator and face mask ± intravenous immunoglobulin or palivizumab Oral: Efficacy in respiratory viral infections is not established but suggested by case series Intravenous: Request through FDA emergency investigational new drug program	Inhaled form: Bronchospasm, respiratory distress, cough Oral form: Hemolytic anemia, neutropenia, thrombocytopenia, GI[c], headache, insomnia, asthenia Intravenous form: Hemolytic anemia	No resistance mutations characterized for RSV

[a]Recommended usage may differ from FDA-approved indications and doses
[b]Dosage information as suggested for normal adults. See full dosing information provided in package insert
[c]GI (gastrointestinal) symptoms include nausea and vomiting (diarrhea less often)
[d]N2 numbering system used for mutations except H275Y
[e]CNS (central nervous system) symptoms include confusion, difficulty concentrating, dizziness, hallucinations, and seizures

ated, with adverse effects limited to nausea and vomiting [78], but controversially associated neuropsychiatric events have been described mainly in children and from Japan [79].

Peramivir is intravenously administered as a single 600 mg dose adjusted for renal function since it has a prolonged duration of neuraminidase inhibitory activity [80]. Reported adverse effects were infrequent, including diarrhea and hypersensitivity reactions.

Zanamivir is administered as a powder for inhalation (Table 54.2) and is not approved for use in young children or patients with underlying chronic lung disease. Less than 20% of the inhaled drug reaches the lung, but the high local concentrations may be an advantage [77]. The drug is renally cleared but no dose adjustment is needed for renal failure given the low systemic bioavailability.

Clinical Applications

Because influenza genotypes evolve in unpredictable ways, efficacy of antiviral drugs against prevailing influenza strains will vary over time. Early and preventive use of antiviral therapy is much more effective than trying to resolve an established viral pneumonia. This may require presumptive treatment pending diagnostic testing.

Oseltamivir, peramivir, and zanamivir are FDA-approved for treatment of influenza A and B within 48 h of onset of symptoms, preferably sooner. Under these conditions, healthy adults and children with laboratory-confirmed influenza are shown to have a 1–2-day reduction in symptoms with any of the three NAIs and a little more if treatment is started within 12 h [77, 78]. Although delayed treatment beyond 48 h is unlikely to be statistically effective in normal hosts [81], treatment is recommended in transplant recipients regardless of duration of illness when diagnosed, because of the greater likelihood of prolonged viral replication and severe disease [82, 83]. Depending on clinical response and severity of illness, extension of treatment beyond the FDA-approved 5-day course may be warranted. No controlled studies have shown a mortality benefit from antiviral treatment of influenza, but low-confidence observational studies taken together appear to support a meaningful impact of oseltamivir on mortality if treated within 48 h and possibly later [81]. Comparison of oseltamivir and IV peramivir treatment showed similar outcomes in hospitalized adults with seasonal influenza [84].

As prophylaxis, oseltamivir, and zanamivir are recommended for use as shown in Table 54.2, in conjunction with vaccination [8]. Effectiveness has been shown when started within 2 days of exposure to symptomatic influenza [85] or within 36 h of exposure for zanamivir [86], with reduction in incidence of symptomatic infection of about 80% in institutional and household contacts. Heightened surveillance of acute illness and prompt initiation of therapy has been proposed to address the concern for selection of resistant viruses during prophylaxis [83].

Drug Resistance

Drug resistance is a major determinant of the utility of NAIs against circulating influenza strains. Because information changes rapidly, updated information is regularly posted to the CDC web site (http://www.cdc.gov/flu). As an example of evolving trends, the presently circulating seasonal H3N2 influenza A strain is generally susceptible to oseltamivir, while the seasonal H1N1 influenza A prevalent in 2008 became almost 100% resistant, leading to a recommendation not to use this drug [82]. In 2009, a pandemic strain of H1N1 influenza A susceptible to oseltamivir rapidly displaced the previous H1N1 strain, thus making the drug again widely suitable for presumptive therapy and prophylaxis.

Neuraminidase mutations conferring drug resistance may involve residues that form a framework for the enzyme or catalytic residues that contact sialic acid substrates [87]. The most common mutation H275Y, or H274Y in N2 nomenclature, detected in H1N1 and H5N1 strains is a framework mutation, which confers high-level oseltamivir and peramivir resistance but retains susceptibility to zanamivir. Depending on the genetic context, this mutation may have little adverse effect on viral growth and can easily be transmitted without continued drug exposure, as shown by the 2008 seasonal H1N1 strains. H3N2 influenza A strains tend to develop the framework mutation E119V and a variety of catalytic mutations such as R292K. Zanamivir resistance characteristically involves the framework mutation E119G which confers low-grade cross-resistance to oseltamivir. Resistance to zanamivir is so far less common than resistance to oseltamivir. Phenotypic determination of influenza drug resistance can be performed in cell culture or by enzymatic assays, with significant interassay variability, or more practically by genotypic assays which should test for the range of reported mutations (Table 54.2) rather than just the signature mutations such as H275Y [87].

Amantadine and Rimantadine

These adamantanes act by blocking the function of the M2 ion channel involved in viral uncoating and ribonucleoprotein release for nuclear entry and initiation of replication. This antiviral mechanism is valid only for influenza A because influenza B does not have the same M2 protein. Unfortunately M2 mutations, typically S31 N, can easily develop with little growth penalty, enabling the worldwide spread of resistant influenza A, to the point of making this drug class therapeutically ineffective [88]. The last prevalent strain for which amantadine susceptibility was observed was the 2008 seasonal H1N1 strain. The drugs were administered orally for influenza A prophylaxis and early therapy, with cautions for neurologic side effects (Table 54.2).

Ribavirin

Ribavirin is FDA-approved for oral use as adjunctive therapy for hepatitis C virus (HCV) and aerosol use for severe pediatric RSV bronchiolitis. Its use in transplant recipients is controversial, because the typical inhalation mode of delivery is not FDA-approved, insufficiently evidence-based, and involves extraordinary costs and logistical complexity [89, 90]. Evidence for efficacy of oral or intravenous ribavirin for respiratory viral infections is inconclusive at best.

No single antiviral mechanism of action has been established for ribavirin. It is a carboxamide triazole riboside, which can be considered a synthetic nucleoside analog that is converted to a triphosphate by cellular enzymes. Several mechanisms of action have been proposed [91] (see Table 54.2). The claimed spectrum of antiviral activity of ribavirin is very broad, covering many RNA viruses and some DNA viruses such as adenovirus and poxviruses [91]. Ribavirin is often mentioned as a potential off-label unproven treatment for various life-threatening infections including viral pneumonias and hemorrhagic fevers [92].

Pharmacology

Ribavirin is supplied as a powder for use in making a 20 mg/mL aqueous solution to be delivered using a small particle aerosol generator (SPAG-2 device) (Table 54.2). The substance is teratogenic usually interpreted as requiring a negative pressure ventilated isolation room, and that it may precipitate in ventilator tubing or airways causing mechanical obstruction and respiratory deterioration. Patients may object to the prolonged attachment of a mask. Symptoms include cough, respiratory distress, bronchospasm, or claustrophobia. The delivered dose is unpredictable but systemic toxicity is not expected.

As an oral formulation ribavirin is available as generic capsules and tablets. Oral bioavailability is about 60%, and increases with a high fat meal. For HCV, dosing is weight based, ranging from 800 to 1400 mg total per day; no standard has been set for respiratory viruses. The plasma half-life varies from 79 to 170 h, but ribavirin persists for much longer in other body compartments [93]. It is not protein bound and does not inhibit CYP450 enzymes. Drug interactions prominently include nucleoside antiretroviral drugs, in particular didanosine and zidovudine [94], and azathioprine.

It is renally cleared (61%) and dose adjustments or discontinuation are indicated in patients with renal dysfunction. Hemolytic anemia is the major serious adverse effect; others are as listed in Table 54.2. An IV form of ribavirin has limited availability through an FDA emergency investigational drug protocol [92]. Hemolytic anemia appears to be the main adverse effect of this formulation as well.

Clinical Applications

Aerosol ribavirin for treatment of severe pediatric RSV bronchiolitis was initially supported by controlled trials reporting beneficial effects such as reduction of ventilatory support and hospitalization in normal infants requiring mechanical ventilation [95]. No mortality benefit has been proven in any controlled trial. The reported benefits have been strongly disputed, including negative results in a subsequent controlled trial [96]. In a 2006 guideline [97], the American Academy of Pediatrics suggested that ribavirin might be considered for use in highly selected situations involving severe disease and risk factors for it, but the 2014 updated guideline [98] makes no mention of ribavirin use under any circumstances.

Among hematopoietic cell recipients, lymphopenia is a strong predictor for RSV morbidity and mortality [99]. RSV infection in this population frequently progresses to lower respiratory tract disease and death. The majority of observational studies support a benefit of aerosolized ribavirin treatment in preventing these outcomes, but evidence is of poor quality [90, 100]. An attempted prospective clinical trial was terminated without definitive results because of slow patient accrual [101].

Given the inconclusive data, transplant programs have tended to develop their own clinical protocols, which may involve early use of aerosol ribavirin in an attempt to prevent progression of RSV upper respiratory infection in higher-risk patient subsets such as those with lymphopenia or receiving anti-lymphocyte regimens, or to improve outcomes of established lower respiratory tract disease. Because of the high cost and complexity of aerosol ribavirin administration, use of oral or IV ribavirin as an alternative has been reported, with weak evidence for apparently favorable outcomes [90, 102, 103]. Additional benefit has been attributed to the administration of nonspecific or specific RSV antibody (IVIG or palivizumab) [90], which may be included in institutional protocols for lower respiratory tract disease despite weak data supporting their routine use.

Use of ribavirin to treat other respiratory viral infections such as parainfluenza and metapneumovirus is based on insufficient observational data [104–106]. A review of FDA emergency drug requests for IV ribavirin showed adenovirus to be the most commonly targeted virus, accounting for 55% of all requests, followed by RSV, parainfluenza, influenza, hantavirus, measles (SSPE), and rabies. The reported outcomes were variable [92]. For example, a controlled trial showed no benefit in hantavirus pulmonary syndrome, and published cases of adenovirus infection treated with IV ribavirin had a 63% overall mortality rate [92].

Drug Resistance

No resistance mutations have been described for RSV to support the existence of a specific antiviral drug target for ribavirin despite its tendency to increase the viral mutation rate [107].

Presatovir (GS-5806)

Presatovir (GS-5806) is a small molecule inhibitor of RSV acting on the viral fusion process involved in entry into host cells [102]. It is active against a variety of RSV subtype A and B isolates in vitro, has low cellular cytotoxicity, and is undergoing Phase II clinical trials in lung and hematopoietic cell transplant recipients and in hospitalized adults. Treatment emergent mutations in the RSV F gene such as F140L and T400I have been identified in human subjects treated with 1–3 doses of presatovir, which confer >200-fold increases in EC50 [108].

Hepatitis C Virus Antivirals

Direct-acting small molecule drugs with specific antiviral targets disrupted old treatment paradigms based on interferon and ribavirin and now enable the successful treatment of chronic HCV infection in the vast majority of cases after 8–24 weeks of combination therapy [109]. Clearance of circulating HCV RNA at 12 or 24 weeks after completion of therapy is defined as a sustained virologic response (SVR, SVR12, or SVR24), with nearly all cases of SVR12 achieving SVR24 and essentially a virologic cure [110], thus halting the progression of HCV disease [111], although prior liver damage and its sequelae including hepatocellular carcinoma may persist. The goal of early cure of chronic HCV infection before evidence of liver damage should eventually displace the historical practice of prioritizing patients according to disease severity for receiving older, poorly tolerated therapeutic regimens of dubious efficacy. At present, the high cost of newer treatments is limiting universal access to therapy. In this rapidly evolving field, a joint society (IDSA-AASLD) online resource (http://www.hcvguidelines.org) is available for continuously updated authoritative guidance on treating HCV infection.

HCV therapy (Table 54.3) [112–122] currently involves three antiviral targets, the NS3/NS4A protease, the NS5A accessory protein, and the NS5B viral polymerase. Used in combination the drugs are highly effective in those not previously treated for HCV, with SVR rates routinely exceeding

Table 54.3 Individual direct-acting HCV antiviral agents and amino acid loci of substitutions associated with drug resistance[a]

	HCV genotype						
Antiviral agent	1a	1b	2	3	4	5	6
NS3/4A protease inhibitors							
Glecaprevir	Q80			A166, Y56, Q168			
Grazoprevir	V36, Q80, S122, R155, A156, D168	V36, T54, A156, D168,	V36, A156, D168,	V36, Q168,	V36, R155, A156, D168,	V36, D168	V36, T54, Y56, A156, D168
Paritaprevir	V36, F43, Y56, Q80, R155, D168	Y56, Q80, A156, R155, D168	R155, A156, D168	Y56, R155, A156, D168	Y56, R155, A156	Y56, R155, A156, D168	Y56, A156, D168
Simeprevir	F43, Q80, S122, R155, A156, D168	F43, Q80, S122, R155, D168	S122, R155, A156, D168	D168	R155, A156	R155, D168	R155, A156, D168
Voxilaprevir	V36, Q41, Q80, D168						
NS5A inhibitors							
Daclatasvir	M/L28, Q/R30, L31, P32, H58, Y93	L23, L28, Q/R30, L31, P32, Y93	L30, L31, C92, Y93	L28, A30, L31, Y93	L28, L30, M31, Y93	L31	M28, L31, P32, T58
Elbasvir	Q30, L31, H58, Y93	L28, L31, Y93		A30, L31, Y93	L28, M31, P58, Y93		F28, L31
Ledipasvir	K24, M28, Q30, L31, H58, Y93	Q30, L31, P58, A92, Y93	L31, Y93	M28, A30, L31, Y93	Y93		P32
Ombitasvir	M28, Q30, H58, Y93	L28, R30, L31, P58, Y93	T24, F28, L31, L28, Y93	M28, L31, Y93	L28, M31, Y93	L28, L31	L31, T58
Pibrentasvir	Q30, H58, E62		L31	S24, M28, A30, L31,Y93H			
Velpatasvir	M28, Q30, L31, H58, Y93	L31, Q30, Y93	Y93	M28, A30, Y93	Y93		L31, P32
NS5B inhibitors							
Sofosbuvir	L159, S282	L159, S282, C316	L159, S282, M289	L159, V321, S282	S282	S282	S282
Dasabuvir	C316, M414, Y448, A553, S556	C316, S368, M414, C445, A553, G554, S556, D559		S556	S556	S556	S368, A553, S556

[a]References for resistance substitutions [112–122]

90% [109] (Table 54.4). Some approved regimens require the addition of ribavirin to improve response rates, but with significant ribavirin adverse effects. Further drug development is aimed at optimizing therapy for all genotypes without use of ribavirin, reducing adverse effects and drug interactions, and improving efficacy in difficult situations such as cirrhosis, immune compromise, or failure of prior therapy. Combination therapy directed at multiple viral targets is needed to achieve satisfactory response rates. As with HIV therapy, fixed combinations as tested in clinical trials are offered for treatment convenience but limit the flexibility to use nonstandard combinations for special situations.

HCV NS3/4A Protease Inhibitors

The prototype compounds telaprevir and boceprevir [123, 124], were approved in 2011 for treatment of HCV genotype 1 in combination with Peg-IFN/ribavirin, but were discontinued shortly thereafter because of limited efficacy, unfavorable adverse effects and drug interaction profiles. They have been superseded by newer protease inhibitors including paritaprevir, grazoprevir, glecaprevir, and voxilaprevir (Tables 54.3 and 54.4). Drug interactions with post-transplant immunosuppressive therapy remain an important consideration for use of this drug class. The severe skin rash associated with telaprevir has been less problematic for the newer compounds, which are generally well tolerated, except that no protease inhibitors are approved for use in decompensated cirrhosis (Table 54.4). Although the prototype protease inhibitors were mainly active against genotype 1 (1b more than1a), newer compounds are active against multiple genotypes, which simplifies the formulation of pangenotypic treatment regimens (Table 54.4).

Resistance to earlier generation protease inhibitors developed readily, with NS3 amino acid substitutions typically at codons V36, Y56, Q80, R155, A156, and D168 (Table 54.3) combining to confer high-grade resistance and cross-resistance [112, 121]. Amino acid substitutions conferring drug resistance are found as baseline polymorphisms at

Table 54.4 Approved direct-acting antiviral combinations for HCV therapy (2018)

Trade name (pharmaceutical company)	Components[a]	Approved indications for genotypes[b]	Common adverse reactions
Epclusa (Gilead)	Sofosbuvir Velpatasvir	GT1,2,3,4,5,6: < C[c], C, or DC[d] + RBV (12 week)	Headache, fatigue +ribavirin: see Table 54.2
Harvoni (Gilead)	Sofosbuvir Ledipasvir	GT1: < C (12 week), C (24 week) GT4,5,6: < C or C (12 week) GT1: DC (12 week + RBV) GT1,4: Liver Transplant <C or C (12 week + RBV)	Headache, fatigue, asthenia
Vosevi (Gilead)	Sofosbuvir Velpatasvir Voxilaprevir	GT1,2,3,4,5,6: < C or C (12 week)	Headache, fatigue, diarrhea, nausea
Viekira Pak (Abbvie)	Ombitasvir Paritaprevir Ritonavir Dasabuvir	GT1a: < C 12 week + RBV GT1a: C 24 week + RBV GT1b: < C or C 12 week	Nausea, pruritus, insomnia +ribavirin: see Table 54.2
Zepatier (Merck)	Elbasvir Grazoprevir	GT1,4: < DC, 12 week GT1a with baseline NS5A polymorphisms, retreatment cases may need RBV and 16 week	Headache, fatigue, nausea +ribavirin: see Table 54.2
Mavyret (Abbvie)	Glecaprevir Pibrentasvir	GT1,2,3,4,5,6: < C (8 week), C (12 week) Avoid if previously treated with HCV protease inhibitors	Headache, fatigue
Sovaldi (Gilead) Daklinza (BMS)	Sofosbuvir Daclatasvir +Ribavirin	GT1,3: < C (12 week), or < DC (GT1, 12 week) GT1,3: DC or Liver Tx (12 week with RBV)	Headache, fatigue +ribavirin: see Table 54.2

[a]Dosage for combinations is 1 tablet once daily except for the following: Technvie 2 tablets once daily; Viekira Pak 2 tablets containing ombitasvir/paritaprevir/ritonavir once daily plus 1 tablet dasabuvir twice daily
[b]*GT* genotype, *RBV* ribavirin
[c]*C* cirrhosis, compensated (Child-Pugh class A), <*C* non-cirrhotic
[d]*DC* decompensated cirrhosis (Child-Pugh class B or C), < *DC* non-cirrhotic or compensated cirrhosis

varying frequency across genotypes and geographical regions, an important factor affecting treatment responses [112, 120, 121]. For example, the common baseline HCV genotype 1a polymorphism Q80K reduces susceptibility to simeprevir and combines with the easily selected substitution R155K to confer high-grade resistance associated with a lower SVR rate reported in some clinical trials [118, 120, 125]. Thus, simeprevir was not recommended for treatment of genotype 1a when Q80K is present at baseline [126], and its marketing has since been discontinued. NS3 resistance mutations usually fade or disappear after inhibitor therapy is withdrawn, but the mutations may be archived to affect responses to retreatment [127]. However, newer protease inhibitors have been successful in salvage regimens. Voxilaprevir added to a previously approved combination of sofosbuvir and velpatasvir enabled the successful salvage therapy of those who failed prior direct-acting antiviral therapy [128], as did a combination of glecaprevir and the NS5A inhibitor pibrentasvir [129].

HCV NS5A Inhibitors

The viral NS5A gene product is involved in viral replication and assembly and interacts with the NS5B polymerase and cellular proteins [130]. In general, NS5A inhibitors add few adverse effects and have important roles as part of 2- or 3-drug combinations (Table 54.4). The currently approved drugs ledispasvir, daclatasvir, ombitasvir, velpatasvir, pibrentasvir and elbasvir tend to be potent against multiple genotypes. However, viral genetic changes present at baseline or readily selected after drug exposure can confer high-grade resistance and cross-resistance to other NS5A inhibitors, the same weakness reported for protease inhibitors (Table 54.3). Commonly involved NS5A codons include 28, 30–32, 58, and 93 [112, 120, 121]. For example, NS5A substitution Y93H, as a baseline polymorphism or drug-selected variant, factors in high-grade resistance to almost all of the NS5A inhibitors listed above, producing a >100-fold increase in EC50. Pibrentasvir, a newer NS5A inhibitor, also selected for Y93H in vitro, but the mutation conferred only low-grade resistance (< ten-fold EC50 increase) [131]. Unlike NS3 resistance mutations, NS5A mutations may persist long after treatment is withdrawn [120].

HCV NS5B Inhibitors

HCV NS5B inhibitors target the RNA-dependent RNA polymerase and may be categorized as nucleoside/nucleotide or non-nucleoside [132]. The nucleotide phosphoramidate prodrug sofosbuvir shows high potency against most genotypes, but less for genotype 3 [109]. It is a key component of several effective multi-drug treatment regimens in combination with ledipasvir, daclatasvir, or velpatasvir and voxilaprevir [109] (Table 54.4). Sofosbuvir is well tolerated in combination therapies, but caution is required for those with renal failure or taking interacting cardiac medications. Lack of interaction with cyclosporine and tacrolimus is an advantage. For those with severe renal impairment, alternative regimens should be selected such as elbasvir-grazoprevir or glecaprevir-pibrentasvir. Sofosbuvir has a relatively high barrier to resistance; resistant mutants selected after drug exposure such as S282T have low growth fitness [132]. Non-nucleoside NS5B inhibitors tend to have a more restricted genotype range, lower potency, and lower barrier to resistance. An example is dasabuvir, with activity limited to genotype 1 (with ribavirin added for genotype 1a), but it has achieved high SVR rates in combination with ombitasvir and ritonavir-boosted paritaprevir [133–135], including in liver transplant recipients [136]. NS5B amino acid substitutions such as C316Y confer high-grade dasabuvir resistance resulting in 1000-fold or more increased EC50, but S556G, which confers ~30-fold increased EC50 for genotype 1a, was more commonly encountered in treated individuals [116].

Drug Resistance Testing

Drug resistance testing is expected to have a limited role in the management of HCV therapy as potent pangenotypic regimens with a better barrier to resistance become available, because high rates of SVR have been achieved even in treatment-experienced subjects. Diagnostic HCV genotyping technology is not well standardized for the representative amplification and accurate detection of mutations in the specimen being tested [120]. Deep sequencing approaches may enable the detection of smaller subpopulations (<15%) of mutant sequences than conventional Sanger sequencing, but has no proven added benefit in optimization of therapy [120]. If reliable diagnostic genotyping services are available, it is appropriate to screen for baseline mutations or polymorphisms that may affect response to drugs under consideration, for example, NS3 Q80K for simeprevir or NS5A amino acid substitutions at codons listed above for elbasvir [120, 126]. Findings may influence decisions on selection and duration of therapy and use of ribavirin. Resistance testing may have a larger role when evaluating retreatment regimens in those who have failed prior therapy.

Hepatitis B Antivirals

The virion of HBV contains a small partially double-stranded circular 3.2 kb DNA genome, which becomes a covalently closed circular (cccDNA) molecule in the infected cell [137]. Replication of the genome occurs through an RNA intermediate and is carried out by a virus-encoded reverse transcriptase. This enzyme is the target of HBV-specific antiviral drugs as well as some HIV-1 reverse transcriptase inhibitors. These drugs are approved for chronic hepatitis B (CHB) infection. Antiviral therapy is unable to eliminate the cccDNA, which persists indefinitely in the nucleus of infected cells and serves as the template for viral rebound when therapy is terminated. Consequently, there are ongoing drug-screening efforts to identify molecules that inhibit production of cccDNA [138].

Drugs approved for CHB antiviral therapy fall into 2 classes: (1) standard and pegylated IFN-α2; and (2) four available nucleoside/nucleotide analog (NA) reverse transcriptase inhibitors, counting tenofovir as one drug with two formulations (Table 54.5). Therapeutic algorithms are based on HBe antigen (positive or negative), HBV DNA levels, and status of liver disease [139, 140]. The goal of HBV antiviral therapy is durable suppression of viral replication and decreased risk of cirrhosis, liver decompensation, and hepatocellular carcinoma [139]. In contrast to HCV, indefinite NA maintenance therapy may be needed to prevent relapse in those patients who have not cleared hepatitis B surface antigen (HBsAg), thus favoring regimens that minimize the emergence of drug resistance. Entecavir and tenofovir disoproxil fumarate (TDF) or tenofovir alafenamide (TAF) are preferred drugs because of a higher genetic barrier to resistance. In those receiving liver transplants for HBV-related liver failure, antiviral treatment may be given prior to transplantation to suppress circulating viral loads, followed by use of hepatitis B immunoglobulin (HBIG) and antivirals post-transplant. This strategy was initially proven successful using lamivudine and later improved by use of entecavir or tenofovir instead, to the extent that HBIG use can be reduced or eliminated [141].

Pegylated Interferon

Peg-IFN-α2 therapy offers the possibility of a durable virologic response with no antiviral resistance, but many do not respond optimally [140]. Given the significant adverse effects that limit its use in those with advanced disease, comorbidities and post-transplant immunosuppressive therapy, patient selection is important. Additional factors to consider are age, transaminase levels, HBV genotype, levels of HBV DNA, and HBsAg [139, 140]. Peg-IFN has been studied in combination with lamivudine, but the superiority of the combination over Peg-IFN alone has not been demonstrated [142].

Lamivudine

Lamivudine was initially developed for HIV-1 and was the first NA to be approved for treatment of CHB, a major

Table 54.5 Antiviral agents approved for HBV therapy (2018)

Antiviral agent	Structure and mechanism of action	Therapeutic uses and doses[a]	Adverse effects	Resistance
Adefovir dipovoxil	Diester prodrug of adenosine monophosphate analog requires intracellular enzymatic activation Inhibition of HBV reverse transcriptase (RT). Viral DNA chain terminator	Chronic HBV > age 12 Oral administration: 10 mg, 1×/day	Nephrotoxicity, asthenia, gastrointestinal symptoms, lactic acidosis and severe hepatomegaly with steatosis, exacerbation of hepatitis on discontinuation of therapy	Reverse transcriptase (RT): N236 T, A181T/V Intermediate genetic barrier to resistance
Entecavir	Guanosine analog Inhibition of 3 functions of HBV RT DNA: priming, negative strand reverse transcription, positive strand synthesis. Non-obligate chain terminator	Chronic HBV in adults with evidence of active viral replication Oral administration Treatment naïve: 0.5 mg 1×/day Previous exposure to lamivudine or telbivudine or decompensated disease: 1 mg 1×/day	Mild GI[b] and CNS[c] symptoms, acute, lactic acidosis and severe hepatomegaly with steatosis, exacerbation of hepatitis on discontinuation of therapy	RT: M204V/I with or without L180M, V173L, L80I, T184G, S202I, M250V (multiple mutations required for high-level resistance) High genetic barrier to resistance
Lamivudine	Dideoxycytidine analog DNA chain terminator, Inhibition of HBV RT polymerization	Chronic HBV in adults with evidence of active viral replication Oral administration: 100 mg once/day	Minimal toxicity. Lactic acidosis, severe hepatomegaly with steatosis, acute exacerbation of hepatitis with termination of therapy	RT: M204V/I,L180M, V173L, L80M, A181T/V cross-resistance to adefovir, entecavir, and telbivudine Low genetic barrier to resistance
Pegylated interferon 2a (PEG-IFN2a)	Covalent conjugate of IFN-α 2a and branched polyethylene glycol (PEG) chains; molecular mass 60,000 Da Binds to cell receptors, induces innate immune response, stimulates IFN response genes, and inhibits viral replication in infected cells. Broad biological effects on uninfected cells	Chronic HBV Subcutaneous injection: 180 μg/week	Fever, myalgia, headache, fatigue, neuropsychiatric disorders[d]	Unknown
Interferon alpha 2b	Unconjugated IFN-α 2b molecular mass 19,271 Da Mechanism same as PEG-IFN-α	Chronic HBV Subcutaneous or intramuscular injection 10 million IU 3×/ week for 16 weeks	Fever, headache, chills, myalgia neuropsychiatric disorders[d]	Unknown
Tenofovir disoproxil fumarate (TDF)	Diester prodrug of acyclic analog of adenosine monophosphate Competitive inhibitor of adenosine triphosphate, DNA chain terminator	Treatment of chronic HBV Oral administration 300 mg 1×/day	GI[b] and CNS[c] symptoms, nephrotoxicity, reduced bone density, lactic acidosis, severe hepatomegaly with steatosis, acute exacerbation of hepatitis with termination of therapy	No TDF-specific mutations identified Reduced susceptibility to ADV, LdT, and 3TC-resistant isolates (A181V/T, N236T, M204I/V) High genetic barrier to resistance
Tenofovir alafenamide fumarate (TAF)	Phosphonamidate prodrug of tenofovir. Acyclic analog of adenosine monophosphate Competitive inhibitor of adenosine triphosphate, DNA chain terminator	Treatment of chronic HBV Oral administration 25 mg (one tablet) 1×/day	GI[b], headache, cough, fatigue, back pain, lactic acidosis, severe hepatomegaly with steatosis, acute exacerbation of hepatitis with termination of therapy Lower reduction of bone density compared to TDF	No TAF-specific mutations identified High genetic barrier to resistance

[a]Dosage information includes only most common applications. See full dosing information provided by pharmaceutical company package insert
[b]GI (gastrointestinal) symptoms include diarrhea, nausea, and vomiting
[c]CNS (central nervous system) symptoms include confusion, difficulty concentrating, dizziness, hallucinations, and seizures
[d]Neuropsychiatric disorders include suicide, depression, and self-injury

advance in therapy at the time. Although lamivudine has been shown to decrease the rate of development of fibrosis as well as the incidence of HCC [143], HBV antiviral resistance develops in 65% of cases after 5 years and is associated with clinical relapse [144]. Thus, it is no longer a preferred treatment. The characteristic amino acid substitution M204V/I that develops in the YMDD motif of the HBV DNA polymerase confers very-high-level lamivudine resistance (>10,000-fold increased IC50) and is followed by the development of L180M that increases viral fitness [145].

Adefovir Dipovoxil

Adefovir is administered as a prodrug that is converted intracellularly to the active adefovir diphosphate. Adefovir treatment resulted in biochemical and histologic improvement in patients with HBeAg-negative CHB with sustained treatment, but evidence of resistance mutations were identified in 6% at 3 years and 29% after 5 years of therapy [146]. Because of the intermediate genetic barrier to resistance, adefovir is not a preferred drug for long-term therapy. Adefovir resistance mutations differ from those of lamivudine and mainly involve polymerase amino acid substitutions A181V and N236T [146].

Telbivudine

Telbivudine is a thymidine nucleoside analog and a stronger inhibitor of HBV than lamivudine but likewise has a low genetic barrier to resistance. It selects for amino acid substitution M204I (YMDD motif), which also confers cross-resistance to lamivudine [147]. While it performed better than lamivudine [148] or adefovir [149] in comparison trials of CHB treatment, telbivudine was withdrawn from marketing after 2016. Telbivudine cannot be combined with Peg-IFN because of increased risk of neuropathy [150].

Entecavir

Entecavir undergoes intracellular anabolism to the active deoxyguanosine triphosphate analog, which has a 3′-hydroxyl group that makes it a nonobligate chain terminator of HBV DNA synthesis. It inhibits three polymerase functions: priming, reverse transcription, and second-strand synthesis [151]. Entecavir has a relatively high genetic barrier for drug resistance, requiring multiple mutations that reduce viral fitness. Selection of DNA polymerase substitution M204V ± L180M from previous lamivudine therapy facilitates entecavir resistance through additional substitutions T184G/L, S202G, and M250V [152], but the reported rate of resistance after entecavir therapy is only 1.2% after 5 years [151]. It remains a first-line agent for CHB antiviral therapy, although tenofovir-based therapy would be a better option in those previously exposed to lamivudine or telbivudine [139].

Tenofovir Disoproxil Fumarate (TDF)

This prodrug undergoes intracellular hydrolysis followed by phosphorylation to an adenosine triphosphate analog. It has become a first-line drug for CHB therapy, because it has a high genetic barrier to resistance and potent antiviral activity [139, 140]. TDF resistance has not been observed after up to 8 years of therapy [153]. TDF therapy is generally well tolerated but requires periodic monitoring for renal toxicity. TDF is also available as a combined formulation (Truvada) with the nucleoside analog emtricitabine, which has anti-HBV activity similar to lamivudine [154]. This combined formulation has been investigated for treatment of CHB, but did not perform any better than TDF alone in patients with lamivudine-resistant infection [155]. Emtricitabine monotherapy is not recommended, because it has the same low genetic barrier to resistance and resistance profile (M204V/I with or without L180M) as lamivudine [156].

Tenofovir Alafenamide (TAF)

Tenofovir alafenamide (TAF) was approved for treatment of CHB in 2016. This alternative prodrug formulation of tenofovir achieves equally effective intracellular levels of the active tenofovir diphosphate at much lower doses of 300 mg for TDF vs. 25 mg for TAF and lower plasma tenofovir levels with less consequent toxicity [157]. In a comparison trial, TAF was non-inferior to TDF for the treatment of CHB, with fewer adverse changes in bone mineral density and renal function detected in the TAF group [158, 159]. TAF may be preferable to TDF in older subjects and those with renal function impairment or bone mineral disorders [139].

Summary

A basic principle of antiviral therapy in immunosuppressed hosts is to anticipate and screen for infections that can be prevented or treated early before irreversible damage from invasive disease. For herpesviruses, guanosine nucleoside analogs acyclovir and ganciclovir, selectively activated by viral kinases and ultimately targeting the viral DNA polymerase, have long been preferred antivirals. Orally bioavailable prodrugs valacyclovir, famciclovir, and valganciclovir greatly simplify outpatient management and are suitable for mild to moderate disease and extended prophylactic use.

Acyclovir and related prodrugs have a superior safety profile for use in herpes simplex and varicella-zoster infections, but are insufficiently active against cytomegalovirus, for which ganciclovir and valganciclovir are used instead, with monitoring for bone marrow suppression. Long-term use with incomplete viral suppression may select for drug resistance mutations, typically in the viral kinase gene that initially phosphorylates these drugs. Foscarnet and cidofovir are alternative herpesvirus treatments that evade drug resistance resulting from kinase mutations, but viral DNA polymerase mutations can confer cross-resistance. They are available for intravenous use only and have significant dose-limiting toxicity. Orally bioavailable drugs with alternative viral targets are being introduced for cytomegalovirus infection, such as the terminase inhibitor letermovir.

Neuraminidase inhibitors available for oral, intravenous, and inhalation use are the current treatments of choice for influenza infections. Optimum benefit requires early diagnosis and presumptive treatment or post-exposure prophylaxis, whereas it is difficult to show a mortality benefit of antiviral therapy for any viral pneumonia that has caused respiratory failure. Ribavirin in aerosolized or systemic form has been proposed for treatment of respiratory syncytial virus with a lesser evidence base and lack of clarity in balance of risks and benefits.

Hepatitis C virus is a leading cause of liver failure requiring transplantation. The complexity and toxicity of previous interferon and ribavirin regimens for this virus required careful evaluation of treatment indications and risks, but newer direct-acting antivirals targeting the protease and viral replication proteins offer far higher cure rates with shorter combination regimens applicable to a wider range of viral genotypes and disease states. Therapeutic options are being further improved with potent, pangenotypic, ribavirin-free regimens that can be applied to populations with historically lower treatment response rates.

Treatment of chronic hepatitis B is primarily directed at the viral DNA polymerase (reverse transcriptase). Current antivirals such as tenofovir offer good potency and adequately high genetic barrier to the development of drug resistance, but are unable to clear the covalently closed circular form of viral DNA responsible for viral persistence. Strategies to overcome this limitation are in development.

References

1. Meng Q, Hagemeier SR, Fingeroth JD, Gershburg E, Pagano JS, Kenney SC. The Epstein-Barr virus (EBV)-encoded protein kinase, EBV-PK, but not the thymidine kinase (EBV-TK), is required for ganciclovir and acyclovir inhibition of lytic viral production. J Virol. 2010;84(9):4534–42.
2. Talarico CL, Burnette TC, Miller WH, Smith SL, Davis MG, Stanat SC, et al. Acyclovir is phosphorylated by the human cytomegalovirus UL97 protein. Antimicrob Agents Chemother. 1999;43(8):1941–6.
3. Earnshaw DL, Bacon TH, Darlison SJ, Edmonds K, Perkins RM, Vere Hodge RA. Mode of antiviral action of penciclovir in MRC-5 cells infected with herpes simplex virus type 1 (HSV-1), HSV-2, and varicella-zoster virus. Antimicrob Agents Chemother. 1992;36(12):2747–57.
4. Laskin OL, de Miranda P, King DH, Page DA, Longstreth JA, Rocco L, et al. Effects of probenecid on the pharmacokinetics and elimination of acyclovir in humans. Antimicrob Agents Chemother. 1982;21(5):804–7.
5. Smith JP, Weller S, Johnson B, Nicotera J, Luther JM, Haas DW. Pharmacokinetics of acyclovir and its metabolites in cerebrospinal fluid and systemic circulation after administration of high-dose valacyclovir in subjects with normal and impaired renal function. Antimicrob Agents Chemother. 2010;54(3):1146–51.
6. Tyring SK, Baker D, Snowden W. Valacyclovir for herpes simplex virus infection: long-term safety and sustained efficacy after 20 years' experience with acyclovir. J Infect Dis. 2002;186(Suppl 1):S40–6.
7. Bell WR, Chulay JD, Feinberg JE. Manifestations resembling thrombotic microangiopathy in patients with advanced human immunodeficiency virus (HIV) disease in a cytomegalovirus prophylaxis trial (ACTG 204). Medicine (Baltimore). 1997;76(5):369–80.
8. Tomblyn M, Chiller T, Einsele H, Gress R, Sepkowitz K, Storek J, et al. Guidelines for preventing infectious complications among hematopoietic cell transplantation recipients: a global perspective. Biol Blood Marrow Transplant. 2009;15(10):1143–238.
9. Ullmann AJ, Schmidt-Hieber M, Bertz H, Heinz WJ, Kiehl M, Kruger W, et al. Infectious diseases in allogeneic haematopoietic stem cell transplantation: prevention and prophylaxis strategy guidelines 2016. Ann Hematol. 2016;95(9):1435–55.
10. Pergam SA, Limaye AP. Varicella zoster virus in solid organ transplantation. Am J Transplant. 2013;13(Suppl 4):138–46.
11. Wilck MB, Zuckerman RA. Herpes simplex virus in solid organ transplantation. Am J Transplant. 2013;13(Suppl 4):121–7.
12. Slifkin M, Doron S, Snydman DR. Viral prophylaxis in organ transplant patients. Drugs. 2004;64(24):2763–92.
13. Piret J, Boivin G. Antiviral drug resistance in herpesviruses other than cytomegalovirus. Rev Med Virol. 2014;24(3):186–218.
14. Sauerbrei A, Deinhardt S, Zell R, Wutzler P. Phenotypic and genotypic characterization of acyclovir-resistant clinical isolates of herpes simplex virus. Antivir Res. 2010;86(3):246–52.
15. Andrei G, Topalis D, Fiten P, McGuigan C, Balzarini J, Opdenakker G, et al. In vitro-selected drug-resistant varicella-zoster virus mutants in the thymidine kinase and DNA polymerase genes yield novel phenotype-genotype associations and highlight differences between antiherpesvirus drugs. J Virol. 2012;86(5):2641–52.
16. Sarisky RT, Quail MR, Clark PE, Nguyen TT, Halsey WS, Wittrock RJ, et al. Characterization of herpes simplex viruses selected in culture for resistance to penciclovir or acyclovir. J Virol. 2001;75(4):1761–9.
17. Bacon TH, Levin MJ, Leary JJ, Sarisky RT, Sutton D. Herpes simplex virus resistance to acyclovir and penciclovir after two decades of antiviral therapy. Clin Microbiol Rev. 2003;16(1):114–28.
18. Topalis D, Gillemot S, Snoeck R, Andrei G. Distribution and effects of amino acid changes in drug-resistant alpha and beta herpesviruses DNA polymerase. Nucleic Acids Res. 2016;44(20):9530–54.
19. Crumpacker CS. Ganciclovir. N Engl J Med. 1996;335(10):721–9.
20. Field AK, Davies ME, DeWitt C, Perry HC, Liou R, Germershausen J, et al. 9-([2-hydroxy-1-(hydroxymethyl)ethoxy]methyl)guanine: a selective inhibitor of herpes group virus replication. Proc Natl Acad Sci U S A. 1983;80(13):4139–43.
21. Gentry BG, Drach JC. Metabolism of cyclopropavir and ganciclovir in human cytomegalovirus-infected cells. Antimicrob Agents Chemother. 2014;58(4):2329–33.
22. Lischka P, Hewlett G, Wunberg T, Baumeister J, Paulsen D, Goldner T, et al. In vitro and in vivo activities of the novel anticy-

tomegalovirus compound AIC246. Antimicrob Agents Chemother. 2010;54(3):1290–7.
23. Pescovitz MD, Pruett TL, Gonwa T, Brook B, McGory R, Wicker K, et al. Oral ganciclovir dosing in transplant recipients and dialysis patients based on renal function. Transplantation. 1998;66(8):1104–7.
24. Danziger-Isakov L, Mark BG. Hematologic complications of anti-CMV therapy in solid organ transplant recipients. Clin Transpl. 2009;23(3):295–304.
25. Salzberger B, Bowden RA, Hackman RC, Davis C, Boeckh M. Neutropenia in allogeneic marrow transplant recipients receiving ganciclovir for prevention of cytomegalovirus disease: risk factors and outcome. Blood. 1997;90(6):2502–8.
26. Shepp DH, Dandliker PS, de Miranda P, Burnette TC, Cederberg DM, Kirk LE, et al. Activity of 9-[2-hydroxy-1-(hydroxymethyl) ethoxymethyl]guanine in the treatment of cytomegalovirus pneumonia. Ann Intern Med. 1985;103(3):368–73.
27. McGavin JK, Goa KL. Ganciclovir: an update of its use in the prevention of cytomegalovirus infection and disease in transplant recipients. Drugs. 2001;61(8):1153–83.
28. Paya C, Humar A, Dominguez E, Washburn K, Blumberg E, Alexander B, et al. Efficacy and safety of valganciclovir vs. oral ganciclovir for prevention of cytomegalovirus disease in solid organ transplant recipients. Am J Transplant. 2004;4(4):611–20.
29. Kotton CN, Kumar D, Caliendo AM, Asberg A, Chou S, Danziger-Isakov L, et al. Updated international consensus guidelines on the management of cytomegalovirus in solid-organ transplantation. Transplantation. 2013;96(4):333–60.
30. Humar A, Lebranchu Y, Vincenti F, Blumberg EA, Punch JD, Limaye AP, et al. The efficacy and safety of 200 days valganciclovir cytomegalovirus prophylaxis in high-risk kidney transplant recipients. Am J Transplant. 2010;10(5):1228–37.
31. Asberg A, Humar A, Rollag H, Jardine AG, Mouas H, Pescovitz MD, et al. Oral valganciclovir is noninferior to intravenous ganciclovir for the treatment of cytomegalovirus disease in solid organ transplant recipients. Am J Transplant. 2007;7(9):2106–13.
32. Lurain NS, Chou S. Antiviral drug resistance of human cytomegalovirus. Clin Microbiol Rev. 2010;23(4):689–712.
33. Chou S, Ercolani RJ, Vanarsdall AL. Differentiated levels of ganciclovir resistance conferred by mutations at Codons 591 to 603 of the Cytomegalovirus UL97 Kinase Gene. J Clin Microbiol. 2017;55(7):2098–104.
34. Komatsu TE, Pikis A, Naeger LK, Harrington PR. Resistance of human cytomegalovirus to ganciclovir/valganciclovir: a comprehensive review of putative resistance pathways. Antivir Res. 2014;101:12–25.
35. Wagstaff AJ, Bryson HM. Foscarnet. A reappraisal of its antiviral activity, pharmacokinetic properties and therapeutic use in immunocompromised patients with viral infections. Drugs. 1994;48(2):199–226.
36. Bacigalupo A, Boyd A, Slipper J, Curtis J, Clissold S. Foscarnet in the management of cytomegalovirus infections in hematopoietic stem cell transplant patients. Expert Rev Anti-Infect Ther. 2012;10(11):1249–64.
37. Avery RK, Arav-Boger R, Marr KA, Kraus E, Shoham S, Lees L, et al. Outcomes in transplant recipients treated with foscarnet for ganciclovir-resistant or refractory cytomegalovirus infection. Transplantation. 2016;100(10):e74–80.
38. Reusser P, Einsele H, Lee J, Volin L, Rovira M, Engelhard D, et al. Randomized multicenter trial of foscarnet versus ganciclovir for preemptive therapy of cytomegalovirus infection after allogeneic stem cell transplantation. Blood. 2002;99(4):1159–64.
39. De Clercq E. Clinical potential of the acyclic nucleoside phosphonates cidofovir, adefovir, and tenofovir in treatment of DNA virus and retrovirus infections. Clin Microbiol Rev. 2003;16(4):569–96.
40. Ljungman P, Deliliers GL, Platzbecker U, Matthes-Martin S, Bacigalupo A, Einsele H, et al. Cidofovir for cytomegalovirus infection and disease in allogeneic stem cell transplant recipients. The Infectious Diseases Working Party of the European Group for Blood and Marrow Transplantation. Blood. 2001;97(2):388–92.
41. Scott RA, Pavesio C. Ocular side-effects from systemic HPMPC (Cidofovir) for a non-ocular cytomegalovirus infection. Am J Ophthalmol. 2000;130(1):126–7.
42. Painter W, Robertson A, Trost LC, Godkin S, Lampert B, Painter G. First pharmacokinetic and safety study in humans of the novel lipid antiviral conjugate CMX001, a broad-spectrum oral drug active against double-stranded DNA viruses. Antimicrob Agents Chemother. 2012;56(5):2726–34.
43. Marty FM, Winston DJ, Rowley SD, Vance E, Papanicolaou GA, Mullane KM, et al. CMX001 to prevent cytomegalovirus disease in hematopoietic-cell transplantation. N Engl J Med. 2013;369(13):1227–36.
44. Ljungman P, Ribaud P, Eyrich M, Matthes-Martin S, Einsele H, Bleakley M, et al. Cidofovir for adenovirus infections after allogeneic hematopoietic stem cell transplantation: a survey by the Infectious Diseases Working Party of the European Group for Blood and Marrow Transplantation. Bone Marrow Transplant. 2003;31(6):481–6.
45. Florescu DF, Pergam SA, Neely MN, Qiu F, Johnston C, Way S, et al. Safety and efficacy of CMX001 as salvage therapy for severe adenovirus infections in immunocompromised patients. Biol Blood Marrow Transplant. 2012;18(5):731–8.
46. Duan R, de Vries RD, Osterhaus AD, Remeijer L, Verjans GM. Acyclovir-resistant corneal HSV-1 isolates from patients with herpetic keratitis. J Infect Dis. 2008;198(5):659–63.
47. Frobert E, Burrel S, Ducastelle-Lepretre S, Billaud G, Ader F, Casalegno JS, et al. Resistance of herpes simplex viruses to acyclovir: an update from a ten-year survey in France. Antivir Res. 2014;111:36–41.
48. van der Beek MT, Vermont CL, Bredius RG, Marijt EW, van der Blij-de Brouwer CS, Kroes AC, et al. Persistence and antiviral resistance of varicella zoster virus in hematological patients. Clin Infect Dis. 2013;56(3):335–43.
49. Fisher CE, Knudsen JL, Lease ED, Jerome KR, Rakita RM, Boeckh M, et al. Risk factors and outcomes of ganciclovir resistant cytomegalovirus infection in solid organ transplant recipients. Clin Infect Dis. 2017;65(1):57–63.
50. Sahoo MK, Lefterova MI, Yamamoto F, Waggoner JJ, Chou S, Holmes SP, et al. Detection of cytomegalovirus drug resistance mutations by next-generation sequencing. J Clin Microbiol. 2013;51(11):3700–10.
51. Chou S, Boivin G, Ives J, Elston R. Phenotypic evaluation of previously uncharacterized cytomegalovirus DNA polymerase sequence variants detected in a valganciclovir treatment trial. J Infect Dis. 2014;209(8):1219–26.
52. Chou S, Ercolani RJ, Sahoo MK, Lefterova MI, Strasfeld LM, Pinsky BA. Improved detection of emerging drug-resistant mutant cytomegalovirus subpopulations by deep sequencing. Antimicrob Agents Chemother. 2014;58(8):4697–702.
53. James SH, Larson KB, Acosta EP, Prichard MN. Helicase-primase as a target of new therapies for herpes simplex virus infections. Clin Pharmacol Ther. 2015;97(1):66–78.
54. Weller SK, Kuchta RD. The DNA helicase-primase complex as a target for herpes viral infection. Expert Opin Ther Targets. 2013;17(10):1119–32.
55. Tyring S, Wald A, Zadeikis N, Dhadda S, Takenouchi K, Rorig R. ASP2151 for the treatment of genital herpes: a randomized, double-blind, placebo- and valacyclovir-controlled, dose-finding study. J Infect Dis. 2012;205(7):1100–10.
56. Wald A, Corey L, Timmler B, Magaret A, Warren T, Tyring S, et al. Helicase-primase inhibitor pritelivir for HSV-2 infection. N Engl J Med. 2014;370(3):201–10.

57. Wald A, Timmler B, Magaret A, Warren T, Tyring S, Johnston C, et al. Effect of pritelivir compared with valacyclovir on genital HSV-2 shedding in patients with frequent recurrences: A randomized clinical trial. JAMA. 2016;316(23):2495–503.
58. Chono K, Katsumata K, Kontani T, Shiraki K, Suzuki H. Characterization of virus strains resistant to the herpes virus helicase-primase inhibitor ASP2151 (Amenamevir). Biochem Pharmacol. 2012;84(4):459–67.
59. Field HJ, Biswas S. Antiviral drug resistance and helicase-primase inhibitors of herpes simplex virus. Drug Resist Updat. 2011;14(1):45–51.
60. Edlefsen PT, Birkmann A, Huang ML, Magaret CA, Kee JJ, Diem K, et al. No evidence of pritelivir resistance among herpes simplex virus type 2 isolates after 4 weeks of daily therapy. J Infect Dis. 2016;214(2):258–64.
61. Biron KK, Harvey RJ, Chamberlain SC, Good SS, Smith AA 3rd, Davis MG, et al. Potent and selective inhibition of human cytomegalovirus replication by 1263 W94, a benzimidazole L-riboside with a unique mode of action. Antimicrob Agents Chemother. 2002;46(8):2365–72.
62. Chou S, Van Wechel LC, Marousek GI. Effect of cell culture conditions on the anticytomegalovirus activity of maribavir. Antimicrob Agents Chemother. 2006;50(7):2557–9.
63. Marty FM, Ljungman P, Papanicolaou GA, Winston DJ, Chemaly RF, Strasfeld L, et al. Maribavir prophylaxis for prevention of cytomegalovirus disease in recipients of allogeneic stem-cell transplants: a phase 3, double-blind, placebo-controlled, randomised trial. Lancet Infect Dis. 2011;11(4):284–92.
64. Winston DJ, Saliba F, Blumberg E, Abouljoud M, Garcia-Diaz JB, Goss JA, et al. Efficacy and safety of maribavir dosed at 100 mg orally twice daily for the prevention of cytomegalovirus disease in liver transplant recipients: a randomized, double-blind, multicenter controlled trial. Am J Transplant. 2012;12(11):3021–30.
65. Avery RK, Marty FM, Strasfeld L, Lee I, Arrieta A, Chou S, et al. Oral maribavir for treatment of refractory or resistant cytomegalovirus infections in transplant recipients. Transpl Infect Dis. 2010;12(6):489–96.
66. Strasfeld L, Lee I, Tatarowicz W, Villano S, Chou S. Virologic characterization of multidrug-resistant cytomegalovirus infection in 2 transplant recipients treated with maribavir. J Infect Dis. 2010;202(1):104–8.
67. Chou S. Cytomegalovirus UL97 mutations in the era of ganciclovir and maribavir. Rev Med Virol. 2008;18(4):233–46.
68. Chou S, Ercolani RJ, Marousek G, Bowlin TL. Cytomegalovirus UL97 kinase catalytic domain mutations that confer multidrug resistance. Antimicrob Agents Chemother. 2013;57(7):3375–9.
69. Bigley TM, Reitsma JM, Terhune SS. Antagonistic relationship between human cytomegalovirus pUL27 and pUL97 activities during infection. J Virol. 2015;89(20):10230–46.
70. Chou S. Diverse cytomegalovirus UL27 mutations adapt to loss of viral UL97 kinase activity under maribavir. Antimicrob Agents Chemother. 2009;53(1):81–5.
71. Goldner T, Hewlett G, Ettischer N, Ruebsamen-Schaeff H, Zimmermann H, Lischka P. The novel anticytomegalovirus compound AIC246 (Letermovir) inhibits human cytomegalovirus replication through a specific antiviral mechanism that involves the viral terminase. J Virol. 2011;85(20):10884–93.
72. Neuber S, Wagner K, Goldner T, Lischka P, Steinbrueck L, Messerle M, et al. Mutual Interplay between the Human Cytomegalovirus Terminase Subunits pUL51, pUL56, and pUL89 Promotes Terminase Complex Formation. J Virol. 2017;91(12):e02384-16.
73. Chemaly RF, Ullmann AJ, Stoelben S, Richard MP, Bornhauser M, Groth C, et al. Letermovir for cytomegalovirus prophylaxis in hematopoietic-cell transplantation. N Engl J Med. 2014;370(19):1781–9.
74. Chou S. Rapid in vitro evolution of human cytomegalovirus UL56 mutations that confer letermovir resistance. Antimicrob Agents Chemother. 2015;59(10):6588–93.
75. Goldner T, Hempel C, Ruebsamen-Schaeff H, Zimmermann H, Lischka P. Geno- and phenotypic characterization of human cytomegalovirus mutants selected in vitro after letermovir (AIC246) exposure. Antimicrob Agents Chemother. 2014;58(1):610–3.
76. Lischka P, Michel D, Zimmermann H. Characterization of cytomegalovirus breakthrough events in a Phase 2 prophylaxis trial of letermovir (AIC246, MK 8228). J Infect Dis. 2016;213(1):23–30.
77. Moscona A. Neuraminidase inhibitors for influenza. N Engl J Med. 2005;353(13):1363–73.
78. Dobson J, Whitley RJ, Pocock S, Monto AS. Oseltamivir treatment for influenza in adults: a meta-analysis of randomised controlled trials. Lancet. 2015;385(9979):1729–37.
79. Toovey S, Prinssen EP, Rayner CR, Thakrar BT, Dutkowski R, Koerner A, et al. Post-marketing assessment of neuropsychiatric adverse events in influenza patients treated with oseltamivir: an updated review. Adv Ther. 2012;29(10):826–48.
80. McLaughlin MM, Skoglund EW, Ison MG. Peramivir: an intravenous neuraminidase inhibitor. Expert Opin Pharmacother. 2015;16(12):1889–900.
81. Hsu J, Santesso N, Mustafa R, Brozek J, Chen YL, Hopkins JP, et al. Antivirals for treatment of influenza: a systematic review and meta-analysis of observational studies. Ann Intern Med. 2012;156(7):512–24.
82. Harper SA, Bradley JS, Englund JA, File TM, Gravenstein S, Hayden FG, et al. Seasonal influenza in adults and children--diagnosis, treatment, chemoprophylaxis, and institutional outbreak management: clinical practice guidelines of the Infectious Diseases Society of America. Clin Infect Dis. 2009;48(8):1003–32.
83. Kumar D, Morris MI, Kotton CN, Fischer SA, Michaels MG, Allen U, et al. Guidance on novel influenza A/H1N1 in solid organ transplant recipients. Am J Transplant. 2010;10(1):18–25.
84. Ison MG, Hui DS, Clezy K, O'Neil BJ, Flynt A, Collis PJ, et al. A clinical trial of intravenous peramivir compared with oral oseltamivir for the treatment of seasonal influenza in hospitalized adults. Antivir Ther. 2013;18(5):651–61.
85. Welliver R, Monto AS, Carewicz O, Schatteman E, Hassman M, Hedrick J, et al. Effectiveness of oseltamivir in preventing influenza in household contacts: a randomized controlled trial. JAMA. 2001;285(6):748–54.
86. Hayden FG, Gubareva LV, Monto AS, Klein TC, Elliot MJ, Hammond JM, et al. Inhaled zanamivir for the prevention of influenza in families. Zanamivir Family Study Group. N Engl J Med. 2000;343(18):1282–9.
87. Pizzorno A, Abed Y, Boivin G. Influenza drug resistance. Semin Respir Crit Care Med. 2011;32(4):409–22.
88. van der Vries E, Schutten M, Boucher CA. The potential for multidrug-resistant influenza. Curr Opin Infect Dis. 2011;24(6):599–604.
89. Li L, Avery R, Budev M, Mossad S, Danziger-Isakov L. Oral versus inhaled ribavirin therapy for respiratory syncytial virus infection after lung transplantation. J Heart Lung Transplant. 2012;31(8):839–44.
90. Shah JN, Chemaly RF. Management of RSV infections in adult recipients of hematopoietic stem cell transplantation. Blood. 2011;117(10):2755–63.
91. Graci JD, Cameron CE. Mechanisms of action of ribavirin against distinct viruses. Rev Med Virol. 2006;16(1):37–48.
92. Riner A, Chan-Tack KM, Murray JS. Original research: Intravenous ribavirin--review of the FDA's Emergency Investigational New Drug Database (1997–2008) and literature review. Postgrad Med. 2009;121(3):139–46.
93. Preston SL, Drusano GL, Glue P, Nash J, Gupta SK, McNamara P. Pharmacokinetics and absolute bioavailability of ribavirin in

healthy volunteers as determined by stable-isotope methodology. Antimicrob Agents Chemother. 1999;43(10):2451–6.
94. Perronne C. Antiviral hepatitis and antiretroviral drug interactions. J Hepatol. 2006;44(1 Suppl):S119–25.
95. Smith DW, Frankel LR, Mathers LH, Tang AT, Ariagno RL, Prober CG. A controlled trial of aerosolized ribavirin in infants receiving mechanical ventilation for severe respiratory syncytial virus infection. N Engl J Med. 1991;325(1):24–9.
96. Guerguerian AM, Gauthier M, Lebel MH, Farrell CA, Lacroix J. Ribavirin in ventilated respiratory syncytial virus bronchiolitis. A randomized, placebo-controlled trial. Am J Respir Crit Care Med. 1999;160(3):829–34.
97. American Academy of Pediatrics Subcommittee. Diagnosis and management of bronchiolitis. Pediatrics. 2006;118(4):1774–93.
98. Ralston SL, Lieberthal AS, Meissner HC, Alverson BK, Baley JE, Gadomski AM, et al. Clinical practice guideline: the diagnosis, management, and prevention of bronchiolitis. Pediatrics. 2014;134(5):e1474–502.
99. Boeckh M. The challenge of respiratory virus infections in hematopoietic cell transplant recipients. Br J Haematol. 2008;143(4):455–67.
100. Waghmare A, Campbell AP, Xie H, Seo S, Kuypers J, Leisenring W, et al. Respiratory syncytial virus lower respiratory disease in hematopoietic cell transplant recipients: viral RNA detection in blood, antiviral treatment, and clinical outcomes. Clin Infect Dis. 2013;57(12):1731–41.
101. Boeckh M, Englund J, Li Y, Miller C, Cross A, Fernandez H, et al. Randomized controlled multicenter trial of aerosolized ribavirin for respiratory syncytial virus upper respiratory tract infection in hematopoietic cell transplant recipients. Clin Infect Dis. 2007;44(2):245–9.
102. Burrows FS, Carlos LM, Benzimra M, Marriott DJ, Havryk AP, Plit ML, et al. Oral ribavirin for respiratory syncytial virus infection after lung transplantation: Efficacy and cost-efficiency. J Heart Lung Transplant. 2015;34(7):958–62.
103. Gorcea CM, Tholouli E, Turner A, Saif M, Davies E, Battersby E, et al. Effective use of oral ribavirin for respiratory syncytial viral infections in allogeneic haematopoietic stem cell transplant recipients. J Hosp Infect. 2017;95(2):214–7.
104. Ison MG, Michaels MG. RNA respiratory viral infections in solid organ transplant recipients. Am J Transplant. 2009;9(Suppl 4):S166–72.
105. Liu V, Dhillon GS, Weill D. A multi-drug regimen for respiratory syncytial virus and parainfluenza virus infections in adult lung and heart-lung transplant recipients. Transpl Infect Dis. 2010;12(1):38–44.
106. McCurdy LH, Milstone A, Dummer S. Clinical features and outcomes of paramyxoviral infection in lung transplant recipients treated with ribavirin. J Heart Lung Transplant. 2003;22(7):745–53.
107. Aljabr W, Touzelet O, Pollakis G, Wu W, Munday DC, Hughes M, et al. Investigating the influence of ribavirin on human respiratory syncytial virus RNA synthesis by using a high-resolution transcriptome sequencing approach. J Virol. 2016;90(10):4876–88.
108. Jordan R, Stray K, Anderson F, Perron M, Mackman R, Miller M, et al. Analysis of GS-5806 resistance emergence in human healthy adult subjects experimentally infected with respiratory syncytial virus (RSV). IDWeek; 2015; San Diego, Abstract 1189.
109. Li G, De Clercq E. Current therapy for chronic hepatitis C: the role of direct-acting antivirals. Antivir Res. 2017;142:83–122.
110. Burgess SV, Hussaini T, Yoshida EM. Concordance of sustained virologic response at weeks 4, 12 and 24 post-treatment of hepatitis C in the era of new oral direct-acting antivirals: A concise review. Ann Hepatol. 2016;15(2):154–9.
111. Simmons B, Saleem J, Heath K, Cooke GS, Hill A. Long-term treatment outcomes of patients infected with hepatitis C virus: A systematic review and meta-analysis of the survival benefit of achieving a sustained virological response. Clin Infect Dis. 2015;61(5):730–40.
112. Bagaglio S, Uberti-Foppa C, Morsica G. Resistance mechanisms in hepatitis C virus: implications for direct-acting antiviral use. Drugs. 2017;77(10):1043–55.
113. Cuypers L, Li G, Libin P, Piampongsant S, Vandamme AM, Theys K. Genetic diversity and selective pressure in hepatitis C virus genotypes 1–6: significance for direct-acting antiviral treatment and drug resistance. Viruses. 2015;7(9):5018–39.
114. Esposito I, Trinks J, Soriano V. Hepatitis C virus resistance to the new direct-acting antivirals. Expert Opin Drug Metab Toxicol. 2016;12(10):1197–209.
115. Krishnan P, Beyer J, Mistry N, Koev G, Reisch T, DeGoey D, et al. In vitro and in vivo antiviral activity and resistance profile of ombitasvir, an inhibitor of hepatitis C virus NS5A. Antimicrob Agents Chemother. 2015;59(2):979–87.
116. Krishnan P, Tripathi R, Schnell G, Reisch T, Beyer J, Irvin M, et al. Resistance analysis of baseline and treatment-emergent variants in hepatitis C virus genotype 1 in the AVIATOR study with paritaprevir-ritonavir, ombitasvir, and dasabuvir. Antimicrob Agents Chemother. 2015;59(9):5445–54.
117. Kwo PY, Poordad F, Asatryan A, Wang S, Wyles DL, Hassanein T, et al. Glecaprevir and pibrentasvir yield high response rates in patients with HCV genotype 1-6 without cirrhosis. J Hepatol. 2017;67(2):263–71.
118. Lontok E, Harrington P, Howe A, Kieffer T, Lennerstrand J, Lenz O, et al. Hepatitis C virus drug resistance-associated substitutions: state of the art summary. Hepatology. 2015;62(5):1623–32.
119. Patino-Galindo JA, Salvatierra K, Gonzalez-Candelas F, Lopez-Labrador FX. Comprehensive screening for naturally occurring hepatitis C virus resistance to direct-acting antivirals in the NS3, NS5A, and NS5B genes in worldwide isolates of viral genotypes 1 to 6. Antimicrob Agents Chemother. 2016;60(4):2402–16.
120. Pawlotsky JM, Hepatitis C. Virus resistance to direct-acting antiviral drugs in interferon-free regimens. Gastroenterology. 2016;151(1):70–86.
121. Sarrazin C. The importance of resistance to direct antiviral drugs in HCV infection in clinical practice. J Hepatol. 2016;64(2):486–504.
122. Welzel TM, Bhardwaj N, Hedskog C, Chodavarapu K, Camus G, McNally J, et al. Global epidemiology of HCV subtypes and resistance-associated substitutions evaluated by sequencing-based subtype analyses. J Hepatol. 2017 Aug;67(2):224–36.
123. Jacobson IM, McHutchison JG, Dusheiko G, Di Bisceglie AM, Reddy KR, Bzowej NH, et al. Telaprevir for previously untreated chronic hepatitis C virus infection. N Engl J Med. 2011;364(25):2405–16.
124. Poordad F, McCone J Jr, Bacon BR, Bruno S, Manns MP, Sulkowski MS, et al. Boceprevir for untreated chronic HCV genotype 1 infection. N Engl J Med. 2011;364(13):1195–206.
125. Lenz O, Verbinnen T, Fevery B, Tambuyzer L, Vijgen L, Peeters M, et al. Virology analyses of HCV isolates from genotype 1-infected patients treated with simeprevir plus peginterferon/ribavirin in Phase IIb/III studies. J Hepatol. 2015;62(5):1008–14.
126. Molino S, Martin MT. Hepatitis C virus resistance testing in genotype 1: the changing role in clinical utility. Ann Pharmacother. 2017;51(9):811–6.
127. Kan H, Imamura M, Uchida T, Hiraga N, Hayes CN, Tsuge M, et al. Protease inhibitor resistance remains even after mutant strains become undetectable by deep sequencing. J Infect Dis. 2016;214(11):1687–94.
128. Bourliere M, Gordon SC, Flamm SL, Cooper CL, Ramji A, Tong M, et al. Sofosbuvir, velpatasvir, and voxilaprevir for previously treated HCV infection. N Engl J Med. 2017;376(22):2134–46.
129. Poordad F, Felizarta F, Asatryan A, Sulkowski MS, Reindollar RW, Landis CS, et al. Glecaprevir and pibrentasvir for 12 weeks for hepatitis C virus genotype 1 infection and prior direct-acting antiviral treatment. Hepatology. 2017;66(2):389–97.
130. Pawlotsky JM. NS5A inhibitors in the treatment of hepatitis C. J Hepatol. 2013;59(2):375–82.

131. Ng TI, Krishnan P, Pilot-Matias T, Kati W, Schnell G, Beyer J, et al. In Vitro antiviral activity and resistance profile of the next-generation hepatitis C virus NS5A inhibitor pibrentasvir. Antimicrob Agents Chemother. 2017;61(5):e02558-16.
132. Scheel TK, Rice CM. Understanding the hepatitis C virus life cycle paves the way for highly effective therapies. Nat Med. 2013;19(7):837–49.
133. Feld JJ, Kowdley KV, Coakley E, Sigal S, Nelson DR, Crawford D, et al. Treatment of HCV with ABT-450/r-ombitasvir and dasabuvir with ribavirin. N Engl J Med. 2014;370(17):1594–603.
134. Ferenci P, Bernstein D, Lalezari J, Cohen D, Luo Y, Cooper C, et al. ABT-450/r-ombitasvir and dasabuvir with or without ribavirin for HCV. N Engl J Med. 2014;370(21):1983–92.
135. Zeuzem S, Jacobson IM, Baykal T, Marinho RT, Poordad F, Bourliere M, et al. Retreatment of HCV with ABT-450/r--ombitasvir and dasabuvir with ribavirin. N Engl J Med. 2014;370(17):1604–14.
136. Kwo PY, Mantry PS, Coakley E, Te HS, Vargas HE, Brown R Jr, et al. An interferon-free antiviral regimen for HCV after liver transplantation. N Engl J Med. 2014;371(25):2375–82.
137. Levrero M, Pollicino T, Petersen J, Belloni L, Raimondo G, Dandri M. Control of cccDNA function in hepatitis B virus infection. J Hepatol. 2009;51(3):581–92.
138. Durantel D, Zoulim F. New antiviral targets for innovative treatment concepts for hepatitis B virus and hepatitis delta virus. J Hepatol. 2016;64(1 Suppl):S117–31.
139. European Association for the Study of the Liver. EASL 2017 clinical practice guidelines on the management of hepatitis B virus infection. J Hepatol. 2017;67(2):370–98.
140. Martin P, Lau DT, Nguyen MH, Janssen HL, Dieterich DT, Peters MG, et al. A treatment algorithm for the management of chronic hepatitis B virus infection in the United States: 2015 update. Clin Gastroenterol Hepatol. 2015;13(12):2071–87.
141. Saab S, Chen PY, Saab CE, Tong MJ. The management of hepatitis B in liver transplant recipients. Clin Liver Dis. 2016;20(4):721–36.
142. Lau GK, Piratvisuth T, Luo KX, Marcellin P, Thongsawat S, Cooksley G, et al. Peginterferon Alfa-2a, lamivudine, and the combination for HBeAg-positive chronic hepatitis B. N Engl J Med. 2005;352(26):2682–95.
143. Liaw YF, Sung JJ, Chow WC, Farrell G, Lee CZ, Yuen H, et al. Lamivudine for patients with chronic hepatitis B and advanced liver disease. N Engl J Med. 2004;351(15):1521–31.
144. Lok AS, Lai CL, Leung N, Yao GB, Cui ZY, Schiff ER, et al. Long term safety of lamivudine treatment in patients with chronic hepatitis B. Gastroenterology. 2003;125(6):1714–22.
145. Allen MI, Deslauriers M, Andrews CW, Tipples GA, Walters KA, Tyrrell DL, et al. Identification and characterization of mutations in hepatitis B virus resistant to lamivudine. Lamivudine Clinical Investigation Group Hepatology. 1998;27(6):1670–7.
146. Hadziyannis SJ, Tassopoulos NC, Heathcote EJ, Chang TT, Kitis G, Rizzetto M, et al. Long-term therapy with adefovir dipivoxil for HBeAg-negative chronic hepatitis B for up to 5 years. Gastroenterology. 2006;131(6):1743–51.
147. Nash K. Telbivudine in the treatment of chronic hepatitis B. Adv Ther. 2009;26(2):155–69.
148. Liaw YF, Gane E, Leung N, Zeuzem S, Wang Y, Lai CL, et al. 2-year GLOBE trial results: telbivudine is superior to lamivudine in patients with chronic hepatitis B. Gastroenterology. 2009;136(2):486–95.
149. Chan HL, Heathcote EJ, Marcellin P, Lai CL, Cho M, Moon YM, et al. Treatment of hepatitis B e antigen positive chronic hepatitis with telbivudine or adefovir: a randomized trial. Ann Intern Med. 2007;147(11):745–54.
150. Marcellin P, Wursthorn K, Wedemeyer H, Chuang WL, Lau G, Avila C, et al. Telbivudine plus pegylated interferon alfa-2a in a randomized study in chronic hepatitis B is associated with an unexpected high rate of peripheral neuropathy. J Hepatol. 2015;62(1):41–7.
151. Tenney DJ, Rose RE, Baldick CJ, Pokornowski KA, Eggers BJ, Fang J, et al. Long-term monitoring shows hepatitis B virus resistance to entecavir in nucleoside-naive patients is rare through 5 years of therapy. Hepatology. 2009;49(5):1503–14.
152. Walsh AW, Langley DR, Colonno RJ, Tenney DJ. Mechanistic characterization and molecular modeling of hepatitis B virus polymerase resistance to entecavir. PLoS One. 2010;5(2):e9195.
153. Liu Y, Corsa AC, Buti M, Cathcart AL, Flaherty JF, Miller MD, et al. No detectable resistance to tenofovir disoproxil fumarate in HBeAg+ and HBeAg- patients with chronic hepatitis B after 8 years of treatment. J Viral Hepat. 2017;24(1):68–74.
154. Saag MS. Emtricitabine, a new antiretroviral agent with activity against HIV and hepatitis B virus. Clin Infect Dis. 2006;42(1):126–31.
155. Fung S, Kwan P, Fabri M, Horban A, Pelemis M, Hann HW, et al. Tenofovir disoproxil fumarate (TDF) vs. emtricitabine (FTC)/TDF in lamivudine resistant hepatitis B: A 5-year randomised study. J Hepatol. 2017;66(1):11–8.
156. Lim SG, Ng TM, Kung N, Krastev Z, Volfova M, Husa P, et al. A double-blind placebo-controlled study of emtricitabine in chronic hepatitis B. Arch Intern Med. 2006;166(1):49–56.
157. Ray AS, Fordyce MW, Hitchcock MJ. Tenofovir alafenamide: a novel prodrug of tenofovir for the treatment of Human Immunodeficiency Virus. Antivir Res. 2016;125:63–70.
158. Chan HL, Fung S, Seto WK, Chuang WL, Chen CY, Kim HJ, et al. Tenofovir alafenamide versus tenofovir disoproxil fumarate for the treatment of HBeAg-positive chronic hepatitis B virus infection: a randomised, double-blind, phase 3, non-inferiority trial. Lancet Gastroenterol Hepatol. 2016;1(3):185–95.
159. Buti M, Gane E, Seto WK, Chan HL, Chuang WL, Stepanova T, et al. Tenofovir alafenamide versus tenofovir disoproxil fumarate for the treatment of patients with HBeAg-negative chronic hepatitis B virus infection: a randomised, double-blind, phase 3, non-inferiority trial. Lancet Gastroenterol Hepatol. 2016;1(3):196–206.

Pharmacokinetics and Pharmacodynamics of Antiviral Drugs in Special Population

55

Marco R. Scipione and John Papadopoulos

Introduction

Viral infections are a serious public health concern and can contribute significantly to patients' morbidity and mortality. It is estimated that there are 350 million people worldwide who are carriers of the hepatitis B virus (HBV) and 17,000 new cases per year of hepatitis C (HCV) are identified [1]. Herpes viruses remain a threat with an estimated 50% seroprevalence of herpes simplex virus type-1 (HSV-1) and 20% seroprevalence of HSV-2 among adults in the United States [2]. Influenza is also a global health problem with thousands of deaths each year and specifically 18,500 confirmed deaths worldwide from the 2009 influenza A H1N1 pandemic alone [3, 4]. It is imperative that clinicians have an intimate knowledge of any medication used in their practice and a working knowledge base of pharmacokinetics (PK) and pharmacodynamics (PD) is especially true in the discipline of infectious diseases. This chapter will review in detail the pharmacokinetic and pharmacodynamic parameters of antiviral agents utilized to treat selected viral infections in the immunosuppressed transplant population.

Anti-herpes Virus Agents

Acyclovir

Mechanism of Action and Resistance

Acyclovir is a synthetic purine nucleoside analogue with in vitro and in vivo inhibitory activity against herpes simplex virus type 1 (HSV-1), herpes simplex virus type 2 (HSV-2), and varicella zoster virus (VZV) [5]. Acyclovir competitively inhibits viral DNA polymerase, incorporates and terminates the growing viral DNA chain, and inactivates viral DNA polymerase only after it has been phosphorylated by the enzyme thymidine kinase (TK) encoded by HSV and VZV. This enzyme converts acyclovir into acyclovir monophosphate, which is then further converted into diphosphate by a cellular guanylate kinase and finally into a triphosphate, which exerts its antiviral activity [6]. Resistance to acyclovir is due to mutations on the UL23 gene that encodes the TK enzyme, or the UL30 gene that encodes for viral DNA polymerase [2]. Approximately 95% of clinical isolates with acyclovir resistance have a UL23 gene mutation. Mutations in the UL30 gene are less common in clinical isolates [2]. The concentration of acyclovir needed to inhibit viral plaques by 50% in vitro is 0.01 μg/mL to 2.7 μg/mL for HSV-1 and 0.01 μg/mL to 4.4 μg/mL for HSV-2. The concentration of acyclovir needed for inhibition of VZV in vitro is 0.17 μg/mL to 26 μg/mL [7].

Pharmacokinetics

Plasma protein binding of acyclovir ranges from 9% to 33% with an average plasma elimination half-life ($t_{1/2}$) of 2.5–3.3 h after oral administration [8, 9] (Table 55.1). The bioavailability of acyclovir is low, with only 10–20% bioavailability after administration of enteral acyclovir, and proportional increases in dose do not provide proportional increases in plasma acyclovir concentrations [7]. Peak plasma concentrations (C_{max}) at steady state after multiple doses of oral acyclovir are approximately 0.83 μg/mL after 200 mg, 1.21 μg/mL after 400 mg, and 1.61 μg/mL after 800 mg [9]. The C_{max} after intravenous (IV) administration of acyclovir 5 mg/kg every 8 hours is 9.8 μg/mL, and the trough concentration (C_{min}) is 0.7 μg/mL [9, 10]. After 10 mg/kg every 8 h of IV acyclovir, the C_{max} is 20.7 μg/mL, and the C_{min} is 2.3 μg/mL [9, 10]. Food does not affect the rate or extent of oral acyclovir absorption. Plasma elimination $t_{1/2}$ and total body clearance (Cl_{total}) are dependent on renal function, and Cl_{total} is markedly reduced in anuric patients [10, 11]. Renal excretion is the major route of elimination and is dependent on

M. R. Scipione (✉)
Department of Pharmacy, Memorial Sloan Kettering Cancer Center, New York, NY, USA

J. Papadopoulos
Department of Pharmacy, Division of Pharmacotherapy, NYU Langone Medical Center, New York, NY, USA
e-mail: john.papadopoulos@nyumc.org

A. Safdar (ed.), *Principles and Practice of Transplant Infectious Diseases*, https://doi.org/10.1007/978-1-4939-9034-4_55

Table 55.1 Pharmacokinetics of antiviral agents for treatment of herpes viruses

	Acyclovir	Valacyclovir[a]	Ganciclovir	Valganciclovir[a]	Famciclovir[a]	Cidofovir	Foscarnet
Maximum concentration (μg/mL)	*200 mg* 0.83 *400 mg* 1.21 *800 mg* 1.61	*500 mg* 3.7 ± 0.87 *1000 mg* 4.96 ± 0.64	*5 mg/kg* 8.27 ± 1.02 to 9.0 ± 1.4	5.61 ± 1.52	*250 mg* 1.6 *500 mg* 3.3 *1000 mg* 6.6	*Without probenecid:* *3 mg/kg* 7.3 ± 1.4 *5 mg/kg* 11.5 *With probenecid:* *3 mg/kg* 9.8 ± 3.7 *5 mg/kg* 19.6 ± 7.2	*60 mg/kg q8h* 589 ± 192 *90 mg/kg q12h* 623 ± 132
Minimum concentration (μg/mL)	*200 mg* 0.46 *400 mg* 0.63 *800 mg* 0.83	ND	ND	ND	ND	ND	*60 mg/kg q8h* 114 ± 91 *90 mg/kg q12h* 63 ± 57
AUC (μg*h/mL)	ND	*500 mg* 9.88 ± 2.01 *1000 mg* 15.7 ± 2.27	*5 mg/kg* 22.1 ± 3.2 to 26.8 ± 6.1	29.1 ± 9.7	*250 mg* 4.48 *500 mg* 8.95 *1000 mg* 17.9	*Without probenecid:* *3 mg/kg* 20 ± 2.3 *5 mg/kg* 28.3 *With probenecid:* *3 mg/kg* 25.7 ± 8.3 *5 mg/kg* 40.8 ± 9.0	ND
Clearance	ND	ND	*Total clearance* 3.52 ± 0.80 mL/min/kg *Renal clearance* 3.20 ± 0.8 mL/min/kg	ND	ND	*Without probenecid:* *Total clearance* 179 ± 23.1 mL/min/1.73m^2 *Renal clearance* 150 ± 26.9 mL/min/1.73m^2 *With probenecid:* 148 ± 39 mL/min/1.73m^2 *Renal clearance* 98.6 ± 27.9 mL/min/1.73m^2	*60 mg/kg q8h* 6.2 ± 2.1 L/h *90 mg/kg q12h* 7.1 ± 2.7 L/h
Volume of distribution (V_d)	ND	ND	0.74 ± 0.15 L/kg	ND	1.08 ± 0.17 L/kg	*Without probenecid:* 537 ± 126 mL *With probenecid:* 410 ± 102 mL	*60 mg/kg q8h* 0.41 ± 0.13 *90 mg/kg q12h* 0.52 ± 0.2
Half-life ($t_{1/2}$)	2.5–3.3 h	2.5–3.3 h	*IV* 3.5 h *PO* 4.8 h	4 h	2.3 h	ND	*60 mg/kg q8h* 4 h *90 mg/kg q12h* 3.3 h
Protein binding	9–33%	14–18%	1–2%	ND	<20%	ND	14–17%
Bioavailability	10–20%	55%	5%	59%	77%	ND	ND

ND no data available
[a]Data related to acyclovir, ganciclovir, or penciclovir

active tubular secretion [10, 12]. As a result, the dose of acyclovir should be adjusted based on renal function. Acyclovir concentrations are decreased by 60% after a 6-h hemodialysis (HD) period, and less than 10% of acyclovir is removed during peritoneal dialysis [13, 14].

Acyclovir is extensively distributed in a wide variety of tissues and body fluids. After administration of IV acyclovir, the level in cerebral spinal fluid (CSF) is approximately 50% of plasma concentration; however, one study estimated the penetration ratio which ranges from 13% to 52% of plasma, with a mean value of 31% [10, 15]. The concentration of acyclovir in aqueous humor is 3.26 μmol/L [16]. Concentrations in amniotic fluid of 1.3 μg/mL are higher than corresponding maternal plasma concentrations of 0.2 μg/mL at the time of labor in pregnant women taking acyclovir three times daily [17]. There is minimal systemic absorption seen after application of topical acyclovir 5% cream or ointment on intact skin [18].

Pharmacokinetics in Pediatric Patients

The pharmacokinetics of acyclovir in pediatric patients is similar to adults, with a $t_{1/2}$ of 2.6 h after oral administration of acyclovir and a bioavailability of 12% [19]. The peak concentrations after IV acyclovir doses of 250 mg/m^2 and 500 mg/m^2 in children are 10 μg/mL and 21 μg/mL, respectively [10]. In neonates the $t_{1/2}$ of acyclovir is 3.8 h, and the C_{max} is 30 μg/mL after a 5 mg/kg dose, 61 μg/mL after a 10 mg/kg dose, and 86 μg/mL after a 15 mg/kg dose [20].

Dosing and Drug Interactions

The dose of IV acyclovir for the treatment of HSV encephalitis or VZV in immunocompromised hosts is 10–15 mg/kg given every 8 h (Table 55.2). The dose of oral acyclovir depends on the indication with 400 mg every 8 h recommended for treatment of the first episode of genital HSV or 400 mg five times daily if the patient is immunocompromised. For VZV, the oral dose of acyclovir is 800 mg five times daily. Acyclovir concentrations are increased when used in combination with probenecid due to decreased renal tubular secretion (Table 55.3). Combination of acyclovir and zidovudine may cause lethargy (Table 55.4).

Valacyclovir

Mechanism of Action and Resistance

Valacyclovir is the L-valyl ester of acyclovir which is rapidly converted to acyclovir and L-valine by first-pass metabolism [21]. Plasma concentrations of unconverted valacyclovir are low and undetectable 3 h after oral administration [22]. Valacyclovir plasma concentrations are 0.5 μg/mL, 0.4 μg/mL, and 0.8 μg/mL after a single administration of 1000 mg of valacyclovir in patients with hepatic dysfunction, renal dysfunction, and health volunteers, respectively [23, 24]. Once valacyclovir is converted to acyclovir, it undergoes the same phosphorylation to triphosphate as acyclovir to exert its antiviral activity [6]. As valacyclovir is rapidly converted to acyclovir, aforementioned mechanisms of drug resistance remain identical.

Pharmacokinetics

The absolute bioavailability of acyclovir after administration of valacyclovir is approximately 55% after a 1000 mg dose (Table 55.1). Similar to oral acyclovir, increases in acyclovir C_{max} and area under the curve (AUC) after single and multiple doses of valacyclovir are not proportional to increases in dose. The C_{max} is 3.3 μg/mL and the AUC is 11.6 μg*h/mL after a single dose of 500 mg of valacyclovir compared to a C_{max} and AUC of 5.7 μg/mL and 19.5 μg*h/mL, respectively, after a single dose of 1000 mg of valacyclovir [25]. Plasma protein binding of valacyclovir ranges from 14% to 18%.

Forty-one percent of acyclovir is recovered in urine after a single dose of 1000 mg of valacyclovir. In patients with end-stage renal disease, the acyclovir $t_{1/2}$ increases from 2 to 3 h to approximately 14 h after administration of valacyclovir [24]. In patients undergoing hemodialysis (HD), approximately 33% of acyclovir gets removed during a 4-h dialysis session [26]. Since valacyclovir needs to get converted to acyclovir by first-pass intestinal or hepatic metabolism, there is a concern that patients with moderate to severe liver disease may not have adequate conversion to acyclovir after administration of valacyclovir [27]. However, the rate and not the extent of conversion of valacyclovir to acyclovir is reduced, and the $t_{1/2}$ is not affected [28].

Distribution of acyclovir after administration of valacyclovir is similar to the distribution seen after administration of IV or oral acyclovir. After administration of 1000 mg of valacyclovir every 8-h regimen, the concentration of acyclovir in CSF is 2.5 μmol/L at 2 h and 2.3 μmol/L at 8 hours [29]. In patients with normal renal function the AUC in CSF to AUC in serum ratio is approximately 19% after administration of 1000 mg of valacyclovir every 8 h and 25% after administration of 2000 mg of valacyclovir every 6 h [29, 30].

Pharmacokinetics in Pediatric Patients

The pharmacokinetics of acyclovir has been evaluated in pediatric patients after administration of valacyclovir oral suspension. The C_{max} and AUC are 7.0 μg/mL and 27.6 μg*h/mL in children 1–2 months old, 5.2 μg/mL and 17.7 μg*h/mL in children 3–5 months old, 4.9 μg/mL and 14.1 μg*h/mL in children 6–11 months, and 4.7 μg/mL and 15.3 μg*h/mL in children 12–23 months after doses of 25 mg/kg of valacyclovir [31]. In children 2–5 years old who received 20 mg/kg of valacyclovir, the C_{max} and AUC were 3.8 μg/mL and 10.1 μg*h/mL; and in children 6–11 years, the C_{max} and AUC were 4.7 μg/mL and 13.1 μg*h/mL [31].

Table 55.2 Dose of antiviral agents for treatment of herpes viruses

Virus	Agent	Route	Usual adult dosage	Duration
Herpes simplex virus (HSV)				
Genital first episode	Acyclovir	IV	5 mg/kg q8h[a,b]	5 days[c]
		PO	400 mg q8h[a,d]	7–10 days[e]
		PO	200 mg five times daily[a,d,f]	7–10 days
		Topical	Apply q3h (6 times per day)	7 days
	Valacyclovir	PO	1000 mg q12h[a,d,g]	7–10 days[e]
	Famciclovir	PO	250 mg q8h[a,f]	7–10 days
		PO	500 mg q12h[a]	5–14 days
Genital recurrent episode	Acyclovir	PO	800 mg q8h[a,b]	2 days
		PO	400 mg q8h[a,b]	5 days[e]
		PO	200 mg five times daily[a]	5 days
	Valacyclovir	PO	500 mg q12h[a,b,f]	3 days
		PO	1000 mg q24h[a,b,f]	5 days
		PO	1000 mg q12h[a,b,g]	7–10 days
	Famciclovir	PO	125 mg q12h[a,b]	5 days
		PO	500 mg × 1 followed by 250 mg q12h[a,b]	2 days
		PO	1000 mg q12h[a,b]	1 day
Genital suppression	Acyclovir	PO	400 mg q12h[a]	12 months
		PO	200 mg q8h[a,f]	12 months
	Valacyclovir	PO	500 mg q24h[a,h]	12 months
		PO	1000 mg q24h[a,i]	12 months
		PO	250 mg q12h[a]	12 months
		PO	500 mg q12h[a]	12 months
Encephalitis	Acyclovir	IV	10–15 mg/kg q8h[a]	14–21 days
Mucocutaneous in immunocompromised patients	Acyclovir	IV	5–10 mg/kg q8h[a,j]	7–14 days
		PO	400 mg five times daily[a]	7–14 days
	Valacyclovir	PO	500 mg q12h[a]	7–10 days
		PO	1000 mg q12h[a]	7–10 days
	Famciclovir	PO	500 mg q12h[a]	7–10 days
	Foscarnet	IV	40 mg q8h[a]	14–21 days
		IV	60 mg q12h[a]	14–21 days
Orolabial	Acyclovir	PO	400 mg q8h[a]	5–10 days
		Topical	Apply five times daily	4 days
	Valacyclovir	PO	2000 mg q12h[a]	1 day
	Famciclovir	PO	500 mg q12h[a]	5–10 days
		PO	1500 mg × 1	1 day
	Penciclovir	Topical	Apply q2h while awake	4 days
Varicella zoster virus (VZV)				
Herpes zoster (shingles) in normal host	Acyclovir	PO	800 mg five times daily[a]	7–10 days
	Valacyclovir	PO	1000 mg q8h[a]	7 days
	Famciclovir	PO	500 mg q8h[a]	7 days
Herpes zoster (shingles) in immunocompromised host	Acyclovir	IV	10 mg/kg q8h[a,c]	7–10 days
		PO	800 mg five times daily[a,k]	7–10 days
	Valacyclovir	PO	1000 mg q8h[a,k]	7–10 days
	Famciclovir	PO	500 mg q8h[a,k]	7 days
Cytomegalovirus (CMV)				
Retinitis	Ganciclovir	IV	5 mg/kg q12h[a] (induction)	21 days
		IV	5 mg/kg q24h[a] (maintenance)	
	Valganciclovir	PO	900 mg q12h[a] (induction)	21 days
		PO	900 mg q24h[a] (maintenance)	
	Cidofovir	IV	5 mg/kg once weekly × 2 then 5 mg/kg every other week	
	Foscarnet	IV	60 mg/kg q8h[a] Or 90 mg/kg q12h[a] (induction)	21 days
		Iv	90–120 mg/kg q24h[a,l] (maintenance)	

Table 55.2 (continued)

[a]Dose adjustment required for renal insufficiency
[b]Start within 24 h of onset of symptoms
[c]Therapy may be completed with oral acyclovir for a total of 10 days
[d]Start within 48 h of onset of symptoms
[e]Duration for patients with HIV should be 5–14 days
[f]Do not use for immunocompromised patients or patients with HIV
[g]Dose of 1000 mg PO q12h should be used for treatment of all initial and recurrent episodes in patients with HIV
[h]If <10 episodes per year
[i]If ≥10 episodes per year
[j]Acyclovir 10 mg/kg should be reserved for progressive infections
[k]Oral therapy should only be used in patients with an acute localized dermatome
[l]Chronic suppression may be necessary with valganciclovir 900 mg PO q24h

Table 55.3 Pharmacokinetic drug-drug interactions with antiviral agents

Object antiviral agent	Increased levels of object antiviral agent	Decreased levels of object antiviral agent	Increased levels *due* to object antiviral agent	Decreased levels *due* to object antiviral agent
Acyclovir	Probenecid: Decreased renal tubular secretion			
Adefovir	Ibuprofen: Increased bioavailability			
Amantadine	Quinidine, quinine, triamterene, trimethoprim: Decreased renal tubular secretion			
Boceprevir: *Strong inhibitor of CYP4503A4 and p-glycoprotein*	Amiodarone, voriconazole: Decreased hepatic metabolism	Carbamazepine, efavirenz, dexamethasone, fosphenytoin, phenobarbital, phenytoin, rifabutin, rifampin, ritonavir, St. John's wort: Increased hepatic metabolism	Alfuzosin, alprazolam, amiodarone, colchicine, conivaptan, cyclosporine,dronedarone, eplerenone, felodipine, flecainide, lovastatin, methadone, midazolam, nicardipine, nifedipine, propafenone, ranolazine, rivaroxaban, sildenafil, simvastatin, sirolimus, tacrolimus, tadalafil, ticagrelor, tolvaptan, triazolam, vardenafil, voriconazole, warfarin: Decreased hepatic metabolism Digoxin, rivaroxaban: Decreased p-glycoprotein-mediated elimination	
Cidofovir	–	–	–	–
Entecavir	–	–	–	–
Famciclovir	Probenecid: Decreased renal tubular secretion			
Foscarnet	–	–	–	–
Ganciclovir	Probenecid: Decreased renal tubular secretion			
Interferon alpha *Inhibits CYP4501A2*			Theophylline, zidovudine: Decreased hepatic metabolism	
Lamivudine	Trimethoprim: Decreased renal tubular secretion			

(continued)

Table 55.3 (continued)

Object antiviral agent	Increased levels of object antiviral agent	Decreased levels of object antiviral agent	Increased levels *due* to object antiviral agent	Decreased levels *due* to object antiviral agent
Oseltamivir	Probenecid: Decreased renal tubular secretion			
Ribavirin	–	–	–	–
Rimantadine	–	–	–	–
Telaprevir *Inhibitor of CYP4503A4 and p-glycoprotein*	Amiodarone, voriconazole: Decreased hepatic metabolism	Carbamazepine, efavirenz, dexamethasone, fosphenytoin, phenobarbital, phenytoin, rifabutin, rifampin, ritonavir, St. John's wort: Increased hepatic metabolism	Alfuzosin, alprazolam, amiodarone, bosentan, colchicine, conivaptan, cyclosporine,dronedarone, eplrenenone, felodipine, flecainide, lovastatin, methadone, midazolam, nicardipine, nifedipine, propafenone, ranolazine, rivaroxaban, sildenafil, simvastatin, sirolimus, tacrolimus, tadalafil, tenofovir, ticagrelor, tolvaptan, triazolam, vardenafil, voriconazole, warfarin: Decreased hepatic metabolism Digoxin, rivaroxaban: Decreased p-glycoprotein-mediated elimination	
Tenofovir *Inhibitor of CYP4501A2 and inducer of p-glycoprotein*			Didanosine: Increased bioavailability Theophylline, zidovudine: Decreased hepatic metabolism	Dabigatran, linagliptin: Increased elimination by p-glycoprotein induction
Valacyclovir	Probenecid: Decreased renal tubular secretion			
Valganciclovir	Probenecid: Decreased renal tubular secretion			
Zanamivir	–	–	–	–

Dosing and Drug Interactions

The dose of valacyclovir for treatment of the first episode of HSV is 1000 mg every 12 h and 500 mg every 12 h for any recurrent episodes (Table 55.2). The dose of valacyclovir is 1000 mg every 8 h for the treatment of VZV. Similar to acyclovir, valacyclovir concentrations are increased when used concurrently with probenecid, and the combination of valacyclovir and zidovudine may cause lethargy (Table 55.3).

Ganciclovir

Mechanism of Action and Resistance

Ganciclovir is an acyclic nucleoside analogue of 2′-deoxyguanosine that inhibits replication of cytomegalovirus (CMV), HSV, and VZV [32]. In order to exhibit its antiviral activity, ganciclovir similar to acyclovir must be phosphorylated. The phosphorylation unlike acyclovir does not depend on viral TK; in fact it is mediated via CMV-encoded (UL97 gene) protein kinase homologue [32]. After conversion to ganciclovir monophosphate, it is converted to di- and triphos-

Table 55.4 Pharmacodynamic drug-drug interactions with antiviral agents

	Increased pharmacodynamics (drug effect)
Acyclovir	Interferon Additive antiviral effect Zidovudine May cause lethargy
Adefovir	Aminoglycosides, amphotericin, cyclosporine, tacrolimus, vancomycin Increased nephrotoxicity Ribavirin Increased hepatotoxicity
Amantadine	Anticholinergic agents Additive anticholinergic effects May prolong the QT interval Use with caution with other agents that prolong the QT interval
Boceprevir	
Cidofovir	Aminoglycosides, amphotericin B, foscarnet, pentamidine Increased nephrotoxicity
Entecavir	Ribavirin Increased hepatotoxicity
Famciclovir	

Table 55.4 (continued)

	Increased pharmacodynamics (drug effect)
Foscarnet	May prolong the QT interval Use with caution with other agents that prolong the QT interval Can cause significant electrolyte disturbances (hypokalemia, hypocalcemia, hypomagnesemia, hypophosphatemia) Use with caution with aminoglycosides, amphotericin B, diuretics, and pentamidine Aminoglycosides, amphotericin B, cidofovir, pentamidine Increased nephrotoxicity
Ganciclovir	Azathioprine, cyclosporine, didanosine, zidovudine Increased hematological toxicity Ganciclovir may antagonize the effect of didanosine and zidovudine against HIV Aminoglycosides, amphotericin B, cidofovir, foscarnet, pentamidine Increased nephrotoxicity Imipenem-cilastatin Increased seizure risk
Interferon alpha	Aldesleukin Increased myocardial and renal toxicity
Lamivudine	Ribavirin Increased hepatotoxicity
Oseltamivir	
Ribavirin	Adefovir, entecavir, lamivudine
Rimantadine	
Telaprevir	
Tenofovir	Adefovir May diminish therapeutic effect
Valacyclovir	Interferon Additive antiviral effect Zidovudine May cause lethargy
Valganciclovir	Azathioprine, cyclosporine, didanosine, zidovudine Increased hematological toxicity Aminoglycosides, amphotericin B, cidofovir, foscarnet, pentamidine Increased nephrotoxicity Imipenem-cilastatin Increased seizure risk
Zanamivir	–

phate forms by cellular kinases. Ganciclovir triphosphate concentrations are 100-fold greater in CMV-infected cells than uninfected cells [33]. Ganciclovir triphosphate inhibits viral DNA synthesis by competitive inhibition of viral DNA polymerases and incorporation into viral DNA, resulting in slowing of viral DNA elongation [33]. Resistance to ganciclovir is commonly a result of a mutation in the UL97 gene; mutation in DNA polymerase is a less common mechanism of viral drug resistance [34]. The 0.1–1.6 μg/mL ganciclovir concentration leads to inhibit 50% of viral plaques in cell line CMV cultures [32].

Pharmacokinetics

After administration of 5 mg/kg IV ganciclovir, the C_{max} ranges from 8.0 to 9.0 μg/mL, and the AUC ranges from 22.1 to 26.8 μg*h/mL [35] (Table 55.1). The bioavailability of oral ganciclovir is only 5–8%, with a C_{max} of 1.2 μg/mL and AUC of 15.4 μg*h/L [35]. Intravenous ganciclovir exhibits linear pharmacokinetics up to 5 mg/kg and oral ganciclovir exhibits linear pharmacokinetics up to 4000 mg/day [36]. Protein binding of ganciclovir is only 1–2%, and the average $t_{1/2}$ is 3.5 h following IV administration and 3–7 h following oral administration [37, 38]. The volume of distribution (V_d) of IV ganciclovir is 0.7 L/kg. Ganciclovir is also available as a 0.15% ophthalmic gel and 4.5 mg intraocular implant for treatment of CMV retinitis. The estimated daily dose of ganciclovir that is obtained after administration of the 0.15% ophthalmic gel is 0.04% and 0.1% of the oral and IV doses, respectively, limiting the systemic exposure [39]. After insertion of the intraocular implant, the release rate of ganciclovir and the mean vitreous ganciclovir level are 1.4 μg/h and 4.1 μg/mL, respectively [40].

The renal clearance (Cl_{renal}) of ganciclovir is 3.2 mL/min/kg, which accounts for 91% of Cl_{total} in patients with normal renal function [41, 42]. The major route of elimination of ganciclovir is unchanged drug by glomerular filtration and active renal tubular secretion. The $t_{1/2}$ of ganciclovir increases from 3.6 h in patients with normal renal function to 11.5 h in patients with renal insufficiency after receiving 5 mg/kg of IV ganciclovir [43]. In patients undergoing HD, plasma concentrations of ganciclovir are reduced by approximately 50% [43]. The concentration obtained in CSF 3.5 hours after administration of IV ganciclovir 2.5 mg/kg is 0.7 μg/mL, while the serum concentration is 2.2 μg/mL [44].

Pharmacokinetics in Pediatric Patients

The C_{max} after IV doses of 4 mg/kg or 6 mg/kg of ganciclovir are 5.5 μg/mL and 7.0 μg/mL in neonates aged 2–49 days, respectively [45, 46]. The $t_{1/2}$ is 2.4 h for both dosing regimens. In pediatric patients aged 6 months to 17 years, the C_{max} is 6.6 μg/mL after doses of 5 mg/kg IV ganciclovir [47].

Dosing and Drug Interactions

The dose of IV ganciclovir for the treatment of CMV retinitis is 5 mg/kg every 12 h for 14–21 days followed by 5 mg/kg every 24 h (Table 55.2). Oral ganciclovir should not be used for the treatment of CMV due to poor bioavailability. Ganciclovir concentrations increase with concurrent probenecid use (Table 55.3). Hematological toxicities may be increased when ganciclovir is used in combination with azathioprine, cyclosporine, didanosine, or zidovudine. Ganciclovir may antagonize the effects of didanosine and zidovudine against HSV. Caution should be used when ganciclovir is combined with aminoglycosides, amphotericin B, cidofovir, foscarnet, or pentamidine due to the increased risk of nephrotoxicity (Table 55.4). The combination of ganciclovir and imipenem-cilastatin may increase the risk of seizures.

Valganciclovir

Mechanism of Action and Resistance

Valganciclovir is the L-valyl ester of ganciclovir and exists as a mixture of two diastereomers, which are rapidly converted to ganciclovir by intestinal and hepatic esterases [33, 48]. Plasma concentrations of unconverted valganciclovir are low with an AUC of 1% and C_{max} of 3% of ganciclovir [49]. Once valganciclovir is converted to ganciclovir, it is phosphorylated by the same mechanism in order to inhibit viral DNA synthesis [33, 48].

Pharmacokinetics

The bioavailability of ganciclovir after administration of 900 mg once daily of enteral valganciclovir in healthy subjects was 59%, which is significantly higher than the 5% bioavailability after administration of oral ganciclovir [50–52] (Table 55.1). The time to C_{max} after administration of oral valganciclovir is 1–2 h [51]. The ganciclovir AUC increases by 30% and the C_{max} increases by 14% when valganciclovir is administered with a high fat meal; however, there is no change in the time to C_{max} [49]. The $t_{1/2}$ of valganciclovir and IV ganciclovir is 4 h and 3.8 h, respectively [38, 49]. Similarly, AUC for oral valganciclovir and IV ganciclovir are comparable (24.8 μg*h/mL vs. 26.5 μg*h/mL), although valganciclovir C_{max} is 30% lower compared to IV ganciclovir (6.1 μg/mL vs. 9.0 μg/mL) [35, 51]. The pharmacokinetics of ganciclovir after administration of oral valganciclovir has been evaluated in solid organ transplant patients. The AUC, C_{max}, and $t_{1/2}$ of ganciclovir after administration of valganciclovir are similar regardless of type of solid organ transplantation including heart, liver, and kidney organ graft transplants [53].

Valganciclovir is mainly eliminated by renal excretion as ganciclovir through glomerular filtration and active tubular secretions. The elimination $t_{1/2}$ is increased and Cl_{total} of ganciclovir is reduced following administration of valganciclovir in patients with renal impairment. The $t_{1/2}$ of ganciclovir increases from 4.9 h in patients with creatinine clearance (CrCl) 51–70 mL/min to 22 h and 68 h in patients with CrCl 11 to 20 mL/min and ≤10 mL/min, respectively [54]. Hemodialysis reduces plasma concentrations of ganciclovir by 50% following valganciclovir administration [54].

Pharmacokinetics in Pediatric Patients

The bioavailability of ganciclovir after administration of oral valganciclovir is slightly lower in children at 42–54% compared to adults at 60%, and clearance is related to body surface area and renal function [53, 55, 56]. A lower C_{min} may be seen in younger children with mean age of 4.5 years compared to older children with a mean age of 11 years [56, 57]. The pharmacokinetics of oral valganciclovir was compared to IV ganciclovir in neonates >7 days to 3 months of age with congenital CMV infection of the CNS. After 6 weeks of therapy with 14–20 mg/kg twice-daily oral valganciclovir solution, the AUC_{0-12h} was 27.4 μg*h/mL which is similar to the AUC_{0-12h} of 25.4 μg*h/mL achieved from 5 mg/kg of IV ganciclovir [55, 58].

Dosing and Drug Interactions

The dose of valganciclovir for the treatment of CMV retinitis is 900 mg every 12 h for 21 days followed by 900 mg every 24 h (Table 55.2). Drug interactions with valganciclovir are the same as those seen with ganciclovir (Table 55.3).

Foscarnet

Mechanism of Action and Resistance

Foscarnet is an organic analogue of inorganic pyrophosphate that inhibits replication of herpes virus by selective inhibition at the pyrophosphate binding site on virus-specific DNA polymerases at concentrations that do not affect cellular DNA polymerases [59]. Unlike acyclovir, valacyclovir, ganciclovir, or valganciclovir, foscarnet does not require phosphorylation by TK or other kinases such as UL97. As a result, foscarnet has activity against HSV, VZV, and CMV including TK deficient mutants and CMV UL97 mutants [59]. Foscarnet resistance has been identified and is a result of single base substitutions in conserved and nonconserved regions of the DNA polymerase [2]. Some of these isolates can retain susceptibility to acyclovir; however, mutants with alterations in both TK and DNA polymerase would result in resistance to both acyclovir and foscarnet [2]. The concentrations of foscarnet needed to inhibit viral plaques in cell line cultures were 0.4 μmol/mL to 3.5 μmol/L for HSV-1 and 0.6 μmol/L to 22 μmol/L for HSV-2. The concentration of foscarnet needed for inhibition of VZV in cultures was 0.4 μmol/L, and for CMV inhibition it was 0.3 μmol/L [59].

Pharmacokinetics

The pharmacokinetics of foscarnet has been established during induction therapy in AIDS patients with CMV retinitis (Table 55.1). After administration of 60 mg/kg IV q8h, the C_{max} is 589 μmol/L, and C_{min} is 114 μmol/L at steady state [60, 61]. The V_d is 0.31 to 0.74 L/kg and the plasma $t_{1/2}$ is 4 h [62–64]. After administration of 90 mg/kg IV every 12 h, the C_{max} and C_{min} are 623 μmol/L and 63 μmol/L, respectively, while the V_d is 0.52 L/kg with a plasma $t_{1/2}$ of 3 hours and Cl_{total} of 7.0 L/h [62–64]. A total of 14–17% of foscarnet is protein bound. Although not approved in the United States, foscarnet has been given as an intravitreal injection for treatment of acute retinal necrosis [65–67].

The Cl_{total} of foscarnet is 6.2 L/h, with 78–86% of this agent cleared via renal elimination [62–64]. The clearance of foscarnet is significantly reduced with reduced renal function and the elimination $t_{1/2}$ increases by ten-fold [68]. As a result of the reduced clearance, the $t_{1/2}$ of foscarnet increases from 2 hours in patients with a mean CrCl of 108 mL/min to 3.4 h in patients with a mean CrCl of 68 mL/min to 13 and 25 h in patients with a mean CrCl of 34 mL/min and 20 mL/min, respectively [68]. It is mportant to note that foscarnet terminal $t_{1/2}$ based on urinary excretion is 88 h, which is significantly higher than the plasma $t_{1/2}$, and this possibly in part reflects release of foscarnet from the bone [62, 64, 68].

Dosing and Drug Interactions

The dose of foscarnet for the treatment of CMV is 60 mg/kg every 8 h followed by 90–120 mg/kg every 24 h (Table 55.2). An alternative dosing regimen of 90 mg/kg every 12 hours has also been used. Chronic suppression with oral valganciclovir may still be necessary. As foscarnet may prolong the QT interval, caution should be taken when it is used with other agents that may also prolong the QT interval (Table 55.4). Caution should be used when foscarnet is used with aminoglycosides, amphotericin B, diuretics, and pentamidine due to the risk of significant electrolyte abnormalities including hypokalemia, hypocalcemia, hypomagnesemia, and hypophosphatemia. There is also an increased risk of nephrotoxicity when foscarnet is used concurrently with aminoglycosides, amphotericin B, cidofovir, or pentamidine.

Cidofovir

Mechanism of Action and Resistance

Cidofovir is a nucleoside analogue, which suppresses viral replication by selective inhibition of viral DNA synthesis. Cidofovir must be phosphorylated by cellular enzymes to cidofovir diphosphate, which is the active intracellular metabolite. Incorporation of cidofovir into the growing viral DNA chain results in reductions in viral DNA synthesis [69]. Cidofovir is active against HSV, VZV, and CMV, including acyclovir and ganciclovir resistant isolates, as cidofovir does not require activation by TK or UL97 [34]. Mutations in DNA polymerase can cause resistance to cidofovir. Almost all DNA polymerase mutations that confer ganciclovir resistance will also confer cidofovir resistance [34]. Ganciclovir-resistant isolates due to mutations in UL97 genes retain susceptibility to cidofovir [69]. The concentrations of cidofovir needed to inhibit viral plaques by 50% in cell cultures were 12.7–31.7 μmol/L for HSV-1 and HSV-2. The concentrations of cidofovir needed for inhibition of VZV and CMV were 0.79 μmol/L and 0.5 μmol/L to 2.8 μmol/L, respectively [70].

Pharmacokinetics

Pharmacokinetics of cidofovir has been evaluated in patients who received cidofovir with or without probenecid in HIV-infected patients. Less than 6% of cidofovir is protein bound [71]. Probenecid competitively inhibits the renal tubular secretion of cidofovir, reducing the Cl_{renal} to a level consistent with glomerular filtration [72]. In patients who receive cidofovir without probenecid, the C_{max} and AUC are 7.3 μg/mL and 20 μg*h/mL after 3 mg/kg and 11.5 μg/mL and 28.3 μg*h/mL after 5 mg/kg dose [71]. After administration of 5 mg/kg of IV cidofovir without probenecid, the V_d is 556 L/kg, the Cl_{total} is 177 mL/h/kg, and the Cl_{renal} is 149 mL/h/kg, which is greater than glomerular filtration [71]. When probenecid is administered along with cidofovir, the C_{max} and AUC increase to 9.8 μg/mL and 25.7 μg*h/mL after 3 mg/kg and 19.6 μg/mL and 40.8 μg*h/mL after 5 mg/kg [69, 72]. The V_d decreases to 388 L/kg, and the Cl_{total} decreases to 138 mL/h/kg, and the Cl_{renal} is reduced to 96 mL/h/kg, which is consistent with glomerular filtration [72].

In patients with normal renal function, 80–100% of the cidofovir dose is recovered unchanged in the urine within 24 h [71]. Approximately 70 to 85% of the cidofovir dose is excreted unchanged in the urine when it is administered with probenecid [69]. Cidofovir's renal tubular secretion and renal clearance decrease proportionally to glomerular filtration CrCl [73]. Hemodialysis reduces serum cidofovir levels by 75% [73]. Due to therapy-related renal failure, cidofovir bladder irrigation has been used for treatment of polyomavirus-associated hemorrhagic cystitis; however, there is only limited data on its use in this situation [74]. Topical cidofovir gel has been used successfully for the treatment of cutaneous acyclovir- and foscarnet-resistant herpes virus; however, there is limited information regarding the pharmacokinetics of this dosage form [75]. As there is no commercially available product, topical cidofovir must be prepared using specific compounding instructions [75]. Topical eye drops with cidofovir have also been used for the treatment of viral conjunctivitis [76].

Dosing and Drug Interactions

The dose of cidofovir for the treatment of CMV is 5 mg/kg once weekly for two doses followed by 5 mg/kg every other week (Table 55.2). There is a potential for increased nephrotoxicity when cidofovir is used concurrently with aminoglycosides, amphotericin B, foscarnet, and pentamidine (Table 55.4).

Famciclovir

Mechanism of Action and Resistance

Famciclovir is the diacetyl 6-deoxy analogue of the active antiviral agent penciclovir. After oral administration, famciclovir is rapidly converted to penciclovir, along with other inactive metabolites including 6-deoxy penciclovir (5%), monoacetylated penciclovir (<0.5%), and 6-deoxy-monoacetylated penciclovir (<0.5%) by aldehyde oxidase with little to no famciclovir detected [77]. Similar to acyclovir, penciclovir undergoes phosphorylation to the active form penciclovir triphosphate [77]. Resistance to penciclovir is due to mutations in the UL23 gene, encoding the TK enzyme, with cross-resistance noted between penciclovir and acyclovir [2]. The concentration of penciclovir needed to inhibit viral plaques by 50% in vitro was 0.6 μg/mL to 0.8 μg/mL for HSV-1 and 2.2 μg/mL to 2.4 μg/mL for HSV-2 [78].

Pharmacokinetics

The bioavailability of penciclovir after administration of 500 mg of oral famciclovir is 77% [79] (Table 55.1). Unlike acyclovir and valacyclovir, penciclovir concentrations are proportionally increased with increasing doses of famciclovir. The C_{max} and AUC of penciclovir are 1.6 mg/L and 4.3 mg*h/L after a single dose of 250 mg famciclovir, and the C_{max} and AUC increase to 3.3 mg/L and 9.3 mg*h/L, respectively, after a single dose of 500 mg. After a single dose of 750 mg famciclovir, the C_{max} of penciclovir is 5.1 mg/L and the AUC is 14.1 mg*h/L [79]. Plasma protein binding of penciclovir is <20%, and the V_d is 1.5 L/kg in healthy males after a single IV dose of penciclovir [80]. The $t_{1/2}$ of penciclovir is approximately 2 h in healthy male volunteers after oral administration of famciclovir [79–81]. Famciclovir is not available as a topical preparation; however, there is a topical penciclovir 1% cream that is commercially available for the treatment of herpes labialis [82].

Approximately 94% of penciclovir is recovered in the urine over 24 hours with 83% of the dose recovered in the first 6 hours after administration of IV penciclovir [83]. After administration with 500 mg of oral famciclovir, 73% of the dose is recovered in the urine with penciclovir and 6-deoxy penciclovir accounting for 82% and 7%, respectively [81]. Only 27% of the administered dose of famciclovir is recovered in the feces [79]. Clearance of penciclovir after administration of famciclovir is via renal elimination with active tubular secretion, a contributing factor [79, 81]. The clearance of penciclovir decreases linearly with declining renal function [81]. The $t_{1/2}$ of penciclovir increases from 2.2 h in patients with no renal impairment to 2.5 h, 3.9 h, and 9.9 h in patients with mild (CrCl 60 to 80 mL/min), moderate (CrCl 30 to 59 mL/min), and severe (CrCl 5 to 29 mL/min) renal impairment, respectively [81].

Patients with mild to moderate hepatic impairment have no effect on the AUC of penciclovir following 500 mg of famciclovir dose, although the C_{max} was reduced by 43% and the time to C_{max} was increased by 0.75 h [84]. The pharmacokinetics of penciclovir after administration of famciclovir has not been studied in patients with severe hepatic impairment.

Dosing and Drug Interactions

The treatment dose for HSV of famciclovir is 250 mg every 8 h for the first episode and 125 mg every 8 h for any recurrent episodes (Table 55.2). In immunocompromised patients with HSV the dose of famciclovir is 500 mg every 12 h and the dose for treatment of VZV is 500 mg every 8 h. Concentrations of famciclovir will increase with concurrent use of probenecid due to decreased renal tubular secretion (Table 55.3).

Anti-influenza Agents

Amantadine

Mechanism of Action and Resistance

Amantadine is a symmetric tricyclic amine that inhibits the replication of influenza A virus isolates and has very little to no activity against influenza B [85]. Amantadine prevents the release of viral nucleic acid into the host cell by interfering with the function of the transmembrane domain of the viral M2 protein [86, 87]. Amantadine resistance has limited its use, as resistance can emerge after 2–4 days of treatment due to an amino acid substitution in the M2 protein [88, 89].

Pharmacokinetics

Amantadine is well absorbed. Oral bioavailability, which is 86–92%, and C_{max} are directly related to doses up to 200 mg/day (Table 55.5). In subjects given doses above 200 mg/day, greater increases in C_{max} may occur [85]. An N-acetylated metabolite accounts for 5–15% of the administered dose found in urine. Following 200 mg dose of amantadine, plasma acetylamantadine accounted for 80% of the concurrent amantadine plasma concentration in 5 healthy volunteers, while 7 volunteers did not have any acetylamantadine detected [85]. The C_{max} of amantadine is 0.29 μg/mL, and the time to C_{max} is 1–12 h with a $t_{1/2}$ of 10–45 h [85, 90]. Amantadine Cl_{plasma} is 7–22 L/h and the V_d is 3–12 L/kg and amantadine is 67% plasma protein bound [85, 90, 91].

Amantadine is primarily excreted unchanged in the urine by glomerular filtration and tubular secretion. The Cl_{plasma} is reduced and $t_{1/2}$ and plasma concentrations are increased in elderly patients compared to young adults [85, 92]. These changes could be a result of a decrease in renal function. The Cl_{plasma} of amantadine is reduced and the $t_{1/2}$ increase by 2 to 3 times when CrCl <40 m L/min/1.73m^2 [90]. The $t_{1/2}$ increases

Table 55.5 Pharmacokinetics of antiviral agents for treatment of influenza viruses

	Rimantadine	Amantadine	Oseltamivir	Zanamivir
Maximum concentration (ng/mL)	*Single dose* *100 mg* 74	*Single dose* *100 mg* 220 ± 30 *200 mg* 510 ± 140 *Steady state* *100 mg q12h* 240 ± 40	*Oseltamivir* 65 *Oseltamivir carboxylate* 348	17 to 142
Minimum concentration (ng/mL)	*Steady State* *100 mg q12h* 118 to 468	ND	ND	ND
Time to maximum concentration	*Single dose* *100 mg* 6 h	*Single dose* *100 mg* 3.3 ± 1.5 h *Steady state* 2–4 h	ND	1–2 h
AUC (ng*h/mL)	*Steady state* *100 mg q12h* 30% > single dose	ND	*Oseltamivir* 112 *Oseltamivir carboxylate* 2719	111 to 1364
Clearance (L/h/kg)	ND	*IV* 0.2–0.3	ND	ND
Volume of distribution (V_d)	ND	*IV* 3–8 L/kg	*Oseltamivir carboxylate* 23–26 L	ND
Half-life ($t_{1/2}$)	*Single dose* *100 mg* 25.4 ± 6 h	16–17 h	*Oseltamivir* 1–3 h *Oseltamivir carboxylate* 6–10 h	2.5–5 h
Protein binding	40%	67%	*Oseltamivir* 42% *Oseltamivir carboxylate* 3%	<10%
Bioavailability	ND	ND	ND	4–17%

ND no data available

to 8 days and amantadine is not removed in anuric patients receiving HD with less than 5% removed during a 4-h HD session [90]. After a single 200 mg dose, the maximum nasal mucus concentrations of amantadine after 1, 4, and 8 h were 0.15 μg/g, 0.28 μg/g, and 0.39 μg/g with a C_{max} of 0.42 μg/g, which is 31%, 59%, 95%, and 71% of the plasma concentrations, respectively [92].

Dosing and Drug Interactions

The dose of amantadine for the treatment of influenza A is 100 mg every 12 h for 5 days (Table 55.6). Amantadine should not be used for the treatment of influenza B. Amantadine levels increase when used concurrently with quinidine, quinine, triamterene, or trimethoprim due to decreased renal tubular secretion (Table 55.3). Caution should be taken when amantadine is used with anticholinergic agents due to additive anticholinergic effects (Table 55.4). Furthermore, amantadine should be used with caution when given with agents that prolong the QT interval.

Rimantadine

Mechanism of Action and Resistance

Rimantadine is a symmetric tricyclic amine that inhibits the replication of influenza A virus isolates and has very little to no activity against influenza B [93, 94]. The mechanism of action is similar to amantadine as it prevents the release of viral nucleic acid in the host cell by interfering with the function of the transmembrane domain of the viral M2 protein [88, 89].

Pharmacokinetics

Approximately 90% of a rimantadine dose is absorbed, the C_{max} after a single 100 mg dose of rimantadine is 0.074 μg/mL, and the time to C_{max} is 6 h [95] (Table 55.5). The $t_{1/2}$ after a single dose ranges from 25 to 37 h [95]. In elderly patients aged 71–79 years old, the $t_{1/2}$ is 32 h [95]. Similar to $t_{1/2}$ the AUC also increases by 20–30% in elderly patients.

Rimantadine is metabolized in the liver and only 25% is excreted in the urine as unchanged drug [95]. There are no

Table 55.6 Dose of antiviral agents for treatment of respiratory viruses

Virus	Agent	Route	Usual adult dosage	Duration
Influenza A	Rimantadine	PO	100 mg q12h[a]	7 days[b]
	Amantadine	PO	100 mg q12h[a,c]	5 days[b]
	Oseltamivir	PO	75 mg q12h[a,d]	5 days[b]
	Zanamivir	Oral inhalation	10 mg q12h[e]	5 days[b]
Influenza B	Oseltamivir	PO	75 mg q12h[a,d]	5 days[b]
	Zanamivir	Oral inhalation	10 mg q12h[e]	5 days[b]
Respiratory syncytial virus or human metapneumovirus	Ribavirin	Inhalation	6 g/day[f]	7–10 days

[a]Dose adjustment required for renal insufficiency
[b]Duration prophylaxis for influenza should be continued for at least 10 days following known exposure
[c]Amantadine 200 mg PO q24h can also be used for influenza A
[d]Oseltamivir 75 mg PO q24h for 10 days should be used for prophylaxis of influenza A or B virus
[e]Zanamivir 10 mg inhaled orally q24h for 10 days should be used for prophylaxis of influenza A or B virus
[f]Should be given as 2 g over 2–3 h every 8 h or 6 g over 18 h continuously. Must be administered via Small Particle Aerosol Generator-2 (SPAG-2)

differences in C_{max}, C_{min}, and AUC in patients with normal renal function compared to patients with mild to moderate renal insufficiency (CrCl 30–80 mL/min). However, there is an increase in C_{max} by 75%, C_{min} by 82%, and AUC by 81% in patients with severe renal impairment (CrCl 5–29 mL/min) [95]. In HD patients the $t_{1/2}$ increases by 1.6-fold, and there is a 40% decrease in clearance after a single 200 mg oral dose [95]. Nasal fluid concentrations of rimantadine are 1.5 times higher than plasma concentrations [95].

Dosing and Drug Interactions

The dose of rimantadine for the treatment of influenza A is 100 mg every 12 hours for 5 days (Table 55.6). Rimantadine should not be used for the treatment of influenza B. There are no significant drug-drug interactions with rimantadine (Table 55.3).

Oseltamivir

Mechanism of Action and Resistance

Oseltamivir is an ethyl ester prodrug that requires ester hydrolysis to convert it to the active form, oseltamivir carboxylate, which inhibits influenza virus neuraminidase affecting the release of viral particles [96]. Oseltamivir is absorbed from the GI tract and is converted by hepatic esterases to oseltamivir carboxylate, with less than 5% remaining as oseltamivir [97]. Approximately 75% of the oral dose is found as oseltamivir carboxylate in the systemic circulation [97, 98]. Reduced susceptibility of influenza virus to oseltamivir carboxylate may be due to amino acid substitutions in viral neuraminidase and/or hemagglutinin [99, 100]. Substitutions in hemagglutinin amino acids may reduce viral dependency on neuraminidase activity but do not confer resistance to oseltamivir on their own [99, 101]. Cross-resistance has been observed between zanamivir and oseltamivir; however, some oseltamivir resistance-associated substitutions do not reduce susceptibility to zanamivir [102–105]. There has not been a single amino acid substitution that confers cross-resistance between neuraminidase inhibitors and the M2 ion channel inhibitors, although two separate substitutions may be present in a single virus [101].

Pharmacokinetics

Following multiple doses of oseltamivir 75 mg twice daily, the C_{max} and AUC_{0-12} of oseltamivir are 65 ng/mL and 112 ng*h/mL, and the C_{max} and AUC_{0-12} of oseltamivir carboxylate are 348 ng/mL and 2719 ng*h/mL [97] (Table 55.5). The V_d at steady state of oseltamivir carboxylate following IV administration is 23 to 26 L, and the protein binding is only 3% [97, 98]. The protein binding of oseltamivir is 42%. Approximately 90% of oseltamivir is converted to oseltamivir carboxylate. The $t_{1/2}$ of oseltamivir is 1–3 h, and the $t_{1/2}$ of oseltamivir carboxylate is 6–10 h [96, 97, 106].

Almost all (>99%) of oseltamivir carboxylate is eliminated unchanged in the urine [97]. Oseltamivir carboxylate is removed via renal tubular secretion as well as glomerular filtration [97]. As elimination of oseltamivir carboxylate is via renal clearance, the exposure of oseltamivir carboxylate is inversely proportional to declining renal function. The C_{max} of oseltamivir carboxylate is 494 µg/L in patients with normal renal function (CrCl >90 mL/min) compared to 4052 µg/L in patients with a CrCl <30 mL/min after receiving oseltamivir 100 mg every 12 h. The AUC_{0-12} of oseltamivir carboxylate also increases from 4187 µg*h/L to 43,086 µg*h/L [97]. In patients undergoing HD the C_{max} for oseltamivir carboxylate is 943 ng/mL after a single dose and 1120 ng/mL after repeated doses [107]. Oseltamivir carboxylate exposure is not different in patients with mild to moderate hepatic impairment [98, 108].

Pharmacokinetics in Pediatric Patients

Pediatric patients clear oseltamivir and oseltamivir carboxylate faster than adults, resulting in lower drug exposure [109]. The Cl_{total} of oseltamivir carboxylate decreases linearly with increasing age up to 12 years. The pharmacokinetics of oseltamivir carboxylate in children >12 years old is similar to adults [109].

Dosing and Drug Interactions

The dose of oseltamivir for the treatment of influenza A or B is 75 mg every 12 h and the dose for prophylaxis is 75 mg every 24 h (Table 55.6). Oseltamivir levels may be increased if used with probenecid due to decreased renal tubular secretion (Table 55.3).

Zanamivir

Mechanism of Action and Resistance

Zanamivir is an orally inhaled inhibitor of influenza virus neuraminidase that affects the release of viral particles [110]. Reduced susceptibility in cell culture to zanamivir is associated with mutations that result in amino acid changes in the viral neuraminidase, viral hemagglutinin, or both [101]. Cross-resistance has been observed between some zanamivir-resistant and oseltamivir-resistant influenza viruses [101]. The Q136K zanamivir resistance-associated substitution observed in N1 neuraminidase confers resistance to zanamivir but not oseltamivir [101].

Pharmacokinetics

After inhalation, approximately 13% of the dose is deposited in the lungs and 78% in the oropharynx [111] (Table 55.5). The C_{max} in serum occurs within 2 h after an inhaled dose of zanamivir [112]. Zanamivir has limited protein binding of <10%, and 90% of the drug is excreted unchanged in the urine after intravenous administration, whereas only 4% of the dose is recovered in the urine after intranasal administration [112]. The $t_{1/2}$ of zanamivir after inhalation is 3.6 h [112].

Pharmacokinetics in Pediatric Patients

Serum zanamivir concentrations in pediatric patients ≤5 years of age was similar to adults after administration of inhaled zanamivir 10 mg (183 ng*h/L vs. 194 ng*h/L, respectively) [113].

Dosing and Drug Interactions

The dose of zanamivir for the treatment of influenza A or B is 10 mg via inhaler every 12 h and the dose for prophylaxis is 10 mg via inhaler every 24 h (Table 55.6). There are no significant drug-drug interactions with zanamivir (Table 55.3).

Anti-hepatitis Virus Agents

Adefovir Dipivoxil

Mechanism of Action and Resistance

Adefovir is an acyclic nucleotide analogue of adenosine monophosphate. Once phosphorylated by cellular kinases to the active metabolite, adefovir diphosphate, it inhibits *Hepatitis B virus* (HBV) DNA polymerase and reverse transcriptase, by competing with deoxyadenosine triphosphate causing DNA chain termination after incorporation into viral DNA [114]. Adefovir dipivoxil is a prodrug and is rapidly converted to the active agent adefovir. Amino acid substitutions rtN236T and rtA181T/V are the primary mutations that are associated with adefovir resistance causing a two- to ninefold decrease in susceptibility to adefovir [115–118]. Adefovir resistance-associated substitution rtA181V is also associated with decreased susceptibility to lamivudine [116].

Pharmacokinetics

The bioavailability of adefovir after administration of adefovir dipivoxil is 59% [114]. The C_{max} of adefovir is 18 to 19 ng/mL after a single oral dose of 10 mg of adefovir dipivoxil, and the time to C_{max} is 2 h [114, 119] (Table 55.7). The AUC of adefovir is 204 ng*h/mL and the $t_{1/2}$ is 7.1–7.5 h [114, 119]. The plasma protein binding of adefovir is <4%. The V_d at steady state is 392 mL/kg after IV administration of 1 mg/kg/day of adefovir and 352 mL/kg after 3 mg/kg/day [114].

Adefovir is excreted by glomerular filtration and active renal tubular secretion; 40–45% of the adefovir dipivoxil dose was recovered as adefovir in the urine 24 h after administration [114, 119, 120]. In patients who receive 10 mg/day of adefovir dipivoxil suspension with a CrCl 50–79 mL/min, the C_{max} is 34 ng/mL and the AUC is 361 ng*h/mL at 48 weeks [121]. In patients with CrCl 20–49 mL/min who receive 5 mg/day, the C_{max} is 20 ng/mL and the AUC is 277 ng*h/mL at 48 weeks [121]. For patients undergoing HD who receive 1 mg × 1 followed by 0.5 mg three times weekly, the C_{max} is 10 ng/mL at week 12 and the AUC is 213 ng*h/mL. Plasma concentrations of adefovir decrease by 70–90% after HD [121].

Pharmacokinetics in Pediatric Patients

The pharmacokinetics of adefovir dipivoxil has been evaluated in pediatric patients with chronic hepatitis B [122]. In children aged 2–6 years, the C_{max} and AUC were 15 ng/mL and 105 ng*h/mL, respectively, following 0.14 mg/kg of adefovir dipivoxil dose. The C_{max} and AUC were 27 ng/mL and 224 ng*h/mL, respectively following 0.3 mg/kg of adefovir dipivoxil. In children aged 7–11 years who receive 0.14 mg/kg dose, the C_{max} was 14 ng/mL, and the AUC was 129 ng*h/mL compared to 33 ng/mL and 292 ng*h/mL for children who receive 0.3 mg/kg, respectively. For adolescents aged 12–17 years who were given 10 mg dose, the C_{max} was 23 ng/mL, and the AUC was 237 ng*h/mL and was similar to parameters noted in adults [122].

Dosing and Drug Interactions

The dose of adefovir for the treatment of chronic HBV is 10 mg every 24 h (Table 55.8). The use of ibuprofen with adefovir may increase the bioavailability of adefovir (Table 55.3). The combination of adefovir and ribavirin may increase the risk of hepatotoxicity and the use of adefovir with aminoglycosides, amphotericin B, cyclosporine, tacrolimus, or vancomycin may enhance the risk for nephrotoxicity (Table 55.4).

Table 55.7 Pharmacokinetics of antiviral agents for treatment of hepatitis viruses

	Adefovir	Entecavir	Lamivudine	Tenofovir	Telaprevir	Boceprevir	Ribavirin	Interferons
Maximum concentration (ng/mL)	*Single dose* *10 mg* 18.4 ± 6.26	*Steady state* *0.5 mg* 4.2 *1 mg* 8.2	*Single dose* *100 mg* 1280 ± 560	*Single dose* *300 mg* 300 ± 90	*Steady state* *75 0 mg* 3510 ± 1280	*Steady state* *800 mg* 1723	*Single dose* *600 mg* 782 *Steady state* *1200 mg/day* 2748 ± 8118	ND
Minimum concentration (ng/mL)	ND	ND	ND	ND	*Steady state* 2030 ± 930	*Steady state* 88	*Steady state* *800 mg/day* 1662 ± 545 *1200 mg/day* 2112 ± 810	ND
Time to maximum concentration	0.58–4 h	0.5–1.5 h	0.5–2 h	1 h	4–5 h	ND	1.7–2 h	*Nonpegylated* 3–12 hours *Pegylated* *Alfa-2b* 15–44 h *Alfa-2a* 72–96 h
AUC (ng*h/mL)	220 ± 70	27.9	*Single dose* *100 mg* 4300 ± 1400 *Steady state* 4700 ± 1700	*Single dose* 2290 ± 690	*Steady state* 22,300 ± 8650	*Steady state* 5408	*Single dose* *600 mg* 13,400 *Steady state* *1200 mg/day* 25,361 ± 7110	ND
Clearance	ND	ND	*Renal clearance* 199.7 ± 56.9 mL/min	ND	ND	*Total clearance* 161 L/h	*Total clearance* 26 L/h	*Pegylated* 94 mL/h
Volume of distribution (V_d)	*Steady state* *1 mg/kg/day IV* 392 mL/kg *3 mg/kg/day IV* 352 ± 9 mL/kg	ND	1.3 ± 0.4 L/kg	*Steady state* *1 mg/kg IV infusion* 1.13 ± 0.6 L/kg *3 mg/kg IV infusion* 1.32 L/kg	252 L	*Steady state* 772 L	ND	*Nonpegylated* 31 L
Half-life ($t_{1/2}$)	7.5 h	128–149 h	ND	ND	*Single dose* 4–4.7 h *Steady state* 9–11 h	3	*Single dose* 120–170 h	*Nonpegylated* 2–3 h *Pegylated* 160 h
Protein binding	<4%	13%	<36%	7%	59–76%	75%	ND	ND
Bioavailability	59%	ND	*150 mg* 86%	25%	ND	ND	64%	*Nonpegylated* 90%

ND no data available

Table 55.8 Dose of antiviral agents for treatment of hepatitis viruses

Virus	Agent	Route	Usual adult dosage	Duration
Chronic hepatitis C	Telaprevir[a,b]	PO	750 mg q8h[c]	12 weeks[d]
	Boceprevir[a,b]	PO	800 mg q8h	Based on virologic response[e]
	Ribavirin	PO	800–1400 mg/day in 2 divided doses[f,g,h]	48 weeks[i]
		PO	800–1200 mg/day in 2 divided doses[f,g,j,k]	48 weeks[i]
	Peg-interferon-alfa-2a	SQ	180 μg weekly[f,l]	48 weeks[i]
	Peg-interferon-alfa-2b	SQ	1.5 μg weekly[f,l]	48 weeks[i]
Chronic hepatitis B	Adefovir dipivoxil	PO	10 mg q24h[f]	
	Entecavir	PO	0.5–1 mg q24h[f,m]	
	Lamivudine	PO	100 mg q24h[f]	
	Tenofovir	PO	300 mg q24h[f]	

[a]Telaprevir and boceprevir should only be used in patients infected with Hepatitis C Virus genotype-1
[b]Should always be used in combination with peg-interferon-alfa and ribavirin
[c]No data is available regarding use in renal insufficiency
[d]Continued treatment with peg-interferon-alfa and ribavirin is based on clinical response. The three-drug regimen should be discontinued at week 4 or 12 if viral RNA levels are ≥1000 international units/mL. Peg-interferon-alfa and ribavirin should be discontinued if viral RNA levels are detectable at week 24
[e]Boceprevir should be added to peg-interferon-alfa and ribavirin after 4 weeks of treatment. The three-drug regimen should be discontinued at week 12 if viral RNA levels ≥100 international units/mL or at week 24 if confirmed detectable viral-RNA levels
[f]Dose adjustment required for renal insufficiency
[g]Should be used in combination with interferon-alfa ± boceprevir or telaprevir
[h]Rebetol® dose is based on weight and is approved for use in combination with peg-interferon-alfa-2b for patients following prior treatment failure in compensated liver disease
[i]Duration of therapy should be 24 weeks for patients infected with HCV-genotype-2 or -3
[j]Copegus® should be used in combination with peg-interferon-alfa-2a for interferon-alfa naïve patients with compensated liver disease
[k]Ribavirin dose should be 1000–1200mg/day for HCV-genotype-1 or -4, and 800mg/day for HCV-genotype-2
[l]Should be used in combination with ribavirin +/- boceprevir or telaprevir
[m]Entecavir 1mg PO q24h should be used for lamivudine-refractory or -resistant HCV or for patients with decompensated liver disease

Entecavir

Mechanism of Action and Resistance

Entecavir is a guanine nucleoside analogue with activity against HBV reverse transcriptase. Entecavir must be phosphorylated to the active triphosphate form, which competes with the natural substrate deoxyguanosine triphosphate to functionally inhibit base priming, reverse transcription of the negative strand from the pregenomic messenger RNA, and synthesis of the positive strand of HBV DNA [123–125]. Entecavir is also a weak inhibitor of cellular DNA polymerases and mitochondrial DNA polymerase [123–125]. There is a slight reduction in entecavir susceptibility observed for lamivudine-resistant strains [126]. A reduction in entecavir susceptibility is seen in the presence of rtM204I/V substitutions with or without rtL180M. Additional substitutions at rt184, rtS202, and rtM250, or a combination of these may also reduce susceptibility to entecavir [127].

Pharmacokinetics

The C_{max} of entecavir at steady state is 4.2 ng/mL following a 0.5 mg dose and 8.2 ng/mL after a 1 mg dose [128, 129] (Table 55.7). The C_{max} occurs between 0.5 and 1.5 h after the dose [129]. The C_{max} and AUC at steady state increase proportionally to the dose. Administration of entecavir with a high fat containing meal or a light meal causes a delay in absorption, a decrease in C_{max} of 45%, and a decrease in AUC of 20% [129]. Protein binding of entecavir is 13%, and the apparent V_d is in excess of total body water [129]. The terminal $t_{1/2}$ of entecavir is approximately 128–149 h [128, 129].

Entecavir is primarily cleared by the kidneys; 62–73% of unchanged drug was recovered in urine [129]. Entecavir undergoes both glomerular filtration and net tubular secretion [128]. The C_{max} of entecavir increases to 10.4 ng/mL in patients with CrCl 50–80 mL/min, 15.3 ng/mL in patients with CrCl of <30 mL/min, and 15.4 ng/mL in patients undergoing HD [128]. The pharmacokinetics of entecavir is similar in patients with normal hepatic function compared to patients with moderate or severe hepatic dysfunction [129].

Dosing and Drug Interactions

The dose of entecavir for the treatment of chronic HBV is 0.5 mg every 24 h (Table 55.8). Entecavir 1 mg every 24 h should be used for patients with lamivudine resistant or refractory HBV infection or those with hepatic decompensation. The use of entecavir and ribavirin may increase the risk of hepatotoxicity (Table 55.4).

Lamivudine

Mechanism of Action and Resistance

Lamivudine is a synthetic nucleoside analogue, which is phosphorylated to its active 5′-triphosphate metabolite, lamivudine triphosphate [130]. The monophosphate form is incorporated into viral DNA by HBV reverse transcriptase that results in DNA chain termination. Lamivudine triphosphate also inhibits the RNA- and DNA-dependent DNA polymerase activities of HIV-1 reverse transcriptase [130]. Lamivudine resistance results from M204 V/I substitution in the viral reverse transcriptase [131]. HBV containing lamivudine resistance-associated substitutions may still retain susceptibility to adefovir dipivoxil; however, such viral strains may have a 30-fold reduced susceptibility to entecavir [131]. The substitution rtA181T will also result in decreased response to entecavir [131]. Entecavir-resistance HBV exhibit 1000-fold reduced susceptibility to lamivudine [131].

Pharmacokinetics

Lamivudine is rapidly absorbed after oral administration with a C_{max} in HBV infected patients of 1.3 μg/mL following a single dose of 100 mg [132] (Table 55.7). The time to C_{max} occurs between 0.5 and 2 hours after the dose is administered [132]. The AUC following a single 100 mg dose of lamivudine is 4.3 μg*h/mL, and the AUC at steady state following repeated doses is 4.7 μg*h/mL [132]. There is no difference in AUC in fasting or fed states, although C_{max} may be lower. The bioavailability of lamivudine is 86% after a dose of 150 mg tablet and 87% after 10 mg/mL oral solution with a $t_{1/2}$ of approximately 5 hours [133, 134]. Plasma protein binding is <36%, and the V_d after IV administration of lamivudine in HIV patients is 1.3 L/kg, which suggests that it distributes widely into extravascular space [132, 133]. Five to ten percent of a 300 mg dose of lamivudine is excreted as a trans-sulfoxide metabolite in the urine [132]. The serum concentration of the trans-sulfoxide metabolite has not been measured [132].

Lamivudine is eliminated in the urine as unchanged drug by active cationic secretion Cl_{renal} accounting for 71% of total drug clearance [135]. Compared to patients with normal renal function, patients with moderate to severe renal impairment have 4- to 13-fold increases in AUC and a 1.2- to 1.8-fold longer half-life [132, 135]. A 4-hour HD session does not affect the overall exposure of lamivudine due to the large V_d even though 50% of lamivudine is extracted from plasma [132, 136]. The pharmacokinetic parameters of lamivudine are not significantly altered by reduced hepatic function. After a single dose of 300 mg of lamivudine, the C_{max} is 2.6 μg/mL in patients with normal hepatic function compared to 2.9 μg/mL in patients with moderate hepatic impairment and 3.1 μg/mL patients with severe hepatic impairment. The AUC is also similar between patients with normal hepatic function (11.8 μg*h/mL) and moderate (11.4 μg*h/mL) to severe (12.8 μg*h/mL) hepatic impairment [137].

Pharmacokinetics in Pediatric Patients

In neonates, the median $t_{1/2}$ of lamivudine is 6 h, the C_{max} is 1969 μg/L, and the AUC is 16,883 μg*h/L when a dose of 4 mg/kg every 12 h is administered for 1 week [138]. In infants and adolescents, lamivudine is rapidly absorbed with a time to C_{max} of 0.5 to 1 h. The C_{max} and AUC of lamivudine are proportional to the dose for patients aged 2–12 years; however, the absolute bioavailability is reduced by 59% [132, 139]. The mean AUC in patients <12 years old receiving 4 mg/kg is 5056 μg*h/L, which is roughly half of the adult dose [132, 139].

Dosing and Drug Interactions

The dose of lamivudine for the treatment of chronic HBV is 100 mg every 24 h (Table 55.6). Use of trimethoprim with lamivudine may increase the levels of lamivudine due to decreased renal tubular secretions (Table 55.3). Lamivudine given along with ribavirin may increase the risk for hepatotoxicity (Table 55.4).

Tenofovir Disoproxil Fumarate

Mechanism of Action and Resistance

Tenofovir disoproxil fumarate (TDF) is an acyclic nucleoside phosphate diester analogue of adenosine monophosphate. TDF requires initial diester hydrolysis for conversion to tenofovir and subsequent phosphorylation by cellular enzymes to form tenofovir diphosphate [140]. Tenofovir diphosphate inhibits the activity of HBV reverse transcriptase by competing with the natural substrate deoxyadenosine 5′-triphosphate and incorporates into DNA causing chain termination [141]. Tenofovir has demonstrated the highest barrier to resistance in clinical studies [142, 143]. Tenofovir has been shown to be effective in patients with lamivudine resistance and in patients with an incomplete response to adefovir, but not necessarily in all patients with adefovir resistance [142, 144].

Pharmacokinetics

The oral bioavailability of tenofovir in fasting patients was 25%, and the C_{max} after a single dose in HIV-1 infected individuals was 0.2 μg/mL to 0.3 μg/mL, which is reached in 1 h, and the AUC is 2.3–2.5 μg*h/mL [141, 145, 146] (Table 55.7). Protein binding of tenofovir is 7% and the V_d at steady state is 1.3 L/kg [141]. After a single oral dose, the $t_{1/2}$ of tenofovir was 17 h, whereas intracellular half-life was 95 hours [147]. Administration of TDF with a high-fat meal increases oral bioavailability, and AUC and C_{max} are increased by 40% and 14%, respectively. Albeit, administration of light meal has not affected the bioavailability of the drug [141, 145].

Approximately 70–80% of the tenofovir dose is recovered unchanged in the urine within 72 h after IV administration [148]. Tenofovir is eliminated via a combination of glomerular filtration and active tubular secretion [141]. After a single dose of 300 mg of TDF, the C_{max} is 0.34 µg/mL in patients with CrCl ≥80 mL/min, 0.33 µg/mL in patients with CrCl 50–80 mL/min, 0.37 µg/mL in patients with CrCl 30–49 mL/min, and 0.60 µg/mL in patients with CrCl 12–29 mL/min [146]. The AUC is 2.2 µg*h/mL in patients CrCl >80 mL/min compared to 3.1 µg*h/mL in patients with CrCl of 50–80 mL/min, 6.0 µg*h/mL in patients with CrCl 30–49 mL/min, and 15.9 µg*h/mL in patients with CrCl 12–29 mL/min [146]. Approximately 10% of tenofovir is removed during a 4-hour HD session following a single 300 mg dose of TDF [149]. There are no differences in tenofovir pharmacokinetics in patients with moderate or severe hepatic impairment [146, 149].

Pharmacokinetics in Pediatric Patients

Tenofovir exposure in pediatric patients aged 2–18 is similar to adult patients with a C_{max} of 0.27 µg/mL and an AUC of 2.2 µg*h/mL [150].

Dosing and Drug Interactions

The dose of TDF for the treatment of HBV is 300 mg every 24 h (Table 55.8). Tenofovir is an inhibitor of CYP 450 1A2; therefore, tenofovir will decrease the hepatic metabolism of theophylline and zidovudine causing increased concentrations of these agents (Table 55.3). Tenofovir is also an inducer of p-glycoprotein (P-gp), which may thereby increase dabigatran and linagliptin elimination.

Telaprevir

Mechanism of Action and Resistance

Telaprevir is an inhibitor of the hepatitis C Virus (HCV) NS3/4A serine protease, necessary for the proteolytic cleavage of the HCV-encoded polyprotein into mature forms of the NS4A, NS4B, NS5A, and NS5B proteins and essential for viral replication. In a biochemical assay, telaprevir inhibits the proteolytic activity of the recombinant HCV NS3 protease domain [151]. Resistance to telaprevir is due to genetic changes in the RNA that codes for the amino acid residues of the NS3/NS4A protease active site [152–154]. In treatment naïve patients, high levels of HCV variants conferring telaprevir resistance were uncommon. However, resistance may develop in patients undergoing treatment, although the incidence is low in patients receiving combination therapy with ribavirin and peg-interferon-alfa [152, 155, 156].

Pharmacokinetics

The pharmacokinetic properties of telaprevir have been evaluated in healthy adult individuals and in patients with chronic HCV infection (Table 55.7). After multiple doses of telaprevir (750 mg every 8 h) in combination with peg-interferon-alfa and ribavirin in treatment-naïve subjects with genotype 1 with chronic HCV infection, the C_{max} is 4036–4523 ng/mL, C_{min} is 2476 to 2624 ng/mL, and the AUC is 80,420 to 85,890 ng*h/mL [157, 158]. Telaprevir is absorbed from the small intestine, there is no evidence of absorption in the colon [151, 158]. Plasma C_{max} after a single oral dose were generally achieved after 4–5 h. Exposure to telaprevir is higher during coadministration with peg-interferon-alfa and ribavirin compared with telaprevir given alone [151]. The AUC of telaprevir increases by 237% when it was administered with a standard fat meal compared to fasting conditions [151, 159]. When telaprevir is administered with a low-fat meal, the AUC increases by 117% compared to 330% with a meal high in fat content [151, 159]. Protein binding of telaprevir was 59–76% and it binds primarily to alpha 1-acid glycoprotein and albumin. Protein binding was concentration dependent, decreasing with higher telaprevir concentrations [151, 159]. The V_d after oral administration of telaprevir was 252 L [151, 159]. The $t_{1/2}$ after a 750 mg single oral dose ranged from 4.0 to 4.7 h and at steady state, the $t_{1/2}$ was 9 to 11 h [151, 159]. Telaprevir is extensively metabolized in the liver with multiple active and inactive metabolites detected in feces, plasma, and urine. Cytochrome p450 3A4 (CYP3A4) is responsible for telaprevir metabolism; however, non-CYP-mediated metabolism may play a role after multiple doses. Telaprevir is also a substrate of P-glycoprotein (P-gp) [151, 159].

Approximately 82% of telaprevir is recovered within 96 h in feces and only 1% in urine after a single 750 mg dose. Unchanged drug accounts for 32% of the recovered dose, while 19% is the R-diastereomer [151, 159]. The AUC of telaprevir decreases by 46% in HCV-negative patients with moderate hepatic impairment (Child-Pugh Class B) compared to healthy patients. In patients with mild hepatic impairment (Child-Pugh Class A), the AUC is only reduced by 15% in HCV-negative subjects [151, 159]. Patients with cirrhosis have similar pharmacokinetic parameters compared to those without cirrhosis in whom telaprevir was used in combination with peg-interferon-alfa and ribavirin. Compared with healthy adults, in patients with CrCl of <30 mL/min, C_{max} and AUC increased by 3% and 21%, respectively, after a single 750 mg telaprevir dose [151, 159].

Dosing and Drug Interactions

The dose of telaprevir for the treatment of HCV is 750 mg every 8 h in combination with peg-interferon-alfa and ribavirin (Table 55.8). Telaprevir is a substrate of CYP450 3A4; therefore, concurrent use with CYP450 3A4 inhibitors, such as amiodarone and voriconazole, will result in increased telaprevir levels (Table 55.3). A reduced telaprevir concentration may occur when given with CYP450 3A4 inducers, such as carbamazepine, efavirenz, rifampin, and phenytoin. Telaprevir is also an inhibitor of CYP450 3A4 and p-glycoprotein; therefore the use of telaprevir with substrates of either enzymes will cause increased concentrations of those substrates due to reduced hepatic metabolism.

Boceprevir

Mechanism of Action and Resistance

Boceprevir is an inhibitor of the HCV NS3/4A protease that is necessary for the proteolytic cleavage of the HCV encoded polyprotein into mature forms [160, 161]. Boceprevir forms a covalent, yet reversible bond to the NS3 protease active serine site to inhibit viral replication in HCV-infected cells [160, 161]. Monotherapy with NS3/4 protease inhibitors results in rapid selection of resistant viral strains [162, 163]. The activity of boceprevir against the HCV NS3/4A protease or genotype 1b is reduced by amino acid substitutions in the NS3 protease domain [162, 164]. Patients who filed to respond to boceprevir therapy are more likely to have boceprevir-resistant mutants at the end of treatment [162]. Treatment-emergent NS3 amino acid substitutions detected in boceprevir-treated subjects, in whom SVR was not achieved, demonstrate a reduced activity of other HCV NS3/4A protease inhibitors [162, 165, 166].

Pharmacokinetics

Boceprevir capsules contain a 1:1 mixture of two diastereomers, which change to a 2:1 ratio, favoring the active diastereomer in plasma. Boceprevir demonstrates linear pharmacokinetics and the oral bioavailability is 26–34% in animals [167] (Table 55.7). After a single dose of boceprevir 400 mg, the C_{max} and AUC are 557 ng/mL and 2020 ng*h/mL in healthy subjects [168]. After receiving 400 mg every 8 h for 7 days, the AUC and C_{max} of boceprevir in HCV-positive patients were 1990 ng*h/mL and 523 ng/mL, respectively [169]. In subjects who receive monotherapy with 800 mg every 8 h, the AUC was 5408 ng*h/mL, and the C_{max} was 1723 ng/mL [162]. The time to C_{max} after oral administration was 2 h; AUC, C_{max}, and C_{min} all increase in a less-than-dose-proportional manner, indicating decreased absorption at higher dose concentrations [162, 167]. The AUC of boceprevir when administered as 800 mg every 8 h is 65% higher when it is given with food compared to given in a fasting state [162]. However, there is no difference whether it is given with a high or low fat meal [162]. The V_d at steady state was 772 L and 75% protein binding after a single dose [167]. The $t_{1/2}$ of boceprevir is approximately 3 h with a Cl_{total} of 161 L/h [162].

The primary mechanism of metabolism of boceprevir is through the aldo-keto reductase (AKR)-mediated pathway, which produces inactive metabolites [162, 168, 170]. Boceprevir also undergoes oxidative metabolism mediated by CYP3A4/5, although this is to a lesser extent [161, 168, 169]. Approximately 79% of the boceprevir dose is excreted in feces compared to only 9% in urine [162]. The mean AUC of the active diastereomer of boceprevir is 2050 ng*h/mL and 2690 ng*h/mL in subjects with moderate (Child-Pugh 7–9) and severe (Child-Pugh 10–12) hepatic impairment compared to 2020 ng*h/mL in normal patients following a single 400 mg dose of boceprevir [168]. Subjects with mild hepatic impairment have similar active diastereomer exposure as subjects with normal hepatic function. The mean AUC of boceprevir is 10% lower in subjects undergoing HD relative to subjects with normal renal function after a single dose of 800 mg of boceprevir [168]. Hemodialysis removes less than 1% of the boceprevir dose.

Dosing and Drug Interactions

The dose of boceprevir for the treatment of HCV is 800 mg every 8 h in combination with peg-interferon-alfa and ribavirin (Table 55.8). Boceprevir is a substrate of CYP450 3A4 therefore concurrent use with CYP450 3A4 inhibitors will cause an increase in boceprevir levels and concurrent use with CYP450 3A4 inducers will result in decrease boceprevir concentration (Table 55.3). Boceprevir is a strong inhibitor of CYP450 3A4, and concomitant boceprevir use with amiodarone, cyclosporine, simvastatin, tacrolimus, voriconazole, and warfarin will reduce their hepatic metabolism and potentially lead to toxic drug concentration unless appropriate dose adjustment has been undertaken. Boceprevir is also an inhibitor of p-glycoprotein, causing increases in digoxin and rivaroxaban concentrations.

Ribavirin

Mechanism of Action and Resistance

Ribavirin has direct antiviral activity in tissue culture against many RNA viruses, and increases the frequency of genomic mutation among several RNA viruses. Ribavirin triphosphate inhibits HCV polymerase in a biochemical reaction; the precise mechanism that confers antiviral activity of ribavirin is not known [171–173]. The combination of peg-interferon-alfa-2a and ribavirin is more effective at inhibiting HCV RNA replication than either agent alone [171]. Several studies have suggested that ribavirin has immunomodulatory effects, and HCV-specific T-cell responses have been observed in patients on combination therapy with interferon; however, this effect may be due to the reduction in viral load [171, 174]. Evidence of immunomodulation by ribavirin acting synergistically with interferon is lacking, but the loss of infected HCV cells by immune-mediated damage is thought to underlie the second phase decline in HCV RNA following interferon use [171, 175–177]. Ribavirin has been shown to enhance this second phase decline, suggesting that it also has an immunomodulatory effect [171, 176, 178]. It is suggested that the faster decline in HCV RNA with combination therapy may be related to ribavirin-induced restoration of hosts' immune response and perhaps independent of concurrent interferon use [171, 177]. This suggests that ribavirin may garner hosts' anti-HCV immune response; however, mechanism and immune pathways to support this hypothesis remain evasive [171].

Pharmacokinetics

After a single dose of 600 mg of ribavirin, the C_{max} and AUC were 782 ng/mL and 13,400 ng*h/mL, respectively, and time to C_{max} was 1.7 h [171, 179, 180] (Table 55.7). The $t_{1/2}$ after a single oral dose of ribavirin was 120–170 h and ribavirin tends to accumulate, therefore the C_{max} is higher after multiple doses [171]. Following multiple 600 mg twice-daily doses of ribavirin, C_{max} was 3677 ng/mL, a fivefold increase compared to single-dose therapy [171, 180]. The AUC after multiple doses also increased to 227,867 ng*h/mL, and the terminal $t_{1/2}$ was higher (274–298 h) [171, 173]. The absolute bioavailability of ribavirin after oral administration was 64% [171, 181]. When a single dose of ribavirin was given with a meal high in fat content the time to C_{max} was extended. The $AUC_{0\text{-}192h}$ and C_{max} increased by 42%, and 66%, respectively, when given with a high fat meal compared to fasting state [182]. Administration of ribavirin with antacids caused a 14% reduction in the AUC after a single dose [182]. Ribavirin is not a substrate of CYP450 enzymes, and the exact mechanism of elimination and metabolism is not known [171].

Ribavirin is also available as an aerosol for inhalation for treatment of respiratory syncytial virus (RSV) and human metapneumovirus (hMNV) [183]. After administration of aerosolized ribavirin by facemask for 2.5 h three times daily, the plasma concentrations ranged from 0.44 to 1.55 μmol/L after 3 days of therapy. When administered by facemask or mist tent for 20 h each day, the plasma concentration ranged from 1.5 to 14.3 μmol/L after 5 days of therapy [184].

The clearance of ribavirin is reduced in subjects with CrCl of ≤50 mL/min, including those undergoing HD. The clearance is reduced by approximately 30% compared to subjects with normal renal function. In patients with end-stage kidney disease on HD who were given a 200 mg daily dose, the ribavirin exposure was 20% lower compared to patients with normal renal function who received standard ribavirin dose [182]. Approximately 50% of plasma ribavirin is removed by HD; however, the plasma exposure should not change with HD because of the large V_d of ribavirin [182]. Hepatic dysfunction (Child-Pugh A, B, or C) has no effect on ribavirin AUC when compared to patients with intact liver function [171, 179].

Pharmacokinetics in Pediatric Patients

The pharmacokinetics of ribavirin is similar in adults and pediatric patients. The C_{max} and AUC were 3275 ng/mL and 29,774 ng*h/mL, respectively, after 15 mg/kg daily dose given in two divided doses [185]. The 2-h time to C_{max} was also similar [185].

Dosing and Drug Interactions

The dose of ribavirin for the treatment of HCV ranges from 1000 to 1200 mg daily given in combination with peg-interferon-alfa (Table 55.8). The dose of ribavirin for treatment of RSV is 6 g per day administered via a Small Particle Aerosol Generator-2 (SPAG-2) nebulizer. The use of oral ribavirin with adefovir, lamivudine, or entecavir may increase the risk of hepatotoxicity (Table 55.4).

Interferon

Mechanism of Action and Resistance

Interferons exert a vast array of biological functions, including development of innate immunity, and cellular and humoral adaptive immune responses, as well as exhibiting direct antiviral activity [186]. Interferons bind to high-affinity receptors on the surface of virus-infected cells, which activate an intracellular signal transduction pathway that results in rapid activation of gene transcription for proteins that inhibit viral protein translation and RNAases leading to inhibit of viral replication [187–189]. In addition to the direct antiviral effect, interferons cause an upregulation of major histocompatibility complex (MHC) class-I and class-II molecules; an increase in IL-10, IL-12, and TNF-α production; and activation of dendritic cells [190–194].

Pharmacokinetics

After subcutaneously administered, approximately 80% of the interferon-alfa dose is absorbed [195] (Table 55.7). The C_{max} occurs after 1–8 h, followed by a measureable concentration for 4–24 h after administration [195]. The V_d of interferon-alfa is 12–40 L with a terminal $t_{1/2}$ of 4–16 h [195]. Wide fluctuations in serum concentrations of interferon-alfa have been observed, which may result in impaired suppression of viral replication [196]. The development of pegylated interferon (peg-interferon) has greatly improved the poor pharmacokinetic profile of nonpegylated conventional interferon, delaying its clearance and allowing it to be given less frequently while ensuring effective concentrations [196].

The V_d for peg-interferon-alfa-2a was 4–16 L, and it distributes primarily in the blood and interstitial fluid resulting in high concentrations in the liver [196]. A single dose of peg-interferon-alfa-2a produces a C_{max} of 14.2 mg/L in a mean duration of 78 h [197]. After administration of multiple doses of peg-interferon-alfa-2a to patients with chronic

HCV infection, the C_{max} was 25.6 mg/L in a mean duration of 45 h [197]. Peg-interferon-alfa-2a has a low peak to trough ratio indicating less fluctuation in the serum concentration of the drug during the weekly dosing interval. Peg-interferon-alfa-2a is cleared by both the kidney and the liver; due to its large size, the pharmacokinetics of the drug is unaffected in patients with renal failure [197].

Peg-interferon-alfa-2b has a smaller polymer attached causing it to have a slightly different pharmacokinetic profile to peg-interferon-alfa-2a. Peg-interferon-alfa-2b reaches a C_{max} after 15–44 h, which is sustained for 48–72 h after the dose [196]. Peg-interferon-alfa-2b had a V_d of 0.99 L/kg [187]. The absorption $t_{1/2}$ of peg-interferon-alfa-2b was 4–5 h compared to 50 h for peg-interferon-alfa-2a [187]. Free interferon-alfa-2b is released from the pegylated form soon after administration and undergoes renal excretion, whereas interferon-alfa-2a does not get released and the pegylated form interacts with cell surface receptors. The C_{max} and AUC of peg-interferon-alfa-2b increases in a dose-related manner and week 48, and C_{min} is threefold higher than C_{min} observed at week 4 [198]. Renal elimination accounts for 30% of the clearance of peg-interferon-alfa-2b [198].

Pharmacokinetics in Pediatric Patients

The clearance of peg-interferon-alfa-2a in children is nearly fourfold lower compared to the clearance reported in adults, although the steady-state trough levels in children with a body surface area (BSA)-adjusted dosing are similar to trough levels observed in adults given 180 μg fixed dosing [199]. Time to reach the steady state in children is approximately 12 weeks, whereas in adults, steady state is reached within 5–8 weeks. In children receiving the BSA-adjusted dose, the AUC during the dosing interval is 25–70% higher than that observed in adults receiving 180 μg fixed dosing [199].

Dosing and Drug Interactions

The dose of peg-interferon-alfa-2a for the treatment of HCV in adults is 180 μg subcutaneously once weekly in combination with ribavirin, while the dose for peg-interferon-alfa-2b is 1.5 μg/kg subcutaneously once weekly in combination with ribavirin (Table 55.8). The use of interferon-alfa with aldesleukin can cause increased myocardial and renal toxicity (Table 55.4). Interferon-alfa is an inhibitor of CYP450 1A2; therefore, the concentrations of theophylline and zidovudine will increase due to reduced hepatic metabolism, when used concurrently with interferon-alfa (Table 55.3).

Summary

Intense research has led to introduction of a number of new agents available to treat infections caused by major viral pathogens among the highly susceptible patients undergoing hematopoietic stem cell and solid organ transplantation. Clinicians caring for such patients face ongoing challenge in selection of the best drug therapy of various viral illness. The understanding and application of pharmacokinetics and pharmacodynamics principles may improve selection of appropriate agent or regimens, dose optimization, minimization for potential drug-drug interaction, and avoidance of drug toxicity when possible in the vulnerable transplant population.

References

1. Wasley A, Grytdal S, Gallagher K. Surveillance for acute viral hepatitis—United States, 2006. MMWR Morb Mortal Wkly Rep. 2008;57(SS-2):1–24.
2. Piret J, Boivin G. Resistance of herpes simplex viruses to nucleoside analogues: mechanisms, prevalence, and management. Antimicrob Agents Chemother. 2011;55(2):459–72.
3. Estimates of deaths associated with seasonal influenza—United States, 1976–2007. MMWR Morb Mortal Wkly Rep. 2010;59(33):1057–89.
4. Dawood FS, Iuliano AD, Reed C, Meltzer MI, Shay DK, Cheng P-Y, et al. Estimated global mortality associated with the first 12 months of 2009 pandemic influenza A H1N1 virus circulation: a modelling study. Lancet Infect Dis. 2012;12(9):687–95.
5. Information P. Zovirax (Acyclovir). Research Triangle Park: GlaxoSmithKline; 2007.
6. Elion GB. Mechanism of action and selectivity of acyclovir. Am J Med. 1982;73(1A):7–13.
7. Wagstaff AJ, Faulds D, Goa KL. Aciclovir. A reappraisal of its antiviral activity, pharmacokinetic properties and therapeutic efficacy. Drugs. 1994;47(1):153–205.
8. Laskin OL. Clinical pharmacokinetics of acyclovir. Clin Pharmacokinet. 1983;8(3):187–201.
9. de Miranda P, Blum MR. Pharmacokinetics of acyclovir after intravenous and oral administration. J Antimicrob Chemother. 1983;12(Suppl B):29–37.
10. Blum MR, Liao SH, de Miranda P. Overview of acyclovir pharmacokinetic disposition in adults and children. Am J Med. 1982;73(1A):186–92.
11. Laskin OL, Longstreth JA, Whelton A, Krasny HC, Keeney RE, Rocco L, et al. Effect of renal failure on the pharmacokinetics of acyclovir. Am J Med. 1982;73(1A):197–201.
12. Laskin OL, Longstreth JA, Saral R, de Miranda P, Keeney R, Lietman PS. Pharmacokinetics and tolerance of acyclovir, a new anti-herpesvirus agent, in humans. Antimicrob Agents Chemother. 1982;21(3):393–8.
13. Krasny HC, Liao SH, de Miranda P, Laskin OL, Whelton A, Lietman PS. Influence of hemodialysis on acyclovir pharmacokinetics in patients with chronic renal failure. Am J Med. 1982;73(1A):202–4.
14. Seth SK, Visconti JA, Hebert LA, Krasny HC. Acyclovir pharmacokinetics in a patient on continuous ambulatory peritoneal dialysis. Clin Pharm. 1985;4(3):320–2.
15. Lycke J, Andersen O, Svennerholm B, Appelgren L, Dahlof C. Acyclovir concentrations in serum and cerebrospinal fluid at steady state. J Antimicrob Chemother. 1989;24(6):947–54.
16. Hung SO, Patterson A, Rees PJ. Pharmacokinetics of oral acyclovir (Zovirax) in the eye. Br J Ophthalmol. 1984;68(3):192–5.
17. Kimberlin DF, Weller S, Whitley RJ, Andrews WW, Hauth JC, Lakeman F, et al. Pharmacokinetics of oral valacyclovir and acyclovir in late pregnancy. Am J Obstet Gynecol. 1998;179(4):846–51.
18. Information P. Zovirax (Acyclovir Ointment) 5%. Research Triangle Park: GlaxoSmithKline Inc; 2001.

19. Tod M, Lokiec F, Bidault R, De Bony F, Petitjean O, Aujard Y. Pharmacokinetics of oral acyclovir in neonates and in infants: a population analysis. Antimicrob Agents Chemother. 2001;45(1):150–7.
20. Hintz M, Connor JD, Spector SA, Blum MR, Keeney RE, Yeager AS. Neonatal acyclovir pharmacokinetics in patients with herpes virus infections. Am J Med. 1982;73(1A):210–4.
21. Information P. Valtrex (Valacyclovir). Research Triangle Park: GlaxoSmithKline; 2011.
22. Wang LH, Schultz M, Weller S, Smiley ML, Blum MR. Pharmacokinetics and safety of multiple-dose valaciclovir in geriatric volunteers with and without concomitant diuretic therapy. Antimicrob Agents Chemother. 1996;40(1):80–5.
23. Beutner KR. Valacyclovir: a review of its antiviral activity, pharmacokinetic properties, and clinical efficacy. Antivir Res. 1995;28(4):281–90.
24. Soul-Lawton J, Seaber E, On N, Wootton R, Rolan P, Posner J. Absolute bioavailability and metabolic disposition of valaciclovir, the L-valyl ester of acyclovir, following oral administration to humans. Antimicrob Agents Chemother. 1995;39(12):2759–64.
25. Weller S, Blum MR, Doucette M, Burnette T, Cederberg DM, de Miranda P, et al. Pharmacokinetics of the acyclovir pro-drug valaciclovir after escalating single- and multiple-dose administration to normal volunteers. Clin Pharmacol Ther. 1993;54(6):595–605.
26. Kambhampati G, Pakkivenkata U, Kazory A. Valacyclovir neurotoxicity can be effectively managed by hemodialysis. Eur J Neurol. 2011;18(3):e33.
27. MacDougall C, Guglielmo BJ. Pharmacokinetics of valaciclovir. J Antimicrob Chemother. 2004;53(6):899–901.
28. Rolan P. Pharmacokinetics of new antiherpetic agents. Clin Pharmacokinet. 1995;29(5):333–40.
29. Lycke J, Malmestrom C, Stahle L. Acyclovir levels in serum and cerebrospinal fluid after oral administration of valacyclovir. Antimicrob Agents Chemother. 2003;47(8):2438–41.
30. Smith JP, Weller S, Johnson B, Nicotera J, Luther JM, Haas DW. Pharmacokinetics of acyclovir and its metabolites in cerebrospinal fluid and systemic circulation after administration of high-dose valacyclovir in subjects with normal and impaired renal function. Antimicrob Agents Chemother. 2010;54(3):1146–51.
31. Kimberlin DW, Jacobs RF, Weller S, van der Walt JS, Heitman CK, Man CY, et al. Pharmacokinetics and safety of extemporaneously compounded valacyclovir oral suspension in pediatric patients from 1 month through 11 years of age. Clin Infect Dis. 2010;50(2):221–8.
32. Crumpacker CS. Ganciclovir. N Engl J Med. 1996;335(10):721–9.
33. Cheng YC, Grill SP, Dutschman GE, Nakayama K, Bastow KF. Metabolism of 9-(1,3-dihydroxy-2-propoxymethyl)guanine, a new anti-herpes virus compound, in herpes simplex virus-infected cells. J Biol Chem. 1983;258(20):12460–4.
34. Lurain NS, Chou S. Antiviral drug resistance of human cytomegalovirus. Clin Microbiol Rev. 2010;23(4):689–712.
35. Anderson RD, Griffy KG, Jung D, Dorr A, Hulse JD, Smith RB. Ganciclovir absolute bioavailability and steady-state pharmacokinetics after oral administration of two 3000-mg/d dosing regimens in human immunodeficiency virus- and cytomegalovirus-seropositive patients. Clin Ther. 1995;17(3):425–32.
36. Zhou XJ, Gruber W, Demmler G, Jacobs R, Reuman P, Adler S, et al. Population pharmacokinetics of ganciclovir in newborns with congenital cytomegalovirus infections. NIAID Collaborative Antiviral Study Group. Antimicrob Agents Chemother. 1996;40(9):2202–5.
37. DeArmond B. Future directions in the management of cytomegalovirus infections. J Acquir Immune Defic Syndr. 1991;4(Suppl 1):S53–6.
38. Spector SA, Busch DF, Follansbee S, Squires K, Lalezari JP, Jacobson MA, et al. Pharmacokinetic, safety, and antiviral profiles of oral ganciclovir in persons infected with human immunodeficiency virus: a phase I/II study. AIDS Clinical Trials Group, and Cytomegalovirus Cooperative Study Group. J Infect Dis. 1995;171(6):1431–7.
39. Information P. Zirgan (Ganciclovir ophthalmic gel) 0.15%. Tampa: Sirion Therapeutics, Inc; 2009.
40. Information P. Vitrasert (Ganciclovir Intravitreal Implant). Irvine: Chiron Vision Corporation; 1997.
41. Lake KD, Fletcher CV, Love KR, Brown DC, Joyce LD, Pritzker MR. Ganciclovir pharmacokinetics during renal impairment. Antimicrob Agents Chemother. 1988;32(12):1899–900.
42. Jacobson MA, de Miranda P, Cederberg DM, Burnette T, Cobb E, Brodie HR, et al. Human pharmacokinetics and tolerance of oral ganciclovir. Antimicrob Agents Chemother. 1987;31(8):1251–4.
43. Sommadossi JP, Bevan R, Ling T, Lee F, Mastre B, Chaplin MD, et al. Clinical pharmacokinetics of ganciclovir in patients with normal and impaired renal function. Rev Infect Dis. 1988;10(Suppl 3):S507–14.
44. Fletcher C, Sawchuk R, Chinnock B, de Miranda P, Balfour HH Jr. Human pharmacokinetics of the antiviral drug DHPG. Clin Pharmacol Ther. 1986;40(3):281–6.
45. Marshall BC, Koch WC. Antivirals for cytomegalovirus infection in neonates and infants: focus on pharmacokinetics, formulations, dosing, and adverse events. Paediatr Drugs. 2009;11(5):309–21.
46. Trang JM, Kidd L, Gruber W, Storch G, Demmler G, Jacobs R, et al. Linear single-dose pharmacokinetics of ganciclovir in newborns with congenital cytomegalovirus infections. NIAID Collaborative Antiviral Study Group. Clin Pharmacol Ther. 1993;53(1):15–21.
47. Frenkel LM, Capparelli EV, Dankner WM, Xu J, Smith IL, Ballow A, et al. Oral ganciclovir in children: pharmacokinetics, safety, tolerance, and antiviral effects. The Pediatric AIDS Clinical Trials Group. J Infect Dis. 2000;182(6):1616–24.
48. Martin JC, Dvorak CA, Smee DF, Matthews TR, Verheyden JP. 9-[(1,3-Dihydroxy-2-propoxy)methyl]guanine: a new potent and selective antiherpes agent. J Med Chem. 1983;26(5):759–61.
49. Brown F, Banken L, Saywell K, Arum I. Pharmacokinetics of valganciclovir and ganciclovir following multiple oral dosages of valganciclovir in HIV- and CMV-seropositive volunteers. Clin Pharmacokinet. 1999;37(2):167–76.
50. Information P. Valcyte (Valganciclovir). Nutley: Roche Laboratories Inc; 2001.
51. Jung D, Dorr A. Single-dose pharmacokinetics of valganciclovir in HIV- and CMV-seropositive subjects. J Clin Pharmacol. 1999;39(8):800–4.
52. Pescovitz MD, Rabkin J, Merion RM, Paya CV, Pirsch J, Freeman RB, et al. Valganciclovir results in improved oral absorption of ganciclovir in liver transplant recipients. Antimicrob Agents Chemother. 2000;44(10):2811–5.
53. Wiltshire H, Hirankarn S, Farrell C, Paya C, Pescovitz MD, Humar A, et al. Pharmacokinetic profile of ganciclovir after its oral administration and from its prodrug, valganciclovir, in solid organ transplant recipients. Clin Pharmacokinet. 2005;44(5):495–507.
54. Czock D, Scholle C, Rasche FM, Schaarschmidt D, Keller F. Pharmacokinetics of valganciclovir and ganciclovir in renal impairment. Clin Pharmacol Ther. 2002;72(2):142–50.
55. Acosta EP, Brundage RC, King JR, Sanchez PJ, Sood S, Agrawal V, et al. Ganciclovir population pharmacokinetics in neonates following intravenous administration of ganciclovir and oral administration of a liquid valganciclovir formulation. Clin Pharmacol Ther. 2007;81(6):867–72.
56. Vethamuthu J, Feber J, Chretien A, Lampe D, Filler G. Unexpectedly high inter- and intrapatient variability of ganciclovir levels in children. Pediatr Transplant. 2007;11(3):301–5.
57. Zhang D, Lapeyraque AL, Popon M, Loirat C, Jacqz-Aigrain E. Pharmacokinetics of ganciclovir in pediatric renal transplant recipients. Pediatr Nephrol. 2003;18(9):943–8.
58. Kimberlin DW, Acosta EP, Sanchez PJ, Sood S, Agrawal V, Homans J, et al. Pharmacokinetic and pharmacodynamic assessment of oral

valganciclovir in the treatment of symptomatic congenital cytomegalovirus disease. J Infect Dis. 2008;197(6):836–45.
59. Crumpacker CS. Mechanism of action of foscarnet against viral polymerases. Am J Med. 1992;92(2A):3S–7S.
60. Aweeka F, Gambertoglio J, Mills J, Jacobson MA. Pharmacokinetics of intermittently administered intravenous foscarnet in the treatment of acquired immunodeficiency syndrome patients with serious cytomegalovirus retinitis. Antimicrob Agents Chemother. 1989;33(5):742–5.
61. Taburet AM, Katlama C, Blanshard C, Zorza G, Gazzard D, Dohin E, et al. Pharmacokinetics of foscarnet after twice-daily administrations for treatment of cytomegalovirus disease in AIDS patients. Antimicrob Agents Chemother. 1992;36(9):1821–4.
62. Fletcher CV, Collier AC, Rhame FS, Bennett D, Para MF, Beatty CC, et al. Foscarnet for suppression of human immunodeficiency virus replication. Antimicrob Agents Chemother. 1994;38(3):604–7.
63. Sjovall J, Bergdahl S, Movin G, Ogenstad S, Saarimaki M. Pharmacokinetics of foscarnet and distribution to cerebrospinal fluid after intravenous infusion in patients with human immunodeficiency virus infection. Antimicrob Agents Chemother. 1989;33(7):1023–31.
64. Sjovall J, Karlsson A, Ogenstad S, Sandstrom E, Saarimaki M. Pharmacokinetics and absorption of foscarnet after intravenous and oral administration to patients with human immunodeficiency virus. Clin Pharmacol Ther. 1988;44(1):65–73.
65. Lee MY, Kim KS, Lee WK. Intravitreal foscarnet for the treatment of acyclovir-resistant acute retinal necrosis caused by varicella zoster virus. Ocul Immunol Inflamm. 2011;19(3):212–3.
66. Wong R, Pavesio CE, Laidlaw DA, Williamson TH, Graham EM, Stanford MR. Acute retinal necrosis: the effects of intravitreal foscarnet and virus type on outcome. Ophthalmology. 2010;117(3):556–60.
67. Ausayakhun S, Watananikorn S, Ngamtiphakorn S, Prasitsilp J. Intravitreal foscarnet for cytomegalovirus retinitis in patients with AIDS. J Med Assoc Thail. 2005;88(1):103–7.
68. Aweeka FT, Jacobson MA, Martin-Munley S, Hedman A, Schoenfeld P, Omachi R, et al. Effect of renal disease and hemodialysis on foscarnet pharmacokinetics and dosing recommendations. J Acquir Immune Defic Syndr Hum Retrovirol. 1999;20(4):350–7.
69. Cundy KC. Clinical pharmacokinetics of the antiviral nucleotide analogues cidofovir and adefovir. Clin Pharmacokinet. 1999;36(2):127–43.
70. Safrin S, Cherrington J, Jaffe HS. Clinical uses of Cidofovir. Rev Med Virol. 1997;7:145–56.
71. Cundy KC, Petty BG, Flaherty J, Fisher PE, Polis MA, Wachsman M, et al. Clinical pharmacokinetics of cidofovir in human immunodeficiency virus-infected patients. Antimicrob Agents Chemother. 1995;39(6):1247–52.
72. Lalezari JP, Holland GN, Kramer F, McKinley GF, Kemper CA, Ives DV, et al. Randomized, controlled study of the safety and efficacy of intravenous cidofovir for the treatment of relapsing cytomegalovirus retinitis in patients with AIDS. J Acquir Immune Defic Syndr Hum Retrovirol. 1998;17(4):339–44.
73. Brody SR, Humphreys MH, Gambertoglio JG, Schoenfeld P, Cundy KC, Aweeka FT. Pharmacokinetics of cidofovir in renal insufficiency and in continuous ambulatory peritoneal dialysis or high-flux hemodialysis. Clin Pharmacol Ther. 1999;65(1):21–8.
74. Mackey MC. Intravesicular cidofovir for the treatment of polyomavirus-associated hemorrhagic cystitis. Ann Pharmacother. 2012;46(3):442–6.
75. Muluneh B, Dean A, Armistead P, Khan T. Successful clearance of cutaneous acyclovir-resistant, foscarnet-refractory herpes virus lesions with topical cidofovir in an allogeneic hematopoietic stem cell transplant patient. J Oncol Pharm Pract. 2013;19(2):181–5
76. Skevaki CL, Galani IE, Pararas MV, Giannopoulou KP, Tsakris A. Treatment of viral conjunctivitis with antiviral drugs. Drugs. 2011;71(3):331–47.
77. Gill KS, Wood MJ. The clinical pharmacokinetics of famciclovir. Clin Pharmacokinet. 1996;31(1):1–8.
78. Weinberg A, Bate BJ, Masters HB, Schneider SA, Clark JC, Wren CG, et al. In vitro activities of penciclovir and acyclovir against herpes simplex virus types 1 and 2. Antimicrob Agents Chemother. 1992;36(9):2037–8.
79. Pue MA, Pratt SK, Fairless AJ, Fowles S, Laroche J, Georgiou P, et al. Linear pharmacokinetics of penciclovir following administration of single oral doses of famciclovir 125, 250, 500 and 750 mg to healthy volunteers. J Antimicrob Chemother. 1994;33(1):119–27.
80. Fowles SE, Pierce DM, Prince WT, Staniforth D. The tolerance to and pharmacokinetics of penciclovir (BRL 39,123A), a novel antiherpes agent, administered by intravenous infusion to healthy subjects. Eur J Clin Pharmacol. 1992;43(5):513–6.
81. Boike SC, Pue MA, Freed MI, Audet PR, Fairless A, Ilson BE, et al. Pharmacokinetics of famciclovir in subjects with varying degrees of renal impairment. Clin Pharmacol Ther. 1994;55(4):418–26.
82. Information P. Denavir (Penciclovir cream 1%). Parsippany: Novartis Consumer Health Inc; 2002.
83. Filer CW, Allen GD, Brown TA, Fowles SE, Hollis FJ, Mort EE, et al. Metabolic and pharmacokinetic studies following oral administration of 14C-famciclovir to healthy subjects. Xenobiotica. 1994;24(4):357–68.
84. Boike SC, Pue M, Audet PR, Freed MI, Fairless A, Ilson BE, et al. Pharmacokinetics of famciclovir in subjects with chronic hepatic disease. J Clin Pharmacol. 1994;34(12):1199–207.
85. Aoki FY, Sitar DS. Clinical pharmacokinetics of amantadine hydrochloride. Clin Pharmacokinet. 1988;14(1):35–51.
86. Dourmashkin RR, Tyrrell DA. Electron microscopic observations on the entry of influenza virus into susceptible cells. J Gen Virol. 1974;24(1):129–41.
87. Skehel JJ, Hay AJ, Armstrong JA. On the mechanism of inhibition of influenza virus replication by amantadine hydrochloride. J Gen Virol. 1978;38(1):97–110.
88. Krumbholz A, Schmidtke M, Bergmann S, Motzke S, Bauer K, Stech J, et al. High prevalence of amantadine resistance among circulating European porcine influenza A viruses. J Gen Virol. 2009;90(Pt 4):900–8.
89. Higgins RR, Eshaghi A, Burton L, Mazzulli T, Drews SJ. Differential patterns of amantadine-resistance in influenza A (H3N2) and (H1N1) isolates in Toronto. J Clin Virol. 2009;44(1):91–3.
90. Horadam VW, Sharp JG, Smilack JD, McAnalley BH, Garriott JC, Stephens MK, et al. Pharmacokinetics of amantadine hydrochloride in subjects with normal and impaired renal function. Ann Intern Med. 1981;94(4 pt 1):454–8.
91. Deleu D, Northway MG, Hanssens Y. Clinical pharmacokinetic and pharmacodynamic properties of drugs used in the treatment of Parkinson's disease. Clin Pharmacokinet. 2002;41(4):261–309.
92. Hayden FG, Minocha A, Spyker DA, Hoffman HE. Comparative single-dose pharmacokinetics of amantadine hydrochloride and rimantadine hydrochloride in young and elderly adults. Antimicrob Agents Chemother. 1985;28(2):216–21.
93. Betts RF. Amantadine and rimantadine for the prevention of influenza A. Semin Respir Infect. 1989;4(4):304–10.
94. Belshe RB, Burk B, Newman F, Cerruti RL, Sim IS. Resistance of influenza A virus to amantadine and rimantadine: results of one decade of surveillance. J Infect Dis. 1989;159(3):430–5.
95. Wintermeyer SM, Nahata MC. Rimantadine: a clinical perspective. Ann Pharmacother. 1995;29(3):299–310.
96. Moscona A. Neuraminidase inhibitors for influenza. N Engl J Med. 2005;353(13):1363–73.
97. He G, Massarella J, Ward P. Clinical pharmacokinetics of the prodrug oseltamivir and its active metabolite Ro 64-0802. Clin Pharmacokinet. 1999;37(6):471–84.
98. Dutkowski R, Thakrar B, Froehlich E, Suter P, Oo C, Ward P. Safety and pharmacology of oseltamivir in clinical use. Drug Saf. 2003;26(11):787–801.

99. Abed Y, Bourgault AM, Fenton RJ, Morley PJ, Gower D, Owens IJ, et al. Characterization of 2 influenza A(H3N2) clinical isolates with reduced susceptibility to neuraminidase inhibitors due to mutations in the hemagglutinin gene. J Infect Dis. 2002;186(8):1074–80.
100. McKimm-Breschkin JL. Resistance of influenza viruses to neuraminidase inhibitors – a review. Antivir Res. 2000;47(1):1–17.
101. Pizzorno A, Abed Y, Boivin G. Influenza drug resistance. Semin Respir Crit Care Med. 2011;32(4):409–22.
102. Moscona A. Oseltamivir resistance – disabling our influenza defenses. N Engl J Med. 2005;353(25):2633–6.
103. Sheu TG, Deyde VM, Okomo-Adhiambo M, Garten RJ, Xu X, Bright RA, et al. Surveillance for neuraminidase inhibitor resistance among human influenza A and B viruses circulating worldwide from 2004 to 2008. Antimicrob Agents Chemother. 2008;52(9):3284–92.
104. Kiso M, Mitamura K, Sakai-Tagawa Y, Shiraishi K, Kawakami C, Kimura K, et al. Resistant influenza A viruses in children treated with oseltamivir: descriptive study. Lancet. 2004;364(9436):759–65.
105. Mishin VP, Hayden FG, Gubareva LV. Susceptibilities of antiviral-resistant influenza viruses to novel neuraminidase inhibitors. Antimicrob Agents Chemother. 2005;49(11):4515–20.
106. Wattanagoon Y, Stepniewska K, Lindegardh N, Pukrittayakamee S, Silachamroon U, Piyaphanee W, et al. Pharmacokinetics of high-dose oseltamivir in healthy volunteers. Antimicrob Agents Chemother. 2009;53(3):945–52.
107. Robson R, Buttimore A, Lynn K, Brewster M, Ward P. The pharmacokinetics and tolerability of oseltamivir suspension in patients on haemodialysis and continuous ambulatory peritoneal dialysis. Nephrol Dial Transplant. 2006;21(9):2556–62.
108. Snell P, Dave N, Wilson K, Rowell L, Weil A, Galitz L, et al. Lack of effect of moderate hepatic impairment on the pharmacokinetics of oral oseltamivir and its metabolite oseltamivir carboxylate. Br J Clin Pharmacol. 2005;59(5):598–601.
109. Oo C, Barrett J, Hill G, Mann J, Dorr A, Dutkowski R, et al. Pharmacokinetics and dosage recommendations for an oseltamivir oral suspension for the treatment of influenza in children. Paediatr Drugs. 2001;3(3):229–36.
110. Woods JM, Bethell RC, Coates JA, Healy N, Hiscox SA, Pearson BA, et al. 4-Guanidino-2,4-dideoxy-2,3-dehydro-N-acetylneuraminic acid is a highly effective inhibitor both of the sialidase (neuraminidase) and of growth of a wide range of influenza a and B viruses in vitro. Antimicrob Agents Chemother. 1993;37(7):1473–9.
111. Cass LM, Brown J, Pickford M, Fayinka S, Newman SP, Johansson CJ, et al. Pharmacoscintigraphic evaluation of lung deposition of inhaled zanamivir in healthy volunteers. Clin Pharmacokinet. 1999;36(Suppl 1):21–31.
112. Cass LM, Efthymiopoulos C, Bye A. Pharmacokinetics of zanamivir after intravenous, oral, inhaled or intranasal administration to healthy volunteers. Clin Pharmacokinet. 1999;36(Suppl 1):1–11.
113. Hedrick JA, Barzilai A, Behre U, Henderson FW, Hammond J, Reilly L, et al. Zanamivir for treatment of symptomatic influenza A and B infection in children five to twelve years of age: a randomized controlled trial. Pediatr Infect Dis J. 2000;19(5):410–7.
114. Rivkin AM. Adefovir dipivoxil in the treatment of chronic hepatitis B. Ann Pharmacother. 2004;38(4):625–33.
115. Qi X, Xiong S, Yang H, Miller M, Delaney WE 4th. In vitro susceptibility of adefovir-associated hepatitis B virus polymerase mutations to other antiviral agents. Antivir Ther. 2007;12(3):355–62.
116. Ghany MG, Doo EC. Antiviral resistance and hepatitis B therapy. Hepatology. 2009;49(5 Suppl):S174–84.
117. Villeneuve JP, Durantel D, Durantel S, Westland C, Xiong S, Brosgart CL, et al. Selection of a hepatitis B virus strain resistant to adefovir in a liver transplantation patient. J Hepatol. 2003;39(6):1085–9.
118. Angus P, Vaughan R, Xiong S, Yang H, Delaney W, Gibbs C, et al. Resistance to adefovir dipivoxil therapy associated with the selection of a novel mutation in the HBV polymerase. Gastroenterology. 2003;125(2):292–7.
119. Kearney BP, Ramanathan S, Cheng AK, Ebrahimi R, Shah J. Systemic and renal pharmacokinetics of adefovir and tenofovir upon coadministration. J Clin Pharm Ther. 2005;45(8):935–40.
120. Cundy KC, Barditch-Crovo P, Walker RE, Collier AC, Ebeling D, Toole J, et al. Clinical pharmacokinetics of adefovir in human immunodeficiency virus type 1-infected patients. Antimicrob Agents Chemother. 1995;39(11):2401–5.
121. Shiffman ML, Pol S, Rostaing L, Schiff E, Thabut D, Zeuzem S, et al. Efficacy and pharmacokinetics of adefovir dipivoxil liquid suspension in patients with chronic hepatitis B and renal impairment. J Clin Pharm Ther. 2011;51(9):1293–301.
122. Sokal EM, Kelly D, Wirth S, Mizerski J, Dhawan A, Frederick D. The pharmacokinetics and safety of adefovir dipivoxil in children and adolescents with chronic hepatitis B virus infection. J Clin Pharm Ther. 2008;48(4):512–7.
123. Seifer M, Hamatake RK, Colonno RJ, Standring DN. In vitro inhibition of hepadnavirus polymerases by the triphosphates of BMS-200475 and lobucavir. Antimicrob Agents Chemother. 1998;42(12):3200–8.
124. Gish RG. Clinical trial results of new therapies for HBV: implications for treatment guidelines. Semin Liver Dis. 2005;25(Suppl 1):29–39.
125. Honkoop P, De Man RA. Entecavir: a potent new antiviral drug for hepatitis B. Expert Opin Investig Drugs. 2003;12(4):683–8.
126. Sherman M, Yurdaydin C, Sollano J, Silva M, Liaw YF, Cianciara J, et al. Entecavir for treatment of lamivudine-refractory, HBeAg-positive chronic hepatitis B. Gastroenterology. 2006;130(7):2039–49.
127. Tenney DJ, Levine SM, Rose RE, Walsh AW, Weinheimer SP, Discotto L, et al. Clinical emergence of entecavir-resistant hepatitis B virus requires additional substitutions in virus already resistant to Lamivudine. Antimicrob Agents Chemother. 2004;48(9):3498–507.
128. Yan JH, Bifano M, Olsen S, Smith RA, Zhang D, Grasela DM, et al. Entecavir pharmacokinetics, safety, and tolerability after multiple ascending doses in healthy subjects. J Clin Pharmacol. 2006;46(11):1250–8.
129. Sims KA, Woodland AM. Entecavir: a new nucleoside analog for the treatment of chronic hepatitis B infection. Pharmacotherapy. 2006;26(12):1745–57.
130. Cammack N, Rouse P, Marr CL, Reid PJ, Boehme RE, Coates JA, et al. Cellular metabolism of (−) enantiomeric 2′-deoxy-3′-thiacytidine. Biochem Pharmacol. 1992;43(10):2059–64.
131. Information P. Epivir-HBV (Lamivudine). Research Triangle Park: GlaxoSmithKline; 2011.
132. Johnson MA, Moore KH, Yuen GJ, Bye A, Pakes GE. Clinical pharmacokinetics of lamivudine. Clin Pharmacokinet. 1999;36(1):41–66.
133. van Leeuwen R, Lange JM, Hussey EK, Donn KH, Hall ST, Harker AJ, et al. The safety and pharmacokinetics of a reverse transcriptase inhibitor, 3TC, in patients with HIV infection: a phase I study. AIDS. 1992;6(12):1471–5.
134. Yuen GJ, Morris DM, Mydlow PK, Haidar S, Hall ST, Hussey EK. Pharmacokinetics, absolute bioavailability, and absorption characteristics of lamivudine. J Clin Pharmacol. 1995;35(12):1174–80.
135. Heald AE, Hsyu PH, Yuen GJ, Robinson P, Mydlow P, Bartlett JA. Pharmacokinetics of lamivudine in human immunodeficiency virus-infected patients with renal dysfunction. Antimicrob Agents Chemother. 1996;40(6):1514–9.
136. Johnson MA, Verpooten GA, Daniel MJ, Plumb R, Moss J, Van Caesbroeck D, et al. Single dose pharmacokinetics of lamivudine in subjects with impaired renal function and the effect of haemodialysis. Br J Clin Pharmacol. 1998;46(1):21–7.

137. Johnson MA, Horak J, Breuel P. The pharmacokinetics of lamivudine in patients with impaired hepatic function. Eur J Clin Pharmacol. 1998;54(4):363–6.
138. Moodley J, Moodley D, Pillay K, Coovadia H, Saba J, van Leeuwen R, et al. Pharmacokinetics and antiretroviral activity of lamivudine alone or when coadministered with zidovudine in human immunodeficiency virus type 1-infected pregnant women and their offspring. J Infect Dis. 1998;178(5):1327–33.
139. Lewis LL, Venzon D, Church J, Farley M, Wheeler S, Keller A, et al. Lamivudine in children with human immunodeficiency virus infection: a phase I/II study. The National Cancer Institute Pediatric Branch-Human Immunodeficiency Virus Working Group. J Infect Dis. 1996;174(1):16–25.
140. Grim SA, Romanelli F. Tenofovir disoproxil fumarate. Ann Pharmacother. 2003;37(6):849–59.
141. Jenh AM, Thio CL, Pham PA. Tenofovir for the treatment of hepatitis B virus. Pharmacotherapy. 2009;29(10):1212–27.
142. Zoulim F. Hepatitis B virus resistance to antiviral drugs: where are we going? Liver Int. 2011;31(Suppl 1):111–6.
143. Reijnders JG, Deterding K, Petersen J, Zoulim F, Santantonio T, Buti M, et al. Antiviral effect of entecavir in chronic hepatitis B: influence of prior exposure to nucleos(t)ide analogues. J Hepatol. 2010;52(4):493–500.
144. van Bommel F, de Man RA, Wedemeyer H, Deterding K, Petersen J, Buggisch P, et al. Long-term efficacy of tenofovir monotherapy for hepatitis B virus-monoinfected patients after failure of nucleoside/nucleotide analogues. Hepatology. 2010;51(1):73–80.
145. Barditch-Crovo P, Deeks SG, Collier A, Safrin S, Coakley DF, Miller M, et al. Phase i/ii trial of the pharmacokinetics, safety, and antiretroviral activity of tenofovir disoproxil fumarate in human immunodeficiency virus-infected adults. Antimicrob Agents Chemother. 2001;45(10):2733–9.
146. Kearney BP, Flaherty JF, Shah J. Tenofovir disoproxil fumarate: clinical pharmacology and pharmacokinetics. Clin Pharmacokinet. 2004;43(9):595–612.
147. Delaney WE, Ray AS, Yang H, Qi X, Xiong S, Zhu Y, et al. Intracellular metabolism and in vitro activity of tenofovir against hepatitis B virus. Antimicrob Agents Chemother. 2006;50(7):2471–7.
148. Deeks SG, Barditch-Crovo P, Lietman PS, Hwang F, Cundy KC, Rooney JF, et al. Safety, pharmacokinetics, and antiretroviral activity of intravenous 9-[2-(R)-(Phosphonomethoxy)propyl]adenine, a novel anti-human immunodeficiency virus (HIV) therapy, in HIV-infected adults. Antimicrob Agents Chemother. 1998;42(9):2380–4.
149. Kearney BP, Yale K, Shah J, Zhong L, Flaherty JF. Pharmacokinetics and dosing recommendations of tenofovir disoproxil fumarate in hepatic or renal impairment. Clin Pharmacokinet. 2006;45(11):1115–24.
150. Hazra R, Balis FM, Tullio AN, DeCarlo E, Worrell CJ, Steinberg SM, et al. Single-dose and steady-state pharmacokinetics of tenofovir disoproxil fumarate in human immunodeficiency virus-infected children. Antimicrob Agents Chemother. 2004;48(1):124–9.
151. Kim JJ, Culley CM, Mohammad RA. Telaprevir: an oral protease inhibitor for hepatitis C virus infection. Am J Health Syst Pharm. 2012;69(1):19–33.
152. Smith LS, Nelson M, Naik S, Woten J. Telaprevir: an NS3/4A protease inhibitor for the treatment of chronic hepatitis C. Ann Pharmacother. 2011;45(5):639–48.
153. Welsch C, Domingues FS, Susser S, Antes I, Hartmann C, Mayr G, et al. Molecular basis of telaprevir resistance due to V36 and T54 mutations in the NS3-4A protease of the hepatitis C virus. Genome Biol. 2008;9(1):R16.
154. Sarrazin C, Zeuzem S. Resistance to direct antiviral agents in patients with hepatitis C virus infection. Gastroenterology. 2010;138(2):447–62.
155. Forestier N, Reesink HW, Weegink CJ, McNair L, Kieffer TL, Chu HM, et al. Antiviral activity of telaprevir (VX-950) and peginterferon alfa-2a in patients with hepatitis C. Hepatology. 2007;46(3):640–8.
156. Kieffer TL, Sarrazin C, Miller JS, Welker MW, Forestier N, Reesink HW, et al. Telaprevir and pegylated interferon-alpha-2a inhibit wild-type and resistant genotype 1 hepatitis C virus replication in patients. Hepatology. 2007;46(3):631–9.
157. Reesink HW, Zeuzem S, Weegink CJ, Forestier N, van Vliet A, van de Wetering de Rooij J, et al. Rapid decline of viral RNA in hepatitis C patients treated with VX-950: a phase Ib, placebo-controlled, randomized study. Gastroenterology. 2006;131(4):997–1002.
158. Marcellin P, Forns X, Goeser T, Ferenci P, Nevens F, Carosi G, et al. Telaprevir is effective given every 8 or 12 hours with ribavirin and peginterferon alfa-2a or -2b to patients with chronic hepatitis C. Gastroenterology. 2011;140(2):459–68 e1; quiz e14.
159. Information P. Incivek (Telaprevir). Cambridge, MA: Vertex Pharmaceuticals Inc; 2012.
160. Malcolm BA, Liu R, Lahser F, Agrawal S, Belanger B, Butkiewicz N, et al. SCH 503034, a mechanism-based inhibitor of hepatitis C virus NS3 protease, suppresses polyprotein maturation and enhances the antiviral activity of alpha interferon in replicon cells. Antimicrob Agents Chemother. 2006;50(3):1013–20.
161. Gale M Jr, Foy EM. Evasion of intracellular host defence by hepatitis C virus. Nature. 2005;436(7053):939–45.
162. Klibanov OM, Vickery SB, Olin JL, Smith LS, Williams SH. Boceprevir: a novel NS3/4 protease inhibitor for the treatment of hepatitis C. Pharmacotherapy. 2012;32(2):173–90.
163. Kuntzen T, Timm J, Berical A, Lennon N, Berlin AM, Young SK, et al. Naturally occurring dominant resistance mutations to hepatitis C virus protease and polymerase inhibitors in treatment-naive patients. Hepatology. 2008;48(6):1769–78.
164. Curry S, Qiu P, Tong X. Analysis of HCV resistance mutations during combination therapy with protease inhibitor boceprevir and PEG-IFN alpha-2b using TaqMan mismatch amplification mutation assay. J Virol Methods. 2008;153(2):156–62.
165. Mo H, Lu L, Pilot-Matias T, Pithawalla R, Mondal R, Masse S, et al. Mutations conferring resistance to a hepatitis C virus (HCV) RNA-dependent RNA polymerase inhibitor alone or in combination with an HCV serine protease inhibitor in vitro. Antimicrob Agents Chemother. 2005;49(10):4305–14.
166. Lin C, Gates CA, Rao BG, Brennan DL, Fulghum JR, Luong YP, et al. In vitro studies of cross-resistance mutations against two hepatitis C virus serine protease inhibitors, VX-950 and BILN 2061. J Biol Chem. 2005;280(44):36784–91.
167. Foote BS, Spooner LM, Belliveau PP. Boceprevir: a protease inhibitor for the treatment of chronic hepatitis C. Ann Pharmacother. 2011;45(9):1085–93.
168. Treitel M, Marbury T, Preston RA, Triantafyllou I, Feely W, O'Mara E, et al. Single-dose pharmacokinetics of boceprevir in subjects with impaired hepatic or renal function. Clin Pharmacokinet. 2012;51(9):619–28.
169. Sarrazin C, Rouzier R, Wagner F, Forestier N, Larrey D, Gupta SK, et al. SCH 503034, a novel hepatitis C virus protease inhibitor, plus pegylated interferon alpha-2b for genotype 1 nonresponders. Gastroenterology. 2007;132(4):1270–8.
170. Kempf DJ, Klein C, Chen HJ, Klein LL, Yeung C, Randolph JT, et al. Pharmacokinetic enhancement of the hepatitis C virus protease inhibitors VX-950 and SCH 503034 by co-dosing with ritonavir. Antivir Chem Chemother. 2007;18(3):163–7.
171. Dixit NM, Perelson AS. The metabolism, pharmacokinetics and mechanisms of antiviral activity of ribavirin against hepatitis C virus. Cell Mol Life Sci. 2006;63(7–8):832–42.
172. Sidwell RW, Huffman JH, Khare GP, Allen LB, Witkowski JT, Robins RK. Broad-spectrum antiviral activity of Virazole:

1-beta-D-ribofuranosyl-1,2,4-triazole-3-carboxamide. Science. 1972;177(4050):705–6.
173. Streeter DG, Witkowski JT, Khare GP, Sidwell RW, Bauer RJ, Robins RK, et al. Mechanism of action of 1- -D-ribofuranosyl-1,2,4-triazole-3-carboxamide (Virazole), a new broad-spectrum antiviral agent. Proc Natl Acad Sci U S A. 1973;70(4):1174–8.
174. Cramp ME, Rossol S, Chokshi S, Carucci P, Williams R, Naoumov NV. Hepatitis C virus-specific T-cell reactivity during interferon and ribavirin treatment in chronic hepatitis C. Gastroenterology. 2000;118(2):346–55.
175. Neumann AU, Lam NP, Dahari H, Gretch DR, Wiley TE, Layden TJ, et al. Hepatitis C viral dynamics in vivo and the antiviral efficacy of interferon-alpha therapy. Science. 1998;282(5386): 103–7.
176. Layden-Almer JE, Ribeiro RM, Wiley T, Perelson AS, Layden TJ. Viral dynamics and response differences in HCV-infected African American and white patients treated with IFN and ribavirin. Hepatology. 2003;37(6):1343–50.
177. Herrmann E, Lee JH, Marinos G, Modi M, Zeuzem S. Effect of ribavirin on hepatitis C viral kinetics in patients treated with pegylated interferon. Hepatology. 2003;37(6):1351–8.
178. Pawlotsky JM, Dahari H, Neumann AU, Hezode C, Germanidis G, Lonjon I, et al. Antiviral action of ribavirin in chronic hepatitis C. Gastroenterology. 2004;126(3):703–14.
179. Glue P, Schenker S, Gupta S, Clement RP, Zambas D, Salfi M. The single dose pharmacokinetics of ribavirin in subjects with chronic liver disease. Br J Clin Pharmacol. 2000;49(5):417–21.
180. Khakoo S, Glue P, Grellier L, Wells B, Bell A, Dash C, et al. Ribavirin and interferon alfa-2b in chronic hepatitis C: assessment of possible pharmacokinetic and pharmacodynamic interactions. Br J Clin Pharmacol. 1998;46(6):563–70.
181. Preston SL, Drusano GL, Glue P, Nash J, Gupta SK, McNamara P. Pharmacokinetics and absolute bioavailability of ribavirin in healthy volunteers as determined by stable-isotope methodology. Antimicrob Agents Chemother. 1999;43(10):2451–6.
182. Information P. Copegus (Ribavirin). South San Francisco: Genentech USA Inc; 2011.
183. Shah JN, Chemaly RF. Management of RSV infections in adult recipients of hematopoietic stem cell transplantation. Blood. 2011;117(10):2755–63.
184. Information P. Virazole (Ribavirin for inhalation solution). Aliso Viejo: Valeant Pharmaceuticals; 2008.
185. Information P. Rebetol (Ribavirin). Kenilworth: Schering Plough Corporation; 2003.
186. Theofilopoulos AN, Baccala R, Beutler B, Kono DH. Type I interferons (alpha/beta) in immunity and autoimmunity. Annu Rev Immunol. 2005;23:307–36.
187. Bruno R, Sacchi P, Cima S, Maiocchi L, Novati S, Filice G, et al. Comparison of peginterferon pharmacokinetic and pharmacodynamic profiles. J Viral Hepat. 2012;19(Suppl 1):33–6.
188. Baron S, Tyring SK, Fleischmann WR Jr, Coppenhaver DH, Niesel DW, Klimpel GR, et al. The interferons. Mechanisms of action and clinical applications. JAMA. 1991;266(10):1375–83.
189. Sen GC. Viruses and interferons. Annu Rev Microbiol. 2001;55:255–81.
190. Tamir A, Jordan WJ, Ritter M, Habib N, Lechler RI, Foster GR, et al. Interferon-alpha2a is sufficient for promoting dendritic cell immunogenicity. Clin Exp Immunol. 2005;142(3):471–80.
191. Barnes E, Salio M, Cerundolo V, Medlin J, Murphy S, Dusheiko G, et al. Impact of alpha interferon and ribavirin on the function of maturing dendritic cells. Antimicrob Agents Chemother. 2004;48(9):3382–9.
192. Pachiadakis I, Pollara G, Chain BM, Naoumov NV. Is hepatitis C virus infection of dendritic cells a mechanism facilitating viral persistence? Lancet Infect Dis. 2005;5(5):296–304.
193. Ji X, Cheung R, Cooper S, Li Q, Greenberg HB, He XS. Interferon alfa regulated gene expression in patients initiating interferon treatment for chronic hepatitis C. Hepatology. 2003;37(3):610–21.
194. Luik A, Knapp S, Thursz M, Thomas HC, Schlaak JF. Autoregulatory role of interleukin-10 in hepatitis C patients treated with IFN-alpha. J Interf Cytokine Res. 2004;24(10):585–93.
195. Wills RJ. Clinical pharmacokinetics of interferons. Clin Pharmacokinet. 1990;19(5):390–9.
196. Rumi M, Aghemo A, Prati GM. Comparative trials of peginterferon alpha2a and peginterferon alpha2b for chronic hepatitis C. J Viral Hepat. 2012;19(Suppl 1):37–41.
197. Noureddin M, Ghany MG. Pharmacokinetics and pharmacodynamics of peginterferon and ribavirin: implications for clinical efficacy in the treatment of chronic hepatitis C. Gastroenterol Clin N Am. 2010;39(3):649–58.
198. Information P. Pegintron (Peg-interferon-alfa-2b). Whitehouse Station: Merck & Co, Inc; 2011.
199. Information P. Pegasys (Peg-interferon-alfa-2a). South San Francisco: Genentech USA, Inc; 2011.

Antimycobacterial Consideration in Transplantation Including Drug Non-susceptibility and Resistance: Tuberculosis and Nontuberculous Mycobacterial Disease

56

Julie V. Philley and David E. Griffith

Introduction

The increasing availability and success of solid organ transplant (SOT) programs are an unequivocal success story for contemporary medicine and for the thousands of patients who receive SOT. A large part of that success is due to potent immunosuppressive drugs that prevent the body from rejecting transplanted organs. The highly desirable effect of immunosuppression is unfortunately accompanied by the predictable and inevitable risk of infection as a consequence of immunosuppression. Tuberculosis (TB) and nontbuerculous mycobacteria (NTM) are two important infections that can occur in this setting. Tuberculosis is an especially important concern because of its public health implications. Additionally, because of the increasingly international background of SOT participants, donors, and recipients, the risk of drug-resistant TB is also increasingly apparent. In this chapter we will discuss the mechanisms of mycobacterial drug resistance, the epidemiology of drug-resistant mycobacteria, the clinical presentation of mycobacterial disease in SOT recipients, the treatment options for drug-resistant mycobacterial pathogens, and the strategies for avoiding drug-resistant mycobacterial infection. Because of the overarching public health importance of TB as well as the greater risk for TB in SOT versus NTM infection, the emphasis of this chapter will be on TB.

J. V. Philley
University of Texas Health Science Center at Tyler, Department of Pulmonary and Critical Care Medicine, Tyler, TX, USA
e-mail: julie.philley@uthct.edu

D. E. Griffith (✉)
University of Texas Health Science Center, Tyler, TX, USA

Heartland National TB Center, Tyler, TX, USA
e-mail: david.griffith@uthct.edu

Mechanisms of Mycobacterial Drug Resistance

Resistance to antituberculous drugs occurs during selective multiplication of drug-resistant mycobacteria which spontaneously emerge in any population of *M. tuberculosis*. These resistant mutants are able to proliferate and replace the wild-type strains most frequently when there are a suboptimal number of effective companion medications. For instance, organisms with spontaneous mutations in the rpoβ gene conferring rifamycin resistance can flourish if rifampin is used as monotherapy with elimination of the rifamycin susceptible organisms. This phenomenon is the basis for the well-known admonishment that TB patients should never be treated with a single antituberculosis drug or with inadequate companion drugs to protect against the emergence of drug-resistant organisms. Molecular epidemiology indicates that multidrug-resistant TB (MDR-TB) strains arise by sequential accumulation of resistance mutations for individual drugs as a consequence of inadequate or inappropriate TB medication regimens [1]. In that context, it is noteworthy that clinically apparent drug-resistant TB did not exist until antituberculosis drugs were introduced with subsequent selection of the naturally occurring resistant strains. Resistance is not linked between classes of antituberculous drugs. Drug resistance which develops during or after a course of treatment has been called "acquired drug resistance" (the name that will be used in this chapter) but is also now referred to as "resistance among previously treated cases" by the World Health Organization (WHO) [2]. Similarly, drug resistance which develops when there is no history of TB treatment has been labeled as "primary drug resistance" but is now also called "resistance among new cases" [2]. For *Mycobacterium tuberculosis* isolates, there is generally good and predictable correlation between in vitro susceptibility results and in vivo response to the antimycobacterial agents. There are potent bactericidal agents for treating TB so that drugs can be tested individually in patients over short time periods, not long

A. Safdar (ed.), *Principles and Practice of Transplant Infectious Diseases*, https://doi.org/10.1007/978-1-4939-9034-4_56

enough to result in acquired mutational resistance, which allows reasonable assurance that in vitro findings will translate into in vivo results.

Multidrug-resistant TB (MDR-TB), caused by strains resistant to at least isoniazid and rifampin [2], is difficult to treat effectively and requires medications that are expensive, toxic, and less effective than first-line antituberculosis therapy [2]. Extensively drug-resistant TB (XDR-TB) is defined as TB resistant to isoniazid, rifampin, second-line injectable drug (kanamycin, amikacin, or capreomycin), and any fluoroquinolone [2]. MDR- and XDR-TB strains are resistant to the most potent antituberculous medications that are predictably associated with successful outcomes.

The origins of drug resistance for NTM are more complicated and include both innate and acquired drug resistance mechanisms. For *Mycobacterium avium* complex (MAC), the only antibiotics that show a correlation between in vitro MIC and in vivo response are clarithromycin, azithromycin, and amikacin [3, 4]. This observed concordance between in vitro susceptibility and in vivo response has a genetic correlate with the development of 23S rRNA gene mutations for macrolide resistance and 16S rRNA gene mutations for amikacin resistance [3, 4]. In this regard, MAC behaves like TB so that acquired mutational resistance to macrolides and to amikacin can occur if these drugs are used improperly [4, 5]. This correlation has not been established for any other agents used for treating MAC which means that the in vitro MICs for drugs like ethambutol, the rifamycins, and the fluoroquinolones do not help guide therapeutic choices [3]. For instance, ethambutol appears to be a critically important agent for protecting against the emergence of acquired mutational macrolide resistance regardless of the in vitro MIC, while there is no apparent role for fluoroquinolones in the therapy of MAC regardless of the MIC [5]. It is assumed that innate resistance factors, independent of the MIC of the drug for that organism, govern the response of MAC to these antibiotics [6].

For *M. abscessus* subsp. *abscessus*, it is even more complicated. *Mycobacterium abscessus* subsp. *abscessus* has an active inducible macrolide resistance gene or erm gene [7]. Because of the erm gene, these isolates may appear macrolide susceptible with low macrolide MICs on initial in vitro testing, but with macrolide exposure, the MICs increase to resistant levels. This is perhaps the best described type of innate mycobacterial drug resistance. Innate resistance likely accounts for the majority of in vivo drug resistance seen with many NTM. The *erm* gene is probably just the tip of the NTM drug resistance iceberg. To add a further complicating factor, some *M. abscessus* isolates have an *erm* gene mutation that inactivates the *erm* gene rendering the isolate macrolide susceptible [8]. In this circumstance, if a macrolide is used inappropriately, the isolates can still develop acquired mutational macrolide resistance (23S rRNA gene).

Preventing the emergence of drug-resistant TB and NTM isolates is paramount and requires familiarity with the individual mycobacterial organisms and their sometimes unpredictable behavior. It remains critically important to have adequate laboratory services in transplant recipients for adequate drug susceptibility testing and to identify molecular mechanisms of resistance.

Tuberculosis

Solid organ transplant recipients are at a 36- to 74-fold higher risk of developing TB risk of developing infection with *Mycobacterium tuberculosis* compared with the general population [9–16]. Infection may come from the transplant donor and recipient or be community acquired. Posttransplant TB has been reported to be more common in lung recipients than in liver transplant patients although the variation may depend on the local incidence of infection rather than the organ transplanted [17, 18]. The incidence of posttransplant TB varies greatly depending on the local prevalence of TB infection ranging from 1% in Germany to 13.7% in India [12, 13]. Studies in the United States and Europe suggest that 0.35–6.6% of SOT recipients develop TB and 4% of those cases are donor derived [13]. Most patients develop TB infection in the first year post transplantation, but a bimodal distribution has also been observed, with the incidence of TB at a peak 2 years after SOT [12].

While the majority of SOT patients develop pulmonary TB, the risk of disseminated infection and death due to TB is higher in transplant recipients than in the general population [12–16]. The high incidence of disseminated infections is up to tenfold greater than in immunocompetent TB patients [12–14]. Tuberculosis mortality in SOT recipients is variable but ranges from 9.5 to 17% [12–16]. Because of the nonspecific clinical manifestations of extrapulmonary and disseminated MAC which is also associated with a lack of clearly diagnostic symptoms, the diagnosis may be problematic and elusive [12–14]. The delayed diagnosis results in a delayed therapeutic intervention with attendant excess morbidity and mortality.

The majority of posttransplant TB cases occur secondary to reactivation in recipients with unrecognized or untreated latent TB infection (LTBI) although transmission of TB through the allograft can also occur [12–16]. One study reported that 20–25% of all TB diagnosed post transplantation was in people who had positive TST before transplantation [15]. Donor-derived TB is often unrecognized especially in areas of low TB prevalence contributing to significant morbidity and mortality [12–14]. Global travel and immigration have resulted in an increasingly diverse transplant donor population in lower-incidence countries, while organ transplantation has increased in some of the higher-incidence regions, both factors affecting the overall incidence of donor-derived TB and the risk for drug-resistant TB. The United States is among the nations with the lowest rates of TB, approximately 3 cases per 100,000 population, with the majority of cases occurring in individuals born outside the United States [19]. Thus in the United States, it is more likely that donor-derived TB may be associated with a donor who is foreign born or has lived for significant period of time in TB-endemic countries. In several of the reported SOT, TB transmission events, the donor was born in an area of high TB endemicity; in most cases the transmitted TB could be typed to a strain from the area where the donor was born [17, 18].

Epidemiology

Because of the increasing impact of international patients on SOT as well as TB epidemiology in the United States, it is absolutely essential to understand global TB trends in general and global trends for drug-resistant TB in particular. Global TB rates declined at the slow pace of 1.5% from 2014 to 2015. Based on a limited number of countries reporting longitudinal TB drug resistance data, the WHO concludes that during that time period, there was a slight trend for an increase in MDR-TB cases as a proportion of all TB cases in the reporting countries [2]. The estimates for the number of incident rifampin-resistant (RR-TB), MDR-TB and XDR-TB, cases increased to a combined total of 580,000 [2]. The inclusion of rifampin-resistant cases is the result of increasing the use of GeneXpert technology in the developing world which identifies TB isolates with rpoβ mutations and is frequently an indication of MDR-TB isolates [2].

The prognosis for MDR-TB and XDR-TB worldwide is very poor. In 2015 a total of 125,000 (20%) of the estimated 580,000 patients with MDR-/RR-TB were enrolled in treatment [2]. The treatment success rate in the 2013 cohort (cured or completed therapy) was only 52%. Patients with XDR-TB who started on treatment in 2013 had successful completion of therapy (28%), death (27%), and treatment failure (21%) or were lost to follow-up (23%) [2].

Overall, the percentage of MDR-TB cases in the United States decreased slightly from 1.4% (96 cases) in 2013 to 1.3% (91 cases) in 2014 [19]. Of the total number of reported MDR-TB cases, the proportion occurring among foreign-born persons increased from 31% (149 of 484) in 1993 to 88% (80 of 91) in 2014 [19]. There were no reported cases of XDR-TB in 2014 [19].

Knowing the country of origin for SOT donors and recipients is an essential information for determining the risk of drug-resistant TB. Of the estimated 580,000 cases of MDR-/RR-TB that emerged in 2015, over 45% were in India (130,000), the People's Republic of China (70,000), and the Russian Federation (60,000) [2]. Other countries with large numbers of cases include Indonesia (32,000), Nigeria (29,000), Pakistan (26,000), Ukraine (20,000), and South Africa (20,000) [2]. The top 30 countries with the highest number of TB cases accounted for nearly 90% of MDR-/RR-TB [2]. These countries are primarily in sub-Saharan Africa, Southeast Asia, and Eastern Europe. The estimated percentage of new MDR-/RR-TB cases for the 30 high-burden countries was 4.3% for new cases and 22% for previously treated cases [2].

Diagnosis of LTBI and Active TB

All potential transplant donors and recipients should be screened for LTBI and active TB. The sometimes precipitous nature of organ availability precludes rigorous evaluation of some donors, but an effort must be made to assess the risk of LTBI or active TB despite often rapidly evolving circumstances as with deceased donors. When there is adequate time, a deliberate and thorough evaluation should be undertaken. While current screening and diagnostic modalities were designed primarily to identify cases of LTBI, it is, of course, essential that screening protocols identify donors with unrecognized active TB, to facilitate diagnosis and management of TB and improve transplantation outcome.

The current method for donor screening for both latent and active TB includes history and symptom assessment (prior TB exposures, history of active TB, travel or residence in endemic regions, history of pneumonia, fever, weight loss, and past tuberculin skin test results), physical examination (cachexia or lymphadenopathy), cultures, and thoracic imaging. For living donors, the tuberculin skin test (TST) or interferon-gamma release assay (IGRA) screening should also be used. Cultures may be helpful when active TB is suspected although cultures can take up to 6 weeks before turning positive and thus may occur post transplantation. Nucleic acid amplification tests (NAAT) will identify *Mycobacterium tuberculosis* in clinical specimens with active infection and should be obtained routinely from sputum of pulmonary TB suspects.

The major risk factors for likelihood of TB infection in the United States are recent TB exposure and prior residence in a country with high TB endemicity. Once infected, patients undergoing immunosuppression following SOT are at very high risk for progression from LTBI to active TB. It is also clear that treatment of LTBI among high-risk groups reduces the risk of progression from LTBI to active tuberculosis [19].

The currently FDA-approved screening methods for LTBI in the United States include the tuberculin skin test (TST) and the IGRA and QuantiFERON-TB gold in-tube (QFT-GIT) assay and T-SPOT.TB test (T-SPOT). None of these tests are definitive for diagnosing LTBI, and none of these tests differentiate active from latent TB. As many as 10–25% of people with active TB do not react to TST with 5 mm or greater of induration, and patients with disseminated TB have a false-negative test rate of approximately 50% [20].

IGRAs are primarily a reflection of CD4 T-cell immune response to mycobacterial antigens manifested by the clonal expansion of antigens specific T cells. Effector memory T cells respond to subsequent antigen exposure which is characterized by the release of cytokines, including interferon gamma, and further cellular expansion. IGRA reflect the presence of these antigen-specific memory T cells. Currently there are two commercially available IGRA platforms that measure interferon-gamma release in response to *M. tuberculosis*-specific antigens. The QuantiFERON-TB gold in-tube (QFT-GIT) assay and T-spot. TB test (T-spot). The QFT measures interferon-gamma plasma concentration using an enzyme-linked immunoabsorbant assay (ELISA), while the T-spot assay enumerates T cells releasing interferon gamma using an enzyme-linked immunospot assay.

The IGRAs offer advantages over the TST for several reasons. Importantly, they require only one patient encounter to perform the test. The IGRAs also eliminate the need for technical skill required for TST placement and the subjectivity associated with manual reading of the TST. A main strength of the IGRAs is that they are not influenced by BCG vaccination and therefore have increased specificity compared with a TST in BCG-vaccinated patients due to the use of highly specific antigens that were derived from *Mycobacterium tuberculosis* which are absent in all strains of BCG and most NTM [20]. Thus a specific T-cell response toward those antigens is a more specific marker for true *M. tuberculosis* infection and then a TST response toward purified protein derivative (PPD). In people from TB-endemic areas where BCG vaccination is common, IGRAs have clear advantages over TST because of increased specificity of the results. This is an especially important performance characteristic of the IGRAs in the United States with the preponderance of TB including resistant TB, occurring in BCG-vaccinated patients born out outside of the United States. Problems associated with the IGRAs include indeterminate/invalid IGRA responses, poor reproducibility of IGRA results (especially in low-risk populations), and frequent discordance between the IGRAs and the TST [20].

Studies have compared the TST and IGRAs in immunocompromised patients [20–27]. Both diagnostic tests have diminished sensitivity in this setting, but data suggest that IGRAs are at least as sensitive as TST in the setting of HIV infection [26, 27]. Studies have been done comparing IGRAs with TST in populations that are heterogeneous with respect to the type of underlying immunocompromised [20–27]. These studies demonstrate significant discordance between TST an IGRA results. Overall it does not appear that there are sufficient data to recommend a preference for either a TST or an IGRA as the first-line diagnostic test in individuals likely to be infected with TB or have a high risk of progression to TB disease, such as organ transplant patients receiving immunosuppressive drugs to prevent allograft rejection [20]. The exception is for patients who have had BCG vaccination where the IGRA is clearly preferred to the TST. Both TST and IGRAs are less sensitive in the diagnosis of new TB exposure after solid organ transplant.

While TST is not feasible in deceased donor site due to the delay in development of a reaction, IGRA testing in deceased donors is possible [12]. In a deceased donor, it is important to assess whether antigen-presenting cells and T cells are functional enough to produce an appropriate immune response. Therefore, an advantage of IGRAs in the deceased donor setting is that specific stimulation reactions are accompanied both by a negative control that allows assessment of nonspecific background reactivity and also by a mitogen stimulus that is used as a positive control to assess general T-cell responsiveness. This may allow for interpretable results. Unfortunately, there are no data on the clinical utility or test performance of IGRAs in the deceased donor population. It is also unknown whether brain death may impact the performance of the assays.

Another issue about testing for LTBI in the deceased donor population is that the donor may be from a potentially low-risk population. Positive tests in a low-risk population may represent a false-positive result rather than a true latent TB infection [20]. Donors with an indeterminate or positive IGRA should not be excluded from donation although they should be carefully screened for active disease. In these cases it may be advantageous to procure tissue and blood for additional testing.

The epidemiologic history is more reliable compared with currently available tests for living donors who are generally healthy but may be from an area of high TB prevalence or have received BCG vaccine. Either IGRA or TST is routinely recommended to screen for LTBI in living donors with the exception of BCG-vaccinated individuals who should be tested with an IGRA. For living kidney and liver donors, transplant can often be delayed until a full evaluation of possible latent or active TB is performed. Although there are no formal studies of TST or IGRAs in the living donor population, test characteristics in living donors should be similar to those of healthy adults.

There is no specific guidance for patients with a severe immunocompromised state such as those who have undergone SOT who undergo both TST and IGRA. Some experts recommend that if either test is positive, then treatment for presumed LTBI would be appropriate regardless of the BCG status of the patient if the patient is from a country highly endemic for TB.

Treatment of LTBI

It is absolutely essential to exclude the presence of active TB disease in any patient with a positive TST or IGRA, either donor or recipient. The initiation of LTBI therapy in a patient with active disease would likely result in the development of drug-resistant TB.

There are several approved and effective treatment regimens for LTBI. The treatment regimen supported by the most experience and evidence of efficacy is INH monotherapy administered for at least 9 months [28]. Isoniazid LTBI therapy is effective for preventing active TB in both pre- and post-renal transplant recipients even in TB-endemic areas [29]. Isoniazid is also effective for preventing reactivation TB in liver transplant patients [30]. The problems with this regimen include the long duration of treatment and the risk for hepatic toxicity [28]. For patients who are awaiting transplant, there may not be adequate time to complete 9 months of INH therapy prior to the transplant. A recent meta-analysis of INH in renal transplant patients reported that the risk of developing liver dysfunction among those who received TB prophylaxis was 59% higher than those who received no chemoprophylaxis [29]. However, most reported instances of liver dysfunction were mild and reversible and did not warrant discontinuation of treatment. Liver transplant recipients present a high risk of hepatotoxicity with INH therapy including the need for emergency transplantation [31]. Other investigators have not reported increased hepatotoxicity associated with INH in the liver transplant population [32–35]. Clinicians may still be reluctant to use this approach for patients with impending hepatic failure who are waiting for liver transplantation or for patients who have recently received a liver transplant. The advantage of this regimen is the relatively low risk for significant drug-drug interactions with immunosuppressive agents to prevent allograft rejection compared to rifamycins. Specifically the interaction between INH with calcineurin inhibitors is limited [36] (see Table 56.1).

The second regimen involves rifampin monotherapy for 4 months [20]. The major problem with this regimen is the drug-drug interactions that are encountered with multiple immunosuppressive agents because of the stimulation by rifampin of hepatic cytochrome P450 enzymes (CYP3A4) that increase metabolism of the antirejection drugs [36]. When rifamycins are used, levels of immunosuppressive drugs should be closely monitored, and the dose of calcineurin inhibitors, mTOR, and corticosteroids should be increased. The advantages of rifampin in this setting are shorter duration of therapy and decreased risk of hepatic toxicity than with INH although the risk of hepatotoxicity is not completely avoided. The 5-month difference in regimen duration may allow some patients awaiting transplantation to complete LTBI therapy before transplantation. The use of rifamycins in the treatment of active TB is discussed below.

The challenges and benefits of LTBI therapy in SOT patients was recently reported in a study of 189 SOT patients with LTBI who were initially prescribed isoniazid (73%), rifampin (12.7%), or another regimen (14.3%) [37]. Adequate LTBI therapy occurred in 122 (64.5%). Patients who were liver transplant candidates or recipients were less likely to complete therapy than nonliver transplant patients as were patients treated in the posttransplant phase. Liver enzyme elevation led to discontinuation of therapy more often in liver transplant candidates and recipients and posttransplant treatment. After a mean follow-up of 4.9 year/patient, there were no cases of active TB.

A third and more recent approach involves 12 weekly doses of INH and rifapentine [38–40] given by directly observed therapy. The major problems with this approach are the potential for hepatic toxicity with isoniazid and the potential for drug-drug interactions with rifapentine, although the stimulation of hepatic cytochrome P450 enzymes with rifa-

Table 56.1 Mycobacterial disease and transplant drug-drug interactions

Drug and mechanism	Cyclosporin drug levels available	Mycophenolate	Sirolimus drug levels available	Tacrolimus drug levels available	Prednisone
Rifampin Cytochrome P450 inducer RIF > RPT > RBT	↑ Drug clearance ↓ Serum drug levels	↑ Drug clearance ↓ Serum drug levels	↑ Drug clearance ↓ Serum drug levels	↑ Drug clearance ↓ Serum drug levels	↑ Drug clearance ↓ Serum drug levels
Isoniazid Cytochrome P450 inhibitor	↓ Drug clearance ↑ Serum drug levels		↓ Drug clearance ↑ Serum drug levels	↓ Drug clearance ↑ Serum drug levels	
Clarithromycin Cytochrome P450 inhibitor	↓ Drug clearance ↑ Serum drug levels		↓ Drug clearance ↑ Serum drug levels	↓ Drug clearance ↑ Serum drug levels	
Ethambutol	NS[a]	NS[a]	NS[a]	NS[a]	NS[a]
Aminoglycosides	Possible additive or synergistic risk of renal impairment			Possible additive or synergistic risk of renal impairment	

[a]*NS* no significant interaction

pentine may be somewhat less than with rifampin. This regimen has been shown to be associated with fewer instances of hepatic toxicity than INH alone in both HIV seropositive and seronegative populations [38–40]. A major advantage of this approach is the relatively rapid completion of therapy for LTBI (3 months vs. 4 months for rifampin and 9 months for INH) and a demonstrably improved completion rate compared with INH. Because of the short duration and association with improved treatment completion, this regimen appears to be superior to the alternative regimens.

As discussed in detail in the section on multidrug-resistant TB (MDR-TB), fluoroquinolone monotherapy is another choice [41]. An advantage of this approach is the relative safety of fluoroquinolones from a hepatic perspective. The major drawback to this regimen is the lack of conclusive data demonstrating its efficacy in the setting of either drug-susceptible or drug-resistant TB. In patients exposed to drug-resistant TB isolates, there is also the risk of developing fluoroquinolone resistance if there is occult active disease, which could transform a patient with MDR-TB into one with XDR-TB.

From the risk/benefit perspective related to TB, any patient with LTBI should receive therapy. Each patient must be assessed individually so that the best and most appropriate LTBI regimen can be chosen.

A major concern for treating LTBI and active TB is the drug-drug interactions that may occur between the antimycobacterial medications, especially the rifamycins, and the immunosuppressive antirejection agents. The following discussion about these interactions is pertinent to both LTBI and active TB therapy.

Significant drug-drug interactions can occur with antimycobacterial medications and most immunosuppressive agents used to deter allograft rejection (Table 56.2). The rifamycins

Table 56.2 Recommended treatment regimens for TB and NTM

Organism and resistance	Recommended regimen	Extent/duration of therapy
No first-line drug resistance	RIF 10 mg/kg daily INH 5 mg/kg daily PZA 20–25 mg/kg daily initial 2 months)	6–9 months
INH resistance	RIF 10 mg/kg daily EMB 15 mg/kg daily PZA, 20–25 mg/kg daily	Rifampin + at least two other drugs, 6–9 months Extensive Add LEVO 1000–1500 mg daily or Amikacin *or* capreomycin 15 mg/kg 5×/week
RIF Resistance	EMB 15 mg/kg daily PZA, 20–25 mg/kg daily LEVO, 750–1000 mg daily[b] Amikacin *or* capreomycin 15 mg/kg 5×/week	Amikacin or capreomycin, 5×/week until culture conversion and then 3×/week for at least 6 months Oral drugs for 18 months Extensive Amikacin or capreomycin, 5×/week for 6 months and then 3×/week for 6–12 months Oral drugs for 18–24 months
MDR-TB INH RIF Rifabutin	Amikacin *or* capreomycin 15 mg/kg 5×/week LEVO, 750–1000 mg daily[b] PZA, 20–25 mg/kg daily EMB, 15 mg/kg daily Ethionamide, 500–750 mg daily B_6, 100 mg daily	Primary or limited Amikacin or capreomycin, 5×/week for 4–6 months and then 3×/week for 6–12 months Oral drugs for 18–24 months Extensive Amikacin or capreomycin, 5×/week for 4–6 months and then 3×/week until culture negative for 12 months Oral drugs for 24 months PAS or cycloserine may be added
XDR-TB		
INH RIF Rifabutin Kanamycin and/ or amikacin and/or capreomycin Ofloxacin ±Others	Use any new fluoroquinolone that is sensitive Use any injectable that may be active Any first-line drug available Linezolid, 600 mg daily Ethionamide if available PAS, 6–8 g daily Cycloserine, 500–750 mg daily Other third-line drugs if needed to have at least five drugs available[b]	Primary or limited Amikacin (capreomycin or kanamycin), if available, 5×/week for 6 months and then 3×/week until culture negative for 12 months Include linezolid for entire 24 months Oral drugs, at least four or five, for 24 months Extensive Amikacin (capreomycin or kanamycin), if available, 5×/week for 6 months and then 3×/week until culture negative for 12 months Include linezolid for entire 24 months Oral drugs, at least four or five, for 24 months
MAC[c] Macrolide susceptible	Azithromycin 250 mg/day or clarithromycin 500 mg BID EMB 15 mg/kg daily RIF 10 mg/kg daily	Extensive, cavitary, or severe Amikacin, 5×/week for 6 months and then 3×/week until culture negative for 12 months

Table 56.2 (continued)

Organism and resistance	Recommended regimen	Extent/duration of therapy
MAC Macrolide resistant	EMB 15 mg/kg daily RBT 150–300 mg daily Amikacin, 5×/week for 6 months and then 3×/week until culture negative for 12 months	Extensive or severe disease, consider: Clofazimine 100 mg daily Linezolid 300–600 mg/daily Bedaquiline
M. abscessus subsp. *abscessus*	Amikacin, 5×/week for 6 months and then 3×/week until culture negative for 12 months Tigecycline 25–50 mg daily Cefoxitin 3–4 mg twice daily Imipenem 500–1000 mg twice daily Clofazimine 100 mg daily	

[a]Treatment should always be in consultation with an expert in management of MDR-TB, XDR-TB, macrolide-resistant MAC, or *M. abscessus* subsp. *abscessus*. Extensive disease consists of extensive infiltrates, cavities, or pulmonary destruction

[b]We usually prefer LEVO (with a dosage of at least 750 mg daily), but patients with decreased renal failure or those with possible resistance to LEVO should receive moxifloxacin (see text)

[c]Mycobacterium avium complex

are the major concern, but isoniazid also has the potential to alter the pharmacokinetics of several agents as well. The interactions between the antituberculosis drugs and the anti-rejection immunosuppressive drugs is mediated primarily through the hepatic cytochrome P450 enzyme system (CYP3A4) with either stimulation (rifamycins) or inhibition (isoniazid) of the hepatic enzymes resulting in either decreased or increased serum drug levels, respectively. Among the rifamycins, rifampin is the most potent cytochrome P450 enzyme stimulant followed by rifapentine and then rifabutin. It is important to remember that the rifamycins, especially rifampin, are the best and most effective drugs for treating TB disease. If a rifamycin is not included in a TB treatment regimen, the shortest duration of therapy becomes 12 months with likely exposure to more hepatotoxic drugs such as INH. Maintaining rifamycins in a TB treatment regimen is a very high priority, and abandoning rifamycins in a post SOT patient should only be done as a last resort. The rifamycins are generally less important for the treatment of NTM pathogens, with the exception of *M. kansasii*. Mycophenolate levels are significantly reduced in the presence of rifampin [36]. Isoniazid does not apparently have a significant effect on mycophenolate metabolism. Cyclosporin is metabolized by hepatic cytochrome P450 enzymes, and stimulation of these enzymes by rifampin significantly increases metabolism and clearance of cyclosporin with subsequent decrease in cyclosporin serum concentrations. Inhibition of the cytochrome P450 enzymes by INH diminishes metabolism and clearance of cyclosporin with subsequent increase in serum cyclosporin concentrations and the potential for cyclosporin toxicity. Similarly clarithromycin can increase serum cyclosporin concentrations. The rifamycins also increase the metabolism of tacrolimus and sirolimus through stimulation of cytochrome P450 enzymes. The effect of INH is not as clear as with cyclosporin. Clarithromycin also decreases the metabolism and clearance of the drugs and increases the serum concentration with the potential for nephrotoxicity. The rifamycins also increase prednisone metabolism but do not have a significant effect on Imuran metabolism. Serum levels are available for mycophenolate, cyclosporin, tacrolimus, and sirolimus which may be helpful for guiding therapy with concomitant use of a rifamycin.

Diagnosis of Active TB

Although primary pulmonary TB can be a presenting illness in the recipient, fever of unknown origin, sepsis, and organ dysfunction are more typical of transmission from non-pulmonary organs or in a donor site with disseminated disease at the time of donation. About one third to one half of all active TB cases after transplantation are disseminated or occur at extrapulmonary sites, compared to about 15% of cases in immunocompetent persons [12–14]. Any SOT patient with unexplained pulmonary densities should be suspected of having active TB. Any SOT patient with unexplained fever or evidence of multi-organ involvement should be suspected of having active TB. False-negative TST and IGRA results may occur with miliary or disseminated disease [19, 42]. Therefore, neither IGRA nor TST should be relied upon to exclude active TB disease.

Clinicians should be aware of the risk of donor-derived reactivation and an occult infection and when clinically indicated test for disease in the allograft and elsewhere, using cultures, NAAT, radiology, pathology, and clinical acumen, maintaining a low threshold to diagnose this disease clinically. In several transmission events, appropriate cultures for TB were collected but became positively well after the transplants had occurred [12].

Early recognition of risk factors for drug resistance is important. Drug resistance should be suspected in those who were born or lived in countries with a high rate of drug resistance, were exposed to a person with drug resistance, or have a history of prior TB treatment, TB treatment failure, or if treatment was not directly observed, the regimen was inadequate, medication supply was inconsistent, or there was poor adherence.

For any AFB smear- or culture-positive specimen from an SOT donor or recipient, a GeneXpert® analysis should be requested. The GeneXpert utilizes both an NAAT for determining the presence of *M. tuberculosis* and is a screening test for rifampin resistance by evaluating the presence of rpoβ mutations that confer rifampin resistance [20, 43]. Pretest preparation of samples with this technology is minimal, and the results are available within hours. The sensitivity and specificity of the GeneXpert for detecting rifampin-resistant *M. tuberculosis* isolates from AFB smear-positive respiratory specimens are >95% [20, 43]. As previously noted, the presence of rifampin resistance is strongly associated with MDR-TB especially in high-incidence countries. In the setting of SOT, a positive smear or culture specimen must be evaluated by GeneXpert to screen for rifampin resistance. Standard in vitro susceptibility testing is also always mandatory because both false-positive and false-negative results can occur with GeneXpert, although rare. In most instances of discordant GeneXpert and phenotypic drug susceptibility results, the GeneXpert result is most predictive of treatment response [20].

If a specimen appears rifampin resistant by GeneXpert, it should be referred to the Centers for Disease Control and Prevention (CDC) for molecular detection of drug resistance (MDDR) which analyzes mutations that are associated with resistance to other antimycobacterial agents [44]. For drugs other than rifampin, MDDR is approximately 80–85% sensitive depending on the drug in question [45]. Results are typically available within 48 h after receipt of the specimen by the CDC. Standard phenotypic in vitro drug susceptibility testing is always necessary for confirmation of results, again because of the potential for false-positive or false-negative MDDR results.

The two major concerns for treating active mycobacterial disease after transplantation are the immunosuppression necessary to avoid allograft rejection which may hinder effective treatment response and the drug-drug interactions that may occur between the antimycobacterial medications, especially the rifamycins, and the immunosuppressive agents. The first concern is a strong argument for inclusion of rifamycins in the treatment regimen of SOT TB patients. The use of rifampin with multiple antirejection medications can increase the risk of acute rejection [46, 47]. Conversely, a study evaluating the impact of rifampin-based anti-TB regimens found that neither rejection rate nor mortality after TB differed between those treated with and without rifampin [48]. Another study also demonstrated similar graft rejection and mortality between rifampin-containing and levofloxacin-containing groups [49]. Additionally few rejections were reported in SOT recipients with TB treated with rifampin [50, 51]. Given the importance of rifampin in the treatment of TB, some experts prefer the use of rifampin for SOT with TB with at least twofold to fivefold increase of doses of calcineurin inhibitors and close monitoring of their serum levels [52, 53].

Examples of TB treatment regimens based on in vitro drug susceptibility results are given in Table 56.1. The importance of rapid identification of drug-resistant *M. tuberculosis* disease cannot be overstated. Because of the risks of treatment failure posed by the extreme immunosuppression following SOT, the risks for allograft rejection posed by drug-drug interactions between immunosuppressive drugs (Table 56.2), and the risks for drug toxicity posed by the antimycobacterial drugs and TB drug, especially second-line TB drug, empiric TB therapy is extremely difficult and fraught with potential pitfalls.

Treatment for MDR-TB should be guided by an expert in the management of MDR-TB and should preferably begin with six but not fewer than four new drugs with proven susceptibility, two of which should be bactericidal [2, 54]. A standard approach is to (a) use any first-line drugs to which the isolate remains susceptible; (b) add a second-line injectable drug (SLID) such as streptomycin, kanamycin, amikacin, and capreomycin unless the patient has specific contraindications to the use of these drugs such as over age 60, baseline chronic kidney disease, baseline hearing loss, young children, or persons with decreased body mass (an SLID is recommended for 8 months of treatment, unless contraindicated; this period defines the intensive phase); (c) add a fluoroquinolone (high-dose levofloxacin or moxifloxacin); and (d) choose additional remaining drugs to bring the number of drugs in the regimen to at least five, preferably six, if all susceptibility tests are not yet available. Initial consideration should be given to linezolid and high-dose PZA. The remaining drugs should be chosen from the weaker second-line oral agents such as ethionamide, cycloserine, clofazimine, and PAS. In interactions with transplant rejections, medications must be considered, adjusted, and monitored through the treatment course. The recent WHO guidelines allow for extension of the intensive phase when treatment response has been slow, when there is extensive pulmonary or extrapulmonary TB disease, and when patients have failed prior treatment for MDR-TB [2]. At least three, preferably four, effective medications are recommended in the continuation phase of therapy. This phase is extended 12 months past the initial phase for a total duration of therapy of 20 months in most patients. However, in patients with extensive cavitary disease, longer therapy, i.e., at least 12 months of the injectable after conversion of cultures to negative and 24–26 months of treatment with the oral regimen, is likely to be needed to decrease the incidence of relapse [2, 54].

Short Course MDR-TB Treatment Regimens

Standardized short-course treatment regimens, lasting 12 months or less, are a new treatment option recommended by the 2016 WHO Guidelines for any patient with MDR-TB who has not previously been treated with second-line TB drugs for greater than 1 month and whose *M. tuberculosis* isolate is proven or thought likely to be susceptible to all medications in the regimen [2]. The isolate should be shown to be susceptible to at least the fluoroquinolones and SLID agents prior to starting the regimen.

The WHO short-course regimen is standardized and divided into two phases. The initial intensive phase is 4 months (which can be extended to 6 months if sputum conversion is slow) and includes high-dose gatifloxacin (or moxifloxacin), kanamycin, ethionamide (or prothionamide), clofazimine, high-dose INH, PZA, and ethambutol. This is followed by the 5-month-long continuation phase of treatment which includes high-dose gatifloxacin (or moxifloxacin), clofazimine, PZA, and ethambutol. The applicability of this approach for SOT recipients is unknown and as with any MDR-TB treatment regimen should only be undertaken with consultation from experts.

Just as treatment for MDR-TB is largely based on expert opinion and observational studies, so is treatment for XDR-TB. Treatment is even more difficult, as there is less information available to guide providers. It is essential to have both first- and second-line drug susceptibility tests, including tests for all injectable agents, ethionamide, and a newer-generation fluoroquinolone in order to maximize the therapeutic regimen. Treatment should be guided by an expert in the management of MDR- and XDR-TB.

Treatment of XDR-TB is based on the same principles as is the treatment of MDR-TB [2]. The treatment regimen is built the same way. It is especially important to include any first-line drug to which the isolate remains susceptible. An injectable should always be used if any is identified as effective. Testing should be done against each SLID, kanamycin, amikacin, and capreomycin, as inclusion of an injectable to which the isolate is susceptible will improve treatment outcomes. If susceptibility to levofloxacin or moxifloxacin is determined, one of these should be used. Additional second- and third-line drugs should be added to bring the number of drugs in the regimen to at least six. Usually, treatment with both the injectable and the oral drug regimen should be longer and more aggressive than for MDR-TB, although definite guidelines do not exist [2].

Treatment regimens for MDR- and XDR-TB include drugs with significant toxicity [2, 54, 55]. Patients should be warned to expect some adverse effects but encouraged that once they complete treatment, most drug-related side effects and toxicities will resolve. Suggestions for monitoring TB medication toxicity are provided in Table 56.3.

Table 56.3 Commonly used antimycobacterial drugs: toxicity, side effects, and monitoring

Drug	Side effects, toxicity[a,b]	Drug monitoring
Rifampin, rifapentine	Orange staining of body fluids, GI discomfort, flu-like symptoms, hepatotoxicity, renal failure, hemolytic anemia, thrombocytopenia	Baseline and monthly liver enzymes, bilirubin, creatinine, CBC
Rifabutin	Leukopenia, thrombocytopenia, skin discoloration, hepatotoxicity, arthralgias, anterior uveitis	Baseline and monthly liver enzymes and bilirubin, CBC Drug interactions
Isoniazid (INH)	Hepatitis, peripheral neuropathy, optic neuritis, arthralgias, drug-induced lupus	Clinical monitoring for hepatotoxicity is essential. Baseline and monthly liver enzymes and bilirubin
Ethambutol	Retrobulbar neuritis, visual acuity and color vision loss, peripheral neuropathy	Baseline and monthly visual acuity and color vision checks
PZA	Hepatotoxicity, arthralgias, photosensitivity, nausea, abdominal discomfort, gout	Baseline and monthly liver enzymes and bilirubin. Baseline uric acid then as dictated by symptoms
Amikacin, streptomycin	Nephrotoxicity, ototoxicity, vestibular toxicity, electrolyte imbalances (hypokalemia, hypocalcemia, hypomagnesemia)	Baseline and monthly creatinine, electrolytes, magnesium, calcium Baseline and monthly audiometry and vestibular exams
Levofloxacin, moxifloxacin	Nausea, headache, dizziness, insomnia, arthralgia, tendonitis, rarely tendon rupture, QTc prolongation	Symptomatic monitoring No routine laboratory monitoring recommended
Linezolid	Myelosuppression, diarrhea, nausea, optic and peripheral neuropathy	Symptomatic monitoring Baseline and monthly CBC, visual acuity, and color vision testing
Clofazimine	Discoloration of skin, nausea, photosensitivity, GI bleeding, and bowel obstruction	Symptomatic monitoring No routine laboratory, monitoring recommended
Cefoxitin	Abdominal discomfort, leukopenia	Baseline and monthly CBC
Imipenem	Diarrhea, nausea, vomiting, seizure	Symptomatic monitoring
Tigecycline	Nausea and vomiting	Symptomatic monitoring No routine laboratory monitoring
Clarithromycin	Diarrhea, nausea, abnormal taste, abdominal pain, hepatotoxicity, hearing loss	Symptomatic monitoring No routine laboratory monitoring is recommended

[a]All drugs used for treating mycobacterial infections have the potential for causing hypersensitivity reactions
[b]All drugs require clinical monitoring on at least a monthly basis

Medications Recommended for MDR-TB

Injectable agents include streptomycin, amikacin, and kanamycin, which are aminoglycosides, and the closely related polypeptide capreomycin act at the 30S ribosome to inhibit protein synthesis [54]. Adverse events include ototoxicity, nephrotoxicity, and rare neuromuscular blockade. Aminoglycoside and capreomycin use may be complicated by reductions in serum calcium, magnesium, and potassium [54, 55]. Cross resistance is not seen between streptomycin and amikacin, so unless patients have had prior treatment with either kanamycin or amikacin, these isolates are generally sensitive to amikacin. Isolates which are kanamycin resistant are usually resistant to amikacin (Table 56.4).

Fluoroquinolones including ciprofloxacin, ofloxacin, levofloxacin, and moxifloxacin are bactericidal against both extracellular rapidly multiplying bacteria and intracellular nonmultiplying bacteria [56–59]. They inhibit bacterial DNA gyrase, an enzyme that is essential for the maintenance of DNA supercoils, which are needed for chromosomal replication [54]. The fluoroquinolones penetrate well into tissues (alveolar macrophages), respiratory secretions, and body fluids, with concentrations equal to or higher than those in serum. Central nervous system (CNS) penetration is good, allowing these drugs to be used for tuberculous meningitis [54]. Despite the absence of prospective clinical trials using fluoroquinolones for MDR-TB, because of considerable experience with levofloxacin and moxifloxacin, they are regarded as critical to good treatment outcomes [2, 54].

Fluoroquinolone resistance develops as a two-step process, and higher serum levels protect against selection of mutants [60, 61]. Resistance to fluoroquinolones develops rapidly when they are used as monotherapy [60]. Single-fluoroquinolone prescriptions for community-acquired pneumonia in a Canadian study were not associated with development of resistant *M. tuberculosis*, whereas multiple-fluoroquinolone prescriptions were [61]. Cross resistance within the class of fluoroquinolones was previously felt to be complete. Recent anecdotal experience noted ofloxacin resistance but retained in vitro susceptibility to the newer agents [54]. Toxicity with the fluoroquinolone class of drugs most commonly is reported as gastrointestinal upset such as nausea and bloating. Myalgia is relatively common, and, rarely, tendon rupture has been reported [54]. Prolongation of the QT interval has been noted in patients taking moxifloxacin, but a detrimental clinical impact of that observation has not been demonstrated.

Most reports note that 20–30% or more of MDR-TB isolates retain sensitivity to rifabutin [62]. Rifabutin is bactericidal, with an MIC for TB less than or equal to 2 μg/ml regarded as susceptible. Although peak serum levels are 1 μg/ml, the drug has excellent activity and penetrates into polymorphonuclear leukocytes, lymphocytes, and macrophages. Tissue levels are significantly higher than serum levels. In the lungs, tissue levels are five to ten times higher than

Table 56.4 Key recommendations

It is imperative to test potential transplant recipient and donors for LTBI as early in the process as possible. That means testing potential SOT candidates for LTBI as soon as the possibility of SOT is considered, hopefully well before the patient is put on a transplant list.
The TST or IGRA are acceptable tests for screening for LTBI. In the case of discrepant results, any positivity (unless related to a documented BCG vaccination) should be considered for treatment of LTBI.
Prior to the initiation of LTBI therapy, it is imperative to exclude active TB.
It is imperative to treat LTBI in potential transplant recipient site and donors as expeditiously as possible, preferably completing that therapy prior to transplantation but if necessary, continuing therapy posttransplant.
Options for treating LTBI include INH for 9 months, rifampin for 4 months, and INH/rifapentine for 3 months. The optimal regimen for each patient must be determined individually.
It is imperative to assess carefully the risk of both LTBI and active TB in deceased donors especially those from areas of high TB endemicity.
Patients who are posttransplant must be assessed very carefully for active TB prior to initiation of LTBI therapy. Mycobacterial disease, especially TB, should be suspected in posttransplant patients with unexplained fever or evidence of disease dissemination. In the presence of active TB, LTBI therapy could result in the development of acquired drug resistance.
Cultures and NAAT from suspected sites of TB diseases are necessary for confirming the diagnosis.
Invasive techniques such as bronchoscopy with transbronchial biopsy for pulmonary disease or direct sampling from an extrapulmonary site of involvement should be performed if routine evaluation is not diagnostic.
For severe forms of TB or disseminated TB, the use of a rifamycin (rifampin or rifabutin) should be considered.
When rifamycins are used, levels of immunosuppressive drugs should be closely monitored, and the dose of calcineurin inhibitors, mTOR, and corticosteroids should be increased.
Treatment of drug-resistant TB, including multidrug-resistant TB (MDR-TB), should be managed by an expert in TB treatment.
Diagnosis of NTM pulmonary disease requires fulfilling four criteria, (a) a compatible clinical presentation, (b) radiographic abnormalities consistent with NTM disease, (c) exclusion of other diagnoses, and (d) isolation of a pathogenic NTM species from sputum (at least two positive cultures), bronchoalveolar lavage, or tissue biopsy (one positive culture).
Diagnosis of extrapulmonary disease requires isolation of a pathogenic NTM from a normally sterile body site such as blood, cerebrospinal fluid, or other sterile fluids.
Treatment of NTM disease should be managed by an expert in NTM treatment.

in plasma [54]. Patients whose *M. tuberculosis* isolates are rifampin resistant but rifabutin susceptible should receive rifabutin as part of their MDR-TB treatment regimen [2].

Ethionamide is structurally similar to isoniazid and also appears to inhibit cell wall mycolic acid synthesis [54]. The drug is bactericidal, well absorbed orally, and widely distributed. The most frequent adverse effect is gastrointestinal intolerance, including nausea, epigastric pain, and metallic taste. Significant hepatitis occurs in about 4.3% of patients, but transient abnormalities in liver tests are more common. Hypothyroidism develops in a significant number of patients treated with ethionamide.

Cycloserine is bacteriostatic for mycobacteria, acting to inhibit cell wall synthesis [54]. It is rapidly absorbed after oral administration and is widely distributed. The most common side effects pertain to the CNS seizures, psychosis, mania, depression, other emotional disturbances, and drowsiness. Neurotoxicity appears to be dose dependent and is rarely seen if serum drug levels remain below 30 μg/ml.

Clofazimine is a riminophenazine dye compound used to treat *Mycobacterium leprae* with activity against TB [54]. The mechanism of action is unknown but may involve DNA binding. Concentrated in macrophages, clofazimine has proven effective in a murine TB model. Generally well tolerated except for occasional gastrointestinal complaints, the most frequent patient concern is reversible skin darkening due to drug deposition.

Linezolid is an oxazolidinone antibacterial agent that blocks ribosomal protein synthesis. It acts by binding to the 50S bacterial ribosomal subunit, which prevents formation of the initiation complex for protein synthesis [54]. The drug has good in vitro activity against *Mycobacterium tuberculosis*, with modest early bactericidal activity and minimal extended bactericidal activity during days 2–7 [63].

In observational studies linezolid in multidrug regimens has been associated with improved outcomes in patients with MDR- and XDR-TB even when added to a chronically failing regimen as salvage therapy [63–68]. The dosage of linezolid for bacterial infections is 600 mg twice daily, but most studies have used 600 mg once daily for treatment of TB, in an effort to limit toxicity and cost. Serum drug levels are sufficiently above the MIC with this dosage [67].

Unfortunately, administration of 600 mg daily has not shown significant reduction in toxicity [65–67]. More recently, good outcomes with less frequent and severe toxicity have been reported for small series of patients treated with linezolid at 300 mg daily [66]. Most reports show frequent serious adverse events occur in a significant proportion of patients treated with linezolid and may lead to discontinuation of the drug. These reactions, which are caused by inhibition of mitochondrial protein synthesis, include myelosuppression, peripheral and optic neuropathy, and lactic acidosis [69–72]. Peripheral neuropathy has been especially concerning, as it may persist after stopping treatment [72]. Toxicity is related to duration of therapy. Hematological toxicity may occur in the first weeks to months of therapy, but neurologic toxicity usually occurs after 3–4 months. Lactic acidosis occurs during the initial weeks of therapy [72]. Linezolid is associated with the serotonin syndrome in up to 25% of patients given selective serotonin reuptake inhibitors or other medications that increase serotonin concentrations in the CNS [72]. Patients should also be counseled to avoid foods, dietary supplements, and beverages high in tyramine. The toxicity of linezolid is significant, and patients must be monitored carefully and the risks and benefits repeatedly reviewed and discussed with the patients [73].

Treatment of Latent Infection Possibly Due to MDR-TB

All persons identified as MDR-TB contacts are at risk and should be quickly evaluated for latent infection and active disease. The optimal management of established LTBI is a matter of debate. No regimen has been proved unequivocally effective, and it is unlikely that a definitive study will be done to guide management. Those who are tuberculin skin test positive are close contacts of an MDR-TB case, have no history of a previously positive tuberculin test, and can be considered for treatment of latent MDR-TB. Most clinicians agree that LTBI treatment should be offered to tuberculin skin test-positive, immunosuppressed individuals with documented exposure to MDR-TB. If assessment indicates the likelihood of exposure to drug-susceptible TB, isoniazid therapy may be preferred.

The selection of agents should be guided by the susceptibility profile of the index case. One possible regimen is a combination of pyrazinamide (25–30 mg daily) and ethambutol (15–25 mg daily). If fluoroquinolone susceptibility is documented, a regimen that combines ofloxacin (800 mg), levofloxacin (750 mg), or moxifloxacin (400 mg) daily with pyrazinamide might be used. A pyrazinamide-fluoroquinolone combination appears to result in enhanced activity within the macrophage [74]. The pyrazinamide-based regimens have been associated with high levels of hepatotoxicity [75]. A fluoroquinolone also can be combined with ethambutol. There is preliminary data that suggests fluoroquinolone administration alone prevents early disease progression in patients with LTBI who are contacts to MDR-TB patients [41]. The fluoroquinolones are also relatively nontoxic to the liver. Some experts recommend fluoroquinolone monotherapy, although emergence of fluoroquinolone resistance is a concern. LTBI treatment with fluoroquinolone is usually prescribed for 6–12 months (see above).

Nevertheless, it is important to monitor all persons with presumed latent MDR-TB for at least 2 years following the exposure. Periodic assessments should include clinical exams and chest radiographs every 3 months for persons with HIV or other immunosuppressing illness and every 6 months for all others [54].

Nontuberculous Mycobacteria

The pathophysiology of nontuberculous mycobacterial lung disease is not well-known, and specifically it is not known if there is a latent infection stage similar to that of *Mycobacterium tuberculosis*. There are no tests similar to the TST and IGRAs to evaluate the possibility of latent nontuberculous mycobacterial infection. Therefore, there is no possibility of screening for latent nontuberculous mycobacterial infection in SOT donors or recipients. The diagnosis of nontuberculous mycobacterial disease can only be made on the basis of positive cultures and by clinical history. There are no surrogate markers of infection or disease. A positive culture from biopsy is usually adequate for diagnosis of nontuberculous mycobacterial infection, but diagnoses of nontuberculous mycobacterial lung disease are more difficult due to the possibility of respiratory specimen contamination by NTM.

In contrast to MTB, DST for NTM remains controversial and problematic providing less reliable therapeutic guidance. For many species such as the *Mycobacterium avium* complex (MAC), the correlation between in vitro DST results and in vivo response to antimycobacterial medications remains inconsistent and unpredictable. An important example is MAC where the only antimicrobial agents for which a correlation between in vitro DST for MAC and clinical response has been demonstrated in controlled clinical trials are the macrolides (clarithromycin and azithromycin) and amikacin.

This frustrating phenomenon is due to multiple factors unrelated to resistance factors not tested by DST and MICs. Natural resistance to antimicrobial drugs is conferred by a variety of mechanisms that interfere with uptake of the drug, enable it biotransformation in the cell, or decrease the affinity with the drug target. The most frustrating aspect of these natural drug resistance mechanisms is that they are generally not reflected in the in vitro MIC of specific drugs utilized for treatment of NTM. Natural drug resistance likely determines a large part of the multidrug resistance that is commonplace in NTM. This multidrug resistance, in turn, is a likely explanation of the limited efficacy of current treatment regimens for NTM disease. Testing the susceptibility of individual clinical isolates is of limited value for drugs to which natural resistance occurs. Ultimately, for most drugs used for treating NTM pathogens, there is no clear correlation between in vitro activity and the outcome of treatment, in vivo.

In contrast to MTB, DST of NTM should be performed on the initial isolate only for clinically significant isolates that exhibit variability in susceptibility to clinically useful antimicrobial agents and/or significant risk of acquired mutational resistance to one or more of these agents. For slowly growing NTM such as MAC, DST should be performed using a broth-based method, either macrodilution or microdilution.

Molecular analysis of MAC isolates that have developed resistance to macrolides in vitro has shown that these isolates have acquired a point mutation for the 23S rRNA gene. DST is indicated for clinically significant MAC isolates from patients on prior macrolide therapy, isolates who develop bacteremia while on macrolide prophylaxis, and isolates from patients who relapse while on macrolide therapy or initial isolates to establish baseline values. DST should be repeated after 3 months of treatment for patients with disseminated disease and after 6 months of treatment for patients with pulmonary disease if the patient shows either no clinical improvement or clinical deterioration while on therapy.

Other important NTM species that exhibit poor correlation between in vitro susceptibility and in vivo response to therapy include *M. xenopi*, *M. malmoense*, *M. marinum* and *M. szulgai*, and *M. simiae*.

M. kansasii is a clinically significant slowly growing mycobacterium which can cause disease resembling TB. For *M. kansasii*, the MICs for rifampin, INH, and ethambutol for untreated strains fall within a narrow range, and routine susceptibility testing is generally not needed. Treatment failure can occur and is invariably associated with resistance to rifampin. Given that treatment failure is associated with rifampin resistance and drug treatment histories are generally unavailable, susceptibility to the single drug rifampin is the only one currently recommended for primary testing. Susceptibility testing should be repeated for patients who fail initial therapy or remain AFB culture positive after 3 months of therapy. For secondary drug testing of isolates resistant to rifampin, a total of eight drugs could be tested including macrolides and fluoroquinolones.

For rapidly growing mycobacteria, broth microdilution testing of pathogenic RGM requires skill acquired through experience with the test method and knowledge of the expected susceptibility patterns of different species. Therefore, in general, for laboratories that encounter these organisms infrequently, referring those isolates for which susceptibility testing is indicated to an established reference laboratory is recommended. Susceptibility testing is indicated for any RGM that is considered clinically significant. These organisms may cause pulmonary disease, but they also may be recovered as a contaminant so that not all RGM recovered from sputum is clinically significant. Isolates recovered in low numbers from only one of multiple sputum specimens are not likely to cause disease and therefore do not warrant susceptibility testing. Agents that should be tested against the RGM are amikacin, cefoxitin, ciprofloxacin, clarithromycin, doxycycline, imipenem, sulfamethoxazole, and tobramycin. Other drugs that should be considered include linezolid, tigecycline, and moxifloxacin.

While macrolides have traditionally been used in this role, recent studies have questioned the importance of macrolides in the treatment of *Mycobacterium abscessus* subsp. *abscessus* as the organism contains the erm(41) gene [76]. This is an inducible gene so that when the organism is incubated in the presence of clarithromycin, induction occurs and the organism rapidly acquires macrolide resistance. In contrast, *M. massiliense* has a nonfunctional copy of the gene, so macrolide resistance is not induced in the presence of clarithromycin. Patients infected with *M. massiliense* are more likely to improve clinically, radiographically, and bacteriologically with macrolide-based therapy than those with *M. abscessus* [77]. Limited data suggest that azithromycin may be more effective against *M. abscessus* than clarithromycin [78].

Species identification discriminating between *M. abscessus* and *M. massiliense* informs clinicians about the presence of an active erm gene and presumptive antibiotic choices but is frequently not available from reference laboratories. However, the presence of an active *erm* gene can be ascertained in most mycobacteriology laboratories in a relatively short time frame and is the critical information needed by the clinician to guide antibiotic therapy for isolates initially identified as *M. abscessus*.

M. chelonae is an RGM that causes skin and soft tissue disease similar to that of *M. abscessus*. Unlike *M. abscessus* and *M. fortuitum*, *M chelonae* does not carry an *erm* gene, and therefore effective therapy with a macrolide may be more obtainable in these individuals. Isolates of *M. chelonae* are susceptible to doxycycline (25% of isolates), ciprofloxacin (25% of isolates), tobramycin (100% of isolates), clarithromycin (100% of isolates), imipenem (70% of isolates), clofazimine, and linezolid (65% of isolates). *M. chelonae* is resistant to cefoxitin.

M. fortuitum is also a rapid grower similar to that of *M. abscessus*. It is recognized as a rare cause of lung disease, almost always associated in patients with gastroesophageal issues and/or achalasia [3]. It is also a cause of skin and soft tissue disease. Multidrug therapy with agents shown to be susceptible in vitro, including amikacin, newer quinolones, tetracyclines, and trimethoprim/sulfamethoxazole, should be given for 12 months or until clinical resolution of disease recognizing that without therapy for the underlying gastrointestinal disorder, symptoms rarely improve. *M. fortuitum* isolates are usually susceptible to fluoroquinolones, doxycycline and minocycline (50%), sulfonamides and trimethoprim/sulfamethoxazole, amikacin, imipenem, and tigecycline, and approximately one half of the isolates are susceptible to cefoxitin. Most *M. fortuitum* isolates have a functional *erm* gene so most are macrolide resistant.

References

1. Ramaswamy S, Musser JM. Molecular genetic basis of antimicrobial agent resistance in Mycobacterium tuberculosis: 1998 update. Tuber Lung Dis. 1998;79(1):3–29.
2. World Health Organization (WHO) global TB report, 2016.
3. Griffith DE, Aksamit T, Brown-Elliott BA, Catanzaro A, Daley C, Gordin F, ATS Mycobacterial Diseases Subcommittee; American Thoracic Society; Infectious Disease Society of America, et al. An official ATS/IDSA statement: diagnosis, treatment, and prevention of nontuberculous mycobacterial diseases. Am J Respir Crit Care Med. 2007;175(4):367–416. Review. Erratum in: Am J Respir Crit Care Med. 2007 Apr 1;175(7):744–5. Dosage error in article text.
4. Brown-Elliott BA, Iakhiaeva E, Griffith DE, Woods GL, Stout JE, Wolfe CR, et al. In vitro activity of amikacin against isolates of Mycobacterium avium complex with proposed MIC breakpoints and finding of a 16S rRNA gene mutation in treated isolates. J Clin Microbiol. 2013;51(10):3389–94. Erratum in: J Clin Microbiol. 2014;52(4):1311.
5. Griffith DE, Brown-Elliott BA, Langsjoen B, Zhang Y, Pan X, Girard W, et al. Clinical and molecular analysis of macrolide resistance in Mycobacterium avium complex lung disease. Am J Respir Crit Care Med. 2006;174(8):928–34.
6. van Ingen J, Boeree MJ, van Soolingen D, Mouton JW. Resistance mechanisms and drug susceptibility testing of nontuberculous mycobacteria. Drug Resist Updat. 2012;15(3):149–61.
7. Nash KA, Brown-Elliott BA, Wallace RJ Jr. A novel gene, erm(41), confers inducible macrolide resistance to clinical isolates of Mycobacterium abscessus but is absent from Mycobacterium chelonae. Antimicrob Agents Chemother. 2009;53(4):1367–76.
8. Brown-Elliott BA, Vasireddy S, Vasireddy R, Iakhiaeva E, Howard ST, Nash K, et al. Utility of sequencing the erm(41) gene in isolates of Mycobacterium abscessus subsp. abscessus with low and intermediate clarithromycin MICs. J Clin Microbiol. 2015;53(4):1211–5. Erratum in: J Clin Microbiol. 2016;54(4):1172.
9. Singh N, Paterson DL. Mycobacterium tuberculosis infection in solid-organ transplant recipients: impact and implications for management. Clin Infect Dis. 1998;27(5):1266–77.
10. Queipo JA, Broseta E, Santos M, Sánchez-Plumed J, Budía A, Jiménez-Cruz F. Mycobacterial infection in a series of 1261 renal transplant recipients. Clin Microbiol Infect. 2003;9(6):518–25.
11. Muñoz P, Rodríguez C, Bouza E. Mycobacterium tuberculosis infection in recipients of solid organ transplants. Clin Infect Dis. 2005;40(4):581–7. Review.
12. Meije Y, Piersimoni C, Torre-Cisneros J, Dilektasli AG, Aguado JM, ESCMID Study Group of Infection in Compromised Hosts. Mycobacterial infections in solid organ transplant recipients. Clin Microbiol Infect. 2014;20(Suppl 7):89–101.
13. Morris MI, Daly JS, Blumberg E, Kumar D, Sester M, Schluger N, et al. Diagnosis and management of tuberculosis in transplant donors: a donor-derived infections consensus conference report. Am J Transplant. 2012;12(9):2288–300.
14. Bumbacea D, Arend SM, Eyuboglu F, Fishman JA, Goletti D, Ison MG, et al. The risk of tuberculosis in transplant candidates and recipients: a TBNET consensus statement. Eur Respir J. 2012;40(4):990–1013.
15. Klote MM, Agodoa LY, Abbott K. Mycobacterium tuberculosis infection incidence in hospitalized renal transplant patients in the United States, 1998-2000. Am J Transplant. 2004;4(9):1523–8.
16. Abbott KC, Klote MM. Update on guidelines for prevention and management of mycobacterium tuberculosis infections after transplant. Am J Transplant. 2005;5(5):1163.
17. Morales P, Briones A, Torres JJ, Solé A, Pérez D, Pastor A. Pulmonary tuberculosis in lung and heart-lung transplantation: fifteen years of experience in a single center in Spain. Transplant Proc. 2005;37(9):4050–5.

18. Clemente WT, Faria LC, Lima SS, Vilela EG, Lima AS, Velloso LF, et al. Tuberculosis in liver transplant recipients: a single Brazilian center experience. Transplantation. 2009;87(3):397–401.
19. Scott C, Kirking HL, Jeffries C, Price SF, Pratt R, Centers for Disease Control and Prevention (CDC). Tuberculosis trends--United States, 2014. MMWR Morb Mortal Wkly Rep. 2015;64(10):265–9.
20. Lewinsohn DM, Leonard MK, LoBue PA, Cohn DL, Daley CL, Desmond E, Keane J, et al. Official American Thoracic Society/Infectious Diseases Society of America/Centers for disease control and prevention clinical practice guidelines: diagnosis of tuberculosis in adults and children. Clin Infect Dis. 2017;64(2):111–5.
21. Redelman-Sidi G, Sepkowitz KA. IFN-γ release assays in the diagnosis of latent tuberculosis infection among immunocompromised adults. Am J Respir Crit Care Med. 2013;188(4):422–31. Review
22. Pai M, Zwerling A, Menzies D. Systematic review: T-cell-based assays for the diagnosis of latent tuberculosis infection: an update. Ann Intern Med. 2008;149(3):177–84. Review
23. Sester U, Wilkens H, van Bentum K, Singh M, Sybrecht GW, et al. Impaired detection of Mycobacterium tuberculosis immunity in patients using high levels of immunosuppressive drugs. Eur Respir J. 2009;34(3):702–10.
24. Diel R, Loddenkemper R, Meywald-Walter K, Niemann S, Nienhaus A. Predictive value of a whole blood IFN-gamma assay for the development of active tuberculosis disease after recent infection with Mycobacterium tuberculosis. Am J Respir Crit Care Med. 2008;177(10):1164–70.
25. Mancuso JD, Mazurek GH, Tribble D, Olsen C, Aronson NE, Geiter L, et al. Discordance among commercially available diagnostics for latent tuberculosis infection. Am J Respir Crit Care Med. 2012;185(4):427–34.
26. Cattamanchi A, Smith R, Steingart KR, Metcalfe JZ, Date A, Coleman C, et al. Interferon-gamma release assays for the diagnosis of latent tuberculosis infection in HIV-infected individuals: a systematic review and meta-analysis. J Acquir Immune Defic Syndr. 2011;56(3):230–8.
27. Talati NJ, Seybold U, Humphrey B, Aina A, Tapia J, Weinfurter P, et al. Poor concordance between interferon-gamma release assays and tuberculin skin tests in diagnosis of latent tuberculosis infection among HIV-infected individuals. BMC Infect Dis. 2009;9:15.
28. Targeted tuberculin testing and treatment of latent tuberculosis infection. American Thoracic Society. MMWR Recomm Rep. 2000;49(RR-6):1–51.
29. Adamu B, Abdu A, Abba AA, Borodo MM, Tleyjeh IM. Antibiotic prophylaxis for preventing post solid organ transplant tuberculosis. Cochrane Database Syst Rev. 2014;3:CD008597.
30. Holty JE, Gould MK, Meinke L, Keeffe EB, Ruoss SJ. Tuberculosis in liver transplant recipients: a systematic review and meta-analysis of individual patient data. Liver Transpl. 2009;15(8):894–906.
31. Aguado JM, Torre-Cisneros J, Fortún J, Benito N, Meije Y, et al. Tuberculosis in solid-organ transplant recipients: consensus statement of the group for the study of infection in transplant recipients (GESITRA) of the Spanish Society of Infectious Diseases and Clinical Microbiology. Clin Infect Dis. 2009;48(9):1276–84.
32. Stucchi RS, Boin IF, Angerami RN, Zanaga L, Ataide EC, Udo EY. Is isoniazid safe for liver transplant candidates with latent tuberculosis? Transplant Proc. 2012;44(8):2406–10.
33. Singh N, Wagener MM, Gayowski T. Safety and efficacy of isoniazid chemoprophylaxis administered during liver transplant candidacy for the prevention of posttransplant tuberculosis. Transplantation. 2002;74(6):892–5.
34. Agoglia L, Balbi E, Halpern M, Roma J, Carius L, Martinho JM, Moreira LP. Tuberculosis in liver transplant recipients: prophylaxis in an endemic area. Transplant Proc. 2011;43(1):199–202.
35. Moon HH, Park SY, Kim JM, Park JB, Kwon CHD, Peck KR, et al. Isoniazid prophylaxis for latent tuberculosis infections in liver transplant. Recipients in a tuberculosis-endemic area. Ann Transplant. 2017 [revised 2017 Jan 1];22:338–345.
36. Trofe-Clark J, Lemonovich TL. AST infectious diseases Community of Practice. Interactions between anti-infective agents and immunosuppressants in solid organ transplantation. Am J Transplant. 2013;13(Suppl 4):318–26.
37. Sidhu A, Verma G, Humar A, Kumar D. Outcome of latent tuberculosis infection in solid organ transplant recipients over a 10-year period. Transplantation. 2014;98(6):671–5.
38. Sterling TR, Scott NA, Miro JM, Calvet G, La Rosa A, Infante R, Tuberculosis Trials Consortium, the AIDS Clinical Trials Group for the PREVENT TB Trial (TBTC Study 26ACTG 5259) The investigators of the TB Trials Consortium and the AIDS Clinical Trials Group for the PREVENT TB Trial are listed in the Supplement, item 17, et al. Three months of weekly rifapentine and isoniazid for treatment of Mycobacterium tuberculosis infection in HIV-coinfected persons. AIDS. 2016;30(10):1607–15.
39. Sterling TR, Villarino ME, Borisov AS, Shang N, Gordin F, Bliven-Sizemore E, TB Trials Consortium PREVENT TB Study Team, et al. Three months of rifapentine and isoniazid for latent tuberculosis infection. N Engl J Med. 2011;365(23):2155–66.
40. Martinson NA, Barnes GL, Moulton LH, Msandiwa R, Hausler H, Ram M, et al. New regimens to prevent tuberculosis in adults with HIV infection. N Engl J Med. 2011;365(1):11–20.
41. Bamrah S, Brostrom R, Dorina F, Setik L, Song R, Kawamura LM, et al. Treatment for LTBI in contacts of MDR-TB patients, Federated States of Micronesia, 2009-2012. Int J Tuberc Lung Dis. 2014;18(8):912–8.
42. Sester M, Sotgiu G, Lange C, Giehl C, Girardi E, Migliori GB, et al. Interferon-γ release assays for the diagnosis of active tuberculosis: a systematic review and meta-analysis. Eur Respir J. 2011;37(1):100–11. Erratum in: Eur Respir J. 2012;39(3):793.
43. Steingart KR, Schiller I, Horne DJ, Pai M, Boehme CC, Dendukuri N. Xpert® MTB/RIF assay for pulmonary tuberculosis and rifampicin resistance in adults. Cochrane Database Syst Rev. 2014;1:CD009593.
44. Tans-Kersten J, Grace Lin SY, Desmond E, Warshauer D. Evaluating shared laboratory services: detecting mycobacterium tuberculosis complex and drug resistance using molecular and culture-based methods. Public Health Rep. 2016;131(1):117–25.
45. Yakrus MA, Driscoll J, Lentz AJ, Sikes D, Hartline D, Metchock B, Starks AM. Concordance between molecular and phenotypic testing of Mycobacterium tuberculosis complex isolates for resistance to rifampin and isoniazid in the United States. J Clin Microbiol. 2014;52(6):1932–7.
46. Bhaloo S, Prasad GV. Severe reduction in tacrolimus levels with rifampin despite multiple cytochrome P450 inhibitors: a case report. Transplant Proc. 2003;35(7):2449–51.
47. Offermann G, Keller F, Molzahn M. Low cyclosporin A blood levels and acute graft rejection in a renal transplant recipient during rifampin treatment. Am J Nephrol. 1985;5(5):385–7.
48. Sun HY, Munoz P, Torre-Cisneros J, Aguado JM, Lattes R, Montejo M, et al. Tuberculosis in solid-organ transplant recipients: disease characteristics and outcomes in the current era. Prog Transplant. 2014;24(1):37–43.
49. Ha YE, Joo EJ, Park SY, Wi YM, Kang CI, Chung DR, et al. Tacrolimus as a risk factor for tuberculosis and outcome of treatment with rifampicin in solid organ transplant recipients. Transpl Infect Dis. 2012;14(6):626–34.
50. Hsu MS, Wang JL, Ko WJ, Lee PH, Chou NK, Wang SS, et al. Clinical features and outcome of tuberculosis in solid organ transplant recipients. Am J Med Sci. 2007;334(2):106–10.
51. Chou NK, Wang JL, Chi NH, Wu IH, Huang SC, Chen YS, et al. Tuberculosis after heart transplantation: twenty years of experience in a single center in Taiwan. Transplant Proc. 2008;40(8):2631–3.

52. Sun HY. Treating tuberculosis in solid organ transplant recipients. Curr Opin Infect Dis. 2014;27(6):501–5.
53. EBPG Expert Group on Renal Transplantation. European best practice guidelines for renal transplantation. Section IV: long-term management of the transplant recipient. Nephrol Dial Transplant. 2002;17(Suppl 4):1–67.
54. Drug-resistant tuberculosis: a survival guide for clinicians. 3rd ed. Curry Center; 2016.
55. Shin S, Furin J, Alcántara F, Hyson A, Joseph K, Sánchez E, Rich M. Hypokalemia among patients receiving treatment for multidrug-resistant tuberculosis. Chest. 2004;125(3):974–80.
56. Gillespie SH, Kennedy N. Fluoroquinolones: a new treatment for tuberculosis? Int J Tuberc Lung Dis. 1998;2(4):265–71. Review
57. Ginsburg AS, Grosset JH, Bishai WR. Fluoroquinolones, tuberculosis, and resistance. Lancet Infect Dis. 2003;3(7):432–42. Review
58. Peloquin CA, Hadad DJ, Molino LP, Palaci M, Boom WH, Dietze R, Johnson JL. Population pharmacokinetics of levofloxacin, gatifloxacin, and moxifloxacin in adults with pulmonary tuberculosis. Antimicrob Agents Chemother. 2008;52(3):852–7.
59. Yew WW, Chan CK, Leung CC, Chau CH, Tam CM, Wong PC, Lee J. Comparative roles of levofloxacin and ofloxacin in the treatment of multidrug-resistant tuberculosis: preliminary results of a retrospective study from Hong Kong. Chest. 2003;124(4):1476–81.
60. Devasia RA, Blackman A, Gebretsadik T, Griffin M, Shintani A, May C, et al. Fluoroquinolone resistance in Mycobacterium tuberculosis: the effect of duration and timing of fluoroquinolone exposure. Am J Respir Crit Care Med. 2009;180(4):365–70.
61. Long R, Chong H, Hoeppner V, Shanmuganathan H, Kowalewska-Grochowska K, Shandro C, et al. Empirical treatment of community-acquired pneumonia and the development of fluoroquinolone-resistant tuberculosis. Clin Infect Dis. 2009;48(10):1354–60.
62. Lee CN, Lin TP, Chang MF, Jimenez MV, Dolfi L, Olliaro P. Rifabutin as salvage therapy for cases of chronic multidrug-resistant pulmonary tuberculosis in Taiwan. J Chemother. 1996;8(2):137–43.
63. Dietze R, Hadad DJ, McGee B, Molino LP, Maciel EL, Peloquin CA, et al. Early and extended early bactericidal activity of linezolid in pulmonary tuberculosis. Am J Respir Crit Care Med. 2008;178(11):1180–5.
64. Condos R, Hadgiangelis N, Leibert E, Jacquette G, Harkin T, Rom WN. Case series report of a linezolid-containing regimen for extensively drug-resistant tuberculosis. Chest. 2008;134(1):187–92.
65. Migliori GB, Eker B, Richardson MD, Sotgiu G, Zellweger JP, Skrahina A, TBNET Study Group, et al. A retrospective TBNET assessment of linezolid safety, tolerability and efficacy in multidrug-resistant tuberculosis. Eur Respir J. 2009;34(2):387–93.
66. Koh WJ, Shim TS. Daily 300 mg dose of linezolid for the treatment of intractable multidrug-resistant and extensively drug-resistant tuberculosis—authors' response. J Antimicrob Chemother. 2009;64(5):1119–20. https://doi.org/10.1093/jac/dkp344.
67. Yew WW, Chang KC, Chau CH. What is the optimal dosage of linezolid in treatment of complicated multidrug-resistant tuberculosis? Eur Respir J. 2009;34(6):1492–4.
68. Schecter GF, Scott C, True L, Raftery A, Flood J, Mase S. Linezolid in the treatment of multidrug-resistant tuberculosis. Clin Infect Dis. 2010;50(1):49–55.
69. Beekmann SE, Gilbert DN, Polgreen PM, IDSA Emerging Infections Network. Toxicity of extended courses of linezolid: results of an Infectious Diseases Society of America Emerging Infections Network survey. Diagn Microbiol Infect Dis. 2008;62(4):407–10.
70. Garrabou G, Soriano A, López S, Guallar JP, Giralt M, Villarroya F, et al. Reversible inhibition of mitochondrial protein synthesis during linezolid-related hyperlactatemia. Antimicrob Agents Chemother. 2007;51(3):962–7.
71. McKee EE, Ferguson M, Bentley AT, Marks TA. Inhibition of mammalian mitochondrial protein synthesis by oxazolidinones. Antimicrob Agents Chemother. 2006;50(6):2042–9.
72. Narita M, Tsuji BT, Yu VL. Linezolid-associated peripheral and optic neuropathy, lactic acidosis, and serotonin syndrome. Pharmacotherapy. 2007;27(8):1189–97. Review
73. Bishop E, Melvani S, Howden BP, Charles PG, Grayson ML. Good clinical outcomes but high rates of adverse reactions during linezolid therapy for serious infections: a proposed protocol for monitoring therapy in complex patients. Antimicrob Agents Chemother. 2006;50(4):1599–602.
74. Papastavros T, Dolovich LR, Holbrook A, Whitehead L, Loeb M. Adverse events associated with pyrazinamide and levofloxacin in the treatment of latent multidrug-resistant tuberculosis. CMAJ. 2002;167(2):131–6.
75. Younossian AB, Rochat T, Ketterer JP, Wacker J, Janssens JP. High hepatotoxicity of pyrazinamide and ethambutol for treatment of latent tuberculosis. Eur Respir J. 2005;26(3):462–4.
76. Koh WJ, Stout JE, Yew WW. Advances in the management of pulmonary disease due to Mycobacterium abscessus complex. Int J Tuberc Lung Dis. 2014;18(10):1141–8.
77. Koh WJ, Jeon K, Lee NY, Kim BJ, Kook YH, Lee SH, et al. Clinical significance of differentiation of Mycobacterium massiliense from Mycobacterium abscessus. Am J Respir Crit Care Med. 2011;183(3):405–10.
78. Choi GE, Shin SJ, Won CJ, Min KN, Oh T, Hahn MY, et al. Macrolide treatment for Mycobacterium abscessus and Mycobacterium massiliense infection and inducible resistance. Am J Respir Crit Care Med. 2012;186(9):917–25.

Adaptive Immunotherapy for Opportunistic Infections

57

Aspasia Katragkou, Thomas J. Walsh, and Emmanuel Roilides

Introduction

Infectious complications of viral, bacterial, fungal, or parasitic origin are a major cause of morbidity and mortality in patients undergoing solid organ or stem cell transplantation [1–3]. The risk of infection after transplantation is a dynamic interplay between the intensity of immunosuppression and the patient's exposure to infectious organisms. The latter include mainly the patient's endogenous opportunists: the organisms transferred along with the transplant organ and pathogens from the exogenous hospital or community environment [4]. The incidence of opportunistic infections after transplantation varies from center to center, and, according to the classical perception, it is maximal during the first months after transplantation. Moreover, severe infections could occur late after transplantation in patients with particular risk factors such as acute rejection in the early period, chronic graft malfunction, reoperation, previous infections, or lung transplantation [5].

Almost all transplant recipients require lifelong immunosuppression as donor-specific immunotolerance is hard to achieve [6]. Most of the currently used immunosuppressive agents inhibit activation and proliferation of T-cells, weaken antibody response, and cause leucopenia. Conventional anti-infective therapeutic modalities are often compromised by the emergence of bacterial resistance, their side effects, or the emergence of pathogens like *Fusarium* spp. or *Scedosporium* spp., which are intrinsically resistant to most available antifungal agents. Therefore, the current developments in the management and care of transplanted patients have not proven to be a panacea. Knowing the limitations of the current anti-infective armamentarium, approaches that target the host through manipulations to augment the host immune response without increasing the risk of rejection provide a helpful aid to conventional treatment options.

A substantial body of evidence has demonstrated that strategies aiming to stimulate immune response could be feasible approaches that would benefit immunocompromised patients. In the present chapter, we present the immunomodulatory therapeutic and prophylactic approaches that have received interest and have clinical implications in the transplantation field. In particular, we discuss adoptive T-cell immunotherapy and administration of cytokines.

Adoptive T-Cell Therapy After Transplantation

Adoptive immunotherapy typically involves infusion of donor-derived lymphocytes or antibodies to patients suffering from a specific deficiency. T-cells are the most common lymphocytes infused as they play a critical role in controlling viral and fungal infections. The selective restoration of cellular immunity has been a particularly attractive strategy

A. Katragkou
Transplantation-Oncology Infectious Diseases Program, New York-Presbyterian/Weill Cornell Medical Center, New York, NY, USA

3rd Department of Pediatrics, Aristotle University, Hippokration Hospital, Thessaloniki, Greece

Nationwide Children's Hospital, Department of Pediatric Infectious Diseases, Columbus, OH, USA

T. J. Walsh
Transplantation-Oncology Infectious Diseases Program, New York-Presbyterian/Weill Cornell Medical Center, New York, NY, USA

Department of Pediatrics, New York-Presbyterian/Weill Cornell Medical Center, New York, NY, USA

Department of Microbiology and Immunology, New York-Presbyterian/Weill Cornell Medical Center, New York, NY, USA

Transplant Infectious Diseases Program, Division of Infectious Diseases, Weill Cornell Medical Center, New York, NY, USA
e-mail: thw2003@med.cornell.edu

E. Roilides (✉)
3rd Department of Pediatrics, Hippokration Hospital, School of Health Sciences, Aristotle University of Thessaloniki, Thessaloniki, Greece
e-mail: roilides@med.auth.gr

A. Safdar (ed.), *Principles and Practice of Transplant Infectious Diseases*, https://doi.org/10.1007/978-1-4939-9034-4_57

in the context of hematopoietic stem cell transplantation (HSCT) for the treatment of hematologic malignancies and the prophylaxis or treatment of opportunistic infections. For immunotherapy against infections, peripheral blood lymphocytes of the donor containing pathogen-specific T-cells are stimulated in vitro and then transfused into the patient resulting in control of the specific pathogen replication (Fig. 57.1). An important limitation of this kind of therapy is the potential fatal complication caused by the alloreactive T-cells that are also present in the donor lymphocyte infusion and the low concentration of pathogen-specific T-cells in the donor lymphocyte preparation. However, enrichment of pathogen-specific T-cell by in vitro culture before transfer reduces the risk of graft-versus-host disease (GVHD) [7].

After the pioneering work by Riddell et al. and Walter et al. showing, in the hematopoietic setting, that adoptive transfer of CMV-specific CD8+ T-cell clones into patients at risk protects them from CMV-related complications, Einsele et al. have shown that the adoptively transferred donor-derived CMV-specific T-cell lines have a therapeutic effect, too [8–10]. The most recent single-arm open-label phase I/II trial has shown that the translation of cellular therapy into clinic could be feasible and effective in restoring anti-CMV immunity in patients after HSCT [11]. There are no data available for solid organ transplant recipients for the prophylactic or therapeutic effect of adoptively transferred donor-derived CMV-specific T-cell lines. As recommended by the Transplantation Society International CMV consensus group, this strategy may be an experimental strategy for CMV disease in those who are unresponsive to standard therapies [12].

Polyclonal donor-derived T-cell lines specific for EBV have been used either to treat EBV-associated posttransplant lymphoproliferative disease (PTLD) or to prevent EBV-related immunoblastic lymphoma in HSCT patients [13, 14]. Among the six PTLD-treated patients, five showed complete regression, and the one failure involved a patient with the resolution of immunoblastic lymphoma [14]. The prophylactic administration of T-cell lines in 39 pediatric HSCT patients proved effective as it elicited an immediate decrease in the EBV DNA load, and none of the infused patients developed PTLD [13]. Similar results have been reported by other independent investigators [15–17]. The therapeutic potential of EBV-specific T-cells against EBV-associated PTLD has been investigated in

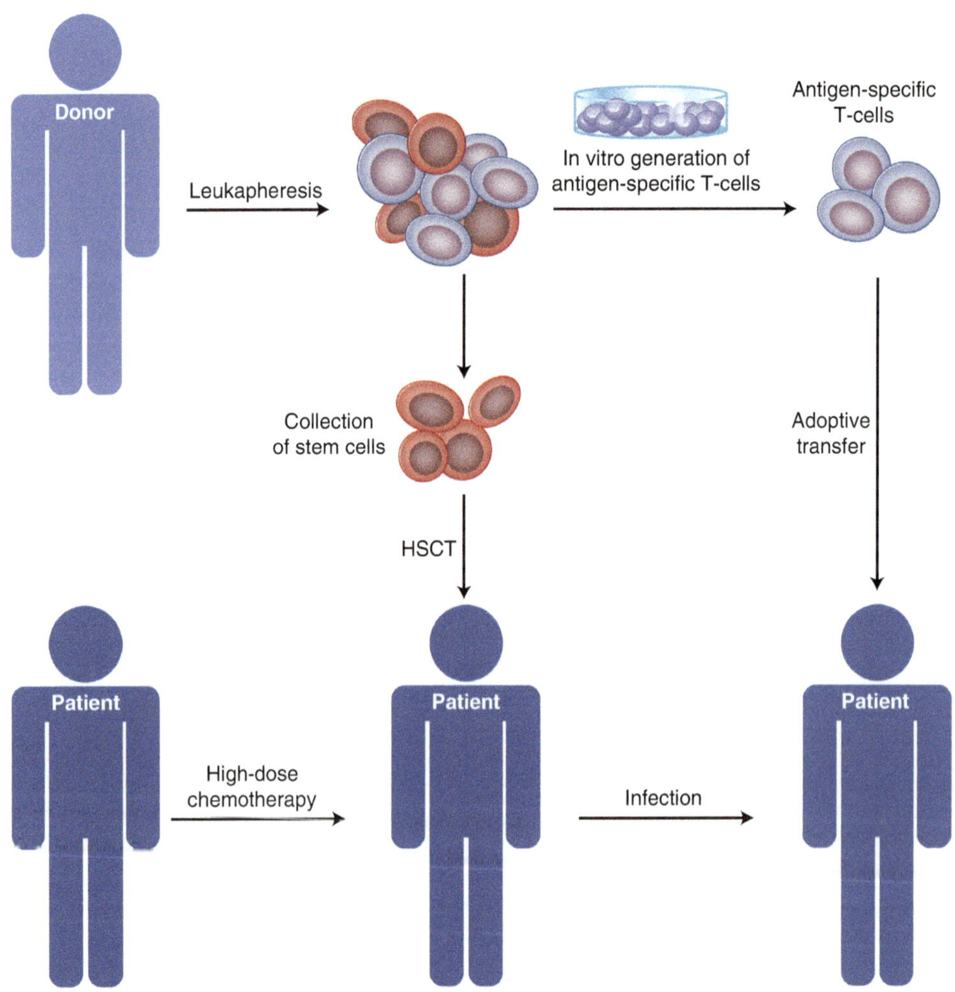

Fig. 57.1 Concept of adoptive T-cell therapy for infections (viral, fungal) after allogeneic hematopoietic stem cell transplantation. HSCT, hematopoietic stem cell transplantation [31]. (Adapted from Tramsen et al. [31])

solid organ transplant recipients. EBV T-cell-specific preparations either derived from the patients themselves or selected on the basis of the best HLA class I antigen match from a bank of such preparations that has been generated and cryopreserved from healthy allogeneic donors [18–22]. The feasibility and effectiveness of adoptive T-cell transfer have been applied for other viral infections such as adenovirus, varicella for HSCT recipients, or BK virus in renal transplant recipients [23–25]. Collectively, all these proof-of-principle studies have shown encouraging results about the safety and efficacy of adoptive T-cell therapy against viral infections which, if could be verified in clinical trials, then would represent an appreciable prophylactic and therapeutic modality for transplanted patients. However, technical requirements and regulatory burdens do not make adoptive T-cell therapy widely popular in the transplant community.

Concerning fungal infections, the first successful adoptive transfer of donor-derived *Aspergillus*-specific T-cells after haplo-identical HSCT without triggering GVHD has been described by Perruccio et al. [26]. The basis of adoptive immunotherapeutic strategies has been studied for *Aspergillus* [27], *Candida* [28], and *Zygomycetes* [29]. Nevertheless, as the therapeutic approach of fungal infections in the posttransplant setting is complicated, future clinical trials assessing the potential of antifungal adoptive immunotherapies should be able to answer questions as which patient subpopulation would benefit from adoptive immunotherapy or whether the prophylactic or therapeutic strategy is related with better outcome [30, 31].

Colony-Stimulating Factors: Preclinical Data

Colony-stimulating factors (CSFs) are a group of pleiotropic glycoproteins that stimulate the growth of specific blood cells and were considered to be a therapeutic "breakthrough" during the early 1990s. Three CSFs with activity on white blood cells have been developed and used clinically: granulocyte colony-stimulating factor (G-CSF), granulocyte-macrophage colony-stimulating factor (GM-CSF), and macrophage colony-stimulating factor (M-CSF).

Granulocyte Colony-Stimulating Factor (G-CSF)

Granulocyte colony-stimulating factor (G-CSF) is produced by macrophages, fibroblasts, and endothelial cells in virtually all organs in the body. It exerts its biological actions by binding to its specific cell surface receptors, which are expressed mainly on precursors as well as on mature neutrophils. In particular, G-CSF accelerates the maturation and differentiation of neutrophil precursors and delays the apoptosis of mature neutrophils, hence increasing the number of circulating neutrophils [32]. G-CSF effects not only neutrophil production but also their functions including promotion of chemotaxis, phagocytosis, priming of neutrophil respiratory burst, as well as antibody-dependent cell-mediated cytotoxicity [33]. Moreover, G-CSF has been shown in vitro to promote antibacterial and antifungal activities of mature neutrophils [34–36]. Especially in transplant recipients, ex vivo studies have demonstrated that incubation with G-CSF enhanced the impaired respiratory burst response of neutrophils against *Candida* and *Cryptococcus* [37]. G-CSF, in addition to increasing and activating neutrophils, modulates the inflammatory response exerting anti-inflammatory effects. Ex vivo studies have shown that G-CSF attenuates the capacity of neutrophils to release pro-inflammatory cytokines, such as tumor necrosis factor (TNF)-α, interferon (IFN)-γ, interleukin (IL)-6, IL-1β, and IL-12, whereas it increases the production of the anti-inflammatory soluble TNF receptor p55 and p75, IL-1 receptor antagonist (IL-1ra), and prostaglandin E2 [38–40]. This type of G-CSF-induced immunomodulatory effect has been proven in animal transplantation models to be advantageous for the control of acute graft-versus-host disease and for acute graft rejection reactions. Pretreatment of either the donor before organ retrieval [41, 42] or the recipient [43–45] with G-CSF has been shown to significantly facilitate organ acceptance. Simultaneously, this G-CSF-induced host immune hyporesponsiveness could reduce immunosuppressive agents' requirement and their subsequent adverse events [46].

Granulocyte-Macrophage Colony-Stimulating Factor (GM-CSF)

Granulocyte-macrophage colony-stimulating factor (GM-CSF) is produced by T lymphocytes, monocytes, macrophages, fibroblasts, and endothelial cells [34]. Like G-CSF, GM-CSF stimulates numerous activities of mature effector cells, including neutrophils, monocytes, macrophages, and dendritic cells, such as the respiratory burst in vitro and their antibacterial and antifungal activities [47–49]. GM-CSF, however, does not seem to play a significant role in normal neutrophil development and, unlike G-CSF, raises the number of neutrophils by redistributing them and increasing the number of cells from other hematopoietic lineages. The latter finding has raised a theoretical concern of an augmented adaptive immune response and, thus, an increased risk of allograft rejection in transplant recipients or of more severe infections due to intracellular organisms [50]. Nevertheless, in vitro, ex vivo, and in vivo studies have shown that GM-CSF therapy has a differential immune restoration potential. GM-CSF selectively boosts the innate immune response improving host's resistance against infections upon transplantation while simultaneously suppressing

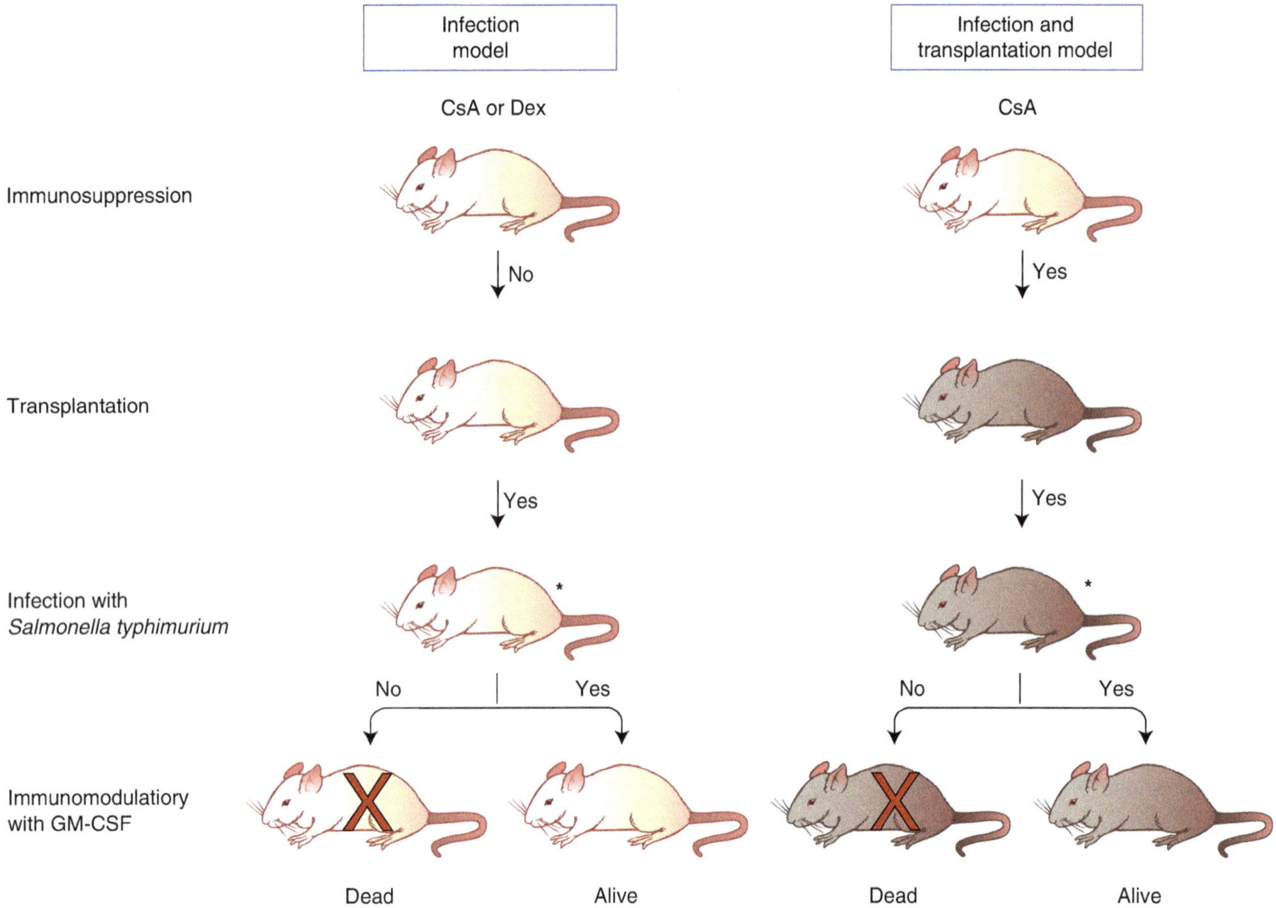

	Innate Immunity	Adaptive Immunity	Response to infection	Graft rejection
Normal Host	~	~	~	NA
Immunosuppressed Host (Dex, CsA)	↓	↓	↓	↓
Immunomodulated Host (GM-CSF)	↑	↓	↑	↓

Fig. 57.2 Panel A: Survival of lethal bacterial (*Salmonella typhimurium*) infection of immunosuppressed mice (CBA/Ca) treated with GM-CSF. Mice were immunosuppressed with dexamethasone (Dex) or cyclosporine (CsA). GM-CSF treatment allowed immunosuppressed mice to survive the lethal bacterial infection without inducing graft rejection. Panel B: GM-CSF differential immune restoration potential. In immunocompromised organ transplant recipients GM-CSF has the capacity of supporting the anti-infectious defense (innate immunity) while continuing the suppression of the adaptive immune response, preventing, thus rejection [51, 52]. (Adapted from Xu et al. [51, 52]). ~, normal; NA, not applicable; ↑, increased; ↓, decreased; Dex, dexamethasone; CsA, cyclosporine A

the adaptive immune response and thus preventing rejection [51, 52] (Fig. 57.2). Moreover, in ex vivo experiments from immunosuppressed or liver transplant blood donors, GM-CSF treatment restored the production of TNF without inducing IL-2 production and T-cell proliferation. Moreover, gene array technology was able to identify the differential reconstitution capacity of GM-CSF after immunosuppression. Namely, gene array experiments demonstrated that in addition to the TNF gene, the reconstitution potential of GM-CSF extends to more genes encoding transcription factors, involved in the innate inflammatory response such as NF-κB (p65 subunit), the stress-activated protein kinase (SAPK)/c-JUN N-terminal kinase (JNK), mitogen-activated protein kinase 38, IL-6, IL-8, and platelet-activating factor receptor. On the contrary, GM-CSF has not been shown to reactivate genes involved to adaptive immunity, such as IL-2, CD27, and T-cell-specific RANTES (regulated upon activation, normally T-cell expressed and presumably secreted) production, T-cell proliferation, and mixed leukocyte reaction [51, 52]. Collectively, these preclinical findings showing the differential pharmacological profile of GM-CSF able to improve host defense resistance to infection without compromising the graft are in favor of GM-CSF clinical use in the transplantation setting.

Macrophage Colony-Stimulating Factor (M-CSF)

Macrophage colony-stimulating factor (M-CSF) is produced by monocytes/macrophages, fibroblasts, and endothelial cells. M-CSF accelerates proliferation and differentiation of the monocyte/macrophage lineage, recruits mononuclear cells to sites of infection, and activates macrophages. Some effects of M-CSF may also be through indirect mechanisms, comprising stimulation of other cytokines (G-CSF, GM-CSF, interleukin-1, tumor necrosis factor-α) which may further stimulate activities against infecting organisms [34, 35]. In vitro, M-CSF augmented antifungal and antibacterial activity of monocytes and tissue macrophages against *C. albicans* [53], *Trichosporon asahii* [54], *Aspergillus fumigatus* [55], *Penicillium marneffei* [56], and *Staphylococcus aureus* [57] partly by enhancing oxidation-dependent mechanisms. Accordingly, in animal models with yeast infections, M-CSF showed a favorable effect in terms of improved survival and reduced fungal burden [58–60]. Administration of high-dose M-CSF has been shown to significantly prolong skin graft survival in mice through inhibition of TNF-α production [61].

Clinical Applications of CSFs in Opportunistic Infections

CSFs have been evaluated by an appreciable amount of randomized controlled studies in oncologic settings [62–65]. These studies have concluded that G-CSF and GM-CSF reduce the duration of neutropenia, length of hospitalization, and duration of parenteral antimicrobial therapy and permit intensification of chemotherapy [65].

Data concerning CSF clinical utility in the prevention or treatment of opportunistic infections in transplant recipients are relatively scarce. On the basis of the above preclinical data, two clinical applications of CSFs as adjunctive anti-infective therapy have been proposed: first to increase the production of neutrophils in neutropenic patients and second to enhance the function of existing neutrophils in non-neutropenic patients.

G-CSF

Prophylaxis During Neutropenia

Neutropenia has long been considered a significant risk factor for infection especially in immunocompromised patients. In transplant recipients, neutropenia could be due to immunosuppressive agents as well as to viral infections (most commonly cytomegalovirus) and antiviral therapy (ganciclovir and related agents) [66]. Given that immunosuppression is intentional and critical for a successful transplantation and antiviral agents should be used, on many occasions, either prophylactically or therapeutically for prolonged periods, the benefit of factors like CSFs able to raise circulating neutrophils appears a viable strategy to prevent opportunistic infections.

In HSCT, G-CSF has been used before transplantation for stem cell priming and after transplantation for better stem cell engraftment to minimize the morbidity and mortality associated with prolonged neutropenia [67]. Administration of G-CSF in the posttransplant period has been associated with an accelerated rate of neutrophil engraftment, shorter duration of hospitalization, and decreased incidence of febrile episodes [68–71]. According to the most recent guidelines of the American Society of Clinical Oncology (ASCO), the use of G-CSF is recommended after autologous but not after allogeneic HSCT [72]. The rationale behind this recommendation is that while among autologous HSCT recipients posttransplant G-CSF use has been associated with shortened duration of hospitalization and savings in the overall medical costs [70], the same has not been noted for allogeneic transplant recipients [73]. Moreover, the use of G-CSF after allogeneic HSCT has been associated with increased incidence of severe GVHD and mortality [74]. However, it should be clarified that G-CSF is safe and effective in patients undergoing allogeneic transplantation when they receive peripheral blood stem cells. In the bone marrow transplantation setting, G-CSF use is not recommended as there are no adequate studies to allow firm conclusions about its safety and efficacy [67]. The optimal time to start G-CSF is a controversial issue in the autologous stem cell setting. The ASCO guidelines recommend G-CSF to be administered between day 1 and 5 after high-dose chemotherapy and continued until neutrophils are 2000–3000/μl [72]. However, several studies have shown that initiation of G-CSF beyond day 5 results in comparable engraftment [75–77]. Additionally, the number of CD34+ cells infused per kg used as a criterion for G-CSF administration is not indicated in autologous recipients [67].

Neutropenia after solid organ transplantation is relatively common and together with other secondary disorders such as operative trauma, blood transfusion, or hypersplenism render transplant recipients vulnerable to infection [78, 79]. However, there are no guidelines for the management of neutropenia in solid organ recipients. The current clinical practice, in many transplantation centers worldwide, is to reduce or discontinue the agents causing neutropenia and in selected patients use G-CSF. Contrary to oncologic patients where G-CSF is widely accepted, similar studies in solid organ transplant recipients are limited. Extrapolating treatment of neutropenia from oncologic patients to solid organ transplant recipients is not feasible due to different degrees and durations of immunosuppression and different patterns of infections [80]. In a national cohort of 41,705 renal transplant recipients from the United States Renal Data System database, neutropenia developed in 14.5% of them and was related with an increased risk of allograft loss and death. In this study G-CSF was used in 12% of the neutropenic patients, and its use was not related with increased risk of allograft loss [81]. The safety and efficacy of G-CSF in solid organ recipients have been described in few case reports and retrospective studies [79, 80, 82–88]. In a retrospective study of 102 adult kidney and/or pancreas transplant recipients followed for over 1 year, Hartmann, et al. found that treating patients with a short course (mean 3.1 doses) of G-CSF is safe and effective [80]. In a retrospective study of 50 liver and kidney transplant recipients who received G-CSF due to neutropenia, Turgeon et al. noted that the effectiveness of G-CSF was indication-related. G-CSF successfully reversed CMV and ganciclovir-associated neutropenia; however, its effectiveness was particularly poor for the subgroup of patients receiving G-CSF for sepsis-associated neutropenia [83]. Other studies have shown that G-CSF could achieve reversal of leucopenia in all renal allograft recipients and, in most cases, after a single-dose administration [82].

Despite the encouraging results of these studies, their usefulness is limited by their retrospective design, the small number of participating patients with heterogeneous demographics and underlying pathology, different leucopenia definitions, and varying G-CSF dosage and duration regimens. Until further prospective studies are carried out to evaluate the use of G-CSF in solid organ transplant recipients with neutropenia, G-CSF should be used cautiously.

Therapy of Non-neutropenic Patients

The most extensive experience with G-CSF in non-neutropenic solid organ transplants was reported by Foster et al. in a pilot clinical trial with 37 primary liver allograft recipients who received daily G-CSF for the first 7–10 days after transplantation. These were compared with 49 historical controls who did not receive G-CSF. The two groups of patients had no differences regarding the risk factors for sepsis and rejection. G-CSF-treated patients had a decreased number of sepsis episodes per patient (0.92 versus 2.18), a lower percentage of sepsis-related deaths (8% versus 22%), and a decreased incidence of acute rejection episodes (22% versus 51%) [89]. These promising effects of G-CSF to reduce bacterial and fungal sepsis as well as its concurrent antirejection potential in liver transplant recipients have not been subsequently confirmed. Thus, a randomized, placebo-controlled, double-blind, multicenter trial involving 194 liver transplant patients has shown that G-CSF had no beneficial effect on infection, rejection, or survival. Moreover, G-CSF-treated patients had more biopsy-proven rejections and nosocomial pneumonias compared with placebo-treated patients [90]. The reasons proposed for these discrepancies were differences in study design, immunosuppressive agents, antimicrobial prophylaxis, and definitions of infection as well as improvement of care of transplant patients since the Foster trial used historical controls. Consequently, although G-CSF appears to be safe in this patient population, there is no evidence that it prevents or treats infections when used as an adjunct to standard antimicrobial or antifungal therapy.

GM-CSF

Like G-CSF, the predominant clinical use of GM-CSF concerns oncologic patients aiming to accelerate marrow recovery after chemotherapy [34]. Regarding the transplantation setting, GM-CSF efficacy has been mainly evaluated in patients undergoing bone marrow or peripheral hematopoietic stem cell transplantation to accelerate or sustain neutrophil recovery or reduce the incidence of opportunistic infections (Table 57.1) [91–99]. The ASCO guidelines have

Table 57.1 Clinical studies on GM-CSF use according to the type of transplantation [89–96, 99–101]

Transplantation type	Study type	Indication	GM-CSF dose	Ref
Bone marrow transplantation	Phase II/non randomized historical controls	Accelerate neutrophil recovery	60 μg/m²/day	[89]
	Phase II/non randomized	Accelerate neutrophil recovery	100–400 μg/m²/day	[90]
	Cohort evaluation	Sustain neutrophil recovery	3–10 μg/kg/day	[91]
	Phase III/randomized, double-blind, multicenter	Accelerate neutrophil recovery	10 μg/kg/day	[92]
	Randomized, double-blind	Accelerate neutrophil recovery	250 μg/m²/day	[93]
	Cohort evaluation	Enhance peripheral progenitor cell yield	250 μg/m²/day	[94]
	Phase I, II, III, retrospective, historical controls	Reduce fungal, bacterial infections, pulmonary infections	30–250 μg/m²/day	[96]
Stem cell transplantation	Phase III/double-blind	Accelerate myeloid recovery, decrease incidence of bacterial infections	10 μg/kg/day	[95]
Solid organ transplantation	Comparison of cases historical controls (renal transplants)	Increase neutrophil count, decrease infections	5 μg/kg/day	[99]
	Safety and efficacy (orthotopic liver transplantation)	Increase neutrophil count, beneficial for severe bacterial infections and sepsis	5 μg/kg/day	[100]
	Randomized, unblinded, placebo-controlled, prospective study (non-neutropenic patients)	Absence of organ failure or mortality	3 μg/kg/day	[101]

provided recommendations for the use of CSFs (either G-CSF or GM-CSF) in patients after bone marrow or stem cell transplantation without commenting on their equivalency [72].

In solid organ transplant recipients, the potential role of GM-CSF has been proposed by few case reports [99, 100] and a limited number of clinical studies with relatively small number of patients [101–103]. GM-CSF combined with appropriate antiviral or antimicrobial treatment proved effective against complicated varicella zoster infection or ecthyma gangrenosum in renal transplant recipients [99, 100]. A single center experience has yielded promising results about the safety and efficacy of GM-CSF in pediatric liver transplant recipients. GM-CSF was used in 13 cases; of these 9 cases were neutropenic and 10 infected and 3 had severe sepsis without neutropenia among the 430 pediatric orthotropic liver transplantation recipients age ranged between 1 and 15 years of age. Not only was the administration of GM-CSF safe and well tolerated, but all patients with sepsis were cured [102]. Patients on tacrolimus did not appear to benefit from GM-CSF contrary to patients with EBV infections [102, 104]. Corroborative were the results of a small study with seven leukopenic renal transplant recipients; three patients with CMV infection being treated with ganciclovir who had a reduced rate of infection and mortality compared with seven historical controls [101]. In a large study of the utility of GM-CSF in adult non-neutropenic patients, including seven solid organ transplant recipients, fulfilling the criteria of systemic inflammatory response syndrome, GM-CSF despite its pro-inflammatory properties, did not cause progression to circulatory shock or other organ failures [103].

Most data on the use of GM-CSF as adjuvant therapy for transplant recipients with opportunistic infections are encouraging, with the caveat that these data are not based on prospective randomized trials and the potential for long-term adverse events cannot be ruled out. Preclinical data show that this cytokine has a good potential, whereas many issues remain to be resolved, like the optimal dose or time to administer as it seems to be a "treatment window." Table 57.1 provides an overview of representative clinical studies on GM-CSF use according to the type of transplantation.

M-CSF

Compared to G-CSF and GM-CSF, clinical experience with M-CSF is limited basically due to its specificity for cells of the monocytic lineage. The efficacy of adding M-CSF to standard antifungal treatment was examined in a retrospective study involving 46 bone marrow transplant patients with documented invasive fungal infection. Survival of patients who received M-CSF was greater (27%) compared to historical controls (5%) [105]. However, the favorable effect of M-CSF treatment on patients' survival was attributed to less severe infection and better functional status in a subgroup of treated patients. Further evolution of critical care techniques may influence the results as M-CSF-treated patients were compared with historical controls [105]. No prospective, randomized, controlled clinical trials of M-CSF for adjunctive therapy of opportunistic infections in transplant recipients have been published.

Toxicity and Adverse Events of CSFs

At present, the licensed CSFs in the USA and Europe are recombinant human G-CSF, GM-CSF, and more recently a pegylated form of G-CSF [106–108]. The commercially available preparations for G-CSF are filgrastim (a non-glycosylated protein expressed in *Escherichia coli*) and lenograstim (a glycosylated protein expressed in Chinese hamster ovarian cells in vitro) and for GM-CSF, molgramostim (a non-glycosylated protein expressed in *Escherichia coli*), sargramostim (a glycosylated protein expressed in *Saccharomyces cerevisiae*), and regramostim (a glycosylated protein expressed in mammalian cells). The pegylated form of G-CSF, available as pegfilgrastim, is a large size molecule that prevents renal clearance. Thus, the drug is eliminated predominantly through a neutrophil self-regulating, "feedback-loop-like" mechanism that allows stimulation of neutrophil production when neutrophil counts are low and rapid clearance as neutrophil counts recover.

Safety data from several clinical settings show an acceptable safety profile of G-CSF with the most commonly reported side effects being mild to moderate bone and musculoskeletal pain observed in approximately 10–20% of recipients depending on the dose administered [109]. However, the incidence of untoward side effects appears to be greater with GM-CSF [110]. This may be attributed to actions on macrophages with GM-CSF priming macrophages for increased formation and release of inflammatory cytokines, whereas G-CSF induces production of anti-inflammatory factors, such as IL-1 receptor antagonist and soluble TNF receptors [108]. GM-CSF's expression system included yeasts, bacteria, or mammalian cells, and its glycosylation status, whether or not it is glycosylated, influenced its clinical toxicity. In general, the reported frequency of adverse events, such as fluid retention, dyspnea, fever, myalgias, bone pains, and rash, was higher in patients treated with *E. coli*-derived GM-CSF [103, 111]. First dose reactions like flushing, tachycardia, hypotension, musculoskeletal pain, dyspnea, nausea, vomiting, and arterial oxygen desaturation have been reported in approximately 5% of the patients receiving intravenous GM-SCF.

On the other hand, the glycosylated form appears to be more antigenic than the non-glycosylated forms, and 1% of patients develop antibodies to the agent [92]. Administration of CSFs involves the theoretical risk of malignant transformation, but, nevertheless, there is no supporting evidence for this [112]. Another concern is the possibility for aggravating the inflammatory response in patients with pre-existing infections resulting in clinical deterioration. However, this does not constitute a contraindication to CSF administration, since it is rather based on anecdotal reports than on comprehensive studies [113].

There is a theoretical concern that G-CSF use may be harmful for organ graft survival as the G-CSF-induced monocyte, i.e., antigen-presenting cells rise may be the cause of transplant rejection. The use of G-CSF has been associated in some reports with a worsening in graft function [114]; however, in most series, it was not associated with an increased incidence of rejection episodes in solid organ transplant recipients.

Interferon-Gamma (IFN-γ)

IFN-γ is produced endogenously primarily by T-cells and NK cells and is a potent activator of monocytes/macrophages and neutrophils. In vitro, IFN-γ has been shown to enhance the neutrophil and/or macrophage activity against a number of bacteria, fungi, and protozoa [34, 47]. In addition, IFN-γ plays a regulatory role in the cytotoxic function of macrophages and the killing of intracellular pathogens like *Mycobacterium*, *Leishmania*, *Rickettsia*, *Legionella*, and *Chlamydia* species [34, 115, 116]. IFN-γ plays an important role in regulating BK virus infection by exerting a potent inhibitory effect on BK virus expression both at the level of transcription and at the level of translation and viral progeny production in primary cultures of renal tubular epithelial cells proximal [117]. Further studies using a BK infection mouse model provide evidence that IFN-γ directly depresses viral replication and contribute to the antiviral control of BK infection in the host [118]. In animal models, IFN-γ enhances host resistance against invasive *Candida* or *Aspergillus* infection [119, 120].

In clinical trials, IFN-γ has been primarily used in children with chronic granulomatous disease (CGD) [121]. In 1990, IFN-γ was approved for prophylactic use in individuals with CGD for the prevention of bacterial and fungal infections [34].

IFN-γ has never been systematically studied for the treatment or prevention of opportunistic infections in transplant recipients. The safety of IFN-γ was evaluated in a retrospective study of 32 HSCT recipients. Not only was the administration of IFN-γ tolerated without serious adverse events but in high-risk allogeneic transplantation recipients with GVHD the cytokine led to the amelioration of both acute and chronic GVHD [122]. In general, IFN-γ is well tolerated, and adverse events occur only with higher doses [34].

Conclusions

Despite the advantages on our current understanding of the immunopathogenesis of infections in immunocompromised patients, the outcome of opportunistic infections in transplant recipients remains poor. In this regard, the concept of immunomodulatory therapies constitutes a rational approach aiming to selectively restore the innate immunity while keeping the adaptive immune response, which is implicated in graft rejection, suppressed. Among the immunotherapeutic strategies studied in transplant recipients aiming to enhance the adaptive immune response are the adoptive transfer of T lymphocytes and the use of cytokines such as G-CSF, GM-CSF, M-CSF, or IFN-γ. Despite some encouraging results in in vitro and in vivo studies currently available, clinical evidence on the use of these approaches is too limited to allow firm recommendations. Many questions, however, regarding various immunomodulatory approaches, such as safety, efficacy, timing of intervention, dosing, or eligible patients will need appropriately designed and powered clinical trials in order to be answered.

Disclosure of Potential Conflict of Interest None of the authors of this manuscript have potential conflict of interest.

References

1. Patel R, Paya CV. Infections in solid-organ transplant recipients. Clin Microbiol Rev. 1997;10:86–124.
2. Centers for Disease Control and Prevention; Infectious Disease Society of America; American Society of Blood and Marrow Transplantation. Guidelines for preventing opportunistic infections among hematopoietic stem cell transplant recipients. MMWR Recomm Rep. 2000;49:1–125, CE1-7.
3. Munoz P, Fernandez NS, Farinas MC. Epidemiology and risk factors of infections after solid organ transplantation. Enferm Infecc Microbiol Clin. 2012;30(Suppl 2):10–8.
4. Fishman JA. Infection in solid-organ transplant recipients. N Engl J Med. 2007;357:2601–14.
5. San Juan R, Aguado JM, Lumbreras C, et al. Incidence, clinical characteristics and risk factors of late infection in solid organ transplant recipients: data from the RESITRA study group. Am J Transplant. 2007;7:964–71.
6. Yu X, Carpenter P, Anasetti C. Advances in transplantation tolerance. Lancet. 2001;357:1959–63.
7. Moss P, Rickinson A. Cellular immunotherapy for viral infection after HSC transplantation. Nat Rev Immunol. 2005;5:9–20.
8. Riddell SR, Watanabe KS, Goodrich JM, Li CR, Agha ME, Greenberg PD. Restoration of viral immunity in immunodeficient humans by the adoptive transfer of T cell clones. Science. 1992;257:238–41.
9. Walter EA, Greenberg PD, Gilbert MJ, et al. Reconstitution of cellular immunity against cytomegalovirus in recipients of allogeneic bone marrow by transfer of T-cell clones from the donor. N Engl J Med. 1995;333:1038–44.
10. Einsele H, Roosnek E, Rufer N, et al. Infusion of cytomegalovirus (CMV)-specific T cells for the treatment of CMV infection not responding to antiviral chemotherapy. Blood. 2002;99:3916–22.

11. Peggs KS, Thomson K, Samuel E, et al. Directly selected cytomegalovirus-reactive donor T cells confer rapid and safe systemic reconstitution of virus-specific immunity following stem cell transplantation. Clin Infect Dis. 2011;52:49–57.
12. Kotton CN, Kumar D, Caliendo AM, et al. International consensus guidelines on the management of cytomegalovirus in solid organ transplantation. Transplantation. 2010;89:779–95.
13. Rooney CM, Smith CA, Ng CY, et al. Infusion of cytotoxic T cells for the prevention and treatment of Epstein-Barr virus-induced lymphoma in allogeneic transplant recipients. Blood. 1998;92: 1549–55.
14. Rooney CM, Smith CA, Ng CY, et al. Use of gene-modified virus-specific T lymphocytes to control Epstein-Barr-virus-related lymphoproliferation. Lancet. 1995;345:9–13.
15. Papadopoulos EB, Ladanyi M, Emanuel D, et al. Infusions of donor leukocytes to treat Epstein-Barr virus-associated lymphoproliferative disorders after allogeneic bone marrow transplantation. N Engl J Med. 1994;330:1185–91.
16. Gustafsson A, Levitsky V, Zou JZ, et al. Epstein-Barr virus (EBV) load in bone marrow transplant recipients at risk to develop post-transplant lymphoproliferative disease: prophylactic infusion of EBV-specific cytotoxic T cells. Blood. 2000;95:807–14.
17. Doubrovina E, Oflaz-Sozmen B, Prockop SE, et al. Adoptive immunotherapy with unselected or EBV-specific T cells for biopsy-proven EBV+ lymphomas after allogeneic hematopoietic cell transplantation. Blood. 2012;119:2644–56.
18. Haque T, Wilkie GM, Taylor C, et al. Treatment of Epstein-Barr-virus-positive post-transplantation lymphoproliferative disease with partly HLA-matched allogeneic cytotoxic T cells. Lancet. 2002;360:436–42.
19. Savoldo B, Goss J, Liu Z, et al. Generation of autologous Epstein-Barr virus-specific cytotoxic T cells for adoptive immunotherapy in solid organ transplant recipients. Transplantation. 2001;72:1078–86.
20. Khanna R, Bell S, Sherritt M, et al. Activation and adoptive transfer of Epstein-Barr virus-specific cytotoxic T cells in solid organ transplant patients with posttransplant lymphoproliferative disease. Proc Natl Acad Sci U S A. 1999;96:10391–6.
21. Comoli P, Labirio M, Basso S, et al. Infusion of autologous Epstein-Barr virus (EBV)-specific cytotoxic T cells for prevention of EBV-related lymphoproliferative disorder in solid organ transplant recipients with evidence of active virus replication. Blood. 2002;99:2592–8.
22. Haque T, Taylor C, Wilkie GM, et al. Complete regression of posttransplant lymphoproliferative disease using partially HLA-matched Epstein Barr virus-specific cytotoxic T cells. Transplantation. 2001;72:1399–402.
23. Feuchtinger T, Matthes-Martin S, Richard C, et al. Safe adoptive transfer of virus-specific T-cell immunity for the treatment of systemic adenovirus infection after allogeneic stem cell transplantation. Br J Haematol. 2006;134:64–76.
24. Blyth E, Gaundar SS, Clancy L, et al. Clinical-grade varicella zoster virus-specific T cells produced for adoptive immunotherapy in hemopoietic stem cell transplant recipients. Cytotherapy. 2012;14:724–32.
25. Blyth E, Clancy L, Simms R, et al. BK virus-specific T cells for use in cellular therapy show specificity to multiple antigens and polyfunctional cytokine responses. Transplantation. 2011;92:1077–84.
26. Perruccio K, Tosti A, Burchielli E, et al. Transferring functional immune responses to pathogens after haploidentical hematopoietic transplantation. Blood. 2005;106:4397–406.
27. Beck O, Topp MS, Koehl U, et al. Generation of highly purified and functionally active human TH1 cells against Aspergillus fumigatus. Blood. 2006;107:2562–9.
28. Tramsen L, Beck O, Schuster FR, et al. Generation and characterization of anti-Candida T cells as potential immunotherapy in patients with Candida infection after allogeneic hematopoietic stem-cell transplant. J Infect Dis. 2007;196:485–92.
29. Schmidt S, Tramsen L, Perkhofer S, et al. Characterization of the cellular immune responses to Rhizopus oryzae with potential impact on immunotherapeutic strategies in hematopoietic stem cell transplantation. J Infect Dis. 2012;206:135–9.
30. Lehrnbecher T, Schmidt S, Koehl U, et al. Adoptive antifungal T cell immunotherapy--into the clinic? Med Mycol. 2011;49(Suppl 1):S164–9.
31. Tramsen L, Schmidt S, Roeger F, Koehl U, Lehrnbecher T. Challenges and prospects of adoptive immunotherapy in prevention and treatment of opportunistic mycoses in hematologic transplant recipients. Curr Infect Dis Rep. 2010;12:444–9.
32. Anderlini P, Champlin RE. Biologic and molecular effects of granulocyte colony-stimulating factor in healthy individuals: recent findings and current challenges. Blood. 2008;111:1767–72.
33. Dale DC, Liles WC, Summer WR, Nelson S. Review: granulocyte colony-stimulating factor--role and relationships in infectious diseases. J Infect Dis. 1995;172:1061–75.
34. Hubel K, Dale DC, Liles WC. Therapeutic use of cytokines to modulate phagocyte function for the treatment of infectious diseases: current status of granulocyte colony-stimulating factor, granulocyte-macrophage colony-stimulating factor, macrophage colony-stimulating factor, and interferon-gamma. J Infect Dis. 2002;185:1490–501.
35. Roilides E, Walsh T. Recombinant cytokines in augmentation and immunomodulation of host defenses against Candida spp. Med Mycol. 2004;42:1–13.
36. Roilides E, Uhlig K, Venzon D, Pizzo PA, Walsh TJ. Enhancement of oxidative response and damage caused by human neutrophils to Aspergillus fumigatus hyphae by granulocyte colony-stimulating factor and gamma interferon. Infect Immun. 1993;61:1185–93.
37. Pursell K, Verral S, Daraiesh F, et al. Impaired phagocyte respiratory burst responses to opportunistic fungal pathogens in transplant recipients: in vitro effect of r-metHuG-CSF (Filgrastim). Transpl Infect Dis. 2003;5:29–37
38. Boneberg EM, Hareng L, Gantner F, Wendel A, Hartung T. Human monocytes express functional receptors for granulocyte colony-stimulating factor that mediate suppression of monokines and interferon-gamma. Blood. 2000;95:270–6.
39. Hartung T, Docke WD, Gantner F, et al. Effect of granulocyte colony-stimulating factor treatment on ex vivo blood cytokine response in human volunteers. Blood. 1995;85:2482–9.
40. von Aulock S, Boneberg EM, Diterich I, Hartung T. Granulocyte colony-stimulating factor (filgrastim) treatment primes for increased ex vivo inducible prostanoid release. J Pharmacol Exp Ther. 2004;308:754–9.
41. Hayamizu K, Egi H, Ohmori I, Kitayama T, Asahara T. Improvement of heart allograft acceptability by pretreatment of donors with granulocyte colony-stimulating factor. Transplant Proc. 2002;34:2732.
42. Hayamizu K, Yahata H, Shinozaki K, Tanji H, Strober S, Asahara T. Granulocyte colony-stimulating factor-mobilized donor monocytes facilitate heart allograft acceptance. Transplant Proc. 2000;32:2068–9.
43. Foster PF, Kociss K, Shen J, et al. Granulocyte colony-stimulating factor immunomodulation in the rat cardiac transplantation model. Transplantation. 1996;61:1122–5.
44. Egi H, Hayamizu K, Kitayama T, Ohmori I, Okajima M, Asahara T. Downregulation of both interleukin-12 and interleukin-2 in heart allografts by pretransplant host treatment with granulocyte colony-stimulating factor and tacrolimus. Cytokine. 2002;18:164–7.
45. Ohmori I, Hayamizu K, Kitayama T, Egi H, Aihaiti X, Asahara T. Downregulation of interleukin-12p35 and upregulation of interleukin-12p40 mRNA expression in heart allografts by blood transfusion from granulocyte colony-stimulating factor-treated donors. Cytokine. 2003;21:27–31.

46. Kitayama T, Hayamizu K, Egi H, Ohmori I, Yoshimitsu M, Asahara T. Facilitation of tacrolimus-induced heart-allograft acceptability by pretransplant host treatment with granulocyte colony-stimulating factor: interleukin-12-restricted suppression of intragraft monokine mRNA expression. Transplantation. 2003;75:553–6.
47. Gil-Lamaignere C, Simitsopoulou M, Roilides E, Maloukou A, Winn RM, Walsh TJ. Interferon- gamma and granulocyte-macrophage colony-stimulating factor augment the activity of polymorphonuclear leukocytes against medically important zygomycetes. J Infect Dis. 2005;191:1180–7.
48. Weisbart RH, Golde DW, Clark SC, Wong GG, Gasson JC. Human granulocyte-macrophage colony-stimulating factor is a neutrophil activator. Nature. 1985;314:361–3.
49. Dale DC, Liles WC, Llewellyn C, Price TH. Effects of granulocyte-macrophage colony-stimulating factor (GM-CSF) on neutrophil kinetics and function in normal human volunteers. Am J Hematol. 1998;57:7–15.
50. Page AV, Liles WC. Granulocyte colony-stimulating factor, granulocyte-macrophage colony-stimulating factor, and other immunomodulatory therapies for the treatment of infectious diseases in solid organ transplant recipients. Curr Opin Organ Transplant. 2008;13:575–80.
51. Xu J, Lucas R, Schuchmann M, et al. GM-CSF restores innate, but not adaptive, immune responses in glucocorticoid-immunosuppressed human blood in vitro. J Immunol. 2003;171:938–47.
52. Xu J, Lucas R, Wendel A. The potential of GM-CSF to improve resistance against infections in organ transplantation. Trends Pharmacol Sci. 2004;25:254–8.
53. Roilides E, Lyman CA, Sein T, Gonzalez C, Walsh TJ. Antifungal activity of splenic, liver and pulmonary macrophages against Candida albicans and effects of macrophage colony-stimulating factor. Med Mycol. 2000;38:161–8.
54. Sasaki E, Tashiro T, Kuroki M, et al. Effects of macrophage colony-stimulating factor (M-CSF) on anti-fungal activity of mononuclear phagocytes against Trichosporon asahii. Clin Exp Immunol. 2000;119:293–8.
55. Roilides E, Sein T, Holmes A, et al. Effects of macrophage colony-stimulating factor on antifungal activity of mononuclear phagocytes against Aspergillus fumigatus. J Infect Dis. 1995;172:1028–34.
56. Roilides E, Lyman CA, Sein T, Petraitiene R, Walsh TJ. Macrophage colony-stimulating factor enhances phagocytosis and oxidative burst of mononuclear phagocytes against Penicillium marneffei conidia. FEMS Immunol Med Microbiol. 2003;36:19–26.
57. Roilides E, Lyman CA, Mertins SD, et al. Ex vivo effects of macrophage colony-stimulating factor on human monocyte activity against fungal and bacterial pathogens. Cytokine. 1996;8:42–8.
58. Cenci E, Bartocci A, Puccetti P, Mocci S, Stanley ER, Bistoni F. Macrophage colony-stimulating factor in murine candidiasis: serum and tissue levels during infection and protective effect of exogenous administration. Infect Immun. 1991;59:868–72.
59. Vitt CR, Fidler JM, Ando D, Zimmerman RJ, Aukerman SL. Antifungal activity of recombinant human macrophage colony-stimulating factor in models of acute and chronic candidiasis in the rat. J Infect Dis. 1994;169:369–74.
60. Kuhara T, Uchida K, Yamaguchi H. Therapeutic efficacy of human macrophage colony-stimulating factor, used alone and in combination with antifungal agents, in mice with systemic Candida albicans infection. Antimicrob Agents Chemother. 2000;44:19–23.
61. Nishina T, Naomoto Y, Gouchi A, et al. Macrophage colony-stimulating factor inhibits tumor necrosis factor production and prolongs skin graft survival. Transplantation. 2004;77:456–9.
62. Rowe JM, Andersen JW, Mazza JJ, et al. A randomized placebo-controlled phase III study of granulocyte-macrophage colony-stimulating factor in adult patients (> 55 to 70 years of age) with acute myelogenous leukemia: a study of the Eastern Cooperative Oncology Group (E1490). Blood. 1995;86:457–62.
63. Antman KS, Griffin JD, Elias A, et al. Effect of recombinant human granulocyte-macrophage colony-stimulating factor on chemotherapy-induced myelosuppression. N Engl J Med. 1988;319:593–8.
64. Gerhartz HH, Engelhard M, Meusers P, et al. Randomized, double-blind, placebo-controlled, phase III study of recombinant human granulocyte-macrophage colony-stimulating factor as adjunct to induction treatment of high-grade malignant non-Hodgkin's lymphomas. Blood. 1993;82:2329–39.
65. Lyman GH, Kuderer NM, Djulbegovic B. Prophylactic granulocyte colony-stimulating factor in patients receiving dose-intensive cancer chemotherapy: a meta-analysis. Am J Med. 2002;112:406–11.
66. Fishman JA, Emery V, Freeman R, et al. Cytomegalovirus in transplantation – challenging the status quo. Clin Transpl. 2007;21:149–58.
67. Trivedi M, Martinez S, Corringham S, Medley K, Ball ED. Optimal use of G-CSF administration after hematopoietic SCT. Bone Marrow Transplant. 2009;43:895–908.
68. Ozcan M, Ustun C, Akcaglayan E, et al. Recombinant human granulocyte colony-stimulating factor (rh-G-CSF) may accelerate hematopoietic recovery after HLA-identical sibling allogeneic peripheral blood stem cell transplantation. Bone Marrow Transplant. 2001;27:499–505.
69. Bishop MR, Tarantolo SR, Geller RB, et al. A randomized, double-blind trial of filgrastim (granulocyte colony-stimulating factor) versus placebo following allogeneic blood stem cell transplantation. Blood. 2000;96:80–5.
70. McQuaker IG, Hunter AE, Pacey S, Haynes AP, Iqbal A, Russell NH. Low-dose filgrastim significantly enhances neutrophil recovery following autologous peripheral-blood stem-cell transplantation in patients with lymphoproliferative disorders: evidence for clinical and economic benefit. J Clin Oncol. 1997;15:451–7.
71. Klumpp TR, Mangan KF, Goldberg SL, Pearlman ES, Macdonald JS. Granulocyte colony-stimulating factor accelerates neutrophil engraftment following peripheral-blood stem-cell transplantation: a prospective, randomized trial. J Clin Oncol. 1995;13:1323–7.
72. Smith TJ, Khatcheressian J, Lyman GH, et al. 2006 update of recommendations for the use of white blood cell growth factors: an evidence-based clinical practice guideline. J Clin Oncol. 2006;24:3187–205.
73. Stinson TJ, Adams JR, Bishop MR, Kruse S, Tarantolo S, Bennet CL. Economic analysis of a phase III study of G-CSF vs placebo following allogeneic blood stem cell transplantation. Bone Marrow Transplant. 2000;26:663–6.
74. Ringden O, Labopin M, Gorin NC, et al. Treatment with granulocyte colony-stimulating factor after allogeneic bone marrow transplantation for acute leukemia increases the risk of graft-versus-host disease and death: a study from the Acute Leukemia Working Party of the European Group for blood and marrow transplantation. J Clin Oncol. 2004;22:416–23.
75. Faber E, Pytlik R, Slaby J, et al. Individually determined dosing of filgrastim after autologous peripheral stem cell transplantation in patients with malignant lymphoma--results of a prospective multicentre controlled trial. Eur J Haematol. 2006;77:493–500.
76. Piccirillo N, Sica S, Laurenti L, et al. Optimal timing of G-CSF administration after CD34+ immunoselected peripheral blood progenitor cell transplantation. Bone Marrow Transplant. 1999;3:1245–50.
77. Bence-Bruckler I, Bredeson C, Atkins H, et al. A randomized trial of granulocyte colony-stimulating factor (Neupogen) starting day 1 vs day 7 post-autologous stem cell transplantation. Bone Marrow Transplant. 1998;22:965–9.
78. Zafrani L, Truffaut L, Kreis H, et al. Incidence, risk factors and clinical consequences of neutropenia following kidney transplantation: a retrospective study. Am J Transplant. 2009;9:1816–25.

79. Ishizone S, Makuuchi M, Kawasaki S, et al. Effect of granulocyte colony-stimulating factor on neutropenia in liver transplant recipients with hypersplenism. J Pediatr Surg. 1994;29:510–3.
80. Hartmann EL, Gatesman M, Roskopf-Somerville J, Stratta R, Farney A, Sundberg A. Management of leukopenia in kidney and pancreas transplant recipients. Clin Transpl. 2008;22:822–8.
81. Hurst FP, Belur P, Nee R, et al. Poor outcomes associated with neutropenia after kidney transplantation: analysis of United States Renal Data System. Transplantation. 2011;92:36–40.
82. Schmaldienst S, Bekesi G, Deicher R, Franz M, Horl WH, Pohanka E. Recombinant human granulocyte colony-stimulating factor after kidney transplantation: a retrospective analysis to evaluate the benefit or risk of immunostimulation. Transplantation. 2000;69: 527–31.
83. Turgeon N, Hovingh GK, Fishman JA, et al. Safety and efficacy of granulocyte colony-stimulating factor in kidney and liver transplant recipients. Transpl Infect Dis. 2000;2:15–21.
84. Tajima A, Aso Y, Kawabe K, et al. Colony-stimulating factor for treatment of leukopenia after kidney allografting. Transplant Proc. 1991;23:1369–70.
85. Peddi VR, Hariharan S, Schroeder TJ, First MR. Role of granulocyte colony stimulating factor (G-CSF) in reversing neutropenia in renal allograft recipients. Clin Transpl. 1996;10:20–3.
86. Colquhoun SD, Shaked A, Jurim O, Colonna JO, Rosove MH, Busuttil RW. Reversal of neutropenia with granulocyte colony-stimulating factor without precipitating liver allograft rejection. Transplantation. 1993;56:1593–5.
87. Atici AE, Bostanci EB, Ozer I, Ulas M, Akdogan M, Akoglu M. Use of granulocyte colony-stimulating factor for neutropenia after orthotopic liver transplantation: report of two cases. Transplant Proc. 2011;43:909–11.
88. Birkeland SA, Elbirk A, Rohr N, Jorgensen KA. Severe neutropenia after renal transplantation and its reversal with granulocyte colony-stimulating factor. Transplant Proc. 1994;26:3098–9.
89. Foster PF, Mital D, Sankary HN, et al. The use of granulocyte colony-stimulating factor after liver transplantation. Transplantation. 1995;59:1557–63.
90. Winston DJ, Foster PF, Somberg KA, et al. Randomized, placebo-controlled, double-blind, multicenter trial of efficacy and safety of granulocyte colony-stimulating factor in liver transplant recipients. Transplantation. 1999;68:1298–304.
91. Taylor KM, Jagannath S, Spitzer G, et al. Recombinant human granulocyte colony-stimulating factor hastens granulocyte recovery after high-dose chemotherapy and autologous bone marrow transplantation in Hodgkin's disease. J Clin Oncol. 1989;7: 1791–9.
92. Devereaux S, Linch DC, Gribben JG, McMillan A, Patterson K, Goldstone AH. GM-CSF accelerates neutrophil recovery after autologous bone marrow transplantation for Hodgkin's disease. Bone Marrow Transplant. 1989;4:49–54.
93. Klingemann HG, Eaves AC, Barnett MJ, et al. Recombinant GM-CSF in patients with poor graft function after bone marrow transplantation. Clin Invest Med. 1990;13:77–81.
94. Greenberg P, Advani R, Keating A, et al. GM-CSF accelerates neutrophil recovery after autologous hematopoietic stem cell transplantation. Bone Marrow Transplant. 1996;18:1057–64.
95. Gorin NC, Coiffier B, Hayat M, et al. Recombinant human granulocyte-macrophage colony-stimulating factor after high-dose chemotherapy and autologous bone marrow transplantation with unpurged and purged marrow in non-Hodgkin's lymphoma: a double-blind placebo-controlled trial. Blood. 1992;80: 1149–57.
96. Ho AD, Haas R, Korbling M, Dietz M, Hunstein W. Utilization of recombinant human GM-CSF to enhance peripheral progenitor cell yield for autologous transplantation. Bone Marrow Transplant. 1991;7(Suppl 1):13–7.
97. Advani R, Chao NJ, Horning SJ, et al. Granulocyte-macrophage colony-stimulating factor (GM-CSF) as an adjunct to autologous hemopoietic stem cell transplantation for lymphoma. Ann Intern Med. 1992;116:183–9.
98. Nemunaitis J, Buckner CD, Dorsey KS, Willis D, Meyer W, Appelbaum F. Retrospective analysis of infectious disease in patients who received recombinant human granulocyte-macrophage colony-stimulating factor versus patients not receiving a cytokine who underwent autologous bone marrow transplantation for treatment of lymphoid cancer. Am J Clin Oncol. 1998;21:341–6.
99. Vales-Albertos LJ, Andrade-Sierra J, Gomez-Navarro B, et al. Nonspecific immunoglobulin and granulocyte-macrophage colony-stimulating factor use in complicated varicella zoster: the first case report in a renal transplant recipient. Transplantation. 2006;81:809–10.
100. Gregorini M, Castello M, Rampino T, et al. GM-CSF contributes to prompt healing of ecthyma gangrenosum lesions in kidney transplant recipient. J Nephrol. 2012;25:137–9.
101. Hashmi A, Hussain M, Hussain Z, et al. Use of rHu GM-CSF in renal-transplant patients developing leukopenia. Transplant Proc. 1997;29:3053.
102. Trindade E, Maton P, Reding R, et al. Use of granulocyte macrophage colony stimulating factor in children after orthotopic liver transplantation. J Hepatol. 1998;28:1054–7.
103. Rosenbloom AJ, Linden PK, Dorrance A, Penkosky N, Cohen-Melamed MH, Pinsky MR. Effect of granulocyte-monocyte colony-stimulating factor therapy on leukocyte function and clearance of serious infection in nonneutropenic patients. Chest. 2005;127:2139–50.
104. Sokal EM, Caragiozoglou T, Lamy M, Reding R, Otte JB. Epstein-Barr virus serology and Epstein-Barr virus-associated lymphoproliferative disorders in pediatric liver transplant recipients. Transplantation. 1993;56:1394–8.
105. Nemunaitis J, Shannon-Dorcy K, Appelbaum FR, et al. Long-term follow-up of patients with invasive fungal disease who received adjunctive therapy with recombinant human macrophage colony-stimulating factor. Blood. 1993;82:1422–7.
106. Antachopoulos C, Roilides E. Cytokines and fungal infections. Br J Haematol. 2005;129:583–96.
107. Kamrokji RS, Lyman GH. The colony-stimulating factors: use to prevent and treat neutropenia and its complications. Expert Opin Biol Ther. 2004;4:1897–910.
108. Roilides E, Lamaignere CG, Farmaki E. Cytokines in immunodeficient patients with invasive fungal infections: an emerging therapy. Int J Infect Dis. 2002;6:154–63.
109. Welte K, Gabrilove J, Bronchud MH, Platzer E, Morstyn G. Filgrastim (r-metHuG-CSF): the first 10 years. Blood. 1996;88:1907–29.
110. Root RK, Dale DC. Granulocyte colony-stimulating factor and granulocyte-macrophage colony-stimulating factor: comparisons and potential for use in the treatment of infections in nonneutropenic patients. J Infect Dis. 1999;179(Suppl 2):S342–52.
111. Rodriguez-Adrian LJ, Grazziutti ML, Rex JH, Anaissie EJ. The potential role of cytokine therapy for fungal infections in patients with cancer: is recovery from neutropenia all that is needed? Clin Infect Dis. 1998;26:1270–8.
112. Ohno R, Tomonaga M, Kobayashi T, et al. Effect of granulocyte colony-stimulating factor after intensive induction therapy in relapsed or refractory acute leukemia. N Engl J Med. 1990;323:871–7.
113. Pappas PG, Bustamante B, Ticona E, et al. Recombinant interferon- gamma 1b as adjunctive therapy for AIDS-related acute cryptococcal meningitis. J Infect Dis. 2004;189:2185–91.
114. Minguez C, Mazuecos A, Ceballos M, Tejuca F, Rivero M. Worsening of renal function in a renal transplant patient

treated with granulocyte colony-stimulating factor. Nephrol Dial Transplant. 1995;10:2166–7.
115. Gallin JI, Farber JM, Holland SM, Nutman TB. Interferon-gamma in the management of infectious diseases. Ann Intern Med. 1995;123:216–24.
116. Murray HW. Interferon-gamma and host antimicrobial defense: current and future clinical applications. Am J Med. 1994;97: 459–67.
117. Abend JR, Low JA, Imperiale MJ. Inhibitory effect of gamma interferon on BK virus gene expression and replication. J Virol. 2007;81:272–9.
118. Wilson JJ, Lin E, Pack CD, et al. Gamma interferon controls mouse polyomavirus infection in vivo. J Virol. 2011;85:10126–34.
119. Nagai H, Guo J, Choi H, Kurup V. Interferon-gamma and tumor necrosis factor-alpha protect mice from invasive aspergillosis. J Infect Dis. 1995;172:1554–60.
120. Kullberg BJ, van 't Wout JW, Hoogstraten C, van Furth R. Recombinant interferon-gamma enhances resistance to acute disseminated Candida albicans infection in mice. J Infect Dis. 1993;168:436–43.
121. A controlled trial of interferon gamma to prevent infection in chronic granulomatous disease. The International Chronic Granulomatous Disease Cooperative Study Group. N Engl J Med. 1991;324:509–16.
122. Safdar A, Rodriguez G, Ohmagari N, et al. The safety of interferon-gamma-1b therapy for invasive fungal infections after hematopoietic stem cell transplantation. Cancer. 2005;103: 731–9.

Immunotherapy for Invasive Mold Disease in Transplant Patients: Dendritic Cell Immunotherapy, Interferon Gamma, Recombinant Myeloid Growth Factors, and Healthy Donor Granulocyte Transfusions

58

William K. Decker, Matthew M. Halpert, Vanaja Konduri, Dan Liang, Christopher N. Hampton, and Amar Safdar

Introduction

In the healthy individual, the incidence of fungal infection is low due to efficient mitigation by appropriate immune responses. Infection is acquired through the inhalation of microconidia or fungal spores, and primary infection takes hold in the lungs where the conidia swell and germinate to produce the hyphal growth pattern typically associated with mold. This is followed by contiguous spread and hematologic dissemination to the brain, kidney, and other organ systems if unchecked [1, 2]. Alveolar macrophages and neutrophils are quick to respond and phagocytose the fungal threat via several different internalization mechanisms, followed by an adaptive response carried out by dendritic cells (DC) and T cells primed for an optimal T_H1 response [3–6]. Despite high efficiency clearance of fungal infections in immunocompetent individuals, there has been a steady rise in opportunistic fungal infections since the 1960s due to the increased incidence of patients with sub-par immune responses mostly due to the advent of solid organ and hematopoietic stem cell transplantation (HSCT), the increased use of chemotherapy and biologic immunosuppressive treatment regimens, and the epidemic of advanced HIV disease [7–13].

W. K. Decker (✉) · M. M. Halpert · V. Konduri · D. Liang
Department of Pathology and Immunology, Baylor College of Medicine, Houston, TX, USA
e-mail: decker@bcm.edu; halpert@bcm.edu; konduri@bcm.edu; dan_liang@hms.harvard.edu

C. N. Hampton
Department of Pathology and Immunology, Baylor College of Medicine, Huffington Center on Aging, Houston, TX, USA
e-mail: christopher.hampton@bcm.edu

A. Safdar
Clinical Associate Professor of Medicine, Texas Tech University Health Sciences Center El Paso, Paul L. Foster School of Medicine, El Paso, TX, USA
e-mail: amar.safdar@cidimmunology.com

As the number of immunocompromised patients in hospitals rises, so do the incidence and mortality associated with invasive fungal diseases. In severely immunocompromised patients, invasive aspergillosis (IA) is caused predominantly by *Aspergillus fumigatus* followed by *A. flavus*, *A. terreus*, *A. nidulans*, and *A. niger.* These species represent important filamentous mold pathogens as they are relatively prevalent and exhibit a high mortality rate approaching 45% to 80% despite antifungal therapy [14–16]. Many of the systemic antifungal therapies that work reasonably well within the general population are far less satisfactory in the immunocompromised setting. The extensive use of empiric antifungal therapies is now a growing concern given the development of drug resistance, including the emergence of the azole-resistant strains of *A. fumigatus* [17]. Additionally, these drugs have numerous limitations, including high toxicity, limited efficacy, and complex drug interactions. Though the immune system is capable of handling a fungal threat when competent, there is currently a dearth of clinically approved vaccines, despite the fact that a 1967 review article cited 32 publications showing preclinical efficacy of various fungal vaccines [18].

Historically, severe and prolonged neutropenia has been the predominant risk factor when assessing who may succumb to IA, though more recent studies have shed light on a broader breadth of relevant antifungal immune responses. For example, IA in allogeneic stem cell graft recipients is more frequently seen late after undergoing transplantation in non-neutropenic patients and often occurs during treatment for chronic graft-versus-host disease [19, 20]. Additionally, IA in patients following solid organ allograft transplantation is an opportunistic disease that is noted in the absence of severe neutropenia [21, 22]. It is important to note that heterozygous nude mice survive intravenous fungal microconidia infection while homozygous nude mice succumb to the disease, indicating an important and non-redundant role for the

A. Safdar (ed.), *Principles and Practice of Transplant Infectious Diseases*, https://doi.org/10.1007/978-1-4939-9034-4_58

adaptive immune response in fungal clearance [23]. Indeed, both the innate and the adaptive immune response are necessary for proper and efficient fungal clearance and survival of the host [5, 24, 25]. Recently, an increased understanding of the reasons why some patients survive IA and others do not has suggested the use of therapeutic interventions that utilize adaptive immunity as IA survivors typically have a significant proliferation of antigen-specific, IFN-γ-producing T cells, and generally robust T_H1 immune responses [6, 26]. After intranasal challenge of *A. fumigatus*, there occurs a vigorous secretion of pro-inflammatory T_H1 cytokines including IL-12, IFN-γ, TNF-α, and IL-18, and mice deficient for T_H1 cytokines exhibit considerable deficits in effective fungal clearance [3, 4]. Many of these T_H1 cytokines are thought to be produced by type I polarized $CD4^+$ T cells, raising concerns that antifungal immunotherapy may be ineffective in CD4-deficient hosts; however, there also exists encouraging evidence that these patients can be successfully vaccinated and that $CD8^+$ T cells can subsume the roles of $CD4^+$ cells in the development of vaccine-induced adaptive immunity [27–29].

A broad variety of immune-based approaches, some experimental in nature, have been considered for the treatment of invasive fungal disease. Experimental approaches like dendritic cell immunotherapy will be considered first, whereas more clinically relevant approaches such as patient mobilization with recombinant growth factors and granulocyte transfusion are considered later in the chapter.

Dendritic Cell Immunotherapy

Dendritic cells are important mediators of T_H1 responses and orchestrate global antifungal immunity in the lungs [2, 30–33]. Plasmacytoid dendritic cells (pDC), a lymphoid subset of DC that support T_H1 immunity through the production of type I interferons, have been observed to respond to nucleic acids from *A. fumigatus* via TLR-9 activation [34]. However, a majority of antifungal vaccine studies have focused on the use of conventional myeloid DC subsets which have shown a remarkable ability to discern between the conidia and hyphal forms of the emerging fungus [2, 35, 36]. Under physiologic conditions, lung dendritic cells engulf conidia within hours, traffic to the regional lymph nodes and spleen, and prime efficient cytotoxic T-cell (CTL) responses [2]. This concept has been adapted in animal vaccine studies in which vaccination with DC pulsed with *Aspergillus* or transfected with microconidial RNA increased the survival of mice after HSCT, when subsequently challenged with conidial inoculums, from 0% to 95% [31]. This effect could be further enhanced when DC were concurrently pulsed with fungal extracts and transfected with an IL-12-producing adenoviral vector, although there exist more conventional methods that stimulate physiologic secretion of IL-12 [32]. Importantly, the responses appeared to be antigen-specific and most robust when loaded DC were administered directly in contrast to adoptive transfer of pathogen-specific T lymphocytes [31, 32] Fungus-pulsed DC or DC transfected with fungal mRNA have also elicited a reasonable rate of immune efficiency against other types of fungi, including *Candida* [37]. In contrast to the anti-conidia T_H1 immune response, hyphae appear to promote a T_H2-skewed response using both hyphae-pulsed DC and DC-transfected hyphal RNA [2, 33]. Though an ideal antifungal vaccine would exhibit multigenera cross-reactivity, current preclinical vaccines are genus specific, exhibiting little antigenic overlap between genus or species [31].

Interferon Gamma (IFN-γ)

Interferon gamma is the only member of the type II class of interferons. It is a homodimerized soluble cytokine critical for innate and adaptive immune responses against nearly all types of pathogens including viruses, bacteria, protozoa, and fungi [38]. IFN-γ activates macrophages and upregulates MHC class I expression on a broad variety of different cell types. Produced by NK, NKT, CD4, and CD8 cells, IFN-γ both inhibits viral replication and activates macrophages, permitting more effective killing of intracellular organisms.

Preclinical Experience

IFN-γ activation of macrophages via T_H1 cell stimulation induces macrophages to overcome inhibition of phagolysosome maturation caused by mycobacteria [39], and experimental work in vitro suggests that the addition of IFN-γ increases killing of microbes by upregulating T_H1 responses through polymorphonuclear leukocytes, monocytes, and macrophages [40]. IFN-γ appears to prime macrophages for enhanced microbial killing and inflammatory activation through the toll-like receptor pathway [41]. Immune cell activation by IFN-γ is dependent on STAT1 activation which in turn activates interferon-stimulated genes. IFN-γ is also responsible for altering epigenetic governance of macrophages, inducing and priming enhancers to increase transcriptional output in response to TLR signaling [42]. Davis and colleagues demonstrated that IFN-γ prevents fungal inhibition of lysosomal activity, enhancing and maintaining the ability of the macrophage to destroy *Cryptococcus* [39]. Stevens and colleagues demonstrated that pulmonary macrophage and neutrophil function may be upregulated by IFN-γ, including respiratory burst killing of intra- and intercellular fungal infections. Stevens further demonstrated that cytokines themselves are very weakly active, even when administered in combination with antifungal drugs, yet significant synergy occurs when effector cells, cytokines, and antifungal drugs are combined [43]. IFN-γ was approved by the US Food and Drug Administration in February of 2000 to treat chronic granulomatous disease, a genetically diverse disorder characterized by a defect in oxygen metabolite production in phagocytic cells [44]. Marketed as ACTIMMUNE (IFN-γ-1b), this product was authorized by the FDA for treatment of CGD even without evidence of increased superoxide production as a result of treatment. Granulomas include *Aspergillus*, especially *A. fumigatus*, and *Candida* species. Filiz and colleagues subsequently demonstrated that IFN-γ indeed improves the oxidative burst activity of neutrophils in specific subtypes of CGD in vitro, particularly with respect to the gp91^{phox} subgroup [45].

Adjunct Clinical Use

Clinical case reports in HIV-infected and diabetic children with chronic fungal infections have been published, describing the use of IFN-γ in conjunction with various colony-stimulating factors to combat these infections. While this approach was not found to be curative, it did help to stabilize chronic infections over a course of several years [46]. Other clinical reports describe the use of IFN-γ as a curative agent in the treatment of invasive fungal infections following kidney transplant with only a limited, 6-week treatment cycle [47]. Here, it was hypothesized that standard immunosuppressive therapies predispose patients to fungal infection by specifically targeting and downregulating the function of T_H1 cell populations. This results in an inadequate IFN-γ-driven response to fungal insult, allowing the microbes to expand relatively unchallenged. In six of seven reported subjects, otherwise lethal infections were cleared, and long-term follow-ups have remained clear; the remaining patients' blood samples became negative for *C. albicans* 5 days after starting IFN-γ treatment and remained clear for 20 consecutive days until unexpected death from noninfectious causes (*ibid*). Delsing and colleagues report on case studies using recombinant IFN-γ for 2 weeks with partial restoration of immunologic function in the treatment of patients with *Candida* and *Aspergillus* infections. These experimental results showed general leukocyte responses primarily reflected by increased ex vivo IL-1β or TNF-α inflammatory responses as well as increased IL-17 and IL-22 cytokine secretion. This stimulation was however accompanied by concomitant decrease in granulocyte populations [48].

Safety of adjuvant recombinant interferon gamma-1b was assessed in 32 HSCT recipients at a comprehensive cancer center. Among these 32 patients, 81% had undergone allogeneic stem cell graft transplantation. In this retrospective analysis, interferon gamma-1b was mostly administered at a dose of 50 micrograms subcutaneously every other day. Six median doses ranged between 1 and 29 doses among the 32 patients. The median cumulative dose was 487 micrograms and ranged between 35 and 2175 micrograms. Fever was noted in 28% of subjects, and one patient developed reversible, new-onset lymphocytopenia while on cytokine adjunct therapy. None of the patients exhibited interferon gamma-1b-related neutropenia, thrombocytopenia, anemia, or hepatic dysfunction. It was important to note that treatment with recombinant cytokine did not precipitate nor exacerbate existing acute or chronic graft-versus-host disease. Among the 26 patients with aspergillosis, 54% died. It was considered encouraging that 60% of patients with disseminated aspergillosis after HSCT had a favorable response to antifungals and adjuvant interferon gamma-1b therapy. Multicenter clinical trials are needed to evaluate the efficacy of this cytokine therapy in highly susceptible transplant recipients with difficult-to-treat invasive mold disease [49]. Salvage combination cytokine therapy in severely immunocompromised patients with non-*Aspergillus* mold disease such as disseminated *Fusarium* spp. infection has also been reported to result in a favorable response. The authors suggested further clinical development to determine safety and therapeutic feasibility of interferon gamma-1b plus recombinant GM-CSF in highly susceptible allogenic stem cell graft recipients with life-threatening invasive fungal disease [50].

Recombinant Myeloid Growth Factors

Solid tumors, lymphomas, leukemias, and multiple myelomas exhibit similar risks of infectious complications. Myeloablative treatments for oncologic diseases including chemotherapy and/or radiation therapy are often complicated by myelosuppression prominently presenting as severe neutropenia which renders patients susceptible to potentially lethal infections. Gram-negative bacteria including *Pseudomonas aeruginosa* as well as systemic candidiasis and invasive disease due to *Aspergillus fumigatus* are serious and potentially life-threatening complications that are often encountered in patients with prolonged and severe neutropenia [51]. Antimicrobial chemoprophylaxis against bacteria, fungi, and viruses in transplant populations has predictably been largely ineffective even though a marked reduction in the risk for such infections has resulted in their routine implementation in various transplant protocols [52].

Myeloid cells are important in the prevention of fungal infections. In an experimental model of HSCT with post-transplant infection by *A. fumigatus* similar to what is observed in clinical practice, cotransplanation of common myeloid progenitor/granulocyte progenitor (CMP/GMP) cells prevented the establishment of lethal fungal infection in mice, and survival was significantly increased with addition of granulocyte colony-stimulating factor (G-CSF) [53]. Granulocyte-CSF is a glycoprotein which promotes the proliferation and differentiation of granulocyte precursors and their mobilization into the bloodstream. Currently available recombinant human G-CSF drugs (rhG-CSF) include lenograstim (glycosylated G-CSF), filgrastim (non-glycosylated G-CSF produced in *Escherichia coli*), and pegfilgrastim (pegylated filgrastim). Granulocyte macrophage colony-stimulating factor (GM-CSF) is another glycoprotein which promotes the production of both granulocytes and monocytes and plays an important role in the immune/inflammatory cascade and provides robust defense against systemic infections. The pharmaceutical analogs include glycoprotein produced in Chinese hamster ovary cells (regramostim), *Escherichia coli* (molgramostim), or yeast (sargramostim).

rG-CSF is widely used to mobilize transplanted hematopoietic stem cells [54, 55]. In a multicenter randomized controlled trial in southwestern China, high-risk acute myeloid leukemia (HR-AML) patients receiving HLA-haploidentical HSCT who underwent primary conditioning with rhG-CSF exhibited a lower rate of relapse than those conditioned without rhG-CSF [56]. More importantly, the administration of rG-CSF to healthy individuals induced earlier peak neutrophil counts [57] and has been shown to prevent chemotherapy-induced neutropenia [58]. These observations were mirrored in randomized, multicenter trials in patients with advanced soft tissue sarcoma, small-cell lung cancer (SCLC), non-Hodgkin's lymphoma (NHL), multiple myeloma, acute myeloid leukemia (AML), and others [55, 59–66]. These growth factors also accelerated the recovery of neutrophils following bone marrow (BMT) and $CD34^+$ peripheral blood stem cell (PBSC) transplantation [62, 64, 65, 67–75]. In a trial of patients with de novo AML undergoing HSCT, a regimen of G-CSF and high-dose cytarabine provided optimized disease-free survival (DFS) and low treatment-related mortality (TRM) [70]. Within a group of 221 pediatric patients receiving an allogeneic or autologous bone marrow or peripheral blood progenitor cell (PBPC) transplant, rG-CSF treatment significantly accelerated neutrophil recovery in all groups [76]. The ability of rG-CSF and rGM-CSF to stimulate myelopoiesis was essential to their anti-infectious capabilities [77]. In some trials, time of hospitalization due to infection or antibacterial treatment regimen was significantly shorter with lenograstim than in patients given placebo. In a cohort of German adults with multiple myeloma or lymphoma who received high-dose chemotherapy and PBSC transplantation, G-CSF (lenograstim 263 μg) was given after chemotherapy to all patients, and leukocyte peak was seen 12 hours after the cytokine was administered. The degree to which patient neutrophil counts peaked in response to G-CSF mobilization was negatively correlated with length of neutropenia, infections following PBSC infusion, and the duration of antibiotic therapy. Serious infections such as pneumonia or enterocolitis were less frequent in individuals with a good response, whereas invasive fungal infections were seen only among poor responders [78].

Both G-CSF and GM-CSF have been shown by several investigators to mediate direct, anti-infective activities mediated by granulocytes. Phagocytic and microbicidal functions of granulocytes against *Staphylococcus aureus* (although not against *Candida albicans*) were significantly increased by 50–70% following 1000–4000 units/ml of G-CSF preincubation [79]. On the other hand, GM-CSF protected neutropenic mice from lethal infections caused by *Pseudomonas aeruginosa*, *Staphylococcus aureus*, and *C. albicans* and also neutropenic rats from lung injury and mortality caused by *C. albicans* [80, 81]. These effects were not observed among G-CSF-treated animals. GM-CSF also stimulates human monocyte fungicidal activity for *C. albicans* [82–84], and GM-CSF together with IL-3 protected patients receiving high-dose chemotherapy from systemic fungal infections when administered with or without autologous stem cell support [85].

At a comprehensive cancer center, 66 patients in whom GM-CSF was given in conjunction with systemic antifungal therapy were assessed retrospectively. Severe neutropenia (77%) and refractory/relapsed cancer (65%) were common in the group. Prior to GM-CSF therapy, 15% of patients received high-dose corticosteroids for a median duration of 30 days with a median cumulative GM-CSF dose of 1184 mg. Nine patients received systemic steroids during GM-CSF therapy for a median of 16 days. In 9% of patients, modest adverse events were noted. None of the 66 patients exhibited moderate or severe systemic adverse events or cardiopulmonary toxicity. In this cohort, nearly half (48%) of the patients died due to progressive IFD. The probability of death was significantly increased in patients receiving high-dose corticosteroids prior to GM-CSF treatment commenced (odds ratio [OR] = 24.0), and GM-CSF started in the intensive care unit (OR = 10.0). GM-CSF adjunct therapy was well tolerated in these severely immunocompromised patients with opportunistic fungal disease. Antifungal treatment failure remained a challenge in patients treated with high-dose systemic corticosteroids [86].

Normal Donor Granulocyte Transfusion

Advances in leukapheresis technology in the late 1960s and early 1970s established the use of healthy donor granulocyte transfusion (GTx) for the treatment of infections in canine models and severely neutropenic patients [87–92]. However, because the advent of this therapeutic modality was not underpinned by randomized, placebo-controlled trials, the utility of GTx for the treatment of invasive fungal disease has remained controversial [93] for decades despite widespread adoption of the technique and evidence that neutrophil recovery is associated with local and systemic control of infection [94]. In a 1984 case-controlled study, only granulocytopenia was identified as a significant risk factor associated with the development of invasive pulmonary aspergillosis, whereas sinus disease, history of smoking, recurrent leukemia, chemotherapy, and corticosteroid administration were not significant predictors for this complication. Additionally, others have shown that risk of invasive aspergillosis proportionally rises with the extended duration of granulocytopenia [95].

Early studies of GTx in HSCT populations that were largely inconclusive and relied upon positive anecdotal reports [96, 97] were counterbalanced by larger, retrospective studies indicating little or no benefit [98]. These confounding series of events underscored the need for better-controlled or prospective studies. In 1997, a meta-analysis of eight prophylactic granulocyte transfusion trials performed between 1970 and 1995 identified both granulocyte dose and serum compatibility as important factors for clinical success, demonstrating significantly reduced risk of infection (RR = 0.075), death (RR = 0.224), and death from infection (RR = 0.168) among patients treated with GTx and well-matched control population [99]. This finding was important at the time as the recent contemporaneous advent of recombinant growth factors began to routinely enable increased yields of granulocytes to be harvested from mobilized normal donors. In 2013, Martinez et al. published the results of a well-designed animal study in which neutropenic mice treated concomitantly with antibiotics to prevent bacterial sepsis were inoculated with infectious doses of *Aspergillus* microconidia. In this model system, i.v. administration of 10^7 PMNs derived from syngeneic mobilized donors reduced post-infection mortality from 70% to 10% and completely cleared the infection in up to 50% of survivors as determined by analysis of fungal colony-forming units in the lungs of infected animals. Survival was shown to be correlated directly with the dose of neutrophils administered [100]. In another case control analysis at the MD Anderson Cancer Center, the impact of high-dose GTx (mean 5.5×10^{10} cells) was assessed. Twenty-nine patients with candidemia had received GTx, and 462 patients with candidemia in whom GTx was not given and who were comparable in age, gender, APACHE II score, recent treatment with antineoplastic chemotherapy, broad-spectrum antibiotics, systemic corticosteroids, radiotherapy, presence of intravascular catheter, and concordant antifungal therapy served as concomitant controls [101]. The patients who received granulocyte transfusions had a significantly higher incidence of persistent neutropenia (59% vs. 18%, $P < 0.001$), non-*Candida albicans* species candidemia (including 35% *Candida glabrata* and 31% *Candida krusei*, 90% vs. 67%, $p = 0.01$), and invasive antifungal breakthrough disease (62% vs. 23%, $p < 0.001$). The median duration of neutropenia in GTx group was 28 days compared with 10 days among the control group ($p < 0.001$), and 28% in the GTx group had received HSCT compared with 13% in patients among the control group ($p = 0.03$). Similarly, stays in critical care units were more prominent in the GTx group (62%) vs. patients in the control cohort (40%, $P = 0.02$). The overall attributable mortality rate was 48% in adjunct GTx group vs. 45% among 254 evaluable patients in the control group. On the basis of a reduced multivariate model, a significantly increased risk of candidemia-associated death was found for patients with HSCT (OR 2.51), for patients with persistent neutropenia (OR = 4.57), for patients with leukemia who also had prolonged candidemia (OR = 3.59), for those with disseminated candidiasis (OR = 5.19), and for patients with non-*C. albicans* species candidemia (OR = 5.02). Despite the presence of multiple predictors for significantly higher probability of candidemia-attributable death, recipients of healthy donor-derived, high-dose GTx adjunct therapy were associated with better than expected survival rates in this single center observation.

With increasing acceptance of the basic premise of GTx, subsequent studies were able to focus on the development of best practices including the means by which to increase granulocyte yield, identification of optimal granulocyte storage conditions, and the safe use of unrelated community donors [102–104]. In 2001, Lee et al. attempted to establish an optimal normal donor mobilization regimen for GTx therapy, though the study was successful only in identifying greater utility of GTx for the treatment of fungal or Gram-negative infections. Interestingly, protection was not evident for infections due to Gram-positive bacteria [105]. Additionally, clinicians became increasingly willing to attempt GTx for the treatment of invasive fungal infections such as rhinosinusitis [106], *Candida* septicemia [101, 107], nasal aspergillosis [108], *Candida* meningitis, central nervous system *Aspergillus* infection, and *Absdia* mucormycosis involving the upper airway [109]. Use of GTx for the management of mycoses in neutropenic pediatric populations became commonplace as well [110], and, as with the adults, the data were not without considerable controversy. A review of 66 pediatric trials published by van de Wetering et al. in 2007 reported no evidence of benefit and urged caution absent the future completion of a well-designed, randomized trial in children [111]. Subsequent pediatric studies suggested, as with adults, that cell dose is critical in achieving good clinical outcome [112]. Despite a broad and general contemporary acceptance of GTx efficacy for the treatment of infections in the neutropenic host, there remain advocates of large, randomized, placebo-controlled trials to firmly establish GTx efficacy. The fact that a conclusive study has not been performed in nearly 50 years of clinical experience with GTx indicates that this idealized goal is likely to remain both logistically and morally unfeasible in practice. Because of these practical and ethical realities, informative data derived from well-designed animal studies may have to suffice for the foreseeable future. Data derived from prophylactic studies of GTx administration are more clear and less equivocal with regard to preventative efficacy [113]; however, prophylactic GTx can often not be justified given the relative paucity of neutropenic patients who ultimately develop serious infections despite traditional antifungal prophylaxis in comparison to the significant costs associated with GTx.

Results of the most contemporary evidence-based approaches indicate that continuous flow centrifugation leukapheresis (CFCL) is the optimal method by which to isolate normal donor granulocyte populations. As opposed to earlier methodologies of isolation and harvest based on adherence, CFCL does not prematurely activate granulocytes thereby contributing to better functional activity and enhanced longevity in vivo following infusion [114]. Because the dose of the transfusion product is so critical to functional efficacy ($>1 \times 10^{10}$ granulocytes/dose in a variety of different studies) [114, 115], it is critical to mobilize donor granulocytes into peripheral circulation prior to leukapheresis and harvest. Optimal donor mobilization in many centers consists of synergistic administration of both corticosteroids such as dexamethasone and recombinant G-CSF, the combination of which produces a 10- to 13.5-fold increase in donor peripheral blood absolute neutrophil count [114, 116–118]. The use of single-agent CXCR4-antagonist plerixafor [119–122] is also under investigational study for use as a neutrophil mobilization agent among GTx donors [114].

Despite limited evidence for efficacy, GTx is also used to prevent and treat opportunistic infections in patients with severe and prolonged neutropenia. In one retrospective study, 373 GTx given to 74 patients were assessed. It was interesting to note that GTx was discontinued because of clinical improvement more often in patients with severe infections than in patients without severe infections (27 vs. 12%, $p \leq 0.002$), whereas deaths resulted in discontinuation of GTx therapy less often in patients with severe infections than in patients without severe infections (8 vs. 39%, $p \leq 0.002$). Patients who died by 12 weeks after GTx initiation were more likely to have not recovered from neutropenia ($p < 0.0001$) and to have started GTx during a critical care unit stay ($p < 0.001$). Concomitant uses of G-CSF ($p \leq 0.02$) and IFN-γ ($p \leq 0.04$) were also more common in patients who survived. It was important to recognize that probability of failure was significantly higher in patients in whom granulocyte transfusion was given if they had pre-existing medical comorbidities (OR 12.6), in whom therapy commenced while the patients were in critical care unit (OR 8.8), or in whom hyperbilirubinemia developed by the end of GTx therapy (OR 2.1). The possibility that a niche neutropenic population, such as those with severe systemic infections administered adjunct recombinant myeloid growth factor plus IFN-γ, might benefit from GTx requires further assessment [123].

The response to antifungal therapy alone often is suboptimal in patients with refractory neutropenia, and even donor-derived GTx has not consistently shown favorable outcomes. At a tertiary cancer center, 20 patients were given high-dose (approximately 5.5×10^{10} neutrophils per transfusion) healthy primed donor-derived GTx and adjunct IFN-gamma1b. Most patients (90%) had recurrent or refractory cancer, and 30% had undergone allogeneic stem cell graft transplantation. The median duration of GTx plus IFN-gamma1b was 26 days and ranged between 12 and 372 days after transplantation. Seventy percent of patients had proven or probable invasive fungal disease. Systemic corticosteroids during GTx plus IFN-gamma1b therapy were given in 40% of the patients in this study. The median doses of GTx were 8 transfusions that ranged between 4 and 28 transfusions, whereas IFN-gamma1b median doses were 9 and ranged between 1 and 28 doses with a cumulative IFN dose of 400 +/− 2621 micrograms. Other concomitant cytokines included G-CSF in 75% of patients, and 70% also received GM-CSF. Fever was the most common adverse event noted in 20% of patients in this group, and 10% developed skin rash. Reversible liver dysfunction in 15% and tachycardia in a single patient were also attributed to IFN-gamma1b therapy, whereas transient dyspnea was considered as a GTx toxicity. Four weeks after therapy started, 45% of patients exhibited complete or partial resolution of infection, and in another 15%, invasive fungal disease had become stable. These results were indicative of tolerability of GTx and adjunct cytokine therapy among this highly vulnerable patient population. IFN-gamma1b immune enhancement in patients being treated with high-dose healthy donor GTx for systemic fungal infections appears an attractive approach and needs further validation trials [124].

In addition, off-the-shelf neutrophil-like cells can be generated and expanded from hematopoietic progenitors [114, 125–129]; however, these largely hypothetical efforts are unlikely to impact clinical medicine in the near future. Given the lack of definitive indications for GTx, only clinically driven suggestions should govern justification for the use of GTx in the treatment of infections among patients with severe and prolonged neutropenia, particularly those with evidence of severe systemic infection such as invasive fungal diseases who fail monotherapeutic antimicrobial therapy [114].

Summary

In summary, while cell therapy and recombinant growth factors appear to play important and relevant roles in the management of posttransplant invasive fungal disease, the use of such agents remains somewhat controversial. In some cases, definitive evidence of efficacy can only be found in the research literature. In others, adoption of treatment procedures in the absence of randomized, placebo-controlled trials has created an environment in which clinicians are reasonably certain of efficacy and therefore lack the moral authority to withhold such treatments, as would be necessitated by administration of a placebo. As the field grapples with these issues, the development of innovative statistical methods and retrospective studies will likely be necessary to definitively confirm what is already anecdotally known. And in spite of the controversy, there are few who doubt the genuine efficacy of GTx and growth factor administration under appropriate clinical circumstances and fewer still who call for a complete re-evaluation of these treatment regimens in routine management. Nonetheless, future studies are certain to be beneficial in satisfying the needs of evidence-based approaches [130–133].

References

1. Kurup VP. Interaction of Aspergillus fumigatus spores and pulmonary alveolar macrophages of rabbits. Immunobiology. 1984;166:53–61.
2. Bozza S, Gaziano R, Spreca A, et al. Dendritic cells transport conidia and hyphae of Aspergillus fumigatus from the airways to the draining lymph nodes and initiate disparate Th responses to the fungus. J Immunol. 2002;168:1362–71.
3. Cenci E, Mencacci A, Del Sero G, et al. Interleukin-4 causes susceptibility to invasive pulmonary aspergillosis through suppression of protective type I responses. J Infect Dis. 1999;180:1957–68.
4. Chotirmall SH, Al-Alawi M, Mirkovic B, et al. Aspergillus-associated airway disease, inflammation, and the innate immune response. Biomed Res Int. 2013;2013:723129.
5. Cenci E, Mencacci A, Fe d'Ostiani C, et al. Cytokine- and T helper-dependent lung mucosal immunity in mice with invasive pulmonary aspergillosis. J Infect Dis. 1998;178:1750–60.
6. Grazziutti ML, Rex JH, Cowart RE, et al. Aspergillus fumigatus conidia induce a Th1 type cytokine response. J Infect Dis. 1997;176:1579–83.
7. Singh N, Paterson DL. Aspergillus infections in transplant recipients. Clin Microbiol Rev. 2005;18:44–69.
8. Patterson TF, Kirkpatrick WR, White M, et al. Invasive aspergillosis. Disease spectrum, treatment practices, and outcomes. I3 Aspergillus Study Group. Medicine. 2000;79:250–60.
9. Armstrong D. Infections with Pseudomonas aeruginosa, Aspergillus species and Mucoraceae. Int J Radiat Oncol Biol Phys. 1976;1:297–9.
10. Chamilos G, Luna M, Lewis RE, et al. Invasive fungal infections in patients with hematologic malignancies in a tertiary care cancer center: an autopsy study over a 15-year period (1989–2003). Haematologica. 2006;91:986–9.
11. Romani L. Cell mediated immunity to fungi: a reassessment. Med Mycol. 2008;46:515–29.
12. Kontoyiannis DP, Marr KA, Park BJ, et al. Prospective surveillance for invasive fungal infections in hematopoietic stem cell transplant recipients, 2001-2006: overview of the Transplant-Associated Infection Surveillance Network (TRANSNET) Database. Clin Infect Dis. 2010;50:1091–100.
13. Pagano L, Caira M, Candoni A, et al. Invasive aspergillosis in patients with acute myeloid leukemia: a SEIFEM-2008 registry study. Haematologica. 2010;95:644–50.
14. Perlroth J, Choi B, Spellberg B. Nosocomial fungal infections: epidemiology, diagnosis, and treatment. Med Mycol. 2007;45:321–46.
15. Tekaia F, Latge JP. Aspergillus fumigatus: saprophyte or pathogen? Curr Opin Microbiol. 2005;8:385–92.
16. Perea S, Patterson TF. Invasive Aspergillus infections in hematologic malignancy patients. Semin Respir Infect. 2002;17:99–105.
17. Steinmann J, Hamprecht A, Vehreschild MJ, et al. Emergence of azole-resistant invasive aspergillosis in HSCT recipients in Germany. J Antimicrob Chemother. 2015;70:1522–6.
18. Kong YC, Levine HB. Experimentally induced immunity in the mycoses. Bacteriol Rev. 1967;31:35–53.
19. Marr KA, Carter RA, Boeckh M, Martin P, Corey L. Invasive aspergillosis in allogeneic stem cell transplant recipients: changes in epidemiology and risk factors. Blood. 2002;100:4358–66.
20. Grow WB, Moreb JS, Roque D, et al. Late onset of invasive aspergillus infection in bone marrow transplant patients at a university hospital. Bone Marrow Transplant. 2002;29:15–9.
21. Marr KA, Patterson T, Denning D. Aspergillosis. Pathogenesis, clinical manifestations, and therapy. Infect Dis Clin N Am. 2002;16:875–94.
22. Denning DW, Follansbee SE, Scolaro M, et al. Pulmonary aspergillosis in the acquired immunodeficiency syndrome. N Engl J Med. 1991;324:654–62.
23. Williams DM, Weiner MH, Drutz DJ. Immunologic studies of disseminated infection with Aspergillus fumigatus in the nude mouse. J Infect Dis. 1981;143:726–33.
24. Roilides E, Katsifa H, Walsh TJ. Pulmonary host defences against Aspergillus fumigatus. Res Immunol. 1998;149:454–65.
25. Cenci E, Mencacci A, Bacci A, et al. T cell vaccination in mice with invasive pulmonary aspergillosis. J Immunol. 2000;165:381–8.
26. Hebart H, Bollinger C, Fisch P, et al. Analysis of T-cell responses to Aspergillus fumigatus antigens in healthy individuals and patients with hematologic malignancies. Blood. 2002;100:4521–8.
27. Fierer J, Waters C, Walls L. Both CD4+ and CD8+ T cells can mediate vaccine-induced protection against Coccidioides immitis infection in mice. J Infect Dis. 2006;193:1323–31.
28. Wuthrich M, Filutowicz HI, Warner T, Deepe GS Jr, Klein BS. Vaccine immunity to pathogenic fungi overcomes the requirement for CD4 help in exogenous antigen presentation to CD8+ T cells: implications for vaccine development in immune-deficient hosts. J Exp Med. 2003;197:1405–16.
29. Zheng M, Ramsay AJ, Robichaux MB, et al. CD4+ T cell-independent DNA vaccination against opportunistic infections. J Clin Invest. 2005;115:3536–44.
30. Bozza S, Clavaud C, Giovanni G, et al. Immune sensing of Aspergillus fumigatus proteins, glycolipids, and polysaccharides and the impact on Th immunity and vaccination. J Immunol. 2009;183:2407–14.
31. Bozza S, Perruccio K, Montagnoli C, et al. A dendritic cell vaccine against invasive aspergillosis in allogeneic hematopoietic transplantation. Blood. 2003;102:3807–14.
32. Shao C, Qu J, He L, et al. Dendritic cells transduced with an adenovirus vector encoding interleukin-12 are a potent vaccine for invasive pulmonary aspergillosis. Genes Immun. 2005;6:103–14.
33. Bozza S, Gaziano R, Lipford GB, et al. Vaccination of mice against invasive aspergillosis with recombinant Aspergillus proteins and CpG oligodeoxynucleotides as adjuvants. Microbes Infect. 2002;4:1281–90.
34. Ramirez-Ortiz ZG, Specht CA, Wang JP, et al. Toll-like receptor 9-dependent immune activation by unmethylated CpG motifs in Aspergillus fumigatus DNA. Infect Immun. 2008;76:2123–9.
35. Feldmesser M. Prospects of vaccines for invasive aspergillosis. Med Mycol. 2005;43:571–87.

36. Stevens DA, Clemons KV, Liu M. Developing a vaccine against aspergillosis. Med Mycol. 2011;49:S170–6.
37. Bacci A, Montagnoli C, Perruccio K, et al. Dendritic cells pulsed with fungal RNA induce protective immunity to Candida albicans in hematopoietic transplantation. J Immunol. 2002;168:2904–13.
38. Gray PW, Goeddel DV. Structure of the human immune interferon gene. Nature. 1982;298:859–63.
39. Davis MJ, Eastman AJ, Qiu Y, et al. Cryptococcus neoformans-induced macrophage lysosome damage crucially contributes to fungal virulence. J Immunol. 2015;194:2219–31.
40. Liles WC. Immunomodulatory approaches to augment phagocyte-mediated host defense for treatment of infectious diseases. Semin Respir Infect. 2001;16:11–7.
41. Su X, Yu Y, Zhong Y, et al. Interferon-gamma regulates cellular metabolism and mRNA translation to potentiate macrophage activation. Nat Immunol. 2015;16:838–49.
42. Ostuni R, Piccolo V, Barozzi I, et al. Latent enhancers activated by stimulation in differentiated cells. Cell. 2013;152:157–71.
43. Stevens DA, Brummer E, Clemons KV. Interferon-γ as an Antifungal. J Infect Dis. 2006;194:S33–7.
44. www.fda.gov/Drugs/DevelopmentApprovalProcess/HowDrugsareDevelopedandAproved/ApprovalApplications/TherapeuticBiologicApplications/ucm080426.htm
45. Filiz S, Uygun DFK, Köksoy S, Şahin E, Yeğin O. In vitro interferon γ improves the oxidative burst activity of neutrophils in patients with chronic granulomatous disease with a subtype of gp91phox deficiency. Cent Eur J Immunol. 2015;40:54–60.
46. Abzug MJ, Walsh TJ. Interferon-gamma and colony-stimulating factors as adjuvant therapy for refractory fungal infections in children. Pediatr Infect Dis J. 2004;23:769–73.
47. Armstrong-James D, Teo IA, Shrisvastava S, et al. Exogenous interferon-gamma immunotherapy for invasive fungal infections in kidney transplant patients. Am J Transplant. 2010;10:1796–803.
48. Delsing CE, Gresnigt MS, Leentjens J, et al. Interferon-gamma as adjunctive immunotherapy for invasive fungal infections: a case series. BMC Infect Dis. 2014;14:166.
49. Safdar A, Rodriguez G, Ohmagari N, et al. The safety of interferon-gamma-1b therapy for invasive fungal infections after hematopoietic stem cell transplantation. Cancer. 2005;103(4):731–9.
50. Lewis R, Hogan H, Howell A, Safdar A. Progressive fusariosis: unpredictable posaconazole bioavailability, and feasibility of recombinant interferon-gamma plus granulocyte macrophage-colony stimulating factor for refractory disseminated infection. Leuk Lymphoma. 2008;49(1):163–5.
51. Weinberger M, Elattar I, Marshall D, et al. Patterns of infection in patients with aplastic anemia and the emergence of Aspergillus as a major cause of death. Medicine. 1992;71:24–43.
52. Giles FJ. Monocyte-macrophages, granulocyte-macrophage colony-stimulating factor, and prolonged survival among patients with acute myeloid leukemia and stem cell transplants. Clin Infect Dis. 1998;26:1282–9.
53. Andrew B, Stacy MB, David T, et al. Myeloid progenitors protect against invasive aspergillosis and Pseudomonas aeruginosa infection following hematopoietic stem cell transplantation. Blood. 2002;100:4660–7.
54. Simone C, Andrea GZ, Stefano F, et al. A phase II study on the safety and efficacy of a single dose of pegfilgrastim for mobilization and transplantation of autologous hematopoietic stem cells in pediatric oncohematology patients. Transfusion. 2011;51:2480–7.
55. Gillian MK. Lenograstim. Drugs. 2011;7:679–707.
56. Lei G, Qin W, Xinghua C, et al. Effects of priming with recombinant human granulocyte colony-stimulating factor on conditioning regimen for high-risk acute myeloid leukemia patients undergoing human leukocyte antigen-haploidentical hematopoietic stem cell transplantation: a multicenter randomized controlled study in Southwest China. Biol Blood Marrow Transplant. 2014;20:1932–9.
57. Paolo A, Richard EC. Biologic and molecular effects of granulocyte colony-stimulating factor in healthy individuals: recent findings and current challenges. Blood. 2008;111:1767–72.
58. Riccardo R, Giulio C, Ilaria S, et al. Pegfilgrastim: current and future perspectives in the treatment of chemotherapy-induced neutropenia. Future Oncol. 2006;2:667–76.
59. Bui BN, Chevallier B, Chevreau C, et al. Efficacy of lenograstim on hematologic tolerance to MAID chemotherapy in patients with advanced soft tissue sarcoma and consequences on treatment dose-intensity. J Clin Oncol. 1995;13:2629–36.
60. Chevreau C, Bui BN, Chevallier B, et al. Phase I-II trial of intensification of the MAID regimen with support of lenograstim (rHuG-CSF) in patients with advanced soft-tissue sarcoma (STS). Am J Clin Oncol. 1999;22:267–72.
61. Gatzemeier U, Kleisbauer JP, Drings P, et al. Lenograstim as support for ACE chemotherapy of small-cell lung cancer: a phase III, multicenter, randomized study. Am J Clin Oncol. 2000;23:393–400.
62. Takahashi S. Recombinant human G-CSF combined regimen for allogeneic BMT in myeloid leukemias. Rinshō ketsueki. 1997;38:489–95.
63. Geissler RG, Schulte P, Ganser A. Treatment with growth factors in myelodysplastic syndromes. Pathol Biol. 1997;45:656–67.
64. Tabbara IA, Ghazal CD, Ghazal HH. The role of granulocyte colony-stimulating factor in hematopoietic stem cell transplantation. Cancer Investig. 1997;15:353–7.
65. Greenberg P, Advani R, Keating A, et al. GM-CSF accelerates neutrophil recovery after autologous hematopoietic stem cell transplantation. Bone Marrow Transplant. 1996;18:1057–64.
66. Day SJO, Rabinowe SN, Neuberg D, et al. A phase II study of continuous infusion recombinant human granulocyte-macrophage colony-stimulating factor as an adjunct to autologous bone marrow transplantation for patients with non-Hodgkin's lymphoma in first remission. Blood. 1994;83:2707–14.
67. Battiwalla M, McCarthy PL. Filgrastim support in allogeneic HSCT for myeloid malignancies: a review of the role of G-CSF and the implications for current practice. Bone Marrow Transplant. 2009;43:351–6.
68. Kobbe G, Bruns I, Fenk R, Czibere A, Haas R. Pegfilgrastim for PBSC mobilization and autologous haematopoietic SCT. Bone Marrow Transplant. 2009;43:669–77.
69. Piccirillo N, Matteis SD, Vita SD, et al. Kinetics of peg-filgrastim after high-dose chemotherapy and autologous peripheral blood stem cell transplantation. Bone Marrow Transplant. 2007;40:579–83.
70. Takehiko M, Yoshinobu A, Reiko W, et al. Long-term follow-up of allogeneic hematopoietic stem cell transplantation for de novo acute myelogenous leukemia with a conditioning regimen of total body irradiation and granulocyte colony-stimulating factor-combined high-dose cytarabine. Biol Blood Marrow Transplant. 2008;14:651–7.
71. Clifford L, Craig W, Aaron PR, Alister CW. Granulocyte colony-stimulating factor receptor: stimulating granulopoiesis and much more. Int J Biochem Cell Biol. 2009;41:2372–5.
72. Ian MW, Olga M, Leah B, et al. Sequential administration of sargramostim and filgrastim in pediatric allogeneic stem cell transplantation recipients undergoing myeloablative conditioning. Pediatr Transplant. 2009;13:464–74.
73. Takahashi S, Oshima Y, Okamoto S, et al. Recombinant human granulocyte colony-stimulating factor (G-CSF) combined conditioning regimen for allogeneic bone marrow transplantation (BMT) in standard-risk myeloid leukemia. Am J Hematol. 1998;57:303–8.
74. Teshima H, Ishikawa J, Kitayama H, et al. Clinical effects of recombinant human granulocyte colony-stimulating factor in leukemia patients: a phase I/II study. Exp Hematol. 1989;17:853–8.
75. Asano S, Masaoka T, Takaku F. Clinical effect of recombinant human granulocyte colony-stimulating factor in bone marrow

transplantation. The Japan rhG-CSF Clinical Study Group. Gan To Kagaku Ryoho. 1990;17:1201–9.
76. Sandro D, Roberto R, Chiara M, et al. Clinical benefits of granulocyte colony-stimulating factor therapy after hematopoietic stem cell transplant in children: results of a prospective randomized trial. Haematologica. 2002;87:1274–80.
77. César Gómez R, Alvaro Pinto M, Manuel González B. Colony-stimulating factors: clinical evidence for treatment and prophylaxis of chemotherapy-induced febrile neutropenia. Clin Transl Oncol. 2006;8:729–34.
78. Christian S, Michael S, Hans S, et al. Testing G-CSF responsiveness predicts the individual susceptibility to infection and consecutive treatment in recipients of high-dose chemotherapy. Blood. 2011;117:2121–8.
79. Roilides E, Walsh TJ, Pizzo PA, Rubin M. Granulocyte colony-stimulating factor enhances the phagocytic and bactericidal activity of normal and defective human neutrophils. J Infect Dis. 1991;163:579–83.
80. Lechner AJ, Lamprech KE, Potthoff LH, Tredway TL, Matuschak GM. Recombinant GM-CSF reduces lung injury and mortality during neutropenic Candida sepsis. Am J Phys. 1994; 266:8.
81. Mayer P, Schütze E, Lam C, Kricek F, Liehl E. Recombinant murine granulocyte-macrophage colony-stimulating factor augments neutrophil recovery and enhances resistance to infections in myelosuppressed mice. J Infect Dis. 1991;16:584–90.
82. Smith PD, Lamerson CL, Banks SM, et al. Granulocyte-macrophage colony-stimulating factor augments human monocyte fungicidal activity for Candida albicans. J Infect Dis. 1990;161: 999–1005.
83. Djeu JY, Blanchard DK, Halkias D, Friedman H. Growth inhibition of Candida albicans by human polymorphonuclear neutrophils: activation by interferon-gamma and tumor necrosis factor. J Immunol. 1986;137:2980–4.
84. Weisbart RH, Golde DW, Clark SC, Wong GG, Gasson JC. Human granulocyte-macrophage colony-stimulating factor is a neutrophil activator. Nature. 1985;314:361–3.
85. Peters BG, Adkins DR, Harrison BR, et al. Antifungal effects of yeast-derived rhu-GM-CSF in patients receiving high-dose chemotherapy given with or without autologous stem cell transplantation: a retrospective analysis. Bone Marrow Transplant. 1996;18: 93–102.
86. Safdar A, Rodriguez G, Zuniga J, Al Akhrass F, Georgescu G, Pande A. Granulocyte macrophage colony-stimulating factor in 66 patients with myeloid or lymphoid neoplasms and recipients of hematopoietic stem cell transplantation with invasive fungal disease. Acta Haematol. 2013;129(1):26–34.
87. Graw RG Jr, Herzig G, Perry S, Henderson ES. Normal granulocyte transfusion therapy: treatment of septicemia due to gram-negative bacteria. N Engl J Med. 1972;287:367–71.
88. Raubitschek AA, Levin AS, Stites DP, Shaw EB, Fudenberg HH. Normal granulocyte infusion therapy for aspergillosis in chronic granulomatous disease. Pediatrics. 1973;51:230–3.
89. Debelak KM, Epstein RB, Andersen BR. Granulocyte transfusions in leukopenic dogs: in vivo and in vitro function of granulocytes obtained by continuous-flow filtration leukapheresis. Blood. 1974;43:757–66.
90. Dale DC, Reynolds HY, Pennington JE, et al. Experimental pneumonia die to Pseudomonas in dogs: controlled trial of granulocyte transfusion therapy. J Infect Dis. 1974;130:S143–4.
91. Lowenthal RM, Grossman L, Goldman JM, et al. Granulocyte transfusions in treatment of infections in patients with acute leukaemia and aplastic anaemia. Lancet. 1975;1:353–8.
92. Gercovich FG, Richman SP, Rodriguez V, et al. Successful control of systemic Aspergillus niger infections in two patients with acute leukemia. Cancer. 1975;36:2271–6.
93. Petersen FB, Buckner CD, Clift RA, et al. Prevention of nosocomial infection sin marrow transplant patients: a prospective randomized comparison of systemic antibiotics versus granulocyte transfusions. Infect Control. 1986;7:586–92.
94. Goering P, Berlinger NT, Weisdorf DJ. Aggressive combined modality treatment of progressive sinonasal fungal infections in immunocompromised patients. Am J Med. 1988;85:619–23.
95. Gerson SL, Talbot GH, Hurwitz S, et al. Prolonged granulocytopenia: the major risk factor for invasive pulmonary aspergillosis in patients with acute leukemia. Ann Intern Med. 1984;100: 345–51.
96. Clarke K, Szer J, Shelton M, Coghlan D, Grigg A. Multiple granulocyte transfusions facilitating successful unrelated bone marrow transplantation in a patient with very severe aplastic anemia complicated by suspected fungal infection. Bone Marrow Transplant. 1995;16:723–6.
97. Catalano L, Fontana R, Scarpato N, et al. Combined treatment with amphotericin-B and granulocyte transfusion with G-CSF-stimulated donors in an aplastic patient with invasive aspergillosis undergoing bone marrow transplantation. Haematologica. 1997;82:71–2.
98. Bhatia S, McCullough J, Perry EH, et al. Granulocyte transfusions: efficacy in treating fungal infections in neutropenic patients following bone marrow transplantation. Transfusion. 1994;34:226–32.
99. Vamvakas EC, Pineda AA. Determinants of the efficacy of prophylactic granulocyte transfusions: a meta-analysis. J Clin Apher. 1997;12:74–81.
100. Martinez M, Chen V, Tong A-J, et al. Experimental evidence that granulocyte transfusions are efficacious in treatment of neutropenic hosts with pulmonary aspergillosis. Antimicrob Agents Chemother. 2013;57:1882–7.
101. Safdar A, Hanna HA, Boktour M, et al. Impact of high-dose granulocyte transfusions in patients with cancer with candidemia: retrospective case-control analysis of 491 episodes of Candida species bloodstream infections. Cancer. 2004;101(12):2859–65.
102. Hubel K, Dale DC, Liles WC. Granulocyte transfusion therapy: update on potential clinical applications. Curr Opin Hematol. 2001;8:161–4.
103. Yeghen T, Devereux S. Granulocyte transfusion: a review. Vox Sang. 2001;81:87–92.
104. Hubel K, Carter RA, Liles WC, et al. Granulocyte transfusion therapy for infections in candidates and recipients of HPC transplantation: a comparative analysis of feasibility and outcome for community donors versus related donors. Transfusion. 2002;42:1414–21.
105. Lee JJ, Chung IJ, Park MR, et al. Clinical efficacy of granulocyte transfusion therapy in patients with neutropenia-related infections. Leukemia. 2001;25:203–7.
106. Samadi DS, Goldberg AN, Orlandi RR. Granulocyte transfusion in the management of fulminant invasive fungal rhinosinusitis. Am J Rhinol. 2001;15:263–5.
107. Illerhaus G, Wirth K, Dwenger A, et al. Treatment and prophylaxis of severe infections in neutropenic patients by granulocyte transfusions. Ann Hematol. 2002;81:273–81.
108. Piccaluga PP, Ricci P, Martinelli G, et al. Prompt resolution of nasal aspergillosis with intranasal instillation of liposomal amphotericin-B (amBisome) and granulocyte transfusions. Leuk Lymphoma. 2004;45:637–8.
109. Grigull L, Beilken A, Schmid H, et al. Secondary prophylaxis of invasive fungal infections with combination antifungal therapy and G-CSF-mobilized granulocyte transfusions in three children with hematological malignancies. Support Care Cancer. 2006;14:783–6.
110. Sachs UJ, Reiter A, Walter T, Bein G, Woessmann W. Safety and efficacy of therapeutic early onset granulocyte transfusions

in pediatric patients with neutropenia and severe infections. Transfusion. 2006;46:1909–14.
111. van de Wetering MD, Weggelaar N, Offringa M, Caron HN, Kuijpers TW. Granulocyte transfusions in neutropaenic children: a systematic review of the literature. Eur J Cancer. 2007;43:2082–92.
112. Seidel MG, Minkov M, Witt V, et al. Granulocyte transfusions in children and young adults: does the dose matter? J Pediatr Hematol Oncol. 2009;31:166–72.
113. Kerr JP, Liakopolou E, Brown J, et al. The use of stimulated granulocyte transfusions to prevent recurrence of past severe infections after allogeneic stem cell transplantation. Br J Haematol. 2003;123:114–8.
114. Marfin AA, Price TH. Granulocyte transfusion therapy. J Intensive Care Med. 2015;30:79–88.
115. Massey E, Paulus U, Doree C, Stanworth S. Granulocyte transfusion for preventing infections in patients with neutropenia or neutrophil dysfunction. Cochrane Database Syst Rev. 2009;1:CD005341.
116. Liles WC, Rodger E, Dale DC. Combined administration of G-CSF and dexamethasone for the mobilization of granulocytes in normal donors: optimization of dosing. Transfusion. 2000;40: 642–4.
117. Liles WC, Huang JE, Llewellyn C, et al. A comparative trial of granulocyte-colony stimulating factor and dexamethasone, separately and in combination, for the mobilization of neutrophils in the peripheral blood of normal volunteers. Transfusion. 1997;37:182–7.
118. Ikemoto J, Yoshihara S, Fujioka T, et al. Impact of the mobilization regimen and the harvesting technique on the granulocyte yield in health donors for granulocyte transfusion therapy. Transfusion. 2012;52:2646–52.
119. Bendinger WI. Allogeneic transplantation: peripheral blood vs. bone marrow. Curr Opin Oncol. 2012;24:191–6.
120. Liles WC, Broxmeyer H, Rodger E, et al. Mobilization of hematopoietic progenitor cells in healthy volunteers by AMD 3100, a CXCR4 antagonist. Blood. 2003;102:2728–30.
121. McDermott DH, Liu Q, Ulrick J, et al. The CXCR4 antagonist plerixafor corrects panleukopenia in patients with WHIM syndrome. Blood. 2011;118:4957–62.
122. Dale DC, Bolyard AA, Kelley ML, et al. The CXCR4 antagonist plerixafor is a potential therapy for myelokathexis, WHIM syndrome. Blood. 2011;119:4963–6.
123. Safdar A, Rodriguez G, Zuniga J, Al Akhrass F, Pande A. Use of healthy-donor granulocyte transfusions to treat infections in neutropenic patients with myeloid or lymphoid neoplasms: experience in 74 patients treated with 373 granulocyte transfusions. Acta Haematol. 2014;131(1):50–8.
124. Safdar A, Rodriguez GH, Lichtiger B, et al. Recombinant interferon gamma1b immune enhancement in 20 patients with hematologic malignancies and systemic opportunistic infections treated with donor granulocyte transfusions. Cancer. 2006;106(12):2664–71.
125. Hino M, Suzuki K, Yamane T, et al. Ex vivo expansion of mature human neutrophils with normal functions from purified peripheral blood CD34+ haematopoietic progenitor cells. Br J Haematol. 2000;109:314–21.
126. McNiece I, Briddell R. Ex vivo expansion of hematopoietic progenitor cells and mature cells. Exp Hematol. 2001;29:3–11.
127. Marturana F, Timmins NE, Nielsen LK. Short-term exposure of umbilical cord blood CD34+ cells to granulocyte-macrophage colony stimulating factor early in culture improves ex vivo expansion of neutrophils. Cytotherapy. 2011;13:366–77.
128. Dick EP, Prince LR, Sabroe I. Ex vivo-expanded bone marrow CD34+ derived neutrophils have limited bactericidal ability. Stem Cells. 2008;26:2552–63.
129. Brunck MEG, Nielsen LK. Concise review: next-generation cell therapies to prevent infection in neutropenic patients. Stem Cells Transl Med. 2014;3:541–8.
130. Safdar A. Immunotherapy for invasive mold disease in severely immunosuppressed patients. Clin Infect Dis. 2013;57(1):94–100.
131. Safdar A. Immunomodulation therapy for invasive aspergillosis: discussion on myeloid growth factors, recombinant cytokines, and antifungal drug immune modulation. Curr Fungal Infect Rep. 2010;4(1):1–7.
132. Safdar A. Antifungal immunity and adjuvant cytokine immune enhancement in cancer patients with invasive fungal infections. Clin Microbiol Infect. 2007;13(1):1–4.
133. Safdar A. Strategies to enhance immune function in hematopoietic transplantation recipients who have fungal infections. Bone Marrow Transplant. 2006;38(5):327–37.

Antimicrobial Stewardship: Considerations for a Transplant Center

59

Susan K. Seo and Graeme N. Forrest

Introduction

In this era of multidrug-resistant organisms (MDRO), clinicians are facing difficult-to-treat infections with a dearth of novel antimicrobial agents in the pipeline [1, 2]. In order to optimize the use of currently available anti-infective drugs, antimicrobial stewardship encompassing all patient populations has been advocated [3], and the 2015 *National Action Plan for Combating Antibiotic-Resistant Bacteria* has stipulated that all United States (US) acute care hospitals should develop a formal antimicrobial stewardship program (ASP) by 2020 [4]. However, antimicrobial stewardship efforts in immunocompromised patients can be challenging due to the complexity of cases, difficulty with making timely diagnoses, and the high morbidity and mortality associated with invasive bacterial, viral, and fungal infections [5]. While there are limited data for hematopoietic cell transplant (HCT) and none for solid organ transplant (SOT) to date, cost-savings and other benefits of ASPs in the care of transplant recipients are thought to be feasible [6]. The purpose of this chapter is to explore several features of coordinating an ASP at a transplant center. While basic stewardship tenets are applicable [7], there are also unique aspects to consider in the management of transplant patients.

Implementation of ASPs

Effective antimicrobial stewardship is defined as the optimal selection, dose, and duration of an antibiotic, resulting in the cure of an infection with minimal toxicity to the patient and minimal impact on the selection of MDRO [8]. In 2016, the Infectious Diseases Society of America (IDSA) and the Society for Healthcare Epidemiology of America (SHEA) updated an evidence-based guideline for the development of a formal ASP by healthcare institutions [7]. Although many major medical centers in the US have an institutional ASP, not all of these established programs are inclusive of adult and pediatric transplant patients, showing that there is still work to be done [9]. How an ASP is implemented will vary depending on the institution's size and resources, but a comprehensive approach with a full-time dedicated multidisciplinary team can lead to increased infection cures, reduced treatment failures, and cost-savings [10]. From a practical standpoint, the Centers for Disease Control and Prevention (CDC) have summarized the seven core elements for building a successful ASP: administrative support, physician leader responsible for program outcomes, designated personnel with appropriate anti-infective expertise, selection of stewardship strategies, regular audits, prescriber feedback, and education to healthcare providers about resistance and optimal prescribing [11].

The transplant center though represents a distinctive entity, and formation of an ASP should take into account issues that are unique to such a place, such as local susceptibility patterns and the intricacies of managing patients with compromised host defenses. Advances in SOT [12] and HCT [13] have prolonged survival and increased probability of cure in patients with previously untreatable conditions. However, infections continue to be a major threat to the success of transplantation. As a consequence, antimicrobials are commonly prescribed for prolonged periods of time to either prevent or treat infectious complications in transplant recipients. It is not surprising then to find that units caring for SOT and HCT patients have some of the highest rates of antibacterial and antifungal use within hospitals [14, 15].

There is a well-established association between antimicrobial use and emergence of drug resistance and *Clostridium difficile* infection (CDI). At the patient level, the longer the duration of exposure to antimicrobials the greater is the

S. K. Seo (✉)
Department of Medicine, Infectious Disease Service, Memorial Sloan-Kettering Cancer Center, New York, NY, USA
e-mail: seos@mskcc.org

G. N. Forrest
Division of Infectious Diseases, Portland VA Medical Center and Oregon Health and Science University, Portland, OR, USA
e-mail: forrestg@ohsu.edu

A. Safdar (ed.), *Principles and Practice of Transplant Infectious Diseases*, https://doi.org/10.1007/978-1-4939-9034-4_59

likelihood of colonization with resistant organisms; at the communal level, areas within hospitals with the highest rates of antimicrobial use are likely to have the highest rates of drug resistance [8]. While quinolone prophylaxis has been beneficial in reducing infection and mortality, breakthrough infections have been connected to quinolone use in HCT recipients [16–18]. An increasing trend of infections caused by methicillin-resistant *Staphylococcus aureus* (MRSA) [19], vancomycin-resistant enterococci (VRE) [20, 21], and multidrug-resistant (MDR) Gram-negative bacteria [21–23] in febrile, neutropenic patients irrespective of quinolone prophylaxis has also been reported.

Colonization and infection by resistant organisms have also been recognized in SOT recipients. The potential for infection by a resistant organism can complicate selection of appropriate initial treatment, and similar to studies in other patient groups, a delay in adequate empiric antibiotic therapy has been correlated with increased mortality among SOT patients [24]. VRE infection has been reported to occur between 4% and 11% among liver and kidney recipients [25, 26] with the majority of infections happening within the first month following transplantation. VRE infections in SOT are often severe and have been associated with persistent and recurrent bacteremia, prolonged hospitalization, and higher risk of death [27]. Data suggest that extended-spectrum beta-lactamase (ESBL)-producing bacteria commonly colonize the gastrointestinal tract of liver and intestinal transplant recipients [28, 29], and sporadic nosocomial outbreaks have occurred in intensive care units managing transplant patients, as well as in liver and renal transplant units [28, 30–32]. At least one group in Spain has found increased morbidity associated with ESBL-producing and Amp C beta-lactamase Gram-negative organisms in a population of kidney recipients [33]. Persistent colonization and infections with MDR *Achromobacter*, *Pseudomonas*, *Stenotrophomonas*, and *Burkholderia* species have been most frequently reported for lung transplant recipients, particularly in those with cystic fibrosis, and their detection seems to have prognostic significance [34]. The presence of *Pseudomonas aeruginosa* might adversely impact survival of lung transplant recipients by favoring the development of bronchiolitis obliterans following transplantation [35], and post-transplant survival among patients colonized with *Burkholderia* hinges on which infecting species is present [36, 37].

Aside from bacterial pathogens, invasive fungal infections (IFIs) occur disproportionately more in patients with compromised host defenses and are associated with considerable morbidity and mortality. The difficulty in diagnosing IFIs often results in the prolonged use of empiric antifungal therapy [38]. The overuse of these agents not only results in increased costs, but also has associated toxicities in this population [39]. Serum and bronchoalveolar lavage galactomannan antigen and the serum (1–3)-β-D-glucan assay, which is non-specific, have improved the ability to diagnose IFIs in SOT and HCT recipients [40, 41], but should these tests be performed off-site, the increased turnaround time lessens the potential to shorten or stop unnecessary antifungal therapy. Even a negative result has to be assessed in the clinical context of the host and radiologic factors to determine whether therapy can be discontinued.

Three potential targets for antimicrobial stewardship in transplant patients are antibacterial prophylaxis, empiric treatment of specific infectious conditions (e.g., fever and neutropenia, pneumonia, sepsis), and prevention and therapy of IFIs. ASP teams can craft practice guidelines with input by their transplant colleagues. However, ASP personnel should be knowledgeable about a wide spectrum of anti-infective agents and also be on the lookout for alternative therapies, including investigational agents, when breakthrough infections occur [42].

Multidisciplinary Collaboration

Antimicrobial stewardship entails a multidisciplinary approach with designated oversight by an ASP team. Core ASP members include an infectious disease (ID) physician and one or more clinical pharmacists with ID specialty training [8]. These members generally have dedicated time expressly for the purpose of antibiotic management and are compensated accordingly. Because antimicrobial stewardship relates to patient safety and is considered to be a medical staff function, the program is usually directed by the ID specialist [8]. In addition, the ASP should have administrative backing; prescriber acceptance; and strong working relationships with information technology (IT), Pharmacy and Therapeutics (P&T) committee, pharmacy, microbiology, and infection control to be successful [11].

A computer-based infrastructure facilitates stewardship efforts. Utilization of healthcare IT in the form of electronic medical records (EMR), computer order entry (COE), and clinical decision support has the potential to improve prescribing and reduce medication errors, as demonstrated by LDS Hospital in Salt Lake City, UT [43–46]. While the computer surveillance and decision-support system of LDS Hospital is ideal, adoption of such technology by individual institutions on a broader scale has been slow. Depending on the IT resources available, the ASP can still find ways to efficiently follow local susceptibilities, monitor antimicrobial use, and target antimicrobial interventions [8]. Several reports confirming the usefulness of COE in reducing the use of a target antibiotic like linezolid [47] or improving compliance with surgical prophylaxis guidelines [48] seem to indicate that hospitals are showing interest in investing in IT support.

Because of the nature of SOT and HCT care, the transplant center is well suited for multidisciplinary collaboration. However, there needs to be a sense by the transplant physicians and surgeons of a shared appreciation for the complexities of caring for immunocompromised patients. Recognizing the heterogeneity of patients is one key way. The net state of immunosuppression can vary greatly among immunocompromised individuals and even in the same person at different times, so being able to assess the degree and type of immunosuppression requires a level of expertise on the part of stewardship personnel working in such a setting [42].

Another way is to share data and demonstrate good outcomes in order to build trust with future interventions [42]. To illustrate, antibacterial prophylaxis was not routine prior to 2006 at a tertiary cancer center in New York City, but the prevention of pre-engraftment viridans streptococcal bacteremia (VSB) in allogeneic HCT became a high priority due to an incidence of 7.4% and an attributable mortality of 21% [49]. Vancomycin-based prophylaxis was instituted in 2006 and was subsequently associated with elimination of VSB and reduced staphylococcal bacteremia in a joint antimicrobial stewardship, ID, and transplant service analysis [50]. Since then, VRE has emerged as the leading cause of pre-engraftment bacteremia, so ongoing surveillance is being conducted at the center [50].

Combining forces to develop local guidelines is a further means to get transplant backing for ASP work. Although evidence-based national guidelines (e.g., management of febrile, neutropenic patients [51]; prevention of opportunistic infections in HCT recipients [52]; surgical transplant prophylaxis [53]) are available, these should be modified within the context of an institution's specific patient characteristics and local epidemiologic factors. The ASP can be an invaluable resource to assist transplant teams in these efforts. Time and energy should then be spent to educate, monitor implementation, assess compliance and outcomes, and update guidelines accordingly [42]. While complete adherence is not likely to occur, improved clinical outcomes have been demonstrated if guidelines are followed [54, 55].

Another important function of the ASP is to assist in the management and update of the hospital's formulary alongside the P&T committee to ensure that appropriate antimicrobial agents are available to support transplant patients [56]. One challenge that has not abated is shortages of drugs that are either first-line agents or the only drugs available to treat specific infections (e.g., foscarnet, the recommended agent for ganciclovir-intolerant patients or ganciclovir-resistant viruses; intravenous (IV) trimethoprim-sulfamethoxazole, the treatment of choice for *Pneumocystis jiroveci* and *Stenotrophomonas maltophilia* infections) [57]. The ASP can be an invaluable asset during contingency planning by working with pharmacy to assess the drug supply and usage, modify service- or hospital-wide guidelines, and communicate with healthcare providers, as described in one ASP's efforts to manage a critical pentamidine shortage [58].

The use of extended interval (EI) dosing of antibiotics for the treatment of serious Gram-negative infections, especially *P.* aeruginosa, has become a major intervention of the clinical pharmacist. The drugs most commonly considered for EI include piperacillin-tazobactam, cefepime, doripenem, and meropenem [59–61]. The use of EI is especially important for nosocomial and MDR Gram-negative infections, a major problem in transplant patients. Monte Carlo simulation models and clinical studies have suggested that EI can achieve or maintain concentrations of the antibiotic greater than the minimal inhibitory concentration of the organism [60]. Clinical outcomes suggest that use of EI can reduce mortality and length-of-stay (LOS), as well as drug use and costs when compared to conventional dosing schedules [59, 62, 63]. Implementation of an EI policy does require effort to establish and maintain adherence and does tie up intravascular access for several hours; this may complicate other IV therapies and even patient transfers for radiology or procedures [64].

A close relationship between the ASP and the microbiology laboratory is essential. The timely identification of pathogens and selective reporting of susceptibilities helps the ASP in making recommendations for appropriate therapy to clinicians [8, 65]. However, the outsourcing of infrequently ordered microbiologic tests to reference laboratories as part of cost-containment and quality-control efforts is a problematic trend [66]. Since these tests may be disproportionately requested for transplant recipients, clinical decision-making may be affected, particularly if there is a lag in receiving results. Although there is limited evidence that they can lead to improved empiric therapy, location-specific antibiograms should be considered since stratification can reveal differences in susceptibilities of pathogenic bacteria in transplant units as opposed to the rest of the hospital [67]. In addition to bacterial infections, opportunistic infections (e.g., viral, fungal) occur frequently in transplant recipients. Testing for antifungal susceptibilities of *Candida* species should be made available since azole prophylaxis is commonly used in immunocompromised patients [68]. Results of antifungal susceptibility testing can improve treatment selection (e.g., patients with fluconazole-resistant isolates) as well as assist in de-escalation (e.g., echinocandin to azole, IV-to-oral switch) [69, 70].

The role of rapid molecular testing for transplant patients has not been clearly established, but one potential advantage is the rapid return of accurate results over standard culture methods. There are many available technologies and not all will be suited to every center. Such assays include non-culture-based methods (e.g., procalcitonin (PCT),T2Candida panel) and pre-Gram stain diagnostics (e.g., direct polymerase chain reaction (PCR) from whole blood), but the most frequently used are post-Gram stain tests (e.g., real-time (RT)-PCR, broad-based nucleic acid microarrays, matrix-assisted laser desorption/ionization-time of flight mass spectrometry (MALDI-TOF MS), and peptide nucleic acid fluorescence in situ hybridization (PNA FISH)) [71–75].

PCT is a precursor of calcitonin and is a specific and sensitive marker of bacterial sepsis in non-neutropenic hosts. The results are non-specific with regard to which bacterial pathogen is the cause of infection, but an elevation above 0.5 ng/mL is indicative of sepsis and for the purposes of an ASP, no elevation is consistent with a non-bacterial process [72]. Furthermore, results can be reported back to the treating team within an hour if the test is performed at the institution. There are very few studies in neutropenic hosts. One report evaluated PCT in patients with leukemia and found that the sensitivity of PCT to detect bacteremia was 60% and specificity 82% with the cut-off value of 0.8 ng/mL [76]. Koivula et al. did serial monitoring in febrile, neutropenic patients and found that PCT had a sensitivity of 70% and specificity of 77% at 0.5 ng/mL to predict Gram-negative bacteremia after the onset of fever [77]. There are little data in transplant patients and PCT may actually be more useful for streamlining of antibiotics if results are serially negative [78].

The T2Candida Panel (T2 Biosystems), a US Food and Drug Administration (FDA)-cleared test, can detect five species of *Candida* directly from whole blood without the need for culture within 3–5 h. Mylonakis et al. performed a clinical study using the T2Candida panel with 1801 consecutive blood specimens from patients and showed that the median time-to-identification was 4 h and was 99% specific based on spiked blood bottles [79]. This technology is also being developed for rapid bacterial identification from blood.

Direct PCR from the blood for the diagnosis of bacterial and fungal septicemia is commercially available in Europe. The Septifast™ test (Roche, Basel, Switzerland) can identify 25 common bloodstream pathogens using a multiplex PCR format with a turnaround time of 4–8 h [73, 74]. This is a pre-Gram stain test that is drawn at the same time as blood cultures. The current data are mixed on its benefit in immunocompromised hosts. Results suggest that this assay cannot replace blood cultures in the workup of fever and neutropenia although it may be helpful in situations when the blood cultures are negative (e.g., during antimicrobial therapy or in IFI) [80, 81]. However, this is of limited utility for an ASP given the expense of the test and the low barrier to initiation of antimicrobial therapy in this patient population.

The use of RT-PCR in blood cultures with positive Gram stain and for the diagnosis of CDI offers a more targeted benefit for antimicrobial stewardship in both treatment and de-escalation of antibiotics [73, 82, 83]. The currently available commercial PCR tests are only approved for the diagnosis of methicillin-sensitive *S. aureus* (MSSA), MRSA, and coagulase negative staphylococci (CNS) and have a turnaround time of 2 h [73, 82]. This allows for the possibility of reducing vancomycin usage, LOS, hospital costs, and perhaps even the emergence of VRE [82]. The future development of other PCR tests in this area is critically important, especially for Gram-negative organisms and resistance genes.

The use of PCR testing for *C. difficile* has greatly enhanced the diagnosis of this serious infection in the transplant population. Not only is PCR more sensitive than the cytotoxic assay, but it can also identify the NAP1/B1/027 hypervirulent strain. It also is much faster with results attained within 2 h; this provides important information for ASP and infection control [83]. In Europe, a two-step approach is currently recommended with testing for the antigen and then performing PCR if positive or indeterminate [84, 85]. The benefits to an ASP are that it can reduce unnecessary oral vancomycin use and limit costs and emergence of VRE in the stool from its overuse [86, 87].

There are several nucleic acid microarrays that can rapidly identify organisms from blood cultures. In the US, there are two FDA-cleared platforms, the Verigene® Gram-Positive Blood Culture (BC-GP) and Gram-Negative Blood Culture (BC-GN) tests (Nanosphere, Inc., Northbrook, IL) and the FilmArray® BCID panel (bioMerieux, Durham, NC). These technologies can identify within 2 h over 20 Gram-positive and Gram-negative organisms that commonly cause bacterial sepsis, and the FilmArray® BCID panel even detects *Candida* species. The unique feature of these multi-array platforms is the detection of resistance genes such as mecA in *S. aureus* and vanA and vanB in enterococcus, as well as KPC, NDM, CTX-M, VIM, IMP, and OXA genes in Gram-negatives [75]. The impact of early identification of bacteria with their resistance genes has been demonstrated on the Verigene® platform in which a large multicenter prospective study of the BC-GN assay showed improvements in time-to-optimal therapy, antimicrobial cost-savings, and one of the first to show a survival benefit [88]. A prospective randomized controlled trial found that use of the FilmArray® assay was associated with less treatment of contaminant blood cultures, less broad-spectrum antibiotic use, and shorter time-to-appropriate antibiotic escalation and de-escalation [89].

MALDI-TOF MS (Bruker Biotyper, Billerica, MA and bioMerieux MS, bioMerieux, Inc., Durham, NC) can rapidly identify a large number of organisms including bacteria and yeast recovered from cultures of different body sites within 15–20 min [75]. By using MALDI-TOF as recommended in conjunction with an active ASP, Perez et al. demonstrated that they could reduce LOS (average of 2.6 days) and costs (average of $19,547) but were unable to show a reduction in mortality [90]. The inability to identify resistance genes within bacteria is a current limitation of MALDI-TOF MS. There are further studies ongoing to address this need.

PNA FISH (AdvanDx, Woburn, MA) utilizes a DNA mimic to target 16S ribosomal targets in bacteria and yeast. There are multiple probes currently available for staphylococci, enterococci, *Candida* species, *Klebsiella*, *Pseudomonas*, and *Escherichia coli* [71, 91]. The turnaround time after Gram stain is normally 90 min, but recently has been reduced to 30 min [91]. It identifies the selected bacteria to species level but does not detect resistance and requires the use of antibiograms to direct therapy [71]. Several studies have shown that PNA FISH can identify species faster, reduce costs, and vancomycin usage, and with enterococci, reduce mortality [92–94]. All of these studies were performed in conjunction with an active ASP to obtain the best results, as, without their interventions, there are no benefits to performing the testing [95].

Hospital infection control interfaces with the ASP by analyzing the relationship between antibiotic use and trends in bacterial resistance. Monitoring epidemiology of nonbacterial infections is also important since emergent viral and fungal resistance while less prevalent is also being recognized [96–100]. The risks and benefits of prophylaxis also need to be continually weighed, as illustrated by reports of an increased incidence of zygomycosis occurring at transplant centers possibly linked to voriconazole use [101, 102]. Finally, there is a rapidly expanding armamentarium of novel chemotherapeutic and immunomodulatory biologic agents being used in oncology, transplant, and other fields of medicine. It has also been recognized that patients receiving these medications can develop unintended and sometimes fatal infectious consequences, such as hepatitis B reactivation in rituximab recipients [103, 104], cytomegalovirus (CMV), and other opportunistic infections in HCT recipients who received alemtuzumab for lymphoproliferative disorders [105], and invasive aspergillosis in lung transplant patients on daclizumab [106]. Minimizing such infectious complications requires vigilance on the part of the ASP and clinicians caring for these patients [107].

Strategies to Improve Antimicrobial Prescribing

In general, the ASP team should understand their hospital culture in terms of prescribing practice and choose stewardship strategies that fit within the institutional framework. The 2016 IDSA/SHEA guideline for implementing an ASP advocates pre-authorization (also called prior approval) and/or prospective audit and feedback (PAF) over no such intervention [7]. These are not mutually exclusive and can be enhanced with supplemental strategies.

The first core strategy, pre-authorization, is associated with a restricted formulary. The American Society of Health-System Pharmacists (ASHP) has put forth a guideline on how hospital P&T committees can effectively evaluate whether a drug would be suitable for inclusion on the formulary [56]. A well-structured formulary reflects local susceptibilities, minimizes the number of agents available for successful therapy, and avoids duplication [56]. Furthermore, restriction of certain agents with the condition that prescribers call an ID physician or clinical pharmacist for approval has been reported to be effective in reducing inappropriate use and expenditures without detriment to patient care [108–111]. At the Hospital of the University of Pennsylvania (HUP) in Philadelphia, ASP recommendations were more likely to be in accordance with prescribing guidelines (87% vs. 47%, $P < 0.001$) and to result in clinical cure (64% vs. 42%, $P = 0.007$) compared to ID fellows [10]. The HUP findings highlight the need for scheduled time to engage thoughtfully in the approval process as well as staffing by practitioners with expertise in using antibiotics. The downsides of this approach include perceived loss of prescriber autonomy, delay in therapy (while awaiting approval), potential for manipulating the system (e.g., team presents the request to the ASP in a biased way to get approval), and influence on primarily empiric (and not definitive) therapy [7].

In PAF, patients already on empiric therapy are identified by computer-generated screening and targeted for evaluation. When an intervention is deemed necessary, the ASP team communicates with the primary service, either verbally or electronically. Examples of interventions include ensuring appropriate dosing, narrowing coverage (also called streamlining or de-escalation), modifying duration, or stopping antibiotics altogether if there is no evidence for infection. Success of this core strategy is contingent on how feedback is delivered to the prescribers, whether IT support is available, and whether prescribers demonstrate willingness to modify therapy [7].

The report by Schentag et al. was one of the earliest to show that clinical pharmacy specialists in conjunction with ID support could effectively handle streamlining and IV-to-oral conversion [112]. By linking the pharmacy and microbiology computer systems, patients could be screened for inappropriate dosing as well as for mismatches between pathogens and drugs. No adverse outcomes were noted in patients whose regimens were modified or stopped, and antibiotic expenditures declined from 31% of the total pharmacy budget to 21.5% within 1 year. Improvements in antimicrobial use with associated cost-savings have also been reported by other centers [113, 114]. Moreover, Carling et al. noted concomitant decreases in nosocomial infections due to *C. difficile* or resistant Enterobacteriaceae [114]. A significant impact can even be demonstrated at resource-limited hospitals [115].

Much of the literature on antimicrobial stewardship has been on single-center experiences. In 2012, Cosgrove et al. reported on the first multicenter trial in which PAF was implemented using a standardized approach across five academic medical centers, of which one was a Manhattan tertiary cancer center with a preexisting ASP [116]. Results showed that PAF could reduce broad-spectrum and total antimicrobial use although its efficacy seemed to be more robust at institutions that had invested resources for an ASP. The finding that antimicrobial utilization could decrease at hospitals with the most stringent restriction policies also suggests that combining pre-authorization with PAF may lead to better optimization.

Supplemental strategies include, but are not limited to, education, development of local guidelines, streamlining, and IV-to-oral conversion. Depending on the personnel and available institutional resources, an ASP can combine one or more of these with at least one core stewardship strategy to augment program activities. A full, detailed explanation of these other supplemental strategies is beyond the scope of this chapter, but can be found in other published reviews and guidelines [7, 8, 117, 118].

Briefly, education is the most basic strategy by which to influence clinicians to adopt and maintain good prescribing practices. Initiatives range from one-on-one instruction to formal didactics. Although education is the cornerstone of any ASP, its effectiveness is dependent on the motivation of the clinician to make a behavioral change [119, 120]. Without the incorporation of active intervention, education alone is marginally effective and has not demonstrated a sustained impact on prescribing practices [121–123], and thus the 2016 IDSA/SHEA guideline suggests against relying solely on education for stewardship work [7].

The development of peer-reviewed, evidence-based guidelines simplifies the process of antibiotic selection for prophylaxis or treatment but should be coupled with a plan for dissemination and implementation [7]. Examples of national guidelines that would be of relevance to a transplant center include empiric treatment for fever and neutropenia [51], prevention of opportunistic infections in HSCT recipients [52], treatment of aspergillosis [124], treatment of candidiasis [125], and surgical prophylaxis [53]. Standardized antimicrobial order forms, automatic stop orders, and computerized systems can ease the implementation of guidelines [44, 118].

Streamlining is a process that ensures that antimicrobial therapy is matched to culture and susceptibility data within 48–72 h after initiation of treatment. The objective is thus to avoid prolonged, excessively broad treatment. As seen in the management of ventilator-associated pneumonia (VAP), antimicrobial therapy may be shortened [126] or even stopped based on clinical criteria and negative culture results [127, 128]. Singh et al. also found that the rate of subsequent antibiotic-resistant infections was lower in the group receiving short-course treatment for suspected VAP compared to those receiving standard duration (15% vs. 35%, $P = 0.017$) [127]. An economic benefit has also been derived from this strategy. In one report, recommendations for streamlining occurred in 54% of antibiotic courses over 7 months, resulting in a projected annual savings of $107,637 [129]. In another report, a pharmacist-based intervention to discontinue unnecessary agents was successful in 134 (98%) of 137 episodes [130]. Potential drug cost savings and reduction in redundant antibiotic combination days were $10,800 and 584 days, respectively.

Finally, a systematic plan for IV-to-oral conversion can decrease hospital LOS and healthcare costs. The excellent oral bioavailability of several antimicrobial classes, including the fluoroquinolones, azoles, and oxazolidinones, makes this approach quite reasonable. In contrast to oral formulations, IV medications are generally more expensive and can be associated with adverse events like phlebitis and catheter-related infections. Patients also benefit since oral treatment is convenient and easy [131]. This strategy, however, is reserved for those who are hemodynamically stable, have improved clinically within 48 h of prior IV therapy, and have functioning gastrointestinal tracts. Individuals with severe immunodeficiency states or infections like meningitis and endocarditis are not candidates [131, 132]. Representative studies report a positive experience with IV-to-oral conversion in terms of clinical effectiveness and cost savings [133–137].

What Can Be Accomplished?

Effective ASPs can reduce antibiotic use, improve patient care, and be financially self-supporting in both large academic institutions and small community hospitals [10, 113–115, 138]. While much of the published literature has focused on general patient populations, established stewardship strategies, such as PAF and antimicrobial de-escalation, can be effectively performed in cancer patients [116, 139]. In addition, the disproportionate use of antifungal drugs in immunocompromised patients has led to an emerging literature on antifungal stewardship. Several institutions have successfully used a multi-pronged approach that included PAF, education, and development of local guidelines to improve antifungal prescribing [140–143]. Making available appropriate diagnostic testing for IFI, review of drug–drug interactions, and therapeutic drug monitoring for mold-active azoles are other key components for antifungal stewardship [144].

What is the current state of antimicrobial stewardship for transplant patients? In a recent survey of US medical centers performing SOT and/or HCT, the majority of respondents had an institutional ASP [9]. Yet, of the 62 ASPs, the proportion performing stewardship activities was 46 (74%) for adult SOT, 44 (71%) for adult HCT, 29 (47%) for pediatric SOT, and 31 (50%) for pediatric HCT [9]. This finding shows that there is a sizeable number of ASPs that need to think about how to incorporate transplant patients. This same study found that ASPs that did oversee anti-infective utilization in the transplant setting employed a variety of strategies, including formulary restriction, guideline development, education, antimicrobial de-escalation, and IV-to-oral conversion in combination with at least one core strategy, of which PAF had a slight edge over pre-authorization [9]. Perceived challenges to antimicrobial stewardship in transplant include undefined duration for certain infections, diagnostic uncertainty, the tendency for prescribers to want to escalate therapy, prescriber opposition, and expensive drugs [9, 145]. Another challenge is the lack of published data on stewardship effectiveness in transplant, which may be due to the lack of robust monitoring in this patient group with the exception of *C. difficile* rates and antimicrobial costs [9]. Tracking antimicrobial utilization, as well as both process and outcome metrics, has been emphasized in the 2016 IDSA/SHEA guideline [7]. Efforts examining whether antimicrobial stewardship interventions are effective in the transplant setting should thus be encouraged.

Conclusion

The emergence and spread of MDR pathogens coupled with a meager antimicrobial pipeline have led to the realization that optimization of currently available agents is an important priority. Advocacy by the ID professional societies has led to a national call that all healthcare institutions create an ASP that encompasses all patients, including transplant. Transplant recipients are very important targets for antimicrobial stewardship since they are exposed to prolonged courses of prophylactic and therapeutic anti-infectives, and because they receive multi-faceted care, multidisciplinary collaboration between an ASP and the transplant team is feasible. While it is anticipated that transplant patients can benefit, studies pertaining to stewardship efforts in the transplant setting and their measured outcomes are needed.

References

1. Spellberg B, Powers JH, Brass EP, Miller LG, Edwards JE Jr. Trends in antimicrobial drug development: implications for the future. Clin Infect Dis. 2004;38(9):1279–86.
2. Boucher HW, Talbot GH, Bradley JS, et al. Bad bugs, no drugs: no ESKAPE! An update from the Infectious Diseases Society of America. Clin Infect Dis. 2009;48(1):1–12.
3. Society for Healthcare Epidemiology of America, Infectious Diseases Society of America, Pediatric Infectious Diseases Society. Policy statement on antimicrobial stewardship by the Society for Healthcare Epidemiology of America (SHEA), the Infectious Diseases Society of America (IDSA), and the Pediatric Infectious Diseases Society (PIDS). Infect Control Hosp Epidemiol. 2012;33(4):322–7.
4. National action plan for combating antibiotic-resistant bacteria. The White House website. https://www.whitehouse.gov/the-press-office/2015/03/27/fact-sheet-obama-administration-releases-national-action-plan-combat-ant. Published 2015. Accessed 6 June 2016.
5. Abbo LM, Ariza-Heredia EJ. Antimicrobial stewardship in immunocompromised hosts. Infect Dis Clin N Am. 2014;28(2):263–79.
6. Aitken SL, Palmer HR, Topal JE, Gabardi S, Tichy E. Call for antimicrobial stewardship in solid organ transplantation. Am J Transplant. 2013;13(9):2499.
7. Barlam TF, Cosgrove SE, Abbo LM, et al. Implementing an antibiotic stewardship program: guidelines by the Infectious Diseases Society of America and the Society for Healthcare Epidemiology of America. Clin Infect Dis. 2016;62(10):e51–77.
8. Dellit TH, Owens RC, JE MG Jr, et al. Infectious Diseases Society of America and the Society for Healthcare Epidemiology of America guidelines for developing an institutional program to enhance antimicrobial stewardship. Clin Infect Dis. 2007;44(2):159–77.
9. Seo SK, Lo K, Abbo LM. Current state of antimicrobial stewardship at solid organ and hematopoietic cell transplant centers in the United States. Infect Control Hosp Epidemiol. 2016;37(10):1195–200.
10. Gross R, Morgan AS, Kinky DE, Weiner M, Gibson GA, Fishman NO. Impact of a hospital-based antimicrobial management program on clinical and economic outcomes. Clin Infect Dis. 2001;33(3):289–95.
11. Core elements of hospital antibiotic stewardship programs. The Centers for Disease Control and Prevention website. http://www.cdc.gov/getsmart/healthcare/implementation/core-elements.html. Updated 2016. Accessed 6 June 2016.
12. Kahan BD. Forty years of publication of Transplantation Proceedings--the fourth decade: globalization of the enterprise. Transplant Proc. 2011;43(1):3–29.
13. Appelbaum FR. Hematopoietic-cell transplantation at 50. N Engl J Med. 2007;357(15):1472–5.
14. Polk RE, Hohmann SF, Medvedev S, Ibrahim O. Benchmarking risk-adjusted adult antibacterial drug use in 70 US academic medical center hospitals. Clin Infect Dis. 2011;53(11):1100–10.
15. Meyer E, Schwab F, Gastmeier P, Ruden H, Heininger A. Antifungal use in intensive care units. J Antimicrob Chemother. 2007;60(3):619–24.
16. Bonadio M, Morelli G, Mori S, Riccioni R, Papineschi F, Petrini M. Fluoroquinolone resistance in hematopoietic stem cell transplant recipients with infectious complications. Biomed Pharmacother. 2005;59(9):511–6.
17. Mikulska M, Del Bono V, Raiola AM, et al. Blood stream infections in allogeneic hematopoietic stem cell transplant recipients: reemergence of Gram-negative rods and increasing antibiotic resistance. Biol Blood Marrow Transplant. 2009;15(1):47–53.
18. Therriault BL, Wilson JW, Barreto JN, Estes LL. Characterization of bacterial infections in allogeneic hematopoietic stem cell transplant recipients who received prophylactic levofloxacin with either penicillin or doxycycline. Mayo Clin Proc. 2010;85(8):711–8.
19. Morris PG, Hassan T, McNamara M, et al. Emergence of MRSA in positive blood cultures from patients with febrile neutropenia--a cause for concern. Support Care Cancer. 2008;16(9):1085–8.
20. Weinstock DM, Conlon M, Iovino C, et al. Colonization, bloodstream infection, and mortality caused by vancomycin-resistant enterococcus early after allogeneic hematopoietic stem cell transplant. Biol Blood Marrow Transplant. 2007;13(5):615–21.
21. Irfan S, Idrees F, Mehraj V, Habib F, Adil S, Hasan R. Emergence of Carbapenem resistant Gram negative and vancomycin resistant Gram positive organisms in bacteremic isolates of febrile neutropenic patients: a descriptive study. BMC Infect Dis. 2008;8:80.

22. Oliveira AL, de Souza M, Carvalho-Dias VM, et al. Epidemiology of bacteremia and factors associated with multi-drug-resistant gram-negative bacteremia in hematopoietic stem cell transplant recipients. Bone Marrow Transplant. 2007;39(12):775–81.
23. Gudiol C, Tubau F, Calatayud L, et al. Bacteraemia due to multidrug-resistant Gram-negative bacilli in cancer patients: risk factors, antibiotic therapy and outcomes. J Antimicrob Chemother. 2011;66(3):657–63.
24. Hamandi B, Holbrook AM, Humar A, et al. Delay of adequate empiric antibiotic therapy is associated with increased mortality among solid-organ transplant patients. Am J Transplant. 2009;9(7):1657–65.
25. Patel R, Allen SL, Manahan JM, et al. Natural history of vancomycin-resistant enterococcal colonization in liver and kidney transplant recipients. Liver Transpl. 2001;7(1):27–31.
26. McNeil SA, Malani PN, Chenoweth CE, et al. Vancomycin-resistant enterococcal colonization and infection in liver transplant candidates and recipients: a prospective surveillance study. Clin Infect Dis. 2006;42(2):195–203.
27. Munoz P. Multiply resistant gram-positive bacteria: vancomycin-resistant enterococcus in solid organ transplant recipients. Am J Transplant. 2009;9(Suppl 4):S50–6.
28. Green M, Barbadora K. Recovery of ceftazidime-resistant Klebsiella pneumoniae from pediatric liver and intestinal transplant recipients. Pediatr Transplant. 1998;2(3):224–30.
29. Paterson DL, Singh N, Rihs JD, Squier C, Rihs BL, Muder RR. Control of an outbreak of infection due to extended-spectrum beta-lactamase--producing Escherichia coli in a liver transplantation unit. Clin Infect Dis. 2001;33(1):126–8.
30. Rebuck JA, Olsen KM, Fey PD, Langnas AN, Rupp ME. Characterization of an outbreak due to extended-spectrum beta-lactamase-producing Klebsiella pneumoniae in a pediatric intensive care unit transplant population. Clin Infect Dis. 2000;31(6):1368–72.
31. Martins IS, Moreira BM, Riley LW, Santoro-Lopes G. Outbreak of extended-spectrum beta-lactamase-producing Klebsiella pneumoniae infection among renal transplant recipients. J Hosp Infect. 2006;64(3):305–8.
32. Zarate MS, Gales AC, Picao RC, Pujol GS, Lanza A, Smayevsky J. Outbreak of OXY-2-Producing Klebsiella oxytoca in a renal transplant unit. J Clin Microbiol. 2008;46(6):2099–101.
33. Linares L, Cervera C, Cofan F, et al. Risk factors for infection with extended-spectrum and AmpC beta-lactamase-producing gram-negative rods in renal transplantation. Am J Transplant. 2008;8(5):1000–5.
34. van Delden C, Blumberg EA. Multidrug resistant gram-negative bacteria in solid organ transplant recipients. Am J Transplant. 2009;9(Suppl 4):S27–34.
35. Botha P, Archer L, Anderson RL, et al. Pseudomonas aeruginosa colonization of the allograft after lung transplantation and the risk of bronchiolitis obliterans syndrome. Transplantation. 2008;85(5):771–4.
36. Alexander BD, Petzold EW, Reller LB, et al. Survival after lung transplantation of cystic fibrosis patients infected with Burkholderia cepacia complex. Am J Transplant. 2008;8(5):1025–30.
37. Murray S, Charbeneau J, Marshall BC, LiPuma JJ. Impact of burkholderia infection on lung transplantation in cystic fibrosis. Am J Respir Crit Care Med. 2008;178(4):363–71.
38. Ananda-Rajah MR, Slavin MA, Thursky KT. The case for antifungal stewardship. Curr Opin Infect Dis. 2012;25(1):107–15.
39. Luong ML, Hosseini-Moghaddam SM, Singer LG, et al. Risk factors for voriconazole hepatotoxicity at 12 weeks in lung transplant recipients. Am J Transplant. 2012;12(7):1929–35.
40. Luong ML, Clancy CJ, Vadnerkar A, et al. Comparison of an Aspergillus real-time polymerase chain reaction assay with galactomannan testing of bronchoalvelolar lavage fluid for the diagnosis of invasive pulmonary aspergillosis in lung transplant recipients. Clin Infect Dis. 2011;52(10):1218–26.
41. Nguyen MH, Leather H, Clancy CJ, et al. Galactomannan testing in bronchoalveolar lavage fluid facilitates the diagnosis of invasive pulmonary aspergillosis in patients with hematologic malignancies and stem cell transplant recipients. Biol Blood Marrow Transplant. 2011;17(7):1043–50.
42. Seo SK. Antimicrobial stewardship in challenging patient populations. Available at: http://www.medscape.org/viewarticle/767072. Accessed 6 June 2016.
43. Pestotnik SL, Classen DC, Evans RS, Burke JP. Implementing antibiotic practice guidelines through computer-assisted decision support: clinical and financial outcomes. Ann Intern Med. 1996;124(10):884–90.
44. Evans RS, Pestotnik SL, Classen DC, et al. A computer-assisted management program for antibiotics and other antiinfective agents. N Engl J Med. 1998;338(4):232–8.
45. Evans RS, Pestotnik SL, Classen DC, Burke JP. Evaluation of a computer-assisted antibiotic-dose monitor. Ann Pharmacother. 1999;33(10):1026–31.
46. Mullett CJ, Evans RS, Christenson JC, Dean JM. Development and impact of a computerized pediatric antiinfective decision support program. Pediatrics. 2001;108(4):E75.
47. Po JL, Nguyen BQ, Carling PC. The impact of an infectious diseases specialist-directed computerized physician order entry antimicrobial stewardship program targeting linezolid use. Infect Control Hosp Epidemiol. 2012;33(4):434–5.
48. Rodrigues JF, Casado A, Palos C, Santos C, Duarte A, Fernandez-Llimos F. A computer-assisted prescription system to improve antibacterial surgical prophylaxis. Infect Control Hosp Epidemiol. 2012;33(4):435–7.
49. Jaffe D, Jakubowski A, Sepkowitz K, et al. Prevention of peritransplantation viridans streptococcal bacteremia with early vancomycin administration: a single-center observational cohort study. Clin Infect Dis. 2004;39(11):1625–32.
50. Seo SK, Xiao K, Huang YT, et al. Impact of peri-transplant vancomycin and fluoroquinolone administration on rates of bacteremia in allogeneic hematopoietic stem cell transplant (HSCT) recipients: a 12-year single institution study. J Infect. 2014;69(4):341–51.
51. Freifeld AG, Bow EJ, Sepkowitz KA, et al. Clinical practice guideline for the use of antimicrobial agents in neutropenic patients with cancer: 2010 update by the Infectious Diseases Society of America. Clin Infect Dis. 2011;52(4):427–31.
52. Tomblyn M, Chiller T, Einsele H, et al. Guidelines for preventing infectious complications among hematopoietic cell transplantation recipients: a global perspective. Biol Blood Marrow Transplant. 2009;15(10):1143–238.
53. Bratzler DW, Dellinger EP, Olsen KM, et al. Clinical practice guidelines for antimicrobial prophylaxis in surgery. Am J Health Syst Pharm. 2013;70(3):195–283.
54. Zuckermann J, Moreira LB, Stoll P, Moreira LM, Kuchenbecker RS, Polanczyk CA. Compliance with a critical pathway for the management of febrile neutropenia and impact on clinical outcomes. Ann Hematol. 2008;87(2):139–45.
55. Pagano L, Caira M, Offidani M, et al. Adherence to international guidelines for the treatment of invasive aspergillosis in acute myeloid leukaemia: feasibility and utility (SEIFEM-2008B study). J Antimicrob Chemother. 2010;65(9):2013–8.
56. Tyler LS, Cole SW, May JR, et al. ASHP guidelines on the pharmacy and therapeutics committee and the formulary system. Am J Health Syst Pharm. 2008;65(13):1272–83.
57. Griffith MM, Gross AE, Sutton SH, et al. The impact of anti-infective drug shortages on hospitals in the United States: trends and causes. Clin Infect Dis. 2012;54(5):684–91.

58. Paskovaty A, Lucarelli CD, Patel P, et al. Antimicrobial stewardship efforts to manage a pentamidine shortage. Am J Health Syst Pharm. 2014;71(23):2014–8.
59. Lodise TP Jr, Lomaestro B, Drusano GL. Piperacillin-tazobactam for Pseudomonas aeruginosa infection: clinical implications of an extended-infusion dosing strategy. Clin Infect Dis. 2007 Feb;44(3):357–63.
60. Nicolau DP. Pharmacodynamic optimization of beta-lactams in the patient care setting. Crit Care. 2008;12(Suppl 4):S2.
61. Bulik CC, Nicolau DP. In vivo efficacy of simulated human dosing regimens of prolonged-infusion doripenem against carbapenemase- producing Klebsiella pneumoniae. Antimicrob Agents Chemother. 2010;54(10):4112–5.
62. Xamplas RC, Itokazu GS, Glowacki RC, Grasso AE, Caquelin C, Schwartz DN. Implementation of an extended-infusion piperacillin-tazobactam program at an urban teaching hospital. Am J Health Syst Pharm. 2010;67(8):622–8.
63. Yost RJ, Cappelletty DM, RECEIPT Study Group. The Retrospective Cohort of Extended-Infusion Piperacillin-Tazobactam (RECEIPT) study: a multicenter study. Pharmacotherapy. 2011;31(8):767–75.
64. Heinrich LS, Tokumaru S, Clark NM, Garofalo J, Paek JL, Grim SA. Development and implementation of a piperacillin-tazobactam extended infusion guideline. J Pharm Pract. 2011;24(6):571–6.
65. Struelens MJ. Multidisciplinary antimicrobial management teams: the way forward to control antimicrobial resistance in hospitals. Curr Opin Infect Dis. 2003;16(4):305–7.
66. Procop GW, Winn W. Outsourcing microbiology and offsite laboratories. Implications on patient care, cost savings, and graduate medical education. Arch Pathol Lab Med. 2003;127(5):623–4.
67. Binkley S, Fishman NO, LaRosa LA, et al. Comparison of unit-specific and hospital-wide antibiograms: potential implications for selection of empirical antimicrobial therapy. Infect Control Hosp Epidemiol. 2006;27(7):682–7.
68. Forrest G. Role of antifungal susceptibility testing in patient management. Curr Opin Infect Dis. 2006;19(6):538–43.
69. Shah DN, Yau R, Weston J, et al. Evaluation of antifungal therapy in patients with candidaemia based on susceptibility testing results: implications for antimicrobial stewardship programmes. J Antimicrob Chemother. 2011;66(9):2146–51.
70. Bal AM, Shankland GS, Scott G, Imtiaz T, Macaulay R, McGill M. Antifungal step-down therapy based on hospital intravenous to oral switch policy and susceptibility testing in adult patients with candidaemia: a single centre experience. Int J Clin Pract. 2014;68(1):20–7.
71. Forrest GN. PNA FISH: present and future impact on patient management. Expert Rev Mol Diagn. 2007;7(3):231–6.
72. Faix JD. Using procalcitonin to diagnose sepsis and the potential for improved antibiotic stewardship. MLO Med Lab Obs. 2008;40(11):25–6.
73. Mancini N, Carletti S, Ghidoli N, Cichero P, Burioni R, Clementi M. The era of molecular and other non-culture-based methods in diagnosis of sepsis. Clin Microbiol Rev. 2010;23(1):235–51.
74. Tsalik EL, Jones D, Nicholson B, et al. Multiplex PCR to diagnose bloodstream infections in patients admitted from the emergency department with sepsis. J Clin Microbiol. 2010;48(1):26–33.
75. Avdic E, Carroll KC. The role of the microbiology laboratory in antimicrobial stewardship programs. Infect Dis Clin N Am. 2014;28(2):215–35.
76. Gac AC, Parienti JJ, Chantepie S, et al. Dynamics of procalcitonin and bacteremia in neutropenic adults with acute myeloid leukemia. Leuk Res. 2011;35(10):1294–6.
77. Koivula I, Hamalainen S, Jantunen E, et al. Elevated procalcitonin predicts Gram-negative sepsis in haematological patients with febrile neutropenia. Scand J Infect Dis. 2011;43(6–7):471–8.
78. Koivula I, Juutilainen A. Procalcitonin is a useful marker of infection in neutropenia. Leuk Res. 2011;35(10):1288–9.
79. Mylonakis E, Clancy CJ, Ostrosky-Zeichner L, et al. T2 magnetic resonance assay for the rapid diagnosis of candidemia in whole blood: a clinical trial. Clin Infect Dis. 2015;60(6):892–9.
80. von Lilienfeld-Toal M, Lehmann LE, Raadts AD, et al. Utility of a commercially available multiplex real-time PCR assay to detect bacterial and fungal pathogens in febrile neutropenia. J Clin Microbiol. 2009;47(8):2405–10.
81. Lamoth F, Jaton K, Prod'hom G, et al. Multiplex blood PCR in combination with blood cultures for improvement of microbiological documentation of infection in febrile neutropenia. J Clin Microbiol. 2010;48(10):3510–6.
82. Bauer KA, West JE, Balada-Llasat JM, Pancholi P, Stevenson KB, Goff DA. An antimicrobial stewardship program's impact with rapid polymerase chain reaction methicillin-resistant Staphylococcus aureus/S. aureus blood culture test in patients with S. aureus bacteremia. Clin Infect Dis. 2010;51(9):1074–80.
83. O'Horo JC, Jones A, Sternke M, Harper C, Safdar N. Molecular techniques for diagnosis of Clostridium difficile infection: systematic review and meta-analysis. Mayo Clin Proc. 2012;87(7):643–51.
84. Crobach MJ, Dekkers OM, Wilcox MH, Kuijper EJ. European Society of Clinical Microbiology and Infectious Diseases (ESCMID): data review and recommendations for diagnosing Clostridium difficile-infection (CDI). Clin Microbiol Infect. 2009;15(12):1053–66.
85. Knetsch CW, Bakker D, de Boer RF, et al. Comparison of real-time PCR techniques to cytotoxigenic culture methods for diagnosing Clostridium difficile infection. J Clin Microbiol. 2011;49(1):227–31.
86. Dubberke ER, Wertheimer AI. Review of current literature on the economic burden of Clostridium difficile infection. Infect Control Hosp Epidemiol. 2009;30(1):57–66.
87. Nerandzic MM, Mullane K, Miller MA, Babakhani F, Donskey CJ. Reduced acquisition and overgrowth of vancomycin-resistant enterococci and Candida species in patients treated with fidaxomicin versus vancomycin for Clostridium difficile infection. Clin Infect Dis. 2012;55(Suppl 2):S121–6.
88. Suzuki H, Hitomi S, Yaguchi Y, et al. Prospective intervention study with a microarray-based, multiplexed, automated molecular diagnosis instrument (Verigene system) for the rapid diagnosis of bloodstream infections, and its impact on the clinical outcomes. J Infect Chemother. 2015;21(12):849–56.
89. Banerjee R, Teng CB, Cunningham SA, et al. Randomized trial of rapid multiplex polymerase chain reaction-based blood culture identification and susceptibility testing. Clin Infect Dis. 2015;61(7):1071–80.
90. Perez KK, Olsen RJ, Musick WL, et al. Integrating rapid pathogen identification and antimicrobial stewardship significantly decreases hospital costs. Arch Pathol Lab Med. 2013;137(9):1247–54.
91. Deck MK, Anderson ES. Buckner RJ,et al. Multicenter evaluation of the Staphylococcus QuickFISH method for simultaneous identification of Staphylococcus aureus and coagulase-negative staphylococci directly from blood culture bottles in less than 30 minutes. J Clin Microbiol. 2012;50(6):1994–8.
92. Forrest GN, Mehta S, Weekes E, Lincalis DP, Johnson JK, Venezia RA. Impact of rapid in situ hybridization testing on coagulase-negative staphylococci positive blood cultures. J Antimicrob Chemother. 2006;58(1):154–8.
93. Forrest GN, Mankes K, Jabra-Rizk MA, et al. Peptide nucleic acid fluorescence in situ hybridization-based identification of Candida albicans and its impact on mortality and antifungal therapy costs. J Clin Microbiol. 2006;44(9):3381–3.
94. Forrest GN, Roghmann MC, Toombs LS, et al. Peptide nucleic acid fluorescent in situ hybridization for hospital-acquired entero-

coccal bacteremia: delivering earlier effective antimicrobial therapy. Antimicrob Agents Chemother. 2008;52(10):3558–63.
95. Holtzman C, Whitney D, Barlam T, Miller NS. Assessment of impact of peptide nucleic acid fluorescence in situ hybridization for rapid identification of coagulase-negative staphylococci in the absence of antimicrobial stewardship intervention. J Clin Microbiol. 2011;49(4):1581–2.
96. Frobert E, Burrel S, Ducastelle-Lepretre S, et al. Resistance of herpes simplex viruses to acyclovir: an update from a ten-year survey in France. Antivir Res. 2014;111:36–41.
97. Tramontana AR, George B, Hurt AC, et al. Oseltamivir resistance in adult oncology and hematology patients infected with pandemic (H1N1) 2009 virus, Australia. Emerg Infect Dis. 2010;16(7):1068–75.
98. Chou S. Approach to drug-resistant cytomegalovirus in transplant recipients. Curr Opin Infect Dis. 2015;28(4):293–9.
99. Pfaller MA. Antifungal drug resistance: mechanisms, epidemiology, and consequences for treatment. Am J Med. 2012;125(1 Suppl):S3–13.
100. van der Linden JW, Arendrup MC, Melchers WJ, Verweij PE. Azole resistance of Aspergillus fumigatus in immunocompromised patients with invasive aspergillosis. Emerg Infect Dis. 2016;22(1):158–9.
101. Marty FM, Cosimi LA, Baden LR. Breakthrough zygomycosis after voriconazole treatment in recipients of hematopoietic stem-cell transplants. N Engl J Med. 2004;350(9):950–2.
102. Pongas GN, Lewis RE, Samonis G, Kontoyiannis DP. Voriconazole-associated zygomycosis: a significant consequence of evolving antifungal prophylaxis and immunosuppression practices? Clin Microbiol Infect. 2009;15(Suppl 5):93–7.
103. Dervite I, Hober D, Morel P. Acute hepatitis B in a patient with antibodies to hepatitis B surface antigen who was receiving rituximab. N Engl J Med. 2001;344(1):68–9.
104. Tsutsumi Y, Tanaka J, Kawamura T, et al. Possible efficacy of lamivudine treatment to prevent hepatitis B virus reactivation due to rituximab therapy in a patient with non-Hodgkin's lymphoma. Ann Hematol. 2004;83(1):58–60.
105. Martin SI, Marty FM, Fiumara K, Treon SP, Gribben JG, Baden LR. Infectious complications associated with alemtuzumab use for lymphoproliferative disorders. Clin Infect Dis. 2006;43(1):16–24.
106. Iversen M, Burton CM, Vand S, et al. Aspergillus infection in lung transplant patients: incidence and prognosis. Eur J Clin Microbiol Infect Dis. 2007;26(12):879–86.
107. Koo S, Marty FM, Baden LR. Infectious complications associated with immunomodulating biologic agents. Infect Dis Clin N Am. 2010;24(2):285–306.
108. Woodward RS, Medoff G, Smith MD, Gray JL 3rd. Antibiotic cost savings from formulary restrictions and physician monitoring in a medical-school-affiliated hospital. Am J Med. 1987;83(5):817–23.
109. Coleman RW, Rodondi LC, Kaubisch S, Granzella NB, O'Hanley PD. Cost-effectiveness of prospective and continuous parenteral antibiotic control: experience at the Palo Alto Veterans Affairs Medical Center from 1987 to 1989. Am J Med. 1991;90(4):439–44.
110. Maswoswe JJ, Okpara AU. Enforcing a policy for restricting antimicrobial drug use. Am J Health Syst Pharm. 1995;52(13):1433–5.
111. White AC Jr, Atmar RL, Wilson J, Cate TR, Stager CE, Greenberg SB. Effects of requiring prior authorization for selected antimicrobials: expenditures, susceptibilities, and clinical outcomes. Clin Infect Dis. 1997;25(2):230–9.
112. Schentag JJ, Ballow CH, Fritz AL, et al. Changes in antimicrobial agent usage resulting from interactions among clinical pharmacy, the infectious disease division, and the microbiology laboratory. Diagn Microbiol Infect Dis. 1993;16(3):255–64.
113. Fraser GL, Stogsdill P, Dickens JD Jr, Wennberg DE, Smith RP Jr, Prato BS. Antibiotic optimization. An evaluation of patient safety and economic outcomes. Arch Intern Med. 1997;157(15):1689–94.
114. Carling P, Fung T, Killion A, Terrin N, Barza M. Favorable impact of a multidisciplinary antibiotic management program conducted during 7 years. Infect Control Hosp Epidemiol. 2003;24(9):699–706.
115. LaRocco A Jr. Concurrent antibiotic review programs--a role for infectious diseases specialists at small community hospitals. Clin Infect Dis. 2003;37(5):742–3.
116. Cosgrove SE, Seo SK, Bolon MK, et al. Evaluation of postprescription review and feedback as a method of promoting rational antimicrobial use: a multicenter intervention. Infect Control Hosp Epidemiol. 2012;33(4):374–80.
117. Paskovaty A, Pflomm JM, Myke N, Seo SK. A multidisciplinary approach to antimicrobial stewardship: evolution into the 21st century. Int J Antimicrob Agents. 2005;25(1):1–10.
118. Bearden DT, Allen GP. Impact of antimicrobial control programs on patient outcomes. Pharmacy perspective. Dis Manag Health Out. 2003;11(11):723–36.
119. Grimshaw JM, Shirran L, Thomas R, et al. Changing provider behavior: an overview of systematic reviews of interventions. Med Care. 2001;39(8 Suppl 2):II2–45.
120. Gray J. Changing physician prescribing behaviour. Can J Clin Pharmacol. 2006;13(1):e81–4.
121. Girotti MJ, Fodoruk S, Irvine-Meek J, Rotstein OD. Antibiotic handbook and pre-printed perioperative order forms for surgical antibiotic prophylaxis: do they work? Can J Surg. 1990;33(5):385–8.
122. Bantar C, Sartori B, Vesco E, et al. A hospitalwide intervention program to optimize the quality of antibiotic use: impact on prescribing practice, antibiotic consumption, cost savings, and bacterial resistance. Clin Infect Dis. 2003;37(2):180–6.
123. Belongia EA, Knobloch MJ, Kieke BA, Davis JP, Janette C, Besser RE. Impact of statewide program to promote appropriate antimicrobial drug use. Emerg Infect Dis. 2005 Jun;11(6):912–20.
124. Patterson TF, Thompson GR 3rd, Denning DW, et al. Practice guidelines for the diagnosis and management of aspergillosis: 2016 update by the Infectious Diseases Society of America. Clin Infect Dis. 2016;63(4):e1–e60.
125. Pappas PG, Kauffman CA, Andes DR, et al. Clinical practice guideline for the management of candidiasis: 2016 update by the Infectious Diseases Society of America. Clin Infect Dis. 2016;62(4):e1–50.
126. Chastre J, Wolff M, Fagon JY, et al. Comparison of 8 vs 15 days of antibiotic therapy for ventilator-associated pneumonia in adults: a randomized trial. JAMA. 2003;290(19):2588–98.
127. Singh N, Rogers P, Atwood CW, Wagener MM, Yu VL. Short-course empiric antibiotic therapy for patients with pulmonary infiltrates in the intensive care unit. A proposed solution for indiscriminate antibiotic prescription. Am J Respir Crit Care Med. 2000;162(2. Pt 1):505–11.
128. Kollef MH, Kollef KE. Antibiotic utilization and outcomes for patients with clinically suspected ventilator-associated pneumonia and negative quantitative BAL culture results. Chest. 2005;128(4):2706–13.
129. Briceland LL, Nightingale CH, Quintiliani R, Cooper BW, Smith KS. Antibiotic streamlining from combination therapy to monotherapy utilizing an interdisciplinary approach. Arch Intern Med. 1988;148(9):2019–22.
130. Glowacki RC, Schwartz DN, Itokazu GS, Wisniewski MF, Kieszkowski P, Weinstein RA. Antibiotic combinations with redundant antimicrobial spectra: clinical epidemiology and pilot intervention of computer-assisted surveillance. Clin Infect Dis. 2003;37(1):59–64.
131. Lelekis M, Gould IM. Sequential antibiotic therapy for cost containment in the hospital setting: why not? J Hosp Infect. 2001;48(4):249–57.

132. Drew RH. Programs promoting timely sequential antimicrobial therapy: an American perspective. J Infect. 1998;37(Suppl 1):3–9.
133. Amodio-Groton M, Madu A, Madu CN, et al. Sequential parenteral and oral ciprofloxacin regimen versus parenteral therapy for bacteremia: a pharmacoeconomic analysis. Ann Pharmacother. 1996;30(6):596–602.
134. Sevinc F, Prins JM, Koopmans RP, et al. Early switch from intravenous to oral antibiotics: guidelines and implementation in a large teaching hospital. J Antimicrob Chemother. 1999;43(4):601–6.
135. Ramirez JA, Bordon J. Early switch from intravenous to oral antibiotics in hospitalized patients with bacteremic community-acquired Streptococcus pneumoniae pneumonia. Arch Intern Med. 2001;161(6):848–50.
136. Wong-Beringer A, Nguyen KH, Razeghi J. Implementing a program for switching from i.v. to oral antimicrobial therapy. Am J Health Syst Pharm. 2001;58(12):1146–9.
137. Jones M, Huttner B, Madaras-Kelly K, et al. Parenteral to oral conversion of fluoroquinolones: low-hanging fruit for antimicrobial stewardship programs? Infect Control Hosp Epidemiol. 2012;33(4):362–7.
138. Lutters M, Harbarth S, Janssens JP, et al. Effect of a comprehensive, multidisciplinary, educational program on the use of antibiotics in a geriatric university hospital. J Am Geriatr Soc. 2004;52(1):112–6.
139. Paskovaty A, Pastores SM, Gedrimaite Z, Kostelecky N, Riedel ER, Seo SK. Antimicrobial de-escalation in septic cancer patients: is it safe to back down? Intensive Care Med. 2015;41(11):2022–3.
140. Standiford HC, Chan S, Tripoli M, Weekes E, Forrest GN. Antimicrobial stewardship at a large tertiary care academic medical center: cost analysis before, during, and after a 7-year program. Infect Control Hosp Epidemiol. 2012;33(4):338–45.
141. Lopez-Medrano F, San Juan R, Lizasoain M, et al. A non-compulsory stewardship programme for the management of antifungals in a university-affiliated hospital. Clin Microbiol Infect. 2013;19(1):56–61.
142. Mondain V, Lieutier F, Hasseine L, et al. A 6-year antifungal stewardship programme in a teaching hospital. Infection. 2013;41(3):621–8.
143. Micallef C, Aliyu SH, Santos R, Brown NM, Rosembert D, Enoch DA. Introduction of an antifungal stewardship programme targeting high-cost antifungals at a tertiary hospital in Cambridge, England. J Antimicrob Chemother. 2015;70(6):1908–11.
144. Hamdy RF, Zaoutis TE, Seo SK. Antifungal stewardship considerations for adults and pediatrics. Virulence. 2017;8(6):658–72.
145. Wolf J, Sun Y, Tang L, et al. Antimicrobial stewardship barriers and goals in pediatric oncology and bone marrow transplantation: a survey of antimicrobial stewardship practitioners. Infect Control Hosp Epidemiol. 2016;37(3):343–7.

60 The Use of Palliative Care in Organ Transplant Patients and End-of-Life Issues

Jenny S. Ayala and Joseph Lowy

Introduction

Patients suffering from organ failure experience a reduction in quality of life with a burden of symptoms which are physical, psychosocial, and spiritual. Since the first solid organ transplant in the 1950s, great advances have been made in the field. Organ transplantation can be life-saving but the surgery and postoperative medications have their own complications. More patients are being considered for transplantation but the demand far outstrips the supply and many organ transplant candidates may become too sick to transplant or die waiting.

The transplant team consists of transplant coordinators, physicians, nurses, social workers, psychologists, and financial coordinators. It is rare for a palliative care provider to be involved until the patient is near terminal. Palliative care has been shown to improve quality of life and even prolong life in patients with certain types of malignancy. The provision of palliative care has consistently shown a reduction in cost of care and improved patient satisfaction. Several studies have now demonstrated a beneficial impact of palliative care on the transplant patient.

Dame Cicely Saunders first introduced the concept of caring for the terminally ill in London back in the mid-1950s. This became known as hospice care, and by the 1970s, the state of Connecticut founded its first hospice facility in Branford. While hospice provides care for patients whose survival is expected to be less than 6 months, palliative care is specialized care for the patient with serious illness and can be provided at any stage of the disease. All transplant candidates, by definition, qualify. Like transplant medicine, palliative care is also interdisciplinary. It is person/family centered and provides support along with aggressive symptom management. Patients are screened for pain and other physical symptoms as well as for psychosocial and spiritual distress. Palliative care also fosters communication between the patient/family and health-care providers. The patient's values and principles are elicited so that concordant medical care is provided. Implementing palliative care (sometimes referred to as supportive care) early in the disease trajectory has helped transition patients into hospice care once curative options have been exhausted.

This chapter will elucidate why patients with organ failure who are candidates for transplantation or patients suffering from complications of transplantation are excellent candidates for palliative care and why a palliative care provider should be part of the transplant interdisciplinary team.

Organ Transplantation: The Facts

The field of solid organ transplantation has soared to great heights since the first kidney was transplanted back in 1954. The successful transplantation of kidney, heart, lung, liver, pancreas, and small intestine is now routine. However, the success of organ transplantation has caused a demand and supply mismatch. The number of patients waiting for an organ far exceeds the number of deceased and living donors available. As of November 2017, there were over 116,000 people in need of a life-saving organ transplant [1]. Candidates include all ethnicities and ages, as young as <1 year old to older than 65 years old [1]. Survival rates vary depending on the organ transplanted and whether the organ was from a deceased or a living donor as seen with kidney and liver transplants. Lung transplants have the lowest rate of patient survival [1] (Fig. 60.1) due to primary graft failure and infections [2].

Transplant candidacy depends on organ, extent of the disease, risk of mortality, response to treatment, and individual factors. Patients who are referred for organ transplant have to undergo an extensive evaluation by the transplant team composed of clinical transplant coordinators, transplant physicians, financial coordi-

J. S. Ayala
Hospice and Palliative Medicine, Jacobi Medical Center, Bronx, NY, USA

J. Lowy (✉)
Palliative Care, NYU Langone Health, New York, NY, USA
e-mail: joseph.lowy@nyumc.org

A. Safdar (ed.), *Principles and Practice of Transplant Infectious Diseases*, https://doi.org/10.1007/978-1-4939-9034-4_60

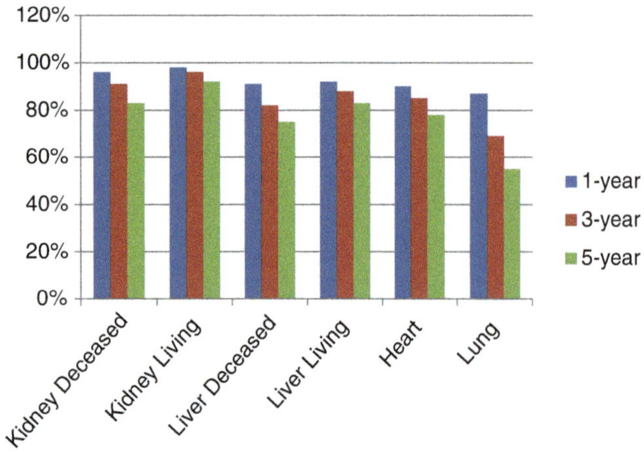

Fig. 60.1 Survival rates for organ recipients between years 2008 and 2015 [1]

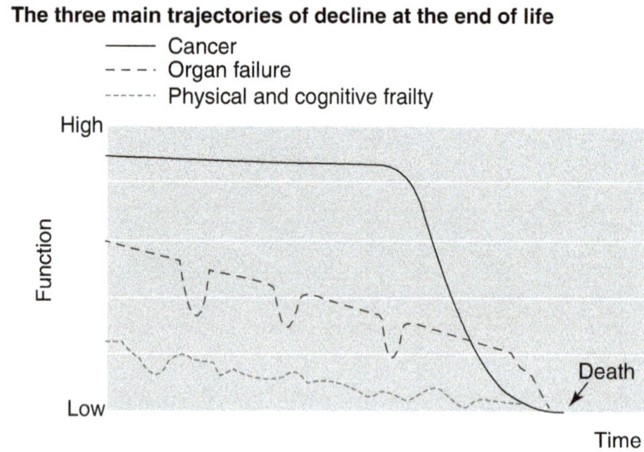

Fig. 60.2 Three main trajectories of decline at end of life [8]. Reprinted with permission from Palliative care in heart failure: a position statement from the palliative care workshop of the Heart Failure Association of the European Society of Cardiology, Jaarsma et al. [8], © 2009, with permission from John Wiley and Sons

nators, and social workers. Waiting time for organs can be days to months to years and is based on the level of urgency and organ availability. Different organ allocation systems have been established that take into account the level of acuity of disease and mortality rate if not transplanted [1, 2]. Kidney and pancreas transplants are exceptions as their allocation system is solely based on genetic compatibility and waiting time.

Organ Transplantation and the Role of Palliative Care

Patients diagnosed with end-stage organ failure may feel similarly to patients with terminal cancer. The symptom burden that patients live with greatly affects their quality of life as well as their families and the people around them. Studies have shown that implementation of early palliative care alongside cancer treatment improves quality of life and mood [3, 4]. These improvements are the result of having a team that specializes in delineating realistic goals of care, symptom control, quality of life, and emotional well-being, while acting as a bridge of communication between patients, family, and medical doctors without altering appropriate treatment plans [5]. Prognosis of patients with cancer is related to their performance status based on the Karnofsky Performance Status (KPS) [6] and Palliative Performance Scale (PPS) [7], which measure the physical function and ability to self-care. See Appendix for full description.

Patients with end-stage organ failure have a more unpredictable disease trajectory marked by periods of symptom exacerbation and disease progression [8] (Fig. 60.2).

Several studies suggest benefit from the integration of palliative care in end-stage heart, lung, liver, and kidney failure [9–12]. Palliative care integration has become part of the guidelines for treatment of end-stage heart and lung failure, as it has shown to improve patients' quality of life and clarify end-of-life wishes and goals [9, 10].

Physicians should understand that the goal of palliative care is to minimize suffering from physical and emotional symptom burden for all patients going through a life-threatening illness, regardless of their diagnosis and should not be considered exclusively as an alternative to curative plans, limited to end-of-life care, or only for non-transplant candidates. Patients living with life-threatening illnesses have identified five domains that they consider important when discussing quality of life [13]:

- *Adequate pain and symptom management*
- *Avoidance of inappropriate prolongation of dying*
- *Achievement of a sense of control*
- *Relief of the burden of their disease on others*
- *Strengthening of relationships with loved ones*

Therefore, it is essential to provide patients living with end-stage organ failure a sense that they are not alone, that we will continue to care for them whether or not they are transplant candidates ("non-abandonment"), and that we will strive to understand their concerns and help them achieve realistic goals.

> The good physician treats the disease; the great physician treats the patient who has the disease. (William Osler)

Understanding the Difference Between Palliative Care and Hospice Care

It is important to differentiate between palliative care and hospice care in order to provide the patient with the right service at the right time. Patients, families, and health-care providers may have the misconception that palliative care equals hospice care, signifying the care of the terminally ill. As stated previously, palliative care may be introduced early in the disease trajectory and alongside curative treatments. However, this is not the same for hospice care. Both specialties embrace the principles of lessening symptom burden and improving quality of life, but hospice focuses specifically on end-of-life care goals and needs of the patient and family. The family of a dying patient may feel significant stress and anxiety. Hospice social workers and pastoral care provide support and counseling to the patient and to the family before and after the death of a loved one. Hospice nurses and physicians provide symptom control and assist with decision-making when patients are home or in an institutionalized setting [14]. If palliative care is implemented early in the disease process and all curative alternatives have been exhausted (e.g., transplantation), but the disease has continued to progress, patients may easily be transitioned into hospice care. While all patients with advanced disease can receive palliative care, not all patients can receive hospice care. There are specific criteria set forth by Medicare and private insurers that must be met in order to qualify for coverage. These include the following: (1) disease is far advanced and alternatives for curative treatment have been exhausted; (2) based on the disease progression, patient has a prognosis of less than 6 months if the disease is allowed to take its natural course; and (3) patient agrees to forgo any further curative therapies and focus on comfort measures only [15]. Hospice care may be provided in multiple settings, such as home, nursing home, hospice inpatient unit, or hospital. Studies have shown that patients, as well as families, prefer home hospice to dying in institutionalized settings; they feel that the needs of the patient are better met at home with hospice care services and family support [14, 16]. It is very important that physicians are aware of the distinction between palliative care and hospice so that patients and their families may receive the appropriate level of treatment and care to which they are entitled.

Hospice care provides palliative care, but all palliative care is not hospice care. (Ministry Health Care)

Review of End-Stage Organ Failure Diseases and the Role of Palliative Care

End-Stage Heart Failure

Cardiovascular disease remains the number one killer in patients older than 65 years, accounting for 27% of total deaths in the USA [17]. Among cardiovascular diseases, heart failure has a high mortality and morbidity risk, and the number of people affected by the disease continues to increase. Latest data shows over 6.5 million Americans are living with heart failure [18]. The New York Heart Association and American College of Cardiology/American Heart Association have classified heart failure into four stages based on symptom severity. The most advanced stage, IV/D, includes patients who are symptomatic at rest living with ~50% 1-year survival rate. Patients at this stage are considered to have end-stage organ failure and require more specialized and, often, invasive treatments in order to prolong survival and improve quality of life. Treatments available for this stage include intravenous inotrope infusion, mechanical circulatory support devices, such as the left ventricular assist device (LVAD), and, ultimately, cardiac transplantation, if feasible [19]. Patients living with stage IV HF have a very poor quality of life due to overwhelming symptoms of fatigue, shortness of breath, depression, and pain [20–22]. A model used to predict survival in heart failure patients using clinical and laboratory data is the Seattle Heart Failure model. It predicts the 1-, 2-, and 3-year survival and can be individualized to each patient by adding the use of devices or certain heart failure medications [23]. It has also proven to be helpful in combination with the Heart Failure Survival Score when referring patients for transplantation [24].

When the disease reaches a point when it is refractory to any type of treatment other than LVAD or cardiac transplantation and the patient is not a candidate for these measures or refuses, the disease will take its course, inevitably ending in death. Currently, there are over 3000 patients on the waiting list for a heart with the average waiting time being 1–2 years [1]. Ten percent of the patients die while waiting and 12% are removed from the list because the patient becomes too sick to transplant [1]. Because of the symptom burden, quality of life issues, and high mortality rate of advanced heart failure, the ACC/AHA have modified their guidelines to include palliative and hospice care as a Class I Recommendation. The goal is to educate the patient and family regarding the services that can be offered by palliative and hospice care to assist in alleviating symptom burden, discussing prognosis, decision-making including setting realistic goals, and, when necessary, end-of-life care [25]. Schwarz et al. studied patients referred for cardiac transplantation who were evaluated by a palliative care team. This intervention resulted in better symptom management with less use of pain medications. Goals of care, advance care planning, and end-of-life goals were discussed actively, and patients' spiritual and psychosocial needs were met either by referral to chaplaincy, psychiatry or through the use of pharmacology [26].

End-Stage Pulmonary Disease

Respiratory insufficiency may be defined as the inability to maintain adequate gas exchange and is classified according to the Global Initiative for Chronic Obstructive Lung Disease. Severity of disease is based on spirometry assessment post bronchodilator, and patients with a FEV1 (Forced Expiratory Volume in 1 s) <30% are considered to have very severe disease causing significant impairment in the daily life [27].

Chronic lower respiratory disease is the third leading cause of death in the USA [17]. End-stage lung failure, seen in patients with class 4, can be seen in multiple pulmonary conditions, but the most common is chronic obstructive pulmonary disease (COPD). About 15 million Americans suffer from COPD and over 11,000 people die annually [17]. Patients suffering from COPD are classified based on the decline of the FEV1 using the GOLD criteria. Those with GOLD IV have an FEV1/FVC < 0.70 and FEV1 < 30% predicted [28] and tend to suffer greater number of exacerbations as compared to lower stages [29]. It has also been shown that patients who suffer repeated COPD exacerbations, especially those who require hospitalization, have a more rapid decline in lung function and higher mortality risk [30–33]. In addition, their post exacerbation quality of life changes for the worse as they become more dependent on others and require more medical interventions [32]. Patients living with severe COPD suffer from a number of symptoms, such as dyspnea, fatigue, pain, cough, weight loss, depression, and decreased functional status. When compared to lung cancer patients, patients with COPD receive significantly less treatment for these symptoms [34]. This difference in intervention is especially evident for dyspnea and pain, symptoms that respond to the use of opioids. Unfortunately, there are many barriers to the utilization of these medications, including the misconception of hastening death [35].

Palliative care has been shown to have significant impact on quality of life in patients with end-stage COPD, shown in a study of home-base palliative care, where the main goal was symptom management and pain relief. Through these interventions, patients had improved quality of life and fewer emergency room visits and hospitalizations [36]. The American Thoracic Society now promotes and recommends the integration of this service as part of the management of any chronic pulmonary disease, especially COPD [37]. Patients whose disease has become refractory to treatment may be candidates for lung transplant. In the last year, about 2,000 lung transplants were performed in the USA, and the number of patients waiting for a transplant continues to exceed the number of donor lungs available [1]. Currently, there are about 1400 patients on the waiting list, and as the number of patients continues to increase so does the number of patients being removed due to death of the patient (10%) or because the patient becomes too sick to transplant (12%) [1]. Although lung transplantation provides resolution of symptoms with improved quality of life, survival rates remain a limitation, averaging only a 54% 5-year survival rate which is significantly lower than the rates for heart, liver, and kidney transplantation [1] (Fig. 60.1). Physicians caring for end-stage COPD patients should make an effort to educate patients about their disease process, symptoms, treatment option, prognosis, and end-of-life goals. This will lead to proper symptom management and appropriate referral to palliative care and hospice for medical, emotional, and psychosocial needs.

End-Stage Liver Disease

Cirrhosis is the common final pathway in chronic liver disease (CLD). The liver is known to be one of the only organs with the ability to regenerate itself after acute injury. However, when cirrhosis has taken place, regeneration is no longer possible and the damage becomes permanent leading to End-Stage Liver Disease (ESLD). CLD and cirrhosis rank as the 12th leading cause of death in the USA and kills over 30,000 patients annually [17]. There are multiple causes for ESLD including hepatitis, drug toxicity, and genetic errors, but chronic alcohol use is responsible for approximately 50% of cases [17]. Patients diagnosed with ESLD have no available curative options other than liver transplant. Treatment is focused on managing the complications rather than reversing the disease process. While there are patients with "compensated cirrhosis" who live for many years and are asymptomatic, many patients with "decompensated cirrhosis" are consumed by the many complications that arise from this condition such as ascites, hepatic encephalopathy, spontaneous bacterial peritonitis, esophageal variceal bleeding, and hepato-renal syndrome. Patients presenting with decompensated cirrhosis require hospitalization. Despite treatment, a patient's 1-year mortality risk increases to about 20% [38]. Hepatorenal syndrome (HRS) is the most severe complication of ESLD and is associated with a 2-week mortality risk of 80% in patients presenting with Type I [39], defined as the rapid deterioration of renal function in less than 2 weeks, with the serum creatinine doubling by >2.5 mg/dL or a 50% reduction in the 24-h creatinine clearance to <20 mL/min [40]. Common causes include systemic bacterial infections, paracentesis with significant volume loss, or bleeding. Type II also occurs in ESLD but its progression is much slower [40]. ESLD like other end organ failure conditions, have a very unpredictable disease trajectory, marked by periods of decompensation and return to baseline. For this reason, integrating palliative care early in the disease process is beneficial even if the patient is referred for transplantation. Patients referred for liver transplant have to deal with the stress and uncertainty of whether and when they would receive an organ. Currently, over 13,500 patients are on the waiting list, and 10,000 patients are removed from the list annually, most commonly for death and for being "too sick" to transplant [1]. Because the number of candidates far exceeds the available donor organs, an allocation system was developed to prioritize those patients who are acutely ill and have a high mortality risk based on the MELD score. This model uses laboratory values of serum bilirubin and creatinine and international normalized ratio (INR) to predict a 3-month mortality in patients with ESLD; the higher the MELD score, the higher the mortality risk present [41].

In a study, Lamba et al. incorporated a palliative care approach into the care of liver transplant patients in the ICU and showed an increase in discussion of goals of care, resuscitation preferences, improved symptom management, and better communication with the family and among the physicians involved in the patient's care [42]. Patients with ESLD suffer from multiple physical, emotional, and psychological issues that have a profound negative impact on quality of life [43–45]. Among these are fatigue, insomnia, lethargy, and depression. The latter is associated with higher mortality rates among patients with cirrhosis awaiting a transplant [45]. For this reason, and the ones mentioned before, we must continue to work hard to integrate services that will help patients living with ESLD improve their quality of life by focusing on every aspect of the disease and its impact on the patient.

End-Stage Kidney Failure

There are 3.9 million patients living with kidney disease today, and annually more than 48,000 patients die from this condition making it the ninth leading cause of death in the USA [17]. Chronic kidney disease (CKD) is classified into five different stages. Stage 5 ESRD is defined as having a GFR <15 mL/min/1.73 m^2 [46]. There are multiple causes of CKD, but the most common are diabetes, hypertension, polycystic kidney disease, and irreversible drug-induced kidney injury. Like many other end organ failure conditions, the treatment options are limited. When a patient reaches end stage of the disease, the only treatments available are maintenance dialysis or kidney transplantation. For this reason, the Kidney Disease Outcomes Quality Initiative (KDOQI) [46] recommends that patients with a GFR <30 mL/min/1.73 m^2 should be educated about disease progression so that they and their families understand the options and avoid having to make decisions when the patient becomes cognitively impaired by uremic encephalopathy. Depending on quality of life and goals of care, the choices would include permanent access for dialysis, "preemptive kidney transplantation" (kidney transplantation prior to starting dialysis) or hospice.

Patients who are started on maintenance dialysis have been found to have a greater decline in their physical, mental, emotional, and social functioning as well as an annual 25% mortality risk compared to those who are not started on dialysis [47, 48]. Dialysis patients also experience a profound symptom burden, the most common being fatigue, pruritus, insomnia, depression, and pain [49–52]. Depression impacts quality of life and is associated with increased mortality risk among maintenance dialysis patients [53]. Other complications of renal failure, such as anemia, low albumin, poor nutritional status, and worsening co-morbidities, also negatively impact quality of life in dialysis patients [54–56]. Over 16,000 transplants are done annually. As is the case for other organs, the number of candidates exceeds the number of available kidneys suitable for transplant [1]. The median waiting time is between 2 and 4 years depending on the blood type and HLA typing [1]. Over 25,000 patients are removed from the waiting list annually for death of the patient (16%) or for the patient being too sick to transplant (8%) [1]. Preemptive kidney transplantation leads to a 25% reduction in graft failure and a 26% reduction in patient mortality as compared to patients who have been on maintenance dialysis before referral [57]. Patients undergoing kidney transplantation before the initiation of dialysis, a term referred as pre-emptive transplantation, has shown improvement in functional status and improved quality of life compared to those who are started on dialysis and undergo transplantation after [58]. Given the high symptom burden and quality of life issues in ESRD, nephrologists and palliative care specialists must work together to address patient and family needs and concerns so that medical decisions and treatments can be implemented appropriately.

Bone Marrow Transplantation

Hematopoietic stem cell transplantation was pioneered by E. Donall Thomas in 1957. Since then, its use has evolved beyond treatment for acute leukemia and aplastic anemia to include many other hematopoietic diseases and the number of transplants performed annually has continued to increase in number (Figs. 60.3 and 60.4) [59].

Transplantation may be autologous or allogenic (related and unrelated donors) and donor stem cells may be derived from bone marrow, umbilical cord, or peripheral blood. Nonmalignant and malignant blood disorders can qualify patients for transplantation (Figs. 60.3 and 60.4) [59]. Indications for transplantation in malignant blood disorders include failure of chemoradiation therapy and multiple relapses. Referral guidelines can be obtained at http://www.asbmt.org [60]. Patients who undergo bone marrow transplant (BMT) are prone to multiple complications. Before undergoing BMT, patients are given chemotherapy along with total body irradiation in order to destroy the residual marrow cells and allow for the transplant to "engraft". Post-transplant patients remain in the hospital for weeks to months to recover

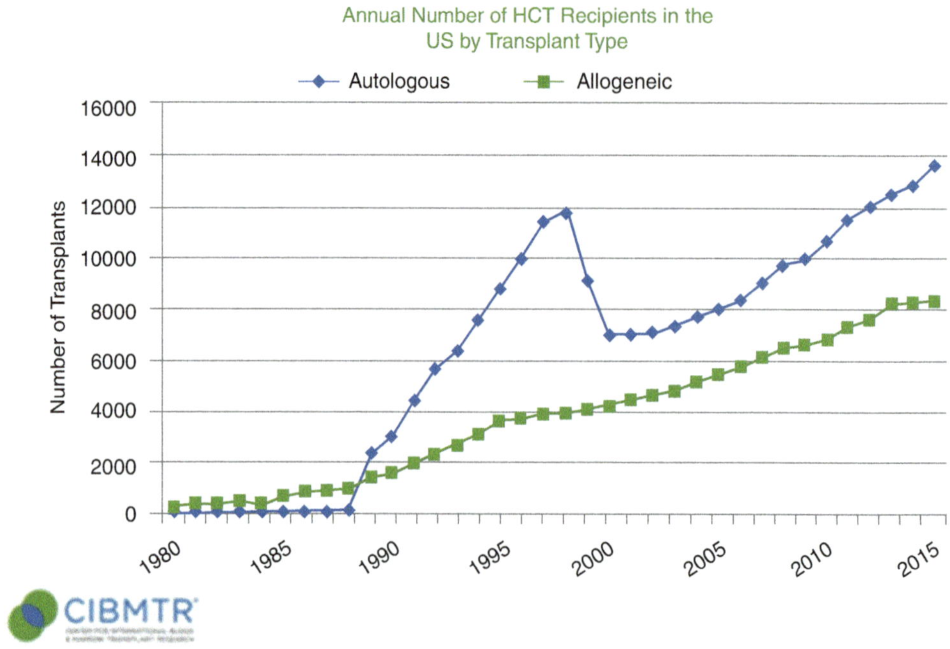

Fig. 60.3 Annual number of HCT recipients in the US by transplant type [59]. Reprinted from D'Souza and Zhu [59]

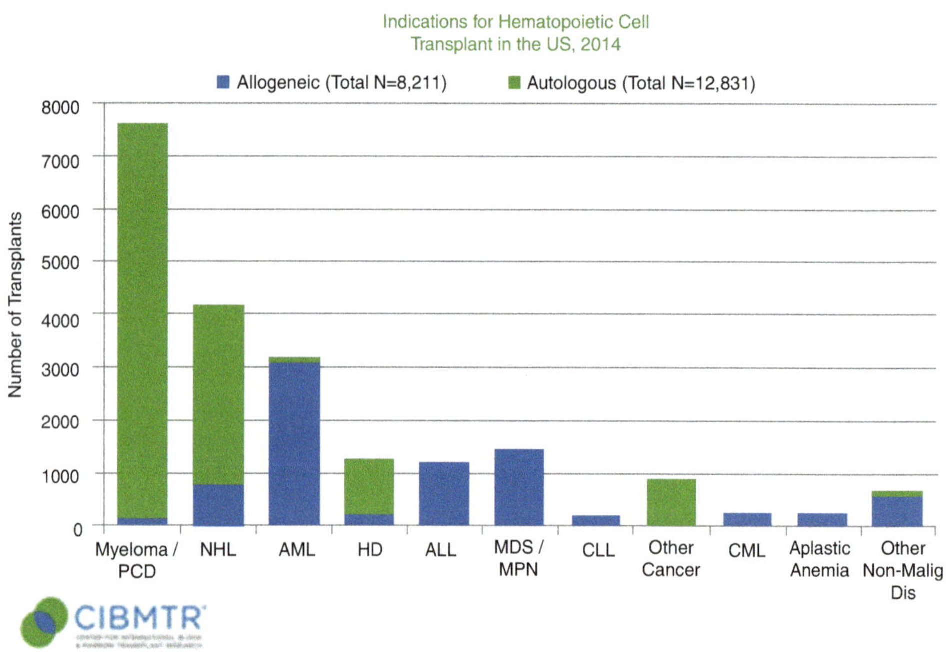

Fig. 60.4 Indications for hematopoietic cell transplant in the US, 2014 [59]. Reprinted from D'Souza and Zhu [59]

as they are susceptible to opportunistic infections. Common side effects due to chemotherapy and irradiation include mucositis, diarrhea, nausea, vomiting, loss of hair, infertility and organ toxicity. Patients are placed under strict isolation, which, in turn, can cause emotional distress. Osama et al. followed post-BMT patients for 1 year after transplant and found they suffered from severe psychological distress as a result of fear of cancer recurrence (68%) and development of new cancer (58%) as opposed to those who did not undergo transplant [61]. Patients also expressed high levels of depression, pain, and decreased coping skills post-transplant [61]. Patients suffer the most stress and fear of uncertainty during the period of initial hospitalization when enduring intensive therapy composed of chemotherapy, total body irradiation, patient isolation, and decreased physical activity [62, 63]. The level of anxiety, depression, anger, and uncertainty are greater at this time compared to any other [64]. Studies have shown that there is a significant emotional cost as a result of loss of personal control in the period prior to transplant and 1 year thereafter. Subsequently, sense of personal control improved, as did emotional symptoms [64, 65] El-Jawahri et al. (2016) demonstrated that inpatient integration of palliative care in this patient population leads to improvement in depression and PTSD symptoms at 6 months post-transplant [66].

Importance of Prognostication

Clinical prognostication involves "foreseeing", that is, formulating the prediction of a medical outcome, and "foretelling", that is, communicating the prediction to the patient [67]. Medical education focuses on the identification and treatment of disease and the return to health. While some patients may respond to treatment, there are many who do not, and the disease may progress even in those who are able to recover from an acute exacerbation. Studies show that patients want to know their prognosis in order to make informed decisions regarding the type of treatment they choose [68, 69]. All patients should complete a health-care proxy so that a health-care agent is identified if and when the patient loses the capacity to make decisions. The health-care agent is morally and legally bound to follow the patient's directives. For the minority of patients who do not want to know their prognosis, the health-care agent should be informed of the status, prognosis, and range of available treatment options so that they can make decisions that are based on the patient's known wishes, best interest, values, and principles. Physicians vary in their ability to "communicate bad news". This is a skill that is an essential part of medical school training but can be learned or improved at any point in a physician's career. Communication of prognosis is essential for patients who suffer from end-stage organ failure. While many patients are able to undergo transplantation, there are still a greater number of patients who succumb to their disease because they are not transplant candidates or do not survive to get a transplant. Patients often undergo a prolonged and painful death, involving uncomfortable, invasive and expensive care because of lack of communication between providers and the patient/family about realistic prognosis and goals when they could understand and make informed decisions about treatment options [70].

Many different prognostic tools have been developed to aid physicians in the task of formulating a prognosis. Tools commonly include the Karnofsky Performance Status (KPS), Palliative Performance Scale (PPS), the Palliative Prognostic Index (PPI), and the Palliative Prognostic Score (PaP). Palliative care consultation is often requested to help with communication of prognosis, goals of care, and advance directives, as the primary care physician often fails to initiate such discussions beforehand [71]. Prognosis for survival is not communicated as a specific amount of time, but rather as a timeframe that is meaningful to the patient and family, such as hours to days, days to weeks or weeks to months [72]. Physician surveys have indicated that among generalists and specialists, "professional norms of prognostication" are often followed which consist of providing limited information to patients and families because of uncertainty of the prediction, being optimistic, and not sharing prognosis/prediction unless asked. There is also a fear of being judged by the patient, family, or other clinicians if their prognostication is incorrect [73]. For this reason, communication of prognosis has become a core clinical skill for palliative care physicians.

Palliative Performance Scale (PPS)

The PPS is one of the most used tools available for clinicians to evaluate a patient's clinical status. It is based on ambulation, activity, self-care, intake, and level of consciousness. The scale ranges from 10% (totally bedbound, unable to do any activity, extensive disease, drowsy to comatose) to 100% (fully ambulatory, normal level of activity, no evidence of disease, fully conscious). A PPS of <50% generally represents loss of ability to perform activities of daily living independently [7]. This tool was modified from the KPS to include intake and level of consciousness, which the KPS does not take into account. This scale is not limited to cancer patients nor to end of life. It can be used in patients living with chronic illness who are experiencing progression of disease to assist in prognosticating survival. PPS cores have been used in cancer and non-cancer patients and across settings including hospital and nursing homes and correlate well with survival and symptom distress [74–77]. In a study involving Japanese patients admitted to a palliative care unit and stratified according to PPS, overall median survival was as follows: PPS 10–20%, median survival 6 days; PPS 30–50%, median survival 41 days; and PPS 60–70%, median survival of 108 days [78]. A similar correlation between PPS and survival was seen in a large community-based hospice center [77].

Prognosticating Survival in Non-cancer Patients

While there have been multiple tools developed to accurately prognosticate survival in cancer patients, these patients tend to undergo a more predictable decline compared to non-cancer patients. Patients with chronic illnesses, such as those with end-stage organ failure, often suffer multiple periods of exacerbations followed by stabilization until finally culminating in death [8] (Fig. 60.2).

For this reason, formulating an accurate prognosis becomes a real challenge to the treating physician. In an emergency room study, physicians identified 17% of patients admitted with CHF exacerbation to have a 10% chance of surviving 90 days when, in fact, 67% did not survive [79]. Palliative care specialists are trained to assess the status and prognosis of patients with serious and chronic illness and to communicate this information in a compassionate way to patient and family so that they may make an informed decision with regard to options for care. One of these options is hospice, a Medicare and insurance benefit for patients who are not expected to survive more than 6 months given the natural history of the disease. Patients with end-stage organ failure who are on the list for organ transplantation are often denied the opportunity to have palliative care services because of the misconception that palliative care is equivalent to hospice care and end-of-life care. As noted previously, palliative care may be introduced into the care of patients with serious illness concurrent with curative attempts such as transplantation. This would provide improved symptom control as well as increased support for their emotional and spiritual needs.

The National Hospice and Palliative Care Organization (NHPCO) developed guidelines that can aid a physician in formulating a prognosis, when the disease has become far advanced, so that they may communicate with patients and families regarding realistic treatment goals at the end-of-life. According to the NHPCO: "A life-limiting condition with evidence of either disease progression and/or impaired nutritional status indicated by an involuntary weight loss greater than 10% of body weight in past 6 months. The goal of treatment should be relief of symptoms, not cure." [80] (Table 60.1).

Table 60.1 Guidelines for prognosis in selected non-cancer diseases [81]

Heart disease	Recurrent symptoms of heart failure or angina at rest, discomfort with any activity (NYHA IV) Patient already optimally treated with diuretics and vasodilators
Pulmonary disease	Disabling dyspnea at rest Progressive pulmonary disease (e.g. increasing emergency department visits of hospitalizations for pulmonary infections and/or respiratory failure) Hypoxemia at rest on supplemental oxygen O_2 $pO_2 \leq 55$ mmHg on supplemental O_2 O_2 sat $-\leq 88\%$ on supplemental O_2 or Hypercapnia: $pCO_2 \geq 50$ mmHg
Liver disease	End-stage cirrhosis; not a candidate for liver transplant PT > 5 s over control or INR > 1.5 and serum albumin < 2.5 g/dL At least one of the following: Ascites despite treatment Spontaneous peritonitis Hepatorenal syndrome Hepatic encephalopathy despite treatment Recurrent variceal bleeding
Renal disease	Chronic renal failure; coming off or not a candidate for dialysis Creatinine clearance <10 cc/min (for diabetics <15 cc/min) Serum creatinine >8.0 mg/dL (for diabetics >6.0 mg/dL) Signs and symptoms associated with renal failure Uremia: nausea, pruritus, confusion, or restlessness Oliguria: output <400 cc/24 h Intractable hyperkalemia serum >7.0 Uremic pericarditis Hepatorenal syndrome Intractable fluid overload

Used with permission from Taylor and Francis and the National Hospice and Palliative Care Organization [81]

Symptom Management in Chronic Illness and the Role of Palliative Care

While the field of palliative medicine enhances the treatment of emotional, spiritual, and psychosocial suffering of patients with serious illness, it also focuses on pain and non-pain symptom management. By integrating palliative care along with curative care early in the disease trajectory, chronically ill patients nearing the end of life reported improved satisfaction with care and demonstrated fewer acute interventions [82]. Patients suffering from chronic illness have a longer life trajectory that is complicated by an intensifying symptom burden, which is similar to the symptoms experienced by cancer patients [83] (Table 60.2). The patient's illness progression and symptom burden can guide the clinician as to the best time to introduce palliative care, though one can argue that it is never too early, even if it is only to address goals of care, help establish advance directives, and most of all, serve as a bridge of communication between patient, families, and treating physicians.

Table 60.2 Symptoms common to malignant and non-malignant conditions [83]

Physical	Social	Psychosocial	Existential
Pain Breathlessness Anorexia Immobility Constipation	Loss of employment Role change Fear for dependants	Depression Fear and anxiety Uncertainty Guilt	Religious Nonreligious Meaning of life Why?

Reproduced from O'Brien et al. [83], copyright 1998, with permission from BMJ Publishing Group Ltd.

In a systematic review of symptom burden in end-stage organ failure, it was reported that daily symptom burden is likely to be high, irrespective of the underlying disease [84]. The most common symptoms experienced by patients with end-stage organ failure are fatigue, dyspnea, insomnia, and pain [84, 85]. Management of these symptoms must be specific to the underlying disease and patient, as response to and tolerance of medications varies.

End-of-Life Care for Transplant Patients

While palliative care addresses much more than end-of-life issues, primary care physicians and staff often consult the palliative care service to assist with the care of patients who are actively dying. As the disease progresses, symptoms increase and curative options (such as transplantation or re-transplantation) are exhausted, patients and families should receive the additional support they need. While it is recommended that goals of care (including end-of-life care) be discussed early in the disease trajectory or when patients are listed for organ transplantation, it is not often done because of both physician and patient barriers to these discussions. A study by Schickedanz et al. showed that discussions of end-of-life advance care planning were primarily impeded by the perception of irrelevance by the patient/family, lack of relationship between patient and family, patient's personal problems, and physician time constraints [86]. When end-of-life issues are addressed early, while the patient is still able to discuss his/her wishes and preferences, the patient's quality of life can improve [87, 88]. A study of bereaved family members demonstrated that they were satisfied with life-sustaining interventions but not with the lack of communication and pain control. Of the 461 patients studied, 46% of the discussions involved patients directly, 14% involved discussion with family members of a patient who lacked decision-making capacity, 6% involved discussion with the family of patient who had capacity, and 23% had no discussion at all [89]. Wright et al. suggest a number of strategies for initiating the topic of advance care planning at the end of life to help overcome many physicians' reticence due to lack of experience or fear (Table 60.3) [87].

Palliative care physicians must continue to work collaboratively with the primary care physicians and specialists involved in a patient's care in order to provide the patient with end-of-life plans that are acceptable and in keeping with their principles and values. When organ transplantation is no longer an option or if a patient is clearly dying despite prior transplantation, it is the palliative care physician's duty to communicate with patients and families about the option of death in hospice (in home or inpatient) surrounded by family and friends rather than in isolation on artificial life support.

Table 60.3 Strategies for Initiating conversation with patients about advance care planning for end of life [87]

Acknowledge emotions "Is talking about these issues difficult for you?"
Legitimize the feelings "Of course, talking about this makes you sad- it wouldn't be normal if it didn't"
Offer support "No matter what the road holds ahead. I'm going to be there with you"
Explore "You just mentioned feeling scared. Can you tell me more about what scares you the most?"
Hope for the best but prepare for the worst "Have you thought about what might happen if things don't go as you wish? Sometimes having a plan that prepares you for the worst makes it easier to focus on what you hope for the most" "I wish too that this transplant had lasted longer. If we cannot do another transplantation, what other short-term goals might we work toward?" "What sorts of things are left undone for you? Let's talk about how we might be able to make these happen"

Reprinted from Wright et al. [87]

Appendix

Karnofsky Performance Status

100	Normal, no complaints, no evidence of disease
90	Able to carry on normal activity, some minor symptoms of disease
80	Normal activity with effort: some symptoms of disease
70	Able to care for self but unable to carry on normal activity or active work
60	Requires occasional assistance but is able to care for most of personal needs
50	Requires considerable assistance and frequent medical care
40	Disabled: requires special care and assistance
30	Severely disabled: hospitalization is indicated, death not imminent
20	Very sick, hospitalization necessary: active treatment necessary
10	Moribund, fatal processes progressing rapidly
0	Death

Palliative Performance Scale (PPSv2) [87] Reprinted with permission from Victoria Hospice Society, BC, Canada (2001) www.victoriahospice.org

	Ambulation	Activity and evidence of disease	Self-Care	Intake	Conscious level
100%	Full	Normal activity and work. No evidence of disease	Full	Normal	Full
90%	Full	Normal activity and work. Some evidence of disease	Full	Normal	Full
80%	Full	Normal activity *with* effort. Some evidence of disease	Full	Normal or reduced	Full
70%	Reduced	Unable normal job/work. Significant disease	Full	Normal or reduced	Full
60%	Reduced	Unable hobby/house work. Significant disease	Occasional assistance necessary	Normal or reduced	Full or confusion
50%	Mainly sit/lie	Unable to do any work. Extensive disease	Considerable assistance required	Normal or reduced	Full or confusion
40%	Mainly in bed	Unable to do most activity. Extensive disease	Mainly assistance	Normal or reduced	Full or drowsy +/− confusion
30%	Totally bed bound	Unable to do any activity. Extensive disease	Total care	Normal or reduced	Full or drowsy +/− confusion
20%	Totally bed bound	Unable to do any activity. Extensive disease	Total care	Minimal to sips	Full or drowsy +/− confusion
10%	Totally bed bound	Unable to do any activity. Extensive disease	Total care	Mouth care only	Drowsy or coma +/− confusion
0%	Death	–	–	–	–

Instructions for Use of PPS (See also Definition of Terms)

1. PPS scores are determined by reading horizontally at each level to find a "best fit" for the patient which is then assigned as the PPS% score.
2. Begin at the left column and read downwards until the appropriate ambulation level is reached, then read across to the next column and downwards again until the activity/evidence of disease is located. These steps are repeated until all five columns are covered before assigning the actual PPS for that patient. In this way, "leftward" columns (columns to the left of any specific column) are "stronger" determinants and generally take precedence over others.

   Example 1: A patient who spends the majority of the day sitting or lying down due to fatigue from advanced disease and requires considerable assistance to walk even for short distances but who is otherwise fully conscious level with good intake would be scored at PPS 50%.

   Example 2: A patient who has become paralyzed and quadriplegic requiring total care would be PPS 30%. Although this patient may be placed in a wheelchair (and perhaps seem initially to be at 50%), the score is 30% because he or she would be otherwise totally bed bound due to the disease or complication if it were not for caregivers providing total care including lift/transfer. The patient may have normal intake and full conscious level. Example 3: However, if the patient in example 2 was paraplegic and bed bound but still able to do some self-care such as feed themselves, then the PPS would be higher at 40 or 50% since he or she is not "total care".
3. PPS scores are in 10% increments only. Sometimes, there are several columns easily placed at one level but one or two which seem better at a higher or lower level. One then needs to make a "best fit" decision. Choosing a

"half-fit" value of PPS 45%, for example, is not correct. The combination of clinical judgment and "leftward precedence" is used to determine whether 40 or 50% is the more accurate score for that patient.

4. PPS may be used for several purposes. First, it is an excellent communication tool for quickly describing a patient's current functional level. Second, it may have value in criteria for workload assessment or other measurements and comparisons. Finally, it appears to have prognostic value.

Definition of Terms for PPS

As noted below, some of the terms have similar meanings with the differences being more readily apparent as one reads horizontally across each row to find an overall "best fit" using all five columns.

1. *Ambulation*

   The items *mainly sit/lie*, *mainly in bed*, and *totally bed bound* are clearly similar. The subtle differences are related to items in the self-care column. For example, "totally bed 'bound' at PPS 30% is due to either profound weakness or paralysis such that the patient not only can't get out of bed but is also unable to do any self-care. The difference between 'sit/lie' and 'bed' is proportionate to the amount of time the patient is able to sit up vs need to lie down."

   Reduced ambulation is located at the PPS 70% and PPS 60% level. By using the adjacent column, the reduction of ambulation is tied to inability to carry out their normal job, work occupation or some hobbies or housework activities. The person is still able to walk and transfer on their own but at PPS 60% needs occasional assistance.

2. *Activity and Extent of disease*

   Some, *significant*, and *extensive* disease refer to physical and investigative evidence which shows degrees of progression. For example in breast cancer, a local recurrence would imply "some" disease; one or two metastases in the lung or bone would imply "significant" disease, whereas multiple metastases in the lung, bone, liver, brain, hypercalcemia, or other major complications would be "extensive" disease. The extent may also refer to progression of disease despite active treatments. Using PPS in AIDS, "some" may mean the shift from HIV to AIDS, and "significant" implies progression in physical decline, new or difficult symptoms, and laboratory findings with low counts. "Extensive" refers to one or more serious complications with or without continuation of active antiretrovirals, antibiotics, etc.

   The above extent of disease is also judged in context with the ability to maintain one's work and hobbies or activities. Decline in activity may mean the person still plays golf but reduces from playing 18 holes to 9 holes, or just a par 3, or to backyard putting. People who enjoy walking will gradually reduce the distance covered, although they may continue trying, sometimes even close to death (e.g., trying to walk the halls).

3. *Self-Care*

   Occasional assistance means that most of the time patients are able to transfer out of bed, walk, wash, go to toilet, and eat by their own means but that on occasion (perhaps once daily or a few times weekly) they require minor assistance.

   Considerable assistance means that regularly every day, the patient needs help, usually by one person, to do some of the activities noted above. For example, the person needs help to get to the bathroom but is then able to brush his or her teeth or wash at least hands and face. Food will often need to be cut into edible sizes but the patient is then able to eat of his or her own accord.

   Mainly assistance is a further extension of "considerable." Using the above example, the patient now needs help getting up but also needs assistance washing his face and shaving, but can usually eat with minimal or no help. This may fluctuate according to fatigue during the day.

   Total care means that the patient is completely unable to eat without help, go to toilet, or do any self-care. Depending on the clinical situation, the patient may or may not be able to chew and swallow food once prepared and fed to him or her.

4. *Intake*

   Changes in intake are quite obvious with *normal intake* referring to the person's usual eating habits while healthy. *Reduced* means any reduction from that and is highly variable according to the unique individual circumstances. *Minimal* refers to very small amounts, usually pureed or liquid, which are well below nutritional sustenance.

5. *Conscious Level*

   Full consciousness implies full alertness and orientation with good cognitive abilities in various domains of thinking, memory, etc. *Confusion* is used to denote presence of either delirium or dementia and is a reduced level of consciousness. It may be mild, moderate or severe with multiple possible etiologies. *Drowsiness* implies either fatigue, drug side effects, delirium, or closeness to death and is sometimes included in the term stupor. *Coma* in this context is the absence of response to verbal or physical stimuli; some reflexes may or may not remain. The depth of coma may fluctuate throughout a 24-h period.

replaces the first PPS published in 1996 [J Pall Care 9(4): 26-32]. It cannot be altered or used in any way other than as intended and described here. Programs may use PPSv2 with appropriate recognition. Available in electronic Word format by email request to edu.hospice@viha.ca

Correspondence should be sent to Director Education and Research, Victoria Hospice Society, 1952 Bay Street, Victoria, BC, V8R 1J8, Canada

References

1. Health Resources and Services Administration, Organ Procurement and Transplantation Network. Available at: https://optn.transplant.hrsa.gov/data/view-data-reports/national-data/
2. Bloom RD, Goldberg LR, Wang AY, et al. An overview of solid organ transplantation. Clin Chest Med. 2005;26:529–43.
3. Temel JS, Greer JA, Muzikansky A, et al. Early palliative care for patients with metastatic non-small cell lung cancer. N Engl Med. 2010;363(8):733–42.
4. Bakitas M, Lyons KD, Hegel MT, et al. Effects of a palliative care intervention on clinical outcomes in patients with advanced cancer: the project ENABLE II randomized controlled trial. JAMA. 2009;302:741–9.
5. World Health Organization. Available at: http://www.who.int/cancer/palliative/definition/en/
6. Karnofsky DA, Abelmann WH, Craver LF, Burchenal JH. The use of the nitrogen mustards in the palliative treatment of carcinoma – with particular reference to bronchogenic carcinoma. Cancer. 1948;1(4):634–56.
7. Palliative Performance Scale (PPSv2) version 2. Medical Care of the Dying, 4th ed., p. 121. ©Victoria Hospice Society, 2006.
8. Jaarsma T, Beattie JM, Ryder M, Rutten FH, McDonagh T, Mohacsi P, Advanced Heart Failure Study Group of the HFA of the ESC, et al. Palliative care in heart failure: a position statement from the palliative care workshop of the heart failure Association of the European Society of Cardiology. Eur J Heart Fail. 2009;11:433–43. European Society of Cardiology.
9. Adler ED, Goldfinger JZ, Kalman J, et al. Contemporary reviews in cardiovascular medicine. Palliative care in the treatment of advanced heart failure. Circulation. 2009;120:2597–606.
10. Hardin KA, Meyers M, Louie S. Integrating palliative Care in Severe Chronic Obstructive Lung Disease. COPD. 2008;5(4):207–20.
11. Hope AA, Morrison RS. Integrating palliative care with chronic liver disease care. J Palliat Care. 2011;27(1):20–7.
12. Holley JL. Palliative care in end-stage renal disease: illness trajectories, communication, and hospice use. Adv Chronic Kidney Dis. 2007;14(4):402–8.
13. Singer PA, Martin DK, Kelner M. Quality end-of-life care: patents' perspectives. JAMA. 1999;281:163–8.
14. Teno JM, Clarridge BR, Casey V, et al. Family perspectives on end-of-life care at the last place of care. JAMA. 2004;291(1):88–93.
15. Medicare part A: medicare hospice benefits. Available at: http://www.medicare.gov/Pubs/pdf/02154.pdf
16. Higginson IJ, Sen-Gupta GJ. Place of care in advanced cancer qualitative systematic literature review of patient preferences. J Palliat Med. 2000;3(3):287–300.
17. Murphy SL, Xu J, et al. Deaths: final data for 2015. National vital statistics report Vol 66. No 6 November 27, 2017.
18. Benjamin EJ, Virani SS, Callaway CW, et al. Heart disease and stroke statistics-2017 update: a report from the American Heart Association. Circulation. 2018;137(25)
19. American Heart Association. Classes of heart failure. Available at: http://www.heart.org/HEARTORG/Conditions/HeartFailure/AboutHeartFailure/Classes-of-Heart-Failure_UCM_306328_Article.jsp
20. Blinderman CD, Homel P, Billings JA, Portenoy RK, Tennstedt SL. Symptom distress and quality of life in patients with advanced heart failure. J Pain Symptom Manag. 2008;35(6):594–603.
21. Levenson JW, McCarthy EP, Lynn J, et al. The last six months of life for patients with congestive heart failure. J Am Geriatr Soc. 2000;48(5 Suppl):S101–9.
22. Nordgren L, Sörensen S. Symptoms experienced in the last six months of life in patients with end-stage heart failure. Eur J Cardiovasc Nurs. 2003;2:213–7.
23. Levy WC, Mozaffarian D, Linker DT, et al. The seattle heart failure model: prediction of survival in heart failure. Circulation. 2006;113(11):1424–33.
24. Goda A, Williams P, Manicini D, et al. Selecting patients for heart transplantation: comparison of the Heart Failure Survival Score (HFSS) and the Seattle heart failure model (SHFM). J Heart Lung Transplant. 2011;30(11):1236–43.
25. Yancy CW, Jessup M, Bozkurt B, Butler J, Casey DE Jr, Colvin MM, et al. 2017 ACC/AHA/HFSA focused update of the 2013 ACCF/AHA guideline for the management of heart failure: a report of the American College of Cardiology/American Heart Association Task Force on Clinical Practice Guidelines and the Heart Failure Society of America. Circulation. 2017;136(6):e137–61.
26. Schwarz ER, Baraghoush A, Morrissey RP, et al. Pilot study of palliative care consultation in patients with advanced heart failure referred for cardiac transplantation. J Palliat Med. 2012;15(1):12–5.
27. Global Initiative for Chronic Obstructive Lung Disease. Global strategy for the diagnosis, management, and prevention of chronic obstructive pulmonary disease. 2018 report. www.goldcopd.org. Accessed 25 Sept 2018.
28. GOLD. 2017 Global strategy for the diagnosis, management and prevention of COPD. http://goldcopd.org
29. Hurst JR, Vestbo J, Anzueto A, et al. Susceptibility to exacerbation in chronic obstructive pulmonary disease. N Engl J Med. 2010;363:1128–38.
30. Halpin DM, Decramer M, Celli B, Kesten S, Liu D, Tashkin DP. Exacerbation frequency and course of COPD. Int J Chron Obstruct Pulmon Dis. 2012;7:653–61.
31. Soler-Cataluna JJ, Martinez-Garcia MA, Sanchez PR. Severe acute exacerbations and mortality in patients with chronic obstructive pulmonary disease. Thorax. 2005;60:925–31.
32. Connors AF, Dawson NV, Thomas C, et al. Outcomes following acute exacerbation of severe chronic obstructive lung disease. Am J Respir Crit Care Med. 1996;154:959–67.
33. Donaldson GC, Seemungal TA, Bhowmik A, Wedzicha JA. Relationship between exacerbation frequency and lung function decline in chronic obstructive pulmonary disease. Thorax. 2002;57:847–52.
34. Gore JM, Brophy CJ, Greenstone MA. How well do we care for patients with end stage chronic obstructive pulmonary disease (COPD)? A comparison of palliative care and quality of life in COPD and lung cancer. Thorax. 2000;55(12):1000–6.
35. Connor SR, Pyenson B, Flitch K, et al. Comparing hospice and nonhospice patient survival among patients who die within a three year window. J Pain Symptom Manage. 2007;33(3):238–46.
36. Brumley R, Enguidanos S, Cherin D. Effectiveness of a home-base palliative care program for end-of-life. J Palliat Med. 2003;6:715–72438.
37. Lanken PN, Terry PB, Delisser HM, Fahy BF, Hansen-Flaschen J, Heffner JE, et al. ATS end-of-life care task force. An official American Thoracic Society clinical policy statement: palliative

care for patients with respiratory diseases and critical illness. Am J Respir Crit Care Med. 2008;177(8):912–27.
38. Zipprich A, Garcia-Tsao G, Rogowski S. Prognostic indicators of survival in patients with compensated and decompensated cirrhosis. Liver Int. 2012;32(9):1407–14.
39. Llach J, Ginès P, Arroyo V, Rimola A, Tito L, Badalamenti S, et al. Prognostic value of arterial pressure, endogenous vasoactive systems, and renal function in cirrhotic patients admitted to the hospital for the treatment of ascites. Gastroenterology. 1988;94:482–7.
40. Arroyo V, Gine SP, Alexander L. Definition and diagnostic criteria ascites and hepatorenal syndrome in cirrhosis. Hepatology. 1996;23(1):164–76.
41. Kamath PS, Wiesner RH, Malinchoc M, et al. A model to predict survival in patients with end-stage liver disease. Hepatology. 2001;33(2):464–70.
42. Lamba S, Murphy P, McVicker S. Changing end-of-life care practice for liver transplant service patients: structured palliative care intervention in the surgical intensive care unit. J Pain Symptom Manag. 2012;44(4):508–19.
43. Singh N, Gayowski T, Wagener MM. Depression in patients with cirrhosis: impact on outcome. Dig Dis Sci. 1997;42(7):1421–7.
44. Marchesini G, Bianchi G, Amodio P, et al. Factors associated with poor health-related quality of life of patients with cirrhosis. Gastroenterology. 2001;120(1):170–8.
45. Roth K, Lynn J, Zhong Z, et al. Dying with end stage liver disease with cirrhosis: insights from SUPPORT. Study to understand prognoses and preferences for outcomes and risks of treatment. J Am Geriatr Soc. 2000;48(5 Suppl):S122–30.
46. KDOQI clinical practice guidelines and clinical practice recommendations for 2006 updates: hemodialysis adequacy, peritoneal Dialysis adequacy and vascular access. Am J Kidney Dis. 2006;48(suppl 1):S1–322.
47. Perlman RL, Finkelstein FO, Liu L, et al. Quality of life in chronic kidney disease (CKD): a cross-sectional analysis in the Renal Research Institute-CKD study. Am J Kidney Dis. 2005;454(4):658–66.
48. The 2008 United States Renal Data System (USRDS) annual data report. Bethesda: National Institutes of Health, National Institute of Diabetes and Digestive and Kidney Diseases.
49. Merkus MP, Jager KJ, Dekker FW, de Haan RJ, Boeschoten EW, Krediet RT. Physical symptoms and quality of life in patients on chronic dialysis: results of The Netherlands Cooperative Study on Adequacy of Dialysis (NECOSAD). Nephrol Dial Transplant. 1999;14:1163–70.
50. Lee BO, Lin CC, Chaboyer W, Chiang CL, Hung CC. The fatigue experience of hemodialysis patients in Tai- wan. J Clin Nurs. 2007;16:407–13.
51. McCann K, Boore JR. Fatigue in persons with renal failure who require maintenance haemodialysis. J Adv Nurs. 2000;32:1132–42.
52. Kimmel PL, Emont SL, Newmann JM, Danko H, Moss AH. ESRD patient quality of life: symptoms, spiritual beliefs, psychosocial factors, and ethnicity. Am J Kidney Dis. 2003;42:713–21.
53. Kimmel PL, Peterson RA, Weihs KL, Simmens SJ, Alleyne S, Cruz I, Veis JH. Multiple measurements of depression predict mortality in a longitudinal study of chronic hemodialysis outpatients. Kidney Int. 2000;57:2093–8.
54. Moreno F, Lopez Gomez JM, Sanz-Guajardo D, et al. Quality of life in dialysis patients. A Spanish multicentre study. Spanish Cooperative Renal Patients Quality of Life Study Group. Nephrol Dial Transplant. 1996;11(Suppl 2):125–9.
55. Mingardi G, Cornalba L, Cortinovis E, et al. Health-related quality of life in dialysis patients. A report from an Italian study using the SF-36 Health Survey. DIA-QOL Group. Nephrol Dial Transplant. 1999;14(6):1503–10.
56. Valderrabano F, Jofre R, Lopez-Gomez JM. Quality of life in end stage renal disease patients. Am J Kidney Dis. 2001;38(3):443–64.
57. Kasiske BL, Snyder JJ, Matas MD, Ellison MD, Gill JS, Kausz AT. Preemptive kidney transplantation: the advantage and the advantaged. J Am Soc Nephrol. 2002;13:1358–64.
58. Abecassis M, Bartlett ST, et al. Kidney transplantation as primary therapy for end-stage renal disease: a National Kidney Foundation/ Kidney Disease Outcomes Quality Initiative (NKF/KDOQI™) conference. Clin J Am Soc Nephrol. 2008;3(2):471–80.
59. D'Souza A, Zhu X. Current uses and outcomes of Hematopoietic Cell Transplantation (HCT): CIBMTR summary slides; 2016. Available at: http://www.cibmtr.org
60. American Society for Blood and Marrow Transplantation. Transplant referral guidelines. Available at: http://www.asbmt.org
61. Saleh US, Brockopp DY. Quality of life one year following bone marrow transplantation: psychometric evaluation of the quality of life in bone marrow transplant survivors tool. Oncol Nurs Forum. 2001;28(9):1457–64.
62. Andrykowski MA. Psychiatric and psychological aspects of bone marrow transplantation. Psychosomatics. 1994;35:13–24.
63. Lesko LM. Psychiatric aspects of bone marrow transplantation: part I. Special issues during pre-transplant assessment and hospitalization. Psychooncology. 1993;2:161–83.
64. Fife BL, Huster GA, Cornetta KG, Kennedy VN, Akard LP, Broun ER. Longitudinal study of adaptation to the stress of bone marrow transplantation. J Clin Oncol. 2000;18(7):1539–49.
65. Baker F, Marcellus D, Zabora J, et al. Psychological distress among adult patients being evaluated for bone marrow transplantation. Psychosomatics. 1997;38:10–9.
66. El-Jawahri A, LeBlanc T, VanDusen H, Traeger L, Greer JA, Pirl WF, et al. Effect of inpatient palliative care on quality of life 2weeks after hematopoietic stem cell transplantation. JAMA. 2016;316(20):2094–103.
67. Lamon EB, Christakis NA. Some elements of prognosis in terminal cancer. Oncology (Willston Park). 1999;13(8):1165–70.
68. Heyland DK, Allan DE, Rocker G, et al. Discussing prognosis with patients and their families near the end of life: impact on satisfaction with end-of-life care. Open Med. 2009;3(2):e101–10.
69. Repetto L, Piselli P, Raffaele M, et al. Communicating cancer diagnosis and prognosis: when the target is the elderly patient-a GIOGER study. Eur J Cancer. 2009;45(3):374–83.
70. SUPPORT Principal Investigators. A controlled trial to improve care for seriously ill hospitalized patients. JAMA. 1995;274:1591–8.
71. Homsi J, Walsh D, Nelson KA, et al. The impact of palliative medicine consultation service in medical oncology. Support Care Cancer. 2002;10(4):337–42.
72. Rich A. How long have I got? Prognostication and palliative care. Eur J Palliat Care. 1999;6:179–82.
73. Christakis N. Death Foretold: prophecy and prognosis in medical care. Chicago: Chicago University Press; 1999.
74. Virik K, Glare P. Validation of the palliative performance scale for inpatients admitted to a palliative care unit in Sydney, Australia. J Pain Symptom Manag. 2002;23(6):455–7.
75. Olajide O, Hanson L, Usher BM, Qaqish BF, Schwartz R, Bernard S. Validation of the palliative performance scale in the acute tertiary care hospital setting. J Palliat Med. 2007;10(1):111–7.
76. Harrold J, Rickerson E, Carroll JT, McGrath J, et al. Is the palliative performance scale a useful predictor of mortality in a heterogeneous hospice population? J Palliat Med. 2005;8(3):503–9.
77. Head B, Ritchie CS, Smoot TM. Prognostication in hospice care: can the palliative performance scale help? J Palliat Med. 2005;8(3):492–502.
78. Morita T, Tsunod J, Inoue S, et al. Validity of the palliative performance scale from a survival perspective. J Pain Symptom Manag. 1999;18(1):2–3.

79. Poses RM, Smith WR, McClish DK, et al. Physicians' survival predictions for patients with acute congestive heart failure. Arch Intern Med. 1997;157(9):1001–7.
80. National Hospice and Palliative Care Organization (NHPCO). https://www.nhpco.org/
81. National Hospice and Palliative Care Organization. Medical guidelines for determining prognosis in selected non-cancer diseases, 2nd ed. Arlington: National Hospice Organization; 1997, J Pain Palliat Care Pharmacother. 1996;11(2).
82. Brumley RD, Enguidanos S, Cherin DA. Effectiveness of a home-based palliative care program for end-of-life. J Palliat Med. 2003;6:715–24.
83. O'Brien T, Welsh J, Dunn FG. ABC of palliative care. Non malignant conditions. BMJ. 1998;316(7127):286–9.
84. Janssen DJ, Spruit MA, Wouters EF, Schols JM. Daily symptom burden in end-stage chronic organ failure: a systematic review. Palliat Med. 2008;22:938–48.
85. Solano JP, Gomes B, Higginson IJ. A comparison of symptom prevalence in far advanced cancer, AIDS, heart disease, chronic obstructive pulmonary disease and renal disease. J Pain Symptom Manag. 2006;31:58–69.
86. Schickedanz A, Schillinger D, Landefeld CS. A clinical framework for improving the advance care planning process: start with patient' self-identified barriers. J Am Geriatr Soc. 2009;57(1):31–9; quiz 62.
87. Wright L, Pape D, Ross K, Campbell M, Bowman K. Approaching end-of-life care in organ transplantation: the impact of transplant patients' death and dying. Prog Transplant. 2007;17(1):57–61.
88. Gourdji I, McVey L, Purden M. A quality end of life from a palliative care patient's perspective. J Palliat Care. 2009;25(1):40–50.
89. Hanson LC, Danis M, Garrett J. What is wrong with end-of-life care? Opinions of bereaved family members. J Am Geriatr Soc. 1997;45(11):1339–44.

Part VI

Infection Prevention

Infection Control Strategies in Transplant Populations

61

S. Cutro, M. Phillips, and H. W. Horowitz

Introduction

The immunocompromised host presents both routine and unique challenges from an infection control and prevention perspective. Cell-mediated and humoral immune deficiencies in the pre-transplant and post-transplant periods lead to increased susceptibility to a wide variety of viral, bacterial, parasitic, and fungal pathogens: some endogenous and others originating from the host's environment. Innate immune defects including severe neutropenia during the pre-engraftment period and secondary graft loss due to cancer recurrence, drug toxicity, or myelosuppressive viral opportunistic infections are also of significant concern in transplant patients. The "net state of immunosuppression" is helpful in stratifying patients' risk for developing infections and is determined in large part by the nature of the immune suppression employed. However, environmental factors, preexisting immune deficits, metabolic derangements, and antimicrobial exposure all play a role in determining the risk for infection [1]. The use of prophylactic antimicrobials, including antibacterial, antiviral, antiparasitic, and antifungal agents, has led to a reduction in all-cause mortality, infection-related mortality, and risk of clinically and microbiologically documented infections [2–4]. However, despite prophylaxis, infections remain a significant threat in this patient population.

Autologous and allogeneic stem cell transplant (SCT) recipients carry the greatest risk for post-transplant infection, with anywhere from 35% to 100% of adult SCT recipients developing infections after transplant [5, 6]. Infection-related mortality among SCT recipients ranges from 5% to 33% and is the leading cause of death in 8% of autologous and 17–20% of allogeneic SCT recipients. This difference is due in large part to greater immune suppression employed in allogeneic transplantation versus autologous transplantation [6, 7]. Among solid organ transplant (SOT) recipients, infectious complications are also of significant concern, with bacterial infections occurring in 33–68% of liver, 21–30% of heart, 35% of pancreas, 47% of kidney, and 54% of lung transplant recipients [8]. Cytomegalovirus (CMV) infection occurs in 44–85% of kidney, heart, and liver transplant recipients, while varicella-zoster virus (VZV) reactivation occurs in 5–13% of SOT recipients [8]. Systemic fungal infection occurs in 5–17% of heart, 14–22% of heart-lung, 2–42% of liver, and 2–14% of kidney transplant recipients [8]. In the SOT population, infection is the leading cause of death among patients receiving lung, intestine, and liver transplants [9, 10].

A temporal relationship exists between the development of particular infections and the time of transplantation and engraftment as outlined in Table 61.1. This chapter considers potentially preventable infections using infection control practice in the context of time from transplantation/engraftment and focuses specifically on the most common infections that transplant patients are at risk to develop during the various stages of transplantation: pre-transplant period, early post-solid organ transplant/pre-engraftment period, intermediate post-solid organ transplant/early post-engraftment period, and late post-solid organ transplant/late post-engraftment period. Antimicrobial prophylaxis and pre-/post-transplant vaccinations are discussed elsewhere in this book and are beyond the scope of this chapter.

S. Cutro (✉)
Department of Infectious Diseases, The Southeast Permanente Medical Group, Kaiser Permanente, Atlanta, GA, USA

M. Phillips
New York University School of Medicine, Division of Infectious Diseases and Immunology, New York, NY, USA
e-mail: michael.phillips@nyumc.org

H. W. Horowitz
Department of Medicine, Division of Infectious Diseases, New York Presbyterian-Brooklyn Methodist Hospital, Weill Cornell Medical College, Brooklyn, NY, USA
e-mail: hwh2002@med.cornell.edu

A. Safdar (ed.), *Principles and Practice of Transplant Infectious Diseases*, https://doi.org/10.1007/978-1-4939-9034-4_61

Table 61.1 Common pathogens in transplant patients based on time relative to transplant/engraftment and type of transplant [7, 88, 89]

SOT	*Timeframe*	Pre-transplant	Early post-transplant (<1 month)	Intermediate post-transplant (1–6 months)	Late post-transplant (>6 months)
	Pathogens	Typical community organisms if no recent healthcare exposures Nosocomial pathogens if recent healthcare exposures Endemic infections	Gram-positive organisms (including MRSA and VRE) *C. difficile* *Aspergillus*, *Candida*	*Listeria*, *Nocardia* HSV, CMV, HBV, HCV, EBV, BK virus *Toxoplasma*, *Strongyloides*, *PCP*, *TB*, *Leishmania*	Typical community organisms CMV *Aspergillus*, dermatophytes
SCT	*Timeframe*	Pre-transplant	Pre-engraftment (15–45 days post-transplant)	Early post-engraftment (30–100 days post-transplant)	Late post-engraftment (>100 days post-transplant)
	Pathogens	Typical community organisms if no recent healthcare exposures Nosocomial pathogens if recent healthcare exposures Endemic infections	Gram-negative rods, gram-positive organisms, gastrointestinal *Streptococcus* spp. HSV, respiratory and enteric viruses *Aspergillus*, *Candida*	Gram-positive organisms, gram-negative rods (lower frequency), gastrointestinal *Streptococcus* spp. HSV, CMV, HHV, EBV, respiratory/enteric viruses *Aspergillus*, *Candida*, PCP	Encapsulated bacteria HSV, VZV, HHV, EBV, respiratory and enteric viruses *Aspergillus*, PCP

SOT solid organ transplantation, *SCT* stem cell transplantation

While there are many unique infection control and prevention considerations in this patient population, standard hand hygiene, disinfection of medical equipment and surfaces in patient rooms, and isolation precautions should be applied to transplant patients per established guidelines [11–13]. Some hospitals may choose to place all transplant recipients on isolation precautions even in the absence of active infection or colonization with organisms of interest. However, evidence-based guidelines to support this approach do not exist, and studies to determine the most effective isolation precaution strategies in immune compromised patients are needed. Infection control and prevention practices should be implemented to prevent device-related infections such as central line-associated bloodstream infection (CLABSI), catheter-associated urinary tract infection (CAUTI), and ventilator-associated pneumonia (VAP). Routine hand hygiene and use of antiseptic handwash/rub should be stressed as in non-transplant populations [14]. Standard perioperative antimicrobial prophylaxis should be used and other recommended procedures and processes should be followed to minimize surgical site infections [15].

Pre-transplant Period

The home and work environments are the primary sources of infection that clinicians and transplant candidates must consider during the pre-transplant period. Community-acquired organisms, colonization with nosocomial pathogens due to recent healthcare exposure, and exposures to environmentally endemic pathogens are all of great concern during this period. Clinicians should identify and treat active infections, review available microbiological data for previous infection/colonization with methicillin-resistant *Staphylococcus aureus* (MRSA), vancomycin-resistant *Enterococcus* (VRE), and multidrug resistant (MDR) gram-negative rods, and screen candidates for the presence of latent infections that may reactivate with subsequent immune suppression. Understanding previous infection/colonization history is important in order to risk-stratify patients for post-transplant prophylaxis and to help guide future empiric antimicrobial therapy decisions. Clinicians should counsel transplant candidates to avoid certain environmental situations that may predispose them to infections [16]. Some daily activities such as gardening, pigeon rearing, farming, drinking well water, spelunking, potholing, and traveling may expose patients to endemic bacterial, fungal, and parasitic organisms that manifest in severe infection after transplantation. Serologic testing for Chagas disease, *Coccidioides*, *Histoplasma*, *Cryptococcus* spp., *Strongyloides stercoralis*, *Schistosoma* spp., and human T-lymphotropic virus (HTLV) 1/2 should be considered based upon initial risk factor assessment for potential exposure and therefore at-risk individuals [17, 18].

A complete medical history, including country of origin, travel history (both within and outside of the United States), pet exposure, risk factors for tuberculosis (TB), family history, work history, and social history should be obtained. History of recent/prior hospitalizations also should be obtained, with a particular focus on any infections and the name/type of antimicrobials received. For both SCT and SOT candidates, serologic screening for herpes simplex virus (HSV), VZV, CMV, human immunodeficiency virus (HIV), hepatitis B virus (HBV), hepatitis C virus (HCV), Epstein-Barr virus (EBV), and *Toxoplasma gondii* are recommended [7, 19, 20]. Potential SCT donors are also screened for potentially communicable diseases in accordance with published guidelines, and this topic is covered elsewhere in this book [21].

Table 61.2 High-risk foods that should be avoided in transplant recipients, with pathogens of concern and acceptable alternatives [7, 90–92]

Food group	Unacceptable foods	Pathogens of concern	Acceptable alternatives
Dairy	Nonpasteurized or raw milk Cheeses containing uncooked vegetables Cheeses with molds (Bleu, Stilton, Roquefort, gorgonzola)	*Listeria monocytogenes* *Salmonella enteritidis* *E. coli*	Pasteurized milk and milk products Commercially packaged hard and semisoft cheeses (cheddar, mozzarella, etc.)
Meat	Raw or undercooked meat, poultry, fish, game, tofu Raw or undercooked eggs, nonpasteurized egg substitutes (including certain preparations of hollandaise sauce and Caesar dressing) Raw or undercooked seafood Deli-style ready-to-eat meats and poultry Uncooked hot dogs or sausage Uncooked smoked seafood (salmon/lox) Tempeh products	*E. coli* O157:H7 *Salmonella enteritidis* *Campylobacter jejuni* *Clostridium perfringens* *Toxoplasma gondii* *Vibrio* spp. *Listeria monocytogenes*	Well-done meats, cooked to safe minimum cooking temperatures Eggs cooked until both white and yolk are firm Canned meats Pasteurized eggs and egg substitutes Cooked hot dogs or sausage Refrigerated smoked seafood if cooked to 160°F
Fruits and nuts	Unwashed raw fruits Nonpasteurized fruit and vegetable juices Fresh fruit salsas Unroasted raw nuts or nuts in shells	*E. coli* O157:H7 *Salmonella enteritidis* Norovirus Hepatitis A virus *Shigella* *Cryptosporidium* *Giardia*	Well-washed raw and frozen fruit Cooked, canned, and frozen fruit Pasteurized juices and frozen juice concentrates Dried fruits Canned or bottled roasted nuts Commercially packaged nut butters
Vegetables and soups	Unwashed raw vegetables or herbs Fresh nonpasteurized vegetable salsa Raw vegetable sprouts (alfalfa, clover, etc.) Salads Miso products (soups, paste)	*E. coli* O157:H7 *Salmonella enteritidis* Norovirus Hepatitis A virus *Shigella* *Cryptosporidium* *Giardia*	Well-washed raw and frozen vegetables Cooked fresh/frozen/canned vegetables Shelf-stable bottled salsa Cooked vegetable sprouts Fresh, well-washed herbs and dry herbs used in cooked foods
Others	Raw honey	*Clostridium botulinum*	Commercial "Grade A" honey

Originally published in Cutro et al. [92]

Clinicians should also screen transplant candidates for latent tuberculosis infection (LTBI) using an interferon gamma release assay (IGRA) or tuberculin skin test (TST). TB incidence among SOT recipients in non-endemic countries ranges from 1.2% to 6.4% and most commonly occurs within the first year after transplantation, while the incidence of TB in SCT recipients in the United States ranges from 0.0014% to 3% [22–24]. In SOT candidates, pre-transplant treatment of LTBI has been shown to decrease the risk of reactivation to 0% and therefore should be strongly considered [23]. TST is often unreliable in immunosuppressed patients and may underestimate the prevalence of LTBI in these high-risk patients. IGRAs tend to have increased sensitivity in immunosuppressed patients but can generate frequent "indeterminate" results in this population, especially among patients with end-stage liver disease, high Model for End-Stage Liver Disease (MELD) scores, and end-stage renal disease [23, 25, 26]. In patients from TB-endemic regions, combination testing using TST and IGRA can be considered.

Primary infection with and reactivation of CMV are of great concern in transplant populations, especially in SCT recipients. In addition to serologic screening for CMV, SCT candidates should avoid sharing cups, glasses, and eating utensils with others and should use latex condoms with new sexual partners or known partners that are CMV-sero-discordant to decrease the risk of CMV transmission [7, 27]. Similarly, candidates should avoid contact with oral and genital HSV lesions during the pre-transplant period, especially among candidates with no serologic evidence of HSV 1 or 2. Transplant candidates should also avoid contact with persons who developed a post-vaccination rash after receiving varicella/zoster vaccines until resolution of the rash/skin lesions [27]. Avoidance of areas of high dust exposure such as construction sites, chicken coops, caves, and activities that disturb soil is recommended in the pre-transplant period [27, 28]. Certain high-risk foods, including raw fruits and vegetables, shellfish, and undercooked meats, should be avoided. Some of these high-risk foods, with pathogens of concern, and acceptable alternatives are outlined in Table 61.2.

Early Post-Solid Organ Transplant (<1 Month)/Pre-engraftment (Days 15–45 Post-SCT) Period

Early infections in transplant recipients arise almost exclusively in the hospital setting and are most often attributed to surgical complications, compromise of normal mucosal barriers, the presence of invasive devices such as central venous catheters (CVCs), environmental exposures within the hospital, and/or ill healthcare workers (HCWs) or visitors. During this period, bacterial pathogens (including MRSA, VRE, gram-negative rods, and *Clostridium difficile*), viruses, and fungal species (*Aspergillus* and *Candida*) are of greatest concern for SOT and SCT patients (Table 61.1).

Hospital Exposures and Healthcare Workers

This period typically represents the first extensive exposure to HCWs and the hospital environment for transplant recipients, so targeting potentially preventable infections is critical. Hospitals should enact a comprehensive vaccination policy that adheres to Centers for Disease Control and Prevention (CDC)/Advisory Committee on Immunization Practices (ACIP)/Healthcare Infection Control Practices Advisory Committee (HICPAC) recommendations to decrease the transmission of infectious diseases from HCWs to patients [29]. Ideally, HCWs should receive inactivated vaccines instead of live vaccines to minimize the risk of transmission of vaccine virus to transplant recipients. Although transmission of live attenuated influenza virus from intranasal influenza vaccine has not been reported in healthcare settings, this vaccine is contraindicated for HCWs caring for transplant recipients. HCWs who receive this vaccine inadvertently should avoid contact with transplant recipients, although the duration of avoidance has not been determined [29]. Vaccine-strain poliovirus in oral polio vaccine (OPV) can be transmitted from person-to-person. Therefore, OPV administration is contraindicated for HCWs caring for transplant recipients as well as household contacts of transplant recipients. If OPV is inadvertently administered, the vaccine recipient should avoid contact with transplant recipients for 4–6 weeks [30]. HCWs, family members, close contacts, and visitors who do not have a documented history of varicella infection or who are seronegative should receive varicella vaccine before being allowed to visit or have direct contact with a transplant recipient, and vaccination should be completed at least 4 weeks prior to commencement of the transplant process [30].

In accordance with published guidelines, every effort should be made to restrict/minimize direct patient contact between HCWs with potentially transmissible infections and transplant candidates/recipients [31]. Hospitals should also develop screening policies for visitors to transplant units, especially during respiratory virus season, to reduce exposure to pathogens such as influenza and respiratory syncytial virus (RSV). While these respiratory viruses are primarily transmitted via respiratory droplets, dispersion by airborne droplets is possible under certain circumstances [32, 33]. Visitors and HCWs with infectious symptoms or with recent exposure to communicable infections should avoid direct contact with transplant candidates/recipients [34]. While guidelines exist for organisms and syndromes that require droplet isolation precautions, some transplant centers choose to place all transplant recipients on droplet isolation precautions during respiratory virus season [11].

Screening for Carriage of Bacterial Pathogens

There is insufficient evidence to recommend routine MRSA screening of all transplant recipients and insufficient evidence to support decolonization of these patients [7]. However, routine surveillance cultures can be considered in certain settings such as intensive care units to help reduce the incidence of MRSA infections [35]. A study of liver transplant recipients and candidates found that patients colonized with MRSA were more likely to develop subsequent MRSA infection, while those colonized with VRE had an increased risk of subsequent VRE infection and death [36]. At another liver transplant center, implementation of a multi-faceted infection control protocol, which included active surveillance for MRSA, contact precautions for those colonized with MRSA, cohorting patients with culture-positive MRSA, and nasal decolonization of those colonized with MRSA, led to decreased rates of new MRSA nasal carriage and decreased rates of *Staphylococcus aureus* infection and bacteremia [37]. Extended-spectrum β-lactamase (ESBL)-producing organisms and carbapenem-resistant *Enterobacteriaceae* (CRE) and *Acinetobacter* spp. present significant challenges for transplant patients, and asymptomatic carriage of these organisms has been associated with subsequent infection [38, 39]. Importantly, it has been reported that transplant recipients colonized with ESBL/CRE organisms may introduce these organisms into hospital settings, presenting an ongoing challenge for hospital-wide infection control departments [38, 39]. While active surveillance of MRSA, VRE, and other MDR organisms may be considered, no current guidelines support this approach in transplant populations.

Isolation Precautions

Likewise, no transplant-specific evidence-based guidelines exist regarding initiation and discontinuation of isolation precautions. Until additional studies are performed in this patient population, adherence to HICPAC guidelines for isolation precautions is recommended [11, 13]. At some transplant centers, patients with a history of VRE infection/colonization are presumptively placed on contact isolation precautions during subsequent hospital admissions. Although there are insufficient data to guide discontinuation of contact precautions in these patients, individual transplant centers may implement local criteria for discontinuation of these precautions [7, 11, 13, 40]. Interestingly, the results of a 2008 survey of European SCT centers showed significant variability in the nature and level of isolation precautions implemented at individual centers. This variability reiterates the need for additional studies on which to base the development of guidelines for severely immunocompromised populations [41]. Readmitted patients with a history of MRSA, VRE, or MDR/CRE infection/colonization represent a challenge to clinicians and infection control practitioners alike, given the potential long-term carriage of resistant organisms among these patients. Unfortunately, the exact duration of carriage of these organisms has not been adequately studied in transplant patients. Data do exist, however, regarding carriage following hospital discharge in the general population. One study found MRSA carriage can persist on average 566 days in patients readmitted at least once and longer persistence is associated with a greater number of colonized anatomical sites [42]. Among discharged patients found to have VRE colonization, median duration of VRE culture positivity from time of discharge was found to be 5.57 weeks [43]. The risk of prolonged carriage was increased if patients received inpatient antibiotics, surgery, or dialysis, and if patients were discharged to a nursing home [43]. For CRE, prior fluoroquinolone use, history of inter-facility transfer, and time interval ≤3months from last positive CRE screen were associated with a greater probability of positive CRE screen on readmission. Persistence of CRE carriage was on average 387 days following hospital discharge, with 78, 65, and 39% of patients retaining CRE carriage at 3, 6, and 12 months, respectively [44, 45]. Because transplant recipients may have longer carriage periods for these organisms, hospitals may consider placing all patients with a history of infection/colonization with MRSA, VRE, or MDR/CRE on contact isolation precautions should they be readmitted to the hospital [40].

Protective Environment Rooms and Hospital Facilities Management

Despite an absence of robust data, use of a protective environment (PE) room is recommended for allogeneic SCT recipients, and can also be considered in patients with profound immunosuppression including autologous SCT recipients, those with prolonged neutropenia, and during episodes of graft-versus-host disease (GVHD) [7, 34, 46]. Allogeneic SCT recipients should ideally be placed in a PE room that includes: ≥12 air exchanges per hour, central or point-of-use high-efficiency particulate air (HEPA) filters (with 99.97% efficiency for removing particles ≥0.3 μm in diameter), directed air flow so that air intake occurs at one side of the room and exhaust occurs at the opposite end, consistent positive air pressure differential between the patient's room and hallway >0.19 mmHg, well-sealed rooms, continuous pressure monitoring, and self-closing doors to maintain constant pressure differentials [34]. Laminar air flow rooms have been used in the past, but aside from some benefit in reducing cases of *Aspergillus* linked to construction, they are not routinely recommended for SCT recipients [28, 47]. Scrupulous maintenance of air supply systems is critical. The hospital facilities department should ensure that filter banks are inspected and routinely changed, water incursion into heating, ventilation, and air conditioning (HVAC) ducts is prevented, and air intakes into the system are kept free of conditions which may result in patient exposure to environmental pathogens (e.g., birds' nests containing *Cryptococcus* spp.). Backup electrical and ventilation systems should be in place for transplant units during emergencies and scheduled downtimes. Anterooms are optional except in the case of SCT recipients requiring airborne precautions for infections such as TB, measles, varicella, or disseminated zoster [34]. Fresh, cut, or potted flowers/plants should not be permitted in PE rooms due to the risk of acquiring infection due to *Aspergillus* spp. and water-borne bacteria that colonize plants [28, 48, 49]. The necessity of PE rooms for allogeneic SCT recipients and other severely immunocompromised hosts is becoming increasingly controversial, and several studies have suggested that morbidity and mortality are not significantly different between patients who were placed in PE rooms and those who were either discharged to their home environments or who did not utilize PE rooms in the hospital setting [50–53]. Further studies should help to elucidate the optimal timing of and nature of isolation precautions for SCT recipients and the role of PE rooms [46].

During hospital construction/renovation, an infection control risk assessment (ICRA) should be performed for each construction site. The ICRA should specify the appropriate environmental controls enacted to minimize dust generation and reduce the risk of fungal dispersion [54]. In addition to routine inspections to ensure the measures outlined in the ICRA are followed, infection control personnel should ensure patients in the vicinity of the construction site are placed in rooms which minimize risk; the use of negative pressure/airborne isolation rooms is avoided unless indicated by the patient's condition [55]. Transplant recipients should avoid construction areas in the hospital if possible and should wear an N95 respirator or a powered air-purifying respirator (PAPR) when being transported outside of the PE room if they are unable to avoid these areas [28]. However, it should be noted that neither of these methods has been specifically tested and proven to decrease the risk of *Aspergillus* infection in this patient population [27, 34]. Surgical masks do not protect patients from airborne particles and their efficacy in preventing exposure to environmental mold spores is unknown. Floor surfaces in SCT units should be smooth and non-porous to facilitate cleaning/disinfection. Furthermore, carpeting and other materials that may harbor mold must be avoided in transplant units. Daily wet dusting of horizontal surfaces using cloths moistened with hospital disinfectant/detergents should be performed in transplant units and cleaning methods that disperse dust should be avoided.

Avoidance of Central Line-Associated Bloodstream Infections

Because of the high utilization of CVCs in transplant patients due to the frequent need for total parenteral nutrition, maintenance of reliable intravenous access, and infusion-related complications when using peripheral catheters, adherence to evidence-based guidelines for preventing CLABSI is crucial [56, 57]. The CLABSI rate (infections per 1000 central line days) for SCT recipients ranges from 2.5 for permanent catheters to 3.0 for temporary catheters, while the infection rate ranges from 0.3 for permanent catheters to 1.2 for temporary catheters in SOT recipients [57]. In comparison, CLABSI rates in general medical or medical/surgical floors range from 0.9 to 1.4 [57]. If implementation of standard practices such as "bundles" during CVC insertion is not effective in reducing the infection rate or if the CLABSI rate is >1, the use of CVCs impregnated with either chlorhexidine/silver sulfadiazine or minocycline/rifampin can be considered [56]. In one study of cancer patients, the use of minocycline/rifampin-impregnated catheters led to a CLABSI rate of 0.25 compared to patients with non-impregnated catheters who had a rate of 1.28 [58]. Another study among patients receiving chemotherapy followed by SCT demonstrated that chlorhexidine/silver sulfadiazine-impregnated CVCs had decreased catheter colonization and a nonstatistically significant trend toward decreased bloodstream infections as compared to non-impregnated CVCs [59]. Utilization of chlorhexidine/silver sulfadiazine-impregnated CVCs has also led to decreased bacterial colonization of catheters and concomitant infections in SOT recipients [60]. While antibiotic lock therapy may be an encouraging approach for line salvage, it is not currently recommended for routine prophylaxis in transplant populations [7]. Although not specifically studied in the transplant population, chlorhexidine-impregnated dressings/sponges at the CVC insertion site should be considered in transplant patients, as they have proven effective in reducing the incidence of CLABSIs and exit-site/tunnel infections among non-transplant recipients with CVCs [61, 62]. Practices to minimize the risk of contamination of CVCs during use, such as disinfection of IV valve devices whenever IV tubing is connected, routine replacement of IV valves, use of alcohol-impregnated caps and scheduled changes of IV tubing must be standardized and rigorously followed. Most importantly, as in all patients, the CVC should be removed as soon as clinically feasible.

Respiratory Viruses

Nosocomial transmission of respiratory viruses has been well-reported [63]. SOT and SCT recipients are at higher risk for developing significant complications related to exposure to respiratory viruses including influenza, RSV, adenovirus, parainfluenza, and human metapneumovirus [64, 65]. Exposure prevention is a key component in reducing the risk for respiratory virus illness in transplant patients because many of these viruses have no treatment options other than supportive care. HCWs and visitors with upper respiratory tract infection (URI) symptoms must avoid contact with SOT and SCT recipients. Active surveillance for URI signs/symptoms should be performed daily in all transplant recipients and their visitors during respiratory virus season [27]. If URI signs/symptoms are present, the patient should be placed on droplet and contact precautions until the precise infectious etiology of signs/symptoms is determined using rapid molecular-based technologies if available [11, 27]. Future studies in transplant patients are needed to define optimal isolation precautions for respiratory viruses owing to the potential for airborne transmission of these viruses [32, 33]. Immunocompromised patients may shed respiratory viruses for weeks to months after initial infection. Therefore, continuing isolation precautions for the duration of the hospitalization should be considered during respiratory virus season [66]. Because pre-engraftment SCT recipients carry the greatest risk of developing severe RSV pneumonia, early diagnosis and treatment are critical when URI symptoms are present in this population. Among SOT recipients, especially lung and renal transplant recipients, influenza infection has been associated with a greater risk of acute transplant rejection [66]. The risk of influenza is highest among lung transplant recipients (41.8 cases/1000 person-years), followed by liver transplant recipients (4.3 cases/1000 person-years), and renal transplant recipients (2.8 cases/1000 person-years) [66]. HCWs, family members, and other close contacts with transplant recipients, should receive seasonal influenza vaccination. If the vaccine is received during an outbreak, antiviral chemoprophylaxis for 2 weeks can be considered for these close contacts of transplant recipients until an appropriate vaccine response is achieved. In the setting of an institutional influenza outbreak, antiviral chemoprophylaxis is recommended for transplant patients in accordance with CDC/ACIP guidelines [67].

Gastrointestinal Infections

Transplant recipients experiencing symptoms consistent with gastrointestinal infection, including nausea, vomiting, and diarrhea, must be considered infectious until an alternative explanation for these symptoms is identified. Prolonged viral shedding of norovirus and other viruses has been reported in transplant recipients even when gastrointestinal symptoms have resolved, therefore, we advocate symptom-based instead of laboratory-based initiation of isolation precautions in these patients [68–71]. While norovirus, rotavirus, and astrovirus have been associated with outbreaks in transplant populations, making a laboratory-based diagnosis is often challenging. The advent of newer molecular techniques for GI pathogen detection offers the promise of improved differentiation between infectious and non-infectious causes of diarrhea; however, their use in transplant recipients has been limited. Due to prolonged and varied viral shedding in transplant recipients, hospitals may consider initiating contact isolation precautions among patients who have a history of gastrointestinal infection if they are readmitted to the hospital even in the absence of gastrointestinal symptoms at the time of readmission.

Varicella Zoster Virus

While VZV is more commonly seen in the late post-transplant period, clinicians must remain vigilant during the early post-transplant period because VZV infection during this period frequently presents as disseminated disease, capable of airborne spread and transmission to susceptible patients and hospital staff [11]. Contact and airborne precautions for VZV should be continued until all lesions are dried and crusted over. Transplant recipients with potential VZV exposure while in the hospital, including being in an enclosed air space with a contagious source patient or having close contact with a contagious source patient in an open area, should be placed on airborne precautions from days 8 to 21 after exposure unless the patient has been given varicella zoster immunoglobulin (VZIG) or acyclovir postexposure chemoprophylaxis, in which case airborne precautions should continue from days 8 to 28 after exposure [11, 72].

Institutional Food and Beverages

Food and beverages consumed in the hospital setting are also potential sources for infection in transplant recipients. Efforts to serve "sterile" food have been unsuccessful, due in large part to lack of palatability of the food [73]. "Low-bacteria" or "neutropenic diets," with highly variable definitions in the literature and in practice, have been used at many institutions. However, data are not convincing that these diets lead to fewer infectious complications and improved clinical outcomes. In fact, one study found a higher rate of infections in transplant recipients who received a "neutropenic diet" as compared to those receiving a general diet [74]. Institutional food handling should adhere to federal, state, and local regulations. Several published guidelines describe safe and unsafe foods for SCT and SOT recipients, and these recommendations are outlined in Table 61.2 [7, 10, 27, 75]. Given the risk of cryptosporidiosis, SCT and SOT recipients should avoid tap water during the early post-transplant period and should only drink bottled water that has been processed to remove *Cryptosporidium* by reverse osmosis, distillation, or 1 μm particulate absolute filtration [7]. Transplant recipients should also avoid fountain beverages and ice made from tap water, as rare instances of nosocomial legionellosis have been reported. An aggressive water-testing program in hospital areas housing susceptible patients should be implemented. Hyperchlorination, silver/copper ionization, and/or superheating should be employed to reduce *Legionella* spp. in the water supply in accordance with published recommendations [7, 48, 76].

Intermediate Post-Solid Organ Transplant (1–6 Months)/Early Post-Engraftment Period (30–100 Days)

Patients often spend the intermediate post-SOT period and the early post-engraftment periods within the hospital environment. Pathogens of concern vary with ongoing immune reconstitution. SOT recipients are at higher risk of developing listeriosis and *Nocardia* infections during this period, while SCT recipients carry higher risks of developing gram-positive infections and respiratory/enteric viral illness (Table 61.1). Both SOT and SCT recipients have a greater likelihood of acquiring or reactivating herpesvirus infections such as HSV, CMV, and EBV during this period. During ongoing and/or recurrent hospitalizations, previously described infection control practices should be followed to minimize exposure to healthcare-associated pathogens.

Blood Products and Cytomegalovirus

Patients in this period frequently require transfusion of blood and blood products due to anemia and thrombocytopenia. CMV-seronegative allogeneic SCT recipients with CMV-seronegative donors (R-D-) should only receive leukocyte-reduced/CMV-seronegative red blood cells or leukocyte-reduced platelets to prevent transfusion-associated CMV infection [27]. However, insufficient evidence exists to support this strategy in CMV-seronegative recipients with CMV-seropositive donors (R-D+) [27]. In CMV-seronegative autologous SCT recipients, CMV-seronegative red blood cells and leukocyte-reduced platelets can be used but are not routinely recommended [7]. In addition to blood products, a comprehensive CMV prevention strategy should continue for SCT patients through first 100 days after transplantation. This strategy should include antiviral prophylaxis, aggressive and regular CMV screening, and use of gloves by HCW when handling blood products or other potentially contaminated biologic materials to prevent transmission of CMV to susceptible SCT recipients. Among SOT recipients, CMV-seronegative donor/recipient pairs (D-R-) should receive only leukocyte reduced/CMV-seronegative blood products [77].

Late Post-Solid Organ Transplant (>6 Months)/Late Post-Engraftment Period (>100 Days)

Patients spend most of the late post-SOT period and late post-engraftment period outside the hospital environment, with the majority of healthcare contacts occurring during outpatient clinic visits. CDC has recently published an infection control and prevention framework for outpatient oncology settings, and these recommendations should also serve as a basis for outpatient transplant clinics [78]. Although still immune suppressed, the spectrum of infectious complications during this period changes dramatically. For SOT recipients, bacterial pathogens from the community predominate. There is also a second peak of invasive *Aspergillus* infections [16]. For SCT and SOT recipients, CMV remains a concern and transmission in the home environment can occur from many sources. Transplant recipients and their household contacts must be educated to practice good hand hygiene, especially if handling soiled diapers and when in contact with nasal secretions so that they prevent exposure to CMV and respiratory viruses. Several guidelines and expert opinions to reduce household exposure to infectious pathogens following transplantation have been published for SCT and SOT recipients [7, 79–81]. Despite the absence of strong evidence, most published reports agree that SCT and SOT recipients have the greatest risk of infection in the first 6 months after transplantation and when immune suppression is augmented to prevent rejection [27, 81]. Allogeneic SCT recipients with chronic GVHD, those with cancer recurrence, and those with secondary graft loss or graft compromise remain at highest risk for infections during this period. Among SOT recipients, recurrence of the primary malignancy, namely liver and kidney, and patients receiving antineoplastic therapy for late-onset neoplasms remain at highest risk for development of infections during this period.

Avoidance of Infections After Transplantation

While avoidance of potentially infectious organisms is paramount, appropriate vaccination of transplant recipients is also important during this period as discussed elsewhere in this book. A thorough discussion with the patient and their close contacts regarding the risks of infections developing outside the hospital environment is crucial and must take into account the desire for the transplant recipient to regain a sense of normalcy post-transplant. Most infectious organisms in this period are acquired through direct contact, ingestion, or inhalation. Hand hygiene is a key component of reducing infectious risk: hands should be washed before preparing food, eating, and touching mucous membranes. Good hand hygiene needs to be followed after transplant recipients handle or clean up after pets, garden or touch plants/soil, change diapers, and touch secretions/excretions and after touching items that have had contact with human or animal feces [27, 81]. Gloves should be worn during outdoor activities when handling soil, moss, or manure, walking barefoot should be avoided, and long-sleeved shirts/long pants should be worn while performing yard work to minimize abrasions and cuts from bushes and shrubs. These efforts will decrease exposure to potentially invasive fungal diseases such as sporotrichosis [28, 79]. To minimize the risk of respiratory illness, transplant recipients should avoid close contact with persons with respiratory illnesses and crowded areas during respiratory virus season. Frequent use of alcohol-based handwash/rub may decrease the risk of infection [14]. Tobacco smoking and marijuana should be avoided to decrease the risk for respiratory virus infection and exposure to *Aspergillus* spp., respectively [28, 82, 83].

Transplant recipients may also need to consider changes in their occupation and consider delaying return to work until after the critical 6-month period post-transplant has elapsed. If delayed return to employment is not possible, patients should be counseled extensively regarding protective measures if their occupation places them at risk for particular infections. Some such workplace risks include airborne mold (construction), TB (healthcare), or respiratory virus infection (education, retail, healthcare, or office settings). In addition, transplant recipients who work with animals should avoid this work environment if possible for the first 6 months after transplantation. SCT recipients living in or visiting areas with endemic levels of coccidiomycosis should avoid or minimize exposure to disturbed soil, while recipients living in or visiting areas with endemic levels of histoplasmosis should avoid chicken coops or other bird-roosting sites and caves during the first 6 months after transplantation [27]. While exercise and outdoor activities are recommended and may be beneficial for transplant recipients, some activities including hunting, camping, fishing, spelunking, and canoeing can be associated with the development of invasive fungal disease in immunocompromised hosts. Therefore, these activities should be limited at least for the first 6 months after transplantation or during times of increased immunosuppression [79].

Counseling about sexual behaviors is also important in the late post-transplant period for SCT and SOT recipients. Latex condoms should be used to reduce the chance of exposure to HIV, HBV, HCV, HSV, and CMV. Sexual partners of transplant recipients could also consider receiving serologic testing for CMV to better characterize risks of transmission [7].

During periods of maximal immune suppression, especially during the first 6 months after transplantation, transplant recipients should avoid contact with domesticated animals that have diarrheal illness and should wash hands regularly after handling pets. Transplant recipients should avoid cleaning bird cages and litter boxes, handling animal feces including bird droppings, and should wear gloves when cleaning aquariums or designate another household member to perform this task [16]. If avoidance of the above activities is not possible, transplant recipients should wear disposable gloves and wash hands with soap and water for 15 s after removing gloves. Transplant recipients should avoid stray animals, animal bites, and contact with nonhuman primates. Transplant recipients and clinicians should be mindful of infectious risks posed by certain animals: rodents (lymphocytic choriomeningitis virus), young cats (*Bartonella henselae*), all cats (*Toxoplasma gondii*), and reptiles/chickens/ducklings (*Salmonella* spp.) [81]. Finally, recipients should defer obtaining a new pet until 1 year after transplantation and when on a stable immunosuppressive regimen.

Consumption of contaminated water or inadvertent ingestion of water during recreational activities may increase the chance of developing infections after transplantation. *Cryptosporidium* has been identified as a cause of severe diarrhea in both SCT and SOT populations [81]. Unlike other organisms, *Cryptosporidium* is not killed by chlorine. Therefore, even treated water supplies cannot be assuredly free of this organism. In order to eliminate the risk of *Cryptosporidium*, transplant recipients can boil water for at least 1 min or use filtered/bottled water as described earlier in this chapter. Well, lake, and river water should not be ingested. In addition, transplant recipients should avoid swimming in water likely to be contaminated with human or animal waste. Hot tubs should be avoided to reduce the risk of *Pseudomonas* folliculitis, legionellosis, and nontuberculous mycobacterial infections (NTM). "Hot tub lung" caused by *Mycobacterium avium* complex and *Mycobacterium kansasii* can present with significant cough, fever, and hypoxia, while exposure to other NTM such as *Mycobacterium chelonae* (cutaneous infections), *Mycobacterium abscessus* (pulmonary and cutaneous infections), and *Mycobacterium marinum* (cutaneous infections) can lead to a diverse presentation of illnesses. Water leaks within the home or basement should be promptly repaired and water-damaged materials should be removed within 48 hours if still damp to avoid mold growth [81]. Guidelines regarding foods to be avoided have been published and are described in Table 61.2 [7, 10, 27]. The FDA has published a practical patient handout for transplant recipients describing food safety practices in the home environment [84].

Transplant recipients and clinicians need to be aware of geographic risk factors associated with travel to or residence in various parts of the world where the risk for endemic infections may differ from their location of origin. This issue is paramount during times of significant immune suppression. In general, allogeneic SCT recipients should not travel to developing countries for 6–12 months after transplantation, while autologous SCT recipients should defer travel for 3–6 months after transplantation [16, 27]. SOT recipients should defer travel to developing countries until 3–6 months after transplantation [80]. All transplant recipients should avoid regions with visceral leishmaniasis (Kala-Azar) and trypanosomiasis and rural parts of Africa, Mexico, South and Central America, and Asia to avoid potential exposure to various diseases including rabies. A hallmark of disease prevention when traveling to the developing world is appropriate vaccination, which is outlined elsewhere in this book as well as in CDC's Yellow Book published online [85]. The Yellow Book also provides detailed information about geographic risks for endemic pathogens. A recent review summarizes risks of fungal infections in immunocompromised travelers [86]. Transplant recipients should consider evaluation at a travelers' health clinic prior to such travel, as each destination presents unique geographic risk factors. Diarrheal illness is common among travelers and may lead to dehydration and acute kidney injury, which can subsequently lead to increased levels and toxicity of immunosuppressive agents. Transplant recipients should be cautioned to consume only boiled or bottled water/beverages and to avoid raw food and food sold by street vendors while abroad. Transplant recipients should bring antibiotics, typically fluoroquinolones or azithromycin, to treat empirically for infectious diarrhea while traveling. Clinicians should inform patients that azithromycin might increase the levels of cyclosporine and tacrolimus [80]. The risk of influenza varies based on travel location: in tropical climates, influenza is seen year-round; in the northern hemisphere, influenza peaks between October and April; and in the southern hemisphere, influenza peaks between May and October. Malarial prophylaxis should be considered when traveling to an endemic area, but clinicians should note the potential drug-drug interactions between antimalarial medications and immunosuppressive medications. Additional discussion of travel-related zoonoses and malaria can be found in other sections of this book.

Conclusion

Infection control and prevention in transplant populations presents challenges to clinicians and infection control practitioners in both the pre-transplant and post-transplant periods.

Guidelines and recommendations in this population are frequently based on small studies and historical experiences, and often more questions than answers are generated by clinicians owing to lack of conclusive evidence in this field [87]. However, despite the absence of definitive studies in this population, standard precautions, appropriate antimicrobial prophylaxis, and avoidance of potential sources of infection should be emphasized throughout the entire transplantation process to reduce the likelihood of infections in this vulnerable population.

References

1. Fishman JA. Infections in immunocompromised hosts and organ transplant recipients: essentials. Liver Transplant. 2011;17(Suppl 3):S34–7.
2. Gafter-Gvili A, Fraser A, Paul M, Vidal L, Lawrie T, van de Wetering M, et al. Antibiotic prophylaxis for bacterial infections in afebrile neutropenic patients following chemotherapy. Cochrane Database Syst Rev. 2012;1:CD004386.
3. Goodman JL, Winston DJ, Greenfield RA, Chandrasekar PH, et al. A controlled trial of fluconazole to prevent fungal infections in patients undergoing bone marrow transplantation. N Engl J Med. 1992;326(13):845–51.
4. Goodrich J, Bowden R, Fisher L, et al. Ganciclovir prophylaxis to prevent cytomegalovirus disease after allogeneic marrow transplant. Ann Intern Med. 1993;118:173–8.
5. Sepkowitz K. Antibiotic prophylaxis in patients receiving hematopoietic stem cell transplant. Bone Marrow Transplant. 2002;29:367–71.
6. Busca ASE, Giacchino M, et al. Analysis of early infectious complications in pediatric patients undergoing bone marrow transplantation. Support Care Cancer. 1999;7:253–9.
7. Tomblyn M, Chiller T, Einsele H, Gress R, Sepkowitz K, Storek J, et al. Guidelines for preventing infectious complications among hematopoietic cell transplantation recipients: a global perspective. Biol Blood Marrow Transplant. 2009;15(10):1143–238.
8. Patel R, Paya C. Infections in solid-organ transplant recipients. Clin Microbiol Rev. 1997;10(1):86.
9. Taylor AL, Watson CJ, Bradley JA. Immunosuppressive agents in solid organ transplantation: mechanisms of action and therapeutic efficacy. Crit Rev Oncol Hematol. 2005;56(1):23–46.
10. Obayashi PA. Food safety for the solid organ transplant patient: preventing foodborne illness while on chronic immunosuppressive drugs. Nutr Clin Pract. 2012;27(6):758–66.
11. Siegel JD, Rhinehart E, Jackson M, Chiarello L, the Healthcare Infection Control Practices Advisory Committee. 2007 guideline for isolation precautions: preventing transmission of infectious agents in healthcare settings; 2007.
12. Magauran C, Salgado C. Challenges and advances in infection control of hematopoietic stem cell transplant recipients. Infect Disord Drug Targets. 2011;11:18–26.
13. Siegel JD, Rhinehart E, Jackson M, Chiarello L, the Healthcare Infection Control Practices Advisory Committee. Management of multidrug-resistant organisms in healthcare settings; 2006. https://www.cdc.gov/mrsa/pdf/mdroGuideline2006.pdf
14. Guideline for Hand Hygiene in Health-Care Settings: Recommendations of the Healthcare Infection Control Practices Advisory Committee and the HICPAC/SHEA/APIC/IDSA Hand Hygiene Task Force MMWR: Centers for Disease Control and Prevention; 2002. p. RR-16.
15. Bratzler DW, Dellinger EP, Olsen KM, Perl TM, Auwaerter PG, Bolon MK, et al. Clinical practice guidelines for antimicrobial prophylaxis in surgery. Am J Health Syst Pharm. 2013;70(3):195–283.
16. Kusnea S, Krystofiak S. Infection control issues after bone marrow transplantation. Curr Opin Infect Dis. 2001;14:427–31.
17. Morris M. Pre-transplant recipient evaluation & management. http://www.antimicrobe.org/final/t33.asp. Cited 14 Aug 2016.
18. Fishman JA, Issa NC. Infection in organ transplantation: risk factors and evolving patterns of infection. Infect Dis Clin N Am. 2010;24(2):273–83.
19. Avery RK. Recipient screening prior to solid-organ transplantation. Clin Infect Dis. 2002;35:1513–9.
20. Shaffner A. Pretransplant evaluation for infections in donors and recipients of solid organs. Clin Infect Dis. 2001;33(Suppl 1):S9–14.
21. Services USDoHaH. Guidance for industry: eligibility determination for donors of human cells, tissues, and cellular and tissue-based products (HCT/Ps). In: Administration FaD, editor; 2007.
22. Casas S, Muñoz L, Moure R, Castellote J, Guerra MR, Gonzalez L, et al. Comparison of the 2-step tuberculin skin test and the quantiFERON-TB gold in-tube test for the screening of tuberculosis infection before liver transplantation. Liver Transplant. 2011;17(10):1205–11.
23. Theodoropoulos N, Lanternier F, Rassiwala J, McNatt G, Preczewski L, DeMayo E, et al. Use of the QuantiFERON-TB Gold interferon-gamma release assay for screening transplant candidates: a single-center retrospective study. Transplant Infect Dis. 2012;14(1):1–8.
24. Russo RL, Dulley FL, Suganuma L, Franca IL, Yasuda MA, Costa SF. Tuberculosis in hematopoietic stem cell transplant patients: case report and review of the literature. Int J Infect Dis. 2010;14(Suppl 3):e187–91.
25. Ferrara G, Losi M, D'Amico R, Roversi P, Piro R, Meacci M, et al. Use in routine clinical practice of two commercial blood tests for diagnosis of infection with Mycobacterium tuberculosis: a prospective study. Lancet. 2006;367(9519):1328–34.
26. Kim SY, Jung GS, Kim SK, Chang J, Kim MS, Kim YS, et al. Comparison of the tuberculin skin test and interferon-gamma release assay for the diagnosis of latent tuberculosis infection before kidney transplantation. Infection. 2013;41(1):103–10.
27. Guidelines for preventing opportunistic infections among hematopoietic stem cell transplant recipients: recommendations of CDC, the Infectious Disease Society of America, and the American Society of Blood and Marrow Transplantation. MMWR: Centers for Disease Control and Prevention; 2000.
28. Partridge-Hinckley K, Liddell GM, Almyroudis NG, Segal BH. Infection control measures to prevent invasive mould diseases in hematopoietic stem cell transplant recipients. Mycopathologia. 2009;168(6):329–37.
29. Immunization of Health-Care Personnel Recommendations of the Advisory Committee on Immunization Practices (ACIP). MMWR: Centers for Disease Control and Prevention; 2011. p. 1–46.
30. Ljungman P, Cordonnier C, Einsele H, Englund J, Machado CM, Storek J, et al. Vaccination of hematopoietic cell transplant recipients. Bone Marrow Transplant. 2009;44(8):521–6.
31. Bolyard E, Tablan O, Williams W, Pearson ML, Shapiro C, Deitchman S, et al. Guideline for infection control in healthcare personnel. Infect Control Hosp Epidemiol. 1998;19:407–63.
32. Bischoff WE, Swett K, Leng I, Peters TR. Exposure to influenza virus aerosols during routine patient care. J Infect Dis. 2013;207(7):1037–46.
33. Noti JD, Lindsley WG, Blachere FM, Cao G, Kashon ML, Thewlis RE, et al. Detection of infectious influenza virus in cough aerosols generated in a simulated patient examination room. Clin Infect Dis. 2012;54(11):1569–77.
34. Yokoe D, Casper C, Dubberke E, Lee G, Munoz P, Palmore T, et al. Infection prevention and control in health-care facilities in which

hematopoietic cell transplant recipients are treated. Bone Marrow Transplant. 2009;44(8):495–507.
35. Huang S, Yokoe D, Hinrichsen V, et al. Impact of routine intensive care unit surveillance cultures and resultant barrier precautions on hospital-wide methicillin-resistant Staphylococcus aureus bacteremia. Clin Infect Dis. 2006;43:971–8.
36. Russell DL, Flood A, Zaroda TE, Acosta C, Riley MM, Busuttil RW, et al. Outcomes of colonization with MRSA and VRE among liver transplant candidates and recipients. Am J Transplant. 2008;8(8):1737–43.
37. Singh N, Squier C, Wannstedt C, et al. Impact of an aggressive infection control strategy on endemic Staphylococcus aureus infection in liver transplant recipients. Infect Control Hosp Epidemiol. 2006;27:122–6.
38. Patel G, Perez F, Bonomo RA. Carbapenem-resistant Enterobacteriaceae and Acinetobacter baumannii: assessing their impact on organ transplantation. Curr Opin Organ Transplant. 2010;15(6):676–82.
39. Bert F, Larroque B, Paugam-Burtz C, Dondero F, Durand F, Marcon E, et al. Pretransplant fecal carriage of extended-spectrum beta-lactamase-producing Enterobacteriaceae and infection after liver transplant, France. Emerg Infect Dis. 2012;18(6):908–16.
40. Banach D, Bearman G, Barnden M, Hanrahan J, Leekha S, Morgan D, Wiemken T. Duration of contact precautions for acute-care settings. Infect Control Hosp Epidemiol. 2018;39(2):127–44. https://doi.org/10.1017/ice.2017.245
41. Hicheri Y, Einsele H, Martino R, Cesaro S, Ljungman P, Cordonnier C. Environmental prevention of infection in stem cell transplant recipients: a survey of the Infectious Diseases Working Party of the European Group for Blood and Marrow Transplantation. Transpl Infect Dis. 2013;15(3):251–8.
42. Mattner F, Biertz F, Ziesing S, Gastmeier P, Chaberny IF. Long-term persistence of MRSA in re-admitted patients. Infection. 2010;38(5):363–71.
43. Sohn KM, Peck KR, Joo EJ, Ha YE, Kang CI, Chung DR, et al. Duration of colonization and risk factors for prolonged carriage of vancomycin-resistant enterococci after discharge from the hospital. Int J Infect Dis. 2013;17(4):e240–6.
44. Schechner V, Kotlovsky T, Tarabeia J, Kazma M, Schwartz D, Navon-Venezia S, et al. Predictors of rectal carriage of carbapenem-resistant Enterobacteriaceae (CRE) among patients with known CRE carriage at their next hospital encounter. Infect Control Hosp Epidemiol. 2011;32(5):497–503.
45. Zimmerman FS, Assous MV, Bdolah-Abram T, Lachish T, Yinnon AM, Wiener-Well Y. Duration of carriage of carbapenem-resistant Enterobacteriaceae following hospital discharge. Am J Infect Control. 2013;41(3):190–4.
46. Hayes-Lattin B, Leis JF, Maziarz RT. Isolation in the allogeneic transplant environment: how protective is it? Bone Marrow Transplant. 2005;36(5):373–81.
47. Cornet M, Levy V, Fleury L, Lortholary J. Efficacy of prevention by high-efficiency particulate air filtration or laminar airflow against aspergillus airborne contamination during hospital renovation. Infect Control Hosp Epidemiol. 1999;20(7):508–13.
48. Sehulster LM, Chinn RYW, Arduino MJ, Carpenter J, Donlan R, Ashford D, Besser R, Fields B, McNeil MM, Whitney C, Wong S, Juranek D, Cleveland J. Guidelines for environmental infection control in health-care facilities. Recommendations from CDC and the Healthcare Infection Control Practices Advisory Committee (HICPAC); 2004. www.cdc.gov/ncidod/hip/enviro/guidehtm
49. Walsh T, Dixon D. Nosocomial aspergillosis: environmental microbiology, hospital epidemiology, diagnosis, and treatment. Eur J Epidemiol. 1989;5:131–42.
50. Russell J, Chaudhry A, Booth K. Early outcomes after allogeneic stem cell transplantation for leukemia and myelodysplasia without protective isolation: a 10-year experience. Biol Blood Marrow Transplant. 2000;6(2):109–14.
51. Fernandez-Aviles F, Carreras E, Urbano-Ispizua A, Rovira M, Martinez C, Gaya A, et al. Case-control comparison of at-home to total hospital care for autologous stem-cell transplantation for hematologic malignancies. J Clin Oncol. 2006;24(30):4855–61.
52. Russell J, Poon M-C, Jones A, Woodman R, Ruether B. Allogeneic bone-marrow transplantation without protective isolation in adults with malignant disease. Lancet. 1992;339:38–40.
53. Svahn BM, Remberger M, Myrback KE, Holmberg K, Eriksson B, Hentschke P, et al. Home care during the pancytopenic phase after allogeneic hematopoietic stem cell transplantation is advantageous compared with hospital care. Blood. 2002;100(13):4317–24.
54. Mayhall CG. Hospital epidemiology and infection control. Philadelphia: Lippincott Williams & Wilkins; 2012.
55. Novosad SA, Vasquez A, Nambiar A, et al. Notes from the field. probable mucormycosis among adult solid organ transplant recipients at an acute care hospital—Pennsylvania, 2014–2015. MMWR Morb Mortal Wkly Rep. 2016;65:481–2.
56. O'Grady NP, Alexander M, Burns LA, Dellinger EP, Garland J, Heard SO, et al. Guidelines for the prevention of intravascular catheter-related infections. Am J Infect Control. 2011;39(4. Suppl 1):S1–34.
57. National Healthcare Safety Network (NHSN) report, data summary for 2010, device-associated module. Centers for Disease Control and Prevention; 2010.
58. Hanna H, Benjamin R, Chatzinikolaou I, Alakech B, Richardson D, Mansfield P, et al. Long-term silicone central venous catheters impregnated with minocycline and rifampin decrease rates of catheter-related bloodstream infection in cancer patients: a prospective randomized clinical trial. J Clin Oncol. 2004;22(15):3163–71.
59. Maaskant JM, De Boer JP, Dalesio O, Holtkamp MJ, Lucas C. The effectiveness of chlorhexidine-silver sulfadiazine impregnated central venous catheters in patients receiving high-dose chemotherapy followed by peripheral stem cell transplantation. Eur J Cancer Care. 2009;18(5):477–82.
60. George S, Vuddamalay P, Boscoe M. Antiseptic impregnated central venous catheters reduce the incidence of bacterial colonization and associated infection in immunocompromised transplant patients. Eur J Anaesthesiol. 1997;14:428–31.
61. Timsit JF, Mimoz O, Mourvillier B, Souweine B, Garrouste-Orgeas M, Alfandari S, et al. Randomized controlled trial of chlorhexidine dressing and highly adhesive dressing for preventing catheter-related infections in critically ill adults. Am J Resp Crit Care Med. 2012;186(12):1272–8.
62. Chambers ST, Sanders J, Patton WN, Ganly P, Birch M, Crump JA, et al. Reduction of exit-site infections of tunnelled intravascular catheters among neutropenic patients by sustained-release chlorhexidine dressings: results from a prospective randomized controlled trial. J Hosp Infect. 2005;61(1):53–61.
63. Aitken C, Jeffries DJ. Nosocomial spread of viral disease. Clin Microbiol Rev. 2001;14(3):528–46.
64. Weigt SS, Gregson AL, Deng JC, Lynch JP 3rd, Belperio JA. Respiratory viral infections in hematopoietic stem cell and solid organ transplant recipients. Semin Respir Crit Care Med. 2011;32(4):471–93.
65. Raboni SM, Nogueira MB, Tsuchiya LR, Takahashi GA, Pereira LA, Pasquini R, et al. Respiratory tract viral infections in bone marrow transplant patients. Transplantation. 2003;76(1):142–6.
66. Martin ST, Torabi MJ, Gabardi S. Influenza in solid organ transplant recipients. Ann Pharmacother. 2012;46(2):255–64.
67. Antiviral agents for the treatment and chemoprophylaxis of influenza. Recommendations of the Advisory Committee on Immunization Practices (ACIP). MMWR: Centers for Disease Control and Prevention; 2011.

68. Roos-Weil D, Ambert-Balay K, Lanternier F, Mamzer-Bruneel MF, Nochy D, Pothier P, et al. Impact of norovirus/sapovirus-related diarrhea in renal transplant recipients hospitalized for diarrhea. Transplantation. 2011;92(1):61–9.
69. Henke-Gendo C, Harste G, Juergens-Saathoff B, Mattner F, Deppe H, Heim A. New real-time PCR detects prolonged norovirus excretion in highly immunosuppressed patients and children. J Clin Microbiol. 2009;47(9):2855–62.
70. Schorn R, Hohne M, Meerbach A, Bossart W, Wuthrich RP, Schreier E, et al. Chronic norovirus infection after kidney transplantation: molecular evidence for immune-driven viral evolution. Clin Infect Dis. 2010;51(3):307–14.
71. Bok K, Green KY. Norovirus gastroenteritis in immunocompromised patients. N Engl J Med. 2012;367(22):2126–32.
72. Zuckerman RA, Limaye AP. Varicella zoster virus (VZV) and herpes simplex virus (HSV) in solid organ transplant patients. Am J Transplant. 2013;13(Suppl 3):55–66; quiz.
73. Donnelly JP. Infection prevention – protected environment and infection control. In: Safdar A, editor. Principles and practice of cancer infectious diseases. New York: Humana Press; 2011. p. 541–50.
74. Trifilio S, Helenowski I, Giel M, Gobel B, Pi J, Greenberg D, et al. Questioning the role of a neutropenic diet following hematopoetic stem cell transplantation. Biol Blood Marrow Transplant. 2012;18(9):1385–90.
75. FDA food code: US Food and Drug Administration; 2013. Available from: http://www.fda.gov/downloads/Food/GuidanceRegulation/RetailFoodProtection/FoodCode/UCM374510.pdf. Cited 24 Aug 2016.
76. O'Connor KA, Kingston M, O'Donovan M, Cryan B, Twomey C, O'Mahony D. Antibiotic prescribing policy and Clostridium difficile diarrhoea. QJM. 2004;97(7):423–9.
77. Kotton CN, Kumar D, Caliendo AM, Asberg A, Chou S, Snydman DR, et al. International consensus guidelines on the management of cytomegalovirus in solid organ transplantation. Transplantation. 2010;89(7):779–95.
78. Basic infection control and prevention plan for outpatient oncology settings: Centers for Disease Control and Prevention; 2011. Available from: http://www.cdc.gov/HAI/settings/outpatient/basic-infection-control-prevention-plan-2011/index.html. Cited 14 Aug 2016.
79. Sipsas NV, Kontoyiannis DP. Occupation, lifestyle, diet, and invasive fungal infections. Infection. 2008;36(6):515–25.
80. Kotton CN, Ryan ET, Fishman JA. Prevention of infection in adult travelers after solid organ transplantation. Am J Transplant. 2005;5(1):8–14.
81. Avery RK, Michaels MG. Strategies for safe living following solid organ transplantation. Am J Transplant. 2009;9(Suppl 4):S252–7.
82. Cescon DP, AV; Richardson S, Moore MJ. Invasive pulmonary aspergillosis associated with marijuana use in a man with colorectal cancer. J Clin Oncol. 2008;26(13):2214–5.
83. Szyper-Kravitz M, Lang R, Manor Y, Lahav M. Early invasive pulmonary aspergillosis in a leukemia patient linked to aspergillus contaminated marijuana smoking. Leuk Lymphoma. 2001;42:1433–7.
84. Food safety for transplant recipients: US Food and Drug Administration; 2011. Available from: http://www.fda.gov/Food/ResourcesForYou/Consumers/SelectedHealthTopics/ucm312570.htm. Cited 14 Aug 2016.
85. The Yellow Book: Centers for Disease Control and Prevention; 2012. Available from: http://wwwnc.cdc.gov/travel/yellowbook/2012/chapter-2-the-pre-travel-consultation/the-pre-travel-consultation.htm. Cited 14 Aug 2016.
86. Lortholary O, Charlier C, Lebeaux D, Lecuit M, Consigny PH. Fungal infections in immunocompromised travelers. Clin Infect Dis. 2013;56(6):861–9.
87. Kontoyiannis DP. Preventing fungal disease in chronically immunosuppressed outpatients: time for action? Ann Intern Med. 2013;158(7):555–7.
88. Fishman JA. Infection in solid-organ transplant recipients. N Engl J Med. 2007;357:2601–14.
89. Wingard JR, Hsu J, Hiemenz JW. Hematopoietic stem cell transplantation: an overview of infection risks and epidemiology. Hematol Oncol Clin North Am. 2011;25(1):101–16.
90. Guides for people at risk of foodborne illness: food and drug administration; 2012. Available from: http://www.fda.gov/Food/ResourcesForYou/Consumers/SelectedHealthTopics/default.htm
91. Lund BM, O'Brien SJ. Microbiological safety of food in hospitals and other healthcare settings. J Hospital Infect. 2009;73(2):109–20.
92. Cutro SR, Dean R, Phillips MS. Implementation of a restricted foods policy at a large academic medical center. Infect Control Hosp Epidemiol. 2014;35(6):749–51.

Travel and Transplantation

62

Camille Nelson Kotton and José G. Montoya

Introduction

Transplant recipients are growing in number, and as their overall health improves, they are more likely to engage in foreign travel and experience exposures to endemic pathogens. Transplant recipients are at higher risk of complications from travel-related infections and are less likely to respond to vaccines; furthermore, vaccines containing live attenuated strains are contraindicated in the subset of severely immunocompromised recipients. This review will summarize the medical literature regarding travel medicine and travel-related vaccines in the adult transplant recipient population. In addition, the infectious disease risks of "transplant tourism" that includes travel by either the donor or recipient for the express purpose of undergoing organ transplantation will be discussed.

A travel medicine specialist who is familiar with patients' immunocompromised state and medications should see transplant recipients who wish to travel. Optimizing their care should include excellent and comprehensive advice and education on travel medicine and vaccinations. Travel medicine specialists for complex patients should confer with the travelers' other physicians as needed to develop an appropriate plan. Three recent surveys of transplant centers found significant rates of illness in transplant recipients during foreign travel and insufficient rates of pre-travel counseling and interventions. In one survey of 267 solid organ transplant recipients at the University of Toronto, 36% indicated that they had recently traveled outside Canada and the United States; 66% of travelers sought pre-travel advice, primarily from their transplant physician. In general, many of the recommended preventative measures were overlooked: 63% traveled to areas where hepatitis A was endemic, but only 5% had received hepatitis A immunization; 50% traveled to dengue- and malaria-endemic areas, but only 25% adhered to mosquito prevention measures; and 10% reported behaviors that exposed them to blood or body fluids [1]. A review at the Mayo Clinic, Rochester, Minnesota, found that of 1130 solid organ transplant recipients, 27% had reported travel outside of the United States or Canada after undergoing transplantation; 16% had traveled to destinations at higher risk for infectious diseases, and travelers to these destinations were more likely to be men (73% vs 54% of low-infection risk travelers; $P = 0.018$) or born outside the United States or Canada (29% vs 6%; $P < 0.0001$) [2]. Liver recipients were more likely to travel than other organ recipients. Ninety-six percent of travelers reported that they did not seek specific pre-travel healthcare consul before foreign trip; 8% of travelers required medical attention because of illness, and illness was significantly more likely among travelers to high-infection risk (18%) than low-risk (6%) destinations ($P = 0.004$). Another cross-sectional, descriptive study of 290 Dutch kidney transplant recipients evaluated their travel health knowledge, attitudes, and practices while staying abroad. Thirty-four percent had traveled outside Western Europe and Northern America; 22% of these travelers did not seek pre-travel health advice, and 29% were ill during their most recent journey [3]. Transplant physicians were most frequently (53%) consulted for the pre-travel advice. Four of 17 ill recipients (24%) needed hospitalization, reflecting the high morbidity of travel-related diseases in the susceptible transplant population.

C. N. Kotton
Transplant and Immunocompromised Host Infectious Diseases, Division of Infectious Diseases, Massachusetts General Hospital, Travelers' Advice and Immunization Center, Division of Infectious Diseases, Massachusetts General Hospital, Harvard Medical School, Boston, MA, USA
e-mail: ckotton@partners.org

J. G. Montoya (✉)
Division of Infectious Diseases and Geographic Medicine, Stanford University School of Medicine, Stanford, CA, USA

Palo Alto Medical Foundation Toxoplasma Serology Laboratory, National Reference Center for the Study and Diagnosis of Toxoplasmosis, Palo Alto, CA, USA
e-mail: gilberto@stanford.edu

A. Safdar (ed.), *Principles and Practice of Transplant Infectious Diseases*, https://doi.org/10.1007/978-1-4939-9034-4_62

Planning Travel

Numerous factors can alter the risks of travel, as outlined in Table 62.1. Timing of travel can be an important decision. Significantly immunocompromised hosts include those who underwent hematopoietic stem cell transplantation (HSCT) within the past 2 years or recipients of solid organ transplant (SOT) within a year after transplantation [4, 5] (Table 62.1) Additional factors associated with higher levels of immune suppression include patients with recent treatment for rejection after SOT or significant doses of immunosuppressive medications for treatment of graft-versus-host disease (GVHD), AIDS with low CD4 counts, active leukemia or lymphoma, metastatic solid organ malignancy, aplastic anemia, congenital immunodeficiency, or persons who have received recent radiation therapy [4]. Patients with chronic hepatic disease due to cirrhosis and alcoholism, chronic renal disease, poorly controlled diabetes, asplenia, and nutritional deficiencies could be considered moderately to severely immunosuppressed, depending on the details of their disease [4]. Transplant recipients more than 2 years after HSCT and who are not on immunosuppressive drugs and without GVHD or solid organ transplant recipients more than 1 year after transplant on standard low-dose antirejection medications without recent allograft rejection episode are less immunocompromised and could be better able to face the risks associated with foreign travel.

Table 62.1 Travel planning and educational topics for travel medicine in immunocompromised hosts

Travel planning: Defining and moderating risk
Timing after transplant (> 1 year for destinations with infection risk) [4]
Net state of immunosuppression
Delay travel after treatment of rejection or periods of higher immunosuppression
Location of travel
Risk of specific infection(s); esp. yellow fever zones
Availability of good healthcare/medications
Rich country vs tropical poor country
Type and length of travel
Visiting friends and relatives (VFR) conveys risk of infection
Luxury versus backpacking
Short stay versus relocation
Educational topics
Food and water precautions
Mosquito precautions
Blood-/sex-borne infection precautions
Sun and altitude precautions
Traveler's diarrhea
Every patient travels with antibiotics
Respiratory, skin, other infections
Plan if sick in foreign country
Medical evacuation insurance

Location of travel is another important decision. Certain regions may convey a higher risk of specific infections, i.e., as with meningococcal disease and yellow fever virus. Immunocompromised hosts should be encouraged to defer travel during outbreaks of dengue fever, chikungunya, Eastern equine encephalitis, Zika virus endemic regions, and viral hemorrhagic illness such as Ebola virus disease. Regional outbreaks of novel respiratory tract infection such as Middle East respiratory syndrome (MERS) may cause serious illness in the immunosuppressed transplant recipients and should be avoided. The availability of good healthcare, medications, and other resources may improve outcomes. Also, the overall level of risk of infection in developed compared with developing or underdeveloped tropical countries may be lower.

Type and length of travel can also impact risk for acquiring an infection. Visiting friends and relatives (VFR) conveys a higher risk of numerous infections. Similarly, luxury travel is less likely to result in infection, compared with travel, e.g., involving backpacking. Short-stay travel for less than 2 weeks of tourism also conveys a lower risk compared with a month or longer stays.

Non-vaccine Preventable Illness

Diarrhea is the most common illness of travelers, affecting 10–60% of travelers with suppressed immune function. Dehydration may compromise renal function and markedly increase nephrotoxicity of calcineurin inhibitors such as tacrolimus; further worsening in renal function promotes systemic toxicity of these drugs due to unintended rise in serum drug concentration. Complications of diarrhea may include altered intestinal absorption and metabolism of oral immunosuppressive medications, as well as intestinal translocation of bacteria and less commonly yeasts resulting in hematogenous dissemination and seeding of distant body sites. Prior to international travel, organ recipients should be instructed in appropriate food and water precautions [6]. In general, SOT recipients should be cautioned to drink boiled or bottled water and other beverages, to avoid food sold by street vendors and raw foods with the exception of fruit and vegetables that can be peeled after thoroughly washing them in previously boiled water, and to be cautious about the cleanliness of the source of their food. If transplant recipients develop diarrhea for more than 2 days while traveling, especially with fever, vomiting, and/or bloody stools, patients should consider seeking medical attention; they should carry appropriate self-treatment oral medications such as ciprofloxacin or azithromycin. Due to microbial resistance, trimethoprim-sulfamethoxazole is generally ineffective against travelers' diarrhea. There are no data regarding the use of antimotility agents in transplant recipients with diarrhea; however, such agents may delay clearance of toxins from the gut. Transplant recipients with an acute decline in renal function may be at a higher risk for salicylate toxicity; in the gastrointestinal tract, bismuth subsalicylate commercially available as Pepto-Bismol is converted to salicylic acid and insoluble bismuth salts. Prophylaxis against bacterial traveler's diarrhea with daily antibiotics is very rarely indicated and should only be considered for short-term use, after considering the risks of antibiotic resistance, *Clostridium difficile* colitis, microbiome alterations, potential for drug interactions, and side effects.

Respiratory infections are the second most common infection affecting travelers [7]. Endemic fungal pulmonary infections, such as histoplasmosis, coccidioidomycosis, and blastomycosis in North America, paracoccidioidomycosis in Central and South America, and talaromycosis (formerly known as penicilliosis) due to *Talaromyces (formerly known as Penicillium) marneffei* infection in Southeast Asia, could be acquired during travel [8, 9]. SOT recipients are at higher risk for invasive fungal infection and should avoid activities such as spelunking and excavating, activities that have been associated with exposure to *Cryptococcus neoformans* or *Histoplasma capsulatum*. The appropriate use of masks may be helpful.

Malaria and dengue fever are the most common arthropod-borne illnesses of travelers. Most cases of dengue fever are self-limited in the normal host; the risk for complications in transplant recipients is not well understood. In a series of eight renal transplant recipients with dengue fever living in India, three developed dengue hemorrhagic shock syndrome and died [10]. In a 20-year retrospective study of 1917 renal transplant recipients, 13 (0.7%) recipients were diagnosed with laboratory-confirmed dengue with a median age of 39 years (interquartile ranges [IQR], 22–46); 54% were males [83]. All patients resolved without complications, except one had hemophagocytic lymphohistiocytosis. Ten (76.9%) patients experienced eGFR reduction with a median of 13.7 mL/min/1.73 m^2 (IQR, 8.3–20.5); eight (80%) had a full allograft function recovery. Authors concluded that although a transient decline in allograft function can occur, the overall clinical and allograft outcomes seem to be favorable [83]. Malaria is a significant risk for all travelers to endemic areas. Prophylaxis against malaria should be based on the travel itinerary; the CDC Yellow Book provides country-specific guidelines (wwwnc.cdc.gov/travel/destinations/list.htm wwwnc.cdc.gov/travel/destinations/list.htm) [6]. Transplant recipients should be instructed on ways to minimize insect bites, including the use of repellents containing DEET (N,N-diethyl-3-methylbenzamide), bed nets, protective clothing, and permethrin-impregnated clothing [6].

Travelers to endemic regions may contract parasitic infections such as *Strongyloides stercoralis* infections, when larvae from contaminated soil penetrate skin or mucous membranes. Unlike other intestinal parasites, *Strongyloides* can replicate inside the human host, which allows the perpetuation of autoinfection. *Strongyloides* infection may persist for decades and can flourish in the setting of immunosuppression, resulting in life-threatening hyperinfection and disseminated infection. Travelers should wear socks and shoes to avoid contact with this and other pathogens. Swimmer's itch due to *Schistosoma* spp., cryptosporidiosis, and other parasitic infections can be prevented by avoiding swims in non-chlorinated freshwater ponds, lakes, and rivers.

The large African snail invasion in South America has heightened the concerns for accidental infection due to rat lungworm or *Angiostrongylus cantonensis*. Travelers to South America (or to other areas of world known to host *A. cantonensis* such Asia, Pacific Islands, and Africa) should be counseled regarding *A. cantonensis* infection and the risk for potentially life-threatening eosinophilic meningitis. These infections are acquired by intentional and inadvertent consumption of raw or undercooked intermediate hosts of the parasite such as snails or slugs. Infection can also be transmitted via consumption of poorly prepared or raw freshwater shrimp, crabs, and frogs that are not essential for the parasites' life cycle but may serve as paratenic host. Consumption of snails and uncooked shellfish is not recommended for transplant recipients and must always be avoided.

Echinococcosis is caused by the ingestion of eggs of either the *Echinococcus granulosus* or *Echinococcus multilocularis*. *E. granulosus* is a parasite of domestic dogs that causes hydatid or unilocular cystic disease, whereas *E. multilocularis* is a parasite of wild canines that causes alveolar cyst disease. Patients with hydatid cysts are usually asymptomatic for years. Echinococcosis is not uncommon in rural India, rural Mexico, Alaska, and other regions of the developing world. Transplant patients with severe B-cell dysfunction, especially those receiving aggressive anti-B-cell therapy for allograft rejection, may present echinococcosis with highly unusual accelerated growth and rapidly enlarging tumor-like mass lesion [11]. Transplant patients should avoid travel to the rural endemic regions and keep their essential travel to a brief stay. Furthermore, contact with all non-domesticated canines should be avoided.

Acute toxoplasmosis acquired in certain areas of Latin America may have unusual and more severe manifestations than when acquired in Europe or the United States and Canada. Transplant physicians should entertain the possibility of acute toxoplasmosis in travelers returning from Latin America who present with fever of unknown origin, severe headaches, acute community-acquired pneumonia, hepatitis, chorioretinitis, brain abscesses, myositis, and myocarditis. In order to decrease the possibility of acquiring *T. gondii*, patients should be advised to avoid ingestion of raw or undercooked meat or shellfish; consumption of untreated water or unwashed vegetables of fruits; exposure to soil or feces of domestic, wild, or stray cats; and eating food that has been prepared in surfaces where raw meat was manipulated.

Transplant recipients have a markedly increased risk of skin cancer that correlates with the intensity of sun exposure, and it is important to recommend the use of hats, sunglasses, protective clothing which are also useful for prevention of arthropod-borne infections, and sun protection lotions with ultraviolet A and B protection.

Travelers who rapidly ascend to altitude are at risk for altitude sickness. Acetazolamide accelerates acclimatization and decreases the risk of altitude sickness [12]; its use in organ transplant recipients is unstudied. Travelers to high attitude should be advised to avoid vigorous activities for the first few days at high altitudes. Acetazolamide should be offered to those travelers ascending rapidly to greater than 2500 meters since there is at least a 15–25% risk of altitude sickness. Small series suggests that selected and well-prepared transplant recipients can perform strenuous physical activities and tolerate exposure to high altitude similar to normal healthy people [13, 14].

Drug interactions are of particular concern in transplant recipients, and they should be cautioned about using new medications that may be given by unknowledgeable practitioners or purchased "over the counter." Online drug interaction calculators may be helpful to savvy travelers. Chloroquine can increase serum levels of cyclosporine and perhaps sirolimus and tacrolimus. Data are limited regarding other possible interactions between travel-associated drugs and immunosuppressive medications (Table 62.2). Short courses of ciprofloxacin or azithromycin for travelers' diarrhea seem unlikely to have a major impact on cyclosporine levels (Table 62.2).

Acquisition of new viruses should be avoided, via safer sex practices, use of clean needles and syringes, or avoidance, if possible, of blood transfusions in foreign countries. Sterile needles and syringes may be given to a traveling transplant recipient with a physician's letter stating they are for medical use. Patients with end-stage renal disease, either prior to or after organ transplant, and who undergo hemodialysis in resource-limited countries, where suboptimal infection control policies pose a risk of exposure to blood-borne viruses, are at significant risk of acquiring new viral infections. A number of cases of hepatitis C have been reported in Western travelers to the Indian subcontinent, Tenerife, Egypt, Saudi Arabia, Singapore, and Slovakia [15, 16]. Such exposures may have an impact on policies in transplant centers regarding evaluation of those on the waiting list for solid organ transplants [17].

Vaccination and Response

In general, many of the indications for vaccination are the same in immunocompromised and non-immunocompromised hosts, with a few exceptions. When possible, vaccination for travel should be started several months before the trip, to allow time for further serologic evaluation and possible additional booster doses, as needed. Emergency travel may present a potentially high-risk situation in which passive immunization could be used, such as administration of intramuscular immunoglobulin to protect against hepatitis A virus infection. To optimize the immunologic response, immunocompromised hosts should be vaccinated during periods of no or low exogenous immunosuppression when possible, such as before undergoing solid organ or hematopoietic stem cell transplantation. When possible, vaccination should be avoided in the initial 3–6 months after solid organ or hematopoietic stem cell transplant, since during this period, vaccine response will be significantly stunted due to the severity of immune suppression [18] and also to avoid confusion with early graft dysfunction or rejection. Whether

Table 62.2 Interactions between transplant and travel-related medications

	Calcineurin trimethoprim/ inhibitors (CNI)	Sirolimus	Sulfamethoxazole
Azithromycin	May ↑ CNI levels		
Mefloquine	May ↑ CNI levels	May ↑ sirolimus levels	May increase risk of cardiac toxicity, QT prolongation, torsades de pointes or cardiac arrest
Atovaquone			May increase risk of proguanil of bone marrow toxicity
Doxycycline	May ↑ CNI levels	May ↑ sirolimus levels	
Chloroquine	May ↑ CNI levels		May increase risk of cardiac toxicity, QT prolongation, torsades de pointes or cardiac arrest
Primaquine	May ↑ CNI levels		
Sulfadoxine/ pyrimethamine	May ↓ CNI levels		May increase risk of bone marrow toxicity
Acetazolamide	May ↑ CNI levels		

Adapted from MicroMedex® DrugReax® interactive drug interactions and Lexi-Comp OnlineTM interaction analysis

Significant interactions of travel medicines and azathioprine, mycophenolate mofetil, and corticosteroids have not been reported; significant interactions of transplant medicines and levofloxacin, diphenoxylate hydrochloride, and atropine sulfate tablets or loperamide have not been reported; minimal data available vaccinations could contribute to acute rejection or GVHD has been an area of debate, although this does not seem likely based on the available data. In a study of 20 autologous stem cell transplant recipients who were serially vaccinated with the diphtheria-tetanus-poliomyelitis, pneumococcal, and conjugated *Haemophilus influenzae*, type B (Hib) vaccines showed that a minimum threshold level of CD19(+) cells was needed to generate adequate vaccine response [19].

The measure of antibody titers following immunization may prove useful in certain settings. In general, a fourfold increase in titer is often considered evidence of seroconversion, and titers above certain levels are considered evidence of seroprotection; both of these concepts were derived from data in normal hosts. Transplant recipients are less likely to have a significant immunologic response, although this does not mean that they are not at least partially protected. In addition, immune responses to vaccination may wane more rapidly. Booster doses of vaccine are occasionally administered to those with lower or undetectable antibody titers, but such practices have not been subjected to rigorous trials nor evaluated for protective efficacy. The efficacy of vaccine adjuvants, such as aluminum hydroxide and incomplete Freund's adjuvant, as well as experimental agents, has been variable in limited studies in transplant recipients [20–22]; until more is known, it may be prudent to avoid adjuvants, especially in allogeneic transplant recipients where they could abrogate the delicate immunologic tolerance and potentially increasing the risk for allograft rejection [23].

Table 62.3 Vaccination in transplant recipients

Vaccine	Recommendation
Routine vaccines	
Influenza-parenteral	Yearly
Influenza-intranasal[a]	Contraindicated in patients/ family members
Pneumococcal polysaccharide	Recommended, with booster after 5 years
Tetanus/diphtheria/pertussis	Recommended
Human papilloma virus	Recommended
MMR[a]	Contraindicated
Varicella[a]	Contraindicated
	Contraindicated
Vaccines for selected transplant recipient travelers when indicated by destination and/or circumstances	
Bacille Calmette-Guerin[a]	Contraindicated
Cholera	Recommended when indicated/available
Hepatitis A	Recommended when indicated
Hepatitis B	Recommended when indicated
Japanese encephalitis	Recommended when indicated
Meningococcal polysaccharide	Recommended when indicated
Meningococcal conjugate	Recommended when indicated
Polio (OPV)[a] (oral)	Contraindicated in patients/ family members
Polio (IPV) (injectable)	Recommended when indicated
Rabies	Recommended when indicated
Salmonella typhi Ty21a[a] (oral)	Contraindicated
Typhim vi (injectable)	Recommended when indicated
Yellow fever[a]	Contraindicated

Adapted from the Centers for Disease Control "Recommended Adult Immunization Schedule—United States"[26], "Advising Travelers with Specific Needs: The Immunocompromised Traveler" in Centers for Disease Control's "Health Information for International Travel" [4], and "Guidelines for vaccination of solid organ transplant candidates and recipients" [27]

[a]Live, attenuated

Routine Vaccines

Adults often miss standard recommended vaccines [24], and transplant recipients are no exception [25]. Some physicians, perhaps concerned about causing harm, may elect to skip vaccination of this vulnerable population. Annual recommendations for routine adult vaccinations, including immunizations for immunocompromised individuals, are available through the Centers for Disease Control and Prevention [26]; additional publications also have helpful travel-related guidelines for immunocompromised hosts [5, 27–33]. Table 62.3 includes recommendations on both routine and travel-related vaccinations in immunocompromised hosts (Table 62.3).

Hematopoietic stem cell transplant recipients lose immunologic memory of exposure to infectious agents and vaccines and therefore need to be revaccinated. Standard guidelines for revaccination after HSCT were developed through collaboration between numerous international groups [34]. Standard recommendations for revaccination after hematopoietic stem cell transplant include diphtheria and tetanus toxoids, pertussis vaccine, *Haemophilus influenza* type B conjugate, 23-valent pneumococcal polysaccharide, inactivated influenza and polio vaccine, and live attenuated measles-mumps-rubella vaccine, as well as other vaccines [35]. Re-immunization protocols may vary among transplant centers but should be considered in all recipients. Vaccination either primary or booster in allogeneic stem cell graft donor can be effective [36] and should occur well before stem cells are harvested. In a study, antibody levels among recipients of allogeneic HSCT correlated most with recipient pre-transplant antibody levels, whereas donor antibody levels prior to obtaining the stem cell graft had less of a correlation; other factors such as patient or donor age, total body irradiation, and presence of GVHD or its treatment did not appear to have an effect, suggesting that immunization of the recipient and the donor before transplant may be more effective in improving antibody-mediated immunity after transplantation compared with managing GVHD, altering preparatory conditioning regimens, or increasing the number of lymphocytes in the HSCT graft [37].

Tetanus is rare in the industrialized world, where vaccination rates are quite good; it has a much higher prevalence in resource-poor regions, although is still rare among travelers. Tetanus boosters are routinely recommended for SOT and HSCT recipients and should be up to date before traveling. Diphtheria is common in resource-poor regions with 5–10% mortality among normal hosts, despite therapy. A diphtheria antibody level of >0.1 IU/mL suggests adequate protection. Patients with a lower titer and those vaccinated more than 10 years prior to travel should be revaccinated before entering an area in which diphtheria is endemic or resurgent. For immunocompromised travelers entering high-risk areas, diphtheria antibody levels may be measured a month or more after vaccination. There has been an increased amount of disease activity in the United States due to pertussis in recent times, and recommendations are for more adults to be vaccinated [38]. Prior pertussis vaccines caused significant side effects in adults, which largely precluded their use. A new acellular pertussis vaccine is now available for adults and is included in the vaccine for tetanus and diphtheria, called Tdap. This has not been studied in immunocompromised hosts thus far but could be considered for use in the appropriate setting.

Vaccination against influenza should occur annually in most immunocompromised hosts. In a recent study, 616 transplant patients from 20 centers in the United States, Canada, and Spain with microbiologically confirmed influenza (477 SOT; 139 HSCT) were prospectively studied [84]. The receipt of influenza vaccine in the same season was associated with a decrease in disease severity as determined by the presence of pneumonia (odds ratio [OR], 0.34 [95% confidence interval {CI}, 0.21–0.55], $P < 0.001$) and ICU admission (OR, 0.49 [95% CI, 0.26–0.90], $P = 0.023$). In patients with influenza A, pneumonia, ICU admission, and not being immunized were also associated with higher viral loads at presentation ($P = 0.018$, $P = 0.008$, and $P = 0.024$, respectively). Early antiviral treatment (within 48 h) was also associated with improved outcomes. Annual influenza vaccination and early antiviral therapy are clearly associated with a significant reduction in influenza-associated morbidity and should be emphasized as strategies to improve outcomes of transplant recipients [84]. Those who underwent transplantation, treatment of rejection, or other profound immune suppression in the past few months may be an exception, in whom vaccination should be delayed, balancing the risks of infection with the likelihood of developing an immune response, for example, in North America, deferring such a vaccine from early October to December after a kidney transplant performed in August may allow for a better immune response (immunogenicity) and better protection against influenza (vaccine efficacy) [23]. Given the year-round influenza activity in the tropics, it may be prudent to vaccinate all immunocompromised travelers to those areas if they were not vaccinated within the past year. Influenza immunity wanes, and it is not known whether such travelers should be given booster vaccines prior to travel. An alternative strategy to the conventional one-dose influenza vaccine is the booster strategy proposed from the results of a recent study [85]. A total of 499 SOTR were enrolled. Although seroconversion at 10 weeks did not meet significance in the modified intention-to-treat population, seroconversion rates were significantly higher in the booster arm for the per-protocol population (53.8% vs 37.6% for influenza A(H1N1); 48.1% vs 32.3% for influenza A(H3N2); and 90.7% vs 75% for influenza B; $P < 0.05$). Moreover, seroprotection at 10 weeks was higher in the booster group: 54% vs 43.2% for A(H1N1), 56.9% vs 45.5% for A(H3N2), and 83.4% vs 71.8% for influenza B ($P < 0.05$). Clinical efficacy (99.2% vs 98.8%) and serious adverse events (6.4% vs 7.5%) were similar for both groups. Authors concluded that in solid organ transplant recipients, a booster strategy 5 weeks after standard influenza vaccination can be safe and effective in inducing increased antibody responses compared with standard (single dose) influenza vaccination [85]. Pneumococcal vaccine should be given to immunocompromised hosts, optimally at times of less immune suppression, and it may be sensible to vaccinate before travel. Data suggests that immunity to pneumococcal vaccine wanes more rapidly in renal transplant recipients, and conjugate vaccines do not improve the durability of response when compared with the pure polysaccharide vaccine [39].

Measles is a global illness, with approximately 30 million cases annually, resulting in approximately 750,000 deaths. Measles vaccination in the United States is usually performed with a trivalent live viral vaccine including measles, mumps, and rubella (MMR). Live vaccines are generally contraindicated in immunocompromised individuals [6, 30, 40–42]. In a small study of 18 pediatric patients vaccinated with MMR after liver transplantation, immunity developed in 7 children by serologic criteria, and there were no complications attributed directly to immunization [43]. Prior to travel to endemic areas, serologic evidence of immunity against measles, mumps, rubella, and varicella should be evaluated in transplant recipients. Immune globulin should be considered for measles-susceptible, severely immunosuppressed travelers who travel to measles-endemic countries and are at risk for exposure. In general, MMR could be given 24 months after HSCT in patients with no evidence of chronic GVHD or those not receiving systemic immunosuppressive therapy [34].

Immunization against hepatitis B before travel may be indicated for certain immunocompromised hosts, including those with new sexual partners while traveling and those living in endemic areas for extended periods or who are likely to need transfusions or medical procedures while traveling. Compared to the immune response following immunization pre-transplantation [30, 40], the efficacy of standard hepatitis B vaccination is reduced when the vaccine is administered post-transplantation with severely diminished response rates of 5–15% [44]. In comparison, 20 liver transplant patients given extra doses of hepatitis B vaccine with 1 of 2 new adjuvants demonstrated a serologic response rate of 80% [45]. A group of 24 renal transplant patients who did not respond to intramuscular vaccine had an overall response rate of 63% to a series of 8 intradermal vaccinations followed by an intramuscular vaccination [46]. For immunocompromised adults, some authorities recommend immunization with a vaccine containing 40 mcg of hepatitis B surface antigen such as two 1 ml Engerix-B® vaccines, each containing 20 mcg, or a special formulation of Recombivax-HB® given at one site, in a three- or four-dose schedule [38], although this regimen has been predominantly evaluated in dialysis patients. HSCT recipients are at higher risk for hepatitis B acquisition given their exposure to blood products, and it would be prudent to vaccinate them. In a cohort of 292 recipients of unrelated or related allogeneic stem cell allografts given recombinant hepatitis B vaccine, 64% of patients seroconverted; in multivariate analyses, response was adversely affected by age older than 18 years and history of prior chronic GVHD but not by donor type or by use of T-cell depletion, adoptive immunotherapy, or treatment with rituximab [47]. It was interesting to note that 89% of the nonresponders mounted a threefold or greater rise in polio titers following three doses of inactivated poliovirus vaccine, demonstrating that response to vaccination can be highly variable.

Varicella is less common in childhood in the tropics, especially in rural areas, and thus it is more common for an adult to have chickenpox than in the higher latitudes. Varicella (Varivax®) and varicella zoster (Zostavax®) vaccines have lower and higher doses, respectively, of the attenuated live Oka strain of varicella, and, in general, their use should be deferred in transplant recipients until there is more data regarding their safety. When possible, patients who are seronegative for varicella should be vaccinated with two separate doses of varicella vaccine at least 1–3 months before undergoing exogenous immunosuppression, as in pre-SOT assessment. There are several small studies in carefully selected pediatric SOT recipients given varicella vaccine, but similar data has not yet been shown in adult SOT recipients. One pilot study of nine autologous HSCT recipients who were seropositive for varicella and who were vaccinated 3–4 months after HSCT with the Oka strain demonstrated a boost in varicella-specific cellular immunity as measured by lymphocyte proliferation, without significant systemic side effects [48]. A recombinant zoster vaccine (Shingrix®) has been recently approved by the US FDA for healthy adults 50 years and older, two doses separated by 2–6 months [86]. This recombinant zoster vaccine provides strong protection against shingles and postherpetic neuralgia (PHN) in healthy adults and should be considered the zoster vaccine of choice over the live attenuated vaccine (Zostavax®) since it is not contraindicated in transplant recipients unless recipients are undergoing immunosuppression thought to interfere with an effective and durable immune response. Studies of the recombinant zoster vaccine in transplant recipient have not been published yet in peer review literature.

Immunization for Travel-Associated Infections

Hepatitis A

The risk of hepatitis A in nonimmune travelers in resource-poor regions has been estimated to be 1 in 1000 per week for those on a usual tourist route and 1 in 200 for those on more adventuresome travel [7]. A recent Swiss study showed much lower rates, with an actual incidence of hepatitis A in travelers to countries of high or intermediate risk of transmission of 3–11 per 100,000 person-months abroad for all travelers [49]. Hepatitis A could be a devastating illness in immunocompromised hosts. Pooled immunoglobulins, given as intramuscular gamma globulin, are 85–90% effective at protecting against hepatitis A infection, although this effect only lasts for 3–6 months and dependent on the dose given; new recommendations suggest a larger dose be routinely used [87]. Prior to development of hepatitis A vaccine, gamma globulin was the standard for hepatitis A protection. Some transplant recipients with hypogammaglobulinemia are given routine immunoglobulin repletion with intravenous immunoglobulin (IVIG); this dose is much higher (0.66 mL/kg, delivering at least ~100 mg/kg immunoglobulin) than the dose used for gamma globulin (0.02 mL/kg, the dose recommended for 3-month protection against hepatitis A, which delivers ~3 mg/kg immunoglobulin), and such patients would not need additional antibody protection. The preparations are similar, although IVIG has had immune aggregates removed such that it can safely be given intravascularly

Hepatitis A vaccine is less effective in solid organ transplant recipients. In a study of 37 hepatitis A seronegative liver transplant recipients who were given hepatitis A vaccine 6 months apart, only 8% had seroconverted at 1 month following vaccination and only 26% at 7 months, 1 month after the second vaccination [50]. In another study, zero of eight liver transplant recipients responded to the two doses of vaccine given 2 months apart [51]. In a third trial, liver and renal transplant recipients, 39 in each group, received 2 doses of hepatitis A vaccine 6 months apart [52]; response after the primary dose occurred in 41% of the liver transplant patients and 24% of the renal transplant patients, while after the second dose, the respective conversion rates were 97% and 72%. Discrepancies between studies may be explained by differences in patient selection, severity of liver disease, immunosuppressive medications, and type of vaccine used.

Organ transplant recipients have a more rapid antibody decline than controls: 2 years after vaccination, only 59% of liver transplant and 26% of renal transplant recipients who seroconverted retained protective titers [53], while mathematical models of vaccination in normal hosts have predicted antibodies to persist for at least 20–25 years [54]. Hepatitis A vaccine has not been well studied in the HSCT population.

Overall, immunologic response to hepatitis A vaccine among transplant recipients shows attenuated rates and shortened durability. Use of higher or more doses of hepatitis A vaccine has not been studied in the immunocompromised population. If there is enough time before travel, it may be useful to vaccinate SOT recipient travelers with two doses of hepatitis A vaccine 6–12 months apart when the transplant recipients are at least a year after the transplantation procedure and are on a modest dose immunosuppressive regimen; titers should be checked to assess seroconversion. SOT recipients who do not have adequate time before travel or do not respond to immunization should be given intramuscular immunoglobulin prior to travel [6].

Salmonella enterica serovar Typhi

An estimated 16–33 million cases of typhoid fever and 500,000–600,000 related deaths occur worldwide each year [55]. Approximately 300–400 cases of typhoid fever are reported in the United States each year, and most cases are related to international travel. Severe complications can occur in immunocompromised individuals during infection with *Salmonella enterica* serovar Typhi, and they should be immunized against typhoid prior to travel to endemic areas. There are currently two vaccines commonly available: the injectable polysaccharide vaccine (TyphimVi®, Aventis Pasteur SA) and the oral live, attenuated vaccine Ty21a (Vivotif®, Berna). The live oral typhoid vaccine has not been shown to cause disseminated disease; however, for theoretical reasons, the inactive parenteral vaccine should preferentially be administered to immunocompromised individuals. Immune response in immunocompromised hosts to either typhoid vaccine is usually poor, and data are minimal in immunocompromised hosts. As a relatively well-tolerated vaccine in general [56], and given the significant morbidity and mortality with typhoid fever, it may be prudent to vaccinate transplant recipients with the injectable vaccine when they travel to endemic areas.

Polio

Poliomyelitis caused by wild-type poliovirus has been eradicated from the Western hemisphere; wild-type virus exists in sub-Saharan Africa and South Asia. Outbreaks of vaccine-associated poliomyelitis occasionally occur, due to neuro-virulent reversion of live attenuated poliovirus from the oral polio vaccine. Vaccine-associated outbreaks of poliomyelitis have recently occurred in Hispaniola (Haiti and the Dominican Republic), the Philippines, Madagascar, and Cape Verde. Worldwide, two forms of the polio vaccine are available: the orally administered, live, attenuated virus (OPV or Sabin) and the injected inactivated poliovirus vaccine (IPV or Salk). Since attenuated vaccine strain polioviruses may spread through fecal-oral contact, transplant recipients and household contacts of immunocompromised individuals should not receive OPV. OPV is no longer distributed in the United States and Canada. Travelers should have received a primary series of polio vaccine during childhood and at least one booster as an adult. Some authorities recommend booster immunization if more than 10 years have elapsed since administration of the last polio vaccine, especially for individuals traveling to areas of the world with a polio outbreak or with circulating wild-type polio viruses; waning immunity in transplant recipients may require more frequent immunization.

The longevity of the response to revaccination with poliovirus after allogeneic stem cell transplant was studied in 134 patients who were given three doses of trivalent inactivated polio vaccine starting 12 months after HSCT and who survived at least 5 years after vaccination with a mean follow-up of 8 years (range, 1–19 years) [57]. Twenty-one patients (15.6%) became seronegative to at least one of the poliovirus serotypes during follow-up; in multivariate analysis, the only risk factor for loss of immunity was younger patient age, and there was a strong trend for patients with chronic GVHD to lose immunity more rapidly. All 14 patients given a booster dose of an inactivated poliovirus vaccine responded. Poliovirus immunity was thus shown to be retained long term after revaccination in most patients after allogeneic SCT. Response to vaccination after SOT has not been well studied but should be considered in anyone traveling to an endemic region.

Meningococcus

Meningococcal disease has high case-fatality rates of 5–15%. In the United States, a quadrivalent polysaccharide vaccine against *Neisseria meningitidis* A, C, Y, W-135 strains has traditionally been used; a similar protein conjugate vaccine is also available. Two new vaccines (MenB) have been approved for the prevention of disease caused by serogroup B. Meningococcal vaccines (ACYW-135 vaccine and B vaccine) are indicated for individuals traveling to areas of the world with known outbreaks of invasive meningococcal disease, those traveling to the meningitis belt of sub-Saharan

Africa, especially during the dry winter months from December through June, and for those traveling to Saudi Arabia for the Muslim pilgrimages of *Hajj* or *Umrah*, where proof of vaccination is required. There are no published data regarding the response of solid organ transplant recipients to immunization with the polysaccharide or protein conjugate meningococcal vaccine.

A recent study of the tetravalent protein-conjugated meningococcal vaccine (MCV4) in 46 recipients of related and unrelated allogeneic HSCT found a poor response to a single MCV4 vaccination is poor and recommended that administration of a 2-dose series, as currently recommended for patients with asplenia, complement deficiency, and HIV infection, should be evaluated in this patient population [58]. The majority of 44 patients who were given the polysaccharide vaccine 8 or 20 months after HSCT had significant immune responses to serogroups A and C; these responses were higher in individuals 20 months after transplantation than 8 months after transplantation and declined sharply over the first 6–12 months after vaccination suggesting revaccination should be considered for those at risks of exposure to meningococcal infection [59]. As transplant recipients are more likely to have significant morbidity and mortality from meningococcal disease, vaccination would seem prudent for those with potential exposure; safety and efficacy remain to be ascertained. The CDC website has information on areas with frequent epidemics of meningococcal meningitis at http://wwwnc.cdc.gov/travel/images/map3-13-frequent-epidemics-meningococcal-meningitis.jpg [60].

Yellow Fever

Yellow fever, a mosquito-borne viral hemorrhagic fever with a high case-fatality rate, occurs in tropical regions of South America and sub-Saharan Africa and kills an estimated 30,000 people every year. The CDC says transplant patients should not travel to yellow fever zones; if they must, they should travel with waivers, which must be completed and signed by a physician in the Medical Contraindications to Vaccination section of the International Certificate of Vaccination or Prophylaxis, which can only be given by approved yellow fever immunization centers [61]. Case fatality may surpass 20%; no specific treatment exists. Yellow fever may be a risk for travelers to endemic countries. The yellow fever vaccine contains a live attenuated viral strain and is distributed only through the Department of Public Health-certified vaccination centers, including travel clinics and some county health departments. A listing of approved yellow fever vaccination centers is available from local Departments of Public Health and the US CDC (available at http://wwwnc.cdc.gov/travel/yellow-fever-vaccination-clinics/search.htm) [62].

As a general rule, the yellow fever vaccine should not be given to immunosuppressed individuals [30, 42, 63–66]. While a few mildly immunosuppressed travelers have tolerated the vaccine including individuals with early HIV infection or a distant history of hematological malignancy not currently being treated with antineoplastic therapy [67–70], vaccine complications including death have been reported in immunosuppressed individuals [42, 71]. Optimally, the immunocompromised traveler should avoid regions where yellow fever is endemic or decrease risk by avoiding travel to those regions during peak season like January through March in Brazil and July through October in rural West Africa [42].

A travel physician who has decided to issue a waiver must complete and sign the Medical Contraindications to Vaccination section of the International Certificate of Vaccination or Prophylaxis, which can only be given by approved yellow fever immunization centers. The clinician should also give the traveler a signed and dated exemption letter on the physician's letterhead stationery, clearly stating the contraindications to vaccination and bearing the stamp used by the yellow fever vaccination center. Transplant recipients must understand the increased risk for yellow fever infection associated with non-vaccination and how to minimize this risk by avoiding mosquito bites. Some countries may still deny entry without immunization. To improve the likelihood that the waiver will be accepted at the destination country, clinicians may suggest that the traveler before beginning travel should obtain specific and authoritative advice from the embassy or consulate of the destination country or countries and request documentation of their requirements for waivers and retain this information along with their waiver. Further information is available from the Centers for Disease Control website (wwwnc.cdc.gov/travel/destinations/list.htm) [42]. Family members of immunosuppressed persons may receive yellow fever vaccine.

Rabies

Many travelers are at an increased risk of exposure to rabid animals while traveling. Long-term travelers, individuals expecting intense exposure to animal, and individuals who plan to be far from medical care should be considered candidates for pre-travel immunization against rabies. Since transplant recipients may not mount adequate antibody responses to the rabies vaccine, titers >0.5 IU/ml are considered adequate, some authorities recommend administration of human rabies immunoglobulin (HRIG) after all at-risk exposures; normally, HRIG is only given to previously nonimmunized individuals [72]. Intradermal administration of rabies vaccines may result in variable immune responses even in immunocompetent individuals and is not recommended by most authorities. Data are minimal in

SOT and HSCT recipients. One study of seven HIV + patients with low CD4 T lymphocyte counts (<200 cells/uL) found poor neutralizing antibody responses to pre- and post-exposure rabies vaccination even with doubling of the intradermal doses of cell culture rabies vaccine. Three HIV-infected patients with higher CD4 T lymphocyte counts ranging between 295 and 472 cell/uL tended to have better antibody responses to post-exposure rabies vaccination [73]. Since transplant recipients may be less likely than others to participate in adventure travel or to spend long duration of time away from civilization, vaccination should be considered in those with significant risks factors such as significant animal, exposure, and prolonged stays in endemic regions, and careful post-exposure prophylaxis is strongly advised.

Japanese Encephalitis

Japanese encephalitis (JE) may cause up to 10,000 deaths annually in Asia. Immunization against Japanese encephalitis should be considered for individuals with intense rural travel in areas of Asia endemic for JE, especially during periods of increased transmission [6, 74]. The JE vaccine is a killed viral vaccine and estimated to be 80– 90% effective. Hypersensitivity reactions in immunocompetent individuals occur in 0.6% of recipients and include generalized urticaria and angioedema or both. Neurologic adverse reactions including acute disseminated encephalomyelitis may rarely occur. The efficacy of the JE vaccine is not studied in SOT and HSCT recipients. In a study of HIV-infected Thai children who were given 2 doses of JE vaccine at 12 months of age, 5 of 14 (36%) HIV-infected children and 18 of 27 (67%) uninfected children had positive JE antibody titers after immunization [75]. In another study of HIV+ Thai children with immune recovery on HAART and who were seronegative for JE, 88% developed protective antibody after JE revaccination [76]. Since this vaccine is more likely to elicit systemic toxicity, careful observation after administration with an eye to transplant graft function would be prudent.

Bacille Calmette-Guerin

Bacille Calmette-Guerin (BCG) is one of the most commonly administered vaccines in the world; a live, attenuated strain of *M. bovis*, it is used to prevent tuberculosis, especially in infants and children. BCG is rarely given in the travel medicine setting and is contraindicated in immunocompromised hosts, as they can develop a disseminated infection. No specific prophylaxis other than infection control measures have been shown to be helpful in the immunocompromised population. Patients with compromised immune system may wish to wear masks when in healthcare settings in areas endemic for tuberculosis. Pre- and post-travel tuberculosis skin tests with the purified protein derivative (PPD) or gamma-interferon-based testing may be helpful, although PPD is more likely to be falsely negative in the immunocompromised population.

Cholera Vaccine

The oral cholera vaccine, available outside of the United States, has not been studied in immunocompromised hosts but has been safe in populations of healthy people and may provide protection. Two oral vaccines are available outside the United States: Dukoral (Crucell, the Netherlands) and Shanchol (Shantha Biotechnics, India)/mORCVAX (Vabiotech, Vietnam). Compared with the previously licensed injectable vaccine, these vaccines appear to be safe, provide better immunity, and have fewer adverse effects. However, CDC does not recommend these vaccines for most travelers because of the low risk of cholera to US travelers and the incomplete immunity that the vaccines confer [6]. No country or territory requires vaccination against cholera as a condition for entry.

Vaccination of Close Contacts of Immunocompromised Hosts

Close contacts of transplant recipients could transmit some live, attenuated vaccine strains to the immunocompromised host. In general, certain live viral vaccines such as oral polio, nasal influenza, and smallpox should be deferred from use in close contacts of immunocompromised hosts. Administration of other live vaccines such as measles, mumps, rubella, yellow fever, oral Salmonella, varicella (Varivax®) [77], and zoster (Zostavax®) vaccines are much less likely to be transmitted and may be given to close contacts of immunocompromised hosts. If a rash develops with varicella vaccine, the immunocompromised host should avoid direct contact with the rash.

Post-travel Evaluation

For routine, short-stay travel, most patients do not need to be evaluated afterward, unless they are ill. Clinicians seeing transplant recipients who are ill after travel should consider both routine and atypical, geographic-, and travel-related infections. Travel destinations are associated with the probability of the diagnosis of certain diseases, which can guide clinicians diagnostically; destination-specific information can be obtained from the Centers for Disease Control

Travelers Health website (available at wwwnc.cdc.gov/travel/destinations/list.htm [78]. A report from 30 GeoSentinel sites that specialized travel or tropical medicine clinics on 6 continents found that dengue and malaria were among the most frequent causes of systemic febrile illness among travelers [79]. Travelers from all regions except Southeast Asia presented with parasite-induced diarrhea more often than with bacterial diarrhea. Among travelers returning from sub-Saharan Africa, rickettsial infection, primarily tick-borne spotted fever, occurred more frequently than typhoid or dengue.

Recent case reports of travel-related infections in transplant recipients include visceral *Leishmania* in a pancreas and kidney transplant recipient who traveled to Greece [80], disseminated histoplasmosis in a renal transplant recipient after traveled to Bangladesh [81], disseminated *Penicillium marneffei* infection in an Australian renal transplant patient who presented shortly after a 10-day holiday to Vietnam [9], and *Vibrio parahaemolyticus* septicemia in a liver transplant recipient who traveled to the Gulf of Mexico [82]. Transplant recipients may manifest unusual infections or unusual manifestations of routine infections, and clinicians caring for them should be prepared for broad array of diagnostics and treatment.

Conclusions

Every year there are more transplant recipients with an increasing variety of immunosuppression. As their health improves, they may wish to travel more frequently. Research on vaccines and transplant recipients in recent years has been quite helpful in eliciting the potential immunogenicity and safety of various vaccines in this population. Hopefully within the next 5 years, we will begin to understand more of the immunology in these hosts, which should allow for better vaccination. Improved vaccines, the ability to safely give adjuvants to boost immunogenicity, and more selective immunosuppression may allow for better protection of travelers in this vulnerable population.

In summary:

- Transplant recipients are increasing in number, as is the extent of global travel; thus this issue will continue to expand. Further studies are needed and will help guide clinical management. Prior to foreign travel, it is prudent to have transplant recipients seen by travel medicine specialists familiar with this complex and vulnerable population. Travel vaccines should be guided by the details of the travel in combination with details of the immunosuppressive regimen.
- Transplant recipients are more vulnerable to infection and are less likely to have a strong immunologic response to immunization. Vaccination either before undergoing immunosuppression or optimizing the time of vaccination after immunosuppression may help optimize the immunologic response.
- Routine immunization is important to consider and may have been overlooked or avoided in this population. Routine immunization should be considered before patients undergo solid organ or stem cell transplant. In addition, booster doses should be considered, especially after HSCT.
- Although not generally evidence based, additional or higher doses of certain vaccines may result in better protection, as has been demonstrated with hepatitis B vaccine in immunocompromised hosts.
- Immunoglobulin may provide protection against hepatitis A, measles, and other illnesses when the recipient is less likely to have an immunologic response, vaccination is contraindicated, or does not have enough time to develop protection.
- Evaluation of serologic response after vaccination may provide an index of seroprotection and may help guide the use of additional vaccinations. Serologic response is primarily a measure of humoral immunity and does not generally include information on cellular immunity. Even in situations where the antibody titers are low or undetectable, these subjects may be more protected than those that were never vaccinated (i.e., even minimal immunity may be better than none).

References

1. Boggild AK, Sano M, Humar A, Salit I, Gilman M, Kain KC. Travel patterns and risk behavior in solid organ transplant recipients. J Travel Med. 2004;11(1):37–43.
2. Uslan DZ, Patel R, Virk A. International travel and exposure risks in solid-organ transplant recipients. Transplantation. 2008;86(3):407–12.
3. Roukens AH, van Dissel JT, de Fijter JW, Visser LG. Health preparations and travel-related morbidity of kidney transplant recipients traveling to developing countries. Clin Transpl. 2007;21(4):567–70.
4. Kotton CN, Kroger AT, Feedman D. Immunocompromised Travelers – Chapter 8 – 2018 Yellow Book | Travelers' Health | CDC. https://wwwnc.cdc.gov/travel/yellowbook/2018/advising-travelers-with-specific-needs/immunocompromised-travelers. Published 2017.
5. The immunocompromised traveller. An Advisory Committee Statement (ACS). Can Commun Dis Rep. 2007;33(ACS-4):1–24.
6. Centers for Disease Control Health Information for International Travel. Atlanta, GA; 2018 [cited 2019 April 22]. Available from: https://wwwnc.cdc.gov/travel/page/yellowbook-home.
7. Ryan ET, Kain KC. Health advice and immunizations for travelers. N Engl J Med. 2000;342(23):1716–25.
8. Panackal AA, Hajjeh RA, Cetron MS, Warnock DW. Fungal infections among returning travelers. Clin Infect Dis. 2002;35(9):1088–95.
9. Hart J, Dyer JR, Clark BM, McLellan DG, Perera S, Ferrari P. Travel-related disseminated *Penicillium marneffei* infection in a renal transplant patient. Transpl Infect Dis. 2012;14:434–9.
10. Prasad N, Bhadauria D, Sharma RK, Gupta A, Kaul A, Srivastava A. Dengue virus infection in renal allograft recipi-

ents: a case series during 2010 outbreak. Transpl Infect Dis. 2012;14(2):163–8.
11. Geyer M, Wilpert J, Wiech T, Theilacker C, Stubanus M, Kramer-Zucker A, et al. Rapidly progressive hepatic alveolar echinococcosis in an ABO-incompatible renal transplant recipient. Transpl Infect Dis. 2011;13:278–84.
12. Hackett PH, Roach RC. High-altitude illness. N Engl J Med. 2001;345(2):107–14.
13. Pirenne J, Van Gelder F, Kharkevitch T, Nevens F, Verslype C, Peetermans WE, et al. Tolerance of liver transplant patients to strenuous physical activity in high-altitude. Am J Transplant. 2004;4(4):554–60.
14. Roi GS, Mosconi G, Capelli I, Cuna V, Persici E, Parigino M, et al. Alpine skiing and anaerobic performance in solid organ transplant recipients. Transplant Proc. 2010;42(4):1029–31.
15. Ghafur A, Raza M, Labbett W, Chawla A, Smith C, Ngui SL, et al. Travel-associated acquisition of hepatitis C virus infection in patients receiving haemodialysis. Nephrol Dial Transplant. 2007;22(9):2640–4.
16. Coward RA, Garrues M, Solomon LR, Gibson SP. Hepatitis C and holiday dialysis. A postal survey of UK renal units. Nephrol Dial Transplant. 2000;15(10):1715.
17. Parsons D, Coward RA, Woywodt A. Travel-associated acquisition of hepatitis C-- implications for the renal transplant waiting list. Nephrol Dial Transplant. 2008;23(6):2104; author reply –5
18. Fishman JA. Infection in solid-organ transplant recipients. N Engl J Med. 2007;357(25):2601–14.
19. van der Velden AM, Claessen AM, van Velzen-Blad H, de Groot MR, Kramer MH, Biesma DH, et al. Vaccination responses and lymphocyte subsets after autologous stem cell transplantation. Vaccine. 2007;25(51):8512–7.
20. Magnani G, Falchetti E, Pollini G, Reggiani LB, Grigioni F, Coccolo F, et al. Safety and efficacy of two types of influenza vaccination in heart transplant recipients: a prospective randomised controlled study. J Heart Lung Transplant. 2005;24(5):588–92.
21. Nevens F, Zuckerman JN, Burroughs AK, Jung MC, Bayas JM, Kallinowski B, et al. Immunogenicity and safety of an experimental adjuvanted hepatitis B candidate vaccine in liver transplant patients. Liver Transpl. 2006;12(10):1489–95.
22. Rosenau J, Hooman N, Rifai K, Solga T, Tillmann HL, Grzegowski E, et al. Hepatitis B virus immunization with an adjuvant containing vaccine after liver transplantation for hepatitis B-related disease: failure of humoral and cellular immune response. Transpl Int. 2006;19(10):828–33.
23. Kumar D, Blumberg EA, Danziger-Isakov L, Kotton CN, Halasa NB, Ison MG, et al. Influenza vaccination in the organ transplant recipient: review and summary recommendations(dagger). Am J Transplant. 2011;11(10):2020–30.
24. Roush SW, Murphy TV. Historical comparisons of morbidity and mortality for vaccine-preventable diseases in the United States. JAMA. 2007;298(18):2155–63.
25. Henning KJ, White MH, Sepkowitz KA, Armstrong D. A national survey of immunization practices following allogeneic bone marrow transplantation. JAMA. 1997;277(14):1148–51.
26. Recommended Adult Immunization Schedule for ages 19 years or older, United States 2019, Available at: https://www.cdc.gov/vaccines/schedules/hcp/imz/adult.html. MMWR Morb Mortal Wkly Rep. 2019;68(5):115–8.
27. Danziger-Isakov L, Kumar D, AST ID Community of Practice. Vaccination of solid organ transplant candidates and recipients: guidelines from the American Society of Transplantation Infectious Diseases Community of Practice. Clin Transplant. 2019;19:e13563.
28. Avery RK, Michaels M. Update on immunizations in solid organ transplant recipients: what clinicians need to know. Am J Transplant. 2008;8(1):9–14.
29. Ballout A, Goffin E, Yombi JC, Vandercam B. Vaccinations for adult solid organ transplant recipient: current recommendations. Transplant Proc. 2005;37(6):2826–7.
30. Duchini A, Goss JA, Karpen S, Pockros PJ. Vaccinations for adult solid-organ transplant recipients: current recommendations and protocols. Clin Microbiol Rev. 2003;16(3):357–64.
31. Kotton CN, Ryan ET, Fishman JA. Prevention of infection in adult travelers after solid organ transplantation. Am J Transplant. 2005;5(1):8–14.
32. Kotton CN. Vaccination and immunization against travel-related diseases in immunocompromised hosts. Expert Rev Vaccines. 2008;7(5):663–72.
33. Buchan CA, Kotton CN, AST Infectious Diseases Community of Practice. Travel medicine, transplant tourism, and the solid organ transplant recipient-Guidelines from the American Society of Transplantation Infectious Diseases Community of Practice. Clin Transplant. 2019:e13529.
34. Ljungman P, Cordonnier C, Einsele H, Englund J, Machado CM, Storek J, et al. Vaccination of hematopoietic cell transplant recipients. Bone Marrow Transplant. 2009;44(8):521–6.
35. Machado CM. Reimmunization after hematopoietic stem cell transplantation. Expert Rev Vaccines. 2005;4(2):219–28.
36. Leung AY, Chow HC, Kwok JS, Lui CK, Cheng VC, Yuen KY, et al. Safety of vaccinating sibling donors with live-attenuated varicella zoster vaccine before hematopoietic stem cell transplantation. Bone Marrow Transplant. 2007;39(11):661–5.
37. Storek J, Viganego F, Dawson MA, Herremans MM, Boeckh M, Flowers ME, et al. Factors affecting antibody levels after allogeneic hematopoietic cell transplantation. Blood. 2003;101(8):3319–24.
38. Sever MS, Kazancioglu R, Yildiz A, Turkmen A, Ecder T, Kayacan SM, et al. Outcome of living unrelated (commercial) renal transplantation. Kidney Int. 2001;60(4):1477–83.
39. Kumar D, Welsh B, Siegal D, Chen MH, Humar A. Immunogenicity of pneumococcal vaccine in renal transplant recipients--three year follow-up of a randomized trial. Am J Transplant. 2007;7(3):633–8.
40. Avery RK, Ljungman P. Prophylactic measures in the solid-organ recipient before transplantation. Clin Infect Dis. 2001;33(Suppl 1):S15–21.
41. Molrine DC, Hibberd PL. Vaccines for transplant recipients. Infect Dis Clin N Am. 2001;15(1):273–305. xii
42. Gershman M, Staples JE. Chap. 3: Infectious diseases related to travel: yellow fever. 2012 Health Information for International Travel (available at wwwnccdcgov/travel/yellowbook/2012/chapter-3-infectious-diseases-related-to-travel/yellow-feverhtm). 2012 ed. Atlanta: Centers for Disease Control and Prevention. 2012.
43. Rand EB, McCarthy CA, Whitington PF. Measles vaccination after orthotopic liver transplantation. J Pediatr. 1993;123(1):87–9.
44. Hayney MS, Welter DL, Reynolds AM, Francois M, Love RB. High-dose hepatitis B vaccine in patients waiting for lung transplantation. Pharmacotherapy. 2003;23(5):555–60.
45. Bienzle U, Gunther M, Neuhaus R, Vandepapeliere P, Vollmar J, Lun A, et al. Immunization with an adjuvant hepatitis B vaccine after liver transplantation for hepatitis B-related disease. Hepatology. 2003;38(4):811–9.
46. Choy BY, Peiris JS, Chan TM, Lo SK, Lui SL, Lai KN. Immunogenicity of intradermal hepatitis B vaccination in renal transplant recipients. Am J Transplant. 2002;2(10):965–9.

47. Jaffe D, Papadopoulos EB, Young JW, O'Reilly RJ, Prockop S, Kernan NA, et al. Immunogenicity of recombinant hepatitis B vaccine (rHBV) in recipients of unrelated or related allogeneic hematopoietic cell (HC) transplants. Blood. 2006;108(7):2470–5.
48. Ljungman P, Wang FZ, Nilsson C, Solheim V, Linde A. Vaccination of autologous stem cell transplant recipients with live varicella vaccine: a pilot study. Support Care Cancer. 2003;11(11):739–41.
49. Mutsch M, Spicher VM, Gut C, Steffen R. Hepatitis A virus infections in travelers, 1988–2004. Clin Infect Dis. 2006;42(4):490–7.
50. Arslan M, Wiesner RH, Poterucha JJ, Zein NN. Safety and efficacy of hepatitis A vaccination in liver transplantation recipients. Transplantation. 2001;72(2):272–6.
51. Dumot JA, Barnes DS, Younossi Z, Gordon SM, Avery RK, Domen RE, et al. Immunogenicity of hepatitis A vaccine in decompensated liver disease. Am J Gastroenterol. 1999;94(6):1601–4.
52. Stark K, Gunther M, Neuhaus R, Reinke P, Schroder K, Linnig S, et al. Immunogenicity and safety of hepatitis A vaccine in liver and renal transplant recipients. J Infect Dis. 1999;180(6):2014–7.
53. Gunther M, Stark K, Neuhaus R, Reinke P, Schroder K, Bienzle U. Rapid decline of antibodies after hepatitis A immunization in liver and renal transplant recipients. Transplantation. 2001;71(3):477–9.
54. Rendi-Wagner P, Korinek M, Winkler B, Kundi M, Kollaritsch H, Wiedermann U. Persistence of seroprotection 10 years after primary hepatitis A vaccination in an unselected study population. Vaccine. 2007;25(5):927–31.
55. World Health Organization: Initiative for Vaccine Research: Typhoid Fever. [cited April 27, 2008]; Available from: http://www.who.int/vaccine_research/diseases/diarrhoeal/en/index7.html.
56. Begier EM, Burwen DR, Haber P, Ball R. Postmarketing safety surveillance for typhoid fever vaccines from the Vaccine Adverse Event Reporting System, July 1990 through June 2002. Clin Infect Dis. 2004;38(6):771–9.
57. Ljungman P, Aschan J, Gustafsson B, Lewensohn-Fuchs I, Winiarski J, Ringden O. Long-term immunity to poliovirus after vaccination of allogeneic stem cell transplant recipients. Bone Marrow Transplant. 2004;34(12):1067–9.
58. Mahler MB, Taur Y, Jean R, Kernan NA, Prockop SE, Small TN. Safety and immunogenicity of the tetravalent protein-conjugated meningococcal vaccine (MCV4) in recipients of related and unrelated allogeneic hematopoietic stem cell transplantation. Biol Blood Marrow Transplant. 2012;18(1):145–9.
59. Parkkali T, Kayhty H, Lehtonen H, Ruutu T, Volin L, Eskola J, et al. Tetravalent meningococcal polysaccharide vaccine is immunogenic in adult allogeneic BMT recipients. Bone Marrow Transplant. 2001;27(1):79–84.
60. CDC Website. Available from http://wwwnc.cdc.gov/travel/images/map3-13-frequent-epidemics-meningococcal-meningitis.jpg.
61. CDC Website. Available from https://wwwnc.cdc.gov/travel/yellowbook/2018/infectiousdiseases-related-to-travel/yellow-fever.
62. CDC Website. Available from http://wwwnc.cdc.gov/travel/yellow-fever-vaccination-clinics/search.htm.
63. Cetron MS, Marfin AA, Julian KG, Gubler DJ, Sharp DJ, Barwick RS, et al. Yellow fever vaccine. recommendations of the Advisory Committee on Immunization Practices (ACIP), 2002. MMWR Recomm Rep. 2002;51(RR-17):1–11. quiz CE1–4.
64. Fishman JA. Smallpox and live-virus vaccination in transplant recipients. Am J Transplant. 2003;3(7):786–93.
65. Ljungman P. Vaccination of transplant recipients. In: RA Bowden PL, Paya CV, editors. Transplant infections. Philadelphia: Lippincott Williams & Wilkins; 2003. p. 611–24.
66. Mileno M. Preparation of immunocompromised travelers. In: JS Keystone PK, Freedman DP, Nothdurft HD, Connor BA, editors. Travel medicine. 1st ed. Edinburgh: Mosby; 2004. p. 249–55.
67. Gowda R, Cartwright K, Bremner JA, Green ST. Yellow fever vaccine: a successful vaccination of an immunocompromised patient. Eur J Haematol. 2004;72(4):299–301.
68. Receveur MC, Thiebaut R, Vedy S, Malvy D, Mercie P, Bras ML. Yellow fever vaccination of human immunodeficiency virus-infected patients: report of 2 cases. Clin Infect Dis. 2000;31(3):E7–8.
69. Tattevin P, Depatureaux AG, Chapplain JM, Dupont M, Souala F, Arvieux C, et al. Yellow fever vaccine is safe and effective in HIV-infected patients. AIDS. 2004;18(5):825–7.
70. Ho YL, Enohata T, Lopes MH, De Sousa Dos Santos S. Vaccination in Brazilian HIV-infected adults: a cross-sectional study. AIDS Patient Care STDs 2007.
71. Kengsakul K, Sathirapongsasuti K, Punyagupta S. Fatal myeloencephalitis following yellow fever vaccination in a case with HIV infection. J Med Assoc Thail. 2002;85(1):131–4.
72. Gibbons RV, Rupprecht CE. Postexposure rabies prophylaxis in immunosuppressed patients. JAMA. 2001;285(12):1574–5.
73. Tantawichien T, Jaijaroensup W, Khawplod P, Sitprija V. Failure of multiple-site intradermal postexposure rabies vaccination in patients with human immunodeficiency virus with low CD4+ T lymphocyte counts. Clin Infect Dis. 2001;33(10):E122–4.
74. Inactivated Japanese encephalitis virus vaccine. Recommendations of the Advisory Committee on Immunization Practices (ACIP). MMWR Recomm Rep. 1993;42(RR-1):1–15.
75. Rojanasuphot S, Shaffer N, Chotpitayasunondh T, Phumiamorn S, Mock P, Chearskul S, et al. Response to JE vaccine among HIV-infected children, Bangkok, Thailand. Southeast Asian J Trop Med Public Health. 1998;29(3):443–50.
76. Puthanakit T, Aurpibul L, Yoksan S, Sirisanthana T, Sirisanthana V. Japanese encephalitis vaccination in HIV-infected children with immune recovery after highly active antiretroviral therapy. Vaccine. 2007;25(49):8257–61.
77. Marin M, Guris D, Chaves SS, Schmid S, Seward JF. Prevention of varicella: recommendations of the Advisory Committee on Immunization Practices (ACIP). MMWR Recomm Rep. 2007;56(RR-4):1–40.
78. Centers for Disease Control Travelers Health website. Available at wwwnc.cdc.gov/travel/destinations/list.htm.
79. Freedman DO, Weld LH, Kozarsky PE, Fisk T, Robins R, von Sonnenburg F, et al. Spectrum of disease and relation to place of exposure among ill returned travelers. N Engl J Med. 2006;354(2).119–30.
80. Aardema H, Sijpkens YW, Visser LG. Pancytopenia in a simultaneous pancreas and kidney transplant recipient: an unexpected cause – a case of visceral leishmaniasis in a transplant recipient. Clin Nephrol. 2009;71(4):460–2.
81. Rappo U, Beitler JR, Faulhaber JR, Firoz B, Henning JS, Thomas KM, et al. Expanding the horizons of histoplasmosis: disseminated histoplasmosis in a renal transplant patient after a trip to Bangladesh. Transpl Infect Dis. 2010;12(2):155–60.
82. Fernando RR, Krishnan S, Fairweather MG, Ericsson CD. Vibrio parahemolyticus septicaemia in a liver transplant patient: a case report. J Med Case Rep. 2011;5:171.
83. Pinsai S, Kiertiburanakul S, Watcharananan SP, Kantachuvessiri S, Boongird S, Bruminhent J. Epidemiology and outcomes of dengue in kidney transplant recipients: a 20-year retrospective analysis and comparative literature review. Clin Transplant. 2019;33(1):e13458.
84. Kumar D, Ferreira VH, Blumberg E, Silveira F, Cordero E, Perez-Romero P, Aydillo T, Danziger-Isakov L, Limaye AP, Carratala J, Munoz P, Montejo M, Lopez-Medrano F, Farinas MC, Gavalda J, Moreno A, Levi M, Fortun J, Torre-Cisneros J, Englund JA, Natori Y, Husain S, Reid G, Sharma TS, Humar A. A 5-year prospective

multicenter evaluation of influenza infection in transplant recipients. Clin Infect Dis. 2018;67(9):1322–9.

85. Cordero E, Roca-Oporto C, Bulnes-Ramos A, Aydillo T, Gavaldà J, Moreno A, Torre-Cisneros J, Montejo JM, Fortun J, Muñoz P, Sabé N, Fariñas MC, Blanes-Julia M, López-Medrano F, Suárez-Benjumea A, Martinez-Atienza J, Rosso-Fernández C, Pérez-Romero P. TRANSGRIPE 1–2 Study Group. Two doses of inactivated influenza vaccine improve immune response in solid organ transplant recipients: results of TRANSGRIPE 1-2, a randomized controlled clinical trial. Clin Infect Dis. 2017;64(7):829–38. https://doi.org/10.1093/cid/ciw855.
86. [No authors listed]. Shingrix – an adjuvanted, recombinant herpes zoster vaccine. Med Lett Drugs Ther. 2017;59(1535):195–6. PMID: 29186082
87. Nelson NP. Updated dosing instructions for immune globulin (human) GamaSTAN S/D for hepatitis A virus prophylaxis. MMWR Morb Mortal Wkly Rep. 2017;66:959–60. https://doi.org/10.15585/mmwr.mm6636a5.

Vaccination in Organ Transplant Patients

63

Lara Danziger-Isakov and Camille Nelson Kotton

Introduction

Vaccination has saved more lives than any other therapeutic modality in medicine, yet this remains an overlooked and underutilized tool for protection in immunocompromised hosts, especially adults. According to the 2015 National Health Interview Survey (NHIS), pneumococcal vaccination coverage in high-risk adults aged 19–64 years was only 23% and 74% in adults ≥65 years; zoster was only 31% of those ≥60 years, and 62% of adults have had tetanus boosters [1]. Pediatric patients tend to be much better vaccinated than adults, although some of those with chronic illness may have missed vaccines, and pediatric transplant patients have been documented to miss numerous vaccines [2]. With the rise in vaccine avoidance and alternative vaccination strategies for children due to unfounded concerns regarding potential side effects, the need for vaccines in immunocompromised children is even more acute as herd immunity to common vaccine-preventable diseases is waning as evidenced by recent outbreaks of measles and mumps. Studies from Iran, Brazil, and Switzerland have shown that pediatric solid organ transplant candidates have incomplete vaccination status prior to transplantation [2–4]. A single center survey of adult solid organ transplant (SOT) recipients found that more than half had received no information on vaccination [5]. Routine adult and pediatric vaccine schedules appear on the CDC website [6]. A summary of vaccines that can be used in transplant recipients appears in Table 63.1.

This lack of vaccination in immunocompromised hosts stems, in part, from concerns about potentially doing harm in the setting of a suppressed immune system. While live vaccines should be avoided in immunosuppressed hosts, most other vaccines are well tolerated and do not have significant adverse effects. Live vaccines that should generally be avoided (or used very cautiously, as discussed below and in the chapter on "Travel Medicine") include those against varicella, zoster, measles, mumps, rubella, rotavirus, polio or *Salmonella typhi* (for the last two, avoid oral vaccine; injectable is not live), tuberculosis (as attenuated *Mycobacterium bovis* or *Bacillus* Calmette-Guérin (BCG)), yellow fever, and smallpox; some are highlighted as contraindicated in immunocompromised hosts in Table 63.1. While there is some emerging data that influenza vaccine may be associated with de novo alloantibody formation and/or augmented cellular alloimmunity [7, 8], the long-term impact remains unknown, and vaccination has never been clearly associated with a risk of acute or chronic organ transplant rejection.

In general, vaccination in immunocompromised hosts is at least partly protective and may attenuate disease severity, if not prevent it all together [9]. Studies show a broad array of response to vaccination; overall responses to influenza vaccination have ranged from 15% to 93% with lower responses seen in lung transplant and greater responses several years after kidney transplant [10]. Factors that contribute to a reduced immunologic response to vaccination include exogenous immunosuppression, including both induction agents (i.e., thymoglobulin, alemtuzumab, belatacept, rituximab) and those used for chronic immunosuppression (i.e., mycophenolate mofetil, cyclosporine, tacrolimus, prednisone, sirolimus, azathioprine, and others); underlying disease states (lupus, rheumatoid arthritis, vasculitides); comorbidities (diabetes, human immunodeficiency virus (HIV), renal or hepatic insufficiency, obesity); hypogammaglobulinemia; age; and numerous other factors. Whether

L. Danziger-Isakov (✉)
Pediatric Infectious Diseases, Immunocompromised Host Infectious Disease, Cincinnati Children's Hospital Medical Center & University of Cincinnati, Cincinnati, OH, USA
e-mail: lara.danziger-isakov@cchmc.org

C. N. Kotton
Transplant and Immunocompromised Host Infectious Diseases, Division of Infectious Diseases, Massachusetts General Hospital, Travelers' Advice and Immunization Center, Division of Infectious Diseases, Massachusetts General Hospital, Harvard Medical School, Boston, MA, USA
e-mail: ckotton@partners.org

A. Safdar (ed.), *Principles and Practice of Transplant Infectious Diseases*, https://doi.org/10.1007/978-1-4939-9034-4_63

Table 63.1 Summary of vaccines that can be used in transplant recipients

Vaccine	Vaccine type	Recommended pretransplant		Recommended posttransplant	
		Pediatric	Adult	Pediatric	Adult
Influenza, injectable	Inactivated	Yes	Yes	Yes	Yes
Influenza, nasal	Live, attenuated	Yes	Yes	No	No
Pneumococcal	Conjugated (polysaccharide or protein)	Yes	Yes	Yes	Yes
Meningococcal	Conjugated (polysaccharide or protein)	Yes[b]	Yes[b]	Yes[b]	Yes[b]
Varicella	Live, attenuated	Yes	Yes[a]	No	No
Zoster	Live, attenuated	No	Yes	No	No
Tetanus, diphtheria, pertussis (Td/Tdap)	Toxoid	Yes	Yes	Yes	Yes
Hepatitis B	Subunit	Yes	Yes	Yes	Yes
Hepatitis A	Inactivated	Yes	Yes[b]	Yes	Yes[b]
Human papillomavirus (HPV)	Inactivated	Yes	Yes	Yes	Yes
Measles, mumps, rubella (MMR)	Live, attenuated	Yes	Yes[a]	No	No

[a]Nonimmune or nonvaccinated individuals
[b]With specific risk factors

specific immunosuppressive agents have an impact on response to vaccination remains poorly understood, as studies have been variable and sometimes contradictory. Response rates to specific vaccines are discussed in further detail below.

To improve response to vaccination, transplant clinicians may wish to vaccinate during periods of lower immunosuppression. Pretransplant vaccination is likely to result in higher levels of protection, especially for those recipients not yet on immunosuppression, and this is an excellent window of opportunity for vaccination, especially since live vaccines could be given then (assuming at least a 1-month washout period before immunosuppression is begun) [11]. Routine vaccines, as outlined on the Centers for Disease Control and Prevention (CDC) website [6], should be updated during the pretransplant period. Experts would generally avoid vaccination during the first few months after transplant, when immunosuppression is generally most potent [12]. A group of transplant infectious disease experts recently recommended that influenza vaccines should be given no earlier than 3 months after transplantation or intensified immunosuppression for rejection, although during periods of pandemic or high influenza activity, vaccine can be given as early as 1 month posttransplant with the caveat that incomplete protection may be achieved and that if influenza activity is still significant, it may be a reasonable approach to reimmunize children and adults who received early vaccination (i.e., at <3 months posttransplant) [10]. The Infectious Disease Society of America's recommendations in immunocompromised hosts suggest waiting at least 2 months after SOT for influenza vaccination [13].

Household contacts of severely immunocompromised patients may be given live-virus vaccines such as yellow fever, measles-mumps-rubella (MMR), or varicella/zoster vaccines [14], but should not be given transmissible vaccine such as oral polio or smallpox vaccines [13, 15]. Live-attenuated influenza vaccine (LAIV) should be avoided if possible but has been used for household contacts in circumstances where inactivated injectable influenza vaccine is not available. Whether rotavirus can safely be given to infants in homes with immunocompromised hosts is unknown; the virus has been shown to cause diarrhea in infants with severe combined immunodeficiency [16], and the vaccine strain has been shown to shed for up to 9 days after vaccination [17]. However, transmission vaccine-strain rotavirus from a recently vaccinated infant to immunocompromised caretaker has not been reported, and standard precautions when handling potentially infectious materials are recommended. Clinicians must weigh the risks of vaccination of household contacts with the benefits of protection and avoiding active disease with potentially higher rates of transmission of wild-type disease to the immunocompromised host. Pet owners should be aware of the risk of transmission to them of live vaccines such as *Bordetella bronchiseptica*, which has been transmitted to immunocompromised hosts resulting in clinical infection [18, 19].

Patients may be considered for an accelerated vaccination series prior to transplant, given the improved efficacy of vaccination prior to transplant, although such vaccination has not been systematically evaluated in adult pediatric transplant candidates. Accelerated vaccination schedules for traveling infants have been published and include MMR vaccine from 6 months of age and meningococcal vaccine from 9 months of age [20]. Catch-up vaccination schedules for children who have missed or delayed vaccines are reviewed biannually and updated by the ACIP and available on the CDC website.

Adverse reactions to vaccines should be reported so that other providers can be aware of the potential risk. Reporting can be done in the United States either by filling out the Vaccine Adverse Event Reporting System (VAERS) form on the VAERS website (http://www.vaers.hhs.gov) or by calling 1-800-822-7967; reporting in other countries varies.

Specific Vaccines

Influenza

Influenza is an orthomyxovirus with three types, A, B, or C. Influenza A viruses are further divided into subtypes on the basis of their surface hemagglutinins (17 types) and neuraminidases (10 types). Combinations of the hemagglutinin and neuraminidase determine the circulating strains (e.g., H1N1 or H3N2). Influenza B does not have subtypes but can be subdivided into strains (Yamagata and Victoria lineages), and neither influenza B nor influenza C are reported to cause epidemics. Historically, around 40–50% of respiratory tract infections have been attributed to influenza in solid organ transplant recipients during the winter months with the current literature suggesting that 1–4% of recipients are infected annually [16, 21–24].

Influenza can cause significant morbidity and mortality in solid organ transplant (SOT) recipients. The recent 2009 H1N1 influenza pandemic provided an opportunity to delineate risk factors for severe illness. Kumar and colleagues reported recent augmentation of immune suppression, lymphopenia, infancy, diabetes, and delay in the initiation of antiviral therapy as risks for more severe diseases [16]. While 4% of adult patients died, mortality in pediatric patients did not occur in this cohort which is significantly decreased from a prior pediatric cohort from the early 1990s with a 23% mortality [16, 25, 26]. Early institution of antiviral therapy appears to substantially affect outcome [16].

Influenza vaccines were first available in 1945 but have evolved with improved immunogenicity, efficacy, and safety profiles. Current formulations include standard-dose intramuscular, high-dose intramuscular, adjuvanted vaccine, and live-attenuated influenza vaccine (LAIV) [10]. Specific content of these formulations is adjusted annually based on the predictions for circulating viral strains and usually contains antigens for influenza A (two strains) and influenza B (one strain in trivalent vaccine, two in quadrivalent vaccine). Live-attenuated vaccines are cold adapted and should not replicate at 37°C; however, due to the small theoretical risk of replication, LAIV is not recommended after transplant [10]. The pediatric age group is unique in that two doses of vaccine are recommended for first-time vaccine recipients under the age of 9 regardless of immunologic status.

Adult

Vaccination of adult transplant recipients is recommended by national and transplant groups [11, 13, 27]. Various nuances of influenza vaccination are covered in Table 63.2. Trials regarding immunogenicity of influenza vaccine all vary with

Table 63.2 Recommendations for influenza vaccine graded according to strength of recommendation and quality of evidence [10]

Seasonal inactivated influenza vaccine should be recommended for annual administration in pre- and posttransplant recipients (recommendation supported by WHO, ACIP, AST) (strong, moderate)
The benefit of vaccination outweighs any theoretical safety concerns related to rejection[a]
LAIV is not recommended for posttransplant recipients (strong, moderate)
Influenza vaccine should be given no earlier than 3 months after transplantation or intensified immunosuppression for rejection (weak, moderate)
During periods of pandemic or high influenza activity, vaccine can be given as early as 1 month posttransplant, although incomplete protection may be achieved (strong, low)
If influenza activity is still significant, a reasonable approach is to reimmunize children and adults who received early vaccination (i.e., at <3 months posttransplant) (weak, low)
There are insufficient data to recommend
High-dose influenza vaccine
Adjuvanted vaccine
Intradermal vaccine
Booster doses of vaccine within the same season
Close contacts of transplant patients should be immunized (strong, moderate)
Inactivated vaccine is preferred if available (strong, low)
HCW including those working with transplant patients should be immunized (strong, moderate)
Inactivated vaccine is preferred if available (strong, low)
Organs from donors who recently received LAIV (in the past 7 days) (including lung transplant donors) can be transplanted (strong, low)
Influenza vaccination for children should follow the standard age and dose recommendation
At this time, vaccine dosing and the number of doses should follow age-appropriate recommendations as for nontransplant patients.
Vaccine is not approved for administration to children younger than 6 months of age.
Two doses 4 weeks apart are recommended for children younger than 9 years of age who have not been previously vaccinated against influenza (strong, high).
Persons with known severe allergic reactions to chicken or egg protein should not receive influenza vaccine; it can be considered to give vaccine under the supervision of an allergy expert (strong, high).

Modified from Ref. [10]

WHO World Health Organization, *ACIP* Advisory Committee on Immunization Practices, *AST* American Society of Transplantation, *LAIV* live-attenuated influenza vaccine, *HCW* health-care workers

[a]Excluding vaccine-related history of Guillain-Barre syndrome

respect to host, vaccine dose and type, adjuvant use, and evaluation of immunologic outcome [28]. Nonetheless, they are notable for a trend toward diminished immune response in organ transplant recipients, with some minor augmentation of immune response in those given multiple vaccine doses. Use of adjuvant or multiple doses did not necessarily impact immunogenicity across various studies. Given the enhanced complexity of double vaccination (patients returning for a second visit, cost, etc.) conclusive recommendations cannot yet be made regarding the optimal number of vaccine doses. Durability of protection against influenza is also diminished; whether a second, appropriately timed dose might provide longer coverage remains to be determined and could be considered for certain higher risk transplant recipients. The role of adjuvants to augment response to vaccination of transplant patients is somewhat controversial; there are safety concerns that adjuvants may increase the risk of organ rejection by immune stimulation, although this has never been proven, and some vaccines are not commercially available without adjuvants.

Optimal timing of vaccination after solid organ transplant is likely to be very important in optimizing the immunologic response. Unfortunately, there are few trials that analyze optimal timing with respect to vaccination response. Most vaccine trials exclude patients who underwent organ transplant within the past 2 to 6 months. The potent immunosuppression given at the time of organ transplant is likely to result in muted immunologic response to vaccination for at least several months. Many programs defer vaccination of their transplant patients in the first few months after transplantation. One early study of mixed organ transplant recipients saw no difference in the time after transplant in vaccine nonresponders versus responders [29]. In a series of 51 liver transplant recipients who underwent influenza vaccination, vaccine response corresponded to the length of time after transplant: within 4 months of transplantation, 1/7 (14%) responded; within 4–12 months, 6/9 (67%); and after 12 months, 30/35 (86%) subjects responded to the H1 strain; overall, more than 55% of the subjects vaccinated 4–12 months posttransplantation had adequate antibody seroconversion to the three strains of the influenza vaccine [30]. Another study showed lower antibody titers in kidney transplant recipients vaccinated within 6 months of transplantation [31]. One third of the 53 transplant recipients were 6 months or less from the time of kidney transplantation. The muted response to vaccination was more marked with response to seroresponse (fourfold increase in antibody titer) than with seroprotection (antibody titer $\geq$1:32).

There have been reports of human leukocyte antigen (HLA) and donor-specific antibody (DSA) production after influenza vaccination. Thus far, there is no rejection or graft dysfunction following immunization reported in studies that have specifically looked at this outcome (summarized in Kumar et al. [10]). In a retrospective case-control series of 60 heart transplant patients, of whom 15 had been vaccinated with H1N1 virus antigen with ASO3 adjuvant vaccine within 21 days, the overall rate of all grades of cellular rejection was not statistically different between groups; however, acute cellular rejection, >/=grade 2 (1990 ISHLT criteria), was more frequent among those who were recently vaccinated (control: 1/45 vs. 6/15, $p = 0.001$) [7].

In the absence of strong data to drive the clinical decision regarding timing, many programs develop local protocols. A survey of 239 transplant programs showed that the majority of the respondents began posttransplant vaccination within the first 6 months, with 42% of programs giving influenza vaccine within the first 3 months, 43% at 3–6 months, 13% at 6–12 months, and 3% more than 12 months after transplant [32]. Guidelines from the American Society of Transplantation Infectious Diseases Community of Practice suggest restarting vaccination 3–6 months after transplant, while Infectious Diseases Society of America (IDSA) guidelines suggest starting as early as 2 months posttransplant [11, 13]. Expert guidelines based on the 2009 H1N1 pandemic experience suggested that transplant recipients begin to receive influenza vaccine during a pandemic as soon as 1 month after transplant [33].

Pediatrics

As in adults, vaccination for pediatric solid organ transplant recipients is recommended beginning 3–6 months after transplantation [11]; however, earlier administration in pediatrics has been considered in pediatric lung recipients and reported after pediatric heart transplantation [34, 35]. Compared to studies in adult transplant recipients, studies of influenza vaccine safety, immunogenicity, and efficacy in pediatric transplant recipients are limited. Many of these studies were performed in the 1990s when immunosuppressive regimens differed significantly from current use although data from the 2009 H1N1 pandemic regarding vaccination has been emerging.

Seasonal influenza vaccination prior to 2009 in both pediatric liver and renal transplant recipients demonstrated seroprotective responses ranging from 15% to 85% depending on the influenza antigen used with lower responses to influenza B antigens as has been reported in healthy controls [36–38]. In liver transplant recipients, younger age and time closer to transplant have been associated with decreased influenza vaccine responses, and repeat vaccination did not significantly improve responses in some studies [37, 39]. While most studies focus on humoral responses, Madan and colleagues showed similar seroprotection and seroconversion in a cohort of long-term pediatric liver transplant, but interferon gamma production was decreased compared to healthy sibling controls [36].

Data on 2009 pandemic H1N1 influenza vaccine responses in pediatric transplant patients have also emerged. In Germany,

Goldschmidt et al. retrospectively evaluated the efficacy of an adjuvanted 2009 H1N1 vaccination in pediatric liver transplant recipients without measuring seroresponses; they reported higher rates of H1N1 infection in unvaccinated (25%) compared to vaccinated (4%) individuals [40]. In pediatric renal transplant recipients, Esposito et al. detailed 81–100% seroprotection with 2009 A/H1N1 MF59-adjuvanted influenza vaccine [41]. Five pediatric heart transplant recipients received adjuvanted vaccine between 5 and 23 weeks after transplant with 60% developing seroprotection despite recent induction with antithymocyte globulin [35]. Conversely, fewer than 50% of pediatric transplant recipients, predominantly renal, developed seroprotection after administration of nonadjuvanted vaccination [42]. Haller and colleagues reported increased seroprotection from 66.6% to 89.5% after a second dose of nonadjuvanted 2009 H1N1 influenza vaccine unlike previous reports for seasonal vaccination [37, 39, 43]; the authors concluded that a two-dose regimen should be considered in pediatric liver transplant recipients in the pandemic setting. Further, a recent study suggested that high-dose vaccination (60 µg) may have improved immunogenicity compared to routine dosing (15 µg) for pediatric transplant recipients [44]. Importantly, significant side effects from vaccination including acute rejection were not found in studies of seasonal or pandemic influenza vaccines in the pediatric population.

Pneumococcal (Polysaccharide/Protein Conjugate Vaccines)

Pneumococcal disease is among the most common infections, and a broad range of hosts should be vaccinated according to guidelines, including transplant recipients [27]. Transplant recipients who remain on trimethoprim/sulfamethoxazole may be protected against *Streptococcus pneumoniae* infections, as well as other infections; pneumococcal vaccination would still be recommended. The vaccine comes in the traditional polysaccharide 23-valent form (PPV23, commercially known as Pneumovax) and protein-conjugate forms. The 7-valent (PCV7, marketed under the trade name Prevnar) has recently been replaced by the 13-valent (PCV13, marketed under the trade name Prevnar 13, which in addition to the 7 serotypes included in the original PCV7 contains the 6 pneumococcal serotypes responsible for 63% of invasive pneumococcal disease cases now occurring in children younger than 5 years; PCV13 is replacing PCV7). While PCV7 is no longer available in the United States, PCV13 has not yet been studied in transplant recipients, and subsequent studies of conjugate vaccines discussed were performed with PCV7. Clinicians should be aware that PCV7 and PCV13 provide a narrower spectrum of coverage (7 and 13 serotypes, respectively), while PPV23 covers 23 serotypes. Use of both together is recommended.

Response to vaccination in SOT recipients is generally adequate, although lower than controls [45]. A trial of 43 adult kidney transplant recipients immunized with PPV23 demonstrated a significant increase in total antibody concentration against the 14 serotypes tested, from a median of 12.1 mg/L (range: 2.6–124.0) before vaccination to 51.9 mg/L (4.0–160.7) 4 weeks after vaccination, as well as a significant increase in the number of serotypes recognized, from a median of 9 (0–13) to 13 (3–14) [46]. Antibody responses after vaccination were only slightly lower than in a published cohort of vaccinated healthy controls. The estimated glomerular filtration rate correlated with response to vaccination. In another trial of PPV23 in renal transplant recipients, almost all antipneumococcal IgG titers were greater than the protective titer recommended by the World Health Organization (WHO) [47]. A trial of adult kidney transplant recipients comparing a single dose of PPV23 or PCV7 found a response rate was not significantly different between groups; there was a trend toward enhanced immunogenicity for PCV7 by ELISA; however, functional antibody responses were not different [48].

Multiples studies have investigated the utility of serial dosing of different pneumococcal vaccine formulations, i.e., PCV7 prior to PPV23, and the optimal dosing strategy for pneumococcal vaccine in transplant recipients remains uncertain due to conflicting reports in the literature. A trial of 113 adult liver transplant recipients given either PCV7 followed by a PPV23 booster 8 weeks later or placebo followed by a standard single dose of PPV23 found similar results with respect to response to at least 1 serotype, mean number of serotypes to have a response, and functional antibody titers (measured by opsonophagocytic assay); the authors concluded that administration of a single dose of PPV23 should continue to be the standard of care for adult liver transplant recipients [49]. A pediatric study in which 81 pneumococcal vaccine-naive transplant recipients (31 heart, 18 liver, 5 lung, and 27 kidney) were given 3 doses of PCV7 at 8-week intervals, followed 8 weeks later by a dose of PPV23, demonstrated that PCV7 was safe and immunogenic and that PPV23 when administered more than a year after transplant was useful in boosting antibody responses in recipients demonstrating lower rates of responsiveness [50]. Two doses of PCV7 induced ≥ twofold increases in geometric mean concentrations in all organ groups; cardiac and lung recipients demonstrated additional benefit from a third dose of PCV7. Gattringer et al. evaluated serial vaccination with PCV7 followed by PPV23 in 26 adult heart or lung transplant recipients; while PCV7 was immunogenic in these patients, PPV23 did not further augment the immune response to those 7 serotypes but did provide protection against other serotypes [51].

The timing of vaccination after SOT has not been well studied. In one study of 158 recipients of allogeneic bone marrow transplant, PCV7 vaccination at 3 months after stem cell transplantation was found to be not inferior to PCV7 vaccination at 9 months after transplantation, at 79% versus 82%; the authors suggested that the durability of protection might be shorted in this population [52]. Whether such data is transferrable to SOT recipients is not known; perhaps earlier vaccination of naïve patients, with a plan to repeat, may provide better protection than a delay (and possible omission).

Repeat vaccination may be indicated to provide optimal protection; however, unlike other vaccines, a booster effect is not generally seen with pneumococcal vaccination. One-time revaccination 5 years after the first dose is recommended for persons 19 through 64 years of age with immunocompromising conditions, and those who received PPV23 before age 65 years for any indication should receive another dose of the vaccine at age 65 years or later if at least 5 years have passed since their previous dose; no further doses are needed for persons vaccinated with PPV23 at or after age 65 years [27]. In normal hosts, both primary vaccination and revaccination with PPV23 induce antibody responses that persist during 5 years of observation [53]. Concerns about hyporesponsiveness with multiple doses of pneumococcal vaccine have not borne out in all trials and has not been studied in transplant recipients. A trial in adults of single-dose PPV23 given to 14 dialysis and 37 kidney transplant recipients demonstrated a response of 96% at 4 weeks, 94% at 6 months, and 85% 1 year after transplant; authors postulate that such a decline may warrant more frequent vaccination [54]. In general, testing for pneumococcal antibody response is not clinically useful, and clinicians should be the revaccination timing on the net state of immunosuppression and predicted response and durability of vaccination, as well as ease of administration.

Meningococcal (Polysaccharide/Protein Conjugate)

Neisseria meningitidis can cause a life-threatening meningitis or disseminated disease (meningococcemia), both in normal and immunocompromised hosts, and less commonly carditis, septic arthritis, or pneumonia. Patients who have undergone splenectomy are at higher risk for infection from these encapsulated bacteria, and vaccination is recommended before and periodically after splenectomy. The previously used polysaccharide vaccine (Menomune) has mostly been replaced by the meningococcal conjugate vaccines (Menactra and Menveo) containing groups A, C, Y, and W-135 along with diphtheria toxoid due to better immunogenicity in normal hosts. Experts expect that this will provide better protection in immunocompromised hosts as well [55]. Meningococcal B vaccination was also recently approved (Bexsero and Trumemba) to cover the additional Group B; however, no studies in transplant recipients have been reported to date.

Meningococcal vaccine is poorly studied in SOT recipients, although it is generally recommended. One study in 10 pediatric SOT recipients showed that a single dose of conjugate meningococcus C vaccine resulted in all patients demonstrating an increase of serum bactericidal antibody titers after vaccination; a significant decrease in titers was seen after 6 months; however, all patients maintained protective titers ($\geq$ 1:8) [56]. Until we have better data, this vaccine should be used as per standard guidelines (available at https://www.cdc.gov/vaccines/schedules/ [6]), especially in vulnerable teenagers and those after splenectomy, perhaps with more frequent booster doses in SOT recipients [11, 55].

Varicella/Zoster

Varicella-zoster virus (VZV) is an α-herpesvirus that establishes latency in sensory ganglia [57–59]. Primary VZV infection, often called chickenpox, presents with a disseminated vesiculopapular rash, fever, and transaminitis. Herpes zoster (HZ), the reactivation of VZV, is usually characterized by a painful or prutitic rash which follows the dermatome of the affected nerve [60, 61]; it sometimes causes disseminated disease. The largest series of pediatric transplant recipients with VZV infection, reported from the prevaccination era, revealed infection in approximately one of every seven solid organ transplant recipients; primary chickenpox and herpes zoster were equally represented [62]. VZV infection has been reported despite the postexposure prophylactic use of acyclovir and varicella-immunoglobulin in naïve recipients.

Varicella vaccines are live-attenuated varicella virus derived from the Oka strain. Several formulations are available including Varivax (Merck, NJ, USA) and Okavax (Biken, Osaka, Japan) for over 12 months of age and Varilrix (GlaxoSmithKline, Rixensart, Belgium) for over 9 months of age. A combination vaccine with MMR (Proquad, Merck, NJ, USA) is also available. Additionally, Zostavax (Merck, NJ, USA) targeted to reduce HZ infections is approved for immunocompetent patients over 50 years of age. In immunocompetent individuals, varicella vaccine has excellent seroconversion in naïve individuals, with 94–99% of children and 94% of adults responding after two doses [63–65]. Quadrivalent vaccination (VZV-MMR, Proquad) showed seroprotection of >90% after one dose and 99% after two doses equivalent to concomitant dosing of individual varicella vaccine [66]. Approximately 64–85% of adults maintained seroprotective titers for 1–6 years postvaccination [65]. Even one dose of varicella vaccine prevented typical chickenpox and drastically reduced the incidence of breakthrough infections to <5% within 3 years of vaccination [67].

Pediatrics (Varicella Vaccine)

In pediatric transplant recipients, varicella vaccine given prior to transplant has been shown to be effective in preventing posttransplant infection. Vaccination is recommended in pediatric solid organ transplant candidates if no other contraindications to vaccination exist; however, as a live-virus vaccine, it is not routinely recommended after transplant [11]. Pediatric renal transplant recipients who had received vaccination prior to transplant developed significantly fewer varicella infections after transplant (12%) compared to those without a history of varicella vaccine or infection (45%) [68]. In pediatric heart transplant recipients vaccinated a median of 16 months pretransplant, the majority (> 80% of those evaluated) had sustained vaccine responses up to 1 year after transplant [50].

Although live-viral vaccines are not recommended after transplantation, several groups have evaluated their administration in pediatric liver and kidney recipients as seropositivity against varicella has been shown to decline after transplant [69]. Eleven living donor liver transplant recipients received varicella vaccination with 87% seroconversion rate, although three had also received vaccination prior to transplant [70]. Khan and colleague retrospectively identified 35 pediatric liver transplant recipients who had received varicella vaccination after transplant; seroconversion occurred in 65% without any significant safety events [71]; this mirrors the response rate of 6 pediatric kidney transplant recipients and 7 additional liver transplant recipients who were also vaccinated in other studies [72, 73]. Another 16 VZV-naïve pediatric liver and/or intestine transplant recipients showed 87% seroconversion, but four developed fever and rash remote from the injection site and three were treated with oral acyclovir for this postvaccine reaction [74]. Further, prospective evaluation of 79 pediatric liver transplant recipients received varicella vaccination in a controlled study that showed safety and immunogenicity, including humoral and cellular responses, to vaccination in this population [75]. Overall, in selected populations of stable liver and kidney pediatric transplant recipients, varicella vaccination after transplantation could be considered but should not be routinely recommended. Routine evaluation for declining antibody titers should be performed, however, to assess potential risk of VZV exposure in immunocompromised pediatric solid organ transplant recipients. Similarly, nonimmune adults should be vaccinated prior to transplant whenever possible.

Adults (Zoster Vaccine)

Zoster occurs in one third of adults and at much high rates in SOT recipients, with an estimated incidence in SOT recipients that is 10- to 100-fold higher than the general population [76]. The vast majority (≥95%) of adults have had prior VZV infection and are at risk for reactivation as clinical zoster, either dermatomal or disseminated [76]. Zostavax®, a higher dose of the attenuated Oka varicella vaccine strain, is Food and Drug Administration (FDA) approved for healthy adults ≥50 years old; there are no published data on its safety and efficacy among immunocompromised patients. The goal of the zoster vaccine is to boost prior immunity, which wanes with time, age, and immunosuppression, increasing the risk of developing clinical zoster. SOT recipients could be vaccinated before transplant, in hopes of decreasing the risk of zoster before and after transplant; there are no data as to whether this is efficacious in this setting and whether it might be helpful in younger transplant patients (i.e., below the FDA-approved age of 50), although a clinical trial is underway to evaluate this. The vaccine is contraindicated after transplant when they are on active immunosuppression [14]. A new nonlive zoster vaccine is being developed and may be in useful in immunocompromised patients [77].

Tetanus, Diphtheria, and Pertussis

Protection against three disparate bacterial diseases—tetanus, diphtheria, and pertussis—is often grouped together in combination vaccines. Tetanus ("lockjaw") and diphtheria (involving thick membranes in the throat) remain relatively rare diseases in the developed world. Pertussis ("whooping cough") is an upper respiratory infection caused by the *Bordetella pertussis* or *Bordetella parapertussis* bacteria, which may lead to coughing with emesis; periodic epidemics occur every 3 to 5 years, with frequent outbreaks. Whether transplant recipients are more susceptible to these infections is not known. A clinical case of severe tetanus in a renal transplant recipient in Brazil has been reported, with autonomic dysfunction, requiring intensive care unit (ICU) care and mechanical ventilation, tetanus-induced acute kidney injury, and sepsis; he was discharged after 37 days of hospitalization with recovered renal function, and authors highlight the importance of vaccination [78].

The vaccine components often include diphtheria and tetanus toxoids (Td), sometimes with acellular pertussis (in DTaP and Tdap). Prior versions contained killed whole cells of the organism that causes pertussis, which was much more reactogenic and less well tolerated. Pertussis outbreaks have occurred in recent years in the United States and elsewhere, and although the vaccine has not yet been studied in this population, it would seem prudent to protect transplant recipients. Currently, the American guidelines recommends a single dose of Tdap as a booster for adults whose last Td was >10 years ago, for health-care workers and for persons who are in close contact with infants <12 months of age. Tdap can be given as soon as 2 years (or shorter intervals) after Td vaccine in high-risk persons [27]. Vaccination is generally felt to be safe and is recommended before and after SOT [11, 55]. A single-center survey of vaccination practices in 464 transplant recipients found that seroprotection rates against tetanus were fairly high in liver (85.3%) and renal (86.8%) transplant recipients and lower for diphtheria (73% and 60%, respectively) (pertussis was not measured), with considerably lower rates for hepatitis A and influenza [5]. Huzly et al. compared 164 renal transplant recipients with healthy controls before and after tetanus vaccination and found that all patients developed protective tetanus antibody levels that remained protective for at least 1 year after immunization [79]. Diphtheria antitoxin titers before and after booster vaccination were lower in transplant recipients than in controls: 88.5% of patients versus 96.2% of controls developed protective diphtheria antibody titers, and 12 months after vaccination, diphtheria antitoxin values were below the protective level (0.1 IU/ml) in 38% of patients. Neither rejection episodes nor change in renal function was noted after immunization, suggesting that vaccination was safe in this population.

There is little information on the incidence or severity of pertussis or diphtheria in transplant recipients. Another species, *Bordetella bronchiseptica*, the etiologic agent of "kennel cough" in dogs, has caused serious respiratory illness in patients who undergo pediatric lung transplantation [80], heart transplantation [81], and hematopoietic stem cell transplantation (HSCT) [82, 83]. Several of these case patients had pet dogs. The "kennel cough" live vaccine, which contains a mixture of parainfluenza virus and *B. bronchiseptica*, has the potential to cause human *B. bronchiseptica* infection [84]; transplant recipients should be aware of the risk of transmission to them from their pets.

Hepatitis B

Transplant recipients tend to be poorly protected against hepatitis B; in one series of liver, heart, and kidney transplant recipients, 76% were seronegative [85]. This is likely due to multiple factors, including oversight (most commonly), lack of immune response, and insufficient time prior to transplant to give the multiple doses required for sustained seroconversion. In pediatrics, recommendations for hepatitis B vaccination range from universal vaccination of all infants in the United States, Australia, and Switzerland to targeted vaccination of high-risk infants in other European countries including Denmark and the United Kingdom [86–88]. Canada utilizes targeted vaccination in infancy based on the provincial prevalence of hepatitis B and universal vaccination during adolescence in low-prevalence provinces [89]. Regardless, all children undergoing transplant evaluation should be vaccinated [11]. American guidelines recommend vaccination in adults for those with end-stage renal disease, chronic liver disease, and diabetics younger than 60 years as soon as feasible after diagnosis (those over 60 should be vaccinated at the discretion of their clinician), as well as other at-risk populations [27]. High-titer antibody to hepatitis B surface antigen before liver transplantation has been shown to prevent de novo hepatitis B infection, which is especially important in endemic regions; in a pediatric study in Taiwan, 8 of 9 de novo hepatitis B virus (HBV)-infected recipients had anti-HB titers <200 mIU/mL [90].

High-dose vaccine has been more successful in various populations with organ insufficiency. The American guidelines recommend that adult patients receiving hemodialysis or with other immunocompromising conditions receive 1 dose of 40 μg/mL (Recombivax HB) administered on a 3-dose schedule or 2 doses of 20 μg/mL (Engerix-B) administered simultaneously on a 4-dose schedule at 0, 1, 2, and 6 months [27]. Nonetheless, response is still not soaring; a study of 138 immunosuppressed patients (86 with cirrhosis, 42 dialysis patients, 10 allogeneic hematopoietic cell transplants) and 26 healthy subjects as controls who were vaccinated utilizing a high-dose vaccine (40 mcg) and a shortened immunization schedule showed that while 98% of controls responded, only 48% of the immunosuppressed patients seroconverted ($p < 0.001$) [91].

Hepatitis B vaccination is less likely to be effective after SOT. In a series of liver, heart, and kidney transplant recipients who underwent vaccination against hepatitis B (40 ucg dose), 73/98 (74.5%) responded to vaccination; response correlated with more doses (> 4) of vaccine and age less than 52 years old [85]. In another trial, only 3 of 17 liver transplant recipients responded who had undergone transplant for HBV-related disease and were subsequently vaccinated using intramuscular doses (40 ucg) of recombinant vaccine at month 0, 1, and 2, followed, in nonresponders, by a second cycle of 6 intradermal 10 ucg doses every 15 days [92]. Hepatitis B vaccination is less likely to be effective in those with prior hepatitis B exposure. A study of recipients of HBV cAb+ donors showed that none of the 15 chronic HBV carriers succeeded in maintaining HBsAb titers, yet 5 of 6 non-HBV patients with HBcAb-positive donors achieved HBsAb >100 IU/l [93]. This may relate to various genetic issues that decrease their immunologic response to HBV and their ability to clear virus, increasing their risk of developing chronic HBV disease.

As more children and adults are vaccinated against HBV prior to immunosuppression, the population will be more protected at baseline and in less need of complex vaccination schedules before or after SOT. When needed for poor seroconverters, clinicians can consider using multiple and higher vaccine doses, intradermal administration, and sometimes the use of adjuvants to boost immune response. Adjuvants are generally discouraged after SOT, given concerns about immunostimulation and potentially abrogating tolerance, thus elevating the risk of rejection [92].

Hepatitis A

Hepatitis A is relatively rare in the United States, although recently outbreaks have occurred. About half of cases are associated with foreign travel; a recent survey of cases from 2005 to 2007 demonstrated that risk factors were international travel (45.8%), contact with a case (14.8%), employee or child in a daycare center (7.6%), exposure during a food- or waterborne common-source outbreak (7.2%), illicit drug use (4.3%), and men who had sex with men (3.9%) [94]. Universal vaccination of children was recently added to the US national guidelines, but other countries employ prevalence-based (Australia) and individual risk-based administration (Canada) for hepatitis A [87, 89, 95]. Vaccination of adults focuses on those with risk, including men who have sex with men, and persons who use injection drugs, persons working with HAV-infected primates or with HAV in a research laboratory setting, persons with chronic liver disease, persons who receive clotting factor concentrates, persons traveling to or working in countries that have high or intermediate endemicity of hepatitis A, and unvaccinated persons who anticipate close personal contact (e.g., household or regular babysitting) with a recent international adoptee from a country with high or intermediate endemicity [27].

Whether organ transplant recipients (especially liver transplant) are at higher risk for complications from hepatitis A is not known. There have been case reports of recurrent hepatitis A after initial liver transplant for fulminant hepatitis A [96]. With recommendations to protect patients with chronic hepatitis B [97] and hepatitis C [98] against hepatitis A given the potentially augmented risk of fulminant hepatic failure in this population, it would seem prudent to vaccinate liver transplant recipients prior to transplant, as well as any other patients with risk factors for acquiring hepatitis A; whether all transplant recipients should be vaccinated has not been determined but may be reasonable and is currently recommended by most experts [11, 13].

Hepatitis A vaccine is less effective in solid organ transplant recipients. In a study of 37 hepatitis A seronegative liver transplant recipients who were given hepatitis A vaccine 6 months apart, only 8% had seroconverted at 1 month following vaccination and only 26% at 7 months (1 month after the second vaccination) [99]. In another study, none of the eight liver transplant recipients vaccinated responded to the two doses of vaccine given 2 months apart [100]. In a third trial, liver and renal transplant recipients (39 in each group) received 2 doses of hepatitis A vaccine 2 months apart [101]; response after the primary dose occurred in 41% of the liver transplant patients and 24% of the renal transplant patients, while after the second dose, the respective conversion rates were 97% and 72%. In a series of liver, heart, and kidney transplant recipients who underwent vaccination against hepatitis A, 13/17 (76%) responded to vaccination [85]. In a small pediatric study, among 18 patients who had been immunized with one dose before transplant, only seven of 18 (39%) had anti-HAV antibodies 1 year after transplant [2]. A study of 34 children with chronic liver disease found the seroconversion rate 4 weeks after primary hepatitis A immunization to be 76% (94% in controls); 1 month after second dose (6 months later), the seroconversion rates were 97% and 100%, respectively [102]. Discrepancies between studies may be explained by differences in patient selection, severity of liver disease, immunosuppressive medications, and type of vaccine used. In addition, organ transplant recipients have a more rapid antibody decline than controls: 2 years after vaccination, only 59% of liver transplant and 26% of renal transplant recipients who seroconverted retained protective titers [103], while mathematical models of vaccination in normal hosts have predicted antibodies to persist for at least 20–25 years [104]. Use of higher, more than two, or booster doses of hepatitis A vaccine has not been studied in the immunocompromised population but could be considered in the individual patient. SOT recipients who do not have adequate time before higher risk exposure such as travel or do not respond to immunization should be given intramuscular immunoglobulin prior to travel [15]; for more information, see Chap. 62 on "Travel and Transplantation."

Haemophilus Influenzae Type B

Haemophilus influenzae type b (Hib) is an encapsulated pleomorphic gram-negative coccobacillus that causes pneumonia, meningitis, bacteremia, epiglottitis, cellulitis, osteomyelitis, and otitis media among others in healthy children and adults. In the prevaccination era, pneumonia and bacteremia from Hib were reported in solid organ transplant recipients [105, 106].

Hib vaccinations are Hib capsular polysaccharides conjugated to carrier proteins. Hib vaccine has been available in the United States since 1987 with universal infant vaccination recommended since 1990. Since the institution of vaccination in the United States and elsewhere, meningitis, bacteremia, and other invasive infections due to Hib have significantly decreased with up to 95% decreases reported in children under 5 years of age [107, 108]; however, in areas where vaccination is not routine, like much of Africa, Hib continued to cause over 30% of meningitis in the past decade [109].

Stable adult kidney transplant recipients tolerated vaccination with Hib and showed excellent responses regardless of immunosuppressive strategy [110]. In pediatrics, Hib vaccine is routinely recommended as part of routine childhood vaccinations and in the pretransplant setting [11, 13, 111]. In one study, all 42 children under 5 years with chronic renal failure who received Hib vaccination developed protective responses [112]. Compared to the HSCT population, few studies have assessed the seroprotection against Hib after solid organ transplant. Nearly 100% of pediatric cardiac recipients regardless of the age at which they were transplanted responded to conjugated Hib vaccine after transplant [113]. Further, Urschel and colleagues recently studied 46 pediatric cardiothoracic transplant recipients and reported that only 17.4% had titers below protective levels without booster dosing [114].

Polio

Polio, an enterovirus, has been the focus of a worldwide eradication program. Polio which is spread by the fecal-oral and respiratory routes occurs only in humans. While nearly 95% of infection are asymptomatic, other presentations include aseptic meningitis, sore throat, and fever or, in less than 1% of cases, rapid onset of flaccid paralysis and areflexia. Polio vaccines have eradicated disease in most of the world, with the last reported case of wild-type polio infection acquired in the United States in 1979. Since that time, imported infection or vaccine-associated infections have occurred rarely. Polio vaccines are available in two formulations, an inactivated poliovirus vaccine (IPV) and a live-virus vaccine (OPV). IPV is available alone or in combined formulations with DTaP, Hib, or HBV. OPV can cause vaccine-associated paralytic polio in infants and immunocompromised individuals; therefore, only IPV is recommended in transplant candidates and recipients [11, 13].

Polio vaccination responses have been evaluated in both adult and pediatric transplant recipients. In adult kidney transplant recipients, prevaccination responses to serotype 2 were decreased compared to healthy controls, but seroprotection rates for all three serotypes were equivalent after the booster vaccination [79]. Diana and colleagues reported on a Swiss cohort for which only 43% of pediatric liver transplant candidates had received recommended number of polio vaccine doses [2]. An evaluation of pediatric liver and kidney transplant recipients compared to healthy controls and those with underlying liver or kidney disease assessed geometric mean titer responses to polio serotypes 1, 2, and 3 [115]. Responses were decreased in pediatric kidney transplant recipients compared to pediatric liver recipients and controls.

Measles, Mumps, and Rubella

Measles, mumps, and rubella are all RNA viruses that cause infections that were common in childhood prior to vaccine development. Measles is characterized by the development of cough, coryza, conjunctivitis, and erythematous maculopapular rash that causes acute encephalitis in approximately 1 in every 1000 cases. Mumps is characterized by fever and swelling of salivary glands including parotids, aseptic meningitis, and orchitis. Rubella is generally a subclinical infection but can cause fever, lymphadenopathy, and erythematous maculopapular rash. Encephalitis with rubella is rare (fewer than 1:5000 cases). All three have become less common since vaccination was introduced.

While the first measles vaccine was developed in 1958, a commercially available vaccine was not approved until 1963. The combination vaccine with mumps and rubella was introduced in 1971, and the strains have been refined over time. MMR vaccine led to significant declines in infection rates; however, outbreaks still occur despite vaccination in some cases [116–120]. Single-antigen components are not currently produced in the United States. Quadrivalent vaccine that includes MMR and VZV (Proquad, Merck, NJ, USA) was licensed in the United States in 2005 and showed >90% seroprotection equivalent to concomitant dosing of individual vaccine components [66].

MMR vaccination prior to transplant in children with chronic renal or liver disease has been evaluated. Eight infants with chronic renal disease vaccinated at a mean of 11.6 months old showed 88–100% response to each of the vaccine components comparable to healthy children [121], while ten toddlers (15–33 months of age) on dialysis showed 80%, 50%, and 80% responses to measles, mumps, and rubella, respectively [122]. Forty-two older children awaiting renal transplant had a 98% seroconversion rate with measles vaccination [123]. When single-antigen components were administered to liver transplant candidates, response rates were 82%, 90%, and 100% to measles, mumps, and rubella, respectively [73].

Adults born before 1957 are generally considered immune to measles. Those born after 1957 until about 1980 were less well protected by the measles vaccines and are considered at risk for infection. Transplant clinicians may wish to check antibody titers before transplant in this vulnerable population and use this preimmunosuppression phase to vaccinate nonimmune hosts [11]. After transplant, the vaccine is contraindicated, as it could cause life-threatening disseminated disease including encephalitis, for which there are no specific antiviral agents. Nonimmune (or those at high risk for being nonimmune) SOT recipients at risk for being exposed or who have been exposed to measles should be given immune globulin for protection [15].

Again, live-viral vaccines are not routinely recommended after transplantation; however, their administration after pediatric liver and kidney transplantation has been studied as seropositivity against measles has been shown to decline or be absent after liver and thoracic transplant [69, 114]. The earliest report of posttransplant MMR vaccination occurred when 7 of 18 liver transplant recipients had at least transient seroconversion in 1993 [124]. Additional studies in liver transplant recipients including over 50 patients revealed seroconversion rates ranging from 73 to 100% for MMR components without significant safety events [70, 71, 73]. Reports of MMR vaccination after other pediatric solid organ transplantation are lacking.

Human Papillomavirus (HPV)

Human papillomaviruses are generally clinically unremarkable; however, some cause clinically apparent epithelial proliferation (warts), and others are associated with anogenital dysplasia and cancers (HPV 16 and 18). Estimates in the United States report over 6.2 million new acquisitions of genital HPV and 11,100 new cases of cervical cancer yearly [125]. The prevalence of an anogenital malignancy in a large cohort of renal transplant recipients was 1.6%, and the majority were associated with a high-risk HPV types [126]. Furthermore, using Medicare billing, Kasiske and colleagues report a five-fold increase in cervical and vulvovaginal cancers in female kidney transplant recipients compared to the general population in the United States [127]. Similar increases in cervical cancer and cervical intraepithelial neoplasia have been reported in heart and lung transplant cohorts, respectively [128, 129].

Human papillomavirus vaccines currently available include the bivalent (Cervarix; GlaxoSmithKline Biologicals, Rixensart, Belgium with HPV 16 and 18) and nonavalent (Gardasil; Merck & Co Inc., West Point, PA, USA with HPV 6, 11, 16, 18, 31, 33, 45, 52, and 58) which cover up to 90% of the oncogenic strains leading to cervical and anogenital cancers. Both vaccines are given in series and are approved in the United States in both young women since 2006 and men since 2009. Vaccines were shown to be efficacious against the acquisition and persistence of HPV infection as well as progression to cervical or anogenital disease in multiple randomized double-blind placebo-controlled trials [125, 130–133].

Limited data in transplant recipients exist; however, Kumar and colleagues reported data on 47 transplant recipients vaccinated with the quadivalent vaccine showing both vaccine safety and vaccination response between 50 and 70% depending on the HPV serotype. Further, decreased responses were seen early after transplant, in lung transplant recipients, and with increased tacrolimus levels. In addition, vaccine responses waned by 12 months postvaccination [134].

Conclusions

Vaccination of transplant recipients is a power tool for protection of this vulnerable population and yet remains an underutilized resource. The majority of vaccines are safe and well tolerated. Live viral vaccines should not generally be used in immunocompromised hosts, and there should be at least a one-month lag time after vaccination and before transplant. Additional research regarding optimal doses, number of vaccines, use of adjuvants, impact of immunosuppressive regimens, and timing of vaccination is much needed in solid organ transplant recipients.

References

1. Williams WW, Lu PJ, O'Halloran A, Kim DK, Grohskopf LA, Pilishvili T, et al. Surveillance of vaccination coverage among adult populations – United States, 2015. Morb Mortal Wkly Rep Surveill Summ. 2017;66(11):1–28.
2. Diana A, Posfay-Barbe KM, Belli DC, Siegrist CA. Vaccine-induced immunity in children after orthotopic liver transplantation: a 12-yr review of the Swiss national reference center. Pediatr Transplant. 2007;11(1):31–7.
3. Chaves TS, Pereira LM, De Santos SS, David-Neto E, Lopes MH. Evaluation of the vaccination status in pediatric renal transplant recipients. Pediatr Transplant. 2008;12(4):432–5.
4. Dehghani SM, Shakiba MA, Ziaeyan M, Imanieh MH, Haghighat M, Bahador A, et al. Vaccination status in pediatric liver transplant candidates. Pediatr Transplant. 2009;13(7):820–2.
5. Chesi C, Gunther M, Huzly D, Neuhaus R, Reinke P, Engelmann HB, et al. Immunization of liver and renal transplant recipients: a seroepidemiological and sociodemographic survey. Transpl Infect Dis. 2009;11(6):507–12.
6. CDC Website Immunization Schedules available from https://www.cdc.gov/vaccines/schedules/
7. Katerinis I, Hadaya K, Duquesnoy R, Ferrari-Lacraz S, Meier S, van Delden C, et al. De novo anti-HLA antibody after pandemic H1N1 and seasonal influenza immunization in kidney transplant recipients. Am J Transplant. 2011;11(8):1727–33.
8. Danziger-Isakov L, Cherkassky L, Siegel H, McManamon M, Kramer K, Budev M, et al. Effects of influenza immunization on humoral and cellular alloreactivity in humans. Transplantation. 2010;89(7):838–44.
9. Agarwal N, Ollington K, Kaneshiro M, Frenck R, Melmed GY. Are immunosuppressive medications associated with decreased responses to routine immunizations? A systematic review. Vaccine. 2012;30(8):1413–24.
10. Kumar D, Blumberg EA, Danziger-Isakov L, Kotton CN, Halasa NB, Ison MG, et al. Influenza vaccination in the organ transplant recipient: review and summary recommendations. Am J Transplant. 2011;11(10):2020–30.
11. Danziger-Isakov L, Kumar D, Practice ASTIDCo. Vaccination in solid organ transplantation. Am J Transplant. 2013;13(Suppl 4):311–7.
12. Fishman JA. Infection in solid-organ transplant recipients. N Engl J Med. 2007;357(25):2601–14.
13. Rubin LG, Levin MJ, Ljungman P, Davies EG, Avery R, Tomblyn M, et al. 2013 IDSA clinical practice guideline for vaccination of the immunocompromised host. Clin Infect Dis. 2014;58(3):309–18.
14. Harpaz R, Ortega-Sanchez IR, Seward JF. Prevention of herpes zoster: recommendations of the Advisory Committee on Immunization Practices (ACIP). MMWR Recomm Rep. 2008;57(RR-5):1–30; quiz CE2-4
15. Centers for Disease Control Health Information for International Travel. Atlanta, GA2012 [cited 2012 April 14]. Available from: https://wwwnc.cdc.gov/travel

16. Kumar D, Michaels MG, Morris MI, Green M, Avery RK, Liu C, et al. Outcomes from pandemic influenza A H1N1 infection in recipients of solid-organ transplants: a multicentre cohort study. Lancet Infect Dis. 2010;10(8):521–6.
17. Yen C, Jakob K, Esona MD, Peckham X, Rausch J, Hull JJ, et al. Detection of fecal shedding of rotavirus vaccine in infants following their first dose of pentavalent rotavirus vaccine. Vaccine. 2011;29(24):4151–5.
18. Gisel JJ, Brumble LM, Johnson MM. Bordetella bronchiseptica pneumonia in a kidney-pancreas transplant patient after exposure to recently vaccinated dogs. Transpl Infect Dis. 2010;12(1):73–6.
19. Kotton CN. Zoonoses in solid-organ and hematopoietic stem cell transplant recipients. Clin Infect Dis. 2007;44(6):857–66.
20. CDC. Recommended immunization schedule for persons aged 0 through 6 years 2012 [cited 2012 June 15]. Available from: https://www.cdc.gov/vaccines/schedules/easy-to-read/child.html
21. Gottlieb J, Schulz TF, Welte T, Fuehner T, Dierich M, Simon AR, et al. Community-acquired respiratory viral infections in lung transplant recipients: a single season cohort study. Transplantation. 2009;87(10):1530–7.
22. Hopkins P, McNeil K, Kermeen F, Musk M, McQueen E, Mackay I, et al. Human metapneumovirus in lung transplant recipients and comparison to respiratory syncytial virus. Am J Respir Crit Care Med. 2008;178(8):876–81.
23. Ison MG, Sharma A, Shepard JA, Wain JC, Ginns LC. Outcome of influenza infection managed with oseltamivir in lung transplant recipients. J Heart Lung Transplant. 2008;27(3):282–8.
24. Vilchez RA, McCurry K, Dauber J, Lacono A, Griffith B, Fung J, et al. Influenza virus infection in adult solid organ transplant recipients. Am J Transplant. 2002;2(3):287–91.
25. Kim DK, Riley LE, Harriman KH, Hunter P, Bridges CB. Advisory Committee on Immunization Practices Recommended Immunization Schedule for Adults Aged 19 Years or Older - United States, 2017. MMWR Morb Mortal Wkly Rep. 2017;66(5):136–8.
26. Robinson CL, Romero JR, Kempe A, Pellegrini C. Advisory Committee on Immunization Practices Child/Adolescent Immunization Work G. Advisory Committee on Immunization Practices Recommended Immunization Schedule for Children and Adolescents Aged 18 Years or Younger – United States, 2017. MMWR Morb Mortal Wkly Rep. 2017;66(5):134–5.
27. Recommended Adult Immunization Schedule for United States 2012 available at www.cdc.gov/vaccines/recs/schedules/downloads/adult/mmwr-adult-schedule.pdf. Morbidity and Mortality Weekly Report (MMWR). 2012;61(04). The 2018 version is on the website at https://www.cdc.gov/vaccines/schedules/ or https://www.cdc.gov/vaccines/schedules/downloads/adult/adult-schedule-easy-read-bw.pdf
28. Kotton CN. Optimizing the immunogenicity of pandemic H1N1 2009 influenza vaccine in adult organ transplant patients. Expert Rev Vaccines. 2012;11(4):423–6.
29. Blumberg EA, Albano C, Pruett T, Isaacs R, Fitzpatrick J, Bergin J, et al. The immunogenicity of influenza virus vaccine in solid organ transplant recipients. Clin Infect Dis. 1996;22(2):295–302.
30. Lawal A, Basler C, Branch A, Gutierrez J, Schwartz M, Schiano TD. Influenza vaccination in orthotopic liver transplant recipients: absence of post administration ALT elevation. Am J Transplant. 2004;4(11):1805–9.
31. Birdwell KA, Ikizler MR, Sannella EC, Wang L, Byrne DW, Ikizler TA, et al. Decreased antibody response to influenza vaccination in kidney transplant recipients: a prospective cohort study. Am J Kidney Dis. 2009;54(1):112–21.
32. Chon WJ, Kadambi PV, Harland RC, Thistlethwaite JR, West BL, Udani S, et al. Changing attitudes toward influenza vaccination in U.S. Kidney transplant programs over the past decade. Clin J Am Soc Nephrol. 2010;5(9):1637–41.
33. Kumar D, Morris MI, Kotton CN, Fischer SA, Michaels MG, Allen U, et al. Guidance on novel influenza A/H1N1 in solid organ transplant recipients. Am J Transplant. 2010 Jan;10(1):18–25.
34. Benden C, Danziger-Isakov LA, Astor T, Aurora P, Bluemchen K, Boyer D, et al. Variability in immunization guidelines in children before and after lung transplantation. Pediatr Transplant. 2007;11(8):882–7.
35. Altamirano-Diaz L, West L, Humar A, Ely L, Urschel S, Gubbay J, et al. Early post-transplant vaccination with pandemic influenza A/H1N1 vaccine in pediatric heart transplant recipients. Pediatr Transplant. 2011;15(2):172–5.
36. Madan RP, Tan M, Fernandez-Sesma A, Moran TM, Emre S, Campbell A, et al. A prospective, comparative study of the immune response to inactivated influenza vaccine in pediatric liver transplant recipients and their healthy siblings. Clin Infect Dis. 2008;46(5):712–8.
37. Hojsak I, Avitzur Y, Mor E, Shamir R, Haimi-Cohen Y, Zakay-Rones Z, et al. Antibody response to influenza vaccine in pediatric liver transplant recipients. Pediatr Infect Dis J. 2011;30(6):491–4.
38. Nailescu C, Xu X, Zhou H, Hall H, Wilson AC, Leiser JD, et al. Influenza vaccine after pediatric kidney transplant: a Midwest Pediatric Nephrology Consortium study. Pediatr Nephrol. 2011;26(3):459–67.
39. Mack DR, Chartrand SA, Ruby EI, Antonson DL, Shaw BW Jr, Heffron TG. Influenza vaccination following liver transplantation in children. Liver Transpl Surg. 1996;2(6):431–7.
40. Goldschmidt I, Pfister ED, Becker M, Hackl S, Bott OJ, Baumann U, et al. Acceptance and adverse events of the 2009 H1N1 vaccination in immunosuppressed pediatric liver transplant recipients. J Pediatr. 2011;158(2):329–33.
41. Esposito S, Meregalli E, Daleno C, Ghio L, Tagliabue C, Valzano A, et al. An open-label, randomized clinical trial assessing immunogenicity, safety and tolerability of pandemic influenza A/H1N1 MF59-adjuvanted vaccine administered sequentially or simultaneously with seasonal virosomal-adjuvanted influenza vaccine to paediatric kidney transplant recipients. Nephrol Dial Transplant. 2011 Jun;26(6):2018–24.
42. Long CB, Ramos I, Rastogi D, Manwani D, Janow G, Del Rio M, et al. Humoral and cell-mediated immune responses to monovalent 2009 influenza A/H1N1 and seasonal trivalent influenza vaccines in high-risk children. J Pediatr. 2012;160(1):74–81.
43. Haller W, Buttery J, Laurie K, Beyerle K, Hardikar W, Alex G. Immune response to pandemic H1N1 2009 influenza a vaccination in pediatric liver transplant recipients. Liver Transpl. 2011;17(8):914–20.
44. GiaQuinta S, Michaels MG, McCullers JA, Wang L, Fonnesbeck C, O'Shea A, et al. Randomized, double-blind comparison of standard-dose vs. high-dose trivalent inactivated influenza vaccine in pediatric solid organ transplant patients. Pediatr Transplant. 2015;19(2):219–28.
45. Blumberg EA, Brozena SC, Stutman P, Wood D, Phan HM, Musher DM. Immunogenicity of pneumococcal vaccine in heart transplant recipients. Clin Infect Dis. 2001;32(2):307–10.
46. Lindemann M, Witzke O, Lutkes P, Fiedler M, Kreuzfelder E, Philipp T, et al. ELISpot assay as a sensitive tool to detect cellular immunity following influenza vaccination in kidney transplant recipients. Clin Immunol. 2006;120(3):342–8.
47. Willcocks LC, Chaudhry AN, Smith JC, Ojha S, Doffinger R, Watson CJ, et al. The effect of sirolimus therapy on vaccine responses in transplant recipients. Am J Transplant. 2007;7(8):2006–11.
48. Kumar D, Rotstein C, Miyata G, Arlen D, Humar A. Randomized, double-blind, controlled trial of pneumococcal vaccination in renal transplant recipients. J Infect Dis. 2003;187(10):1639–45.
49. Kumar D, Chen MH, Wong G, Cobos I, Welsh B, Siegal D, et al. A randomized, double-blind, placebo-controlled trial to evaluate the

prime-boost strategy for pneumococcal vaccination in adult liver transplant recipients. Clin Infect Dis. 2008;47(7):885–92.
50. Barton M, Wasfy S, Melbourne T, Hebert D, Moore D, Robinson J, et al. Sustainability of humoral responses to varicella vaccine in pediatric transplant recipients following a pretransplantation immunization strategy. Pediatr Transplant. 2009;13(8):1007–13.
51. Gattringer R, Winkler H, Roedler S, Jaksch P, Herkner H, Burgmann H. Immunogenicity of a combined schedule of 7-valent pneumococcal conjugate vaccine followed by a 23-valent polysaccharide vaccine in adult recipients of heart or lung transplants. Transpl Infect Dis. 2011;13(5):540–4.
52. Ljungman P, de la Camara R, Perez-Bercoff L, Abecasis M, Nieto Campuzano JB, Cannata-Ortiz MJ, et al. Outcome of pandemic H1N1 infections in hematopoietic stem cell transplant recipients. Haematologica. 2011;96(8):1231–5.
53. Romero-Steiner S, Musher DM, Cetron MS, Pais LB, Groover JE, Fiore AE, et al. Reduction in functional antibody activity against Streptococcus pneumoniae in vaccinated elderly individuals highly correlates with decreased IgG antibody avidity. Clin Infect Dis. 1999;29:281–8.
54. Pourfarziani V, Ramezani MB, Taheri S, Izadi M, Einollahi B. Immunogenicity of pneumococcal vaccination in renal transplant recipients and hemodialysis patients: a comparative controlled trial. Ann Transplant. 2008;13(3):43–7.
55. Avery RK, Michaels M. Update on immunizations in solid organ transplant recipients: what clinicians need to know. Am J Transplant. 2008;8(1):9–14.
56. Zlamy M, Elias J, Vogel U, Frosch M, Jeller V, Cortina G, et al. Immunogenicity of conjugate meningococcus C vaccine in pediatric solid organ transplant recipients. Vaccine. 2011;29(37):6163–6.
57. Cohen JI, Brunell PA, Straus SE, Krause PR. Recent advances in varicella-zoster virus infection. Ann Intern Med. 1999;130(11):922–32.
58. Gnann JW. Herpes simplex and varicella-zoster virus infection after hematopoietic stem cell or solid organ transplantation. In: Bowden R, Ljungman P, Snydman D, editors. Transplant infections. 3rd ed. Philadelphia: Lippincott Williams & Wilkins; 2010. p. 391–410.
59. Heininger U, Seward JF. Varicella. Lancet. 2006;368(9544):1365–76.
60. Dworkin RH, Johnson RW, Breuer J, Gnann JW, Levin MJ, Backonja M, et al. Recommendations for the management of herpes zoster. Clin Infect Dis. 2007;44(Suppl 1):S1–26.
61. Gnann JW Jr, Whitley RJ. Clinical practice. Herpes zoster. N Engl J Med. 2002;347(5):340–6.
62. Pandya A, Wasfy S, Hebert D, Allen UD. Varicella-zoster infection in pediatric solid-organ transplant recipients: a hospital-based study in the prevaricella vaccine era. Pediatr Transplant. 2001;5(3):153–9.
63. Weibel RE, Neff BJ, Kuter BJ, Guess HA, Rothenberger CA, Fitzgerald AJ, et al. Live attenuated varicella virus vaccine. Efficacy trial in healthy children. N Engl J Med. 1984;310(22):1409–15.
64. Weibel RE, Kuter BJ, Neff BJ, Rothenberger CA, Fitzgerald AJ, Connor KA, et al. Live Oka/Merck varicella vaccine in healthy children. Further clinical and laboratory assessment. JAMA. 1985;254(17):2435–9.
65. Gershon AA, Steinberg SP, LaRussa P, Ferrara A, Hammerschlag M, Gelb L. Immunization of healthy adults with live attenuated varicella vaccine. J Infect Dis. 1988;158(1):132–7.
66. Shinefield H, Black S, Digilio L, Reisinger K, Blatter M, Gress JO, et al. Evaluation of a quadrivalent measles, mumps, rubella and varicella vaccine in healthy children. Pediatr Infect Dis J. 2005;24(8):665–9.
67. Scheifele DW, Halperin SA, Diaz-Mitoma F. Three-year follow-up of protection rates in children given varicella vaccine. Can J Infect Dis. 2002;13(6):382–6.
68. Broyer M, Tete MJ, Guest G, Gagnadoux MF, Rouzioux C. Varicella and zoster in children after kidney transplantation: long-term results of vaccination. Pediatrics. 1997;99(1):35–9.
69. Warmington L, Lee BE, Robinson JL. Loss of antibodies to measles and varicella following solid organ transplantation in children. Pediatr Transplant. 2005;9(3):311–4.
70. Shinjoh M, Miyairi I, Hoshino K, Takahashi T, Nakayama T. Effective and safe immunizations with live-attenuated vaccines for children after living donor liver transplantation. Vaccine. 2008;26(52):6859–63.
71. Khan S, Erlichman J, Rand EB. Live virus immunization after orthotopic liver transplantation. Pediatr Transplant. 2006;10(1):78–82.
72. Chaves Tdo S, Lopes MH, de Souza VA, Dos Santos SS, Pereira LM, Reis AD, et al. Seroprevalence of antibodies against varicella-zoster virus and response to the varicella vaccine in pediatric renal transplant patients. Pediatr Transplant. 2005;9(2):192–6.
73. Kano H, Mizuta K, Sakakihara Y, Kato H, Miki Y, Shibuya N, et al. Efficacy and safety of immunization for pre- and post- liver transplant children. Transplantation. 2002;74(4):543–50.
74. Weinberg A, Horslen SP, Kaufman SS, Jesser R, Devoll-Zabrocki A, Fleckten BL, et al. Safety and immunogenicity of varicella-zoster virus vaccine in pediatric liver and intestine transplant recipients. Am J Transplant. 2006;6(3):565–8.
75. Posfay-Barbe KM, Pittet LF, Sottas C, Grillet S, Wildhaber BE, Rodriguez M, et al. Varicella-zoster immunization in pediatric liver transplant recipients: safe and immunogenic. Am J Transplant. 2012;12(11):2974–85.
76. Miller GG, Dummer JS. Herpes simplex and varicella zoster viruses: forgotten but not gone. Am J Transplant. 2007;7(4):741–7.
77. Lal H, Cunningham AL, Godeaux O, Chlibek R, Diez-Domingo J, Hwang SJ, et al. Efficacy of an adjuvanted herpes zoster subunit vaccine in older adults. N Engl J Med. 2015;372(22):2087–96.
78. Lima EQ, Silva RG, Fernandes IM, Abbud-Filho M, Burdmann EA. Tetanus-induced acute kidney injury in a renal transplant recipient. Am J Trop Med Hyg. 2007;77(2):400–2.
79. Huzly D, Neifer S, Reinke P, Schroder K, Schonfeld C, Hofmann T, et al. Routine immunizations in adult renal transplant recipients. Transplantation. 1997;63(6):839–45.
80. Ner Z, Ross LA, Horn MV, Keens TG, MacLaughlin EF, Starnes VA, et al. Bordetella bronchiseptica infection in pediatric lung transplant recipients. Pediatr Transplant. 2003;7(5):413–7.
81. Chauncey JB, Schaberg DR. Interstitial pneumonia caused by Bordetella bronchiseptica in a heart transplant patient. Transplantation. 1990;49(4):817–9.
82. Choy KW, Wulffraat NM, Wolfs TF, Geelen SP, Kraaljeveld CA, Fleer A. Bordetella bronchiseptica respiratory infection in a child after bone marrow transplantation. Pediatr Infect Dis J. 1999;18(5):481–3.
83. Bauwens JE, Spach DH, Schacker TW, Mustafa MM, Bowden RA. Bordetella bronchiseptica pneumonia and bacteremia following bone marrow transplantation. J Clin Microbiol. 1992;30(9):2474–5.
84. Berkelman RL. Human illness associated with use of veterinary vaccines. Clin Infect Dis. 2003;37(3):407–14.
85. Perez-Padilla R, de la Rosa-Zamboni D, Ponce de Leon S, Hernandez M, Quinones-Falconi F, Bautista E, et al. Pneumonia and respiratory failure from swine-origin influenza A (H1N1) in Mexico. N Engl J Med. 2009;361(7):680–9.
86. CDC. Hepatitis B Information for Health Professionals [cited 2012 January 30]. Available from: http://www.cdc.gov/hepatitis/HBV/index.htm
87. Australian Government Department of Health and Ageing: Immunise Australia Program [cited 2012 January 30]. Available from: http://www.immunise.health.gov.au/internet/immunise/publishing.nsf/Content/nips2.
88. Report on First survey of Immunisation Programs in Europe. 2007 April 2007. VENICE project.
89. Public Health Agency of Canada: Immunizations & Vaccines [cited 2012 January 30]. Available from: http://www.phac-aspc.gc.ca/im/index-eng.php.

90. Su WJ, Ho MC, Ni YH, Chen HL, Hu RH, Wu YM, et al. High-titer antibody to hepatitis B surface antigen before liver transplantation can prevent de novo hepatitis B infection. J Pediatr Gastroenterol Nutr. 2009;48(2):203–8.
91. Idilman R, Colantoni A, De Maria N, Ustun C, Sam R, Ing TS, et al. Impaired antibody response rates after high dose short interval hepatitis B virus vaccination of immunosuppressed individuals. Hepato-Gastroenterology. 2003;50(49):217–21.
92. Angelico M, Di Paolo D, Trinito MO, Petrolati A, Araco A, Zazza S, et al. Failure of a reinforced triple course of hepatitis B vaccination in patients transplanted for HBV-related cirrhosis. Hepatology. 2002;35(1):176–81.
93. Ishigami M, Kamei H, Nakamura T, Katano Y, Ando H, Kiuchi T, et al. Different effect of HBV vaccine after liver transplantation between chronic HBV carriers and non-HBV patients who received HBcAb-positive grafts. J Gastroenterol. 2011;46(3):367–77.
94. Klevens RM, Miller JT, Iqbal K, Thomas A, Rizzo EM, Hanson H, et al. The evolving epidemiology of hepatitis A in the United States: incidence and molecular epidemiology from population-based surveillance, 2005–2007. Arch Intern Med. 2010;170(20): 1811–8.
95. CDC. Hepatitis A Information for Health Professionals [cited 2012 January 30]. Available from: https://www.cdc.gov/hepatitis/hav/
96. Park GC, Hwang S, Yu YD, Park PJ, Choi YI, Song GW, et al. Intractable recurrent hepatitis A virus infection requiring repeated liver transplantation: a case report. Transplant Proc. 2010;42(10):4658–60.
97. Lok AS, McMahon BJ. Chronic hepatitis B: update 2009. Hepatology. 2009;50(3):661–2.
98. Ghany MG, Strader DB, Thomas DL, Seeff LB. Diagnosis, management, and treatment of hepatitis C: an update. Hepatology. 2009;49(4):1335–74.
99. Arslan M, Wiesner RH, Sievers C, Egan K, Zein NN. Double-dose accelerated hepatitis B vaccine in patients with end-stage liver disease. Liver Transpl. 2001;7(4):314–20.
100. Dumot JA, Barnes DS, Younossi Z, Gordon SM, Avery RK, Domen RE, et al. Immunogenicity of hepatitis A vaccine in decompensated liver disease. Am J Gastroenterol. 1999;94(6):1601–4.
101. Stark K, Gunther M, Neuhaus R, Reinke P, Schroder K, Linnig S, et al. Immunogenicity and safety of hepatitis A vaccine in liver and renal transplant recipients. J Infect Dis. 1999;180(6):2014–7.
102. Ferreira CT, da Silveira TR, Vieira SM, Taniguchi A, Pereira-Lima J. Immunogenicity and safety of hepatitis A vaccine in children with chronic liver disease. J Pediatr Gastroenterol Nutr. 2003;37(3):258–61.
103. Gunther M, Stark K, Neuhaus R, Reinke P, Schroder K, Bienzle U. Rapid decline of antibodies after hepatitis A immunization in liver and renal transplant recipients. Transplantation. 2001;71(3):477–9.
104. Rendi-Wagner P, Korinek M, Winkler B, Kundi M, Kollaritsch H, Wiedermann U. Persistence of seroprotection 10 years after primary hepatitis A vaccination in an unselected study population. Vaccine. 2007;25(5):927–31.
105. Schroter GP, West JC, Weil R 3rd. Acute bacteremia in asplenic renal transplant patients. JAMA. 1977;237(20):2207–8.
106. Mermel LA, Maki DG. Bacterial pneumonia in solid organ transplantation. Semin Respir Infect. 1990;5(1):10–29.
107. Haemophilus influenzae invasive disease among children aged <5 years – California, 1990–1996. MMWR Morb Mortal Wkly Rep. 1998;47(35):737–40.
108. Progress toward elimination of Haemophilus influenzae type b disease among infants and children – United States, 1987–1995. MMWR Morb Mortal Wkly Rep. 1996;45(42):901–6.
109. Pediatric bacterial meningitis surveillance – African region, 2002–2008. MMWR Morb Mortal Wkly Rep. 2009;58(18):493–7.
110. Sever MS, Yildiz A, Eraksoy H, Badur S, Yuksel-Onel D, Gorcin B, et al. Immune response to Haemophilus influenzae type B vaccination in renal transplant recipients with well-functioning allografts. Nephron. 1999;81(1):55–9.
111. Furth SL, Neu AM, Sullivan EK, Gensler G, Tejani A, Fivush BA. Immunization practices in children with renal disease: a report of the North American Pediatric Renal Transplant Cooperative Study. Pediatr Nephrol. 1997;11(4):443–6.
112. Laube GF, Berger C, Goetschel P, Leumann E, Neuhaus TJ. Immunization in children with chronic renal failure. Pediatr Nephrol. 2002;17(8):638–42.
113. Gennery AR, Cant AJ, Spickett GP, Walshaw D, Hunter S, Hasan A, et al. Effect of immunosuppression after cardiac transplantation in early childhood on antibody response to polysaccharide antigen. Lancet. 1998;351(9118):1778–81.
114. Urschel S, Cremer S, Birnbaum J, Dallapozza R, Fuchs A, Jager G, et al. Lack of serologic immunity against vaccine-preventable diseases in children after thoracic transplantation. Transpl Int. 2010;23(6):619–27.
115. Balloni A, Assael BM, Ghio L, Pedrazzi C, Nebbia G, Gridelli B, et al. Immunity to poliomyelitis, diphtheria and tetanus in pediatric patients before and after renal or liver transplantation. Vaccine. 1999;17(20–21):2507–11.
116. Hospital-associated measles outbreak – Pennsylvania, March–April 2009. MMWR Morb Mortal Wkly Rep. 2012;61(2):30–2.
117. Chen TH, Kutty P, Lowe LE, Hunt EA, Blostein J, Espinoza R, et al. Measles outbreak associated with an international youth sporting event in the United States. Pediatr Infect Dis J. 2007;29(9):794–800.
118. Greenland K, Whelan J, Fanoy E, Borgert M, Hulshof K, Yap KB, et al. Mumps outbreak among vaccinated university students associated with a large party, the Netherlands, 2010. Vaccine. 2012 Jun 29;30(31):4676–80.
119. Marin M, Quinlisk P, Shimabukuro T, Sawhney C, Brown C, Lebaron CW. Mumps vaccination coverage and vaccine effectiveness in a large outbreak among college students – Iowa, 2006. Vaccine. 2008;26(29–30):3601–7.
120. Zipprich J, Winter K, Hacker J, Xia D, Watt J, Harriman K, et al. Measles outbreak – California, December 2014–February 2015. MMWR Morb Mortal Wkly Rep. 2015;64(6):153–4.
121. Flynn JT, Frisch K, Kershaw DB, Sedman AB, Bunchman TE. Response to early measles-mumps-rubella vaccination in infants with chronic renal failure and/or receiving peritoneal dialysis. Adv Perit Dial. 1999;15:269–72.
122. Schulman SL, Deforest A, Kaiser BA, Polinsky MS, Baluarte HJ. Response to measles-mumps-rubella vaccine in children on dialysis. Pediatr Nephrol. 1992;6(2):187–9.
123. Mori K, Kawamura K, Honda M, Sasaki N. Responses in children to measles vaccination associated with perirenal transplantation. Pediatr Int. 2009;51(5):617–20.
124. Rand EB, McCarthy CA, Whitington PF. Measles vaccination after orthotopic liver transplantation. J Pediatr. 1993;123(1):87–9.
125. Markowitz LE, Dunne EF, Saraiya M, Lawson HW, Chesson H, Unger ER. Quadrivalent human papillomavirus vaccine: recommendations of the Advisory Committee on Immunization Practices (ACIP). MMWR Recomm Rep. 2007;56(RR-2):1–24.
126. Meeuwis KA, Melchers WJ, Bouten H, van de Kerkhof PC, Hinten F, Quint WG, et al. Anogenital malignancies in women after renal transplantation over 40 years in a single center. Transplantation. 2012 May 15;93(9):914–22.
127. Kasiske BL, Snyder JJ, Gilbertson DT, Wang C. Cancer after kidney transplantation in the United States. Am J Transplant. 2004;4(6):905–13.
128. Kellerman L, Neugut A, Burke B, Mancini D. Comparison of the incidence of de novo solid malignancies after heart transplantation to that in the general population. Am J Cardiol. 2009;103(4):562–6.

129. Malouf MA, Hopkins PM, Singleton L, Chhajed PN, Plit ML, Glanville AR. Sexual health issues after lung transplantation: importance of cervical screening. J Heart Lung Transplant. 2004;23(7):894–7.
130. Koutsky LA, Ault KA, Wheeler CM, Brown DR, Barr E, Alvarez FB, et al. A controlled trial of a human papillomavirus type 16 vaccine. N Engl J Med. 2002;347(21):1645–51.
131. Mao C, Koutsky LA, Ault KA, Wheeler CM, Brown DR, Wiley DJ, et al. Efficacy of human papillomavirus-16 vaccine to prevent cervical intraepithelial neoplasia: a randomized controlled trial. Obstet Gynecol. 2006;107(1):18–27.
132. Villa LL, Costa RL, Petta CA, Andrade RP, Ault KA, Giuliano AR, et al. Prophylactic quadrivalent human papillomavirus (types 6, 11, 16, and 18) L1 virus-like particle vaccine in young women: a randomised double-blind placebo-controlled multicentre phase II efficacy trial. Lancet Oncol. 2005;6(5):271–8.
133. Villa LL, Costa RL, Petta CA, Andrade RP, Paavonen J, Iversen OE, et al. High sustained efficacy of a prophylactic quadrivalent human papillomavirus types 6/11/16/18 L1 virus-like particle vaccine through 5 years of follow-up. Br J Cancer. 2006;95(11):1459–66.
134. Kumar D, Unger ER, Panicker G, Medvedev P, Wilson L, Humar A. Immunogenicity of quadrivalent human papillomavirus vaccine in organ transplant recipients. Am J Transplant. 2013;13(9):2411–7.

Prevention of Fungal Disease

64

Shirish Huprikar and John R. Wingard

Introduction

Invasive fungal infections (IFIs) are serious complications associated with significant morbidity and mortality in solid organ transplant (SOT) and hematopoietic cell transplant (HCT) recipients. The recent epidemiology of IFIs in SOT and HCT recipients in the United States was described by the Transplant-Associated Infection Surveillance Network (TRANSNET), a consortium of 23 transplant centers in the United States that prospectively identified IFIs in SOT recipients [1] and HCT recipients [2]. The 1-year incidence of first IFIs in SOT patients was as follows: small bowel transplant (11.6%), lung (8.6%), liver (4.7%), heart (4%), pancreas (3.4%), and kidney (1.3%). The 1-year incidence of first IFIs in HCT patients was as follows: mismatched related donor (8.1%), matched unrelated donor (7.7%), matched related donor (5.8%), and autologous (1.2%). The most common IFIs in SOT recipients were invasive candidiasis (IC) (53%), invasive aspergillosis (IA) (19%), cryptococcosis (8%), endemic IFIs (5%), and mucormycosis (2%). The median onset of IC and IA was 103 and 184 days, respectively. In contrast, the median onset of cryptococcosis was 575 days after transplantation. The most common IFIs in HCT recipients were IA (43%), IC (28%), and mucormycosis (8%). The median times of onset of IC and IA were 61 and 99 days, respectively.

Strategies to prevent early IFIs in SOT and HCT recipients are generally advocated in patients with established risk factors. In this chapter, we review the literature regarding antifungal prevention in the various transplant types and consensus antifungal prophylaxis guidelines that may exist (Table 64.1).

Liver Transplantation

Current guidelines recommend antifungal prophylaxis with fluconazole to target *Candida* in high-risk liver transplant recipients with ≥2 of the following risk factors: prolonged or reoperation, re-transplantation, renal failure, ≥ 40 blood product units, choledochojejunostomy, and perioperative *Candida* colonization [3]. Although no definitive recommendation for duration exists, it is reasonable to continue prophylaxis until risk factors have resolved. Some experts will also consider antifungal prophylaxis with a lipid formulation of amphotericin B or an echinocandin to target *Aspergillus* in patients with ≥1 of the following risk factors: re-transplantation, renal replacement therapy, reoperation, and fulminant hepatic failure [4].

Antifungal prophylaxis is a very common practice in liver transplant centers in North America. A survey study conducted in 2006 and 2007 indicated that 91% of responding centers used either universal (28%) or targeted (72%) antifungal prophylaxis [5] Although the antifungal choice and duration were quite variable, universal or targeted fluconazole prophylaxis was the preferred approach in the majority of centers. The most common indications for targeted prophylaxis were re-transplantation (78%), dialysis (72%), re-exploration (61%), and colonization with *Candida* (57%). Other indications included prolonged intensive care unit (ICU) stay or mechanical assisted ventilation, high transfusion requirements, and receipt of T cell-depleting agents. Recent studies also demonstrate MELD score as a risk factor for IFI after liver transplantation [6].

Universal Antifungal Prophylaxis Strategies

Universal prophylaxis strategies with both amphotericin B formulations and azoles have been extensively explored in liver transplant recipients. In an observational study, 58 liver transplant recipients received 1 mg/kg of AmBisome for 7 days [7, 8]. There was one *Candida* infection and three fatal *Aspergillus* infections.

S. Huprikar (✉)
The Mount Sinai Hospital, Icahn School of Medicine at Mount Sinai, New York, NY, USA
e-mail: shirish.huprikar@mountsinai.org

J. R. Wingard
University of Florida, Division of Hematology/Oncology, Department of Medicine, Gainesville, FL, USA
e-mail: wingajr@ufl.edu

A. Safdar (ed.), *Principles and Practice of Transplant Infectious Diseases*, https://doi.org/10.1007/978-1-4939-9034-4_64

Table 64.1 Summary of antifungal prophylaxis in stem cell and solid organ transplantation

Transplant type	Preferred antifungal regimens	Alternative antifungal regimens	Relative cost (least expensive to most expensive)	Comments
Allogeneic HCT, standard risk	FLU MICA	ITRA VORI L-AmB	FLU ITRA VORI, POSA MICA/L-AmB	FLU lacks mold activity - monitoring important ITRA, VORI, and POSA should not be used concomitantly with cyclophosphamide and vincristine; doses of concomitant calcineurin inhibitors should be adjusted; blood concentrations may vary so monitoring may be necessary Most experts deem the ECH as therapeutically equivalent
Allogeneic HCT, high risk	VORI POSA	MIC ITRA FLU L-AmB	FLU ITRA VORI, POSA MICA, L-AmB	Definitions of high risk vary but generally include mismatched or unrelated donor transplants, cell-depleting maneuvers, cord blood grafts, older age, acute myelogenous leukemia, and GVHD Randomized trials show strong (usually nonsignificant) trends for reduced rates of IA with anti-mold agents in this subset although an alternative approach would be anti-yeast prophylaxis with close monitoring, including galactomannan screening and aggressive evaluation of syndromes suspected to be fungal in origin with preemptive antifungal therapy
Allogeneic or autologous HCT with prior IFI	VORI If prior IFI was *Aspergillus*, ECH or FLU if prior IFI was *Candida*, L-AmB if prior IFI was mucormycosis	Any agent that is active against the prior IFI	FLU ITRA VORI, POSA MICA, L-AmB	There are no randomized trials, but retrospective case series suggest strong protective effect with secondary prophylaxis; most experience is with VORI
Autologous HCT	FLU	MICA	FLU ITRA VORI, POSA MICA, L-AmB	The most common IFI risk is Candida, in conditioning regimens that cause mucosal damage The risk for aspergillus and other molds is low
Liver, High risk	FLU	ECH, L-AmB	FLU ECH, L-AmB	No indication for prophylaxis in low-risk patients
Lung	Ae-AmB	VORI	Ae-AmB, ITRA VORI	No randomized placebo-controlled trials for ae-AmB
Heart, High risk	ITRA Ae-AmB		ITRA, ae-AmB	
Pancreas, High risk	FLU			
Small bowel	FLU	ECH	FLU ECH	

HCT hematopoietic stem cell transplant, *FLU* fluconazole, *MICA* micafungin, *ITRA* itraconazole, *VORI* voriconazole, *L-AmB* lipid formulation of amphotericin B, *POSA* posaconazole, *ECH* echinocandin, IFI invasive fungal infection, *Ae-AmB* aerosolized amphotericin B.

The first randomized controlled study of universal antifungal prophylaxis in liver transplant recipients was conducted in 86 consecutive liver transplant recipients in a single center [9]. Patients were randomized to either 1 mg/kg of liposomal amphotericin B (L-AmB) or placebo for 5 days. The overall incidence of IFIs was 0% vs. 16%, respectively ($p < 0.01$), but there was no difference in mortality. There were five *Candida albicans* infections and one *Aspergillus niger* pneumonia in the placebo arm.

There is another single-center randomized, double-blind, placebo-controlled study in 212 liver transplant recipients who received fluconazole prophylaxis (400 mg daily) or placebo for 10 weeks [10]. Overall IFIs were observed in 45 (43%) of the placebo arm compared to 10 (9%) of the fluconazole group ($p < 0.001$). Significantly fewer IFIs were observed in the fluconazole group (6% vs. 23%; $p < 0.001$). The majority were *Candida* infections. Risk factors for IFI were assignment to placebo, United Network Organ Sharing classification 1, baseline fungal colonization, and re-transplantation. In low-risk patients without a risk factor; there was no difference in IFIs between the groups. Furthermore, there was no difference in overall mortality although there were fewer deaths attributed to IFIs in the fluconazole group (2% vs. 13%; $p = 0.003$).

In a multicenter randomized controlled study, 143 liver transplant recipients were randomized to daily oral fluconazole (100 mg) or nystatin for 28 days [11]. Lower rates of *Candida* colonization (25% vs. 53%, $p = 0.04$) and *Candida* infections (13% vs. 34%, $p = 0.022$) were observed in the fluconazole group. However, most of the *Candida* infections were superficial infections; there was no difference in invasive *Candida* infections or mortality.

Another single-center randomized, double-blind, placebo-controlled study [12] was performed in 71 liver transplant recipients who were randomized to either itraconazole 5 mg/kg orally preoperatively and 2.5 mg/kg orally twice daily postoperatively or placebo for a maximum of 56 days or until discharge from the hospital or treatment with systemic antifungal therapy for a proven, suspected, or superficial IFI. Fewer "fungal infection endpoints" were observed in the itraconazole group (4% vs. 24%; $p = 0.04$); however, none of these patients had a proven IFI. Furthermore, there was no difference in mortality.

In another single-center randomized controlled study, 188 evaluable liver transplant recipients were randomized to oral itraconazole solution 200 mg every 12 hr. or fluconazole given 400 mg every 24 hr for 10 weeks [13]. Proven IFIs were observed in 9% of the itraconazole group and 4% of the fluconazole group ($p = 0.25$) with no difference in mortality. Fungal pathogens included *Candida glabrata* (4), *Candida albicans* (3), and *Aspergillus* species (2) in the itraconazole group and *Candida glabrata* (2), *Candida krusei* (1), and *Aspergillus* species (1) in the fluconazole group. There were more gastrointestinal side effects in the itraconazole group.

In another single-center randomized placebo-controlled study of universal antifungal prophylaxis, 131 patients were randomized to one of three arms: 1 mg/kg of AmBisome for 7 days followed by 200 mg of itraconazole for 3 weeks; 400 mg of fluconazole for 7 days followed by 200 mg of itraconazole for 3 weeks; and placebo [14]. There were no significant differences in infection or mortality between the groups, and the authors concluded that routine use of antifungal prophylaxis is not justified.

Targeted Antifungal Prophylaxis Strategies

Observational studies demonstrate lower rates of IFIs with targeted antifungal prophylaxis with amphotericin B or fluconazole in high-risk liver transplant recipients when compared to historical data [15–18]. Furthermore, in the previously mentioned study that compared universal prophylaxis with itraconazole versus fluconazole, a trend favoring fluconazole was observed in high-risk liver transplant recipients with at least one risk factor such as UNOS classification 1, fungal colonization at the time of transplantation, or repeat transplantation [13].

Dosing of prophylactic amphotericin B was explored in a single-center observational study targeting high-risk liver transplant recipients [19]. All patients received nystatin for 3 months, and patients with risk factors including fulminant hepatic failure, re-transplantation, or ICU treatment also received fluconazole prophylaxis (100 mg daily). Consecutive patients requiring mechanical ventilation or continuous venovenous hemofiltration for ≥5 days after transplantation received additional prophylaxis with Abelcet until discharge from ICU or death (5 mg/kg daily for the first 10 patients, 2.5 mg/kg daily for the next 10 patients, and 1 mg/kg daily for the last 10 patients). Median duration of Abelcet prophylaxis in these 30 patients was 7 days and ranged from 1 to 37 days. There were no proven IFIs observed within 12 months of follow-up in all survivors. Of the six deaths, there was no histologic evidence of IFI in three who underwent postmortem examination.

In another single-center retrospective study of 186 consecutive liver transplant recipients, the incidence of IFIs was significantly higher in patients who required renal replacement therapy [20]. Among the patients requiring renal replacement therapy, the incidence of IFI was significantly lower (0%) in those who received prophylaxis with a lipid formulation of amphotericin B compared with those who received no prophylaxis (36%). Antifungal prophylaxis was independently associated with prevention of IFIs but not reduction in mortality.

Another single-center retrospective study examined targeted prophylaxis in 280 consecutive liver transplant recipients [21]. Starting in 1998, prophylaxis with a lipid formulation of amphotericin B was administered to patients with ≥4 of the following risk factors: > 30 units of packed red blood cells, renal failure, dialysis requirement, re-transplantation, surgical re-intervention, positive cytomegalovirus antigenemia or disease, acute rejection, mold colonization, > 5 days of antibiotic therapy, and ICU stay before transplantation. There was a trend toward fewer IFIs with preemptive amphotericin B prophylaxis compared to no prophylaxis in patients with >4 risk factors (14% vs. 36%; $p = 0.07$).

A single-center randomized controlled study [22] compared prophylaxis with conventional amphotericin B 15 mg daily or AmBisome 50 mg daily in 92 high-risk patient episodes based on ICU stay >4 days following transplant, fulminant hepatic failure, or readmission to ICU within 3 months of transplantation. IFIs were uncommon including 5 *Candida* infections and didn't differ between the groups. However, there was a significant difference in survival to ICU discharge favoring the AmBisome arm, 60% vs. 80% ($p = 0.038$).

In a single-center prospective observational study of 100 consecutive liver transplant recipients [23], 21 were identified as high risk and received 1 mg/kg of AmBisome for 7–10 days based on the presence of >1 of the following risk factors: acute liver failure, > 7 days of mechanical ventilation, re-transplantation, re-laparotomy, > 14 days of antibiotic therapy, > 20 packed red blood cell units, and biliary leak. No difference in the rate of IFIs was observed between the low-risk (5/79) and high-risk groups (2/21). Both infections in the high-risk group were due to *Aspergillus* species.

A randomized, double-blind controlled study [24] compared liposomal amphotericin B and fluconazole prophylaxis in high-risk liver transplant recipients with ≥2 of the following risk factors: choledochojejunostomy anastomosis; re-transplantation; ≥ 40 units of intraoperative blood product; reoperation for bleeding, anastomotic leak, or vascular insufficiency; renal insufficiency; and *Candida* colonization. Patients were randomized to either 2 mg/kg of liposomal amphotericin B or 400 mg of fluconazole daily for 14 days. Ten of 71 patients developed proven or probable invasive IFIs due to intra-abdominal *Candida* infection (n = 6), *Candida* bloodstream infection (n = 3), and *Cryptococcus* (n = 1); however, there were no differences between the two groups in rates of IFI or death.

The use of echinocandins for prophylaxis in liver transplant recipients has also been explored [25, 26]. In a multicenter prospective observational study [25], high-risk patients with ≥1 major criteria such as re-transplantation, renal replacement therapy, or fulminant hepatic failure or ≥ 2 minor criteria including renal failure, ≥ 40 intraoperative blood product units, choledochojejunosotomy, ≥ 2 surveillance cultures with *Candida*, or reoperation within 5 days of liver transplant received caspofungin for 21 days. Only two (2.8%) of the 71 patients developed IFIs at the surgical site due to *Candida albicans* and *Mucor* spp. infection.

In a multicenter prospective double-blind trial [26], 200 high-risk liver transplant recipients were randomized to either anidulafungin or fluconazole prophylaxis. The overall incidence of IFI was similar: 5.1% in anidulafungin and 8% in fluconazole treated patients. Anidulafungin prophylaxis was associated with favorable trends in preventing *Aspergillus* colonization and infection, lower breakthrough IFIs in patients with pretransplant fluconazole exposure, and fewer cases of antifungal resistance. There were no differences in graft rejection, fungal-free survival, or mortality.

The safety of withholding prophylaxis in low-risk liver transplant recipients has been described in two studies [27, 28]. In a prospective multicenter observational study [27], low-risk recipients were identified with ≤1 of the following risk factors: choledochojejunostomy anastomosis; re-transplantation; ≥ 40 units of intraoperative blood product; reoperation for bleeding, anastomotic leak, or vascular insufficiency; renal insufficiency; and *Candida* colonization. Of the 192 eligible patients, only 7 (4%) developed invasive IFIs. Only 3 (2%) were early *Candida* infections that were potentially preventable with fluconazole prophylaxis. In a cohort study of 12 Spanish hospitals [28], 799 low-risk liver transplant recipients were identified without risk factors such as renal failure in the first 15 days after transplant, urgent transplant, re-transplant, or choledochojejunostomy. Three hospitals performed universal prophylaxis with fluconazole for a minimum of 7 days. There were 11 episodes of IFI in 10 patients but no differences in the incidence of IFI between the patients receiving versus not receiving prophylaxis (4/206 or 1.9% vs. 6/593 or 1%; p-0.36).

Two meta-analyses have evaluated antifungal prophylaxis in liver transplant recipients [29, 30]. Cruciani, et al. [29] evaluated 698 patients from six randomized studies that compared fluconazole, itraconazole, or liposomal amphotericin B with placebo or oral nystatin and demonstrated that prophylaxis was associated with reduced fungal colonization, proven superficial and invasive infections, and mortality attributable to IFI but was not associated with overall mortality. Playford, et al. [30] evaluated 1106 patients from ten randomized studies comparing any antifungal prophylactic regimen with either no prophylaxis or another regimen and also demonstrated that antifungal prophylaxis reduced the rate of IFIs but not mortality.

Lung Transplantation

According to current guidelines [4], antifungal prophylaxis for up to 1 year is considered reasonable in lung transplant recipients with pre- or posttransplant *Aspergillus* colonization and also may be considered if ≥1 of the following risk factors is present: early airway ischemia, induction with alemtuzumab or thymoglobulin, single lung transplant, CMV infection, rejection and augmented immunosuppression, or acquired hypogammaglobulinemia. A meta-analysis and systematic review of controlled studies demonstrated no significant reduction in invasive aspergillosis or *Aspergillus* colonization with universal prophylaxis [31].

Antifungal prophylaxis strategies in lung transplantation have evolved over time with significant variation in practices. In a survey of 37 lung transplant centers in the United States that was conducted in 2001 [32], 76% of the centers provided posttransplant antifungal prophylaxis with targeted prophylaxis in 24% of these centers. Aerosolized amphotericin B was the most preferred agent (61%) followed by itraconazole (46%), parenteral amphotericin B formulations (25%), and fluconazole (21%). The median duration of prophylaxis was 3 months and ranged between <1 month and lifetime. In an international survey of 43 lung transplant centers between September 2002 and February 2003 [33], 69% provided universal antifungal prophylaxis. Aerosolized AmBd alone or in combination with itraconazole was the preferred strategy in 56% of the centers. The median duration of aerosolized AmBd and itraconazole was 1 month and 3 months, respectively. In a recent international survey of 58 lung transplant centers in 2009–2010 [34], universal prophylaxis was used in the majority of centers (58.6%) with nearly all of these centers (97.1%) targeting *Aspergillus*. The preferred first-line agents were voriconazole alone or in combination with inhaled amphotericin B. Preemptive or targeted approaches were used in 36.2% of centers. Of these, 90.5%

targeted *Aspergillus* and favored voriconazole prophylaxis. The survey also noted the use of posaconazole and echinocandins as first-line prophylactic agents in some centers.

The safety of aerosolized amphotericin B formulations has been demonstrated in a number of studies [35–40]. The most frequent adverse effects include cough, bronchospasm, nausea, and change of taste; however, discontinuation due to adverse effects is uncommon. A few studies have explored the pharmacokinetics of aerosolized amphotericin B formulations. A study of 12 lung transplant recipients demonstrated that delivery of aerosolized amphotericin B lipid complex (ABLC) is well distributed in the lungs although delivery to the native lung was suboptimal in some cases [41]. Another prospective study in 35 lung transplant recipients demonstrated that aerosolized ABLC administered daily for 4 days achieved concentrations in epithelial lining fluid above the minimum inhibitory concentration of *Aspergillus* up to 168 hours after that last dose [40].

There are no randomized placebo-controlled studies regarding the efficacy of aerosolized formulations of amphotericin B in lung transplant recipients; however, a number of observational studies [35, 36, 38, 39, 42] and one randomized controlled comparative study [43] have been published. In an early single-center study of lung, heart-lung, and predominantly heart transplant recipients [35], aerosolized amphotericin B deoxycholate (AmBd) was administered three times daily during the hospital stay. The incidence of *Aspergillus* infection was significantly decreased compared to a historic control group ($p < 0.005$). In another single-center study of 55 lung transplant recipients, 44 received nebulized AmBd three times daily for 120 days and then once daily for life [36]. Eighteen (33%) developed *Aspergillus* infection after a mean of 8.8 months including 14/18 (78%) within 2 months of transplantation. In multivariate analysis, nebulized AmBd was independently associated with a decreased risk of *Aspergillus* infection.

The efficacy of aerosolized ABLC was assessed in a prospective single-center study of 51 lung or heart-lung transplant recipients who were treated daily for 4 days and then weekly thereafter for up to 2 months [42]. The overall rate of pulmonary IFI included two (4%) anastomotic infections, no fungal pneumonia, and 8% with extrapulmonary IFI. One year survival was 78%. The treatment was subjectively well tolerated in 98%, and fewer than 5% developed worsening of pulmonary mechanics.

The efficacy of aerosolized L-AmB was assessed in an observational study of 104 consecutive lung transplant recipients in two centers [38]. Aerosolized L-AmB was administered three times per week up to day 60 followed by once weekly until day 180 and then every other week for life. IFIs were observed in only two patients with invasive pulmonary aspergillosis and tracheobronchitis. Outcomes were similar in 49 historic controls who received AmBd three times daily for 120 days and then daily for life thereafter.

A single-center prospective, randomized double-blind study comparing aerosolized ABLC and AmBd was conducted in 100 lung transplant recipients [43]. Patients received prophylaxis daily for 4 days and then weekly for 7 weeks. There were no fungal pneumonias observed. Other IFIs within 2 months included anastomotic and pleural space infections as well as candidemia, but there was no difference between the groups. More adverse events were observed in the AmBd group vs. ABLC including shortness of breath (19.9% vs. 2.1%), cough (10.6% vs. 2.1%), and change in taste (10.6% vs. 7.7%), respectively. Treatment discontinuation was also more frequent in the AmBd group (12.2% vs. 5.9% in ABLC group). Another retrospective single-center study compared aerosolized liposomal amphotericin B (L-AmB) and AmBd in 38 patients and found no difference in risk for IFIs or adverse effects [44].

The efficacy of aerosolized amphotericin B in combination with azoles has also been explored in observational studies. In a retrospective single-center study of 52 lung transplant recipients who received fluconazole 400 mg daily and aerosolized AmBd for at least 1 month [45], no IFIs were observed during the follow-up period. This was compared to a rate of 23% in a historical cohort from the same center. In another retrospective single-center study, there were 16 cases of invasive aspergillosis among 88 lung transplant recipients without prophylaxis compared to 4 cases among 81 recipients who received prophylaxis with aerosolized amphotericin B followed by itraconazole (18.2% vs. 4.9%; $p < 0.05$) [46]. In a retrospective study of 60 lung transplant recipients in 2 centers who received aerosolized ABLC once every 2 days for 2 weeks and then weekly for ≥13 weeks in addition to fluconazole (200 mg) for 21 days, there was only one patient with possible IFI, likely *Aspergillus fumigatus* colonization in the 6-month follow-up period, and only four patients experienced nausea and vomiting but without treatment discontinuation [39].

Observational studies have also explored the prophylactic use of azoles without aerosolized amphotericin B. In a single-center retrospective study of lung transplant recipients, invasive aspergillosis occurred in only 2/82 (2%) after implementing a prophylaxis strategy with voriconazole in patients with pretransplant *Aspergillus* colonization compared to 6/75 (8%) who had received itraconazole prophylaxis [47]. In a single-center retrospective study of 40 lung transplant recipients who received oral itraconazole 200 mg twice daily for 6 months, there were no *Candida* infections and only two *Aspergillus* infections, both occurring after itraconazole prophylaxis had been discontinued [48].

Low rates of invasive aspergillosis have been observed in patients receiving voriconazole prophylaxis. In a single-center nonrandomized study [49], 65 lung transplant recipients received universal voriconazole prophylaxis, while 30 received either fluconazole (200 mg) prophylaxis for 3 months or targeted prophylaxis with itraconazole +/− inhaled amphotericin B for 4–6 months in patients with pre- or posttransplant *Aspergillus* colonization except *A. niger*. The rates of IA at 1 year were 1.5% and 23% ($p = 0.001$), respectively. Rates of non-IA IFI were also lower in the voriconazole group (3% vs. 23%; $p = 0.004$). Voriconazole prophylaxis was more frequently associated with elevations in liver enzymes. In another retrospective single-center study, 32 lung transplant recipients received itraconazole prophylaxis (200 mg twice daily) for 3 months and 35 received voriconazole prophylaxis (200 mg twice daily) for 3 months plus inhaled amphotericin B for 2 weeks [50]. There were four IFIs in the itraconazole group compared to one IFI in the voriconazole arm. However, there was more hepatotoxicity with voriconazole (12/35 vs. 0/32); $p < 0.001$). Another single-center retrospective study compared itraconazole and voriconazole prophylaxis [51]. Forty lung transplant recipients received itraconazole, and 20 received voriconazole for 3 months. There were no differences in invasive IFIs, but tacrolimus dosing required greater dose reduction with itraconazole than voriconazole.

Heart Transplantation

Antifungal prophylaxis targeting *Candida* is not routinely recommended in heart transplant recipients [3]. Risk factors for *Aspergillus* infection include isolation of *Aspergillus fumigatus* from bronchoalveolar lavage, reoperation, CMV disease, hemodialysis, and an episode of IA in the program 2 months before or after heart transplant [52–54]. Current guidelines recommend targeted prophylaxis with itraconazole or voriconazole in heart transplant recipients with ≥1 of these risk factors [4]. In a single-center study, oral itraconazole prophylaxis was associated with fewer cases of IA and better 1-year survival [53]. In another study, prophylaxis with either oral itraconazole or inhaled amphotericin B for 3 months was associated with fewer episodes of IA [55]. Targeted antifungal prophylaxis in high-risk patients following heart transplantation is associated with reduction in invasive aspergillosis [56].

Pancreas and Kidney Transplantation

Risk factors for invasive candidiasis in pancreas transplant recipients include enteric drainage, vascular thrombosis, and post-perfusion pancreatitis [57], and current guidelines suggest that prophylactic fluconazole should be considered if risk factors are present [3]. In one study, intra-abdominal IFIs occurred in 6% of pancreas transplant recipients who received fluconazole prophylaxis for 7 days compared to 10% in those without prophylaxis [57]. Graft and patient survival were significantly worse in patients with IFI. In another study, fluconazole prophylaxis was associated with fewer IFIs [58]. Since rates of invasive IFIs in isolated kidney transplantation are low, antifungal prophylaxis is not recommended [3].

Small Bowel Transplantation

Although clinical trials are lacking, current guidelines recommend antifungal prophylaxis in small bowel transplantation due to high rates of *Candida* infections in these patients [3]. Local epidemiology should guide the choice between fluconazole and echinocandins. The appropriate duration of prophylaxis is not established, but some experts recommend a minimum of 4 weeks or until complete healing of the anastomosis [3]. In the setting of rejection and intensified immunosuppression, continued prophylaxis should be considered.

Allogeneic HCT

Invasive candidiasis historically was the chief pathogen accounting for IFI after allogeneic HCT; IC rates of 16–18% were observed [59, 60]. Oral nystatin or amphotericin B was routinely used as prophylaxis in many HCT centers but without demonstrable efficacy. With the introduction of fluconazole, clinical trials demonstrated a marked reduction in IC.

In a randomized double-blind trial of fluconazole 400 mg once daily versus placebo in 356 patients undergoing HCT comprising of half allogeneic and half autologous where prophylaxis was begun at the start of the conditioning regimen and continued until engraftment, fewer systemic IFIs were noted in the fluconazole group (3% versus 16% in placebo arm) [59]. Also noted were fewer superficial IFIs and lower rates of *Candida* colonization. Deaths due to IFIs were less, but overall survival was similar. Of note, there were few IA cases in both arms, in keeping with the observations of multiple studies that most episodes of IA occur later in the course of HCT after engraftment; the interval of the trial was pre-engraftment. Fluconazole was well tolerated. Unfortunately, the analysis did not break down if there were differences between allogeneic and autologous HCT as to efficacy and toxicity.

A second randomized trial of fluconazole versus placebo in 300 patients undergoing allogeneic HCT was conducted with prophylaxis extending to 75 days after transplant, encompassing both the neutropenic pre-engraftment and GVHD risk periods [60]. Fewer IFIs were noted in the fluconazole group (7% vs. 18%) due principally to fewer invasive *Candida* infections in the fluconazole arm. There were also fewer superficial IFIs, less use of empiric antifungal therapy for suspected IFIs, and no increase in non-albicans *Candida* infections. Overall survival was significantly higher in the fluconazole arm. Fluconazole was well tolerated without increased toxicity. A follow-up study demonstrated enduring benefit with fewer late *Candida* deaths and an enduring overall survival benefit [61]. Interestingly, there was less gastrointestinal involvement by GVHD in patients receiving fluconazole.

On the basis of such trials demonstrating both safety and efficacy, consensus guidelines recommend the routine use of fluconazole prophylaxis [62]. One trial examined the optimal dose of fluconazole and found 200 mg once daily was as effective as 400 mg daily [63]. One concern has been the risk for emergence of fluconazole-resistant *Candida* species and an increase in mold infections. Despite some single-center reports raising these concerns, fluconazole has remained effective for two decades without substantive resistance in this population. Today, IFIs due to *Candida* are infrequently encountered after HCT. Attention has shifted to IA and other mold pathogens. During the 1990s, greater numbers of IA were noted [64].

The echinocandins have an advantage over fluconazole with a broader spectrum of activity against several non-*albicans* species less susceptible to fluconazole, such as *C. krusei* and *C. glabrata*, as well as activity against *Aspergillus*. Micafungin at a once daily dose of 50 mg was compared to fluconazole as prophylaxis in 882 allogeneic or autologous HCT recipients administered from the start of the conditioning until time of engraftment in a randomized, blinded trial [65]. Both study drugs were well tolerated. Success, defined as no suspected or documented IFI, was greater in micafungin than fluconazole (80% vs. 74%). The greater success rate with micafungin was driven largely by fewer courses of empiric antifungal therapy for suspected IFI. Rates of candidemia were similar. There was a trend to fewer IAs (0.2% vs. 1.5%), but the rate of IA was low in both arms as would be expected in the pre-engraftment phase after HCT. This trial established the echinocandins as suitable alternatives to fluconazole for prophylaxis after HCT.

Since the echinocandins require intravenous administration, they are not well suited for prolonged administration in the outpatient setting to cover the later phases of HCT after engraftment in which IA is most likely to occur. The extended spectrum azoles available in oral formulations are particularly well suited for prolonged administration. They also have the attractive attribute of having both *Candida* and *Aspergillus* activity. Itraconazole, posaconazole, and voriconazole have been evaluated for antifungal prophylaxis.

In a randomized open-label trial, itraconazole at a dose of 200 mg twice daily was compared with fluconazole as antifungal prophylaxis in 140 patients undergoing allogeneic HCT [66]. Both were initially given intravenously and then changed to oral as tolerated. The study drug was started after completion of the conditioning on day 1 of transplant and continued to day 100. There were fewer proven IFIs in the itraconazole arm (9% versus 25%). The rates of superficial IFIs were similar in the two groups. There was an imbalance in factors associated with the risk for IFI in the two study arms, suggesting that the fluconazole group was overall at greater risk, and this may in part explain the very high rate of IFI in the fluconazole arm, much higher than would be expected in this patient population, even without any antifungal prophylaxis. Adjusting for risk factors known to be associated with IFI, itraconazole remained associated with fewer IFIs, but the small sample size of the trial makes such adjustments difficult to truly compensate for imbalances. There were more adverse events in the itraconazole arm and a greater proportion of patients who had discontinuation of study drug due to adverse events or death in the itraconazole arm. There was a trend to more deaths in the itraconazole arm, and overall there was no improvement in patients alive and free of IFI at 6 months in the itraconazole group.

A larger randomized, open-label comparison between itraconazole and fluconazole was conducted in 304 allogeneic HCT patients in a single center [67]. This trial had several important design differences from the Winston trial. Study drugs were initiated prior to the conditioning regimen; duration of prophylaxis was 180 days; dosing was 2.5 mg/kg three times daily; itraconazole drug levels were assessed because of the known variability in absorption after oral administration; and doses were adjusted to reach a predetermined level thought to be associated with antifungal efficacy (0.5 ug/ml). In this trial, more patients receiving itraconazole developed hepatotoxicity and nephrotoxicity, and more were discontinued due to gastrointestinal intolerance or toxicity (36% vs. 16%). Overall, there was no reduction in the rate of IFI (13% vs. 16%) with itraconazole. However, for patients who were able to tolerate study drug, there were fewer IFIs (7% versus 15%). This protective effect was due to fewer mold infections, with a similar protection against yeast pathogens. There was a trend toward a lower rate of fungal-free survival in the itraconazole arm (61% vs. 69%). Patients who received cyclophosphamide were noted to have greater toxicity with itraconazole, leading to a protocol amendment to initiate study drug after completion of the conditioning regimen. A subsequent analysis indicated an increase in toxic metabolites of cyclophosphamide potentiated by concomitant itraconazole [68]. The lingering concerns regarding tolerance and drug interaction-related toxicity with itraconazole have dampened widespread adoption of itraconazole, but the suggestions of reduction in invasive mold infections encouraged further testing with other extended spectrum azoles.

Recognizing the association of GVHD with a higher risk for IFI, posaconazole was tested in a randomized double-blinded comparison with fluconazole in 600 allogeneic HCT recipients with GVHD [69]. Study drugs were given for 16 weeks. Posaconazole was dosed 200 mg three times daily. There was a trend to fewer IFIs of all types (5% vs. 9%) and a significant reduction in IA (2% vs. 7%) with posaconazole. There were fewer deaths due to IFI in the posaconazole group (1% vs. 4%), but overall survival was similar in both study groups. Both all and severe treatment-related adverse events occurred at similar rates. An important observation in this study was that serum galactomannan assays were performed at study entry and 51 patients were positive. The galactomannan results were not used in the trial but analyzed afterward. The group with negative baseline galactomannan tests did not benefit from posaconazole (IFI rates, 5% vs. 8%); a reduction in IFI was observed in the patients given posaconazole who had positive galactomannan test results (10% vs. 23%). This suggests that the benefit of posaconazole was evident in patients who had incipient IA. Thus, an alternative interpretation of the results of this trial is that these findings are supportive of a preemptive treatment of early IA.

Two trials tested voriconazole as prophylaxis in allogeneic HCT recipients. The dose of voriconazole used in the two trials was 200 mg twice daily. There were several important design differences in the two trials. In one trial, the comparator was fluconazole, the study drugs were blinded, the endpoint was free from IFI or death at 6 months, and the sample size was 600 subjects [70]. In the second trial, the comparator was itraconazole; the study drugs were administered in an open-label fashion; the endpoint was free from IFI, death, and interruption of study drug for more than 2 weeks; and the sample size was 489 subjects [71]. In the first trial, there was no difference in fungal-free survival or overall survival at 6 months [70]. There were trends to fewer IFIs (7% vs. 11%), fewer cases of IA, and fewer empiric trials of antifungal therapy (24% vs. 30%) with voriconazole. There were no differences in adverse events. In a post hoc analysis, there were fewer IFIs and a higher rate of fungal-free survival in the subgroup of patients who were transplanted for AML. In the second trial, there was a higher rate of success with voriconazole compared to itraconazole (49% vs. 33%) [71]. The rates of IFI (1% vs. 2%) and survival (82% vs. 81%) were similar at 6 months. There were fewer empiric trials of empiric antifungal therapy (30% vs. 42%) with voriconazole. The tolerance of study drug was much better with voriconazole than itraconazole (54% vs. 39%) and accounted for the higher success rates of voriconazole.

Several single-center reports suggested an increase in IFIs due to the agents of mucormycosis with voriconazole prophylaxis [72–74]. It is important to note that voriconazole was not uniformly used in a standardized approach and presumably clinicians chose to use voriconazole in patients who were at high risk for all types of mold IFIs; thus, elimination of IA might open the door for mucormycosis. The prospective voriconazole prophylaxis multicenter trials did not show any increase in the risk for mucormycosis in patients given voriconazole [70, 71].

These two voriconazole prophylaxis trials suggest that the rates of IFI after standard-risk allogeneic HCT may not be sufficiently high to either demonstrate a benefit for anti-mold prophylaxis and to warrant the routine use of anti-mold therapy. However, there still remains the issue as to whether or not anti-mold prophylaxis has a role in higher-risk HCT patients. The trends in patients transplanted for AML (at higher risk for IFI and in whom lower IFI rates were seen with voriconazole)[70] and the trends for fewer IFI in the GVHD trial [69] suggest there may be a protective role in such individuals. An important group of high-risk HCT patients are those with prior IFI before HCT. Earlier studies have shown a high rate of reactivation of IFI even when they had been brought under control prior to HCT [75]. Indeed, the high risk of fungal deaths after HCT in patients with prior IFI subsequently led to many transplant centers excluding patients from consideration for transplant. However, several observational studies indicate that secondary prophylaxis prevents secondary recurrence [76, 77] and now many such patients can proceed to transplant.

Autologous HCT

The risk for IFI is lower in autologous transplants. Since the duration of neutropenia after autologous transplant was similar to that of allogeneic HCT, especially if bone marrow is used as the source of stem cells and the conditioning regimens were similar, a number of the earlier prophylaxis trials testing anti-yeast prophylaxis included both allogeneic and autologous HCT patients [59]. Although often not analyzed separately, it was assumed the risk for IFI was similar in the two types of transplant. Some trials included autologous HCT patients with patients undergoing induction therapy for AML [78]. In general, a benefit accrued to fluconazole. Other antifungal agents, including amphotericin B formulations, were also studied as prophylaxis, but toxicity of amphotericin B deoxycholate, the high cost of the lipid formulations of amphotericin B, the lack of clear superiority over the azoles, the lack of rigor of many of the studies, and the much lower risk for invasive mold infections have led most clinicians to not see a need for routine use of these other agents. Today, the conditioning regimens for autologous HCT are more heterogeneous. Since one of the major risk factors for IFIs due to *Candida* is mucosal injury, which allows gut *Candida* easier entry into the bloodstream, the risk for *Candida* IFI varies according to conditioning regimen. Additionally, there is a shorter time to engraftment today with optimization of stem cell grafts using G-CSF and apheresis collections of peripheral blood progenitor cells.

Thus, the routine use of antifungal prophylaxis to prevent *Candida* IFIs in autologous HCT remains uncertain.

Immune reconstitution after engraftment is more rapid than after allogeneic HCT since immunosuppressive medications are not necessary and there is no risk for GVHD. Thus, the risk for IA or other molds is low compared to allogeneic HCT. Thus, there is no substantial risk for IA after engraftment.

Coccidioides and Other Endemic Mycoses in SOT and HCT Recipients

Current guidelines recommend targeted lifelong fluconazole prophylaxis in SOT recipients with a history of coccidioidomycosis or with positive serologies, which are known risk factors for reactivation after transplantation [79, 80]. Prophylaxis is also recommended if the donor has infection or positive serologies. Although randomized, controlled trials are lacking, prophylaxis has decreased the risk of reactivation [81–84]. Some experts have recently recommended universal antifungal prophylaxis in liver and lung transplant recipients who reside in endemic areas [85, 86].

Antifungal prophylaxis for blastomycosis is not recommended as there are no sensitive or specific assays to detect latent or active blastomycosis and clinical trials are lacking [79]. Since the risk of reactivated histoplasmosis is low after transplantation [87], pretransplant screening is not routinely recommended [79].

The role of antifungal prophylaxis for endemic fungal pathogens has not been studied in HCT recipients. Currently, there are no consensus guidelines regarding these pathogens in HCT recipients. However, for allogeneic HCT recipients who are on active immunosuppressive therapy, similar approaches to those taken for SOT are sensible.

Summary

Routine or targeted antifungal prevention strategies are considered standard of care in both solid organ and stem cell transplant recipients. Future studies should continue to explore the safest and most cost-effective strategies.

References

1. Pappas PG, Alexander BD, Andes DR, et al. Invasive fungal infections among organ transplant recipients: results of the Transplant-Associated Infection Surveillance Network (TRANSNET). Clin Infect Dis. 2010;50(8):1101–11.
2. Kontoyiannis DP, Marr KA, Park BJ, et al. Prospective surveillance for invasive fungal infections in hematopoietic stem cell transplant recipients, 2001-2006: overview of the Transplant-Associated Infection Surveillance Network (TRANSNET) Database. Clin Infect Dis. 2010;50(8):1091–100.
3. Silveira FP, Kusne S, ASTIDCo P. Candida infections in solid organ transplantation. Am J Transplant. 2013;13(Suppl 4):220–7.
4. Singh N, Husain S, ASTIDCo P. Aspergillosis in solid organ transplantation. Am J Transplant. 2013;13(Suppl 4):228–41.
5. Singh N, Wagener MM, Cacciarelli TV, Levitsky J. Antifungal management practices in liver transplant recipients. Am J Transplant. 2008;8(2):426–31.
6. Saliba F, Delvart V, Ichai P, et al. Fungal infections after liver transplantation: outcomes and risk factors revisited in the MELD era. Clin Transpl. 2013;27(4):E454–61.
7. Braun F, Ruchel R, Lorf T, et al. Is liposomal amphotericin B (ambisome) an effective prophylaxis of mycotic infections after liver transplantation? Transplant Proc. 1998;30(4):1481–3.
8. Lorf T, Braun F, Ruchel R, Muller A, Sattler B, Ringe B. Systemic mycoses during prophylactical use of liposomal amphotericin B (Ambisome) after liver transplantation. Mycoses. 1999;42(1–2):47–53.
9. Tollemar J, Hockerstedt K, Ericzon BG, Jalanko H, Ringden O. Liposomal amphotericin B prevents invasive fungal infections in liver transplant recipients. A randomized, placebo-controlled study. Transplantation. 1995;59(1):45–50.
10. Winston DJ, Pakrasi A, Busuttil RW. Prophylactic fluconazole in liver transplant recipients. A randomized, double-blind, placebo-controlled trial. Ann Intern Med. 1999;131(10):729–37.
11. Lumbreras C, Cuervas-Mons V, Jara P, et al. Randomized trial of fluconazole versus nystatin for the prophylaxis of Candida infection following liver transplantation. J Infect Dis. 1996;174(3):583–8.
12. Sharpe MD, Ghent C, Grant D, Horbay GL, McDougal J, David Colby W. Efficacy and safety of itraconazole prophylaxis for fungal infections after orthotopic liver transplantation: a prospective, randomized, double-blind study. Transplantation. 2003;76(6):977–83.
13. Winston DJ, Busuttil RW. Randomized controlled trial of oral itraconazole solution versus intravenous/oral fluconazole for prevention of fungal infections in liver transplant recipients. Transplantation. 2002;74(5):688–95.
14. Biancofiore G, Bindi ML, Baldassarri R, et al. Antifungal prophylaxis in liver transplant recipients: a randomized placebo-controlled study. Transpl Int. 2002;15(7):341–7.
15. Mora NP, Klintmalm G, Solomon H, Goldstein RM, Gonwa TA, Husberg BS. Selective amphotericin B prophylaxis in the reduction of fungal infections after liver transplant. Transplant Proc. 1992;24(1):154–5.
16. Kung N, Fisher N, Gunson B, Hastings M, Mutimer D. Fluconazole prophylaxis for high-risk liver transplant recipients. Lancet. 1995;345(8959):1234–5.
17. Decruyenaere J, Colardyn F, Vogelaers D, et al. Combined use of fluconazole and selective digestive decontamination in the prevention of fungal infection after adult liver transplantation. Transplant Proc. 1995;27(6):3515–6.
18. Hellinger WC, Bonatti H, Yao JD, et al. Risk stratification and targeted antifungal prophylaxis for prevention of aspergillosis and other invasive mold infections after liver transplantation. Liver Transplant. 2005;11(6):656–62.
19. Singhal S, Ellis RW, Jones SG, et al. Targeted prophylaxis with amphotericin B lipid complex in liver transplantation. Liver Transplant. 2000;6(5):588–95.
20. Singh N, Paterson DL, Gayowski T, Wagener MM, Marino IR. Preemptive prophylaxis with a lipid preparation of amphotericin B for invasive fungal infections in liver transplant recipients requiring renal replacement therapy. Transplantation. 2001;71(7):910–3.
21. Fortun J, Martin-Davila P, Moreno S, et al. Prevention of invasive fungal infections in liver transplant recipients: the role of prophylaxis with lipid formulations of amphotericin B in high-risk patients. J Antimicrob Chemother. 2003;52(5):813–9.

22. Shah T, Lai WK, Gow P, Leeming J, Mutimer D. Low-dose amphotericin for prevention of serious fungal infection following liver transplantation. Transpl Infect Dis. 2005;7(3–4):126–32.
23. Castroagudin JF, Ponton C, Bustamante M, et al. Prospective interventional study to evaluate the efficacy and safety of liposomal amphotericin B as prophylaxis of fungal infections in high-risk liver transplant recipients. Transplant Proc. 2005;37(9):3965–7.
24. Hadley S, Huckabee C, Pappas PG, et al. Outcomes of antifungal prophylaxis in high-risk liver transplant recipients. Transpl Infect Dis. 2009;11(1):40–8.
25. Fortun J, Martin-Davila P, Montejo M, et al. Prophylaxis with caspofungin for invasive fungal infections in high-risk liver transplant recipients. Transplantation. 2009;87(3):424–35.
26. Winston DJ, Limaye AP, Pelletier S, et al. Randomized, double-blind trial of anidulafungin versus fluconazole for prophylaxis of invasive fungal infections in high-risk liver transplant recipients. Am J Transplant. 2014;14(12):2758–64.
27. Pappas PG, Andes D, Schuster M, et al. Invasive fungal infections in low-risk liver transplant recipients: a multi-center prospective observational study. Am J Transplant. 2006;6(2):386–91.
28. San-Juan R, Aguado JM, Lumbreras C, et al. Universal prophylaxis with fluconazole for the prevention of early invasive fungal infection in low-risk liver transplant recipients. Transplantation. 2011;92(3):346–50.
29. Cruciani M, Mengoli C, Malena M, Bosco O, Serpelloni G, Grossi P. Antifungal prophylaxis in liver transplant patients: a systematic review and meta-analysis. Liver Transplant. 2006;12(5):850–8.
30. Playford EG, Webster AC, Sorrell TC, Craig JC. Systematic review and meta-analysis of antifungal agents for preventing fungal infections in liver transplant recipients. Eur J Clin Microbiol Infect Dis. 2006;25(9):549–61.
31. Bhaskaran A, Mumtaz K, Husain S. Anti-Aspergillus prophylaxis in lung transplantation: a systematic review and meta-analysis. Curr Infect Dis Rep. 2013;15(6):514–25.
32. Dummer JS, Lazariashvilli N, Barnes J, Ninan M, Milstone AP. A survey of anti-fungal management in lung transplantation. J Heart Lung Transplant. 2004;23(12):1376–81.
33. Husain S, Zaldonis D, Kusne S, Kwak EJ, Paterson DL, McCurry KR. Variation in antifungal prophylaxis strategies in lung transplantation. Transpl Infect Dis. 2006;8(4):213–8.
34. Neoh CF, Snell GI, Kotsimbos T, et al. Antifungal prophylaxis in lung transplantation--a world-wide survey. Am J Transplant. 2011;11(2):361–6.
35. Reichenspurner H, Gamberg P, Nitschke M, et al. Significant reduction in the number of fungal infections after lung-, heart-lung, and heart transplantation using aerosolized amphotericin B prophylaxis. Transplant Proc. 1997;29(1–2):627–8.
36. Monforte V, Roman A, Gavalda J, et al. Nebulized amphotericin B prophylaxis for Aspergillus infection in lung transplantation: study of risk factors. J Heart Lung Transplant. 2001;20(12):1274–81.
37. Monforte V, Ussetti P, Lopez R, et al. Nebulized liposomal amphotericin B prophylaxis for Aspergillus infection in lung transplantation: pharmacokinetics and safety. J Heart Lung Transplant. 2009;28(2):170–5.
38. Monforte V, Ussetti P, Gavalda J, et al. Feasibility, tolerability, and outcomes of nebulized liposomal amphotericin B for Aspergillus infection prevention in lung transplantation. J Heart Lung Transplant. 2010;29(5):523–30.
39. Borro JM, Sole A, de la Torre M, et al. Efficiency and safety of inhaled amphotericin B lipid complex (Abelcet) in the prophylaxis of invasive fungal infections following lung transplantation. Transplant Proc. 2008;40(9):3090–3.
40. Husain S, Capitano B, Corcoran T, et al. Intrapulmonary disposition of amphotericin B after aerosolized delivery of amphotericin B lipid complex (Abelcet; ABLC) in lung transplant recipients. Transplantation. 2010;90(11):1215–9.
41. Corcoran TE, Venkataramanan R, Mihelc KM, et al. Aerosol deposition of lipid complex amphotericin-B (Abelcet) in lung transplant recipients. Am J Transplant. 2006;6(11):2765–73.
42. Palmer SM, Drew RH, Whitehouse JD, et al. Safety of aerosolized amphotericin B lipid complex in lung transplant recipients. Transplantation. 2001;72(3):545–8.
43. Drew RH, Dodds Ashley E, Benjamin DK Jr, Duane Davis R, Palmer SM, Perfect JR. Comparative safety of amphotericin B lipid complex and amphotericin B deoxycholate as aerosolized antifungal prophylaxis in lung-transplant recipients. Transplantation. 2004;77(2):232–7.
44. Lowry CM, Marty FM, Vargas SO, et al. Safety of aerosolized liposomal versus deoxycholate amphotericin B formulations for prevention of invasive fungal infections following lung transplantation: a retrospective study. Transpl Infect Dis. 2007;9(2):121–5.
45. Calvo V, Borro JM, Morales P, et al. Antifungal prophylaxis during the early postoperative period of lung transplantation. Valencia Lung Transplant Group. Chest. 1999;115(5):1301–4.
46. Minari A, Husni R, Avery RK, et al. The incidence of invasive aspergillosis among solid organ transplant recipients and implications for prophylaxis in lung transplants. Transpl Infect Dis. 2002;4(4):195–200.
47. Mattner F, Chaberny IF, Weissbrodt H, et al. Surveillance of invasive mold infections in lung transplant recipients: effect of antimycotic prophylaxis with itraconazole and voriconazole. Mycoses. 2005;48(Suppl 1):51–5.
48. Shitrit D, Ollech JE, Ollech A, et al. Itraconazole prophylaxis in lung transplant recipients receiving tacrolimus (FK 506): efficacy and drug interaction. J Heart Lung Transplant. 2005;24(12):2148–52.
49. Husain S, Paterson DL, Studer S, et al. Voriconazole prophylaxis in lung transplant recipients. Am J Transplant. 2006;6(12):3008–16.
50. Cadena J, Levine DJ, Angel LF, et al. Antifungal prophylaxis with voriconazole or itraconazole in lung transplant recipients: hepatotoxicity and effectiveness. Am J Transplant. 2009;9(9):2085–91.
51. Kramer MR, Amital A, Fuks L, Shitrit D. Voriconazole and itraconazole in lung transplant recipients receiving tacrolimus (FK 506): efficacy and drug interaction. Clin Transpl. 2011;25(2):E163–7.
52. Berenguer J, Munoz P, Parras F, Fernandez-Baca V, Hernandez-Sampelayo T, Bouza E. Treatment of deep mycoses with liposomal amphotericin B. Eur J Clin Microbiol Infect Dis. 1994;13(6):504–7.
53. Munoz P, Rodriguez C, Bouza E, et al. Risk factors of invasive aspergillosis after heart transplantation: protective role of oral itraconazole prophylaxis. Am J Transplant. 2004;4(4):636–43.
54. Munoz P, Alcala L, Sanchez Conde M, et al. The isolation of Aspergillus fumigatus from respiratory tract specimens in heart transplant recipients is highly predictive of invasive aspergillosis. Transplantation. 2003;75(3):326–9.
55. Paniagua Martin MJ, Marzoa Rivas R, Barge Caballero E, et al. Efficacy and tolerance of different types of prophylaxis for prevention of early aspergillosis after heart transplantation. Transplant Proc. 2010;42(8):3014–6.
56. Munoz P, Valerio M, Palomo J, et al. Targeted antifungal prophylaxis in heart transplant recipients. Transplantation. 2013;96(7):664–9.
57. Benedetti E, Gruessner AC, Troppmann C, et al. Intra-abdominal fungal infections after pancreatic transplantation: incidence, treatment, and outcome. J Am Coll Surg. 1996;183(4):307–16.
58. Humar A, Kandaswamy R, Granger D, Gruessner RW, Gruessner AC, Sutherland DE. Decreased surgical risks of pancreas transplantation in the modern era. Ann Surg. 2000;231(2):269–75.
59. Goodman JL, Winston DJ, Greenfield RA, et al. A controlled trial of fluconazole to prevent fungal infections in patients undergoing bone marrow transplantation. N Engl J Med. 1992;326(13):845–51.
60. Slavin MA, Osborne B, Adams R, et al. Efficacy and safety of fluconazole prophylaxis for fungal infections after marrow transplantation--a prospective, randomized, double-blind study. J Infect Dis. 1995;171(6):1545–52.

61. Marr KA, Seidel K, Slavin MA, et al. Prolonged fluconazole prophylaxis is associated with persistent protection against candidiasis-related death in allogeneic marrow transplant recipients: long-term follow-up of a randomized, placebo-controlled trial. Blood. 2000;96(6):2055–61.
62. Tomblyn M, Chiller T, Einsele H, et al. Guidelines for preventing infectious complications among hematopoietic cell transplantation recipients: a global perspective. Biol Blood Marrow Transplant. 2009;15(10):1143–238.
63. MacMillan ML, Goodman JL, DeFor TE, Weisdorf DJ. Fluconazole to prevent yeast infections in bone marrow transplantation patients: a randomized trial of high versus reduced dose, and determination of the value of maintenance therapy. Am J Med. 2002;112(5):369–79.
64. Marr KA, Carter RA, Crippa F, Wald A, Corey L. Epidemiology and outcome of mould infections in hematopoietic stem cell transplant recipients. Clin Infect Dis. 2002;34(7):909–17.
65. van Burik JA, Ratanatharathorn V, Stepan DE, et al. Micafungin versus fluconazole for prophylaxis against invasive fungal infections during neutropenia in patients undergoing hematopoietic stem cell transplantation. Clin Infect Dis. 2004;39(10):1407–16.
66. Winston DJ, Maziarz RT, Chandrasekar PH, et al. Intravenous and oral itraconazole versus intravenous and oral fluconazole for long-term antifungal prophylaxis in allogeneic hematopoietic stem-cell transplant recipients. A multicenter, randomized trial. Ann Intern Med. 2003;138(9):705–13.
67. Marr KA, Crippa F, Leisenring W, et al. Itraconazole versus fluconazole for prevention of fungal infections in patients receiving allogeneic stem cell transplants. Blood. 2004;103(4):1527–33.
68. Marr KA, Leisenring W, Crippa F, et al. Cyclophosphamide metabolism is affected by azole antifungals. Blood. 2004;103(4):1557–9.
69. Ullmann AJ, Lipton JH, Vesole DH, et al. Posaconazole or fluconazole for prophylaxis in severe graft-versus-host disease. N Engl J Med. 2007;356(4):335–47.
70. Wingard JR, Carter SL, Walsh TJ, et al. Randomized, double-blind trial of fluconazole versus voriconazole for prevention of invasive fungal infection after allogeneic hematopoietic cell transplantation. Blood. 2010;116(24):5111–8.
71. Marks DI, Pagliuca A, Kibbler CC, et al. Voriconazole versus itraconazole for antifungal prophylaxis following allogeneic haematopoietic stem-cell transplantation. Br J Haematol. 2011;155(3):318–27.
72. Marty FM, Cosimi LA, Baden LR. Breakthrough zygomycosis after voriconazole treatment in recipients of hematopoietic stem-cell transplants. N Engl J Med. 2004;350(9):950–2.
73. Siwek GT, Dodgson KJ, de Magalhaes-Silverman M, et al. Invasive zygomycosis in hematopoietic stem cell transplant recipients receiving voriconazole prophylaxis. Clin Infect Dis. 2004;39(4):584–7.
74. Kontoyiannis DP, Lionakis MS, Lewis RE, et al. Zygomycosis in a tertiary-care cancer center in the era of Aspergillus-active antifungal therapy: a case-control observational study of 27 recent cases. J Infect Dis. 2005;191(8):1350–60.
75. Martino R, Subira M, Rovira M, et al. Invasive fungal infections after allogeneic peripheral blood stem cell transplantation: incidence and risk factors in 395 patients. Br J Haematol. 2002;116(2):475–82.
76. Cordonnier C, Maury S, Pautas C, et al. Secondary antifungal prophylaxis with voriconazole to adhere to scheduled treatment in leukemic patients and stem cell transplant recipients. Bone Marrow Transplant. 2004;33(9):943–8.
77. Cordonnier C, Rovira M, Maertens J, et al. Voriconazole for secondary prophylaxis of invasive fungal infections in allogeneic stem cell transplant recipients: results of the VOSIFI study. Haematologica. 2010;95(10):1762–8.
78. Rotstein C, Bow EJ, Laverdiere M, Ioannou S, Carr D, Moghaddam N. Randomized placebo-controlled trial of fluconazole prophylaxis for neutropenic cancer patients: benefit based on purpose and intensity of cytotoxic therapy. The Canadian Fluconazole Prophylaxis Study Group. Clin Infect Dis. 1999;28(2):331–40.
79. Proia L, Miller R. Endemic fungal infections in solid organ transplant recipients. Am J Transplant. 2009;9. Suppl 4:S199–207.
80. Blair JE, Logan JL. Coccidioidomycosis in solid organ transplantation. Clin Infect Dis. 2001;33(9):1536–44.
81. Blair JE, Douglas DD, Mulligan DC. Early results of targeted prophylaxis for coccidioidomycosis in patients undergoing orthotopic liver transplantation within an endemic area. Transpl Infect Dis. 2003;5(1):3–8.
82. Braddy CM, Heilman RL, Blair JE. Coccidioidomycosis after renal transplantation in an endemic area. Am J Transplant. 2006;6(2):340–5.
83. Blair JE, Kusne S, Carey EJ, Heilman RL. The prevention of recrudescent coccidioidomycosis after solid organ transplantation. Transplantation. 2007;83(9):1182–7.
84. Keckich DW, Blair JE, Vikram HR, Seville MT, Kusne S. Reactivation of coccidioidomycosis despite antifungal prophylaxis in solid organ transplant recipients. Transplantation. 2011;92(1):88 93.
85. Vucicevic D, Carey EJ, Blair JE. Coccidioidomycosis in liver transplant recipients in an endemic area. Am J Transplant. 2011;11(1):111–9.
86. Vikram HR, Dosanjh A, Blair JE. Coccidioidomycosis and lung transplantation. Transplantation. 2011;92(7):717–21.
87. Vail GM, Young RS, Wheat LJ, Filo RS, Cornetta K, Goldman M. Incidence of histoplasmosis following allogeneic bone marrow transplant or solid organ transplant in a hyperendemic area. Transpl Infect Dis. 2002;4(3):148–51.

Antimicrobial Drug Prophylaxis: Challenges and Controversies

65

Gaurav Trikha, Marcio Nucci, John R. Wingard, and Amar Safdar

Introduction

Prevention is the best way to manage an infection, especially in the susceptible transplant population. In these patients, the diagnosis is usually difficult, and response to treatment is often suboptimal. Antimicrobial drugs are the cornerstone for the prevention of opportunistic and other routine infections during the high-risk periods following solid organ and hematopoietic stem cell transplantation (SOT, and HSCT, respectively). However, there are many controversies associated with antimicrobial prophylaxis. These include (a) an appropriate selection of the subgroup of transplant recipients at a greater risk for infection, (b) selection of effective antimicrobial drugs, and, importantly, (c) how long such preventive interventions should be given. In general, antimicrobial prophylaxis is beneficial during periods when risk of a particular infection is higher due to a well-recognized complication following transplantation procedure. In a number of other situations, a clear benefit from such innervation is not certain. In this chapter, a comprehensive discussion regarding antimicrobial prophylaxis in recipients of HSCT and SOT is presented with a focus on controversies associated with such practices in the prevention of bacterial, fungal, and viral infections.

G. Trikha
Division of Infectious Diseases, University of Florida College of Medicine, Gainesville, FL, USA

University of Florida Health Shands Hospital, Division of Hematology/Oncology, Department of Medicine, Gainesville, FL, USA
e-mail: gaurav.trikha@medicine.ufl.edu

M. Nucci
University Hospital, Universidade Federal do Rio de Janeiro, Rio de Janeiro, RJ, Brazil

Hospital Universitário Clementino Fraga Filho, Department of Internal Medicine – Hematology, Rio de Janeiro, RJ, Brazil
e-mail: mnucci@hucff.ufrj.br

J. R. Wingard
University of Florida, Division of Hematology/Oncology, Department of Medicine, Gainesville, FL, USA
e-mail: wingajr@ufl.edu

A. Safdar (✉)
Clinical Associate Professor of Medicine, Texas Tech University Health Sciences Center El Paso, Paul L. Foster School of Medicine, El Paso, TX, USA
e-mail: amar.safdar@cidimmunology.com

Antibacterial Prophylaxis

Hematopoietic Cell Transplantation

Bacterial infections are common after HSCT and may significantly influence morbidity and patients' survival. There are other potential effects of bacterial infection on transplant biology. During a systemic bacterial infection, in some patients release of proinflammatory cytokines in excess may accentuate tissue damge; this phenotypic differential in cytokine response to a systemic bacterial infection has been speculated as a possible trigger for the onset of graft-versus-host disease (GVHD) or exacerbation of existing GVHD. Stem cell allograft recipients may experience systemic bacterial infections during the following periods at a significantly higher rate: a) pre- and post-engraftment severe neutropenia (ANC < 500 cells/mm); b) acute and chronic GVHD.

Neutropenia during the pre-engraftment and less commonly post-engraftment period is approached in a similar manner as patients with severe neutropenia while undergoing antineoplastic therapy for acute myeloid leukemia (AML) [1, 2]. There is limited data regarding efficacy and feasibility of antibiotic prophylaxis in HSCT population during the pre-engraftment neutropenia. Furthermore, no prospective trials have been conducted to assess this intervention in patients who may develop severe neutropenia after stem cell engraftment that is frequently seen in patients with relapsed cancer; drug-induced or viral myelosuppression potentially resulting in the loss of hematopoietic stem cell graft [3]. Several stud-

A. Safdar (ed.), *Principles and Practice of Transplant Infectious Diseases*, https://doi.org/10.1007/978-1-4939-9034-4_65

ies suggest that there may be unique issues that are clinically relevant in the transplant population compared with non-transplant patients receiving induction chemotherapy for acute leukemia. Antibiotics and antineoplastic therapy are now increasingly recognized to have a direct impact on the hosts' gut microbiota [4]. For example, in pediatric patients with AML, treatment with daunorubicin and etoposide may reduce the growth of anaerobic and aerobic microbes, whereas cytarabine therapy resulted in no such effect. There is also a differential effect of various drugs on the growth of different bacterial species. The antineoplastic and immune modulator agents commonly used for preparatory conditioning and the prevention of GVHD in allogeneic HSCT protocols appears to have a variable impact on the hosts' gut micorflora compared to the anticancer agents. Routine use of oral, absorbable, and nonabsorbable antibiotics given for prophylaxis to patients following transplantation may further complicate the aberration in physiologic composition of the gut microbiome in ways that are still not well understood.

Fluoroquinolones are generally chosen for prophylaxis during neutropnia. A report in allogeneic HSCT patients compared an earlier experience with ceftazidime prophylaxis subsequently switched to prophylaxis with levofloxacin [5]. Patients who received levofloxacin experienced more episodes of fever and need for a change in antibiotic regimen; however in this group, less bacteremia episodes, unchanged spectrum of bacterial pathogens, and low costs were encouraging findings. Such data may suggest that different prophylactic antibiotics may have variable effect on gut microflora and consequently subsequent risk for invasive disease, i.e., ciprofloxacin has greater anti-*Pseudomonas* activity but poor activity against *Streptococcus* and *Enterococcus* spp., whereas levofloxacin has protective activity against important Gram-positive pathogens including *Streptococcus* spp. including *Streptococcus pneumoniae*; beta-hemolytic streptococci like *Streptococcus pyogenes* and *Streptococcus agalactiae* among others. A major limitation of levofloxacin coverage includes limited activity against *Enterococcus* spp. and *Streptococcus* viridans group. Moxifloxacin has activity against common clinical anaerobes. How use of these antibiotics for extended periods given for prevention of infection may have a variable impact on hosts' commensal microbiota and overtime the risk of breakthrough systemic bacterial infections; yeast overgrowth and risk for subsequent invasive candidiasis as a consequence of antibacterial prophylaxis remains uncertain. These influences may playout differently as purturbation in homeostatsis of patients' microflora is widely diverse; probably representing a culmunation and permutation among a number of intrinsic i.e., genetic haecciety and external influences that may include household environment and diet, travel-related exposure, treatment with antineoplastic and immunosuppressive drugs, and prolonged exposure to hospital microenvironment, among others.

The role of antibiotic prophylaxis in the autologous HSCT setting is less clear. Some studies have demonstrated benefit [6]. There are many different conditioning regimens used in autologous HSCT, and the degree of mucosal injury, an important risk factor for neutropenic fever and bacteremia, varies considerably depending on the preparatory regimen used. Therefore, it stands to reason that the risk for neutropenic bacterial infections may also be different. Unfortunately, none of these issues have been studied in depth. Additionally, drugs given to patients to treat cancer prior to undergoing transplantation such as rituximab, an anti-B-cell antibody commonly used in treatment of B-cell lymphoma, or purine analogues that affect T-cell immunity, and corticosteroids that additionally affect neutrophil, monocyte, macrophage functions and T-cell immune response. Furthermore iron and other heavy metal overload conditions may exist in patients prior to transplantation, which may also influence a protean risk for infection in patients undergoing transplantation procedure.

The emergence and spread of antibiotic resistance accompanied by a shift in inherent less drug susceptible bacterial species such as *Stenotrophomonas maltophilia, Achromobacter xylosoxidans,* and *Burkholderia cepacia*, to name a few is a well-recognized concern with routine antibacterial prophylaxis. In some transplant centers, high frequency of drug resistant bacterial infections has led to a serious reevaluation of routine practices in antibiotic prophylaxis. A vigilant approach and continued surveillance for monitoring trends in drug resistance and emergence of infections due to difficult-to-treat bacterial species are recommended for hospital units caring for patients undergoing transplantation.

Clostridium difficile-associated diarrhea (CDAD) has become a serious and potentially life-threatening complication in transplant recipients [7, 8]. Various novel approaches and perspectives in CDAD risk mitigation CDAD **[delet "CDAD"]** include prophylaxis with fidaxomycin and antitoxin antibodies [9, 10]. Such interventions, if effective and routinely introduced in this population, are bound to alter hosts' intestinal microflora. It remains to be seen what degree of alteration in microbiota may occur and for how long it may persist plus the influence of such changes may have on the risk of subsequent bacterial and, possibly fungal infections. It is important to note that this risk may be accentuated in recipients of HSCT and solid organ allograft transplantation who are routinely given immunosuppressive drugs like systemic corticosteroids to prevent and treat GVHD and allograft rejection, respectively.

Animals transplanted in a germ-free environment had superior outcomes in experiments assessing relationship between infection and GVHD [11, 12]. It is believed that bacterial by-products, such as lipopolysaccharides, entering the bloodstream across a damaged gut mucosa stimulate the production of proinflammatory cytokines such as TNF and IL6 that in turn upregulate cellular mediators of GVHD [13]. A general hypothesis, now several decades old, was developed that suppression of bacterial flora and infection by antibiotics coupled with a protective environment may reduce the risk for GVHD and may improve survival following HSCT. A number of studies conducted at one institution have indicated a potential benefit from such an approach [14], whereas others were not able to reproduce this benefit from adherence to rigorous protective environment. The ongoing pyrosequencing studies of bacterial 16S rRNA genes to examine the composition of gut microbiota and the changes that may happen over time after HSCT and its impact on hosts' inflammatory response, risk for infection, and risk for GVHD are of great interest [15, 16]. These studies we hope will provide further insight into what appears to be a complex relationship between the host and its resident microbiota; new strategies may then be devised to harness and exploit such interactions for the benefit of patients who are undergoing evaluation for future transplantation procedures.

Presence of chronic GVHD, hypogammaglobulinemia, or IgG subclass deficiencies are particularly problematic; and so are impaired reticuloendothelial function including functional asplenia or hyposplenism. Susceptibility to infection by encapsulated bacteria is higher than general population, and so is the risk for devastating uncontrolled disseminated bacterial infection that often carries a greater risk of death. Although no randomized trials have been conducted, antibiotic prophylaxis has been shown to improve survival when compared with the results from older studies [17]. The consensus guidelines recommend institution of appropriate antibacterial prophylaxis in such patients [18]. The optimum choice of antibiotic, duration, or dose schedule is not validated; furthermore, increasing prevalence of community *S. pneumoniae* isolates that have become resistant to penicillin, erythromycin, azolides, and other antibiotics complicates the selection of appropriate agent in this setting. Moreover, the duration of risk is not well understood. In allogeneic HSCT patients with chronic GVHD, antibiotic prophylaxis is frequently discontinued as chronic GVHD subsides and patients are taken off anti-GVHD therapy. However, the immune deficits may persist for a long duration; studies to assess the duration of such immune defects after resolution of chronic GVHD are needed. It will be of interest to validate and incorporate immune reconstitution assays as a surrogate guidance for the decision as to the optimal timing to stop antibacterial prophylaxis in patients, in whom chronic GVHD has improved or resolved. Formal parameters for immune restitution-based guidance in stopping antibiotic prophylaxis will require prospective validation studies.

Alternatively, antibiotic prophylaxis may be supplanted by the emerging, and much desired interventions to boost hosts' immune response. The periodic administration of intravenous immunoglobulins in patients with hypogammaglobulinemia is regarded as standard-of-care for decades [19]. However, due to infusion-related toxicity, high cost, and no durable benefit, this intervention is selected for patients with severe and prolonged hypogammaglobulinemia with recurrent disabling sinopulmonary and less commonly, skin and skin structure infections [20, 21]. Targeted use of IVIG may also benefit patients with chronic GVHD, in whom chronic airway damage resulting from bronchiolitis obliterans and bronchiectasis leads to irreversible loss of pulmonary function; there is a growing consensus that such an intervention may lead to preservation of pulmonary function [22].

Immunization against *S. pneumoniae*, *H. influenzae*, and *N. meningitidis* is recommended for all patients undergoing HSCT [18]. Waiting to vaccinate until 12 months after transplantation is being revisited. Earlier immunization, especially with newer conjugated vaccines (Prevnar13) with higher immunogenicity, albeit limited serotype protection compared with older pneumococcal capsular polysaccharide vaccine (Pneumovax) that is marginally immunogenic; immunization with conjugate vaccines can be given as early as 3 months after HSCT [23]. However, responses to early immunizations may not be durable, and a booster dose is recommended for individuals with low antibody titers between 6 to 12 months after the first immunization. It was also encouraging that concomitant use of systemic corticosteroids or presence of GVHD did not severely impede in developing response to new-generation vaccines using conjugate protein construct. Further studies are needed. Pneumovax, a 23-valent capsular polysaccharide vaccine, has a broad spectrum of pneumococcal serotype coverage; however, due to pure polysaccharide construct, it has low immune stimulatory potential, especially in patients undergoing stem cell allograft transplantation. Some experts recommend an initial series of 2 to 3 Prevnar doses given at 3-month intervals followed by a single dose of Pneumovax 12 months after HSCT [24]. The newer Prevnar 13 does somewhat mitigate the concern regarding limited coverage compared with the earlier iteration of conjugate Prevnar 7 vaccine [25].

Solid Organ Transplantation

Bacterial infections in this population involves surgical site wounds, deep surgical bed infections, infections of the transplanted organ allografts site, deep tissue infected seroma or hematoma, infections involving the urinary tract, respiratory tract, and vascular-access devices, among others. In the pretransplant period, patients with end-stage heart, lung, liver and kidney disease and those with severe intestinal failure, are exposed to extensive antibiotics due to greater susceptibility for local and systemic infections and recurrent episodes of sepsis. However, the overall risk of bacterial infection from the donor allograft remains low [26], with the exception of patients undergoing lung transplantation [27]. Except for an organ procured from a donor with bacterial meningitis, simple bacteremia, or complicated bloodstream infection with or without endovascular source of infection; there is no convincing evidence that the recipient should be given antibacterial prophylaxis that is commonly started intraoperatively and continued during early posttransplant period.

Standard surgical antibiotic prophylaxis is recommended for all organ transplant procedures. Choice of drug(s) may vary with the type of organ transplantation being performed. Colonization with Gram-positive bacteria or *Candida* spp. needs appropriate coverage, but no consensus or evidence exists for the management of Gram-negative bacterial colonization, with the exception of patient with ESLD with high MELD score and presence of sepsis or complicated peritonitis. Patients with LVAD infections undergoing heart transplant and those with cyctic fibrosis during and after early lung transplant period, the choice of primary and secondary antibacterial prophylaxis is varied and center-specific protocols are generally implemented.

During the first 6 months after transplant, there is no consensus or evidence for using antibacterial prophylaxis. Trimethoprim-sulfamethoxazole (TMP-SMX) is routinely given for the prevention of *Pneumocystis jirovecii* pneumonia. The ancillary benefit of TMP-SMX prophylaxis similar to that seen in patients with HIV/AIDS, provide added protection against *Streptococcus pneumoniae*, *Listeria monocytogenes*, and *Nocardia* spp. infections. A recent systematic review and meta-analysis of renal transplant patients receiving antibacterial prophylaxis showed no significant reduction in all-cause mortality or adverse events; results were conflicting regarding the development of bacterial drug resistance following prolonged exposure to antibiotics [28]. These findings underscore the need for randomized controlled trials to assess ideal prophylactic antibacterial regimen and its optimum duration in this population.

Antifungal Prophylaxis

Hematopoietic Cell Transplantation

The use of antifungal agents to prevent the occurrence of invasive fungal disease (IFD) in HSCT recipients is appealing for the following reasons: the incidence of IFD is high, timely diagnosis is fraught with uncertainty, and high risk for death. Despite a number of randomized clinical trials, antifungal prophylaxis continues to generate controversies. Allogeneic HSCT recipients are at high risk for IFD in the early neutropenic pre-engraftment period with treatment-induced mucosal damage; the other two high-risk periods coincide with the development of acute and chronic GVHD. The risk for IFD during the latter two risk periods involves T-cell immune defects, whereas unlike pre-engraftment neutropenia, most patients have adequate number and functional peripheral blood neutrophils. Invasive candidiasis and aspergillosis account for the majority of IFD in this population. In the autologous HSCT, the risk for IFD is almost completely limited to the early posttransplant period, which coincides with the duration of profound neutropenia and severity of mucositis; invasive systemic candidiasis being the main concern. In addition, severe T-cell immunodeficiency may exist in heavily pretreated patients with refractory, relapsed lymphoma, or multiple myeloma, in whom autologous stem cell transplantation may also heighten the risk for invasive mold disease such as invasive aspergillosis (IA). Most patients who respond to an initial episode of IFD, especially those with a mold infection, require secondary suppressive antifungal therapy.

Two randomized clinical trials showed that fluconazole reduced the rate of superficial and systemic candidiasis, as well as infection-related mortality in patients undergoing allogeneic HSCT [29, 30]. Fluconazole was given until day 75 after HSCT in one trial; a post hoc analysis revealed prolonged protection against invasive candidiasis resulting from an extended fluconazole prophylaxis [31]. Prophylaxis with fluconazole has become the standard of care for the prevention of invasive *Candida* spp. infection in patients undergoing allogeneic HSCT. In autologous stem cell transplant recipients, routine use of fluconazole, especially beyond periods of severe neutropenia, remains controversial. It is recommended to give fluconazole prophylaxis to autologous HSCT recipients, in whom severe and prolonged mucositis is expected [32]. The problem is accurately predicting severity mucositis prior to transplant procedure. There is also a debate regarding the optimum dose of fluconazole (200 mg vs. 400 mg/day) in patients undergoing allogeneic HSCT; in one trial, no clear advantage was noted with higher 400 mg daily dose [33]. Most experts recommend giving 400 mg daily fluconazole dose as this was the dose chosen for the major prospective validation trials [32]. Still, the optimal duration of prophylaxis with fluconazole in allogeneic HSCT recipients with various posttransplant complications is not clearly defined.

In addition to fluconazole, other antifungal agents have been studied following allogeneic HSCT for the prevention of invasive candidiasis and include micafungin [34], oral itraconazole solution [35, 36], and voriconazole [37]. Posaconazole is another potential option; it was only assessed for post-engraftment high-risk periods [38]. These agents, especially mold-active azole-based drugs and echinocandins, are particularly useful in the following two situations: (a) high incidence of invasive candidiasis due to fluconazole resistant or nonsusceptible *Candida* spp. such as *C. glabrata* and *Candida krusei, respectively* and (b) if anti-*Aspergillus* coverage is needed.

Use of anti-mold prophylaxis in HSCT recipients still generates controversy.

Due to IA-associated devastating illness in HSCT recipients, effective prevention is highly sought after [39]. However, the results of randomized clinical trials are not as clear as they were with fluconazole prophylaxis for the prevention of invasive candidiasis. Oral itraconazole solution was compared with fluconazole in two randomized clinical trials [35, 36]. In both these studies, prophylaxis was given during pre- and post-engraftment periods. In one trial, the overall incidence of IFD was lower in the itraconazole arm [35], whereas in the other, itraconazole was associated with less invasive mold infections; however, this benefit did not extend in prevention of invasive candidiasis [36]. In both studies, gastrointestinal intolerance noted in one fourth of itraconazole-treated patients was the main limitation. Prophylactic posaconazole was compared with fluconazole in allogeneic HSCT patients with GVHD [38]). The primary endpoint including incidence of IFD on day 112 of prophylaxis showed no significant advantage for posaconazole use ($p = 0.07$); however, there was a significant reduction in the incidence of IA among patients given posaconazole (2.3%) vs. fluconazole (7%;$p = 0.006$). The fourth study compared voriconazole with fluconazole, given during pre- and post-engraftment periods [37]. The primary endpoint was fungal infection-free survival 180 days after HSCT; there was no difference in either group (75% in fluconazole vs. 78% in voriconazole; $p = 0.49$). Therefore, despite the fact that voriconazole is considered the drug of choice for the treatment of IA and that itraconazole and posaconazole showed benefit in reducing the incidence of IA, voriconazole failed to show superiority over fluconazole.

A careful analysis of the study design of these different trials, including procedures during protocol, population of patients, and endpoints, may in part explain these unexpected puzzling results. For example, when analyzing the incidence of IA, there was a trend for a benefit for voriconazole use over fluconazole (9 vs. 17 IA cases; $p = 0.09$). The study population in the posaconazole vs. fluconazole trial was allogeneic HSCT recipients with moderate to severe (stage II to IV) acute GVHD or extensive chronic GVHD, or substantial number of patients receiving intensive immunosuppressive therapies, or a select population at the highest risk for IA. In the voriconazole vs. fluconazole trial, most allogeneic HSCT enrollees did not end up developing GVHD. Furthermore, studies had different endpoints, and therefore it is difficult to compare results obtained from these trials despite all of the trials having a similar objective: to determine what is the most effective agent for IFD prophylaxis.

The important differences in the procedures that patients were submitted during the study period are outlined as follows. In the voriconazole vs. fluconazole trial [37], all patients were monitored biweekly until day 60 and then weekly from day 60 to day 100 after HSCT, including serial serum galactomannan monitoring. Empiric antifungal therapy was initiated in the event that patients developed a positive galactomannan assay and found to have radiographic and/or clinical features consistent with IFD. Therefore, another way of looking at the results of this trial would be that fluconazole prophylaxis plus a structured galactomannan monitoring for appropriate initiation of antifungal therapy was as good as prophylaxis with voriconazole in susceptible HSCT population. Important to note is that the trial enrolled "standard risk" HSCT patients, excluding those at high risk for transplant complications. Patients at higher risk for transplant complications such as GVHD are also at higher risk for IFD; therefore, it is possible that anti-mold prophylaxis may have a protective role in such patients. Important to note is that there were 3 risk factors for IFD in multivariate analysis [37]: older age, GVHD, and transplant for AML as the underlying disease. In the group transplanted for AML, a post hoc analysis showed there were fewer IFDs in those receiving voriconazole (8.5% vs. 21% in fluconazole); there was no protective effect in older patients or those with GVHD [37].

Due to all these variables in validation, randomized trial recommendations for anti-*Aspergillus* prophylaxis in allogeneic HSCT recipients remain controversial, for example, selection of at-risk subpopulation among all allogeneic HSCT recipients who would benefit the most from effective anti-*Aspergillus* prophylaxis. A group identified using the well-established risk factors for such susceptibility as illustrated in Table 65.1 may lend to a more focused and targeted approach towards anti-*Aspergillus* prophylaxis. As a general rule, the higher the risk is, the more likely prophylaxis will be of benefit. Another topic that should be considered is the potential for the emergence of drug resistance. For *Candida* spp. infection, there is little doubt that fluconazole use has resulted in a shift from highly susceptible *Candida* spp. such as *C. albicans*, *C. parapsilosis*, and *C. tropicalis* to less susceptible or inherently drug-non-susceptible species such as *C. glabrata* and *C. krusei*, respectively [40]. Recent studies have reported an alarming trend of the emergence of azole-resistant *Aspergillus* isolates in England and the Netherlands [41, 42]. Azole-resistant *Aspergillus* strains presently do not pose a clinical problem; however, a future potential for the development of resistance among disease-causing mold isolates following prolonged exposure to azole-based drugs given for prophylaxis does exist. The authors recommend a close monitoring of pathogen susceptibility trends and potential benefit of prophylaxis vs. the alarming risk of potential drug resistance among clinical fungal isolates be constantly assessed.

Another topic of controversy regarding anti-*Aspergillus* prophylaxis in allogeneic HSCT recipients is the optimal duration of prophylaxis. While in the pre-engraftment period the risk of IA is related to neutropenia and the period for such risk can be estimated, the same is not true for assessing

Table 65.1 Factors to take into consideration for deciding for anti-*Aspergillus* prophylaxis in allogeneic hematopoietic cell transplantation

Factor	Prophylaxis	No prophylaxis
Pre-engraftment period		
Type of transplant	Myeloablative	Non-myeloablative
Type of room	No HEPA filter and positive pressure	HEPA filter and positive pressure
Building construction or renovation	Yes	No
Local incidence	High	Low
Stem cell source	Bone marrow or cord blood	Peripheral blood
Post-engraftment period		
GVHD	Acute and/or chronic	No GVHD
Donor relatedness and HLA compatibility	Unrelated and/or HLA mismatch	HLA-matched related
All phases		
Serial serum galactomannan testing	Nonavailable	Available
Immunogenetics: MBL deficiency, TLR polymorphisms	Present	Absent
Comorbidities: iron overload, smoking, chronic sinusitis, or lung disease	Present	Absent

HEPA high efficiency particulate air, *GVHD* graft-versus-host disease, *HLA* human leukocyte antigen, *MBL* mannose-binding lectin, *TLR* toll-like receptor

risk during the post-engraftment period. It is reasonable to assume that once prophylaxis is initiated for patients receiving intensive immunosuppressive regimens for the treatment of severe GVHD, it should be maintained as long as severe immunodeficiency persists. The problem is that objective parameters to evaluate the severity of immune defect(s) are mostly available for research purposes and not widely used in patient care. Once sophisticated immune testing becomes clinically feasible, this will, as expected, substantially improve optimization of the duration of anti-*Aspergillus* prophylaxis during the post-engraftment period.

Finally, patients undergoing autologous HSCT may develop IA in the setting of extensive prior exposure to antineoplastic therapy for refractory multiple myeloma [43]; for such patients, currently there is no recommendation to initiate anti-*Aspergillus* prophylaxis.

Solid Organ Transplantation

The incidence and specific etiology of IFD vary in frequency according to the type of organ transplant procedure and the transplant center [44, 45]. A multicenter, prospective surveillance data showed 1-year cumulative incidences of the initial posttransplant IFD were 11.6% in recipients of small bowel transplantation, followed by 8.6% in lung, 4.7% in liver, 4.0% in heart, and 3.4% in pancreas and 1.3% after kidney transplantation [46]. The 1-year incidence was highest for invasive candidiasis (1.95%) followed by aspergillosis (0.65%). *Candida* spp. infections were a significant complication in liver and pancreas transplant recipients, whereas the impact of IA was high after heart and lung transplantations. An estimated 9.3% of deaths in lung transplant recipients and 16.9% in liver recipients are due to IA [47].

In liver transplant recipients, aspergillosis when present is notable during early post-transplant period; patients are uniquely predisposed to disseminated *Aspergillus* infection beyond the lungs and involvement of the central nervous system is not uncommon.**[the pargraph below belongs here]**

The overall, disseminated extrapulmonary disease has been described in 50–60% of liver transplant recipients with IA [47]. Liver transplant recipients are also recognized to have high risk for invasive candidiasis. Longer operation time, blood loss, repeated operations, re-transplantation, broad-spectrum antibiotic use, and renal failure are prominent risk factors for invasive candidiasis in this population [44].**[the following paragraph belong here]**

In a Cochrane database review, it was found that fluconazole prophylaxis significantly reduces the incidence of IFDs with no definite mortality benefit. Given a 10% incidence of IFD, 14 liver transplant recipients would require fluconazole prophylaxis to prevent one infection. In transplant centers where the incidence of IFD is high, or in situations where the individual patient's risk is greater, antifungal prophylaxis should be considered [48].

Antifungal prophylaxis is routinely used in most lung transplant programs during the early postoperative period. The duration for antifungal prophylaxis varies from center to center [49]. To prevent the occurrence of pulmonary aspergillosis, multiple strategies have been used including oral itraconazole, voriconazole, or aerosolized amphotericin B (AMB), used alone or in combination. Aerosolized drug delivery bypasses systemic circulation, mitigating concerns for drug-drug interaction and systemic toxicity [50]. Several centers have reported safety of aerosolized AMB deoxycholate in a variety of dosing regimens for patients undergoing heart, heart-lung or lung transplantation [51–53]. Aerosolized AMB lipid formulations have also been used successfully in this setting [53–55]. Monforte et al. have demonstrated that aerosolized deoxycholate AMB and lipid preparations of AMB are safe and achieve high concentrations in the bronchoalveolar lavage fluid within the first 24 h and 14 days, respectively. These lipid formulations allow a delayed administration every 7–14 days. With respect to oral prophylaxis, a recent study examined efficacy and toxicity of universal antifungal prophylaxis with voriconazole [56]. In this study, the overall rate of IA at 1-year interval was reduced to

1.5% in patients treated with prophylactic voriconazole compared with 23.5% rate in patients given a targeted prophylaxis approach. Interestingly, the rate of *Candida* colonization particularly that of non-*albicans* spp. in the voriconazole group was significantly higher [56]. In the cohort given voriconazole prophylaxis, 27% of the lung transplant recipients had normal liver enzymes during the course of the study. The main limitation of using voriconazole in lung transplant recipients was a potentially serious interaction with antirejection medication; therefore, in such patients, a preemptive dose reduction of calcineurin inhibitors is recommended along with a close monitoring of serum drug levels. Of interest, universal voriconazole prophylaxis was not associated with an increased rate of non-*Aspergillus* IFD including mucormycosis. Most transplant centers now use universal prophylaxis during the first 3 months after transplantation. After 3 months, a variety of permutations exist among transplant centers in the choice of agent used and how long such measures are continued. In patients who exhibit a higher risk of IA after undergoing lung transplantation such as (a) patients with chronic rejection and (b) those with *Aspergillus* spp. colonization of the respiratory tract, effective antifungal prophylaxis is recommended, and often given for a duration of 6 months [57]. In certain high-risk subgroups, anti-IA prophylaxis may have to be continued indefinitely.

Given the uncertain clinical benefits of prophylaxis, expense of drug cost, potential drug-drug interactions, and drug toxicity plus a concern for the emergence of resistant organisms, antifungal prophylaxis may not be routinely administered to all solid organ transplant recipients. Transplant centers use a targeted approach, i.e., prophylaxis is introduced only for patients at an increased risk of IFD and continued for a duration that coincides with the presence of precipitating risk factor(s) [58, 59]. The 2009 Infectious Diseases Society of America guidelines for the management of candidiasis recommend fluconazole (200–400 mg [3–6 mg/kg] daily) or liposomal AMB (1–2 mg/kg intravenously daily) prophylaxis for at least 7–14 days in patients undergoing liver, pancreas, and small bowel transplantation that are considered high risk of invasive fungal infection [60].

Antiviral Prophylaxis

Hematopoietic Cell Transplantation

Several viral infections that are commonly inconsequential in most immunocompetent patients pose serious threat to patients undergoing HSCT. In this regard, viruses belonging to *Herpesviridae* family of DNA viruses are common. Effective and safe prophylaxis with acyclovir or valaciclovir has dramatically reduced recrudescence of often severe herpes simplex virus (HSV) and varicella-zoster virus (VZV) infections. Furthermore, emergence of drug resistant breakthrough viral infection after prolonged exposure to antiviral drugs is not a significant problem, in most cases.

Cytomegalovirus (CMV) reactivation and/or rarely adult-onset acute CMV infection is a well-recognized serious life-threatening complication in patients undergoing allogeneic HSCT. Three decades ago, nearly one in four CMV-seropositive HSCT recipients died as a result of CMV disease; this changed after routine CMV control strategies were realized. Despite extensive research and debate, CMV infection continues to pose a serious challenge in providing optimized management for highly susceptible individuals after stem cell allograft transplantation.

With the development of effective antiviral therapy and the use of anti-CMV prophylaxis or preemptive therapy, infection rates have fallen and early posttransplant CMV disease rates have declined to nearly 3% [61, 62]. Ganciclovir or valganciclovir prophylaxis is effective in prevention of CMV end-organ disease and considered superior to monitoring and exercise in preemptive treatment approach. Routine use of these drugs with potential for myelotoxicity is fraught with increase morbidity due to myelosuppression, and overall survival benefits from their routine use are difficult to demonstrate. Presumably, antiviral benefits are offset by a higher frequency of secondary bacterial and fungal infections that may result from drug-induced myelosuppression. There remains an urgent need for effective, oral, and, importantly, less toxic antiviral drug(s). Maribavir appeared to be safe and effective in a randomized phase 2 trial; however, in phase 3 trial, it did not meet the criteria for efficacy [62]. Study design issues may have been the culprit in undoing of this promising anti- CMV drug include suboptimal dose schedule, delayed initiation of the study drug until after engraftment, exclusion of high risk patients with severe GVHD, and the regulatory agency's requirement at that time to demonstrate a reduction in CMV disease, which is an infrequent event, rather than a reduction in a more clinically relevant endpoint like CMV viremia [63, 64]. The requirement of regulatory oversight at that time was predicated on the assumption that a prophylaxis trial must demonstrate a reduction in CMV end-organ disease, an endpoint that now is seldom (<3%) seen in allogeneic HSCT recipients. This posesan impediment in demonstrating efficacy for new prophylaxis drugs and novel vaccine trials. This could dampen the enthusiasm for R&D in new technology that could eventually be licensed for clinical use. In recent years, there is a more receptive posture to accept surrogate markers with an aim to improve feasibility of clinical trials in the high-risk transplant population. Another promising antiviral agent under investigation is CMX001 (brincidofovir), a lipid conjugate of cidofovir with oral bioavailability[65]. The phase 3 study did not find a benefit, noting problems with diarrhea as a limiting toxicity [66], which may have overlapped with intestinal GVHD and may have confounded drug efficacy evaluation. Brincidofovir has a broad spectrum of antiviral coverage against a number of clinically relevant viral pathogens, including adenovirus and BK and JC polyomaviruses. Letermovir (AIC246) another agent in clinical trials has promising activity against laboratory and clinical strains of CMV [67]; in phase 3 trial it has demonstrated a significant reduction in CMV viremia [68].

Preemptive therapy with ganciclovir was associated with survival benefits, which could not be demonstrated in the case of routine anti-CMV prophylaxis [69]. The reasons for this puzzling observation remain unclear; limited exposure to this potentially myelotoxic drugs may well be the contributing factor. Most HSCT centers, therefore, have adopted preemptive therapy approach over routine long-term prophylaxis with ganciclovir. Patients undergoing cord blood stem cell transplantation are a notable exception due to a high risk for CMV infection and end-organ disease compared with other allograft HSCTprocedures; in such patients, intensified program of anti-CMV prophylaxis with ganciclovir before transplantation and high-dose acyclovir after transplant has been effective rather than a preemptive anti-CMV treatment approach [70].

An increase in late onset CMV disease is a clear limitation for preemptive therapy [71]. Risk factors for late CMV disease include early viremia, GVHD, and lymphopenia; patients at risk should be monitored and considered for preemptive therapy [72], although the benefit of preemptive therapy for late CMV disease in transplant population is also not certain. The limited ability to monitor CMV reactivation in patients dispersed to communities far from the transplant center may impede correct estimation of the true frequency and hands-on management of this serious complication. This continues to be a major challenge for which, the authors currently do not have good solutions, although boosting immunity to reduce the risk of late CMV disease; perhaps once effective vaccine becomes available may address this unmet need.

Resistance to antivirals is not a common problem in patients following HSCT; however, it is recognized as an evolving issuein the recipients of SOT [73]. New antiviral drugs are urgently needed. Maribavir is a benzimidazole that has activity against drug-resistant CMV strains, due to a novel mechanism by binding to the UL97 viral protein kinase, thereby inhibiting encapsidation and nuclear egress [74]. Maribavir was shown to successfully treat infections due to drug-resistant CMV infections in transplant recipients [75]. Leflunomide, a protein kinase and pyrimidine inhibitor, has long been considered as a promising therapy for ganciclovir-resistant CMV [64, 76]; however, there is limited clinical efficacy data to support its routine use. Letermovir, AIC246, has a novel mechanism that blocks UL56-mediated DNA processing or packaging; it is active against both drug-sensitive and drug-resistant strains [68]. New drug development remains an area of high and urgent priority.

Cellular immunotherapy has long been noted as a promising modality for prevention and treatment of opportunistic infections in the severely immunosuppressed patients. The ultimate control of CMV infection requires restoration of CMV-specific cytotoxic natural killer cells and T lymphocytes [77, 78]. Adoptive immunotherapy generated ex vivo from donor-derived, target-specific cytotoxic T lymphocytes is an area of interest and active research in prevention and treatment of CMV reactivation among at risk stem cell transplant population [79]. Recently, other targets include NK cells [78] and T cells armed with anti-CD3- and anti-CMV-specific antibodies [80]. These cell preparations have potential advantages over conventional T cells as they do not require analogous HLA and low risk for GVHD. The main advantage of immunotherapy approach is the efficacy against all viral strains independent of drug susceptibility. However, the daunting obstacle in development of cellular immunotherapy and availability for clinical use is technical complexity and high cost [81].

New vaccines are also promising. Glycoprotein B vaccines was found to boost both antibody and cellular responses in women with chronic viral infection [82]. Boosted antibody response and shortened viremic episodes in renal and liver transplant recipients are also encouraging [83]. A DNA vaccine was found to induce immune responses and to reduce viremia after HSCT in a randomized phase 2 trial [84]; phase 3 trial is underway. Effective immunization holds an enormous promise in preventing CMV infection and end-organ disease. As mentioned earlier, with drug prophylaxis trials, endpoint selection will be a crucial element in study design to assess clinical feasibility for such vaccines. Clear benefit in garnering protective immune response, a favorable impact on frequency and duration of CMV viremia, and avoidance, or short duration preemptive antiviral therapy were noted in randomized phase 2 trials; there may not be a reduction on the elusive, now a rare endpoint of CMV end-organ disease; if this remains as a requisite to measure success of phase 3 trials. Of interest, in the event CMV vaccines are effective, the need for drug prophylaxis will certainly lessen. However, since it is unlikely that a vaccine will be fully protective in all HSCT recipients, monitoring and preemptive therapy will still be needed, albeit less frequently.

Relationship between polymorphisms in innate immune response genes and the inherent risk for CMV infection (viremia) and potential for organ disease is an exciting new field. The ability to identify subgroup of patients with a higher propensity for viral disease, when available, will allow a more personalized approach for infection prevention, viral monitoring, and selective allocation of preemptive therapy. A study identified certain polymorphisms in genes encoding chemokine receptor 5, interleukin 10, and monocyte chemoattractant protein 1 that corroborated with CMV reactivation and CMV organ disease, even when controlled for well-established risk factors such as T-cell depletion or CD34 selection and/or presence of GVHD [85]. Importantly, these gene-products serve as virtual targets of the virus in its quest to suppress host antiviral immune response [86]. Additional, larger studies are needed to confirm these early observations, however there is considerable excitement that we are on the threshold of a new era of constructing individualized risk profiles and customizing prophylaxis based on such attributes.

Although CMV reactivation may occur frequently in recipients of autologous HSCT, it is seldom that these patients will present with end-organ CM disease. Accordingly, prophylaxis has not been considered in this patient population. Removal of T cells or CD34+ cell selection from the stem cell graft may increase the risk for CMV disease [87]. Several recent reports suggest that patients with multiple myeloma who underwent tandem autologous transplants and those who have received bortezomib are at higher risk for CMV disease just as they are at an increased risk for VZV reactivation. This may mean that in the future some patients undergoing autologous HSCT will be candidates for anti-CMV prophylaxis. With the growing use of purine analogues and an increasing array of monoclonal antibodies in use for lymphoma therapy may accentuate the net state of immune suppression among certain autologous transplant recipients; the likelihood of these emerging antineoplastic treatment advances on the risk for CMV disease in this traditionally low risk transplant group need to be seen.

EBV is a major pathogen after HSCT and can cause febrile syndrome; however, posttransplant lymphoproliferative disease (PTLD), infrequent albeit, a serious complication associated with this virus. Primary EBV infection in seronegative patients carries a high risk. Patients most vulnerable for the development of PTLD are those with profound T-cell deficiency; risk factors include mismatched or cord blood stem cell transplants, T cell depleted graft, use of ATG, or prolonged high-dose corticosteroid therapy. Monitoring EBV DNA by a blood EBV quantitative PCR can identify those at risk, and rise in viral titers typically occur several weeks prior to the clinical manifestation of lymphoproliferative disease. Drug prophylaxis is not effective, and immune modulation remains the mainstay of prevention and therapy. Preemptive reduction in iatrogenic immune suppression when possible, or treatment with anti-CD20 rituximab may prevent PTLD in high risk patients [18]. Alternatively, unselected donor lymphocyte infusions or infusions of donor-expanded, EBV-specific T cells or third-party EBV-specific cytotoxic T-cell lines (CTLs) can be given prophylactically or as therapy [88]. Unselected donor cells are appealing due to their simplicity of not requiring ex vivo manipulation, although they do carry a greater risk for GVHD [89]. The optimal strategy and refined parameters to identify at risk subgroupsare the goals for ongoing study.

HHV6 is associated with viral pneumonitis, encephalitis, myelosuppression, and infectious cause of graft compromise along with a variety of other syndromes like viral hepatitis, enterocolitis during post allogeneic transplant period. The relationship between HHV6 reactivation and its potential to cause end-organ disease remains a topic of controversy [90]. Ultimately, it will take a prophylaxis trial to determine if prevention of HHV6 reactivation leads to reduction in such clinical syndromes. Currently there is no generally accepted effective HHV6 prophylaxis strategy.

Solid Organ Transplantation

CMV infection remains one of the most common opportunistic viral infections in solid organ transplant patients despite availability of effective antiviral drugs [91]. Acute infection may occur via allograft from CMV + donor given to a seronegative recipient, or by reactivation of recipients' latent CMV infection. Seronegative patients who acquire organs from seropositive donors are at the greatest risk for developing infection; these primary infections tend to be most severe [92]. In addition to the direct impact of viral end-organ infection and organ damage, CMV infection appears to enhance the overall level of host immunosuppression, promoting risk for other opportunistic infections and malignancies. More insidiously, CMV infection is linked to chronic allograft dysfunction and risk for allograft loss [93]. The risk for CMV disease persists for life, although most cases occur shortly after antiviral prophylaxis is discontinued, and seen within the first year after transplantation [94].

In an attempt to minimize the adverse impact of CMV infection during the posttransplantation course, emphasis has shifted from premeptive therapy to preventive strategies. Numerous prospective randomized trials, summarized in several reviews and in one met analysis, have documented the efficacy of antiviral prophylaxis in reducing the risk of CMV infection and end-organ disease [93–96]. Valganciclovir is an effective anti-CMV agent for prophylaxis and treatment of CMV disease that is widely used in providing care for patients undergoing solid organ allograft transplantation [97–100]. Universal prophylaxis of all seronegative recipients with grafts from seropositive donor is recommended due to the amplified risk and prospect of CMV disease [101, 102]. A meta-analysis of 17 universal prophylaxis trials and 9 preemptive therapy trials demonstrated that both universal antiviral prophylaxis and preemptive strategies were equally effective in reducing the incidence of CMV end-organ disease [103]. However, only universal prophylaxis favorably influenced patient survival, reduced graft rejection, incidence of posttransplant opportunistic infections and PTLD; therefore, this strategy is preferred for at-risk SOT populations [103, 104].

The risk of CMV disease is significantly lower in seropositive organ allograft recipients, independent of donor CMV status; it has been argued that universal prophylaxis in this group leads to overtreatment, increasing the cost of care, and unduly exposing patients to the risk of drug toxicity and drug-drug interaction. In this population, preemptive strategies using targeted antivirals exclusively for patients demonstrating a rising CMV viral load are being developed [102, 105].

Emergence of ganciclovir-resistant strains of CMV threatens to unravel the therapeutic gains made in the past few decades. Across all populations, CMV donor-positive and recipient-negative status confers greatest risk for developing viral drug resistance, which probably is a reflection on high-grade viremia associated with primary CMV infection during a period of recently introduced, boosted drug-induced immune suppression seen in the early post-transplant period [106, 107]. Other risk factors include the use of potent immunosuppressive agents such as antilymphocyte antibodies, use of daclizumab, and prolonged exposure to ganciclovir [106, 107]. Unpredictable bioavailability of oral ganciclovir vs. valganciclovir, and therefore, prolonged potential under-exposure to ganciclovir is of particular significance in promoting viral drug resistance mutants [108]. Foscarnet is the agent of choice for the treatment of ganciclovir-resistant end organ disease; however, potentially serious drug-induced nephrotoxicity may limit its use. In patients undergoing lung transplantation, CMV disease due to ganciclovir-resistant virus is an important predictor for poor survival [107].

Conclusions

Antimicrobial prophylaxis is a common and an important practice in the management of infectious complications among transplant recipients. However, despite many clinical trials in different scenarios, controversies regarding the appropriate use of such intervention continue to exist. Use of antimicrobial prophylaxis has been of great benefit in the prevention of serious and life-threatening infections after transplantation. However, it is imperative to periodically assess the potential benefit versus limitations of existing practices in antimicrobial prophylaxis including (a) drug safety, tolerabilty and toxicity profile; (b) potential for drug-drug interaction, (c) novel transplant procedures and protocols, (d) changes in hosts' susceptibility for infection, and (e) shifts in the causative pathogens including emergence and reemergence of less drug susceptible pathogens; change in prevalence of drug-resistant microorganisms, and exposure to novel pathogens among patients undergoing transplantation.

References

1. Freifeld AG, Bow EJ, Sepkowitz KA, Boeckh MJ, Ito JI, Mullen CA, et al. Clinical practice guideline for the use of antimicrobial agents in neutropenic patients with cancer: 2010 update by the Infectious Diseases Society of America. Clin Infect Dis. 2011;52(4):427–31.
2. Wingard JR, Elmongy M. Strategies for minimizing complications of neutropenia: prophylactic myeloid growth factors or antibiotics. Crit Rev Oncol Hematol. 2009;72(2):144–54.
3. Wingard JR, Eldjerou L, Leather H. Use of antibacterial prophylaxis in patients with chemotherapy-induced neutropenia. Curr Opin Hematol. 2012;19(1):21–6.
4. van Vliet MJ, Tissing WJ, Dun CA, Meessen NE, Kamps WA, de Bont ES, et al. Chemotherapy treatment in pediatric patients with acute myeloid leukemia receiving antimicrobial prophylaxis leads to a relative increase of colonization with potentially pathogenic bacteria in the gut. Clin Infect Dis. 2009;49(2):262–70.
5. Guthrie KA, Yong M, Frieze D, Corey L, Fredricks DN. The impact of a change in antibacterial prophylaxis from ceftazidime to levofloxacin in allogeneic hematopoietic cell transplantation. Bone Marrow Transplant. 2010;45(4):675–81.
6. Eleutherakis-Papaiakovou E, Kostis E, Migkou M, Christoulas D, Terpos E, Gavriatopoulou M, et al. Prophylactic antibiotics for the prevention of neutropenic fever in patients undergoing autologous stem-cell transplantation: results of a single institution, randomized phase 2 trial. Am J Hematol. 2010;85(11):863–7.
7. Cornely OA, Crook DW, Esposito R, Poirier A, Somero MS, Weiss K, et al. Fidaxomicin versus vancomycin for infection with Clostridium difficile in Europe, Canada, and the USA: a double-blind, non-inferiority, randomised controlled trial. Lancet Infect Dis. 2012;12(4):281–9.
8. Louie TJ, Miller MA, Mullane KM, Weiss K, Lentnek A, Golan Y, et al. Fidaxomicin versus vancomycin for Clostridium difficile infection. N Engl J Med. 2011;364(5):422–31.
9. Cornely OA, Miller M, Fantin B, Mullane K, Kean Y, Gorbach S. Clinical outcomes for cancer patients with Clostridium difficile infection. In: 22nd European congress of clinical microbiology and infectious diseases; 2012.
10. Lowy I, Molrine DC, Leav BA, Blair BM, Baxter R, Gerding DN, et al. Treatment with monoclonal antibodies against Clostridium difficile toxins. N Engl J Med. 2010;362(3):197–205.
11. van Bekkum DW, Roodenburg J, Heidt PJ, van der Waaij D. Mitigation of secondary disease of allogeneic mouse radiation chimeras by modification of the intestinal microflora. J Natl Cancer Inst. 1974;52(2):401–4.
12. Jones JM, Wilson R, Bealmear PM. Mortality and gross pathology of secondary disease in germfree mouse radiation chimeras. Radiat Res. 1971;45(3):577–88.
13. Ferrara JL, Levine JE, Reddy P, Holler E. Graft-versus-host disease. Lancet. 2009;373(9674):1550–61.
14. Storb R, Prentice RL, Buckner CD, Clift RA, Appelbaum F, Deeg J, et al. Graft-versus-host disease and survival in patients with aplastic anemia treated by marrow grafts from HLA-identical siblings. Beneficial effect of a protective environment. N Engl J Med. 1983;308(6):302–7.
15. Jenq RR, Ubeda C, Taur Y, Menezes CC, Khanin R, Dudakov JA, et al. Regulation of intestinal inflammation by microbiota following allogeneic bone marrow transplantation. J Exp Med. 2012;209(5):903–11.
16. Taur Y, Xavier JB, Lipuma L, Ubeda C, Goldberg J, Gobourne A, et al. Intestinal domination and the risk of bacteremia in patients undergoing allogeneic hematopoietic stem cell transplantation. Clin Infect Dis. 2012;55:905.
17. Bowden R, Myers JD. Infection complicating bone marrow transplantation. In: Rubin RH, Young LS, editors. Clinical approach

to infection in the compromised host. New York: Plenum; 1994. p. 601–28.
18. Tomblyn M, Chiller T, Einsele H, Gress R, Sepkowitz K, Storek J, et al. Guidelines for preventing infectious complications among hematopoietic cell transplant recipients: a global perspective. Preface. Bone Marrow Transplant. 2009;44(8):453–5.
19. Sullivan KM, Kopecky KJ, Jocom J, Fisher L, Buckner CD, Meyers JD, et al. Immunomodulatory and antimicrobial efficacy of intravenous immunoglobulin in bone marrow transplantation. N Engl J Med. 1990;323(11):705–12.
20. Bass EB, Powe NR, Goodman SN, Graziano SL, Griffiths RI, Kickler TS, et al. Efficacy of immune globulin in preventing complications of bone marrow transplantation: a meta-analysis. Bone Marrow Transplant. 1993;12(3):273–82.
21. Sullivan KM, Storek J, Kopecky KJ, Jocom J, Longton G, Flowers M, et al. A controlled trial of long-term administration of intravenous immunoglobulin to prevent late infection and chronic graft-vs.-host disease after marrow transplantation: clinical outcome and effect on subsequent immune recovery. Biol Blood Marrow Transplant. 1996;2(1):44–53.
22. Holland HK, Wingard JR, Beschorner WE, Saral R, Santos GW. Bronchiolitis obliterans in bone marrow transplantation and its relationship to chronic graft-v-host disease and low serum IgG. Blood. 1988;72(2):621–7.
23. Cordonnier C, Labopin M, Chesnel V, Ribaud P, de la Camara R, Martino R, et al. Randomized study of early versus late immunization with pneumococcal conjugate vaccine after allogeneic stem cell transplantation. Clin Infect Dis. 2009;48(10):1392–401.
24. Cordonnier C, Labopin M, Chesnel V, Ribaud P, Camara RL, Martino R, et al. Immune response to the 23-valent polysaccharide pneumococcal vaccine after the 7-valent conjugate vaccine in allogeneic stem cell transplant recipients: results from the EBMT IDWP01 trial. Vaccine. 2010;28(15):2730–4.
25. Centers for Disease Control and Prevention (CDC). Licensure of 13-valent pneumococcal conjugate vaccine for adults aged 50 years and older. MMWR Morb Mortal Wkly Rep. 2012;61:394–5.
26. Len O, Gavalda J, Blanes M, Montejo M, San JR, Moreno A, et al. Donor infection and transmission to the recipient of a solid allograft. Am J Transplant. 2008;8(11):2420–5.
27. Ruiz I, Gavalda J, Monforte V, Len O, Roman A, Bravo C, et al. Donor-to-host transmission of bacterial and fungal infections in lung transplantation. Am J Transplant. 2006;6(1):178–82.
28. Green H, Rahamimov R, Gafter U, Leibovitci L, Paul M. Antibiotic prophylaxis for urinary tract infections in renal transplant recipients: a systematic review and meta analysis. Transpl Infect Dis. 2011;13(5):441–7.
29. Goodman JL, Winston DJ, Greenfield RA, Chandrasekar PH, Fox B, Kaizer H, et al. A controlled trial of fluconazole to prevent fungal infections in patients undergoing bone marrow transplantation. N Engl J Med. 1992;326(13):845–51.
30. Slavin MA, Osborne B, Adams R, Levenstein MJ, Schoch HG, Feldman AR, et al. Efficacy and safety of fluconazole prophylaxis for fungal infections after marrow transplantation--a prospective, randomized, double-blind study. J Infect Dis. 1995;171(6):1545–52.
31. Marr KA, Seidel K, Slavin MA, Bowden RA, Schoch HG, Flowers ME, et al. Prolonged fluconazole prophylaxis is associated with persistent protection against candidiasis-related death in allogeneic marrow transplant recipients: long-term follow-up of a randomized, placebo-controlled trial. Blood. 2000;96(6):2055–61.
32. Marr KA, Bow E, Chiller T, Maschmeyer G, Ribaud P, Segal B, et al. Fungal infection prevention after hematopoietic cell transplantation. Bone Marrow Transplant. 2009;44(8):483–7.
33. MacMillan ML, Goodman JL, DeFor TE, Weisdorf DJ. Fluconazole to prevent yeast infections in bone marrow transplantation patients: a randomized trial of high versus reduced dose, and determination of the value of maintenance therapy. Am J Med. 2002;112(5):369–79.
34. van Burik JA, Ratanatharathorn V, Stepan DE, Miller CB, Lipton JH, Vesole DH, et al. Micafungin versus fluconazole for prophylaxis against invasive fungal infections during neutropenia in patients undergoing hematopoietic stem cell transplantation. Clin Infect Dis. 2004;39(10):1407–16.
35. Winston DJ, Maziarz RT, Chandrasekar PH, Lazarus HM, Goldman M, Blumer JL, et al. Intravenous and oral itraconazole versus intravenous and oral fluconazole for long-term antifungal prophylaxis in allogeneic hematopoietic stem-cell transplant recipients. A multicenter, randomized trial. Ann Intern Med. 2003;138(9):705–13.
36. Marr KA, Crippa F, Leisenring W, Hoyle M, Boeckh M, Balajee SA, et al. Itraconazole versus fluconazole for prevention of fungal infections in patients receiving allogeneic stem cell transplants. Blood. 2004;103(4):1527–33.
37. Wingard JR, Carter SL, Walsh TJ, Kurtzberg J, Small TN, Baden LR, et al. Randomized, double-blind trial of fluconazole versus voriconazole for prevention of invasive fungal infection after allogeneic hematopoietic cell transplantation. Blood. 2010;116(24):5111–8.
38. Ullmann AJ, Lipton JH, Vesole DH, Chandrasekar P, Langston A, Tarantolo SR, et al. Posaconazole or fluconazole for prophylaxis in severe graft-versus-host disease. N Engl J Med. 2007;356(4):335–47.
39. Kontoyiannis DP, Marr KA, Park BJ, Alexander BD, Anaissie EJ, Walsh TJ, et al. Prospective surveillance for invasive fungal infections in hematopoietic stem cell transplant recipients, 2001–2006: overview of the Transplant-Associated Infection Surveillance Network (TRANSNET) Database. Clin Infect Dis. 2010;50(8):1091–100.
40. Marr KA, Seidel K, White TC, Bowden RA. Candidemia in allogeneic blood and marrow transplant recipients: evolution of risk factors after the adoption of prophylactic fluconazole. J Infect Dis. 2000;181(1):309–16.
41. Howard SJ, Cerar D, Anderson MJ, Albarrag A, Fisher MC, Pasqualotto AC, et al. Frequency and evolution of Azole resistance in Aspergillus fumigatus associated with treatment failure. Emerg Infect Dis. 2009;15(7):1068–76.
42. van der Linden JW, Snelders E, Kampinga GA, Rijnders BJ, Mattsson E, Debets-Ossenkopp YJ, et al. Clinical implications of azole resistance in Aspergillus fumigatus, the Netherlands, 2007–2009. Emerg Infect Dis. 2011;17(10):1846–54.
43. Nucci M, Nouer SA, Grazziutti M, Kumar NS, Barlogie B, Anaissie E. Probable invasive aspergillosis without prespecified radiologic findings: proposal for inclusion of a new category of aspergillosis and implications for studying novel therapies. Clin Infect Dis. 2010;51(11):1273–80.
44. Silveira FP, Husain S. Fungal infections in solid organ transplantation. Med Mycol. 2007;45(4):305–20.
45. Gavalda J, Len O, San JR, Aguado JM, Fortun J, Lumbreras C, et al. Risk factors for invasive aspergillosis in solid-organ transplant recipients: a case-control study. Clin Infect Dis. 2005;41(1):52–9.
46. Pappas PG, Alexander BD, Andes DR, Hadley S, Kauffman CA, Freifeld A, et al. Invasive fungal infections among organ transplant recipients: results of the Transplant-Associated Infection Surveillance Network (TRANSNET). Clin Infect Dis. 2010;50(8):1101–11.
47. Paterson DL, Singh N. Invasive aspergillosis in transplant recipients. Medicine (Baltimore). 1999;78(2):123–38.
48. Playford EG, Webster AC, Sorell TC, Craig JC. Antifungal agents for preventing fungal infections in solid organ transplant recipients. Cochrane Database Syst Rev. 2004;3:CD004291.
49. Husain S, Zaldonis D, Kusne S, Kwak EJ, Paterson DL, McCurry KR. Variation in antifungal prophylaxis strategies in lung transplantation. Transpl Infect Dis. 2006;8(4):213–8.
50. Drew R. Potential role of aerosolized amphotericin B formulations in the prevention and adjunctive treatment of invasive fungal infections. Int J Antimicrob Agents. 2006;27(Suppl 1):36–44.

51. Reichenspurner H, Gamberg P, Nitschke M, Valantine H, Hunt S, Oyer PE, et al. Significant reduction in the number of fungal infections after lung-, heart-lung, and heart transplantation using aerosolized amphotericin B prophylaxis. Transplant Proc. 1997;29(1–2):627–8.
52. Calvo V, Borro JM, Morales P, Morcillo A, Vicente R, Tarrazona V, et al. Antifungal prophylaxis during the early postoperative period of lung transplantation. Valencia Lung Transplant Group. Chest. 1999;115(5):1301–4.
53. Monforte V, Roman A, Gavalda J, Lopez R, Pou L, Simo M, et al. Nebulized amphotericin B concentration and distribution in the respiratory tract of lung-transplanted patients. Transplantation. 2003;75(9):1571–4.
54. Drew RH, Dodds AE, Benjamin DK Jr, Duane DR, Palmer SM, Perfect JR. Comparative safety of amphotericin B lipid complex and amphotericin B deoxycholate as aerosolized antifungal prophylaxis in lung-transplant recipients. Transplantation. 2004;77(2):232–7.
55. Palmer SM, Drew RH, Whitehouse JD, Tapson VF, Davis RD, McConnell RR, et al. Safety of aerosolized amphotericin B lipid complex in lung transplant recipients. Transplantation. 2001;72(3):545–8.
56. Husain S, Paterson DL, Studer S, Pilewski J, Crespo M, Zaldonis D, et al. Voriconazole prophylaxis in lung transplant recipients. Am J Transplant. 2006;6(12):3008–16.
57. Symoens F, Knoop C, Schrooyen M, Denis O, Estenne M, Nolard N, et al. Disseminated Scedosporium apiospermum infection in a cystic fibrosis patient after double-lung transplantation. J Heart Lung Transplant. 2006;25(5):603–7.
58. Fortun J, Martin-Davila P, Moreno S, de Vicente E, Nuno J, Candelas A, et al. Risk factors for invasive aspergillosis in liver transplant recipients. Liver Transpl. 2002;8(11):1065–70.
59. Hellinger WC, Bonatti H, Yao JD, Alvarez S, Brumble LM, Keating MR, et al. Risk stratification and targeted antifungal prophylaxis for prevention of aspergillosis and other invasive mold infections after liver transplantation. Liver Transpl. 2005;11(6):656–62.
60. Pappas PG, Kauffman CA, Andes D, Benjamin DK Jr, Calandra TF, Edwards JE Jr, et al. Clinical practice guidelines for the management of candidiasis: 2009 update by the Infectious Diseases Society of America. Clin Infect Dis. 2009;48(5):503–35.
61. Boeckh M, Nichols WG, Papanicolaou G, Rubin R, Wingard JR, Zaia J. Cytomegalovirus in hematopoietic stem cell transplant recipients: current status, known challenges, and future strategies. Biol Blood Marrow Transplant. 2003;9(9):543–58.
62. Marty FM, Ljungman P, Papanicolaou GA, Winston DJ, Chemaly RF, Strasfeld L, et al. Maribavir prophylaxis for prevention of cytomegalovirus disease in recipients of allogeneic stem-cell transplants: a phase 3, double-blind, placebo-controlled, randomised trial. Lancet Infect Dis. 2011;11(4):284–92.
63. Marty FM, Boeckh M. Maribavir and human cytomegalovirus-what happened in the clinical trials and why might the drug have failed? Curr Opin Virol. 2011;1(6):555–62.
64. Snydman DR. Leflunomide: a small step forward in meeting the urgent need for treatment of drug-resistant cytomegalovirus infection. Transplantation. 2010;90(4):362–3.
65. Marty FM, Winston DJ, Rowley SD, et al. CMX001 to prevent cytomegalovirus disease in hematopoietic-cell transplantation. N Engl J Med. 2013;369:1227.
66. Marty FM, Winston DJ, Chemaly RF, et al. Brincidofovir for prevention of cytomegalovirus (CMV) after allogeneic hematopoietic cell transplantation (HCT) in CMV-seropositive patients: a randomized, double-blind, placebo-controlled, parallel-group phase 3 trial. Biol Blood Marrow Transplant. 2016;22(3, Suppl1):S23. (abstr 5)
67. Marty FM, Winston D, Rowley SD, Boeckh M, Vance E, Papanicolaou G, et al. CMX001 for prevention and control of CMV infection in CMV-seropositive allogeneic stem-cell transplant recipients: a phase 2 randomized, double-blind, placebo-controlled, dose-escalation trial of safety, tolerability and antiviral activity. Biol Blood Marrow Transplant. 2012;18(2):S203–4.
68. Marschall M, Stamminger T, Urban A, Wildum S, Ruebsamen-Schaeff H, Zimmermann H, et al. In vitro evaluation of the activities of the novel anticytomegalovirus compound AIC246 (letermovir) against herpesviruses and other human pathogenic viruses. Antimicrob Agents Chemother. 2012;56(2):1135–7.
69. Einsele H, Ehninger G, Hebart H, Wittkowski KM, Schuler U, Jahn G, et al. Polymerase chain reaction monitoring reduces the incidence of cytomegalovirus disease and the duration and side effects of antiviral therapy after bone marrow transplantation. Blood. 1995;86(7):2815–20.
70. Milano F, Pergam SA, Xie H, Leisenring WM, Gutman JA, Riffkin I, et al. Intensive strategy to prevent CMV disease in seropositive umbilical cord blood transplant recipients. Blood. 2011;118(20):5689–96.
71. Boeckh M, Leisenring W, Riddell SR, Bowden RA, Huang ML, Myerson D, et al. Late cytomegalovirus disease and mortality in recipients of allogeneic hematopoietic stem cell transplants: importance of viral load and T-cell immunity. Blood. 2003;101(2):407–14.
72. Peggs KS, Preiser W, Kottaridis PD, McKeag N, Brink NS, Tedder RS, et al. Extended routine polymerase chain reaction surveillance and preemptive antiviral therapy for cytomegalovirus after allogeneic transplantation. Br J Haematol. 2000;111(3):782–90.
73. Snydman DR. Why did maribavir fail in stem-cell transplants? Lancet Infect Dis. 2011;11(4):255–7.
74. Biron KK, Harvey RJ, Chamberlain SC, Good SS, Smith AA III, Davis MG, et al. Potent and selective inhibition of human cytomegalovirus replication by 1263W94, a benzimidazole L-riboside with a unique mode of action. Antimicrob Agents Chemother. 2002;46(8):2365–72.
75. Avery RK, Marty FM, Strasfeld L, Lee I, Arrieta A, Chou S, et al. Oral maribavir for treatment of refractory or resistant cytomegalovirus infections in transplant recipients. Transpl Infect Dis. 2010;12(6):489–96.
76. Sudarsanam TD, Sahni RD, John GT. Leflunomide: a possible alternative for gangciclovir sensitive and resistant cytomegalovirus infections. Postgrad Med J. 2006;82(967):313–4.
77. Quinnan GV Jr, Kirmani N, Rook AH, Manischewitz JF, Jackson L, Moreschi G, et al. Cytotoxic t cells in cytomegalovirus infection: HLA-restricted T-lymphocyte and non-T-lymphocyte cytotoxic responses correlate with recovery from cytomegalovirus infection in bone-marrow-transplant recipients. N Engl J Med. 1982;307(1):7–13.
78. Foley B, Cooley S, Verneris MR, Pitt M, Curtsinger J, Luo X, et al. Cytomegalovirus reactivation after allogeneic transplantation promotes a lasting increase in educated NKG2C+ natural killer cells with potent function. Blood. 2012;119(11):2665–74.
79. Walter EA, Greenberg PD, Gilbert MJ, Finch RJ, Watanabe KS, Thomas ED, et al. Reconstitution of cellular immunity against cytomegalovirus in recipients of allogeneic bone marrow by transfer of T-cell clones from the donor. N Engl J Med. 1995;333(16):1038–44.
80. Lum LG, Ramesh M, Thakur A, Mitra S, Deol A, Uberti JP, et al. Targeting cytomegalovirus-infected cells using T cells armed with anti-CD3 x anti-CMV Bispecific antibody. Biol Blood Marrow Transplant. 2012;18(7):1012–22.
81. Norkin M, Wingard JR. Armed killers face off against cytomegalovirus. Biol Blood Marrow Transplant. 2012;18(7):977–8.
82. Sabbaj S, Pass RF, Goepfert PA, Pichon S. Glycoprotein B vaccine is capable of boosting both antibody and CD4 T-cell responses to cytomegalovirus in chronically infected women. J Infect Dis. 2011;203(11):1534–41.
83. Griffiths PD, Stanton A, McCarrell E, Smith C, Osman M, Harber M, et al. Cytomegalovirus glycoprotein-B vaccine with MF59 adjuvant in transplant recipients: a phase 2 randomised placebo-controlled trial. Lancet. 2011;377(9773):1256–63.

84. Kharfan-Dabaja MA, Boeckh M, Wilck MB, Langston AA, Chu AH, Wloch MK, et al. A novel therapeutic cytomegalovirus DNA vaccine in allogeneic haemopoietic stem-cell transplantation: a randomised, double-blind, placebo-controlled, phase 2 trial. Lancet Infect Dis. 2012;12(4):290–9.
85. Loeffler J, Steffens M, Arlt EM, Toliat MR, Mezger M, Suk A, et al. Polymorphisms in the genes encoding chemokine receptor 5, interleukin-10, and monocyte chemoattractant protein 1 contribute to cytomegalovirus reactivation and disease after allogeneic stem cell transplantation. J Clin Microbiol. 2006;44(5):1847–50.
86. Boeckh M, Geballe AP. Cytomegalovirus: pathogen, paradigm, and puzzle. J Clin Invest. 2011;121(5):1673–80.
87. Holmberg LA, Boeckh M, Hooper H, Leisenring W, Rowley S, Heimfeld S, et al. Increased incidence of cytomegalovirus disease after autologous CD34-selected peripheral blood stem cell transplantation. Blood. 1999;94(12):4029–35.
88. Doubrovina E, Oflaz-Sozmen B, Prockop SE, Kernan NA, Abramson S, Teruya-Feldstein J, et al. Adoptive immunotherapy with unselected or EBV-specific T cells for biopsy-proven EBV+ lymphomas after allogeneic hematopoietic cell transplantation. Blood. 2012;119(11):2644–56.
89. Heslop HE. Equal-opportunity treatment of EBV-PTLD. Blood. 2012;119(11):2436–8.
90. Zerr DM, Boeckh M, Delaney C, Martin PJ, Xie H, Adler AL, et al. HHV-6 reactivation and associated sequelae after hematopoietic cell transplant. Biol Blood Marrow Transplant. 2012;18(11):1700–8.
91. Aguado JM, Navarro D, San JR, Caston JJ. Cytomegalovirus infection in solid organ transplantation. Enferm Infecc Microbiol Clin. 2012;30(Suppl 2):57–62.
92. Akalin E, Sehgal V, Ames S, Hossain S, Daly L, Barbara M, et al. Cytomegalovirus disease in high-risk transplant recipients despite ganciclovir or valganciclovir prophylaxis. Am J Transplant. 2003;3(6):731–5.
93. Sia IG, Patel R. New strategies for prevention and therapy of cytomegalovirus infection and disease in solid-organ transplant recipients. Clin Microbiol Rev. 2000;13(1):83–121.
94. Gupta S, Mitchell JD, Markham DW, Mammen PP, Patel PC, Kaiser P, et al. High incidence of cytomegalovirus disease in D+/R- heart transplant recipients shortly after completion of 3 months of valganciclovir prophylaxis. J Heart Lung Transplant. 2008;27(5):536–9.
95. Couchoud C, Cucherat M, Haugh M, Pouteil-Noble C. Cytomegalovirus prophylaxis with antiviral agents in solid organ transplantation: a meta-analysis. Transplantation. 1998;65(5):641–7.
96. Kotton CN. Management of cytomegalovirus infection in solid organ transplantation. Nat Rev Nephrol. 2010;6(12):711–21.
97. Said T, Nampoory MR, Pacsa AS, Essa S, Madi N, Fahim N, et al. Oral valgancyclovir versus intravenous gancyclovir for cytomegalovirus prophylaxis in kidney transplant recipients. Transplant Proc. 2007;39(4):997–9.
98. Diaz-Pedroche C, Lumbreras C, Del VP, San JR, Hernando S, Folgueira D, et al. Efficacy and safety of valgancyclovir as preemptive therapy for the prevention of cytomegalovirus disease in solid organ transplant recipients. Transplant Proc. 2005;37(9):3766–7.
99. Pescovitz MD, Rabkin J, Merion RM, Paya CV, Pirsch J, Freeman RB, et al. Valganciclovir results in improved oral absorption of ganciclovir in liver transplant recipients. Antimicrob Agents Chemother. 2000;44(10):2811–5.
100. Luan FL, Chopra P, Park J, Norman S, Cibrik D, Ojo A. Efficacy of valganciclovir in the treatment of cytomegalovirus disease in kidney and pancreas transplant recipients. Transplant Proc. 2006;38(10):3673–5.
101. Singh N. Preemptive therapy versus universal prophylaxis with ganciclovir for cytomegalovirus in solid organ transplant recipients. Clin Infect Dis. 2001;32(5):742–51.
102. Rubin RH. Prevention and treatment of cytomegalovirus disease in heart transplant patients. J Heart Lung Transplant. 2000;19(8):731–5.
103. Small LN, Lau J, Snydman DR. Preventing post-organ transplantation cytomegalovirus disease with ganciclovir: a meta-analysis comparing prophylactic and preemptive therapies. Clin Infect Dis. 2006;43(7):869–80.
104. Kalil AC, Levitsky J, Lyden E, Stoner J, Freifeld AG. Meta-analysis: the efficacy of strategies to prevent organ disease by cytomegalovirus in solid organ transplant recipients. Ann Intern Med. 2005;143(12):870–80.
105. van der Bij W, Speich R. Management of cytomegalovirus infection and disease after solid-organ transplantation. Clin Infect Dis. 2001;33(Suppl 1):S32–7.
106. Limaye AP, Corey L, Koelle DM, Davis CL, Boeckh M. Emergence of ganciclovir-resistant cytomegalovirus disease among recipients of solid-organ transplants. Lancet. 2000;356(9230):645–9.
107. Bhorade SM, Lurain NS, Jordan A, Leischner J, Villanueva J, Durazo R, et al. Emergence of ganciclovir-resistant cytomegalovirus in lung transplant recipients. J Heart Lung Transplant. 2002;21(12):1274–82.
108. Fishman JA. Infection in solid-organ transplant recipients. N Engl J Med. 2007;357(25):2601–14.

Index

A. Safdar (ed.), *Principles and Practice of Transplant Infectious Diseases*, https://doi.org/10.1007/978-1-4939-9034-4

B

D

E

I

S

T